AMA
DRUG
EVALUATIONS
FOURTH EDITION

Prepared by the
AMA
DEPARTMENT
OF DRUGS

In Cooperation with the
American Society for
Clinical Pharmacology
and Therapeutics

Not For Resale

American Medical Association
Chicago, Illinois

First Edition - January 1971
Second Edition - September 1973
Third Edition - March 1977
    Second Printing - August 1977
Fourth Edition - February 1980
    Second Printing - October 1980

Printed in the United States of America

International Standard Book Number: 0-89970-004-7
Library of Congress Catalog Card Number: 76-9254

NEA:79-717A:25M:10/80

Preface

The fourth edition of *AMA Drug Evaluations* (AMA-DE) continues the successful joint cooperative effort between the AMA Department of Drugs and the American Society for Clinical Pharmacology and Therapeutics (ASCPT). As in the previous edition, the text for the fourth edition was written by the professional staff of the AMA Department of Drugs or outside contributors, reviewed by several hundred distinguished consultants, and then subjected to final review by members or other selected experts for the American Society for Clinical Pharmacology and Therapeutics. Thus, this publication is a joint scientific contribution to the field of applied therapeutics by the AMA and ASCPT. The introductions and evaluations contained therein represent a distillation of the current scientific literature plus the combined wisdom of many experienced clinicians.

Since its first edition in 1971, the goal of AMA-DE has been to provide physicians and other health care professionals with up-to-date, unbiased information on the *clinical* use of drugs. Thus, AMA-DE is not intended to serve as a textbook of basic pharmacology but, rather, as a reference source for practical drug therapy. Basic pharmacologic information, pharmacokinetics, and pathogenesis of disease are presented only to the extent deemed necessary to understand drug use in patients.

Probably no field of medicine changes as rapidly as drug therapy. Thus, even though only three years have elapsed since the last edition, most of the text of this fourth edition has been completely rewritten or rigorously revised to reflect the latest information and expert consensus on the most effective use of therapeutic agents. Evaluations of 57 new drugs marketed since the third edition, plus expanded information on important investigational agents and new uses of older drugs, have been added. There is a reorganized table of contents for the 87 chapters, including new chapters on Immunomodulators, Antiviral Agents, Parenteral and Enteral Nutrition, and Agents Used to Treat Infertility.

The format of AMA-DE has evolved considerably since the first edition. In an effort to be responsive to reader comment and criticism, a questionnaire was included with later press runs of the last edition. The very gratifying response by many thousands of readers has provided many suggestions for improving the format and usefulness of this fourth edition. The page layout and typography have been redesigned for ease of reading and quick reference. This edition contains expanded general discussion on use of drugs in special groups (pediatric patients, geriatric patients, pregnant and lactating women, patients with renal impairment), adverse reactions, drug interactions, and drug response variation. An innovation is the use of outlines at the beginning of each chapter to aid the reader in determining chapter organization quickly. The use of tables has also been expanded for easy access to information. The multiple indexes of previous editions have been consolidated into a single comprehensive index that includes drug names (both generic and trademark), indications, and adverse reactions. The index also includes selected Canadian trade names with their nonproprietary names. There is also an expanded listing of available dosage forms and sizes of generic products in addition to trademark preparations. Finally, in response to requests by users of previous editions, a listing of selected references has been added to the end of the chapters; this should not be interpreted as a bibliography of the literature consulted in preparation of the text but merely a guide for readers interested in further reading.

AMA-DE continues to describe uses, routes of administration, or dosages that may not be found in the "package insert." FDA-approved labeling limits the use of drugs for purposes of marketing and advertising but does not constrain a physician's use of the drug for individual patients. Furthermore, FDA may not be current in approving new uses, routes, or dosages of older drugs. Accordingly, AMA-DE describes all scientific, recognized uses of drugs, irrespective of their status in approved labeling in the "package insert."

The American Medical Association is grateful to the American Society for Clinical Pharmacology and Therapeutics for invaluable assistance rendered in the preparation of this book and hopes that AMA-DE will continue to be a valuable and useful reference source for the medical profession and others working in the field of medical care.

James H. Sammons, M. D.
Executive Vice President
American Medical Association

Contents

Acknowledgments

Appreciation is expressed to the following members of the professional staff of the Department of Drugs for their assistance in the preparation of the text and coordination of the consultants' and final reviewers' comments:

Donald R. Bennett, M.D., Ph.D.
Charles B. Clayman, M.D.
Mary Ellen Kosman, Ph.D.
John Reed Lewis, Ph.D.
Barbara F. Murphy, M.S.
Carol M. Proudfit, Ph.D.
Donald O. Schiffman, Ph.D.

The editorial and technical aid furnished by the following members of the Department staff is also gratefully acknowledged and appreciated:

Hermese Bryant
Joaquin Chang
Marilyn A. Krause
Sandra McVeigh
Marsha Meyer
Beverly J. Rodgers
Patti J. Stone
Yuriko Takemoto
Wanda Wade

Special Contributors

Saul Krugman, M.D.
    New York University Medical Center
    New York
Hans B. Nevinny, M.D.
    Weiss Memorial Hospital
    Chicago
John A. Robinson, M.D.
    Loyola University Medical Center
    Maywood, Illinois

Charles W. Roscoe, Ph.D.
    University of the Pacific
    Stockton, California
Edward M. Sellers, M.D., Ph.D.
    Addiction Research Foundation
    University of Toronto
    Toronto, Canada
Professor Doctor M. Verstraete
    Catholieke Universiteit Leuven
    Leuven, Belgium

Consultants

The Department of Drugs expresses its appreciation to the following individuals for their cooperation and assistance in reviewing the content of this edition of *AMA Drug Evaluations*.

George N. Aagard, M.D.
Louis M. Aledort, M.D.
Harvey J. Alter, M.D.
Richard D. Amelar, M.D.
Richard P. Ames, M.D.
Navin P. Amin, M.D.
Douglas R. Anderson, M.D.
Jack R. Anderson, M.D.
Jeffrey L. Anderson, M.D.
Lawrence J. Anderson, M.D.
Terence W. Anderson, M.D.
William C. Andrews, M.D.
David F. Archer, M.D.
Kenneth Arndt, M.D.
Harry Arnold, Jr., M.D.
Wilbert S. Aronow, M.D.
Richard H. Aster, M.D.
Robert Austrian, M.D.
William R. Barclay, M.D.
Roger M. Barkin, M.D.
Frederic C. Bartter, M.D.
Doris G. Bartuska, M.D.
John V. Basmajian, M.D.
D. J. Bauer, M.A., Ph.D., M.B.
John Baum, M.D.
Jules Baum, M.D.
J. Weldon Belleville, M.D.
Henrik Holt Bendixen, M.D.
John E. Bennett, M.D.
William M. Bennett, M.D.
I. Leonard Bernstein, M.D.
C. Warren Bierman, M.D.
Paul A. Blake, M.D.
Saul S. Bloomfield, M.D.
Robert E. Bolinger, M.D.
Jeanne R. Bonar, M.D.
David Botero R., M.D.
Robert F. Bradley, Jr., M.D.
Lloyd L. Brandborg, M.D.
A. David Brandling-Bennett, M.D.
George A. Bray, M.D.
Rubin Bressler, M.D.
Frank P. Brooks, M.D., Sc.D.
Henry Brown, M.D.
Anthony Bryceson, M.D.
Maurice B. Burg, M.D.
W. Arthur Burke, Pharm. D.
Robert P. Burns, M.D.

James R. Busvine, D.Sc., M.I. Biol.
John J. Canary, M.D.
Craig J. Canfield, M.D.
Paul J. Cannon, M.D.
Harold E. Carlson, M.D.
William Chin, M.D.
Robert E. Christensen, M.D.
David Clyde, M.D.
William E. Cobb, M.D.
Joseph Cochin, M.D., Ph.D.
Jay D. Coffman, M.D.
Sidney Cohen, M.D.
Jay N. Cohn, M.D.
Franklin R. Cole, Ph.D.
Harold O. Conn, M.D.
Elizabeth B. Connell, M.D.
Marcel E. Conrad, M.D.
Allan R. Cooke, M.D.
Denis Craddock, M.D.
John J. Cronin, Jr., M.D.
William H. Crosby, Jr., M.D.
Donald J. Dalessio, M.D.
Lawrence J. D'Angelo, M.D.
Daniel Danahy, M.D.
W. A. Daniel, Jr., M.D.
Leslie J. DeGroot, M.D.
Thomas J. DeKornfeld, M.D.
Daniel Deykin, M.D.
Richard P. Dickey, M.D., Ph.D.
Ananias C. Diokno, M.D.
Joseph R. DiPalma, M.D.
Robert G. Dluhy, M.D.
J. E. Doherty, M.D.
John Doull, M.D., Ph.D.
Daniel B. Drachman, M.D.
Stephen M. Drance, M.D.
F. E. Dreifus, M.D.
Victor A. Drill, M.D., Ph.D.
Thomas D. DuBose, M.D.
Carlos A. Dujovne, M.D.
Roger C. Duvoisin, M.D.
Joseph Dwek, M.D.
George Ehrlich, M.D.
Philip P. Ellis, M.D.
Robert J. Ellis, Ph.D.
Andrew G. Engel, M.D.
Mary Allen Engle, M.D.
Stephen E. Epstein, M.D.

William L. Epstein, M.D.
Laurence Farer, M.D.
Richard S. Farr, M.D.
Robert J. Fass, M.D.
F. Robert Fekety, Jr., M.D.
Roger A. Feldman, M.D.
James A. Ferrendelli, M.D.
Ronald R. Fieve, M.D.
Maxwell Finland, M.D.
Mieczyslaw Finster, M.D.
Delbert A. Fisher, M.D.
John S. Fordtran, M.D.
Walter B. Forman, M.D.
Charles L. Fox, Jr., M.D.
Joseph A. Franciosa, M.D.
David W. Fraser, M.D.
Edward D. Freis, M.D.
Joseph French, M.D.
Arnold P. Friedman, M.D.
Henry G. Friesen, M.D.
Edward D. Frohlich, M.D.
Lawrence A. Frohman, M.D.
J. Lester Gabrilove, M.D.
Charles M. Gaitz, M.D.
John T. Galambos, M.D.
Jerry D. Gardner, M.D.
Kenneth D. Gardner, Jr., M.D.
Erwin W. Gelfand, M.D.
Gabriel Genkins, M.D.
Ray W. Gifford, Jr., M.D.
J. Christian Gillin, M.D.
Charles J. Glueck, M.D.
Leon Goldberg, M.D.
R. B. Goldrick, M.D.
Richard E. Goldsmith, M.D.
Robert E. Goldstein, M.D.
Joseph W. Goldzieher, M.D.
Sherwood L. Gorbach, M.D.
W. Morton Grant, M.D.
Robert Graw, M.D.
Harry L. Greene, M.D.
William H. Greene, M.D.
Tibor J. Greenwalt, M.D.
Alfred Grindon, M.D.
David Grob, M.D.
Isabel Guerrero, M.D.
Rolf M. Gunnar, M.D.
Clifford W. Gurney, M.D.
W. Dallas Hall, M.D.
Lawrence M. Halpern, Ph.D.
Charles B. Hammond, M.D.
John W. Hare, M.D.
Donald C. Harrison, M.D.

James T. Hartford, M.D.
Robert A. Hatcher, M.D.
William S. Haubrick, M.D.
William H. Havener, M.D.
William M. Heller, Ph.D.
Owen J. Hendley, M.D.
Paul Henkind, M.D., Ph.D.
Victor Herbert, M.D., J.D.
Alfred D. Hernandez, M.D.
Ernest C. Herrmann, Jr., M.D.
John Hetherington, Jr., M.D.
Margaret W. Hilgartner, M.D.
Alan R. Hinman, M.D.
Paul D. Hoeprich, M.D.
Stephen L. Hoffman, M.D.
James M. Holman, M.D.
Edward W. Holmes, Jr., M.D.
George R. Honig, M.D., Ph.D.
Sibley W. Hoobler, M.D.
David L. Horwitz, M.D.
H. Dunbar Hoskins, Jr., M.D.
Frank M. Howard, Jr., M.D.
A. S. P. Hua, M.B., B.S., M.R.A.C.P.
James M. Hughes, M.D.
George W. Hunter, III, Ph.D.
Richard S. Irwin, M.D.
Jon I. Isenberg, M.D.
Robert R. Jacobson, M.D.,Ph.D.
Sheldon Jacobson, M.D.
Joseph Jarabak, M.D., Ph.D.
Graham H. Jeffries, M.D.
Joseph B. Jerome, Ph.D.
Joseph E. Johnson, III, M.D.
Judith K. Jones, M.D., Ph.D.
Richard J. Jones, M.D.
Rodney C. Jung, M.D., Ph.D.
Dennis D. Juranek, D.V.M., M.Sc.
Thomas Kahn, M.D.
Mitchell V. Kaminski, Jr., M.D.
Norman M. Kaplan, M.D.
Karl D. Kappus, Ph.D.
Lester Karafin, M.D.
Raja W. Abdul-Karim
John E. Kasik, M.D.
Herbert E. Kaufman, M.D.
Charles Y. Kawada, M.D.
B. H. Kean, M.D.
Robert J. Keim, M.D.
A. Richard Kendall, M.D.
Theodore M. King, M.D.
Joseph B. Kirsner, M.D., Ph.D.
Harold L. Klawans, M.D.
Francis J. Kleeman, M.D.

Stuart A. Kleit, M.D.
James R. Klinenberg, M.D.
David Knox, M.D.
Delbert D. Konnor, Pharm. M.D.
Stanley G. Korenman, M.D.
Dorothy T. Kreiger, M.D.
Saul Krugman, M.D.
Leslie A. Kuhn, M.D.
Calvin M. Kunin, M.D.
Richard L. Landau, M.D.
Rene Langou, M.D.
Jack Lapides, M.D.
James E. Lebensohn, M.D., Ph.D.
Garrett Lee, M.D.
Robert S. Lees, M.D.
Howard Leibowitz, M.D.
Irving H. Leopold, M.D., D.Sc.
Simmons Lessell, M.D.
Irving M. Levine, M.D.
Robert I. Levy, M.D.
Lawrence M. Lichtenstein, M.D.
Theodore W. Lieberman, M.D.
William Likoff, M.D.
Robert D. Lindeman, M.D.
Mortimer B. Lipsett, M.D.
Samuel Livingston, M.D.
R. Bruce Logue, M.D.
Matilda MacIntyre, Ph.D.
Howard I. Maibach, M.D.
Dennis G. Maki, M.D.
Juan R. Malaglada, M.D.
Philip D. Marsden, M.D.
John R. Marshall, M.D.
Maurice J. Martin, M.D.
William R. Martin, M.D.
R. Michael Massanari, M.D.
Barry J. Materson, M.D.
Kenneth P. Mathews, M.D.
Richard H. Mattson, M.D.
A. Edward Maumenee, M.D.
George H. McCracken, Jr., M.D.
Edwin M. Meares, Jr., M.D.
James C. Melby, M.D.
Joseph L. Melnick, M.D.
Wallace B. Mendelson, M.D.
Arlen D. Meyers, M.D.
Myron Miller, M.D.
Joel S. Mindel, M.D.
Daniel R. Mishell, Jr., M.D.
Drogo K. Montague, M.D.
Arnold S. Monto, M.D.
Neil C. Moran, M.D.
Karl M. Morgenstein, M.D.

Arnold M. Moses, M.D.
Harry Most, M.D.
Gilbert H. Mudge, M.D.
John F. Mueller, M.D.
John D. Nelson, M.D.
Stephen R. Newmark, M.D.
S. H. Ngai, M.D.
Murray Nussbaum, M.D.
Gary K. Oakes, M.D.
Harold A. Oberman, M.D.
Paul O'Keefe, M.D.
Jack H. Oppenheimer, M.D.
Robert A. O'Reilly, M.D.
Milton Orkin, M.D.
Jack Orloff, M.D.
John A. Owen, Jr., M.D.
Lot B. Page, M.D.
Ogelsby Paul, M.D.
David F. Paulson, M.D.
Harold E. Paulus, M.D.
George J. Pazin, M.D.
J. Kiffin Penry, M.D.
Edward L. Pesanti, M.D.
Thomas H. Pettit, M.D.
Thomas L. Petty, M.D.
Alan L. Plummer, M.D.
Steven M. Podos, M.D.
Bernard S. Pogorel, M.D.
Irvin P. Pollack, M.D.
William B. Pratt, M.D.
Stephen R. Preblud, M.D.
Irving Pruce, B.S., R.Ph.
Harry Quigley, M.D.
Herbert Rakatansky, M.D.
Judith L. Rapoport, M.D.
Howard Rasmussen, M.D, Ph.D.
A.S. Rebuck, M.D.
Samuel Refetoff, M.D.
Warren Richards, M.D.
Alan G. Robinson, M.D.
John A. Robinson, M.D.
Robert L. Rosenfield, M.D.
Edward C. Rosenow, III, M.D.
Norman O. Rothermich, M.D.
Arthur Rubenstein, M.D.
Barry H. Rumack, M.D.
Henry I. Russek, M.D.
Lester B. Salans, M.D.
Paul Sandor, M.D.
Joel R. Saper, M.D.
Felix A. Sarubbi, M.D.
Joseph Sataloff, M.D.
Deborah A. Saunders, Pharm. D.

Michael A. Savin, M.D.
Jane G. Schaller, M.D.
Martin Scharf, M.D.
Irwin J. Schatz, M.D.
Steven Schenker, M.D.
Maurice Schiff, M.D.
Lawrence B. Schonberger, M.D.
Robert W. Schrier, M.D.
Harold Schulman, M.D.
Myron G. Schultz, D.V.M., M.D.
Franklin D. Schwartz, M.D.
Herbert A. Selenkow, M.D.
Sarah H. Wood Sell, M.D.
Nasrollah T. Shahidi, M.D.
Maurice E. Shils, M.D., Sc.D.
David Shoch, M.D.
Roy G. Shorter, M.D.
Sheldon C. Siegel, M.D.
Fredric J. Silverblatt, M.D.
Fred Simmons, M.D.
R. A. Simpson, M.D.
Carroll N. Smith, Ph.D.
R. Brian Smith, M.D.
J. Graham Smith, Jr., M.D.
William J. Snape, Jr., M.D.
Frederic Solomon, M.D.
Lester F. Soyka, M.D.
Gershon J. Spector, M.D.
Sheldon L. Spector, M.D.
Leon Speroff, M.D.
Roy T. Steigbigel, M.D.
Frederick Steigmann, M.D.
Jay H. Stein, M.D.
E. Richard Stiehm, M.D.
Emanuel M. Steindler, M.S.
Gordon J. Strewler, M.D.
M. Stuart Strong, M.D.
Charles D. Swartz, M.D.
J. Clyde Swartzwelder, Ph.D.
Ewart A. Swinyard, Ph.D.
John H. Talbott, M.D.

Robert C. Tarazi, M.D.
Howard F. Taswell, M.D.
James J. Tennenbaum, M.D.
Helen M. Tepperman, Ph.D.
Steven M. Teutsch, M.D.
E. Clinton Texter, Jr., M.D.
David L. Thomson, M.D.
Michael Thorner, M.D.
Donald R. Tredway, M.D., Ph.D.
Ross M. Tucker, M.D.
John S. Turner, M.D.
John P. Utz, M.D.
Professor Doctor M. Verstraete
Stanley L. Wallace, M.D.
Stanley Wallach, M.D.
Morton Ward, M.D.
Albert J. Wasserman, M.D.
D. Robert Webb, M.D.
Donald E. Weidhaas, Ph.D.
Max H. Weil, M.D, Ph.D.
Alan J. Wein, M.D.
Harvey J. Weiss, M.D.
Nathan S. Weiss, M.D.
Anne C. Wentz, M.D.
Stanford Wessler, M.D.
Robert Whang, M.D.
Philip L. White, Sc.D.
Richard J. Whitley, M.D.
B. J. Wilder, M.D.
John T. Wilson, III, M.D.
Charles L. Winek, Ph.D.
Roger A. Winkel, M.D.
William Winkler, D.V.M.
G. L. Wollam, M.D.
Colin R. Woolf, M.D., F.R.C.P.
Sumner J. Yaffe, M.D.
Ts' ai-fan Yu, M.D.
Dewey K. Ziegler, M.D.
Douglas P. Zipes, M.D.
Thomas T. Zsotér, M.D.
Frederick P. Zuspan, M.D.

Reviewers for the American Society for Clinical Pharmacology and Therapeutics

Jeffrey L. Anderson, M.D.
  Ann Arbor, Michigan
Daniel L. Azarnoff, M.D.
  Chicago, Illinois
William T. Beaver, M.D.
  Washington, D.C.
Henrik Holt Bendixen, M.D.
  New York, New York

Henry J. Binder, M.D.
  New Haven, Connecticut
Barry Blackwell, M.D.
  Dayton, Ohio
Robert E. Bolinger, M.D.
  Kansas City, Kansas
George A. Bray, M.D.
  Torrance, California

W. Arthur Burke, Pharm.D.
  Wilmington, Delaware
Robert P. Burns, M.D.
  Columbia, Missouri
Harold E. Carlson, M.D.
  Los Angeles, California
Edward A. Carr, Jr., M.D.
  Buffalo, New York
Jay D. Coffman, M.D.
  Boston, Massachusetts
Jay N. Cohn, M.D.
  Minneapolis, Minnesota
Benjamin G. Covino, M.D., Ph.D.
  Boston, Massachusetts
William H. Crosby, Jr., M.D.
  La Jolla, California
Tapas K. DasGupta, M.D., Ph.D.
  Chicago, Illinois
Robert A. Davidoff, M.D.
  Miami, Florida
John M. Davis, M.D.
  Chicago, Illinois
Ghislain Devroede, M.D.
  Quebec, Canada
Daniel Deykin, M.D.
  Boston, Massachusetts
Ananias C. Diokno, M.D.
  Ann Arbor, Michigan
Alan K. Done, M.D.
  Detroit, Michigan
F. E. Dreifuss, M.D.
  Charlottesville, Virginia
Roger C. Duvoisin, M.D.
  New York, New York
Philip P. Ellis, M.D.
  Denver, Colorado
F. Robert Fekety, Jr., M.D.
  Ann Arbor, Michigan
Charles L. Fox, Jr., M.D.
  New York, New York
Daniel X. Freedman, M.D.
  Chicago, Illinois
Edward D. Freis, M.D.
  Washington, D.C.
Milo Gibaldi, Ph.D.
  Seattle, Washington
Ray W. Gifford, Jr., M.D.
  Cleveland, Ohio
Robert E. Goldstein, M.D.
  Bethesda, Maryland
David Y. Graham, M.D.
  Houston, Texas

David J. Greenblatt, M.D.
  Boston, Massachusetts
Tibor J. Greenwalt, M.D.
  Washington, D.C.
Rolf M. Gunnar, M.D.
  Maywood, Illinois
Robert A. Hatcher, M.D.
  Atlanta, Georgia
Stephen L. Hoffman, M.D.
  San Diego, California
Alan F. Hofmann, M.D.
  San Diego, California
William W. Hofmann, M.D.
  Palo Alto, California
David L. Horwitz, M.D.
  Chicago, Illinois
H. Dunbar Hoskins, Jr., M.D.
  San Francisco, California
Carl C. Hug, Jr., M.D., Ph.D.
  Atlanta, Georgia
Anthony Kales, M.D.
  Hershey, Pennsylvania
Fred E. Karch, M.D.
  Rochester, New York
John E. Kasik, M.D.
  Oakdale, Iowa
Arthur S. Keats, M.D.
  Houston, Texas
Theodore M. King, M.D.
  Baltimore, Maryland
Frederick A. Klipstein, M.D.
  Rochester, New York
Stuart Krauss, M.D.
  Chicago, Illinois
Jack Lapides, M.D.
  Ann Arbor, Michigan
Gerhard Levy, Pharm.D.
  Amherst, New York
Robert I. Levy, M.D.
  Bethesda, Maryland
Abraham N. Lieberman, M.D.
  New York, New York
Theodore W. Lieberman, M.D.
  New York, New York
Mortimer B. Lipsett, M.D.
  Bethesda, Maryland
Armand Littman, M.D., Ph.D.
  Hines, Illinois
Howard I. Maibach, M.D.
  San Francisco, California
Kenneth P. Mathews, M.D.
  Ann Arbor, Michigan

Myron Miller, M.D.
  Syracuse, New York
John D. Nelson, M.D.
  Dallas, Texas
Harold E. Paulus, M.D.
  Los Angeles, California
Bernard S. Pogorel, M.D.
  Los Angeles, California
Albert W. Pruitt, M.D.
  Atlanta, Georgia
Howard Rasmussen, M.D., Ph.D.
  New Haven, Connecticut
Karl Rickels, M.D.
  Philadelphia, Pennsylvania
Harris D. Riley, Jr., M.D.
  Oklahoma City, Oklahoma
Donald S. Robinson, M.D.
  Huntington, West Virginia
John A. Robinson, M.D.
  Maywood, Illinois
Alan Rosenbaum, M.D.
  Rochester, Minnesota
Marvin E. Rosenthale, Ph.D.
  Raritan, New Jersey
Norman O. Rothermich, M.D.
  Columbus, Ohio
Felix A. Sarubbi, M.D.
  Chapel Hill, North Carolina
D. R. Saunders, M.D.
  Seattle, Washington
Myron G. Schultz, D.V.M., M.D.
  Atlanta, Georgia

Edward M. Sellers, M.D., Ph.D.
  Toronto, Canada
Maurice E. Shils, M.D., Sc.D.
  New York, New York
J. Graham Smith, Jr., M.D.
  Augusta, Georgia
Lester F. Soyka, M.D.
  Burlington, Vermont
Gershon J. Spector, M.D.
  St. Louis, Missouri
Leon Speroff, M.D.
  Portland, Oregon
R. W. Summers, M.D.
  Iowa City, Iowa
Steven M. Teutsch, M.D.
  Atlanta, Georgia
Miles M. Weinberger, M.D.
  Iowa City, Iowa
Anne C. Wentz, M.D.
  Memphis, Tennessee
Stanford Wessler, M.D.
  New York, New York
Philip L. White, Sc.D.
  Wilmette, Illinois
Colin R. Woolf, M.D., F.R.C.P.
  Toronto, Canada
Melvin D. Yahr, M.D.
  New York, New York
Hyman J. Zimmerman, M.D.
  Washington, D.C.

The contributions of those pharmaceutical companies that supplied information on products of their manufacture to assist in the preparation of the evaluative statements in this volume are acknowledged.

JOHN C. BALLIN, Ph.D.
Director
Department of Drugs

New Drugs Evaluated
For Fourth Edition

Drug	Indication or Classification
Asparaginase [Elspar]	Antineoplastic
Azatadine Maleate [Optimine]	Antihistamine
Baclofen [Lioresal]	Skeletal muscle relaxant
Beclomethasone Dipropionate [Beclovent, Vanceril]	Adrenal corticosteroid for bronchoconstriction
Bretylium Tosylate [Bretylol]	Antiarrhythmic
Bromocriptine Mesylate [Parlodel]	Dopaminergic
Butorphanol Tartrate [Stadol]	Analgesic
Calcitriol [Rocaltrol]	Vitamin D metabolite
Carboprost Tromethamine [Prostin/M15]	Uterine stimulant
Carmustine [BiCNU]	Antineoplastic
Cefaclor [Ceclor]	Cephalosporin
Cefadroxil Monohydrate [Duricef]	Cephalosporin
Cefamandole Nafate [Mandol]	Cephalosporin
Cefoxitin Sodium [Mefoxin]	Cephamycin
Chlorhexidine Gluconate [Hibiclens] [Hibitane Tincture]	Dermatologic Antimicrobial skin cleaner Preoperative preparation of patient's skin
Cimetidine [Tagamet]	Gastrointestinal ulcer therapy
Cisplatin [Platinol]	Antineoplastic
Clemastine Fumarate [Tavist]	Antihistamine
Colestipol Hydrochloride [Colestid]	Hypolipidemic
Cyclobenzaprine Hydrochloride [Flexeril]	Skeletal muscle relaxant
Desmopressin Acetate [DDAVP]	Antidiuretic
Desoximetasone [Topicort]	Topical corticosteroid
Dextranomer [Debrisan]	Nonenzymatic preparation for wound debridement
Diflorasone Diacetate [Florone]	Topical corticosteroid
Diloxanide Furoate [Furamide]	Amebicide
Dinoprostone [Prostin E2]	Uterine stimulant
DMSO (dimethyl sulfoxide) [Rimso-50]	Interstitial cystitis
Disopyramide Phosphate [Norpace]	Antiarrhythmic
Dobutamine Hydrochloride [Dobutrex]	Inotropic agent

Etidocaine Hydrochloride [Duranest]	Local anesthetic
Etidronate Disodium [Didronel]	Paget's disease
Hepatitis B Immune Globulin [H-BIG, Hep-B-Gammagee]	Antiserum
Hymenoptera Venom Allergenic Extracts [Albay, Pharmalgen]	Immunotherapeutic agent
Intralipid	Intravenous fat emulsion
Lactulose [Cephulac, Duphalac]	Portal-systemic encephalopathy
Lomustine [CeeNU]	Antineoplastic
Loperamide Hydrochloride [Imodium]	Antidiarrheal
Lorazepam [Ativan]	Antianxiety
Metoclopramide [Reglan]	Gastrointestinal motility stimulant
Metoprolol Tartrate [Lopressor]	Antihypertensive
Microfibrillar Collagen Hemostat [Avitene]	Hemostatic
Minoxidil [Loniten]	Antihypertensive
Nalbuphine [Nubaine]	Analgesic
Pneumococcal Vaccine, Polyvalent [Pneumovax]	Immunologic
Prazepam [Verstran]	Antianxiety
Prazosin Hydrochloride [Minipress]	Antihypertensive
Probucol [Lorelco]	Hypolipidemic
Protirelin [Relefact TRH, Thypinone]	Thyroid function diagnosis
Sincalide [Kinevac]	Gastrointestinal agent
Somatropin [Asellacrin]	Human growth hormone
Sulindac [Clinoril]	Antiarthritic
Tamoxifen Citrate [Nolvadex]	Antineoplastic
Ticarcillin Disodium [Ticar]	Penicillin
Ticrynafen [Selacryn]	Antihypertensive-Diuretic
Timolol Maleate [Timoptic]	Antiglaucoma drug
Trimipramine Maleate [Surmontil]	Antidepressant
Urokinase [Abbokinase]	Anticoagulant
Valproic Acid [Depakene]	Anticonvulsant
Vidarabine [Vira-A]	Antiviral

Investigational Drugs Discussed in Fourth Edition

Drug	Indication or Classification
Anti-Human Lymphocyte Globulin	Immunomodulator
Azacitidine	Antineoplastic
Captopril	Antihypertensive
Chenodiol (Chenodeoxycholic Acid) [Chenix]	Gallstone therapy
Clofazimine [Lamprene]	Antimycobacterial (leprosy)
Daunorubicin Hydrochloride	Antineoplastic
Deprenyl	Antiparkinsonism
Domperidone	Antiemetic
Etomidate	General anesthetic (intravenous)
Flunitrazepam [Rohypnol]	General anesthetic (intravenous)
Ftorafur	Antineoplastic
Haemophilius Influenzae Type B Vaccine	Vaccine
Hepatitis B Vaccine Inactivated	Vaccine
Hexamethylmelamine	Antineoplastic
Isoflurane [Forane]	General anesthetic (inhalant)
Isophosphamide	Antineoplastic
Isotretinoin (13-*cis*-retinoic acid)	Dermatologic (acne)
Levamisole	Immunomodulator
Mitolactol	Antineoplastic
Penfluridol [Semap]	Antipsychotic
Porfiromycin	Antineoplastic
Propiram Fumarate [Dirame]	Analgesic
Razoxane	Antineoplastic
Ritodrine	Uterine relaxant
Saralasin	Antihypertensive
Semustine	Antineoplastic
Streptozocin [Zanosar]	Antineoplastic
Teprotide	Antihypertensive
Tetrabenazine	Antichorea
Varicella-Zoster Vaccine Live Attenuated	Vaccine
Zomepirac Sodium [Zomax]	Analgesic

Scope and Organization of Evaluations | 1

As with the previous editions of *AMA Drug Evaluations*, this fourth edition has been organized into chapters that are based, insofar as possible, on therapeutic classifications. All chapters have been updated from the third edition; some also have been reorganized, expanded, and renamed, and some new chapters (eg, antiviral agents, immunomodulators) have been added. Most chapters contain an introduction that presents a general discussion of the uses of the drugs within the therapeutic category. When possible, the introduction includes comparative evaluations and a statement on drugs of choice within the class. This is followed by evaluations for individual drugs. Drugs selected for individual evaluations include virtually all therapeutic agents in the official compendia, *United States Pharmacopeia* (U.S.P.) and *National Formulary* (N.F.); the drugs, including mixtures, most commonly prescribed or administered by physicians in the United States; and other agents, including some investigational drugs, which are judged to be of particular importance to complete a discussion of a therapeutic category. Other nationally distributed preparations that are not evaluated individually are listed and indexed to give information about their therapeutic category, composition, and availability. Although most drugs listed or described are dispensed exclusively or principally by prescription, many, of course, *can* be sold without prescription and these are so indicated.

Drug evaluations have been based upon the most recent information available but, in a project of this scope, it is inevitable that some products have been omitted inadvertently; such omissions are regretted. Also, some drugs may no longer be marketed when this edition appears in print. Updating of information has continued as near as possible to the time of publication. In addition, efforts have been made to include drugs newly introduced to the market as near the publication date as practicable, and drugs that have investigational status are so indicated in the chapter introductions and evaluations.

The inclusion of a particular drug in *AMA Drug Evaluations* does not imply endorsement by the American Medical Association, nor should it be a criterion for approving use of that drug in any institution or for any other purpose. The principal purpose of this volume is to provide the medical profession with evaluations of selected drugs based on the available evidence. An evaluation may be favorable, unfavorable, or a combination of both, and it only represents a statement of the general merits of the preparation, not its specific usefulness in a given patient. The physician should determine in each individual case the relevancy of the limitations, adverse reactions, contraindications, or precautions given in the text.

The evaluative or interpretive information in the book, particularly on controversial matters, may disagree with opinions from other sources. Statements are based on the convergent trend of information available from scientific literature, unpublished data, the advice of consultants, and the opinion of reviewers from the American Society for Clinical Pharmacology and Therapeutics. Because the indications approved for labeling by the Food and Drug Administration may lag behind both the world literature and good medical practice, uses other than those included in the approved labeling for many drugs are discussed in order to provide more complete information. The information on *adverse reactions* and *precautions* usually has been condensed and represents that considered most essential to the physician's use of the drugs. Accordingly, such information as rare, minor, or unconfirmed reactions or precautions that relate to obvious or remote situations are sometimes omitted. For other information, for basic data, and even for varying points of view, the physician is encouraged to consult and compare the statements made in this text with those appearing in the many other sources of information on drugs.

The *usual dosage* information presented in this text falls within the ranges given in official compendia, those suggested by manufacturers, or those considered appropriate by other authorities. For many drugs, however, the correct dose depends upon the size, age, and condition of the patient; response to treatment; sensitivity or tolerance; and the possible synergistic or antagonistic effect of concomitant medication. If the clinical situation permits, establishment of the dose should be cautious and exploratory unless a wide margin of safety prevails. However, if immediate disaster threatens because of therapeutic failure, treatment should be aggressive. In either situation, the physician should remember that improper dosage with the proper drug is probably as common a cause of inadequate response or complete therapeutic failure as the use of an improper drug. Accordingly, many usual doses are stated as ranges. Even the limits of these ranges are not inviolable. The upper limits given for most ranges, however, do suggest that

larger amounts either may increase the risks of toxicity beyond what is ordinarily acceptable or may fail to provide a significant degree of additional therapeutic effect; similarly, the lower limits often indicate that smaller doses could not be expected to provide full therapeutic effects for most patients. In the individual evaluations of some drugs, a collateral statement may make it clear that, on the basis of the evaluation, no dosage is suggested for that drug.

The *preparations* listed for each drug, including those available generically, appear at the end of each evaluation. However, published reports of clinical experience often are limited to the products of one or only a few manufacturers. Adequate clinical comparisons of all brands of the same drug are rarely available. For this reason, a valid comparison of brands has rarely been possible and seldom attempted. Physicians should bear in mind that all brands and generically labeled forms of the same drug are not necessarily equivalent therapeutically. Differences in pharmaceutical formulations (coatings, binders, particle size, rate of disintegration and dissolution, purity of ingredients, and other factors) can lead to variations in absorption and biological availability of the drug. Also, the degree of consistency from batch to batch depends upon the manufacturer's quality control procedures. In vitro tests designed to demonstrate product uniformity do not assure in vivo effectiveness. How frequently significant differences occur among various brands of allegedly equivalent products is difficult to estimate. Nevertheless, the fact that differences sometimes do occur should be recognized by the prescribing physician in appraising the information in this book and in writing prescriptions that may be filled with a product from any of several manufacturers.

Physicians are urged to become informed about the quality and purity of drug products available from multiple sources and to supplement medical considerations with cost considerations when selecting the drug of choice for a particular patient. Pharmacy and Therapeutic Committees of local hospitals, which often base their review of products for inclusion in the hospital's formulary on literature reports, experiences of local physicians, availability, and cost in their region, can serve as a source of information and guidance.

Timed-release preparations, which are formulated to release a drug slowly after oral administration in order to increase its duration of action, deserve special consideration because of their potential variability in action. The general term, "timed-release," used to describe these oral preparations in this text is synonymous with the term, "controlled-release," used by the Food and Drug Administration and includes formulations variously known as "delayed-action," "extended-release," "prolonged-action," "sustained-action," or "repeat-action," but does not include tablets specifically identified as "enteric-coated."

Data on which to base an evaluation of effectiveness are inadequate or unavailable for many timed-release forms; however, some have been tested for effectiveness, and these are indicated in the individual evaluations. No precise product specifications have been established by the official compendia for timed- release preparations. These preparations are listed in this book to provide information on their availability; as with all product information, such listing does not imply endorsement.

Drugs that are rapidly metabolized or excreted, but whose effects must be maintained steadily for prolonged periods, can be inconvenient to use because of the need for repeated administration at short intervals. Therefore, some timed- release preparations may provide a certain convenience and may improve compliance over more frequent administration--provided they actually deliver the medication in the even, measured manner that is intended. On the other hand, the use of timed-release preparations of drugs that have inherently long half-lives generally is not warranted. However, for those patients who eliminate these drugs rapidly, a timed-release preparation may be useful to prolong the duration of action if an effective plasma concentration of drug is achieved.

In *parenteral* preparations, sustained release is achieved by using relatively insoluble salts or esters of the active drug or a special vehicle from which the drug is slowly absorbed. It is doubtful that such techniques can ever deliver a dosage that is as precisely controlled as with intravenous infusion. Nevertheless, when some latitude in the range of the safe and effective blood level is permissible, substitution of slowly released preparations for repeated injections may provide a somewhat more uniform blood concentration, and this type of preparation is certainly more convenient. The depot preparation of benzathine penicillin G is an outstanding example of a useful sustained-release formulation. In some serious infections, of course, continuous intravenous infusion is still needed. Insulin is another excellent example of a drug which, even though dosage requirements are critical, has been prepared in sustained-release forms that have greatly simplified the management of diabetes. Reasonably satisfactory formulations for parenteral use also are available for various corticosteroids, androgens, estrogens, and a few other agents.

In response to requests of users of previous editions, a list of *Selected References* is included at the end of each chapter. In some instances, specific statements in the evaluations are cited, but in general the references have been selected to provide sources of additional information that the reader may wish to consult.

Doses and Use of Drugs In Certain Groups of Patients | 2

PEDIATRIC PATIENTS

There are many difficulties in choosing the most appropriate drugs and determining the dosage in pediatric patients. Whether children and infants will respond to a particular drug in the same manner as adults can be determined only through research and experience. Indeed, their responses to many drugs are known to be different. Factors that affect drug dosage in pediatric patients include the age and size of the individual as well as the disease state. Pediatric patients are usually divided into three age groups: newborn, 0 to 4 weeks (perinatal, first week, or first two weeks in premature infants); infant, 5 to 52 weeks; child, 1 to 16 years (adolescent, 12 to 16 years).

The pharmacokinetics of many drugs change with the continuing development of several physiologic functions as age increases. Many of the metabolic mechanisms in premature and newborn infants are not fully developed, and toxic blood concentrations of drugs may accumulate if dosage is based upon the traditional criteria for conversion from the amount given to adults. In fact, the infant's response to drugs during the first weeks of life probably varies more, overall, from that of a one-year-old than the response of a one-year-old varies from that of an adult.

Although an increasing number of studies are being conducted on the pharmacokinetics of drugs in pediatric patients, data on which to base dosage recommendations for specific drugs are limited. Consequently, most marketed drugs do not have established doses for infants and children. Nevertheless, some generalizations can be made on the basis of the information available, and these can be used as guides to determine the appropriateness of certain drugs and their dosage in pediatric patients.

The basic pharmacokinetic functions (absorption, distribution, metabolism, and excretion) affect a drug's disposition and concentration at receptor sites and hence its actions. The effects of these functions on a drug's actions at various ages should be considered when treating pediatric patients.

Absorption: Differences in gastrointestinal function that may affect the absorption of drugs occur primarily in the newborn and infant. (In general, there are no important differences in gastrointestinal absorption between the healthy child and adult.) Peristalsis is irregular during the first several weeks, gastric emptying is prolonged until about 6 to 12 months of age, and gastric pH fluctuates and does not reach adult values until about 3 years of age. Delayed oral absorption of nalidixic acid, gentamicin, phenytoin, and acetaminophen has been noted in neonates, and absorption of phenobarbital is delayed and reduced during the first two weeks. Because gastric acidity is decreased in the neonatal period, there is increased absorption of acid-labile penicillins in infants and children up to 3 years. In older infants and children, the rate of absorption of several anticonvulsants (phenobarbital, ethosuximide, valproic acid, clonazepam, diazepam) and imipramine is increased; thus, the frequency of administration of these drugs should be reduced. It should be kept in mind that diseases of the gastrointestinal tract may alter the absorption rate of orally administered drugs.

Intramuscular absorption in infants may be decreased and erratic, but percutaneous absorption occurs more rapidly and to a greater extent in infants than in adults because of anatomic differences in skin thickness.

Distribution: The distribution of drugs in neonates and infants may differ from that in older children and adults because body composition varies markedly with age. The proportion of body water (total and extracellular) is greater in the newborn but gradually decreases to adult values at about 12 months. The relative mass of subcutaneous tissue also varies; it is greatest at 9 months, decreases until about 6 years, and increases again in adolescence. These changes affect distribution of lipid-soluble drugs.

Another factor affecting drug disposition is plasma protein binding, which is decreased for some drugs in the newborn, but adult values are reached in about 10 to 12 months. Drugs for which decreased protein binding in infants has been reported include salicylates, penicillins, sulfonamides, phenytoin, phenylbutazone, phenobarbital, and imipramine. The protein binding of diazepam and digoxin is similar in infants and adults. In infants 1 to 6 months of age with congenital heart disease, digoxin has been found to have increased binding to the myocardium, which probably accounts for the increased dosage requirements in these patients. In neonates with hyperbilirubinemia, drugs that are highly bound to plasma proteins (eg, sulfonamides, salicylates, phenytoin) may displace bilirubin, resulting in toxic concentrations in the brain.

Metabolism: In general, the capacity of the infant's liver to metabolize drugs is low, but it varies for different drugs depending upon which enzymes are involved, since not all enzyme systems are affected to the same degree and do not attain adult values at the same rate. Drugs dependent on hepatic metabolism for elimination have longer apparent plasma half-lives in infants; thus, the interval between doses should be increased and the daily dose decreased. In addition, some drugs administered to the mother during pregnancy may affect metabolism in the newborn through induction of hepatic enzymes. For example, phenytoin and carbamazepine have shorter half-lives in neonates who were exposed to the drug prenatally. In addition, an inducing agent given to the mother may affect its own plasma half-life and that of certain other drugs given to the infant. Therefore, the possibility of a previous exposure to an inducing agent should be considered when administering drugs to a newborn infant. Although data on specific drugs are limited, longer apparent plasma half-life in infants has been reported for diazepam, digoxin, indomethacin, nalidixic acid, nortriptyline, acetaminophen, phenylbutazone, phenobarbital, phenytoin, salicylates, and tolbutamide. Conversely, in older children, theophylline, phenylbutazone, and most anticonvulsants are metabolized faster than in adults. It should be kept in mind that hepatic disease may affect the liver's metabolizing ability in children as well as in adults.

Excretion: Renal function is greatly reduced in neonates and infants but approaches adult values in about 6 to 12 months. Drugs that depend upon renal excretion for elimination are disposed of slowly in infants and have longer apparent half-lives. Therefore, the dosage of these drugs must be adjusted to avoid accumulation and toxic reactions. Dosage schedules for several antibiotics (eg, penicillins, gentamicin, kanamycin) that are eliminated by the kidney have been developed (see the appropriate chapters). Other drugs that are excreted at reduced rates include indomethacin, salicylic acid, acetaminophen, and sulfonamides. The renal clearance of digoxin is low at 1 month of age but increases to within the adult range at about 6 months. (See the section on Doses for Patients with Renal Impairment.)

Calculation of Doses for Children: It must be emphasized that any method devised to calculate drug dosage for both children and adults provides an estimate only, to be verified or corrected by clinical experience and by the response of the individual patient. Usually, the dose for children is given in terms of mg/kg of body weight or as a fraction proportionate to the weight of the child in comparison with that of an average adult. However, the dose of many drugs is not a simple linear function of body weight, and to calculate the dose as so much per kilogram of body weight is often inaccurate. Another common practice in determining a child's dose has been to give some fraction of an adult dose, using the age of the patient as a rough guide. Because of the great variation in size among children of the same age, this method can be satisfactory only if the drug has a wide margin of safety. Experience has shown that the dose of many drugs is more nearly proportionate to weight to the 0.7 power ($Wt^{0.7}$). The surface area of the body (in square meters) also may be calculated approximately by Wt (lb)$^{0.7} \times 0.055$. Although the validity of this method has been criticized because body surface area

TABLE 1.
DETERMINATION OF CHILDREN'S DOSES
FROM ADULT DOSES ON THE BASIS OF BODY SURFACE AREA

Age	Weight* (Kg.)	Weight* (lb.)	Surface area* (sq. M.)	Fraction of adult dose†
	2.0	4.4	0.15	0.09
Birth	3.4	7.4	0.21	0.12
3 weeks	4.0	8.8	0.25	0.14
3 months	5.7	12.5	0.29	0.17
6 months	7.4	16	0.36	0.21
9 months	9.1	20	0.44	0.25
1 year	10	22	0.46	0.27
1½ years	11	25	0.50	0.29
2 years	12	27	0.54	0.31
3 years	14	31	0.60	0.35
4 years	16	36	0.68	0.39
5 years	19	41	0.73	0.42
6 years	21	47	0.82	0.47
7 years	24	53	0.90	0.52
8 years	27	59	0.97	0.56
9 years	29	65	1.05	0.61
10 years	32	71	1.12	0.65
11 years	36	78	1.20	0.70
12 years	39	86	1.28	0.74

*Approximate average for age.
†Based on adult surface area of 1.73 sq. M.
From Done AK: Drugs for children, in Modell W (ed): *Drugs of Choice 1972-1973*. St Louis, CV Mosby Co, 1972.

may not be related directly to physiologic and metabolic function, it does provide a practical and useful basis for the estimation of drug dosage in children. Thus, dosage expressed as grams or milligrams of a given drug per square meter of surface area rather than per unit of body weight may provide a more accurate method of adjusting the dosage to the age or size of the patient.

Statements of pediatric doses for individual drugs in this book follow the method of conversion that has been developed for that particular drug. Thus, some conversions are based upon age, some upon weight, and some upon body surface area. If adequate dosage information based on actual pediatric use is either nonexistent or not readily available, suggested dosage guidelines sometimes are furnished even though it is recognized that more data would be desirable; for some drugs, lack of data has been specifically acknowledged. When the dosage for children has been established, it is given in the text and should be used in preference to any calculated dose. When information is inadequate, it is suggested that the body surface area be taken as the criterion —*provided there is no evidence that a child will react to the drug differently from an adult*. Calculation of a fractional exponential function of weight is too forbidding for practical use, but the task may be simplified by employing a table (see Table 1).

GERIATRIC PATIENTS

Elderly patients also should be given special consideration when determining the dosage of certain drugs. Because they use relatively more drugs than other age groups, the appropriate choice of drugs and dosage is of primary importance in their health care. Although a specific age cannot be applied to define this group, patients over 60 or 65 are usually included. However, it should be kept in mind that the aging process occurs at different rates in different people; thus, each patient must be evaluated individually. A patient's mental and physical state should be the primary consideration and not the chronologic age.

When prescribing drugs for an elderly patient, special attention should be given to several general principles:

(1) The physician should ascertain what other medications, including OTC products, the patient is taking. Elderly people often take many drugs, some of which may not be needed and should be discontinued. The patient should receive as few drugs as possible.

(2) The dosage schedule should be as simple as possible, and the dosage form should be easily self-administered. Directions for taking the medication should be understood by the patient; written instructions are more desirable than oral.

(3) Patients should be followed closely to determine compliance, drug efficacy, and adverse effects.

(4) Any physiologic or pathologic changes that may affect the dosage and response to the drug must be considered. However, these factors are often difficult to identify and studies on the pharmacokinetics of drugs in the elderly have been limited. Nevertheless, available evidence indicates that changes in several physiologic functions occur with aging and these may affect the actions of certain drugs.

Absorption: There is little evidence that the absorption of drugs, which are absorbed by passive diffusion, is diminished, except indirectly. Other factors are usually responsible for altered drug effects in the elderly. However, conditions such as decreased gastric acidity and gastrointestinal motility, which reduce gastric emptying, may delay or impair drug absorption. Drugs that affect these functions (eg, antacids, anticholinergics) may affect the absorption of other agents. In contrast to drugs, the absorption of nutrients, vitamins, and minerals may be impaired in the elderly. For example, it has been reported that iron absorption is decreased and, thus, larger doses may be necessary to correct iron deficiency anemia.

Distribution: Alterations in circulation and changes in body composition may affect the distribution of drugs. Total body weight may decrease, especially in the very elderly, but the ratio of fat to lean is usually greater, which may affect the distribution and accumulation of lipid-soluble agents. In addition, the total circulating plasma albumin level may be decreased; thus, drugs that are highly protein bound (eg, warfarin) will have more unbound (active) drug available. Because warfarin or other anticoagulants may have an enhanced effect in geriatric patients, therapy should be monitored carefully. Furthermore, since displacement of one drug by another from protein-binding sites is one mechanism of drug-drug interaction (see Chapter 5), it is particularly important to consider this possibility in the elderly.

Metabolism: The metabolism of drugs by hepatic enzymes may be reduced in the elderly, but few studies indicate that this is clinically significant unless liver function is seriously impaired as a result of disease. There appears to be greater individual variability among the elderly than the young. The response to enzyme inducers may be reduced in the elderly. The half-lives of chlordiazepoxide and diazepam are prolonged in these patients, thus increasing central nervous system depression; however, metabolic clearance is reduced only for the former drug. Increased half-life may result from altered protein binding or a change in apparent distribution. The plasma half-life of phenylbutazone also is increased in the elderly, presumably due to decreased hepatic enzyme activity.

Excretion: Because renal function decreases with age, the elimination of drugs excreted by the kidney is reduced in the elderly. In addition, most individuals over 60 years of age have some renal pathology, which further reduces renal function. Therefore, it is important to consider the patient's renal function when selecting doses of certain drugs. Doses should be reduced or given at longer intervals to prevent accumulation, and the patient should be monitored carefully. Drugs excreted by the kidney that are used commonly in elderly patients include digoxin, quinidine, aminoglycoside antimicrobials, penicillins, tetracyclines, amantadine, and lithium. The evaluations on these drugs should be consulted for dosages in patients with decreased renal function. See also the section on Doses for Patients with Renal Impairment.

Sensitivity: Elderly patients apparently are more sensitive to some drug effects. However, the mechanism involved is not known. Increased receptor sensitivity is difficult to determine and explain pharmacologically. Changes in hormone, adrenergic, and biogenic amine receptors have been shown to be associated with aging, but their clinical significance with respect to drug action has not yet been determined. In general, the elderly are more sensitive to narcotics: Morphine produces increased pain relief but more variable serum levels, and meperidine has a longer half-life and causes an increased incidence of adverse reactions. Barbiturates cause erratic and paradoxical effects; their half-lives are prolonged but the mechanism is unknown. The tricyclic antidepressants cause confusion and disorientation, which may result from increased sensitivity to their anticholinergic effects. The incidence of extrapyramidal reactions and orthostatic hypotension caused by phenothiazines may be increased. The thiazides also cause more orthostatic hypotension, which may result from an impaired compensatory action. Also, they may cause hypokalemia that potentiates the effects of digitalis. Potassium-sparing diuretics appear to cause a greater incidence of hyperkalemia, possibly as a result of impaired renal function. The elderly may have increased susceptibility to hypoglycemia with use of the sulfonylureas. With aspirin, there may be a higher incidence of occult blood loss, which may lead to iron deficiency anemia, and thus larger doses of iron than usual may be required because of decreased absorption.

DOSES FOR PATIENTS WITH RENAL IMPAIRMENT

Drugs that are excreted unchanged by the kidney or whose pharmacologically active metabolites are eliminated by renal excretion may produce adverse effects in patients with impaired renal function if usual doses are administered. To prevent drug accumulation and toxic effects caused by increased plasma levels of the drug or metabolite, it is necessary to reduce the rate of drug administration so that the desired plasma concentration of the drug will be maintained. This can be accomplished by reducing the size of the dose and maintaining the usual interval between doses or increasing the interval between doses while using the standard dosage. In either case, the mean steady state plasma concentration of the drug will be decreased; however, decreasing the dose reduces the peak drug plasma concentration proportionately more than the trough plasma concentration of the drug, whereas the reverse occurs when the dose interval is lengthened. For example, drugs with a high toxic peak level (eg, digoxin) should be given in reduced doses, and for aminoglycoside antibiotics, the interval usually is increased. In some instances, it may be preferable to give reduced doses at increased intervals to prevent toxic peak levels or subtherapeutic trough levels.

Dosage adjustment is most important if renal function is less than 50% of normal, if the percentage of drug excreted unchanged is above 50%, or if active metabolites are extensively eliminated by the kidney.

Since changes in the renal clearance of a drug generally correspond to changes in endogenous creatinine clearance, determination of the latter value can be used in conjunction with the percentage of drug or metabolite(s) excreted to calculate the dosage adjustment. If creatinine clearance cannot be obtained, it can be estimated from the serum creatinine value if age and body weight are considered and renal function and serum creatinine are at steady state. Nomograms to facilitate the determination of this conversion have been published, but it also may be calculated from the following equation (Cockcroft and Gault, 1976):

$$\text{Creatinine Clearance} = \frac{(140 - \text{age}) \times (\text{body weight in kg})}{72 \times \text{serum creatinine}}$$

An overestimation of creatinine clearance may be obtained in certain patients (eg, pregnant women, patients with markedly reduced renal function [10 ml/min]) but, for purposes of altering dosage, the degree of overestimation is probably not important.

The dosage adjustment factor can be calculated with the following formula:

$$\text{Dosage Adjustment Factor} = \frac{1}{F(kf - 1) + 1}$$

F = fraction of drug excreted unchanged
kf = relative kidney function, calculated by dividing creatinine clearance by 120 ml/min

TABLE 2.
DOSAGE-ADJUSTMENT FACTORS

% Excreted Unchanged in Urine	Creatinine Clearance (ml/min)						
	0	10	20	40	60	80	120
10	1.1	1.1	1.1	1.1	1.1	1.0	1.0
20	1.3	1.2	1.2	1.1	1.1	1.1	1.0
30	1.4	1.3	1.3	1.2	1.2	1.1	1.0
40	1.7	1.6	1.5	1.4	1.3	1.1	1.0
50	2.0	1.8	1.7	1.5	1.3	1.2	1.0
60	2.5	2.2	2.0	1.7	1.4	1.3	1.0
70	3.3	2.8	2.3	1.9	1.5	1.3	1.0
80	5.0	3.7	3.0	2.1	1.7	1.4	1.0
90	10.0	5.7	4.0	2.5	1.8	1.4	1.0
100	∞	12.0	6.0	3.0	2.0	1.5	1.0

From Drugs and renal disease, in Bochner F, et al (eds): *Handbook of Clinical Pharmacology.* Boston, Little, Brown and Company, 1978, 28-35.

or it may be determined from a table, which has been derived from this formula (see Table 2).

The dosage adjustment factor can be used to reduce the size of the dose given at the usual interval or to increase the time between administration of doses given to patients with normal renal function. To determine an adjusted dose given at the same interval, the usual dose is divided by the dosage adjustment factor. To calculate the increased interval between usual doses, the normal interval is multiplied by the dosage adjustment factor. Although conditions usually do not exist for exact application of this factor, a reasonable dosage modification is generally possible. Guidelines for specific dosage adjustments for many drugs have been published (Bennett et al, 1977) and some are included in the individual evaluations.

USE OF DRUGS DURING PREGNANCY

Drugs are used during pregnancy primarily to treat maternal disease, but the fetus also becomes a drug recipient. Consequently, medication prescribed during pregnancy may result in unexpected and occasionally tragic effects in the developing fetus, for whom the drug was not intended in the first place.

Placental transport of maternal substances to the fetus and from the fetus to the mother is established at about the fifth week of embryonic life. In view of the ease with which substances in the mother's blood stream pass into the fetus, the earlier concept of a placental barrier is now recognized as a myth. Any drug or chemical substance administered to the mother is able to penetrate the placenta to some extent unless it is destroyed or altered during passage. Hence, administration of a drug to a pregnant woman presents a unique problem to the physician: Not only must he consider maternal pharmacologic mechanisms for drug action and disposition, but he also must be constantly aware of the fetus as a potential recipient of the drug.

It is essential that the physician have information concerning the potential risk to the fetus so that he may weigh this against the potential benefit to be gained from therapeutic treatment of the mother. Unfortunately, this information is seldom available. Although laboratory experiments have yielded considerable information on the embryopathic effects of drugs, these experimental findings cannot be extrapolated from animals to man. Thus, the preclinical evaluation of fetal toxicity that is routinely included in the investigation of new drugs does not provide reliable information that can be translated into clinical usage. It also is apparent from animal testing that a single teratogen can produce a variety of malformations and, conversely, the same malformations can be caused by a variety of teratogens. Because of this lack of specificity of both cause and effect, it is difficult to establish in man a relationship between events during pregnancy and malformations manifested after birth. The fact that a drug has been given during pregnancy without recognized untoward effects is not proof that it will be safe in all instances. Nevertheless, a drug that has a long history of safety tends to be more acceptable for use in pregnant women than a newer similar drug or one that has been associated with reported fetal injury.

Relatively few drugs are recognized as definitely or potentially teratogenic, that is, capable of affecting organogenesis when administered during the first several months of pregnancy. Among these are the folic acid antagonists, aminopterin and methotrexate. These agents are also abortifacients and, if they fail as such, the liveborn infant is likely to be severely malformed. Synthetic progestins and androgens can cause masculinization of the female fetus when given during early pregnancy. Progestational agents given in large doses over prolonged periods, usually to treat threatened abortion, account for the majority of cases, but the incidence of masculinization under these circumstances is probably less than 1%. A delayed effect of diethylstilbestrol has been the occurrence of vaginal adenosis and cervical adenocarcinoma in female offspring 15 to 20 years after their mothers had received this drug during pregnancy. Abnormalities of the genitourinary tract in male offspring also have been reported. A syndrome characterized by minor deformities of craniofacial structures, limbs, and other tissues, as well as microcephaly and mental deficiency, has been reported in infants of epileptic mothers receiving phenytoin alone or with phenobarbital. Congenital malformations have occurred in infants born to mothers receiving trimethadione.

In addition to the above drugs, others have sometimes been regarded as potentially teratogenic on the basis of only one or a few reports in the literature. These include amphetamine, diazepam, lithium, radioactive iodine, and warfarin. However, the evidence suggests only a slight risk and the great majority of children are normal.

Although not commonly considered a drug, alcohol has produced a pattern of congenital malformations, termed the fetal alcohol syndrome, in children born to mothers who drank heavily during the first six months of pregnancy.

Drugs given to the mother after the first trimester also may affect fetal function. These effects are usually noted at the time of delivery, but they may be evanescent and not recognized until later in life. For example, large doses of strong analgesics, inhalation or local anesthetics, and barbiturates may depress the fetal central nervous system so that respiration is not adequately established at birth. Dependence of the mother on opiates, barbiturates, other hypnotics, diazepam, or alcohol may result in withdrawal symptoms (eg, hyperirritability, vomiting, shrill cry) in the baby after delivery. The administration of diazepam to the mother may cause hypothermia and hypotonia in the infant. Atropine may exert a sympathomimetic effect, and succinylcholine may result in temporary ileus. Reserpine may cause nasal congestion associated with excessive mucus production, lethargy, and bradycardia. Antithyroid drugs and potassium iodide may cause goiter and thyroid dysfunction in the newborn. Cigarette smoking during pregnancy

has been associated with smaller babies and an increased incidence of abortion, stillbirth, and neonatal death.

Absolute safety for the fetus can be guaranteed only by practicing therapeutic nihilism for all women between the ages of 14 and 40. However, this would deny women medications necessary for the treatment of serious disease. An appreciation by the physician of the potential effects of drugs upon the embryo and fetus, together with curtailment in drug prescribing, appears to be a more sensible approach.

In this book, an effort has been made to include information on known or reasonably assumed hazards if drugs are given during pregnancy. With many drugs, and particularly with most new ones, little or no information is available on use in man. Accordingly, it often has been necessary to warn that a drug should be given only if the expected benefits exceed the risks both to mother and fetus. This warning is not too helpful when inadequate data exist to know what risks, if any, are present; however, it does serve as a reminder that unless a systemically absorbed drug has been studied extensively in pregnant women, it should be given only if an appropriate need exists, and the possibility of fetal toxicity should be borne in mind.

USE OF DRUGS DURING BREAST FEEDING

The increased popularity of breast feeding in the United States has led to increased questioning of the physician concerning the potential toxicity of drugs taken by lactating women that may appear in breast milk. Answers to these questions are not readily apparent. Our knowledge concerning both the short- and long-term effects and safety of maternally ingested drugs upon the suckling infant is woefully inadequate.

The mechanisms that determine the concentration of a drug in breast milk are similar to those existing elsewhere within the organism. Drugs traverse membranes generally by passive diffusion, and the concentration finally achieved is dependent not only upon the existing concentration gradient but also upon lipid solubility, degree of ionization, and extent of drug-protein interaction. Since breast milk is more acid (pH 7.0) than plasma (pH 7.4), weak bases that become more ionized with decreasing pH will have equal or higher concentrations in milk than in plasma. This results from the greater degree of ionization of the weak base in the more acidic milk than in plasma with consequent "trapping" of the relatively membrane-impermeable ionized form of the drug within breast milk. The opposite situation occurs with weak acids. Thus, theoretically, lincomycin, erythromycin, most antihistamines, theophylline, propylthiouracil, tetracyclines, streptomycin,

lithium, phenytoin, cycloserine, chloramphenicol, and isoniazid should have equal or higher concentrations in milk than in plasma. On the other hand, many barbiturates, organic acids, sulfonamides, diuretics, and penicillins (all weak acids) should have lower concentrations in milk than in plasma. Many reports of milk/plasma ratios are available to support these theoretical considerations. These ratios signify only that the drug is present in the milk. They indicate nothing about the total amount absorbed by the infant and the possibility of adverse effects in the infant —questions that are of concern to the practicing physician in individual patients. It is now quite clear that, with very few exceptions, all drugs present in the maternal circulation

TABLE 3.
DRUGS EXCRETED IN BREAST MILK AFFECTING THE INFANT

Drug(s) Ingested by Mother	Effect in Infant
Anthraquinone-type laxatives	Effect on gastrointestinal tract in infant in addition to mother
Anticoagulants, oral	Bleeding episodes after surgery or trauma
Anticonvulsants (carbamazepine, phenobarbital, phenytoin)	Potentially may cause adverse effect of these drugs and modify activity of hepatic enzymes
Antineoplastic agents	Contraindicated in pregnant women
Antithyroid preparations (iodide, thiouracils)	Effect on thyroid hormone synthesis and release
Atropine	Anticholinergic effects may occur
Barbiturates and other hypnotics (large doses)	Sedation; induction of hepatic metabolizing enzymes also may occur
Bromides	Drowsiness, rashes
Chloramphenicol	Adverse reactions typical of chloramphenicol
Diazepam	Lethargy and weight loss; metabolite accumulation with resulting reactions and neonatal jaundice also possible
Dihydrotachysterol	Possible hypercalcemia
Diuretics	Although there have been no reports of toxic effects in infants, electrolyte disturbances and thrombocytopenia are potential effects
Ergot alkaloids in migraine preparations	Signs of ergotism common
Lithium	Hypotonia, hypothermia, cyanosis, ECG changes
Metronidazole	High concentration in milk; possible carcinogen
Nalidixic acid, Sulfonamides	Hemolytic anemia in infants deficient in G6PD
Oral contraceptives containing estrogens and progestins	Gynecomastia; long-term effects upon nursing infant (physiologic and behavioral) unknown
Tetracyclines	Staining of teeth possible but has not been reported, possibly because calcium in the milk complexes with the tetracycline

will be transferred into milk. In the following sections, substances excreted into breast milk have been divided into two main groupings: those associated with undesirable adverse effects and those that are not.

Examples of Drugs Causing Adverse Effects: Some drugs that produce adverse effects are only of historical interest (eg, bromides, which cause drowsiness and rash). The use of lead nipple shields with the occurrence of lead encephalopathy in the infant also is a historical fact today. On the other hand, environmental pollutants are a very modern concern and two documented disasters were caused by them. In Turkey, severe porphyria followed ingestion of the fungicide, hexachlorobenzene. This also was noted in infants who were breast feeding. In Japan, Minamata disease, a severe form of mercury poisoning, was produced by ingestion of contaminated fish in adults and breast milk in babies.

Drugs listed in Table 3 should not be given to mothers who are breast feeding unless their use is absolutely essential for the management of maternal illness; in such instances, artificial formula should be substituted for breast feeding.

Examples of Drugs Not Ordinarily Considered Hazardous to the Infant: This classification includes several compounds that are either not excreted in breast milk (heparin) or are not absorbed by the infant (kaolin, pectin, insulin, corticotropin, epinephrine). Mild analgesics are used very commonly by nursing women. No adverse effects have been reported following use of aspirin or propoxyphene in analgesic doses. In fact, the amount of aspirin absorbed by the newborn infant constitutes less than 1% of the dose absorbed by the mother. Although narcotic analgesics are excreted in milk, the amount is not sufficient to affect the infant. Antibiotics pass into breast milk in small concentrations. If absorbed, the blood levels in the infant are not significant except, perhaps, for the antibiotics mentioned in Table 3.

There have been no reports of toxic effects in the infant after the maternal use of antihistamines, propranolol, digoxin, or small doses of antianxiety agents.

In addition to the drugs mentioned above, there is a large gray area of compounds whose safety in the nursing infant is unknown. These include many psychotherapeutic agents administered in large doses, corticosteroids, theophylline, reserpine, aspirin in large doses, streptomycin, and quinidine. Caution is advised with the administration of these drugs, since they may be toxic to the nursing infant if taken by the mother in large doses or over a prolonged period in the usual doses.

It is clear that the long-term safety of drugs ingested in breast milk is unknown. Objective evaluation of the safety and efficacy of drugs in breast milk should be undertaken. Until these data are available, the physician should always weigh the benefits versus the risks when prescribing any medication. He also should consider whether medication is necessary in nursing mothers rather than whether the medicated mother should nurse. Sometimes drugs are prescribed to the nursing mother for relief of symptoms that do not require drug therapy.

Selected References

Pediatric

Done AK, et al: Pediatric clinical pharmacology and the "therapeutic orphan." *Annu Rev Pharmacol Toxicol* 17:561-573, 1977.

George SL, Gehan EA: Methods for measurement of body surface area. *J Pediatr* 94:342, 1979.

Haycock GB, et al: Geometric method for measuring body surface area: Height-weight formula validated in infants, children, and adults. *J Pediatr* 93:62-66, 1978.

Morselli PL: Clinical pharmacokinetics in neonates. *Clin Pharmacokinet* 1:81-98, 1976.

Rane A, Wilson JT: Clinical pharmacokinetics in infants and children. *Clin Pharmacokinet* 1:2-24, 1976.

Udkow G: Pediatric clinical pharmacology: Practical review. *Am J Dis Child* 132:1025-1032, 1978.

Yaffe SJ: Modifying drug dosages in children. *Drug Ther* 9:165-170, (Jan) 1979.

Yaffe SJ, Danish M: Problems of drug administration in pediatric patient. *Drug Metab Rev* 8:303-318, 1978.

Geriatric

Briant RH: Drug treatment in the elderly: Problems and prescribing rules. *Drugs* 13:225-229, 1977.

Crooks J, et al: Pharmacokinetics in the elderly. *Clin Pharmacokinet* 1:280-296, 1976.

Hollister LE: Prescribing drugs for the elderly. *Geriatrics* 32:71-73, (Aug) 1977.

Lamy PP: Considerations in drug therapy of the elderly. *J Drug Issues* 9:27-45, 1979.

Richey DP, Bender AD: Pharmacokinetic consequences of aging. *Annu Rev Pharmacol Toxicol* 17:49-65, 1977.

Wallace DE, Watanabe AS: Drug effects in geriatric patients. *Drug Intell Clin Pharm* 11:597-603, 1977.

Ward M, Blatman M: Drug therapy in the elderly. *Am Fam Physician* 19:143-152, (Feb) 1979.

Renal Impairment

Bennett WM: Drug prescribing in renal failure. *Drugs* 17:111-123, 1979.

Bennett WM, et al: Guidelines for drug therapy in renal failure. *Ann Intern Med* 86:754-783, 1977.

Cheigh JS: Drug administration in renal failure. *Am J Med* 62:555-563, 1977.

Cockcroft DW, Gault MH: Prediction of creatinine clearance from serum creatinine. *Nephron* 16:31-41, 1976.

Dettli L: Drug dosage in renal disease. *Clin Pharmacokinet* 1:126-134, 1976.

Drayer DE: Pharmacologically active drug metabolites: Therapeutic and toxic activities, plasma and urine data in man, accumulation in renal failure. *Clin Pharmacokinet* 1:426-443, 1976.

Henrich WL, Anderson RJ: Drug use in renal failure. *Postgrad Med* 64:153-162, (Nov) 1978.

Pregnancy

Committee on Drugs, American Academy of Pediatrics: Effect of medication during labor and delivery on infant outcome. *Pediatrics* 62:402-403, 1978.

Hill RM, Stern L: Drugs in pregnancy: Effects on fetus and newborn. *Drugs* 17:182-197, 1979.

O'Brien TE, McManus CE: Drugs and human fetus. *US Pharmacist* 37-57, (Aug) 1977.

Yaffe SJ: Drug use during pregnancy. *Drug Ther* 8:137-146, (June) 1978.

Lactation

Anderson PO: Drugs and breast feeding —Review. *Drug Intell Clin Pharm* 11:208-223, 1977.

O'Brien TE: Excretion of drugs in human milk. *Am J Hosp Pharm* 31:844-854, 1974.

Rivera-Calimlim L: Drugs in breast milk. *Drug Ther* 7:59-63, (Dec) 1977.

Vorherr H: Drug excretion in breast milk. *Postgrad Med* 56:97-104, (Oct) 1974.

Prescription Practices and Regulatory Agencies | 3

PRESCRIPTION LABELING AND RELATED MATTERS

The American Medical Association encourages physicians to instruct the pharmacist to put information on the label by including on the prescription the direction, "Label as such," "L.A.S.," or merely "Label." Exceptions should be made only when such disclosure would be inadvisable for psychological reasons or detrimental to the welfare of the patient. The reasons for believing that prescription drugs should be labeled with their names and strength have been set forth repeatedly: (1) The patient has the right to be informed about his illness and the medications prescribed. (Many physicians are remiss in not discussing the details of therapy with their patients.) (2) In emergencies, such as accidental poisoning, overdosage, or attempted suicide, immediate identification of a prescription drug from the label may be lifesaving. (3) The information is valuable when the patient changes physicians, moves to another locality, or contacts the prescribing physician at a time when his records are not readily available. (4) The information on the label is of value in group practices in which the patient may not always have the same attending physician. (5) It is advisable that patients with allergies know what is being prescribed. (6) Identification on the label helps to avoid confusion between two or more drugs being taken concurrently or between

medications being taken by different members of the family. (7) If it becomes necessary to issue a warning against the use of a particular drug, the name on the label serves as a danger signal to those who have been given prescriptions for the product.

A related matter involves that of refills. Restrictions on refills are controlled by law for certain drugs under the Controlled Substances Act (see the discussion on Prescribing Controlled Psychotropic Drugs). However, for other drugs also it is advisable for the physician to designate the number of refills, if any, he wishes the patient to have and to prescribe only the number of doses usually required for the specific condition, since adjustments in dosage often are necessary. Prescriptions may not legally be refilled without the physician's authorization. When this authorization is given in advance (on the prescription at the time of writing), the physician would be well advised to place some time limit on the authorization. The very fact that a drug is dispensed by prescription implies the need for professional control. Yet prescriptions with open-end authorization for refills, especially if marked "refill p.r.n." or "ad lib," remain valid indefinitely. It is not unusual for prescriptions to be refilled repeatedly for years after the prescriber has retired, moved away, or even has long been dead. However, in some circumstances, a large-quantity prescription is appropriate. If a patient is expected to take a drug for a prolonged period, if his correct dosage has been established, and if he can be trusted to follow instructions properly, a prescription for a large quantity often is more economical than repeated prescriptions or refills for small quantities.

An additional matter that pertains to practically any drug that may be prescribed for administration at home is the possibility of accidental poisoning. Although the physician's control over this hazard is often limited, he can at least caution patients against improvising in their dosage, against carelessness in reading labels, and against leaving medicines accessible to small children.

PRESCRIBING CONTROLLED PSYCHO-TROPIC DRUGS

Because of the proliferation of psychotropic substances, the physician should guard against contributing to drug abuse through injudicious prescribing practices or by acquiescing to the demands of some patients for instant chemical solutions to their problems. The physician should convey to patients through his own attitude and manner that drugs, no matter how helpful, are only one part of an overall plan of treatment and management. In essence, he can play a preventive role in his practice by exercising good judgment in administering and prescribing psychotropic drugs, so that diversion to illicit use is avoided and the development of drug dependence is minimized or prevented. Psychotropic drugs likely to be abused are subject to the provisions of the Federal Comprehensive Drug Abuse Prevention and Control Act of 1970.

In managing an illness for which no cure is available, the physician should attempt to keep his patient as comfortable and symptom-free as possible. Treatment frequently includes administration of a psychotropic drug, such as a narcotic for relief of pain in terminal illness or a hypnotic for insomnia. Symptomatic relief is a legitimate goal in medical practice, but the prescription of many psychotropic drugs requires caution because of their abuse potential and dependence-producing capability. Patients should be warned about possible adverse effects caused by interactions with other drugs, including alcohol.

Even when sound medical indications have been established for using a psychotropic drug, three additional factors should be weighed in deciding on the dosage and duration of therapy: (1) the severity of symptoms in terms of the patient's ability to accommodate them; (2) the patient's reliability in taking medication, noted through observation and careful history taking; and (3) the dependence liability of the drug. The physician should assess the susceptibility of the patient to drug abuse before prescribing any psychotropic drug and weigh the benefits against the hazards. With periodic check-ups and family consultations, he can monitor the possible development of dependence in patients on long-term therapy.

Opiates (Opioids): Morphine and morphine-like drugs have legitimate clinical usefulness, and the physician should not hesitate to consider prescribing them when they are indicated for the comfort and well-being of patients who require analgesia or other symptomatic relief. Such drugs are useful for moderate to severe pain that cannot be alleviated by non-narcotic analgesics.

For patients with chronic or incurable painful conditions, it is legitimate practice to administer morphine-like drugs for prolonged periods when all reasonable alternative procedures, including the administration of other analgesics, have failed. The comfort of the patient should be the principal concern of the physician. Prolonged administration of morphine-like drugs is most frequently required in patients with terminal disorders but, in unusual circumstances, long-term use also may be indicated in nonfatal illnesses. It should be recognized, however, that prolonged administration, especially parenteral use, may result in tolerance to the therapeutic effects of the drug and some degree of dependence.

Strong analgesics generally should not be used to treat mild or moderate pain, particularly when caused by benign conditions, or to treat pain that can be relieved satisfactorily by non-narcotic analgesics. However, narcotics should not be withheld for short-term therapy if their use for relief of moderate to severe pain is warranted by the patient's needs. Severe pain (eg, that associated with biliary, renal, or ureteral colic or acute myocardial infarction) can be relieved best by morphine or its potent congeners.

Other indications for morphine-like agents, in low doses, include insomnia when sleeplessness is due to pain or cough, preoperative sedation in anesthesia, control of cough, relief of certain forms of dyspnea, and control of diarrhea.

Although codeine is less potent than morphine on a milligram basis, it has a higher oral/parenteral potency ratio. It is, therefore, commonly used orally to relieve mild to moderate pain. It also is widely used as an antitussive. Because it is an opium derivative, codeine is classified as a Schedule II drug under the Controlled Substances Act; however, combination products containing codeine (eg, aspirin, phenacetin, and caffeine with codeine) are classified as Schedule III drugs. The dependence liability of codeine is less than that of morphine, and physical dependence seldom occurs from its use as an oral analgesic. However, abuse of the drug, particularly in the form of cough syrup, is not uncommon.

The adverse reactions associated with the therapeutic use of the morphine-like drugs are discussed in Chapter 6, General Analgesics.

Abuse Potential and Dependence Liability: Ordinarily, morphine and morphine-like drugs should be given in the smallest effective doses and as infrequently as possible to minimize the development of tolerance and physical dependence. This is particularly true when treating chronic diseases or conditions that might lead to drug abuse. The development of tolerance with prolonged use of morphine-like drugs varies from patient to patient; some appear to develop little tolerance to the effects of these drugs, whereas others require increasing doses. An increased need for the drug expressed by the patient should, therefore, be evaluated in relation to the clinical situation to determine if it is caused by an increase in the severity of pain, development of tolerance to the effects of the drug, or by the anxiety of the patient.

The fact that these drugs have actions other than analgesia (eg, relief of anxiety or depression) may lead to abuse by some patients. Such responses should be recognized and use of the drug monitored to prevent abuse and dependence. Most patients given a morphine-like drug for analgesia are able to discontinue its use without difficulty; even though they have developed mild degrees of dependence, they rarely become compulsive abusers. A careful history will be helpful in determining which patients need to be followed closely.

Special attention should be given to patients with a morphine-type drug dependence or a history of such dependence who also have other medical or surgical problems. If there is a genuine symptomatic need demonstrated by adequate diagnostic evaluation, it is the physician's responsibility to prescribe analgesic medication as he would for any other patient. The physician must, however, remain constantly alert in such situations to certain considerations: (1) the patient may be simulating a disease condition in order to request a dependence-producing drug; (2) the effective dose level will vary, depending upon tolerance; and (3) abrupt withdrawal can increase morbidity or result in death if the patient with an established dependence on a morphine-like drug undergoes major medical or surgical trauma. Drug dependence can be maintained until the patient begins to recover from the other illness. Then a regimen of gradual withdrawal should be considered.

Benzodiazepines, Barbiturates, and Other Hypnotic and Antianxiety Agents:

The antianxiety and hypnotic agents produce varying degrees of central nervous system depression. The principal object of therapy with these drugs is to relieve symptoms of anxiety and insomnia without producing dependence. Although some patients may respond equally well to properly selected doses of nonbenzodiazepine drugs, the benzodiazepines are most often the drugs of choice when an antianxiety, sedative, or hypnotic action is required because of their better benefit/ risk ratio. The development of drug tolerance and dependence, drug interactions, and lethality associated with overdose is less with the benzodiazepine group of drugs.

The benzodiazepine derivatives, chlordiazepoxide, clorazepate, diazepam, flurazepam, lorazepam, oxazepam, and prazepam, are used primarily to control moderate to severe anxiety and insomnia. Although seldom used for anxiety, flurazepam is the most frequently prescribed drug for insomnia. Lorazepam is used for insomnia associated with anxiety. Certain benzodiazepines are used to treat skeletal muscle hyperactivity (ie, spasticity, localized spasm generally caused by trauma).

The specific indications for barbiturates vary considerably among the agents available. Phenobarbital is used to manage some convulsive disorders as well as for hypnosis and daytime sedation to reduce awareness, spontaneous activity, and mild anxiety; butabarbital also is used as a hypnotic and sedative. Amobarbital, secobarbital, and pentobarbital are used principally for insomnia. These drugs are not analgesics. When given to patients in pain without concomitant use of analgesics, they may produce paradoxical excitement.

Chloral hydrate is used as a hypnotic instead of the benzodiazepines and barbiturates in selected patients. Ethchlorvynol, ethinamate, glutethimide, methaqualone, and methyprylon are no more effective for this indication than the benzodiazepines or barbiturates; furthermore,

when overdose or a suicide attempt occurs, these drugs produce toxicity as severe as that seen with the barbiturates.

Meprobamate is given only to treat mild to moderate anxiety and localized muscle spasm; however, it is not as effective as the benzodiazepines for severe anxiety and has a greater potential for producing physical dependence. Hydroxyzine also is used to treat mild to moderate apprehension and anxiety, especially if antihistaminic and antiemetic actions are also desired. The potential for physical dependence is not as great as that of meprobamate.

The hypnotic and antianxiety agents are not recommended for use in those with minor distress or discomfort. The physician should attempt to diagnose and treat underlying disorders before relying on these drugs for symptomatic relief.

For a discussion on the adverse reactions, precautions, and drug interactions associated with use of these agents, see Chapter 11, Drugs Used for Anxiety and Insomnia.

Abuse Potential and Dependence Liability: Prolonged, uninterrupted use of barbiturates may result in tolerance and either physical or psychological dependence or both. Although physical dependence is seldom induced by therapeutic doses of barbiturates, other hypnotics, and antianxiety agents, psychological dependence can result, in part, from therapeutic use of these drugs. This may lead to continued use of increased doses after medical indications for therapy no longer prevail. Self-medication with large doses may constitute a chronic abuse problem and eventually produces physical dependence. Because nonbarbiturate hypnotics other than the benzodiazepines also have a high abuse potential, substituting one of those drugs for a barbiturate does not necessarily reduce the risk of drug dependence.

The longer-acting barbiturates, such as phenobarbital, have a slow absorption rate and penetrate the brain slowly. It is probably for this reason that they do not produce the "high" sought by those who take drugs for nonmedical, recreational purposes. Thus, their abuse potential is comparatively low.

Shorter-acting barbiturates have a greater abuse potential because of their rapid onset of action and the comparatively high intensity of their psychoactive effects. They are included in Schedule II of the Controlled Substances Act, as is methaqualone.

Unlike dependence of the morphine type, dependence of the barbiturate type does not follow a typical dose-related curve. Moderate doses (less than 300 mg/day) of even short-acting barbiturates do not produce detectable physical dependence; it usually requires large doses (more than 600 mg/day) administered regularly and continuously for at least six to seven weeks. Tolerance becomes important as the patient increases the self-administered dose.

Abrupt withdrawal in a person with strong physical dependence of the barbiturate type is followed in two or three days by a severe withdrawal syndrome that usually is more serious than the opiate withdrawal syndrome. Convulsions, delirium, fever, and even coma and death may result. When physical dependence on a sedative-hypnotic other than a benzodiazepine is suspected, substitution of phenobarbital is recommended for withdrawal, with gradual reduction of dosage. The use of a benzodiazepine for withdrawal in barbiturate-dependent patients is inadvisable.

Long-term administration of larger than usual therapeutic doses of the benzodiazepines or meprobamate also may cause physical dependence. Symptoms are similar to those produced by chronic intoxication with barbiturates or alcohol. Withdrawal reactions may develop if the drug is discontinued abruptly. These reactions, which are also similar to those produced by barbiturate withdrawal, may appear within 36 hours to one week, depending on the drug's half-life and whether or not it is converted to an active metabolite. To avoid withdrawal reactions, it is advisable to reduce the dosage of these drugs gradually. Because dependence occurs, although relatively infrequently, these drugs

are included in Schedule IV of the Controlled Substances Act.

Amphetamines and Other Stimulants: Amphetamines and several chemically related drugs are central nervous system stimulants. Small doses give the user a feeling of increased mental alertness and a sense of well being. As doses are increased, apprehension, decreased appetite, volubility, tremor, and excitement occur. Because tolerance and psychological dependence can develop rather quickly with large doses, the physician should prescribe amphetamines and other stimulants only for a limited time for a specific purpose. In an attempt to reduce the abuse problem with some of these agents, many physicians have stopped prescribing amphetamines altogether.

The major medical uses of amphetamines are to control symptoms of narcolepsy and certain hyperkinetic behavioral disorders in children. Amphetamines also have been widely used as anorexiants to help some patients limit their food intake and facilitate weight loss. However, because their efficacy over a long period has not been demonstrated and because of their high abuse potential, this use of the amphetamines is not advocated. Other drugs and nondrug programs are preferable in the treatment of obesity. Although amphetamines have been suggested for the diagnosis and treatment of depression, neither suggested indication is supported by the results of controlled studies. Amphetamines have been reported to be useful in combination with scopolamine to prevent motion sickness; in conjunction with morphine to potentiate analgesic action; and in conjunction with some anticonvulsants to counteract their sedative effects.

It is emphasized that the use of amphetamines to allay fatigue is unjustifiable except under the most extraordinary circumstances; they are not to be regarded as an instant source of extra mental or physical energy. They serve only to impel the user to a greater expenditure of his own resources, sometimes to a hazardous point of fatigue of which he is not aware.

The prolonged administration of stimulants to alcohol- and barbiturate-dependent individuals is not appropriate therapy because such use can induce the patient to take increasing amounts of depressant drugs. Amphetamine-type drugs also are contraindicated for other dependence-prone individuals, and their regular use to counteract the "hangover" effects of excessive use of alcohol or barbiturates is hazardous.

The stimulant action of cocaine makes this drug popular among drug abusers, but its medical use is limited to topical anesthesia and, under certain surgical circumstances, nasal decongestion. Prolonged use for the latter indication may cause ischemic damage to the nasal mucosa. Tolerance does not develop, but psychological dependence can.

Methylphenidate, a mild central nervous system stimulant, is useful in the management of hyperkinetic children and in the treatment of narcolepsy. Like the amphetamines, it has a potential for abuse and thus should be used with the same degree of caution. Pemoline is another stimulant used to treat the hyperkinetic syndrome in children.

The untoward effects produced by the amphetamines and similar agents are related to their spectrum of pharmacologic actions. For a discussion of their adverse reactions and drug interactions, see Chapter 14, Drugs Used in Nonpsychotic Mental Disorders, and Chapter 56, Agents Used in Obesity.

Abuse Potential and Dependence Liability: Amphetamine-type drugs were in widespread use before their dependence-producing properties were recognized; as a result, several countries experienced epidemics of stimulant abuse. Under the Controlled Substances Act of 1970, amphetamines, phenmetrazine, and methylphenidate are included among the Schedule II drugs; other stimulants and anorexiants are classed as Schedule III or IV drugs.

The physician who prescribes stimulants for any indication must always be alert to their dependence-producing potential and recognize that some patients may seek other sources of supply, either illegally or from another physician. There also is the danger that the efficacy of a stimulant in helping a person achieve a time-limited goal may predispose that person to regard amphetamine-type drugs as being desirable rather than dangerous substances and thus may encourage future abuse. Dependence-prone persons who have been introduced to stimulants as anorexiants or to combat fatigue or depression can become chronic abusers.

Amphetamine abuse is manifested in several ways. The chosen route of administration may be oral or intravenous. The drug of choice may be an amphetamine, but substituting methylphenidate or another stimulant is not uncommon when the preferred drug is not readily available.

Polydrug abuse, especially concomitant use of amphetamines with sedative-hypnotics (including alcohol), is frequent. (Uppers in the morning and downers at bedtime is one abuse pattern of the polydrug type.) In fact, problems associated with the secondary drug may bring the patient to the physician's attention and mask the amphetamine abuse.

Amphetamine abuse can cause three kinds of medical problems: (1) chronic medical complications associated with drug effects, such as exacerbation of hypertension and development of arrhythmias or self-induced strokes and retinal damage due to intense vasospasm, or with drug administration, such as septicemia and endocarditis from unclean needles; (2) emergency conditions, such as hyperthermia and convulsions arising from use of toxic doses or acute amphetamine psychosis; and (3) signs and symptoms during the abstinence period following regular use that are indicative of drug dependence.

Federal Comprehensive Drug Abuse Prevention and Control Act of 1970: The Federal Comprehensive Drug Abuse Prevention and Control Act is designed to improve the administration and regulation of the manufacturing, distribution, and dispensing of controlled substances by providing a "closed" system for legitimate handlers of these drugs. Every person not specifically exempted who manufactures, distributes, prescribes, administers, or dispenses any controlled substance must register annually with the Attorney General. Accurate records of drugs purchased, distributed, and dispensed must be maintained and kept on file for two years by all persons legitimately involved in the handling of controlled substances who regularly dispense and charge for such drugs in the course of their practice.

The Act establishes five schedules of controlled drugs, with varying degrees of control for each schedule. Each drug or substance subject to control is assigned to a schedule depending upon the drug's potential for abuse, its medical usefulness, and the degree of dependence if abused. These schedules and the drugs included in them are:

Schedule I: Drugs and other substances having a high potential for abuse and no current accepted medical usefulness. Included are certain opium derivatives (eg, heroin), opiates (synthetic narcotics), and hallucinogenic substances (eg, LSD).

Schedule II: Drugs having a high potential for abuse and accepted medical usefulness; abuse leads to severe psychological or physical dependence. In general, drugs in this schedule were previously controlled under the Narcotic Acts, eg, opium and its derivatives, opiates (synthetic narcotics), cocaine. Other stimulants, such as amphetamine and related compounds and the short-acting barbiturates, also are in this schedule.

Schedule III: Drugs having a lesser degree of abuse potential and accepted medical usefulness; abuse leads to moderate dependence. Included in this schedule are certain other stimulants and depressants (eg, barbiturates not included in another schedule), as well as preparations containing limited quantities of certain narcotic drugs.

Schedule IV: Drugs having a low abuse potential, accepted medical usefulness, and limited dependence. Included in this schedule are certain depressants not in

another schedule (eg, chloral hydrate, phenobarbital).

Schedule V: Drugs having a low abuse potential, accepted medical usefulness, and limited dependence. Mixtures containing limited quantities of narcotic with non-narcotic drugs as active ingredients are included in this schedule.

The Act also provides that no prescription order for drugs in Schedule II can be renewed. Emergency telephone prescriptions for drugs in this schedule may be dispensed if the practitioner furnishes a written, signed prescription order to the pharmacy within 72 hours, provided the drug prescribed is limited to the amount needed to treat the patient during the emergency period. Prescription orders for drugs in Schedules III and IV may be redispensed up to five times within six months after the date of issue if authorized by the prescriber. Prescription orders for Schedule V drugs may be redispensed only as expressly authorized by the practitioner on the prescription.

Responsibility for administration of the Federal Comprehensive Drug Abuse Prevention and Control Act of 1970 is assigned to the Drug Enforcement Administration (DEA). This Act replaces the former Narcotic Acts and the Drug Abuse Control Amendments of 1965. The DEA issues the physician registration and order forms. *A Manual for the Medical Practitioner*, which explains the provisions of the Controlled Substances Act, may be obtained from the Drug Enforcement Administration, U.S. Department of Justice, Attention: Voluntary Compliance Programs, Washington, D.C. 20537. As a convenience, the *U.S.P.* includes the latest DEA regulations that affect practicing physicians and pharmacists.

Many states have controlled substances acts patterned after the federal law. Because there may be differences in the scheduling of drugs, however, physicians are urged to acquaint themselves with the exact provisions of the statutes and regulations in their local jurisdictions.

Precautions for Controlled Substances: The physician should take the following precautions to minimize the chances of controlled substances being procured illegally:

Keep prescription blanks where they can't be stolen easily. Never sign them in advance and don't use them for writing notes or memos.

When prescribing a controlled substance, write out the actual amount in addition to giving an arabic number or roman numeral in order to discourage alterations in written prescription orders.

Avoid writing prescription orders for large quantities of controlled drugs unless such amounts are absolutely necessary.

Maintain an accurate record of controlled drugs dispensed, as required by the Controlled Substances Act of 1970.

Maintain only a minimum stock of controlled drugs in the medical bag, which should not be left unattended.

Assist any pharmacist who telephones to verify information about a written prescription order.

OFFICIAL AND REGULATORY AGENCIES

There are several official governmental and quasi-official voluntary bodies concerned with standards, distribution, labeling, and advertising of drug products. To acquaint the reader with the functions of these agencies and their spheres of influence as they pertain to medicinal agents, following are brief descriptions of their organization and duties.

The United States Pharmacopeial Convention, Inc.: Under the General Committee of Revision, the United States Pharmacopeial Convention, Inc. issues the *United States Pharmacopeia (U.S.P.)* and the *National Formulary (N.F.)* at five-year intervals with cumulative annual *Supplements* and *Interim Revisions* as needed. This is a private body incorporated in the District of Columbia and is composed of representatives from medical and pharmacy schools, state medical and pharmaceutical associations, the American Medical Association, the American Pharmaceutical Association, the American Chemical Society, many other scientific and trade associations, and various interested federal bureaus and departments.

Under authority of the Federal Food, Drug and Cosmetic Act, the standards for the products described in *U.S.P.* and *N.F.* are official. Articles are admitted by the Committee of Revision on the basis of demonstrated therapeutic value, extent of use, or pharmaceutic necessity.

The Pharmacopeial Convention also publishes separately the annual publication, *USP Dispensing Information*, which includes guidelines on consultation with patients on drug use, an expansion of such information formerly included in the official compendia; and *USAN and the USP Dictionary of Drug Names*, an annual cumulation of United States Adopted Names and other names for drugs, both current and retrospective.

The Food and Drug Administration: The FDA regulates the availability and distribution of drugs, including biological products, in interstate commerce. It is concerned with the safety, effectiveness, and reliability of drugs; the standardization of drug names; the labeling of drugs; and the advertising of prescription drugs. To ensure the safety, identity, strength, quality, and purity of drugs, adequate quality control measures are required in all manufacturing plants. In addition, certification procedures conducted by the FDA itself are applied to antibiotics intended for use in man, as well as to insulin.

The Secretary of Health, Education and Welfare is given the authority to designate an established name for any drug if he determines that such action is necessary or desirable in the interest of usefulness and simplicity. This name then is to be used in any subsequent issue of any official compendium as the only official title for that drug. In practice, the official name will probably be one that has been recommended by the USAN Council (see the following discussion). Such an official established name is the only nonproprietary or generic name, other than the chemical name or chemical formula, that may appear on the label of a drug. The label for a prescription drug must state the quantities of all active ingredients, and the established drug name for each active ingredient must appear both on the label and in conjunction with the brand name in other labeling. The label for an over-the-counter drug also must disclose the active ingredients but unfortunately is not required to give the quantities or ratios of these ingredients.

The Federal Food, Drug and Cosmetic Act provides that the labeling for any drug must not be false or misleading. Also, the advertising of prescription drugs must conform to the labeling in specified ways. Standards also exist for advertising over-the-counter drugs, but this is regulated by the Federal Trade Commission rather than the FDA.

To market a new drug in interstate commerce, a manufacturer must have approval, through a New Drug Application (NDA), from the FDA. Among other things, the application must provide for the labeling under which the drug will be distributed. For prescription drugs, this labeling includes a document, commonly called a package insert, addressed to physicians and containing, among other information, the recommended uses and dosage as well as disclosure of the possible adverse reactions, warnings, and recommended precautions in using the drug. If it is deemed possible to write directions for use of a drug by the layman, such directions *must* be written as part of the manufacturer's labeling, and the drug is not entitled to bear the prescription legend. A physician may, of course, prescribe the drug if he chooses, but the manufacturer may not *restrict* it to prescription sale. For selected drugs (eg, oral contraceptives), informational brochures that discuss the uses and possible adverse reactions of the drug have been prepared for patients.

Another of the many components of an NDA is the clinical data that have been developed during premarketing investigation of the drug. These data must support the claims made for the drug in the labeling, and they must be adequate to prove safety and efficacy to the satisfaction of the government. The law and regulations set forth many requirements and procedures that must be followed during the investigational stage of the development of a drug prior to submission or approval of the NDA.

After a new drug has been marketed under specific approved labeling, the FDA generally requires further proof of safety and efficacy if the labeling is to be changed to add a new therapeutic indication or a variation in dosage. As a general rule, *whether new claims are added to labeling depends upon whether the pharmaceutical company has sufficient interest in the matter to follow the necessary procedures to obtain approval.* However, manufacturers are required to submit to the FDA all reports of adverse effects, other clinical experience, and other relevant data on drugs on the market. The agency can require updating of labeling to keep precautionary information current. It also can take steps to have claims deleted that it considers no longer warranted, or even to suspend (ie, revoke) an NDA and remove the drug from the market if evidence discloses the drug not to be safe and effective, as originally believed. Legal remedies are available by which manufacturers may contest such actions if they disagree.

The FDA's jurisdiction over uses of marketed drugs, doses, and related matters extends only to what the manufacturer may recommend and must disclose in its labeling and advertising. The jurisdiction does not extend to the way a physician uses the drug in the normal course of his practice.

The physician is well advised to be *aware* of what is in a package insert and to give it due weight. However, his decision on how to use a drug must be based on what is good medicine and best for the patient. This statement is both true and legally sound whether his use of a drug conforms to a package insert or departs from it. In a malpractice suit, such drug labeling *may* have evidentiary weight for or against a physician, but the evidence is subject to refutation; drug labeling, *per se*, does not set the standard for what is good medical practice.

The FDA does not have jurisdiction over extemporaneous drugs that the physician may devise for use in the normal course of his practice, provided the physician does not introduce these drugs into interstate commerce. Such drugs include those he has compounded from separate ingredients or certain readily available chemicals or other nonpharmaceutical products that can be used therapeutically. The physician and pharmacist, of course, are responsible for the suitability of the preparations for the use chosen, but the FDA would not be involved.

The Federal Trade Commission: The Federal Trade Commission (FTC) is an independent agency of the federal government directly responsible to the President. The Commission administers several laws, the principal one being the Federal Trade Commission Act, which deals mainly with the regulation of trade practices.

The principal power of the FTC with respect to drugs is contained in Section 15 of the Federal Trade Commission Act: This Act gives the Commission broad power to prevent the dissemination of false or misleading advertising of foods, drugs, and cosmetics to the general public. This power is circumscribed with respect to advertisements directed to the medical profession. Regulation of prescription drug advertising is the responsibility of the FDA. For drugs sold over the counter to the public, the FTC relies upon FDA determinations and has taken action against advertising claims that are inconsistent with these.

Department of Justice: Responsibility for administration of the Federal Comprehensive Drug Abuse Prevention and Control Act of 1970 is assigned to the Drug Enforcement Administration (DEA) in the Department of Justice (see the section on Prescribing Controlled Psychotropic Drugs).

The USAN Council: The United States Adopted Names (USAN) Council, an agency formed to adopt appropriate nonproprietary names for all new drugs, was organized in January, 1964 and was preceded by the AMA-USP Nomenclature Committee. It is sponsored by the American Medical Association, the American Pharmaceutical Association, and the United States Pharmacopeial Convention, Inc. The Council is a five-member group, with one member appointed by each sponsor, one member-at-large who must be approved by all three sponsors, and one member from the Food and Drug Administration.

The primary functions of the USAN Council are: (1) to negotiate with pharmaceutical manufacturers in the selection of meaningful and distinctive nonproprietary names for new drug entities; (2) to publicize the adopted names, the guiding principles used in devising these names, and the procedures involved in their adoption; and (3) to cooperate with other national and international agencies, particularly the World Health Organization, in standardizing, as much as possible, the nonproprietary nomenclature for drugs.

New USAN are published in *The Journal of the American Medical Association* promptly after adoption and are cumulated annually. The current version of The Guiding Principles for Coining United States Adopted Names for Drugs appears in the annual cumulative publication, *USAN and the USP Dictionary of Drug Names.*

Drug Response Variation | 4

PHARMACOGENETIC DETERMINANTS

Individual variation in response to a drug is often a major obstacle to rapid delivery of optimum drug therapy. *Endogenously* induced variation is caused by genetic differences, age, and disease. Exposure to environmental nondrug chemicals, diet, and drugs are responsible for most *exogenously* induced variation.

Ultimately, all drug response variation is based on a few fundamental characteristics and processes. These include the physicochemical characteristics of the drug (ie, ionization, molecular size, chemical reactivity, solubility), the biochemical kinetic processes (ie, binding, transport, enzyme and enzyme-regulating activity), drug receptor activity, and physiologic status of the individual. These factors underlie the main elements of both pharmacokinetics (ie, absorption, distribution, biotransformation, excretion) and pharmacodynamic receptor action.

Variability among individuals in their pharmacokinetic response to drugs is due in part to genetic differences (Chapman, 1977; Meyer, 1978; Vesell, 1979). Genetic differences also may affect pharmacodynamic receptor sensitivity to certain drugs, and individuals with genetic variants may fail to respond or may experience adverse effects with usual therapeutic doses of drugs.

Genetic Differences in Drug Biotransformation: Since most drugs are biotransformed before they are excreted, genetic variations in metabolic pathways or rate of biotransformation may have important clinical implications.

Drug oxidation appears to be controlled by genes located at more than one place on the chromosomes (polygenic inheritance). The disposition of oral anticoagulants, tricyclic antidepressants, phenytoin, and phenylbutazone has been studied in twins and in families, and most of the variability in response to these drugs is apparently due to genetic rather than environmental factors.

Several drugs are biotransformed by acetylation; the metabolite may be inactive (eg, isoniazid) or active (eg, N-acetyl-procainamide). The general population can be divided into slow or fast inactivators. Because of these genetic differences, individualization of therapy based on acetylator phenotype and drug response may help avoid therapeutic failure or toxic reactions. Rapid inactivators are homozygous or heterozygous for a gene controlling an "acetylating" enzyme, while slow inactivation is a homozygous recessive trait. Approximately one-half of American whites and blacks are slow inactivators of isoniazid, but this trait occurs infrequently among Japanese and rarely in Eskimos. Liver damage is more common in rapid acetylators, apparently because a larger percentage of a dose is converted to a hepatotoxic metabolite in these individuals. In slow acetylators, the relatively high level of isoniazid may interfere with the biotransformation of other drugs (eg, phenytoin) and may predispose to dose-related toxicity.

Slow acetylators of hydralazine and sulfasalazine, but probably not phenelzine, experience adverse effects more frequently than do fast acetylators, and usual doses may be less effective in the latter. The rate of onset of procainamide-induced lupus erythematosus also may be related to rapid acetylation; a metabolite of procainamide may be responsible for this adverse reaction.

The neuromuscular blocking agent, succinylcholine, ordinarily has a short duration of action because of its rapid hydrolysis by plasma cholinesterase, but some individuals experience prolonged paralysis and apnea after standard doses of the drug and require artificial ventilation for a longer period prior to recovery. This increased sensitivity usually is associated with genetic variants of plasma cholinesterase that inactivate succinylcholine less rapidly. The variants are controlled by at least four allelic autosomal genes. The "atypical" variant has been studied most extensively. In most North American populations having this enzyme type, the homozygous state (which is associated with succinylcholine sensitivity) occurs in about 1 in 2,500 individuals.

Hereditary Diseases Causing Altered Drug Response: Hereditary diseases in which symptoms of the disease and/or other adverse effects are precipitated by specific drugs are good examples of the influence of genetic factors on drug response. In other genetic disorders, the response to certain drugs is enhanced, diminished, or abnormal, and these agents may be useful to diagnose or detect heterozygotes.

A number of drugs can produce *hemolytic anemia* in individuals with an inherited deficiency of the enzyme, glucose-6-phosphate dehydrogenase (G6PD). Enzyme-deficient cells cannot protect themselves as efficiently as normal erythrocytes against the effects of oxidant drugs or their metabolites; in the presence of these agents, essential cell components are oxidized and hemolysis occurs. This inborn error of metabolism is frequently called "primaquine sensitivity," because it was originally observed in patients receiving antimalarial drugs (primaquine, pamaquine, pentaquine). Hemolytic anemia also has developed in susceptible individuals after administration of some sulfonamides, nitrofurans, sulfones, antipyretic-analgesics (acetanilid, phenacetin, and, in some extreme variants, aspirin), chloramphenicol, aminosalicylic acid, quinidine, methylene blue, and vitamin K. It also has occurred after contact with naphthalene or ingestion of fava beans. Most individuals with G6PD deficiency do not have hematologic symptoms unless they are exposed to these agents.

G6PD deficiency is transmitted by a sex-linked gene. The trait gains full expression in the affected hemizygous male ($\overline{X}Y$) and homozygous female ($\overline{XX}$). In populations with a high frequency of the gene, homozygous females are not extremely rare. Because only one X chromosome is active in each cell of a female, heterozygous women ($\overline{XX}$) have two red cell populations: one deficient and one normal. For this reason, symptoms are generally less severe in female heterozygotes than in male hemizygotes. However, because of the random nature of X inactivation and because of postzygotic selection, a substantial number of heterozygous females may have an essentially normal or an essentially deficient red cell population.

The geographical distribution of G6PD deficiency closely follows the distribution of *Plasmodium falciparum* malaria, which suggests that the trait provides some selective advantage against this disease. It appears most frequently in populations of African and Mediterranean descent and occurs in about 10% to 13% of black American males. Oxidant drugs or their metabolites often cause more severe symptoms in whites with G6PD deficiency than in affected blacks. Also, hemolysis may be induced in whites by agents that have no hemolytic effect on enzyme-deficient blacks (eg, chloramphenicol, aminosalicylic acid, fava beans).

Oxidant drugs also may cause hemolysis in individuals with a deficiency of glutathione (GSH) in the erythrocytes, an uncommon inborn error of metabolism. Another rare recessive metabolic disorder, *hereditary methemoglobinemia* (NADH diaphorase deficiency), is characterized by a chronically high level of methemoglobin in the blood. Individuals with this disorder develop severe methemoglobinemia after nitrites and sulfonamides are administered. The methemoglobin can be converted to hemoglobin by methylene blue or ascorbic acid.

Hemoglobinopathies, biochemical variants in the hemoglobin molecule, are produced by genetically controlled differences in amino acid sequences in the globin structure. Although, many variants are not associated with any known pathology, others are characterized by hematologic disorders that may be precipitated by drugs.

Sickle cell disease is one of the most common hemoglobinopathies. In the homozygous state, red cells contain approximately 80% Hb S and 20% fetal hemoglobin (Hb F); no normal adult hemoglobin (Hb A) is present, and patients have chronic hemolytic anemia. In the heterozygous state (sickle cell trait), 55% to 80% of the hemoglobin present is Hb A, while the remainder is Hb S; little or no Hb F is present. Individuals with sickle cell trait generally are asymptomatic unless they are exposed to reduced oxygen tension.

Patients with sickle cell disease must be treated cautiously during general anesthesia with any anesthetic because hypoxia, diminished tissue blood flow, dehydration, acidosis, or hypothermia may induce a sickling crisis. Local infiltration or nerve block anesthesia is preferred, and a preoperative transfusion may be indicated. There is no strong evidence that individuals with sickle cell trait are at greater risk than normal persons; nevertheless, care should be taken to avoid hypoxia, dehydration, and acidosis.

Some hemoglobin variants are easily oxidized to methemoglobin, which cannot transport oxygen. As a result, severe methemoglobinemia and hemolysis may develop after administration of certain drugs. Hemoglobin H disease occurs in individuals with an inherited defect in hemoglobin synthesis (thalassemia and certain related disorders). Patients with this disease generally have 10% to 35% abnormal hemoglobin and have chronic anemia because the mean life span of erythrocytes is reduced by one-half. Acute hemolytic anemia may develop in these individuals after administration of sulfonamides, nitrites, or methylene blue. Hemoglobin Zürich is associated with chronic compensated hemolytic disease; severe methemoglobinemia and hemolytic crisis may occur after administration of sulfonamides and probably after other methemoglobin-forming drugs.

Porphyrias are hereditary disorders of porphyrin and heme production. The hepatic forms (acute intermittent porphyria, porphyria variegata, and hereditary coproporphyria) are characterized by elevated levels of porphyrins and porphyrin precursors and presumably are caused by increased activity of the hepatic enzyme, delta-aminolevulinic acid (ALA) synthetase. These disorders are transmitted as autosomal dominant traits and are aggravated by drugs that induce ALA synthetase.

Acute intermittent porphyria is characterized by periodic attacks of severe abdominal pain, usually accompanied by neurologic and psychotic symptoms. Attacks may be precipitated by various drugs, including many of those which induce drug biotransforming hepatic enzymes. Those reported to produce attacks most frequently include barbiturates, sulfonamides, estrogens, and griseofulvin.

Porphyria variegata occurs in about 1% of the white population of South Africa. The skin of individuals with this defect tends to erode and form bullae after exposure to sunlight or mechanical trauma. These patients occasionally have attacks similar to acute intermittent porphyria, usually in association with the use of barbiturates, sulfonamides, or alcohol; cutaneous signs and jaundice have been precipitated by oral contraceptives. The symptoms and drug sensitivity of hereditary coproporphyria resemble porphyria variegata.

Familial nonhemolytic jaundice (Crigler-Najjar syndrome) is a rare, recessive hereditary defect causing severe postnatal jaundice and kernicterus. Most homozygotes are severely affected and die within the early weeks or months of life. Survivors may have no obvious abnormality except for jaundice, but elimination of drugs that normally undergo glucuronidation is slowed. Decreased glucuronidation of salicylates, adrenal corticosteroids, menthol, and trichloroacetic acid has been found in affected individuals. Excretion of these drugs by heterozygotes is intermediate between the normal level and that of homozygotes. This disease should not be confused with another hereditary disease (Gilbert's syndrome), which also is characterized by intermittent jaundice, unconjugated hyperbilirubinemia, but normal glucuronidation of drugs.

Dubin-Johnson syndrome is an auto-somal recessive disorder associated with chronic, mild conjugated hyperbilirubinemia, intermittent bilirubinuria, and dark pigment deposits in liver cells. The condition is frequently asymptomatic, but various environmental factors can exacerbate the hyperbilirubinemia, causing overt jaundice. Asymptomatic women with this genetic defect have developed clinical jaundice during the last trimester of pregnancy and after using oral contraceptives.

A rare and often fatal complication of general anesthesia, *malignant hyperpyrexia* is characterized by a rapid rise in body temperature to above 106 F, tachycardia, tachypnea, cyanosis, and severe acidosis, usually accompanied by skeletal muscle rigidity. The syndrome has occurred most frequently after exposure to potent anesthetics and muscle relaxants, although psychotropic, narcotic, and anticholinergic agents have been implicated occasionally.

Many cases of malignant hyperpyrexia appear to have a genetic basis and may be associated with subclinical myopathy that is transmitted as an autosomal dominant trait. Abnormally high levels of serum creatine phosphokinase (CPK) have been found in some patients and their relatives, and tissue studies suggest a calcium storage defect in muscle cells of individuals with this genetic disorder.

The thiazide and loop diuretics tend to produce asymptomatic *hyperuricemia*, which is caused by both decreased tubular secretion and increased tubular reabsorption of uric acid. In patients with a hereditary predisposition to gout, these diuretics may precipitate an acute attack.

Hereditary fructose intolerance is a rare autosomal recessive trait causing fructose-1-phosphate aldolase deficiency. In patients with this genetic deficit, fructose can cause hypoglycemia, nausea, vomiting, tremors, coma, and convulsions. These patients should avoid foods, parenteral solutions, or medicinal syrups containing fructose.

When corticosteroids are applied topically to the eye, *glaucoma* occurs in some individuals. This response is genetically determined and occurs most frequently in patients with primary open-angle glaucoma, their relatives, in myopes with no family history of glaucoma, and in diabetics.

Topically applied mydriatics (anticholinergic and adrenergic agents) may precipitate an attack of *acute angle-closure glaucoma* in eyes with narrow angles and shallow anterior chambers; this angle configuration is hereditary. Rarely, systemically administered anticholinergic agents have induced angle-closure glaucoma in susceptible individuals.

AGE DETERMINANTS

The patient's age often may be responsible for variations in drug response; the very old and very young are the most vulnerable. Special considerations regarding dose and dosage schedules for patients in these groups are presented in Chapter 2.

Transport, enzymatic, and protein binding processes gradually deteriorate with advancing age. Absorption, gastrointestinal transit time, plasma albumin level, metabolizing capability, glomerular filtration, and tubular secretion decrease, and there is a selective loss of receptors for some drugs. Total or regional blood flow also may be depressed. Thus, pharmacokinetic and pharmacodynamic mechanisms are affected by age, and the gradual depression of compensatory homeostatic reflexes may result in adverse responses to drugs that might have been averted in younger individuals. Because the rate of aging differs widely among individuals, studies show considerable variability depending upon the range of ages of the individuals studied. As a general rule, the effective and toxic doses of drugs decrease with age due to alteration of these processes.

Infants, especially preterm neonates, are vulnerable to the actions of many drugs. Incomplete maturation of transport, metabolizing, enzymatic, and protein binding processes, together with immature cardiovascular systems are frequently responsible. The maturation pattern is not always uniform (eg, conjugation mechanisms for glucuronidation but not sulfation may be incompletely developed). Altered transport processes may enhance absorption, which suggests that the normal adult barrier is not completely developed. The latter may account for the increased sensitivity of the very young to narcotics and tetracycline. However, experience with one drug cannot be extrapolated to other drugs. For instance, nondepolarizing muscle relaxants are more effective in the very young, but depolarizing relaxants are much less effective.

DISEASE DETERMINANTS

Of all the factors that affect the response to a drug, the influence of disease is least understood (Benet, 1976). Although diseases alter normal functions which, in turn, affect the response to a drug, research has been delayed because there are few good animal models for the study of human disease. The technical and ethical limitations on clinical drug investigation preclude rigorous studies in patients. Moreover, there are difficulties in separating drug response variation caused by age and disease. It must be remembered that much pharmacokinetic data are obtained in ambulatory, young, low fat/lean ratio, healthy volunteers, whereas most drugs are used in elderly patients with chronic illnesses.

Pharmacokinetic data on humans with impaired renal function have been quite fruitful, and guidelines have been developed for adjusting dose and dosage schedules in patients receiving drugs that are eliminated principally through the kidney (Jusko, 1976; Bennett et al, 1977). Dosage guidelines for drugs that are metabolized principally by the liver in patients with impaired hepatic function are still being developed (Closson, 1977; Bond, 1978).

Examples of disease-induced alterations

in drug effects other than depressed elimination include the following: The half-lives of antithyroid agents (eg, propylthiouracil, methimazole) may be lengthened gradually twofold to threefold during the course of therapy as abnormally accelerated drug metabolism returns to normal.

Hypoproteinemia in patients with severe cirrhosis, nephrosis, and extensive burns can alter drug distribution, especially for drugs that are highly bound to protein (Tillement et al, 1978). In hyperlipidemias, circulating lipids may bind various drugs that also bind to protein and act as additional reservoirs for lipid drugs (Benet, 1976). Changes in drug binding alter the volume of distribution of drugs and emphasize the need to develop methods that measure free, rather than total, drug levels in the blood.

Certain diseases limit total cardiac output or regional blood flow and affect elimination processes which are limited by perfusion. Edema can alter transport processes at many sites. Gastrointestinal mucosal edema significantly depresses the absorption of drugs such as quinidine, procainamide, and hydrochlorothiazide in patients with congestive heart failure.

Modification of receptor sensitivity or actual destruction of acetylcholine receptor sites which occurs in myasthenia gravis and loss of dopaminergic receptors which develops in parkinsonism illustrate the considerable range of disease effects on the pharmacodynamic response to a drug.

It is likely that most diseases have multiple effects on drug pharmacokinetics. For example, diabetes could decrease permeability, metabolism, and blood flow as well as increase circulating lipids and the fat/lean ratio.

ENVIRONMENTAL CHEMICAL DETERMINANTS

Excessive noise, heat, and crowded conditions can produce stress which, in turn, alters neuroendocrine responsiveness and can lead to variation in drug response. However, examples of physical factors that produce clinically relevant changes in drug responsiveness are uncommon.

Chemical determinants include food, drugs, and nondrug chemicals; the latter group includes chemicals associated with diet, household use, incidental environmental exposure, occupation, and social activities (eg, alcohol, nicotine). Drug interaction is a term used broadly by some authors to describe altered drug effects caused by other drugs, food, or an environmental chemical (Alvares, 1978; Alvares et al, 1979). *Food-drug interaction* specifically describes only those examples related to food, whereas *drug-drug interaction* specifically refers to interactions between drugs (whether prescription or nonprescription) but, by definition, excludes nondrug chemicals. More information on interactions, especially drug-drug interactions that are encountered most commonly in clinical practice, is presented in Chapter 5, Drug Interactions and Adverse Drug Reactions.

Diet can have significant effects on the absorption, distribution, biotransformation, and elimination of drugs. A non-nutritious diet may cause serious vitamin and protein deficiencies which can affect drug biotransformation. Dietary intake of fat, even without excessive caloric intake, can alter the absorption of lipid-soluble drugs (eg, griseofulvin).

Most food-drug interactions depress the rate or extent of drug absorption. Some are clinically relevant but generally modest in intensity. If indicated, certain drugs may be administered at different times to avoid interaction. Variation in absorption can be minimized by taking almost all drugs on an empty stomach with an adequate amount (150 to 200 ml) of fluid (Welling, 1977). In a few instances, giving certain drugs with food may avoid irritation (eg, iron preparations, doxycycline, oral steroids) or enhance absorption (eg, griseofulvin, lithium). This information is included in the drug evaluations.

The average individual in the United States is exposed to numerous nondrug chemicals yearly in the form of food additives and food contaminants. In addition, occupational or household chemical exposures orally, dermally, or by inhalation must be taken into account. The clinical relevance of this chemical burden on altered drug responsiveness is unknown, but the physician must remember that he is giving drugs to patients who are exposed to nondrug chemicals. Since most nondrug chemicals do not appear in patient histories or drug profiles, the suspicion and identification of an occupational or household chemical exposure may help explain an adverse drug reaction or therapeutic failure.

Cigarette smoke contains polycyclic hydrocarbons which induce mixed-function hepatic oxidases. Because of this action, cigarette smoking decreases the bioavailability of phenacetin and increases dosage requirements for theophylline by enhancing their rate of metabolism, and plasma levels of the tricyclic antidepressant, imipramine, and the investigational drug, antipyrine, are decreased. Other hydrocarbons (eg, chlorinated hydrocarbons in pesticides such as DDT and lindane, the flame retardant polychlorinated biphenyls, polycyclic hydrocarbons generated in the charcoal broiling of meat) also can increase the biotransformation of antipyrine, theophylline, and phenacetin.

Alcohol has numerous actions that can alter the response to many drugs. Because of its widespread use, it has the most clinically significant drug interaction capacity of any single nondietary nondrug chemical. Its actions are variable and depend upon the degree and duration of intake. Acute alcohol ingestion may inhibit the biotransformation of numerous drugs. Conversely, chronic alcohol use induces microsomal oxidation enzymes which metabolize many drugs. In the absence of acute intoxication, the chronic alcoholic metabolizes some substances, such as the barbiturates, more rapidly and thus shows considerable tolerance to such agents. Conversely, in later stages of hepatic necrosis, the chronic alcoholic may become extremely sensitive to drugs that depend upon hepatic metabolism for elimination.

PHARMACOKINETIC TERMINOLOGY

Pharmacokinetics is the study of concentrations and amounts of a drug and metabolite(s) in biological fluids, tissues, and excreta over time, and their relationship to pharmacologic response. Most parameters are derived from data relating time to plasma or urinary concentrations of drug and/or metabolite. Drug and metabolite concentrations in other tissues or body fluids generally are determined only in research studies.

To determine how individual and environmental determinants influence an individual's pharmacokinetic response to a specific drug, it is necessary to extrapolate broadly from controlled, small-population studies. (Suitable mathematical models are developed for various pharmacokinetic parameters to define a "normal" range for comparison with individual patient data.) Although these studies are usually inadequate for confident extrapolation to individual patients, extensive pharmacokinetic information is becoming more available. Adverse drug reactions, particularly those arising from drug interactions, may occur less frequently when physicians are cognizant of the factors that can alter a drug's pharmacokinetic profile.

Pharmacokinetic data do not substitute for careful clinical evaluation of a patient's response to therapy, but they can raise a suspicion of or confirm clinical underdosage or overdosage, and they are helpful in developing therapeutic plans for chronic therapy.

Pharmacokinetic reference sources consist of introductory clinical reviews (Jusko, 1972, 1976; Greenblatt and Koch-Weser, 1975; Gibaldi and Levy, 1976; Sjöqvist, 1976, Rowland, 1978), extensive discussions or special reviews (Wagner, 1975; Krüger-Thiemer, 1977; Hug, 1978; Atkinson and Kushner, 1979), or compilations of pharmacokinetic data such as drug half-lives (Pagliaro and Benet, 1975; Done, 1977), volumes of distribution (Done, 1978), and drug plasma concentrations (Winek, 1977).

The following pharmacokinetic terms are defined because they may be encountered in the drug evaluations and recommended references. Terminology in this new, rapidly expanding discipline is in a state of flux; the following abbreviations and current definitions include those pharmacokinetic parameters most frequently used (Zathurecky, 1977). Certain definitions are meaningful only if corollary assumptions are understood; therefore, the reader also should note the assumptions at the end of the definitions.

Terms	Abbreviations	Units
Absorption fraction	F	fraction
Absorption rate constant	K_a	hr^{-1}
Area under the curve	AUC	$\dfrac{mg \times hr}{L}$
Bioavailability		
Biopharmaceutics		
Biotransformation		
Clearance	Cl	L/hr or L/hr/kg
Clearance, renal	Cl_R	L/hr/kg
Clearance, nonrenal	Cl_{NR}	L/hr/kg
Clearance, total body	Cl_T	L/hr/kg
Compartment		
Disintegration		
Disposition		
Dissolution		
Distribution		
Dose	D	mg/kg
Dosing interval	τ	hr
Dose, loading	LD	mg/kg
Dose, maintenance	MD	mg/kg
Dosing rate, mean	DR	mg/kg/hr
Elimination rate constants, specific	k	hr^{-1}
Elimination rate constant, overall	K_e	hr^{-1}
First Pass Effect		
Half-life, biological	$t_{\frac{1}{2}}$	hr
Plasma concentration	C or C_p	mg/L
Plasma concentration, initial	C_0	mg/L
Plasma concentration, mean steady state	C_{ss}	mg/L
Plasma concentration, maximum steady state	$C_{ss\ max}$	mg/L
Plasma concentration, minimum steady state	$C_{ss\ min}$	mg/L
Volume of distribution	V or V_d	L/kg

Definitions

Biopharmaceutics: The study of the influence of product formulation on a drug's therapeutic activity. Alternatively, it is defined by many investigators as a study of the relationship of the physical and chemical properties of the drug and its formulations to the biological effects observed following administration of the drug in its various dosage forms.

Bioavailability: The rate and extent to which the active ingredient in the administered dose is delivered to the general circulation.

Biotransformation: The chemical alteration of a drug, if any, that occurs by virtue of the length of time the drug remains in a biological system.

D (Dose): The amount of drug expressed in mass units, usually micrograms or milligrams.

LD (loading dose; initial or priming dose): The larger than maintenance dose (MD) given at the initiation of therapy in order to attain a therapeutically effective drug plasma concentration more rapidly.

Disintegration: The breaking up of tablet or capsule into granules or aggregates in aqueous fluid.

Dissolution: The dissolving of active ingredient released after or concurrently with product disintegration into the fluid present at the ingested or injected site.

K_a: The overall absorption rate constant for the transfer of drug through any biological membrane (eg, skin, gastrointestinal mucosa, intramuscular injection site). Units refer to fraction of drug absorbed per unit of time.

F: The fraction of a dose that reaches the general circulation following administration by any route except intravenous. The term is synonymous with systemic availability and, when correlated with K_a, reflects bioavailability. F is determined experimentally from the area under the plasma concentration-time curve (AUC) following an oral dose compared to the same parameter following an intravenous dose.

C: Plasma concentration of drug expressed as mg/liter. (The entity C_p also is used occasionally to specify plasma concentration.) Ideally, plasma concentration refers only to the portion of drug that is in true solution. Total concentration is the term that denotes bound as well as free drug; however, plasma concentration more commonly refers to total concentration because of the difficulty in measuring free drug.

C_0: Initial plasma concentration of drug immediately after an intravenous bolus at time 0.

AUC: Area under the plasma concentration-time curve from zero to infinite time, which reflects the total amount of drug present in the body. Alternatively, this can be determined by $AUC = F/Cl_T$ or $AUC = F/K_e \times V$.

Distribution: The dispersing of the total amount of drug absorbed from the blood to extravascular tissues. The overall distributive rate constant is composed of a set of specific rate constants for drug entering and leaving the various organs and tissues from the blood.

Disposition: The processes (distribution, metabolism, and excretion) involved from the time a drug reaches the circulation to the time when it and/or its metabolites leave the body in urine, feces, expired air, sweat, or milk or are biotransformed.

Compartment: A fictitious space in which the drug is homogeneously distributed and all parts of which exchange the drug with the other compartments at the same rate.

V: Apparent volume of distribution of drug (also designated V_d). The hypothetical volume of body fluid required to dissolve the amount of drug in the body to give the concentration found in plasma $V = D/C$. Lipid solubility and the degree of plasma and tissue binding of a drug are principal determinants of the volume of distribution. Low values of V generally reflect drugs that are highly bound to plasma protein, while drugs that are highly lipid soluble and able to penetrate into fatty tissue exhibit a large V.

First pass effect: Orally administered drugs are absorbed from the gastrointestinal tract into the portal circulation prior to reaching the systemic circulation. A first pass effect refers to that fraction of an oral dose that undergoes hepatic or gastrointestinal biotransformation during the process of absorption and therefore fails to reach the systemic circulation.

$t_{1/2}$ (biological half-life): The time (in hours) during a first order elimination process that is required for the unchanged drug concentration in the blood, plasma, or serum to be reduced by one-half, measured after input has ceased and distribution equilibrium is attained. It can be measured graphically or determined by $t_4 = 0.693/K_e$. The value listed in the literature is often determined in normal healthy volunteers. It sometimes can be ascertained in the individual patient during therapy by determining the plasma decay curve during a dose interval or by omitting the next dose to attain more data if needed.

K_e: The overall elimination rate constant expressed as the fraction of drug eliminated per unit of time. Elimination is essentially the sum of all biotransformation and excretory processes causing the disappearance of the drug from the body. K_e is calculated from the terminal slope (beta slope) of a linear semilogarithmic plot of the unchanged drug concentration in the central compartment versus time after absorption is terminated and distribution equilibrium is attained.

k_r, k_b, k_m: Specific elimination rate constants. The overall elimination rate constant, K_e, is a summation of all renal and biliary excretory and metabolic biotransformation processes; these are described individually as k_r (renal), k_b (biliary), and k_m (metabolic).

Cl (clearance): A hypothetical volume of fluid completely cleared of contained drug per unit of time.

Cl_T (total or whole body clearance): The hypothetical volume of biological fluid cleared of unchanged drug per unit of time, which represents the sum of all elimination processes, including metabolism and excretion. Cl_T is expressed as liter/hour and, because it is a ratio of the dose absorbed to the total area under the plasma concentration-time curve from zero to infinity, is determined by $Cl_T = F/AUC$ or, alternatively, by $Cl_T = K_e \times V$.

Cl_R (renal clearance): The hypothetical volume of biological fluid cleared per unit of time by urinary excretion of unchanged drug. Cl_R = urinary excretion rate of unchanged drug divided by the plasma concentration.

Cl_{NR} (nonrenal clearance): Because current clinical capabilities to measure hepatic, pulmonary, and metabolic clearances directly are inadequate, nonrenal clearance is generally determined by subtracting the renal clearance from the total body clearance of that drug. It includes all clearance of the drug by metabolic and excretory processes other than renal.

T: The dosing interval, tau, usually expressed in hours, between two successive drug doses. Intervals are chosen to assure that the minimum plasma concentration does not fall below the known effective level and the peak plasma concentration does not reach toxic levels. This interval often approximates the biological half-life of the drug. Shorter intervals may be chosen when it is necessary to minimize the difference between $C_{ss\ max}$ and $C_{ss\ min}$.

$\overline{DR}$: Hypothetical mean dose rate during multiple dose therapy that is determined by dividing the dose (in mg) by the dose interval (in hours) and expressed as mg/kg/hr. When the drug is administered by constant intravenous infusion (zero order input), the term infusion rate or dosage flow is used and is expressed as mg/unit time. $\overline{DR} = MD/T$.

$\overline{C}_{ss}$: The mean plasma concentration determined under steady state conditions. For intravenous administration via constant infusion, C_{ss} = Infusion Rate (mg/hr)/Total Clearance (L/hr) and for oral administration $C_{ss} = F \times (\overline{DR})/Cl_T$ or $F \times (MD)/Cl_T \times T$ The mean plasma concentration usually rises proportionately with increasing dose, but saturation of metabolic or elimination processes causes a disproportionate increase in plasma concentration. A useful general rule is that, exclusive of loading dose, a drug reaches $0.5\ \overline{C}_{ss}$ in one biological half-life but requires five

biological half-lives to attain greater than $0.95\ \overline{C}_{ss}$.

$C_{ss\ max}$: Maximum plasma concentration determined under steady state conditions.

$C_{ss\ min}$: Minimum plasma concentration determined under steady state conditions.

MD (maintenance dose): One of the doses following the loading dose in a multiple-dose regimen designed to maintain a certain drug concentration in blood or tissues. MD = desired $\overline{C}_{ss} \times Cl_T \times T/F$ or desired $\overline{C}_{ss} \times V \times K_e \times T/F$.

Assumptions

1. With most drugs, absorption and elimination kinetics are independent of dose (first order), ie, the rates of drug absorption, biotransformation, and excretion are proportional to the amount or concentration at the site where the process occurs, and half-life remains constant regardless of dose. With a small number of drugs (eg, ethanol, phenytoin, salicylates), larger doses exceed the capacity (saturate) to absorb, metabolize, or excrete the substance and thus, a constant amount of drug may be gained or lost over a given time regardless of dose. The latter situation is described as zero order kinetics (a limiting case of Michaelis-Menten kinetics), and the time required to eliminate one-half the amount of drug in the body increases with dose. When the elimination capacity is saturated, a drug exhibits zero order kinetics and predictions based on first order kinetics do not apply. Constant intravenous infusion is a classic example of zero order input.

2. Assuming patient compliance, systemic availability is dependent upon a complex series of events: drug product disintegration and dissolution, possible drug deterioration or degradation, blood flow to the site of absorption, and extent and rate of absorption. Increased gastrointestinal activity and/or increased first-pass elimination through the portal circulation may diminish systemic availability following oral administration. It should not be assumed that intramuscular absorption is faster than oral absorption, since intramuscular absorption of diazepam, chlor-

diazepoxide, digoxin, phenytoin, and lidocaine, for example, is usually slower, more erratic, and more incomplete than oral absorption.

3. The pharmacokinetic parameters given for any drug reflect properties of the parent drug. This is significant when metabolism and elimination are quite different for the parent drug and its metabolites, as they are for diazepam and oxazepam, and may be even more significant when the metabolites also are active drugs as they are for procainamide, lidocaine, and sulindac.

4. Drug concentration in certain drug-avid tissues is only very slowly reversible and may persist even when drug plasma concentrations are low or undetectable after stopping the drug. Examples are tetracycline in bone, quinacrine in skin, digitoxin in ventricular muscle, phenothiazines in neuronal endings, and an antimalarial agent in the retina. Drug in such a tissue is not rapidly accessible via dialysis.

5. Pharmacokinetic parameters are dependent upon blood flow or enzymes associated with transport, metabolic, and elimination processes. Either immaturity (eg, neonates) or suboptimal function of these systems (eg, the elderly, patients with certain diseases) can markedly change drug response.

6. Expressions of pharmacokinetic parameters on a per kilogram or square meter basis are preferred for comparative purposes.

7. Pharmacologic actions generally correlate best with the amount of free drug in the plasma. Routine plasma level determinations usually reflect both protein bound and free drug. Improved analytical techniques, including radioimmunoassay, mass spectrometry, nuclear magnetic resonance, and gas-liquid chromatography, are helpful to measure free drug levels.

DRUG PLASMA CONCENTRATIONS

Knowledge of blood, plasma, or serum concentrations of drugs is usually unneces-sary in uncomplicated cases or when the toxic potential of the drug is not great, especially when information on well-defined clinical endpoints is available (eg, blood pressure, blood sugar, prothrombin time, urine output, ventilatory function). Drug plasma concentrations may be helpful (Gugler and Azarnoff, 1976; Sjöqvist, 1977): (1) to confirm suspicions of under-dosage or overdosage (eg, to distinguish between symptoms of nausea and vomiting attributable to either digitalis intoxication or progressing congestive heart failure); (2) when initiating long-term therapy in chronic diseases (eg, epilepsy, congestive heart failure); (3) to establish optimum dosage schedules in complicated situations; (4) when multiple therapy is planned and drug interactions are likely; (5) to identify selected cases of noncompliance, errors of medication, development of tolerance, lack of bioavailability, or an unusual pharmacogenetically based reaction; and (6) to monitor the results of antidotal treatment in selected cases of toxicity; nonlinear kinetics, which often develop with overdosage, can be detected with multiple sampling, allowing the physician to establish the severity of the toxicity and providing an index for monitoring the efficacy and duration of therapy.

Total clearance and biological half-life often form the basis for dosage schedules in order to avoid periods of insufficient or excessive plasma concentrations. The maintenance dose interval usually should not exceed the biological half-life of the drug. Half-life also serves as an index for determining the most satisfactory times to measure the mean steady state drug plasma concentration. For drugs with short half-lives (ie, four to six hours or less), blood samples are taken at zero time, one hour after the dose, and at two to three equally distributed times thereafter to the end of the dosing interval. Conversely, for drugs with a long distributive phase and a long half-life (ie, at least eight hours), blood samples should be drawn at least six hours after administration to avoid values nearer to the maximum steady state plasma concentration rather than the mean steady state plasma concentration. When no loading dose is administered, it is important not to sample for the mean steady state plasma concentrations until five half-lives have elapsed in order to attain at least the 0.95 $\bar{C}_{ss}$ value.

Selected References

Alvares AP: Interactions between environmental chemicals and drug biotransformation in man. *Clin Pharmacokinet* 3:462-477, 1978.

Alvares AP, et al: Regulation of drug metabolism in man by environmental factors. *Drug Metab Rev* 9:185-205, 1979.

Atkinson AJ, Kushner W: Clinical pharmacokinetics. *Annu Rev Pharmacol Toxicol* 19:105-127, 1979.

Benet LZ (ed): *The Effect of Disease States on Drug Pharmacokinetics*. Washington, DC, American Pharmaceutical Association, 1976.

Bennett WM, et al: Guidelines for drug therapy in renal failure. *Ann Intern Med* 86:754-783, 1977.

Bond WS: Clinical relevance of effect of hepatic disease on drug disposition. *Am J Hosp Pharm* 35:406-414, 1978.

Chapman CJ: Drugs and genes: Therapeutic implications. *Drugs* 14:120-127, 1977.

Closson RG: Terminal half-lives of drugs studied in patients with hepatic diseases. *Am J Hosp Pharm* 34:520-524, 1977.

Done AK: Toxic emergency: Pharmacokinetics. *Emergency Med* 10:67-81, (June) 1978.

Done AK: Toxic emergency: Helpful half-life. *Emergency Med* 9:211-220, (Jan) 1977.

Gibaldi M, Levy G: Pharmacokinetics in clinical practice. I. Concepts. II. Applications. *JAMA* 235:1864-1867, 1987-1992, 1976.

Greenblatt DJ, Koch-Weser J: Clinical pharmacokinetics, parts I and II. *N Engl J Med* 293:702-705, 964-970, 1975.

Gugler R, Azarnoff DL: Clinical use of plasma drug concentrations. *Ration Drug Ther* 10:1-7, (Nov) 1976.

Hug CC Jr: Pharmacokinetics of drugs administered intravenously. *Anesth Analg* 57:704-723, 1978.

Jusko WJ: Drug dosage adjustments in diseased patients. *Ration Drug Ther* 10:1-7, (June) 1976.

Jusko WJ: Pharmacokinetic principles in pediatric pharmacology. *Pediatr Clin North Am* 19:81-100, 1972.

Krüger-Thiemer E: Pharmacokinetics: Kinetic aspects of absorption, distribution, and elimination of drugs, in van Rossum JM (ed): *Kinetics of Drug Action*. New York, Springer-Verlag, 1977, 63-123.

Meyer UA: Role of genetic factors in rational use of drugs, in Melmon KL, Morrelli HF (eds): *Clinical Pharmacology*, ed 2. New York, Macmillan Publishing Co, Inc, 1978, 913-929.

Pagliaro LA, Benet LZ: Pharmacokinetic data: Critical compilation of terminal half-lives, percent excreted unchanged, and changes of half-life in renal and hepatic dysfunction for studies in humans with references. *J Pharmacokinet Biopharm* 3:333-383, 1975.

Rowland M: Drug administration and regimens, in Melmon KL, Morrelli HF (eds): *Clinical Pharmacology*, ed 2. New York, Macmillan Publishing Co, Inc, 1978, 25-70.

Sjöqvist F: Clinical use of drug plasma level determinations, in Azarnoff DL, et al (eds): *Year Book of Drug Therapy*. Chicago, Year Book Medical Publishers, Inc, 1977, 13-20.

Sjöqvist F, et al: Fundamentals of clinical pharmacology, in Avery GS (ed): *Drug Treatment: Principles and Practice of Clinical Pharmacology and Therapeutics*. Littleton, Mass, Publishing Sciences Group, Inc, 1976, 1-42.

Tillement JP, et al: Diseases and drug protein binding. *Clin Pharmacokinet* 3:144-154, 1978.

Vesell ES: Pharmacogenetics: Multiple interactions between genes and environment as determinants of drug response. *Am J Med* 66:183-187, 1979.

Wagner JG: *Fundamentals of Clinical Pharmacokinetics*. Washington, DC, Drug Intelligence Publications, 1975.

Welling PG: How food and fluid affect drug absorption: Results of initial studies. *Postgrad Med* 62:73-82, (July) 1977.

Winek CL: Drug and chemical blood level data, in Lewis AJ (ed): *Modern Drug Encyclopedia*, ed 14. New York, Yorke Medical Books, 1977, xii-xvi.

Zathurecky L: Developing a standard terminology in biopharmaceutics and pharmacokinetics. *Drug Intell Clin Pharm* 11:281-296, 1977.

Drug Interactions and Adverse Drug Reactions | 5

DRUG INTERACTIONS

Many drug interactions cause undesirable effects and may account for a significant number of documented adverse drug reactions. They also can limit bioavailability or block desired drug effects to cause therapeutic failures. However, drug interactions also can be clinically valuable: Probenecid prolongs and increases the effectiveness of penicillin in the therapy of gonorrhea, diuretics enhance the therapeutic action of other antihypertensive drugs, and certain drugs are used as antidotes in drug overdosage (eg, chelating agents for metals, leucovorin for methotrexate, protamine for heparin). All combination therapies utilize beneficial drug interactions, and these are the most common interactions in clinical practice.

Mechanisms

Except for the category of drug interactions attributed to physical *incompatibilities*, drug interactions are either pharmacokinetically based, ie, one drug affecting the *absorption, distribution, biotransformation,* and *excretion* of a second drug or pharmacodynamically based, ie, one drug altering *receptor activity* of a second drug. Most drug interactions are classified by the mechanism of the interaction (Kristensen, 1976). Many of them have been attributed to a mechanism that is either incorrect or only one of several responsible mechanisms. Unfortunately, such inaccuracies persist in the literature.

Incompatibility: This includes the direct physical or chemical inactivation of drugs. Examples include the degradation of amphotericin B by light, adsorption of insulin by glass, the preferential binding of some drugs by intravenous in-line filters and protein hydrolysates, and the neutralization of certain drugs when they are put into the same intravenous bottle (eg, kanamycin and methicillin). Incompatibility reduces bioavailability because less active drug is available following administration (Bergman, 1977). Most hospital pharmacists have incompatibility information for parenterally administered drugs to help avoid the serious consequences of such interactions.

Absorption: The extent and rate of absorption can be affected independently by drugs. Those with long half-lives are usually not affected by changed rates of absorption, but changes in the fraction absorbed may be important. Large doses of antacids or large amounts of milk or phytic acid (which is present in cereals and grains) may decrease the total amount of iron absorbed orally. Milk and antacids decrease absorption of tetracycline. Cholestyramine resin reduces the bioavailability of digoxin, thyroid hormone, and warfarin; administering cholestyramine two to three hours before or after the other drugs will avoid this interaction.

Drugs with short half-lives are affected by changes in not only extent but also rate of absorption. Altered rate is especially important when rapid attainment of peak blood level may be critical. Classic examples include the concomitant oral administration of agents used in infectious diseases. Food decreases the rate of sulfonamide absorption without decreasing the extent of absorption. In fact, sulfadiazine is absorbed more slowly but more completely when taken with food. Interactions involving alterations in the rate of absorption after oral administration are easily avoided by adjusting the dosage schedule to avoid meals or a second drug.

Gastrointestinal transit time may be altered by drugs administered orally. Enhanced transit time induced by cathartics is beneficial in terminating intestinal absorption of poisons; however, the use of cathartics or even the routine use of laxatives can interfere with the desired absorption of drugs. Delayed transit time induced by anticholinergic drugs can increase the fraction of drug absorbed (eg, that of slow-dissolving tablets of digoxin). Such an effect is not always predictable, however, for anticholinergic drugs depress the rate but not the fraction of acetaminophen absorbed.

Distribution: For most drugs, free-drug plasma concentration correlates with clinical response. The effects of drugs that are avidly bound in certain tissue compartments may persist even at low or undetectable plasma levels after terminating drug administration. Bound drugs may be displaced by chemicals or other drugs, but clinically relevant interactions are unlikely unless the original drug is at least 85% bound. With this high degree of binding, small changes in displacement can temporarily double or triple the free drug concentration until compensation takes place. The rate and extent of compensation depends upon biotransformation and/or elimination of the drug. For example, adequate compensation occurs quickly if the excess free drug is rapidly eliminated or widely distributed (ie, the drug is characterized by a large volume of distribution). These compensatory mechanisms probably explain the less serious interactions noted when a protein-bound drug is displaced. Conversely, a serious interaction may occur when a highly bound drug that is not widely distributed and requires biotransformation is displaced in a patient with impaired metabolic or renal function. Displacement of warfarin by phenylbutazone can produce serious hemorrhage, and their concurrent use should be avoided.

Biotransformation: Many environmental chemicals and drugs administered to animals on a subchronic or chronic basis have been shown to increase the synthesis or activity of drug metabolizing enzymes (enzyme induction). Because enzyme activity is determined genetically, there is considerable variation in the degree of enzyme induction. Many drugs are not given for sufficient periods in large enough doses to produce clinically significant enzyme induction in man. Nevertheless, those that are enzyme inducers can markedly alter the response to a second drug, especially when they are used for prolonged periods. Common examples include the barbiturates (especially phenobarbital), phenytoin, phenylbutazone, meprobamate, and glutethimide. Since multiple mechanisms are operating simultaneously, interactions predicted from animal studies may not be observed clinically. For example, phenylbutazone induces drug metabolizing enzymes in animals but, in man, it also simultaneously inhibits their activity.

Drug metabolizing processes are also susceptible to *enzyme inhibition* involving oxidative, reductive, hydrolytic, and conjugative chemical reactions. Compensatory mechanisms, such as increased enzyme synthesis, may diminish the effects of enzyme inhibition, although this does not always occur (eg, no compensation occurs with the inhibition of tolbutamide oxidation by sulfaphenazole).

A number of these mechanisms are useful therapeutically. Allopurinol blocks xanthine oxidase metabolism of purines to uric acid, and it increases blood levels of mercaptopurine (6-MP) by the same mechanism. Azathioprine may be anticipated to react similarly to mercaptopurine, but this has not been documented. The therapeutic use of disulfiram is based on its ability to block the oxidation of acetaldehyde.

Chloramphenicol and dicumarol may cause serious drug interactions in man by inhibiting drug-metabolizing enzymes, eg, the half-life of dicumarol is prolonged by chloramphenicol and can result in bleeding, the half-life of phenytoin is prolonged by dicumarol or by disulfiram and is expressed clinically as phenytoin toxicity.

The principal drug disposition function of the liver is biotransformation. Generally, routine liver function tests correlate poorly with defects in drug biotransformation; thus, only severe liver impairment as determined by routine laboratory tests is associated with a clinically significant effect on biotransformation. Other determinants of hepatic function (age, genetic profile, nutritional status and plasma drug binding,

disease, and hepatic blood flow) may predispose to interactions when one drug is a hepatotoxin and the second drug requires hepatic biotransformation. Therefore, patient monitoring, determination of drug plasma concentrations (if indicated), and individualization of dosage are especially important to avoid such interactions.

Excretion: Drug-induced alterations in renal blood flow, glomerular filtration, tubular reabsorption, or tubular secretion can result in drug interaction. Aminoglycoside antibiotics administered with other potentially nephrotoxic drugs (eg, cephalothin, polymyxin, ethacrynic acid, furosemide) can produce additive impairment of renal function. Tubular reabsorption can be especially sensitive to tubular fluid pH, and both reabsorption and secretion are affected by competing normal metabolites (eg, uric acid) or exogenous chemicals. Tubular secretory mechanisms are either anionic or cationic. The cationic transport system has greater specificity than the anionic system. Many anionic metabolites or drugs (eg, uric acid, salicylates, sulfonamides, sulfates, glycine and glucuronide conjugates, penicillin, probenecid, thiazides) are eliminated via the same transport system and thus can competitively block each other's excretion.

Drugs that affect gastrointestinal excretory processes (eg, laxatives, cathartics, antacids, drugs with anticholinergic or constipating activities) can be the basis for interactions. In addition, colonic flora enzymatically biotransform and alter the absorption of some drugs; therefore, antibiotic-induced changes in colonic microorganisms may alter the clinical response to other drugs.

Receptor Action: Certain drug responses are mediated by activating specific receptors. When two drugs are given concurrently, activation of one drug's receptor may enhance or decrease the response of the second drug's receptor. This type of interaction may involve the same or two active receptors. Although these response-producing receptors are sometimes considered a specialized compartment of distribution, this drug interaction is usually categorized as pharmacodynamic rather than pharmacokinetic. The anticholinergic effects of tricyclic antidepressants, quinidine, antihistamines, and certain phenothiazines operate through the same muscarinic cholinergic receptor, while the potentiation of central nervous system depression with combined administration of a narcotic and a barbiturate operates through different active receptors. Naloxone's ability to antagonize respiratory depression induced by an opiate drug is a beneficial drug interaction in which the same receptor is affected by the antagonist and agonist.

Examples of pharmacodynamic drug interactions are numerous. Additive pharmacologic or toxicologic effects of two drugs are more common than antagonistic effects.

Potentially Serious Drug Interactions

Drug-drug interactions can cause therapeutic failure by decreasing drug bioavailability, increasing clearance, or negating the desired effect. Drug absorption interactions in the gastrointestinal tract and drug incompatibilities account for most examples of interaction-induced limited bioavailability. Generally, incompatibilities are relatively easy to avoid by careful and appropriate preparation and administration of parenteral drugs, and absorption interactions may be avoided by staggering the times of oral administration of the two interacting drugs.

Administering two drugs that act on the same physiologic system to produce an additive effect (or, less often, an antagonistic effect) commonly leads to an adverse

EXAMPLES OF POTENTIALLY SERIOUS DRUG INTERACTIONS THAT RESULT IN THERAPEUTIC FAILURE[1] OR AN ADVERSE DRUG REACTION[2]

Drugs[3] and Action			Comment
Alcohol	central sedation additive with	**CNS Depressants:** Analgesics, opiate and opioid Antianxiety Drugs Anticholinergics, centrally acting Anticonvulsants Antihistamines Antipsychotics Central Skeletal Muscle Relaxants Clonidine Hypnotics Magnesium Salts (Parenteral) Methyldopa Reserpine Tricyclic Antidepressants	Warn patient to avoid or limit alcohol intake and of potential danger of driving or operating machinery. Patients receiving any combination of drugs with the potential for producing CNS depression should be observed more frequently, especially during the initiation of such combined therapy.
Aminoglycoside Antibiotics: Amikacin **Gentamicin** Kanamycin Neomycin Streptomycin Tobramycin	nephrotoxicity additive with	**Cephalothin** Other Cephalosporins **Polymyxins**	Aminoglycoside antibiotics administered concurrently with cephalosporins or polymyxins have the potential to produce additive renal injury, especially in patients with impaired renal function. Avoid concurrent use, if possible or monitor renal function frequently.

[1]*Limited bioavailability or antagonism of desired effect.*

[2]*Additive or potentiated toxic effect.*

[3]*Drugs in boldface type and regular type represent well- and less well-documented examples of drug antagonism, respectively.*

drug reaction. Additive central nervous system depression, anticholinergic activity, nephrotoxicity, ototoxicity, hypotensive activity, gastric irritation, and neuromuscular depression are well-documented examples. Less common but often more serious drug interaction adverse reactions result from potentiation of toxicity. One drug's interference with the biotransformation and/or elimination of a second drug may potentiate the second drug's toxicity, especially when liver or kidney function is compromised by age or disease. Adverse drug reactions resulting from these types of interactions can be avoided or minimized by selecting an alternative drug, altering the dose or dosage schedule initially, and/or periodic clinical or laboratory monitoring.

Specific information on clinically relevant drug interactions is included in the chapter introductions and individual evaluations in this text. The Table in this chapter provides examples of drug interactions that are potentially serious, ie, clinical situations in which (1) a time interval is recommended between the administration of two drugs when both drugs are given orally, (2) alternative drug therapy should be considered if possible, (3) it is highly desirable to alter initial doses, and/or (4) a symptom, laboratory test, or physical sign should be monitored periodically (especially quantitatively) to assure a good therapeutic response without drug toxicity.

EXAMPLES OF POTENTIALLY SERIOUS DRUG INTERACTIONS THAT RESULT IN THERAPEUTIC FAILURE[1] OR AN ADVERSE DRUG REACTION[2]

Drugs[3] and Action			Comment
Aminoglycoside Antibiotics: Amikacin Gentamicin **Kanamycin** Neomycin Streptomycin Tobramycin	ototoxicity additive with	**Ethacrynic Acid** Furosemide	Avoid this combination if possible, especially in patients with renal damage. If combination is required, periodic monitoring of hearing is recommended.
Aminoglycoside and Polymyxin Antibiotics Lincomycin Clindamycin	neuromuscular depression additive with	**Neuromuscular Blocking Agents**	To avoid respiratory depression, extreme caution is necessary if drugs from these two classes are given together during surgery or the postoperative period.
Anticholinergics	peripheral and CNS anticholinergic action additive with	**Other Drugs with Anticholinergic Activity:** Antispasmodics Antiparkinson Drugs Antihistamines Antipsychotics Disopyramide Quinidine Tricyclic Antidepressants	Not only are the peripheral anticholinergic effects of dryness of the mouth, blurred vision, acute glaucoma, constipation, and urinary retention probably additive but a central anticholinergic toxic psychosis also is a potential danger, especially in the elderly and children. Monitor and adjust dosage or select alternative medication when necessary.

EXAMPLES OF POTENTIALLY SERIOUS DRUG INTERACTIONS
THAT RESULT IN THERAPEUTIC FAILURE[1]
OR AN ADVERSE DRUG REACTION[2]

Drugs[3] and Action		Comment
Anticoagulants, Oral	anticoagulant action potentiated by	**Allopurinol** **Anabolic Steroids** **Aspirin** **Chloral Hydrate** **Chloramphenicol** **Clofibrate** **Disulfiram** **Hypoglycemics, Oral** **Phenylbutazone** **Quinidine** **Sulfonamides** **Thyroid Hormones** **Ticrynafen**	Severe hemorrhage is observed when anticoagulant drugs are given with aspirin or phenylbutazone; therefore, their concurrent use is not recommended. Bleeding and/or prolonged prothrombin times have been reported with concomitant administration of an anticoagulant and one of the other drugs listed; however, their combined use is not contraindicated providing periodic examination for bleeding and prothrombin measurements are determined and appropriate adjustments in dosage are made.
Anticoagulants, Oral	anticoagulant action antagonized by	**Glutethimide** **Griseofulvin** **Phenobarbital** **Phytonadione** **Rifampin**	Concurrent administration of the vitamin K preparation, phytonadione, should be avoided unless it is needed to antagonize the anticoagulant effect. The enzyme inducers listed should not be discontinued abruptly if they have been administered with an oral anticoagulant, for severe bleeding may occur.
Antidepressants, Tricyclic	cardiotoxicity additive with	**Quinidine** **Procainamide**	Avoid the combination. The quinidine-like cardiotoxicity of tricyclic antidepressants, especially with large doses (overdosage), is additive with that of quinidine and procainamide.
Antihypertensive Drugs	hypotensive action additive with	Antianginals Antiarrhythmics Antidepressants Antipsychotics	Combination antihypertensive drug therapy that includes a diuretic is desirable because it allows the use of lower doses of each agent which minimizes the risk of adverse events; however, the potential hypotensive action of numerous psychopharmacologic, antiarrhythmic, and antianginal drugs administered with antihypertensive medications can cause serious undesirable hypotension. The elderly and debilitated are most susceptible.
Aspirin	gastric irritation additive with	**Alcohol** See Anticoagulants, Oral; Heparin; Methotrexate; and Sulfinpyrazone	Concurrent use should be avoided, especially in patients with a history of gastric irritation or bleeding after use of either agent. Acetaminophen is a useful alternative for analgesia or antipyresis.
Chlorpromazine	antipsychotic action antagonized by	**Levodopa**	The antagonism is reciprocal; if it is necessary to use the drugs simultaneously, the effectiveness of both should be monitored periodically.

EXAMPLES OF POTENTIALLY SERIOUS DRUG INTERACTIONS
THAT RESULT IN THERAPEUTIC FAILURE[1]
OR AN ADVERSE DRUG REACTION[2]

Drugs[3] and Action			Comment
Chlorpromazine Promazine	antipsychotic action antagonized by	**Phenobarbital**	Prolonged administration of phenobarbital can decrease the effectiveness of chlorpromazine. Other antipsychotic drugs may interact with phenobarbital, but there is no documentation for this action for other barbiturates.
Cholestyramine Resin Colestipol	decreases bioavailability of	**Digoxin Thyroid Hormones Warfarin**	A 3-hour interval between the oral administration of cholestyramine resin and drugs listed is recommended.
Dicumarol	anticoagulant action antagonized by	**Phenytoin**	Avoid the combination. Warfarin is less likely to interact, but it is essential to monitor prothrombin times and signs of phenytoin toxicity (see phenytoin-dicumarol interaction) for possible dosage adjustment of either or both drugs.
Digoxin	bioavailability decreased by	**Antacids**	A 1- to 2-hour interval between the oral administration of digoxin and an antacid is recommended.
Digoxin Other Digitalis Glycosides	cardiotoxicity potentiated by potassium depleting action of	**Thiazide Diuretics Amphotericin B Chlorthalidone Corticosteroids Ethacrynic Acid Furosemide Mercurial Diuretics**	Potassium supplementation is recommended for patients receiving digoxin and a potassium-depleting diuretic but only if determination of a baseline serum potassium concentration, followed by periodic monitoring to avoid hyperkalemia, is part of the management program. Potassium-sparing diuretics (spironolactone or triamterene) may be a better alternative in selected patients.
Digoxin	cardiotoxicity potentiated by	**Quinidine**	Quinidine increases plasma levels of digoxin, and a reduction of digoxin dosage is suggested when the drugs are given concurrently.
Epinephrine Other Direct-Acting Alpha-Adrenergic Amines	cardiovascular actions potentiated by	Tricyclic Antidepressants: Amitriptyline Desipramine Doxepin **Imipramine** Nortriptyline Protriptyline	The infusion of epinephrine and other direct-acting adrenergic amines in patients receiving tricyclic antidepressants concurrently exaggerates the cardiovascular actions (arrhythmias, hypertension, tachycardia) of epinephrine. Monitoring of cardiovascular status is recommended if combination therapy is necessary; doxepin may be a better alternative since it is less potent in blocking the uptake of epinephrine. The actions of indirect-acting alpha-adrenergic amines may be antagonized by tricyclic antidepressants.

EXAMPLES OF POTENTIALLY SERIOUS DRUG INTERACTIONS THAT RESULT IN THERAPEUTIC FAILURE[1] OR AN ADVERSE DRUG REACTION[2]

Drugs[3] and Action			Comment
Ether Cyclopropane Halothane Methoxyflurane Nitrous Oxide	neuromuscular depression additive with	**Neomycin** Other Aminoglycoside Antibiotics Polymyxins	Depression of neuromuscular transmission has been reported after intraperitoneal administration of the antibiotic. The interaction is especially likely to occur in children or those who are elderly, debilitated, or receiving neuromuscular blocking drugs such as tubocurarine, pancuronium, gallamine, decamethonium, or succinylcholine.

Furazolidone	potentiates
	the hypertensive
	action of
		Amphetamine
		Alpha-Adrenergic
		  Amines,
		  Indirect-Acting
			Avoid concurrent administration. A metabolite of furazolidone possesses monoamine oxidase inhibiting activity that intensifies the hypertensive action of these amines. See the monoamine oxidase inhibitor-alpha adrenergic amine interaction.

Furazolidone	potentiates the toxicity of	**Alcohol**	A disulfiram-like action of furazolidone may occur with alcohol ingestion. The patient should be warned of this possibility.
Griseofulvin	bioavailability decreased by	**Phenobarbital**	Select a nonbarbiturate or monitor effectiveness and/or serum level of griseofulvin.
Guanethidine	antihypertensive action antagonized by	Butyrophenones **Chlorpromazine** Other Phenothiazines Thioxanthenes	Select another antihypertensive drug.
Guanethidine	antihypertensive action antagonized by	Amitriptyline **Desipramine** Imipramine Nortriptyline Protriptyline	Select another antihypertensive drug or a trial with the tricyclic antidepressant, doxepin (no more than 100 mg/day) may obviate the interaction.
Guanethidine	antihypertensive action antagonized by	**Dextroamphetamine** Other Amphetamines Ephedrine Methylphenidate Phenylpropanolamine	Select another antihypertensive drug or avoid the concurrent use of guanethidine and listed drugs.

Halothane
Cyclopropane
Enflurane
Methoxyflurane
	potentiates
	cardiotoxicity of
		Epinephrine
		Other Direct-Acting
		  Alpha-Adrenergic
		  Agents
			Arrhythmias induced by the rapid intravenous administration of epinephrine in the presence of certain inhalation anesthetics can be life-threatening. The dosage of epinephrine must be reduced if it must be used. Indirect-acting sympathomimetic agents (eg, phenylephrine) are less likely to be potentiated.

Heparin	anticoagulant action potentiated by	**Aspirin**	Because aspirin inhibits platelet function, it should be used only with caution in patients receiving heparin; acetaminophen, sodium salicylate, or other analgesics are suggested as substitutes.

EXAMPLES OF POTENTIALLY SERIOUS DRUG INTERACTIONS
THAT RESULT IN THERAPEUTIC FAILURE[1]
OR AN ADVERSE DRUG REACTION[2]

Drugs[3] and Action			Comment
Hypoglycemics, Oral: Acetohexamide (Possible) **Chlorpropamide** Tolazamide (Possible) **Tolbutamide**	hypoglycemic action potentiated by	**Alcohol** **Chloramphenicol** **Clofibrate** **Dicumarol** **Monoamine Oxidase Inhibitors** **Phenylbutazone** **Sulfaphenazole** **Sulfinpyrazone**	The listed drugs may prolong the half-life of tolbutamide and chlorpropamide, even with short-term use of therapeutic doses. Blood glucose determinations are recommended to monitor the presence and severity of this adverse reaction so that the offending drug may be avoided or the dose of the oral hypoglycemic agent reduced. Although less information is available on acetohexamide and tolazamide, they also should be used cautiously.
Insulin	hypoglycemic action antagonized by	**Chlorpromazine** Other Phenothiazines	The interaction occurs only with use of large doses of chlorpromazine (more than 100 mg/day) for prolonged periods (months). Appropriate periodic monitoring for hyperglycemia is recommended.
Insulin Oral Hypoglycemics	hypoglycemic action potentiated by	Guanethidine **Isocarboxazid** **Phenelzine** **Propranolol** Tranylcypromine	Avoid the concurrent use of insulin and monoamine oxidase inhibitors if possible. The potential of propranolol or guanethidine to interfere with carbohydrate metabolism may necessitate adjustment of insulin or oral hypoglycemic dosage. Periodic monitoring of serum glucose is recommended.
Kaolin	decreases bioavailability of	**Lincomycin**	Avoid kaolin with this antibiotic.
Levodopa	antiparkinsonism action antagonized by	**Chlorpromazine** Related Antidopaminergic Drugs	The antagonism is reciprocal; the effectiveness of both drugs should be monitored periodically if they must be used simultaneously.
Levodopa	antiparkinsonism action antagonized by	**Pyridoxine**	Since carbidopa is not affected by pyridoxine, its substitution for levodopa is recommended in patients who require pyridoxine supplementation.
Levodopa	dopamine hypertensive action potentiated by	Isocarboxazid **Phenelzine** Tranylcypromine	Levodopa, when converted to dopamine, may increase the blood pressure in the presence of monoamine oxidase inhibitors or within two weeks following termination of use of the latter. Avoid combination, select a tricyclic antidepressant, or use carbidopa if necessary.
Lincomycin Clindamycin	bactericidal activity antagonized by	Chloramphenicol **Erythromycin**	Avoid combination.

EXAMPLES OF POTENTIALLY SERIOUS DRUG INTERACTIONS
THAT RESULT IN THERAPEUTIC FAILURE[1]
OR AN ADVERSE DRUG REACTION[2]

Drugs[3] and Action			Comment
Lithium	cardio- and neurotoxicity potentiated by	**Chlorothiazide** Other Thiazide Diuretics Chlorthalidone	Caution is suggested in the use of this combination; monitor serum lithium levels periodically. The potassium-sparing diuretics, spironolactone and triamterene, or the loop diuretic, furosemide, may be safer alternative diuretics when use of lithium is necessary.
Lithium	hypothyroid action additive with	**Iodine Compounds**	Avoid all iodine-containing drugs, including nonprescription products.
Meperidine Other Narcotic Analgesics	analgesic and respiratory depressant actions potentiated by	**Chlorpromazine** Other Phenothiazines **Hydroxyzine** Promethazine	Respiratory depression may occur unless the narcotic dose is decreased by 25% to 50% when phenothiazines, promethazine, or hydroxyzine are administered concurrently. Naloxone reverses the respiratory depression.
Meperidine Other Related Analgesics	unusual CNS toxicity caused by	**Isocarboxazid** **Phenelzine** **Tranylcypromine**	The monoamine oxidase inhibitors can cause central nervous system toxicity (excitement, convulsions, hyperpyrexia or severe respiratory depression) with meperidine. The combination has caused fatalities and avoidance is recommended even though the interaction does not always occur. The cautious use of small doses of morphine is recommended if a narcotic analgesic is required.
Mercaptopurine Azathioprine	toxicity potentiated by	**Allopurinol**	The dose of mercaptopurine or azathioprine should be reduced by one-third to one-fourth if allopurinol is administered concurrently. Maintenance doses are adjusted on the basis of clinical response.
Methotrexate	toxicity potentiated by	**Aspirin**	Avoid the combination if possible. Acetaminophen (for analgesia and antipyresis) and indomethacin (for anti-inflammatory action) appear to be acceptable alternatives to aspirin.
Monoamine Oxidase Inhibitors: Isocarboxazid Phenelzine Tranylcypromine	potentiate the hypertensive action of	**Alpha-Adrenergic Amines, Indirect-Acting**	Anorexiants, amphetamines, ephedrine, phenylephrine, phenylpropanolamine, pseudoephedrine, methylphenidate, tyramine-containing foods, and nonprescription drugs containing such sympathomimetic amines have been reported most often to be responsible for this interaction. Avoidance of these drugs, a diet low in tyramine, and, if needed, cautious substitution of direct-acting alpha-adrenergic sympathomimetic agents are recommended.

EXAMPLES OF POTENTIALLY SERIOUS DRUG INTERACTIONS
THAT RESULT IN THERAPEUTIC FAILURE[1]
OR AN ADVERSE DRUG REACTION[2]

Drugs[3] and Action			Comment
Monoamine Oxidase Inhibitors	toxicity potentiated by	**Antidepressants, Tricyclic**	The concurrent use of these drugs is not contraindicated; however, see the evaluations of both classes of drugs before combination therapy is undertaken.
Nitrofurantoin	urinary antibacterial action antagonized by and toxicity potentiated by	**Probenecid** Sulfinpyrazone	Avoid combination. Probenecid diminishes the renal excretion of nitrofurantoin and can, therefore, inhibit its effectiveness in urinary tract infections. In addition, the combination increases the serum concentration of nitrofurantoin, which causes polyneuropathies and even degeneration of sensory and motor nerves. The action may be most pronounced in patients with impaired renal function.
Penicillin G Other Penicillins	bactericidal action antagonized by	**Chlortetracycline** Other Tetracyclines	Avoid combination, especially when the rapid bactericidal activity of penicillin is required.
Phenobarbital	sedation potentiated by	**Valproic Acid**	Valproic acid is reported to increase the plasma concentration of phenobarbital, resulting in excessive sedation. It may be necessary to reduce the dose of phenobarbital when these drugs are administered concurrently.
Phenytoin Phenobarbital Primidone	decreases bioavailability of	**Folic Acid**	CNS symptoms of folic acid deficiency may develop with long-term use of phenytoin, especially during pregnancy. Folic acid supplementation may be necessary.
Phenytoin	antagonizes effects of	**Vitamin D**	Sufficient dietary intake of vitamin D and exposure to sunlight or vitamin D supplements may be indicated in patients receiving phenytoin for prolonged periods, especially those susceptible to the development of osteomalacia and rickets.
Phenytoin	toxicity potentiated by	**Chloramphenicol** Oxyphenbutazone **Phenylbutazone** **Sulfamethizole**	When the listed drugs are administered to a patient receiving phenytoin, the serum phenytoin concentration may increase within one to three days and result in CNS toxicity. Avoid concurrent use if possible or monitor serum phenytoin concentrations for four days after initiating therapy.
Phenytoin	toxicity potentiated by	**Dicumarol**	Anticoagulant action of dicumarol is also diminished. Warfarin is less likely to interact, but it is essential to monitor prothrombin times and observe patient for signs of phenytoin toxicity; adjustment of dosage of either or both drugs may be necessary.

EXAMPLES OF POTENTIALLY SERIOUS DRUG INTERACTIONS THAT RESULT IN THERAPEUTIC FAILURE[1] OR AN ADVERSE DRUG REACTION[2]

Drugs[3] and Action			Comment
Phenytoin Primidone	toxicity potentiated by	**Disulfiram**	Avoid combination if possible. Otherwise, monitor for signs of phenytoin toxicity and determine phenytoin serum concentration; adjust dosage if necessary.
Phenytoin Primidone	toxicity potentiated by	**Isoniazid**	Patients who are slow inactivators of isoniazid are most susceptible to this interaction. It is necessary to monitor for signs of phenytoin toxicity and possibly determine phenytoin serum concentrations; adjust dosage if necessary.
Spironolactone **Triamterene**	potassium-sparing action potentiated by	**Potassium Chloride**	This interaction can be considered beneficial; however, concurrent use of these agents increases the risk of hyperkalemia and their combined use is not recommended in most instances. Periodic monitoring of serum potassium is strongly recommended if concurrent therapy is employed.
Succinylcholine	respiratory depression potentiated by	**Lidocaine** Magnesium Salts (Parenteral)	Inadequate ventilation due to the neuromuscular blocking action of succinylcholine is enhanced by the central respiratory depressant action of lidocaine and magnesium. Careful attention to adequate ventilation is recommended after concurrent use of these agents.
Sulfinpyrazone Probenecid	uricosuric action antagonized by	**Aspirin**	The uricosuric action of sulfinpyrazone and probenecid is reduced in the presence of aspirin. Another analgesic is recommended.
Tetracyclines	bioavailability decreased by	**Antacids** **Dairy Products**	This interaction occurs with all tetracyclines except doxycycline and perhaps minocycline. Dairy products containing calcium and laxatives containing magnesium also interfere with action of tetracycline. If concurrent use is necessary, oral administration should be separated by an interval of at least 3 hours.
Tetracyclines	bioavailability decreased by	**Ferrous Salts**	This interaction occurs with all tetracyclines. A 3-hour interval is recommended between the oral administration of each agent.
Tetracyclines	nephrotoxicity additive with	**Methoxyflurane**	Alternative antibiotic is recommended for patients who will be or recently have been anesthetized with methoxyflurane.

ADVERSE DRUG REACTIONS

Definition and Classification: The broad WHO definition of an adverse drug reaction is "any response to a drug that is noxious and unintended and that occurs at doses used in man for prophylaxis, diagnosis or therapy." Effects caused by medication errors are not included since the routine, appropriate use of the drug is implied. Inadequate doses or problems of bioavailability that result in failure to accomplish the intended purpose (therapeutic failure) are also excluded. Drug abuse, patient noncompliance, and accidental or suicidal poisoning are other drug-related adverse events that are not classified as adverse drug reactions. Drug interactions can be classified as adverse drug reactions when the circumstances and clinical outcome meet the criteria specified in the WHO definition. Adverse drug reactions are not always caused by the main, active ingredient of a product; impurities formed during manufacture, preservatives, vehicles, or degradation products in the formulation may be responsible.

Adverse reactions to any drug include *known* and as yet *unknown* actions that produce predictable minor (side effects) and major (serious injury) toxicity, as well as unpredictable idiosyncratic and hypersensitivity reactions. Adverse reaction information is always incomplete when a drug is first introduced into clinical use. The full range of toxicity may not be known until a drug has been widely used for several years. A high index of suspicion is required to detect and distinguish adverse drug reactions from other adverse events. This is especially true with new drugs. The potential for adverse drug reactions is relatively high among the elderly and newborn (see the section on Age Determinants in Chapter 4, Drug Response Variation).

Notification and Identification: An Adverse Drug Reaction Monitoring Program has been established by the Department of Drug Experience of the Food and Drug Administration, Parklawn Building, Rockville, MD, 20857. The Program also encourages the reporting of drug experi-ences other than adverse drug reactions that indicate problems in bioavailability (Lee and Groth, 1977; Lee and Turner, 1978). Two report forms, FD-1639, a 25-element data form, and FD-1639a, a shorter 13-element form (periodically attached to the *Food and Drug Bulletin* sent to most health-care professionals), are distributed by the Food and Drug Administration, Department of Health, Education and Welfare, Washington, DC, 20204. Practicing physicians, hospital pharmacists, and selected nursing personnel are in key positions to contribute to the success of this monitoring program.

Proving that a specific drug is responsible for an adverse event in an individual can be extremely difficult (Karch and Lasagna, 1975). The clinical assessment is often complicated by multiple drug exposures and underlying illnesses.

Criteria have been developed in the form of an algorithm (Irey, 1976; Karch and Lasagna, 1977) and are utilized by the FDA Department of Drug Experience to help identify causality of adverse drug reactions. These criteria include the following: (1) the temporal relationship between the suspected drug and the adverse reaction; (2) the presence or absence of dechallenge or improvement after removal of the individual drug; (3) the presence or absence of rechallenge, ie, recurrence of the adverse reaction if the drug is purposely or inadvertently restarted; and (4) the likelihood that the concomitant disease would cause the same type of disorder. After causality has been assessed, the adverse reaction is classified as definite, probable, possible, or remote as follows:

Definite: A reaction that follows a reasonable temporal sequence from administration of the drug or in which the drug level has been established in body fluids or tissues; that follows a known response pattern to the suspected drug; and that is confirmed by improvement on stopping or reducing the dosage of the drug (dechallenge), and reappearance of the reaction on repeated exposure (rechallenge).

Probable: A reaction that follows a reasonable temporal sequence from administration of the drug; that follows a known response pattern to the suspected drug; that is confirmed by dechallenge; and that could not be reasonably explained by the known characteristics of the patient's clinical state.

Possible: A reaction that follows a reasonable temporal sequence from administration of the drug; that follows a known response pattern to the suspected drug; but that could have been produced by the patient's clinical state or other modes of therapy administered to the patient.

Remote: Any reaction that does not meet the criteria above.

Avoiding Adverse Drug Reactions: Almost all drugs cause known and reasonably predictable toxic reactions in excessive doses; however, some drugs must be given in doses that approach or reach the toxic range for some patients. If a drug must be administered with another drug in a situation in which drug interaction is likely, appropriate observations are needed to detect the approach or onset of toxicity, to reverse it, and to avoid its progression to intolerable proportions.

The most important information that a physician can have about adverse drug reactions is knowing which reactions to anticipate from each drug prescribed. When a drug is known to cause serious organ damage relatively frequently, relevant baseline studies and a program of periodic surveillance for pre-specified toxic endpoints are recommended. Serious toxicity can often be avoided by teaching patients to be alert for early signs of drug toxicity. In this book, the usual custom has been to warn of reactions but not to attempt detailed advice on monitoring them. Suggestions for periodic evaluation of symptoms, signs, and laboratory test results are ordinarily reserved for situations in which these are of definite value. More commonly, reliance is placed upon the physician's discretion and judgment in determining the details of monitoring treatment. Even when advice to perform laboratory tests is indicated, it seldom has been practical to specify frequency, for it is impossible to devise a precise routine that is ideal for all patients.

Vital organs, such as the hematopoietic system, the liver, and the kidneys, can be adversely affected by drugs. When toxic reactions occur gradually or their overt manifestations appear slowly, laboratory test abnormalities may precede the appearance of symptoms and warn of toxicity. For example, drugs that may cause megaloblastic anemia with prolonged use, such as some anticonvulsants and folic acid antagonists, warrant monitoring by periodic blood studies. This reaction progresses gradually, may be detected well in advance of symptoms, and can be controlled by proper management. This precaution is particularly significant during pregnancy, because megaloblastic anemia may damage the fetus if allowed to progress. On the other hand, much routine laboratory testing done in the absence of symptoms or signs is wasteful and may lead to a false sense of security, as when efforts are made to anticipate reactions that occur precipitously. Warning the patient to alert the physician to any significant untoward event is more important in guarding against agranulocytosis than prodigious numbers of hemograms. If such an event occurs (eg, infection), immediate laboratory evaluation is indicated, in spite of a recent normal hemogram.

Drug-induced liver disease of an allergic or hypersensitivity type presents the greatest problem in early detection. Using laboratory tests to monitor therapy is valuable for drugs known to produce gradual, subtle, and serious hepatotoxic injury. Fortunately, few modern drugs have such potential. Nevertheless, many can produce liver damage (without apparent relation to dosage) in hypersensitive patients, and serious hypersensitivity reactions tend to develop precipitously. Evidence that such reactions can be diagnosed in a substantial number of patients by performing routine liver function tests before symptoms develop is scanty. Although such diagnoses might occasionally be made, minor abnormalities are often difficult to assess in terms of cause or importance, and striking ones seldom precede symptoms by a significant length of time. The most important precaution is to observe the patient for malaise, abdominal discomfort, anorexia, dark urine, and jaundice and to perform proper laboratory studies if any of these reactions occur. Cholestatic reactions are typically less dangerous than the hepatocellular type, but either must be regarded as potentially serious.

Occasionally, drug-induced nephrotoxicity occurs with dramatic suddenness. Usually, however, drugs that cause kidney damage produce it subtly and well before the patient develops symptoms. When such a drug is given for prolonged periods, periodic urinalyses, serum creatinine, and an occasional creatinine clearance test may be useful for early detection.

The following suggestions are recommended to lessen the incidence of adverse drug reactions, including those that arise from interactions.

Individualize drug therapy based on an individual assessment of the endogenous and exogenous determinants that alter drug responsiveness. Thus, an adequate history and physical examination to identify hereditary diseases and present health status is required. Assessing exogenous determinants includes occupational or environmental chemical exposures, dietary intake, and particularly the use of alcohol, tobacco, and other drugs (both prescription and nonprescription).

Refer to a literature source on drug interactions (Cohen and Armstrong, 1974; American Pharmaceutical Association, 1976 and 1978; Avery, 1977; Davies, 1977; Hansten, 1979; *Medical Letter*, 1979), particularly if the drug(s) intended for use has not been prescribed recently. Avoid compendia that make no attempt to establish the clinical relevance of the drug interactions listed. The clinical relevance of drug interactions requires perspective. A considerable number of reported interactions are of no clinical relevance because they are based on (1) animal studies not confirmed in humans, (2) limited studies (eg, case reports) not substantiated by well-controlled studies, (3) hypothetical situations, or (4) minor changes that are insignificant clinically. Even among confirmed, clinically relevant drug interactions, benefit/risk perspective evaluated in each individual case is more appropriate than blanket avoidance.

Anticipate that patients requiring prolonged drug therapy (eg, those with heart disease, hypertension, diabetes, epilepsy, psychoses) are most likely to react adversely when new therapy is initiated or terminated. Adverse reactions occurring at termination of part or all of a therapeutic program are often overlooked. During such periods, it is important to schedule more frequent visits, offer additional patient education, and monitor symptoms, signs, and laboratory tests. Teach patients to identify the early signs of drug toxicity and to notify the physician as soon as possible. Serious toxicity often can be avoided when the patient knows what to anticipate.

Optimize drug therapy, giving the least number of drugs that achieve the desired effect; the risk of an adverse drug reaction is directly proportional to the number of drugs prescribed.

Selected References

Adverse interactions of drugs. *Med Lett Drugs Ther* 21:5-12, 1979.

Evaluations of Drug Interactions, ed 2. Washington, DC, American Pharmaceutical Association, 1976.

Evaluations of Drug Interactions, ed 2 (supplement). Washington, DC, American Pharmaceutical Association, 1978.

Avery GS: Drug interactions that really matter: Guide to major important drug interactions. *Drugs* 14:132-146, 1977.

Bergman HD: Incompatibilities in large volume parenterals. *Drug Intell Clin Pharm* 11:346-360, 1977.

Cohen SN, Armstrong MF: *Drug Interactions: A Handbook for Clinical Use*. Baltimore, Williams & Wilkins Company, 1974.

Davies DM: *Textbook of Adverse Drug Reactions*. New York, Oxford University Press, 1977.

Hansten PD: *Drug Interactions*, ed 4. Philadelphia, Lea & Febiger, 1979.

Irey NS: Adverse drug reactions and death: Review of 827 cases. *JAMA* 236:575-578, 1976.

Karch FE, Lasagna L: Toward operational identification of adverse drug reactions. *Clin Pharmacol Ther* 21:247-254, 1977.

Karch FE, Lasagna L: Adverse drug reactions. Critical review. *JAMA* 234: 1236-1241, 1975.

Kristensen MB: Drug interactions and clinical pharmacokinetics. *Clin Pharmacokinet* 1:351-372, 1976.

Lee B, Groth P: Drug reaction alerts. *Am J Hosp Pharm* 34:694-695, 1977.

Lee B, Turner WM: Food and Drug Administration's adverse drug reaction monitoring program. *Am J Hosp Pharm* 35:929-932, 1978.

General Analgesics | 6

Analgesic drugs discussed in this chapter are divided into two groups depending upon whether they interact with opiate receptors: (1) the opiates and related drugs (opioids), which bind to opiate receptors, and (2) the nonopiates (analgesic-antipyretics), which have no affinity for these receptors. Although drugs in both groups have analgesic properties, their other pharmacologic actions differ and they are discussed in separate sections of this chapter. Because many combination products contain drugs from each group, these are discussed in a third section. The classification of analgesics used in previous editions of this book was based upon the severity of pain that the drugs were capable of relieving. Those given primarily to relieve moderate to severe pain were designated strong analgesics, while those given

to relieve mild to moderate pain were designated mild analgesics.

OPIATES AND OPIOIDS

Drugs considered as opiates include the purified alkaloids of opium such as morphine and codeine and the semisynthetic modifications of morphine (hydromorphone [Dilaudid], nalbuphine [Nubain], oxymorphone [Numorphan], oxycodone [in Percodan]). The opioids include various synthetic compounds that resemble morphine in many of their actions. The latter drugs can be classified by chemical structure as (1) phenylpiperidine derivatives (meperidine [Demerol], alphaprodine [Nisentil], anileridine [Leritine]);

55

(2) morphinan (or phenanthrene) derivatives (levorphanol [Levo-Dromoran], butorphanol [Stadol]); (3) diphenylheptane derivatives (methadone, propoxyphene [Darvon]); (4) a benzomorphan derivative (pentazocine [Talwin]); and (5) a propionamide derivative (propiram [Dirame]). Other available analgesics, which are less widely used and thus are not evaluated in this chapter, include fentanyl [Sublimaze], hydrochlorides of opium alkaloids [Pantopon], hydrocodone [Dicodid], and methotrimeprazine [Levoprome].

The concept of the existence of analgesic receptors that could interact with compounds of various chemical structures to produce analgesia was proposed many years ago, but only recently have specific opiate binding sites been identified as receptors and their anatomical distribution determined. The density of opiate binding sites varies markedly in different regions of the central nervous system. Densities are high in anatomical areas associated with physiologic functions that are altered by opiates, suggesting a correlation between site of action and opiate effect. Neurochemical evidence has indicated that the receptors are associated with synapses of the brain and appear to function as sites for a natural neurotransmitter substance. Endogenous polypeptides, which bind to opioid binding sites and mimic some of the actions of opioids, have been found in brain tissue and identified as a mixture of two pentapeptides, methionine-enkephalin and leucine-enkephalin. A larger peptide with similar activity, beta-endorphin, has been found in the pituitary. Subsequent studies showed that it was comprised of the amino acid sequence 61-91 of the pituitary peptide, beta-lipotropin, which has no opiate activity, and that met-enkephalin was the amino acid sequence 61-65 of the structure of beta-lipotropin (see also Chapter 46, Agents Related to Pituitary and Hypothalamic Function).

It has been postulated that the chemical structure and conformation of the enkephalins and morphine alkaloids are similar, enabling them to interact with the opiate receptors to produce analgesia and other pharmacologic actions characteristic of opiates. Although the opiates and related drugs (opioids) have various chemical structures, they all interact with opiate receptors. Several types of receptors have been postulated to explain the different actions of the various opioids; these have been designated μ, κ, and σ. The μ receptor probably mediates morphine-like analgesia and euphoria. The κ receptor probably mediates pentazocine-like analgesia, sedation, and miosis. The σ receptor mediates dysphoria and hallucinations produced by pentazocine and other drugs with antagonist activity. The relative analgesic potency of these drugs appears to parallel their affinity for these specific binding sites, as determined by in vitro studies. For example, morphine has a greater affinity for opiate binding sites than codeine. Although the discovery of the opiate receptors and the naturally occurring opioids has led to a better understanding of their effects, additional studies are necessary to explain the mechanism of the various actions (analgesia, behavioral effects, dependence) of the opiates and the role of the enkephalins and endorphin in physiologic functions. More detailed discussions on these subjects are presented in many reviews in the literature.

Indications

Morphine is the prototype of the opiates and related analgesics. All have qualitatively similar actions on the central nervous system, but their relative usefulness in a particular clinical situation is determined by differences in the rapidity of onset and duration of effectiveness, oral activity, and type and severity of pain being treated. However, the differences among them are not great and the physician may meet the needs of most patients by becoming familiar with the properties of representative drugs. The availability of several analgesics in this category, including those with "strong or potent" or "weak or mild" activity, as well as those with mixed agonist-antagonist properties, permits the physician to exercise greater latitude in selecting an agent for specific situations.

Acute Pain: Analgesics that relieve moderate to severe pain (strong analgesics) alter the psychological response to pain as well as its perception, probably at a spinal level, and suppress anxiety and apprehension. They act on higher nerve centers without producing loss of consciousness, although fully effective doses usually alter consciousness or behavior somewhat. Small to moderate doses relieve constant dull pain, and moderate to large doses alleviate intermittent sharp pain caused by trauma or of visceral origin. Agents that are weaker than morphine are useful for mild or moderate pain but not for severe pain. Because of their potential for dependence, the stronger analgesics generally should not be used for pain that can be relieved satisfactorily by weaker drugs or nonopiate analgesics. These drugs should not be withheld for short-term therapy if they are indicated to relieve moderate to severe acute pain (eg, that occurring postoperatively or after injuries).

Chronic Pain: The management of chronic pain differs from that of acute pain; the continual use of strong analgesics in patients with the former will result in development of tolerance to these drugs and may lead to complications more debilitating than the pain itself (ie, drug dependence) or conditioned pain behavior may develop. Withdrawal of strong analgesics and a re-evaluation of therapy may be necessary for some patients with chronic pain not associated with malignant disease.

The type of therapy indicated for chronic pain will depend upon its cause. When analgesics are indicated for chronic pain, it often is possible to provide adequate relief initially with a nonopiate (eg, acetaminophen, aspirin, another nonsteroidal anti-inflammatory agent), followed by one of the weaker opiates with low dependence liability, if necessary. Drugs of other classes (eg, antidepressants, sedatives, antianxiety agents) also are frequently useful. The use of strong analgesics should be reserved until necessary, but the advisability of their prolonged administration in chronic pain of nonmalignant etiology is questionable. Other treatment, such as nerve blocks, should be considered in this situation. It may be necessary to refer certain patients to a pain clinic where multidisciplinary attention is available and neurosurgical interruption of the pain pathway may be considered.

The management of patients with chronic pain associated with *neoplastic disease*, especially in its terminal phase, requires special considerations. A primary consideration is maintenance of the patient's comfort, and aspects other than medical (eg, physical, social, mental, spiritual) also must be taken into account in the total care program. The choice of analgesic drug depends upon the status of the disease and the response. It may be necessary to try several compounds to determine the best one for a particular patient and the drug regimen should be changed as required to relieve pain. As for chronic pain in general, a nonopiate (acetaminophen, aspirin, or another nonsteroidal anti-inflammatory drug) should be tried initially. The weaker opiates or an agonist-antagonist drug with low dependence liability should then be given before a strong analgesic is prescribed. It is important to increase the dose as rapidly as possible to reach the therapeutic range and then maintain it. The oral route of administration is preferred and is usually adequate unless the pain is very severe, as may occur in the last few days of the patient's life. Although the oral/parenteral effectiveness ratio of morphine and some closely related drugs is not as favorable as that of other strong analgesics (eg, methadone, levorphanol), they may be effective orally if the dosage is adjusted appropriately.

In the opinion of many authorities, strong analgesics should be administered on a regular fixed time schedule rather than on an as needed basis when used in chronic pain to keep the patient free of pain. The dose, route, and schedule must be individualized in accordance with the potency and duration of action of the drug and the response of the patient. A drug with a long duration of action is preferred in order to reduce the frequency of administration. Although tolerance develops to the strong analgesics, this may not be a serious problem with the appropriate selection of drug and dosage schedule. Further, iatrogenic dependence should not be considered a problem when treating the severe pain of neoplastic disease and must not be a reason to withhold strong analgesics from patients who may benefit from them.

Myocardial Infarction: The aim in treating the severe pain of acute myocardial infarction is to provide adequate relief without undue side effects, especially those affecting the respiratory and cardiovascular systems. Morphine is generally considered to be the drug of choice for this use; when prompt relief is required, a dilute solution may be given intravenously in small divided doses. Its hemodynamic effects are slight and may be beneficial (eg, reduction of left ventricular work index). Although morphine may produce adverse reactions (eg, nausea, vomiting, respiratory depression), it relieves the pain and reduces associated anxiety. Any excessive bradycardia, hypotension, or respiratory depression that occurs may be counteracted with naloxone [Narcan]. Meperidine also is used in myocardial infarction and equieffective analgesic doses have effects similar to those of morphine. Because pentazocine increases the left ventricular workload and myocardial oxygen demands, it is not preferred to morphine.

Obstetric Analgesia: Use of a strong analgesic in the obstetric patient requires considerable experience and judgment in order to provide adequate analgesia for the mother while avoiding interference with the progress of labor and production of respiratory depression in the newborn infant. Meperidine is widely used for this purpose; however, as with all strong analgesics, it crosses the placenta and may depress fetal respiration (see the evaluation). If respiratory depression occurs in the infant, it may be counteracted with naloxone. Administration of an antagonist to the mother prior to delivery to counteract depression in the fetus is not recommended.

Preanesthetic Medication and Anesthesia: Strong analgesics are useful for preanesthetic medication because of their sedative, antianxiety, and analgesic properties which afford smoother induction and maintenance of anesthesia and reduce excitement during emergence. However, hypnotics or antianxiety agents (eg, diazepam) are preferred by some anesthesiologists unless pain is present. Certain strong analgesics (meperidine, morphine, fentanyl, and hydromorphone) are used to supplement the hypnotic and analgesic effects of nitrous oxide. In addition, large doses of morphine (1 to 3 mg/kg of body weight) are administered intravenously in balanced anesthesia, in those undergoing cardiac surgery, and in other poor-risk patients. (See Chapter 21, Adjuncts to Anesthesia and Analeptic Drugs.)

Pulmonary Edema: Patients with dyspnea of pulmonary edema secondary to acute left ventricular failure may obtain relief with administration of morphine. This drug allays anxiety caused by hypoxemia and produces peripheral pooling of blood, which reduces the workload on the heart. However, morphine is indicated only if ventilation is adequately controlled or equipment for artificial ventilation is readily available. It is emphasized that other measures (eg, rotating tourniquets, oxygen and IPPB combined with etiologic management) are necessary to treat pulmonary edema. Although acute left ventricular failure is the most common cause of pulmonary edema, the specific etiology should be determined and treatment instituted accordingly. Morphine generally should not be given to patients with pulmonary edema caused by a chemical respiratory irritant. It should be used very cautiously, if at all, in those with bronchial asthma and should not be given during an asthmatic attack.

Cough: The cough reflex is depressed or abolished by morphine and its congeners, but use of strong analgesics for this purpose should be restricted to patients with painful cough that cannot be controlled by codeine or non-narcotic agents. (See Chapter 31, Agents Used to Treat Cough.) When an active cough reflex is desired along with analgesia, meperidine or oxymorphone may be preferred because of their relative lack of antitussive effect.

Gastrointestinal and Urinary Tract Disorders: Although morphine and related strong analgesics produce undesirable effects on the gastrointestinal tract (eg, nausea, vomiting, constipation), their antiperistaltic effect is useful in the symptomatic treatment of diarrhea (see Chapter 58, Antidiarrheal Agents). However, prolonged use may lead to severe constipation even after therapy is discontinued. Acute severe pain associated with biliary, renal, or ureteral colic can be relieved by use of a strong analgesic; however, antispasmodic therapy also should be considered, since morphine and related agents may increase smooth muscle tone. Strong analgesics should not be administered if pain is necessary for diagnosis.

Arthritis, Migraine: See Chapters 7 and 9, respectively.

Adverse Reactions and Precautions

Despite their effective analgesic action, the opiates and related analgesics cause adverse reactions that limit their usefulness: respiratory depression, nausea, vomiting, constipation, cardiovascular effects (hypotension, bradycardia), histamine release, and, in some patients, increased intracranial (spinal fluid) pressure. Other reactions include miosis, spasm of the biliary and urinary tracts, and, rarely, hypersensitivity phenomena (urticaria, rash, and anaphylactoid reactions with intravenous administration).

Respiratory depression is the most potentially dangerous acute reaction produced by the morphine-like analgesics, although it is rarely severe with administration of usual doses. Dangerously decreased ventilation is most likely to develop in elderly debilitated patients and those with disorders characterized by chronic hypoxia (eg, severe pulmonary diseases). If severe respiratory depression occurs or appears to be imminent after use of a morphine-like analgesic, the repeated intravenous administration of a narcotic antagonist (eg, naloxone) will counteract this effect (see Chapter 86, Specific Antidotes).

These drugs should be used with caution in patients with excessive respiratory secretions (eg, in chronic obstructive lung disease) because they decrease ciliary activity and the cough reflex and increase bronchomotor tone.

A strong analgesic should be given in reduced doses or withheld from patients in shock or those with decreased blood volume, since severe hypotension may develop. Because strong analgesics may cause hypoventilation and hypercapnia resulting in cerebrovascular dilatation and increased intracranial pressure, they must be used with extreme caution, if at all, in patients with head injuries, delirium tremens, and conditions in which intracranial pressure is increased. It should be kept in mind that morphine and other strong analgesics may produce miosis and their use in patients with suspected head injuries or those undergoing intracranial surgery may mask an important diagnostic sign of increased intracranial pressure (ie, dilation of one or both pupils).

Drowsiness and clouding of the sensorium and mental processes are the most prominent central effects of the strong analgesics. Although these effects are desirable in some clinical situations, impairment of the ability to concentrate and think clearly limits the usefulness of these agents in ambulatory patients.

Since these analgesics are metabolized by the liver, they should be used with caution in patients with hepatic insufficiency, for their duration of action may be prolonged.

Strong analgesics are not necessarily contraindicated in patients with impaired renal function, but these drugs decrease urine production directly by acting on the kidney and indirectly by stimulating the release of antidiuretic hormone. Their spasmogenic effect on the sphincter of the urinary bladder produces dysuria and may cause acute urinary retention in patients with prostatic hypertrophy or urethral stricture.

Dosage of the strong analgesics should be individualized and based on the severity of pain. For most rapid onset of effect, these agents must be given parenterally; however, oral administration can produce analgesia equivalent to that achieved after intramuscular injection if the dose is increased in accordance with the oral/parenteral potency ratio for the particular drug. Some synthetic analgesics (eg, levorphanol [Levo-Dromoran], methadone, anileridine [Leritine]) have a more favorable oral/parenteral potency ratio than morphine. Intravenous administration is preferred in some situations, because the onset of action is more rapid and a greater degree of dosage control is possible. Since rapid intravenous injection produces sudden, profound respiratory depression and may cause hypotension, a dilute solution of the drug should be injected over a period of several minutes, and a narcotic antagonist and equipment for artificial ventilation must be available. Patients receiving these drugs parenterally should be confined to bed for a period of time to minimize the incidence of hypotension, dizziness, nausea, and vomiting.

Interactions: The dose of strong analgesics should be reduced in patients with myxedema, hypothyroidism, or hypoadrenalism and in those receiving other drugs that depress the central nervous system (eg, antipsychotic agents, barbiturates, antianxiety agents). Severe adverse reactions have occurred following the administration of meperidine [Demerol] to patients receiving monoamine oxidase inhibitors; these have not been observed with morphine but may occur with analgesics chemically related to meperidine.

Tolerance and Dependence: The development of tolerance with prolonged use of morphine-like drugs varies from patient to patient. Therefore, any increase in dosage requirement should be evaluated to determine if it is caused by an increase in the severity of pain due to progression of the pathologic process or by the development of tolerance.

The fact that strong analgesics have effects on the central nervous system other than analgesia (eg, relief of anxiety or depression) may lead to abuse by some patients. The dependence occurring with use of these drugs may be qualitatively and quantitatively different for certain drugs of the group; it is referred to generally as morphine-type dependence to distinguish it from that produced by alcohol, barbiturates, and other types of drugs. Although results of studies designed to determine dependence liability indicated that butorphanol [Stadol], nalbuphine [Nubain], pentazocine [Talwin], propoxyphene [Darvon], and codeine have an abuse potential less than that of morphine, abuse of pentazocine, propoxyphene, and codeine has occurred. Whether butorphanol and nalbuphine will be abused awaits further experience with these drugs.

The physician should not assume that patients with pathologic pain will experience the same effects from morphine-like drugs as the "street addict" or that iatrogenic dependence will develop consistently. In fact, it is extremely unlikely following the short-term use of even large doses of potent injectable analgesics in patients with acute pain. Anxiety on the part of physicians about the development of dependence should not result in undermedication with strong analgesics for acute pain, as this may cause unnecessary suffering by the patient. Most patients given an opiate or opioid for analgesia are able to discontinue its use without difficulty. However, it should be kept in mind that physical dependence without psychological dependence may develop after prolonged use of a strong analgesic, and it is necessary to reduce the dose slowly after the drug is no longer needed. Although it often is difficult to identify dependence-prone patients, physicians should make every effort to do so. Patients with a character disorder or history of dependence or abuse of other psychotropic agents (including alcohol) and some patients with affective disorders may have a special predisposition for analgesic abuse. The use of an opiate drug should be controlled and monitored very carefully in such patients.

Ordinarily, morphine or its congeners should be given in the smallest effective doses to minimize the development of tolerance and physical dependence. This is particularly true when treating chronic diseases or conditions that may lead to drug abuse. (See also the section on Controlled Psychotropic Drugs in Chapter 3.)

OPIUM ALKALOIDS AND SEMISYNTHETIC DERIVATIVES

MORPHINE SULFATE

Morphine is the prototype of the strong analgesics (see the Introduction for uses, adverse reactions, and contraindications). This analgesic must be given parenterally to assure reliable analgesic effect. Morphine is considerably less effective orally because it is metabolized rapidly by the liver, and only a small percentage of an oral dose reaches the systemic circulation. However, this does not preclude its use by the oral route in the management of cancer pain. Although effects may be noted earlier, maximal analgesic action occurs within one hour after parenteral administration. Analgesia persists for approximately four hours (range, two and one-half to seven hours). The plasma half-life is two to three hours. Elderly patients may be more sensitive to morphine and have higher and more variable serum levels than younger patients, but there is no correlation between half-life and age.

Morphine is classified as a Schedule II drug under the Controlled Substances Act.

ROUTES, USUAL DOSAGE, AND PREPARATIONS. *Intramuscular, Subcutaneous*: *Adults*, 10 mg/70 kg of body weight (range, 5 to 20 mg), depending upon the cause of the pain and the response of the patient; *children* (subcutaneous), 0.1 to 0.2 mg/kg (maximal dose, 15 mg).

Intravenous: *Adults*, 2.5 to 15 mg in 4 to 5 ml of water for injection, administered slowly over a period of four to five minutes. This route of administration is used only rarely but may be useful when prompt onset of action is important. For general anesthesia in cardiac surgery, 1 to 3 mg/kg of body weight may be used.

Drug available generically: Solution 2, 4, 10, and 15 mg in 1 ml containers, 8 and 10 mg/ml in 1 ml and half-filled 2 ml containers, and 15 mg/ml in 1 ml, half-filled 2 ml, and 20 ml containers; tablets (hypodermic) 10, 15, and 30 mg.

Oral: This route is less efficacious and the action is variable, but it is useful in the management of cancer pain. Orally administered morphine is about one-sixth as potent as intramuscular morphine in terms of total effect. After oral use, the peak effect occurs later and the duration of action is longer than after intramuscular injection.

Drug available generically: Tablets (hypodermic) 10, 15, and 30 mg.

CODEINE PHOSPHATE

CODEINE SULFATE

Codeine is used to relieve mild to moderate pain from a variety of causes; it is usually administered orally in combination with nonopiate analgesics (see the section on Mixtures). Results of controlled studies have shown that oral codeine 32 or 65 mg is approximately equivalent to aspirin 650 mg; doses of 15 mg or less usually are

62

ineffective. It has been reported that codeine is less effective than aspirin in postpartum uterine or dental pain, and it has been suggested that inhibition of prostaglandin synthesis and an anti-inflammatory action may play a role in aspirin's superiority for these types of pain. When administered intramuscularly, codeine 120 to 130 mg is approximately equivalent to morphine sulfate 10 mg, but the incidence of adverse reactions increases at this dosage level. For its use as an antitussive, see Chapter 31.

Codeine is absorbed rapidly following oral administration; peak plasma levels occur in about one hour and the plasma half-life is about 3.5 hours. After intramuscular injection, peak plasma levels occur in about 30 minutes and the half-life is about three hours. The oral/parenteral analgesic potency ratio is 1:1.5, which demonstrates that the oral bioavailability of codeine is greater than that of morphine. Codeine is metabolized chiefly in the liver and is excreted in the urine as conjugated products; however, a portion is demethylated to form morphine, which has been postulated to contribute significantly to the analgesic effect. Plasma concentration has not been correlated with brain concentration or relief of pain, however.

The adverse reactions of codeine are similar to those of other morphine-like drugs. Constipation is noted occasionally, but nausea, vomiting, and drowsiness are minimal after usual oral doses; dizziness may occur in ambulatory patients. When the larger doses necessary to relieve more severe pain are used, codeine produces most of the adverse effects of morphine, including respiratory depression. Naloxone antagonizes the respiratory depression caused by overdosage. Large doses of codeine may cause the release of significant quantities of histamine, which may be associated with hypotension, cutaneous vasodilation, urticaria, and, more rarely, bronchoconstriction. It appears to have a more potent histamine-releasing action than morphine in equianalgesic doses; therefore, codeine should not be administered intravenously.

The dependence liability of codeine is somewhat less than that of morphine, and physical dependence occurs only rarely after oral analgesic use; however, abuse of the drug, particularly in the form of cough syrup, is not uncommon. Codeine is classified as a Schedule II drug under the Controlled Substances Act.

ROUTES, USUAL DOSAGE, AND PREPARATIONS. *Oral, Subcutaneous, Intramuscular: Adults,* 30 to 60 mg four to six times daily as necessary; *children,* 0.5 mg/kg of body weight four to six times daily.
CODEINE PHOSPHATE:
Drug available generically: Solution 30 mg/ml in 1, 2, and 20 ml containers and 60 mg/ml in 1 and 2 ml containers; tablets (hypodermic) 15, 30, and 60 mg; tablets (oral) 30 and 60 mg.
CODEINE SULFATE:
Drug available generically: Tablets (hypodermic, oral) 15, 30, and 60 mg.

HYDROMORPHONE HYDROCHLORIDE
[Dilaudid]

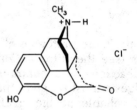

Hydromorphone, a semisynthetic derivative of morphine, has the same actions and uses (see the Introduction). It is about eight times more potent on a milligram basis but has a slightly shorter duration than morphine. This analgesic is about one-fifth as potent orally as intramuscularly; the peak effect occurs later and the duration of action is longer with oral administration. Hydromorphone is more soluble than morphine; thus, higher concentrations may be injected if necessary.

Adverse reactions are the same as those produced by morphine in equianalgesic doses (see the Introduction).

Hydromorphone is classified as a Schedule II drug under the Controlled Substances Act.

ROUTES, USUAL DOSAGE, AND PREPARATIONS.
Intramuscular, Intravenous (slow), Subcutaneous: Adults, 1 to 1.5 mg every four to six hours as required; the dose may be increased for severe pain.

> Drug available generically: Solution 2 mg/ml in 1 ml containers and 2, 3, and 4 mg/ml in 2 ml half-filled containers.
> *Dilaudid* (Knoll). Solution 1, 2, 3, and 4 mg/ml in 1 ml containers; powder in 900 mg containers (for compounding).

Oral: Adults, 2 mg every four hours as required; the dose may be increased if necessary.

> *Dilaudid* (Knoll). Tablets 1, 2, 3, and 4 mg.

Rectal: Adults, 3 mg.

> *Dilaudid* (Knoll). Suppositories 3 mg.

NALBUPHINE HYDROCHLORIDE
[Nubain]

Nalbuphine is chemically related to the opioid analgesic, oxymorphone, and the opioid antagonist, naloxone, and possesses both analgesic and antagonist properties; thus, it resembles pentazocine pharmacologically. The analgesic potency of nalbuphine on a milligram basis is approximately the same as that of morphine and is about three to four times greater than that of pentazocine; its antagonistic potency is about ten times greater than that of pentazocine. The onset of action occurs within 2 to 3 minutes after intravenous administration and within 15 minutes after intramuscular or subcutaneous administration, and the duration of effect is three to six hours.

Results of clinical studies have demonstrated that nalbuphine is effective in relieving moderate to severe pain from a variety of causes (eg, postoperative, trauma, cancer). Nalbuphine (10 to 15 mg) was compared to meperidine (75 to 100 mg) as an obstetric analgesic during labor and it was found that their effects on the mother and the neonate were similar. When used for preanesthetic medication, its analgesic and sedative effects were reported to be comparable to those of morphine. Nalbuphine relieved pain in a small number of patients with renal or biliary colic. Use of this analgesic in patients with chronic pain has been limited, but satisfactory relief of pain was reported and many did not require increasing doses. Results of one study comparing the hemodynamic effects of nalbuphine and morphine in patients with acute myocardial infarction indicated that nalbuphine may have advantages over morphine, since the former relieved pain and reduced myocardial oxygen needs without decreasing blood pressure; however, additional studies are needed to confirm the usefulness of nalbuphine in this condition.

In general, the adverse reactions of nalbuphine are the same as those of morphine and other strong analgesics. The most frequent reaction is sedation, which occurs in about one-third of patients. This effect may be advantageous in some patients but those who are ambulatory should be advised to avoid driving a car or operating machinery while taking the drug. Less frequent reactions include a sweaty clammy feeling, nausea and vomiting, dizziness and vertigo, dryness of the mouth, and headache. Other central nervous system effects (incidence 1% or less) include nervousness, depression, crying, confusion, hallucinations, and dysphoria. The reported incidence of psychotomimetic effects was less than with pentazocine.

Respiratory depresssion may occur with usual doses of nalbuphine, and the degree is comparable to that caused by equianalgesic doses of morphine. However, unlike the latter, the depression is not increased with larger doses of nalbuphine. Naloxone can be used to reverse the respiratory depressant effect when indicated.

Cardiovascular reactions (hypertension, hypotension, bradycardia, tachycardia); gastrointestinal effects (dyspepsia, cramps); and dermatologic reactions (pruritus, burning, urticaria) have been reported infrequently.

Results of studies to determine the abuse potential of nalbuphine showed that it could lead to abuse and would probably be similar to pentazocine in this respect. Although the abuse potential is low, this drug must be prescribed with the same caution as other strong analgesics to prevent its misuse or abuse and the development of physical dependence. The abrupt withdrawal of nalbuphine following prolonged administration causes opiate-like abstinence symptoms, which are milder than those of morphine but more intense than those of pentazocine.

Because of its antagonist property, nalbuphine may precipitate withdrawal symptoms in patients receiving strong analgesics for prolonged periods. Other precautions for the use of nalbuphine are the same as for other strong analgesics (see the Introduction).

Nalbuphine is not classified under the Controlled Substances Act.

ROUTES, USUAL DOSAGE, AND PREPARATIONS. *Subcutaneous, Intramuscular, Intravenous: Adults*, 10 mg, repeated every three to six hours as necessary, depending on the severity of the pain (maximum, 20 mg single dose and 160 mg total daily dose). *Children*, dosage has not been established.
> *Nubain* (Endo). Solution 10 mg/ml in 1, 2, and 10 ml containers.

OXYMORPHONE HYDROCHLORIDE
[Numorphan]

Oxymorphone is a semisynthetic derivative of morphine and is closely related chemically to hydromorphone. This analgesic is about nine to ten times as potent as morphine on a weight basis. Its actions and uses are similar to those of hydromorphone and morphine, except that

it apparently possesses little antitussive activity. When administered by rectal suppository, it is about one-tenth as potent as when injected intramuscularly.

Adverse reactions are similar to those produced by morphine and other narcotic analgesics in equianalgesic doses. See the Introduction for indications and adverse reactions.

Oxymorphone is classified as a Schedule II drug under the Controlled Substances Act.

ROUTES, USUAL DOSAGE, AND PREPARATIONS. *Intramuscular, Subcutaneous: Adults*, 1 to 1.5 mg every four to six hours. For obstetric analgesia, 0.5 to 1 mg intramuscularly.
Intravenous: Adults, 0.5 mg initially.
> *Numorphan* (Endo). Solution 1 mg/ml in 1 ml containers and 1.5 mg/ml in 1 and 10 ml containers.

Rectal: Adults, 5 mg every four to six hours.
> *Numorphan* (Endo). Suppositories 5 mg.

SYNTHETIC COMPOUNDS

Phenylpiperidine Derivatives

MEPERIDINE HYDROCHLORIDE
[Demerol]

Meperidine is the prototype of the phenylpiperidine derivatives. Many of its pharmacologic properties and clinical indications are similar to those of morphine; however, meperidine has little or no effect on the cough reflex. It is one-eighth as potent as morphine on a weight basis. The maximal analgesic effect occurs 30 to 50 minutes after intramuscular injection. The duration of action (two to four hours) is shorter than that of morphine, and the plasma half-life is three to four hours. Meperidine is considerably less effective orally than parenterally; about 50% of an oral dose is metabolized in the first pass through the liver.

This analgesic is widely used, especially for obstetric analgesia. Although it produces satisfactory pain relief, it has a significant respiratory depressant effect on the newborn infant that is proportional to the fetal blood level. To avoid high blood levels, the drug should be given intramuscularly rather than intravenously. Respiratory depression in the infant is less likely to occur if the time between intramuscular administration and birth is less than one hour.

Meperidine may have a spasmogenic effect on intestinal smooth muscle and, like morphine, causes biliary tract spasm. Induration and abscess formation may occur at the injection site after repeated subcutaneous administration, which makes it less desirable than some other analgesics for the treatment of chronic pain.

Adverse reactions most commonly observed include dizziness, nausea, and vomiting (especially in ambulatory patients). Meperidine is less constipating than morphine. Its sedative effect is comparable to that of morphine. Extreme asthenia, hyperhidrosis, syncope, dysphoria, and nightmares also have been observed. Convulsions have occurred following very large doses. Equivalent analgesic doses of meperidine and morphine produce a similar degree of respiratory depression; this effect may be reversed by use of a narcotic antagonist. With prolonged administration, large amounts of normeperidine may accumulate in some patients; this causes excitatory phenomena, including convulsions.

Contraindications to the use of meperidine are similar to those for morphine and other opiate analgesics. They include elevated cerebrospinal pressure and hypersensitivity. Since the drug is inactivated in the liver, the dose should be reduced in patients with severe hepatic insufficiency (see also the Introduction). The dose of meperidine also should be reduced in elderly patients and in those receiving antipsychotic agents, sedative-hypnotics, or other drugs that depress the central nervous system. Severe toxic reactions (eg, restlessness, excitement, fever) have occurred following use of meperidine in patients receiving monoamine oxidase inhibitors.

Meperidine is classified as a Schedule II drug under the Controlled Substances Act.

ROUTES, USUAL DOSAGE, AND PREPARATIONS. *Intramuscular, Intravenous (slow), Oral, Subcutaneous: Adults*, 100 mg (range, 50 to 150 mg). The dose may be repeated at intervals of three to four hours. For obstetric analgesia, 50 to 100 mg intramuscularly or subcutaneously, repeated three or four times at one- to three-hour intervals if necessary. *Children*, 1 to 1.5 mg/kg of body weight (maximal dose, 100 mg) administered intramuscularly, orally, or subcutaneously, repeated at intervals of three to four hours if necessary.

Drug available generically: Solution 25, 75, and 100 mg/ml in 1 and half-filled 2 ml containers and 50 mg/ml in 1, 30, and half-filled 2 ml containers; tablets (oral) 50 and 100 mg.

Demerol (Winthrop). Solution 25, 50, 75, and 100 mg/ml in 1 ml containers, 50 mg/ml in 0.5, 1, 1.5, 2, and 30 ml containers and half-filled 2 ml containers, 75 mg/ml in half-filled 2 ml containers, and 100 mg/ml in 1 ml, half-filled 2 ml, and 20 ml containers; syrup 50 mg/5 ml; tablets (oral) 50 and 100 mg.

ALPHAPRODINE HYDROCHLORIDE
[Nisentil]

This drug is related chemically and pharmacologically to meperidine and has the same uses, but it has a more rapid onset and shorter duration of action. Alphaprodine appears to have no significant advantages over meperidine except that its shorter duration of action may make it useful in certain clinical situations (eg, in obstetrics; in urologic examinations and procedures; preoperatively in major surgery; in minor surgery, especially orthopedic, ophthalmologic, rhinologic, and laryngologic procedures).

Adverse reactions and precautions are similar to those described for meperidine (see that evaluation and the Introduction). Alphaprodine is classified as a Schedule II drug under the Controlled Substances Act.

ROUTES, USUAL DOSAGE, AND PREPARATIONS.
Intravenous: Adults, 0.4 to 0.6 mg/kg of body weight injected slowly over a three- or four-minute period; the initial dose should not exceed 30 mg and the total dose should not exceed 240 mg in 24 hours.
Subcutaneous: Adults, initially, 0.4 to 1.2 mg/kg of body weight (maximum, 60 mg). For obstetrical analgesia, initially, 40 to 60 mg after cervical dilation has begun, repeated at two-hour intervals if necessary. The critical period between the last dose and birth is shorter than with meperidine. The total amount should not exceed 240 mg in 24 hours.

> *Nisentil* (Roche). Solution 40 mg/ml in 1 ml containers and 60 mg/ml in 1 and 10 ml containers.

ANILERIDINE HYDROCHLORIDE
[Leritine]

ANILERIDINE PHOSPHATE
[Leritine]

Anileridine is similar chemically and pharmacologically to meperidine and has the same indications. It is about one-third as potent as morphine and about two and one-half times as potent as meperidine by intramuscular injection. Its onset of action following either parenteral or oral administration is about 15 minutes. The duration of

action is about two to three hours, which is slightly shorter than that of meperidine. Anileridine is relatively more effective when given orally, but otherwise has no advantages over meperidine.

The adverse effects are similar to those produced by meperidine (see that evaluation and the Introduction). Anileridine is classified as a Schedule II drug under the Controlled Substances Act.

ROUTES, USUAL DOSAGE, AND PREPARATIONS.

Oral: Adults, 25 to 50 mg, repeated every four to six hours if necessary.
> ANILERIDINE HYDROCHLORIDE:
> *Leritine* [hydrochloride] (Merck Sharp & Dohme). Tablets 25 mg.

Intramuscular, Subcutaneous: Adults, for moderate pain, 25 to 50 mg repeated every four to six hours if necessary; for severe pain, 75 to 100 mg initially, followed by smaller, more frequent doses if necessary. For obstetric analgesia, 50 mg initially, repeated in three to four hours if necessary. The total amount should not exceed 200 mg in any 24-hour period.

Intravenous (slow): Adults, initially, 5 to 10 mg of well-diluted solution, followed by 0.6 mg/min until the desired amount is given. For rapid action in obstetric analgesia, 10 mg of well-diluted solution may be given intravenously slowly at the same time that 40 mg is injected intramuscularly or subcutaneously.

> ANILERIDINE PHOSPHATE:
> *Leritine* [phosphate] (Merck Sharp & Dohme). Solution 25 mg/ml in 1, 2, and 30 ml containers.

Morphinan Derivatives

LEVORPHANOL TARTRATE
[Levo-Dromoran]

This synthetic analgesic is related chemically and pharmacologically to morphine, and it is used for the same indications (see the Introduction). Levorphanol is four to eight times as potent as morphine by intramuscular injection and has a somewhat longer duration of action. It is relatively more effective orally than morphine, being about one-half as potent orally as intramuscularly.

The adverse reactions and precautions of levorphanol are similar to those of morphine. Although some reports suggest that levorphanol is less likely to cause nausea, vomiting, and constipation, any difference in the incidence of adverse reactions is slight. (See the Introduction.) Levorphanol is classified as a Schedule II drug under the Controlled Substances Act.

ROUTES, USUAL DOSAGE, AND PREPARATIONS.
Oral, Subcutaneous: Adults, 2 to 3 mg.
　　Levo-Dromoran (Roche). Solution 2 mg/ml in 1 and 10 ml containers; tablets (oral) 2 mg.

BUTORPHANOL TARTRATE
　[Stadol]

Although butorphanol is chemically related to levorphanol, it resembles pentazocine pharmacologically since it has both agonist and antagonist properties. Controlled clinical studies have shown that butorphanol provides satisfactory relief of moderate to severe pain; its effectiveness in acute postoperative pain is comparable to that obtained with morphine, meperidine, or pentazocine, but it is 3.5 to 7 times more potent on a weight basis than morphine, 30 to 40 times more potent than meperidine, and 20 times more potent than pentazocine. The peak analgesic effect occurs in about one-half hour and the duration of effect after intramuscular injection is about three to four hours. Butorphanol has

been used to treat severe chronic pain in a relatively small number of patients and, although it was effective and well tolerated when administered over prolonged periods, additional studies are needed to establish its usefulness in chronic pain.

When given to women in active labor, butorphanol was found to be similar to meperidine with respect to pain relief and effects on the neonate; however, further studies also are needed to establish this use for the drug.

In one study of a limited number of patients with ureteral colic, intramuscular doses of 2 mg were found to be as effective in relieving pain as meperidine 80 mg and 4 mg of butorphanol was more effective.

Butorphanol also appears to be comparable to meperidine when used as a preanesthetic medication, except that it produces more sedation. It has been compared to morphine and meperidine as a supplement to balanced anesthesia and was found to be as effective as the older analgesics. Additional studies are required to confirm this analgesic's usefulness in preanesthetic medication and balanced anesthesia.

The respiratory depressant effects of butorphanol are similar to those of morphine in equianalgesic doses. The degree of depression is not increased with larger doses as it is with morphine but the duration of the depression is longer. Naloxone effectively antagonizes respiratory depression caused by butorphanol.

The hemodynamic effects of this drug, as determined in a relatively small number of patients, appear to resemble those of pentazocine more than those of morphine. Butorphanol appears to increase pulmonary arterial pressure and possibly the workload of the heart. However, since its usefulness in myocardial infarction has not been determined, the administration of butorphanol to patients with this condition should be limited to those who cannot tolerate another strong analgesic.

Studies designed to determine dependence liability in animals and a small number of human volunteers indicated that butorphanol has a low potential for dependence. Symptoms resembling those of opiate withdrawal were observed when the drug was discontinued or an antagonist was administered to individuals who had received large doses for several weeks; however, drug-seeking behavior was not exhibited. Subjective effects resembled those produced by morphine but euphoria did not occur and the overall pharmacologic profile resembled that of antagonists more closely than that of morphine. Whether the drug will be abused by patients remains to be seen after its wider use. To prevent or minimize its possible abuse, butorphanol should be prescribed with the same precautions used for opiates and opioids.

Butorphanol is rapidly and essentially completely absorbed after intramuscular injection; peak plasma levels occur in 30 to 60 minutes, and the half-life is about 2.5 to 3.5 hours. It is metabolized primarily to the inactive hydroxybutorphanol which is excreted mainly in the urine, but some is eliminated in the bile. When butorphanol was administered to women in labor, the drug and its glucuronide were found in the serum of the neonate. It is not known whether the drug is excreted in human milk.

The antagonistic potency of butorphanol on a weight basis is about 10 to 30 times that of pentazocine and about one-tenth to one-fortieth that of naloxone, as determined in several animal studies. Results of studies in animals have demonstrated that butorphanol has antitussive activity, but this property has not been studied in man.

The adverse reactions are similar to those produced by other strong analgesics; those reported most frequently are sedation, nausea, and sweating. Other reactions with an incidence of more than 1% include headache, vertigo, feeling of floating, dizziness, lethargy, confusion, and light-headedness. Psychotomimetic effects (eg, hallucinations, unusual dreams, depersonalization) reported with other antagonists have occurred only rarely with butorphanol. Cardiovascular (eg, palpitation) and dermatologic (eg, rash) effects also have been observed only rarely.

Because of its antagonist properties, butorphanol should not be given to patients dependent on opiates. It should be used cautiously in patients with respiratory depression or in conjunction with other drugs that cause respiratory depression; it also should be administered cautiously to patients with hepatic or renal impairment, for these conditions may affect its metabolism and elimination.

Butorphanol is not classified under the Controlled Substances Act.

ROUTES, USUAL DOSAGE, AND PREPARATIONS. *Intramuscular: Adults*, 2 mg, repeated every three to four hours as necessary (range, 1 to 4 mg), depending upon the severity of the pain.
Intravenous: Adults, 1 mg, repeated every three to four hours as necessary (range, 0.5 to 2 mg), depending upon the severity of the pain. *Children*, dosage has not been established.

> *Stadol* (Bristol). Solution 1 mg/ml in 1 ml containers and 2 mg/ml in 1, 2, and 10 ml containers.

Diphenylheptane Derivatives

METHADONE HYDROCHLORIDE
[Dolophine Hydrochloride]

Methadone is a synthetic analgesic that differs chemically from morphine, but its actions and analgesic potency are similar. Following intramuscular injection, the duration of analgesic action is the same as that of morphine. It is approximately one-half as potent orally as intramuscularly and has a longer duration of action relative to its peak effect; this property makes methadone particularly useful in the treatment of chronic painful conditions (eg, cancer). The half-life of methadone averages 25 hours; this comparatively long time may be related to the fact that this drug is extensively bound to plasma proteins. The drug accumulates upon repeated administration. Although methadone depresses the cough reflex, labeling for its use as an antitussive is no longer permitted.

Nausea, vomiting, constipation, dizziness, dryness of the mouth, and mental depression occur more frequently in ambulatory patients. Contraindications are the same as for morphine.

Since methadone can prevent or relieve acute withdrawal symptoms produced by morphine-like drugs, it is useful orally in the detoxification treatment of patients dependent upon these agents. The withdrawal of methadone itself produces symptoms that are less intense but more prolonged than those produced by withdrawal of heroin or morphine, and the syndrome develops more slowly. Methadone also is useful orally in maintenance treatment programs for individuals dependent on heroin or other morphine-like drugs.

The Food and Drug Administration has promulgated regulations providing for strict control over the distribution, use, and dispensing of methadone in order to help reduce the problem of abuse and diversion. Under the conditions established by these regulations, methadone may be used to treat severe pain in hospitalized patients and outpatients, for the detoxification and temporary maintenance treatment of hospitalized narcotic addicts, and for maintenance treatment under approved methadone programs. Methadone is classified as a Schedule II drug under the Controlled Substances Act.

ROUTES, USUAL DOSAGE, AND PREPARATIONS.

Intramuscular, Subcutaneous: Adults, for relief of pain, 2.5 to 10 mg, repeated only when pain returns.

> Dolophine Hydrochloride (Lilly). Solution 10 mg/ml in 1 and 20 ml containers.

Oral: Adults, for relief of pain, 2.5 to 10 mg every six hours.

> Dolophine Hydrochloride (Lilly). Tablets 5 and 10 mg.
> Methadone Hydrochloride (Lilly). Tablets (dispersible) 40 mg.

PROPOXYPHENE HYDROCHLORIDE
[Darvon, Dolene, SK-65]

PROPOXYPHENE NAPSYLATE
[Darvon-N]

Propoxyphene is related chemically to methadone and is used orally to relieve mild to moderate pain. Although this drug is an opioid, its analgesic efficacy with usual doses is less than that of other opioids. It is estimated that the milligram potency of propoxyphene hydrochloride is about one-half to two-thirds that of codeine and 65 mg of propoxyphene hydrochloride is no more effective, and usually less so, than 650 mg of aspirin or acetaminophen. Comparative studies of the two salts of propoxyphene show that equianalgesic effects are produced by equimolar amounts of the salts (100 mg of napsylate is equivalent to 65 mg of hydrochloride).

Propoxyphene does not possess anti-inflammatory or antipyretic actions and has little or no antitussive activity, although the levorotatory isomer has been used for this purpose.

The most common adverse reactions are dizziness, drowsiness, nausea, and vomiting; they are more prominent in ambulatory patients, and some of these reactions may be alleviated if the patient is recumbent. Less common untoward effects include constipation, abdominal pain, rash, and headache. Asthenia, euphoria, dysphoria, and minor visual disturbances have been reported rarely. Concomitant ingestion of alcohol or other central nervous system depressants produces additive depression.

Overdosage is manifested by respiratory depression, extreme somnolence progressing to stupor or coma, pupillary constriction, and acute circulatory failure. In addition to these symptoms characteristic of narcotic poisoning, focal and generalized convulsions are prominent in most cases of propoxyphene poisoning. Arrhythmias and pulmonary edema have been reported occasionally; apnea, cardiac arrest, and death have occurred. The narcotic antagonist, naloxone, is the drug of choice to overcome severe respiratory depression. Resuscitative and supportive therapy also should be initiated as soon as possible. Analeptics or other central nervous system stimulants should not be used, since they may precipitate fatal convulsions.

Propoxyphene should not be prescribed for pregnant women since its safety during pregnancy has not been established. Furthermore, withdrawal symptoms have occurred in the neonate when the drug was used by the mother during pregnancy.

The dependence liability of propoxyphene, as determined in controlled studies, is less than that of codeine; however, abuse of the hydrochloride salt with development of morphine-type dependence has been reported. In recent years it has become apparent that propoxyphene, alone and in combination with alcohol and other central nervous system depressants, is responsible for an alarming number of deaths from drug overdose. Most such fatalities have been associated with suicidal or frankly abusive use of propoxyphene, but some appear to have resulted from accidental overdose. Because propoxyphene may be abused by some patients and death may result from overdosage, physicians should use caution in prescribing this drug (only the number of doses required for a specific condition should be prescribed and the number of refills, if any, should be limited). Propoxyphene is classified as a Schedule IV drug under the Controlled Substances Act.

ROUTE, USUAL DOSAGE, AND PREPARATIONS. *Oral: Adults*, 65 (hydrochloride salt) or 100 mg (napsylate salt) three or four times daily.

PROPOXYPHENE HYDROCHLORIDE:
Drug available generically: Capsules 32 and 65 mg.
Darvon (Lilly). Capsules 32 and 65 mg.
Dolene (Lederle), *SK-65* (Smith Kline & French). Capsules 65 mg.

PROPOXYPHENE NAPSYLATE:
Darvon-N (Lilly). Suspension 50 mg/5 ml; tablets 100 mg.

Benzomorphan Derivative

PENTAZOCINE HYDROCHLORIDE
[Talwin 50]

PENTAZOCINE LACTATE
[Talwin Lactate]

Pentazocine is an analgesic and a weak narcotic antagonist. Thus, it has pharmacologic properties of both agonists of the morphine type and antagonists of the nalorphine type. Results of controlled clinical studies have shown that pentazocine is about one-fourth to one-sixth as potent on a weight basis as morphine, and it is about one-third as potent orally as parenterally.

Pentazocine is effective in relieving moderate pain but may be less effective than morphine in severe pain. Although pentazocine is useful in obstetrics, it causes respiratory depression in the fetus comparable to that produced by meperidine. This drug also is used for preoperative medication. The dependence liability is less than that of morphine, and thus pentazocine is useful to relieve chronic pain when given before the patient has developed appreciable physical dependence on opiates. It also has been used to relieve the pain of myocardial infarction; however, the cardiac workload tends to increase because of an increase in pulmonary arterial and central venous pressure. For this reason, pentazocine is not preferred to morphine for this use, except in hypotensive patients who would benefit from increased aortic pressure.

Following intramuscular injection, maximal analgesia usually occurs within 30 to 60 minutes and lasts two to three hours. Pentazocine has a more rapid onset of action and a shorter duration than morphine; thus, its time-effect curve resembles that of meperidine. After oral ingestion, the peak effect occurs in one to three hours and lasts somewhat longer than after intramuscular injection.

The adverse reactions are generally similar to those produced by other strong analgesics. Nausea, vomiting, and dizziness occur most frequently. Other effects observed occasionally include euphoria, diaphoresis, constipation, urinary retention, and transient hypertension. The repeated injection of pentazocine into a single tissue area can result in sterile abscess formation, ulceration, and scarring of the subcutaneous tissue and muscle. If long-term administration of the drug is required, the injection site should be rotated and only the intramuscular route used.

As with other strong analgesics, pentazocine produces respiratory depression, the degree of which is dose dependent. Although similar in severity, the depression appears to be of shorter duration than that produced by an equianalgesic dose of morphine, and there is some evidence that pentazocine does not cause cumulative respiratory depression following repeated injections.

The degree of drowsiness and sedation caused by pentazocine is approximately the same or greater than that produced by equianalgesic doses of morphine or meperidine.

Psychotomimetic effects (dysphoria, nightmares, feelings of depersonalization, and, most commonly, visual hallucinations) may occur with usual doses but are observed more frequently following larger doses. Epileptiform electroencephalographic abnormalities and grand mal convulsions have been observed rarely after large intravenous doses.

Because of its mixed agonist and antagonist properties, pentazocine has less dependence liability than conventional narcotics; nevertheless, psychic and physical dependence have been reported, primarily after parenteral administration. In most of these individuals, prior dependence on or abuse of other drugs had been established. Thus, pentazocine should be used with caution and carefully monitored in dependence-prone or emotionally unstable individuals. Abrupt withdrawal following prolonged parenteral use has caused abdominal cramps, fever, lacrimation, rhinorrhea, anxiety, and restlessness in some patients. These symptoms rarely require treatment; however, if they are severe, pentazocine can be readministered and the dose reduced gradually. Administration of a benzodiazepine has controlled withdrawal symptoms in some patients. Methadone or other opiates should not be substituted for pentazocine in the treatment of these symptoms because of their potential for dependence. Pentazocine is classified as a Schedule IV drug under the Controlled Substances Act.

Pentazocine is contraindicated if increased intracranial pressure, head injury, or other intracranial lesions are present. The drug should be used with caution in patients with impaired renal or hepatic function, myocardial infarction when nausea and vomiting are present, respiratory depression, and in those undergoing surgery of the biliary tract. Ambulatory patients should be warned not to operate machinery or drive cars while taking the drug.

Pentazocine, like other narcotic antagonists, can precipitate an acute withdrawal syndrome in patients physically dependent on opiates; the severity of the withdrawal reaction is related to the extent of the patient's prior narcotic experience and the dose of pentazocine given.

Naloxone has been reported to be effective in the treatment of overdosage. The narcotic antagonists, levallorphan and nalorphine, are not satisfactory in counteracting respiratory depression or overdosage of pentazocine. Oxygen and other supportive measures should be used as needed.

ROUTES, USUAL DOSAGE, AND PREPARATIONS. (Strengths expressed in terms of the base)

Oral: Adults, 50 mg every three or four hours as necessary, increased to 100 mg if necessary (maximum, 600 mg daily). *Chil-*

dren under 12 years, dosage not established.

PENTAZOCINE HYDROCHLORIDE:

Talwin 50 (Winthrop). Tablets 50 mg.

Intramuscular, Intravenous, Subcutaneous: Adults, 30 mg every three to four hours as necessary; single doses in excess of 30 mg intravenously or 60 mg intramuscularly or subcutaneously are not advisable, and the total daily dose should not exceed 360 mg. The subcutaneous route should not be used unless necessary because of possible tissue damage. (Pentazocine should not be mixed in the same syringe with soluble barbiturates because precipitation will occur.)

For obstetric analgesia, a single intramuscular dose of 20 or 30 mg may be given. When contractions become regular, an intravenous dose of 20 mg may be given and repeated two or three times at two- to three-hour intervals as needed.

Children under 12 years, dosage not established; the amount should be reduced according to weight (see table in Chapter 2).

PENTAZOCINE LACTATE:

Talwin Lactate (Winthrop). Solution 30 mg/ml in 1, 1.5, 2, and 10 ml containers.

Propionamide Derivative

PROPIRAM FUMARATE

[Dirame]

Propiram differs chemically from other analgesics in the opioid group. Its pharmacologic properties are predominantly morphine- like, but it also has slight antagonist activity. It is an effective analgesic for moderate to severe pain when given either parenterally or orally. With parenteral administration, propiram is about one-tenth as potent on a milligram basis as morphine; when given orally, 100 mg of propiram is approximately equivalent to 8 mg of morphine intramuscularly, and 50 mg of propiram is about as effective as 60 mg of codeine and is more effective than 65 mg of propoxyphene.

Adverse reactions are similar to those observed with morphine. Those reported most commonly include drowsiness, sweating, and nausea; vomiting, vertigo, and flushing occur less frequently. Results of studies on the subjective effects of propiram suggested that its euphorigenic effects may be less than those of propoxyphene. The dependence liability of propiram is greater than that of propoxyphene and pentazocine but less than that of morphine.

The same precautions should be observed with use of propiram as with other opiate analgesics.

Dirame (Schering) (Investigational drug).

NONOPIATES (ANALGESIC-ANTIPYRETICS)

The drugs included in this section are classified as nonopiates because they do not bind to opiate receptors. They are not scheduled under the Controlled Substances Act. All relieve mild pain and reduce fever; some also have an anti-inflammatory action.

The exact mechanism of actions of these agents is not known, but evidence from experimental studies in animals has shown that the analgesic action of aspirin and acetaminophen on induced pain is principally a peripheral effect (blockade of pain impulse generation), while the antipyretic action of these agents is thought to be on the hypothalamic nuclei that regulate body temperature.

The anti-inflammatory effect of analgesic-antipyretics possessing this action is peripheral and may result from inhibition of prostaglandin synthesis. Since prostaglandins have been shown to sensitize pain receptors to stimulants, a reduction in prostaglandins would decrease painful impulses. Prostaglandins also have been shown to increase body temperature. It has been suggested that the antipyretic effect of these drugs is exerted by inhibition of prostaglandin synthesis in hypothalamic centers. The neurally mediated peripheral vasodilation that results increases blood flow and sweating and causes heat loss.

Results of recent studies have suggested that dysmenorrhea may be produced by the increased endometrial production of prostaglandin. Thus, several drugs that inhibit prostaglandin synthesis have been tested for effectiveness in relieving dysmenorrhea. Ibuprofen [Motrin], indomethacin [Indocin], mefenamic acid [Ponstel], and naproxen [Naprosyn] (and its sodium salt) are among those found to be effective.

In general, the mild analgesics are effective in alleviating pain of headache, myalgia, and arthralgia and other pain arising from integumental structures. Mild to moderate postoperative and postpartum pain, dysmenorrhea, pain from neoplasms, and some other types of visceral pain also may respond to these drugs. They are generally not useful in severe pain, but large doses may provide relief in some patients. When drug therapy is indicated to reduce fever, an antipyretic selected from this group is preferred.

The choice of analgesic depends upon the effectiveness and adverse reactions of a particular preparation in the individual patient. The most widely used agents of this group are aspirin and acetaminophen. Their analgesic and antipyretic potencies and efficacies are equivalent, but differences in pharmacologic actions and adverse effects may make one preferable to the other for an individual patient. Of the other agents in this group, evidence supporting the analgesic efficacy of mefenamic acid [Ponstel] is limited. It has not been shown to be more effective than aspirin or other similar mild analgesics and has caused a number of serious adverse reactions. Although the newer phenylpropionic acid derivatives and related agents (fenoprofen [Nalfon], ibuprofen, naproxen) have been shown to be effective in a limited number of studies, additional data are needed to establish their usefulness and comparative efficacies. Salicylates other than aspirin and sodium salicylate are discussed in Chapter 7, Antiarthritic Drugs.

Other drugs possessing analgesic and antipyretic properties include indomethacin, phenylbutazone [Azolid, Butazolidin], and oxyphenbutazone [Oxalid, Tandearil], but they are not used as general purpose mild analgesics because of their potential to cause serious adverse reactions; they are discussed in Chapter 7, Antiarthritic Drugs, and Chapter 8, Drugs Used in Gout.

SALICYLATES

ASPIRIN

This prototype of the analgesic-antipyretic group is one of the drugs of choice when a mild analgesic is indicated. It also has an anti-inflammatory effect, which may contribute to relief of pain when inflammation is a factor. Aspirin is more useful in the treatment of headache, neuralgia, myalgia, arthralgia, and other pain arising from integumental structures than in acute severe pain of visceral origin. However, it may be effective in moderate postoperative and postpartum pain or other visceral pain such as that secondary to trauma or cancer. In the latter, aspirin may provide adequate relief and should be tried prior to use of strong analgesics. This drug is the primary agent in the management of some rheumatic diseases (see Chapter 7, Antiarthritic Drugs).

When drug therapy is indicated to reduce fever, aspirin is one of the most effective drugs; however, antipyretic therapy is only symptomatic and the cause of the fever must be sought and treated. In rheumatic fever, the amounts of aspirin required to relieve pain and joint swelling are larger than usual analgesic doses. The inflammatory process is suppressed but progression of the disease is not affected. Penicillin and other appropriate therapy should be administered concomitantly.

Because aspirin inhibits platelet function, it has been tried in various thromboembolic diseases. Results of several trials to date have been encouraging, but additional evidence is needed to determine conclusively whether aspirin prevents arterial thrombosis.

ADVERSE REACTIONS AND PRECAUTIONS.

Serious adverse reactions occur infrequently with usual analgesic doses. Gastrointestinal symptoms of dyspepsia (gastric distress, heartburn) or nausea are most common. Gastric distress may be diminished by taking aspirin with food or a full glass of water. Occult gastrointestinal bleeding occurs in many patients but apparently is not correlated with gastric distress. The amount of blood lost is usually insignificant clinically but, with prolonged administration, it may result in iron deficiency anemia. Aspirin may cause gastric ulcers with long-term use, but there is no evidence that it produces duodenal ulcers. Massive gastrointestinal hemorrhage occurs rarely in relation to the frequency of aspirin use; however, it may be life-threatening. This effect is possibly due to the action of aspirin on the stomach mucosa, platelet dysfunction, or both in susceptible individuals (ie, those with gastric distress, ulcer, or bleeding problems). Aspirin should not be used in those with a recent history of peptic ulcer or gastrointestinal bleeding because it may increase the bleeding. Patients should be advised that alcohol has a synergistic effect with aspirin in causing gastrointestinal bleeding.

Large doses taken for several days can cause hypoprothrombinemia which may be reversed by administration of vitamin K. This effect usually is not clinically significant except in susceptible patients (eg, those receiving anticoagulants). Even usual analgesic doses of aspirin inhibit platelet aggregation and increase bleeding time. Because of the important role of platelets in hemostasis, this effect may be an important factor in gastrointestinal and other bleeding. Aspirin is contraindicated in patients with bleeding disorders (eg, hemophilia). It is advisable to discontinue use of aspirin one week prior to surgery to prevent or minimize excessive postoperative bleeding.

Reversible hepatotoxicity has been reported to be associated with the large doses given to children with rheumatic disease and adults with lupus erythematosus or rheumatoid arthritis. The effect is dependent upon salicylate blood levels, the disease state, and pre-existing liver disease. Therefore, it is advisable to perform periodic liver function tests in patients with these conditions.

In the small percentage of individuals who are hypersensitive to aspirin, even usual doses may cause rash or severe urticarial or asthmatic-type anaphylactic reactions. Those exhibiting an asthmatic-type reaction usually have nasal polyps. This reaction may be related to the inhibition of prostaglandin synthesis, and cross sensitivity to other prostaglandin inhibitors (eg, indomethacin, ibuprofen, phenylbutazone) is common. Salicylic acid, salicylamide, and acetaminophen usually do not show cross sensitivity in this group of patients. Patients who experience cutaneous reactions also appear to be susceptible to anaphylaxis and may have asthma in addition. These reactions may be mediated by an immunologic response, and patients who have them may be more susceptible to cross sensitivity to salicylic acid and acetaminophen. Patients known to be sensitive to aspirin should be advised to avoid products containing it.

The most common sign of chronic aspirin overdosage is tinnitus, which may be reversed by reducing the dose. Reversible deafness also occurs with large doses of aspirin. It should be kept in mind, however, that this symptom will not be reported by patients with pre-existing hearing loss or by infants and young children. It is advisable for physicians to monitor hearing and determine if tinnitus is present in patients receiving large doses for prolonged periods.

Although certain combination products containing aspirin have been implicated as a cause of nephropathy, aspirin alone rarely causes serious renal disease. However, it decreases the glomerular filtration rate and may contribute to or exacerbate chronic or acute renal disease. Thus, it is advisable to perform periodic renal function tests in patients taking large amounts of aspirin.

Acute intoxication from accidental overdosage of aspirin is a common cause of fatal drug poisoning in children, although the number of deaths has been declining in recent years, probably as a result of safety measures and education. Toxic doses cause a disturbance of acid-base balance, usually manifested as metabolic acidosis in infants and young children and as respiratory alkalosis in older children and adults; hyperpyrexia also may occur in infants and young children. The severity of the intoxication is determined by measuring the blood salicylate level. Treatment is aimed at increasing the elimination of salicylate and specific therapy for any of the toxic manifestations. Performance of appropriate laboratory tests for diagnosis, use of alkaline diuresis, and, in severe cases, peritoneal dialysis or hemodialysis are necessary.

Aspirin does not appear to have any teratogenic effects. However, it has been reported that adverse effects were increased in the mother and fetus following chronic ingestion of aspirin. Prolonged pregnancy and labor with increased bleeding before and after delivery, as well as decreased birth weight and increased rate of stillbirth were correlated with high blood salicylate levels. Because of possible adverse effects on the neonate and the potential for increased maternal blood loss, aspirin should be avoided during the last three months of pregnancy.

DRUG INTERACTIONS.

Because aspirin is widely used, its interaction with other drugs must be considered. Large doses of aspirin taken for several days decrease prothrombin production, thus increasing the prothrombin time, and even smaller doses may increase bleeding time by inhibiting platelet aggregation; therefore, aspirin should not be used by patients taking anticoagulants. Salicylates decrease blood glucose levels and may enhance this effect of the oral hypoglycemics; thus, they should not be

given concomitantly or, if this is necessary, the dosage of the hypoglycemic agent must be reduced while the salicylate is given. Although large doses of a salicylate have a uricosuric effect, usual analgesic doses cause uric acid retention, resulting in hyperuricemia in some patients. Salicylates also antagonize the activity of uricosuric agents; thus, patients with gout should avoid their use. Since the incidence of gastric ulceration may be increased if aspirin is given with other ulcerogenic agents, such as corticosteroids, phenylbutazone, or indomethacin, the concurrent use of these agents should be avoided. It has been reported that aspirin can displace methotrexate from protein binding sites, thereby increasing its plasma concentration to toxic levels; however, the therapeutic effect is also increased. If the two drugs are used together, the patient must be carefully monitored. Salicylates also decrease serum protein binding of sulfonamides, which increases the amount of free sulfonamide and potentially increases toxicity.

ABSORPTION, METABOLISM, AND ELIMINATION.

Aspirin is absorbed rapidly following oral administration, partly from the stomach but mostly from the small intestine. It is rapidly hydrolyzed to salicylic acid, which is conjugated with glycine (forming salicyluric acid) and glucuronic acid and excreted largely in the urine. A small fraction of salicylic acid is hydroxylated to gentisic acid and perhaps other metabolites. The pharmacokinetics of salicylate elimination are complex. The half-life of salicylate lengthens as the dose increases: Doses of 300 to 650 mg have a half-life of 3.1 to 3.2 hours; with doses of 1 g, the half-life is increased to 5 hours and with 2 g it is increased to about 9 hours. In addition, as the half-life increases, urinary excretion decreases. Thus, increasing the dose without increasing the interval between doses may result in accumulation of drug and toxic effects. However, there is marked variation in elimination rates among individuals, possibly because of differences in salicyluric acid-forming capacity. Dosage regimens should, therefore, be adjusted individually.

FORMULATIONS.

The rate of absorption or bioavailability of aspirin depends upon its rate of dissolution from the dosage form, the most common of which is unbuffered (plain) tablets. Several studies have shown that differences among various product formulations affect the rate of dissolution and absorption of the drug and thus the levels achieved in the blood. However, the relationship of blood levels to onset and intensity of analgesic effect is not well correlated.

Antacids or buffering ingredients are combined with aspirin in an attempt to reduce gastric irritation. Such a combination is commonly referred to as buffered aspirin. The relatively small amount of antacid present in most products is insufficient to raise the gastric pH significantly; however, the intimate contact of the antacid with the aspirin particle increases the dissolution rate of the aspirin, resulting in its more rapid absorption. Although some individuals claim that they can tolerate the buffered preparations better than plain aspirin, results of controlled clinical studies have been contradictory. As with plain tablets, variation in formulations among different buffered aspirin products affects their dissolution rate and some may be less bioavailable than some unbuffered tablets. Furthermore, it has not been demonstrated conclusively that use of buffered aspirin results in faster onset of action, greater peak intensity, or longer analgesic effect, possibly because of the difficulties and insensitivities of methodology in quantitating analgesic effectiveness.

Aspirin is also available in highly buffered effervescent preparations; when dissolved, the aspirin is present as sodium acetylsalicylate. Results of studies have shown that when aspirin is given in this form, its rate of absorption is faster and the blood salicylate level is higher than with tablet formulations. In addition, highly buffered sodium acetylsalicylate in solution causes less gastric irritation and gastrointestinal bleeding, but the effect on platelets is unchanged. Because effervescent preparations contain more absorbable antacid, repeated use of large doses alkalize the urine, resulting in faster excretion and decreased salicylate blood levels. Nevertheless, because of the rapid absorption of aspirin from effervescent preparations, they are an effective form for occasional use. These preparations should not be taken by patients on a low-sodium diet.

Enteric-coated preparations are sometimes administered to avoid gastric reactions, but increased occult bleeding in sensitive individuals (eg, the elderly) has been reported. In addition, absorption of aspirin is delayed and may be quite variable among different products. Although this type of preparation may be useful when administered repeatedly to treat rheumatoid arthritis, it is not appropriate for prompt relief of pain. Timed-release preparations offer no advantage over the same dose of aspirin in standard tablets.

Rectal suppositories are used in patients unable to take oral medication; however, the absorption of aspirin with rectal administration is variable. It may be slow and incomplete or rapid and cause adverse reactions. Also, aspirin may cause rectal irritation. For these reasons, suppositories are of questionable usefulness and no dosage is suggested.

ROUTE, USUAL DOSAGE, AND PREPARATIONS.

Oral: For analgesia and antipyresis, *adults*, 650 mg every four hours as necessary (maximum, 3.9 g daily). *Children*, 1.5 g/M² of body surface daily in divided doses. For convenience, the following dosage schedule, based on age, may be used:

Age (years)	Dosage (mg)*
2 to under 4	160
4 to under 6	240
6 to under 9	320
9 to under 11	400
11 to under 12	480

*May be repeated every four hours as necessary.

For rheumatic fever, *adults*, 6 to 8 g daily; *children*, 3 g daily (optimum salicylate level, 25 to 30 mg/dl).

> *Note*: Because most manufacturers express dosage sizes of aspirin in grains rather than milligrams, the grain sizes with approximate milligram equivalents are given.
> Drug available generically: Tablets 1 ¼, 5, 7 ½, and 10 gr (80, 300, 500, and 600 mg); tablets (buffered) 5 gr (300 mg); tablets (enteric-coated) 5 and 10 gr (300 and 600 mg); suppositories 1, 2, 3, 5, and 10 gr (60, 125, 200, 300, and 600 mg) (nonprescription).
> Available Trademarks.
> [Examples of various formulations; all nonprescription]
> *Alka-Seltzer* (Miles) (highly-buffered). Each effervescent tablet contains aspirin 324 mg, sodium bicarbonate 1.9 g, and citric acid 1 g.
> *Ascriptin* (Rorer) (buffered). Each tablet contains aspirin 325 mg and magnesium-aluminum hydroxide 150 or 300 [Ascriptin A/D] mg.
> *Bufferin* (Bristol-Myers) (buffered). Each tablet contains aspirin 325 mg, aluminum glycinate 48.6 mg, and magnesium carbonate 97.2 mg.
> *Calurin* (Dorsey). Each tablet contains calcium carbaspirin 414 mg (equivalent to aspirin 300 mg).
> *Cama* (Dorsey) (buffered). Each tablet contains aspirin 600 mg, magnesium hydroxide 150 mg, and aluminum hydroxide dried gel 150 mg.
> *Ecotrin* (Smith Kline & French). Each enteric-coated tablet contains aspirin 300 mg.
> *Measurin* (Breon). Each timed-release tablet contains aspirin 650 mg.

SODIUM SALICYLATE

Sodium salicylate is less effective than equal doses of aspirin in relieving pain and reducing fever. In general, it produces the same adverse reactions as aspirin (see that evaluation); however, individuals who are hypersensitive to aspirin may tolerate sodium salicylate. Sodium salicylate causes less occult gastrointestinal bleeding than aspirin. It does not affect platelet function but, like aspirin, increases prothrombin time. Patients on a low-sodium diet should not take sodium salicylate.

ROUTE, USUAL DOSAGE, AND PREPARATIONS.
Oral: 650 mg every four hours as necessary (range, 325 mg to 4 g daily).

> Drug available generically: Tablets (plain, enteric-coated, timed-release) 300 and 600 mg.

PARA-AMINOPHENOL DERIVATIVE

ACETAMINOPHEN

The efficacy of acetaminophen as an analgesic and antipyretic is equivalent to that of aspirin, and it is also used in the treatment of headache, mild to moderate myalgia, arthralgia, chronic pain from cancer, postpartum pain, postoperative pain, and fever. Acetaminophen, unlike aspirin, has little or no clinically significant antirheumatic effect with usual doses. It is the preferred alternative analgesic-antipyretic to aspirin, particularly in patients allergic to aspirin, those with a coagulation disorder (eg, hemophilia), or individuals with a history of peptic ulcer. Unlike aspirin, acetaminophen does not antagonize the effects of uricosuric agents; thus, it may be used as an analgesic in patients with gouty arthritis who are taking a uricosuric.

Adverse reactions to acetaminophen occur infrequently and hypersensitivity only rarely. Acetaminophen is a metabolite of phenacetin and acetanilid but, unlike these drugs, produces little or no methemoglobinemia and reports of hemolytic anemia have been rare. It does not cause gastrointestinal bleeding. Although large doses have been reported to potentiate the action of oral anticoagulants, small doses have no effect on prothrombin time. It is not known whether prolonged use of acetaminophen can cause the type of renal injury associated with abuse of analgesic mixtures containing phenacetin.

Large doses (15 g as a single dose) of acetaminophen may cause severe hepatic damage and death. Early symptoms of toxicity include nausea, vomiting, diarrhea, diaphoresis, pallor, and abdominal pain. Evidence of hepatic injury is indicated by increased levels of serum transaminases and lactic dehydrogenase, prothrombin time, and serum bilirubin concentrations. Severe hepatic damage may progress to hepatic failure, encephalopathy, coma, and death. The severity of liver damage can be estimated from determinations of serum concentrations and serum half-life of the drug. In addition to instituting appropriate supportive therapy, liver injury may be minimized by administering an agent that acts as a sulfhydryl nucleophil such as acetylcysteine. (For details of treatment, see Chapter 86, Specific Antidotes.)

Acetaminophen is rapidly and almost completely absorbed from the gastrointestinal tract following oral administration; peak plasma levels of 5 to 20 mcg/ml occur in about 30 to 60 minutes with usual analgesic doses, but a correlation between serum level and intensity of analgesic effect has not been demonstrated. Significant binding of acetaminophen to serum protein does not occur with therapeutic doses. The half-life varies from one to three hours. Acetaminophen is metabolized in the liver, largely to glucuronide and sulfate conjugates, and eliminated in the urine. In patients with impaired renal function, the conjugated metabolites accumulate in the blood but the unchanged drug does not. A minor fraction is metabolized to hydroxylates and deacetylated derivatives. It has been suggested that the hydroxylated metabolite is responsible for hepatotoxicity when overdoses are taken.

There is evidence that, in some forms of liver disease, the metabolism (conjugation) of acetaminophen is decreased and the half-life is increased. Whether this increases the potential or severity of hepatotoxicity has not been determined, but the possibility should be considered when giving acetaminophen to patients with pre-existing liver disorders.

ROUTES, USUAL DOSAGE, AND PREPARATIONS.
Oral: *Adults*, 325 to 650 mg at four-hour intervals, if necessary (maximum, 4 g daily). *Children*, same as dosage for aspirin (see the Table in that evaluation).

Rectal: The relative potency of the suppository formulation has been reported to be about one-half that of the oral tablet; however, as with other drugs, the bioavailability of acetaminophen in suppositories may be variable depending upon the composition of the suppository base. Since comparative data of different products are not available, no dosage is suggested.

Drug available generically: Capsules 325, 450, and 500 mg; capsules (timed-release) 500 mg; drops 60 mg/0.6 ml; elixir 120 and 130 mg/5 ml; tablets 60, 300, 325, 500, and 650 mg; suppositories 120, 125, 300, 600, 650, and 900 mg (nonprescription).

Available Trademarks.
Phenaphen (Robins), *Tempra* (Mead Johnson), *Tylenol* (McNeil) (nonprescription).

ANTHRANILIC ACID DERIVATIVE

MEFENAMIC ACID
[Ponstel]

Mefenamic acid is unrelated chemically to other mild analgesics. It is claimed to be useful for relief of pain in condition ordinarily not requiring the use of strong analgesics. Evidence supporting the analgesic efficacy of mefenamic acid is limited. Few well-designed, double-blind clinical trials have been done and results of comparative studies have not shown mefenamic acid to be more effective than aspirin and other mild analgesics. Since its use has been associated with a number of serious adverse reactions, other mild analgesics are preferred. Results of some studies have indicated that mefenamic acid is effective in relieving pain of dysmenorrhea, but additional studies are needed to establish this use.

Gastrointestinal symptoms are the most common adverse effects. Diarrhea occurs in a significant number of patients and usually recurs when mefenamic acid is given a second time. Occult gastrointestinal bleeding is noted less frequently than with aspirin. Dyspepsia, constipation, nausea, abdominal pain, vomiting, headache, drowsiness, vertigo, and dizziness have been observed. Elevated blood urea nitrogen levels were noted in one study on human volunteers. Hemolytic anemia, agranulocytosis, thrombocytopenic purpura, and megaloblastic anemia also have been reported.

If diarrhea or rash occurs, the drug should be discontinued and not used thereafter. Mefenamic acid is contraindicated in patients with gastrointestinal inflammation or ulceration and in those with impaired renal function and should be used with caution in asthmatics because it may exacerbate the condition.

The safety of mefenamic acid for use during pregnancy or in children under 14 years of age has not been established.

ROUTE, USUAL DOSAGE, AND PREPARATIONS. *Oral: Adults and children over 14 years,* 500 mg initially, followed by 250 mg every six hours as needed. The drug preferably should be taken with food. Mefenamic acid should not be used for longer than one week.

    Ponstel (Parke, Davis). Capsules 250 mg.

PHENYLPROPIONIC ACID DERIVATIVES AND RELATED DRUGS

FENOPROFEN CALCIUM
[Nalfon]

Fenoprofen is chemically and pharmacologically similar to ibuprofen. Studies in animals and man have demonstrated that, like aspirin, it has anti-inflammatory, analgesic, and antipyretic properties. Although additional studies are needed to confirm the usefulness of this drug as an analgesic and antipyretic and to establish the dosage, results of a limited number of studies indicated that fenoprofen was similar in effectiveness to aspirin in various painful conditions (eg, trauma, episiotomy, postpartum and postoperative pain). In single or repeated doses of 400 mg, fenoprofen reduced fever associated with acute and chronic respiratory disease. It is effective in rheumatoid arthritis and osteoarthritis and is used primarily in these conditions.

The most common adverse reactions reported have been gastrointestinal effects (eg, dyspepsia, constipation, nausea, vomiting); however, in comparative studies, these reactions occurred less frequently with fenoprofen than with aspirin. The amount of gastrointestinal bleeding was also less than with aspirin. However, since a few cases of ulceration have been observed, the drug should be used with caution in patients with a history of peptic ulcer. (For other adverse reactions, see Chapter 7, Antiarthritic Drugs.)

ROUTE, USUAL DOSAGE, AND PREPARATIONS. *Oral: Adults and children,* dosage for analgesia and antipyresis has not been established.

    Nalfon (Dista). Capsules 300 mg; tablets 600 mg.

IBUPROFEN
[Motrin]

Like aspirin, ibuprofen has analgesic, anti-inflammatory, and antipyretic actions. Its analgesic effectiveness is comparable to that of aspirin in patients with postpartum or episiotomy pain and tension headache. Ibuprofen also has been reported to relieve pain in a limited number of patients with dysmenorrhea or various musculoskeletal disorders.

The antipyretic effect of ibuprofen in doses of 200 or 600 mg was similar to that of 600 mg of aspirin. Thus, ibuprofen might be tried as an antipyretic in patients who cannot tolerate aspirin, but additional studies also are needed to confirm this use.

Ibuprofen is an effective antirheumatic agent and is used primarily in the treatment of rheumatic diseases.

The overall incidence of adverse reactions is low, and this agent appears to be better tolerated than aspirin. The most frequent reactions are nausea and vomiting; diarrhea, constipation, heartburn, and epigastric pain occur less frequently. Patients receiving ibuprofen experienced less gastrointestinal bleeding than those receiving aspirin. However, since ulcer occurred in a few patients, it is advisable to use this agent with caution in those with peptic ulcer or a history of such ulcers. (For other adverse reactions, see Chapter 7.)

ROUTE, USUAL DOSAGE, AND PREPARATIONS.
Oral: Adults, 400 mg every four to six hours as necessary.There is insufficient experience with this drug to establish a dose for *children* or antipyretic use.

  Motrin (Upjohn). Tablets 300, 400, and 600 mg.

NAPROXEN
[Naprosyn]

Naproxen is chemically related to the phenylpropionic acid group of drugs and, like aspirin, has analgesic, anti-inflammatory, and antipyretic actions. This agent has been shown to be effective in the symptomatic treatment of rheumatoid arthritis, degenerative joint disease (osteoarthritis), and ankylosing spondylitis, which are its principal uses. (See Chapter 7, Antiarthritic Drugs.)

The analgesic activity of naproxen in nonrheumatic conditions has been demonstrated in patients with moderate to severe postoperative pain, including that occurring after orthopedic and dental surgery, as well as in postpartum uterine cramps and acute musculoskeletal disorders. In the lat-

ter, naproxen 250 mg was equivalent to indomethacin 50 mg twice daily. Results of several comparative studies showed that the analgesic effectiveness of 400 mg of naproxen is comparable to that of 75 to 150 mg of meperidine given orally; it was greater than that provided by propoxyphene 65 mg in orthopedic pain or aspirin 325 mg with codeine 30 mg in postsurgical dental pain. In postoperative pain, 220 to 330 mg of naproxen provided analgesia equivalent to 600 mg of aspirin, while in postpartum pain, 250 mg of naproxen was equivalent to 650 mg of aspirin and the duration of action was longer. Naproxen and its sodium salt also have been shown to relieve pain in dysmenorrhea; in this condition, the initial dosage was 550 mg, followed by 275 mg every six hours for a maximum of five days.

The most frequent adverse reactions are gastrointestinal effects (eg, heartburn, dyspepsia, abdominal pain, constipation, diarrhea). The gastric mucosa is less severely affected and less gastrointestinal bleeding has been observed than with aspirin; however, the latter reaction occasionally may be severe and ulceration has been reported. Therefore, this drug should be used with caution in patients with a history of peptic ulcer. (For other adverse reactions, see Chapter 7, Antiarthritic Drugs.)

ROUTE, USUAL DOSAGE, AND PREPARATIONS.
Oral: Adults and children, dose for analgesic use has not been established.
  Naprosyn (Syntex). Tablets 250 mg.

ZOMEPIRAC SODIUM
[Zomax]

Zomepirac is a close analogue of tolmetin and has analgesic, anti-inflammatory, and antipyretic actions. Controlled clinical studies have shown that zomepirac 50 and 100 mg is significantly superior to aspirin 650 mg as an analgesic in patients who have undergone oral surgery and in those with postpartum pain. Results of studies assessing the analgesic action after oral surgery and for postoperative pain indicate that zomepirac 100 mg is at least as effective as the combination of two APC tablets plus 60 mg of codeine and, in studies on postoperative pain and chronic cancer, 100 mg of zomepirac orally was shown to be equivalent to 10 mg of morphine given intramuscularly.

Adverse reactions are qualitatively similar to those of other nonsteroidal anti-inflammatory drugs, with gastrointestinal symptoms reported most frequently. The incidence of adverse reactions was significantly less with zomepirac than with aspirin in trials comparing the two drugs. The most frequent adverse reactions are drowsiness, nausea, headache, dizziness, gastrointestinal distress, and diarrhea.

Zomax (McNeil) (Investigational drug).

MIXTURES

Mixtures of analgesic agents or an analgesic with drugs of another class are among the most widely used pharmaceutical products. Most are formulated on the theoretical basis that they will produce a greater analgesic effect, provide broader therapeutic uses, or cause fewer or less severe untoward effects than a single ingredient. Despite the widespread use of these products, relatively few well-controlled studies have been performed to determine their comparative effectiveness.

The various analgesic mixtures are divided into groups on the basis of similarities in their composition. The quantitative formula of some products in each group is listed for information; this does not imply that these products have merit over similar products not listed.

Mixtures of Analgesic-Antipyretic Agents

Many products contain two or more analgesic-antipyretic drugs. Such combinations are alleged to enhance the analgesic action and produce fewer adverse reactions than the individual agents used alone. However, the analgesic effect of a combination is theoretically no greater than the sum of effects of the individual drugs, and few studies have adequately explored this point. Since the common adverse reactions of these agents are not dose related within the therapeutic range, the smaller amount of each agent in the mixture does not necessarily result in fewer or less severe adverse reactions. Moreover, intoxication from acute overdosage of a mixture would not be less dangerous than that of a single agent.

The most frequently used mixture of analgesic drugs is aspirin, phenacetin, and caffeine (APC); however, both aspirin and phenacetin are analgesic-antipyretics and no advantage has been demonstrated by combining them. Furthermore, phenacetin has little anti-inflammatory action. Although the vascular effect of caffeine may be useful in the treatment of migraine headache, there is no evidence that the small amount contained in the usual APC formulation has an analgesic effect or that it affects the activity of the analgesic components. Despite the assumption of many physicians and patients that APC possesses some advantage over aspirin alone, results of well-controlled clinical studies have not supported this belief.

A syndrome termed analgesic nephropathy has been associated with prolonged use of large doses of various analgesic mixtures containing phenacetin and usually aspirin and caffeine. The most common clinical manifestations of the syndrome include sterile pyuria, asymptomatic bacteriuria, and acute pyelonephritis; extrarenal manifestations are dyspepsia, peptic ulcer, anemia, and hypertension. The pathologic changes observed in the kidney are papillary necrosis and interstitial fibrosis. In addition, malignant tumors of the renal pelvis have been reported in some patients with analgesic nephropathy. There is some evidence that renal function often improves if use of analgesics is discontinued. The evidence implicating any single agent as the cause of the renal damage is conflicting; the combination of phenacetin and aspirin appears to be most commonly associated with renal damage. Since there is no conclusive evidence that APC has any advantage over aspirin but may be a cause of renal toxicity, there is no reason to use this traditional mixture in preference to a single analgesic.

Preparations containing aspirin, phenacetin, and caffeine are available under many trademarks and under the name APC.

Mixtures Containing Codeine

Codeine is included in many analgesic preparations to increase the analgesic effectiveness. The combination of codeine with an analgesic- antipyretic appears to be rational because the mechanism of action of each drug differs and results of controlled studies show that their analgesic effects are additive. Thus, use of this combination may provide a greater degree of pain relief than aspirin alone, and the dose of codeine may be smaller than that used when it is given alone. The aspirin component also reduces inflammation and fever. The combination of codeine with acetaminophen provides similar additive analgesic effect, which is comparable to that obtained with codeine plus aspirin.

Codeine also is included in mixtures containing two or more other mild analgesics (eg, codeine with APC); although codeine may enhance their analgesic effect if present in sufficient amount, such complex combinations have no advantages over the simpler mixture of codeine with aspirin.

Examples of available mixtures, which are included in Schedule III of the Controlled Substances Act, include:

Ascriptin with Codeine (Rorer). Each tablet contains aspirin 325 mg, codeine phosphate 16.2 (No. 2) or 32.4 (No. 3) mg, and magnesium-aluminum hydroxide 150 mg.
Empirin with Codeine (Burroughs Wellcome). Each tablet contains aspirin 325 mg, and codeine phosphate 15 mg (No. 2), 30 mg (No. 3), or 60 mg (No. 4).
Empracet with Codeine Phosphate (Burroughs Wellcome). Each tablet contains acetami-

nophen 300 mg and codeine phosphate 30 mg (No. 3) or 60 mg (No. 4).
Phenaphen with Codeine (Robins). Each capsule contains acetaminophen 325 mg and codeine phosphate 15 mg (No. 2), 30 mg (No. 3), or 60 mg (No. 4).
Tylenol with Codeine (McNeil). Each tablet contains acetaminophen 300 mg and codeine phosphate 7.5 mg (No. 1), 15 mg (No. 2), 30 mg (No. 3), or 60 mg (No. 4); each 5 ml of elixir contains acetaminophen 120 mg and codeine phosphate 12 mg.

Mixture Containing Hydrocodone

Hydrocodone, a semisynthetic analogue of codeine, is used as an analgesic and antitussive (see Chapter 31). In combination with acetaminophen, it is used in the same conditions as mixtures containing codeine. Hydrocodone has the same actions as other opiates and, although it is more potent on a milligram basis than codeine, its dependence liability is similar to that of other potent oral narcotics. As with other combinations of an opiate with an analgesic-antipyretic, this mixture appears to provide greater pain relief than either analgesic alone.

The adverse reactions are those of the individual ingredients. Precautions are the same as for other opiate analgesics. The mixture is classified as a Schedule III drug under the Controlled Substances Act.

Vicodin (Knoll). Each tablet contains hydrocodone bitartrate 5 mg and acetaminophen 500 mg.

Mixtures Containing Meperidine

Combinations of meperidine with the mild analgesic mixture, APC (aspirin, phenacetin, and caffeine), and with the mild analgesic-antipyretic, acetaminophen [Demerol APAP], are available for use as oral analgesics. Although these mixtures appear to be rational in that the mechanisms of action of the ingredients differ, no well-controlled studies have been performed to demonstrate the contribution of each ingredient. They may be effective for relief of mild to moderate pain but should not used to relieve severe pain because meperidine is less effective orally than parenterally. Studies comparing them to similar combinations containing codeine have not been published.

Adverse reactions are those of the individual ingredients; the more serious untoward effects are usually produced by meperidine (see the evaluations on Meperidine Hydrochloride and Acetaminophen and the discussion on Mixtures of Analgesic-Antipyretic Agents). The mixtures are included in Schedule II of the Controlled Substances Act.

> *APC with Demerol* (Winthrop). Each tablet contains meperidine hydrochloride 30 mg, aspirin 180 mg, phenacetin 150 mg, and caffeine 30 mg.
> *Demerol APAP* (Breon). Each tablet contains meperidine hydrochloride 50 mg and acetaminophen 300 mg.

Mixtures Containing Oxycodone

Oxycodone, a codeine analogue, has pharmacologic properties similar to those of the morphine-like drugs; it bears the same chemical relationship to codeine that oxymorphone does to morphine. In the United States, oxycodone is available only as an ingredient in mixtures with acetaminophen and APC. Oxycodone is effective orally and, on a milligram basis, its analgesic potency as well as its dependence liability is greater than that of codeine. Dependence on products containing oxycodone has been reported; thus, they should be prescribed with the same caution as other opiates. They are included in Schedule II of the Controlled Substances Act.

Adverse reactions are those of the individual ingredients and are similar to reactions observed with oral codeine preparations (see the evaluation on Codeine). The same precautions should be taken as when other morphine-like drugs are administered (see the Introduction).

> *Percodan* (Endo). Each tablet contains oxycodone hydrochloride 4.5 mg, oxycodone terephthalate 0.38 mg, aspirin 224 mg, phenacetin 160 mg, and caffeine 32 mg; each Percodan-Demi tablet contains oxycodone hydrochloride 2.25 mg, oxycodone terephthalate

0.19 mg, aspirin 224 mg, phenacetin 160 mg, and caffeine 32 mg.
> *Percocet-5* (Endo). Each tablet contains oxycodone hydrochloride 5 mg and acetaminophen 325 mg.
> *Tylox* (McNeil). Each capsule contains oxycodone hydrochloride 4.5 mg, oxycodone terephthalate 0.038 mg, and acetaminophen 500 mg.

Mixture Containing Pentazocine

The mixture of pentazocine with aspirin provides the analgesic action of pentazocine and the analgesic, anti-inflammatory, and antipyretic actions of aspirin. It is indicated for the relief of moderate pain. One controlled comparative clinical study demonstrated that this combination provided greater relief of pain in patients with cancer than aspirin alone; its effectiveness was comparable to that provided by combinations of codeine and aspirin or oxycodone and aspirin.

The adverse effects of this combination are the same as those of the individual ingredients. See the evaluations on Pentazocine and Aspirin.

> *Talwin Compound* (Winthrop). Each tablet contains pentazocine hydrochloride equivalent to 12.5 mg of the base and aspirin 325 mg (Schedule IV).

Mixtures Containing Propoxyphene

The rationale for combining propoxyphene with an analgesic-antipyretic is the same as that for similar combinations containing codeine. Available mixtures contain propoxyphene hydrochloride with aspirin, acetaminophen, or APC and the napsylate salt with aspirin or acetaminophen. Controlled studies with these combinations have been very limited, but results suggest that the analgesic effects of the individual components are additive. However, since propoxyphene is usually less effective than codeine in comparable doses, these combinations may be less effective than similar combinations containing codeine. Preparations containing acetaminophen lack the anti-inflammatory action produced by preparations containing aspirin, although each combination has an antipyretic action.

In addition to being available generically, these combinations are available under the following trademarks and are included as Schedule IV substances under the Controlled Substances Act:

Darvon with A.S.A. (Lilly). Each capsule contains propoxyphene hydrochloride 65 mg and aspirin 325 mg.
Darvon-N with A.S.A. (Lilly). Each tablet contains propoxyphene napsylate 100 mg and aspirin 325 mg.
Darvon Compound (Lilly). Each capsule contains aspirin 227 mg, phenacetin 162 mg, caffeine 32.4 mg, and propoxyphene hydrochloride 32 or 65 mg (Darvon Compound-65).
Darvocet-N (Lilly). Each tablet contains propoxyphene napsylate 50 or 100 mg and acetaminophen 325 or 650 mg.
Dolene Compound 65 (Lederle). Each capsule contains propoxyphene hydrochloride 65 mg, aspirin 227 mg, phenacetin 162 mg, and caffeine 32.4 mg.
SK-65 Compound (Smith Kline & French). Each capsule contains propoxyphene hydrochloride 65 mg, aspirin 227 mg, phenacetin 162 mg, and caffeine 32.4 mg.
Wygesic (Wyeth). Each tablet contains propoxyphene hydrochloride 65 mg and acetaminophen 650 mg.

Mixtures Containing Analgesics With Sedatives

Drugs with a sedative action (sedative-hypnotics, antianxiety agents, centrally acting skeletal muscle relaxants, antihistamines) are components of several widely used analgesic mixtures; they allegedly enhance the analgesic effectiveness of the product and provide relief of muscle spasm or of anxiety accompanying pain.

On theoretical grounds, a sedative might be expected to alter a patient's reaction to pain, and a muscle relaxing action might be useful in patients with tension headache or certain musculoskeletal problems. It has not been definitely shown that the skeletal muscle relaxants have a selective muscle-relaxing action in man that is separate from their sedative effect. (See Chapter 17, Drugs Used to Treat Skeletal Muscle Hyperactivity.) Results of some studies have suggested that a combination of a muscle relaxant and an analgesic provides greater benefit in patients with acute musculoskeletal problems than the analgesic alone; however, few properly controlled studies have been designed to define the patient population that could be expected to benefit from this type of combination.

There is some evidence that a combination containing a barbiturate is more effective in the treatment of tension headache than the analgesic component alone. (See Chapter 9, Drugs Used in Migraine and Other Headaches.) It should be kept in mind that the duration of action of the sedative may differ from that of the mild analgesic, that the actions of the drugs with repeated use might not coincide, and that possible abuse of a preparation containing a barbiturate may occur. It has been reported that meprobamate augments pain but, when given with aspirin, the latter drug antagonizes this effect.

Examples of these products include:

Equagesic (Wyeth). Each tablet contains ethoheptazine citrate 75 mg, aspirin 250 mg, and meprobamate 150 mg (Schedule IV).
Fiorinal (Sandoz). Each tablet or capsule contains aspirin 200 mg, phenacetin 130 mg, caffeine 40 mg, and butalbital 50 mg (Schedule III).
Fiorinal with Codeine (Sandoz). Each capsule contains codeine phosphate 7.5 mg (No. 1), 15 mg (No. 2), or 30 mg (No. 3); aspirin 200 mg; phenacetin 130 mg; caffeine 40 mg; and butalbital 50 mg (Schedule III).
Mepergan (Wyeth). Each millimeter of solution (injection) contains meperidine hydrochloride 25 mg and promethazine hydrochloride 25 mg (Schedule II).
Mepergan Fortis (Wyeth). Each capsule contains meperidine hydrochloride 50 mg and promethazine hydrochloride 25 mg (Schedule II).
Micrainin (Wallace). Each tablet contains aspirin 325 mg and meprobamate 200 mg (Schedule IV).
Norgesic (Riker). Each tablet contains aspirin 225 mg, phenacetin 160 mg, caffeine 30 mg, and orphenadrine citrate 25 mg; each forte tablet contains aspirin 450 mg, phenacetin 320 mg, caffeine 60 mg, and orphenadrine citrate 50 mg.
Parafon Forte (McNeil). Each tablet contains acetaminophen 300 mg and chlorzoxazone 250 mg.
Percogesic (Endo). Each tablet contains acetaminophen 325 mg and phenyltoloxamine citrate 30 mg (nonprescription).

Percogesic with Codeine (Endo). Each tablet contains codeine phosphate 32.4 mg, acetaminophen 325 mg, and phenyltoloxamine citrate 30 mg (Schedule III).
Robaxisal (Robins). Each tablet contains methocarbamol 400 mg and aspirin 325 mg.
Soma Compound (Wallace). Each tablet contains phenacetin 160 mg, caffeine 32 mg, and carisoprodol 200 mg.

Soma Compound with Codeine (Wallace). Each tablet contains codeine phosphate 16 mg, phenacetin 160 mg, caffeine 32 mg, and carisoprodol 200 mg (Schedule III).
Synalgos-DC (Ives). Each capsule contains dihydrocodeine bitartrate 16 mg, aspirin 194.4 mg, phenacetin 162 mg, caffeine 30 mg, and promethazine hydrochloride 6.25 mg (Schedule III).

Selected References

Establishment of a monograph for OTC internal analgesic, antipyretic and antirheumatic products, proposed rules. *Federal Register* 42:35346-35494, (July 8) 1977.

Beaver WT: Analgesic combinations, in Lasagna L (ed): *Combination Drugs: Their Use and Regulation.* New York, Stratton Intercontinental Medical Books, 1975.

Beaver WT: Mild analgesics: Review of their clinical pharmacology, parts I and II. *Am J Med Sci* 250:577-604, 1965; 251:576-599, 1966.

Berkowitz BA: Relationship of pharmacokinetics to pharmacological activity: Morphine, methadone and naloxone. *Clin Pharmacokinet* 1:219-230, 1976.

Bloomfield SS, et al: Aspirin and codeine in two postpartum pain models. *Clin Pharmacol Ther* 20:499-503, 1976.

Bonica JJ (ed): Symposium on pain: parts I and II. *Arch Surg* 112:749-788, 861-902, 1977.

Brogden RN, et al: Pentazocine: Review of its pharmacological properties, therapeutic efficacy and dependence liability. *Drugs* 5:6-91, 1973.

Committee on Drugs, American Academy of Pediatrics: Commentary on acetaminophen. *Pediatrics* 61:108-112, 1978.

Eddy NB, et al: Codeine and its alternates for pain and cough relief. I. Codeine, exclusive of its antitussive action. *Bull WHO* 38:673-741, 1968.

Ferreira SH, Vane JR: New aspects of mode of action of nonsteroid anti-inflammatory drugs. *Annu Rev Pharmacol Toxicol* 14:57-73, 1974.

Finkle BS, et al: National assessment of propoxyphene in postmortem medicolegal investigation, 1972-1975. *J Forensic Sci* 21:706-742, 1976.

Heel RC, et al: Butorphanol: Review of its pharmacological properties and therapeutic efficacy. *Drugs* 16:473-505, 1978.

Kincaid-Smith P, et al: Symposium on analgesic nephropathy. *Kidney Int* 13:1-113, 1978.

Lewis JR: Misprescribing analgesics. *JAMA* 228:1155-1156, 1974.

Loan WB, Morrison JD: Strong analgesics: Pharmacological and therapeutic aspects. *Drugs* 5:108-142, 1973.

Martin WR: Naloxone. *Ann Intern Med* 85:765-768, 1976.

Mather LE, Meffin PJ: Clinical pharmacokinetics pethidine. *Clin Pharmacokinet* 3:352-368, 1978.

Miller RR: Propoxyphene: A review. *Am J Hosp Pharm* 34:413-423, 1977.

Nickander R et al: Nonsteroidal anti-inflammatory agents. *Annu Rev Pharmacol Toxicol* 19:469-490, 1979.

Parkhouse J: Simple analgesics. *Drugs* 10:366-393, 1975.

Rumack BH (ed): Aspirin and acetaminophen: Comparative view for pediatric patient, with particular regard to toxicity, both in therapeutic dose and in overdose. *Pediatrics* 62(suppl): 865-946, (Nov) 1977.

Simon EJ, Hiller JM: Opiate receptors. *Annu Rev Pharmacol Toxicol* 18:371-394, 1978.

Terenius L: Endogenous peptides and analgesia. *Annu Rev Pharmacol Toxicol* 18:189-204, 1978.

Ylikorkala O, Dawood MY: New concepts in dysmenorrhea. *Am J Obstet Gynecol* 130:833-847, 1978.

Antiarthritic Drugs | 7

The drugs discussed in this chapter are used to treat arthritis associated with polyarthritis of unknown etiology (rheumatoid arthritis, juvenile rheumatoid arthritis, ankylosing spondylitis, psoriatic arthritis, and Reiter's syndrome) and osteoarthritis (degenerative joint disease). Such drugs include nonsteroidal anti-inflammatory drugs, analgesics, gold compounds, antimalarial drugs, and immunomodulatory agents, including adrenal corticosteroids. Drug therapy for arthritis associated with some other diseases (eg, gout, rheumatic fever) is discussed in Chapters 8, Drugs Used in Gout; 41, Adrenal Corticosteroids; and 69, Penicillins.

The primary aims in the treatment of arthritis are reduction of pain and inflammation, maintenance of joint mobility, and prevention of deformity. Except for the gold compounds and perhaps penicillamine and immunomodulators, these drugs generally do not affect the ultimate course of disease but provide symptomatic relief of pain and inflammation. Although this discussion is limited to drug therapy, other measures (orthopedic, physiotherapeutic, psychological, nutritional, or surgical) may be of equal or greater importance in managing some rheumatic diseases, especially in restoring lost motion and correcting deformities.

Diseases and Therapy

Rheumatoid Arthritis: This arthropathy, the most common of the chronic inflammatory rheumatic diseases, is a systemic disorder characterized primarily by inflammation of the synovium in and around joints, with secondary involvement of cartilage and bone. The major clinical manifestations are diffuse and prolonged morning stiffness; pain on motion; tenderness and/or swelling of multiple joints, usually symmetrical; subcutaneous nodules; and typical roentgenographic changes.

87

Proper management depends upon accurate diagnosis and is determined by the severity or stage of the disease. The effectiveness of therapy is difficult to evaluate because spontaneous remissions and exacerbations occur. Appropriate treatment requires long-term therapy and the cooperation and motivation of the patient.

In early stages of the disease, a basic conservative program achieves the desired goals in most patients; this includes rest periods, exercise, physical therapy, adequate nutrition, avoidance of extremes in climate, attention to emotional and psychological factors, orthopedic support when indicated, and use of a salicylate or another nonsteroidal anti-inflammatory drug. Although symptoms and signs may be relieved and progression of the disability slowed, the ultimate course of the disease is often unaltered. The patient's status must be re-evaluated periodically and treatment modified accordingly.

Salicylates are the principal basic drugs used in rheumatoid arthritis. Aspirin is preferred because it is the least expensive and most rapidly effective, but larger doses are required to produce an anti-inflammatory effect than are needed for analgesia. Although the former action is most important in the treatment of arthritis, its analgesic action may enhance the therapeutic value. Aspirin should be given in the dosage adequate to control symptoms, and full therapeutic amounts should be taken regularly for as long as synovitis is present. Pain and stiffness are relieved to some degree in more than 90% of patients; objective improvement also can be documented. However, additional therapy is required in more than half of these patients.

As many as 40% of patients cannot tolerate prolonged use of large doses of aspirin. Buffered, enteric-coated, or liquid products (eg, choline salicylate [Arthropan]) or a suppository form may be better tolerated by some patients, although absorption of enteric-coated or rectal preparations may be quite variable. Other salicylates (choline magnesium trisalicylate, magnesium salicylate, salsalate) may be substi-

tuted. Alternatively, one of the newer nonsteroidal anti-inflammatory agents (fenoprofen [Nalfon], ibuprofen [Motrin], naproxen [Naprosyn], sulindac [Clinoril], tolmetin [Tolectin]) may be tried in patients who cannot tolerate or do not respond to aspirin. Like aspirin, these agents have anti-inflammatory, analgesic, and antipyretic actions. Their effectiveness in rheumatoid arthritis appears to be comparable to that of aspirin, and equieffective doses produce fewer gastrointestinal reactions and less gastrointestinal bleeding than aspirin. Because a patient may tolerate or respond better to one drug than another, different drugs and dosages may be tried to determine the optimum regimen for each individual. It should be kept in mind that adequate doses must be given for sufficient periods of time (two to four weeks) to allow evaluation of effects before another drug is substituted.

The use of a mild analgesic in addition to aspirin (eg, acetaminophen, propoxyphene) may provide additional relief of pain in some patients (see Chapter 6, General Analgesics). However, these drugs are not substitutes for aspirin, since they have little or no anti-inflammatory action. Strong analgesics (eg, pentazocine [Talwin]) may relieve severe articular pain, but they should not be used routinely for this purpose.

Additional anti-inflammatory drugs (indomethacin [Indocin] and phenylbutazone [Azolid, Butazolidin] or oxyphenbutazone [Oxalid, Tandearil]) may be needed for patients with moderately severe disease involving multiple joints that cannot be controlled adequately with the basic drugs. However, their use is limited by the adverse reactions they produce. Patients who can tolerate aspirin in anti-inflammatory doses may continue to take it even when other drugs also are required.

Indomethacin is effective in some patients with moderate to severe rheumatoid arthritis, including acute exacerbations of chronic disease. Small doses should be given initially and the amount gradually increased to the level of tolerance (see the evaluations).

Phenylbutazone (or oxyphenbutazone) is effective as an adjunct to physiotherapy or other supportive measures in some patients. If beneficial effects are not observed within one to two weeks, the drug should be discontinued. If more prolonged therapy appears to be warranted, great caution should be exercised because of the potentially serious adverse reactions produced by these agents (see the evaluation).

If the symptoms of active rheumatoid arthritis fail to improve adequately after use of the basic conservative program (including nonsteroidal anti-inflammatory agents), consideration should be given to the addition of gold compounds. They are the only commonly used antiarthritic agents that can stop progression of the disease. Most rheumatologists agree that gold compounds have a definite place in the management of rheumatoid arthritis; some advocate their use early during the course of disease when there is active inflammation, but others prefer to postpone administration until more conservative therapy has failed. In either case, patients should be informed of the potential adverse effects of gold treatment; that frequent, repeated injections are required over a long period; and that beneficial effects may not be observed for 10 to 12 weeks after initiation of therapy. If significant improvement is observed and therapy is tolerated, maintenance injections should be continued for several years and, possibly, indefinitely.

The antimalarial agents, chloroquine and hydroxychloroquine [Plaquenil], may be effective in rheumatoid arthritis, but their use is controversial because of variable and inconsistent results and the potential for visual impairment. These drugs must be given for three to six months before any beneficial effects are noted. It appears that the size of the daily dosage may be the most important factor related to toxicity of these drugs; the risk is greater with larger doses. Small doses can be given for long periods without toxic effects, but ophthalmologic examinations should be performed at intervals of four to six months. Retinal damage may appear or progress even after

the drug is discontinued because chloroquine and hydroxychloroquine have a strong affinity for liver tissue and are deposited therein; thus, many months may be required to eliminate these drugs from the blood stream. If a low-dose schedule does not provide a satisfactory response, agents in another class should be chosen.

Systemic corticosteroid preparations usually improve functional capacity, relieve pain, and control inflammation, although joint destruction may continue. However, their usefulness is limited by their numerous adverse effects. Therefore, systemic use of these drugs should be reserved for patients with moderately severe, rapidly progressing rheumatoid arthritis that does not respond to other antirheumatic agents, for those threatened with severe disability or unemployability, and for those with significant systemic involvement. Prednisone and prednisolone are most commonly used systemically. The minimum dosage that will improve symptoms and signs should be used; complete relief is not sought. The dose should be gradually reduced at frequent intervals, when possible, and the corticosteroid can be withdrawn gradually in many patients. Others require small maintenance doses in order to perform their jobs or household duties or to take care of themselves. Therefore, relief or amelioration of disability may be the major indication for these agents.

When only one or a few joints are affected, pain can be relieved temporarily by injecting corticosteroids intra-articularly. Synovitis can be controlled for about three weeks, depending upon the degree of use and abuse of the joints. Joints should be rested after the injection to enhance the effect of the corticosteroid and, possibly, to reduce the chance of cartilage degeneration. The incidence of rapid joint damage is usually less than 1%. Injections should not be repeated in less than four weeks and the patient should be re-evaluated carefully prior to the injection.

Results of several controlled studies have established the effectiveness of penicillamine [Cuprimine, Depen] in the treatment of rheumatoid arthritis. This agent appears to be as effective as gold compounds or the immunosuppressive agent, azathioprine, and some clinicians prefer it to the latter drugs; however, most rheumatologists reserve penicillamine for patients with long-standing, progressive disease that has not responded adequately to standard drug therapy. Additional controlled and comparative studies are necessary to establish the drug's optimum dosage regimen, relative efficacy, and precise role in the treatment of rheumatoid arthritis. It is not effective in ankylosing spondylitis, psoriatic arthritis, and other HLA-B27 associated arthropathies.

Other drugs that have been used with some success in patients with severe disease include certain immunomodulating agents. Of the immunosuppressive drugs, azathioprine [Imuran] and cyclophosphamide [Cytoxan] have been studied most extensively in the treatment of rheumatoid arthritis, but chlorambucil [Leukeran], methotrexate, and mechlorethamine (nitrogen mustard [Mustargen]) also have been investigated. Although controlled trials have shown that these agents apparently are very beneficial in selected patients, their use is limited by their serious adverse effects, including the possibility of an increased incidence of neoplastic disease. The immunostimulant, levamisole, was shown to be effective in a few controlled trials. Intermittent therapy was as beneficial as continuous therapy and produced fewer adverse reactions (eg, neutropenia, agranulocytosis, epileptic seizures).

The benefit-to-risk ratio of drugs that affect the immune mechanism should be carefully considered for each patient. Additional controlled trials with long-term follow-up are necessary to determine their role in the treatment of rheumatoid arthritis. Because of their many potential serious adverse reactions, at present these agents should be reserved for patients with advanced disease who fail to respond to more conventional management, and their trial must be regarded as investigational only and probably limited to administration by specialists in rheumatology. (See also Chapter 68, Antineoplastic Agents, and Chapter 66, Immunomodulators.)

Juvenile Rheumatoid Arthritis: This disease is divided into three main onset subtypes: (1) systemic (acute febrile), (2) pauciarticular (arthritis in four or fewer joints), and (3) polyarticular (arthritis in five or more joints). The onset subtype is determined by manifestations during the first six months of disease. Each type varies with respect to age at onset, sex ratio, number and distribution of joints affected, results of serologic tests, extra-articular manifestations, and prognosis. It is, therefore, important to recognize these differences in order to establish an accurate diagnosis. For appropriate therapy, juvenile rheumatoid arthritis must be differentiated (usually by exclusion) from several other diseases commonly seen in children (eg, rheumatic fever, ankylosing spondylitis, septic arthritis, trauma, malignancy).

A serious extra-articular manifestation, chronic iridocyclitis, develops in about one-half of patients with the early-onset pauciarticular type during the first ten years of disease. Since this condition is frequently asymptomatic and may be detected only by slit-lamp examination, it is important that children with this type of juvenile rheumatoid arthritis be examined at least every six months so that therapy can be instituted when necessary. Mydriatics and corticosteroids are used in the treatment of iridocyclitis to prevent further complications and loss of vision.

The prognosis for the majority of children with juvenile rheumatoid arthritis is good; overall, more than 75% have remissions without joint damage. However, severe destructive arthritis occurs in more than 50% of patients with polyarticular disease who have positive tests for rheumatoid factor; about 75% of patients in this group also have positive tests for antinuclear antibodies. Severe arthritis develops in only about 10% to 15% of those in the polyarticular, seronegative group and in about 20% of those in the systemic (acute febrile) onset group. Polyarticular disease usually begins in late childhood and resembles severe adult-onset rheumatoid arthritis. The arthritis is only rarely severe in the pauciarticular group, but the subgroup of patients with onset of pauciarticular disease in late childhood have a high incidence (75%) of histocompatibility antigen, HLA-B27, and serologic tests for antinuclear antibodies and rheumatoid factor are negative. There is some evidence that these patients are likely to develop spondylitis or sacroiliitis with increasing duration of disease.

Drug therapy for juvenile rheumatoid arthritis is similar to that employed in the adult form; treatment is most effective when initiated early. Aspirin is preferred initially, regardless of the onset subtype. Beneficial effects may not appear for several days after therapy is started and significant changes may not be observed for several months. The administration of aspirin should be continued for at least six months after articular signs and symptoms have subsided. The drug then may be discontinued gradually, but therapy should be reinstituted if symptoms recur. Since tinnitus, the usual sign of aspirin toxicity, may be difficult to determine in children, serum salicylate concentrations should be monitored to establish optimal dosage; lethargy or episodic hyperpnea are early signs of toxicity. If these occur, aspirin should be discontinued until the signs abate and therapy resumed with a slightly smaller dose. Gastrointestinal disturbances are uncommon in children but, if they occur, other preparations (eg, buffered aspirin, choline salicylate) can be tried. Serum salicylate levels of 20 to 30 mg/dl are generally considered to be safe and effective.

As in adult rheumatoid arthritis, one of the newer, nonsteroidal anti-inflammatory agents may be tried when aspirin is not tolerated; however, children's doses have been established for only some of these agents (see the evaluations). Because of the potentially serious adverse reactions produced by indomethacin, phenylbutazone, oxyphenbutazone, and the antimalarial agents, use of these drugs should be avoided in children.

If polyarticular disease progresses and no improvement is noted after four to six months of salicylate therapy, gold salts may be added to the regimen. Chrysotherapy is of considerable value in many patients, although its effects may not be apparent for several months. Toxic effects are similar to those in adults, and patients should be observed closely and appropriate laboratory tests should be performed prior to each injection (see the evaluation on Gold Compounds).

Antimalarial agents are occasionally useful for children who have failed to respond to other nonsteroidal agents; however, great care must be taken to avoid ocular toxicity or acute, potentially fatal overdosage.

Oral adrenal corticosteroid preparations should not be administered routinely because of their serious adverse reactions and the problems associated with withdrawal. They should be reserved for seriously ill children with the systemic (acute febrile) form of disease who do not respond to aspirin, and the duration of therapy should be limited to a few months. Systemic corticosteroids are recommended in children with myocarditis. Topical corticosteroids are essential in the treatment of chronic iridocyclitis; rarely, locally injected or systemic steroids may be needed if topical administration does not control ocular inflammation. Intra-articular injection may be useful in pauciarticular disease, but no more than three or four injections should be made into the same joint each year to lessen the possibility of cartilage damage.

Ankylosing Spondylitis: This form of arthritis is characterized by involvement of the sacroiliac joints, the spinal apophyseal joints, and the paravertebral soft tissues; the peripheral joints, usually only the hips and shoulders, also may be affected, especially in women (70%). Ankylosing spondylitis occurs most commonly in the second or third decade of life. Onset is usually insidious with primary symptoms of back pain and early morning stiffness; sciatica may occur at onset or later. Symptoms tend to progress and the disease becomes chronic.

The HLA-B27 antigen has been found in about 95% of patients with ankylosing spondylitis. The fact that this antigen is also found in a large percentage of patients with other rheumatic diseases that produce spondylitis (Reiter's syndrome, psoriatic arthritis, some forms of juvenile rheumatoid arthritis) suggests that these diseases have certain common clinical characteristics. Thus, determination of HLA-B27 antigen is useful in the differential diagnosis of rheumatic diseases.

Early recognition and initiation of appropriate therapy is important for successful treatment of ankylosing spondylitis. Although progression of the disease may not be modified by any available therapy, relief of pain and maintenance of function usually are possible. Spontaneous remissions and exacerbations occur, and the prognosis generally is good.

In addition to symptomatic drug therapy, other forms of treatment (eg, rest, exercise, orthopedic measures, management of uveitis) are necessary for the general management of ankylosing spondylitis. Strong and persistent emphasis on maintaining a "military posture" is important in treatment. Although aspirin may be effective for mild attacks, it usually does not provide adequate relief of severe pain. Indomethacin, phenylbutazone, or oxyphenbutazone usually provides symptomatic improvement, but these drugs do not alter the natural course of the disease in most patients. However, although the data are not conclusive, results of some studies suggest that ossification may be retarded by the early administration of indomethacin, phenylbutazone, or oxyphenbutazone in selected patients. Systemic corticosteroids, which are rarely necessary unless iridocyclitis or vasculitis occurs, should be avoided, if possible. Gold compounds are not effective in ankylosing spondylitis, and chloroquine or hydroxychloroquine should not be used to treat this condition. The centrally acting skeletal muscle relaxants are generally ineffective in relieving the muscle spasm of ankylosing spondylitis.

Psoriatic Arthritis: This arthropathy occurs in about 7% of patients with psoriasis.

Onset is insidious and asymmetric inflammation involving only a few joints is common. Any peripheral joint may be affected, but the distal interphalangeal joints of fingers and toes are involved most frequently, often in association with psoriasis of the nails. Sacroiliitis and spondylitis also are commonly observed. An increased frequency of HLA-B27 antigen in patients with psoriatic arthritis has been reported; patients with this antigen have a higher risk of developing spondylitis or sacroiliac disease.

The psoriasis as well as the arthritis must be treated. Remissions of the latter sometimes parallel those of the skin disease. In general, treatment of the arthritic symptoms is similar to that employed for rheumatoid arthritis. Aspirin is sometimes effective for mild or moderately severe cases. Phenylbutazone or oxyphenbutazone is commonly used and has been found to control pain and increase the range of spinal motion; however, the potential serious adverse reactions of these drugs must be kept in mind. Indomethacin may be substituted for phenylbutazone. Gold salts have been beneficial in some patients. Systemic corticosteroids may improve both the skin and joint disease, but the dosage required usually is so large that adverse reactions result and their withdrawal may cause a severe exacerbation of psoriasis. The antimalarial drugs are undesirable because they may aggravate the skin disease. Methotrexate may be useful as a supplement but, because of its toxicity (especially hepatic), it should be reserved for severe, progressive disease and administered only by physicians experienced in its use.

Reiter's Syndrome: This disease occurs primarily in young adult males. Its etiology is unknown, but two epidemiologic forms are recognized: the epidemic form that follows dysentery and the endemic or venereal form that presumably follows sexual contact. The genitourinary, ocular, skeletal, and mucocutaneous systems are affected. There are many similarities between this syndrome and psoriatic arthritis. The HLA-B27 antigen is present in 76% to 96%

of patients with Reiter's syndrome having sacroiliitis.

There is no specific treatment or cure for Reiter's syndrome, but anti-inflammatory drugs are used to suppress the pain of arthritis. Aspirin usually is beneficial when arthritis is mild, but indomethacin and phenylbutazone are more effective. Systemic corticosteroids should be avoided because they are usually less effective, although intra-articular injection may be helpful in some patients. If acute joint inflammation persists, gold salts may be given a trial. Antimalarial agents are ineffective in this disease.

Osteoarthritis: This disease is also referred to as degenerative joint disease, but it is generally agreed that an inflammatory component exists; hence, the term, osteoarthritis, appears to be appropriate. The exact pathogenesis is unknown, although the disorder is characterized by degeneration of articular cartilage and formation of calcium deposits. Episodes of secondary inflammation occur frequently; however, the inflammatory component is much less marked than in rheumatoid arthritis. Osteoarthritis is common in middle-aged and elderly individuals, but it is not necessarily a part of the aging process. The knee and hip joints are most commonly affected; the spine is involved less frequently. Finger joint involvement is limited to the distal interphalangeal joints (Heberden's nodes) and the proximal interphalangeal joints (Bouchard's nodes). In the thumb, the carpometacarpal joints frequently are involved. Symptoms are referable to the joint involved, but the most common is pain that becomes worse with use of the joint; stiffness in the morning and after sitting is also common, but this effect does not last as long as in rheumatoid arthritis.

In addition to drug therapy, physical therapy (including the application of heat or cold to reduce pain), appropriate exercise, and rest are important in the management of this disease. Surgical procedures utilizing total joint replacement are the preferred treatment when the joint deteriorates to instability. The principal objective of drug therapy is to relieve pain.

Anti-inflammatory drugs are generally more effective than a simple analgesic. Aspirin, taken regularly in adequate doses, is the usual initial agent; however, one of the newer nonsteroidal anti-inflammatory agents is preferred by some clinicians. If sufficient relief of pain is not obtained with these agents, indomethacin, phenyl-butazone, or oxyphenbutazone should be used. The latter may be helpful in the treatment of acute exacerbations, and indomethacin is sometimes more effective in degenerative disease of the hip. Other analgesics (eg, acetaminophen, propoxyphene, codeine) are sometimes used, but drugs with abuse liability should be avoided if possible.

Systemic corticosteroids are not indicated in this condition and may cause serious adverse effects when used. The value of intra-articular injections to relieve acute exacerbations is perhaps less than in rheumatoid arthritis; the injections may be beneficial in relieving synovitis but may not affect the development of erosions. If these agents are used to relieve symptoms in a contracted joint in order to permit institution of physical therapy to restore function, the patient should be instructed to use the joint with great care for the first 24 to 48 hours after injection because of the danger of traumatization.

NONSTEROIDAL ANTI-INFLAMMATORY AGENTS

SALICYLATES

The salicylates have a long history of efficacy in relieving pain and stiffness and improving routine task performance in arthropathies; in addition, controlled studies using objective measurements have confirmed their benefits. Of the salicylates, aspirin is the drug of choice. All patients with active rheumatoid arthritis should have an adequate trial with this salicylate. Aspirin is used primarily for its anti-inflammatory effect and must be administered in maximally tolerated doses. If it cannot be tolerated because gastrointestinal disturbances occur, buffered or enteric-coated preparations or another salicylate may be tried; however, there is a paucity of data on comparative antirheumatic efficacies.

Gastrointestinal disturbances are the most common adverse reactions. Nausea, vomiting, and gastric distress occur in 10% to 30% of patients receiving large doses of aspirin; taking the drug with food or use of enteric-coated preparations lessens these reactions. Occult bleeding occurs in about 70% of patients; usually 2 to 6 ml of blood may be lost daily, but some patients lose up to 10 ml daily, which results in iron deficiency anemia. There appears to be no correlation between the incidence of gastric distress and occult bleeding. Blood loss is not decreased by the use of buffered tablets or the simultaneous ingestion of food. Choline salicylate, choline magnesium trisalicylate, and salsalate (salicylsalicylic acid) have been reported to cause less gastrointestinal bleeding than aspirin.

The incidence of peptic ulcer is increased in patients with rheumatoid arthritis who take aspirin for prolonged periods, and the acute use of the drug may activate ulcer and precipitate massive hemorrhage. Therefore, the presence of an active ulcer is a relative contraindication to use of aspirin. The risk of gastric ulceration is increased when alcohol is taken with aspirin.

Tinnitus and hearing loss are the most common initial signs of toxicity (salicylism) in adults and may be used to determine the maximal acceptable daily dose. However, they are not a reliable indication of toxicity in some elderly patients, who may not develop tinnitus even with large doses, or in children. Signs of overdosage in children include hyperventilation with acidosis, increased metabolic rate, and disturbances in carbohydrate and lipid metabolism; the earliest symptoms may be lethargy and episodic hyperpnea. The doses for children and elderly patients should be gradually and cautiously increased, and these patients should be closely observed for early signs of ototoxicity. The ototoxic effects are completely reversible even after administration of large doses for many years.

A very small percentage of patients are hypersensitive to aspirin and may develop rash or an asthmatic-type anaphylactic reaction, which can be life-threatening. The incidence of these reactions is highest in those with asthma, hay fever, or nasal polyps. Hypersensitive patients should avoid aspirin or aspirin-containing products. Some patients sensitive to aspirin also are sensitive to other nonsteroidal anti-inflammatory agents that inhibit prostaglandin synthesis; however, asthmatic-type reactions have not been associated with sodium or magnesium salicylates.

Large doses of salicylates prolong prothrombin time, but this effect is clinically insignificant. Since aspirin (but not sodium salicylate or other nonacetylated salicylates) inhibits platelet aggregation and prolongs bleeding time, it should be avoided in patients receiving heparin and in those with severe liver disease or bleeding disorders (eg, hemophilia) and should be used with caution in patients receiving coumarin anticoagulants. Hepatotoxicity, manifested by abnormal results of liver function studies, has been reported to be common in children with juvenile rheumatoid arthritis receiving prolonged aspirin therapy and in adults with lupus erythematosus. The hepatotoxicity is reversible upon discontinuance of the drug.

The uricosuric effect of probenecid and sulfinpyrazone is diminished by the salicylates. Since the renal clearance of salicylates is increased by corticosteroids, toxicity may occur when corticosteroids are discontinued in patients receiving large doses of salicylates concomitantly.

Patients on a sodium-restricted diet should not be given sodium salicylate. In patients with renal insufficiency, hypermagnesemic toxicity may develop after use of magnesium salicylate.

For additional information on adverse reactions and interactions, see Chapter 6, General Analgesics.

ROUTES, USUAL DOSAGE, AND PREPARATIONS. The dose should be individualized and adjusted to the amount that produces an adequate anti-inflammatory effect. If control of symptoms cannot be achieved with doses below the ototoxic level, the amount should be increased to the point of ototoxicity, then reduced until the level of tolerance is reached. Blood salicylate levels do not correlate well with dose, but a therapeutic effect usually requires a plasma concentration greater than 15 mg/dl; levels above 30 mg/dl are usually toxic. If there is any uncertainty about the adequacy of dosage, toxicity, or patient compliance, plasma salicylate concentrations should be determined.

Oral, Rectal: Adults, 3.6 to 5.4 g of aspirin or the equivalent salicylate daily in divided doses. For juvenile rheumatoid arthritis of pauciarticular or polyarticular onset, *children weighing 25 kg or less*, 100 mg/kg of body weight daily; *children weighing more than 25 kg*, 2.4 to 3.6 g daily. Those with systemic (acute febrile) onset may require larger doses. Since these doses may be toxic for some patients, it is usually advisable to start with about two-thirds of the anticipated optimal dose in order to establish the patient's tolerance, and then gradually increase to the optimal individual dose. The dosage schedule must be adjusted to the patient's living habits. Administration with meals is preferred in order to reduce gastrointestinal disturbances. Milk or a small meal taken at bedtime delays absorption and prolongs the therapeutic effect to allay morning stiffness. Alternatively, a larger dose may be given at bedtime or enteric-coated preparations may be used; however, enteric-coated tablets have a variable rate of absorption.

ASPIRIN:
Drug available generically: Tablets 75, 300, 325, 600, and 650 mg; tablets (enteric-coated) 300, 325, 450, 600, and 650 mg; tablets (buffered) 325 mg; suppositories 60, 120, 125, 200, 300, and 600 mg and 1 and 1.2 g.

Available Trademarks.
Ascriptin A/D (buffered) (Rorer), *Bufferin* (Bristol Myers), Cama (Dorsey), *Ecotrin* (enteric-coated) (Smith Kline & French), *Measurin* (timed-release) (Breon) (nonprescription).

SODIUM SALICYLATE:
Drug available generically: Tablets 300, 325, 600, and 650 mg; tablets (enteric-coated, timed-release) 300 and 600 mg.

CHOLINE SALICYLATE:
Arthropan Liquid (Purdue Frederick). Each 5 ml contains choline salicylate equivalent in salicylate content to 600 mg of aspirin (nonprescription).

CHOLINE MAGNESIUM TRISALICYLATE:
Trilisate (Purdue Frederick). Each tablet contains choline salicylate 293 mg and magnesium salicylate 362 mg to provide 500 mg of salicylate.

MAGNESIUM SALICYLATE:
Drug available generically: Tablets 300 mg.
Magan (Warren-Teed), *Mobidin* (Ascher). Tablets 600 mg (Mobidin) or 650 mg (Magan).

SALSALATE (Salicylsalicylic Acid):
Arcylate (Hauck). Tablets 325 mg.
Disalcid (Riker). Tablets 500 mg.

FENOPROFEN CALCIUM
[Nalfon]

Fenoprofen, a phenylpropionic acid derivative, is chemically and pharmacologically similar to ibuprofen. Studies in animals and man have demonstrated that, like aspirin, it has anti-inflammatory, analgesic, and antipyretic properties. Fenoprofen may be useful as an alternative to aspirin or other nonsteroidal agents in rheumatoid arthritis and osteoarthritis. Results of comparative studies in patients with rheumatoid arthritis indicated that daily doses of 2.4 g of fenoprofen provided relief approximately equivalent to that obtained with 3.9 g of aspirin; in osteoarthritis, the benefit of daily doses of 1.2 to 1.8 g of fenoprofen was similar to that obtained with 2 to 3 g of aspirin and 2 g of fenoprofen with 300 mg of phenylbutazone.

Results of studies in a few patients with ankylosing spondylitis indicated that fenoprofen provided symptomatic relief; however, additional studies are needed to establish its efficacy in this condition. (See also Chapter 6, General Analgesics, and Chapter 8, Drugs Used in Gout, for other uses of fenoprofen.)

Like aspirin, fenoprofen inhibits prostaglandin synthetase, but the significance of this action in relation to the clinical effects produced is not known.

Fenoprofen is rapidly absorbed after oral administration, and peak plasma levels occur within 90 minutes. The plasma half-life is about 160 minutes and does not appear to be dose dependent. Absorption and availability are slightly reduced when this agent is given with food, but are not affected by the concomitant administration of an antacid (aluminum and magnesium hydroxides). Following absorption, fenoprofen is metabolized and excreted almost exclusively in the urine in conjugated form. The drug is highly bound to plasma protein, and it may displace other protein-bound drugs from their binding sites, resulting in drug interactions. The binding of fenoprofen is inhibited by the concomitant administration of indomethacin and phenylbutazone, but not aspirin. The plasma half-life of fenoprofen is decreased by aspirin but not by propoxyphene napsylate.

The most common adverse reactions have been gastrointestinal disturbances (eg, dyspepsia, constipation, nausea, vomiting); however, in comparative studies, these reactions were reported to occur less frequently with fenoprofen than with aspirin. The amount of gastrointestinal bleeding was also less than with aspirin. However, since a few cases of ulceration have been observed, the drug should be used with caution in patients with a history of peptic ulcer.

Central nervous system reactions include drowsiness, dizziness, headache, nervousness, and confusion. Pruritus, rash, sweating, palpitations, tremor, tinnitus, blurred vision, and decreased hearing, as well as sensitivity to the drug, have been reported.

Elevations of serum transaminase, lactic dehydrogenase, and alkaline phosphatase levels have been observed in some patients. A decrease in hemoglobin and hematocrit levels also were noted occasionally. Fenoprofen reduces platelet aggregation and adhesiveness and increases bleeding time. Therefore, it should not be used in patients with bleeding disorders and should be used cautiously in those receiving anticoagulants. Because of the potential for cross sensitivity reactions, fenoprofen should not be given to patients in whom aspirin and other nonsteroidal anti-inflammatory drugs cause symptoms of asthma, rhinitis, or urticaria.

ROUTE, USUAL DOSAGE, AND PREPARATIONS. *Oral: Adults*, initially, 600 mg four times daily for rheumatoid arthritis; 300 to 600 mg four times daily for osteoarthritis. After a satisfactory response is obtained, the dose is adjusted to the patient's needs. The drug should be given 30 minutes before or two hours after meals but, if gastrointestinal reactions occur, it may be given with meals or milk. Dosage for children has not been established.

Nalfon (Dista). Capsules 300 mg; tablets 600 mg.

IBUPROFEN
[Motrin]

$$CH_3CHCH_2 - \!\!\!\!\bigcirc\!\!\!\! - CHCOH$$
$$\quad | \qquad\qquad\qquad | \quad ||$$
$$CH_3 \qquad\qquad\quad CH_3 \quad O$$

Ibuprofen is a phenylpropionic acid derivative that is similar chemically and pharmacologically to fenoprofen. It has analgesic, anti-inflammatory, and antipyretic actions, but its anti-inflammatory effect was demonstrated clinically only with large doses (1.6 to 2.4 g/day). Ibuprofen is effective for the symptomatic treatment of patients with rheumatoid arthritis and osteoarthritis. The number of patients with ankylosing spondylitis treated with ibuprofen has been too small to determine its efficacy. (See Chapter 6, General Analgesics, and Chapter 8, Drugs Used in Gout, for other uses of ibuprofen.)

Doses of 900 mg to 1.6 g provide relief approximately equivalent to that obtained with 3 to 6 g of aspirin, and ibuprofen is similar in effectiveness to phenylbutazone, indomethacin, and tolmetin. Thus, this drug may be useful as an alternative to aspirin or other nonsteroidal anti-inflammatory agents. Ibuprofen may be administered with maintenance doses of gold salts to provide additional symptomatic relief; it also may be given with corticosteroids, but whether it has a steroid-sparing effect has not been determined.

Ibuprofen is rapidly absorbed following oral administration, and peak plasma levels occur after one to two hours. When the drug is taken immediately after meals, absorption is slower and the peak plasma concentration is lower. There is no evidence of drug accumulation. Ibuprofen is rapidly eliminated from plasma; its half-life after single or multiple doses is 1.6 to 2.5 hours. This agent is rapidly metabolized by hydroxylation and carboxylation and is excreted in the urine as unchanged drug and two inactive metabolites. Excretion is essentially complete within 24 hours.

The overall incidence of adverse reactions is low, and ibuprofen appears to be better tolerated than aspirin, indomethacin, or phenylbutazone. The most common reactions are nausea and vomiting; diarrhea, constipation, heartburn, and epigastric pain occur less frequently. In studies designed to measure gastrointestinal bleeding, it was found that patients receiving ibuprofen for as long as one year had less gastrointestinal bleeding than those receiving aspirin. Nevertheless, since ulcer has occurred in a few patients, it is advisable to use this agent with caution in patients with peptic ulcer or a history of such ulcers.

Central nervous system reactions reported occasionally include dizziness, lightheadedness, and headache. Maculopapular, erythematous, or urticarial rashes and generalized pruritus also have occurred.

Toxic amblyopia, characterized by reduced visual acuity and difficulty in color discrimination, has been observed in a few patients. Although a definite cause-and-effect relationship was not established, the symptoms disappeared after ibuprofen was discontinued. Ophthalmologic examination of a large number of patients who received the drug did not reveal any simi-lar cases of visual disturbances. Nevertheless, patients receiving ibuprofen should have a complete ophthalmologic examination if they experience any visual disturbances.

A slight, transient increase in serum transaminase (SGPT) and alkaline phosphatase levels has been observed occasionally during ibuprofen therapy, but jaundice has not been noted. Hyperuricemia also has occurred sporadically. Fluid retention and edema have been reported; therefore, the drug should be used with caution in patients with a history of cardiac decompensation.

Ibuprofen inhibits platelet aggregation, but to a lesser degree than aspirin or indomethacin. A slight, probably clinically insignificant decrease in hemoglobin and hematocrit values has been observed in some patients.

Like aspirin, ibuprofen inhibits prostaglandin synthesis. Since cross sensitivity reactions may occur, ibuprofen should not be used in patients known to be hypersensitive to aspirin or other nonsteroidal anti-inflammatory drugs. Hypersensitivity reactions (eg, fever, rash, nausea, vomiting, abdominal pain, hypotension) and increased serum transaminase levels have been reported in several patients receiving ibuprofen for the treatment of systemic lupus erythematosus.

Coagulation parameters were not affected when doses of up to 2.4 g/day of ibuprofen were given to patients receiving warfarin sodium, but larger amounts may displace warfarin from protein binding sites. The use of ibuprofen with aspirin had no effect on the availability or disappearance of either drug in the plasma in man. Information concerning the potential interactions of ibuprofen with other drugs is not available.

There is no evidence that ibuprofen has any teratogenic effect in rabbits and rats. Since this agent was found in the fetal circulation of animals after administration to the mothers during late pregnancy, it appears to cross the placenta.

Two cases of accidental overdosage in children have been reported; the estimated intake was 120 mg/kg of body weight. The blood level in one child was found to be over 700 mcg/ml, about ten times that found in adults after a single oral dose of 800 mg. However, no apparent ill effects were observed in either child. Since no specific antidote is known, standard supportive treatment for poisoning should be instituted: The stomach should be emptied by induced vomiting or lavage, and urine output should be maintained to ensure excretion of the drug.

ROUTE, USUAL DOSAGE, AND PREPARATIONS. *Oral: Adults*, 400 mg four times daily, preferably on arising in the morning; in midmorning, midafternoon, or both; and at bedtime. Because of the variability in response, the optimal dose for each patient must be determined individually. There is insufficient experience with this drug in children under 14 years to establish a dose.

    Motrin (Upjohn). Tablets 300, 400, and 600 mg.

INDOMETHACIN
  [Indocin]

Indomethacin is a nonsteroidal antiinflammatory compound with analgesic and antipyretic effects. Because of its potential to cause severe adverse effects, this agent is not recommended as a simple analgesic or antipyretic. It is useful as an anti-inflammatory agent in moderate to severe rheumatoid arthritis, ankylosing spondylitis, and osteoarthritis of large joints (hips, knees, shoulders), especially in patients unresponsive to salicylates. Indomethacin also is used to treat attacks of acute gouty arthritis (see Chapter 8, Drugs Used in Gout). It is sometimes administered empirically for bursitis, tendinitis, and traumatic synovitis, although its effi-cacy in these conditions has not been established.

Gastrointestinal disturbances (nausea, vomiting, anorexia, indigestion, epigastric burning, stomatitis, diarrhea) have been observed in 3% to 9% of patients and may be lessened by giving the drug with food. Less common, but more significant, effects are single or multiple ulcerations of the esophagus, stomach, duodenum, or small intestine; perforation and hemorrhage, sometimes fatal, have been reported. Occult bleeding with resultant secondary anemia may occur in the absence of an ulcer. Other gastrointestinal reactions are gastritis and perforation of pre-existing sigmoid lesions. Abdominal cramping and diarrhea occur infrequently and ulcerative colitis and regional enteritis rarely.

Central nervous system effects (headaches, vertigo, dizziness, somnolence) are common during the early weeks of therapy. The headaches, which occur in more than 10% of patients, are usually severe in the morning; if they persist, treatment should be discontinued. Convulsions, peripheral neuropathy, lightheadedness, syncope, confusion, coma, and behavioral disturbances such as depersonalization and depression also have been reported occasionally.

Ocular complications (corneal deposits and retinal disturbances) have been observed in some patients after prolonged use of indomethacin. Blurred vision warrants a thorough ophthalmologic examination. Ototoxic reactions (deafness, tinnitus) occur infrequently.

Leukopenia, hemolytic or aplastic anemia, purpura, bone marrow depression, agranulocytosis, and thrombocytopenia are rarely observed during therapy with indomethacin. Fatal cases of hepatitis and jaundice have been reported. Dermatologic and hypersensitivity reactions (pruritus, urticaria, rash, erythema nodosum, angioedema, angiitis, alopecia, dyspnea, acute respiratory distress, and a rapid fall in blood pressure resembling shock) also may occur.

Like aspirin and other nonsteroidal antiinflammatory agents, indomethacin inhibits platelet aggregation, which may result from its inhibition of prostaglandin synthesis. These effects appear to be related to dose and plasma concentration and have a shorter duration than those produced by aspirin. It is advisable to use indomethacin with caution in patients with coagulation defects. If concomitant administration of indomethacin and an anticoagulant is necessary, the patient should be observed for alterations in prothrombin time and the dose of anticoagulant adjusted accordingly.

The administration of aspirin with indomethacin has been reported to decrease the blood level of indomethacin, but other studies have not confirmed this interaction. However, results of some clinical studies have shown that the concurrent use of these drugs does not produce a better therapeutic effect than indomethacin alone and may increase the incidence of gastrointestinal reactions. The plasma levels of indomethacin may be increased by the concomitant administration of probenecid; thus, lower doses of indomethacin may be used in patients receiving both drugs. Since indomethacin has been reported to reduce the natriuretic and antihypertensive effects of furosemide, patients who receive these two drugs should be observed carefully for possible interactions.

Indomethacin is contraindicated in pregnant women, nursing mothers, infants, and children 14 years of age and under, since safe conditions for use in these patients have not been established. The drug also is contraindicated in patients with active gastrointestinal lesions or a history of recurrent gastrointestinal lesions. Indomethacin should be used with caution in the elderly and in those with epilepsy, parkinsonism, or emotional or psychiatric problems, since it may aggravate these conditions.

ROUTE, USUAL DOSAGE, AND PREPARATIONS.
Oral: For ankylosing spondylitis, osteoarthritis of the hip, and rheumatoid arthritis, *adults*, initially, 25 mg two or three times daily. The daily dose may be increased by increments of 25 or 50 mg at weekly intervals until a maximum of 200 mg daily is reached. Some patients may respond in four to six days while others require up to one month of therapy. In acute exacerbations, it may be necessary to increase the daily dose by 25 mg or, if required, by 50 mg. After the acute phase is under control, attempts to reduce the daily dose should be made until the drug is discontinued.

   Indocin (Merck Sharp & Dohme). Capsules 25 and 50 mg.

NAPROXEN
[Naprosyn]

Naproxen, which is chemically related to the phenylpropionic acid group of drugs, has analgesic, anti-inflammatory, and antipyretic actions. It is effective in the symptomatic treatment of rheumatoid arthritis, osteoarthritis, and ankylosing spondylitis. (See also Chapter 6, General Analgesics, and Chapter 8, Drugs Used in Gout, for other uses of naproxen.)

In patients with rheumatoid arthritis, comparative studies showed that daily doses of 500 mg of naproxen were as efficacious as 3.6 to 4.8 g of aspirin. Studies comparing naproxen to other nonsteroidal anti-inflammatory drugs have indicated that the effectiveness of naproxen is equal to or greater than that of ibuprofen, fenoprofen, or indomethacin. The drug's steroid-sparing effect was demonstrated in a limited number of patients who were also receiving a corticosteroid for rheumatoid arthritis and, when naproxen was given to patients receiving gold therapy, a greater therapeutic effect was observed.

In patients with osteoarthritis, naproxen was found to be as effective as aspirin or indomethacin. In ankylosing spondylitis, results of studies have shown that naproxen relieved symptoms after several months of treatment. It appeared to be more effective than previous therapy with phenylbutazone or indomethacin.

Naproxen is readily absorbed after oral administration; the peak plasma level occurs in one to two hours and the mean plasma half-life is about 13 hours. The drug is excreted largely in the urine in a conjugated form; a small percentage is excreted in the feces. Absorption of the drug is not significantly delayed by the presence of food, but the rate of absorption is slightly decreased by magnesium and aluminum hydroxide and increased by sodium bicarbonate. Naproxen readily crosses the placenta following oral administration to pregnant women and is excreted in the milk of lactating women. Thus, this drug should not be used during pregnancy or lactation.

Naproxen is highly bound to plasma protein and may displace other albumin-bound drugs from their binding sites; thus, patients receiving such drugs (eg, oral anticoagulants, sulfonylureas, hydantoins) should be observed for possible drug interactions. Because there is some evidence that cross sensitivity occurs, naproxen should not be given to patients sensitive to aspirin or other nonsteroidal anti-inflammatory drugs.

Like aspirin, naproxen inhibits platelet aggregation and prolongs bleeding time; however, the mechanism of action on the platelets may be different than that of aspirin. Naproxen also inhibits prostaglandin synthetase.

The most frequent adverse reactions are gastrointestinal disturbances (eg, heartburn, dyspepsia, abdominal pain, constipation, diarrhea). The gastric mucosa is less severely affected and less gastrointestinal bleeding has been observed than with aspirin; however, the latter reaction occasionally may be severe and ulceration has been reported. Therefore, this drug should be used with caution in patients with a history of peptic ulcer.

Central nervous system effects reported occasionally are headache, drowsiness, and dizziness or vertigo. Other adverse reactions occurring occasionally include pruritus, rash, urticaria, sweating, tinnitus, and visual and hearing disturbances.

A few cases of overdosage (four to six times the usual daily dose) have been reported, but no serious toxicity or late sequelae were observed.

ROUTE, USUAL DOSAGE, AND PREPARATIONS. *Oral: Adults,* 500 to 750 mg daily divided into two doses (morning and evening). The dose may be increased or decreased for long-term use, depending upon the patient's response. A dosage for children has not been established.

Naprosyn (Syntex). Tablets 250 mg.

OXYPHENBUTAZONE
[Oxalid, Tandearil]

PHENYLBUTAZONE
[Azolid, Butazolidin]

These drugs have anti-inflammatory, antipyretic, and analgesic properties. They often are more effective in ankylosing spondylitis and acute gouty arthritis than in rheumatoid arthritis and other arthropathies; they are also effective in painful shoulder (bursitis, capsulitis, peritendinitis). However, their usefulness is limited by their potential serious adverse reactions, and generally they should be used only for brief periods.

The most serious adverse reaction is bone marrow depression (eg, leukopenia, pancytopenia, agranulocytosis, aplastic anemia). This occurs only rarely during a one-week trial. Blood counts, including platelet determinations, should be performed regularly during prolonged treatment, but they cannot be depended upon to predict the blood dyscrasia. Therefore, patients should be advised to discontinue the drug and notify their physician immediately if they develop fever, sore throat, or stomatitis.

Rashes, water retention and edema, and gastrointestinal disturbances ranging from mild irritation to ulceration are the most commonly observed adverse reactions; oxyphenbutazone is purported to produce less gastrointestinal irritation than phenylbutazone, but some clinicians doubt that there is any difference between the two drugs. Phenylbutazone is available in combination with antacids, which are claimed to reduce gastrointestinal irritation. Other adverse reactions include jaundice, hepatitis, purpura, and hematuria. Susceptibility to toxic effects increases with age; in elderly patients, phenylbutazone or oxyphenbutazone should be used only for one-week periods and in reduced dosage. Because these drugs sometimes cause severe fluid retention, they should be used with extreme caution, if at all, in patients with borderline or overt congestive heart failure.

These drugs are contraindicated in children 14 years of age and under and in senile patients, since safe conditions for use have not been established; in those with gastrointestinal lesions or a history of recurrent lesions; in those with renal, hepatic, or cardiovascular disease; and in those with a history of blood dyscrasias or drug allergy.

Phenylbutazone and oxyphenbutazone may prolong the prothrombin time in patients receiving coumarin anticoagulants concomitantly and may increase the hypoglycemic effect of insulin and the oral hypoglycemic agents. They also reduce iodine uptake by the thyroid.

ROUTE, USUAL DOSAGE, AND PREPARATIONS.
Oral: *Adults*, initially, 300 to 600 mg daily in three or four equally divided doses. A one-week trial period is considered adequate to determine response. The maintenance dose should not exceed 400 mg daily. If symptoms can be controlled with a maintenance dose of 100 to 200 mg daily, the drug may be given for longer periods under careful supervision.

OXYPHENBUTAZONE:
Oxalid (USV), *Tandearil* (Geigy). Tablets 100 mg.

PHENYLBUTAZONE:
Azolid (USV), *Butazolidin* (Geigy). Tablets 100 mg.

AVAILABLE MIXTURES.
Azolid-A (USV), *Butazolidin alka* (Geigy). Each capsule contains phenylbutazone 100 mg, dried aluminum hydroxide gel 100 mg, and magnesium trisilicate 150 mg.

SULINDAC
[Clinoril]

Sulindac is a substituted indene analogue of indomethacin with similar anti-inflammatory, analgesic, and antipyretic properties. Results of controlled clinical trials have shown that usual doses of sulindac are as effective as aspirin in rheumatoid arthritis. The beneficial results also appear to be comparable to those produced by aspirin and ibuprofen in osteoarthritis and by phenylbutazone in ankylosing spondylitis. In a limited number of patients with acute painful shoulder (bursitis, tendinitis, or capsulitis), a daily dose of 300 to 400 mg of sulindac was found to be as effective as 400 to 600 mg of oxyphenbutazone daily in reducing pain. (See Chapter 8, Drugs Used in Gout, for other uses of sulindac.)

About 90% of a dose is rapidly absorbed following oral administration, and the drug's disposition is complex. The parent drug (sulfoxide) is inactive but is reduced reversibly to the sulfide (active metabolite) and oxidized irreversibly to the sulfone (inactive metabolite). Sulindac and sulfone and their conjugates are excreted in the urine; less than 1% of the administered dose of sulindac appears in the urine as the sulfide metabolite. The sulfide, which is responsible for the biological activities of the parent drug, is eliminated slowly from plasma (half-life, about 18 hours). Results of studies in animals have indicated that sulindac and its metabolites are excreted in the bile to varying degrees; thus, they may be reabsorbed unchanged, biotransformed, or excreted.

The overall incidence of adverse reactions reported is about 25%, but is higher in patients receiving the drug for long-term treatment. The most common reactions are abdominal pain, dyspepsia, nausea, constipation, and diarrhea. Sulindac generally causes a lower incidence of gastrointestinal disturbances than aspirin and about the same as that with ibuprofen. It causes less gastrointestinal bleeding than aspirin; however, because this effect has occurred rarely with use of sulindac, this drug should be used cautiously in patients with a history of gastrointestinal disease and should not be used in those with active gastrointestinal bleeding.

Central nervous system effects include dizziness, drowsiness, and headache; the incidence of these effects is about the same as that with aspirin and ibuprofen. Other adverse reactions reported occasionally are rash, pruritus, anxiety, and stomatitis.

Like aspirin and other nonsteroidal anti-inflammatory drugs, sulindac inhibits platelet aggregation and prolongs bleeding time. Therefore, it should be used cautiously in patients with bleeding disorders.

Although sulindac and its sulfide metabolite are highly bound to plasma protein, no clinically significant interaction with oral anticoagulants or oral hypoglycemic agents has been reported. Plasma levels of the active sulfide were depressed by the concomitant administration of sulindac and aspirin but not acetaminophen or propoxyphene.

ROUTE, USUAL DOSAGE, AND PREPARATIONS. *Oral*: The dosage should be adjusted in accordance with the patient's response. For *adults*, the usual initial dose is 150 mg twice daily with food for rheumatoid arthritis, osteoarthritis, and ankylosing spondylitis and 200 mg twice daily with food for acute painful shoulder. Dosage for *children* has not been established.

   Clinoril (Merck Sharp & Dohme). Tablets 150 and 200 mg.

TOLMETIN SODIUM
   [Tolectin]

This pyrrole-acetic acid derivative differs chemically from aspirin and other nonsteroidal anti-inflammatory agents, but its pharmacologic properties are similar.

Tolmetin alleviates symptoms of rheumatoid arthritis, and its effectiveness has been maintained with long-term use (two years). Results of comparative studies in patients with rheumatoid arthritis indicated that the efficacy of tolmetin was comparable to that of aspirin, indomethacin, ibuprofen, and phenylbutazone. Patients receiving corticosteroid or gold therapy obtained greater relief of symptoms when tolmetin was added to the regimen. Concomitant administration of tolmetin and acetaminophen also has been reported to relieve symptoms more than tolmetin alone, but the combination of tolmetin and aspirin provided no advantage over use of the individual drugs.

This agent also is effective in juvenile rheumatoid arthritis; clinical responses were comparable to those observed with aspirin. The effectiveness of tolmetin in osteoarthritis is similar to that of aspirin, ibuprofen, and indomethacin. In a limited number of studies, the usefulness of tolmetin was found to be comparable to that of indomethacin in ankylosing spondylitis. In addition, it has been reported to be effective in reducing pain in nonarticular and traumatic painful conditions. However, data are insufficient to establish conclusively the usefulness of tolmetin in these conditions.

The drug is rapidly absorbed after oral administration; peak plasma levels occur in 30 to 60 minutes. The plasma half-life is approximately one hour. The pharmacokinetics of tolmetin are not significantly affected by the short-or long-term administration of an antacid mixture of magnesium and aluminum hydroxides. Tolmetin is excreted largely in the urine, primarily as conjugates or metabolites.

Like other nonsteroidal anti-inflammatory agents, tolmetin inhibits prostaglandin synthetase in vitro. It also has been shown to reduce the plasma level of prostaglandin E in man. However, the significance of these actions in relation to the clinical effects is not known.

The most frequently reported adverse reactions are gastrointestinal disturbances; however, they occur less frequently than with aspirin. Epigastric distress (heartburn, dyspepsia, and abdominal pain) was most common; other reactions include nausea, vomiting, and constipation. Gastrointestinal bleeding was reported occasionally; however, results of controlled comparative studies showed that tolmetin caused less occult gastrointestinal bleeding than aspirin with usual doses. In clinical studies, peptic ulcer occurred in approximately 2% of patients, but many of these had a history of peptic ulcer disease. Therefore, it is advisable to use tolmetin cautiously in patients with a history of peptic ulcer.

Central nervous system reactions include headache, dizziness, lightheadedness, nervousness, and drowsiness. These occurred less frequently than with indomethacin. Other reactions observed occasionally are rash or urticaria, pruritus, tinnitus, and mild edema, which is related to sodium retention.

Tolmetin decreases platelet adhesiveness and increases bleeding time; thus, it should not be used in patients with bleeding disorders. Unlike aspirin, this drug has a minimal effect on platelet aggregation. Because the potential exists for cross sensitivity with aspirin and other nonsteroidal anti-inflammatory drugs, tolmetin should not be given to patients in whom aspirin may cause symptoms of asthma, rhinitis, or urticaria. Tolmetin does not affect the anticoagulant activity of warfarin, and, when given to patients receiving insulin or a sulfonylurea, the clinical effects of these agents have not been altered.

Since tolmetin causes pseudoproteinuria in tests involving acid precipitation, other methods for detecting proteinuria should be used in patients receiving this drug.

ROUTE, USUAL DOSAGE, AND PREPARATIONS. *Oral: Adults*, initially, 400 mg three times daily. After a therapeutic response is achieved, the dose is adjusted to the patient's needs; 600 mg to 1.8 g daily is optimal for most patients. *Children over 2 years*, 20 mg/kg of body weight daily in divided doses initially; for maintenance, 15 to 30 mg/kg daily.

   Tolectin (McNeil). Tablets 200 mg (sodium content: 18 mg).

ANTIMALARIAL AGENTS

CHLOROQUINE PHOSPHATE

HYDROXYCHLOROQUINE SULFATE
[Plaquenil Sulfate]

The 4-aminoquinoline compounds, chloroquine and hydroxychloroquine, have similar actions, but hydroxychloroquine is more commonly prescribed. These drugs are used to treat rheumatoid arthritis, usually as second-line therapy; they also are used in lupus erythematosus. Their value is limited by the potential toxicity and the variable beneficial effects obtained; some patients with rheumatoid arthritis experience moderate relief of symptoms while little or no benefit is observed in others. Because clinical improvement is slow, a three- to six-month trial is necessary to obtain maximal benefits and the recommended dosage must not be exceeded. Chloroquine and hydroxychloroquine also have been used in mild, early rheumatoid arthritis, usually with salicylates or small doses of corticosteroids. If no improvement is observed after six months, the antimalarial drug should be discontinued and other therapy used.

Ocular toxicity is the most serious complication; retinopathy appears to be related to the daily dose. The risk is greater with larger doses, even when given for short periods, than with small doses administered over a prolonged period. Serious retinal changes occur infrequently but may result in progressive impairment of vision and eventual blindness, even after the drug is discontinued. The retinopathy appears to affect pigmentation; depigmentation starts in the area of the macula, and increased granularity and edema of the retina are the earliest findings. Regular ophthalmologic examinations (eg, visual fields, color testing, retinal and corneal visualizations) should be performed prior to initiating therapy and every six months during therapy. The drug should be discontinued at the first sign of change in the ocular fundus.

Other adverse reactions include mild headache, gastrointestinal disturbances (diarrhea, nausea, abdominal cramps), rash, and neuropsychiatric disturbances (eg, emotional changes). Acute intermittent porphyria and neuromyopathy also may occur. The skin lesions of psoriasis may be aggravated and exfoliative dermatitis has been reported; therefore, antimalarial agents should not be used in patients with psoriatic arthritis. Patients with glucose-6-phosphate dehydrogenase deficiency should be carefully observed for the development of hemolytic anemia.

These drugs are rapidly absorbed from the gastrointestinal tract and deposited in tissues (eg, lungs, kidney, liver, eyes), where retention is prolonged, as evidenced by their urinary excretion months and even years after therapy is discontinued.

Toxic symptoms may be noted within 30 minutes and death may occur after overdosage. Children are especially sensitive to these drugs; therefore, patients should be warned to keep the drug out of their reach.

ROUTE, USUAL DOSAGE, AND PREPARATIONS.
CHLOROQUINE PHOSPHATE:
Oral: Adults, a maximum of 250 mg once daily with the evening meal or at bedtime. Dosage should be calculated on the basis of body weight and should not exceed 2 mg/lb.
> Drug available generically: Tablets 250 mg.

HYDROXYCHLOROQUINE SULFATE:
Oral: Adults, 200 mg once or twice daily with meals. Dosage should be calculated on the basis of body weight and should not exceed 3.5 mg/lb.
> *Plaquenil Sulfate* (Winthrop). Tablets 200 mg (equivalent to 155 mg of base).

GOLD COMPOUNDS

AUROTHIOGLUCOSE
[Solganal]

GOLD SODIUM THIOMALATE
[Myochrysine]

Active adult and juvenile rheumatoid arthritis are the principal indications for administration of these agents, but beneficial effects also have been obtained in some patients with psoriatic arthritis. Although their exact mechanism of action is not known, the gold compounds exert an anti-inflammatory effect in these disorders and, unlike other antiarthritic drugs, may affect the course of the disease. They should be considered in the treatment of rheumatoid arthritis that progresses despite faithful adherence to a conservative program of salicylates, rest, and physical therapy for several months. Although some physicians advocate their use in early stages of the disease, others prefer to withhold administration until more conservative therapy has been found to be ineffective. The concomitant use of a nonsteroidal anti-inflammatory agent is necessary unless complete remission of arthritis has occurred.

The usefulness of chrysotherapy is limited by toxicity. Dermatitis (ranging from erythema to exfoliative dermatitis) and lesions of the mucous membranes (stomatitis and, more rarely, proctitis and vaginitis) are common and may be serious. Hematologic reactions (eg, eosinophilia, leukopenia, thrombocytopenia, aplastic anemia) are observed rarely; some fatalities have occurred. Effects on the kidney range from proteinuria to the nephrotic syndrome. Cholestatic jaundice has been reported rarely.

Pruritus may signify the early development of a skin reaction. When a pruritic skin lesion whose etiology is not certain appears, gold therapy must be discontinued immediately, for another dose may produce a much more severe skin reaction.

Anaphylactoid or "nitritoid-type" reactions (eg, flushing, syncope, dizziness, sweating) may occur with the thiomalate preparation, but they are probably caused by the vehicle rather than the gold compound. Nausea, vomiting, and weakness may occur.

Toxic effects may be observed after the first injection, during the course of therapy, or several months after chrysotherapy has been discontinued. Their incidence and severity appear to depend upon dosage; although they may occur at any time, severe effects are most common after 300 to 500 mg has been administered. Since the occurrence of these reactions is unpredictable, patients should be questioned about symptoms of toxicity (eg, rash, purple blotches, pruritus, stomatitis, metallic taste) prior to each injection. A complete blood count, including platelet estimation, should be performed every two to three weeks for the first six months, then less often with decreasing dosage. Qualitative urine protein estimates should be performed before every injection. If toxicity develops, gold therapy should be discontinued immediately. Treatment with topical or systemic corticosteroids may be necessary, and the chelating agent, dimercaprol (BAL), may be used to increase the excretion of gold.

Gold compounds should be used with extreme caution in patients with impaired renal or hepatic function, blood disorders, skin rash, or marked hypertension. They are contraindicated in patients with severe debilitation, systemic lupus erythematosus, Sjögren's syndrome, or previous signs of gold toxicity. They are seldom needed during pregnancy but, if their use is contemplated, the benefit/risk ratio should be considered. Diabetes mellitus or congestive heart failure should be under control before initiating gold therapy.

ROUTE, USUAL DOSAGE, AND PREPARATIONS. *Intramuscular (gluteal): Adults,* initially, single weekly injections of 10 mg the first week, 25 mg the second week, 25 or 50 mg the third week, and 50 mg each week thereafter until a total dose of 800 mg to 1 g has been administered. If there is no response after 1 g has been given, the drug should be discontinued. If the patient has improved and no toxic effects have developed, dosage can be reduced to 50 mg every two weeks for four doses, every three weeks for four doses, and then monthly. However, results of recent studies suggest that three weeks should be the maximum interval, and comparative studies have demonstrated that a dose of 10 or 25 mg is as effective as the usual 50-mg dose and that the response is not related to serum level of gold. A remission after one year of maintenance therapy had been considered an indication for complete withdrawal of the drug, but many rheumatologists now feel that gold therapy probably should be continued indefinitely on a reduced dosage schedule. If relapse occurs when the interval between doses is increased or the drug is discontinued, the former schedule should be reinstituted. *Children*, for juvenile rheumatoid arthritis, recommendations of clinicans vary; however, a usual dose is 1 mg/kg of body weight weekly for 20 weeks and the same dose at two- to four-week intervals thereafter for as long as therapy is beneficial and there are no signs of toxicity. Single doses for children and all but the largest adolescents should not exceed 25 mg.

AUROTHIOGLUCOSE:
Solganal (Schering). Suspension 50 mg/ml in sesame oil with aluminum monostearate 2% in 10 ml containers.

GOLD SODIUM THIOMALATE:
Myochrysine (Merck Sharp & Dohme). Solution 10, 25, and 100 mg/ml in 1 ml containers and 50 mg/ml in 1 and 10 ml containers.

ADRENAL CORTICOSTEROIDS

Of the systemic corticosteroids, prednisone and prednisolone are most commonly used in rheumatic disorders and are equally effective when given orally. Others, preferably those with little mineralocorticoid activity, also may be administered in equivalent doses, although their greater potency may make dosage adjustment difficult. The adjunctive use of a nonsteroidal anti-inflammatory agent may permit use of smaller doses of the steroid. For equivalency, adverse reactions, and preparations, see Chapter 41, Adrenal Corticosteroids.

Intra-articular injection of a long-acting corticosteroid is useful for temporary relief of pain when only a few joints are markedly affected. Effects last two weeks to four months, depending upon the preparation used. See Chapter 41 for suitable long-acting preparations and doses.

ROUTE, USUAL DOSAGE, AND PREPARATIONS. PREDNISONE, PREDNISOLONE:
Oral: Adults, dosage must be individualized. Initially, 4 or 5 mg daily, using 1 mg tablets; the amount is increased gradually at three- to seven-day intervals to the maintenance level, depending upon response. Daily doses should not exceed 10 mg except in severely affected patients (eg, those with rheumatoid vasculitis). Even at this low dosage, adverse reactions associated with hypercorticism occur after prolonged use. *Children* with systemic (acute febrile) onset, 0.4 to 1 mg/kg of body weight daily. Alternate-day therapy, in which twice the usual daily dose is given every other morning, can be employed to minimize growth suppression in children during long-term therapy. This dosage schedule can be continued if symptoms are controlled satisfactorily during the day on which no medication is given.

OTHER DRUGS

PENICILLAMINE
[Cuprimine, Depen]

$$CH_3 - \overset{\overset{\displaystyle SH}{|}}{\underset{\underset{\displaystyle CH_3}{|}}{C}} - \overset{\overset{\displaystyle NH_2}{|}}{\underset{\underset{\displaystyle H}{|}}{C}} - \overset{\overset{\displaystyle O}{\|}}{COH}$$

Penicillamine, a chelating drug used in the treatment of Wilson's disease, cystinuria, and heavy metal poisoning, also is effective in rheumatoid arthritis. It is not useful in ankylosing spondylitis, psoriatic arthritis, or other HLA-B27 associated diseases. The mechanism of action is not known, but many of penicillamine's effects are similar to those of the gold compounds. Comparative studies indicate that penicillamine may be as effective as gold or azathioprine.

Because it may cause potentially hazardous adverse reactions, penicillamine should be reserved for patients with longstanding progressive disease that has not responded adequately to standard drug therapy. Physicians who prescribe it should be familiar with its action and should closely supervise patients receiving the drug.

The incidence of adverse reactions is high and may be related to the large doses used in early studies. Some effects are related to the rate of increase of dose and may be prevented by using an appropriate regimen. The most common adverse reactions are pruritus, rash, and an alteration in taste that may be transient. Serious reactions involving the hematologic (thrombocytopenia, leukopenia, agranulocytosis, and aplastic anemia) and renal (proteinuria, hypoalbuminemia, nephrotic syndrome) systems have been observed. Other potentially serious reactions reported occasionally are lupus-like disease, pemphigus, Goodpasture's syndrome, myasthenia gravis, stenosing alveolitis, and polymyositis; if symptoms of toxicity appear, the drug should be discontinued. Blood and urine tests should be performed periodically, and complete blood cell counts, including platelets, must be obtained at two-week intervals during the first six months of treatment and monthly thereafter. Blood urea nitrogen and creatinine levels should be monitored occasionally. Patients over 65 years appear to have a greater risk of developing hematologic toxicity. If urinary protein excretion is greater than 1 g/24 hrs, the dosage should be reduced; this often corrects the proteinuria after several months. Penicillamine must be discontinued if hypoalbuminemia, nephrotic syndrome, or hematuria develops.

ROUTE, USUAL DOSAGE, AND PREPARATIONS. The dose is variable and must be individualized on the basis of the clinical response and adverse reactions. Because of the long latent period before a clinical response is observed, changes in dosage should not be made at intervals of less than two to three months. Other medication, except gold, antimalarial agents, cytotoxic drugs, and phenylbutazone or oxyphenbutazone, should be continued when penicillamine is given; after clinical improvement is observed, the other drugs can be withdrawn gradually. Penicillamine should be given on an empty stomach (about one hour before meals and one hour apart from other food) to ensure maximum absorption and lessen gastrointestinal disturbances.

Oral: Adults, initially, 250 mg/day as a single dose (125 mg/day may be sufficient for some patients); the amount may be increased by increments of 250 mg/day at two- to three-month intervals. The average maintenance dose is 500 to 750 mg/day.

> *Cuprimine* (Merck Sharp & Dohme). Capsules 125 and 250 mg.
> *Depen* (Wallace). Tablets 250 mg.

Selected References

Brogden RN, et al: Sulindac: Review of its pharmacological properties and therapeutic efficacy in rheumatic diseases. *Drugs* 16:97-114, 1978A.

Brogden RN, et al: Tolmetin: Review of its pharmacological properties and therapeutic efficacy in rheumatic diseases. *Drugs* 15:429-450, 1978B.

Brogden RN, et al: Fenoprofen: Review of its pharmacological properties and therapeutic efficacy in rheumatic diseases. *Drugs* 13:241-265, 1977.

Calabro JJ, et al: Juvenile rheumatoid arthritis: General review and report of 100 patients observed for 15 years. *Semin Arthritis Rheum* 5:257-298, 1976.

Ehrlich GE: HLA-B27: Umbrella for a family of rheumatoid variants. *Drug Ther* 6:48-62, (May) 1976.

Ehrlich GE: Rheumatoid arthritis. *Drug Ther* 5:141-156, (Sept) 1975.

Ehrlich GE (ed): *Total Management of the Arthritic Patient*. Philadelphia, JB Lippincott Company, 1973.

Hart FD: Which antirheumatic drug? *Drugs* 11:451-460, 1976.

Hill HFH: Treatment of rheumatoid arthritis with penicillamine. *Semin Arthritis Rheum* 6:361-388, 1977.

Huskisson EC: Osteoarthritis: Changing concepts in pathogenesis and treatment. *Postgrad Med* 65:97-104, (March) 1979.

Jaffe LA: D-penicillamine. *Bull Rheum Dis* 28:948-952, 1977-1978.

Lee P, et al: Evaluation of analgesic action and efficacy of antirheumatic drugs: Study of 10 drugs in 684 patients with rheumatoid arthritis. *J Rheumatol* 3:283-294, 1976.

Levy G: Clinical pharmacokinetics of aspirin. *Pediatrics* 62(suppl):867-872, 1978.

Lewis JR: New antirheumatic agents: Fenoprofen calcium (Nalfon), naproxen (Naprosyn), and tolmetin sodium (Tolectin). *JAMA* 237:1260-1261, 1977.

Lorber A: Monitoring gold plasma levels in rheumatoid arthritis. *Clin Pharmacokinet* 2:127-146, 1977.

Pirofsky B, Baradana EJ Jr: Immunosuppressive therapy in rheumatic disease. *Med Clin North Am* 62:419-437, 1977.

Popert AJ: Chloroquine: A review. *Rheumatol Rehabil* 15:235-238, 1976.

Roe RL: Drug therapy in rheumatic diseases. *Med Clin North Am* 62:405-418, 1977.

Schaller JG: Chronic salicylate administration in juvenile rheumatoid arthritis: Aspirin "hepatitis" and its clinical significance. *Pediatrics* 62(suppl):916-925, 1978.

Scherbel AL: Nonsteroidal antiinflammatory drugs: New alternatives for rheumatic disease. *Postgrad Med* 63:69-74, (March) 1978.

Sharp JT, et al: Comparison of two dosage schedules of gold salts in treatment of rheumatoid arthritis: Relationship of serum gold levels to therapeutic response. *Arthritis Rheum* 20:1179-1187, 1977.

Smyth CJ, Bravo JF: Antirheumatic drugs: Clinical pharmacological and therapeutic aspects. *Drugs* 10:394-425, 1975.

Sonnenblick M, Abraham AS: Ibuprofen hypersensitivity in systemic lupus erythematosus. *Br Med J* 1:619-620, 1978.

Wilkens RF: Use of nonsteroidal anti-inflammatory agents. *JAMA* 240:1632-1635, 1978.

Drugs Used in Gout | 8

Gout is a metabolic disease characterized by hyperuricemia and by episodes of severe, acute arthritis which are frequently monoarticular but sometimes polyarticular, especially later in the course of the disease. The four stages in the natural history of the disease are: (1) asymptomatic hyperuricemia, which infrequently progresses to acute gout, (2) acute gouty arthritis, (3) intercritical (interval) gout, and (4) chronic tophaceous gout (only 30% to 40% of patients with acute gout develop tophi). A serious complication of tophaceous gout is the development of progressive renal failure resulting from the deposition of urate crystals in renal interstitial tissue. Renal calculi also are noted in 20% to 40% of patients with gout.

Gout is commonly classified as (1) primary (familial in about 20% of patients), in which hyperuricemia is attributed to a metabolic error leading to overproduction of uric acid, decreased clearance of uric acid, or both, or (2) secondary, in which hyperuricemia develops during the course of another disease or as a consequence of drug therapy.

Acute or chronic gouty arthritis must be differentiated from other conditions with similar manifestations. For details and procedures of diagnosis, see specialized texts (eg, Talbott and Yu, 1976, and Wyngaarden and Kelley, 1976); for the criteria for the diagnosis of acute arthritis of primary gout developed by the American Rheumatism Association, see Wallace et al, 1977.

Drug Therapy

The principal objectives in the treatment of gout are: (1) to terminate the inflammatory process of an acute attack and prevent its recurrence, and (2) to reduce hyperuricemia in order to promote the resolution of tophi and prevent formation of urate deposits in high-risk patients. The drugs commonly used to treat attacks of acute gouty arthritis include colchicine, phenylbutazone [Azolid, Butazolidin] or oxyphenbutazone [Oxalid, Tandearil], and indomethacin [Indocin]. Corticotropin or systemic corticosteroids may be used in patients refractory to other agents. Drugs used to reduce the miscible pool of uric acid in tophaceous gout and secondary hyperuricemia are probenecid [Benemid] and sulfinpyrazone [Anturane], which increase the renal excretion of uric acid, and allopurinol [Zyloprim], which decreases the formation of uric acid. These agents should not be used to treat acute attacks; they are ineffective and may precipitate an attack. The activity of a new uricosuric agent, ticrynafen [Selacryn], which also has diuretic and antihypertensive properties, appears to be comparable to that of probenecid.

In a limited number of studies, several new nonsteroidal anti-inflammatory agents (eg, fenoprofen [Nalfon], ibuprofen [Motrin], naproxen [Naprosyn], sulindac [Clinoril]) have been shown to be effective in alleviating the pain and inflammation of acute gout. With the exception of sulindac, the number of studies has been insufficient to establish an effective dose for the treatment of acute gouty arthritis. These agents may be considered as alternatives to the older agents, as they are generally better tolerated. Their use in the treatment of other rheumatic diseases is discussed in Chapter 7, Antiarthritic Drugs.

Acute Gouty Arthritis: Colchicine has long been considered the drug of choice for acute gouty arthritis; however, phenylbutazone, oxyphenbutazone, and indomethacin are also effective and are used initially by some clinicians because they are better tolerated than colchicine. If the diagnosis is uncertain, colchicine should be used; if the diagnosis is established, one of the other agents may be employed, the choice of which frequently depends upon the physician's and patient's experience with a certain drug. They are most effective when given early during an acute attack and can be expected to produce beneficial effects within 24 to 48 hours in a large percentage of patients.

Intramuscular administration of corticotropin (ACTH) or intra-articular injection of a corticosteroid rarely may be necessary to treat acute attacks in very severe cases or in patients who fail to respond to the above anti-inflammatory agents. Colchicine should be given concomitantly and after discontinuation of steroids to prevent rebound attacks.

Intercritical (Interval) Gout: Proper management of patients with gout during the intercritical (asymptomatic) period includes not only drug therapy but also attention to diet for control of body weight, excess intake of purines, and hypertriglyceridemia, as well as avoidance of precipitating factors. Many patients do well in the intercritical phase without drug therapy. This discussion is limited to a consideration of appropriate drug therapy.

Small daily doses of colchicine (0.5 to 1.5 mg) prevent acute attacks in a large percentage of patients. After the inflammation of an acute attack has subsided, consideration also should be given to the administration of drugs that decrease the serum uric acid level, although it is important not to decrease serum urate levels suddenly as the rapid mobilization of urate from body pools may precipitate an acute attack. Opinions vary regarding the time in the course of treatment when administration of antihyperuricemic drugs should be started. Although some clinicians prefer to withhold these drugs if hyperuricemia is mild and renal function is normal, most believe that hyperuricemia severe enough to produce one acute attack should be treated.

Since the risk of uric acid stone formation and urate nephropathy, which may be serious complications, is related to the height of serum urate levels and magnitude of urinary uric acid excretion, patients at risk should be given prophylactic antihyperuricemic drug therapy. Thus, a urinary uric acid value persistently above 600 mg/day on a purine-free diet or above 800 to 1,000 mg/day on a nonrestricted diet is generally considered an indication for drug therapy. A uricosuric agent may be used to reduce the serum uric acid level to the normal range if the patient has normal renal function but, in cases of renal insufficiency, allopurinol is preferred. Because it reduces both serum and urinary uric acid values, allopurinol also is preferred for the treatment of nephrolithiasis.

Tophaceous Gout: The objective of treatment of tophaceous gout is to decrease the uric acid content of blood and tissues, thereby reducing tophi and the renal and joint changes that occur in chronic gout. Since allopurinol reduces the load of uric acid excreted by the kidney, it may be the preferred drug in this condition. After tissue stores have been mobilized and excreted, serum levels are usually reduced to normal.

Since uricosuric agents and allopurinol tend to precipitate attacks of acute gouty arthritis during initial administration, prophylactic doses of colchicine should be given concomitantly for 6 to 12 months after the last attack.

Regardless of which drug is used to treat hyperuricemia, serum urate levels should be measured regularly to determine the efficacy of treatment. To help avoid the formation of urate renal calculi, a large flow of urine should be maintained and renal function should be assessed periodically during therapy.

Secondary Hyperuricemia: Secondary hyperuricemia may result from overproduction and/or decreased excretion of uric acid. Overproduction occurs in various myeloproliferative disorders such as polycythemia vera, myeloid metaplasia, leukemia, or lymphoma, as well as during the treatment of these diseases with drugs that cause a breakdown of cellular nucleic acid. Patients with these diseases should be given allopurinol prior to treatment with cytotoxic drugs (see the evaluation on Allopurinol for precautions). Decreased renal excretion of uric acid occurs in such conditions as lead nephropathy, glycogen storage disease, and sickle cell disease; increased endogenous production of uric acid also occurs in the latter two conditions.

Whether it is advisable to treat asymptomatic hyperuricemia is controversial. The risk of developing gouty arthritis and nephropathy is proportional to the degree of hyperuricemia. Mild hyperuricemia with no clinical manifestations of gout need not be treated; however, treatment should be instituted if there is marked overproduction of uric acid as indicated by the urinary excretion of more than 700 or 800 mg daily with rigid purine restriction.

Several drugs, including salicylates in low doses, pyrazinamide, niacin, ethambutol [Myambutol], and alcohol, may produce hyperuricemia. Hyperuricemia also is frequently induced by diuretics widely used in the treatment of hypertension; however, the routine use of drugs to reduce serum uric acid in these patients is unnecessary. Although hypertension is often a problem in patients with gout, antihypertensive therapy should be the primary treatment in such patients. Studies suggest that uncontrolled hypertension may produce more renal disease than uncontrolled hyperuricemia. If indicated, as noted above, the hyperuricemia should be treated with a uricosuric agent or allopurinol (see Chapter 39, Diuretics).

DRUGS USED IN ACUTE GOUTY ARTHRITIS

COLCHICINE

Colchicine is a major drug for reduction of inflammation and relief of pain of acute gouty arthritis. Oral administration should begin at the first sign of an attack and continue until symptoms subside, gastrointestinal distress appears, or the maximal dose is given. If oral administration is contraindicated, the drug may be given intravenously; some clinicians prefer this route to avoid gastrointestinal disturbances. Relief of pain and inflammation usually occurs within 24 to 48 hours after oral therapy and 6 to 12 hours after intravenous injection, but several days may elapse before swelling completely subsides. It may be difficult to obtain prompt relief with nontoxic doses if there is delay in treatment or inconsistency in the dosage schedule.

Use of colchicine prophylactically during the intercritical period may prevent acute attacks or diminish their severity and facilitate treatment. Colchicine also can be given to prevent attacks of acute gouty arthritis that are precipitated during the early stages of administration of uricosurics or allopurinol. The dosage should be adjusted to provide maximal freedom from acute attacks without producing adverse reactions. Patients receiving prophylactic treatment sometimes respond to small therapeutic doses, thus terminating an acute attack without unpleasant reactions.

Colchicine may control acute attacks of pseudogout (chondrocalcinosis articularis), but its effect is less consistent than in gouty arthritis; other anti-inflammatory drugs are more effective.

Colchicine is also effective in the prevention of familial Mediterranean fever. When taken prophylactically, the drug prevents the episodic attacks of painful serositis characteristic of this disease. Alternatively, short courses of colchicine taken at the very onset of symptoms may abort attacks in some patients.

The beneficial effects of colchicine are attributable to its anti-inflammatory action; the precise mechanism of action is not known. Colchicine has several biological effects, most of which do not appear to be related to its anti-inflammatory action.

Following oral administration, colchicine is almost completely absorbed; a mean peak plasma level of about 0.32 mcg/dl is reached in 30 minutes to two hours. The drug is cleared rapidly from the plasma, but it reaches higher concentrations and remains longer in circulating leukocytes. Its metabolism is not completely known, but the half-life is prolonged in patients with renal disease.

Colchicine causes nausea and vomiting or abdominal pain in about 80% of patients, as well as the so-called therapeutic endpoint of diarrhea, especially if maximal doses are given. The warning provided by gastrointestinal intolerance tends to protect the patient from toxic doses. As soon as these symptoms occur, administration should be discontinued, irrespective of the status of activity of joint symptoms. Drugs to control vomiting and diarrhea may be given when indicated. Gastrointestinal distress is uncommon after intravenous administration, but this route is associated with risk of local extravasation that can cause inflammation and necrosis of the skin and soft tissues.

Bone marrow depression with leukopenia and thrombocytopenia, purpura, peripheral neuritis, myopathy, anuria, alopecia, hepatocellular failure, hypersensitivity reactions, and hemorrhagic colitis have been reported infrequently. These reactions generally have been associated with overdosage, liver disease, delayed excretion caused by kidney damage, and especially with combinations of these factors.

Colchicine should be given with special caution to elderly or debilitated patients and to those with hepatic, renal, cardiovascular, or gastrointestinal disease.

ROUTES, USUAL DOSAGE, AND PREPARATIONS. *Oral*: For acute attacks, *adults*, 0.5 or 0.6 mg (one tablet) is administered hourly; alternatively, 1 or 1.2 mg (two tablets) may be given initially, followed by 0.5 or 0.6 mg every two hours until articular symptoms subside or gastrointestinal distress occurs. A maximum dose of 7 or 8 mg may be administered, but most patients cannot tolerate this amount. If the intravenous route is used to complement oral administration, the oral form should be discontinued before 4 mg has been given. For prophylaxis, the dosage depends upon the sensitivity of the patient to gastrointestinal reactions; usually 0.5 to 1 mg daily is given.

Drug available generically: Tablets 0.5 and 0.6 mg.

Intravenous: For acute attacks, *adults*, 1 or 2 mg initially, followed by 0.5 mg every three to six hours until a satisfactory response is achieved. When given promptly, one or two injections (1 to 2 mg) usually terminate an attack. Some clinicians recommend a single dose of 3 mg rather than repeated smaller doses, which increase the risk of extravasation and tissue necrosis. The total dose for one course of treatment should not exceed 4 mg. To minimize sclerosis of the vein, the 2-ml vial should be diluted to 20 ml with sterile normal sodium chloride injection and administered slowly.

Drug available generically: Solution 0.5 mg/ml in 2 ml containers.

CORTICOTROPIN (ACTH)
ADRENAL CORTICOSTEROIDS

Although only rarely needed, corticotropin or systemic corticosteroids may be effective in treating unusually severe acute attacks or in patients refractory to other anti-inflammatory drugs. These agents should not be used for more than a few days and should not be given to treat chronic gout. To prevent rebound attacks, colchicine (0.6 mg two or three times daily) should be given during and for seven days after corticotropin therapy is discontinued.

If the acute attack is limited to a single joint, a corticosteroid injected intra-articularly usually relieves pain. Oral anti-inflammatory drugs should be given concomitantly.

For adverse reactions and precautions, see Chapter 41, Adrenal Corticosteroids, and Chapter 46, Agents Related to Anterior Pituitary and Hypothalamic Function.

ROUTES, USUAL DOSAGE, AND PREPARATIONS.
CORTICOTROPIN:
Intramuscular: Adults, 40 to 80 units every six to eight hours for two to three days; the dose is then gradually reduced until the medication can be withdrawn completely.
Intravenous: Adults, 40 to 80 units diluted in 250 to 500 ml of normal saline may be administered by intravenous drip.

Drug available generically: Powder 25, 40, and 80 units; gel and solution (repository) 25, 40, and 80 units/ml in 5 ml containers.
ACTH (Merrell-National). Solution 20 U.S.P. units/ml in 2 and 10 ml containers.
Acthar (Armour). Powder (lyophilized) 25 and 40 U.S.P. units; gel (repository) 40 and 80 U.S.P. units/ml in 1 and 5 ml containers.
Cortrophin Gel (Organon). Gel (repository) 40 U.S.P. units/ml in 1 and 5 ml containers and 80 U.S.P. units/ml in 5 ml containers.
Cortrophin-Zinc (Organon). Suspension (repository) 40 U.S.P. units of corticotropin with 2 mg of zinc/ml in 5 ml containers.

ADRENAL CORTICOSTEROIDS:
The doses vary greatly depending upon the individual preparation (see Chapter 41 for dosage and preparations).

INDOMETHACIN
[Indocin]

Indomethacin is not specific for gout; however, its anti-inflammatory, antipyretic, and analgesic properties make it useful in the short-term treatment of attacks of acute gouty arthritis. Its effectiveness is comparable to that of colchicine, phenylbutazone, and oxyphenbutazone. Because this agent does not correct hyperuricemia, it is not useful for the treatment of chronic gout. Indomethacin may be beneficial in the treatment of acute pseudogout.

The adverse reactions produced by indomethacin, some of which may be serious, generally are dose and time dependent. The most common reactions are gastrointestinal irritation (nausea, vomiting, and occasional bleeding), dizziness, and headache. Indomethacin should not be given to patients with an active ulcer or history of recurrent gastrointestinal lesions. It causes fluid retention and may worsen congestive heart failure. The drug should be used cautiously in the elderly, since the incidence of adverse reactions appears to be higher in these patients. If indomethacin is administered with probenecid, the latter inhibits the tubular secretion of indomethacin, resulting in increased plasma concentrations, which is usually not clinically important. (See also Chapter 7, Antiarthritic Drugs.)

ROUTE, USUAL DOSAGE, AND PREPARATIONS.
Oral: For attacks of acute gout, *adults*, initially, 50 to 150 mg, followed by 50 mg three times daily until symptoms subside, usually in three to five days. The dose is

then reduced gradually to prevent recurrences. The drug should be taken with food, immediately after meals, or with antacids to reduce gastrointestinal irritation; however, these measures may delay absorption.

 Indocin (Merck Sharp & Dohme). Capsules 25 and 50 mg.

OXYPHENBUTAZONE
[Oxalid, Tandearil]

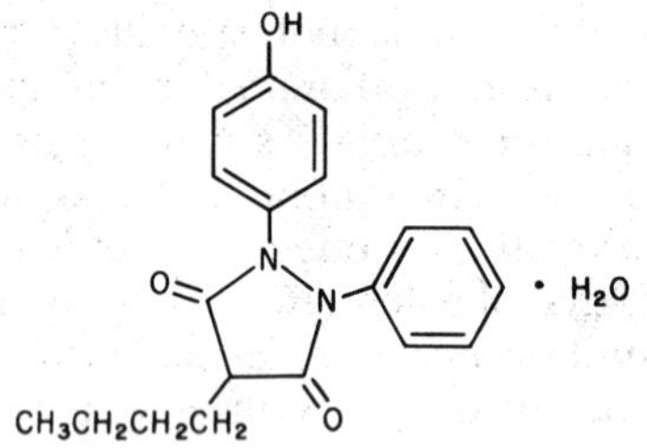

OH

$\cdot$ H$_2$O

CH$_3$CH$_2$CH$_2$CH$_2$

PHENYLBUTAZONE
[Azolid, Butazolidin]

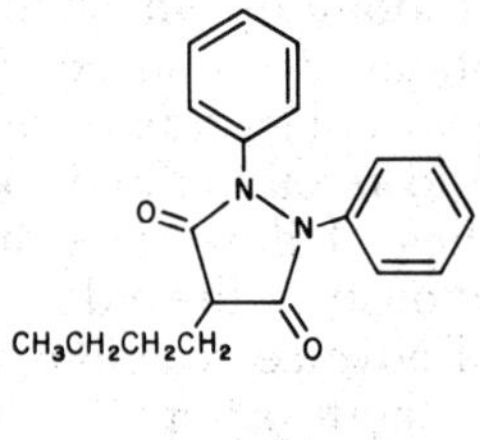

CH$_3$CH$_2$CH$_2$CH$_2$

Phenylbutazone and its analogue, oxyphenbutazone, have the same uses and adverse reactions. Their effectiveness in the treatment of attacks of acute gouty arthritis is comparable to that of colchicine and indomethacin. They have mild uricosuric activity in doses of 600 mg or more daily, but their usefulness in acute gout is from their anti-inflammatory and analgesic actions. Because of their potential to cause adverse reactions, especially with long-term use, these agents should not be used prophylactically or in the treatment of chronic gout.

Adverse reactions are usually minimal with the short- term use required in the treatment of acute attacks. These drugs are better tolerated than colchicine; however, gastrointestinal irritation (nausea, vomiting, or epigastric discomfort) may occur. Fluid retention also is observed occasionally. Because phenylbutazone and oxyphenbutazone may produce serious adverse reactions, particularly hematologic, the patient should be carefully supervised during treatment and therapy should be discontinued immediately if any serious reactions occur. (See also Chapter 7, Antiarthritic Drugs.)

Phenylbutazone and oxyphenbutazone should be used with caution in the elderly; in those with renal, hepatic, or cardiovascular disease; and in those with a history or symptoms of peptic ulcer, drug allergy, or blood dyscrasias. They also should be used cautiously in patients receiving coumarin-type anticoagulants, insulin, phenytoin, or oral hypoglycemic agents because of the danger of potentiating the actions of these agents. Phenylbutazone or oxyphenbutazone should not be given to patients with active peptic ulcer.

ROUTE, USUAL DOSAGE, AND PREPARATIONS. *Oral*: *Adults*, 400 mg initially, followed by 100 mg every four hours until articular inflammation subsides (usually two to three days). Alternatively, 200 mg three or four times the first day, followed by smaller quantities for two or three days, may be given. Therapy should not be continued for more than seven days.

OXYPHENBUTAZONE:
Oxalid (USV), *Tandearil* (Geigy). Tablets 100 mg.

PHENYLBUTAZONE:
Azolid (USV), *Butazolidin* (Geigy). Tablets 100 mg.

AVAILABLE MIXTURES.
Azolid-A (USV), *Butazolidin alka* (Geigy). Each capsule contains phenylbutazone 100 mg, dried aluminum hydroxide gel 100 mg, and magnesium trisilicate 150 mg.

SULINDAC
[Clinoril]

This nonsteroidal anti-inflammatory drug is effective in the treatment of attacks of acute gout. It relieves pain and reduces swelling in the affected joints, usually within 48 to 72 hours. In comparative studies, the efficacy of sulindac (400 mg daily) was found to be comparable to that of phenylbutazone (600 mg daily).

For a discussion of adverse reactions and precautions, see Chapter 7, Antiarthritic Drugs.

ROUTE, USUAL DOSAGE, AND PREPARATIONS.
Oral: Adults, 200 mg twice a day. The dose can be reduced after a satisfactory response has occurred; seven days of therapy are usually sufficient.

> *Clinoril* (Merck Sharp & Dohme). Tablets 150 and 200 mg.

DRUGS USED FOR TOPHACEOUS GOUT AND OTHER HYPERURICEMIAS

ALLOPURINOL
[Zyloprim]

Allopurinol is useful in the treatment of chronic tophaceous gout; it reduces serum urate levels, usually within a few days to two weeks. Prolonged treatment inhibits the formation of tophi and mobilizes stored urates which causes a gradual regression in the size of tophi already formed. Allopurinol is especially useful in chronic gout complicated by renal insufficiency or uric acid renal calculi. The actions of allopurinol differ from those of the uricosuric agents in that renal excretion of uric acid is decreased and its action is not antagonized by salicylates.

Allopurinol also may be used to treat hyperuricemia associated with uric acid overproduction that often occurs in patients with polycythemia vera, myeloid metaplasia, leukemia, lymphoma, or psoriasis, as well as during the treatment of these conditions with cytotoxic agents which cause a breakdown of cellular nucleic acids leading to acute uric acid nephropathy. In addition, allopurinol may be used if indicated to treat drug-induced hyperuricemia, the most common of which is that caused by diuretics; however, most authorities do not treat asymptomatic diuretic-induced hyperuricemia.

Like the uricosurics, allopurinol may increase the frequency of attacks of acute gouty arthritis during the early stages of treatment; therefore, colchicine should be given prophylactically during initial therapy, and patients should receive appropriate treatment if acute attacks do occur. Attacks usually diminish in number and severity after several months of treatment with allopurinol.

The drug decreases the production of uric acid by inhibiting xanthine oxidase, the enzyme that converts hypoxanthine to xanthine and xanthine to uric acid, thereby lowering plasma and urine concentrations of uric acid. In addition to inhibiting xanthine oxidase, allopurinol inhibits de novo purine synthesis through a feedback mechanism, which provides an additional benefit to the patient. This action requires the presence of the enzyme, hypoxanthine-guanine phosphoribosyl transferase. Children with Lesch-Nyhan syndrome, who lack this enzyme, and the few adults with a partial deficiency do not benefit from this effect. Allopurinol is itself metabolized by xanthine oxidase to oxipurinol, which also inhibits xanthine oxidase. Oxipurinol has a considerably longer half-clearance time from plasma than allopurinol (18 to 30 hours and less than 2 hours, respectively), which accounts for the long duration of action of allopurinol and permits use of a single daily dose.

ADVERSE REACTIONS AND PRECAUTIONS.

The most common adverse reaction associated with use of allopurinol is maculopapular rash, frequently preceded by pruritus. Exfoliative, urticarial, and purpuric lesions also have been observed. The incidence of rash occurring after administration of ampicillin is unusually high in patients receiving allopurinol concomitantly. The latter must be discontinued promptly when rash occurs, since this reaction may become serious if treatment is continued after symptoms appear. Allopurinol may act as a haptene, inducing immune complex dermatitis, nephritis, vasculitis, and a polyarteritis syndrome; a few deaths from these reactions have been reported. Although the incidence of vasculitis, nephritis, and death may be low, immune complex skin and liver disease is not rare and is a warning to discontinue the drug. Pruritus is an especially important warning symptom. It may be possible to resume use of allopurinol at a lower dosage after a period of time.

Fever and chills with moderate leukopenia or leukocytosis, eosinophilia, arthralgia, and pruritus, which might represent a hypersensitivity reaction, have been reported in a few patients. Hypersensitivity reactions tend to be severe in patients with renal insufficiency.

Reactions that occur occasionally include nausea, vomiting, diarrhea, abdominal discomfort, drowsiness, headache, and a metallic taste. Other reactions reported rarely, and in which a causal relationship has not been established, include peripheral neuritis, precipitation of peptic ulcer or increase in ulcer symptoms, tachycardia, pancreatitis, pyelonephritis, increased blood urea nitrogen levels, anemia, retinopathy, and macular degeneration. One death associated with bone marrow depression has been reported. Several cases of cataracts have been observed, but careful investigation has shown that they were coincidental with drug use.

Hepatic effects, ranging from alterations in liver function tests (increased serum levels of alkaline phosphatase and transaminases) to hepatitis, have been reported frequently. Although these effects have been reversible, it is advisable to assess liver function monthly in patients on long-term therapy. In addition, rarely, patients with renal insufficiency have developed hepatic dysfunction and progressive renal failure following the administration of allopurinol. Since a number of these patients were also receiving thiazide diuretics, it was suggested that the combination of thiazides and allopurinol occasionally could lead to progressive renal disease. Inhibition of xanthine oxidase by allopurinol does not increase hepatic iron stores in man.

Xanthine renal calculus formation is rare even in patients with Lesch-Nyhan syndrome and has not been reported in those being treated for primary gout.

Because allopurinol inhibits the oxidation of mercaptopurine, the dose of the latter must be reduced to approximately one-third to one-fourth of the usual dose when both drugs are given concomitantly. Since mercaptopurine is a metabolite of azathioprine, similar precautions should be observed when using the latter. Allopurinol inhibits hepatic drug metabolizing enzymes; thus, drugs metabolized by these enzymes (eg, coumarin derivatives) should be given in lower doses. Allopurinol increases the half-life of probenecid, but probenecid increases the excretion of oxipurinol. Allopurinol appears to increase the toxicity of cytotoxic agents (eg, cyclophosphamide).

Studies in animals have shown that allopurinol has no teratogenic effects. However, there is no information on the effects of xanthine oxidase inhibition on the human fetus, and the potential benefits should be weighed against the possible risk to the fetus before allopurinol is used in pregnant women or women of childbearing age.

ROUTE, USUAL DOSAGE, AND PREPARATIONS.

Oral: Dosage should be individualized to obtain the desired serum urate level as determined by frequent measurements. For mild gout, *adults*, 200 to 300 mg daily as a single dose. For more severe gout with tophi, 400 to 600 mg daily; doses greater than 600 mg/day increase the incidence of toxic reactions, and the effect on uric acid production usually is not much greater. For patients with renal insufficiency, 100 to 200 mg daily. Allopurinol is better tolerated if taken after meals. For secondary hyperuricemias, optimal dosage is the smallest amount necessary to maintain serum uric acid levels within the normal range. *Adults*, 100 to 200 mg daily is the minimum effective dose (maximum, 800 mg); *children 6 to 10 years with malignancies*, 300 mg daily; *under 6 years*, 150 mg daily.

Zyloprim (Burroughs Wellcome). Tablets 100 and 300 mg.

PROBENECID
[Benemid]

Probenecid is an effective uricosuric agent used to prevent or reduce the joint changes and tophi that occur in chronic gout. Its uricosuric effect is attributed to inhibition of the tubular reabsorption of filtered urate. Probenecid usually has no significant uricosuric activity when the glomerular filtration rate is less than 30 ml/min, and thus it is not always effective in patients with chronic renal insufficiency. This drug is not useful in acute attacks of gouty arthritis. Probenecid also is used with penicillin preparations to increase their blood levels and prolong their action by blocking their renal tubular secretion.

Acute attacks of gout may occur, especially during the early months of therapy, and colchicine should be given concomitantly for prophylaxis during this period.

A large volume of urine should be maintained to minimize urate precipitation in the urinary tract. Probenecid is contraindicated in patients with a history of renal calculi, especially uric acid stones, because it may aggravate this condition.

Probenecid is readily absorbed following oral administration; the plasma half-life is dose dependent (range, 6 to 12 hours). It is rapidly metabolized and excreted in the urine, principally as the acyl glucuronide and oxidized metabolites; little drug is excreted unchanged.

Probenecid is well tolerated by most patients. Gastrointestinal reactions (anorexia, nausea, vomiting), headache, hypersensitivity reactions, and urinary frequency are the most common adverse reactions. Although serious anaphylactoid reactions, anemia, hemolytic anemia, aplastic anemia, fatal massive necrosis of the liver, and repeated episodes of a reversible nephrotic syndrome have been reported, these reactions are rare.

Since salicylates diminish the effect of probenecid, they should not be used concomitantly. Probenecid inhibits the renal transport of sulfinpyrazone, indomethacin, penicillin, aminosalicylic acid, the sulfonamides (mostly as inactive conjugates), pantothenic acid, iodopyracet and related iodinated organic acids, aminohippuric acid, phenolsulfonphthalein, and sulfobromophthalein. The dosage of these agents therefore should be modified when they are administered with probenecid. Since this agent increases the renal excretion of oxipurinol, inhibition of xanthine oxidase is reduced when probenecid is given with allopurinol. However, in tophaceous gout it can be given with allopurinol for more rapid dissolution of tophi. When probenecid was given with sulindac, the plasma levels of sulindac and its sulfone metabolite were increased but the plasma sulfide levels were only slightly affected.

ROUTE, USUAL DOSAGE, AND PREPARATIONS. *Oral*: Dosage should be determined individually and adjusted to obtain the desired serum urate level. *Adults*, 250 mg two or three times daily for one week or more depending on response, followed by the minimum dose necessary for maintenance.

Drug available generically: Tablets 500 mg.

Benemid (Merck Sharp & Dohme). Tablets 500 mg.

118

SULFINPYRAZONE
[Anturane]

Sulfinpyrazone is a congener of phenyl-butazone, but it lacks the latter's anti-inflammatory, analgesic, and sodium-retaining properties. This effective uricosuric agent is used to treat tophaceous gout; it is more potent than probenecid on a weight basis. It is of no value in treating an acute attack of gouty arthritis.

Because acute attacks of gout may increase in frequency or severity during the early months of therapy with sulfin-pyrazone, colchicine should be given concomitantly. An adequate fluid intake and alkalization of the urine should be maintained to minimize the renal deposition of urate during therapy until the serum urate level is within the normal range. The drug should be used with caution in patients with impaired renal function or a history of renal calculi, especially uric acid stones, because of the possibility of aggravating the condition.

The most frequently reported adverse reactions are abdominal pain and nausea. Since reactivation or exacerbation of peptic ulcer also has been reported, sulfin-pyrazone should be used cautiously in patients with a history of ulcer and is contraindicated in patients with active peptic ulcer. Rash is uncommon; anemia, leukopenia, agranulocytosis, and thrombocytopenia have occurred rarely.

Since sulfinpyrazone inhibits platelet functions, it has been studied as an anti-thrombotic agent. Although the results of some studies have indicated that the drug has a beneficial effect in certain conditions, the evidence from other studies is inconclusive; thus, additional studies are needed to determine the usefulness of sulfin-pyrazone in various thrombotic disorders (see Chapter 63, Anticoagulants and Thrombolytics).

Sulfinpyrazone is rapidly and completely absorbed following oral administration; peak blood levels occur in about one hour and the half- life is one to three hours. It is highly bound to plasma protein. Most of the drug is excreted unchanged in urine; the remainder is metabolized to the parahydroxyl analogue which also has a uricosuric action.

Like probenecid, sulfinpyrazone reduces the renal tubular excretion of p-aminohippuric acid, phenolsulfon-phthalein, and salicylic acid; therefore, diagnostic procedures depending upon measurement of these substances are invalidated by therapy with this drug. Salicylates diminish the effect of sulfinpyrazone, and thus they should not be used concomitantly.

Like phenylbutazone and oxyphenbuta-zone, sulfinpyrazone may potentiate the actions of insulin and oral hypoglycemic agents; therefore, it should be used with caution in patients receiving these drugs. Because of its chemical relationship to phenylbutazone and oxyphenbutazone and the similarity of some adverse effects, sulfinpyrazone should be used cautiously, if at all, in patients known to be sensitive to these drugs; however, serious reactions are less common than with the other two drugs. Sulfinpyrazone has no effect on sodium reabsorption.

ROUTE, USUAL DOSAGE, AND PREPARATIONS. *Oral*: *Adults*, 100 to 200 mg two times daily given with meals or with milk at bedtime. The dose is gradually increased over a one-week period until the dosage (400 to 800 mg daily) required to control blood urate levels is reached. The dose then may be reduced to the minimal effective level; the maintenance dose may be 300 to 400 mg daily given in two divided doses.

Anturane (Ciba). Capsules 200 mg; tablets 100 mg.

TICRYNAFEN
[Selacryn]

Ticrynafen is a uricosuric drug that has been shown to reduce the serum uric acid concentration in patients with hyperuricemia with or without symptoms of gout. The drug also has diuretic and antihypertensive activities (see Chapter 38, Antihypertensive Agents, and Chapter 39, Diuretics). In comparison with probenecid, ticrynafen is more potent on a milligram basis and produces a slightly greater hypouricemic effect. As with other uricosuric agents, ticrynafen may precipitate an attack of acute gout during treatment; thus, colchicine should be used concomitantly for prophylaxis.

The uricosuric activity of ticrynafen is caused by an inhibition of urate resorption in the proximal tubule. It does not inhibit xanthine oxidase or interfere with purine metabolism. Because of its diuretic activity, the formation of renal calculi is minimal with use of ticrynafen.

Like probenecid, ticrynafen decreases the excretion of penicillin, thereby increasing the blood level of the antibiotic. As with other uricosuric drugs, salicylates inhibit the uricosuric action of ticrynafen.

For adverse reactions and precautions, see Chapter 38, Antihypertensive Agents, and Chapter 39, Diuretics.

ADDENDUM: There have been several recent reports of acute renal failure in patients receiving ticrynafen (Selacryn [Smith Kline & French]). Several deaths from hepatic toxicity have also been reported, and the drug was voluntarily removed from the market in January, 1980.

MIXTURE

COLBENEMID

This mixture of probenecid and colchicine is designed to facilitate maintenance therapy of chronic gout, but its usefulness is limited because the amount of each ingredient cannot be individualized. If the usual dosage of probenecid were used, this mixture would provide a greater amount of colchicine than needed by many patients and less than that needed by some.

For adverse reactions and precautions, see the evaluations on Colchicine and Probenecid.

ROUTE, USUAL DOSAGE, AND PREPARATIONS. The dosage is based upon the patient's requirement for the individual ingredients, provided that these have been established individually and are consistent with the ratio present in this preparation. (See the evaluations on Probenecid and Colchicine.)

Mixture available generically: Each tablet contains probenecid 500 mg and colchicine 0.5 mg. *ColBENEMID* (Merck Sharp & Dohme). Each tablet contains probenecid 500 mg and colchicine 0.5 mg.

Selected References

Emmerson BT: Drug control of gout and hyperuricemia. *Drugs* 16:158-166, 1978.

Kelley WN: Current therapy of gout and hyperuricemia. *Hosp Pract* 11:69-76, (May) 1976.

Kelley WN: Effects of drugs on uric acid in man. *Annu Rev Pharmacol Toxicol* 15:327-350, 1975.

Klinenberg JR: Hyperuricemia and gout. *Med Clin North Am* 61:299-312, 1977.

Klinenberg JR (ed): Proceedings of second conference on gout and purine metabolism. *Arthritis Rheum* 18(suppl):659-888, 1975.

Schumacher HR: Gouty arthritis. *Contin Educat Fam Physician* 5:66-71, (Nov) 1976.

Talbott JR, Yu TF: *Gout and Uric Acid Metabolism.* New York, Stratton Intercontinental, 1976.

Wallace SL: Colchicine. *Semin Arthritis Rheum* 3:369-381, 1974.

Wallace SL, et al: Preliminary criteria for classification of acute arthritis of primary gout. *Arthritis Rheum* 20:895-900, 1977.

Wyngaarden JB, Kelley WN: *Gout and Hyperuricemia.* New York, Grune & Stratton, 1976.

Yu TF: Milestones in treatment of gout. *Am J Med* 56:676-685, 1974.

Drugs Used to Treat Migraine and Other Headaches | 9

VASCULAR HEADACHE OF THE MIGRAINE TYPE

Abortive Therapy

Preventive Therapy

MUSCLE-CONTRACTION HEADACHE

INDIVIDUAL EVALUATIONS

MIXTURES

Except for fatigue, headache is the most common symptom experienced by man; however, most headaches occur infrequently and are acute and short-lived. Causative factors include emotional stress (ie, environmental, situational, personality problems); fatigue; chemical sensitivity to certain foods and beverages, including alcohol; medications; and acute illness. Headache also may have no apparent underlying cause. Usually this common type can be treated by self-medication with over-the-counter preparations containing aspirin or acetaminophen and, once relieved, is unlikely to recur.

In contrast, chronic recurrent headache, which may be associated with various medical, neurologic, or psychogenic disorders, is the most common symptom for which patients see physicians. Appropriate therapy depends upon an accurate diagnosis and classification of the type of headache. Several classifications have been proposed, but the principal categories are: (1) vascular headaches of the migraine type, (2) muscle-contraction (tension) headaches, and (3) headaches caused by an underlying disease.

Drugs used in the treatment of the first two classes are considered in this chapter. For those in the third category, the cause should be determined, if possible, and eliminated or treated. This class includes headaches associated with intracranial disturbances (eg, vascular anomalies, tumors, trauma), systemic diseases (eg, allergies; infections; cervical osteoarthritis; disorders of eye, ear, nose, throat), and cranial (eg, trigeminal) neuralgia. Since many of these conditions are serious or even life-threatening, accurate diagnosis is especially important to determine appropriate therapy. The headache usually can be relieved by specific therapy for the underlying disease or organic cause. Surgical correction may be necessary for certain conditions, such as mass lesions, but specific drugs are indicated for others: antibiotics for infections, antirheumatic drugs for osteoarthritis, carbamazepine for trigeminal neuralgia.

Vascular Headache of the Migraine Type

A relatively small percentage of patients with headache have this type, although other conditions may simulate migraine (eg, vascular malformations, aneurysm, temporal arteritis, glaucoma).

Migraine is characterized by recurrent attacks of pain that often is unilateral with associated anorexia and, occasionally, nausea and vomiting. Prodromal aura (visual, sensory, motor, or any combination) are sharply defined in "classic" migraine but may be absent or vague in "common" migraine; the actual headache episode of the latter type frequently persists longer (many hours to days) than that of the classic type. Muscle contraction pain also may occur with a migraine attack.

Another form of vascular headache, termed cluster headache (also called Horton's syndrome, histamine cephalalgia, facial migraine, and migrainous neuralgia), is characterized by brief (30 to 40 minutes), severe, sharp, stabbing frontal and periorbital pain occurring in a series or "cluster" of closely spaced attacks, often at night. Associated signs are conjunctival injection, lacrimation, nasal congestion, facial blanching or flushing, and, occasionally, ptosis and miosis on the side of the pain. "Clusters" generally last 4 to 12 weeks, with intervals of weeks, months, or years between recurrences.

Other less common variants of migraine include hemiplegic, ophthalmoplegic, aphasic, confusional, and hemianopic migraine. In some of these episodes, sensorimotor phenomena persist during and after the headache period.

Although the cause and exact mechanism of a migraine attack have not been determined, the pain has been thought to be of vascular origin. Results of direct measurements of cerebral blood flow suggest the following possible sequence of events: First, a phase of vasoconstriction involving the intracranial arteries with a reduction of blood flow of sufficient degree to produce the initial symptoms, followed by ischemic changes associated with the prodrome of the attack, and a second phase of vasodilatation, primarily of the extracranial arteries, during which the headache occurs. However, since vasodilatation itself is not usually uncomfortable, it has been suggested that mediators of inflammation or vasoactive materials might be elaborated around the pain-dilated arteries that characterize migraine. The direct assessment of the roles of vasoactive materials in patients with migraine is difficult. Studies suggest that the dilated migrainous arteries are hyperpermeable and are involved in a sterile, local inflammatory reaction in which vasoactive substances and platelets participate. The vascular permeability may be influenced by release of vasoactive substances from their reservoirs in the circulation or from tissue sites. Present evidence implicates at least five and possibly more groups of vasoactive substances associated with arterial inflammation and increased permeability, including the catecholamines; other bioactive amines (histamine, tyramine, serotonin); polypeptides (bradykinin and angiotensin); free fatty acids and prostaglandins; and gamma-aminobutyric acid, an inhibitory transmitter.

The management of migraine should combine medical and nonmedical therapy, including the control or elimination, if possible, of underlying factors that precipitate an attack. The pharmacotherapy of migraine consists of symptomatic treatment of the acute attack (abortive) and interval (preventive) therapy to reduce the frequency and severity of the headaches.

Abortive Therapy: A mild analgesic (eg, aspirin, acetaminophen) may provide nonspecific symptomatic relief in mild attacks; strong analgesics (eg, meperidine [Demerol], pentazocine [Talwin]) should be given only when essential because of their potential for abuse and dependence. Some fixed combinations containing sedatives and analgesics are widely prescribed, but they are not specific for migraine. Although they may be helpful in some patients, they should be used carefully because the dose of each ingredient cannot be individualized. Furthermore, since these mixtures are used most commonly by patients with chronic, recurring headaches (who are most liable to abuse sedatives and analgesics), separate prescription, with precautions to prevent abuse, is preferred.

Ergotamine tartrate [Ergomar, Ergostat, Gynergen] is the most effective specific drug for terminating acute attacks and should be administered in adequate dosage early in the attack. It can be given by inhalation, sublingually, parenterally, orally, or rectally (in combination products). It has been shown that absorption of aspirin after oral administration is delayed during an acute attack; since ergotamine may be affected similarly, the most rapidly absorbed form should be administered for optimum effect. Relief after intramuscular injection of 0.5 mg is almost conclusive evidence that the headache is of migrainous origin.

Ergotamine causes peripheral vasoconstriction, especially in the dilated external carotid artery bed. It acts as a vasoconstrictor if the tonus of the vessel is low and as a vasodilator if the tonus is high. In therapeutic doses, ergotamine does not act as an adrenergic blocking agent but potentiates epinephrine and norepinephrine and inhibits the reuptake of these amines after nerve stimulation; thus, a high level of norepinephrine is maintained.

A number of combination products, most of which contain ergotamine tartrate and caffeine and, often, one or more other agents (eg, belladonna alkaloids, sedatives, analgesics) are available. Caffeine, which probably acts as a cerebral vasoconstrictor, is reported to increase absorption of ergotamine, thereby enhancing its effect during the acute attack and permitting use of smaller doses. The belladonna alkaloids are claimed to assist in allaying nausea and vomiting. During the acute attack, sedatives or antianxiety agents may reduce apprehension and reaction to pain and permit sleep. Antiemetics may alleviate nausea and vomiting.

Dihydroergotamine mesylate [D.H.E. 45] also may be given intramuscularly or intravenously; however, its vasoconstrictor action is less pronounced than that of ergotamine and fewer patients respond to it than to ergotamine. Another vasoconstrictor, isometheptene, has been shown to be effective in acute attacks of migraine. It is available only in a combination product (see the section on Mixtures).

The cataclysmic attacks of cluster headaches may be prevented or alleviated by ergotamine preparations, but parenteral or sublingual administration may be required. If attacks occur regularly, ergotamine taken about one hour before an attack is expected may prevent it. Methysergide also may be an effective prophylactic agent. Although corticosteroids have been effective in some patients, headaches recur when this type of drug is discontinued; thus, the risk of long-term steroid therapy does not appear to be justified. It has been reported that the headache can be aborted by inhalation of flowing oxygen (10 L/min in a rebreathing bag mask). Lithium carbonate has been reported to be an effective prophylactic agent for cluster headaches in a limited number of patients. Additional studies are needed to establish its usefulness in this type of headache. For a discussion on other uses and adverse reactions of lithium, see Chapter 13, Drugs Used in Affective Disorders.

Preventive Therapy: Since spontaneous remissions occur, prolonged uninterrupted prophylactic therapy is not advisable. Methysergide [Sansert] is one of the most effective agents for the prophylactic treatment of migraine, but its use must be interrupted after six months to avoid adverse reactions. Its efficacy probably results from the ability to simulate serotonin in maintaining vasoconstriction of scalp arteries. In addition, methysergide inhibits the release of prostaglandins induced by serotonin. It is not effective in the treatment of an acute attack.

The beta-adrenergic blocking agent, propranolol [Inderal], is also useful as a prophylactic agent, especially in patients who cannot take methysergide. Its mechanism of action is not known, but it has been suggested that propranolol prevents vasodilatation and platelet aggregation. Another beta blocker, alprenolol, which is more potent than propranolol, has had little or no effect in reducing the frequency of migraine headache attacks.

Although maintenance doses of ergotamine, alone and in combination products, have been administered for the prophylaxis of migraine, this is generally not advisable because of the drug's potent peripheral vasoconstrictor action, which may produce arterial insufficiency, and because dependence may result from prolonged daily use.

Many other agents have been tried in the prophylaxis of migraine, but none have been more effective than methysergide, although most have produced fewer or less severe adverse reactions.

The monoamine oxidase inhibitors (eg, phenelzine [Nardil], isocarboxazid [Marplan]) increase endogenous serotonin levels and have been beneficial in some patients refractory to other treatment; however, because the response is variable and the adverse effects are potentially severe, these agents are seldom used.

Patients with migraine may also respond to a tricyclic antidepressant. Studies with amitriptyline [Elavil] have shown that the benefit may not be related to the presence of depression. Further controlled studies are necessary to establish the usefulness of these agents in migraine. (See Chapter 13, Drugs Used in Affective Disorders.) Antianxiety agents may be used for short-term prophylaxis to improve the patient's ability to deal with stress.

Cyproheptadine [Periactin], which is a serotonin and histamine antagonist, has been reported to be effective in some patients, but results of controlled studies have demonstrated that it is only slightly better than a placebo. A related compound, pizotyline, which is not available in the United States, also appears to be less effective than methysergide, but it is less toxic. Clonidine [Catapres], an antihypertensive agent, has been tried in the prophylaxis of migraine because it blocks central vasomotor reflexes, which decreases vascular reactivity to both dilator and constrictor stimuli. Results of several studies indicate that it is not uniformly beneficial and additional controlled studies are required to establish whether clonidine is more effective than a placebo.

Among other agents suggested for prophylaxis of migraine, but which have minimal evidence of efficacy, are progestational agents, papaverine, and diuretics, as well as desensitization with histamine.

Muscle-Contraction Headache

The largest percentage (about 90%) of headaches which are described to physicians are muscle-contraction headache. Although this type of headache often is also called tension headache because its occurrence is frequently related to anxiety, such classification is ambiguous in that it may refer either to psychic tension or muscle tension. In addition, it is also classified as psychogenic, which some authors subdivide into tension (anxiety) and depressive; others define psychogenic to include conversion, delusional, and hypochondriacal headaches. Because of the confusion resulting from these various designations, it has been proposed that the use of psychogenic be restricted to headaches without a peripheral pain-inducing mechanism. Although purely psychogenic headache is rare, it is recognized that psychogenic factors may play an important role in various types of headaches.

Certain underlying disorders of muscles or joints (inflammation or infection of the muscles of the head and neck, cervical osteoarthritis, disorders of the temporal-mandibular joint) also are causes of muscle-contraction headache. As with headache in the third primary category, treatment or correction of these underlying conditions is important in the management of these headaches.

If a muscle-contraction headache is of low intensity and occurs only occasionally, a nonopiate analgesic (eg, aspirin, acetaminophen) may be effective. If headaches are more severe and recur at frequent intervals, more potent analgesics may be required; however, if anxiety is a factor, an antianxiety agent (eg, diazepam [Valium]) in addition to an analgesic may be more effective. Certain combination products containing a barbiturate (eg, Fiorinal) or other sedatives (eg, meprobamate) are also effective in this type of headache, but caution must be taken to prevent their abuse. (See also Chapter 6, General Analgesics.)

Many patients with headache have associated depressive reactions, the headache representing a somatization. This type of headache usually has occurred for many years, is often worse in the morning than evening, is generalized rather than localized, and is accompanied by scalp formication and associated with symptoms common in depression, such as sleep disturbances with early and frequent awakening. The antidepressants may be more effective than the common analgesics if such symptoms are present. However, some clinicians believe that antidepressants are effective in chronic muscle-contraction headache independent of the presence of depression. The nighttime dose may be sufficient to relieve both sleeping problems and headache. See also Chapter 13, Drugs Used in Affective Disorders. Psychotherapy also may be necessary as an adjunct to drug therapy for some patients.

INDIVIDUAL EVALUATIONS

ERGOTAMINE TARTRATE
[Ergomar, Ergostat, Gynergen]

Ergotamine, which acts by constricting dilated cranial blood vessels, is the drug of choice in the treatment of acute attacks of migraine. To be most effective, adequate doses must be administered soon after the onset of headache. The dosage should be titrated for each patient to determine an appropriate amount for subsequent attacks. The drug is most rapidly effective when given parenterally, but may be given sublingually or by inhalation; it is poorly absorbed when given orally.

The long-term prophylactic use of ergotamine is generally considered inadvisable because of its potential adverse reactions. However, patients who have daily attacks of cluster headaches may be given the drug for 10 to 14 days to help terminate a bout.

Large doses of ergotamine produce nausea, vomiting, epigastric discomfort, diarrhea, paresthesias of the extremities, cramps and weakness of the legs, myalgia (eg, stiffness of thigh and neck muscles), angina-like precordial pain and distress, transient sinus tachycardia and bradycardia, and, in sensitive patients, localized edema and pruritus. Severe vasoconstriction and endarteritis may occur after long-term, uninterrupted use of ergotamine. Gangrene of the extremities is rare when this agent is given in usual doses in the absence of peripheral vascular disease and other contraindications. Patients taking ergotamine daily for prolonged periods may become dependent on the drug, and an increased dose may be necessary to achieve relief. This may result in a rebound reaction of constriction, vasodilation, and headache. Ergotamine should be discontinued gradually with appropriate treatment of accompanying conditions such as depression, which is common in patients with migraine.

Ergotamine is contraindicated in patients with peripheral vascular disease (eg, Raynaud's disease, thromboangiitis obliterans, thrombophlebitis, marked arteriosclerosis), severe hypertension, ischemic heart disease or a history of anginal pain after exertion, peptic ulcer, renal or hepatic disease, malnutrition, or a history of hypersensitivity to ergot preparations. It should not be used in the presence of infections. Since ergotamine has oxytocic properties, it should not be given to pregnant women.

ROUTES, USUAL DOSAGE, AND PREPARATIONS.
Oral: *Adults*, 1 to 2 mg at onset of attack, followed by 1 to 2 mg every 30 minutes (maximum, 6 mg in 24 hours and 10 mg in one week). For cluster headache, *adults*, 1 to 2 mg at bedtime for 10 to 14 days.
Gynergen (Sandoz). Tablets 1 mg.
Inhalation: *Adults*, single inhalation (0.36 mg) at onset of attack, repeated if necessary at intervals of no less than five minutes to a

total of six inhalations in 24 hours (maximum, 12 mg in one week). It is advisable to monitor patients for compliance, and overdosage should be carefully avoided. The risk of provoking bronchospasm in asthmatic patients should be kept in mind when ergotamine is administered by this route.

> *Medihaler-Ergotamine* (Riker). Solution 9 mg/ml in 2.5 ml containers. Each dose (a single inhalation) contains approximately 0.36 mg of ergotamine tartrate.

Subcutaneous, Intramuscular: *Adults*, 0.25 to 0.5 mg at onset of attack, repeated in 40 minutes, if necessary; no more than 1 mg should be given within a one-week period. If the optimal dose has been determined previously, that amount can be given initially.

> *Gynergen* (Sandoz). Solution 0.5 mg/ml in 0.5 and 1 ml containers.

Sublingual: *Adults*, 2 mg at onset of attack, followed by 2 mg every 30 minutes if necessary (maximum, 6 mg in 24 hours and 10 mg in one week).

> *Ergomar* (Fisons), *Ergostat* (Parke, Davis). Tablets 2 mg.

Intravenous: *Adults*, 0.25 mg initially; no more than 0.5 mg should be given in 24 hours. Use of this route is rarely indicated.

> *Gynergen* (Sandoz). Solution 0.5 mg/ml in 0.5 and 1 ml containers.

DIHYDROERGOTAMINE MESYLATE
[D.H.E. 45]

This preparation is given intramuscularly or intravenously to relieve acute migraine. Although the incidence of gastrointestinal reactions appears to be less than with parenteral forms of ergotamine, the vasoconstrictor effect of dihydroergotamine is less pronounced and a smaller percentage of patients respond to this agent.

For adverse reactions and precautions, see the evaluation on Ergotamine Tartrate.

ROUTES, USUAL DOSAGE, AND PREPARATIONS. *Intramuscular*: *Adults*, 1 mg at onset of attack, repeated if necessary at hourly intervals up to a total of 3 mg. *Intravenous*: For rapid effect, *adults*, 1 mg, repeated if necessary once after one hour. The total dosage should not exceed 2 mg.

> *D.H.E. 45* (Sandoz). Solution 1 mg/ml in 1 ml containers.

METHYSERGIDE MALEATE
[Sansert]

This agent is related chemically to the oxytocic ergot alkaloid derivative, methylergonovine. It is effective as a prophylactic agent in the management of migraine and cluster headaches and is indicated in patients whose vascular headaches are of sufficient frequency and severity to warrant prophylactic therapy. This drug is of no value in treating acute attacks or in preventing or treating muscle contraction-type headaches. Although methysergide is a serotonin antagonist, it may simulate serotonin in constricting scalp arteries. In addition, it potentiates the vasoconstrictor effects of catecholamines and interferes with central vasomotor reflexes; it also inhibits the release of prostaglandins stimulated by serotonin. However, the exact mechanism of action of this agent in preventing migraine has not been definitely established.

ADVERSE REACTIONS AND PRECAUTIONS.

Adverse reactions associated with use of methysergide occur with moderate frequency. Many are mild and disappear with continued use of the drug, but serious reactions necessitate discontinuance of therapy.

Among the serious but uncommon adverse reactions are fibrotic changes in retroperitoneal, pleuropulmonary, and cardiac tissues that may occur with long-term, uninterrupted administration. Retroperitoneal fibrosis may cause obstruction of the urinary tract. Early clinical manifestations are flank pain and dysuria; typical deviation and obstruction of one or both ureters may be demonstrated by intravenous pyelography. Vascular insufficiency of the lower limbs with pain, edema, muscular atrophy, and thrombophlebitis caused by involvement of the aorta, vena cava, and common iliac vessels also may occur.

Usual signs of pleuropulmonary fibrosis are dyspnea, chest pain, and pleural friction rubs or effusion. Murmurs and dyspnea are signs of fibrosis of the aortic and mitral valves and of the root of the aorta.

Administration of methysergide should be discontinued if signs of retroperitoneal, pleuropulmonary, or cardiac fibrosis are noted. Partial and even complete regression of the process may take place after the drug has been discontinued, but surgical treatment may be necessary. Incompetent valves may have to be replaced.

Methysergide, like other ergot derivatives, has vasoconstrictor properties and may cause vascular insufficiency. Angina-like pain has been precipitated or increased. Symptoms of peripheral vascular insufficiency include cold, numb, painful extremities with or without paresthesias and diminished or absent pulse. If these symptoms occur, the drug should be discontinued to prevent severe tissue ischemia.

Methysergide is related chemically to lysergic acid diethylamide (LSD) and may act as a central nervous system stimulant, but it is not psychotomimetic in the usual dosage range. Central nervous system reactions include insomnia, nervousness, euphoria, dizziness, ataxia, rapid speech, difficulty in thinking, feeling of depersonalization, nightmares, and hallucinations. Drowsiness, lethargy, loss of initiative, and mental depression also have been reported.

Gastrointestinal reactions (eg, nausea, vomiting, diarrhea, abdominal pain) are common during early therapy. Administration of methysergide to patients with peptic ulcer has caused pronounced elevations in gastric hydrochloric acid levels. Other adverse reactions include dermatitis, alopecia, peripheral and localized edema, weight gain, arthralgia, and myalgia. Neutropenia and eosinophilia have occurred rarely.

Patients should be seen frequently during therapy with methysergide, and they should be instructed to report symptoms such as chest pain, leg cramps, peripheral edema of ankles or hands, change in skin color, or paresthesias in the extremities. These symptoms can be properly evaluated by careful examination of the blood supply to the extremities, thereby avoiding dangerous sequelae. However, retroperitoneal fibrosis can develop without symptoms or positive results from laboratory studies. Therefore, it is recommended that a urogram be performed initially in all patients who respond favorably to methysergide during a short trial period and who may be candidates for long-term therapy. Urography should then be performed every 6 to 12 months for as long as the patient is taking methysergide to avoid the possible development of a disabling urinary tract disorder.

Contraindications are the same as for ergotamine (see the evaluation). In addition, methysergide should not be used in patients with pulmonary disease, valvular heart disease, rheumatoid arthritis or other collagen diseases, and conditions that tend to progress to fibrosis.

Methysergide should not be used continuously for more than six months without imposing a reasonable drug-free period (three to four weeks). However, the dosage should be reduced gradually during the two to three weeks preceding discontinuation of the drug in order to avoid rebound headache.

ROUTE, USUAL DOSAGE, AND PREPARATIONS. *Oral: Adults,* 4 to 6 mg daily in divided doses, taken with food. The maximal recommended daily dose of 6 mg is smaller

than that suggested by the manufacturer.
Sansert (Sandoz). Tablets 2 mg.

PROPRANOLOL HYDROCHLORIDE
[Inderal]

This beta-adrenergic blocking agent is effective for the prophylaxis of migraine in 50% to 80% of patients. It may be particularly useful in those with frequent attacks who do not respond to or tolerate other agents or who are likely to abuse ergot derivatives or narcotics.

Propranolol is generally well tolerated. Nausea, lightheadedness, fatigue, insomnia, and diarrhea have been reported occasionally. Rarely, mild degrees of mental dulling may occur. It also reduces the heart rate and blood pressure. This drug should not be used in patients with asthma, congestive heart failure, or atrioventricular conduction disturbances.

For a discussion of other uses, adverse reactions, and precautions, see Chapter 35, Antianginal Agents.

ROUTE, USUAL DOSAGE, AND PREPARATIONS. *Oral*: Since therapeutic doses vary widely (160 to 240 mg daily), the dosage must be individualized. Therapy should be started with small doses, usually 20 to 40 mg per day, and increased gradually until a therapeutic effect is observed or adverse reactions occur. Propranolol should be discontinued gradually over a period of two weeks, for abrupt withdrawal may precipitate angina pectoris.

Inderal (Ayerst). Tablets 10, 20, 40, and 80 mg.

MIXTURES

MIXTURES CONTAINING ERGOTAMINE

Several mixtures contain ergotamine tartrate and caffeine and are promoted for relief of the symptoms of migraine headache. Clinical experience and some comparative trials indicate that caffeine increases the effectiveness of ergotamine. Caffeine originally was thought to act as a cranial vasoconstrictor to enhance that action of ergotamine, but recent studies indicate that probably its principal action is to increase the enteral absorption of ergotamine, which is normally poorly absorbed.

A similar enhanced effect appears to occur with rectal administration of the mixture.

In addition to ergotamine and caffeine, some fixed-dose combinations contain other ingredients such as cyclizine, belladonna alkaloids, pentobarbital, or phenacetin. The belladonna alkaloids and cyclizine are claimed to assist in allaying the nausea and vomiting that often accompany a migraine attack or are produced by ergotamine. Although use of a sedative or mild analgesic is beneficial in some patients with migraine, a fixed-dose combination does not permit adjustment of the dose to suit the needs of the patient; thus, it is preferable to prescribe the sedative or analgesic separately.

If a patient cannot tolerate ergotamine orally, a rectal preparation may be tried. (A rectal product containing ergotamine alone is not available.) The rectal route is very fast and effective.

Bellergal contains ergotamine tartrate, belladonna alkaloids, and phenobarbital and is promoted for the preventive treatment of recurrent, throbbing headache. It is not indicated for the treatment of an acute attack of migraine, because the amount of ergotamine in Bellergal is lower than that used to treat migraine. The use of this product is largely empirical and is based on clinical experience. Most authorities believe that it is inadvisable to use ergot preparations continuously over a prolonged period because of their peripheral vasoconstrictor action; however, some specialists treating vascular headaches consider the likelihood of complications a remote possibility in the absence of contraindications. Since the preparation contains a barbiturate, there is potential for abuse with prolonged administration.

Adverse reactions and precautions are those of the ingredients. See also the evaluation on Ergotamine Tartrate.

ROUTES, USUAL DOSAGE, AND PREPARATIONS. CAFERGOT, WIGRAINE:

Oral: Adults, two tablets at the onset of an attack. An additional tablet may be taken every 30 minutes if needed, but the amount generally should be limited to a total of six tablets per attack or no more than 10 tablets per week. *Children*, one-half to one tablet initially, followed by one-half tablet every 30 minutes if necessary (maximum, three tablets).

Mixture of ergotamine and caffeine available generically: Each tablet contains ergotamine tartrate 1 mg and caffeine 100 or 199 mg.
Cafergot (Sandoz). Each tablet contains ergotamine tartrate 1 mg and caffeine 100 mg.
Cafergot P-B (Sandoz). Each tablet contains ergotamine tartrate 1 mg, caffeine 100 mg, levorotatory belladonna alkaloids as malates 0.125 mg, and pentobarbital sodium 30 mg.
Wigraine (Organon). Each tablet contains ergotamine tartrate 1 mg, caffeine 100 mg, levorotatory belladonna alkaloids 0.1 mg, and phenacetin 130 mg.

Rectal: Adults, one-half to one suppository at the onset of an attack. Another suppository may be used in one hour if needed; the total amount should not exceed two suppositories per attack or no more than five suppositories per week.

Cafergot (Sandoz). Each suppository contains ergotamine tartrate 2 mg and caffeine 100 mg.
Cafergot P-B (Sandoz). Each suppository contains ergotamine tartrate 2 mg, caffeine 100 mg, levorotatory belladonna alkaloids as malates 0.25 mg, and pentobarbital 60 mg.
Wigraine (Organon). Each suppository contains ergotamine tartrate 1 mg, caffeine 100 mg, levorotatory belladonna alkaloids 0.1 mg, and phenacetin 130 mg.

BELLERGAL:

Oral: Adults, four tablets daily (one in the morning, one at noon, and two at bedtime) or two timed-release tablets daily (one in the morning and one in the evening).

Bellergal (Dorsey). Each tablet contains ergotamine tartrate 0.3 mg, phenobarbital 20 mg, and levorotatory belladonna alkaloids as malates 0.1 mg.
Bellergal-S (Dorsey). Each tablet (timed-release) contains ergotamine tartrate 0.6 mg,

phenobarbital 40 mg, and levorotatory belladonna alkaloids as malates 0.2 mg.

FIORINAL

This mixture of butalbital and APC is indicated to relieve the symptoms of muscle-contraction (tension) headache. The antianxiety effect of the barbiturate is claimed to supplement the analgesic activity of APC in this type of headache, and the results of some studies have indicated that this mixture gives greater relief of symptoms than the components given separately. However, since the fixed-dose combination does not permit adjustment of dose to suit the needs of the patient, it may be preferable to prescribe the sedative separately for some patients.

The most common adverse reactions are drowsiness and dizziness. Nausea, vomiting, and flatulence occur occasionally. Patients should be cautioned about driving or operating machinery when taking Fiorinal. Other central nervous system depressants taken concomitantly may produce an additive effect with the barbiturate. Precautions should be taken to prevent its abuse.

For other adverse reactions and precautions, see the evaluation on APC in Chapter 6, General Analgesics, and the discussion on barbiturates in Chapter 11, Drugs Used for Anxiety and Insomnia.

ROUTE, USUAL DOSAGE, AND PREPARATIONS. *Oral*: *Adults*, one or two tablets or capsules every four hours (maximum, six daily). Dosage for *children younger than 12 years* has not been established.

Fiorinal (Sandoz). Each capsule or tablet contains butalbital 50 mg, aspirin 200 mg, phenacetin 130 mg, and caffeine 40 mg.

MIDRIN

This mixture contains isometheptene mucate, a sympathomimetic agent; a sedative; and an analgesic. The proposed use of a sympathomimetic drug for the treatment of migraine attacks is based on the claim that this agent causes cranial and cerebral vasoconstriction; however, there is a paucity of data demonstrating this effect. The sedative and analgesic theoretically may provide symptomatic relief, but it is generally preferable to prescribe these types of agents individually. The results of a few controlled studies indicated that the combination was no more effective than isometheptene alone but was slightly better than acetaminophen or a placebo. It appears to be more effective for abortive than preventive treatment. Results of studies comparing this combination product to a mixture of ergotamine and caffeine have been inconsistent. Additional well-controlled comparative studies are necessary to establish the usefulness and comparative effectiveness of this preparation for the treatment of migraine attacks.

Adverse reactions reported include drowsiness, dizziness, feeling of weakness, and palpitations.

ROUTE, USUAL DOSAGE, AND PREPARATIONS.
Oral: Adults, two capsules at the onset of an attack, followed by one capsule every hour until pain is relieved (maximum, five capsules within a 12-hour period).

> *Midrin* (Carnrick). Each capsule contains isometheptene mucate 65 mg, dichloralphenazone 100 mg, and acetaminophen 325 mg.

Selected References

Bille B, et al: Prophylaxis of migraine in children. *Headache* 17:61-63, 1977.

Borgesen SV: Treatment of migraine with propranolol. *Postgrad Med J* 52(suppl 4):163-165, 1976.

Brogden RN, et al: Low-dose clonidine: Review of its therapeutic efficacy in migraine prophylaxis. *Drugs* 10:357-365, 1975.

Dalessio DJ: Mechanisms of headache. *Med Clin North Am* 62:429-442, 1978.

Diamond S: Treatment of migraine with isometheptene, acetaminophen, and dichloralphenazone combination: Double-blind, crossover trial. *Headache* 16:282-287, 1976.

Diamond S: Severe headaches: Understanding types and treatments. *Drug Ther* 5:81-98, (March) 1975.

Diamond S, Medina JL: Double blind study of propranolol for migraine prophylaxis. *Headache* 16:24-27, 1976.

Edmeads J: Cerebral blood flow in migraine. *Headache* 17:148-152, 1977.

Forssman B, et al: Propranolol for migraine prophylaxis. *Headache* 16:238-245, 1976.

Friedman AP: Clinical approach to patient with headache. *Med Clin North Am* 62:443-450, 1978.

Friedman AP: Migraine. *Med Clin North Am* 62:481-494, 1978.

Friedman AP: Migraine and other headaches: Pharmacologic treatment. *Drug Ther* 8:47-58, (Oct) 1978.

Friedman AP: Headache. *Postgrad Med* 53:172-178, (May) 1973.

Hokkanen E, et al: Toxic effects of ergotamine used for migraine. *Headache* 18:95-98, 1978.

Horrobin DF: Hypothesis: Prostaglandins and migraine. *Headache* 17:113-117, 1977.

Janks JF: Oxygen for cluster headaches. *JAMA* 239:191, 1978.

Kallanranta T, et al: Clonidine in migraine prophylaxis. *Headache* 17:169-172, 1977.

Martin MJ: Psychogenic factors in headache. *Med Clin North Am* 62:559-570, 1978.

Medina JL, Diamond S: Drug dependency in patients with chronic headaches. *Headache* 17:12-14, 1977.

Meier J, Schreier E: Human plasma levels of some anti-migraine drugs. *Headache* 16:96-104, 1976.

Rothner AD: Headaches in children: A review. *Headache* 18:169-175, 1978.

Ryan RE Sr, et al: Double blind study of clonidine and placebo for prophylactic treatment of migraine. *Headache* 15:202-206, 1975.

Saper JR: Migraine: I. Classification and pathogenesis. II. Treatment. *JAMA* 239:2380-2383, 2480-2484, 1978.

Saxena RP: Prophylaxis of migraine: Comparative trial of Midrid and Dixarit. *Clin Trials J* 15:132-135, 1978.

Wolff HG: *Headache and Other Head Pain*, ed 3. New York, Oxford University Press, 1972.

Ziegler DK: Tension headache. *Med Clin North Am* 62:495-505, 1978.

The drugs discussed in this chapter are generally more useful than general analgesics in the management of certain specific types of pain, such as that which occurs in central pain syndromes. Some of these syndromes are caused by diseases or injuries affecting portions of the nervous system (eg, tabes dorsalis, postherpetic neuralgia), but the etiology of others (eg, trigeminal neuralgia) remains unexplained. The evaluation of the efficacy of agents used in the treatment of these conditions is very difficult because of the natural history of the disease, the subjective nature of the pain, and the spontaneous remissions that sometimes occur.

Although many reports in the literature claim that a variety of agents are effective for the relief of central pains, only carbamazepine has been conclusively demonstrated to be efficacious in the treatment of trigeminal neuralgia and glossopharyngeal neuralgia. Results of several studies, mostly uncontrolled, have suggested that phenytoin is effective in trigeminal neuralgia, but, in comparison to carbamazepine, it appears to be considerably less efficacious.

In contrast to the episodic variety of some central pain syndromes, which are likely to respond to carbamazepine and phenytoin, constant central pains (eg, in postherpetic neuralgia) usually are not alleviated by these agents, although their trial may be justified. Tricyclic antidepressants (eg, amitriptyline, imipramine) have been reported to be effective in relieving pain of the constant type. Results of recent clinical trials have demonstrated that the combination of amitriptyline and fluphenazine may be effective in relieving the continuous pain of some of the central pain syndromes, particularly peripheral diabetic neuropathy (Davis, 1977). However, additional controlled studies are necessary to establish their role in the treatment of these conditions.

INDIVIDUAL EVALUATIONS

CARBAMAZEPINE
[Tegretol]

Carbamazepine is chemically related to the tricyclic antidepressant drugs, but it does not have the antidepressant activity of these agents. Its pharmacodynamic actions and clinical uses resemble those of phenytoin. Carbamazepine is the drug of choice for the treatment of trigeminal and glossopharyngeal neuralgia. Most patients obtain complete relief of pain within 24 to 72 hours and the effect usually continues as long as the drug is administered. If pain recurs when the drug is withdrawn, retreatment is effective. When a relapse occurs during therapy, relief may be regained by increasing the dose; if this is ineffective, the concomitant administration of phenytoin may be helpful. Some patients may require surgical treatment.

Carbamazepine is also effective in the treatment of the lightning pains of tabes dorsalis, although clinical experience with this use of the drug is more limited than in trigeminal neuralgia. It has been used to relieve pain in multiple sclerosis, acute idiopathic polyneuritis (Guillain-Barré syndrome), peripheral diabetic neuropathy, phantom limb, and post-traumatic paresthesia. This drug also has been reported to improve dystonic symptoms in children, reduce the attack rate of migraine, and eliminate intractable hiccups. Certain forms of epilepsy respond to treatment with carbamazepine (see Chapter 15, Anticonvulsants). In addition, the drug has been shown to have antiarrhythmic activity in animals and a potent antidiuretic effect.

It should be kept in mind that carbamazepine is not a general analgesic but is specific for certain types of pain; thus, it should not be used to treat trivial facial pain or minor pain at other sites. The adverse reactions that occur most commonly during early treatment are drowsiness, dizziness, lightheadedness, ataxia, nausea, and vomiting; these reactions usually subside spontaneously within a week or after a reduction in dose. Their occurrence may be minimized by initiating therapy at a low dose and increasing it gradually. Other neurologic reactions include confusion, headache, fatigue, blurred vision, transient diplopia and oculomotor disturbances, dysphasia, abnormal involuntary movements, peripheral neuritis and paresthesias, depression with agitation, talkativeness, nystagmus, and tinnitus.

Gastrointestinal reactions include gastric distress and abdominal pain, diarrhea, constipation, anorexia, dryness of the mouth, glossitis, and stomatitis.

Dermatologic reactions (pruritic and erythematous rashes, urticaria, Stevens-Johnson syndrome, photosensitivity, alterations in skin pigmentation, exfoliative dermatitis, alopecia, hyperhidrosis, erythema multiforme, erythema nodosum, and aggravation of systemic lupus erythematosus) occur occasionally; if they are severe, it may be necessary to discontinue the drug.

Hematopoietic reactions (leukopenia, agranulocytosis, eosinophilia, leukocytosis, purpura, aplastic anemia, and thrombocytopenia) occur rarely but may be serious. The aplastic anemia and thrombocytopenia may be fatal. Therefore, patients should be advised to discontinue the drug and notify their physician if signs of hematologic toxicity appear (eg, fever, sore throat, aphthous stomatitis, easy bruising, petechial or purpuric hemorrhage).

Cardiovascular, genitourinary, metabolic, hepatic, and miscellaneous reactions have been reported rarely. These include aggravation of hypertension or ischemic heart disease, hypotension, syncope, edema, congestive heart failure, recurrence of thrombophlebitis, urinary frequency, acute urinary retention, albuminuria, glycosuria, elevated blood urea nitrogen levels, microscopic deposits in the urine, impotence, cholestatic and hepatocellular jaundice, fever and chills, adenopathy or lymphadenopathy, myalgia and arthralgia, leg cramps, and conjunctivitis.

It is advisable to obtain pretreatment baseline values of blood and platelet counts, liver function, urinalysis, blood urea nitrogen, and ophthalmologic examination and to repeat these tests at regular intervals during treatment.

Although teratogenicity has not been reported clinically, some teratogenic effects were observed in studies in rats. Therefore, it is advisable to administer carbamazepine to pregnant women only when the benefits outweigh the potential risks. Also, because toxic effects have been reported in nursing rats, mothers taking the drug should not nurse their infants.

Since carbamazepine is chemically related to the tricyclic antidepressants, it should not be administered to patients who are sensitive to these compounds. The possibility of activating latent psychosis or, in elderly patients, of confusion or agitation also exists. Because interactions between tricyclic compounds and monoamine oxidase inhibitors may occur, the latter drugs should be discontinued at least 14 days before carbamazepine is given.

The absorption of carbamazepine from the gastrointestinal tract is slow and variable; reported peak serum concentrations have ranged from 2 to 18 hours. Plasma half-life values have also varied, but the best estimate is 14 to 16 hours. Steady state plasma concentrations are attained in 32 to 40 hours when the drug is given three times daily. Carbamazepine is metabolized in the liver to an epoxide and several other metabolites, which are excreted in the bile and urine. There is some evidence that carbamazepine may induce its own metabolism. The drug is highly bound to plasma albumin, but it is not displaced by acidic drugs as phenytoin is and it does not displace the latter; however, when added to a regimen with phenytoin, the serum concentration of phenytoin falls, probably as a result of enzyme induction.

ROUTE, USUAL DOSAGE, AND PREPARATIONS.
Oral: For trigeminal neuralgia, glossopharyngeal neuralgia, and pain of tabes dorsalis, *adults*, 200 mg to a maximum of 1.2 g daily; small doses should be used initially and increased gradually (eg, 100 mg twice on the first day, increased by increments of 100 mg every 12 hours until freedom from pain is achieved). A pain-free state usually can be maintained with 400 to 800 mg daily. The drug should always be administered at minimal effective doses and with meals. Since many individuals have spontaneous prolonged remissions every few months, occasionally an attempt should be made to discontinue therapy. Similar doses have been used for the treatment of other painful conditions discussed above.
For use in epilepsy, see Chapter 15, Anticonvulsants.
Tegretol (Geigy). Tablets 200 mg.

PHENYTOIN
[Dilantin]

PHENYTOIN SODIUM
[Dilantin]

Phenytoin is sometimes used in the treatment of trigeminal neuralgia, although it is less effective than carbamazepine. It may be tried in patients who do not respond to other treatment, and concomitant use with carbamazepine may be beneficial in some patients. Phenytoin has been reported to be effective in the treatment of several other pain syndromes (eg, peripheral neuralgia, phantom limb pain, Fabry's disease, thalamic pain, dysesthesia, postherpetic neuralgia), but adequate controlled studies to establish its usefulness in these conditions are lacking. One double-blind crossover study showed that phenytoin did not significantly improve symptoms of diabetic symmetric polyneuropathy.

The most common adverse reactions include nausea, dizziness, ataxia, dyspepsia, and nystagmus. Since relief of pain does not correlate with drug blood levels, dosage may be increased until pain is relieved or toxic effects occur. See Chapter 15, Anticonvulsants, for a more detailed discussion of adverse reactions.

ROUTE, USUAL DOSAGE, AND PREPARATIONS.
Oral: For trigeminal neuralgia, *adults*, 300 to 400 mg daily; the dose may be increased if necessary (Loeser, 1975, 1977).
PHENYTOIN:
Dilantin (Parke, Davis). Suspension 125 mg/5 ml.
PHENYTOIN SODIUM:
Drug available generically: Capsules 100 mg.
Dilantin [sodium] (Parke, Davis). Capsules 100 mg.

134

Selected References

Crill WE: Carbamazepine. *Ann Intern Med* 79:844-847, 1973.

Dalessio DJ: Chronic pain syndromes and disordered cortical inhibition: Effects of tricyclic compounds. *Dis Nerv Syst* 28:325-328, 1967.

Davis JL, et al: Peripheral diabetic neuropathy treated with amitriptyline and fluphenazine. *JAMA* 238:2291-2292, 1977.

Levy RH, et al: Pharmacokinetics of carbamazepine in normal man. *Clin Pharmacol Ther* 17:657-668, 1975.

Loeser JD: Management of tic douloureux. *Pain* 3:155-162, 1977.

Loeser JD: Central pains. *Clin Med* 82:24-26, (May) 1975.

Morselli PL, Frigeris A: Metabolism and pharmacokinetics of carbamazepine. *Drug Metab Rev* 4:97-113, 1975.

Penovich PE, Morgan JP: Carbamazepine: A review. *Drug Ther* 6:187-193, (Feb) 1976.

Saudek CD, et al: Phenytoin in treatment of diabetic symmetrical polyneuropathy. *Clin Pharmacol Ther* 22:196-199, 1977.

Walson P, et al: New uses for phenytoin. *JAMA* 233:1385-1389, 1975.

Drugs Used for Anxiety and Insomnia | 11

Anxiety: The cause of anxiety can be entirely intrapsychic or it can occur when distress is caused by generally unpleasant social or interpersonal interactions. Whether it is of endogenous or exogenous etiology, the response to similar distressing situations depends upon the individual and ranges from a feeling of uneasiness through increasingly restricted activities to a complete inability to cope. Psychological symptoms (eg, tension, nervousness, irritability, apprehension, insomnia, inadequacy, indecision) or physiologic signs (eg, tachycardia, tremor, sweating, nausea and anorexia, increased muscle tension) may predominate. If the stigma of anxiety is great and denial is present, the patient's complaints may be principally physiological.

Therapeutic management is based principally upon the type and degree of anxiety present. Uncomplicated anxiety is de-scribed as reactive or free-floating; in the former, the patient recognizes the etiology, whereas in the latter he does not. In reactive anxiety, considered by many physicians to be a variant of the normal reaction to distress, counseling in the physician's office is usually adequate, although antianxiety drugs may be useful adjunctively in severe forms to increase patient confidence and ability to alter behavior. Antianxiety drugs are used to treat the free-floating form; intermittent administration during periods of greatest anxiety is the most rational form of therapy. Patients receiving an antianxiety drug for an extended period of time require periodic follow-up or referral for psychological counseling, behavior modification, environmental alteration, and evaluation of drug efficacy and safety. The efficacy of their continuous use for more than four months has not been evaluated.

Anxiety often is associated with certain other mental disorders. Severe anxiety can occur as a component of phobic neuroses, which generally should be managed with psychological counseling, behavior modification, and the use of antidepressant drug therapy (see Chapter 13, Drugs Used in Affective Disorders). Anxiety occurring as a component of endogenous depression usually responds best to antidepressants, and antianxiety drugs are not necessary routinely. Agitation, which includes not only anxiety but also a marked increase in purposeless motor activity, is usually a component of severe depression or schizophrenia; therefore, antidepressant or antipsychotic drugs rather than antianxiety agents are generally indicated (see Chapters 12 and 13).

Antianxiety drugs are indicated when anxiety causes the patient genuine suffering and interferes with general functioning, job performance, or ability to relate to people. Since these drugs are subject to abuse and their misuse may hinder the development of personal coping strategies or the effective mobilization of social support systems in the family or community, as well as obscure the source of the anxiety, restraint may be necessary in prescribing antianxiety agents. Recent surveys have examined the use of these and other psychotherapeutic medications for psychic distress and life crises (Balter et al, 1974; Mellinger et al, 1978).

Insomnia: Insomnia is the most common sleep disorder. Extensive clinical investigations in sleep laboratories have established that insomnia of any etiology is characterized by difficulty in falling asleep, remaining asleep, early morning final awakening, or a combination of these. The patient's subjective estimate of the inadequacy of his sleep does not always correlate with objectively observed deviations from normal sleep time or electroencephalographic criteria of insomnia. A shortened total sleep time, which occurs with aging, is not considered pathologic.

Transient or situational insomnia is a universal but highly individualized phenomenon; almost everyone has experienced insomnia at one time or another (Soldatos et al, 1979). Transient sleep difficulties may be caused by stresses created in response to the loss of a loved one, job pressures, concerns regarding examinations and anticipation, or reaction to life changes such as marriage or divorce; environmental factors such as overcrowding, excessive noise, and poor bedding or housing conditions; physical restrictions or lack of physical activity; nightshift work and traveling across time zones (jet lag), which are upsetting to internal biological rhythms; and the use of certain drugs (eg, amphetamines, caffeine) or withdrawal of some drugs (eg, alcohol, nicotine).

Insomnia often accompanies medical disorders that are characterized by pain, dyspnea, physical discomfort, fear, anxiety, or depression. Both physical and emotional factors must be considered when insomnia is associated with medical conditions, since there is always an emotional response to a disease process. Medical conditions in which pain and discomfort are primary contributing factors include arthritis, neurogenic pain, various types of headache, and the restless legs syndrome. The pain experienced during the day in these conditions may be greatly magnified when the patient attempts to sleep; there is a decrease in environmental stimuli and consequently more attention is focused internally. In patients with malignancies, in addition to pain being a significant factor, fear and anxiety over the ultimate consequences of their illness are often overwhelming. Patients with angina pectoris and/or cardiac arrhythmias often experience a fear of going to sleep because of a possible attack during the night when they feel most vulnerable and helpless.

Alterations in environment and daily activities (eg, elimination of caffeine-containing beverages, avoidance of strenuous exercise three to four hours before bedtime), behavior modification, relaxation techniques, and psychological counseling obviate the need for drug therapy in many instances.

If drug therapy is indicated, the choice of agent depends principally upon the etiology of the sleeplessness (Hartmann, 1977; Greenblatt and Miller, 1979). If anxiety is the principal cause of insomnia, the bedtime use of a drug that has a high antianxiety/sedation potency ratio may be most appropriate. In some patients, analgesics or sedating antidepressants may be drugs of choice. Thus, the need for a hypnotic should be less frequent if the cause of insomnia is identified and the appropriate management program implemented. Hypnotic drugs are contraindicated in patients who have a suspected diagnosis of sleep apnea.

Sleep laboratory studies have demonstrated that hypnotic doses of most of these agents reduce the amount of time spent in REM (rapid eye movement) sleep, and a number of hypnotics, especially the benzodiazepines, reduce stage IV sleep. The clinical significance of the alteration of any sleep stage is unknown and has yet to be linked to alterations in human behavior.

Withdrawal of most hypnotic drugs can be accompanied by a marked worsening of sleep difficulty. When chronically administered barbiturates are withdrawn abruptly, a disturbance of sleep-dream patterns (REM rebound) also ensues which may disrupt sleep (Kales et al, 1974). Furthermore, an intense degree of insomnia (rebound insomnia) may follow the abrupt withdrawal of benzodiazepines with shorter half-lives than diazepam or flurazepam, even after their use for only a few nights (Kales et al, 1979). However, the rebound insomnia produced by the shorter-acting compounds may be preferable in outpatients compared to flurazepam-induced impairment of daytime skills that require mental alertness and concentration or manual dexterity (Gillin et al, 1979).

The nonbenzodiazepine, nonbarbiturate hypnotics have effects on sleep patterns similar to those of the barbiturates, except for chloral hydrate, which has only a minimal effect (Kales et al, 1977).

Since most hypnotics have been shown to lose much of their effectiveness within two weeks of nightly use (Kales et al, 1977), their use should not be recommended beyond the period of effectiveness demonstrated in well-controlled studies (Kales et al, 1975). Attempts to discontinue medication can result in restless or disturbed sleep which may be mistaken for the original insomnia, thus initiating a chain of dependency. Every effort should be made to avoid these drugs in patients who abuse drugs.

Data on a number of over-the-counter nighttime sleep-aid products recently reviewed by an OTC Sedative, Sleep-Aid and Tranquilizer Panel appointed by the FDA has led the Panel and the FDA Commissioner to conclude the following: (1) that bromide salts and scopolamine are potentially toxic at effective dose levels, and these substances shall be removed from such products; (2) that acetaminophen, salicylic acid, and salicylamide have no sleep-inducing qualities, and their use in such products is irrational; and (3) that short-term use of certain antihistamines (methapyrilene, pyrilamine, and phenyltoloxamine) in such products may be acceptable, although better controlled studies are needed to establish their usefulness and safety (*Federal Register*, 1978). Methapyrilene has since been removed from all nonprescription sleep-aid products by order of the FDA, because data from animal tests indicate that it is carcinogenic.

ANTIANXIETY AND HYPNOTIC DRUGS

Sedation denotes a drug action that diminishes environmental awareness, spontaneity, and motor activity; drowsiness and lethargy are characteristic of more marked sedation, and sleep usually occurs when the sedative dose of a drug is increased. Many psychotropic drugs have sedative properties, and almost all antianxiety, antipsychotic, and antidepressant drugs; antihistamines; centrally acting anticholinergics; and opiate analgesics possess this action to varying degrees, especially at higher dose levels.

Antianxiety and sedation are not synonymous descriptive terms in certain experimental pharmacologic test methods; however, it is often difficult to distinguish between these actions clinically. Although sedatives with minimal antianxiety action may be clinically desirable to diminish awareness and alleviate some types of anxiety (eg, apprehension associated with anticipation of pain [preanesthetic medication]), antianxiety drugs that possess a high antianxiety/low sedative effect are generally preferred to minimize functional impairment in anxious outpatients. The descriptive term antianxiety is preferred clinically to its synonyms (ie, tranquilizing, ataractic) to describe drugs that primarily diminish anxiety.

The drugs available to treat anxiety and insomnia are listed in the Table. Detailed information on biotransformation and other

ANTIANXIETY AND HYPNOTIC DRUGS

	PRINCIPAL USES				
	Anxiety	Insomnia	Preanesthetic Medication	Alcohol Withdrawal	Barbiturate Withdrawal
Benzodiazepines					
Chlordiazepoxide [Libritabs, Librium]	+		+	+	
Clorazepate [Azene, Tranxene]	+			+	
Diazepam [Valium]	+		+	+	
Flurazepam [Dalmane]		+			
Lorazepam [Ativan]	+	+	+		
Oxazepam [Serax]	+	+[2]		+	
Prazepam [Verstran]	+				
Nonbenzodiazepines					
Barbiturates					
Butabarbital [Butisol]	+	+			
Phenobarbital	+	+			+
Amobarbital [Amytal]		+	+		
Pentobarbital [Nembutal]		+	+		
Secobarbital [Seconal]		+	+		
Chloral Derivatives					
Chloral Hydrate		+	+		
Chloral Betaine [Beta-Chlor]		+	+		
Triclofos Sodium [Triclos]		+	+		
Miscellaneous Compounds					
Ethchlorvynol [Placidyl]		+			
Ethinamate [Valmid]		+			
Glutethimide [Doriden]		+			
Hydroxyzine [Atarax, Vistaril]	+		+	+	
Meprobamate [Equanil, Meprospan, Miltown]	+				
Methaqualone [Parest, Quaalude, Sopor]		+			
Methyproylon [Noludar]		+			
Paraldehyde		+		+	

[1]The range of half-lives represents the major active metabolite (ie, desmethyldiazepam for clorazepate, diazepam, and prazepam; N₁ desalkyl flurazepam for flurazepam) but does not represent the active metabolite of chlordiazepoxide, desmethylchlordiazepoxide.

[2]Investigational.

pharmacokinetic data are available for the benzodiazepines (Greenblatt and Shader, 1978 B) and nonbenzodiazepines (Breimer, 1977). Principles of use and drug selection among each of the categories of drugs listed are presented in the following sections. Two drugs not included in the Table, pro-

pranolol [Inderal] and *l*-tryptophan, are being investigated clinically for antianxiety and hypnotic effects, respectively.

Benzodiazepines

The benzodiazepines are the most effective drugs for suppressing the response to

Seizure Disorders	Skeletal Muscle Hyperactivity	Half-Life[1] Hours (Mean or Range)	Parenteral Preparation Available	Controlled Substance Schedule	Generic Form Available	Metabolite
		24 — 48	+	IV	+	Active
		30 — 200	−	IV	−	Active
+	+	48 — 200	+	IV	+	Active
		47 — 100	−	IV	−	Active
		9 — 24	+[2]	IV	−	Inactive
		3 — 21	−	IV	−	Inactive
		30 — 200	−	IV	−	Active
		34 — 42	−	III	+	Inactive
+		72 — 96	+	IV	+	Inactive
+		15 — 34	+	II	+	Inactive
		18 — 48	+	II		Inactive
		19 — 34	+	II	+	Inactive
		7 — 9.5	−	IV	+	Active
		7 — 9.5	−	IV	−	Active
		7 — 9.5	−	IV	−	Active
		5.6	−	IV	−	
			−	IV	−	
		5 — 22	−	III	−	
			+	none	+	
		10	−	IV	+	
			−	II	−	
			−	III	−	
			+	IV	−	

conflict or aggression in animals; they also produce muscle relaxation and control induced seizures in experimental test models. Their mechanism of action remains speculative (Iversen, 1978).

Although some patients may respond equally well to properly selected doses of nonbenzodiazepine drugs, the benzodiazepines are most often the drugs of choice when an antianxiety, sedative, or hypnotic action is required because of their efficacy and safety (Blackwell, 1975; Sellers, 1978; Greenblatt and Shader, 1979). The National Institute on Drug Abuse (NIDA) reviewed the relevant literature and concluded that the benzodiazepines have distinct advantages when compared to nonbenzodiazepines in the following areas: adverse reactions, development of tolerance, drug dependence, drug interactions, and lethality associated with overdose (Cooper, 1978). For more specific information, see the section on Adverse Reactions and Precautions.

A similar review by the Institute of Medicine of the National Academy of Sciences (National Academy of Sciences, 1979; Solomon et al, 1979) agrees in principle with the NIDA Report, but it emphasized the following additional caveats with respect to the use of benzodiazepines as hypnotics: (1) Nightly reliance (not dependence) on drugs for sleep is equally likely with either benzodiazepines or barbiturates. (2) Although less potent than barbiturates on a dose-for-dose basis, the benzodiazepines do produce respiratory depression that can significantly add to that caused by other drugs, including alcohol, to increase the risk of death. (3) An increased likelihood of adverse drug reactions in elderly patients and patients with diminished kidney function is a potentially hazardous attribute not shared by barbiturate hypnotics, and this is, in part, due to the accumulation of active metabolites with long half-lives of certain benzodiazepines. (4) The accumulation of active metabolites also probably explains the greater impairment of visual-motor coordination skills compared to the nonbenzodiazepines (eg, driving, operating dangerous machinery) after a week of use,

especially if alcohol is ingested concomitantly (even after one day of use). With respect to the use of all hypnotics, the report emphasizes the need for clear directions and warnings to the patient about the use of these drugs, frequent clinical reappraisal of diagnosis, and vigilant monitoring for development of either toxic effects or risk factors that would make continuation of the drug hazardous (eg, pregnancy, renal or hepatic disease, alcoholism, depression).

The choice among the benzodiazepines for anxiety and insomnia is less clear. The current extensive usage of the older benzodiazepines (chlordiazepoxide [Libritabs, Librium], diazepam [Valium], and flurazepam [Dalmane]) is based upon considerable clinical experience compared to the limited number of controlled comparative studies available for the more recently introduced drugs in this class. In addition to clinical experience, other factors important in selecting one benzodiazepine over another include the response of the individual patient, desired route of administration, pharmacokinetic profile of the drug, and cost; however, drug interactions and development of tolerance, dependence, and toxicity are not considered major differentiating factors.

All benzodiazepines are absorbed within one to two hours when given orally. Chlordiazepoxide and diazepam also may be given parenterally. Since they are absorbed erratically from intramuscular sites, intravenous use is preferred if parenteral therapy is required. A parenteral formulation of lorazepam, which is reliably absorbed intramuscularly, is being evaluated clinically but has not yet been approved.

The biotransformation of certain benzodiazepines to active metabolites can be important in drug selection. Clorazepate [Azene, Tranxene], chlordiazepoxide, diazepam, flurazepam, and prazepam [Verstran] are transformed to active metabolites, especially to an N-desmethylated product that has a longer half-life than the parent drug; this may be particularly significant in the elderly, newborn, or those with severe liver disease. Only lorazepam [Ativan] and oxazepam [Serax] are directly transformed to inactive glucuronides without passing through intermediate active metabolites, and thus they have the shortest mean half-lives.

There is a thirtyfold variation in plasma concentration among individuals given an equal amount of a benzodiazepine, and individual dosage adjustments and multiple daily doses may be necessary initially until the degree of desired response and severity of untoward effects are established. After the optimum total daily dose is determined, single daily doses may then be instituted in some patients; other patients will continue to require multiple doses daily to control anxiety, even with those benzodiazepines that have a long half-life. The single daily dose or a proportionately larger amount of the multiple daily dose may be given at bedtime to anxious patients who have difficulty in falling asleep.

Other indications for selected benzodiazepines (preanesthetic medication, alcohol withdrawal, seizure disorders, spasticity, localized skeletal muscle spasm, and suppression of certain extrapyramidal movement disorders [akathisia]) are noted in the Table and discussed in the appropriate chapter in this section on Psychopharmacologic Drugs and in the following sections on Neurologic Drugs and Anesthetic Drugs.

Nonbenzodiazepines

Barbiturates: Of the barbiturates, phenobarbital and butabarbital [Butisol] are currently preferred for mild anxiety or insomnia, particularly if daytime sedation also is desirable. These barbiturates are used only infrequently in suicide attempts and are rarely abused. The shorter-acting barbiturates (amobarbital [Amytal], pentobarbital [Nebralin, Nembutal], and secobarbital [Seconal]) are not sufficiently potent or their action specific enough to be used as antianxiety drugs; the safety of the benzodiazepines compared to the barbiturates and the limited effective duration of action of all hypnotic drugs administered repetitively have also tended to reduce the

use of the barbiturates in insomnia. Pentobarbital and secobarbital are still widely used orally, intramuscularly, or intravenously for preanesthetic medication and to provide sedation during regional anesthesia.

Phenobarbital is frequently used for seizure disorders (see Chapter 15, Anticonvulsants) and to control signs and symptoms of withdrawal from other barbiturates, chloral hydrate, ethchlorvynol, ethinamate, glutethimide, methaqualone, methyprylon, paraldehyde, and meprobamate (see the discussion on Drug Dependence, Barbiturates, in the section on Adverse Reactions and Precautions).

Investigations on the use of barbiturates for brain resuscitation in metabolic, toxic, or infectious encephalopathy are continuing in Reye's syndrome (Safar, 1978). It is not certain whether the beneficial effects of the barbiturates are related to a reduction of brain metabolism, cerebral edema, or intracranial pressure.

Chloral Derivatives: Chloral hydrate is a clinically effective sedative and hypnotic. It is not used for anxiety because its antianxiety action is too limited and variable. Its rapid onset of action and short half-life make the drug especially useful in insomnia characterized by difficulty in falling asleep. Some tolerance to the hypnotic action generally develops within five weeks. Although chloral hydrate's benefit/risk ratio is not as good as that of the benzodiazepines, it may be the preferred alternative among the nonbenzodiazepine hypnotics in selected patients with insomnia. The unpleasant taste can be minimized by the use of chilled vehicles, of the capsule form, or of chemical complexes (chloral betaine [Beta-Chlor], triclofos [Triclos]) if the additional cost is acceptable. Chloral hydrate may be administered orally or rectally.

Miscellaneous Compounds: Ethinamate [Valmid], ethchlorvynol [Placidyl], glutethimide [Doriden], methaqualone [Parest, Quaalude, Sopor], and methyprylon [Noludar] have very limited or variable antianxiety action and are marketed only for hypnosis. Ethinamate and ethchlorvynol have low potency and, like chloral hydrate, have a rapid onset and brief duration of action. In some studies, the hypnotic effect was reported to be less predictable than that of chloral hydrate, and their overall safety is judged to be comparable to that of the barbiturates.

The effect of the two piperidinedione derivatives, glutethimide and methyprylon, on electroencephalographic sleep patterns is similar to that of the barbiturates. Management of intoxication with overdosage of these drugs can be very difficult, especially the cardiovascular manifestions. This is also true of the quinazolinone derivative, methaqualone. This drug has been sufficiently abused by drug-dependent individuals to warrant its being classified as a Schedule II controlled substance. Glutethimide, methyprylon, and methaqualone rarely if ever should be considered drugs of choice for the treatment of insomnia.

Paraldehyde formerly was used to treat insomnia; at present, it is used rarely as an alternative to the benzodiazepines in the treatment of selected cases of alcohol withdrawal.

Propranolol [Inderal], a beta-adrenergic blocking drug, suppresses objective autonomic signs of anxiety (eg, palpitations, tachycardia, tremor) but controlled studies reveal that subjective symptoms do not always improve (Whitlock and Price, 1974). Patients with cardiac failure, hypotension, bradycardia, heart block, or asthma are especially prone to the adverse effects of beta-adrenergic blocking drugs.

Since serotonin plays a role in inducing and maintaining normal sleep, *l*-tryptophan has been administered orally to increase brain levels of serotonin. Although 1 g of *l*-tryptophan significantly decreased sleep latency and reduced waking time without alteration of sleep patterns, the hypnotic action is observed only during the early part of the sleep cycle, is unpredictable, and is not characterized by a satisfactory dose-response relationship (Hartmann, 1977). Because the hypnotic action has not been confirmed in other studies, this use of *l*-tryptophan must be considered investigational and it is not recommended in regular clinical practice.

Adverse Reactions and Precautions

BENZODIAZEPINES: Daytime sedation is the most common untoward effect produced by these agents initially at clinically effective dose levels in the treatment of anxiety, but it appears to occur less frequently with the benzodiazepines than with the barbiturates. Sedation may be lessened by starting with relatively small amounts and gradually increasing the dose to produce the desired antianxiety effect without oversedation; however, if considerable tolerance develops, the dosage and use of the drug should be reassessed. Patients should be cautioned to avoid undertaking activities that require mental alertness, judgment, and physical coordination (eg, driving a car, operating dangerous machinery) during initial therapy when sedation may be pronounced or if alcohol is ingested concomitantly. Ataxia, dizziness, and headache are also observed most commonly during the early period of dosage adjustment. Elderly and debilitated patients develop drowsiness and ataxia more often than younger patients. In addition, symptoms of organic brain disease in the elderly may be aggravated if the larger doses appropriate for younger patients are given.

Fatigue, dysarthria, muscle weakness, dryness of the mouth, and gastrointestinal discomfort (nausea and vomiting) also have been reported, but a causal relationship has not been established definitely. The latter may be reduced by administering the drug with or immediately after meals. Rash, chills, fever, and, rarely, blood dyscrasias have been noted.

Paradoxical aggression (increased irritability, insomnia, hyperactivity, and even violent hostile rage reactions) has been reported rarely. An increased frequency of vivid dreams also has been associated with use of or withdrawal from the benzodiazepines.

Caution is required when prescribing these agents for patients with severely impaired renal or hepatic function.

Cumulation occurs with use of benzodiazepines with long plasma half-lives (chlordiazepoxide [Libritabs, Librium], clorazepate [Azene, Tranxene], diazepam [Valium], flurazepam [Dalmane], prazepam [Verstran]) until steady-state concentrations are reached (several days to two weeks). Cumulative clinical effects are not always a consequence, possibly because of tolerance or the fact that benzodiazepine plasma concentrations are often poorly correlated with clinical effects. However, some patients, particularly the elderly, may be subjectively unaware of sedation or impairment of performance, although objectively they are functioning less effectively after a week or two of antianxiety therapy.

For guidelines on the use of benzodiazepines during pregnancy, see the evaluations and Chapter 2, Doses and Use of Drugs in Certain Groups of Patients.

Drug Tolerance: Pharmacodynamic (cellular) tolerance develops with use of the benzodiazepines. Sedation and ataxia decrease with continued administration of the same dose, but it appears that tolerance to the antianxiety action develops at a slower rate. A marked pharmacodynamic tachyphylaxis to the hypnotic, respiratory, and cardiovascular depressant actions associated with overdose of the benzodiazepines does occur. The benzodiazepine blood level may remain well above the normal range associated with sleep or even anesthesia during recovery from overdose when the patient is awake and vital signs are stable. Metabolic tolerance (enzyme induction) does not appear to be of clinical significance.

Drug Poisoning: In the absence of the concomitant use of alcohol and other central nervous system depressants, the benzodiazepines are the safest of all currently available antianxiety and hypnotic agents, and they offer a clinically significant safety margin in cases of overdosage. The treatment of overdosage (ventilatory depression, acute circulatory failure, and coma) with these agents is similar to that for the barbiturates, except that dialysis is of limited value.

Drug Dependence: Long-term administration of larger than usual therapeutic doses of the benzodiazepines may cause physical dependence. However, because it occurs relatively infrequently even though use of these drugs is widespread, the benzodiazepines are classified as Schedule IV agents. Withdrawal symptoms are similar to those produced by dependence on barbiturates or alcohol. The withdrawal reaction may be considerably delayed following cessation of the drug, ie, within 36 hours to one week after the benzodiazepine is withdrawn, depending upon the specific compound's half-life and whether or not it is converted to an active metabolite. If physical dependence has become well established, withdrawal reactions may occur if the drugs are discontinued abruptly; therefore, gradual reduction of dosage is recommended. The physician should maintain close supervision over the duration of use and amount of these drugs prescribed for all patients, especially those with a history of drug dependence.

Drug Interactions: An additive sedative effect may occur with concomitant use of a benzodiazepine and other central nervous system depressants (eg, other antianxiety and hypnotic drugs, alcohol, tricyclic antidepressants, opiate analgesics, antipsychotics, antihistamines). However, this is not necessarily a contraindication to simultaneous use of other drugs, although the dose of the benzodiazepine may require reduction, close follow-up of the patient may be necessary initially, and/or precautionary advice about activities that require alertness should be stressed.

BARBITURATES: Untoward effects commonly observed in sensitive individuals (eg, the elderly, those with severe liver disease) or in patients taking large doses are drowsiness and lethargy; residual sedation ("hangover") is common after hypnotic doses. For these reasons, ambulatory patients should be specifically warned to be cautious of or avoid activities that require mental alertness, judgment, and physical coordination (eg, driving a vehicle, operating dangerous machinery), especially if alcohol is ingested concomitantly.

Reactions noted infrequently include skin eruptions (eg, urticaria, angioedema, generalized morbilliform rash, Stevens-Johnson syndrome, discrete violaceous macules) and gastrointestinal disturbances such as nausea and vomiting. Paradoxical restlessness or excitement and exacerbation of the symptoms of certain organic brain disorders may occur, especially in elderly patients.

Because barbiturates may aggravate symptoms of acute intermittent porphyria by inducing the enzymes responsible for porphyrin synthesis, their use is contraindicated in patients with this disease. Because bilirubin metabolism can be enhanced by barbiturate-induced enzyme induction, phenobarbital is used in some cases of congenital hyperbilirubinemia. Since the major site of degradation of barbiturates is the liver, caution should be observed when these drugs are given initially to patients with hepatic disease. Pulmonary insufficiency is a relative contraindication to the use of barbiturates, for serious ventilatory depression may occur in these patients.

Routine caution should be exercised when barbiturates are used during pregnancy (see Chapter 2).

Great caution should be taken to avoid intra-arterial injection or extravasation of the highly alkaline sodium salts of barbiturates. Accidental injection into an artery provokes intense, prolonged spastic vasoconstriction and ischemia and has caused gangrene of the extremity. Acute excruciating pain, edema, erythema, inflammation, and obliteration of the distal pulse are rapidly evident in the affected limb. For treatment of this complication, see Chapter 20, General Anesthetics.

Drug Tolerance: Two types of tolerance may be observed with the barbiturates. Drug metabolic tolerance may occur when a barbiturate or another drug accelerates hepatic inactivation of the barbiturate. This type of tolerance is most commonly observed with the barbiturates that have half-lives of relatively short duration. Pharmacodynamic tolerance results when the depressant effect on the central nervous system decreases with repeated administration. This is noted most frequently with the long-acting barbiturate, phenobarbital, and with large doses of the shorter-acting barbiturates. Cross tolerance develops among the barbiturates and between these drugs and alcohol. It is important to remember that, although tolerance develops to the hypnotic effects of barbiturates, the lethal dose does not increase significantly.

Drug Poisoning: Barbiturates remain one of the leading causes of fatal drug poisoning. Acute poisoning is usually the result of ingestion for suicidal purposes; some cases have been attributed to a state of drug-induced confusion (automatism) in which the patient forgets having taken the medication and takes more, but there is substantial doubt that this phenomenon exists. The direct or indirect effects of barbiturates and other central nervous system or cardiovascular depressants (eg, alcohol, tricyclic antidepressants, antihistamines, opiates) taken concomitantly can result in death. The usual safeguard is to prescribe small quantities of the drug, but this measure is not invariably effective. Some patients may accumulate a supply of medication until they have enough to attempt suicide.

Overdosage of the barbiturates can cause tachycardia, hypotension, profound shock, ventilatory depression, areflexia, coma, and death due to cardioventilatory failure secondary to depression of the vital medullary centers. Good nursing care is of primary importance in treating barbiturate poisoning, and this may be all that is required if the ventilatory and cardiovascular systems are functioning adequately and there is a positive response to painful stimuli.

If the patient is still conscious and less than four hours have elapsed since ingestion, vomiting may be induced by syrup of ipecac.

Gastric lavage and activated charcoal are used in comatose patients only after an open airway has been secured, if necessary by endotracheal intubation. An adequate airway should be maintained, arterial blood gases should be monitored, and sufficient oxygen should be given to prevent hypoxemia. Controlled ventilation must be instituted if ventilatory failure develops.

Osmotic diuretics significantly increase the renal excretion of phenobarbital; alkalization of the urine also significantly enhances the excretion of phenobarbital.

In severe poisoning, hemodialysis or charcoal hemoperfusion may be lifesaving, especially if a vigorous diuresis cannot be maintained.

The prevention of complications includes changing the patient's position hourly to prevent pressure sores and hypostatic pneumonia, maintaining adequate hydration and nutrition by administering fluids parenterally, and providing all standard supportive therapy.

Drug Dependence: Chronic intoxication occurs most commonly with use of the relatively short-acting barbiturates, and symptoms are similar to those of alcohol intoxication (eg, disorientation, ataxia, euphoria). Prolonged, uninterrupted use of barbiturates (particularly the short-acting drugs), even in therapeutic doses, may result in physical and psychological dependence. Withdrawal reactions have been reported in neonates after maternal ingestion of these drugs.

If a barbiturate appears to have lost its effectiveness after long-term administration, it should be withdrawn slowly. The patient should be warned that unpleasant symptoms (eg, increased frequency and intensity of dreaming, nightmares) may occur. Abrupt withdrawal after several months of therapy (600 mg or more daily of pentobarbital [Nebralin, Nembutal] or secobarbital [Seconal]) may be followed within 24 hours by a severe withdrawal syndrome that is more serious than that caused by opiates. The syndrome usually lasts approximately one week. Status epilepticus may occur with grand mal convulsions (which develop between 12 hours and 12 days after withdrawal), delirium, and, sometimes, progressive hyperpyrexia, coma, and death.

Gradual withdrawal of the offending agent (nonsubstitutive treatment) over a period of ten days to three weeks, depending upon the severity of dependence, is necessary to minimize the signs and symptoms of withdrawal. Because of its long duration of action and, therefore, improved control of withdrawal signs and symptoms, phenobarbital is often used as an alternative treatment (substitutive). It is administered in place of the offending drug until signs and symptoms have stabilized (eg, approximately 30 mg of phenobarbital is substituted for each 100 mg of the shorter-acting barbiturates). The dose of phenobarbital then is reduced gradually by 10% every 24 hours. Phenobarbital also can be used, if substitutive treatment is elected, for patients who are withdrawing from the chloral derivatives, ethchlorvynol, ethinamate, glutethimide, methaqualone, methyprylon, paraldehyde, and meprobamate but not from the benzodiazepines.

Physicians should assess the patient's susceptibility to drug abuse before prescribing any psychoactive drug. In susceptible individuals, psychic dependence leads to frequent self-administration until compulsive abuse becomes an established pattern. The incidence of dependence may be reduced if the physician explains the rationale for use of these drugs to the patient, and if he institutes a follow-up program that includes periodic checkups and family consultations. To reduce the possibility of poisoning and abuse, the physician should caution against storage of the medication within the reach of children or others who might use it either unwittingly or for abuse purposes. The quantity of sedative prescribed should be no greater than that needed for current therapy and less than a potentially lethal dose. Patients also should be counseled on the proper use of the medication (eg, follow directions on label, dispose of old medicine no longer needed for medical reasons, avoid "sharing" prescription drugs). See also Chapter 3, Prescription Practices and Regulatory Agencies.

Amobarbital, pentobarbital, and secobarbital are classified as Schedule II agents. Butabarbital and phenobarbital are classified in Schedules III and IV, respectively, based on their longer half-lives. (See Chapter 3 for additional information.)

Drug Interactions: Doses of barbiturates must be reduced when they are given with other central nervous system depressants (eg, alcohol, other hypnotic and antianxiety agents, tricyclic antidepressants, opiate analgesics, antipsychotics, antihistamines). Barbiturates must be used with caution in patients receiving monoamine oxidase inhibitors (isocarboxazid [Marplan], phenelzine [Nardil], tranylcypromine [Parnate]), since these drugs may potentiate the depressant effects of the barbiturates.

Phenobarbital increases the synthesis and activity of hepatic microsomal enzymes involved in the metabolism of warfarin and dicumarol; the shorter-acting barbiturates are less likely to produce this effect. The benzodiazepines are preferred in patients who are also receiving anticoagulants.

Barbiturates may enhance the metabolism of tricyclic antidepressants, phenytoin, griseofulvin, and adrenal corticosteroids. For example, the administration of phenobarbital to asthmatic patients dependent on corticosteroids has been reported to result in exacerbation of asthma, which was reversed when phenobarbital was discontinued. It may be necessary to adjust the dosage schedule of these drugs to maintain control of the disorder.

CHLORAL DERIVATIVES AND MISCELLANEOUS COMPOUNDS: The adverse reactions for these two classes of drugs are presented in the evaluations.

BENZODIAZEPINES

CHLORDIAZEPOXIDE
[Libritabs]

CHLORDIAZEPOXIDE HYDROCHLORIDE
[Librium]

This benzodiazepine is slightly more effective as an antianxiety agent than nonbenzodiazepines; however, it is less potent than diazepam on a milligram basis and has less anticonvulsant and muscle relaxant activities. Chlordiazepoxide is effective in the treatment of alcohol withdrawal.

Chlordiazepoxide is absorbed more rapidly and predictably after oral than after intramuscular administration; blood levels vary widely among individuals. The half-life is about one to two days, and chlordiazepoxide is converted to the major active metabolite, desmethylchlordiazepoxide; therefore, cumulative effects can occur with repeated daily administration.

Large doses have caused hypotension and syncope, and usual daily oral doses have exacerbated ventilatory failure in patients with chronic bronchitis. Increased or decreased libido, agranulocytosis, jaundice, and a lupus erythematosus-like syndrome have been reported rarely. Chlordiazepoxide also may cause excitement, depression, confusion, and hallucinations.

Long-term use of larger than usual doses may produce psychological and physical dependence. Symptoms of withdrawal develop more slowly than with barbiturates or meprobamate, and convulsions can occur. Withdrawal symptoms have been reported in twin neonates during the third week of life when the mother had taken chlordiazepoxide (20 to 30 mg daily) throughout pregnancy. Chlordiazepoxide has a wide margin of safety unless taken concurrently with alcohol or other central nervous system depressants. Although coma has been reported after ingestion of 300 mg, it has failed to develop after ingestion of as much as 1 g, and patients have recovered after ingesting as much as 2.25 g in a single dose.

See the Introduction and Table for additional information.

ROUTES, USUAL DOSAGE, AND PREPARATIONS. *Oral*: *Adults*, for anxiety, 15 to 100 mg divided into three or four doses or once daily at bedtime; *elderly or debilitated patients*, 5 mg two to four times daily.
Oral, Intramuscular: *Children over 6 years*, 0.5 mg/kg of body weight daily divided into three or four doses. Information is inadequate to establish dosage for *children under 6 years*.
CHLORDIAZEPOXIDE:
Libritabs (Roche). Tablets 5, 10, and 25 mg.
CHLORDIAZEPOXIDE HYDROCHLORIDE:
Drug available generically: Capsules 5, 10, and 25 mg.
Librium (Roche). Capsules 5, 10, and 25 mg.
For parenteral preparations, see below.

Intravenous: *Adults*, for the relief of severe withdrawal symptoms of alcoholism, 50 to 100 mg given cautiously over a period of at least one minute; the dose may be reduced to 25 to 50 mg and administered three or four times daily. The total daily dosage should not exceed 300 mg. Oral administration should be substituted as soon as possible. Chlordiazepoxide also may be given intramuscularly, but absorption is erratic and is usually less than after oral administration. The dosage should be reduced by one-half in elderly or debilitated patients.

> CHLORDIAZEPOXIDE HYDROCHLORIDE:
> *Librium* (Roche). Powder 100 mg in 5 ml containers.

CLORAZEPATE DIPOTASSIUM
[Tranxene]

CLORAZEPATE MONOPOTASSIUM
[Azene]

The actions and uses of both salts of this drug are similar to those of chlordiazepoxide. Controlled studies indicate that clorazepate and diazepam are apparently equally effective antianxiety agents.

Clorazepate undergoes decarboxylation to desmethyldiazepam in liquid, and the rate is accelerated in the presence of a low pH. Therefore, the drug is almost totally converted to desmethyldiazepam in the stomach and is absorbed by the gastrointestinal tract primarily in this form. Cumulation can occur with repeated administration until steady-state concentrations of the major active metabolite, desmethyldiazepam, are reached in the plasma (in about one to two weeks).

The most common adverse effects are similar to those produced by the other benzodiazepines. In addition, blurred vision, euphoria, constipation, hiccups, confusion, and depression occur occasionally.

The benzodiazepines should not be discontinued abruptly, although no serious adverse effects were observed after abrupt discontinuation of clorazepate after a six-week course of 120 mg daily. Long-term therapy with larger than usual doses may produce psychological and physical dependence.

See the Introduction and Table for additional information.

ROUTE, USUAL DOSAGE, AND PREPARATIONS.
Oral: *Adults*, 13 to 52 mg (monopotassium) or 15 to 60 mg (dipotassium) divided into two to four doses or once daily at bedtime; *elderly or debilitated patients*, initially, 6.5 to 13 mg (monopotassium) or 7.5 to 15 mg (dipotassium) daily. Adequate information is not available to establish a dosage for *children under 18 years*.

> CLORAZEPATE DIPOTASSIUM:
> *Tranxene* (Abbott). Capsules 3.75, 7.5, and 15 mg; tablets 11.25 and 22.5 mg (Tranxene-SD).
> CLORAZEPATE MONOPOTASSIUM:
> *Azene* (Endo). Capsules 3.25, 6.5, and 13 mg.

DIAZEPAM
[Valium]

Diazepam is effective in the management of appropriately selected patients with anxiety and has a higher therapeutic index than nonbenzodiazepines. It has been used more extensively and for more indications than any of the other benzodiazepines (see Table).

This drug is absorbed more rapidly and predictably after oral (about 75%) than after intramuscular administration. Cumulative effects can occur with repeated administration until steady-state plasma concentrations are achieved (in about one to two weeks). The half-life ranges from 20 to 100 hours; however, the major active metabolite of diazepam, desmethyldiazepam, has a half-life varying from 48 to 200 hours, depending upon the individual. Another active metabolite, temazepam, has a very short half-life, and it is clinically unimportant after usual therapeutic doses. The half-lives of diazepam and its major active metabolite are usually increased in neonates, the elderly, and those with severe hepatic disorders.

The most common adverse reactions are similar to those observed with the benzodiazepines in general (see the Introduction). Other untoward reactions noted occasionally are blurred vision, diplopia, hypotension, amnesia, slurred speech, tremor, urinary incontinence, and constipation; one case of transitory leukopenia has been reported. Like chlordiazepoxide, diazepam can cause excitement and hallucinations. The appearance of depression most likely represents an undiagnosed concomitant masked depression. Suicidal impulses have been reported in several patients taking 40 to 60 mg daily. Apnea and cardiac arrest have occurred rarely, usually following intravenous administration. This has been observed especially in elderly or severely ill patients, in those receiving other central nervous system depressant drugs, or in those with limited ventilatory reserve. Intravenous injection of diazepam may cause local pain and thrombophlebitis.

Long-term use of larger than usual therapeutic doses may result in psychological and physical dependence. Otherwise, diazepam has a wide margin of safety. Cleft lip, with or without cleft palate, has been associated with the use of diazepam during the first trimester of pregnancy. Diazepam and desmethyldiazepam cross the placenta during labor and are found in the fetus in concentrations exceeding those in the mother. Available evidence suggests that intramuscular or intravenous administration of more than 30 mg of diazepam during the final 15 hours of labor can produce low Apgar scores, apnea, and feeding problems in the newborn infant (the floppy-infant syndrome).

See the Introduction and Table for additional information.

ROUTES, USUAL DOSAGE, AND PREPARATIONS. *Oral*: *Adults*, for anxiety, 4 to 40 mg daily in two to four divided doses or a single dose of 2.5 to 10 mg at bedtime; *elderly or debilitated patients and those taking other central nervous system depressants concomitantly*, initially, 2 to 2.5 mg once or twice daily, increased gradually as needed or tolerated. *Children*, 0.12 to 0.8 mg/kg of body weight daily in three or four divided doses.

Valium (Roche). Tablets 2, 5, and 10 mg.

Intravenous, Intramuscular: The intravenous route is preferred for parenteral administration, because intramuscular absorption is erratic and unpredictable. The intravenous solution should be injected slowly, allowing at least one minute for each 5 mg (1 ml) given, and it should not be mixed or diluted with other solutions or drugs or added to intravenous fluids.

For severe anxiety or severe muscle spasm associated with local trauma, spasticity, akathisia, or tetanus, *adults*, initially, 5 to 10 mg, then 5 to 10 mg in three to four hours if necessary. For tetanus, larger doses may be required. *Children*, 0.04 to 0.2 mg/kg of body weight initially, repeated in three to four hours if necessary.

For status epilepticus and severe recurrent convulsive seizures, *adults*, initially 5 to 10 mg, repeated in 10 to 15 minutes to a maximum of 30 mg; *children*, initially 0.04 to 0.2 mg/kg, repeated in 10 to 15 minutes if necessary to a maximum of 0.6 mg/kg.

For basal sedation for cardioversion and endoscopic procedures, *adults*, the intravenous dosage is adjusted to obtain the desired sedative effect. Generally 10 mg or less is adequate, but up to 20 mg may be given.

For acute alcohol withdrawal symptoms, *adults*, initially 5 to 20 mg intravenously, then 5 to 10 mg in three to four hours if necessary.

Valium (Roche). Solution 5 mg/ml in 2 and 10 ml containers.

FLURAZEPAM HYDROCHLORIDE
[Dalmane]

Flurazepam is chemically and pharmacologically similar to the other benzodiazepines. This drug has been marketed principally for use in insomnia. Results of well-controlled clinical and sleep laboratory studies have shown that flurazepam significantly reduces sleep-induction time, number of awakenings, and time spent awake and increases sleep-duration time. Satisfactory hypnotic effects begin 20 to 45 minutes after oral administration and last seven to eight hours. In a small controlled study, flurazepam has been reported to maintain its effectiveness for up to four weeks. REM sleep may be reduced but REM rebound sleep disturbance does not occur when the drug is discontinued. Flurazepam also markedly suppresses stage IV and increases stage II sleep. After discontinuing therapy, the sleep stage pattern returns to normal. The clinical significance of the alteration in sleep pattern has not been established. Rebound insomnia is not observed with flurazepam as it is with shorter-acting benzodiazepines (Kales et al, 1979).

The advantages of flurazepam and other hypnotic benzodiazepines compared to nonbenzodiazepine hypnotics are: (1) They are essentially ineffective as suicidal agents when used alone. (2) They do not increase the metabolism of oral anticoagulants or tricyclic antidepressants. (3) They appear to have a substantially lower abuse potential than the barbiturates. However, in susceptible individuals, reliance or dependence on flurazepam can be substituted for that on alcohol. The major

metabolite of flurazepam has a long half-life (47 to 100 hours). Cumulation of this active metabolite is probably responsible for increasingly impaired daytime skills; however, its slow elimination on termination of therapy probably accounts for the advantageous lack of rebound insomnia.

Ataxia and vertigo may occur, especially in elderly or debilitated patients. Paradoxical reactions (eg, excitement, nervousness, euphoria, irritability) also have been observed. See the Introduction for additional information.

ROUTE, USUAL DOSAGE, AND PREPARATIONS. *Oral*: For hypnosis, *adults*, 15 or, if needed, 30 mg at bedtime; *elderly or debilitated patients*, 15 mg. Information is inadequate to establish a dosage in *children under 15 years*.

Dalmane (Roche). Capsules 15 and 30 mg.

LORAZEPAM
[Ativan]

Lorazepam is an effective antianxiety and hypnotic agent; because of its amnesic action, it is used as a preanesthetic medication.

Like oxazepam, lorazepam is not metabolized to an active derivative. It is eliminated principally as the inactive glucuronide, and no cumulative effects are noted after daily administration. Among the benzodiazepines, this drug has a relatively short half-life of 15 hours (range, 9 to 24 hours) (Greenblatt et al, 1979). Lorazepam is also similar to oxazepam in that the half-life, volume of distribution, and systemic clearance are reported to be unaltered by age (up to the seventh decade) or by liver disease in patients with associated alcoholic cirrhosis or acute viral hepatitis (Kraus et al, 1978). More pharmacokinetic studies are indicated and, until these data are confirmed, the drug should be used cautiously in elderly patients and those with impaired hepatic function.

Although it is almost completely absorbed, absorption after oral administration is somewhat slow, ie, the peak effect and peak plasma concentrations occur in about two hours. A parenteral formulation is being investigated (Greenblatt et al, 1979) and limited data reveal that, unlike diazepam and chlordiazepoxide, the parenteral formulation is reliably absorbed intramuscularly; however, pain at the injection site has been reported.

The most frequent untoward effects produced by lorazepam are: sedation (15.9%), dizziness (6.9%), weakness (4.2%), and ataxia (3.4%). These reactions abate in over one-half of patients with continued administration; the remainder usually respond to reduced dosages. Other reactions are similar to those reported with most other benzodiazepines (see the Introduction). Only minimal effects on respiration and cardiovascular reflexes have been noted even when large doses were given. Some patients have developed leukopenia and elevated lactic dehydrogenase levels; therefore, periodic monitoring during long-term therapy is suggested. Systematic clinical studies have not been performed to determine whether lorazepam is effective for periods exceeding four months; therefore, longer-term therapy should be based on periodic reassessment of the drug's effectiveness.

Until sufficient clinical experience is available, the drug should be avoided in pregnant and nursing women and in children younger than 12 years.

Based on lorazepam's chemical structure and actions, development of psychological or physical dependence would be expected to be similar to that observed with other benzodiazepines.

See the Introduction and Table for further information.

ROUTE, USUAL DOSAGE, AND PREPARATIONS. *Oral*: *Adults*, for anxiety, initially, 1 to 2 mg two or three times daily; the usual range is 2 to 6 mg daily in divided doses. The dose can be increased gradually if needed to a maximum of 10 mg daily in two or three divided doses. For insomnia associated with anxiety or transient situational stress, a single dose of 2 to 4 mg is given at bedtime. These doses should be reduced by one-half initially in elderly or debilitated patients.

Ativan (Wyeth). Tablets 0.5, 1, and 2 mg.

OXAZEPAM
[Serax]

This drug is similar to the other benzodiazepines in its effectiveness in relieving anxiety. Of the benzodiazepines, oxazepam has the shortest half-life because it, like lorazepam, is not metabolized to active compounds with long half-lives; thus, cumulation is less likely to occur. Because of its lack of active metabolites and short half-life (3 to 21 hours), oxazepam may be indicated in selected patients withdrawing from alcohol, and it is being investigated in selected patients with insomnia characterized by difficulty in falling asleep rather than by early morning awakening.

The drug is eliminated by the kidney as an inactive glucuronide. No metabolically active products are formed, and thus the pharmacokinetic parameters of oxazepam should not be altered by the presence of liver disease (alcoholic cirrhosis, acute viral hepatitis). Nevertheless, until more data are available on possible receptor sensitivity to oxazepam in the elderly and in those with hepatic and renal disorders, this drug should be used cautiously in these patients.

The incidence of adverse reactions is low. Drowsiness is the most common untoward effect and may occur in some individuals after a daily dose of 60 mg. Reactions noted occasionally include rash, nausea, dizziness, syncope, hypotension, tachycardia, edema, nightmares, lethargy, slurred speech, and paradoxical reactions such as excitement and confusion. The incidence of ataxia is less than with related drugs. Leukopenia, eosinophilia, and hepatic dysfunction have occurred rarely. The long-term use of larger than usual therapeutic doses may result in psychological and physical dependence.

See the Introduction and Table for additional information.

ROUTE, USUAL DOSAGE, AND PREPARATIONS. *Oral: Adults,* 30 to 120 mg daily divided into three or four doses. *Elderly patients,* initially, 30 mg daily divided into three doses; if necessary, the dose may be increased cautiously to 45 to 60 mg daily divided into three or four doses. *Children 6 to 12 years,* information is inadequate to establish a dosage; this agent should not be used in *children under 6 years.*

 Serax (Wyeth). Capsules 10, 15, and 30 mg; tablets 15 mg.

PRAZEPAM
 [Verstran]

Prazepam is an effective antianxiety agent (Greenblatt and Shader, 1978 A). Like diazepam and clorazepate, it is converted primarily to desmethyldiazepam, which appears to be the principal active metabolite. This conversion occurs relatively slowly in the liver, and peak levels of desmethyldiazepam are observed approximately six hours following oral administration. A mean half-life of about 60 hours (range, 30 to 200 hours) has been reported, which represents the active metabolite, desmethyldiazepam.

The untoward effects are similar to those seen with other benzodiazepines. Those observed most frequently are fatigue (11.6%), dizziness (8.7%), weakness (7.7%), drowsiness (6.8%), lightheadedness (6.8%), and ataxia (5%).

Based on prazepam's chemical structure, metabolism, and limited data to date, drug tolerance, intoxication, development of dependence, and interactions would be expected to be similar to those observed with other benzodiazepines.

Prazepam is excreted in milk and should be avoided in nursing mothers. It is not recommended for use during pregnancy or in children.

See the Introduction and Table for additional information.

ROUTE, USUAL DOSAGE, AND PREPARATIONS. *Oral: Adults,* initially, 20 mg given as a single dose; if necessary, the dose may be increased to 40 to 60 mg daily in divided amounts or given as a single dose, usually at bedtime. *Elderly or debilitated patients,* 10 to 15 mg.

 Verstran (Parke, Davis). Tablets 10 mg.

NONBENZODIAZEPINES

Barbiturates

PHENOBARBITAL

PHENOBARBITAL SODIUM

Phenobarbital differs from its relatively shorter-acting analogues in that it is used in seizure disorders (see Chapter 15) and occasionally as a daytime sedative or for mild anxiety. This barbiturate is generally given orally, but when oral use is impossible or impractical, it may be administered parenterally. Phenobarbital also is used in the treatment of barbiturate and other nonbenzodiazepine withdrawal syndromes (see the Introduction). Since phenobarbital decreases serum bilirubin levels, it has been used in newborn infants to prevent physiologic jaundice and to treat hyperbilirubinemia, but a hemorrhagic diathesis has been observed occasionally. Phenobarbital also reduces elevated serum bilirubin levels in older children and adults with Gilbert's syndrome (familial nonhemolytic, nonobstructive jaundice). This action may be mediated, at least in part, by the enhanced formation of bilirubin glucuronide.

When phenobarbital is given orally, 80% of the dose is absorbed and peak blood levels occur after 6 to 18 hours; the half-life is three to four days. Ten to thirty percent of the maternal plasma concentration is present in breast milk, and fetal and maternal plasma concentrations are almost equal. A total of 25% of a dose is eliminated unchanged in the urine; the remainder is converted to inactive hydroxylated products that are then conjugated.

Phenobarbital is a potent inducer of hepatic microsomal enzymes and thus can influence the hepatic biotransformation of drugs (eg, oral anticoagulants, chlorpromazine). Pharmacodynamic tolerance may develop in the central nervous system, primarily when large doses are being taken; the mechanism is unknown. Death can occur after ingestion of several grams. The fatal blood level in nontolerant individuals is usually 8 to 12 mg/dl.

Long-term use of larger than usual doses may result in physical and psychological dependence. See the Introduction for adverse reactions, precautions, and information on the use of phenobarbital with other drugs.

ROUTES, USUAL DOSAGE, AND PREPARATIONS.
PHENOBARBITAL:

Oral: For sedation, *adults*, 30 to 120 mg daily in two or three divided doses; *children*, 6 mg/kg of body weight daily in three divided doses. For hypnosis, *adults*, 100 to 320 mg. Since phenobarbital has a very long half-life, timed-release preparations do not offer any significant advantage over ordinary dosage forms.

> Drug available generically: Capsules (timed-release) 60 mg; elixir 20 mg/5 ml; liquid 100 mg/5 ml; tablets 7.5, 15, 30, 60, and 100 mg.
> Available Trademarks.
> *Eskabarb* (Smith Kline & French), *Luminal* (Winthrop), *Solfoton* (Poythress).

PHENOBARBITAL SODIUM:
Intramuscular, Intravenous: These routes should be used only when oral administration is impossible or impractical. For hypnosis, *adults*, 100 to 320 mg; for sedation, same as oral dosage. Patients should be observed carefully during intravenous injection; the rate must not exceed 100 mg (2 ml of 5% solution)/min. Relaxation, drowsiness, yawning, and slowing of speech and motor activity usually indicate that only a small additional amount is necessary; 15 minutes or longer may be required before a peak concentration is attained in the brain.

> Drug available generically: Powder 60, 120, and 130 mg; solution 60 and 130 mg/ml in 1 ml containers and 60 and 150 mg/ml in 2 ml containers.
> Available Trademark.
> *Luminal Sodium* (Winthrop).

Rectal: For sedation, *children*, 6 mg/kg of body weight/day divided into three doses.

> Drug available generically: Suppositories 60 mg.

BUTABARBITAL SODIUM
[Butisol Sodium]

Butabarbital is most commonly used for sedation and mild anxiety. It is used for insomnia when continued daytime sedation is also desirable. This barbiturate is not indicated for seizure disorders. The prolonged administration of butabarbital as a hypnotic is not recommended, since it has not been shown to be effective for more than 14 days. There is some evidence to suggest that the dose should be reduced in those with renal insufficiency.

See the Table and the Introduction for information on adverse reactions, precautions, poisoning, dependence, and the use of barbiturates with other drugs. The fatal blood level is usually 3.5 to 6 mg/dl; adults have survived ingestion of 10 g.

ROUTE, USUAL DOSAGE, AND PREPARATIONS.
Oral: For sedation, *adults*, 50 to 120 mg/day in three or four divided doses; *children*, 6 mg/kg of body weight/day in three divided doses. For hypnosis, *adults*, 50 to 100 mg at bedtime.

> Drug available generically: Capsules 15 and 30 mg; elixir 30 mg/5 ml; liquid; tablets 15, 30, and 100 mg.
> *Butisol Sodium* (McNeil). Capsules 15, 30, 50, and 100 mg [Buticaps]; elixir 30 mg/5 ml (alcohol 7%); tablets 15, 30, 50, and 100 mg.

AMOBARBITAL
[Amytal]

AMOBARBITAL SODIUM
[Amytal Sodium]

Amobarbital is an effective sedative and hypnotic agent that is usually given orally. It is most commonly used as a hypnotic. Its action is comparable to that of secobarbital or pentobarbital but, like similar agents, it may lose its effectiveness by the second week of continued administration. The parenteral routes should be used for insomnia only when oral administration is impossible or impractical.

See the Introduction for adverse reactions, precautions, poisoning, dependence, and information on the use of barbiturates with other drugs. The fatal blood level is usually 3 to 6 mg/dl.

ROUTES, USUAL DOSAGE, AND PREPARATIONS.
AMOBARBITAL:
Oral: Same as oral dosage for sodium salt.

> Drug available generically: Tablets 30, 60, and 100 mg.
> *Amytal* (Lilly). Elixir 44 mg/5 ml (alcohol 34%); tablets 15, 30, 50, and 100 mg.

AMOBARBITAL SODIUM:
Intramuscular: For hypnosis, *adults*, 65 to 500 mg. No more than 5 ml should be injected at any one site.
Intravenous (10% aqueous solution): For hypnosis, *adults and children over 6 years*, 65 to 500 mg; the injection rate should not exceed 1 ml/min. The final dosage is determined largely by the patient's reaction as the dose is titrated.

> Drug available generically: Powder 250 and 500 mg.
> *Amytal Sodium* (Lilly). Powder (sterile) 125, 250, and 500 mg.

Oral: For sedation, *adults and children over 12 years*, 50 to 300 mg daily in divided doses; *children under 12 years*, 6 mg/kg of body weight/day divided into three doses. For hypnosis, *adults and children over 12 years*, 65 to 200 mg at bedtime.

> Drug available generically: Capsules 60 and 180 mg.
> *Amytal Sodium* (Lilly). Capsules 65 and 200 mg.

PENTOBARBITAL
[Nembutal]
PENTOBARBITAL SODIUM
[Nembutal Sodium]

Pentobarbital is an effective, short-acting sedative and hypnotic agent that is usually given orally. Parenteral routes should be used for hypnosis only when oral administration is impossible or impractical. It is used more frequently for hypnosis than for sedation but, like similar agents, may lose its effectiveness by the second week of continued administration.

See the Introduction for adverse reactions, precautions, poisoning, dependence, and information on the use of barbiturates with other drugs. Pentobarbital is commonly abused by drug-dependent individuals. Death can occur after ingestion of more than 3 g; the fatal blood level usually is 1 to 2.5 mg/dl.

ROUTES, USUAL DOSAGE, AND PREPARATIONS.
PENTOBARBITAL:
Oral: Same as oral dosage for sodium salt.

> Drug available generically: Capsules 100 mg.
> *Nembutal* (Abbott). Elixir 20 mg/5 ml (strength expressed in terms of sodium salt).

PENTOBARBITAL SODIUM:

Intramuscular: For hypnosis, *adults*, 150 to 200 mg. No more than 250 mg or 5 ml should be injected at any one site because of possible tissue irritation. Injection should be made only into a large muscle mass, preferably the upper outer quadrant of the gluteus maximus.

Intravenous: For hypnosis, *adults of average weight*, 100 mg initially; when the effect is determined (after at least one minute), additional small incremental doses to a total of 500 mg may be given slowly until the desired effect is obtained. *Children*, 50 mg initially.

> Drug available generically: Solution 50 mg/ml in 1, 2, and 30 ml containers.
> *Nembutal Sodium* (Abbott). Solution 50 mg/ml in 2, 20, and 50 ml containers.

Oral: For sedation, *adults*, 30 mg three or four times daily or 100 mg (as timed-release tablet) in the morning; *children*, 6 mg/kg of body weight daily in three divided doses. For hypnosis, *adults*, 100 mg.

> Drug available generically: Capsules 50 and 100 mg.
> *Nembutal Sodium* (Abbott). Capsules 30, 50, and 100 mg.

Rectal: For sedation or hypnosis, *adults of average weight*, 120 or 200 mg; for sedation, *children*, 6 mg/kg of body weight daily in three divided doses.

> Drug available generically: Suppositories 15, 30, 60, 120, and 200 mg.
> *Nembutal Sodium* (Abbott). Suppositories 30, 60, 120, and 200 mg.

SECOBARBITAL
[Seconal]

SECOBARBITAL SODIUM
[Seconal Sodium]

This barbiturate is comparable in effectiveness to pentobarbital sodium. It is usu-

ally given orally. Parenteral routes should be used for hypnosis only when oral administration is impossible or impractical. Secobarbital is used more frequently for hypnosis than for sedation but, like similar drugs, may lose its effectiveness by the second week of continued administration. For injection, an aqueous solution is preferred to preparations containing polyethylene glycol, since the latter may be irritating to kidneys, especially in patients with renal insufficiency.

See the Introduction for adverse reactions, precautions, poisoning, dependence, and information on the use of barbiturates with other drugs. Secobarbital is commonly abused by drug-dependent individuals. The fatal blood level is usually 1 to 2.5 mg/dl.

ROUTES, USUAL DOSAGE, AND PREPARATIONS.
SECOBARBITAL:

Oral: Same as oral dosage for sodium salt.

> Drug available generically: Capsules 100 mg.
> *Seconal* (Lilly). Elixir 22 mg/5 ml (alcohol 12%).

SECOBARBITAL SODIUM:

Intramuscular: For hypnosis, *adults*, 100 to 200 mg; *children*, 3 to 5 mg/kg of body weight (maximum, 100 mg).

Intravenous: For hypnosis, *adults*, 50 to 250 mg; the injection rate should not exceed 50 mg/15 seconds. Administration should be discontinued as soon as the desired effect is attained.

> Drug available generically: Solution 50 mg/ml in 1, 2, and 30 ml containers.
> *Seconal Sodium* (Lilly). Solution 50 mg/ml with polyethylene glycol in 20 ml containers.

Oral: For hypnosis, *adults*, 100 mg at bedtime. For sedation, *children*, 6 mg/kg of body weight daily in three divided doses.

> Drug available generically: Capsules (plain) 50 and 100 mg.
> *Seconal Sodium* (Lilly). Capsules 50 and 100 mg.

Rectal: For sedation or hypnosis, *adults*, 120 to 200 mg; for sedation, *children*, 6 mg/kg of body weight daily in three divided doses.

> Drug available generically: Suppositories 30, 50, 100, 125, and 200 mg.
> *Seconal Sodium* (Lilly). Suppositories 30, 60, 120, and 200 mg.

Chloral Derivatives

CHLORAL HYDRATE

$$Cl-\underset{\underset{Cl}{|}}{\overset{\overset{Cl}{|}}{C}}-\underset{\underset{OH}{|}}{\overset{\overset{H}{|}}{C}}-OH$$

Chloral hydrate is a relatively safe, rapidly effective, reliable sedative and hypnotic agent, but it may lose its effectiveness by the second week of continued administration. The unpleasant taste and odor of chloral hydrate can be minimized by the use of chilled vehicles, the capsule form, rectal administration, or use of the more costly preparations of chloral betaine and triclofos sodium. Trichloroethanol is the active form of chloral hydrate; it is formed rapidly by a large first-pass hepatic effect and has a half-life of eight hours.

Gastric irritation occurs in some patients. Paradoxical excitement is observed rarely. The continued use of large doses causes peripheral vasodilation, hypotension, ventilatory depression, and some myocardial depression. Overdosage may result in coma, and pinpoint pupils are observed occasionally; neither the pinpoint pupils nor the coma are affected by the narcotic antagonist, naloxone. Chloral hydrate initially potentiates the action of oral anticoagulants in some patients for a few days because its major metabolite displaces the anticoagulants from their protein binding sites. The selection of a benzodiazepine hypnotic might be a better choice in patients receiving oral anticoagulants. Clinically relevant enzyme induction does not occur in man.

Long-term use of larger than usual therapeutic doses may result in psychological and physical dependence. The dose should be reduced in patients with severe hepatic or renal disease. Chloral hydrate is excreted in the urine in part as trichloroethanol glucuronide which may give false-positive results for glucose. See the Introduction and Table for further information on hypnotic drugs.

ROUTES, USUAL DOSAGE, AND PREPARATIONS. *Oral, Rectal*: For sedation, *adults*, 250 mg three times daily after meals; *children*, 25 mg/kg of body weight daily divided into three or four doses. For hypnosis, *adults*, 500 mg to 1 g 15 to 30 minutes before bedtime; *children*, 50 mg/kg. The daily dosage for adults should not exceed 2 g, and no more than 1 g should be given as a single dose in children.

Drug available generically: Capsules 225, 250, 450, and 500 mg; elixir 500 mg/5 ml; syrup 250 and 500 mg/5 ml; suppositories 460 and 500 mg. Available Trademark.
Noctec (Squibb).

CHLORAL BETAINE
[Beta-Chlor]

$$Cl-\underset{\underset{Cl}{|}}{\overset{\overset{Cl}{|}}{C}}-\underset{\underset{OH}{|}}{\overset{\overset{H}{|}}{C}}-OH \cdot CH_3\overset{+}{\underset{\underset{CH_3}{|}}{N}}CH_2\overset{O}{\overset{\|}{C}}O^-$$

This chemical adduct of chloral hydrate and betaine has the same sedative and hypnotic properties, adverse reactions, and contraindications as chloral hydrate; however, it does not exhibit the disagreeable physical properties of the latter (see the evaluation on Chloral Hydrate for further information).

ROUTE, USUAL DOSAGE, AND PREPARATIONS. *Oral*: *Adults and children over 12 years*, for hypnosis, 870 mg to 1.7 g given 15 to 30 minutes before bedtime; for preoperative sedation, the same amounts are given 60 to 90 minutes before surgery. *Children under 12 years*, information is inadequate to establish dosage.

Beta-Chlor (Mead Johnson). Tablets 870 mg (equivalent to 500 mg of chloral hydrate).

TRICLOFOS SODIUM
[Triclos]

$$Cl-\underset{\underset{Cl}{|}}{\overset{\overset{Cl}{|}}{C}}CH_2O\overset{O}{\overset{\|}{\underset{\underset{OH}{|}}{P}}}O^-Na^+$$

This effective sedative and hypnotic agent has the same properties, adverse reactions, and contraindications as chloral hydrate, but it does not exhibit the disagreeable physical properties of the latter.

Triclofos is metabolized principally to trichloroethanol, which is also the active metabolite obtained from chloral hydrate. Peak serum levels of trichloroethanol are produced in about one hour, and the half-life is approximately eight hours. A dose of 1.5 g is equivalent to 1 g of chloral hydrate.

Residual sedation, flatulence, gastric irritation, nausea, vomiting, ataxia, vertigo, lightheadedness, nightmares, and malaise occur infrequently. Tolerance to triclofos may develop, and long-term use of larger than usual therapeutic doses may result in psychological and physical dependence. See the evaluation on Chloral Hydrate for further information.

ROUTE, USUAL DOSAGE, AND PREPARATIONS. *Oral*: For hypnosis, *adults and children over 12 years*, 1.5 g given 15 to 30 minutes before bedtime; *children under 12 years*, for sleep induction in electroencephalography, 20 mg/kg of body weight.

> *Triclos* (Merrell-National). Solution 500 mg/5 ml; tablets 750 mg.

Miscellaneous Compounds

ETHCHLORVYNOL
[Placidyl]

$$CH_3CH_2 \overset{\overset{\displaystyle C\equiv CH}{|}}{\underset{\underset{\displaystyle OH}{|}}{C}} CH=CHCl$$

This drug is a tertiary acetylenic alcohol and is used as a hypnotic agent for short-term therapy. The hypnotic action of ethchlorvynol may be less predictable than that of the benzodiazepines, barbiturates, or chloral hydrate.

Hypotension, nausea or vomiting, aftertaste, blurred vision, dizziness, facial numbness, urticaria, and toxic amblyopia occasionally have been reported. One case of fatal immune thrombocytopenia due to ethchlorvynol has been described.

Although death has occurred following ingestion of single doses of 7 to 50 g, patients have recovered after doses as large as 100 g. Unconsciousness may be prolonged. Pancytopenia and hemolysis have been reported after poisoning with ethchlorvynol. The fatal blood concentration is usually 2 to 5 mg/dl. Because large amounts of ethchlorvynol are taken up by adipose tissue, the blood concentration is a very unreliable indicator of the magnitude of overdose. Charcoal and/or amberlite hemoperfusion may be the most effective means for removal of this drug in cases of overdose.

Long-term use of larger than usual doses may result in psychological and physical dependence. A daily dose of 1.5 g may be sufficient to induce the latter. Withdrawal symptoms, including convulsions, may occur when ethchlorvynol is discontinued abruptly. See the Introduction and Table for further information on hypnotic drugs.

ROUTE, USUAL DOSAGE, AND PREPARATIONS. *Oral*: For hypnosis, *adults*, 500 mg to 1 g at bedtime. This drug should not be used in *children*.

> *Placidyl* (Abbott). Capsules 100, 200, 500, and 750 mg.

ETHINAMATE
[Valmid]

$$\overset{\overset{\displaystyle O}{\overset{\displaystyle \|}{OCNH_2}}}{\underset{\displaystyle C\equiv CH}{}}$$

This carbamic acid ester of alcohol is a relatively weak hypnotic with a rapid onset and brief duration of action; therefore, it is used to induce sleep only in patients who have difficulty in falling asleep. Ethinamate has not been shown to be an effective hypnotic for a period of more than seven days. Minimal pharmacokinetic data are available, and the effects of this compound on REM sleep are unknown. Ethinamate undergoes hepatic hydroxylation and subsequent glucuronide conjugation.

Paradoxical excitement in children, mild gastrointestinal disturbances, and rash occur occasionally. Thrombocytopenic purpura and fever have been reported rarely. Death has occurred after ingestion of 15 g, but survival has been reported after ingestion of 28 g. Long-term use of larger than usual therapeutic doses may result in psychological and physical dependence. Withdrawal symptoms, including convulsions, may occur when ethinamate is discontinued abruptly. See the Introduction for further information on hypnotic drugs.

ROUTE, USUAL DOSAGE, AND PREPARATIONS. *Oral*: As hypnotic, *adults*, 500 mg to 1 g at bedtime; *children*, information is inadequate to establish dosage.

    Valmid (Dista). Capsules 500 mg.

GLUTETHIMIDE
[Doriden]

Glutethimide is an effective hypnotic but, like similar agents, loses its effectiveness by the second week of continued administration. This agent has no therapeutic advantage over the benzodiazepines, barbiturates, or chloral derivatives.

Generalized rash, which usually disappears within two or three days after withdrawal of the drug, may occur. Nausea, residual sedation, paradoxical excitement, blurred vision, acute hypersensitivity reactions, acute intermittent porphyria, thrombocytopenic purpura, aplastic anemia, urticaria, exfoliative dermatitis, and leukopenia have been reported rarely.

If coumarin anticoagulants are used with glutethimide, their metabolism is increased and their dosage may require adjustment, because glutethimide induces hepatic microsomal enzymes. Concurrent ingestion of glutethimide and alcohol may increase blood levels of the latter by approximately 10%, resulting in greater central nervous system depression than when either agent is used alone.

Long-term use of larger than usual doses may result in psychological and physical dependence. A daily dose of more than 2.5 g may be sufficient to cause the latter.

Withdrawal symptoms, including convulsions, may occur when glutethimide is discontinued abruptly. Overdosage (20 to 30 times the usual dose) has caused areflexia, fever, and prolonged coma, sometimes with unilateral clinical findings. Toxic doses produce less respiratory depression than the barbiturates but circulatory depression is more profound. The long duration and variability of the depth of the coma is partly due to the production of a potent active metabolite. Although death has been reported after ingestion of 12 g, patients have recovered after doses as large as 15 g. The fatal blood level is usually 1.5 to 3 mg/dl. This agent is very insoluble in water and catharsis is helpful in removing residual amounts from the intestines. Most authorities feel that peritoneal dialysis or hemodialysis is ineffective in treating overdosage. Because of the drug's low water solubility, lipid dialysis is more effective. Intensive supportive therapy alone frequently yields satisfactory results. See the Introduction and Table for further information on hypnotic drugs.

ROUTE, USUAL DOSAGE, AND PREPARATIONS. *Oral*: For hypnosis, *adults*, 250 to 500 mg at bedtime; the dose may be repeated if necessary, but not less than four hours before arising. Dosage over 1 g daily should be avoided. *Children under 12 years*, information is inadequate to establish dosage.

    Drug available generically: Capsules 500 mg; tablets 250 and 500 mg.

    Doriden (USV). Capsules 500 mg; tablets 250 and 500 mg.

HYDROXYZINE HYDROCHLORIDE
[Atarax, Vistaril]

HYDROXYZINE PAMOATE
[Vistaril]

Hydroxyzine is a less potent antianxiety agent than the benzodiazepines; however, it also possesses antiemetic and antihistaminic effects. Consequently, it is used in motion sickness, preanesthetic medication, and allergic dermatoses, especially when an additional mild antianxiety action is beneficial. The effectiveness of hydroxyzine as an antianxiety agent for long-term use (ie, more than four months) has not been assessed by systematic clinical studies. If narcotics or barbiturates are given with hydroxyzine, it is necessary to reduce their dosage by 50%, because their depressant action on the central nervous system is potentiated.

The incidence of untoward effects appears to be low; drowsiness usually is transient. Fatal overdosage is uncommon and withdrawal reactions have not been associated with use of hydroxyzine. Some teratogenic effects have been reported in animals when doses substantially above the human therapeutic range were administered, but these findings are difficult to evaluate and inconclusive with respect to human pregnancy (see the discussion on Drugs Used During Pregnancy in Chapter 2).

See the Introduction and Table for additional information on antianxiety drugs.

ROUTES, USUAL DOSAGE, AND PREPARATIONS. *Oral*: For anxiety, *adults*, 75 to 400 mg daily divided into four doses. For allergic dermatoses, *adults*, 25 mg three or four times a day; *children under 6 years*, 50 mg daily in divided doses; *over 6 years*, 50 to 100 mg daily in divided doses.

HYDROXYZINE HYDROCHLORIDE:
Drug available generically: Tablets 10, 25, 50, and 100 mg.
Atarax (Roerig). Syrup 10 mg/5 ml; tablets 10, 25, 50, and 100 mg.

HYDROXYZINE PAMOATE:
Drug available generically: Capsules, tablets 25, 50, and 100 mg.
Vistaril [*pamoate*] (Pfizer). Capsules 25, 50, and 100 mg; suspension 25 mg/5 ml (strengths expressed in terms of the hydrochloride salt).

Intramuscular: For severe anxiety, *adults*, 50 to 100 mg initially and every four to six hours as needed.

HYDROXYZINE HYDROCHLORIDE:
Vistaril [*hydrochloride*] (Pfizer). Solution 25 mg/ml in 1 and 10 ml containers and 50 mg/ml in 1, 2, and 10 ml containers.

MEPROBAMATE
[Equanil, Meprospan, Miltown]

$$H_2NCOCH_2\overset{CH_3}{\underset{CH_2CH_2CH_3}{C}}CH_2OCNH_2$$

Meprobamate is useful in the treatment of anxiety, but it appears to be somewhat less effective than the benzodiazepines. Effectiveness coincides with the peak plasma concentration, which occurs about two to three hours after ingestion. Induction of hepatic microsomal enzymes occurs but does not appear to be a problem with usual clinical doses. Consistent bioavailability of the timed-release preparation has been demonstrated; however, since meprobamate has a mean half-life of about ten hours, timed-release preparations do not offer any significant advantage over ordinary dosage forms for most patients.

The most common untoward effect is drowsiness, which develops with doses larger than 1.2 g daily. Thrombocytopenia, leukopenia, dermatitis, urticaria, anaphylactic reactions, hypotension and syncope, blurred vision, weakness of the extremities, and paradoxical reactions of euphoria and anger occur rarely. Agranulocytosis and aplastic anemia have been reported, although no causal relationship has been established.

Long-term use of larger than usual doses may result in psychological and physical dependence. Withdrawal symptoms may occur when meprobamate is discontinued abruptly after the prolonged daily administration of 1.6 to 2.4 g, and convulsions may develop after a daily dose of approximately 6 g. Death has occurred during withdrawal of this drug. Death from poisoning has been reported after ingestion of 12 g of meprobamate, but some patients have survived after ingestion of 40 g.

See the Introduction and Table for additional information on antianxiety drugs.

ROUTE, USUAL DOSAGE, AND PREPARATIONS.
Oral: *Adults*, 1.2 to 1.6 g (maximum, 2.4 g) daily divided into three or four doses. *Children over 6 years*, 25 mg/kg of body weight daily divided into two or three doses; adequate information is not available to establish dosage for *children under 6 years*.

> Drug available generically: Tablets 200 and 400 mg.
> *Equanil* (Wyeth). Capsules 400 mg; tablets 200 and 400 mg; tablets (coated) 400 mg (Wyseals).
> *Meprospan* (Wallace). Capsules (timed-release) 200 and 400 mg.
> *Miltown* (Wallace). Tablets 200, 400, and 600 mg.

METHAQUALONE
[Quaalude, Sopor]

METHAQUALONE HYDROCHLORIDE
[Parest]

Methaqualone is an effective sedative and hypnotic agent but, like similar drugs, may lose its effectiveness by the second week of continued administration. It appears to have no advantage over other hypnotics. This drug is probably safe for use in patients with hereditary porphyria. It has an undeserved reputation as an aphrodisiac.

Methaqualone occasionally produces minor gastric distress (eg, nausea), headache, drowsiness, fatigue, and dryness of the mouth. Acroparesthesia (tingling and numbness of the extremities) has been observed prior to onset of the hypnotic effect, particularly when sleep has not been immediate, and several cases of peripheral neuropathy have been reported.

Methaqualone has been commonly abused by drug-dependent individuals and long-term use of larger than usual therapeutic doses may result in psychological and physical dependence. Tolerance to the drug, not necessarily of metabolic origin, occurs in abusers.

Poisoning is characterized by extrapyramidal signs such as increased muscle tone, hyperreflexia, and myoclonia; however, the incidence of profound, prolonged unconsciousness and serious ventilatory depression may be lower with methaqualone than with the barbiturates. Death has occurred after ingestion of 8 g, but survival has been reported after ingestion of 22 g. The fatal blood level is usually 0.5 to 1.5 mg/dl. Most patients who have ingested excessive amounts of methaqualone respond to intensive supportive therapy, but forced diuresis does not appear to be effective and may induce pulmonary edema. Peritoneal dialysis and hemodialysis should be reserved for only the most severe cases of poisoning; hemodialysis is more effective. Neuromuscular blocking agents and controlled ventilation may be necessary to control muscular hyperactivity.

See the Introduction and Table for further information on hypnotic drugs.

ROUTE, USUAL DOSAGE, AND PREPARATIONS.
Oral: *Adults*, for sedation, 75 mg three or four times daily; for hypnosis, 150 to 400 mg at bedtime. *Children*, information is inadequate to establish dosage.

> METHAQUALONE:
> *Quaalude* (Lemmon), *Sopor* (Arnar-Stone). Tablets 150 and 300 mg.
> METHAQUALONE HYDROCHLORIDE:
> *Parest* (Parke, Davis). Capsules 200 and 400 mg (equivalent to 175 and 350 mg base, respectively).

METHYPRYLON
[Noludar]

Methyprylon is used only as a hypnotic. Dizziness, mild to moderate gastrointestinal upset, headache, paradoxical excitement, and rash have been reported occasionally. Although death has occurred after ingestion of 6 g, patients have recovered after doses as high as 20 g. Long-term use of larger than usual therapeutic doses may result in psychological and physical dependence. Withdrawal symptoms, including convulsions, may occur when methyprylon is discontinued abruptly. See the Introduction and Table for further information on hypnotic agents.

ROUTE, USUAL DOSAGE, AND PREPARATIONS. *Oral*: *Adults*, 200 to 400 mg at bedtime. *Children*, the effective dose varies greatly and, therefore, should be individualized; initially, 50 mg is suggested and the amount may be increased up to 200 mg if required. This drug should not be used in *children under 3 months*.

> *Noludar* (Roche). Capsules 300 mg; tablets 50 and 200 mg.

PARALDEHYDE

This cyclic ether compound is a rapidly effective sedative and hypnotic agent, but it has not been established if this drug is a more efficacious and safe hypnotic than the benzodiazepines, barbiturates, or chloral derivatives. Although paraldehyde has been used in the treatment of alcohol withdrawal symptoms, in spite of its unpleasant taste some chronic alcoholics and drug abusers develop a liking for its psychological effects, and long-term use of larger than usual therapeutic doses may result in psychological and physical dependence. More effective and safer drugs are available for the emergency treatment of convulsive disorders. Although the drug is primarily metabolized by the liver, a small portion is excreted through the lungs, which accounts for the characteristic pungent, disagreeable odor of the patient's breath.

Oral administration is preferred, but gastric irritation may occur; rectal administration is an alternate route. Intravenous administration is not advisable. If paraldehyde is administered intramuscularly, the drug must be injected deep into the gluteus maximus to enhance absorption and to prevent formation of sterile abcesses (permanent sciatic nerve damage has been reported). Only freshly opened preparations should be administered. Paraldehyde reacts with plastic equipment.

The sedative effect may be intensified and prolonged in patients with severe liver damage. See the Introduction for further information on antianxiety-hypnotic drugs.

ROUTES, USUAL DOSAGE, AND PREPARATIONS. *Intramuscular*: For sedation, *adults*, 5 ml; *children*, 0.15 ml/kg of body weight. For hypnosis, *adults*, 10 ml.

> Drug available generically: Liquid 1 g/ml in 2, 5, 10, and 30 ml containers.

Oral, Rectal: For sedation, *adults*, 5 to 10 ml; *children*, 0.15 ml/kg of body weight. For hypnosis, *adults*, 10 to 30 ml; *children*, 0.3 ml/kg.

Paraldehyde must be diluted with an equal or double amount of vegetable oil (eg, olive oil) for rectal administration.

> Drug available generically: Liquid in 30 ml containers.

MIXTURES

Mixtures containing one or more barbiturates, most commonly amobarbital, butabarbital, pentobarbital, phenobarbital, or secobarbital (eg, Ethobral, Qui-A-Zone, S.B.P., Tuinal), or other hypnotic and antianxiety agents (eg, Carbrital) have been used extensively for many years, but any alleged advantage of such combination products is hypothetical. The effects of these mixtures may only be additive, often without any compensating advantage to the patient. Furthermore, fixed-ratio combinations do not permit careful adjustment of the dosage of each drug, which may be important when administering two or more drugs with different durations of action. For these reasons, use of this type of mixture is not recommended.

For the same reasons, fixed-ratio combinations of two or more antianxiety agents or antianxiety agents with anorexiants, antihypertensive agents, estrogens, mild analgesics, antianginal agents, or antispasmodics (eg, Dexamyl, Plexonal, Sedadrops) are not recommended. Such mixtures are marketed for use in the treatment of anxiety, pain, menopausal symptoms, angina pectoris, obesity, hypertension, and musculoskeletal and gastrointestinal disorders.

Selected References

Over-the-counter nighttime sleep-aid and stimulant products, Tentative final orders. *Federal Register* 43:25544-25602, (June 13) 1978.

Balter MB, et al: Cross-national study of extent of anti-anxiety/sedative drug use. *N Engl J Med* 290:769-774, 1974.

Blackwell B: Rational drug use in management of anxiety. *Ration Drug Ther* 9:1-7, (June) 1975.

Breimer DD: Clinical pharmacokinetics of hypnotics. *Clin Pharmacokinet* 2:93-109, 1977.

Cooper JR (ed): Sedative-hynotic drugs: Risks and benefits. Rockville, Md, National Institute on Drug Abuse, National Clearinghouse for Drug Abuse Information, 1978.

Gillin JC, et al: Flurazepam and insomnia. *Science* 205:954-955, 1979.

Greenblatt DJ, Miller RR: Hypnotics, in Miller RR, Greenblatt DJ (eds): *Handbook of Drug Therapy*. New York, Elsevier, 1979, 507-519.

Greenblatt DJ, Shader RI: Antianxiety agents, in Miller RR, Greenblatt DJ (eds): *Handbook of Drug Therapy*. New York, Elsevier, 1979, 520-541.

Greenblatt DJ, Shader RI: Prazepam and lorazepam: Two new benzodiazepines. *N Engl J Med* 299:1342-1344, 1978 A.

Greenblatt DJ, Shader RI: Pharmacokinetic understanding of antianxiety drug therapy. *South Med J* 71(suppl 2):2-9, (Aug) 1978 B.

Greenblatt DJ, et al: Pharmacokinetics and bioavailability of intravenous, intramuscular, and oral lorazepam in humans. *J Pharmaceut Sci* 68:57-63, 1979.

Hartmann E: Drugs for insomnia. *Ration Drug Ther* 11:1-6, (Dec) 1977.

Hartmann E: L-Tryptophan: Rational hypnotic with clinical potential. *Am J Psychiatry* 134:366-370, 1977.

Iversen LL: GABA and benzodiazepine receptors. *Nature* 275:477, 1978.

Kales A, Kales JD: Shortcomings in evaluation and promotion of hypnotic drugs. *N Engl J Med* 293:826-827, 1975.

Kales A, et al: Rebound insomnia: Potential hazard following withdrawal of certain benzodiazepines. *JAMA* 241:1692-1695, 1979.

Kales A, et al: Comparative effectiveness of nine hypnotic drugs: Sleep laboratory studies. *J Clin Pharmacol* 17:207-213, 1977.

Kales A, et al: Chronic hypnotic-drug use: Ineffectiveness, drug-withdrawal insomnia, and dependence. *JAMA* 227:513-517, 1974.

Kraus JW, et al: Effects of aging and liver disease on disposition of lorazepam. *Clin Pharmacol Ther* 24:411-419, 1978.

Mellinger GD, et al: Psychic distress, life crisis, and use of psychotherapeutic medications: National household survey data. *Arch Gen Psychiatry* 35:1045-1052, 1978.

National Academy of Sciences, Institute of Medicine: Sleeping pills, insomnia, and medical practice. Washington, DC, 1979.

Safar P: Brain resuscitation in metabolic-toxic-infectious encephalopathy. *Crit Care Med* 6:68-70, 1978.

Sellers EM: Clinical pharmacology and therapeutics of benzodiazepines. *Can Med Assoc J* 118:1533-1538, 1978.

Soldatos CR, et al: Management of insomnia. *Annu Rev Med* 30:301-312, 1979.

Solomon F, et al: Sleeping pills, insomnia and medical practice. *N Engl J Med* 300:803-808, 1979.

Whitlock FA, Price J: Use of beta-adrenergic receptor blocking drugs in psychiatry. *Drugs* 8:109-124, 1974.

Antipsychotic Drugs | 12

Although antipsychotic (neuroleptic) drugs are not curative, they are useful in the treatment of acute and chronic schizophrenia; schizoaffective disorders; acute psychotic disorders; organic brain syndromes with psychosis; intractable hiccoughs; the chorea of Huntington's disease; ballismus; and Tourette's syndrome.

The chemical classes of drugs having antipsychotic activity are the phenothiazines, thioxanthenes, butyrophenones, dihydroindolones, dibenzoxazepines, and diphenylbutylpiperidines (see the Table). Phenothiazines are divided into three classes (aliphatic, piperidine, and piperazine) on the basis of differences in their chemistry, pharmacologic actions, and potency. The thioxanthene derivatives, chlorprothixene [Taractan] and thiothixene [Navane], are chemically related to the aliphatic and piperazine phenothiazines, respectively. Haloperidol [Haldol], a butyrophenone; molindone [Lidone, Moban], a dihydroindolone; and loxapine [Daxolin, Loxitane], a dibenzoxazepine, are the only representatives of their respective chemical classes available in the United States. They are pharmacologically, but not chemically, related to the piperazine phenothiazines.

ANTIPSYCHOTIC DRUGS

Nonproprietary Drug Name	Chemical Classification	Therapeutically Equivalent Oral Dose (mg)	EFFECTS		
			Sedation	Autonomic[1]	Extrapyramidal Reactions[2]
Fluphenazine Permitil (Schering) Prolixin (Squibb)	Phenothiazine: Piperazine Compound	2	+/++	+	+++
Haloperidol Haldol (McNeil)	Butyrophenone	2	+	+	+++
Thiothixene Navane (Roerig)	Thioxanthene	4	+	+	+++
Trifluoperazine Stelazine (Smith Kline & French)	Phenothiazine: Piperazine Compound	5	++	+	+++
Perphenazine Trilafon (Schering)	Phenothiazine: Piperazine Compound	8	+/++	+	+++
Butaperazine Repoise (Robins)	Phenothiazine: Piperazine Compound	10	++	+	+++
Loxapine Daxolin (Dome) Loxitane (Lederle)	Dibenzoxazepine	10	++	+/++	+++
Molindone Lidone (Abbott) Moban (Endo)	Dihydroindolone	10	++	++	++/+++
Piperacetazine Quide (Dow)	Phenothiazine: Piperidine Compound	10	++	+	++
Prochlorperazine Compazine (Smith Kline & French)	Phenothiazine: Piperazine Compound	15	++	+	+++
Acetophenazine Tindal (Schering)	Phenothiazine: Piperazine Compound	20	++	+	+++
Carphenazine Proketazine (Wyeth)	Phenothiazine: Piperazine Compound	25	++	+	+++
Triflupromazine Vesprin (Squibb)	Phenothiazine: Aliphatic Compound	25	+++	++/+++	++
Mesoridazine Serentil (Boehringer Ingelheim)	Phenothiazine: Piperidine Compound	50	+++	++	+

ANTIPSYCHOTIC DRUGS

Nonproprietary Drug Name	Chemical Classification	Therapeutically Equivalent Oral Dose (mg)	EFFECTS		
			Sedation	Autonomic[1]	Extrapyramidal Reactions[2]
Chlorpromazine Thorazine (Smith Kline & French)	Phenothiazine: Aliphatic Compound	100	+++	++/+++	++
Chlorprothixene Taractan (Roche)	Thioxanthene	100	+++	+++	+/++
Thioridazine Mellaril (Sandoz)	Phenothiazine: Piperidine Compound	100	+++	++/+++	+

[1]*Alpha antiadrenergic and anticholinergic effects*
[2]*Excluding tardive dyskinesia*

Three drugs marketed in Europe are being investigated in the United States. Two diphenylbutylpiperidines, pimozide and penfluridol, have potent antipsychotic properties. Penfluridol is particularly interesting because it is effective orally when given only once a week. Both compounds have a tendency to produce extrapyramidal reactions, but the incidence of autonomic effects is low. The third drug, clozapine [Leponex], a dibenzodiazepine, is unique in that no extrapyramidal reactions have been observed following its use, although sedation and autonomic effects have been noted. However, fatal agranulocytosis has occurred in a few patients and investigational studies are being continued cautiously until the causal relationship and incidence are established.

Reserpine has some antipsychotic activity but is more likely to produce depression and hypotension than the more effective phenothiazines and is no longer used for this purpose. Promazine [Sparine] is obsolete because it has extremely weak antipsychotic activity and the incidence of agranulocytosis is greater than with other phenothiazines.

Dopamine receptors are present in high concentration in the brain and the antipsychotic drugs are believed to control the symptomatology of psychosis by acting as postsynaptic dopamine receptor antag-

onists. Their sites of action are generally thought to be the mesolimbic and mesocortical systems, which influence emotional behavior; similar actions in the nigroneostriatal and tuberoinfundibular systems probably produce extrapyramidal and endocrine adverse reactions, respectively. The site of their antiemetic action is the chemoreceptor trigger zone of the medulla. All antipsychotic drugs have varying degrees of antihistaminic, anticholinergic, and alpha-antiadrenergic activities; it is not known to what extent these actions influence their antipsychotic effects, although they do account for a number of the adverse reactions noted.

Use in Schizophrenia

Schizophrenia represents a group of conditions thought to have some degree of genetic transmission, and the hereditary potential may be activated by environmental or developmental stress (Baldessarini, 1977). The exact biochemical and neurophysiologic abnormalities are unclear. Schizophrenia is characterized primarily by distinctive alterations in concept formations and reality relationships. Symptoms can begin insidiously or acutely at almost any time of life but most often become evident during adolescence or early adulthood.

The primary symptoms are (1) a peculiar thought disorder, manifested as bizarre or vague statements, associated with an otherwise clear sensorium; (2) autism accompanied by social withdrawal and preference for solitary activities; and (3) abnormal affect characterized by illogical emotional responses to environmental stimuli. Secondary behavioral disturbances usually are present in varying degrees; auditory hallucinations, delusions, and abnormal modes of expression (catatonic symptoms) are most common. Primary symptoms must be present to establish the diagnosis. Hyperactivity, anxiety, agitation, paranoia, hostility, hallucinations, and mood disturbances are characteristic of many psychiatric disorders; by themselves, they are not sufficient for diagnosis of schizophrenia. Because no obvious neuropathology or alteration in results of diagnostic tests is evident, schizophrenia must be diagnosed on the basis of symptoms alone. The course of the illness varies widely, ranging from remission to chronicity.

Antipsychotic drugs control most primary and secondary symptoms in many patients; however, symptoms arising from difficulties with complex social tasks (marriage, leaving family of origin, stressful job) are less likely to improve. Antipsychotic drug therapy improves the patient's capacity for adjustment, accelerates remission of psychotic symptoms and deviant behavior, and decreases the period of hospitalization. Controlled studies demonstrate that the relapse rate can be reduced two and one-half times with appropriate drug therapy (Davis and Casper, 1977).

Choice of Drug: Numerous collaborative, well-controlled studies have determined that the patterns of response to any of the antipsychotic drugs are very similar among the various types of schizophrenic patients (eg, paranoid, core, depressed, catatonic). Thus, despite differences in potency, all antipsychotic drugs are equally effective in equivalent doses (Davis, 1975; Davis, 1976; Davis and Casper, 1977; Johnson, 1977). The more sedative drugs often are prescribed for agitated, overactive patients and the less sedative agents for apathetic, withdrawn patients.

Other factors also influence the selection of the appropriate drug for treatment. The history of response to past drug treatment by the patient or close family members is important in drug selection: The patient's or a blood relative's favorable previous response to a particular antipsychotic agent suggests initial treatment with that drug. Conversely, a previously unfavorable response to adequate doses would militate against use of that drug. The patient's age and physical condition, the severity and duration of illness, and the cost of the drug are other significant factors. In addition, the frequency and severity of untoward effects produced by each drug should be taken into account, for the specific adverse reactions the patient is willing to accept is essential in obtaining cooperation. Since sensitivity varies among patients, individualization of dosage and treatment procedures is required. This is usually more important than differences among drugs.

Antipsychotic drugs are arranged in decreasing order of antipsychotic potency in the Table. High-potency drugs have less sedative and autonomic blocking activity but are more likely to produce extrapyramidal reactions (akathisia, dystonia, parkinsonism); with minor exceptions, the reverse is noted as potency decreases. Allergic, endocrine, and oculocutaneous adverse reactions also are more prominent with low-potency drugs. It currently is assumed that all antipsychotic drugs have an equal propensity to produce tardive dyskinesia; there is no evidence to prove that a given antipsychotic drug is more or less dangerous than another in this respect. A rational approach is for the practicing physician to become proficient in the use of at least one low-potency and one high-potency drug (see the Table).

Dosage and Administration: Unless the patient's previous history or current illness dictates the choice, the preferred route of administration is oral. Intramuscular administration is more reliable and assures absorption; the dosage required usually is one-fourth to one-half the oral dose. However, prolonged use of this route is inconvenient and expensive when daily administration is required. Of the oral forms, liquids are absorbed most readily; successively less reliable are tablets and capsules. The mean half-lives of most antipsychotic drugs are prolonged (range, 10 to 30 hours); therefore, the use of timed-release oral preparations offers little advantage for the majority of patients. A few individuals in whom the half-lives of antipsychotics are relatively short (ie, two to six hours) may benefit from their use, but the need for such preparations should be determined on an individual basis. Two injectable forms of fluphenazine (decanoate and enanthate), which can be given every two or three weeks, and the investigational drug, penfluridol, given orally once weekly, are being used increasingly in outpatients and those who are uncooperative. This type of maintenance therapy assures drug intake, but probably should be reserved for use in patients previously stabilized on oral doses. See the evaluation on fluphenazine for a more detailed discussion.

For acutely agitated psychotic patients, aggressive administration of any antipsychotic agent (with appropriate monitoring of response) allows significant reduction of symptoms in a matter of hours. The drug can be given orally as soon as symptoms are controlled.

In the absence of a specific requirement for intramuscular administration, initial oral doses generally should be 200 to 600 mg daily of chlorpromazine or the equivalent; the amount is increased until a response occurs or adverse reactions intervene. The rate of increase depends upon the patient's age, weight, and the severity of symptoms. The range of dosage for chlorpromazine during the latter part of the first week of treatment is generally between 500 mg and 1.5 g. Although the maximum recommended daily dose is 2 g, there is usually little to be gained by giving amounts above 1 to 1.5 g per day. Patients under 40 years of age and those who are hyperactive or have severe psychoses generally require the larger daily doses. Too

gradual increases in dose and inadequate dosage levels are the most frequent causes of drug failure in acutely psychotic patients. No patient should be considered a drug failure without an intensive course of carefully monitored therapy.

The response to initial administration of an antipsychotic agent in newly diagnosed patients varies but should be evident after one to two days of adequate treatment; a few weeks of treatment may be required before the complete response can be judged. If the desired therapeutic effect is not attained after an adequate trial of therapy, substitution of a drug from a different chemical category may be justified. Substitution of a near equivalent dose of the new drug usually can be made without difficulty.

As acute psychotic symptoms subside, the daily dose should be reduced gradually, usually to 200 to 800 mg daily of oral chlorpromazine or the equivalent. The range is necessarily large, since pronounced differences in steady state concentrations of similar doses of the same drug occur among patients. *The maintenance dosage should be the minimum amount that maintains therapeutic response and allows the patient to function best.* This will reduce the potential for the development of tardive dyskinesia. Flexibility of dosage is necessary in order to accommodate periods of increased or decreased symptoms.

Antipsychotic agents are often given in divided amounts to minimize adverse reactions until a satisfactory maintenance dosage has been established. Thereafter, they may be given in one, or occasionally two, doses daily unless adverse reactions increase. It is preferable to give a single dose at bedtime to take advantage of the sedation produced and possibly decrease the incidence of orthostatic hypotension. Often, additional sedation is unnecessary and the patient is less likely to be drowsy during the day. Selected patients may benefit from the daytime sedation produced by daily divided doses.

The patient's progress and drug regimen should be reviewed periodically. Maintenance therapy greatly increases the likelihood that the patient will retain the improvement gained during initial treatment and is more effective if continued surveillance and close contact with the patient and his family is retained. The antipsychotic drugs may be required indefinitely in schizophrenic patients who relapse after drug-free periods. Continuous daily administration may assure better compliance in some patients, but interruptions in treatment (drug holidays) may be advisable for those in whom the drug accumulates or to unmask symptoms of tardive dyskinesia and thus facilitate its early diagnosis.

Combination Therapy: Systematic, well-controlled studies indicate that combination therapy is no more effective than adequate doses of a single antipsychotic agent. The beneficial effects of some antipsychotic agents (eg, thioridazine, fluphenazine) have been reduced when chlordiazepoxide [Librium] was added to the regimen, and schizophrenic symptoms have increased in patients receiving amphetamines concomitantly to overcome the sedation produced by the antipsychotic drug.

Other Therapy for Schizophrenia: There is no substantial evidence from well-controlled studies that niacin (nicotinic acid) or niacinamide (nicotinamide) are efficacious, alone or with large doses of other vitamins, in the treatment of schizophrenia.

Other Indications

Antipsychotic drugs are useful in *acute psychotic disorders* other than schizophrenia. They ameliorate severe disruptive and umanageable excitement, delirium, and violent aggression. These drugs are generally effective regardless of the etiology of the disorder (eg, psychiatric syndromes developing in critical care units following surgery or myocardial infarction, rage reactions, severe agitated endogenous depressions, sensory deprivation syndromes). An antipsychotic is often the drug of choice initially in severe acute mania

inasmuch as specific therapy with lithium has a long latent period before onset of action; as lithium becomes effective, the antipsychotic drug may be discontinued or the dosage reduced.

These drugs usually are given intramuscularly at frequent intervals until symptoms are controlled. Peripheral autonomic and cardiovascular adverse reactions may occur if the dose is not carefully titrated. Currently, the more potent antipsychotic drugs are often employed to treat acute psychotic disorders, although chlorpromazine has been equally effective. The minimal autonomic activity of the more potent piperazine phenothiazines and haloperidol is probably responsible for this trend. Some investigators report that no extrapyramidal reactions occur after use of high-potency antipsychotic drugs for rapid control of symptoms of acute psychoses. Others report that 20% of patients experienced acute dystonic reactions, but these were easily controlled by intramuscular administration of the centrally active anticholinergic, benztropine [Cogentin].

Antipsychotic drugs are beneficial in *schizoaffective disorders*. It may be necessary to combine lithium or another antidepressant with the antipsychotic for complete control of the disorder. (See Chapter 13, Drugs Used in Affective Disorders.)

These agents are useful in the treatment of selected drug-induced toxic psychoses (eg, *amphetamine psychosis*); however, they may increase symptoms in patients who have abused hallucinogens. Toxic delirium caused by drugs with considerable anticholinergic activity may be exacerbated and prolonged by administration of antipsychotic agents, since the latter also have anticholinergic properties.

Paranoia often accompanies toxic (eg, alcohol and amphetamine abuse) or functional psychoses. Treatment of the primary disorder should supersede treatment of paranoia. The prolonged use of antipsychotic drugs has decreased tension and agitation and stabilized some patients with paranoid psychotic illnesses. Paranoia is often resistant to antipsychotic drugs when it occurs as an independent psychotic state, but some patients may respond to low or conventional doses.

The cautious administration of small doses of antipsychotic drugs may be useful in hyperactive patients with acute or chronic *organic brain syndromes with psychosis* (eg, delusions). Phenothiazines have been used to manage behavioral disturbances in epileptics, although the benzodiazepines are preferred because of their anticonvulsant activity. Antipsychotic agents may increase the frequency of seizures, thus requiring an increase in the dose of anticonvulsants.

Antipsychotic agents are reported to be effective occasionally in *mental retardation* not associated with a major psychiatric disorder or in psychosis associated with senility. These drugs may partially alleviate the irritability, disturbed sleep, agitation, hostility, and combativeness, but they do not correct the mental deficiency. Because of the danger of tardive dyskinesia, their use in children and adolescents with behavior disorders other than schizophrenia or autism should be very limited.

Although antipsychotic drugs do not reverse or halt the progress of dementia in *Huntington's disease*, they usually control the chorea. Dopamine-depleting drugs, such as tetrabenazine and reserpine, as well as central acetylcholine precursors, such as choline and lecithin, are also being investigated (see Chapter 16, Drugs Used in Extrapyramidal Movement Disorders).

A few antipsychotic drugs are effective in *ballismus* and *Tourette's syndrome* (multiple tics), which are caused by central motor dysfunction. (See the evaluation on Haloperidol.)

Chlorpromazine is indicated in the treatment of *intractable hiccoughs* and represents one of the rare instances when intravenous administration of a phenothiazine may be necessary.

Because they potentiate the effects of hypnotic, analgesic, and anesthetic agents, some antipsychotic drugs are occasionally used as *adjuncts to anesthesia* (see Chapter 21).

Except for mesoridazine and thiorid-azine, all antipsychotic drugs have a pronounced *antiemetic* action (see Chapter 26, Drugs Used in Vertigo, Motion Sickness, and Vomiting).

Antipsychotic agents have no value in the treatment of acute or chronic alcoholism. They may precipitate seizures during acute alcohol withdrawal reactions, and fatalities have occurred following their intravenous administration. A cautious therapeutic trial of an antipsychotic drug may be justified to calm the rare patient withdrawing from alcohol who is paranoid or not responding adequately to the benzodiazepines.

All antipsychotic drugs produce varying degrees of sedation and suppression of mood. Accordingly, they have been inappropriately termed major tranquilizers and prescribed for patients with anxiety. Antianxiety drugs are more effective, safer, and better tolerated by most anxious patients than even small doses of the antipsychotic drugs. An antidepressant drug may be a better choice than an antianxiety or antipsychotic drug for anxiety associated with depression or for phobic anxiety associated with panic attacks.

Precautions

Patient Reassurance: When a patient is released from the hospital, he and his family should be advised that medication is to be continued even though he feels well, and he should be reassured about fears of addiction. The effects of drowsiness on such tasks as driving or operating machinery also should be stressed, and dosage schedules that minimize interference with the patient's ability to perform these tasks should be employed. The patient should be further warned about the possible additive effects of other drugs (see the discussion on Interactions) and specifically about the concomitant use of alcoholic beverages.

Children: It is possible that antipsychotic agents might retard growth in children, because they have been shown to inhibit release of growth hormone experimentally; linear growth should be measured periodically in young patients on long-term therapy.

Older Patients: The half-life of antipsychotic agents is prolonged in many patients over 55 years of age and, therefore, the incidence of adverse reactions may be greater. To lessen this possibility, the dosage should be reduced to the lowest effective level as quickly as feasible, the patient should be observed closely, and the maintenance regimen should be reviewed periodically.

Since sleep disturbances are more common in elderly patients, the administration of antipsychotic agents once daily at bedtime may be appropriate. However, when higher dosage levels are indicated, smaller doses at more frequent intervals may be necessary, since the drug may not be detoxified quickly enough in these patients to avoid periodic excessive drug plasma concentrations.

Psychiatric syndromes in the elderly can be caused by drugs or organic disease. In these instances, withdrawal of the precipitating drug or treatment of the medical condition should supersede antipsychotic medication and probably will obviate the need for these agents. Since the elderly are particularly prone to develop adverse effects from antipsychotic drugs, these agents should not be used in nonpsychiatric conditions for which other drugs are available.

Drug Interactions: These drugs may enhance the action of other central nervous system depressants, particularly the barbiturates. Doses of other preanesthetic sedatives and general anesthetics may need to be reduced. Antipsychotic agents should be temporarily discontinued if possible in patients receiving spinal or epidural anesthesia to allow time for the remaining drug to be metabolized.

When tricyclic antidepressants are used with antipsychotic drugs, additive central nervous system depression and anticholinergic activity may be expected. Antipsychotic drugs may interfere with the neuronal uptake of guanethidine and clonidine, thereby antagonizing their antihypertensive effects.

Extrapyramidal side effects occurring during treatment (dystonia, akathisia, and parkinsonism) occasionally disappear if the dose of the antipsychotic drug can be reduced without decreasing efficacy. Anticholinergic drugs also may be given for treatment. Although it is agreed that anticholinergic agents can be useful to treat these disorders, some concern exists over whether they should be administered routinely prophylactically. Limited evidence suggests that the concomitant prophylactic use of an antipsychotic and anticholinergic drug reduces the incidence of extrapyramidal effects and may increase compliance; the risks include potential additive anticholinergic toxicity and possibly decreased absorption of the antipsychotic agent. Those who favor prophylactic use note that some extrapyramidal side effects are subtle and may easily be missed by the physician. Avoidance of side effects improves compliance and, in certain special situations such as outpatients who reside at a considerable distance from a physician, prophylactic therapy might prove reasonable. Those who oppose the use of prophylactic treatment emphasize that anticholinergic drugs produce additive toxicity.

Either initial treatment with antipsychotics alone and anticholinergics given if necessary, or initial concomitant treatment with prophylactic anticholinergics is an acceptable alternative. What is most important to remember, regardless of the approach selected, is that dystonia, akathisia, and parkinsonism occur early in treatment. Therefore, if a patient does not exhibit extrapyramidal side effects by the third or fourth month, the dose of the anticholinergic should be reduced gradually (sudden discontinuation may precipitate extrapyramidal symptoms). Reinstitution of therapy may be necessary in a small percentage of patients with recurrent extrapyramidal effects (estimated to be less than 10% despite continued antipsychotic therapy).

Coexisting Medical Problems: A history of liver disease is not an absolute contraindication to use of antipsychotic agents, but smaller doses may be required because metabolic clearance is decreased. The more potent antipsychotics (piperazine phenothiazines, thiothixene [Navane], or haloperidol [Haldol]) are preferred in these patients.

Although tolerance to the hypotensive effect develops with prolonged treatment, caution is required when antipsychotic drugs are given to patients in whom a sudden drop in blood pressure is undesirable.

Antipsychotic agents may be given to epileptics receiving adequate anticonvulsant therapy. The increased incidence of seizures that occurs occasionally may be controlled by increasing the dose of the anticonvulsant. Patients with a family history of seizures or febrile convulsions are more likely to develop seizures than those who have no such history.

Teratogenicity: Although data from controlled studies have shown that there is no increase in the rate of malformations in infants, phenothiazines cross the placenta and have been identified along with their metabolites in maternal and fetal plasma, in amniotic fluid, and in the urine of newborn infants. Prolonged extrapyramidal effects also may appear in the infant. Thus, the use of antipsychotic drugs during pregnancy probably should be restricted to psychotic patients who require continued medication, and drug therapy should be discontinued one to two weeks prior to delivery to avoid neonatal distress. (See also the discussion on use of drugs during pregnancy in Chapter 2.) No adequate data are available on the excretion of antipsychotic drugs in breast milk but, if a mother who needs continuous therapy nurses her infant, close supervision of the infant is mandatory.

Adverse Reactions

All antipsychotic agents produce adverse reactions that are extensions of their pharmacologic effects, although there are differences among the chemical classes of drugs (Charalampous and Keepers, 1978; Zavodnick, 1978). Tolerance appears to be correlated with the severity of the psychosis; adverse subjective feelings may be more uncomfortable and persistent in nonpsychotic patients.

Antipsychotic drugs are remarkably safe in two important aspects: Overdoses are very seldom fatal in adults and addiction does not occur. In children, overdosage may produce serious toxicity, but prompt gastric lavage is an effective counteractant.

Close clinical observation is essential to monitor and treat adverse reactions. Although laboratory profiles are advisable to establish baseline values, frequent laboratory tests are unnecessary and have little predictive value.

Behavioral Effects: Sedation occurs commonly after use of all antipsychotic drugs, but it is especially pronounced after large doses of chlorpromazine, triflupromazine [Vesprin], mesoridazine [Serentil], thioridazine [Mellaril], and chlorprothixene [Taractan] (see Table). It can be minimized by reducing the dose or substituting a less sedating agent. However, the intensity of sedation decreases during long-term treatment and many patients become tolerant to this effect. Daytime somnolence can be avoided in most patients by giving a single dose at bedtime.

It has been suggested that a *toxic psychosis* occurs occasionally that may be difficult to differentiate from deterioration of the schizophrenic state. It is characterized by apparent exacerbation of schizophrenic symptomatology, confusion, insomnia, or marked sedation associated with bizarre dreams and general impairment of psychomotor activity. Reduction of dosage usually ameliorates the condition. Substituting an antipsychotic drug with less anticholinergic activity also may be helpful, particularly if anticholinergic drugs are being prescribed simultaneously.

Extrapyramidal Reactions: Three of these common reactions, dystonia, akathisia, and parkinsonism, occur early during treatment and are most often associated with use of the piperazine phenothiazines, thiothixene [Navane], loxapine [Daxolin, Loxitane], and haloperidol [Haldol]. Thioridazine is least likely to produce these extrapyramidal symptoms. The fourth reaction, tardive dyskinesia, usually is not observed until months to years after initiation of therapy but appears to occur with equal frequency with all antipsychotic drugs. (See Chapter 16, Drugs Used in Extrapyramidal Movement Disorders, for treatment of tardive dyskinesia.)

Acute torsion dystonia is generally the earliest abnormal movement to appear (ie, within hours or a few days). It is characterized primarily by abnormal posturing (ie, spastic torticollis, opisthotonus); perioral spasms (often with protrusion of the tongue), mandibular tics, dysphasia, dysphagia, and oculogyric crisis. These reactions may be accompanied by hyperhidrosis, pallor, fever, and marked anxiety. Dystonic reactions are noted most frequently following parenteral administration, especially in patients under 25 years of age. They probably can be attributed to individual sensitivity as well as to the chemical structure of the compound. Acute dystonic reactions often are bizarre and abrupt in onset; they may be confused with tetanus, hysteria, epilepsy, meningitis, encephalitis, stroke, or strychnine poisoning, and patients have been treated erroneously. Laryngospasm with severe dyspnea has been reported and fatalities have occurred.

Symptoms of dystonia rarely persist. The patient usually adapts with continued antipsychotic medication, although management of this adverse reaction is preferred. If a reduction in dosage is not feasible, the administration of a centrally acting anticholinergic agent (eg, benztropine [Cogentin]) or an antihistamine (eg, diphenhydramine [Benadryl]) alleviates the syndrome and makes antipsychotic drug therapy more tolerable during the adaptive phase.

Akathisia is a feeling of restlessness, and the resultant pacing and agitation may mimic dyskinesia. It commonly appears within a few weeks to a few months after initiation of therapy. Because this condition is often mistaken for psychotic agitation, the dose of the antipsychotic agent is increased unnecessarily and more marked akathisia results. If a reduction in dose is not feasible, central anticholinergic drugs may be used, although it frequently is necessary to add a sedating agent, such as diazepam [Valium], temporarily. After akathisia is controlled, the antipsychotic drug usually can be continued along with anticholinergic medication. If adaptation to this disorder occurs, the antipsychotic drug can be continued alone.

Parkinsonism, consisting of tremors, rigidity, bradykinesia, shuffling gait, postural abnormalities, mask-like facies, and hypersalivation, occurs within a few weeks to a few months after initiating therapy and may be clinically indistinguishable from postencephalitic or idiopathic parkinsonism. These symptoms occur most commonly after parenteral administration of usual doses. Use of a central anticholinergic drug or amantadine orally controls this condition; reducing the dose of antipsychotic drug may be tried if there is no deterioration of schizophrenic symptoms. (See the discussion on Drug Interactions in the section on Precautions.)

Tardive dyskinesias are characterized by choreiform movements of the face, trunk, and extremities resembling Huntington's chorea; axial hyperkinesias or ballistic movements also may be present. All classes of antipsychotic drugs appear to produce these neurologic complications. Their etiology and method of prevention have not been determined, but they may be unmasked or aggravated by sudden discontinuance of antipsychotic drugs and may persist in varying intensity after medication is withdrawn. Tardive dyskinesias may occur in patients of any age but they are most common in older patients, particularly women, and in those with organic brain syndromes. The increased incidence in the elderly may reflect only a longer duration of antipsychotic therapy.

A syndrome resembling tardive dyskinesia has been reported in children when antipsychotic medication was discontinued. Repetitive choreiform movements of the extremities were more common than abnormal movements of the mouth and face, and were reversible several weeks after administration was discontinued.

Because there are no alternative drugs to treat psychosis, tardive dyskinesia may be unavoidable in some patients. However, the risk of this disorder in patients considered for long-term antipsychotic drug therapy may be minimized if (1) antipsychotic agents are used only when clearly indicated; (2) the lowest effective dose is used; and (3) brief drug-free periods are established to unmask symptoms of tardive dyskinesia and thus facilitate its early diagnosis.

Several investigators have observed that early signs of tardive dyskinesia (grimacing or tic-like motions of the head and neck, fine vermicular movements of the tongue) occur, and suggest that the syndrome may not progress if the dosage is reduced gradually. If the antipsychotic agent is withdrawn abruptly, symptoms of tardive dyskinesia may be quite severe and/or psychotic symptoms may be exacerbated. It may be necessary to reinstitute the drug at the lowest dose adequate to control (mask) the symptoms of tardive dyskinesia and then reduce the dose more gradually. Increasing the dose of antipsychotic drugs usually suppresses tardive dyskinesia but, because this masks and may intensify the severity of this disorder, increasingly larger amounts should not be given if possible. (See the section on Precautions and Chapter 16, Drugs Used in Extrapyramidal Movement Disorders.)

Autonomic Nervous System Effects: All antipsychotic agents have both alpha *antiadrenergic* and *anticholinergic* actions to varying degrees (see the Table). These effects are more pronounced after parenteral administration. Autonomic reactions rarely necessitate drug withdrawal, but reduced doses may be advisable if effects are severe.

Orthostatic hypotension is the most troublesome antiadrenergic action but subsides if the patient lies down. It is common after oral administration. Acute hypotensive crises may occur in elderly or debilitated patients or after large parenteral doses. If hypotension is severe, intravenous fluids should be administered to correct hypovolemia. Norepinephrine [Levophed] or phenylephrine [Neo-Synephrine] is seldom required, and vasopressors such as epinephrine are contraindicated, for they may cause a paradoxical worsening of the hypotension. As with other drugs having antiadrenergic actions, the antipsychotic agents, especially thioridazine, may inhibit ejaculation.

Anticholinergic effects include dryness of the mouth, tachycardia, blurred vision, urinary retention, and constipation. Death has resulted from adynamic ileus or fulminating infection of the bladder. Antipsychotic agents impair central thermoregulatory mechanisms.

Allergic and Idiosyncratic Effects: *Cholestatic jaundice*, which occurs in less than 1 of every 200 patients, is noted most often with use of aliphatic phenothiazines, usually within the first four weeks of treatment. This is regarded as an allergic reaction; usually it is mild and self-limited but, if hyperbilirubinemia or jaundice is detected, the drug should be withdrawn immediately and an agent from a different chemical group administered.

Dermal allergic reactions manifested as urticarial, maculopapular, or petechial lesions occur infrequently. Serious reactions (eg, exfoliative dermatitis) have been reported occasionally. If these effects are noted, the drug should be discontinued and therapy resumed later with a drug from a different chemical class.

Photosensitivity is demonstrated by the appearance of a dark purplish-brown pigmentation on exposure to sunlight. This idiosyncratic reaction is the most common dermal reaction, is generally mild, and seldom requires dosage adjustment. It occurs most often when the aliphatic phenothiazines, especially chlorpromazine, are given for prolonged periods in large doses (ie, more than 800 mg daily). Photosensitivity may be irreversible but can be prevented by using the lowest effective dose, avoiding exposure to ultraviolet light, and using protective sunscreen preparations.

See the section on Hematologic Effects for a discussion on agranulocytosis.

Neuroendocrine Effects: Delayed ovulation and menstruation, amenorrhea, and galactorrhea in women and gynecomastia, edema, weight gain, and loss of libido in men have been reported occasionally. These effects are generally transient, dose related, and are considered to be manifestations of neuroendocrine imbalance caused by depressed hypothalamic function.

All neuroleptic drugs produce *hyperprolactinemia* because they block the inhibitory action of dopamine on prolactin secretion (Gruen et al, 1978). Although prolactin increases the incidence and growth of mammary tumors in mice and rats, only a small number of human mammary tumors respond similarly. Results of limited studies conducted to date have not shown an association between long-term adminstration of antipsychotic drugs and the development of mammary tumors in man. Epidemiologic studies are continuing. Until conclusive data are available, breast examination should be performed prior to administration of neuroleptic drugs and during prolonged antipsychotic drug administration, particularly in patients with previously detected breast cancer or in those with a strong family history of breast cancer.

Cardiac Effects: Usual doses of thioridazine may produce electrocardiographic alterations resembling hypokalemia. Similar disturbances in ventricular repolarization have been reported in patients receiving large doses of low-potency drugs.

Ophthalmic Effects: Dose-related *pigmentary keratopathy* and *conjunctival melanosis* have been observed in some patients receiving large doses of chlorpromazine for long periods. Opacities of the cornea and lens due to deposition of fine particulate matter were also detectable on slit-lamp examination. Generally, vision is not impaired and changes regress after withdrawal of therapy. However, chlorpromazine has been implicated in one case of optic atrophy.

Patients receiving large doses of thioridazine have developed *pigmentary retinopathy*, and the loss of visual acuity is sometimes irreversible. For this reason, the maximal recommended dose of thioridazine is 800 mg daily.

Hematologic Effects: Although these reactions occur least frequently with piperazine phenothiazines, they may be associated with use of any phenothiazine. Some *depression of leukopoiesis* is detectable in most patients, particularly with use of low-potency phenothiazines (eg, chlorpromazine, thioridazine), but rarely persists. *Agranulocytosis*, the most serious hematologic complication, is an idiosyncratic reaction not related to dosage and usually appears within the first three months of phenothiazine therapy. Although the incidence is extremely low, mortality is high. Therefore, appearance of fever, sore throat, or cellulitis is an indication for discontinuing the phenothiazine and performing white blood cell and differential counts. After recovery, low doses of nonphenothiazine antipsychotics should be substituted.

INDIVIDUAL EVALUATIONS

All antipsychotic agents have similar efficacy in the treatment of psychoses, and effective daily doses of the various antipsychotic drugs may be equated with 100 mg of chlorpromazine (see the Table). Differences among compounds are related to the presence of other pharmacologic properties, to the prevalence of particular adverse reactions, and variation in individual response.

PHENOTHIAZINE DERIVATIVES

Aliphatic Compounds

CHLORPROMAZINE HYDROCHLORIDE
[Thorazine]

Chlorpromazine was the first antipsychotic agent marketed and remains the reference compound. Intestinal absorption is complete, but this drug may be variably bound or metabolized during its passage through the intestinal wall. Most of a dose of chlorpromazine is metabolized in the liver.

Chlorpromazine has a relatively low milligram potency. It is one of the most sedative antipsychotic drugs; however, tolerance to this effect develops rapidly. This drug should not be employed for its hypnotic effect in nonspychotic patients.

Chlorpromazine probably is best tolerated by patients under 40 years of age. In older patients, the incidence of dizziness, hypotension, ophthalmic changes, and dyskinesias is high.

Chlorpromazine is less likely to cause extrapyramidal symptoms (other than tardive dyskinesia) than some other phenothiazines; parkinsonism occurs more frequently than akathisia or dystonia. Because chlorpromazine has pronounced antiadrenergic and anticholinergic properties, orthostatic hypotension, dryness of the mouth, blurred vision, urinary retention, and constipation are prevalent. These reactions tend to diminish after the first week of continual therapy. Chlorpromazine appears to have the greatest propensity among the phenothiazines for producing agranulocytosis and cholestatic jaundice, but both are rare. Allergic skin reactions are uncommon, but mild photosensitivity occurs relatively frequently and

the patient should be so informed. Patients should be examined periodically for conjunctival melanosis and pigmentary opacities in the cornea and lens. Menstrual irregularities, galactorrhea, gynecomastia, and impotence have been reported occasionally.

For further information on indications, adverse reactions, and precautions, see the Introduction.

ROUTES, USUAL DOSAGE, AND PREPARATIONS. This drug generally should not be used in children under 6 months of age except when it is potentially lifesaving.

Intramuscular: For *acutely psychotic hospitalized adults*, 25 to 100 mg initially, repeated in one to four hours as necessary until control is achieved. It may be necessary to give as much as 1.6 g per day in divided doses to gain control; however, most patients respond to a daily dose of 0.5 to 1 g. *Elderly or debilitated patients*, doses in the lower range for adults are generally sufficient to control symptoms. *Children*, 0.5 mg/kg of body weight every six to eight hours, gradually increasing the dosage until symptoms are controlled; the total daily dose should not exceed 40 mg in children under 5 years or 75 mg in older children. Oral administration should be substituted when symptoms are controlled.

Intravenous: This route is highly irritating and should not be used.

Drug available generically: Solution 25 mg/ml in 1, 2, and 10 ml containers.
Thorazine (Smith Kline & French). Solution 25 mg/ml in 1, 2, and 10 ml containers.

Oral: For severe psychosis, *adults*, initially, 200 to 600 mg daily in divided doses. The dose is increased if necessary until symptoms are controlled or adverse reactions intervene (maximum, 2 g daily). Most patients respond to a daily dose of 500 to 800 mg. *Elderly or debilitated patients*, one-third to one-half the usual adult dose with a more gradual increase in dosage (20- to 25-mg increments). *Children*, 0.5 mg/kg of body weight every four to six hours. For all patients, after two weeks at optimal dosage, the amount should be reduced gradually to the minimum effective level for maintenance. The average oral dose in patients under 40 years is 500 to 800 mg daily. The response of older patients seldom improves with maintenance doses above 300 mg daily. Amounts greater than 1 g daily for prolonged periods usually confer no additional advantage and may produce a higher incidence of adverse reactions in older patients.

> Drug available generically: Liquid (concentrate) 2, 30, and 100 mg/ml; syrup 10 mg/ml; tablets 10, 25, 50, 100, and 200 mg.
> *Thorazine* (Smith Kline & French). Capsules (timed-release) 30, 75, 150, 200, and 300 mg; liquid (concentrate) 30 and 100 mg/ml; syrup 10 mg/5 ml; tablets 10, 25, 50, 100, and 200 mg.

Rectal: *Children*, 1 mg/kg of body weight every six to eight hours.

> *Thorazine* (Smith Kline & French). Suppositories 25 and 100 mg (expressed in terms of the base).

TRIFLUPROMAZINE HYDROCHLORIDE
[Vesprin]

Triflupromazine has the same actions as chlorpromazine and is equally effective (see the Table). For information on indications and adverse reactions, see the Introduction and the evaluation on Chlorpromazine Hydrochloride.

ROUTES, USUAL DOSAGE, AND PREPARATIONS. *Intramuscular*: For acute psychoses in hospitalized patients, *adults*, initially, 60 to 150 mg daily; *elderly or debilitated patients*, 10 to 75 mg daily; *children over 2½ years*, 0.2 to 0.25 mg/kg of body weight (maximum, 10 mg daily). Oral administration should be substituted when symptoms are controlled.

> *Vesprin* (Squibb). Solution 10 mg/ml in 1 and 10 ml containers and 20 mg/ml in 1 ml containers.

Oral: Initially, *adults*, 50 to 150 mg daily in divided doses; *children*, 2 mg/kg of body weight daily in divided doses. When symptoms are controlled, the dosage should be reduced gradually to the minimum effective level for maintenance.

> *Vesprin* (Squibb). Suspension 50 mg/5 ml; tablets 10, 25 and 50 mg.

Piperidine Compounds

THIORIDAZINE HYDROCHLORIDE
[Mellaril]

Thioridazine is one of the most widely used antipsychotic agents. It is the prototype of the piperidine compounds, and its efficacy is similar to that of chlorpromazine with equivalent doses (see the Table). It has almost no antiemetic activity.

Sedative effects and the incidence of orthostatic hypotension with thioridazine are similar to those observed with chlorpromazine. However, the adverse reactions produced are different in some respects than those of other phenothiazine subgroups. The pronounced anticholinergic activity of thioridazine has been suggested as a reason for its low incidence of extrapyramidal reactions other than tardive dyskinesia; however, this explanation is not accepted by all authorities. Large doses may inhibit ejaculation. Electrocardiographic changes have been noted more frequently with thioridazine than with other phenothiazines and may be observed after short-term therapy with daily doses of 300 mg or more. Agranulocytosis occurs only rarely. However, agranulocytosis with hepatitis, which progressed to near-fatal hepatic encephalopathy, has been reported in one patient; jaundice had not been associated previously with thioridazine. Photosensitivity has been reported rarely.

Pigmentary retinopathy is a complication that occurs most often (80%) when doses greater than 800 mg/day are given; diminished visual acuity which may be irreversible has resulted. Some patients receiving smaller daily doses have experienced visual impairment without detectable retinal changes. Because of these ocular reactions, 800 mg/day is the maximum recommended dose; the manufacturer recommends that doses exceeding 300 mg/day be used only in patients with severe psychoses. Thus, if large doses are required for long periods or if doses of 800 mg/day fail to control severely agitated patients, another antipsychotic agent should be substituted.

For further information on indications, adverse reactions, and precautions, see the Introduction.

ROUTES, USUAL DOSAGE, AND PREPARATIONS. *Oral: Adults*, initially, 150 to 300 mg daily in divided doses; this may be increased gradually to 800 mg daily in hospitalized patients. For maintenance therapy, the dose should be reduced gradually to the minimum effective level. *Elderly or debilitated patients*, one-third to one-half the usual adult dosage. *Children 2 years of age or older*, 1 mg/kg of body weight daily in divided doses; *under 2 years*, information is inadequate to establish a dosage.

Mellaril (Sandoz). Liquid (concentrate) 30 and 100 mg/ml; tablets 10, 15, 25, 50, 100, 150, and 200 mg.

MESORIDAZINE BESYLATE
[Serentil]

Mesoridazine, the major active metabolite of thioridazine, is an effective antipsychotic agent and has similar properties (see the Table).

For information on indications and adverse reactions, see the Introduction. Pigmentary retinopathy has not yet been associated with use of mesoridazine.

ROUTES, USUAL DOSAGE, AND PREPARATIONS. *Intramuscular*: For acute psychoses, *adults and children over 12 years*, 25 to 175 mg daily in divided doses. Since in-tramuscular use is irritating, oral administration should be substituted when symptoms are controlled.

Serentil (Boehringer Ingelheim). Solution 25 mg/ml in 1 ml containers.

Oral: Adults and children over 12 years, initially, 150 mg in divided doses. The dose is increased gradually in 50-mg increments until symptoms are controlled. The dose then is reduced gradually to the minimum effective amount for maintenance (range, 100 to 400 mg daily). *Elderly or debilitated patients*, one-third to one-half the usual adult dosage. *Children under 12*, information is inadequate to establish a dosage.

Serentil (Boehringer Ingelheim). Liquid (concentrate) 25 mg/ml; tablets 10, 25, 50, and 100 mg.

PIPERACETAZINE
[Quide]

Although it is technically a piperidine phenothiazine, piperacetazine has pharmacologic actions more closely resembling those of the piperazine compounds. Piperacetazine is less sedating and produces fewer autonomic effects than other piperidine compounds, but is intermediate between them and the piperazine compounds in the frequency of extrapyramidal reactions (see the Table). See also the Introduction.

ROUTE, USUAL DOSAGE, AND PREPARATIONS. *Oral: Adults and children over 12 years*, initially, 20 to 40 mg in divided doses. The amount may be increased gradually in 10-mg increments until symptoms are controlled or adverse effects intervene (maximum, 160 mg daily). After symptoms are stabilized, the dose should be reduced gradually to the minimal effective amount for maintenance. *Elderly or debilitated patients* initially should receive one-third to one-half the usual adult dose. *Children under 12*, information is inadequate to establish a dosage.

Quide (Dow). Tablets 10 and 25 mg.

Piperazine Compounds

TRIFLUOPERAZINE HYDROCHLORIDE
[Stelazine]

Trifluoperazine is the prototype of the piperazine phenothiazines. The piperazines have less sedative activity than other phenothiazines; the incidence of autonomic effects (eg, orthostatic hypotension) is also lower, but extrapyramidal reactions occur more frequently, particularly when large doses are used in patients over 40 years of age. Trifluoperazine has potent antiemetic activity and lowers the convulsive threshold.

Piperazine compounds are less likely to produce blood dyscrasias or jaundice, although transient leukopenia has been reported occasionally. Ocular changes have been reported rarely with trifluoperazine but have not yet been noted with other piperazine compounds. Since no marked electrocardiographic changes have been observed, piperazine compounds may be preferred for use in patients with cardiovascular disease. However, a few patients with angina pectoris have reported increased pain during therapy with trifluoperazine. Therefore, patients with angina should be observed carefully and the drug withdrawn if an unfavorable response occurs.

For further information on indications, adverse reactions, and precautions, see the Introduction.

ROUTES, USUAL DOSAGE, AND PREPARATIONS. *Intramuscular*: For acute psychoses, *adults*, initially 2 to 5 mg, followed by 1 to 2 mg every four to six hours (maximum, 10 mg daily). *Elderly and debilitated patients*, one-third to one-half of the usual adult dose given at less frequent intervals. *Children 6 years of age and older*, 1 mg once or twice daily, with the amount gradually increased by increments of 1 mg; *children under 6 years*, information is inadequate to estab-

lish a dosage. When symptoms are controlled, oral administration should be substituted.

   Stelazine (Smith Kline & French). Solution 2 mg/ml in 10 ml containers.

Oral: Initially, *adults (outpatients)*, 2 to 4 mg daily in divided doses; *(hospitalized)*, 4 to 10 mg daily in divided doses and increased gradually to the optimum amount. *Elderly or debilitated patients*, one-third to one-half the usual adult dose. *Children 6 years or older*, 1 to 2 mg daily, gradually increased to the optimum amount (rarely more than 15 mg daily). When symptoms are controlled, the dosage should be reduced gradually for all patients to the minimum effective amount for maintenance. The liquid concentrate should be diluted in fruit juice or other suitable vehicle just prior to administration.

   Stelazine (Smith Kline & French). Liquid (concentrate) 10 mg/ml; tablets 1, 2, 5, and 10 mg.

ACETOPHENAZINE MALEATE
[Tindal]

See the Introduction and the evaluation on Trifluoperazine Hydrochloride.

ROUTE, USUAL DOSAGE, AND PREPARATIONS. *Oral*: *Adults*, initially, 60 mg in divided doses. The dose may be increased in 20-mg increments until the optimum level (usually 80 to 120 mg daily for hospitalized patients) is reached or adverse effects intervene. Some patients with severe schizophrenia have received doses as high as 600 mg daily. *Elderly or debilitated patients*, one-third to one-half the usual adult dosage. *Children*, information is inadequate to establish a dosage. In all patients, when symptoms have been controlled, the dosage should be reduced gradually to the minimum effective amount for maintenance.

   Tindal (Schering). Tablets 20 mg.

BUTAPERAZINE MALEATE
[Repoise]

See the Introduction and the evaluation on Trifluoperazine Hydrochloride.

ROUTE, USUAL DOSAGE, AND PREPARATIONS. *Oral*: *Adults*, initially, 15 to 30 mg daily in three divided doses, increased gradually by increments of 5 to 10 mg to a maximum daily dose of 100 mg. When symptoms are controlled, the dose should be reduced gradually to the minimum effective level for maintenance. *Elderly or debilitated patients*, one-third to one-half the usual adult dosage. *Children under 12 years*, information is inadequate to establish a dosage.

> *Repoise* (Robins). Tablets 10 and 25 mg (expressed in terms of the base).

CARPHENAZINE MALEATE
[Proketazine]

See the Introduction and the evaluation on Trifluoperazine Hydrochloride.

ROUTE, USUAL DOSAGE, AND PREPARATIONS. *Oral*: *Adults*, initially, 75 to 150 mg daily in three divided doses; the amount may be increased weekly by 25- to 50-mg increments (maximum, 400 mg daily). When symptoms are controlled, the dose should be reduced gradually to the minimum ef-

fective level for maintenance. *Elderly or debilitated patients*, one-third to one-half the usual adult dosage. *Children under 12 years*, information is inadequate to establish a dosage.

> *Proketazine* (Wyeth). Tablets 12.5, 25, and 50 mg.

FLUPHENAZINE DECANOATE
[Prolixin Decanoate]

FLUPHENAZINE ENANTHATE
[Prolixin Enanthate]

FLUPHENAZINE HYDROCHLORIDE
[Permitil, Prolixin]

Fluphenazine has the highest milligram potency of the phenothiazines (see the Table). In addition to its use as an antipsychotic, it has been prescribed concomitantly with an antidepressant for constant central pain syndromes (see Chapter 10).

The duration of action of the parenteral depot forms (sesame oil vehicle), fluphenazine decanoate and fluphenazine enanthate, is approximately two weeks. An interval of four weeks or longer between injections may be adequate in selected patients on maintenance therapy. Depot forms are useful for the management of outpatients with a history of poor cooperation, inadequate absorption of oral medication, or frequent relapses (Groves and Mandel, 1975).

Close supervision and individualization of dosage is required. Patients should be hospitalized initially and stabilized on the short-acting oral form, fluphenazine hydrochloride, then initial doses of a depot form and the intervals between doses should be carefully determined, based on the patient's personal and family drug history. If extrapyramidal reactions have occurred previously (particularly following use of high-potency drugs or those belonging to a chemical class that produces a lower incidence of extrapyramidal symptoms), it is advisable to use a test dose (usual amount, 12.5 mg) and increase the dosage every 10 to 14 days during the first month until a therapeutic response has been attained. After the patient has been stabilized on the optimum dose, the amount should be adjusted to provide administration of the minimum effective maintenance dose as infrequently as possible. Continued supervision and a flexible dosage regimen usually are necessary to achieve an optimum response. In physically healthy schizophrenic patients with refractory, chronic symptoms, optimal doses of parenteral preparations have been used successfully for years without producing severe extrapyramidal reactions.

Excluding tardive dyskinesia, extrapyramidal reactions usually appear during the first few weeks of therapy; however, they may occur even after the patient's condition is stabilized. Occasionally, usual doses of anticholinergic drugs do not adequately control extrapyramidal symptoms, and increased amounts may precipitate toxic psychosis. In such cases, smaller doses or less frequent administration of fluphenazine generally controls symptoms.

Depending upon dosage and individual sensitivity, sedation, anticholinergic side effects, and hypotensive episodes have been observed. Usually these reactions are mild and subside spontaneously without altering dosage. Rarely, jaundice occurs with oral use of fluphenazine; the depot forms have not yet been reported to cause this reaction.

ROUTES, USUAL DOSAGE, AND PREPARATIONS. *Intramuscular, Subcutaneous*: For sustained effects, *adults*, initially 12.5 mg, followed by 25 mg every two weeks to establish appropriate dosage. Adjustment of dosage and intervals must be individualized, but the amount rarely should exceed 100 mg every two to six weeks; if the dose exceeds 50 mg, increases should be made in increments of 12.5 mg. *Debilitated patients or those with a history of extrapyramidal reactions*, initially, 2.5 mg,

followed by 2.5 to 5 mg every 10 to 14 days. *Children*, information is inadequate to establish a dosage.

FLUPHENAZINE DECANOATE:
Prolixin Decanoate (Squibb). Solution 25 mg/ml (in oil) in 1 and 5 ml containers.
FLUPHENAZINE ENANTHATE:
Prolixin Enanthate (Squibb). Solution 25 mg/ml (in oil) in 1 and 5 ml containers.

Intramuscular: For acute psychosis, *adults*, initially 1.25 mg, increased gradually to a total of 2.5 to 10 mg daily in three or four divided doses. When symptoms are controlled, oral administration should be substituted. *Elderly or debilitated patients*, one-third to one-half the usual adult dose. *Children*, information is inadequate to establish a dosage.

FLUPHENAZINE HYDROCHLORIDE:
Prolixin (Squibb). Solution 2.5 mg/ml in 10 ml containers.

Oral: *Adults*, initially, 2.5 to 10 mg, reduced gradually to a usual maintenance dose of 1 to 5 mg daily (doses exceeding 3 mg are rarely necessary). *Elderly or debilitated patients*, 1 to 2.5 mg daily, depending upon response. *Children*, information is inadequate to establish a dosage, although doses of 0.75 to 10 mg/day have been used in children 5 to 12 years of age. Liquid concentrates should be diluted with water, fruit juice, or other suitable vehicle before administration.

FLUPHENAZINE HYDROCHLORIDE:
Permitil (Schering). Liquid (concentrate) 5 mg/ml; tablets 0.25, 2.5, 5, and 10 mg; tablets (timed-release) 1 mg.
Prolixin (Squibb). Elixir 2.5 mg/5 ml; tablets 1, 2.5, 5, and 10 mg.

PERPHENAZINE
[Trilafon]

See the Introduction and the evaluation on Trifluoperazine Hydrochloride.

ROUTES, USUAL DOSAGE, AND PREPARATIONS. *Intramuscular:* Adults, for acute psychoses, initially, 5 to 10 mg; 5 mg may be given every six hours thereafter, but the total amount should not exceed 15 mg daily in ambulatory patients or 30 mg daily in hospitalized patients. *Elderly or debilitated patients*, one-third to one-half the usual adult dose. *Children under 12 years*, information is inadequate to establish a dosage; *over 12 years*, lowest limit of adult dosage. When symptoms are controlled, oral administration should be substituted.

> *Trilafon* (Schering). Solution 5 mg/ml in 1 ml containers.

Oral: Adults, 16 to 64 mg daily in divided doses. When symptoms have been controlled, the dosage should be reduced gradually to the minimum effective level. *Elderly or debilitated patients*, one-third to one-half the usual adult dose. Pediatric dosage has not been established but the following amounts have been given in divided doses: *Children 1 to 6 years*, 4 to 6 mg daily; *6 to 12 years*, 6 mg daily; *over 12 years*, 6 to 12 mg daily. The liquid concentrate should be diluted in fruit juice or other suitable liquid vehicle (tea is not recommended) prior to administration.

> *Trilafon* (Schering). Liquid (concentrate) 16 mg/5 ml; tablets 2, 4, 8, and 16 mg; tablets (timed-release) 8 mg.

PROCHLORPERAZINE EDISYLATE
[Compazine]

PROCHLORPERAZINE MALEATE
[Compazine]

See the Introduction and the evaluation on Trifluoperazine Hydrochloride. This drug is more commonly used as an antiemetic than as an antipsychotic agent.

ROUTES, USUAL DOSAGE, AND PREPARATIONS. *Intramuscular*: For acute psychoses, *adults*, initially, 10 to 20 mg every one to four hours. Information is inadequate to

establish a dosage for *children under 2 years of age* but *children over 2 years* may receive 0.13 mg/kg of body weight daily in three or four divided doses. *Elderly or debilitated patients* are given one-third to one-half the usual adult dose. After symptoms are controlled, oral administration should be substituted.

> PROCHLORPERAZINE EDISYLATE:
> *Compazine [edisylate]* (Smith Kline & French). Solution 5 mg/ml in 2 and 10 ml containers.

Oral: Adults, 15 to 40 mg daily in divided doses, increased by 5 mg every two or three days until symptoms are controlled or adverse reactions intervene. The optimum dosage for moderate psychoses usually is 50 to 75 mg daily and for severe psychoses 100 to 150 mg. *Children over 2 years*, 0.4 mg/kg of body weight daily in divided doses. (The liquid concentrate is not intended for use in children.)

> PROCHLORPERAZINE EDISYLATE:
> *Compazine [edisylate]* (Smith Kline & French). Liquid (concentrate) 10 mg/ml; syrup 5 mg/5 ml.
> PROCHLORPERAZINE MALEATE:
> *Compazine [maleate]* (Smith Kline & French). Capsules (timed-release) 10, 15, 30, and 75 mg; tablets 5, 10, and 25 mg.

THIOXANTHENE DERIVATIVES

CHLORPROTHIXENE
[Taractan]

The chemical structure and pharmacologic actions of chlorprothixene are very similar to those of the aliphatic phenothiazines. For information on indications and adverse reactions, see the Introduction.

ROUTES, USUAL DOSAGE, AND PREPARATIONS. *Intramuscular*: For acute psychoses, *adults and children over 12 years*, 75 to 200 mg daily in divided doses. *Elderly or debilitated patients*, 30 to 100 mg daily in divided doses. When symptoms are controlled, oral administration should be substituted. *Children under 12 years*, information is inadequate to establish a dosage.

>*Taractan* (Roche). Solution 12.5 mg/ml in 2 ml containers.

Oral: Adults, 75 to 200 mg daily in divided doses, increased gradually until symptoms are controlled or adverse reactions intervene. The optimum dose rarely exceeds 600 mg daily. *Elderly or debilitated patients and children over 6 years*, 30 to 100 mg daily in divided doses. When symptoms are controlled, the dosage should be reduced gradually to the minimum effective level. *Children under 6 years*, information is inadequate to establish a dosage.

>*Taractan* (Roche). Liquid (concentrate) 100 mg/5 ml; tablets 10, 25, 50, and 100 mg.

THIOTHIXENE
[Navane]

THIOTHIXENE HYDROCHLORIDE
[Navane Hydrochloride]

The chemical structure and pharmacologic actions of thiothixene are very similar to those of the piperazine phenothiazines. For information on indications and adverse reactions, see the Introduction and the evaluation on Trifluoperazine Hydrochloride.

ROUTES, USUAL DOSAGE, AND PREPARATIONS. *Intramuscular*: For acute psychoses, *adults and children over 12 years*, initially, 4 mg two to four times daily, increased gradually until symptoms are controlled (maximum, 30 mg daily). *Elderly or debilitated patients*, one-third to one-half the usual adult dosage. When symptoms are controlled, oral administration should be substituted. *Children under 12*, information is inadequate to establish a dosage.

>THIOTHIXENE HYDROCHLORIDE:
>*Navane* [*hydrochloride*] (Roerig). Solution 2

mg/ml (expressed in terms of the base) in 2 ml containers.

Oral: Adults, 6 to 10 mg daily in divided doses; the amount may be increased gradually. The usual optimal dose is 20 to 30 mg daily, and doses in excess of 60 mg daily rarely enhance the response. When symptoms are controlled, the dosage should be reduced gradually to the minimum effective level. *Elderly or debilitated patients*, initially, one-third to one-half the usual adult dosage. *Children under 12 years*, information is inadequate to establish a dosage.

>THIOTHIXENE:
>*Navane* (Roerig). Capsules 1, 2, 5, 10, and 20 mg.
>THIOTHIXENE HYDROCHLORIDE:
>*Navane* [*hydrochloride*] (Roerig). Liquid (concentrate) 5 mg/ml (expressed in terms of the base).

BUTYROPHENONE DERIVATIVE

HALOPERIDOL
[Haldol]

Haloperidol is pharmacologically, but not chemically, related to the piperazine phenothiazines. The indications are similar to those of the piperazine phenothiazines (Ayd, 1978), and this drug is a useful substitute in patients who are either hypersensitive or refractory to the phenothiazines. Extrapyramidal reactions are common when haloperidol is given, especially if there is a history of such reactions to other antipsychotic agents. Large doses should be reserved to treat schizophrenia in physically healthy patients. Treatment may be required for four to six months before a maximum effect is demonstrated in chronic schizophrenia.

Haloperidol also has been used successfully in hyperkinetic patients with severe mental retardation to improve social behavior, concentration, and agitation, but no improvement in speech or communication was noted. Because long-term therapy is usually necessary, it should be used only in severe cases. Although haloperidol has been commonly prescribed for this purpose, there is no evidence to suggest that it is superior to other antipsychotic agents.

Haloperidol is the drug of choice for treatment of Tourette's syndrome, a rare disorder manifested by uncontrolled motor tics, barking cries, and explosive outbursts of obscene language (Murray, 1978). However, precise dosage adjustment is difficult in these patients, and the physician must be skilled in the management of adverse reactions to psychotropic drugs.

Ballismus, which is characterized by continual, usually unilateral, purposeless "flinging" movements of the extremities (particularly the arms), responds to haloperidol (Klawans et al, 1978). This extrapyramidal syndrome is almost always produced by acute vascular infarctions of the subthalamic nucleus and has a grave prognosis when untreated, because death often occurs within a month from exhaustion leading to pneumonia and congestive heart failure. Control of the disorder, survival, and even disappearance of the syndrome have occurred in a number of patients within three to six months with doses of 3 to 12 mg of haloperidol daily. Individuals who cannot tolerate haloperidol may be controlled with chlorpromazine (100 to 200 mg daily).

Haloperidol is well absorbed orally and reaches a peak plasma concentration in three to six hours. The half-life is 12 to 22 hours. Approximately 40% of the drug is eliminated in the urine, and the dosage should be adjusted in patients with impaired renal function (see Chapter 2).

Like the piperazine phenothiazines, haloperidol is relatively nonsedating, has a pronounced antiemetic action, and is likely to produce extrapyramidal reactions (see the Table). Akathisia and acute dystonias occasionally may be severe. Persistent extrapyramidal symptoms usually are dose related but have also occurred following use of relatively low doses.

Haloperidol causes fewer autonomic effects than phenothiazines, although transient orthostatic hypotension has been reported occasionally. Also, it does not appear to produce any electrocardiographic changes. Dermatologic reactions have occurred rarely and the risk of adverse hepatic effects is minimal. Mild, transient hematologic changes have occurred, but only one case of agranulocytosis has been reported.

Limb reduction was reported in one infant following maternal use of haloperidol, but epidemiologic studies indicate that the teratogenicity of haloperidol is minimal.

For further information on indications, adverse reactions, and precautions, see the Introduction.

ROUTES, USUAL DOSAGE, AND PREPARATIONS. *Intramuscular*: For acute psychoses, *adults*, initially, 2 to 5 mg. Depending upon response, subsequent doses may be administered as often as every hour (although four- to eight-hour intervals may be satisfactory) until symptoms are controlled; this usually occurs within 72 hours and doses above 15 mg daily seldom are required. Oral administration should then be substituted and the dosage adjusted individually. *Elderly or debilitated patients and children under 12 years*, information is inadequate to establish a dosage.

For mental retardation with hyperkinesia, *adults*, initially, 10 to 15 mg daily in divided doses. The dose may be increased gradually to a total of approximately 60 mg daily. After the patient has been stabilized, oral administration should be substituted. *Elderly or debilitated patients and children under 12 years*, information is inadequate to establish a dosage.

Haldol (McNeil). Solution 5 mg/ml in 1 and 10 ml containers.

Oral: For acute psychoses, *adults and children over 12 years*, initially, 1 to 15 mg in divided doses. When control has been obtained, the dose should be reduced gradually to the minimum effective maintenance level (usually, 2 to 8 mg daily). *Elderly or debilitated patients*, initially, 0.5 to 2 mg, gradually increased in increments of 0.5 mg; the maintenance dose usually is 2 to 4 mg daily.

For chronic refractory schizophrenia, *adults and children over 12 years*, initially, 6 to 15 mg in divided doses gradually increased until control is achieved (100 mg daily may be required) and then gradually reduced to maintenance levels (usually, 15 to 20 mg daily). *Elderly or debilitated patients*, initially, 0.5 to 1.5 mg, increased gradually in small increments. The usual maintenance dose is 2 to 8 mg daily. *Children under 12 years*, information is inadequate to establish dosage.

For severe mental retardation with hyperkinesia (after intramuscular administration), *adults and children over 12 years*, 80 to 120 mg daily, gradually reduced to a maintenance dose of about 60 mg daily. *Elderly or debilitated patients*, initially, 1.5 to 6 mg daily in divided doses, gradually increased in small increments (maximum, 15 mg daily). When control is achieved, the dose is gradually reduced to the minimum effective level for maintenance.

For Tourette's syndrome, *adults and children over 12 years*, initially, 6 to 15 mg daily in divided doses, gradually increased in 2-mg increments until adverse reactions become disabling. After symptoms have been controlled, the dose is gradually reduced to approximately 9 mg daily for maintenance.

   Haldol (McNeil). Liquid (concentrate) 2 mg/ml; tablets 0.5, 1, 2, 5, and 10 mg.

DIBENZOXAZEPINE DERIVATIVE

LOXAPINE HYDROCHLORIDE
   [Daxolin C, Loxitane C]

LOXAPINE SUCCINATE
   [Daxolin, Loxitane]

This dibenzoxazepine derivative represents a new subclass of tricyclic antipsychotic agents that are chemically distinct from the phenothiazines, butyrophenones, and thioxanthenes. It is effective in the treatment of schizophrenia. Its major pharmacological actions do not differ appreciably from the older antipsychotic drugs. Loxapine has sedative, anticholinergic, and alpha-antiadrenergic actions, which are quantitatively intermediate between the aliphatic and piperazine phenothiazines (see the Table). Extrapyramidal reactions other than tardive dyskinesia have been reported frequently after use of this drug. Loxapine has an antiemetic action and decreases the seizure threshold; it should be used with extreme caution in patients with a history of convulsive disorders. Lens opacities and pigmentary retinopathy have not been reported.

For further information on adverse reactions and precautions, see the Introduction.

ROUTE, USUAL DOSAGE, AND PREPARATIONS. *Oral: Adults and adolescents 16 years or older*, initially, 10 mg twice daily to a total of 50 mg daily in severely psychotic patients. Dosage should be increased rapidly over the next week to ten days until control is achieved. For maintenance, dosage should be reduced gradually to the minimum effective level (usually, 60 to 100 mg daily) with a maximum dose of 250 mg daily. *Children under 16*, information is inadequate to establish a dosage. *Elderly and debilitated patients*, initially, one-third to one-half the usual adult dose. The liquid concentrate should be diluted in orange or grapefruit juice prior to administration.

LOXAPINE HYDROCHLORIDE:
Daxolin C (Dome), *Loxitane C* (Lederle). Liquid (concentrate) 25 mg/ml (expressed in terms of the base).
LOXAPINE SUCCINATE:
Daxolin (Dome), *Loxitane* (Lederle). Capsules 5 (Daxolin only), 10, 25, and 50 mg (expressed in terms of the base).

DIHYDROINDOLONE DERIVATIVE

MOLINDONE HYDROCHLORIDE
[Lidone, Moban]

Molindone is chemically unrelated to the phenothiazines, butyrophenones, or thioxanthenes. It is effective in schizophrenia. The extrapyramidal, sedative, anticholinergic, and antiadrenergic actions of molindone are quantitatively intermediate between the aliphatic and piperazine phenothiazines (see the Table). This drug has an antiemetic action and decreases the convulsive threshold experimentally. Lens opacities and pigmentary retinopathy have not been reported.

For further information on adverse reactions and precautions, see the Introduction.

ROUTE, USUAL DOSAGE, AND PREPARATIONS. *Oral*: *Adults*, initially, 5 to 15 mg three or four times daily, gradually increased until symptoms are controlled; the manufacturers' literature indicates that doses as large as 225 mg daily have been used. When symptoms are controlled, the dose should be reduced gradually to the minimum effective level for maintenance. *Elderly or debilitated patients*, initially, one-third to one-half the usual adult dosage. *Children under 12 years*, information is inadequate to establish a dosage.

  Lidone (Abbott). Capsules 5, 10, and 25 mg.
  Moban (Endo). Tablets 5, 10, and 25 mg.

DIPHENYLBUTYLPIPERIDINE DERIVATIVE

PENFLURIDOL

The investigational drug, penfluridol, is chemically unrelated to all other antipsychotic drugs. It is indistinguishable pharmacologically from the piperazine-type phenothiazines and the butyrophenones; however, it is only necessary to administer the drug orally once a week to maintain its effectiveness in chronic schizophrenia. Controlled studies in hospitalized patients and outpatients for a period of one to two years have demonstrated that this drug is as effective as daily administration of fluphenazine hydrochloride (Donlon and Meyer, 1978; Lapierre, 1978).

Penfluridol is rapidly absorbed; a considerable portion of the drug is bound in the liver and, like that fraction of drug in the brain, is released slowly over a period of five to seven days.

The incidence and type of untoward effects are similar to those observed with the piperazine phenothiazines; thus, extrapyramidal movement disorders are more prominent than autonomic signs (dizziness, transient orthostatic hypotension). Sedation, somnolence, weakness, and general malaise were reported occasionally. Muscle aches and spasms, galactorrhea, and an oculogyric episode have occurred, but ocular changes were not observed. Extrapyramidal signs of dystonia and akathisia were controlled with benztropine mesylate or trihexyphenidyl hydrochloride.

In most patients it has been possible to institute penfluridol therapy immediately after discontinuation of another antipsychotic drug. Supplemental doses of antipsychotic drugs are rarely required during the period of drug transfer and stabilization. The most commonly required weekly doses were 60 to 100 mg (range, 20 to 120 mg). Recently completed studies indicated that compliance in patients treated with penfluridol weekly was comparable to that in patients who received the depot fluphenazine preparations parenterally every two weeks (Quitkin et al, 1978).

(Investigational drug)

Selected References

Ayd FJ Jr: Haloperidol: Twenty years' clinical experience. *J Clin Psychiatry* 39:807-814, 1978.

Baldessarini RJ: Schizophrenia. *N Engl J Med* 297:988-995, 1977.

Charalampous KD, Keepers GA: Major side effects of antipsychotic drugs. *J Fam Pract* 6:993-1002, 1978.

Davis JM: Comparative doses and costs of antipsychotic medication. *Arch Gen Psychiatry* 33:858-861, 1976.

Davis JM: Overview: Maintenance therapy in psychiatry: I. Schizophrenia. *Am J Psychiatry* 132:1237-1245, 1975.

Davis JM, Casper R: Antipsychotic drugs: Clinical pharmacology and therapeutic use. *Drugs* 14:260-282, 1977.

Donlon PT, Meyer JE: Twelve month comparison of penfluridol and trifluoperazine in chronic schizophrenic outpatients. *J Clin Psychiatry* 39: 582-587, 1978.

Groves JE, Mandel MR: Long-acting phenothiazines. *Arch Gen Psychiatry* 32:893-900, 1975.

Gruen PH, et al: Prolactin responses to neuroleptics in normal and schizophrenic subjects. *Arch Gen Psychiatry* 35:108-116, 1978.

Johnson DAW: Treatment of chronic schizophrenia. *Drugs* 14:291-299, 1977.

Klawans HL, et al: Combating hemiballismus with neuroleptics. *Drug Ther (Hosp)* 3:65-68, (March) 1978.

Lapierre YD: Controlled study of penfluridol in treatment of chronic schizophrenia. *Am J Psychiatry* 135:956-959, 1978.

Murray TJ: Tourette's syndrome: Treatable tic. *Can Med Assoc J* 118:1407-1410, 1978.

Quitkin F, et al: Long-acting oral vs injectable antipsychotic drugs in schizophrenics: One-year double-blind comparison in multiple episode schizophrenics. *Arch Gen Psychiatry* 35:889-892, 1978.

Zavodnick S: Pharmacological and theoretical comparison of high and low potency neuroleptics. *J Clin Psychiatry* 39:332-336, 1978.

Drugs Used in Affective Disorders | 13

In contrast to the thought disorder of schizophrenia, a mood (affect) disorder characterizes manic and/or depressive illness. Patients may be elated to the extreme of delirious mania or depressed to the other extreme of delusional depression. In most affective disorders, the individual appears to be genetically vulnerable and the condition is activated by environmental stress; the incidence of affective disorders or alcoholism among relatives is also higher. Morbidity and mortality are markedly reduced by psychotherapy and antidepressant drugs, but the impairment remains significant in patients who do not undergo spontaneous remission (usually within 6 to 18 months) or do not receive optimal therapy.

Tricyclic compounds, monoamine oxidase inhibitors, and lithium salts are the principal drugs employed for affective disorders and are used in conjunction with psychotherapy and electroshock (Cain and Cain, 1978; Gelenberg and Klerman, 1978; Hollister, 1978; Rosenbaum et al, 1979).

The mechanism of action of the principal antidepressant drugs is not resolved. Amitriptyline inhibits serotonin uptake while desipramine inhibits norepinephrine uptake in laboratory studies; little, if any, crossover inhibition for these two compounds occurs. However, a metabolite of

187

amitriptyline, nortriptyline, and imipramine affect both types of uptake. Monoamine oxidase inhibitors block intracellular metabolism of these and other biogenic amines, which increases amine concentrations in the nerve terminals. These findings are consistent with the hypothesis that some types of depression result from impaired function of central noradrenergic and/or serotonergic pathways (Sourkes, 1977; Garver and Davis, 1979).

The tricyclic antidepressants block norepinephrine and serotonin uptake shortly after administration. Recent experimental data (Crews and Smith, 1978; Svensson and Usdin, 1978) showed that desipramine and imipramine inhibited presynaptic alpha-adrenergic receptors that regulate norepinephrine release; the net result is an increase in the amount of norepinephrine released per nerve impulse. The time required for development of this action correlates well with the time for onset of action of the tricyclic antidepressants. The onset of action is similar when tricyclic antidepressants are used experimentally to enhance postsynaptic serotonin receptor sensitivity (deMontigny and Aghajanian, 1978).

Increased cholinoceptive activity in the brain has been associated with clinical depression. The central cholinergic blocking action of the tricyclic drugs thus may play a role in their antidepressant action (Davis et al, 1978). The proposed mechanism of action of lithium in manic-depressive illness is not yet firmly established, although the major action is thought to be inhibition of membrane adenyl cyclase which regulates transmitter and metabolic transport across neuroendocrine cells.

Psychomotor stimulants, such as amphetamine and methylphenidate [Ritalin], play a very minor role, if any, in the treatment of depression. They are not recommended for the vast majority of patients with affective disorders. A few physicians employ amphetamine for short-term use in patients with reactive depressions who are intractable to a total psychotherapeutic program that includes other antidepressants or diagnostically to determine more rapidly the probable efficacy of tricyclic antidepressant medication. However, efficacy has not been proven in controlled studies for either the therapeutic or diagnostic indication. Psychomotor stimulants also may produce adverse cardiovascular effects, especially in the elderly.

The antianxiety and hypnotic drugs occasionally may be useful as *adjuncts* in alleviating the anxiety and insomnia often associated with depression. However, since anxiety often results from depression and since some tricyclic antidepressants have a rather pronounced sedative action, adequate therapy with selected antidepressants alone usually resolves most of the anxiety and insomnia that are components of the illness. Therefore, these adjunctive drugs should not be prescribed routinely, substituted inappropriately for antidepressants, or given for longer than two to three weeks without re-evaluation of the disorder. If antianxiety drug therapy is warranted, the benzodiazepines are usually the drugs of choice; compared to the barbiturates, benzodiazepines have a low suicide risk (ie, wide margin of safety with respect to lethality), they cause fewer clinically significant drug interactions, and they do not depress plasma levels of the tricyclic antidepressants. (See Chapter 11, Drugs Used for Anxiety and Insomnia.)

Affective Disorders

Depression: Severe depressive illness is characterized by inability to experience joy or pleasure and feelings of helplessness, worthlessness, and guilt. Somatic signs and symptoms include a blunted affect, tearfulness, mental and motor retardation, hypersomnia or more commonly insomnia of the early morning type but occasionally insomnia on retiring, anorexia but occasionally hyperphagia, weight loss, constipation, apathy, fatigue, and anxiety. The degree of anxiety varies considerably among patients. Ultimately, hallucinations and delusions may lead to an inability to cope with normal social, personal, and work functions. A psychosis caused by morbid preoccupation with depression ensues, resulting in social withdrawal. A feeling of hopelessness is probably most closely linked to suicidal plans and acts.

Depression is one of the most common and clinically heterogeneous psychiatric disorders. Accurate diagnosis is a key factor in determining the need for and choice of therapy. Psychotherapy and, if possible, alteration of the environment are the primary treatment for patients with *affective personality disorders and reactive depressions*. The latter are generally self-limited disorders precipitated by a recognizable loss, disease, or trauma in a normal personality. Reactive depression is similar to a prolonged grief reaction, and patients often have considerable anxiety. A small number of moderately to severely affected individuals are suicide-prone and may benefit from the use of tricyclic antidepressants in addition to the standard therapy.

The tricyclic antidepressants are most useful in *endogenous depression*, which is frequently characterized by the absence of any identifiable precipitating cause and recurrence. Electroshock therapy is especially useful when suicidal plans are well developed in acute endogenous depression or in patients who are refractory to or cannot tolerate tricyclic antidepressants. Rarely, it is necessary to use a tricyclic compound and a monoamine oxidase inhibitor concurrently. In these instances, the dosage regimen is best managed by physicians who have experience in employing such combination therapy.

Many therapeutic agents are known to cause *drug-induced depression*, but the antipsychotics, barbiturates, alcohol, oral contraceptives, and centrally acting antihypertensive agents (eg, reserpine, methyldopa) are most commonly implicated (Whitlock and Evans, 1978). Reducing the dosage or discontinuing therapy and giving psychosupportive care are indicated. Antidepressants are rarely necessary.

Manic-Depressive Disorders: In mania, the patient exhibits euphoria, emotional lability with intolerance to frustration, psychomotor overactivity, lack of need for sleep, flight of ideas with a pressure of speech syndrome, excessive sociability, and extreme self-confidence with delusions of importance and grandiose ideas. Milder forms (hypomania) are less easily recognized; individuals with this disorder may appear to be highly energetic and innovative and often are successful professionally. Pathology does not become obvious until their behavior exceeds rational limits.

Recurrent episodes of primarily mania or primarily depression or alternating episodes of mania and depression (circular type) characterize the three subclasses of *manic-depressive illnesses*.

Up to 85% of patients with the *manic* form respond to lithium, especially when the classic symptoms are present (recurring hyperactivity, elation, and pressure of speech syndrome) with few or no depressive episodes; an antipsychotic drug and lithium are indicated if the mania is severe and psychotic symptoms are present.

The *depressed* type of manic-depressive illness (unipolar depressives) is essentially an endogenous depression and both conditions respond similarly to antidepressant drugs and electroshock.

The *circular* form (bipolar depressives) may respond to lithium alone, although optimum management usually requires concomitant use of a tricyclic drug. Rarely, lithium alone is adequate for maintenance during the first year of stabilization.

The following two specific illnesses have elements of depression and, because they have additional symptomatology, the therapeutic regimen may include an antidepressant or an antipsychotic drug:

Phobic anxiety (agoraphobia), characterized by spontaneous panic attacks, is often associated with depression, and the anxiety that accompanies this syndrome is severe. Moderately or severely affected patients respond to the tricyclic antidepressant, imipramine. A number of clinicians feel that a monoamine oxidase inhibitor also is useful (Ravaris et al, 1978). Phobic anxiety resulting from specific situations and unaccompanied by depression usually responds best to antianxiety drugs.

Patients with *schizoaffective* disorder and paranoid schizophrenia respond to antipsychotic drugs alone or, occasionally, require simultaneous treatment with tricyclic drugs and/or lithium. (See Chapter 12, Antipsychotic Drugs.)

TRICYCLIC ANTIDEPRESSANTS

The available tricyclic antidepressants (amitriptyline [Amitid, Amitril, Elavil, Endep, SK-Amitriptyline], desipramine [Norpramin, Pertofrane], doxepin [Adapin, Sinequan], imipramine [Imavate, SK-Pramine, Tofranil], nortriptyline [Aventyl, Pamelor], protriptyline [Vivactil], and trimipramine [Surmontil]) elevate mood, increase physical activity and mental alertness, improve appetite and sleep patterns, and reduce morbid preoccupation in 60% to 70% of patients with endogenous depression.

A personal or family history of effective use of tricyclic antidepressants and the sedative and anticholinergic activities of a compound are the most influential factors in drug selection (see the Table). The secondary amine-type tricyclic antidepressants have considerably less sedative and anticholinergic actions and are more potent antagonists of the histamine H_2 and alpha-adrenergic receptors than the tertiary amine-type antidepressants. Their H_1 receptor antihistamine activity directly correlates with their sedative activity; amitriptyline and doxepin are at least three to ten times more active on this receptor, depending upon the experimental model used for comparison.

All of these compounds are well absorbed orally, extensively metabolized, highly protein-bound in plasma and tissue, and slowly eliminated; half-lives (in hours) range from 8 to 16 for imipramine, 14 to 76 for desipramine, 17 to 40 for amitriptyline, 18 to 93 for nortriptyline, and approximately two to four days for protriptyline. Much longer half-lives have been reported

and confirmed in older patients, especially those over 55 to 60 years of age (Nies et al, 1977); therefore, modification of the initial dose may be indicated until the clinical response can be assessed. The onset of clinical response is slow (one to three weeks), and parenteral administration does not appreciably accelerate onset of action. Electroshock therapy may, therefore, be the treatment of choice in the severely suicidal patient.

Although tricyclic plasma concentrations correlate reasonably well with efficacy, they vary widely even among responsive patients; therefore, signs and symptoms are used routinely instead to adjust dosage. Because tricyclic plasma concentrations are of limited clinical usefulness in the average patient, they are reserved to aid in optimizing therapy in patients who are difficult to control, to detect noncompliance, and possibly in the management of overdosage.

A curvilinear relationship in the form of an inverted U exists between nortriptyline plasma concentrations and antidepressant efficacy (specifically in responsive patients with endogenous depression), so that maximal efficacy is attained between 50 and 175 ng/ml (Risch et al, 1979). Limited evidence suggests that the relationship between imipramine (plus its active metabolite, desipramine) and amitriptyline (plus its active metabolite, nortriptyline) plasma concentrations and efficacy is linear in endogenous depression; their threshold concentrations are greater than 95 and 120 ng/ml, respectively. Sufficient data are not available to define the type of relationship which exists between plasma concentration and efficacy for protriptyline desipramine, and doxepin; the threshold plasma concentration for protriptyline is approximately 70 ng/ml, while those for desipramine and doxepin await clarification.

Administration and Dosage: Other than inaccurate diagnoses, the administration of inadequate daily doses of tricyclic antidepressants accounts for most treatment failures. Proper initial therapy beginning with carefully graduated doses, especially in outpatients, and reduction of the daily dose if possible in four to six weeks after initial control of depression lessen adverse effects and improve patient compliance. These measures are especially important in elderly, debilitated, or disease-compromised patients.

In institutionalized patients, closer monitoring is possible and the initial daily dose is generally larger than for outpatients; the time needed to attain a maximum daily dose also is usually shorter. The suggested initial daily doses listed in the Table and evaluations do not necessarily reflect the final optimum dose, which must be individualized.

Different schedules are utilized to initiate therapy. One that lessens the intensity of undesirable anticholinergic side effects in outpatients is the administration of imipramine 25 mg twice daily for two days, with an increase in dose to 50 mg twice daily for two days, followed by 75 mg twice daily for the next ten days. After the initial two to three weeks of therapy, a single total daily dose is given at bedtime. Such a divided dosage schedule may be particularly preferable in the aged and those with cardiac disease. Not all patients require 150 mg daily; the doses can be changed proportionately on the divided dose schedule. If insomnia is a prominent symptom, it may be preferable to give the same initial daily doses as a single dose at bedtime to obtain the full benefit of sedation and minimize drowsiness during the day. If little benefit is observed after two or three weeks, the daily dose is increased by 50 mg weekly until satisfactory improvement, intolerable adverse reactions, or the maximum dose of 300 mg is reached. The schedules described for imipramine are also applicable in general to desipramine, amitriptyline, and doxepin. A corresponding proportional dosage for nortriptyline and protriptyline can be determined from the daily and maximum doses given in the Table.

DRUGS USED IN AFFECTIVE DISORDERS

Classification	Drug	Amine Type	Sedative Activity	Anti-cholinergic Activity	Initial* Adult Daily Dose Range (mg)	
					Outpatient	Inpatient
ANTIDEPRESSANTS						
TRICYCLIC COMPOUNDS						
Dibenzazepines	Desipramine Norpramin (Merrell-National) Pertofrane (USV)	Secondary	Minimal	Minimal	75-150	75-300
	Imipramine Imavate (Robins) SK-Pramine (Smith Kline & French) Tofranil (Geigy)	Tertiary	Inter-mediate	Inter-mediate	75-150	100-300
	Trimipramine Surmontil (Ives)	Tertiary	Maximal	Inter-mediate	75-150	100-300
Dibenzocyclo-heptadienes	Protriptyline Vivactil (Merck Sharp & Dohme)	Secondary	Minimal	Inter-mediate	15-40	15-60

DRUGS USED IN AFFECTIVE DISORDERS

Classification	Drug	Amine Type	Sedative Activity	Anti-cholinergic Activity	Initial* Adult Daily Dose Range (mg) Outpatient	Inpatient
	Nortriptyline Aventyl (Lilly) Pamelor (Sandoz)	Secondary	Inter-mediate	Minimal	20-100	40-150
	Amitriptyline Amitid (Squibb) Amitril (Parke, Davis) Elavil (Merck Sharp & Dohme) Endep (Roche) SK-Amitriptyline (Smith Kline & French)	Tertiary	Maximal	Maximal	75-150	100-300
Dibenzoxepin	Doxepin Adapin (Pennwalt) Sinequan (Pfizer)	Tertiary	Maximal	Maximal	75-100	75-300
MONOAMINE OXIDASE INHIBITORS						
Hydrazines	Isocarboxazid Marplan (Roche)				20-30	
	Phenelzine Nardil (Parke, Davis)				45-75	
Nonhydrazine	Tranylcypromine Parnate (Smith Kline & French)				20-40	
ANTIMANIC	Lithium Eskalith (Smith Kline & French) Lithane (Dome) Lithonate (Rowell) Lithonate-S (Rowell) Lithotabs (Rowell)				600-2100 (Acute) 900-1200 (Maintenance)	

*First two to three weeks of therapy.

Since the rates of metabolism and, hence, plasma concentrations of these drugs vary widely, individualization of dose for both efficacy and safety is more important than strict adherence to recommendations for initial, maintenance, and maximum doses. An occasional patient will require more than 300 mg/day; thus, 300 mg should be interpreted as a maximum amount applicable to most but not all patients.

The duration of therapy depends upon the type and severity of depression. In patients with recurrent episodes of depression, maintenance therapy with small total daily doses (eg, 25 to 100 mg of amitriptyline) is reported to have definite prophylactic value. If long-term maintenance therapy is not indicated, the dose should be reduced gradually over a period of a few weeks if there are no symptoms or signs of relapse, and treatment is continued for three to six months.

If patients do not respond to an adequate trial with one tricyclic antidepressant, a trial with a different drug of this class may prove useful.

Imipramine helps to alleviate enuresis in children and adolescents. Since there appears to be no evidence of residual improvement when the drug is discontinued, such therapy may be useful primarily to obtain temporary relief. When given for this purpose, few serious adverse effects occur with the low doses used. (See Chapter 40, Agents Used to Treat Urologic Disorders.)

Amitriptyline and imipramine are being investigated to determine their effectiveness in constant central pain syndromes (see Chapter 10).

Adverse Reactions: The most common adverse reactions of the tricyclic antidepressants are those caused by their anticholinergic and alpha-adrenergic blocking activities: flushing, diaphoresis, dryness of the mouth, blurred vision, and constipation. Tachycardia, orthostatic hypotension, aggravation of angle-closure glaucoma, urinary retention, adynamic ileus, and confusional reactions as part of a toxic delirium may be especially hazardous in elderly patients with other diseases. If gastric irritation is noted, it usually can be managed by taking the drug with food.

Allergic skin reactions and photosensitivity are relatively uncommon, as are agranulocytosis, cholestatic jaundice, leukopenia, leukocytosis, Loeffler's syndrome, eosinophilia, and thrombocytopenia. Hypertension and convulsions have been reported following a course of imipramine in a patient with undiagnosed pheochromocytoma.

Central nervous system effects include sedation (see the Table), fine tremor, speech blockage, and, paradoxically, anxiety or insomnia. Increased appetite with overeating occurs in some patients. These drugs may produce seizures, particularly in those who are prone to such disorders, including patients with a past history of severe alcoholism. Parkinsonism may occur occasionally, especially on abrupt withdrawal of the drug; antidepressants with relatively less anticholinergic activity are most commonly implicated. These drugs are reported to produce tardive dyskinesia (rarely) after prolonged use of large doses, but there are no controlled studies to substantiate this finding. Rarely, hyponatremia resulting in a syndrome of inappropriate secretion of antidiuretic hormone has been observed.

Cardiac reactions are uncommon unless overdosage occurs or these drugs are used in patients with associated cardiac dysfunction. There is some evidence to suggest that the concurrent administration of thyroid hormone may augment the cardiotoxic action of the tricyclic antidepressants. The cardiotoxic effects are similar to the cardiac conduction abnormalities observed with quinidine (particularly conduction disturbances, heart block, and bundle branch blocks). A baseline electrocardiogram prior to initiation of therapy and periodic monitoring, especially to monitor the width of the QRS complex, are recommended for elderly patients or those with prior or existing cardiac impairment.

Precautions: The tricyclic antidepressants should not be used in acutely agitated schizophrenic patients, and they should be used cautiously in those with mixed mania and depression, since they may convert a depression into a mania. Particular attention should be given to patients with suicidal tendencies when they begin to respond to therapy, for the risk of suicide is greatest near the end of the depressive cycle.

These compounds should be used with caution in elderly patients and in those with a history of seizure disorder, renal failure, or severely impaired hepatic function. Close supervision is advised if treatment is considered in patients with angle-closure glaucoma, urinary retention or obstruction, or those at risk of developing ileus.

The risks should be very carefully weighed when tricyclic drugs are used in patients with cardiac disease (eg, congestive failure, angina pectoris, recent myocardial infarction, paroxysmal tachycardia, electrocardiographic changes). It is advisable to monitor the effect of these drugs on blood pressure, especially in patients with hypertension or low normal pressure.

Routine precautions should be followed when these drugs are used during pregnancy (see the discussion in Chapter 2). Since data on the presence and amount of drug secreted in the milk of lactating mothers are sparse and variable, nursing should be avoided.

Overdosage: Overdosage of the tricyclic antidepressants produces symptoms of anticholinergic and cardiac toxicity. Fatal poisoning has been reported in enuretic children or their siblings and in children who have taken pills belonging to their parents. A single oral dose of 1 g of amitriptyline, imipramine, or doxepin produces severe toxic reactions in an adult, and doses in excess of 2 g are often fatal. All patients who have received such overdoses should be hospitalized to permit continuous cardiac monitoring. A widened QRS complex correlates sufficiently well with cardiotoxicity to serve as a presumptive diagnostic sign of probable overdosage. Since the first symptoms usually do not appear for one to four hours after ingestion, patients may be alert when first seen but may become comatose later.

Ventilatory depression, shock, serious atrial and ventricular arrhythmias (ranging from marked bradycardia to supraventricular and ventricular tachycardia), hyperthermia, agitation, ataxia, delirium, and coma may be observed. Other neurologic signs of toxicity include dilated pupils, nystagmus, hyperactive tendon reflexes, tremor, myoclonus, choreoathetosis, bladder and bowel paralysis, and convulsions. Severe poisoning is characterized by coma, seizures, and cardiac arrhythmias.

Treatment consists of general supportive measures, including correction of acidosis. Gastric lavage with charcoal is recom-mended even as late as six to eight hours following ingestion. Continued instillation of activated charcoal via nasogastric tube (with appropriate endotracheal intubation) is indicated for comatose patients, because the parent drug and its active metabolites undergo enterohepatic recirculation. Forced diuresis may not be effective, and hemodialysis, peritoneal dialysis, and exchange transfusion are of no value. If present, hyperpyrexia is managed by physical cooling procedures; however, hypothermia may occur instead. Cardiovascular abnormalities must be monitored carefully and may be particularly difficult to manage. Procainamide and quinidine are contraindicated because of their additive depressive effect on cardiac conduction; lidocaine, propranolol, and phenytoin are the drugs of choice. Physostigmine (1 to 3 mg intravenously in divided doses) may help control myoclonus, choreoathetosis, delirium, coma, and some of the cardiotoxic reactions, but this agent must be used with caution because it can cause potentially serious cholinergic effects, including excessive salivation requiring suction, bradycardia, bronchoconstriction, and convulsions. The course may have to be repeated because physostigmine has a short duration of action. (See Chapter 86, Specific Antidotes.) Cardioversion and/or electrical pacing may be necessary to control the arrhythmias and diazepam may be used to control convulsions. Drugs that may further impair cardiac conduction and depress the central nervous system probably should be avoided.

Drug Interactions: Since drugs used to treat cardiovascular disease and hypertension and those used to treat depression have numerous effects on biogenic amines, there are many interactions between drugs in these classes. Guanethidine [Ismelin] should not be given to patients receiving the tricyclic compounds, since the latter interfere with the action of guanethidine, thus allowing return of the hypertensive state. The effects of clonidine [Catapres] also may be reduced by tricyclic antidepressants.

Direct-acting adrenergic drugs (eg,

epinephrine, certain sympathomimetic amines present in local anesthetics and in some cold remedies) may be potentiated when used with tricyclic antidepressants. Although the action of indirect-acting adrenergic drugs (eg, dextroamphetamine, methylphenidate [Ritalin]) are antagonized by the tricyclic drugs, the former inhibit the metabolism of the latter and cause increased blood concentrations of tricyclic drugs. The nonadrenergic anorexiant, fenfluramine [Pondimin], has sedative properties and markedly potentiates this effect of the tricyclic antidepressants; therefore, the combination should be avoided.

The prominent anticholinergic effects of the tricyclic drugs are additive with those produced by other drugs with a similar action (eg, centrally-acting anticholinergic drugs used in parkinsonism, antihistamines, antipsychotics). A toxic confusional and delirious state may result, particularly in the elderly. Gastric emptying may be delayed in some individuals, thus limiting the rate of bioavailability of some concurrently administered drugs. Physicians are advised to delay administration of other agents one to two hours before or after the tricyclic drugs.

Extreme caution should be exercised if a tricyclic compound is given with or soon after a monoamine oxidase inhibitor, for their concomitant use may produce tremors, excitability, hyperpyrexia, muscle rigidity, generalized clonic convulsions, delirium, and death. Based on theoretical considerations, an interval of several days is suggested after a tricyclic compound is discontinued before the monoamine oxidase inhibitor is given and at least a two-week interval after a monoamine oxidase inhibitor is discontinued before the tricyclic compound is given. Because of reported withdrawal effects, especially with the tricyclic agents, doses of either type of drug should be reduced gradually in patients who have been receiving large amounts; initial dosage of the second drug should be small and the amount increased gradually.

Some reviewers of the literature have concluded that concurrent administration of tricyclic agents and monoamine oxidase inhibitors may not be dangerous if the dosage of each drug is titrated carefully. Combined therapy should be undertaken only by those familiar with the procedure (Ravaris et al, 1978).

The tricyclics with a significant sedative component (ie, doxepin, amitriptyline, protriptyline, imipramine, trimipramine) interact additively with the sedative effect of alcohol when these agents are used concomitantly. Adynamic ileus and excessive hepatic lipid also have been reported after use of this combination. Moderate to heavy alcohol consumption should be avoided, especially if the patient drives or works in a hazardous occupation.

The effectiveness of the tricyclic antidepressants may be reduced by concurrent administration of barbiturates, which induce hepatic microsomal enzymes that hasten the metabolism of the former. The simultaneous administration of barbiturates may be the cause of otherwise unexplained refractoriness to tricyclic drug administration. However, the effects of *toxic* levels of tricyclic compounds may be potentiated in the presence of alcohol and the barbiturates; the mechanism of this interaction is not known.

MONOAMINE OXIDASE INHIBITORS

The monoamine oxidase inhibitors (MAOI) appear to be less effective than the tricyclic antidepressants in patients with endogenous depression, and their use usually requires rigid dietary control; therefore, tricyclic antidepressants are the initial drugs of choice and electroshock is reserved for patients with severe endogenous depression refractory to tricyclic antidepressants (Robinson et al, 1978). Monoamine oxidase inhibitors may be drugs of choice in nonendogenous (atypical) types of depression (eg, agoraphobic, characterological, and hysteroid dysphoric depressions). Unreliable patients who cannot follow a diet or those who are episodic or habitual alcohol drinkers should be excluded, as well as patients with advanced cardiovascular, hepatic, or renal disease and pheochromocytoma (Ravaris et al, 1978).

Before there was an adequate understanding of their hazards, monoamine oxidase inhibitors produced considerable toxicity which limited their clinical investigation and widespread use. Isocarboxazid [Marplan], phenelzine [Nardil], and tranylcypromine [Parnate] are available as antidepressants (see the Table). Those drugs with monoamine oxidase inhibitor activity used to treat hypertension are no longer marketed.

All monoamine oxidase inhibitors, especially tranylcypromine, have amphetamine-like psychomotor stimulant properties, usually manifested only with very large doses. Lower doses produce antidepressant and antiphobic actions. Because these drugs are especially effective when considerable anxiety is present, they are presumed to have antianxiety action also. No antipsychotic effect is evident, and monoamine oxidase inhibitors may produce undesirable stimulation in schizophrenic patients.

The monoamine oxidase inhibitors are well absorbed orally; they are not administered parenterally because their onset of action is delayed (two to three weeks). These drugs are metabolized and excreted relatively rapidly, although the inhibited enzyme requires several weeks for regeneration.

Monoamine oxidase inhibitors may be useful in some patients with migraine syndrome (see Chapter 9, Drugs Used to Treat Migraine and Other Headaches).

Administration and Dosage: At least 80% of monoamine oxidase must be irreversibly inhibited for adequate therapy. The minimal doses cited in the Table reflect that requirement. The principles presented for tricyclic drug administration and dosage are also applicable to monoamine oxidase inhibitor therapy. These drugs should only be administered to patients who can be observed closely, and the ini-

tial dose should be reduced in outpatients. After the dose that relieves symptoms without causing undesirable effects is determined, this amount is then given daily in divided doses. Monoamine oxidase inhibitors may be administered once daily but, because of their mild psychomotor stimulant effect, they should not be given in the evening. The duration of therapy is determined individually based on response. Maintenance doses for those with recurrent depressive episodes have prophylactic value. If the recurrences are part of a manic-depressive illness, concurrent administration of lithium should be considered. Unlike the tricyclic antidepressants, the dose may be terminated abruptly without withdrawal effects. The recommended drug and dietary restrictions should be enforced for two to three weeks. If relapses occur, they will usually be apparent within three to six weeks.

Adverse Reactions: The most common reactions to the monoamine oxidase inhibitors are drowsiness, dryness of the mouth, orthostatic hypotension, blurred vision, dysuria, and constipation. Orthostatic hypotension (dizziness, vertigo) is seldom severe enough to require discontinuation of therapy. Weight gain, insomnia, and jerky movements during sleep are less common. Insomnia associated with euphoria, tremors, and hypomanic agitated behavior may reflect overdosage or individual sensitivity to the drugs. If headache, tachycardia, palpitation, nausea, vomiting, and hypertension occur together, it may indicate paradoxical hypertension caused by drug interaction rather than adverse drug reactions. (See the section on Drug Interactions.) Leukopenia, skin eruptions, photosensitivity, hepatotoxicity, hallucinations, and polyneuropathy have been reported but are rare. Peripheral bilateral edema of the extremities develops rarely and usually responds to thiazide diuretics; if it does not, the monoamine oxidase inhibitor should be discontinued.

Precautions: It is important to educate patients concerning the untoward effects produced by monoamine oxidase inhibitors. Patients should be instructed to inform other physicians treating them and pharmacists that they are taking monoamine oxidase inhibitors. In addition, they should carry a card stating that they are taking these drugs; information on potential interactions also may be included on the card.

Overdosage: Toxic effects may not appear for 12 hours or more after ingestion of the monoamine oxidase inhibitors and are largely adrenergic in nature: agitation, increased ventilatory and cardiac rates, dilated pupils, hyperreflexia, tremors, ataxia, sweating, hyperthermia, heart block, hypotension, delirium, convulsions, and coma. Aggressive supportive therapy to maintain vital functions, physical procedures to lower body temperature, forced diuresis, and acidification of the urine are indicated. Hemodialysis is of little value.

Drug Interactions: Paradoxical hypertension has been associated with the concomitant use of monoamine oxidase inhibitors and foods or beverages with a high tyramine content. These hypertensive crises are characterized by headache, tachycardia, palpitation, hypertension, nausea, and vomiting. Occasionally, pulmonary edema or subarachnoid or intracranial hemorrhage manifested by stiffness of the neck, decreasing levels of consciousness, and syncope occurs. Therefore, patients taking monoamine oxidase inhibitors should be warned that it may be necessary to avoid foods and beverages with a high tyramine content (eg, cheese, particularly strong, aged varieties; red wines; herring, both kippered [dried, salted] and pickled; chicken livers; canned figs; broad beans [fava beans]; chocolate; beer; yeast; meat extracts; game; yogurt). A complete list of such foods and beverages should be given to any patient receiving monoamine oxidase inhibitors.

Other indirect-acting adrenergic drugs (eg, amphetamine, methylphenidate, ephedrine, sympathomimetic amines present in some proprietary cold or asthma remedies) are markedly potentiated and should be avoided. Concurrent administration of direct-acting adrenergic drugs (eg, catecholamines) appears to be safe, because the monoamine oxidase inhibitors do not have a strong catecholamine reuptake blocking action like the tricyclic drugs. Phentolamine [Regitine] and propranolol [Inderal] have been used to counteract the hypertensive crises caused by the concomitant ingestion of monoamine oxidase inhibitors and foods containing tyramine or other indirect-acting adrenergic agents.

Levodopa [Dopar, Larodopa] should be withdrawn two to four weeks prior to institution of treatment with monoamine oxidase inhibitors. Methyldopa [Aldomet], tryptophan, and 5-hydroxytryptophan are also relatively contraindicated.

Severe toxic reactions characterized by excitation and hyperpyrexia may occur when meperidine [Demerol], dextromethorphan, and related analgesics are given to patients receiving monoamine oxidase inhibitors. If emergency surgery is necessary, meperidine should be avoided and the recommended dose of the narcotic chosen should be reduced by one-fourth. The central nervous system depressant action of anesthetics and alcohol is also markedly potentiated.

Furazolidone [Furoxone] and the cancer chemotherapeutic agent, procarbazine [Matulane], act as monoamine oxidase inhibitors when given for more than five days; therefore, caution should be observed if these drugs are administered with other monoamine oxidase inhibitors.

Insulin-dependent patients should be monitored for hypoglycemia at the start of monoamine oxidase inhibitor therapy; the dosage of insulin may need to be adjusted.

Tranylcypromine should be administered with caution to patients receiving disulfiram [Antabuse], because severe toxicity, including convulsions and death, have been noted experimentally.

For drug-drug interactions between tricyclic and monoamine oxidase inhibitor antidepressants, see the section on Tricyclic Antidepressants in this chapter.

STIMULANTS

Psychomotor stimulants (eg, dextroamphetamine, methylphenidate [Ritalin]) are *not* recommended for the vast majority of patients with affective disorders. The potential for tolerance and abuse of these drugs is high, and no controlled studies exist to support their effectiveness in most depressive illnesses. It has been suggested that 10 or 15 mg of dextroamphetamine be given once or twice daily as a diagnostic tool for one or two days to determine more rapidly the probable efficacy of tricyclic antidepressant therapy; however, this technique is not proven in any controlled study.

The reader is advised to consider the adverse reactions, precautions, and suggested dosage for these drugs (see Chapter 14, Drugs Used in Nonpsychotic Mental Disorders).

ANTIMANIC DRUG

Lithium counteracts mood changes without producing sedation and is considered to be the only specific antimanic drug for the prophylaxis and treatment of manic-depressive disorders (Fieve, 1977; Jefferson and Greist, 1977; Goodwin, 1979; Rosenbaum et al, 1979). Lithium alone is preferred to treat mild to moderate mania.

A threshold level in tissues must be reached before lithium is effective (which usually requires three to five days of therapy). Higher initial doses of lithium can shorten the time to clinical response or, because antipsychotic agents control motor hyperactivity, thought disorders, and delusions more rapidly, the latter drugs may be given with lithium in the initial treatment of highly agitated, hyperactive manic patients. When the acute episode is controlled, the antipsychotic agent may be withdrawn gradually and lithium continued as the sole therapeutic agent. Careful adjustment of dosage of both drugs is essential for optimum effectiveness; this also lessens any additive central nervous system toxicity associated with combination therapy (Spring, 1979).

Since lithium decreases the intensity and frequency of successive episodes in cyclic mania and depression, it is clearly indicated in the prophylaxis of circular manic-depressive (bipolar) disorders (Davis, 1976; Ananth and Pecknold, 1978). However, lithium is not effective in all patients; reported failure rates range from 20% to 55%. Therefore, this agent should be given indefinitely only to those patients in whom it reduces the frequency and/or intensity of recurrent manic and depressive episodes. The addition of a tricyclic drug may be necessary in breakthrough depression. Likewise, if mania is observed during use of tricyclic compounds in the treatment of patients with recurring depressive episodes, combination therapy with lithium may be helpful.

At present, there is little agreement on the benefit of lithium in patients with endogenous (unipolar) depressive illness. Not all clinicians feel that the prophylactic effect of lithium in recurrent unipolar depression is significant. Until this issue is clarified, lithium probably should be reserved for use in carefully selected patients with clearly defined recurrences for whom standard therapy is suboptimal. Although lithium is reported to be effective in treating the acute episode of unipolar depression, there is insufficient evidence to recommend its use on a routine basis for this purpose.

Open clinical studies strongly support the fact that lithium is effective for cluster headache (Wyant and Ashenhurst, 1979). This drug is currently under clinical investigation as an immunomodulator (see Chapter 66).

Lithium's role in schizophrenia is investigational. Although it may be effective in schizoaffective disorders with manic signs and symptoms, antipsychotic agents are preferred for agitated patients with this disorder.

Lithium has been proposed for use in a variety of other psychiatric disorders (eg, recurrent alcoholism, socially unacceptable aggressive behavior, obsessive-compulsive neurosis, organic brain syndromes, choreiform disorders, hyperkinesis and other behavior or character disorders in children). However, such uses have not been established or accepted by a majority of physicians.

See the evaluation for dosage and adverse reactions.

Precautions: The use of lithium requires close clinical observation, careful dosage adjustment, and frequent monitoring of blood levels to avoid toxic effects. If the clinical situation permits, a complete physical examination and selected laboratory studies are useful before initiating therapy; this should include tests for cardiovascular, hepatic, thyroid, and renal function; total and differential white blood counts; hemoglobin levels; and complete urinalysis. Serum lithium levels should be determined two to three times weekly during the acute phase and monthly after the maintenance dosage has been established. Blood samples should be drawn 8 to 12 hours after the last dose, and this time interval should remain fairly constant to keep results comparable. Periodic measurements of creatinine clearance, tests for renal concentrating ability, and thyroid function studies are recommended.

Renal function studies are recommended periodically during prolonged therapy for two reasons: Biological variability in some individuals causes enhanced retention of lithium that cannot be detected by measurement of serum lithium concentrations, and lithium may be capable of producing irreversible morphologic changes in the human kidney (Hestbech et al, 1977). However, renal biopsy studies to date have not been designed with adequate controls to prove that renal damage is a definite reproducible complication of lithium therapy. In some studies, the incidence appears to be highest with long-term therapy (ie, 5 to 10 years), although the phenomenon has been reported after less than six months of therapy. Further studies are in progress to define the incidence and risk of hepatotoxicity in patients on long-term lithium therapy. The benefit of lithium in an accurately diagnosed manic-depressive disorder is of sufficient magnitude to recommend its prophylactic use in spite of the risk of renal functional and morphologic involvement. On the other hand, the use of lithium should be avoided in less clearly defined depressive disorders, especially in young individuals.

Since lithium is excreted mainly by the kidneys, its elimination depends upon normal renal function and adequate salt and fluid intake (2.5 to 3 L daily). Lithium usually is relatively contraindicated in patients with renal or cardiac disease (eg, sick sinus syndrome) when interference with excretion is probable (eg, in those with decreased renal blood flow) or when electrolyte imbalance is present. In the presence of sodium deficiency, lithium ion is selectively reabsorbed in the renal tubules and may accumulate to toxic levels because of dehydration and sodium and potassium depletion. Therefore, lithium should be used only with caution in patients receiving diuretics or in those on a "crash" or low-salt diet. If lithium must be used with diuretics, the serum lithium and electrolyte levels should be closely monitored and the dosage of lithium reduced as indicated. Loop diuretics may be less of a problem than other diuretics (Jefferson and Kalin, 1979). If excessive and prolonged diarrhea or vomiting occurs or perspiration is profuse, lithium should be discontinued and supplemental salt and fluid administered. The drug should not be given to debilitated or dehydrated individuals or to those with severe infections.

Special precautions are necessary when lithium is used in the elderly, since the rate of renal excretion tends to decline with age. Use of small doses with very gradual increases and frequent determination of serum lithium levels generally are necessary.

There are reports of an increased rate of congenital abnormalities, especially heart defects, in infants exposed to lithium during early pregnancy. Therefore, its use is relatively contraindicated during the first trimester. If lithium is considered for use after the third month of pregnancy to avoid postpartum psychosis, the risk to the fetus or infant should be weighed against the expected therapeutic benefits. Lithium crosses the placenta and is present in equivalent concentrations in the mother and fetus. Since the half-life of lithium is prolonged in newborn infants, the dose should be decreased or the drug discontinued seven to ten days prior to delivery.

The hemodynamic and metabolic alterations that occur during delivery may cause toxic accumulation of lithium in both mother and infant. During delivery, water deprivation, infusion of hypertonic sodium chloride injection, or injection of pituitary hormones should be avoided. Additionally, lithium appears in breast milk, and mothers taking lithium should not breast-feed their infants.

Although lithium is not contraindicated in diabetics, it has been observed to increase serum insulin levels. Blood sugar and electrolyte levels should be monitored periodically.

The combined use of lithium and iodine should be avoided, for synergistic antithyroid effects have been reported; patients receiving lithium should be warned to avoid medications that contain iodides (eg, cough medicines, multivitamin preparations). One hypothyroid woman receiving lithium gave birth to a hypothyroid infant with a very large goiter and a low plasma concentration of protein-bound iodine.

TRICYCLIC COMPOUNDS

IMIPRAMINE HYDROCHLORIDE
[Imavate, SK-Pramine, Tofranil]

IMIPRAMINE PAMOATE
[Tofranil-PM]

This prototype of the tricyclic compounds is most useful in treating endogenous depression. Although imipramine may reduce the anxiety that sometimes accompanies depression, it is not an anti-anxiety agent in its own right and has only minimal to moderate sedative action at usual therapeutic doses. The pamoate form offers no advantage over the hydrochloride salt, which is inherently long acting.

The untoward effects associated with use of imipramine are characteristic for all tricyclic compounds. Sedation and anticholinergic effects are most common. Cardiac and central nervous system signs and symptoms may be prominent with overdosage. Allergic reactions, blood dyscrasias, endocrine effects, and jaundice are less common.

Abrupt cessation of treatment after long-term therapy may produce withdrawal symptoms (eg, headache, malaise, anorexia, fatigue). An akathisia-like syndrome also has been reported when administration of imipramine (300 mg or more daily) was suddenly stopped. Although most fatal cases of poisoning have occurred after ingestion of more than 1.5 g, death has been reported after ingestion of 500 to 750 mg and recovery after ingestion of 5.4 g.

See the Introduction for a more complete discussion on adverse reactions, precautions, and the use of imipramine with other drugs.

ROUTES, USUAL DOSAGE, AND PREPARATIONS. Doses should be individualized on the basis of clinical response.
Intramuscular: *Adults*, initially, up to 100 mg daily in divided doses. The oral route should be substituted as soon as possible.
IMIPRAMINE HYDROCHLORIDE:
Tofranil (Geigy). Solution 12.5 mg/ml in 2 ml containers.
Oral: *Adults (hospitalized)*, initially, 100 mg daily in divided doses, increased gradually to 200 mg daily; 250 to 300 mg daily may be given if there is no response after two weeks. *Adults (outpatients)*, initially, 75 mg, increased to 150 mg daily in divided doses; for maintenance, 50 to 150 mg daily at bedtime (maximum, 300 mg daily). *Adolescents and elderly patients*, initially, 30 to 40 mg daily (maximum, 100 mg daily).
IMIPRAMINE HYDROCHLORIDE:
Drug available generically: Tablets 10, 25, and 50 mg.
Imavate (Robins). Tablets 25 and 50 mg.
SK-Pramine (Smith Kline & French), *Tofranil*

(Geigy). Tablets 10, 25, and 50 mg.
IMIPRAMINE PAMOATE:
Tofranil-PM (Geigy). Capsules equivalent to 75, 100, 125, and 150 mg of imipramine hydrochloride.

AMITRIPTYLINE HYDROCHLORIDE
[Amitid, Amitril, Elavil, Endep, SK-Amitriptyline]

Amitriptyline is as effective as imipramine in the treatment of depression. The indications, adverse reactions, and precautions with its use are similar to those of the other tricyclic compounds. Effective doses have a moderate to marked sedative action. Because anticholinergic activity may be more pronounced with amitriptyline, the incidence of confusional episodes may be greater, especially in elderly patients. Leukopenia and an increased appetite for carbohydrates with resultant weight gain also have been reported. Although most fatal cases of poisoning have resulted from ingestion of more than 1.3 g, death has been reported after ingestion of 500 mg and recovery after ingestion of almost 4 g.

See the Introduction for a more complete discussion on indications, adverse reactions, precautions, and the use of tricyclic antidepressants with other drugs.

ROUTES, USUAL DOSAGE, AND PREPARATIONS. *Intramuscular: Adults*, initially, 20 to 30 mg four times a day. The oral route should be substituted as soon as possible.
    Drug available generically: Solution 10 mg/ml in 10 ml containers.
    Elavil (Merck Sharp & Dohme). Solution 10 mg/ml in 10 ml containers.
Oral: Adults (hospitalized), initially, 100 mg daily in divided doses, increased gradually to 200 mg daily; some patients may require as much as 300 mg daily. *Adults (outpatients)*, initially, 75 mg, increased to 150 mg daily in divided doses;

for maintenance, 50 to 100 mg once daily at bedtime (maximum, 300 mg daily). *Elderly patients and adolescents*, 10 mg three times daily and 20 mg at bedtime.
    Drug available generically: Tablets 10, 25, 50, 75, 100, and 150 mg.
    Amitid (Squibb). Tablets 10, 25, 50, 75, and 100 mg.
    Amitril (Parke, Davis), *Elavil* (Merck Sharp & Dohme), *Endep* (Roche), *SK-Amitriptyline* (Smith Kline & French). Tablets 10, 25, 50, 75, 100, and 150 mg.

DESIPRAMINE HYDROCHLORIDE
[Norpramin, Pertofrane]

Desipramine, a metabolite of imipramine, has actions and uses similar to those of the other tricyclic compounds. It is as effective as imipramine in the treatment of depression.

Untoward effects are similar to those produced by imipramine but its anticholinergic and sedative actions are less pronounced. See the Introduction for more complete information on indications, adverse reactions, precautions, and the use of tricyclic antidepressants with other drugs.

ROUTE, USUAL DOSAGE, AND PREPARATIONS. *Oral: Adults (hospitalized)*, initially, 75 mg daily in divided doses, increased gradually to 200 mg daily. If necessary, after two weeks, the dosage may be increased gradually to a maximum of 300 mg daily. *Adults (outpatients)*, initially, 75 mg, increased to 200 mg daily in divided doses. For maintenance, the lowest dose that maintains remission should be given; the usual dose is 50 to 100 mg given at bedtime (maximum, 300 mg daily). *Elderly patients and adolescents*, 25 to 50 mg daily, increased to 100 mg in divided doses if necessary.
    Norpramin (Merrell-National). Tablets 25, 50, 75, 100, and 150 mg.
    Pertofrane (USV). Capsules 25 and 50 mg.

DOXEPIN HYDROCHLORIDE
[Adapin, Sinequan]

Doxepin possesses the characteristics of the other tricyclic compounds and is as effective as imipramine and amitriptyline in the treatment of depression. It has a prominent sedative effect.

Untoward effects are similar to those produced by the other drugs in this class. Although most fatal cases of poisoning have resulted from ingestion of more than 1.5 g, death has been reported after ingestion of 850 mg and recovery after ingestion of 5 g.

See the Introduction for additional information on indications, adverse reactions, precautions, and the use of tricyclic antidepressants with other drugs.

ROUTE, USUAL DOSAGE, AND PREPARATIONS. *Oral: Adults (hospitalized)*, initially, 75 to 150 mg daily in divided doses. The dosage may be increased gradually after two weeks to a maximum of 300 mg daily. *Adults (outpatients)*, initially, 75 mg, increased to 150 mg daily in divided doses. For maintenance, 25 to 150 mg daily (maximum, 300 mg daily).

Adapin (Pennwalt). Capsules 10, 25, 50, and 100 mg.
Sinequan (Pfizer). Capsules 10, 25, 50, 75, 100, and 150 mg; solution (concentrate) 10 mg/ml.

NORTRIPTYLINE HYDROCHLORIDE
[Aventyl Hydrochloride, Pamelor]

The actions of nortriptyline are similar to those of other tricyclic compounds, and this drug appears to be as effective as imipramine in the treatment of depression. Plasma levels below 50 ng/ml are generally ineffective, and plasma levels above 175 ng/ml are often associated with a suboptimal response; therefore, excessive dosage, even in the absence of toxicity, may diminish responsiveness. See the Introduction for additional information on indications, adverse reactions, precautions, and the use of tricyclic antidepressants with other drugs.

ROUTE, USUAL DOSAGE, AND PREPARATIONS. *Oral: Adults (hospitalized)*, initially, 40 mg daily in three or four divided doses up to 150 mg daily after two weeks, if necessary. Ordinarily, initial doses are small; after adjustment as needed, the total dose can be given once daily at bedtime. For *outpatients*, initially, 20 to 100 mg daily. *Adolescents and elderly patients*, 30 to 50 mg daily in divided doses. For maintenance, the lowest dose that maintains remission should be given.

Aventyl Hydrochloride (Lilly), *Pamelor* (Sandoz). Capsules equivalent to 10 and 25 mg of base; liquid equivalent to 10 mg of base/5 ml (alcohol 4%, Aventyl Hydrochloride).

PROTRIPTYLINE HYDROCHLORIDE
[Vivactil]

Unlike the other tricyclic antidepressants, protriptyline possesses little, if any, sedative action. Because of this, it may be particularly useful in treating depressed patients whose predominant manifestations of illness are psychomotor retardation, apathy, and fatigue, and it is less beneficial when agitation and anxiety are the most prominent symptoms.

See the Introduction for additional information on indications, adverse reactions, precautions, and the use of tricyclic antidepressants with other drugs.

ROUTE, USUAL DOSAGE, AND PREPARATIONS. *Oral*: *Adults (hospitalized)*, 15 mg daily in three or four divided doses up to 60 mg daily after two weeks, if necessary. Ordinarily, initial doses are small; after adjustment as needed, the total dose can be given once daily at bedtime. For *outpatients*, initially, 15 to 40 mg daily. *Adolescents and elderly patients*, initially, 15 mg daily in three divided doses, increased gradually if necessary. In elderly patients, the cardiovascular system must be monitored closely if the daily dose exceeds 20 mg. For maintenance, the lowest dose that maintains remission should be given.

Vivactil (Merck Sharp & Dohme). Tablets 5 and 10 mg.

TRIMIPRAMINE MALEATE
[Surmontil]

Although trimipramine is the most recently approved tricyclic antidepressant, it has been in use outside the United States for a number of years. Trimipramine is an effective antidepressant similar to the other dibenzazepines in its class (ie, desipramine, imipramine); however, unlike the latter compounds, the sedation produced is equivalent to that observed with amitriptyline and doxepin. The anticholinergic blocking activity is less than with amitriptyline and doxepin but more than with imipramine.

The indications, adverse reactions, and precautions with use of trimipramine are similar to those of the other tricyclic compounds (see the Introduction). There are no adequate and well-controlled studies in pregnant women to assess the potential risk to the fetus.

ROUTES, USUAL DOSAGE, AND PREPARATIONS. *Oral*: *Adults (hospitalized)*, initially, 100 mg daily in divided doses, increased gradually to 200 mg daily; if improvement does not occur in two to three weeks, the dose may be increased to a maximum of 250 to 300 mg. *Adults (outpatients)*, initially, 75 mg daily increased to 150 mg in divided doses; amounts exceeding 200 mg/day are not recommended; for maintenance, dosage should be adjusted to the lowest level required to maintain symptomatic relief. *Elderly and adolescent patients*, initially, 50 mg daily, increased gradually to 100 mg daily, depending upon the response and tolerance.

Surmontil (Ives). Capsules 25 and 50 mg.

MONOAMINE OXIDASE INHIBITORS

PHENELZINE SULFATE
[Nardil]

Phenelzine is effective in the treatment of some depressed patients, particularly outpatients with depressive and phobic neuroses accompanied by anxiety. Like other monoamine oxidase inhibitors, however, phenelzine is probably less effective than the tricyclic drugs in severe endogenous depression, although some patients refractory to the tricyclic drugs respond to phenelzine, especially those with high levels of anxiety. Because all monoamine oxidase inhibitors have the potential for producing serious adverse reactions, patients should be closely supervised and dietary precautions should be observed. Phenelzine is known to be acetylated rapidly or slowly, depending upon the patient's genetic profile; however, no relationship has been demonstrated between acetylator phenotype and therapeutic or adverse effects of phenelzine (Davidson et al, 1978). The dose must be individualized to achieve adequate therapeutic results with minimal adverse effects.

Although several fatal cases of poisoning

have occurred after ingestion of 375 mg to 1.5 g, several other patients have recovered after ingesting doses within this range.

See the Introduction for a discussion on adverse reactions, precautions, and the use of monoamine oxidase inhibitors with other drugs.

ROUTE, USUAL DOSAGE, AND PREPARATIONS. *Oral*: *Adults (outpatients)*, initially, 45 to 75 mg daily in three divided doses. Alternatively, 1 mg/kg of body weight daily may be given initially in three divided doses. The dosage can be increased to 90 mg, but should be decreased if untoward effects develop. A few patients may require more than 90 mg. It is often useful to maintain patients on a therapeutic dose for three to six months after improvement is noted. If maintenance therapy is indicated for recurrent illness, the total daily dose should be reduced to the lowest effective amount. Information is inadequate to establish a dosage for *children under 16 years*.

    Nardil (Parke, Davis). Tablets equivalent to 15 mg of base.

ISOCARBOXAZID
[Marplan]

Isocarboxazid may be useful in some patients who have depressive and phobic neuroses with severe anxiety, but it has not been established that isocarboxazid is as effective as other monoamine oxidase inhibitors or the tricyclic compounds in these conditions. Patients should be closely supervised.

See the Introduction for additional information on indications, adverse reactions, precautions, and the use of monoamine oxidase inhibitors with other drugs. Recovery has been reported after ingestion of 300 to 500 mg of isocarboxazid.

ROUTE, USUAL DOSAGE, AND PREPARATIONS. *Oral*: *Adults (outpatients)*, initially, 20 to 30 mg daily in divided doses; the amount may be increased to 50 mg in hospitalized patients. The dosage should be reduced as soon as clinical improvement is observed; 10 to 20 mg daily or less is the usual amount given for maintenance. Information is inadequate to establish dosage for *children under 16 years*.

    Marplan (Roche). Tablets 10 mg.

TRANYLCYPROMINE SULFATE
[Parnate]

This monoamine oxidase inhibitor has essentially the same actions and uses as phenelzine. Tranylcypromine sulfate is produced from the cyclization of the side chain of amphetamines and may cause psychomotor stimulation, but this usually occurs at doses higher than those used for depression.

Untoward effects are similar to those produced by other monoamine oxidase inhibitors. The incidence of intracranial hemorrhage (sometimes fatal) associated with paradoxical hypertension and severe occipital headache appears to be greater with tranylcypromine than with other monoamine oxidase inhibitors. A significant proportion of a small number of deaths caused by tranylcypromine poisoning occurred with doses over 350 mg; however, patients have survived after ingestion of this amount. Dependence on tranylcypromine has been reported occasionally.

See the Introduction for additional information on indications, adverse reactions, precautions, and the use of monoamine oxidase inhibitors with other drugs.

ROUTE, USUAL DOSAGE, AND PREPARATIONS. *Oral*: *Adults (outpatients)*, initially, 20 to 40 mg daily in two equally divided doses in the morning and afternoon for two weeks. Subsequent doses should be adjusted according to the patient's response; the lowest effective dose should be given in divided amounts. Doses above 30 mg daily are not advisable, although 50 mg has been used in hospitalized patients with severe depression. Information is inadequate to establish a dosage for *children under 16 years*.

Drug available generically: Tablets 10 mg.
Parnate (Smith Kline & French). Tablets equivalent to 10 mg of base.

ANTIMANIC DRUG

LITHIUM CARBONATE
[Eskalith, Lithane, Lithonate, Lithotabs]

LITHIUM CITRATE
[Lithonate-S]

Lithium is effective in the prophylaxis and treatment of manic-depressive disorders. Unlike the antipsychotic or antidepressant drugs, lithium has no specific stimulant effects, has little effect on otherwise healthy patients except for mild sedation, and has no antiadrenergic or anticholinergic action. Its mechanism of action has not been fully elucidated.

Lithium is completely absorbed six to eight hours after oral administration. Since the onset of action is slow (three to five days), parenteral use is of no advantage to hasten the onset of action. Plasma half-life is approximately 7 to 24 hours, and lithium is eliminated almost entirely by the kidneys. About 80% of filtered lithium is reabsorbed. The normal variations in urinary flow rate and dietary sodium intake do not appreciably affect the rate of excretion of lithium. Lithium ion is not protein bound and is distributed in total body water and concentrated in various tissues to different degrees. After a steady state has been achieved, the lithium level in cerebrospinal fluid is about 40% of that in serum, and renal clearance for an individual remains relatively constant.

There is a good correlation between the serum concentration of lithium ion and therapeutic efficacy and toxicity. To prevent toxicity, the dosage should be maintained within a critical and narrow range, for adverse reactions may occur at doses that are close to therapeutic levels. Patients can tolerate larger doses of lithium during acute manic episodes. However, as the attack subsides, dosage should be reduced rapidly to prevent accumulation. *Serum lithium levels should not be permitted to exceed 2.0 (preferably 0.9 to 1.5 for most patients) mEq/L during initial treatment and should be kept within a range of 0.5 to 1.2 mEq/L during maintenance.*

The following general reactions are useful guidelines for evaluating most patients, but dependence on serum lithium levels should not be substituted for clinical observation:

Transient, mild to moderate side effects occur in most patients at serum levels of 1.5 to 2 mEq/L but also may be observed at lower levels, depending upon the tolerance of the patient. The most common reactions include nausea, diarrhea, malaise, and fine hand tremor. Other frequent untoward effects are thirst, polyuria, polydipsia, and fatigue. These symptoms may persist throughout treatment but are reversible when the drug is discontinued. Hand tremor can be controlled with propranolol if it is necessary to maintain dosage for antimanic effectiveness.

Drowsiness, vomiting, muscle weakness, ataxia, dryness of the mouth, abdominal pain, lethargy, dizziness, slurred speech, and nystagmus are early symptoms of intoxication. These reactions may occur at levels above 1.5 mEq/L and are common at concentrations of 2 mEq/L.

Moderate to severe adverse reactions may occur at serum concentrations above 2 mEq/L. At levels of 2 to 2.5 mEq/L, symptoms include anorexia, persistent nausea and vomiting, blurred vision, fasciculations, clonic movements of whole limbs, hyperactive deep tendon reflexes, choreoathetoid movements, epileptiform convulsions, toxic psychosis, syncope, electroencephalographic changes, acute circulatory failure, stupor, and coma. At serum levels above 2.5 mEq/L, symptoms may rapidly progress to generalized convulsions, oliguria, and death.

No specific antidote for lithium poisoning is known. However, when frank symptoms of toxicity occur or serum levels exceed 2 mEq/L, lithium should be discontinued and fluid and electrolyte replacement therapy initiated. Excretion of lithium can be facilitated by alkalization of urine and administration of osmotic diuretics (urea, mannitol), acetazolamide, and theophylline. Electrocardiograms and measurement of serum hematocrit levels should be performed periodically. It may be necessary to administer anticonvulsants if convulsions are present. Peritoneal dialysis is less effective than hemodialysis; the latter may be indicated if renal function is impaired or lithium toxicity is severe (Hansen and Amdisen, 1978).

When the serum lithium level exceeds 1.5 mEq/L or adverse reactions become bothersome, regardless of the serum lithium level the drug generally should be discontinued for 24 hours and therapy resumed at a lower dosage level. The patient and those living in his household should be cautioned to notify the physician immediately if untoward symptoms or unexplained illnesses occur.

Several adverse reactions *not* related to dose or plasma concentrations may develop during prolonged treatment. Diffuse thyroid enlargement with no change in thyroid function or, occasionally, hypothyroidism may occur after long-term treatment. The administration of thyroid hormones controls the glandular enlargement, and thyroid function generally returns to normal when lithium is withdrawn. Thyroid function tests should be performed periodically in all patients on long-term therapy.

A nephrogenic diabetes insipidus-like syndrome has been observed; salt depletion or diuretic therapy should not be instituted, since these measures only enhance lithium toxicity. Polyuria and polydipsia, which are noted early in treatment, are caused by a loss of renal concentrating ability and cannot be corrected by administration of vasopressin. Transient hyperglycemia, leukocytosis, flattened or inverted T waves, headache, peripheral edema, metallic taste, rashes, and other skin reactions (eg, cutaneous ulcers) have been reported infrequently.

A maculopapular cutaneous rash may develop within three weeks after initiating therapy. It may subside spontaneously or require temporary discontinuation of lithium therapy.

Mild leukocytosis (10,000 to 14,000) occurs frequently throughout therapy, but it is reversible when lithium is discontinued. Reversible electrocardiographic alterations (flattening and inversion of T waves and widening of the QRS complex) that does not respond to potassium therapy are also noted in some individuals.

An acute brain syndrome occurs infrequently and is characterized by a toxic confusional state, convulsions, and changes in the electroencephalogram; there are no other signs of lithium toxicity and toxic serum levels are not present. This reaction is observed most commonly within three weeks after initiating therapy and responds rapidly to termination of therapy or reduction of dose. Patients with schizophrenia and organic brain disease may be hypersensitive to this action of lithium.

See also the Introduction for indications, precautions, and drug interactions with lithium.

ROUTE, USUAL DOSAGE, AND PREPARATIONS. *Oral*: Dosage should be individualized on the basis of serum levels and response, and the drug should be discontinued if a satisfactory response is not obtained in a few weeks. *Adults*, for acute mania, initially, 0.6 to 2.1 g daily in three divided doses, increased or decreased daily or every other day by 0.3 g to produce a serum level of 0.8 to 1.5 mEq/L (maximum, 2.4 g). During acute manic episodes, some patients show increased tolerance to ordinarily toxic blood levels. When the acute attack subsides, the dose should be reduced rapidly to obtain a serum level of 0.5 to 1.2 mEq/L. To maintain this level, the usual dosage is 0.9 to 1.2 g daily in three divided doses. Each 5 ml of Lithonate-S syrup contains 8 mEq of lithium ion, equivalent to the amount of lithium in 300 mg of lithium carbonate. The drug should be used cautiously in *debilitated or elderly patients*.

Children under 12, information is inadequate to establish safety and efficacy.

LITHIUM CARBONATE:

Drug available generically: Capsules, tablets 300 mg.

Eskalith (Smith Kline & French), *Lithonate* (Rowell). Capsules 300 mg.

Lithane (Dome), *Lithotabs* (Rowell). Tablets 300 mg.

LITHIUM CITRATE:

Lithonate-S (Rowell). Syrup 8 mEq/5 ml.

MIXTURES

MIXTURES CONTAINING AN ANTIDEPRESSANT AND ANTIPSYCHOTIC DRUG

Combination products containing amitriptyline and perphenazine are available for use in patients with severe agitation and schizoaffective disorders. Most of these patients require only antipsychotic drug therapy, but amitriptyline occasionally may be useful as an adjunct to control symptoms of depression. However, the amounts supplied in fixed-ratio combinations may not be suitable for many patients.

See the section on Tricyclic Antidepressants in this chapter and the evaluation on Perphenazine in Chapter 12, Antipsychotic Drugs, for additional information on indications, adverse reactions, precautions, and the use of tricyclic antidepressants with other drugs.

ROUTE, USUAL DOSAGE, AND PREPARATIONS. The manufacturers' suggested dosage is: *Oral: Adults,* one tablet containing 2 or 4 mg of perphenazine and 25 mg of amitriptyline three or four times daily. The daily dosage should not exceed 16 mg of perphenazine and 100 mg of amitriptyline. In more severely ill patients, initially, two tablets containing 4 mg of perphenazine and 25 mg of amitriptyline three times daily; a fourth dose may be given at bedtime if necessary. *Adolescents and elderly patients,* initially, one tablet containing 4 mg of perphenazine and 10 mg of amitriptyline three or four times daily. The usual maintenance dosage for most patients is one tablet containing 2 or 4 mg of perphenazine and 10 or 25 mg of amitriptyline

two to four times daily. Use of these mixtures in *children* is inadvisable.

Mixture available generically: Tablets containing perphenazine 2 mg and amitriptyline hydrochloride 10 or 25 mg and perphenazine 4 mg and amitriptyline hydrochloride 10 or 25 mg.

Etrafon (Schering), *Triavil* (Merck Sharp & Dohme). Tablets containing perphenazine 2 mg and amitriptyline hydrochloride 10 mg (Etrafon 2-10, Triavil 2-10) or 25 mg (Etrafon, Triavil 2-25); tablets containing perphenazine 4 mg and amitriptyline hydrochloride 10 mg (Etrafon-A, Triavil 4-10), 25 mg (Etrafon-Forte, Triavil 4-25) or 50 mg (Triavil 4-50).

MIXTURE CONTAINING AN ANTIDEPRESSANT AND ANTIANXIETY DRUG

The recent introduction of a combination product containing amitriptyline and chlordiazepoxide is recommended by the manufacturer to improve the rate of response during the first week of therapy in depressed patients with anxiety. Most anxiety accompanying depression is ultimately controlled by an antidepressant drug alone; antianxiety drugs, therefore, are considered adjunctive rather than primary or routine therapy. Combined use for initial therapy is not recommended by most clinicians. Further, antidepressant drugs require individual titration of dose to obtain optimum response, and this is less easily accomplished when the antidepressant is present in a fixed-dose combination. Safe use of Limbitrol during pregnancy and lactation has not been established.

ROUTE, USUAL DOSAGE, AND PREPARATIONS. The manufacturer's suggested dosage is: *Oral: Adults ,* three or four tablets of Limbitrol 10-25 daily in divided doses. This may be increased to six tablets daily as required. Limbitrol 5-12.5 may be substituted in patients who cannot tolerate larger doses.

Limbitrol (Roche). Tablets containing chlordiazepoxide 5 or 10 mg and amitriptyline 12.5 or 25 mg.

Selected References

Ananth J, Pecknold JC: Prediction of lithium response in affective disorders. *J Clin Psychiatry* 39:95-100, 1978.

Cain NN, Cain RM: Compendium of antidepressants. *Drug Ther* 8:114-150, (April) 1978.

Crews FT, Smith CB: Presynaptic alpha-receptor subsensitivity after long-term antidepressant treatment. *Science* 202:322-324, 1978.

Davidson J, et al: Acetylation phenotype, platelet monoamine oxidase inhibition, and effectiveness of phenelzine in depression. *Am J Psychiatry* 135:467-469, 1978.

Davis JM: Overview: Maintenance therapy in psychiatry. II. Affective disorders. *Am J Psychiatry* 133:1-13, 1976.

Davis KL, et al: Cholinergic involvement in mental disorders. *Life Sci* 22:1865-1872, 1978.

deMontigny C, Aghajanian GK: Tricyclic antidepressants: Long-term treatment increases responsivity of rat forebrain neurons to serotonin. *Science* 202:1303-1306, 1978.

Fieve RR: Clinical use of lithium in affective disorders. *Drugs* 13:458-466, 1977.

Garver DL, Davis JM: Biogenic amine hypotheses of affective disorders. *Life Sci* 24:383-394, 1979.

Gelenberg AJ, Klerman GL: Antidepressants: Their use in clinical practice. *Ration Drug Ther* 12:1-7, (April) 1978.

Goodwin FK (ed): Lithium ion: Impact on treatment and research. *Arch Gen Psychiatry* 36:833-916, (July 20) 1979.

Hansen HE, Amdisen A: Lithium intoxication: Report of 23 cases and review of 100 cases from literature. *Q J Med* 47:123-144, 1978

Hestbech J, et al: Chronic renal lesions following long-term treatment with lithium. *Kidney Int* 12:205-213, 1977.

Hollister LE: Tricyclic antidepressants, parts I and II. *N Engl J Med* 299:1106-1109, 1168-1172, 1978.

Jefferson JW, Greist JH: *Primer of Lithium Therapy.* Baltimore, Williams and Wilkins Company, 1977.

Jefferson JW, Kalin NH: Serum lithium levels and long-term diuretic use. *JAMA* 241:1134-1136, 1979.

Nies A, et al: Relationship between age and tricyclic antidepressant plasma levels. *Am J Psychiatry* 134:790-793, 1977.

Ravaris CL, et al: Use of MAOI antidepressants. *Am Fam Physician* 18:105-111, (July) 1978.

Risch SC, et al: Plasma levels of tricyclic antidepressants and clinical efficacy: Review of literature, parts I and II. *J Clin Psychiatry* 40:4-21, 58-69, 1979.

Robinson DS, et al: Clinical pharmacology of phenelzine. *J Clin Psychol* 35:629-635, 1978.

Rosenbaum AH, et al: Drugs that alter mood. I. Tricyclic agents and monoamine oxidase inhibitors. II. Lithium. *Mayo Clin Proc* 54:335-344, 401-407, 1979.

Sourkes TL: Biochemistry of mental depression. *Can Psychiatr Assoc J* 22:467-481, 1977.

Spring GK: Neurotoxicity with combined use of lithium and thioridazine. *J Clin Psychiatry* 40:135-138, 1979.

Svensson TH, Usdin T: Feedback inhibition of brain noradrenaline neurons by tricyclic antidepressants: Alpha-receptor mediation. *Science* 202:1089-1091, 1978.

Whitlock FA, Evans LEJ: Drugs and depression. *Drugs* 15:53-71, 1978.

Wyant GM, Ashenhurst EM: Chronic pain syndromes and their treatment. I. Cluster headache. *Can Anaesth Soc J* 26:38-41, 1979.

Drugs Used in Nonpsychotic Mental Disorders | 14

Pharmacotherapy is of variable benefit in nonpsychotic mental disorders. Drugs discussed in this chapter are used to treat alcoholism, dementia, hyperkinetic syndrome, and narcolepsy, but their administration for these indications is controversial and often yields less than optimum results.

ALCOHOLISM

Ethanol (alcohol) is available as a parenteral preparation that produces long-lasting local anesthetic effects when injected close to selected nerves and as a skin disinfectant or vehicle for many other drugs used on the skin (see Chapter 61, Dermatologic Preparations). It often is an ingredient in medicinal elixirs. Ethanol is most commonly used orally, ostensibly to produce self-relaxation and improve social communication, but intoxication frequently occurs, which is in fact a self-

induced acute organic brain syndrome.

In the fasting state, ethanol is absorbed from the stomach (20%) and small intestine (80%) and is widely distributed. It readily crosses the placenta and moderate to large amounts taken during pregnancy are teratogenic and produce the fetal alcohol syndrome (Clarren and Smith, 1978). Approximately 90% to 98% of a dose undergoes zero-order oxidation to carbon dioxide and water via the intermediate products of acetaldehyde and acetate. Numerous metabolic changes accompany or follow the metabolism of ethanol. Some changes, such as the increase in lactate and fatty acid production and hyperuricemia, seem to be caused by the increased NADH/NAD ratio produced by oxidation of ethanol (Lieber et al, 1971). The liver of a nontolerant individual can metabolize about 180 mg/kg/hr of absolute alcohol (100% or 200 proof); this amount represents approximately one to two ounces of 80 to 100 proof whiskey, a four-ounce glass of wine, or 12 ounces of beer per hour. Alcoholics who have been drinking recently often metabolize ethanol faster, perhaps because of enzyme induction. This effect may be masked in the presence of hepatitis or advanced cirrhosis of the liver. Hyperthyroid patients may metabolize ethanol twice as fast as normal individuals. Ingestion in excess of the individual rate of metabolism will lead to accumulation.

Ethanol is a nonspecific central nervous system depressant. With rising ethanol blood concentrations, reasoning, memory, and coordination are increasingly impaired. Loosening of inhibitions and impaired judgment may lead to dangerous or violent behavior and disregard of social norms. Because of the wide variation in individual susceptibility to the effects of ethanol, based partly on constitutional factors, state of nutrition, and phenomena of acute and chronic tolerance, it is difficult to associate particular blood ethanol concentrations with specific degrees of impairment. In general, if a patient does not abuse ethanol chronically, blood concentrations of 0.2% to 0.3% are associated with slurred speech and ataxia, while concentrations of 0.3% to 0.4% are characterized by stupor, coma, and anesthesia. Blood concentrations of 0.5% to 0.8% are usually lethal; death is due to respiratory depression. However, some chronic alcoholics tolerate concentrations of 0.5% to 0.6% without marked impairment of consciousness.

Hypoglycemia is a serious but uncommon finding in chronic alcoholics during withdrawal after a long bout of drinking (Kallas and Sellers, 1975). This reaction is caused by poor dietary carbohydrate intake, low glycogen stores, and inhibition of gluconeogenesis as a result of an increased NADH/NAD ratio that diverts pyruvic acid to lactic acid. Lactic acidemia and ketoacidosis may occur as well. Much more often, mild to moderate hypoglycemia is observed in intoxicated chronic alcoholics or during withdrawal, probably caused by impaired liver and pancreatic function and perhaps by increased peripheral tissue resistance to the effects of insulin (Nikkilä and Taskinen, 1975).

The chronic excessive intake of alcohol may lead initially to fatty liver. Hepatic necrosis and ultimately cirrhosis are caused by direct toxic effects of alcohol or secondarily by acetaldehyde; hyperlipemia, hyperuricemia, pancreatitis, cardiomyopathy, and hypomagnesemia are additional possible complications (Lieber, 1976). Poor dietary intake and/or malabsorption as a result of gastrointestinal irritation are responsible for the malnutrition that is usually present. Prolonged malnutrition, especially thiamine deficiency, and early cerebral atrophy, possibly due to the direct central nervous system effects of alcohol and its metabolic products, are responsible for producing Wernicke's encephalopathy (confusion, nystagmus, ocular muscle movement abnormalities) and the dysmnesic syndrome (Korsakoff's psychosis) (selective amnesia for events after the onset of the illness, confabulation, and polyneuropathy).

Alcoholism is characterized by the periodic consumption of alcohol which will result in one or more of the following in a given individual: (1) psychological problems (anxiety, depression, loss of control of drinking); (2) social deterioration (decreased performance at work, disrupted family life); (3) physiologic derangement (tremors, amnesic episodes, impaired memory and coordination, alcoholic liver disease). For each alcoholic there is a different conglomerate of biological (genetic, physiologic), psychological (psychosis, character disorder, depression), and social (peer pressure, cultural background, religion) factors that predispose him to alcoholism (Kissin and Begleiter, 1977).

Elevated gamma glutamyl transpeptidase and serum glutamic oxaloacetic transaminase levels are indications of hepatic injury. However, there is no correlation between the magnitude of elevation of serum hepatic enzyme levels and degree of functional impairment or histologic changes in the liver. Only liver biopsy accurately and predictably ascertains the type and extent of liver disease.

Alcohol "dependence" may include components of acquired tolerance, habituation, and physical dependence. Tolerance may be metabolic (due to increased rate of elimination) or neurophysiologic (due to central nervous system adaptation to the presence of ethanol). Initially, both types of tolerance may be found simultaneously. Metabolic tolerance may decrease temporarily in the presence of hepatitis or permanently because of severe cirrhosis. Physical dependence is present when withholding alcohol causes subjective distress and objective signs of withdrawal. On abrupt withdrawal, acquired adaptive neurophysiologic and biochemical changes during the development of tolerance result in hypersensitivity of sensory modalities. Depending upon the degree and duration of tolerance, any or all of the following signs and symptoms are present: irritability, anxiety, insomnia, tremulousness, hyperreflexia, increased muscle tone and tremor, hallucinations, episodic amnesia or blackouts, seizures, delirium (global confusion), and arrhythmias. Withdrawal symptoms in chronic alcoholics may appear even in the presence of blood ethanol levels that would be intoxicating to a nontolerant individual. There can be considerable cross tolerance with certain general anesthetics, hypnotics, and antianxiety drugs (eg, barbiturates, benzodiazepines, meprobamate, chloral hydrate).

Drug Therapy: Treatment of excessive alcohol ingestion can be divided conveniently into three programs of management: acute intoxication, the withdrawal syndrome, and postwithdrawal long-term care.

Drug therapy for even severe acute intoxication is only adjunctive; no drugs are usually required. The essential elements of management include lavage if indicated, mechanical ventilatory support, maintenance of body temperature, and detection and correction of dehydration, acid-base abnormalities, electrolyte imbalance, and hypoglycemia.

Mild sequelae of alcohol withdrawal may be managed adequately with oral benzodiazepines initially, assuming that drug therapy is part of the management program elected. Severe symptoms and signs (delirium tremens) occur in less than 1% of patients during alcohol withdrawal (Whitfield et al, 1978). The peak response occurs about 30 to 36 hours after withdrawal; serious life-threatening signs then gradually disappear over the next 36 hours. The benzodiazepines are drugs of choice because they are at least as efficacious, are less toxic, and have superior anticonvulsant activity compared to ethanol, barbiturates, chloral hydrate, paraldehyde, hydroxyzine, antihistamines, and antipsychotic drugs. Chlordiazepoxide [Librium] and diazepam [Valium] have been used most extensively; however, because of pharmacokinetic considerations, oxazepam [Serax] and lorazepam [Ativan], which are not metabolized to active derivatives and possess relatively shorter half-lives, may be preferred in older patients or those with evidence of severe liver disease (Sellers and Kalant, 1976). Parenteral preparations of chlordiazepoxide and diazepam are available if needed, but since absorption from intramuscular sites is erratic, the intravenous route is preferred. Only lorazepam is well absorbed after intramuscular administration. Transition to oral administration can usually be initiated within 12 hours. Both diazepam and chlordiazepoxide are almost completely absorbed orally, with peak concentrations occurring about 45 minutes after ingestion (Shader and Greenblatt, 1977). For the dosages employed in alcohol withdrawal, see the evaluations in Chapter 11, Drugs Used for Anxiety and Insomnia.

A single oral or parenteral dose of thiamine (100 mg) is recommended early during treatment of withdrawal. In patients with a documented history of seizures during withdrawal, an oral or intravenous loading dose of phenytoin (600 mg) with subsequent maintenance (300 mg daily for five days) prevents recurrence.

Complicated cases may require additional therapy. Intravenous diazepam is indicated if phenytoin does not control seizures; the possibility that seizures have an etiology other than alcohol withdrawal must be ruled out by appropriate investigations. Lidocaine [Xylocaine] or procainamide [Pronestyl] may be needed for arrhythmias; propranolol [Inderal] also is useful for the latter and may be especially effective for uncontrolled, severe tremor. The potent piperazine phenothiazines (eg, fluphenazine) or the butyrophenone, haloperidol [Haldol], may be given for alcoholic hallucinosis or paranoid ideation that does not respond to a benzodiazepine.

Pharmacotherapy plays much less of a role in the long-term management of alcoholic patients than counseling of the patient and his family and a program of rehabilitation. Although the temporary administration of benzodiazepines in gradually diminishing doses during the immediate postwithdrawal period has been tried, it has not been established that such use is beneficial. The long-term effectiveness of disulfiram [Antabuse] in the prevention of alcoholism also has not been established.

Drug Interactions: Alcohol is present to varying degrees in the oral intake profile of one hundred million individuals in the United States. Numerous interactions between alcohol and other drugs have been cited. Those that occur most frequently are based upon additive central nervous system depression. In these instances, the patient should be cautioned against excessive alcohol intake and avoiding hazardous tasks, even with moderate intake. Examples include the following drugs that have considerable sedative action: opiate and opioid analgesics, hypnotic and antianxiety drugs, antihistamines, antipsychotics, tricyclic antidepressants, central skeletal muscle relaxants, centrally acting anticholinergics, anticonvulsants, and certain antihypertensive agents (reserpine, methyldopa, and clonidine).

A less common but significant additive orthostatic hypotensive interaction results from concomitant use of alcohol and drugs with vasodilator activity (eg, reserpine, methyldopa, hydralazine, guanethidine, nitroglycerin).

Metronidazole [Flagyl], furazolidone [Furoxone], and chlorpropamide [Diabinese] have been reported to produce a mild disulfiram-like action when alcohol is ingested; however, controlled studies have not substantiated this finding for metronidazole. Further, acetaldehyde blood levels were not elevated following use of alcohol and chlorpropamide. However, it has been reported (Leslie and Pyke, 1978) that flushing as a result of a chlorpropamide-ethanol interaction is a genetic marker for noninsulin-dependent diabetes even before the onset of glucose intolerance. These adverse reactions should be considered of minor significance since they are much less severe than the disulfiram-ethanol reaction.

Potentially severe interactions occur with ingestion of alcohol and the salicylates, including aspirin; antidiabetic drugs, including insulin; anticonvulsants; and anticoagulants. It is prudent to avoid alcohol when aspirin is prescribed, because of their additive effect in promoting gastrointestinal bleeding. Hypoglycemia may be a dangerous sequel when alcohol is taken with oral hypoglycemic agents or insulin, because the former interferes with their metabolism and produces hypoglycemia in its own right. Conversely, the chronic intake of alcohol can increase the metabolizing activity of enzymes and actually shorten the half-life and reduce the effectiveness of the oral hypoglycemics. Enzyme induction probably accounts for the potentially serious interactions that can occur as a result of the decrease in half-lives of anticoagulants and anticonvulsants. Accordingly, the dosage of the antidiabetic agents, anticonvulsants, and anticoagulants may require adjustment upon initiating and terminating such therapy in chronic alcoholics. Careful monitoring of the patient is essential.

INDIVIDUAL EVALUATION

DISULFIRAM
[Antabuse]

Disulfiram, a thiuram derivative, interferes with aldehyde dehydrogenase. Individuals taking this drug who then ingest alcohol show an increase in the blood acetaldehyde concentration, which produces several uncomfortable symptoms. The unpleasantness of this alcohol-disulfiram reaction is the basis for the drug's use. This reaction may present with symptoms of flushing, dyspnea, nausea, thirst, chest pain, palpitation, and vertigo and may be accompanied by the following signs: hyperventilation, tachycardia, vomiting, hyperhidrosis, hypotension, syncope, and confusion. The blood pressure may fall to a shock level. The reaction usually lasts 30 minutes to several hours. Drowsiness and sleep follow. The intensity of the reaction varies but is generally proportional to the amount of disulfiram and alcohol ingested. In severe reactions, respiratory depression, acute circulatory failure, arrhythmias, myocardial infarction, acute congestive heart failure, syncope, convulsions, and death may occur. The efficacy of disulfiram in the treatment of chronic alcoholism has not been established.

In the absence of alcohol, disulfiram may cause transient mild drowsiness, fatigability, impotence, headache, acneiform eruptions, allergic dermatitis, or a metallic- or garlic-like aftertaste during the first two weeks of therapy. These effects usually disappear spontaneously with continued therapy or reduced dosage. Psychotic reactions have been noted; in most cases, these are attributable to large doses, a drug interaction with isoniazid, or the unmasking of underlying psychosis. Polyneuropathy, peripheral neuritis, and, rarely, optic neuropathy also have occurred. It has been suggested that these reactions may be caused by carbon disulfide, a metabolite of disulfiram (Rainey, 1977).

Recent unconfirmed circumstantial evidence in five patients implicates disulfiram as a hepatotoxin (Ranek and Andreasen, 1977). There was a latent period of 3 to 25 weeks before symptoms of liver disease occurred. Disulfiram hepatotoxicity may have been unnoticed in the past because of the natural tendency to attribute any hepatic involvement to alcohol.

During severe reactions, individuals should be treated as for shock (see Chapter 37). The inhalation of a mixture of 95% oxygen and 5% carbon dioxide and other symptomatic treatment also may be useful. The serum potassium level should be monitored and maintained, particularly in patients receiving digitalis, since hypokalemia has been reported. Because effects persist for up to two weeks after termination of therapy, patients should be warned not to ingest alcohol during this period.

Disulfiram inhibits the metabolism of several drugs in addition to alcohol, and the possible consequences on concomitantly administered drugs should be borne in mind. In particular, toxic levels of phenytoin or its congeners, warfarin, diazepam, or chlordiazepoxide may accumulate when disulfiram is given concomitantly. It may be necessary to adjust the dosage of such drugs when initiating or discontinuing disulfiram therapy. Disulfiram and isoniazid should not be administered together because dizziness, ataxia, incoordination, insomnia, and irritability may develop.

Disulfiram should be used with caution in patients with diabetes mellitus, hypothyroidism, epilepsy, cerebral damage, chronic or acute nephritis, hepatic cirrhosis or insufficiency, and during pregnancy. Its use is contraindicated in patients with ischemic heart disease, coronary thrombosis, psychosis, hypersensitivity, in those recently treated with paraldehyde, and in those who have recently ingested alcohol or an alcohol-containing product (eg, foods, beverages, elixirs, cough syrups). Caution also is advised when using lotions with a high alcohol content that are liberally applied topically. Disulfiram should not be used without the patient's full knowledge and consent.

It may be advisable for those undergoing treatment with disulfiram to carry identification describing the most common symptoms of the disulfiram-alcohol reaction and designating the attending physician. (Identification cards may be obtained from the manufacturer.)

ROUTE, USUAL DOSAGE, AND PREPARATIONS. The patient must not be acutely intoxicated, withdrawing from alcohol, or have used alcohol for at least 12 hours before initiating treatment.

Oral: Adults, initially, 250 mg daily for one to two weeks. For maintenance, 250 mg daily (range, 125 to a maximum of 500 mg) is given for months to years, depending upon the individual. However, in view of potential liver toxicity and unproven efficacy, administration for more than six months at a time is not recommended. Liver enzymes should be monitored at suitable intervals during therapy.

Drug available generically: Tablets 250 and 500 mg.

Antabuse (Ayerst). Tablets 250 and 500 mg.

DEMENTIA

Mental disorders in the elderly may be caused by functional disturbances in the brain, organic brain disease, or both. Impairment of attention span, alertness, memory, cognitive functions, orientation, judgment, and affectivity are the classic signs and symptoms of organic brain syndrome, which help to distinguish it from functional mental disorders.

Chronic organic brain syndrome (senile and presenile [Alzeimer's disease] dementias) are progressive cognitive and behavioral disorders associated with specific degenerative morphologic changes in the brain (Wells, 1978). Dementia may be associated secondarily with encephalitis, trauma, tumor, parkinsonism, nutritional deficiencies, endocrine and metabolic disturbances, normal or low pressure hydrocephalus, functional psychosis, or drug intoxication (eg, alcohol, digitalis, anticholinergic drugs, hypnotics, antianxiety agents, levodopa, antihypertensive drugs that have a prominent central action). Some of these disorders may be potentially reversible with appropriate management; therefore, the physician must ascertain that such is the case before concluding that the dementia is only primary.

Drug therapy is only part of a management program for primary dementia. Psychosocial factors contribute significantly to development of symptoms; therefore, they deserve special attention by the physician. The management program should include improved care and nutrition, treatment of associated physical illness, and attention to problems resulting from impaired vision and hearing, lack of mobility, impairment of daily living activities, lack of occupation, and social isolation. These measures alone may lead to marked improvement, even in patients with significant organic involvement.

When psychotic symptoms and resulting behavioral disturbances accompany dementia, drug therapy can be especially useful. The antipsychotic drugs are used to control agitation and irritability and may clarify thought and improve self-care, cooperation, obstreperousness, and unsociability, even in markedly demented patients. Therapy should be initiated with small doses which should be increased gradually, if needed, because elderly patients are particularly susceptible to severe adverse reactions. Aliphatic and piperidine phenothiazines are used frequently, but if their sedative, hypotensive, or anticholinergic actions are a problem, haloperidol [Haldol] or a piperazine phenothiazine may be indicated. However, the incidence of extrapyramidal reactions is higher with these more potent antipsychotic drugs (see Chapter 12).

Depression is common in geriatric patients and may resemble organic brain syndrome or may be superimposed upon it. The tricyclic antidepressants may be useful in these patients but should be used very cautiously when cardiovascular disease is present.

The benzodiazepines are thought to be useful when anxiety is a primary problem, but other drugs are more appropriate if the anxiety is secondary to depression or psychotic symptoms. Some benzodiazepines may cause paradoxical excitement in elderly patients.

The need for small doses of antipsychotic, antidepressant, and antianxiety drugs in these elderly patients is emphasized. Most responsive patients obtain optimum results with total daily doses of as little as 40 to 200 mg of thioridazine, 25 to 75 mg of amitriptyline, or 2 to 5 mg of diazepam. However, some elderly individuals require essentially the same dose as younger patients; consequently, it may be necessary to increase the dosage cautiously beyond what is adequate for many elderly patients. Because of the increased danger of cumulative toxicity caused by long-acting benzodiazepines in the elderly, it is preferable to prescribe short-acting agents without active metabolites, such as oxazepam [Serax] or lorazepam [Ativan] (see Chapter 11, Drugs Used for Anxiety and Insomnia).

Most studies with cerebral vasodilators have focused on their use in arteriosclerosis, although this condition probably occurs in less than 15% of patients with chronic organic brain syndromes. The presumption is that these vasodilators (papaverine, cyclandelate [Cyclospasmol], and isoxsuprine [Vasodilan]) reduce cerebral vascular resistance and thus improve cerebral blood flow and oxygen supply. However, it is unlikely that dilatation occurs in sclerotic vessels, and there is no evidence that vasodilators prevent progression of arteriosclerotic or organic brain disease or reverse the pathologic process. Furthermore, the vasodilators used to date are not sufficiently specific for cerebral vessels; generalized vasodilatation could actually shunt blood away from involved areas and thus offset their action in the brain. Lastly, cerebral blood flow appears to be adequate in most patients with primary dementia.

Although originally introduced and classified as cerebral vasodilators, the mixture of dihydrogenated ergot alkaloids [Deapril-ST, Hydergine] may have an action on cerebral metabolism as well. Other drugs presumed to exert an effect on cerebral metabolism (naftidrofuryl [Praxilene], hexamethylxanthine [Cosaldron], and pentoxifylline [Trental]) are under investigation in Europe, but it has not yet been established that their actions alter primary dementia. It is extremely difficult to determine if a drug is more effective than a placebo in this type of clinical investigation. Even well-controlled, double-blind, crossover studies are fraught with problems concerning patient selection, monitoring, interpretation, and separation of drug effects from other causative factors in the management of these patients (Caplan, 1977; Yesavage et al, 1979).

In carefully controlled studies carried out for three to six months, the dihydrogenated ergot alkaloids were reported to produce modest improvement of confusion, depression, dizziness, unsociability, and self-care; however, it is difficult to predict which patients will benefit. Positive drug effects were judged better on subjective rating scales than on objective tests of intellectual function and performance, such as those used to determine IQ. A trial course of therapy with this mixture may be indicated in patients with accurately diagnosed primary dementia who are receiving the best nondrug management program possible but who still have clinically significant mental impairment (Gaitz et al, 1977).

The ability of drugs to alter central neurotransmitter metabolism is receiving considerable attention in view of the success of this type of treatment in functional psychoses. The cholinergic system is being investigated most intensively because of the amnesia produced by the centrally acting anticholinergic drug, scopolamine, and the short-term effect of physostigmine [Antilirium] in alleviating memory loss in patients who have suffered central nervous system trauma. However, there may be little relation between these amnesic syndromes and the amnesia of primary dementia. The results achieved in patients with primary dementia who received oral doses of choline are encouraging, but a therapeutic trial is not justified in all patients (Davis and Yamamura, 1978; Yesavage and Hollister, 1978; Ferris et al, 1979). Choline has produced depression in some elderly individuals who received the drug for tardive dyskinesia (see Chapter 16, Drugs Used in Extrapyramidal Movement Disorders).

Hyperbaric oxygen, pentylenetetrazol, and Gerovital H-3 (procaine, benzoic acid, inorganic sodium and potassium salts) have been abandoned by most physicians for the treatment of dementia.

INDIVIDUAL EVALUATION

DIHYDROGENATED ERGOT ALKALOIDS
[Deapril-ST, Hydergine]

This combination of three dihydro de-rivatives of ergot alkaloids is labeled for treatment of "selected symptoms" in the elderly. The dihydrogenated ergot al-kaloids act centrally to reduce vascular tone and slow the heart rate and peripher-ally to block alpha receptors. They lack the marked vasoconstrictor properties of the natural ergot alkaloids. Absorption occurs rapidly, but only 50% of a therapeutic dose gains access to the systemic circulation because of a pronounced first-pass bio-transformation by the liver.

In several short-term studies, this com-bination was judged to be superior to a placebo or papaverine in relieving various mild symptoms attributed to cerebral ar-teriosclerosis (eg, depression, anxiety, un-sociability, confusion). This action is not considered to be due to specific direct cerebrovascular dilatation; instead, an ac-tion on cerebral metabolism is suggested. Recent controlled studies over a 12- to 24-week period suggest that there is mod-est improvement in the cognitive and emo-tional symptoms of nursing home residents (Gaitz et al, 1977).

Adverse reactions include sublingual ir-ritation and transient nausea, vomiting, and gastric disturbances. Sinus bradycardia has occurred rarely.

ROUTES, USUAL DOSAGE, AND PREPARATIONS. The place of this mixture in the therapy of senile dementia has not been established. The manufacturers' suggested dosage is: *Sublingual, Oral: Adults*, 1 mg three times daily.

>Drug available generically: Tablets (oral, sub-lingual) 0.5 and 1 mg.
>*Deapril-ST* (Mead Johnson). Each 1 mg tablet (sublingual) contains dihydroergocornine 0.33 mg, dihydroergocristine 0.33 mg, and dihydro-ergocryptine 0.33 mg as the mesylates.
>*Hydergine* (Sandoz). Each 0.5 mg tablet (sub-lingual) contains dihydroergocornine 0.167 mg, dihydroergocristine 0.167 mg, and dihydroer-gocryptine 0.167 mg as the mesylates; each 1 mg tablet (oral, sublingual) contains dihydroer-gocornine 0.333 mg, dihydroergocristine 0.333

mg, and dihydroergocryptine 0.333 as the mesylates (2:1 ratio of alpha and beta forms).

INDICATIONS FOR CENTRAL NERVOUS SYSTEM STIMULANTS

Hyperkinetic Syndrome: Children with this disorder are of near average, average, or above average general intelligence but have mild to severe behavioral disabilities associated with central nervous system dysfunction. Approximately one-third of these children have learning disabilities. Signs and symptoms include short atten-tion span, distractability, purposeless hyperactivity, impulsiveness, and impaired coordination, perception, and learning. Hyperactivity, short attention span, and impairment of learning are the key diag-nostic features. The prominence of these signs in any individual patient varies con-siderably, and this variation is reflected in the recently suggested revisions in nomenclature of the subclassifications of this disorder (eg, attention deficit disorder with hyperkinesis, hyperkinetic syndrome with learning disorder). The older termi-nology of minimal brain dysfunction or damage is not preferred, because there is considerable variation in symptomatology and organic lesions in the brain generally are not demonstrable. Since there are no objective criteria, diagnosis must be sub-jective and assessment of performance in school may be crucial. Accurate diagnosis is essential for appropriate management. Some authorities believe that the hyper-kinetic syndrome is overdiagnosed and many children are given stimulant drugs without justification (Werry, 1976).

A substantial number of controlled studies utilizing both subjective and objec-tive criteria to judge response indicate that central nervous system stimulants are of benefit over a two-year period in children with hyperkinetic syndrome when they are used as adjuncts to remedial education and counseling on behavioral modification with the parents and child's teachers (Wolraich, 1977). Dextroamphetamine [Dexedrine], methylphenidate [Ritalin], and pemoline

[Cylert] appear to be the most effective drugs; levamfetamine also has been reported to be useful. Although some investigators feel that methylphenidate is the drug of choice, others believe that dextroamphetamine is equally effective. Pemoline is not considered a drug of first choice, because it is less effective than methylphenidate and dextroamphetamine.

The proposed pharmacologic action of these drugs was based on their paradoxical calming effect in children with hyperkinetic syndrome, but it has been shown recently that normal children are affected similarly. There is speculation that a central monoaminergic dysfunction is involved in this disorder, but no firm supporting evidence is available. Although these drugs decrease hyperactivity and prolong attention span, which are thought to improve short-term learning, there are no data which conclusively demonstrate that these drugs alter sustained learning. Long-term follow-up studies indicate that these children may continue to have difficulty in school, behavioral disorders, and a poor self-concept well into adolescence. Drug therapy is not definitive and remains only one component of a program that must include counseling and guidance.

The prolonged use of dextroamphetamine, methylphenidate, and pemoline may limit linear growth and weight, presumably as a result of appetite suppression, decreased food intake, and altered secretion of growth hormone. Therefore, weight gain and linear growth must be monitored closely. A recently completed two-year study showed that methylphenidate had only a slight depressant effect on linear growth in the first year of therapy, which was offset by a greater than expected growth rate in the second year (Satterfield et al, 1979). It was also reported that total dosage and summer drug holidays may influence weight but not height deficits; the use of optimum doses that reduce hyperactivity without suppressing weight is encouraged. Pemoline also depressed longitudinal growth more in the first than the second year of therapy; however, this action was correlated with total

drug dosage in another two-year study (Dickinson et al, 1979).

Deanol [Deaner] was shown to be superior to a placebo but no more effective than the central nervous system stimulants in the hyperkinetic syndrome when single daily doses of 300 to 500 mg were given for two to three weeks, followed by maintenance doses of 100 to 300 mg daily. These findings were not confirmed in other studies.

Antipsychotic and tricyclic drugs are used by some physicians to treat hyperkinetic syndrome. This use should be considered only as investigational alternative therapy in patients who cannot tolerate or do not respond to dextroamphetamine, methylphenidate, and pemoline. Their potential side effects and adverse reactions are much more severe than those of the central nervous system stimulants, and children given these drugs should be monitored closely.

Narcolepsy: The classical diagnostic tetrad of primary symptoms of this sleep disorder (Dement et al, 1976; Parkes, 1977) is: (1) excessive daytime sleepiness with a definite history of falling asleep episodically, rapidly, and often inappropriately while performing a daily task; (2) episodic, cataplectic attacks of muscular weakness precipitated by emotional stimulation (ie, humor, anger, fear, surprise); (3) hypnagogic hallucinations, which may be visual, auditory, or tactile, occurring during the transition from wakefulness to a sleep stage; and (4) sleep paralysis characterized by consciousness and inability to move or cry out also occurring during the transition from wakefulness to a sleep stage. Common secondary signs and symptoms include automatic behavior similar to epileptic absence attacks with complete retrograde amnesia, as well as disturbed nocturnal sleep characterized by frequent awakenings. A polysomnograph showing a transition from wakefulness directly into REM rather than NREM sleep helps to confirm the diagnosis.

Narcolepsy rarely appears after age 40. The most common age of onset is between 15 and 25 years. The disease generally persists for the life of the individual, although some adaptation occurs. Narcolepsy constitutes about 60% of all excessive sleep disorders, and it must be distinguished from sleep apnea, which constitutes about 20% to 25% of these disorders.

Intensive psychological counseling, a schedule of short daytime naps, and pharmacotherapy appear to be most beneficial in the management of narcolepsy, although no controlled studies are available. Methylphenidate, alone or with imipramine, is the principal drug employed. The amphetamines appear to be as effective as methylphenidate. An average daily dose of 20 mg of methylphenidate controls sleepiness but, if cataplexy is severe, imipramine should be added. Initial doses of the latter drug should be small and increased gradually to a total of 100 to 150 mg daily to control the cataplexy as well as the sleep paralysis and hypnagogic hallucinations if these symptoms are also present. The antinarcoleptic action of imipramine is immediate, unlike its antidepressant action. Tolerance develops to both methylphenidate and imipramine; this problem is best obviated by periodic drug holidays, followed by reinstitution of therapy at a lower dose. In one uncontrolled study, the less sedative tricyclic compound, protriptyline [Vivactil], given in a single dose (10 to 20 mg) at bedtime, was considered to be better than imipramine (Schmidt et al, 1977).

It has been reported recently (Kales et al, 1979) that a patient with narcolepsy, which was refractory to treatment with methylphenidate, responded well to propranolol.

Miscellaneous Uses: The amphetamines have been employed in the following disorders.

Dextroamphetamine is helpful in the management of selected patients with petit mal or absence epilepsy to alleviate drowsiness if large doses of phenobarbital or other anticonvulsant sedatives are required. See Chapter 15, Anticonvulsants.

Although amphetamines are effective temporarily in producing slightly more weight loss than control groups, the long-term benefit is clinically insignificant because of the development of tolerance; the potential for abuse is considerable. For these reasons, alternative management programs, preferably nondrug, are strongly recommended and the use of amphetamines is strongly discouraged. See Chapter 56, Agents Used in Obesity.

Concomitant use of scopolamine and dextroamphetamine is effective in severe motion sickness, but such use is not recommended in the management of routine motion sickness. In addition, scopolamine and ephedrine or promethazine and ephedrine are nearly as effective in the management of severe motion sickness. (See Chapter 26, Drugs Used in Vertigo, Motion Sickness, and Vomiting.)

Idiopathic edema occurs almost exclusively in women, and it is diagnosed by exclusion (Streeten, 1978). Most patients experience diurnal fluctuations in the severity of the edema, which is aggravated by prolonged standing and sitting. Dextroamphetamine and methylphenidate have been used experimentally as part of a total management program that also includes diuretic therapy (see Chapter 39), reduction of excessive salt intake, and avoidance of prolonged standing and sitting. Many authorities feel that the use of these drugs for idiopathic edema is entirely inappropriate, because these patients overuse diuretics for psychogenic reasons and may represent a population of potential amphetamine drug abusers (MacGregor et al, 1979).

Short-term use of small doses of dextroamphetamine is recommended by a few physicians (1) for patients with reactive depressions who cannot tolerate other antidepressants (usually the elderly), and (2) in difficult diagnostic situations to determine the probable efficacy of tricyclic drugs. Neither indication is supported by controlled studies. See Chapter 13, Drugs Used in Affective Disorders.

In one controlled study, dextroamphetamine was shown to potentiate morphine analgesia in the treatment of postoperative pain (Forrest et al, 1977). More studies are needed to determine the clinical relevance of this finding.

The use of amphetamines or other stimulants to allay fatigue is unjustifiable except under the most extraordinary circumstances. They are dangerous for drivers and those engaged in comparable activities, and they have no legitimate role in athletics. Indeed, their use may contribute to increased athletic injuries.

INDIVIDUAL EVALUATIONS

DEXTROAMPHETAMINE SULFATE
[Dexedrine]

$$\left[\bigcirc - CH_2 - \overset{\overset{H}{|}}{\underset{\underset{+NH_3}{|}}{C}} - CH_3 \right]_2 SO_4^=$$

Dextroamphetamine is useful primarily in the management of hyperkinetic syndrome and narcolepsy (see the Introduction for miscellaneous uses). All amphetamines are classified as Schedule II drugs under the Controlled Substances Act. Dextroamphetamine is generally preferred over the racemic mixture, amphetamine, because it has less effect on the cardiovascular system.

The amphetamines are well absorbed orally, are not highly bound to protein, and are largely excreted by the kidney. Their half-lives range from 7 to 14 hours (10 ± 1.7 hours) if the urine is acid; however, this may be extended to 30 hours if the urine is alkaline.

ADVERSE REACTIONS AND PRECAUTIONS.

The untoward effects produced by the amphetamines are related to their spectrum of pharmacologic actions, particularly their sympathomimetic effects; thus, these agents may cause nervousness, restlessness, tremors, insomnia, cardiovascular disturbances (eg, tachycardia, arrhythmias, hypertension), dizziness, mydriasis, dryness of the mouth, and gastrointestinal disturbances such as nausea, constipation, and, occasionally, diarrhea. Anorexia and growth retardation have been observed in children. Dosage should not be increased unnecessarily, because larger amounts may produce marked restlessness, irritability, and aggressiveness.

More serious reactions affecting the central nervous system occur rarely and include psychic changes and dystonic movements of the head, neck, and extremities. Serious depressive reactions and toxic psychoses have followed the prolonged use, especially of large doses, of dextroamphetamine.

Generally, the amphetamines should not be prescribed for patients with cardiovascular disease or hyperthyroidism because their sympathomimetic effect may aggravate these conditions. They also should not be given to those known to be susceptible to drug abuse. These drugs should be used with caution in patients who are sensitive to adrenergic agents.

Evidence of teratogenicity has not been observed clinically when amphetamines were taken during pregnancy, although an infant born to a mother who abuses amphetamines may be agitated and have hyperglycemia at birth (see Chapter 2).

Tolerance is a major problem when large doses are administered daily over long periods (eg, in narcolepsy). Occasional drug holidays or withholding therapy during nonworking periods will allow the narcoleptic patient to regain sensitivity to the drug and allow the physician to decrease dosage when therapy is reinstituted.

POISONING.

In general, acute overdosage accentuates the usual pharmacologic effects of excitement, agitation, hypertension, tachycardia, mydriasis, slurred speech, ataxia, tremor, chills, hyperreflexia, tachypnea, fever, headache, and toxic psychoses characterized by auditory and visual hallucinations and paranoid delusions. If these symptoms develop, lavage, sedatives, custodial care, and psychotherapy should be employed when indicated. Excretion can be hastened by acidification of the urine. In severe cases, overdosage may cause hyperpyrexia, chest pain, acute circulatory failure, convulsions, and coma. Chlorpromazine may block the central nervous system effects, but will not block similar signs and symptoms produced by anticholinergic drugs if these have been taken concurrently. Fatalities have occurred in adults after doses of only 100 to 500 mg.

ABUSE.

Susceptible patients may develop marked psychic dependence on amphetamines. Individuals who abuse these drugs frequently inject as much as several grams daily (parenteral commercial products of the amphetamines are not available). In general, the toxic features of chronic abuse include a distinctive amphetamine psychosis characterized by paranoia, stereotyped behavior, picking at the skin, preoccupation with one's own thoughts, and auditory and visual hallucinations.

Reactions occurring after abrupt termination of large doses of amphetamines can mimic symptoms of schizophrenia and may unmask symptoms of chronic fatigue (mental depression, paranoid psychosis, tremors, and gastrointestinal disturbances); in some individuals, the fatigue may be followed by drowsiness and prolonged sleep. Such reactions are considered by many to be a type of abstinence syndrome.

INTERACTIONS.

Amphetamines interfere with the hypotensive effect of guanethidine, and animal studies indicate that they have a similar effect when given with methyldopa. Therefore, they should not be used with these drugs. Amphetamines also are contraindicated in patients receiving monoamine oxidase inhibitors because their use may precipitate a hypertensive crisis. Although the amphetamines are resistant to the action of monoamine oxidase, their actions are potentiated by the monoamine oxidase inhibitors, presumably as a result of the release of biogenic amines. They may initiate arrhythmias through their catecholamine-releasing effect in patients receiving epinephrine-sensitizing anesthetics. Amphetamines and methylphenidate can increase blood levels of the tricyclic antidepressants by interfering with their metabolism. Antipsychotic drugs antagonize most of the central nervous system actions of the amphetamines.

ROUTE, USUAL DOSAGE, AND PREPARATIONS.
Oral: For hyperkinetic syndrome, *children 3 to 5 years*, 2.5 mg daily initially, increased by increments of 2.5 mg at weekly intervals until an optimum response is obtained; *6 years and older*, 5 mg once or twice daily initially, increased by increments of 5 mg daily at weekly intervals until an optimum response is obtained. The effective dosage range is 5 to 20 mg daily (maximum, 40 mg daily).

For narcolepsy, *adults and children over 6 years*, 5 to 60 mg daily in divided doses, depending upon the patient's requirements.

For obesity, see Chapter 56.

> Drug available generically: Capsules 10 and 15 mg; capsules (timed-release) 15 mg; tablets 5 and 10 mg.
> *Dexedrine* (Smith Kline & French). Capsules (timed-release) 5, 10, and 15 mg; elixir 5 mg/5 ml (alcohol 10%); tablets 5 mg.
> Additional Salts and Trademarks.
> Dextroamphetamine Sulfate: *Diphylets*, *Diphylets-T* (Tutag), *Dexampex* (Lemmon).
> Dextroamphetamine Tannate: *Obotan* (Mallinckrodt).

AMPHETAMINE SULFATE
[Benzedrine]

This drug is the racemic form of amphetamine. Because it has less central nervous system activity and a more pronounced effect on the cardiovascular system than the dextrorotatory isomer, the latter is preferred.

See the Introduction to this section and the evaluation on Dextroamphetamine Sulfate for information on adverse reactions and precautions. Amphetamine is classified as a Schedule II drug under the Controlled Substances Act.

ROUTE, USUAL DOSAGE, AND PREPARATIONS.
Oral: The manufacturers' suggested dosage is: For hyperkinetic syndrome, *children 3 to 5 years*, 2.5 mg daily initially, increased by increments of 2.5 mg at weekly intervals until an optimum response is obtained; *6 years and older*, 5 mg once or twice daily initially, increased by increments of 5 mg daily at weekly intervals until an optimum response is obtained.

The effective dosage range is 5 to 20 mg daily (maximum 40 mg daily).

For narcolepsy, *adults and children over 6 years*, 5 to 60 mg daily in divided doses depending upon the patient's requirements.

For obesity, see Chapter 56.

> Drug available generically: Tablets 5 and 10 mg.
> *Benzedrine* (Smith Kline & French). Capsules (timed-release) 15 mg; tablets 5 and 10 mg.

METHAMPHETAMINE HYDROCHLORIDE
[Desoxyn]

Methamphetamine is essentially equivalent to dextroamphetamine in its effect on the central nervous and cardiovascular systems.

The drug has been extensively abused. Large doses can produce psychic and, rarely, physical dependence. It is classified as a Schedule II drug under the Controlled Substances Act. See the Introduction to this section and the evaluation on Dextroamphetamine Sulfate for additional information on adverse reactions and precautions.

ROUTE, USUAL DOSAGE, AND PREPARATIONS.
Oral: For hyperkinetic syndrome, *children over 6 years*, 2.5 to 5 mg once or twice daily initially, increased by increments of 5 mg at weekly intervals until an optimum response is obtained. The usual effective dose is 20 to 25 mg daily.

For obesity, see Chapter 56.

> Drug available generically under the name Desoxyephedrine Hydrochloride: Tablets 10 mg.
> *Desoxyn* (Abbott). Tablets 2.5 and 5 mg; tablets (timed-release) 5, 10, and 15 mg.

METHYLPHENIDATE HYDROCHLORIDE
[Ritalin]

This agent is useful as an adjunct to other remedial measures (psychological, educational, or social) in the management of children with the hyperkinetic syndrome; improvement has been sustained for a period of at least two years as judged by subjective criteria. The drug also may be useful in the treatment of narcolepsy (see the Introduction to this section).

The most common adverse reactions are nervousness, insomnia, and anorexia. Weight loss and growth retardation may occur during prolonged therapy. Occasional reactions include dizziness, dyskinesia, rash, nausea, abdominal pain, hypertension, hypotension, palpitation, changes in the pulse rate, tachycardia, arrhythmias, and headache. Toxic psychosis has been reported rarely. Psychic dependence has occurred after long-term use of large doses. Methylphenidate has been used as a substitute for amphetamines by individuals who abuse drugs. It is classified as a Schedule II drug under the Controlled Substances Act.

This drug is contraindicated in patients with marked anxiety, tension, and agitation and should be used cautiously in epileptic and hypertensive patients or in those taking vasopressors or monoamine oxidase inhibitors. Methylphenidate should be discontinued if seizures occur.

Methylphenidate may potentiate the toxicity of phenytoin and primidone in children. Concurrent administration of a tricyclic antidepressant and methylphenidate may increase the serum level of the former. It may decrease the hypotensive effect of guanethidine. Therefore, the dosage of these agents should be adjusted when they are given with methylphenidate.

ROUTE, USUAL DOSAGE, AND PREPARATIONS.
Oral: For narcolepsy, *adults*, 10 mg two or three times daily (range, 10 to 60 mg daily). For hyperkinetic syndrome, *children 6 years and older*, initially, 5 mg twice daily (before breakfast and lunch); this dose may be gradually increased by increments of 5 or 10 mg at weekly intervals. The usual effective dosage range is 0.3 to 0.5 mg/kg of body weight daily, which represents 10 to 20 mg daily for the average child. The

maximum daily dose is 2 mg/kg or a total of 60 mg. If improvement is not observed after one month of therapy, the drug should be discontinued.

Drug available generically: Tablets 10 mg.
Ritalin (Ciba). Tablets 5, 10, and 20 mg.

PEMOLINE
[Cylert]

This central nervous system stimulant is an oxazolidine. It is indicated as an adjunct in the management program of children with hyperkinetic syndrome. In controlled clinical studies, it improved the condition of hyperkinetic children as judged by physicians, parents, and teachers and by the results of psychological test scores. Pemoline is well absorbed orally, has a half-life of approximately 12 hours, and is excreted principally by the kidney.

In comparative studies, results were similar with pemoline, amphetamines, and methylphenidate, except that the latter drug was statistically superior in some measurements of improvement. The beneficial effects occurred more rapidly with the other stimulants than with pemoline. However, pemoline was administered once daily while the other drugs were given twice daily. As with methylphenidate or dextroamphetamine, the subjective improvement was sustained over a period of two years.

The activity of pemoline in combating depression and fatigue and enhancing performance has been studied, but its effectiveness in these conditions has not been demonstrated.

The most common adverse effects of pemoline are insomnia and anorexia. Insomnia may be transient or it may be severe enough to necessitate adjustment of dosage. Anorexia may result in weight loss, particularly during the early weeks of therapy, but weight gain after approximately three to six months of continued therapy and the weight curve approximate normal. A decrease in expected linear growth has been reported after long-term use (see the Introduction). Onset of puberty was not delayed in the limited number of patients studied to determine this effect.

Other adverse reactions reported infrequently include dizziness, drowsiness, headache, depression, hallucinations, rash, nausea, and gastrointestinal distress. No clinically significant sympathomimetic effects (increased pulse rate or blood pressure) were observed with pemoline. Elevated transaminase levels occurred in a few patients and jaundice has been reported. The enzyme levels returned to normal when the drug was discontinued. This appears to be a hypersensitivity reaction, and it is advisable to determine transaminase levels periodically during therapy. No significant hematologic effects or changes in blood urea nitrogen, uric acid, or bilirubin values were observed in long-term studies.

Although no potential for abuse was found in studies on primates, psychotic symptoms have been reported in adults who misused the drug. Because pemoline has properties similar to other central nervous system stimulants with a potential for abuse, it is classified as a Schedule IV drug.

ROUTE, USUAL DOSAGE, AND PREPARATIONS. *Oral*: For the hyperkinetic syndrome, *children over 6 years*, initially, 37.5 mg daily as a single dose in the morning. The dosage is increased by increments of 18.75 mg at one-week intervals until the desired response is observed. The usual effective range is 56.25 to 75 mg daily (maximum, 112.5 mg daily). Improvement is gradual and may not be observed for three to four weeks.

Cylert (Abbott). Tablets 18.75, 37.5, and 75 mg; tablets (chewable) 37.5 mg.

Selected References

Caplan LR: Drug therapy reviews: Vasodilating drugs and their use in cerebral symptomatology. *Am J Hosp Pharm* 34:1075-1079, 1977.

Clarren SK, Smith DW: Fetal alcohol syndrome. *N Engl J Med* 298:1063-1067, 1978.

Davis KL, Yamamura HI: Cholinergic underactivity in human memory disorders. *Life Sci* 23:1729-1734, 1978.

Dement WC, et al: Narcolepsy: Diagnosis and treatment. *Primary Care* 3:609-623, 1976.

Dickinson LC, et al: Impaired growth in hyperkinetic children receiving pemoline. *J Pediatr* 94:538-541, 1979.

Ferris SH, et al: Long-term choline treatment of memory-impaired elderly patients. *Science* 205:1039-1040, 1979.

Forrest WH Jr, et al: Dextroamphetamine with morphine for treatment of postoperative pain. *N Engl J Med* 296:712-715, 1977.

Gaitz CM, et al: Pharmacotherapy for organic brain syndrome in late life: Evaluation of an ergot derivative vs placebo. *Arch Gen Psychiatry* 34:836-845, 1977.

Kales A, et al: Successful treatment of narcolepsy with propranolol: Case report. *Arch Neurol* 36:650-651, 1979.

Kallas P, Sellers EM: Blood glucose in intoxicated chronic alcoholics *Can Med Assoc J* 112:590-592, 1975.

Kissin B, Begleiter H (eds): *The Biology of Alcoholism, Vol 5: Treatment and Rehabilitation of the Chronic Alcoholic*. New York, Plenum Press, 1977.

Leslie RDG, Pyke DA: Chlorpropamide-alcohol flushing: Dominantly inherited trait associated with diabetes. *Br Med J* 2:1519-1521, 1978.

Lieber CS: Metabolism of alcohol. *Sci Amer* 234:26-33, 1976.

Lieber CS, et al: Effects of ethanol on lipid, uric acid, intermediary and drug metabolism, including pathogenesis of alcoholic fatty liver, in Kissin B, Begleiter H (eds): *The Biology of Alcoholism, Vol 1: Biochemistry*. New York, Plenum Press, 1971, 263-305.

MacGregor GA, et al: Is "idiopathic" oedema idiopathic? *Lancet* 1:397-400, 1979.

Nikkilä EA, Taskinen MR: Ethanol-induced alterations of glucose tolerance, postglucose hypoglycemia, and insulin secretion in normal, obese, and diabetic subjects. *Diabetes* 24:933-934, 1975.

Parkes JD: The sleepy patient. *Lancet* 1:990-993, 1977.

Rainey JM Jr: Disulfiram toxicity and carbon disulfide poisoning. *Am J Psychiatry* 134:371-378, 1977.

Ranek L, Andreasen PB: Disulfiram hepatotoxicity. *Br Med J* 2:94-96, 1977.

Satterfield JH, et al: Growth of hyperactive children treated with methylphenidate. *Arch Gen Psychiatry* 36:212-217, 1979.

Schmidt HS, et al: Protriptyline: Effective agent in treatment of narcolepsy-cataplexy syndrome and hypersomnia. *Am J Psychiatry* 134: 183-185, 1977.

Sellers EM, Kalant H: Alcohol intoxication and withdrawal. *N Engl J Med* 294:757-762, 1976.

Shader RI, Greenblatt DJ: Clinical implications of benzodiazepine pharmacokinetics. *Am J Psychiatry* 134:652-656, 1977.

Streeten DHP: Idiopathic edema: Pathogenesis, clinical features, and treatment. *Metabolism* 27:353-383, 1978.

Wells CE: Chronic brain disease: Overview. *Am J Psychiatry* 135:1-12, 1978.

Werry JS: Medication for hyperkinetic children. *Drugs* 11:81-89, 1976.

Whitfield CL, et al: Detoxification of 1,024 alcoholic patients without psychoactive drugs. *JAMA* 239:1409-1410, 1978.

Wolraich ML: Stimulant drug therapy in hyperactive children: Research and clinical implications. *Pediatrics* 60:512-518, 1977.

Yesavage JA, Hollister LE: Treatment of senile dementia. *Ration Drug Ther* 12:1-6, (Aug) 1978.

Yesavage JA, et al: Vasodilators in senile dementias: Review of literature. *Arch Gen Psychiatry* 36:220-223, 1979.

Anticonvulsants | 15

Convulsions (seizures) are manifestations of a focal or generalized disturbance of the brain. They may be associated with various conditions such as infections, neoplasms, congenital defects or trauma of the central nervous system, fever, metabolic disturbances, anaphylaxis, poisoning, and withdrawal of certain drugs. In most acute conditions, the seizures are transient and do not recur and treatment is directed primarily at the underlying cause. The most common of the convulsive disorders are the epilepsies; these are characterized by a recurrent seizure pattern in which there is a sudden loss or disturbance of consciousness, sometimes in association with motor activity, sensory phenomena, or inappropriate behavior. The exact number of epileptic patients is not known but it has been estimated that approximately 1% of the population has this disorder. Except for those with cerebrovascular disease, probably more individuals have epilepsy than any other serious neurologic disorder.

The current International Classification of Epileptic Seizures divides these central nervous system disorders into four broad groups:

A. *Partial seizures* (focal seizures, seizures beginning locally).

1. Partial seizures with elementary symptomatology (usually consciousness is not impaired), also called cortical focal seizures. These include seizures with motor symptoms (eg, Jacksonian motor epilepsy), special sensory or somatosensory symptoms (eg, Jacksonian sensory epilepsy), autonomic symptoms (sometimes designated nonconvulsive epileptic equivalents), and compound forms.

2. Partial seizures with complex symptomatology (usually consciousness is impaired), also called temporal lobe or psychomotor epilepsy. These seizures are

characterized by confused behavior and a bizarre electroencephalogram.

3. Partial seizures secondarily generalized.

B. *Generalized seizures* (bilateral, symmetrical).

1. Absences (abrupt, brief loss of consciousness), also called petit mal. These seizures are characterized by a blank stare and a three-per-second spike and wave pattern electroencephalogram. There may be clonic movements that vary from simple blinking of the eyelids to violent jerking of the entire body, changes in postural tone, or automatisms.

2. Bilateral massive epileptic myoclonus (usually consciousness is not altered). Isolated clonic jerks and brief bursts of multiple spikes in the electroencephalogram are observed.

3. Infantile spasms (consciousness is lost). This condition is characterized by muscle spasms, a bizarre electroencephalogram, and mental deterioration.

4. Clonic seizures (consciousness is lost). In children, these seizures cause rhythmic contraction of muscle masses with a marked autonomic component.

5. Tonic seizures (consciousness is lost). In children, these seizures cause opisthotonus and marked autonomic manifestations.

6. Tonic-clonic seizures (consciousness is lost), also called grand mal. These seizures are characterized by massive cerebral discharge and contraction of all skeletal muscle masses in a rhythmic tonic-clonic pattern, followed by depression of all central functions.

7. Atonic seizures (consciousness may be lost). These seizures cause a loss of postural tone accompanied by sagging of the head or falling down.

8. Akinetic seizures (consciousness is lost). These seizures produce a complete relaxation of all musculature.

C. *Unilateral seizures* (or seizures that are predominantly unilateral).

D. *Unclassified epileptic seizures* (seizures unclassifiable because of incomplete data).

Aberrant types of seizures may occur, but most epilepsies can be classified in this manner. Categorization according to the older terms, major and minor epilepsy, often led to confusion and was not useful for therapy, since more specific diagnosis was necessary. Epilepsy also may be classified etiologically as idiopathic or symptomatic, the latter implying that a cause has been determined. Most idiopathic epilepsies begin during childhood or adolescence. Epilepsy occurring in infancy usually results from developmental defects, metabolic disease, or birth injury, and epilepsy beginning in adulthood usually is caused by trauma, stroke, tumors, or other recognizable brain disease. Causes for obscure seizures should be sought, since specific underlying illness or focal cerebral lesion may be amenable to definitive treatment.

Drug Therapy

General Principles: The objective of drug therapy is to control seizures as completely as possible without causing intolerable adverse reactions. Since the response to anticonvulsant drugs corresponds most closely to the clinical pattern of seizures, accurate diagnosis and classification are necessary to select the most appropriate agent for each patient.

Anticonvulsant therapy must be individualized; the appropriate dosage of a drug or combination of drugs depends upon the size, age, and condition of the patient, response to treatment, and interactions between concomitantly administered medication. The dose for children is usually somewhat larger on a weight basis than that for adults. The patient should be given a single drug initially in doses within the therapeutic range, with the amount increased gradually until seizures are controlled or until symptoms of overdosage or toxicity make further increases inadvisable. If untoward effects occur, the dose should be reduced to the tolerated level. If serious adverse reactions develop or the frequency of seizures is not reduced, another drug should be substituted. When the initial drug reduces the frequency of seizures but does not provide adequate control, another agent (preferably from a different chemical class) should be added to the .egimen. Any alteration in therapy (substitution or addition) should be made gradually and the effectiveness judged over a long period of time. Medication should not be stopped abruptly. Patients should be warned of the dangers of discontinuing any medication and also should be informed of possible adverse reactions and of the necessity of reporting their occurrence to the physician.

Perhaps the largest number of treatment failures results from noncompliance with the prescribed regimen. It is, therefore, important for the patient to understand and accept his disorder. It is also important for the physician to appreciate the social, psychological, and economic needs of the patient, which may require a multidisciplinary approach. Patient visits should be scheduled regularly in order to evaluate the efficacy and any adverse reactions of medication, to measure drug blood levels when indicated, and to adjust the dosage if necessary.

Because there is a complex relationship between the dose of an anticonvulsant and its plasma level (hence, its therapeutic effects), determination of drug plasma levels may be helpful as a guide to therapeutic and untoward effects. This is particularly useful during the initial adjustment of dosage and to determine patient compliance, if necessary. The usual therapeutic ranges have been determined for most anticonvulsants; however, values vary among different clinics and laboratories, as well as among patients.

Results of some studies have shown that the number of seizures is markedly reduced in most patients when only one drug is given in amounts sufficient to produce usual therapeutic blood levels. A few patients may be controlled with lower levels, while others may not obtain adequate control even with maximally tolerated levels; the latter may benefit from the addition of a second drug.

Epileptic seizures that initially respond to drug therapy sometimes escape from control. When a barbiturate or hydantoin has been used, escape may be due to induction of liver enzymes that increases the rate of metabolism of the drug. This is usually reflected by a decrease in drug concentration in serum, and increasing the dose in such cases re-establishes and maintains control unless the disease itself worsens.

Trauma or emotional stress may increase the dosage requirement. This should particularly be borne in mind if the patient must undergo surgery.

Unless a progressive underlying disease is involved, spontaneous remissions may occur, especially with idiopathic forms that usually begin during childhood. The great majority of absence seizures (petit mal) are limited to childhood. Accordingly, the eventual discontinuation of an anticonvulsant regimen should be considered. When a decision is made to discontinue therapy, the dose of one drug at a time should be reduced very gradually, since sudden withdrawal of any of these agents may precipitate a recurrence of seizures and is one of the most common causes of status epilepticus. Only when a serious adverse reaction occurs should a drug be discontinued abruptly, and another anticonvulsant should be substituted promptly to protect the patient.

Drugs for Various Seizure Types: In general, drugs that are effective in generalized tonic-clonic (grand mal) seizures may be useful in partial seizures with elementary symptomatology (cortical focal), but they have little or no value in absence seizures or myoclonic spasms. Drugs effective in absence seizures usually are ineffective in generalized tonic-clonic, cortical focal, or complex partial (psychomotor) seizures; since the latter may mimic absence seizures, accurate diagnosis is essential.

The initial drug used to treat *generalized tonic-clonic* or *partial (cortical focal) seizures* is usually phenytoin [Dilantin] or phenobarbital. Most neurologists prefer phenytoin, especially for adults, because their experience has indicated that phenytoin is more likely to control the disease when given alone. Carbamazepine [Tegretol] also is useful in these types of seizures. Phenobarbital is more often used initially in children. If a trial with one of these agents fails to control seizures with maximally tolerated blood levels, another drug should be added. Primidone [Mysoline] is chemically related to the barbiturates and is frequently useful alone or with phenytoin. The other long-acting barbiturates, mephobarbital [Mebaral] and metharbital [Gemonil], may be alternatives to phenobarbital; their actions closely resemble those of phenobarbital, but they are less potent anticonvulsants and have no advantages over it. The short-acting barbiturates are not useful prophylactically as anticonvulsants, for their hypnotic action tends to parallel any anticonvulsant effect they might have. The other hydantoins, mephenytoin [Mesantoin] and ethotoin [Peganone], are alternatives to phenytoin, but they have no advantages and may be less effective. Acetazolamide [Diamox] is useful infrequently as an adjunct in generalized tonic-clonic or focal seizures; valproic acid [Depakene] also may be effective adjunctively. The succinimides and oxazolidinediones are ineffective in generalized tonic-clonic seizures and may even precipitate them in susceptible patients. Inorganic bromides (eg, sodium or potassium bromide) also have some anticonvulsant activity in generalized tonic-clonic seizures but, because they are toxic and have limited efficacy, their use has become largely obsolete, although some clinicians still use them in some infants and children.

The anticonvulsants useful in *complex partial seizures* (temporal lobe or psychomotor) include carbamazepine, primidone, and the hydantoins; the barbiturates have limited usefulness. Phenacemide [Phenurone] occasionally is effective against this type of seizure but, because it may produce severe adverse reactions, it should be prescribed only rarely when other drugs are ineffective.

Drugs specifically effective for *absence seizures* include the succinimides, valproic acid, and the oxazolidinediones. Ethosuximide [Zarontin] is usually the drug of choice, but some clinicians prefer valproic acid, which also may be effective in patients refractory to ethosuximide. The other succinimides, methsuximide [Celontin] and phensuximide [Milontin], are alternatives to ethosuximide, but they have no advantages and the latter is less effective. Of the oxazolidinediones, trimethadione [Tridione] is more effective than paramethadione [Paradione]; however, because of its toxicity, it should be reserved for cases refractory to safer drugs. Both typical and *atypical absence seizures* have been treated with the benzodiazepines (diazepam [Valium], clonazepam [Clonopin]) with variable success. These agents should be considered as alternative therapy for absence seizures in patients who do not respond to the succinimides or valproic acid. About one-half of patients with absence seizures also develop generalized tonic-clonic seizures; phenobarbital or phenytoin can be given to prevent this complication. When used alone or as an adjunct, acetazolamide occasionally relieves symptoms of absence seizures. Frequently its effectiveness is only temporary, for tolerance develops rapidly.

Myoclonic seizures occur alone or in association with absence or generalized tonic-clonic seizures and often are refractory to drug therapy. However, valproic acid appears to be particularly effective in this type of epilepsy. Clonazepam also may be useful, but it is probably less effective than valproic acid.

For treatment of *infantile massive spasms*, corticotropin or adrenal corticosteroids are most likely to be effective; the benzodiazepines are occasionally of value but control of seizures, when achieved, is generally temporary. Akinetic seizures and the Lennox-Gastaut syndrome may respond to the benzodiazepines. Valproic acid may be tried in refractory cases.

Status Epilepticus: Status epilepticus of the tonic-clonic type is a serious emergency requiring prompt and vigorous treatment. Diazepam, given intravenously, is the drug of choice for initial control of seizures. After seizures are controlled, a loading dose of phenobarbital sodium or phenytoin sodium should be given intravenously in order to produce a therapeutic plasma concentration as rapidly as possible. (Phenytoin sodium should not be given intramuscularly because the drug crystallizes in the muscle and hence its absorption is erratic and incomplete.) If seizures are not controlled, administration of diazepam may be repeated. If convulsions do not stop within five minutes, parenteral administration of paraldehyde may be tried, although this agent has several disadvantages; it also can be given rectally. If status epilepticus persists, a general anesthetic can be administered. A measure of *last resort* is the slow intravenous infusion of lidocaine [Xylocaine]. When anesthetic agents are necessary, they should be given under the supervision of an anesthesiologist, when possible, and resuscitative equipment should be available. Once status epilepticus has been brought under control, phenytoin sodium should be given intravenously in sufficient amounts to maintain therapeutic plasma levels, followed by transition to an oral maintenance dose or other suitable medication as soon as possible. Treatment of focal motor and complex partial status epilepticus is generally the same as for the tonic-clonic type.

For absence status epilepticus, intravenous diazepam is usually preferred initially. Because its action is transient, an effective serum concentration of ethosuximide should be established as rapidly as possible by using larger than usual oral doses.

Nonepileptic Convulsions: Convulsions per se do not necessarily indicate epilepsy, although seizures occurring in some acute conditions (eg, febrile convulsions in children, convulsion following head trauma) may precede the development of chronic epilepsy.

Other nonepileptic convulsions for which anticonvulsants are used include major motor seizures (usually with severe, protracted clonic convulsions) which are sometimes associated with the withdrawal syndrome in persons physically dependent upon barbiturates, alcohol, or certain other sedatives. In barbiturate and other sedative dependence, gradual discontinuance of the drug is indicated, and substitution of phenobarbital with gradual reduction in the dose helps prevent convulsions (see Chapter 11, Drugs Used for Anxiety and Insomnia). In the treatment of alcohol withdrawal symptoms, diazepam may be used to reduce agitation and prevent or control seizures. Although it is often used, phenytoin has not been conclusively proved to be of value in these conditions.

Adverse Reactions and Precautions

Many minor reactions to anticonvulsants may be overcome by reducing the dose, although this may necessitate the addition of another anticonvulsant to the regimen.

Most anticonvulsants produce gastrointestinal disturbances in some patients, especially during the early stages of treatment. The symptoms may be reduced by administering the drugs after meals or by decreasing the dose.

Many anticonvulsants have sedative effects, and drowsiness is sometimes a significant complaint. This is most noticeable during the early period of treatment and, if it persists, a reduction in dose may be indicated. Sedating drugs may cause alterations in mood, which occasionally are serious (see Chapter 11). Some anticonvulsants also cause mental disturbances; phenacemide [Phenurone] is particularly prone to cause serious personality changes, including psychoses and suicidal depression.

Ataxia is a common dose-related adverse effect with use of the hydantoins and, if it appears, a reduction in dosage is required. There is evidence that these drugs cause cerebellar damage if the amount that produces ataxia is administered for prolonged periods. However, this danger appears remote, since ataxia is so troublesome that dosage adjustment is essential. Very young patients can be exceptions, for drug-induced ataxia may be confused with the natural unsteadiness of the toddler. Ataxia also may occur with use of barbiturates.

Many anticonvulsants commonly cause skin eruptions as a hypersensitivity reaction; the eruptions are usually morbilliform and discontinuance of the drug is necessary. Drug sensitivity reactions cannot be predicted, but skin reactions usually become apparent after 10 to 14 days of therapy. Although rarely associated with anticonvulsant therapy, a skin reaction may precede the development of systemic lupus erythematosus, Stevens-Johnson syndrome, angioedema, serum sickness, or polyarteritis nodosa. Anaphylaxis is extremely rare.

Because the barbiturates and hydantoins are particularly prone to precipitate acute intermittent porphyria, they should not be used in patients with this disease.

Several anticonvulsants may cause reversible visual disturbances such as diplopia and nystagmus; hemeralopia (defective vision in bright light) has been reported with trimethadione [Tridione] and paramethadione [Paradione].

Phenytoin [Dilantin] frequently causes gingival hyperplasia in children, but this seldom occurs with mephenytoin [Mesantoin] and has not been reported with ethotoin [Peganone].

Lymphadenopathies simulating malignant lymphomas have occurred with several anticonvulsants; the hydantoins have been implicated most frequently. Although it is questionable whether phenytoin is as prone to cause these pseudolymphomas as mephenytoin, the incidence is greater since the former drug is more widely used. The signs and symptoms may progress temporarily but usually begin to disappear one to two weeks after therapy is discontinued. A few cases of true lymphoma and Hodgkin's disease have been reported in which a causal relationship to hydantoin therapy seems possible.

Megaloblastic anemias have been observed with several anticonvulsants, particularly the hydantoins, barbiturates, and primidone [Mysoline]. Accordingly, periodic blood studies are indicated in patients receiving these drugs. Usually therapy may be continued if the anemia responds to treatment with folic acid. Even in the absence of anemia, there is some evidence that folic acid depletion induced by anticonvulsants may be manifested by reversible symptoms of mental deterioration. Poor memory, inattentiveness, lethargy, and slow learning may result from other effects of anticonvulsant drugs or may be evidence of brain damage. However, if such symptoms occur in the presence of low folate blood levels, a trial with folic acid may be warranted. Because folic acid increases the rate of metabolism and excretion of phenytoin and thus may decrease its anticonvulsant action, it should not be used routinely for prophylaxis in patients without anemia.

Among the most dangerous reactions that develop during therapy with anticonvulsant drugs are those that result from damage to the bone marrow, liver, and kidneys. Severe blood dyscrasias have been associated most commonly with phenacemide and mephenytoin and rarely with paramethadione, trimethadione, and other anticonvulsants. Baseline blood counts should be performed before initiating treatment with these drugs. Although periodic blood studies during treatment will reveal mild leukopenias, they cannot be relied upon to predict the more serious reactions that occur precipitously (eg, agranulocytosis, thrombocytopenia, aplastic anemia). Since early recognition of the dyscrasia and discontinuance of the offending drug are essential, the patient should be advised to report promptly such symptoms as sore throat, fever, easy bruising, petechiae, epistaxis, or other signs of infection or bleeding tendency. Clinical and laboratory evaluation is necessary if such symptoms occur. Although the risk of blood dyscrasias is diminished after the first year of treatment, the physician should be alert to their possible occurrence. The mortality from aplastic anemia is particularly high and recovery is slow in surviving patients.

Severe, sometimes fatal, hepatitis has occurred with phenacemide and more rarely with other anticonvulsants, including the hydantoins and valproic acid. Before treatment with these drugs is initiated, it is advisable to perform baseline liver function studies, and patients should be instructed to report promptly any symptoms of hepatitis such as jaundice, dark urine, anorexia, abdominal discomfort, or other gastrointestinal symptoms. Since this drug-induced hepatitis is probably idiosyncratic, the value of performing periodic laboratory studies in asymptomatic patients is doubtful. Phenacemide and valproic acid may be exceptions, for there is some evidence that hepatitis can develop insidiously with their use; abnormal results of liver function tests may herald the development of serious disease.

Nephropathies have developed occasionally during treatment with anticonvulsants, especially in patients receiving trimethadione and paramethadione. These reactions may develop insidiously. The development of any significant renal abnormality is an indication for discontinuing the drug.

A frequently cited paradoxical effect of anticonvulsants is the tendency of agents effective for one type of seizure to aggravate or precipitate seizures of another type. However, seizure types tend to be mixed in epileptic disorders, and the apparent aggravation of one type may be a manifestation of the natural course of the disease and reflect the ineffectiveness of the particular drug for that type of seizure. Thus, precipitation of seizures by anticonvulsant drugs probably is rare, and some consultants doubt that it occurs. There is no question, however, that abrupt withdrawal of anticonvulsants can precipitate seizures. When a drug is to be discontinued, the dose should be reduced gradually unless rapid withdrawal and substitution of another drug is mandatory because of a serious adverse reaction.

Use in Pregnancy: Various types of birth defects have been attributed to the use of anticonvulsant drugs during pregnancy. The risk of malformations in infants exposed to anticonvulsants in utero appears to be about twice that of the general population.

Most of the congenital malformations reported have been associated with use of phenytoin and phenobarbital, either alone or in combination. This may reflect their wider use. Trimethadione, which is used less often, has been reported to be a very potent teratogen. Birth defects or spontaneous abortions have occurred in 80% of the reported conceptuses exposed to this agent in utero.

Those abnormalities reported most frequently include cleft lip and/or palate, skeletal anomalies, congenital heart disease, and central nervous system malformations. The pattern of some abnormalities caused by hydantoins and barbiturates is thought to be characteristic, as is that associated with trimethadione, and these have been referred to as the "fetal hydantoin-barbiturate syndrome" and "fetal trimethadione syndrome," respectively. In addition, a depression of clotting factors and neonatal hemorrhages, which are responsive to vitamin K, have been reported in infants exposed to phenytoin or barbiturates in utero. Because of experience with these agents, not only are other agents in the same classes probably teratogenic, but anticonvulsants in other classes also are suspect.

Although the risk of congenital abnormalities with the use of anticonvulsants during pregnancy is small, the benefit versus risk must be carefully considered for each patient. Women of childbearing potential receiving anticonvulsants should be informed that the chance of having a normal child is about 90%, but the risk of a congenital malformation or mental retardation is about two to three times greater than in the general population because of the drug or the disease. Those receiving an oxazolidinedione, hydantoin, or possibly a barbiturate should consider the use of birth control measures. However, the oral contraceptives may be less effective in women receiving anticonvulsants, particularly phenytoin, probably because of the increased rate of estrogen metabolism. If pregnancy occurs during treatment with trimethadione, the patient should have the option of terminating it. Alternatively, consideration may be given to the gradual discontinuation of anticonvulsant medication prior to pregnancy. Although this may be done successfully in some cases, the risks of precipitating seizures or status epilepticus and the potential for fetal damage should a seizure occur must be kept in mind.

Drug Interactions: Some anticonvulsants may interact with other drugs or with each other. Additive effects may occur with alcohol or other central nervous system depressants. The barbiturates, particularly phenobarbital, stimulate the activity of a number of hepatic enzyme systems, thereby affecting the metabolism of many drugs. Thus, phenobarbital has been reported to decrease blood levels of phenytoin by increasing its rate of metabolism. However, phenobarbital is parahydroxylated by the same enzymes and therefore it also competes with phenytoin. The effects of the interactions between these two drugs are variable. Whether the blood level of phenytoin increases or decreases depends upon the level of phenobarbital; a high phenobarbital level increases the phenytoin level whereas it is decreased with a low level of phenobarbital. Thus, when these two drugs are used together, their dosage may require adjustment in accordance with clinical effects and blood levels. When phenytoin and primidone are given together, phenytoin increases the relative phenobarbital level from primidone by increasing the metabolism of the latter drug.

Dicumarol inhibits the metabolism of phenytoin, which may lead to drug accumulation and toxicity. In contrast, the metabolism of coumarin anticoagulants is enhanced by barbiturates, thus necessitating adjustment of anticoagulant dosage when barbiturates are either added to or withdrawn from the regimen.

Interactions between valproic acid and other anticonvulsants (eg, phenobarbital, primidone, phenytoin, carbamazepine) may occur and should be considered when these drugs are given concurrently (see the evaluation on Valproic Acid).

Several other drugs (eg, disulfiram [Antabuse], isoniazid, aminosalicylic acid, chloramphenicol) increase the blood level of phenytoin by interfering with its metabolism. See also the evaluations and Chapter 5, Drug Interactions and Adverse Drug Reactions.

BARBITURATES

PHENOBARBITAL

PHENOBARBITAL SODIUM

Phenobarbital, a long-acting barbiturate, is one of the most widely employed and useful anticonvulsants. Its principal effectiveness is in generalized tonic-clonic (grand mal) and partial (focal motor or sensory) seizures; complex partial and absence seizures do not respond as well. Phenobarbital can be used as the initial drug, particularly in children, although it more commonly is added to the regimen when phenytoin has not completely controlled seizures. Phenobarbital also is useful to control seizures resulting from the withdrawal of barbiturates or alcohol in dependent individuals.

Drowsiness, usually transient, is the most common adverse effect, although some patients become hyperactive. This paradoxical response is particularly common in children and the elderly. Ataxia sometimes occurs; if it persists, a reduction in dosage is required. Skin eruptions are uncommon, but these rarely may progress to exfoliative dermatitis. Megaloblastic anemia is also uncommon.

When the drug is given during pregnancy, the possibility of congenital malformations or a coagulation defect and hemorrhage in the newborn must be considered. Barbiturates are contraindicated in patients with acute intermittent porphyria.

Abrupt termination of therapy may exacerbate seizures, but drug dependence and barbiturate intoxication are unlikely with usual anticonvulsant doses. (See also the Introduction.)

Phenobarbital sodium is used parenterally to treat status epilepticus, although diazepam presently is considered the initial drug of choice. The principal danger when using phenobarbital for this purpose is respiratory depression. Nevertheless, a full anticonvulsant dose should be given initially, for fractional doses may result in the paradoxical situation of drug-induced depression with continued status epilepticus.

ROUTES, USUAL DOSAGE, AND PREPARATIONS. The average plasma half-life is four days; consequently, two to three weeks are required to attain steady state plasma levels. Doubling the dose for the first four days of therapy will provide an effective plasma level more promptly, but sedation is prominent. Serum concentrations of 15 to 40 mcg/ml are usually optimal for the control of epilepsy; concentrations above 40 mcg/ml are often accompanied by overt symptoms of toxicity, but higher levels may be tolerated by some patients. Because of its long half-life, use of timed-release preparations of phenobarbital is unnecessary.

PHENOBARBITAL:

Oral: Adults, 50 to 100 mg two or three times daily; *children*, 15 to 50 mg two or three times daily.
> Drug available generically: Elixir 20 mg/5 ml; tablets 7.5, 15, 30, 60, 90, and 100 mg.
> Available Trademarks.
> *Eskabarb* (timed-release) (Smith Kline & French), *Luminal* (Winthrop).

PHENOBARBITAL SODIUM:

Intramuscular, Intravenous (slow): For status epilepticus, *adults*, 200 to 320 mg, repeated in six hours as necessary; *children* (intramuscular), 3 to 5 mg/kg of body weight.
> Drug available generically: Powder 120 and 130 mg; solution 30, 60, 130, and 150 mg/ml in 1 and 2 ml containers.
> Available Trademark.
> *Luminal Sodium* (Winthrop).

MEPHOBARBITAL
[Mebaral]

Mephobarbital is metabolized to phenobarbital; thus, it has similar properties and uses, but larger doses must be given. However, there is no evidence that it has any advantage over phenobarbital. (See the Introduction and the evaluation on Phenobarbital.)

ROUTE, USUAL DOSAGE, AND PREPARATIONS. The serum levels given for phenobarbital may be used as a guide to adjust the dosage of mephobarbital (see the evaluation).
Oral: Adults, 400 to 600 mg daily in divided doses. *Children under 5 years*, 16 to 32 mg three or four times daily; *over 5 years*, 32 to 64 mg three or four times daily.
> Drug available generically: Tablets 32 and 100 mg.
> *Mebaral* (Breon). Tablets 32, 50, 100, and 200 mg.

DEOXYBARBITURATE

PRIMIDONE
[Mysoline]

Although not a true barbiturate, primidone is considered with this group because of its close chemical relationship. Primidone is converted to two active metabolites, phenobarbital and phenylethylmalonamide (PEMA). Its principal use is in generalized tonic-clonic seizures, partial seizures with elementary symptomatology (cortical focal), and complex partial (temporal lobe) seizures; some clinicians believe that the drug has a specific usefulness in the latter type. Primidone is commonly given with phenytoin. It is not effective in absence seizures.

Sedation is common but often diminishes with continued administration. If the dosage is increased gradually enough, incapacitating drowsiness may be avoided. Ataxia and some of the more minor reactions caused by barbiturates also have been observed with primidone. Skin eruptions such as maculopapular or morbilliform rash are noted occasionally. Megaloblastic anemia, which responds to folic acid, has been reported. When the drug is given during pregnancy, the same considerations should be given as with use of barbiturates (see the Introduction). The contraindication to barbiturates in patients with acute intermittent porphyria also applies to primidone.

ROUTE, USUAL DOSAGE, AND PREPARATIONS. The plasma half-life varies widely (3 to 24 hours), and peak serum concentrations occur in one-half to nine hours. Plasma concentrations of primidone during long-term therapy vary widely but average approximately 1 mcg/ml per mg/kg of daily dose; 5 to 10 mcg/ml is the usual therapeutic range. Plasma concentrations of phenobarbital produced by biotransformation of primidone average 2 mcg/ml per mg/kg of the daily dose of primidone; concentrations of PEMA fall somewhere between the two. The dosage of primidone may be adjusted according to the plasma levels of phenobarbital and the patient's response (see the evaluation). Significant ataxia and lethargy usually occur with concentrations of primidone above 10 mcg/ml. *Oral*: *Adults*, 250 mg daily at bedtime to 2 g daily in divided doses; *children under 8 years*, one-half adult dosage.

Drug available generically: Tablets 250 mg.
Mysoline (Ayerst). Suspension 250 mg/5 ml; tablets 50 and 250 mg.

HYDANTOIN

PHENYTOIN
[Dilantin]

PHENYTOIN SODIUM
[Dilantin Sodium]

Phenytoin (diphenylhydantoin) is useful for treating generalized tonic-clonic, complex partial (temporal lobe), and cortical focal seizures and frequently is chosen for initial therapy, particularly in adults; usually it should be either the first or second agent selected. However, because of some of phenytoin's adverse reactions, phenobarbital is usually the drug of first choice in infants and children. Phenytoin is often used with phenobarbital (or primidone) when a single drug is inadequate. It is ineffective in absence seizures, myoclonic spasms, and akinetic epilepsy.

Phenytoin produces little or no sedation in usual doses. Ataxia occurs with larger doses; if it persists, a reduction in dosage is necessary to avoid cerebellar damage. Ocular signs and symptoms such as nystagmus and diplopia also may necessitate reduction of dosage. Peripheral neuropathy may develop after years of use. Skin eruptions occur frequently but are only rarely serious. Gingival hyperplasia is common and often severe in children. Scrupulous oral hygiene may help prevent secondary inflammatory changes but has little or no effect on the occurrence or severity of this troublesome complication; repeated gingivectomies may be required if use of the drug is continued. Hirsutism is less common but does occur, especially in children. Rare but serious idiosyncratic reactions include hepatitis, bone marrow depression, systemic lupus erythematosus, Stevens-Johnson syndrome, and lymphadenopathy resembling malignant lymphomas. Folic acid depletion may occur and may progress to megaloblastic anemia. Interference with vitamin D metabolism may cause osteomalacia. When the drug is given during pregnancy, the possibility of congenital malformations and a coagulation defect and hemorrhage in the newborn infant must be considered. (See also the Introduction.)

Interactions between phenytoin and other anticonvulsants (phenobarbital, carbamazepine, valproic acid), as well as other agents occur and must be considered with concomitant use. (See the Introduction and the evaluations.)

The sodium salt of phenytoin is sometimes used intravenously to treat status epilepticus but, if administration is too rapid, severe hypotension may occur. The high alkalinity of the drug makes intramuscular injection undesirable for routine or prolonged therapy because local tissue irritation or damage may occur; moreover, the drug crystallizes in muscle and its absorption is erratic. Subcutaneous or perivascular injection of phenytoin must be avoided. Unlike barbiturates, phenytoin seldom depresses respiration.

Phenytoin has been advocated for many other disorders in addition to epilepsy, but conclusive evidence of its effectiveness is inadequate for most proposed indications. However, the intravenous use of the sodium salt in certain arrhythmias has been established (see Chapter 34, Antiarrhythmic Agents). Oral administration has been reported to be effective prophylactically in some patients with migraine, but it is not the drug of choice (see Chapter 9, Drugs Used to Treat Migraine and Other Headaches). In addition, trigeminal neuralgia is sometimes relieved by phenytoin, but carbamazepine is preferred (see Chapter 10, Drugs Used in Central Pain Syndromes). Beneficial effects also have been reported in a variety of psychoses, neuroses, and other psychiatric disorders, but criteria for selecting patients for trial with phenytoin are presently too vague for any firm recommendation. This drug's usefulness in the treatment of convulsions resulting from withdrawal of barbiturates or alcohol has not been proved.

ROUTES, USUAL DOSAGE, AND PREPARATIONS. The plasma half-life averages 24 hours, but wide variations among patients (as much as fourfold) have been reported. Serum concentrations are not linearly related to daily dose, and small increases in dose may greatly alter the serum level, especially near the therapeutic range. Serum concentrations of 10 to 20 mcg/ml are usually optimal. Concentrations at and above the upper level are almost always associated with overt symptoms of toxicity: 20 mcg/ml, nystagmus; 30 mcg/ml, ataxia; and 40 mcg/ml, lethargy. Because of differences in the rate of dissolution and absorption among the various dosage forms and products, it is advisable to maintain patients on one dosage form and one manufacturer's product. If it is necessary to make an alteration, blood levels should be determined and any necessary adjustments in dosage made to maintain optimum blood levels.

Oral: The dosage must be individualized according to the patient's response and the drug blood level; the dose is usually given three times daily. However, because it is released slowly, the capsule preparation made by Parke, Davis may be given once daily. Initially, the drug should be administered in divided doses; after the patient has been stabilized and the optimum blood level determined, the appropriate amount may be given once daily. For patients in whom the drug half-life is short (8 hours), phenytoin should be given more frequently. *Adults*, initially, 300 mg daily; the maintenance dose is usually 300 to 400 mg daily (maximum, 600 mg). *Children*, initially, 5 mg/kg of body weight daily in two or three equally divided doses, with subsequent dosage individualized (maximum, 300 mg daily). A suggested maintenance dose is 4 to 8 mg/kg daily. *Children over 6 years* may require the minimum adult dose (300 mg daily).

PHENYTOIN:
Dilantin (Parke, Davis). Suspension 30 (pediatric) and 125 mg/5 ml; tablets (pediatric) 50 mg.

PHENYTOIN SODIUM:
Drug available generically and under the name Diphenylhydantoin Sodium: Capsules 30 and 100 mg.
Dilantin [*sodium*] (Parke, Davis). Capsules 30 and 100 mg.

Intravenous: For status epilepticus, *adults,* 10 to 15 mg/kg of body weight infused no faster than 50 mg/min, followed by 100 to 150 mg 30 minutes later, if necessary, to produce a therapeutic blood level. *Children,* dosage is reduced. Pediatric dosage may be calculated on the basis of 250 mg/M^2 of body surface. This drug should not be given intramuscularly for status epilepticus.

PHENYTOIN SODIUM:
Drug available generically: Solution 50 mg/ml in 2 and 5 ml containers.
Dilantin [*sodium*] (Parke, Davis). Powder (for solution) containing approximately 50 mg/ml when diluted with the diluent provided in the 100 and 250 mg containers; solution 50 mg/ml in 2 and 5 ml containers.

SUCCINIMIDE

ETHOSUXIMIDE
[Zarontin]

Ethosuximide is usually the drug of choice for absence seizures. It also has been reported to be effective in myoclonic spasms and akinetic epilepsy in some patients, but is generally ineffective in complex partial (temporal lobe) or generalized tonic-clonic seizures.

The most common adverse reactions are gastrointestinal disturbances (eg, nausea, vomiting, anorexia). Drowsiness, ataxia, headache, dizziness, euphoria, hiccup, rash, urticaria, and behavioral changes have been observed occasionally. Serious untoward effects occur less frequently than with trimethadione and paramethadione. Systemic lupus erythematosus, aplastic anemia, thrombocytopenia, leukopenia,

pancytopenia, and eosinophilia have been reported rarely. (See also the Introduction.)

ROUTE, USUAL DOSAGE, AND PREPARATIONS.
The plasma half-life averages 30 hours (range, 24 to 49 hours) in children and 60 hours in adults. The peak plasma level after a single oral dose is reached in one to seven hours. Maximum control of absence seizures is achieved in most patients with serum concentrations of 40 to 80 mcg/ml. Concentrations of up to 160 mcg/ml are sometimes tolerated without excessive adverse reactions, but psychotic reactions may occur with high blood levels.

Oral: Adults and children over 6 years, initially, 500 mg daily; the daily dose may be increased, if necessary, by increments of 250 mg every four to seven days until seizures are controlled or untoward effects develop. Doses exceeding 1 g daily are seldom more effective than smaller doses. *Children 3 to 6 years,* initially, 250 mg daily with incremental increases in dosage as for older patients.

Zarontin (Parke, Davis). Capsules 250 mg; syrup 250 mg/5 ml.

OXAZOLIDINEDIONE

TRIMETHADIONE
[Tridione]

This drug is principally effective in controlling absence seizures. Although trimethadione is among the more effective agents for this purpose, it should be reserved for refractory cases because of its toxicity.

Serious reactions, some of them fatal, include rash that may progress to exfoliative dermatitis or erythema multiforme, nephropathy, hepatitis, and bone marrow depression with aplastic anemia, neutropenia, or agranulocytosis. Pseudolymphomas, systemic lupus erthematosus, and a myasthenia gravis-like syndrome also have been reported. Drowsiness, alopecia, and hiccup may occur during early treatment. Reversible visual disturbances, particularly hemeralopia, are common.

An increase in the incidence of congenital abnormalities has been associated with the use of trimethadione during pregnancy. Accordingly, this drug should be avoided in pregnant women if possible. (See the Introduction.)

ROUTE, USUAL DOSAGE, AND PREPARATIONS. Serum concentrations average 0.6 mcg/ml per mg/kg of the daily dose. The serum concentration of the active metabolite of trimethadione (dimethadione) averages 12 mcg/ml per mg/kg of daily dose and is used as the guide to adjust dosage. Adequate seizure control is usually obtained with dimethadione concentrations above 700 mcg/ml.

Oral: Adults, initially, 900 mg daily in three or four divided doses, increased by increments of 300 mg daily at weekly intervals to a maximum of 2.4 g daily. *Children*, initially, 40 mg/kg of body weight (300 to 900 mg) daily in three or four divided doses.

Tridione (Abbott). Capsules 300 mg; solution 200 mg/5 ml; tablets (chewable) 150 mg.

BENZODIAZEPINES

CLONAZEPAM
[Clonopin]

Clonazepam may be effective alone or with other drugs in absence, myoclonic, and akinetic seizures and in infantile spasms and photosensitive epilepsy. Although this drug is effective in absence seizures, it should be considered an alter-

native to ethosuximide or valproic acid because of the high incidence of adverse reactions associated with its use. Clonazepam also may be effective in generalized tonic-clonic convulsions or complex partial (temporal lobe) epilepsy; it is less effective in focal seizures. However, in some studies, the incidence of generalized tonic-clonic seizures was increased. Clonazepam may be useful in status epilepticus, but diazepam remains the drug of choice for this purpose. Clonazepam also has been tried in the treatment of tardive dyskinesia (see Chapter 16, Drugs Used in Extrapyramidal Movement Disorders). The prolonged use of this drug is limited by the development of tolerance.

The most common adverse reactions affect the central nervous system. Approximately one-half of patients taking clonazepam experience drowsiness, about one-third ataxia, and up to one-quarter personality changes. These effects appear to be dose related, occur early in the course of therapy, and may subside with long-term administration. Other neurologic effects include abnormal eye movements, slurred speech, tremor, vertigo, and confusion. Minor, but sometimes troublesome, reactions involving the cardiovascular, gastrointestinal, and genitourinary systems have been observed. Skin rashes, anemia, leukopenia, thrombocytopenia, and eosinophilia also have occurred. Clonazepam causes respiratory depression and hypersecretion in the upper respiratory passages and, therefore, should be used with caution in individuals with respiratory tract disease. Because clonazepam is excreted by the kidney, it also should be used with care in patients with impaired renal function. This drug is contraindicated in those with a history of sensitivity to the benzodiazepines, significant liver disease, or acute angle-closure glaucoma. In many studies, tolerance was observed after long-term use; accordingly, the initial dosage should be small and increased slowly. Both psychic and physical dependence have been reported with benzodiazepine drugs; withdrawal symptoms similar to those observed for the barbiturates have occurred following sudden withdrawal of clonazepam. This drug is classified as a Schedule IV substance under the Controlled Substances Act.

The effects of clonazepam on the developing fetus and nursing infant are not known; therefore, this drug should be used during pregnancy only if the expected benefits outweigh the potential hazards. Mothers receiving clonazepam should not breast feed their infants.

ROUTE, USUAL DOSAGE, AND PREPARATIONS. The plasma half-life varies between 18 and 50 hours. Seizure control is usually achieved with serum levels of 0.013 to 0.072 mcg/ml.

Oral: *Adults*, initially, 1.5 mg daily in three divided doses. Dosage then may be increased by increments of 0.5 to 1 mg every third day until seizures are adequately controlled or adverse effects intervene (maximum, 20 mg daily). *Infants and children up to 10 years of age or 30 kg of body weight*, 0.01 to 0.03 (maximum, 0.05) mg/kg of body weight daily in two or three divided doses. The total daily dose may be increased by increments of 0.25 to 0.5 mg every third day until a maintenance dose of 0.1 to 0.2 mg/kg/day has been reached.

Clonopin (Roche). Tablets 0.5, 1, and 2 mg.

DIAZEPAM
[Valium]

This benzodiazepine derivative is used primarily as an antianxiety agent, but it also has important anticonvulsant properties. Given intravenously, it is potentially lifesaving in status epilepticus and is the drug of choice for initial control of seizures. When given orally, diazepam is sometimes helpful as an adjunct to other anticonvulsants in myoclonic spasms and akinetic seizures, which often are refractory to other drugs. Diazepam, given intravenously, also may be useful with or as an alternative to magnesium sulfate to control the seizures of eclampsia.

The most common adverse effects with oral use are drowsiness, dizziness, fatigue, and ataxia, which are dose related. Paradoxical excitement or stimulation sometimes occurs. Parenteral administration for status epilepticus requires observation for respiratory depression and hypotension, and the slight possibility of cardiac arrest must be borne in mind. However, the overall safety of the drug appears to compare favorably with that of other agents used for this emergency. The injectable form contains sodium benzoate and benzoic acid as buffers, which have been shown to displace bilirubin from albumin in vitro; thus, the possibility of inducing kernicterus in newborn infants must be considered.

For further information on adverse reactions, precautions, and other uses, see Chapters 11, Drugs Used for Anxiety and Insomnia; 17, Drugs Used to Treat Skeletal Muscle Hyperactivity; and 21, Adjuncts to Anesthesia and Analeptic Drugs. Diazepam is classified as a Schedule IV substance under the Controlled Substances Act.

ROUTES, USUAL DOSAGE, AND PREPARATIONS. Effective plasma levels of diazepam and its active N-demethyl metabolite have not been definitively established. Concentrations between 0.1 and 1 mcg/ml have been reported after long-term oral therapy. Immediately following intravenous injection, the plasma level of diazepam is greater than 0.5 mcg/ml.

Oral: *Adults*, 2 to 10 mg two to four times daily, beginning with a small dose and increasing it gradually; *elderly or debilitated patients*, initially 2 mg. *Children*, initially, 2 to 4 mg daily in divided doses; subsequent doses are less than those used for adults.

Valium (Roche). Tablets 2, 5, and 10 mg.

Intravenous (slow): For status epilepticus, *adults*, initially, 5 to 10 mg given at a rate of 1 ml (5 mg)/min, repeated at 10- to 15-

minute intervals (maximum, 30 mg). This dose may be repeated in two to four hours if necessary. *Infants over 30 days and children under 5 years*, 0.2 to 0.5 mg every two to five minutes (maximum, 5 mg). *Children 5 years or older*, 1 mg every two to five minutes (maximum, 10 mg). Administration is repeated in two to four hours if necessary. If convulsions make slow intravenous injection impossible, intramuscular injection may be substituted. The drug should not be mixed or diluted with other solutions or drugs or added to intravenous fluids.

Valium (Roche). Solution 5 mg/ml in 2 and 10 ml containers.

CHEMICALLY UNRELATED ANTICONVULSANTS

CARBAMAZEPINE
[Tegretol]

Carbamazepine is a tricyclic (iminostilbene) compound which is chemically related to imipramine. It has important anticonvulsant properties and is useful in partial seizures, especially those with complex symptomatology (temporal lobe), and generalized tonic-clonic seizures, as well as in mixed seizures of these types. Its effectiveness appears to be comparable to that of primidone, and most clinicians prefer carbamazepine, especially for children. The drug is ineffective in absence seizures, myoclonic spasms, and akinetic epilepsy. However, it is reported to have a psychotropic action that may increase alertness and elevate mood in many patients with epilepsy; it also reduces the severity of behavioral disorders. For other uses, see Chapter 10, Drugs Used in Central Pain Syndromes.

ADVERSE REACTIONS.

Reactions that occur most commonly during early treatment are drowsiness, dizziness, lightheadedness, ataxia, nausea, and vomiting; these reactions usually subside spontaneously within a week or after a reduction in dose. Their occurrence may be minimized by initiating therapy with a small dose and increasing it gradually. Other reported neurologic reactions include confusion, headache, fatigue, blurred vision, transient diplopia and oculomotor disturbances, dysphasia, abnormal involuntary movements, peripheral neuritis and paresthesias, depression with agitation, talkativeness, nystagmus, and tinnitus.

Gastrointestinal reactions include gastric distress and abdominal pain, diarrhea, constipation, and anorexia. Dryness of the mouth, glossitis, and stomatitis also occur.

Dermatologic reactions (pruritic and erythematous rashes, urticaria, Stevens-Johnson syndrome, photosensitivity, alterations in skin pigmentation, exfoliative dermatitis, alopecia, hyperhidrosis, erythema multiforme, erythema nodosum, and aggravation of systemic lupus erythematosus) occur occasionally; if they are severe, it may be necessary to discontinue the drug.

Hematopoietic reactions (leukopenia, agranulocytosis, eosinophilia, leukocytosis, purpura, aplastic anemia, and thrombocytopenia) occur rarely but may be serious; the aplastic anemia and thrombocytopenia may be fatal. Therefore, patients should be advised to discontinue the drug and notify their physician if signs of hematologic toxicity appear (eg, fever, sore throat, aphthous stomatitis, easy bruising, petechial or purpuric hemorrhage).

Cardiovascular, genitourinary, metabolic, hepatic, and other reactions have been reported rarely. These include aggravation of hypertension or ischemic heart disease, hypotension, syncope, edema, hyponatremia, congestive heart failure, recurrence of thrombophlebitis, urinary frequency, acute urinary retention, albuminuria, glycosuria, elevated blood urea nitrogen levels, microscopic deposits in the urine, impotence, cholestatic and hepatocellular jaundice, fever and chills, adenopathy or lymphadenopathy, myalgia and arthralgia, leg cramps, and conjunctivitis. Water intoxication, which may be related to higher blood levels of carbamazepine, has been reported.

It is advisable to obtain pretreatment baseline values of blood and platelet counts, liver function, urinalysis, and blood urea nitrogen, and ophthalmologic examination should be performed; these tests should be repeated at regular intervals during treatment.

Although teratogenicity has not been reported clinically, some teratogenic effects were observed in studies on rats. Therefore, it is advisable to administer carbamazepine to pregnant women only when the benefits outweigh the potential risks. Also, because toxic effects have been reported in nursing rats, mothers taking the drug should not nurse their infants.

Since carbamazepine is chemically related to the tricyclic compounds, it should not be administered to patients who are sensitive to these drugs. The possibility of activating latent psychosis or inducing confusion or agitation in elderly patients also exists.

The absorption of carbamazepine is variable; reported peak serum concentrations have occurred after 6 to 12 hours. Absorption may be increased when the drug is taken with meals. The plasma half-life also has varied, but the best estimate is 14 to 16 hours. Steady state plasma concentrations are reached in 32 to 40 hours when the drug is given three times daily. Serum concentrations of 1 to 10 mcg/ml are usually attained during long-term therapy (5 to 12 mcg/ml is the usual therapeutic serum level). Carbamazepine is metabolized in the liver to an epoxide and several other metabolites, which are excreted in the bile and urine. There is some evidence that carbamazepine may induce its own metabolism. The drug is highly bound to plasma albumin, but it is not displaced by acidic drugs as phenytoin is and it does not displace the latter; however, when added to a regimen with phenytoin, the serum concentration of phenytoin may decrease, probably as a result of enzyme induction.

ROUTE, USUAL DOSAGE, AND PREPARATIONS. *Oral*: *Children under 6 years*, 100 mg daily; *6 to 12 years*, 100 mg twice daily on the first day. The dose is increased gradually in daily increments of 100 mg and given three or four times daily until the best response is obtained. The usual maximum dose is 1 g. The usual maintenance dose is 400 to 800 mg daily. *Adults and adolescents*, initially, 400 mg divided into two doses on the first day. The dosage is increased gradually in daily increments of 200 mg and administered three or four times daily. The usual maintenance dose is 800 mg to 1.2 g daily. The usual maximum dose is 1 g daily in children 12 to 15 years and 1.2 g in patients over 15 years. Amounts up to 1.6 g daily have been given to adults rarely.

Tegretol (Geigy). Tablets 200 mg.

VALPROIC ACID
[Depakene]

$$CH_3CH_2CH_2\underset{\underset{CH_3CH_2CH_2}{|}}{\overset{\overset{O}{\parallel}}{C}}HCOH$$

Results of clinical trials with valproic acid (as sodium valproate) have shown that this drug reduced the frequency of several types of seizures, but was more effective in generalized than in partial epilepsies. It is most effective in patients with typical absence seizures (simple and complex [petit mal]), especially when three-cycle-per-second spike and wave discharges were demonstrated on electroencephalography, and in photically sensitive seizures. Responses were also promising in the atypical absence type (variant of petit mal). Results in patients with bilateral massive epileptic myoclonus (myoclonic epilepsy) have been similarly favorable; however, additional controlled studies are needed to establish the usefulness of valproic acid in this type of seizure. One investigator considers it the drug of choice, especially in children, because most patients with myoclonic seizures are resistant to other anticonvulsants.

In the majority of patients studied with tonic-clonic seizures (grand mal), sodium valproate was given with other anticonvulsants that were ineffective in maintaining control. Sodium valproate reduced the frequency of seizures by 75% or more in about 50% of these patients, but it was not useful in about 30%. The dosage of other anticonvulsants could be reduced in many patients, and it was possible to discontinue use of other drugs in a few. The efficacy of this agent in those with combination absence and tonic-clonic seizures was about the same as in those with the latter type alone. It was less effective in other mixed types and in atonic or akinetic seizures. The number of patients studied with partial seizures secondarily generalized, infantile spasms, and tonic seizures was too small to establish the effectiveness of the drug. It appeared to be less effective than a benzodiazepine in infantile spasms and the Lennox-Gastaut syndrome.

In one double-blind crossover study, the efficacy of sodium valproate was judged to be comparable to that of ethosuximide in patients with absence seizures alone. Comparative studies of valproic acid with other anticonvulsants have been too limited to determine their relative efficacies.

Since this drug has been found to be useful in some patients who were refractory to all other anticonvulsants, it may warrant a trial in such patients regardless of seizure type.

ADVERSE REACTIONS AND PRECAUTIONS.

Gastrointestinal disturbances, primarily nausea and vomiting, occur in 9% of all patients but in 22% of children; diarrhea, abdominal cramps, and constipation were reported occasionally. Both increased and decreased appetite with accompanying change in weight were observed.

Sedation and drowsiness occurred in about 5% of patients but in only 0.2% of those receiving sodium valproate alone. These effects usually disappeared when the dosage of concurrently administered anticonvulsants was reduced. Central nervous system stimulation and excitement have been observed when the drug was given alone, and aggressiveness and hyperactivity were noted in some children. Other central nervous system effects reported rarely include ataxia, headache, and tremor. Mild postural tremor occurs frequently with larger doses.

Alopecia was reported in 0.5% of patients; this condition was usually temporary and did not necessitate withdrawal of the drug. Rash was observed rarely.

Valproic acid inhibits the secondary phase of platelet aggregation, but this is unlikely to be of clinical significance unless patients are receiving other drugs that affect coagulation. Prolonged bleeding times were reported in some studies, and children appeared to be particularly susceptible. Thrombocytopenia has been observed occasionally.

Increased serum alkaline phosphatase and glutamic oxaloacetic transaminase (SGOT) levels occurred in some patients who received sodium valproate with other anticonvulsants. Recent evidence shows that the elevated liver enzyme levels return to normal when the dose of valproic acid is reduced. However, severe hepatic dysfunction with fatalities has occurred in a few patients during the first six months of treatment with sodium valproate and other anticonvulsants. It is, therefore, advisable to perform baseline hepatic function studies prior to initiating therapy with this drug and periodically thereafter.

The drug has no significant effects on the autonomic and cardiovascular systems, respiration, body temperature, inflammatory responses, smooth muscle contractions, or renal activity.

Because valproic acid may affect platelet aggregation, it is advisable to determine bleeding time prior to initiating therapy, and platelet function should be monitored before major surgery in patients receiving the drug. Caution is recommended when administering drugs that affect coagulation to patients receiving valproic acid, and dosage adjustments should be made when necessary. If other anticonvulsants, particularly the barbiturates, are given concomitantly, serum levels should be determined periodically and the dosage adjusted if necessary to obtain optimum therapeutic levels.

Since valproic acid is partly eliminated as a ketone-containing metabolite, the urine ketone test may show false-positive results.

Studies have demonstrated that valproic acid has teratogenic effects in mice, rats, and rabbits, usually manifested as increased resorption, retarded fetal growth, and major developmental abnormalities, including skeletal defects. The incidence was about the same as that observed when phenytoin was given at similar dose levels. In the few patients reported to have received sodium valproate during pregnancy, no congenital abnormalities were observed. Nevertheless, physicians should carefully consider the possible risk versus benefit when prescribing valproic acid to women of childbearing potential. (See the Introduction.)

OVERDOSAGE.

One case of overdosage of sodium valproate (36 g) taken with phenobarbital (1 g) and phenytoin (300 mg) has been reported. The patient became comatose about four hours after ingesting the drugs but gradually recovered and was discharged from the hospital on the following day. The treatment of overdosage consists of general supportive measures, including maintenance of adequate urinary output in order to facilitate elimination of the drug.

DRUG INTERACTIONS.

An enhanced sedative effect occurs when valproic acid is given with phenobarbital; this may, in part, result from an increase in the serum level of phenobarbital, but the mechanism for this effect is not known. Valproic acid does not induce liver enzymes as do some other anticonvulsants. Increased blood levels of primidone also have been observed when this drug was administered with sodium valproate.

Valproic acid displaces phenytoin from serum proteins. An increase in the free phenytoin plasma level with a decrease of the total phenytoin level was observed. Thus, when the two drugs are administered concurrently, blood levels of phenytoin should be determined and the dose adjusted in accordance with the patient's clinical response. Usually, two or more weeks are required to evaluate effectiveness.

Other interactions between valproic acid and phenobarbital, primidone, phenytoin, and carbamazepine may result from the enzyme-inducing effects of the latter drugs which would reduce the half-life of valproic acid. The half-life was not affected by ethosuximide or the benzodiazepines.

There are reports that absence status epilepticus developed in a few patients receiving clonazepam with valproic acid.

ROUTE, USUAL DOSAGE, AND PREPARATIONS. Valproic acid is absorbed rapidly following oral administration; peak blood levels occur in one to four hours. If taken with food, absorption is delayed but the total amount absorbed is unaffected. Although reports of the plasma half-life of valproic acid have varied, the clinically significant range is about 8 to 12 hours. Serum concentrations vary widely among patients, and the correlation between dose, serum concentration, and clinical efficacy has not been well established. Thus, a therapeutic serum concentration cannot be definitely stated, although ranges between 50 and 100 mcg/ml have been reported most often. The dosage must be individualized.

Oral: *Adults and children*, initially, the usual daily dose is 15 mg/kg of body weight given in divided doses; this may be increased by 5 to 10 mg/kg/day at weekly intervals, depending upon the patient's response and the development of adverse reactions. Doses as high as 60 mg/kg daily may be necessary in some patients.

   Depakene (Abbott). Capsules 250 mg; syrup containing the equivalent of 250 mg valproic acid/5 ml as the sodium salt.

ACETAZOLAMIDE
[Diamox]

This carbonic anhydrase inhibitor has been effective in several forms of epilepsy, most commonly in absence, generalized tonic-clonic, and focal seizures. It is most useful as an adjunct to other drugs; however, its usefulness is limited by the rapid development of tolerance. Acetazolamide is often helpful when intermittent administration is required (eg, in women whose convulsive tendencies increase with menstruation).

For a discussion of adverse reactions and other uses, see Chapter 22, Agents Used to Treat Glaucoma.

ROUTE, USUAL DOSAGE, AND PREPARATIONS. *Oral*: *Adults and children*, 8 to 30 mg/kg of body weight daily in divided doses (range, 375 mg to 1 g daily).

> Drug available generically: Capsules (plain, timed-release) 500 mg; tablets 250 mg.
> *Diamox* (Lederle). Capsules (timed-release) 500 mg; tablets 125 and 250 mg.

PARALDEHYDE

This drug may be used in status epilepticus when other agents are not effective. It should not be given undiluted, and intravenous administration must be slow or severe coughing ensues that may add to the difficulty of administration and may even cause pulmonary hemorrhage. Dilution in sodium chloride injection and administration by drip usually is preferred. Intramuscular injection, although often very irritating, is relatively safe if care is taken to avoid peripheral nerves. Rectal administration also is employed, most commonly in children; however, the dose is more difficult to control by this route. Thrombophlebitis is a frequent complication of intravenous administration.

Fatalities have occurred with use of paraldehyde. Bronchopulmonary disease is a relative contraindication, since a significant amount is excreted by the lungs. The sedative effect may be intensified and prolonged in patients with liver damage. Care must be taken to avoid use of decomposed drug. (See also Chapter 11, Drugs Used for Anxiety and Insomnia.)

ROUTES, USUAL DOSAGE, AND PREPARATIONS. *Intramuscular, Intravenous*: *Adults and children*, for status epilepticus, suggested doses have varied but frequently exceed those given for more benign conditions. The usual dose is 0.15 ml/kg of body weight; sometimes a moderate additional dose may be needed, especially for smaller children. Intravenous injection must be slow, preferably by drip, and the drug should be diluted in sodium chloride injection. Care should be taken to avoid extravasation.

> Drug available generically: Liquid 900 mg/ml in 2, 5, 10, and 30 ml containers.

Rectal: *Children*, 0.3 ml/kg of body weight, with the drug dissolved in an equal quantity of olive oil. Dilution in milk also has been suggested to improve tolerance.

> Drug available generically: Liquid in 30 ml containers.

LIDOCAINE HYDROCHLORIDE
[Xylocaine Hydrochloride]

As an alternative to general anesthesia, this local anesthetic is sometimes infused intravenously in status epilepticus as a last resort after the drugs of choice have failed. However, with overdosage, lidocaine itself is a convulsant and great care is required with its use. (See also Chapter 19, Local Anesthetics, and Chapter 34, Antiarrhythmic Agents.)

ROUTE, USUAL DOSAGE, AND PREPARATIONS. *Intravenous*: An appropriate intravenous solution of lidocaine is administered by continuous infusion at a rate of 1 to 3 mg/min, using a pump if possible. Usually, control of seizures will be achieved with the patient maintaining consciousness. The rate of infusion is reduced periodically until the drug can be discontinued; this

244

may require several days.

Drug available generically: Solution (without preservatives) 1% and 2% in 2 to 50 ml containers.

Xylocaine Hydrochloride (Astra). Solution (without sodium chloride or preservatives) 1 and 2 g additive syringes and single-use vials.

MIXTURES

A small number of fixed-dosage combinations of anticonvulsants are marketed. Two of them are listed below only to acknowledge their availability. Their use for initial therapy is not advisable since, in the management of epilepsy, the dosage of each drug should be established *individually* in accordance with clinical response and drug plasma levels. If this has been done and the concentrations present in a mixture correspond to the ratio and quantities required by a patient, a combination product may be used for convenience until a subsequent dosage adjustment becomes necessary.

Dilantin [sodium] with Phenobarbital (Parke, Davis). Each capsule contains phenytoin sodium 100 mg and phenobarbital 16 or 32 mg.

Phelantin (Parke, Davis). Each capsule contains phenytoin sodium 100 mg, phenobarbital 30 mg, and methamphetamine hydrochloride 2.5 mg.

Selected References

Aird RB, Woodbury DM: *The Management of Epilepsy.* Springfield, Ill, Charles C Thomas Publisher, 1974.

Bertilsson L: Clinical pharmacokinetics of carbamazepine. *Clin Pharmacokinet* 3:128-143, 1978.

Bochner F, Eadie MJ: Treatment of seizure disorders. *Ration Drug Ther* 12:1-6, (Dec) 1978.

Browne TR: Clinical pharmacology of antiepileptic drugs. *Am J Hosp Pharm* 35:1048-1056, 1978.

Browne TR: Drug therapy of status epilepticus. *Am J Hosp Pharm* 35:915-922, 1978.

Browne TR: Clonazepam: Review of new anticonvulsant drug. *Arch Neurol* 33:326-332, 1976.

Bruni J, Wilder BJ: Valproic acid: Review of new antiepileptic drug. *Arch Neurol* 36:393-398, 1979.

Committee on Drugs, American Academy of Pediatrics: Anticonvulsants and pregnancy. *Pediatrics* 63:331-333, 1979.

Dreifuss FE: Use of anticonvulsant drugs. *JAMA* 241:607-609, 1979.

Eadie MJ: Plasma level monitoring of anticonvulsants. *Clin Pharmacokinet* 1:52-66, 1976.

Fishman MA: Febrile seizures: Treatment controversy. *J Pediatr* 94:177-184, 1979.

Hill RM: Fetal malformations and antiepileptic drugs. *Am J Dis Child* 130:923-925, 1976.

Hvidberg EF, Dam M: Clinical pharmacokinetics of anticonvulsants. *Clin Pharmacokinet* 1:161-188, 1976.

Lewis JR: Valproic acid (Depakene). A new anticonvulsant agent. *JAMA* 240:2190-2192, 1978.

Livingston S: Medical treatment of epilepsy, parts I and II. *South Med J* 71:298-310, 432-447, 1978.

Livingston S: *Comprehensive Management of Epilepsy in Infancy, Childhood and Adolescence.* Springfield, Ill, Charles C Thomas Publisher, 1972.

Ludden TM, et al: Individualization of phenytoin dosage regimens. *Clin Pharmacol Ther* 21:287-293, 1977.

Mullen PW: Optimal phenytoin therapy: New technique for individualizing dosage. *Clin Pharmacol Ther* 23:228-232, 1978.

Penry JK (ed): *Epilepsy: The Eighth International Symposium.* New York, Raven Press, 1977.

Penry JK, Newmark ME: Use of antiepileptic drugs. *Ann Intern Med* 90:207-218, 1979.

Richens A: Interactions with antiepileptic drugs. *Drugs* 13:266-275, 1977.

Woo E, Greenblatt DJ: Choosing right phenytoin dosage. *Drug Ther* 7:131-139, (Oct) 1977.

Woodbury DM, et al (eds): *Antiepileptic Drugs.* New York, Raven Press, 1972.

Drugs Used in Extrapyramidal Movement Disorders | 16

PARKINSONISM

Introduction

Drugs with Central Anticholinergic
   Activity

   General Evaluation

   Adverse Reactions and Precautions

Drugs Affecting Brain Dopamine

   Dopamine-Releasing Drug

   Drugs That Increase Brain Levels of
      Dopamine

   Dopaminergic Agonist

CHOREA

   Huntington's Disease

   Tardive Dyskinesia

   Individual Evaluations

Dopamine is believed to act principally as an inhibitory and acetylcholine as an excitatory neurotransmitter within the nigrostriatal pathways of the extrapyramidal motor system. The dopaminergic pathway is the more prominent of the two systems; however, proper balance between the levels of acetylcholine and dopamine in the neostriatum is important for normal function. Imbalance can result in hypokinetic-hypertonic or hyperkinetic-hypotonic movement disorders represented by parkinsonism and chorea, respectively.

PARKINSONISM

The extrapyramidal manifestations of parkinsonism result from dopamine deficiency in the neostriatum, which may be part of a more generalized structural and enzymatic defect. Degeneration of the large pigmented neurons in the substantia nigra is a characteristic neuropathologic change in patients with idiopathic or post-encephalitic parkinsonism, and dopamine depletion is proportional to the amount of cell loss. Treatment of parkinsonism is directed toward enhancement of the dopaminergic system by replenishing striatal dopamine and, to a lesser extent, inhibition of the cholinergic system by blocking central cholinergic receptors (Calne, 1977; Yahr, 1977).

Cognitive, perceptual, and memory deficits and frank clinical dementia occur and cause significant clinical disability in at least one-third of patients (Lieberman,

1979); these symptoms are best correlated with cortical atrophy. Parkinsonian symptoms also may be associated with more extensive central nervous system disorders: progressive supranuclear palsy, Shy-Drager syndrome, olivopontocerebellar atrophy, Wilson's disease, and the juvenile (rigid) form of Huntington's disease. Similar signs and symptoms are produced by midbrain tumors or injury to the central nervous system caused by chronic manganese, carbon monoxide, carbon tetrachloride, or carbon disulfide intoxication. Drug-induced parkinsonism may result from dopamine receptor blockade by the antipsychotic drugs used to treat schizophrenia or depletion of brain dopamine by rauwolfia alkaloids.

The goals in the treatment of parkinsonism are to provide maximum symptomatic relief and to maintain some independence of movement and activity for the patient's lifetime. Therapy is palliative, not curative. Major symptoms (bradykinesia, rigidity, tremor, disorders of posture and equilibrium) can be relieved to varying degrees by drug therapy. The best results are obtained in patients who are willing and able to tolerate some side effects. A total program also should include physiotherapy, exercise, recreation, and psychological support.

The choice of antiparkinsonism drugs (see Table 1) is related principally to the severity of the disease at the time of diagnosis. Relatively inactive patients with

Table 1.
DRUG THERAPY FOR PARKINSONISM

Drug	Comment

CENTRALLY ACTIVE ANTICHOLINERGIC DRUGS
Anticholinergic Agents
   Benztropine [Cogentin]
   Biperiden [Akineton]
   Cycrimine [Pagitane]
   Procyclidine [Kemadrin]
   Trihexyphenidyl [Artane, Tremin]
Antihistamines
   Chlorphenoxamine [Phenoxene]
   Diphenhydramine [Benadryl]
   Orphenadrine [Disipal]
Phenothiazine
   Ethopropazine [Parsidol]
	These drugs are less effective than levodopa, but they are useful in patients with mild involvement in whom anticholinergic therapy is not contraindicated because of age or the presence of illnesses, such as angle-closure glaucoma. They may also be useful as adjuncts to the more potent drugs.

DRUGS AFFECTING BRAIN DOPAMINE Dopamine-Releasing Drug Amantadine [Symmetrel]	This drug is also less effective than levodopa. It can be used as an alternative in patients who cannot tolerate the central anticholinergic drugs or in whom these drugs are contraindicated. It is used occasionally as adjunctive therapy with the latter drugs and/or levodopa in patients who do not respond adequately to therapy.

Drugs That Increase Brain Levels of Dopamine
   Levodopa [Dopar, Larodopa]
   Levodopa and Carbidopa [Sinemet]
	Levodopa is more effective than the central anticholinergic agents or amantadine. It is the drug of choice for productive patients who are moderately affected, especially those with locomotor impairment. The combination of levodopa and the dopa decarboxylase inhibitor, carbidopa, is preferred by many physicians, even for initial levodopa therapy, because higher brain concentrations of levodopa are attained with fewer peripheral side effects than with a comparable dose of levodopa alone.

Table 1.
DRUG THERAPY FOR PARKINSONISM

Drug	Comment
Deprenyl (Investigational)	This drug is a relatively specific inhibitor of type B monoamine oxidase that prolongs the normal degradation of dopamine. The definitive role of deprenyl in parkinsonism therapy is not established.
Dopaminergic Agonist Bromocriptine [Parlodel] (Investigational for treatment of parkinsonism)	This drug is not an initial drug of choice. It is reserved for patients in whom levodopa therapy is contraindicated or not tolerated or it is used with levodopa in patients with severe end-of-dose or on-off adverse reactions.

minimal involvement and no other illness may not require medication. As pathogenesis progresses, use of a drug with central anticholinergic activity should be considered. Amantadine [Symmetrel] may be a better choice for patients in whom drugs with central anticholinergic activity are relatively contraindicated. There is evidence that the combination of an anticholinergic drug and amantadine has an additive effect.

Levodopa [Dopar, Larodopa] is the drug of choice for symptomatic patients without concomitant illness who have locomotor impairment sufficient to limit productivity. Since adverse reactions, particularly those affecting the gastrointestinal tract, are common and often intolerable, therapy usually is initiated with a product combining levodopa and one of two dopa decarboxylase inhibitors (ie, with carbidopa [Sinemet], with benserazide [Madopar]). Sinemet contains carbidopa and levodopa in a ratio of 1:10 (see the evaluation) and Madopar contains benserazide and levodopa in a ratio of 1:4. The latter product is not available in the United States; however, it has been extensively compared with Sinemet. Although some patients may respond better to one preparation than the other, no major differences in efficacy or safety exist between Sinemet and Madopar (Diamond et al, 1978; Lieberman et al, 1978).

The dopaminergic agonist, bromocriptine [Parlodel], is used in the treatment of neuroendocrinologic disorders (see the evaluation), but it is currently being investigated for use in the treatment of parkinsonism. Bromocriptine is not as effective as levodopa in all patients; therefore, it is generally reserved for use when levodopa is contraindicated, cannot be tolerated, or when patients are having significant fluctuations in therapeutic response to levodopa.

After two to five years, responsiveness to the antiparkinsonian action of levodopa gradually diminishes, which is commonly associated with end-of-dose akinesia, on-off phenomena, and/or psychic disturbances; therefore, the prolonged usefulness of levodopa is ultimately limited. Bromocriptine or amantadine has been added to the regimen of these individuals, but neither drug is uniformly effective in reducing the incidence or severity of such adverse reactions or in stabilizing the response for more than a limited period. If current investigational studies are confirmed, relatively specific type B monoamine oxidase inhibitors, such as deprenyl, which prolong the action of dopamine, also may help to alleviate levodopa-induced on-off phenomena.

DRUGS WITH CENTRAL ANTICHOLINERGIC ACTIVITY

General Evaluation: The efficacy of these drugs appears to be related to their central cholinergic blocking action, since quaternary ammonium anticholinergic agents, which do not readily cross the blood-brain barrier, do not alleviate parkinsonian symptoms.

The belladonna alkaloids, atropine and scopolamine, were the first centrally acting anticholinergic agents used in parkinsonism. They have been largely supplanted by synthetic drugs that are equally effective but produce fewer peripheral side effects. These include the piperidyl compounds (trihexyphenidyl [Artane, Tremin] and its analogues, biperiden [Akineton], cycrimine [Pagitane], and procyclidine [Kemadrin]) and the tropanol derivative, benztropine [Cogentin]. The antihistamines (diphenhydramine [Benadryl], chlorphenoxamine [Phenoxene], and orphenadrine [Disipal]) and the phenothiazine derivative, ethopropazine [Parsidol], have some antiparkinson activity that has been attributed to their anticholinergic properties.

When initiating therapy with anti-cholinergic drugs, the dose should be small and increased gradually until maximal benefits are attained or unacceptable untoward effects occur (see Table 2). Patients with postencephalitic parkinsonism may tolerate larger doses than those with the idiopathic form. The dosage should be adjusted gradually, because sudden withdrawal of any agent that has given some degree of relief may cause a marked exacerbation of symptoms. If the initial drug is well tolerated but fails to provide improvement after an adequate trial, another anticholinergic drug may be tried. In most patients not receiving levodopa, the maximal tolerated dose of a single anticholinergic drug often does not provide adequate symptomatic relief. In such instances, a second and, if needed, a third drug from another class may be added; the dose of each drug should be individualized. The duration of action of these anticholinergic drugs differs (see Table 2), and patients may tolerate one drug better

Table 2.
CENTRALLY ACTIVE ANTICHOLINERGIC DRUGS

Drug	Chemical Structure
PIPERIDYL COMPOUNDS Biperiden	
Cycrimine Hydrochloride	
Procyclidine Hydrochloride	

than another. Otherwise, none has any advantages over the others.

Trihexyphenidyl, one of its analogues, or benztropine is usually preferred for initiating therapy. Levodopa or an anticholinergic agent from another class may be added later if needed. When therapy is initiated with levodopa, one of these agents may be added later to achieve maximal improvement. Ethopropazine and the antihistamines, particularly diphenhydramine, are used primarily as adjuncts. In addition to their antiparkinson activity, antihistamines have a sedative effect that helps counteract the insomnia that may follow use of levodopa and the potent anticholinergic drugs. They may be used alone for initial therapy in patients with mild parkinsonism and for maintenance therapy in elderly patients who cannot tolerate the more potent anticholinergic drugs.

After long-term administration of anticholinergic agents, patients frequently become refractory to their effects. This often is caused by progression of the disease, but extraneous factors, such as trauma, unrelated illness, or emotional stress, may exacerbate symptoms. Increasing the dose or substituting a drug from another class may restore responsiveness.

The anticholinergic and antihistamine drugs also are used to control the extrapyramidal reactions, except tardive dyskinesia, induced by the antipsychotic drugs. Diphenhydramine often is preferred because of its low toxicity. Excluding tardive dyskinesia, many drug-induced extrapyramidal reactions have a limited course (three months), but symptoms may recur when anticholinergic drugs are withdrawn after three months of therapy.

Adverse Reactions and Precautions: Most untoward effects are related to the peripheral or central cholinergic blocking activity of these drugs. Adverse effects occur least frequently with the antihistamines and ethopropazine, for their anti-

Usual Dosage	Preparations
Oral: For idiopathic and postencephalitic parkinsonism, *adults,* initially, 2 mg three times daily. The dose may be gradually increased up to 20 mg daily if required and tolerated. For drug-induced extrapyramidal reactions, *adults,* 2 mg one to three times daily.	Akineton (Knoll) Tablets 2 mg [hydrochloride salt]. Solution (for injection) 5 mg in 1 ml containers [lactate salt].
Intramuscular: For drug-induced extrapyramidal reactions, except tardive dyskinesia, *adults,* 2 mg; *children,* 0.04 mg/kg of body weight. This dose may be repeated every one-half hour if required, but no more than four consecutive doses should be given within a 24-hour period.	
Oral: For idiopathic and postencephalitic parkinsonism, *adults,* initially, 1.25 mg three times daily. The dose may be gradually increased to 12.5 to 20 mg daily if required and tolerated.	Pagitane Hydrochloride (Lilly) Tablets 1.25 and 2.5 mg.
Oral: For idiopathic and postencephalitic parkinsonism, *adults,* initially, 5 mg twice daily. The dose may be increased gradually to 20 to 30 mg daily if required and tolerated. For drug-induced extrapyramidal reactions, except tardive dyskinesia, *adults,* initially, 2 to 2.5 mg three times daily. The dose may then be increased by increments of 2 to 2.5 mg daily until symptoms are controlled. Generally, symptomatic relief is obtained with a dose of 10 to 20 mg daily.	Kemadrin (Burroughs Wellcome) Tablets 2 and 5 mg.

Drug	Chemical Structure
Trihexyphenidyl Hydrochloride	
TROPANOL DERIVATIVES Benztropine Mesylate	
ANTIHISTAMINES Chlorphenoxamine Hydrochloride	
Diphenhydramine Hydrochloride	
Orphenadrine Hydrochloride	
PHENOTHIAZINE Ethopropazine	

Usual Dosage	Preparations
Oral: (Tablets or elixir is preferred, as the efficacy of timed-release capsules has not been established.) For idiopathic and postencephalitic parkinsonism, *adults,* initially, 2 mg two or three times daily. The dose is gradually increased until the desired therapeutic effect is obtained or until severe adverse reactions preclude a further increase. Doses larger than 15 to 20 mg daily are rarely required or tolerated, but some patients with postencephalitic parkinsonism may tolerate 40 to 50 mg daily. For drug-induced extrapyramidal reactions, except tardive dyskinesia, *adults,* initially, 1 mg. If symptoms are not controlled within a few hours, subsequent doses are increased until symptoms subside. The usual total daily dose is 5 to 15 mg.	Artane (Lederle) Capsules (timed-release) 5 mg; elixir 2 mg/5 ml; tablets 2 and 5 mg. Tremin (Schering) Tablets 2 and 5 mg.
Oral: For idiopathic and postencephalitic parkinsonism, *adults,* initially, 0.5 to 1 mg at bedtime. Patients with postencephalitic parkinsonism often tolerate an initial dose of 2 mg. The dosage may be gradually increased to 4 to 6 mg daily if required and tolerated. *Oral, Intramuscular, Intravenous:* For drug-induced extrapyramidal reactions, except tardive dyskinesia, *adults,* 1 to 4 mg once or twice daily. In acute dystonic reactions, initially, 2 mg intravenously; to prevent recurrence, 1 to 2 mg orally twice daily.	Cogentin (Merck Sharpe & Dohme) Tablets 0.5, 1, and 2 mg. Solution (for injection) 1 mg/ml in 2 ml containers.
Oral: For idiopathic and postencephalitic parkinsonism, *adults,* initially, 50 mg three times daily. The dosage may be gradually increased to 100 mg two to four times daily if needed.	Phenoxene (Dow) Tablets 50 mg.
Oral: For idiopathic and postencephalitic parkinsonism, *adults,* initially, 25 mg three times daily. The dosage may be gradually increased to 50 mg four times daily if required. *Intramuscular (deep), Intravenous:* For drug-induced extrapyramidal reactions, except tardive dyskinesia, *adults,* 10 to 50 mg. The maximal single dose is 100 mg and the total daily dose should not exceed 400 mg. *Children* (intramuscular), 5 mg/kg of body weight daily. The maximal daily dose should not exceed 300 mg in 24 hours.	Benadryl (Parke, Davis) Capsules 25 and 50 mg; elixir 12.5 mg/5 ml. Solution (for injection) 10 mg/ml in 10 and 30 ml containers and 50 mg/ml in 1 and 10 ml containers.
Oral: For idiopathic and postencephalitic parkinsonism, *adults,* initially, 50 mg three times daily. The dosage may be gradually increased up to 250 mg daily if required and tolerated.	Disipal (Riker) Tablets 50 mg.
Oral: For idiopathic and postencephalitic parkinsonism, *adults,* initially, 50 mg once or twice daily. The dosage may be gradually increased, if required, to a total daily dose of 100 to 400 mg in mild or moderate cases. Patients with severe impairment may require 500 to 600 mg.	Parsidol (Parke, Davis) Tablets 10, 50, and 100 mg.

cholinergic activity is milder. However, some degree of undesirable effects can be expected with use of therapeutic doses of any of these agents.

The most common adverse reactions are dryness of the mouth, mydriasis, cycloplegia, tachycardia, constipation, urinary retention, and psychic disturbances. Patients with prostatic hypertrophy should be observed carefully for signs of urinary retention, and those with gastrointestinal disorders should be monitored for signs of intestinal obstruction. Fatal adynamic ileus has occurred in patients receiving combinations of drugs with anticholinergic properties. Patients with a tendency to develop tachycardia should receive the smallest effective dose. Large doses of anticholinergic drugs can markedly elevate body temperature.

Because of their mydriatic effect, the physician should be aware of the possible occurrence of glaucoma. The anticholinergic drugs could precipitate an attack of acute glaucoma in patients predisposed to angle closure; this has occurred occasionally after parenteral administration of these agents but has been reported only rarely after oral use. Anticholinergic drugs can be given safely to patients with open-angle glaucoma who are receiving miotics.

Mental confusion and excitement may occur with large doses or in susceptible patients (eg, the elderly, patients with existing mental disorders, those taking additional medications that have appreciable anticholinergic activity). Serious mental disturbances include agitation, disorientation, delirium, paranoid reaction, and hallucinations, which may be drug-induced or represent an intensification of existing mental symptoms. These patients should be kept under careful observation, especially at the beginning of treatment or if doses are increased. The antihistamines may be preferred for use in susceptible patients.

The antihistamines have some adverse effects that are unrelated to their anticholinergic action. Drowsiness and dizziness are common with therapeutic doses. Anorexia, nausea, and vomiting may occur. Other reactions reported occasionally include euphoria, hypotension, headache, weakness, tingling, and heaviness of the hands.

Drowsiness, dizziness, inability to concentrate, and confusion are the most common adverse effects of ethopropazine. Mild anticholinergic side effects also have been reported. Muscular cramps, epigastric discomfort, paresthesia, heaviness of the limbs, hypotension, and rash occur occasionally.

Acute anticholinergic withdrawal can cause a rebound worsening of parkinsonism; therefore, anticholinergics should be withdrawn slowly unless they are being discontinued because of acute toxicity.

DRUGS AFFECTING BRAIN DOPAMINE

Dopamine-Releasing Drug

AMANTADINE HYDROCHLORIDE
[Symmetrel]

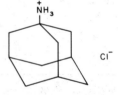

This antiviral agent moderately reduces the severity of signs and symptoms and improves functional capacity in some patients with parkinsonism. It acts by augmenting the release of dopamine and other catecholamines from neuronal storage sites and delaying reuptake of these neurotransmitters into synaptic vesicles. Amantadine is considerably less effective than levodopa, but it produces a more rapid response (two to five days), fewer untoward reactions, and the dosage is easier to adjust. Initial clinical improvement may not be sustained, however, and performance may deteriorate after three to six months of therapy (Timberlake and Vance, 1978).

Amantadine may be used alone for initial therapy but is most useful when given with anticholinergic drugs or levodopa. This agent is particularly beneficial in patients who cannot tolerate maximally effective doses of levodopa or in whom the response to levodopa fluctuates. It also may be helpful when used with levodopa initially to provide immediate therapeutic benefit.

Amantadine is well absorbed orally; the half-life ranges from 10 to 28.5 hours. Since over 90% of this drug is excreted unchanged in the urine, the dosage must be adjusted in patients with renal impairment. Excretion is more rapid in acidic urine.

Amantadine is usually well tolerated. Some of the adverse effects reported occasionally are similar to those produced by anticholinergic agents: dizziness, nervousness, inability to concentrate, ataxia, slurred speech, insomnia, lethargy, blurred vision, dryness of the mouth, gastrointestinal upset, and rash.

Both the peripheral and central adverse effects of anticholinergic drugs are increased by amantadine. In some patients, combined therapy has induced acute psychotic reactions identical to those caused by atropine poisoning. If signs of central toxicity occur during combined therapy, the dose of the anticholinergic drug should be reduced. Results of anecdotal reports indicate that physostigmine may be of value in severe amantadine intoxication. Psychotic reactions also have occurred occasionally in patients receiving amantadine with levodopa.

Livedo reticularis is a relatively common adverse effect in patients (particularly women) receiving amantadine for one month or longer. This reaction may subside during continued administration but can persist throughout the period of administration. It disappeared gradually over a period of 2 to 12 weeks in all patients after amantadine was discontinued. Laboratory studies have not revealed an association between livedo reticularis and any underlying systemic disorder.

Edema of the ankles (usually associated with livedo reticularis) has been noted in some patients. According to the manufacturer's literature, congestive heart failure has developed in some patients receiving amantadine.

ROUTE, USUAL DOSAGE, AND PREPARATIONS. *Oral*: For idiopathic or postencephalitic parkinsonism, *adults*, initially, 100 mg daily after breakfast for five to seven days. If adverse reactions do not occur during this period, an additional 100 mg is given after lunch. In some patients, the dosage has been gradually increased to 500 mg daily, but amounts exceeding 200 mg daily generally provide little additional symptomatic relief and may be associated with increasing toxicity out of proportion to clinical benefit.

Symmetrel (Endo). Capsules 100 mg; syrup 50 mg/5 ml.

Drugs That Increase Brain Levels Of Dopamine

LEVODOPA
[Dopar, Larodopa]

Although dopamine does not enter the brain in sufficient quantities to be of value in the treatment of parkinsonism, levodopa, its immediate precursor, penetrates the blood-brain barrier and is then converted to dopamine by the nonspecific enzyme, L-aromatic amino acid decarboxylase. The amount of this enzyme in peripheral tissues is far in excess of that in the brain and, therefore, large doses of levodopa are required to achieve therapeutic levels of dopamine in the central nervous system.

When administered in gradually increasing doses for an adequate period of time, levodopa relieves symptoms and improves functional capacity in most patients with parkinsonism. It does not halt progression of the disease. This drug is useful in both idiopathic and postencephalitic parkinsonism; patients with the postencephalitic form respond to lower doses.

All major symptoms of parkinsonism may be ameliorated by levodopa, particularly bradykinesia, rigidity, and, to a lesser extent, tremor. Balance, posture, gait, speed, and handwriting improve promptly to a variable degree, mood is often elevated, and seborrhea and drooling may be completely abolished. Although intellectual function may initially return to the premorbid level, mental deterioration and dementia usually develop during long-term therapy. This probably reflects loss of cortical neurons associated with progression of the disease rather than an effect of levodopa.

Although levodopa is more effective than the central anticholinergic drugs and amantadine, it is usually reserved for patients with significant functional impairment. In addition, it may be desirable to withhold levodopa until a later stage of disease because the treatment schedule is demanding, adverse effects are common, and the optimal response may be restricted to the first few years of therapy, regardless of when in the course of illness the drug is given. When initiating levodopa therapy in patients already receiving anticholinergic drugs, the latter medication should not be discontinued or the dosage reduced, for abrupt withdrawal of anticholinergic drugs often causes severe exacerbation of parkinsonian symptoms. If treatment is initiated with levodopa (or levodopa and carbidopa), anticholinergic drugs and/or amantadine may be added later, if needed, to achieve optimal effects. It is best to avoid combining an anticholinergic agent and levodopa, however, if there is a history of psychosis.

In addition to its use in Parkinson's disease, levodopa may be beneficial in other central nervous system disorders in which parkinsonian signs and symptoms are prominent (eg, juvenile form of Huntington's disease, chronic manganese poisoning). Levodopa generally does not reverse parkinsonian symptoms produced by antipsychotic drugs, presumably because this syndrome results from dopamine receptor blockade that cannot be overcome by additional quantities of dopamine.

ADVERSE REACTIONS AND PRECAUTIONS.

Gastrointestinal: Nausea, vomiting, and anorexia occur in most patients if the initial daily dose is large or if dosage is increased too rapidly. To avoid nausea and vomiting, dosage should be titrated slowly or small doses should be given in conjunction with a peripheral dopa decarboxylase inhibitor (eg, carbidopa). Symptoms usually are diminished by temporarily reducing the daily dose, by administering smaller doses more frequently, or by giving the drug with solid, high-protein food and omitting coffee. Nonphenothiazine antiemetics may be tried, but dopamine antagonists (eg, phenothiazines, thioxanthenes, butyrophenones, metoclopramide) should be avoided because they may counteract the therapeutic effect. Other gastrointestinal disturbances occasionally reported, but questionably related to levodopa therapy, include abdominal pain, diarrhea, constipation, and activation of peptic ulcer.

Neurologic: Abnormal involuntary movements often occur just preceding or soon after the optimal therapeutic response is observed and are the major dose-limiting factors in levodopa therapy. Mild, intermittent dyskinesias involving the mouth, tongue, face, and neck are common after a few months of therapy. Some tolerance develops to these dyskinesias, and many patients are willing to tolerate them in order to obtain the beneficial effects of levodopa.

Involuntary choreiform movements of the limbs, particularly the hands, usually appear later. Severe, generalized choreoathetoid movements generally occur after prolonged administration of large doses. They are closely associated with improved control of parkinsonism and may disappear when dosage is reduced, although the symptoms of parkinsonism then may increase. In some patients, involuntary movements recur at progressively lower doses.

Episodes of akinesia, tremor, and rigidity lasting a few minutes to several hours are common in patients receiving levodopa for more than one year. Three forms have been described: (1) End-of-dose akinesia (wearing off effect), which occurs at increasingly shorter intervals between doses and may be improved by reducing the interval between doses. (2) The on-off phenomenon, which appears unexpectedly, bears no relationship to the time of the last dose, and may be relieved by combined therapy with amantadine or bromocriptine in at least 50% of the patients affected. (3) Akinesia paradoxica, which is often precipitated by stress and may develop suddenly during a dyskinetic episode; no satisfactory treatment is available. Some physicians regard all three forms as examples of on-off phenomena.

Headache, peripheral neuropathy, mydriasis, widening of the palpebral fissures, and activation of Horner's syndrome occasionally have been associated with levodopa therapy.

Respiratory abnormalities may develop independent of therapy, most commonly in patients with postencephalitic parkinsonism, although some respiratory abnormalities may develop during drug therapy. Symptoms include coughing, hoarseness, postnasal drip, tachypnea, bradypnea, gasping, panting, sniffing, and feelings of pressure in the chest. These phenomena may represent dyskinesias of the diaphragm and intercostal muscles and are much more common in patients with parkinsonism and autonomic insufficiency (Shy-Drager syndrome). Severe bilateral paresis of vocal cords is common and life-threatening, and tracheostomy should be considered (Williams et al, 1979). Exacerbation of oculogyric crisis has been reported in postencephalitic patients.

Psychiatric: Psychic disturbances are common, particularly in elderly patients receiving other antiparkinsonian drugs, especially anticholinergics, concomitantly. Frequent symptoms are euphoria, restlessness, anxiety, irritability, hyperactivity, insomnia, hallucinations, and vivid dreams. Severe psychic disturbances (agitation, hypomanic and paranoid reactions, delirium, and aggressive or suicidal behavior) have occurred occasionally, most commonly in patients with pre-existing dementia or a history of mental illness; in some cases, the drug may unmask a previously unrecognized dementia. Reactions generally respond to a reduction in dosage but occasionally it may be necessary to discontinue levodopa.

Cardiovascular: If the initial daily dose of levodopa is large or increased too rapidly, the standing systolic and diastolic blood pressures may be reduced by 20 to 30 mm Hg. In most patients, this is well tolerated, but significant orthostatic hypotension may occur. This reaction tends to diminish in time and often can be alleviated by use of elastic bandages or stockings; however, a temporary reduction of dosage may be necessary. Indomethacin [Indocin], used adjunctively, has been reported to help relieve the orthostatic hypotension of this syndrome (Kochar and Itskovitz, 1978). Symptoms also can be alleviated by salt supplementation and, in extreme cases such as the Shy-Drager syndrome, by administration of a salt-retaining steroid; when these measures are employed, the patient should be closely monitored for symptoms of hypervolemia and, possibly, congestive heart failure.

Transient flushing of the skin is common during levodopa therapy. Palpitations may occur but often disappear with continued therapy. Both minor disturbances of cardiac rate and rhythm (tachycardia and premature ventricular contractions) and severe arrhythmias have developed occasionally. It is not clear whether levodopa was a causal factor, but cardiac rhythm should be monitored when dosage is being adjusted. Arrhythmias usually can be controlled by antiarrhythmic drugs and it is seldom necessary to discontinue therapy. No significant difference in the severity of ventricular arrhythmias or in the incidence of orthostatic hypotension occurred in patients receiving carbidopa and levodopa compared to levodopa alone (Leibowitz and Lieberman, 1975). Hypertension, myocardial infarction, and venous thrombosis have been reported occasionally, but there is no evidence that these complications are more common in patients receiving levodopa than in those of a comparable age group not receiving the drug. If myocardial infarction occurs during therapy, modification of the treatment program may be required.

Laboratory Findings: Results of laboratory studies have not revealed evidence of serious hematologic, renal, hepatic, or thyroid dysfunction due to levodopa. Hypokalemia associated with increased plasma levels of aldosterone may be produced by large doses. This effect is substantially reduced by adding carbidopa to the treatment program. Transitory depression of the white blood cell count has occurred in a few patients. A positive Coombs' test has been noted occasionally, and there have been a few reports of reduced hemoglobin and hematocrit levels unrelated to a hemolytic process. Hemolytic anemia of unknown etiology has occurred rarely. Mild, transient elevations of the blood urea nitrogen level may occur and usually can be controlled by increasing fluid intake. Elevation of the serum glutamic oxaloacetic transaminase level has been noted in a few patients, but this usually returned to normal despite continued drug administration. Increases in blood lactic dehydrogenase, bilirubin, and alkaline phosphatase levels have occurred rarely. Elevations of uric acid have been noted using the colorimetric method of measurement but have not been reported in tests using the uricase method. Levodopa increases plasma growth hormone levels and may produce carbohydrate intolerance, but no signs of acromegaly or diabetes mellitus have been found in patients on long-term therapy. Dark-colored sweat and changes in the color of the urine (red-tinged when voiding; black when exposed to air) have been reported but are not indications for discontinuing the drug.

Drug Interactions: Although levodopa is compatible with most drugs, a few adverse interactions have been reported. The therapeutic response to levodopa may be reduced or abolished by administration of pyridoxine in doses as low as 5 mg daily. This has been attributed to the accelerated decarboxylation of levodopa in peripheral tissues. Patients receiving levodopa should avoid multiple vitamin preparations containing more than the minimal daily requirement of pyridoxine (see Chapter 52, Vitamins and Minerals). The effectiveness of levodopa also may be reduced by phenothiazines, butyrophenones, rauwolfia alkaloids, benzodiazepines, and papaverine.

Since a hypertensive crisis may occur if levodopa is given with a nonspecific monoamine oxidase inhibitor, these drugs always should be discontinued two weeks prior to initiation of levodopa therapy. Methyldopa is a weak dopa decarboxylase inhibitor and therefore potentiates all of the central effects of levodopa, including the antiparkinsonian, emetic, and hypotensive effects. Additive hypotensive effects have been noted in patients receiving levodopa and guanethidine.

If general anesthetics are required during therapy, it has been recommended that levodopa be discontinued the night before anesthesia and reinstituted at the same dosage as soon as possible after surgery.

ROUTE, USUAL DOSAGE, AND PREPARATIONS. Levodopa should be given under close medical supervision and the dosage must be carefully individualized. When initiating therapy, individuals in good general health with only moderate neurologic impairment may be treated as outpatients if they are seen at regular intervals and good compliance is anticipated. Hospitalization should be reserved for patients with marked disability, those having co-existing systemic disorders that should be monitored daily, or those for whom drug administration cannot be properly supervised on an outpatient basis. All patients should be seen at regular intervals and the dosage modified as necessary for optimal results.

Oral: Levodopa is administered three to seven times daily during the waking hours. It should be given with food to reduce gastrointestinal disturbances. The initial daily dosage ranges from 300 mg to 1 g, depending upon the patient's tolerance. The daily dose may then be increased by increments of 100 to 500 mg every two or three days, or less frequently in patients who are less tolerant, until the desired therapeutic response is obtained or adverse reactions preclude a further increase. If adverse reactions are severe, the dose should be reduced or the drug discontinued temporarily. Optimal dosage generally is reached in six to eight weeks and usually ranges from 4 to 6 g daily. After several months to a year, a satisfactory clinical response often can be maintained with a lower dose.

Drug available generically: Capsules 125, 250, and 500 mg.
Dopar (Norwich-Eaton). Capsules 100, 250, and 500 mg.
Larodopa (Roche). Capsules and tablets 100, 250, and 500 mg.

LEVODOPA AND CARBIDOPA
[Sinemet]

Approximately 95% of an oral dose of levodopa is decarboxylated in peripheral tissues, leaving a greatly reduced quantity for diffusion across the blood-brain barrier. Thus, large doses are required to achieve therapeutic levels of dopamine in the central nervous system. These large doses frequently cause nausea and vomiting, presumably because of an effect of dopamine on the chemoreceptor trigger zone which is located outside of the blood-brain barrier.

Carbidopa is a dopa decarboxylase inhibitor that does not readily enter the central nervous system when given in small doses. By preventing the extracerebral metabolism of levodopa, carbidopa increases the amount of levodopa available for decarboxylation to dopamine in the brain, thereby enhancing the therapeutic response and reducing side effects caused by peripheral actions of dopamine and other catecholamines. Although carbidopa is available as a single-entity drug [Lodosyn], it is effective only when used with levodopa. Thus, carbidopa is primarily reserved for investigational use and the combination product [Sinemet] is recommended for general use.

Sinemet contains levodopa and carbidopa in a ratio of 10:1. This combination increases the plasma levels and half-life of levodopa. Dosage requirements for levodopa may be decreased by approximately 75%, and the incidence of nausea and vomiting is significantly reduced. Therefore, dosage increments can be added more rapidly and a therapeutic response is usually obtained in a shorter period of time. Sinemet is preferred by many physicians, even for initial therapy, because higher brain concentrations of levodopa are attained with fewer peripheral side effects than with a comparable dose of levodopa alone.

Approximately 15% of patients continue to experience nausea and vomiting; as with levodopa alone, these reactions can be minimized by giving the drug with food. Combined therapy does not significantly decrease the dyskinesias and psychiatric disturbances induced by levodopa alone. In fact, since dosage can be increased rapidly, these reactions may appear earlier and be more severe than with levodopa alone. Although carbidopa prevents the interaction between pyridoxine and levodopa, the amount in the formulations may not be sufficient to fully protect against this interaction in patients receiving supplemental doses of pyridoxine. In other respects, the adverse effects and interactions produced by this combination are similar to those seen with levodopa. No adverse reactions have been attributed to carbidopa alone.

ROUTE, USUAL DOSAGE, AND PREPARATIONS.
Like all fixed-dose combinations, Sinemet may not be suitable for all patients. Dosage must be titrated carefully to obtain the desired therapeutic response with minimal adverse effects. The patient should be carefully observed during dosage adjustment and, if adverse reactions are seen, the dose should be reduced or the compound temporarily discontinued.

Oral: Levodopa should be discontinued at least eight hours before initiating therapy with Sinemet. The initial daily dose should provide approximately 25% of the previous daily dose of levodopa. The suggested initial dosage is one tablet of Sinemet-10/100 three or four times daily for patients who have been maintained on less than 1.5 g of levodopa daily. Patients maintained on larger doses of levodopa may require one tablet of Sinemet-25/250 three or four times daily.

In patients who have not been receiving levodopa, therapy may be initiated with one tablet of Sinemet-10/100 three times daily. The amount may be increased gradually by one tablet every day or every other day up to six tablets daily. If a larger daily dose is needed, one tablet of Sinemet-25/250 three times daily may be given initially. This may be increased, if necessary, by increments of one-half to one tablet daily or every other day. The usual maintenance dosage is three to six tablets of Sinemet-25/250 daily in divided amounts (maximum, eight tablets daily). If further adjustment is indicated, levodopa may be added to the regimen.

> *Sinemet* (Merck Sharp & Dohme). Tablets containing carbidopa 10 mg and levodopa 100 mg [Sinemet-10/100] or carbidopa 25 mg and levodopa 250 mg [Sinemet-25/250].

DEPRENYL

Early clinical trials revealed that monoamine oxidase inhibitors potentiated the antiparkinsonian actions of levodopa, presumably by inhibiting the degradation of dopamine, but their concomitant use produced hypertension. Monoamine oxidase occurs in at least two forms which differ in substrate specificity: Type A is associated principally with the oxidative deamination of noradrenalin and serotonin; type B has similar activity for dopamine in human platelets and brain.

Deprenyl, a relatively specific type B monoamine oxidase inhibitor, is only available investigationally in the United States at present. A double-blind crossover study covering a six-month period was conducted in Europe to determine this drug's role in extending the duration of action and effectiveness of levodopa therapy (Lees et al, 1977). Total daily doses of 5 to 10 mg decreased the amount of levodopa required by an average of 200 mg daily. Deprenyl given with levodopa alone or levodopa plus carbidopa increased the duration of action of levodopa and was beneficial in overcoming early morning immobility and stiffness, but deprenyl relieved only mild on-off disabilities; however, a study in the United States (Yahr, 1978) demonstrated that deprenyl was quite effective in diminishing the incidence of on-off phenomena. Thus, this drug may play a somewhat limited but clinically significant role in the management of parkinsonism.

Deprenyl itself has no antiparkinsonian activity in doses up to 15 mg daily. It has been shown to be extensively metabolized to methamphetamine and amphetamine in man (Reynolds et al, 1978).

The most frequent adverse reaction noted is an increased incidence of dyskinesia which occurs in about one-third of patients and is severe and disabling in one-third of those affected. The incidence of nausea, dryness of the mouth, confusion, and dizziness is 10% to 20% and that of orthostatic hypotension, syncope, circumoral paresthesias, hallucinations, and unpleasant taste is 5% or less. Hypertension following ingestion of tyramine-containing foods and hepatotoxicity have not been observed; however, 1 patient in a group of 32 patients developed hypertension that resolved on cessation of deprenyl therapy.

ROUTE, USUAL DOSAGE, AND PREPARATIONS. *Oral*: The recommended daily dose is 5 mg. The amount may be increased to a maximum of 10 mg daily if no response occurs. Because deprenyl is a potent irreversible type B monoamine oxidase inhibitor, alternate-day treatment can be considered if a good response is obtained.

> *Deprenyl*. Tablets 5 and 10 mg (Investigational drug).

Dopaminergic Agonist

BROMOCRIPTINE MESYLATE
[Parlodel]

The gradual loss of responsiveness to levodopa over a period of one to five years may be caused in part by the continued loss of the nigrostriatal neurons' capacity to synthesize and store dopamine. This clinical assumption reinforced the search for specific drug agonists that act directly on striatal dopamine receptor sites. Bromocriptine, an ergoline derivative of ergot, is the most clinically useful dopaminergic agonist presently available. It is approved for use in neuroendocrinologic disorders, such as amenorrhea and galactorrhea (see Chapter 45, Agents Used To Treat Infertility), and is regarded as an investigational agent in acromegaly (see Chapter 46, Agents Related to Anterior Pituitary and Hypothalamic Function). Its use in parkinsonism also is investigational (Calne, 1978; Yahr, 1978; Lieberman et al, 1979; Parkes, 1979).

Although adequate doses of bromocriptine are more effective than the anticholinergic drugs and amantadine in parkinsonism, this drug is less effective than levodopa alone or with carbidopa; the latter is still the therapy of choice. Approximately 50% to 70% of patients given adequate doses of bromocriptine respond favorably. The remainder show no response or experience adverse effects severe enough to necessitate drug withdrawal.

The primary indications for bromocriptine therapy in parkinsonism are: (1) as an alternative to levodopa if that drug is contraindicated or not tolerated; (2) in patients who are unresponsive to levodopa (not all of these patients should be expected to respond to bromocriptine); and (3) combined with levodopa or levodopa and carbidopa in patients having significant fluctuations in therapeutic response, end-of-dose dystonia, and painful muscle cramps. Regarding the latter indication, this benefit is commonly observed only with larger doses and, therefore, adverse reactions to bromocriptine occur more often. When bromocriptine is used with the combination product, levodopa-carbidopa, the daily dose of the latter should be decreased as the amount of bromocriptine is increased.

There is considerable individual variation in response to bromocriptine. In one study utilizing a mean total daily dose of 10 mg, therapy had to be discontinued in 4 of 24 patients because of intolerable reactions, whereas 3 patients received 40 mg daily without adverse effects. Only careful titration of dose will determine the maximum benefit/risk ratio.

The following adverse reactions occur most commonly with mean total daily doses of 10 to 50 mg: Transient dizziness and nausea occur relatively frequently; administering bromocriptine with food or antacids, reducing the dose, and increasing the daily dose more gradually can be useful in alleviating nausea in more severe cases. Hypotension occurs less frequently but can be severe, even with doses of 2.5 mg, especially when initiating therapy. Colicky abdominal pain, constipation, blurred vision with or without diplopia, frequent extrasystoles, and digital vasospasm in response to cold are observed occasionally. Asymptomatic elevations of serum transaminase and alkaline phosphatase levels have been reported. No other liver function tests or routine laboratory values appear to be affected. Two cases of hepatotoxicity have been reported; the jaundice resolved on discontinuation of bromocriptine (Duvoisin et al, 1979; Lieberman et al, 1979).

More serious adverse reactions that generally occur with mean total daily doses of 50 to 100 mg (and are especially prominent when 100 to 150 mg is given) include erythromelalgia, mental disturbances, and dyskinesias. Erythromelalgia is characterized by red, tender, warm, edematous lower extremities. Mental disturbances may be limited to confusion and vivid dreams or, less frequently, paranoid delusions and visual hallucinations may occur. Dyskinesias are similar to the choreiform movements induced by levodopa. All of these effects are reversible.

ROUTE, USUAL DOSAGE, AND PREPARATIONS. *Oral*: Initially, 2.5 mg three or four times daily. The dose is increased weekly by increments of 2.5 mg over a period of three to eight weeks until beneficial effects or intolerable adverse effects are noted. A total daily dose of 30 mg is generally considered the minimal amount necessary to produce a therapeutic result, and 50 mg is the mean effective daily dose. A few individuals may require up to 100 mg daily (maximum, 150 mg daily).

> *Parlodel* (Sandoz). Tablets 2.5 mg (Investigational drug for treatment of parkinsonism.)

CHOREA

Huntington's Disease

Huntington's disease is a progressive autosomal dominant genetic disorder characterized by choreiform movements and behavioral abnormalities. It most often becomes manifest in the third to fifth decades. The disease is associated with diminished levels of acetylcholine and choline acetylase caused by widespread degenerative changes, principally in cholinergic interneurons in the striatum (Enna et al, 1977), which may result in a relative excess of dopamine. Juvenile-onset (first or second decade) Huntington's disease (the akinetic-rigid form of the disease) is characterized by bradykinesia and muscular hypertonicity which resembles parkinsonism more than chorea. Seizures and mental retardation are present in 10% of patients.

Chorea is the principal locomotor sign in other diseases, such as senile chorea and ballismus. It has been observed in some patients with vitamin B$_{12}$ deficiency, beriberi, hyperthyroidism, hypoparathyroidism, Addison's and Wilson's diseases, polycythemia, and systemic lupus erythematosus.

Drug Therapy: Therapy is aimed at either antagonizing brain dopamine activity or enhancing cholinergic activity. Most cases of adult-onset Huntington's disease are controlled by the antipsychotic agents, which antagonize dopamine. There is no specific drug of choice among the antipsychotic drugs, although those with minimal anticholinergic activity are usually chosen.

Although antipsychotic drugs are effective initially in reducing chorea in Hunt-

ington's disease, their long-term use can produce another form of chorea, tardive dyskinesia. The latter chorea is attributed to the development of supersensitivity to prolonged dopaminergic postsynaptic receptor antagonism. The dopamine-depleting drug, tetrabenazine [Nitoman] is also effective in reducing the chorea of Huntington's disease (de Silva, 1977; Toglia et al, 1978). Since tetrabenazine would not be expected to produce receptor supersensitivity as severe as that induced by postsynaptic dopamine receptor antagonists, it is considered a drug of choice by some physicians in Europe. The drug is not available in the United States.

Choline and deanol acetamidobenzoate [Deaner] have been claimed to enhance cholinergic activity. Deanol is a putative precursor of acetylcholine. Earlier controlled studies did not demonstrate that it has clinically significant antidepressant or cerebral stimulant actions. More recently, deanol has been investigated in the therapy of choreiform disorders. Controlled studies using oral doses up to 2 g daily for prolonged periods failed to demonstrate that the drug has any benefit in either Huntington's chorea or tardive dyskinesia (Caraceni et al, 1978). The ability of deanol to interfere with the transport of choline into the brain in spite of elevating plasma choline levels may explain these clinical failures (Millington et al, 1978). Choline has been reported to be effective in some patients (Davis et al, 1976); poor or absent responses probably reflect a less than normal complement of cholinergic receptors in the late stage of the disease.

Individuals with Huntington's disease experience a widespread loss of brain glutamic acid decarboxylase activity, suggesting a concomitant deficiency of the inhibitory neurotransmitter, gamma-aminobutyric acid (GABA). Baclofen [Lioresal], an analogue of GABA, has not been found to be useful in this disorder or in other types of chorea (see Chapter 17, Drugs Used to Treat Skeletal Muscle Hyperactivity); however, isoniazid produced clinical improvement in an open study of patients with Huntington's disease (Perry et al, 1979). Isoniazid inhibits the enzyme, GABA aminotransferase, and increases the GABA level in experimental animals. The dose required clinically was three to five times that normally used in tuberculosis; therefore, the use of isoniazid in Huntington's disease must be considered investigational and is not without risk.

Levodopa may be of value in juvenile-onset Huntington's disease, but it markedly increases the choreiform activity accompanying adult-onset Huntington's disease (third to fifth decade) and may aggravate the behavioral abnormalities. However, levodopa may be beneficial in adult-onset Huntington's chorea when levels of cerebrospinal fluid homovanillic acid are very low (Loeb et al, 1979). As in Parkinson's disease, drug therapy is palliative and not curative.

Tardive Dyskinesia

In the last decade, there has been an increase in the incidence of iatrogenic choreiform movement disorders. These occur most frequently after the prolonged use of antipsychotic drugs, which are dopamine receptor antagonists. The pathogenesis of this drug-induced disorder, termed tardive dyskinesia, has been attributed to the development of supersensitivity to postsynaptic dopamine receptors rather than to reduction of cholinergic activity as seen in Huntington's chorea. Both defects, however, result in similar brain acetylcholine/dopamine activity imbalances. Tardive dyskinesia is characterized by involuntary repetitive movements of the tongue, mouth, mandible, and face; the trunk and extremities also may be affected. It often follows abrupt cessation of prolonged antipsychotic drug therapy. Patients with primary affective disorders and chronic alcohol abuse may be especially susceptible (Rosenbaum et al, 1977).

Although anticholinergic therapy is useful in dystonia, parkinsonian dyskinesias, and in some patients with akathisia, it does not alleviate tardive dyskinesia. In fact, central anticholinergics tend to unmask or exacerbate tardive dyskinesia. The action is reversible and it may be of value as an aid in the early detection of tardive dyskinesia, and thus warns the physician to reduce antipsychotic dosage if possible (Chouinard et al, 1979).

Drug Therapy: No specific therapy is uniformly effective in all patients with tardive dyskinesia. For guidelines in preventing or lessening this condition, see Chapter 12, Antipsychotic Drugs.

If tardive dyskinesia appears during or after termination of antipsychotic drug therapy, the use of larger doses or reinstitution of drug therapy will usually terminate choreiform activity. Since the cause of tardive dyskinesia is assumed to be related to dopamine receptor supersensitivity, such therapy essentially masks the dyskinesia and is more likely to make it worse when the dose is again reduced. A long-term program (three to four years) designed to desensitize dopamine receptors resulted in the disappearance of tardive dyskinesia in 23 patients, improvement in 26 patients, and no change in 13 patients (Jus et al, 1979). The program included withdrawal, if possible, of central anticholinergic antiparkinsonism drugs; substitution, when indicated, of a sedative phenothiazine for the more potent piperazine phenothiazines with extrapyramidal actions; administration of small doses of either the dopamine depleting agent, reserpine (0.25 to 1 mg daily), or the dopamine antagonist, haloperidol (0.5 to 2 mg daily); then the progressive stepwise decrease of the antipsychotic dose to a level which still allowed adequate control of psychiatric symptoms.

Cholinergic agents have been used to obtain a more favorable acetylcholine/dopamine ratio in the brain; choline has been advocated for this use (Davis et al, 1976). Most studies have not been sufficiently long or doses have not been adequate to demonstrate the potential usefulness and final role of choline in controlling tardive dyskinesia. Since lecithin also has been shown to be effective in tardive dyskinesia and is easier to tolerate than choline, it may replace choline in the management of these disorders (Growdon et al, 1978; Gelenberg et al, 1979).

Experimentally, lithium has been shown to enhance the net transport of choline and the synthesis of acetylcholine in the brain (Millington et al, 1979) and/or to inhibit the development of dopamine receptor supersensitivity (Pert et al, 1978); these actions may explain the beneficial effect of lithium in tardive dyskinesia that has been reported anecdotally.

Although tetrabenazine is considered by some physicians in Europe to be the drug of choice for Huntington's chorea (de Silva, 1977; Toglia et al, 1978), it has not been evaluated sufficiently to determine its value in chorea associated with tardive dyskinesia. Since tetrabenazine is not available in the United States, reserpine in doses of 1 to 5 mg daily has been used as a substitute, but only modest success has been reported in uncontrolled studies. Initial anecdotal reports of the value of combining reserpine (3 to 6 mg daily) with the investigational drug, alpha methyltyrosine (250 mg to 1.5 g every other day), are encouraging.

INDIVIDUAL EVALUATIONS
CHOLINE
CHOLINE BITARTRATE
CHOLINE CHLORIDE
CHOLINE DIHYDROGEN CITRATE

Choline is a lipotropic agent, and 500 to 900 mg is provided by the average daily diet in the United States. It is well absorbed orally and is principally incorporated into phospholipids, lecithin, and sphingomyelin. A smaller amount is converted to acetylcholine, which accounts for its ability to increase the brain acetylcholine/dopamine ratio and thus suppress involuntary extrapyramidal movements.

Choline has been reported to be effective in patients with Huntington's disease (Davis et al, 1976) and choline or lecithin in tardive dyskinesia (Growdon et al, 1978; Gelenberg et al, 1979). Lecithin may be a better choice than choline, although the roles of these agents have not been definitively established in either of these choreas. A diagnostic test to determine the

probable response to choline employs methscopolamine and physostigmine: After pretreatment with 0.5 to 1 mg of methscopolamine bromide, 0.5 mg of physostigmine is given every five minutes until a satisfactory response, intolerable adverse effects, or a total dose of 3 mg has been administered. Lack of response generally indicates advanced neuronal degeneration with markedly reduced cholinoceptive receptors or too little choline acetylase activity. A positive response is an indication for oral choline therapy.

Adverse reactions occur in 5% to 15% of patients and include nausea, dizziness, lacrimation, blurred vision, diarrhea, and possibly a lengthened P-R interval. A peripheral anticholinergic agent may be administered simultaneously to control these reactions. An additional undesirable effect is the presence of a breath and body odor akin to dead fish caused by excretion of trimethylamine in sweat and urine. Clinical depression has been reported on occasion after choline therapy.

ROUTE, USUAL DOSAGE, AND PREPARATIONS. *Oral*: For management of disease- or drug-induced chorea, *adults*, initially, 1 g four times daily, with the amount gradually increased over a three- to eight-week period to a maximum of 4 to 5 g four times daily. Optimum therapy will generally increase the choline plasma level from a mean of 12 to 13 Nmol/ml before treatment to 30 to 40 Nmol/ml.

> Forms available generically: Tablets 250 mg (choline bitartrate); powder (choline chloride, choline dihydrogen citrate).

TETRABENAZINE
[Nitoman]

Although tetrabenazine is not approved or available for any specific use in the United States, a number of controlled studies suggest that this dopamine-depleting agent is effective in controlling the involuntary movements of Huntington's chorea and other hyperkinetic movement disorders (de Silva, 1977; Toglia et al, 1978). It was originally introduced as an antipsychotic drug with actions similar to reserpine, which it resembles pharmacologically. The drug does not possess many of the peripheral actions of reserpine, but it does have the central nervous system catecholamine-depleting activity. More long-term controlled studies are required to evaluate the role of tetrabenazine in the treatment of chorea.

The most frequent adverse reactions are drowsiness and depression. More serious, less frequent adverse reactions include orthostatic hypotension and dysphagia.

ROUTE, USUAL DOSAGE, AND PREPARATIONS. *Oral*: For management of disease- or drug-induced chorea, *adults*, initially, 25 mg four times daily, increased by increments of 25 mg daily every three to four days until the desired response is obtained, intolerable adverse effects occur, or a maximal daily dose of 200 mg is given.

(Investigational drug)

Selected References

Calne DB: Long-term treatment of parkinsonism with bromocriptine. *Lancet* 1:735-738, 1978.

Calne DB: Developments in pharmacology and therapeutics of parkinsonism. *Ann Neurol* 1:111-119, 1977.

Caraceni TA, et al: 2-dimethylaminoethanol (Deanol) in Huntington's chorea. *J Neurol Neurosurg Psychiatry* 41:1114-1118, 1978.

Chouinard G, et al: Tardive dyskinesia and antiparkinsonism medication. *Am J Psychiatry* 136:228-229, 1979.

Davis KL, et al: Choline in tardive dyskinesia and Huntington's disease. *Life Sci* 19:1507-1515, 1976.

de Silva L: Biochemical mechanisms and management of choreiform movement disorders. *Drugs* 14:300-310, 1977.

Diamond SG, et al: Double-blind comparison of levodopa, Madopa, and Sinemet in Parkinson disease. *Ann Neurol* 3:267-272, 1978.

Duvoisin RC, et al: Bromocriptine as adjuvant to levodopa, in Calne DB, Fuxe K (eds): *Dopaminergic Ergot Derivatives and Motor Function*. New York, Pergamon Press, 1979, 329-336.

Enna SJ, et al: Neurobiology and pharmacology of Huntington's disease. *Life Sci* 20:205-212, 1977.

Gelenberg AJ, et al: Choline and lecithin in treatment of tardive dyskinesia: Preliminary results from pilot study. *Am J Psychiatry* 136: 772-776, 1979.

Growdon JH, et al: Lecithin can suppress tardive dyskinesia. *N Engl J Med* 298:1029-1030, 1978.

Jus A, et al: Long term treatment of tardive dyskinesia. *J Clin Psychiatry* 40:72-77, 1979.

Kochar MS, Itskovitz HD: Treatment of idiopathic orthostatic hypotension (Shy-Drager syndrome) with indomethacin. *Lancet* 1:1011-1014, 1978.

Lees AJ, et al: Deprenyl in Parkinson's disease. *Lancet* 2:791-795, 1977.

Leibowitz M, Lieberman A: Comparison of dopa decarboxylase inhibitor (carbidopa) combined with levodopa and levodopa alone on cardiovascular system of patients with Parkinson's disease. *Neurology* 25:917-921, 1975.

Lieberman AN, et al: Dementia in Parkinson disease. *Arch Neurol* 6:355-359, 1979.

Lieberman AN, et al: Bromocriptine in Parkinson disease: Further studies. *Neurology* 29:363-369, 1979.

Lieberman A, et al: Comparative effectiveness of two extracerebral DOPA decarboxylase inhibitors in Parkinson disease. *Neurology* 28:964-968, 1978.

Loeb C, et al: Bromocriptine and dopaminergic function in Huntington disease. *Neurology* 29:730-734, 1979.

Millington WR, et al: Lithium and brain choline levels. *N Engl J Med* 300:196-197, 1979.

Millington WR, et al: Deanol acetamidobenzoate inhibits blood brain barrier transport of choline. *Ann Neurol* 4:302-306, 1978.

Parkes JD: Bromocriptine in treatment of parkinsonism. *Drugs* 17: 365-382, 1979.

Perry TL, et al: Isoniazid therapy of Huntington disease. *Neurology* 29:370-375, 1979.

Pert A, et al: Long-term treatment with lithium prevents development of dopamine receptor supersensitivity. *Science* 201:171-173, 1978.

Reynolds GP, et al: Deprenyl is metabolized to methamphetamine and amphetamine in man. *Br J Clin Pharmacol* 6:542-544, 1978.

Rosenbaum AH, et al: Tardive dyskinesia: Relationship with a primary affective disorder. *Dis Nerv Syst* 38:423-427, 1977.

Timberlake WH, Vance MA: Four-year treatment of patients with parkinsonism using amantadine alone or with levodopa. *Ann Neurol* 3:119-128, 1978.

Toglia JU, et al: Tetrabenazine in treatment of Huntington's chorea and other hyperkinetic movement disorders. *J Clin Psychiatry* 39:81-87, 1978.

Williams A, et al: Vocal cord paralysis in Shy-Drager syndrome. *J Neurol Neurosurg Psychiatry* 42:151-153, 1979.

Yahr MD: Parkinson's disease: Overview of its current status. *Mt Sinai J Med* 44:183-191, 1977.

Yahr MD: Overview of present day treatment of Parkinson's disease. *J Neural Transm* 43:227-238, 1978.

Drugs Used to Treat | 17
Skeletal Muscle Hyperactivity

SPASTICITY

Spasticity, a specific disorder of skeletal muscle tone, affects six million people in the United States (Birkmayer, 1972). The condition is associated with hyperactivity of gamma motoneurons, which tonically control muscle spindle contractile activity (gamma spasticity) (Bishop, 1977). Hyperactivity of alpha motoneurons, which initiate muscle contractile activity (alpha spasticity), also contributes to the increase in muscle tone. The hyperactivity results from a loss of spinal and supraspinal inhibitory influence on the gamma and alpha motoneurons; the effect of excessive supraspinal excitation is less pronounced. Supraspinal inhibitory deficiencies and excitatory excesses produced by upper motoneuron lesions are most commonly caused by central nervous system injuries and strokes. Less frequently, they result from rare neurologic disorders, cerebral palsy, and multiple sclerosis, although moderate to severe spasticity is present in two-thirds of patients with multiple sclerosis.

Transection of the spinal cord is characterized by a marked loss of inhibitory influence. The primary signs of spinal spasticity are hyperactive tendon stretch reflexes, hyperactive stretch reflexes, and clonus. In addition, primitive flexion withdrawal reflexes and a flexed posture are present, since flexor muscles are favored. Varying degrees of spasticity of the bladder and bowel also are noted.

In cerebral spasticity, reflex excitability and increased muscle tone often are less exaggerated, and primitive flexion withdrawal reflexes and flexed posture usually are absent. Supraspinal hyperexcitation of alpha motoneurons may produce a disabling, dystonic posture of flexed, adducted arms and extended legs; the tone is apparently increased in a manner quite different from that induced in the hypertonic state of spinal spasticity. The variable mixture of true spasticity and dystonia occurring in cerebral spasticity determines the response to antispastic drug therapy, for dystonia does not respond well to these drugs. Some athetotic movements that may occur in cerebral spasticity also are relatively resistant to antispastic drugs.

Although patient selection is critical, optimum drug therapy can be achieved only when certain caveats are taken into consideration (Burke, 1975; Bishop, 1977). Use of drugs in spasticity will be beneficial only in patients who are also receiving adequate physical therapy, including an exercise program with muscle cooling and vibratory stimulation when appropriate (eg, contraindicated in multiple sclerosis), as well as re-education to ensure confidence and full use of residual capabilities. A total management program may require corrective orthopedic procedures, selective surgical rhizotomy, and/or stereotactically placed cerebral or cerebellar lesions.

Electromyography and clinical assessment of the musculoskeletal system are the two principal methods employed to monitor alterations in spasticity induced by drug therapy. The former is a more sensitive indicator of change when quantitated and correlated with specific tests in which torque and movement of muscles and joints also are quantitated. However, a statistically significant reduction in spasticity determined by either method does not necessarily correlate with overall functional improvement. Drug therapy may actually be detrimental if reduction of tone unmasks severe muscle weakness, which compromises posture and gait to an intolerable degree.

The three primary antispastic drugs are diazepam [Valium] and baclofen [Lioresal], which represent two chemically different, centrally acting antispastic drugs, and dantrolene [Dantrium], which has a peripheral antispastic action (Davidoff, 1978). Local injection of dilute solutions of procaine or phenol into affected muscles is another form of pharmacotherapy, but the action of the former usually is too brief to be of long-term benefit. These drugs selectively block transmission in small unmyelinated group II afferents and the corresponding gamma motoneuron axons without affecting the heavily myelinated axons of the alpha motoneurons. Neuromuscular depolarizing and nondepolarizing blocking drugs are of no value in spastic disorders. Other than diazepam and the intravenous use of methocarbamol to reduce spasticity in selected patients in preparation for physical therapy, the central skeletal muscle relaxant drugs that are effective in the treatment of localized muscle spasm are not recommended in the treatment of spasticity.

Because spasticity varies considerably from time to time in an individual patient, the positive placebo response is high and only carefully controlled studies are of value in determining patient response to drugs. Results of such studies document the fact that the three primary antispastic drugs (diazepam, baclofen, and dantrolene) are superior to placebos in conditions in which relief of spasticity will restore function and reduce pain. The choice among the three drugs depends upon the condition being treated and its current status, associated illness in the patient, and the drugs' pharmacological action other than antispastic effect. Drug therapy is less satisfactory in cerebral than spinal spasticity; response rates are 65% to 75% in patients with traumatic spinal cord lesions and 30% to 65% in those with multiple sclerosis. Spasticity associated with stroke does not respond to diazepam, although dantrolene occasionally may be beneficial. The efficacy of baclofen in the treatment of spasticity associated with stroke has not been established. These drugs are not effective in rheumatoid arthritis or rigidity associated with parkinsonism. Diazepam and, to a lesser extent, baclofen are less satisfactory in patients with considerable sedation, poor coordination, and/or ataxia associated with marginal cerebellar function, whereas dantrolene tends to be less satisfactory in patients with borderline strength (Schmidt et al, 1976).

Diazepam has had the longest history of successful use; however, baclofen has been prescribed in countries other than the United States for at least a decade and is preferred by some physicians in those countries. Dantrolene has been used for the shortest period of time in the United States and has been reported to be more effective in cerebral spasticity than diazepam or baclofen, but the dose-related incidence of hepatotoxicity has limited its wider use until dosage guidelines for long-term administration can be formulated (see the evaluation). The antispastic action of diazepam does not appear to differ from that of other benzodiazepines, although there are few controlled clinical studies on use of related benzodiazepines in spasticity. There is only one controlled study in which all three drugs have been compared (Levine and Van Brocklin, 1977).

CENTRALLY ACTING DRUGS

BACLOFEN
[Lioresal]

$$H_2NCH_2CHCH_2COH$$

Although baclofen is an analogue of the inhibitory neurotransmitter, gamma aminobutyric acid, its antispastic action is probably unrelated to a direct action on that neurotransmitter's receptor. Baclofen has no direct effect on the neuromuscular junction. This drug diminishes the transmission of monosynaptic extensor and polysynaptic flexor reflexes in the spinal cord. This action may occur presynaptically by hyperpolarizing and thus antagonizing the release of the putative excitatory transmitters, glutamic and aspartic acids, from primary afferent fibers.

Baclofen relieves the primary components of spasticity: involuntary flexor and extensor spasms, resistance to passive movements, and clonus. Patients with spasticity induced by traumatic spinal lesions respond to baclofen more favorably than those with traumatic cerebral spasticity. A controlled study comparing baclofen with dantrolene and diazepam in multiple sclerosis showed baclofen to be the most effective (response rate, up to 65%); in comparison, the placebo response rate was 10% to 30% (Hedley et al, 1975). Controlled studies (Levine et al, 1977; Feldman et al, 1978) comparing placebo and baclofen support the efficacy of baclofen in multiple sclerosis. The degree of response is limited but clinically relevant in terms of improved patient comfort, progression to a more independent state of self-care, and ability to participate in a more aggressive rehabilitation program.

One recent open investigation demonstrated that urethral sphincter spasticity associated with traumatic paraplegia responded to intravenous therapy (Hachen and Krucker, 1977). A nonopiate analgesic action is demonstrable in animals; however, it is not known whether this action is responsible for the relief of spastic-induced pain observed clinically, since doses much higher than those used in man were required. Smooth muscle spasticity generally has not responded to administration of baclofen. Baclofen is not effective in rheumatoid arthritis or the rigidity of parkinsonism; its efficacy and tolerability in the treatment of spasticity associated with stroke is currently being investigated.

The compound is rapidly and well absorbed orally. Absorption is saturable; therefore, peak blood levels are slightly delayed with use of large therapeutic doses (Brogden et al, 1974). The degree of protein binding is low. About 70% to 85% of a dose is eliminated unchanged in the urine. The mean half-life is three to four hours; however, there is a considerable variation in individual response.

Baclofen is relatively well tolerated and severe adverse reactions are uncommon (*Medical Letter,* 1978). The most frequent side effects include drowsiness, lassitude, and dizziness; ataxia occurs even at therapeutic dose levels in some patients. These effects are often transient and may be reduced or eliminated with continued treatment. The incidence of these reactions is reported to be less than with diazepam at equieffective doses and can be reduced appreciably if the initial dose is low and increased gradually. Patients over 40 years of age appear to be more susceptible to these effects.

Severe muscle weakness does not appear to be a direct effect of the drug; more likely it represents existing degrees of paresis unmasked when muscle tone is reduced. This phenomenon frequently is intolerable and is the most common reason for withdrawal from therapy.

Less common side effects, which have a reported incidence of 1% to 10%, are nausea, mild gastrointestinal upset, constipation or diarrhea, insomnia, headache, confusion, asymptomatic hypotension, and urinary frequency. Allergic skin reactions are uncommon. A number of neuropsychiatric signs and symptoms (eg, euphoria, depression, paresthesias, ataxia, muscle pain, impaired coordination, tremor, dystonia, nystagmus, accommodation disorders, hallucinations, seizures, dysuria, enuresis) occur rarely and often are difficult to differentiate causally from the underlying disease.

With overdosage, signs of central nervous system depression are most prominent. Coma is most characteristic but seizures have been observed. It may be necessary to support respiration and cardiovascular function. There is no specific antidote. With intensive support care, one patient survived ingestion of approximately 900 mg.

Baclofen has not been reported to cause abuse or addiction. Auditory and visual hallucinations, paranoid ideation, and agitated behavior have been reported rarely on abrupt termination of the drug; therefore, gradual reduction of the dose over a one- to two-week period is recommended.

There are no absolute contraindications to baclofen therapy other than hypersensitivity. Baclofen should be used with caution when spasticity actually sustains upright posture and balance in locomotion or when spasticity is utilized to obtain increased function. Dosage reduction should be considered in patients with impaired renal function and those receiving other central nervous system depressants concurrently. Occasionally, asymptomatic elevations of the serum glutamic oxaloacetic transaminase, alkaline phosphatase, and blood glucose levels have occurred; therefore, patients with liver disease or diabetes should be monitored periodically to assure that there are no drug-induced alterations of the basic disease process. In a few epileptic patients, control of seizures was affected adversely when baclofen was given. Periodic electroencephalographic monitoring is therefore recommended if this drug is used in patients with a history of seizures. The safety of baclofen therapy during pregnancy and in children under 12 has not been established. It is not known whether the drug is excreted in breast milk.

ROUTE, USUAL DOSAGE, AND PREPARATIONS. Initially, the total daily dose should be low and increased gradually. Administration several times daily appears to control spasticity more evenly with fewer side effects. *Oral: Adults,* 5 mg three times daily for three days, increased by 5 mg three times daily every three days until the optimum effect or a maximum of 25 mg three times daily or 20 mg four times daily has been obtained; the usual optimal dose is 30 to 80 mg daily. At the termination of therapy, the dosage should be reduced gradually over a period of one or two weeks.

Lioresal (Geigy). Tablets 10 mg.

DIAZEPAM
[Valium]

Diazepam has an antispastic action in addition to its sedative, antianxiety, and anticonvulsant properties. It may be useful in a variety of chronic upper motoneuron disorders which have spasticity as a component; the drug also is useful as an adjunct in acute, localized, self-limited traumatic disorders with associated painful muscle spasm.

The muscle relaxant action of diazepam is thought to result from its ability to enhance gamma aminobutyric acid (GABA)-mediated presynaptic inhibition in the spinal cord and to depress neurons in the descending lateral reticular system that are facilitatory to the gamma motoneurons. Unfortunately, diazepam also depresses neurons in the ascending reticular activating system that mediate wakefulness. The resulting sedation and lethargy generally detract from the antispastic effectiveness of diazepam. This drug does not alter the synthesis, release, reuptake, or enzymatic degradation of GABA.

Diazepam is superior to a placebo in the relief of spasticity associated with spinal cord lesions, multiple sclerosis, and cerebral spasticity, although improvement is least satisfactory in disorders in the latter category. Other benzodiazepines probably have similar activity, but few controlled, comparative clinical studies have been published. The development of tolerance to the antispastic action over a number of months may necessitate careful dosage adjustment, drug holidays, or temporary use of an alternate drug to optimize therapy.

A total daily dose of 8 to 20 mg is usually necessary in the average spastic patient, and as much as 60 mg may be necessary in some individuals. Drowsiness thus becomes the primary side effect. Impairment of coordination (hand coordination and speed, walking speed, station stability) will likely be present to a variable degree in this dosage range. These central side effects make the drug less useful in patients with pre-existing sedation and marginal cerebellar function. Unlike dantrolene, diazepam has no peripheral muscle relaxant activity; consequently, less muscle weakness is observed and this drug may be a more appropriate choice for patients with borderline strength. A total daily dose of 2 to 10 mg three or four times daily is generally required for adequate control of localized muscle spasm. Oversedation in the elderly patient may be a problem, even at the lower limits of this dosage range.

Diazepam has been used successfully in the *stiff-man* syndrome to counteract the widespread chronic muscular rigidity, spasm, and pain. It also may be useful in the management of the motor restlessness of *akathisia*, although its antianxiety action is probably of greater significance than its antispastic action in this condition (see Chapter 16, Drugs Used in Extrapyramidal Movement Disorders). When given intravenously, diazepam and clonazepam are useful adjuncts in the treatment of muscle spasms caused by tetanus toxin or strychnine poisoning, although their anticonvulsant rather than antispastic action plays the predominant role.

See the Introduction for additional information on precautions to be observed with diazepam in the treatment of spasticity. For a more complete discussion of the adverse reactions, precautions, and dosage of the benzodiazepines, see Chapter 11, Drugs Used for Anxiety and Insomnia.

ROUTES, USUAL DOSAGE, AND PREPARATIONS. *Oral: Adults*, for spasticity or severe localized muscle spasms, 2 to 10 mg four times daily. *Children*, 0.12 to 0.8 mg/kg of body weight daily divided into three or four doses.

Valium (Roche). Tablets 2, 5, and 10 mg.

Intravenous: Adults, for severe spasticity or acute localized muscle spasm, 2 to 10 mg. The intravenous solution should be injected slowly, allowing at least one minute for each 5 mg (1 ml) given, and it should not be mixed or diluted with other solutions or drugs nor added to intravenous fluids. The dose may be repeated in three to four hours, if necessary. Intravenous diazepam should not be used in the spastic patient with respiratory difficulty. Intramuscular administration is not recommended because absorption is erratic and unpredictable. *Children*, initially, 0.04 to 0.2 mg/kg of body weight (maximum, 0.6 mg/kg in an eight-hour period).

Valium (Roche). Solution 5 mg/ml in 2 and 10 ml containers.

PERIPHERALLY ACTING DRUG

DANTROLENE SODIUM
[Dantrium]

This unique skeletal muscle relaxant reduces muscle tension through its effect at a site beyond the neuromuscular junction where it interferes with the release of calcium ions from the sarcoplasmic reticulum. This action occurs not only in extrafusal skeletal muscle fibers but also in the striated intrafusal muscle fibers surrounding the muscle spindle. With the doses used clinically, dantrolene has little or no effect on cardiac and smooth muscles. The mechanism is somewhat limiting because, unlike the neuromuscular blocking drugs, dantrolene cannot decrease contractile activity more than 50%. The drug has no specific antispastic action on hyperactive neurons.

Dantrolene is superior to a placebo in spasticity induced by spinal cord and cerebral injuries or lesions associated with multiple sclerosis and cerebral palsy. It can be considered for use in spastic patients, especially those with cerebral spasticity, who are in a stable neurologic state and in whom spasticity causes pain, discomfort, or distress or diminishes the ability to utilize residual motor function. It must be given cautiously to ambulatory patients, because relief of spasticity coincides with some degree of weakness that may worsen the patient's overall functional capacity. The benefit of reducing muscle stiffness versus the possible disadvantage of reducing muscle strength must be determined individually. Dantrolene has not been shown to be useful in the treatment of fibrositis, rheumatoid spondylitis, bursitis, arthritis, or acute muscle spasm of local origin. The drug should not be given to patients with amyotrophic lateral sclerosis, for these individuals have a very low tolerance to the muscle weakness induced by dantrolene.

Since dantrolene produces weakness but little drowsiness and incoordination, it may be more beneficial in the already sedated patient with marginal cerebellar function; however, it generally is less useful in patients with only borderline strength.

Side effects generally are transient; those reported most commonly include drowsiness, dizziness, nausea, vomiting, malaise, fatigue, lethargy, and weakness. Less frequently, headache, nervousness, insomnia, and anorexia have occurred. Rarely reported reactions include rash, photosensitivity, visual disturbances, psychotic reaction, and diarrhea. The latter may persist and require treatment, a reduction in dose, or temporary cessation of therapy.

The most serious adverse reaction is an idiosyncratic dose-related hepatocellular injury which has been fatal. The potential is greatest in patients over 30 years, especially women over 35 years, who have received total daily doses of more than 300 mg for 60 days or longer. Total daily doses of 200 mg or less are not likely to cause hepatotoxicity. Most cases (71%) occurred after one to six months of therapy. Therefore, all patients should have routine baseline hepatic function studies prior to therapy, if possible, and SGOT and SGPT levels should be determined monthly during therapy. The lowest effective dose should be prescribed, preferably no more than 300 mg daily if at all possible. Therapy should be continued for more than 60 days only if there has been symptomatic benefit and no evidence of hepatic injury. Hepatotoxicity was not observed in children under 10 years in the largest retrospective study conducted to date (Utili et al, 1977).

Dantrolene is absolutely contraindicated in patients with active hepatic disease. It should be given to patients with impaired respiratory function only with caution; in such instances, frequent monitoring is essential.

No clinically significant drug interactions have been documented and confirmed. The safety of dantrolene during pregnancy has not been established.

ROUTE, USUAL DOSAGE, AND PREPARATIONS. *Oral*: Dosage must be individualized. *Adults*, initially, 25 mg once or twice daily, increased to 25 mg three or four times daily, and then, by increments, to 50 to 100 mg four times daily. Each dosage level should be maintained for four to seven days to determine the patient's response. The dose should not be increased beyond the amount at which the patient receives maximal benefit with an acceptable level of adverse effects. (The manufacturer's literature specifies that most patients will respond to a total dose of 400 mg/day or less;

arely should doses higher than this be
used. *Children*, a similar approach should
be utilized starting with doses of 0.5 mg/kg
of body weight once or twice daily
(maximum, 100 mg four times daily or 3
mg/kg four times daily).

   Dantrium (Norwich-Eaton). Capsules 25, 50,
   75, and 100 mg; suspension 25 mg/5 ml.

SPASM

Spasm is an involuntary contraction of a
muscle or groups of muscles, usually at-
tended by pain and limited function.
Reflex muscle spasm (splinting) occurs
commonly as a protective mechanism in
response to local injury but may be exaggerated beyond its protective value and
require therapeutic intervention. Drug
therapy depends upon the etiology of the
spasm (eg, anticonvulsants for epileptic
myoclonic spasms, calcium for hypocal-
cemic-induced muscle spasm, central
skeletal muscle relaxants for spasm associated with acute and chronic muscular
pain syndromes).

   Most muscle strains and minor injuries
are self-limited and respond rapidly to rest
and physical therapy. Immobilization of
the affected part by use of casts, pressure
bandaging, neck collar, arm slings, or
crutches; cold compresses initially; and
whirlpool baths obviate much of the need
for drugs other than mild analgesics. Occasionally, an anti-inflammatory drug may be
necessary when there is considerable tissue damage and edema.

   Acute or chronic painful skeletal muscle
spasms of local origin may be produced by
musculoskeletal strains and sprains,
trauma, and cervical or lumbar radic-
ulopathy as a result of degenerative osteoarthritis, herniated disc, spondylolysis,
or laminectomy. The spasms are characterized by local pain, tenderness on palpation, increased muscle consistency, and
limitation of motion and daily activities.
There is usually a profound reduction in
electromyographic activity.

   Painful muscle spasms that impair function and do not readily respond to conservative measures usually can be relieved by
skeletal muscle relaxants. The central
skeletal muscle relaxants include carisoprodol [Rela, Soma], chlorphenesin
[Maolate], chlorzoxazone [Paraflex],
diazepam [Valium], methocarbamol
[Delaxin, Robaxin], orphenadrine citrate
[Norflex], and cyclobenzaprine [Flexeril],
which is chemically related to the tricyclic
antidepressants. Although baclofen, dantrolene, and diazepam are useful in spasticity, only the latter is also used in muscle
spasms associated with injury. Diazepam,
methocarbamol, and orphenadrine can be
administered intravenously to relieve severe, acute muscle spasm of local origin
caused by inflammation or trauma. Intravenous methocarbamol also is effective
in reducing spasticity in preparation for
physical therapy in selected patients. Except for diazepam, the skeletal muscle relaxant drugs are, at best, only mildly effective after oral administration in treating
spasticity induced by cerebrospinal
trauma, cerebral palsy, or demyelinating
disorders such as multiple sclerosis; thus,
they are not recommended for oral therapy
in the treatment of spasticity. These drugs
do not possess an anti-inflammatory action,
and they are not recommended for use in
rheumatoid arthritis.

   Comparative, controlled, crossover
studies to identify drugs of choice are difficult to conduct because of the subjective,
variable, and self-limited nature of these
illnesses. However, all of these spasmolytic drugs are superior to a placebo in alleviating the symptoms and signs of localized muscle spasm. Experimentally,
they all depress spinal polysynaptic reflexes preferentially over monosynaptic reflexes, as well as facilitatory and inhibitory
neuronal activity affecting muscle stretch
reflexes, primarily in the lateral reticular
area of the brainstem. All of these drugs
produce some sedation that may reflect
depressed neuronal activity essential for
wakefulness in the medial reticular ascending system. On a milligram basis, cyclobenzaprine and diazepam are the most
potent central muscle relaxants and sedatives. In man, the orally effective doses of
the remaining drugs are well below the

amount required experimentally to elicit muscle relaxant activity; thus, some investigators conclude that their muscle relaxant activity is related only to their sedative effect. However, relief of muscle spasm in patients is not always associated with sedation, which, if present, may contribute to overall improvement in some patients but is considered a side effect in others.

Some central skeletal muscle relaxants are available in combination with analgesics, ie, carisoprodol with phenacetin and caffeine [Soma Compound], chlorzoxazone with acetaminophen [Parafon Forte], methocarbamol with aspirin [Robaxisal], orphenadrine citrate with aspirin, phenacetin, and caffeine [Norgesic, Norgesic Forte] or acetaminophen [X-Otag Plus]. A muscle relaxant and a particular analgesic often are indicated in a specific patient's program to relieve muscle spasm; if both are available in an appropriate fixed-dose combination, then use of the mixture is more convenient and may improve compliance.

ADVERSE REACTIONS AND PRECAUTIONS.

The following adverse reactions and precautions are general in nature and apply to all skeletal muscle relaxant drugs evaluated except cyclobenzaprine. For specific adverse reactions and precautions, see the evaluations.

Drowsiness and dizziness are observed most frequently. Blurred vision, flushing, asthenia, lethargy, and lassitude are more common after intravenous administration than after usual oral doses and are usually transient. Nausea, vomiting, heartburn, abdominal distress, constipation or diarrhea, ataxia, areflexia, flaccid paralysis, respiratory depression, tachycardia, and hypotension occur occasionally after large oral doses. Acute poisoning, which is rarely fatal, is treated in the same manner as barbiturate or benzodiazepine poisoning (see Chapter 11, Drugs Used for Anxiety and Insomnia). Dialysis is of limited value in overdosage of diazepam.

The centrally acting agents should be discontinued if rash, pruritus, or other evidence of hypersensitivity occurs. Serious allergic manifestations (eg, anaphylactic reactions, leukopenia) have been observed rarely.

Patients receiving these drugs should not undertake activities that require mental alertness, judgment, and physical coordination (eg, driving a vehicle, operating dangerous machinery) until it is known that the doses used do not cause drowsiness or other incapacitating effects. Caution is necessary if skeletal muscle relaxants and other central nervous system depressants (eg, alcohol, hypnotics, antianxiety drugs, antipsychotic drugs, antidepressants) are used concomitantly, since their effects may be additive. Symptoms of organic brain disease in elderly patients may be aggravated when doses appropriate for younger patients are given.

Psychic or physical dependence may develop after long-term administration of large doses of some of these agents, especially in patients with a known tendency to abuse drugs. Abrupt discontinuance after long-term use of large doses may produce severe withdrawal symptoms, including convulsions. There is insufficient experience with cyclobenzaprine to determine its abuse potential.

Routine precautions should be followed if these drugs are given during pregnancy (see discussion on use of drugs during pregnancy in Chapter 2). Unless specifically stated in the evaluations, there is no information on the presence of these compounds in the milk of lactating women.

INDIVIDUAL EVALUATIONS

CARISOPRODOL
[Rela, Soma]

$$H_2NCOCH_2\overset{\overset{\displaystyle CH_3}{|}}{\underset{\underset{\displaystyle CH_2CH_2CH_3}{|}}{C}}CH_2OCNHCHCH_3$$

Carisoprodol, a congener of meprobamate, is effective as an adjunct to rest, physical therapy, and other appropriate measures to treat the discomfort produced by localized skeletal muscle spasm. It is not effective in congenital or acquired spastic or dyskinetic movement disorders of central nervous system origin. Onset of action is rapid and the duration is four to six hours. The compound is metabolized in the liver and the resultant products are eliminated in the urine. Carisoprodol is present in the milk of lactating women.

The most common untoward effect is drowsiness. Idiosyncratic reactions (eg, extreme asthenia, transient quadriplegia, dizziness, ataxia, diplopia, agitation, confusion, disorientation) have occurred rarely after the initial administration of carisoprodol. The drug is contraindicated in patients with acute intermittent porphyria. See the Introduction to this section for additional information on adverse reactions and precautions.

ROUTE, USUAL DOSAGE, AND PREPARATIONS.
Oral: Adults, 350 mg four times daily; *children*, information is inadequate to establish a dosage.

> Drug available generically: Tablets 350 mg.
> *Rela* (Schering), *Soma* (Wallace). Tablets 350 mg.

CHLORPHENESIN CARBAMATE
[Maolate]

This analogue of mephenesin is effective as an adjunct to rest, physiotherapy, and other appropriate measures to treat the discomfort produced by skeletal muscle spasm of local origin. It is not effective in congenital or acquired spastic or dyskinetic movement disorders of central nervous system origin. The biological half-life is 3.5 ± 0.2 hours. The compound is conjugated, principally with glucuronic acid, and eliminated in the urine.

The most common untoward effects are drowsiness and dizziness. Adverse reactions noted occasionally include gastrointestinal disturbances, paradoxical stimulation, nervousness, insomnia, headache, and asthenia. Rash, pruritus, and blood dyscrasias occur rarely. See the Introduction to this section for additional information on adverse reactions and precautions.

ROUTE, USUAL DOSAGE, AND PREPARATIONS.
Oral: Adults, initially, 800 mg three times daily until the desired effect is obtained; for maintenance, 400 mg four times daily or less frequently, as required. *Children*, information is inadequate to establish a dosage.

> *Maolate* (Upjohn). Tablets 400 mg.

CHLORZOXAZONE
[Paraflex]

Chlorzoxazone, a benzoxazolidinone, is chemically distinct from all other muscle relaxants. It is effective as an adjunct to rest, physical therapy, and other appropriate measures to treat the discomfort produced by localized skeletal muscle spasm. Chlorzoxazone is not effective in congenital or acquired spastic or dyskinetic movement disorders of central nervous system origin. The drug is rapidly absorbed after oral administration, and peak blood levels are attained in three to four hours; it is extensively metabolized in the liver, conjugated with glucuronic acid, and excreted by the kidney.

The most common side effect observed with use of effective muscle relaxant doses is drowsiness (5%). This agent should be used cautiously in patients with a history of liver disease. Alterations in hepatic function and jaundice have been reported following its use, although it is not possible to establish a causal relationship. Patients should be observed closely for signs of liver damage, and the drug should be discontinued if evidence of hepatic dysfunction develops. Other adverse effects include headache, gastrointestinal irritation, and, rarely, gastrointestinal bleeding and hypersensitivity reactions. See the Introduction to this section for additional information on adverse reactions and precautions.

ROUTE, USUAL DOSAGE, AND PREPARATIONS.
Oral: Adults, 250 to 750 mg three or four
times daily; *children,* 20 mg/kg of body
weight daily in three or four divided doses.
  Paraflex (McNeil). Tablets 250 mg.

CYCLOBENZAPRINE
  [Flexeril]

This tricyclic compound produces central skeletal muscle relaxation in acute and
chronic painful muscle conditions. The
spasmolytic effect begins within one or two
days and is maximal after one to two weeks.
Experimentally, the drug acts primarily at
supraspinal levels where it depresses tonic
neuronal activity; although both gamma
and alpha motoneurons are affected, total
daily doses of 60 mg have not been shown
to affect spinal or cerebral spasticity.

Controlled studies reveal that cyclobenzaprine is superior to a placebo in the
management of spasm produced by acute
painful muscle injuries (Basmajian, 1978)
and in relieving the chronic pain of muscle
spasm secondary to degenerative osteoarthritis (Bercel, 1977). Only a few controlled
studies comparing the effects of cyclobenzaprine with other drugs have been published. These studies suggest that a total
daily dose of 30 mg of cyclobenzaprine or
15 mg of diazepam is necessary to distinguish the effects of these drugs from those
of a placebo.

Pharmacokinetic studies in man (Hucker
et al, 1977) reveal that, although absorption
of oral doses of 5 to 30 mg is rapid, oral
absorption may be saturable with these
amounts. A considerable first-pass effect
occurs in the intestine and/or liver of some
individuals. Cyclobenzaprine is highly
bound to plasma proteins and extensively
metabolized to derivatives that are excreted principally as glucuronide conjugates by the kidney. These effects probably
account, in part, for the large variation in
plasma levels observed among patients.

The most common side effects are
drowsiness (40%), dryness of the mouth
(28%), and dizziness (11%); these reflect
the sedative and anticholinergic activities
of most tricyclic compounds. Tachycardia,
weakness, dyspepsia, paresthesia, unpleasant taste, blurred vision, and insomnia
occur less frequently. The manufacturer
reports that sweating, myalgia, dyspnea,
abdominal pain, constipation, coated
tongue, tremors, dysarthria, euphoria, nervousness, disorientation, confusion,
headache, urinary retention, decreased
bladder tonus, and ataxia have occurred
rarely.

Hepatomegaly and a dose-time related
hepatocyte vacuolation with lipidosis were
observed in rats, but there has been no
clinical documentation of this finding in
man. Presently, the manufacturer recommends limiting treatment to no longer than
two or three weeks.

The dose of cyclobenzaprine used to
treat muscle spasm is much smaller than
that of other tricyclic compounds used as
antidepressants. The real incidence of adverse reactions for cyclobenzaprine in the
low doses used for muscle spasm, compared to the potential adverse reactions
produced by the tricyclic antidepressants,
has not been fully established. For the
general adverse reactions, precautions, and
management of overdosage with tricyclic
antidepressants, see Chapter 13, Drugs
Used in Affective Disorders.

Cyclobenzaprine may interact with
monoamine oxidase inhibitors; enhance
the effects of alcohol and other central
nervous system depressants; enhance the
anticholinergic actions of other drugs; produce cardiotoxicity, especially in patients
with impaired cardiovascular function; and
block the antihypertensive action of
guanethidine and related drugs.

The safe use of cyclobenzaprine during
pregnancy and in nursing mothers and
children younger than 15 has not been
established.

ROUTE, USUAL DOSAGE, AND PREPARATIONS.
Oral: Adults, 10 mg three times daily
(maximum, 60 mg daily).
  Flexeril (Merck Sharp & Dohme). Tablets
  10 mg.

DIAZEPAM
[Valium]

The discussions of the use of this drug in spastic conditions and in discomfort produced by local skeletal muscle spasm are combined and presented in the evaluation in the section on Spasticity in this chapter.

METHOCARBAMOL
[Delaxin, Robaxin]

This analogue of mephenesin is effective as an adjunct to rest and physical therapy to alleviate the discomfort produced by localized skeletal muscle spasm. The drug can be given parenterally in severe cases or when oral administration is not feasible. Methocarbamol is not effective orally in congenital or acquired spastic or dyskinetic movement disorders of central nervous system origin. Pharmacokinetic data are limited.

Dizziness, drowsiness, headache, anorexia, vertigo, and mild nausea occur occasionally after oral administration, and skin eruptions have been reported rarely. Flushing, metallic taste, nausea, nystagmus, diplopia, mild ataxia, hypotension, and bradycardia have been observed after parenteral administration; these untoward effects may be lessened by giving the injection at a rate not exceeding 3 ml/min. Parenteral administration is contraindicated in patients with impaired renal function because the polyethylene glycol-300 vehicle may be nephrotoxic.

ROUTES, USUAL DOSAGE, AND PREPARATIONS. *Oral: Adults*, initially, 1.5 to 2 g four times daily for 48 to 72 hours; for maintenance, 1 g four times daily. *Children*, the safety and effectiveness of this drug in children under 12 are not established.

> Drug available generically: Tablets 500 and 750 mg.
> *Delaxin* (Ferndale). Tablets 500 mg.
> *Robaxin* (Robins). Tablets 500 and 750 mg.

Intramuscular: Adults, 500 mg alternately in each gluteal region every eight hours. *Intravenous: Adults*, 1 to 3 g daily at a rate not exceeding 3 ml/min; some physicians substitute oral administration after 1 or 2 g has been administered. The drug should not be given by this route for more than three days.

> *Robaxin* (Robins). Solution (aqueous) 100 mg/ml with 50% polyethylene glycol-300 in 10 ml containers.

ORPHENADRINE CITRATE
[Norflex]

This drug is an analogue of the antihistamine, diphenhydramine, and is effective as an adjunct to rest, physiotherapy, and other appropriate measures for discomfort produced by localized skeletal muscle spasm. Orphenadrine is not effective orally in congenital or acquired spastic or dyskinetic movement disorders of central nervous system origin. Pharmacokinetic data in man are limited.

The most common side effects of orphenadrine reflect its anticholinergic activity and include blurred vision, dryness of the mouth and skin, and mild excitation. This agent is contraindicated in patients with angle-closure glaucoma or myasthenia gravis, and it should be used with caution in those with tachycardia, cardiac decompensation, or signs of urinary retention. Reduction of dose may be required in the elderly to avoid intolerable side effects. For a more complete discussion of the adverse reactions and precautions of centrally acting anticholinergic drugs, see Chapter 16, Drugs Used in Extrapyramidal Movement Disorders.

Some patients occasionally experience transient episodes of dizziness, lightheadedness, or syncope, which may impair their ability to perform potentially hazardous activities. Hypersensitivity reactions occur rarely.

ROUTES, USUAL DOSAGE, AND PREPARATIONS.
Oral: Adults, 100 mg twice daily.
> Drug available generically: Tablets 100 mg.
> *Norflex* (Riker). Tablets 100 mg.

Intramuscular, Intravenous: Adults, 60 mg twice daily.
> Drug available generically: Solution 30 mg/ml in 2 and 10 ml containers.
> *Norflex* (Riker). Solution (aqueous) 30 mg/ml in 2 ml containers.

Selected References

Baclofen (Lioresal): New muscle relaxant for multiple sclerosis. *Med Lett Drugs Ther* 20:43-44, 1978.

Basmajian JV: Cyclobenzaprine hydrochloride effect on skeletal muscle spasm in lumbar region and neck: Two double-blind controlled clinical and laboratory studies. *Arch Phys Med Rehabil* 59:58-63, 1978.

Bercel NA: Cyclobenzaprine in treatment of skeletal muscle spasm in osteoarthritis of cervical and lumbar spine. *Curr Ther Res* 22:462-468, 1977.

Birkmayer W (ed): *Spasticity: A Topical Survey.* Bern, Switzerland, Hans Huber Publishers, 1972.

Bishop B: Spasticity: Its physiology and management. *Phys Ther* 57:371-401, 1977.

Brogden RN, et al: Baclofen: Preliminary report of its pharmacological properties and therapeutic efficacy in spasticity. *Drugs* 8:1-14, 1974.

Burke DJ: Approach to treatment of spasticity. *Drugs* 10:112-120, 1975.

Davidoff RA: Pharmacology of spasticity. *Neurology* 28:46-51, 1978.

Feldman RG, et al: Baclofen for spasticity in multiple sclerosis: Double-blind crossover and 3-year study. *Neurology* 28:1094-1098, 1978.

Hachen HJ, Krucker V: Clinical and laboratory assessment of efficacy of baclofen (Lioresal) on urethral sphincter spasticity in patients with traumatic paraplegia. *Eur Urol* 3:237-240, 1977.

Hedley DW, et al: Evaluation of baclofen (Lioresal) for spasticity in multiple sclerosis. *Postgrad Med J* 51:615-618, 1975.

Hucker HB, et al: Plasma levels and bioavailability of cyclobenzaprine in human subjects. *J Clin Pharmacol* 17:719-727, 1977.

Levine IM, et al: Lioresal, new muscle relaxant in treatment of spasticity: Double-blind quantitative evaluation. *Dis Nerv Syst* 38:1011-1015, 1977.

Levine MC, Van Brocklin JD: Lioresal (baclofen) treatment of spasticity: Double-blind comparison study with dantrolene and diazepam. *Neurology* 27:391, 1977.

Schmidt RT, et al: Comparison of dantrolene sodium and diazepam in treatment of spasticity. *J Neurol Neurosurg Psychiatry* 39:350-356, 1976.

Utili R, et al: Dantrolene-associated hepatic injury: Incidence and character. *Gastroenterology* 72:610-616, 1977.

Drugs Used in Myasthenia Gravis | 18

Myasthenia gravis is characterized by progressive weakness and rapid fatigability of skeletal muscle due to impaired neuromuscular transmission. This disorder is caused by an autoimmune reaction that reduces the number of available acetylcholine receptors on postsynaptic membranes of the neuromuscular junctions. Hence, the number of interactions between the acetylcholine released by nerve stimulation and the receptors is decreased, which results in a reduction of muscle strength or progressive failure of contraction from repeated nerve stimulation.

Despite recent advances in defining the nature of the neuromuscular defects of myasthenia gravis, its complete pathogenetic mechanisms are not yet fully understood. Circulating antibodies to acetylcholine receptor have been demonstrated in about 90% of patients with myasthenia, although the severity of the disease does not correlate well with the antibody titer. However, the severity of clinical signs increases with an increased proportion of receptors bound by antibody. Decreased antibody titers have been reported after thymectomy and, since thymectomy benefits many myasthenic patients, it has been suggested that clinical improvement is associated with the decreased antireceptor antibody levels that occur over a period of several years. Although the thymus is probably involved in the autoimmune process, its precise role in myasthenia gravis is not known.

Diagnosis: The diagnosis of myasthenia gravis usually can be made on the basis of the patient's history and symptoms. In doubtful cases, the diagnosis can be established and differentiated from some other neuromuscular diseases by the parenteral administration of the short-acting anticholinesterase, edrophonium [Tensilon]. An appropriate endpoint such as ptosis, diplopia, or weakness of a specific muscle group should be selected for evaluation, and the effect of drug administration on it followed closely and quantitatively, if possible. Improvement in muscle strength is usually observed in patients with myasthenia gravis, whereas those with other disorders develop either no increase in strength or even a slight weakness and also may develop fasciculations, especially in the eyelids. If results are equivocal, the test should be repeated at another time or a double-blind test, using one syringe containing saline and another edrophonium, may be helpful. Parenteral administration of pyridostigmine bromide [Mestinon] or neostigmine methylsulfate [Prostigmin Methylsulfate] is less convenient for diagnosis because these drugs have a longer duration of action; therefore, they are used primarily for treatment.

If diagnosis cannot be established with the anticholinesterase compounds, electromyography (EMG) using repetitive motor nerve stimulation may be definitive. Measurements of antiacetylcholine receptor antibodies, which can be performed in a number of institutions, are helpful adjuncts in making the diagnosis of myasthenia gravis.

Treatment: The principal agents used to treat myasthenia gravis are the reversible anticholinesterases, pyridostigmine bromide and neostigmine bromide; ambenonium chloride [Mytelase] is used occasionally. These drugs inhibit acetylcholinesterase, the enzyme that hydrolyzes acetylcholine, thereby increasing the duration of action of acetylcholine released at the motor endplate. Thus, the number of interactions between the transmitter and receptors is increased and the patient's muscular strength and response to repetitive nerve stimulation is improved. However, these agents are not curative in that they have no effect on the primary cause of the disease. Although the anticholinesterases may produce marked improvement in some patients, muscle strength remains below normal in others, and they must learn to live with some disability. Improvement reaches a plateau in most patients; increasing the dosage further does not provide greater benefits but only increases the danger of overdosage. There is some evidence that anticholinesterase drugs have a direct toxic effect on nicotinic acetylcholine receptors. This action may be related to the development of resistance in some patients; thus, the physician must evaluate therapeutic and toxic drug effects.

The maximal muscle strength produced by optimal oral doses of any anticholinesterase is approximately the same, but the dosage required varies greatly among patients. The optimal dosage and timing of administration must be determined empirically for each patient, taking into account fluctuations in strength and variations in the patient's needs. There are no adequately controlled studies that unequivocally document differences in efficacy among the available agents. However, many physicians regard pyridostigmine as the drug of choice for maintenance because it is more acceptable to patients and produces fewer adverse effects than neostigmine or ambenonium.

The dose of anticholinesterase medication often must be increased in the presence of infection and, occasionally, premenstrually. Also, since stress often produces physical fatigue, an increase in dosage may be required. Mild exacerbations of myasthenia are treated by increasing the dose of oral medication very gradually with the patient under careful observation; this should continue as long as symptomatic improvement results. Critically ill patients often are refractory to anticholinesterase medication, however, and responsiveness can sometimes be restored by a temporary reduction in dose or complete withdrawal of medication for 72 hours in the hospital. If ventilatory failure develops, institution of appropriate supportive care, endotracheal intubation, and controlled ventilation should be undertaken. Some authorities believe that if responsiveness is restored after a drug-free period, the symptoms were probably due to overdosage (cholinergic crisis).

Myasthenic weakness may worsen suddenly, often without recognizable cause. Such exacerbations are characterized by decreased responsiveness to drug therapy that cannot be overcome by administration of larger doses and may progress to a myasthenic crisis, characterized by severe muscular weakness with dysphagia and ventilatory insufficiency. Cautious intravenous or intramuscular administration of pyridostigmine bromide or neostigmine methylsulfate may be beneficial. Atropine should not be administered routinely to control the side effects of the anticholinesterase compound on the secretory glands, heart, and gastrointestinal smooth muscle, for masking the muscarinic effects may inadvertently lead to cholinergic crisis.

Overdosage may occur when patients in a refractory phase of myasthenia gravis receive increasing amounts of an anticholinesterase drug in an attempt to control symptoms. In these patients, the maximal strength attained after optimal doses is below normal, and the administration of excessive amounts may convert a myasthenic crisis into a cholinergic crisis. It has been suggested that these agents may occupy the acetylcholine receptors and, when present in excess, may prevent the action of the transmitter; thus, an overdose increases the amount of acetylcholine present but reduces the number of receptors available, thereby increasing muscle weakness. Fasciculations and cholinergic side effects, which are common symptoms of overdosage in normal individuals, may be mild or absent in myasthenic patients; instead, generalized weakness may be the principal sign.

The symptoms of *myasthenic crisis* may be difficult to distinguish from those of *cholinergic crisis*, which is caused by an overdose of the anticholinesterase drug. If the differential diagnosis cannot be made on the basis of signs and symptoms, ventilation must be supported and the patient observed until a diagnosis is possible. Pharmacologic tests should be performed only after endotracheal intubation and controlled ventilation have been instituted. A small intravenous dose (1 to 2 mg) of edrophonium may improve strength temporarily if the patient has not received enough of the anticholinesterase agent, or aggravate the weakness if he has received too much.

If overdosage is confirmed, the anticholinesterase should be discontinued temporarily and 1 to 2 mg of atropine given intravenously; endotracheal intubation, controlled ventilation, and suction also may be necessary. The cholinesterase reactivator, pralidoxime [Protopam], is much less effective against reversible anticholinesterases than the irreversible type and thus is seldom used (see Chapter 86, Specific Antidotes).

For patients who do not respond adequately to anticholinesterase drugs, immunologic therapeutic measures (thymectomy, adrenal corticosteroids) should be considered. Thymectomy results in improvement or remission in many patients. Although the presence of a thymoma is an indication for surgery, opinion is divided on the indications for thymectomy in myasthenic patients with nonthymomatous glands. Thymectomy should not be considered for all patients and should not be considered as an emergency treatment. Some authorities believe steroids should be used in conjunction with thymectomy. Whether steroid therapy is preferred to thymectomy, except for thymoma, is debated. Other literature should be consulted for further discussion of surgical treatment.

Therapy with adrenal corticosteroids has been shown to be beneficial in patients with various degrees of muscle weakness. Treatment must be continued indefinitely, and employment of a high-dose, alternate-day maintenance regimen has minimized adverse effects while improving muscular strength. This regimen appears to prevent lethal weakness and permanent structural damage to the neuromuscular system as long as it is continued. A short-acting steroid (eg, prednisone) is preferred for the alternate-day regimen because it does not interfere with the normal corticotropin-cortisol cycle and will not accumulate as long-acting agents will, thus reducing the likelihood of deleterious effects on the tissues.

When large doses of steroids are used initially, exacerbation of weakness occurs in about 80% of patients. Therefore, treatment should be started with relatively small doses that are then increased gradually, even though this may slow the rate of improvement. Anticholinesterase medication should be continued with the dosage adjusted to optimal levels, especially during initiation of steroid treatment. The need for anticholinesterase drugs may decrease as the patient improves. It has been suggested that patients on alternate-day doses of the steroid receive a high-protein low-carbohydrate, 2 g sodium diet, supplemented with potassium and antacids.

The mechanism of action of the adrenal

corticosteroids in myasthenia gravis has not been precisely determined; however, it is known that they suppress the immune system, which may explain in part their beneficial effects. However, steroid therapy is only suppressive and does not cure the disease, as evidenced by a recurrence of symptoms within three months after such therapy is discontinued.

The employment of current methods of treatment with adrenal corticosteroids (high-dose, alternate-day therapy) may be preferable to the use of corticotropin because the latter produces variable effects and requires parenteral administration and repeated hospitalization.

The immunosuppressive drugs, azathioprine [Imuran] and mercaptopurine [Purinethol], have been reported to be highly effective in a small number of patients. They may be useful in otherwise refractory cases, but their severe toxicity, especially with long-term therapy, limits their usefulness in myasthenia gravis (see Chapter 66, Immunomodulators).

Other measures that have been tried on a small number of patients include plasmapheresis and plasma exchange; these procedures have been useful in some patients with severe myasthenia gravis but produce relatively short-term improvement. Thoracic duct drainage has been tried but is not generally used.

Adverse Reactions and Precautions

The adverse reactions of anticholinesterase agents represent, in part, the effects produced by cholinergic nervous system stimulation and include both muscarinic and nicotinic reactions. The former consist of abdominal cramps, nausea, vomiting, diarrhea, hypersalivation, increased bronchial secretions, lacrimation, miosis, and diaphoresis, all of which may be counteracted by atropine. Nicotinic effects include muscle cramps, fasciculations, and weakness. Some patients cannot tolerate optimal doses of anticholinesterase drugs unless atropine is given; however, atropine

should not be given routinely without indication because it may mask the sudden increase in adverse effects that is the first sign of overdosage and may result in drying and inspissation of bronchial secretions.

The anticholinesterase compounds are contraindicated in the presence of mechanical obstruction of the intestinal or urinary tract. They should be used with extreme caution in patients with bronchial asthma. Those compounds containing the bromide ion (pyridostigmine bromide, neostigmine bromide) should not be used in patients with a history of sensitivity to this ion.

Infection may increase the severity of myasthenia, and any increase in dosage of the anticholinesterase must be carefully supervised. Because aminoglycoside and polymyxin antibiotics and antiarrhythmic drugs affect neuromuscular transmission, they should be used with caution in patients with myasthenia gravis. Myasthenic patients are sensitive to central nervous system depressants; these agents should be used with caution, chiefly because of their inhibitory effects on the respiratory drive.

ANTICHOLINESTERASE AGENTS

PYRIDOSTIGMINE BROMIDE
[Mestinon]

Pyridostigmine, given orally, is the most widely used anticholinesterase agent for the treatment of myasthenia gravis. The drug also may be administered parenterally with great caution for diagnosis, treatment of exacerbations, and management of neonatal myasthenia. The therapeutic response is similar to that observed with neostigmine, but pyridostigmine has a slightly longer duration of action.

Dosage requirements vary widely among patients because of differences in absorption, metabolism, and excretion of the drug; thus, the individual dosage and intervals of administration must be determined empirically. Careful record keeping by the patient is helpful in adjusting the timing of dosages. An early attempt should be made to reduce or eliminate doses during periods of rest or during the night. This approach may help maintain sensitivity to the drug and reduce direct end-plate damage. The syrup is useful for infants, young children, and patients who cannot swallow tablets or whose doses are fractions of the tablets; it may be given by nasogastric tube if necessary. The timed-release preparation is useful for nighttime medication only to maintain strength at night if necessary. Some patients find that a timed-release tablet at night improves their strength in the morning upon awakening.

Because of marked fluctuations in drug blood levels after intramuscular administration, controlled very slow intravenous injection is preferable when parenteral medication is essential.

Adverse effects after therapeutic doses occur less frequently with pyridostigmine than with neostigmine. For a discussion of adverse reactions, see the Introduction.

ROUTES, USUAL DOSAGE, AND PREPARATIONS.
Oral: *Adults*, the dose and frequency of administration vary greatly and must be individualized according to the severity of the disease and the response of the patient. A usual initial dose is 60 to 120 mg every three to four hours; the intervals are shortened or lengthened as necessary on the basis of response. *Children*, 7 mg/kg of body weight daily in divided doses and timed as required.

Mestinon (Roche). Syrup 60 mg/5 ml; tablets 60 mg; tablets (timed-release) 180 mg.

Intramuscular, Intravenous: For exacerbations of myasthenia gravis or when oral dosage is impractical, *adults*, approximately 1/30th of the oral dose. For *newborn infants* of myasthenic mothers, 0.05 to 0.15 mg/kg of body weight.

Mestinon (Roche). Solution 5 mg/ml in 2 ml containers.

NEOSTIGMINE BROMIDE
[Prostigmin Bromide]

NEOSTIGMINE METHYLSULFATE
[Prostigmin Methylsulfate]

Neostigmine bromide may be used orally to treat myasthenia gravis. The therapeutic response is similar to that obtained with pyridostigmine and ambenonium, but neostigmine has a shorter duration of action and is more potent than pyridostigmine; 15 mg of neostigmine is approximately equivalent to 60 mg of pyridostigmine. The methylsulfate salt is administered parenterally for the management of myasthenia gravis in patients who are unable to swallow. It also may be administered for diagnosis.

Adverse effects after therapeutic doses occur more frequently with neostigmine than with pyridostigmine or ambenonium. For adverse reactions and precautions, see the Introduction.

ROUTES, USUAL DOSAGE, AND PREPARATIONS.
NEOSTIGMINE BROMIDE:
Oral: For treatment of myasthenia gravis, the dose and frequency of administration must be individualized according to the severity of the disease and the response of the patient. *Adults*, initially, 15 mg every three to four hours; the dose and frequency of administration are then adjusted in accordance with the patient's requirements. *Children*, 2 mg/kg of body weight daily in divided doses as required.

Drug available generically: Powder; tablets 15 mg.
Prostigmin [bromide] (Roche). Tablets 15 mg.
NEOSTIGMINE METHYLSULFATE:
Intramuscular: For diagnosis of myasthenia gravis, *adults*, 0.022 mg/kg of body weight. To control adverse effects, atropine (0.011 mg/kg intramuscularly) should be given before administration of neostigmine. An improvement in the strength of

myasthenic muscle should appear within 10 minutes and last three to four hours. *Children*, 1.5 mg given with atropine (0.6 mg intramuscularly) to control adverse effects.

For treatment of exacerbations of myasthenia gravis, *adults*, 0.5 mg. Subsequent dosage should be adjusted according to the patient's response.

Intramuscular, Subcutaneous: For treatment of exacerbations of myasthenia gravis, *children or infants*, 0.01 to 0.04 mg/kg of body weight every two to three hours. Atropine (0.01 mg/kg intramuscularly or subcutaneously) can be given with each dose or with alternate doses to control adverse effects.

Intravenous: When parenteral administration is essential, controlled very slow intravenous injection is preferable to intramuscular administration. The amount given orally (or equivalent if receiving pyridostigmine) is dissolved in volume of fluid that would be infused over a course of four hours. For example, 1 mg might be dissolved in 100 ml and infused at a rate of 25 ml/hr.

> Drug available generically: Solution 1:1,000, 1:2,000, and 1:4,000.
>
> *Prostigmin* [methylsulfate] (Roche). Solution 1:1,000, 1:2,000, and 1:4,000.

AMBENONIUM CHLORIDE
[Mytelase Chloride]

Ambenonium is given orally to treat myasthenia gravis. It produces fewer cholinergic side effects than neostigmine, but may have a longer duration of action and a greater tendency to accumulate. Ambenonium is used less commonly than pyridostigmine or neostigmine but may be preferred in patients who cannot tolerate these drugs because of sensitivity to the bromide ion.

For adverse reactions and precautions, see the Introduction.

ROUTE, USUAL DOSAGE, AND PREPARATIONS.
Oral: The dose and frequency of administration vary greatly and must be individualized according to the severity of the disease and response of the patient. *Adults* initially, 5 mg three or four times daily increased as required; the dosage should be adjusted at intervals of one to two days to avoid accumulation of the drug. *Children*, initially, 0.3 mg/kg of body weight daily in divided doses increased, if necessary, to 1.5 mg/kg daily in divided doses.

> *Mytelase Chloride* (Winthrop). Tablets 10 mg.

EDROPHONIUM CHLORIDE
[Tensilon]

Edrophonium is used in the diagnosis of myasthenia gravis. It has a more rapid onset and shorter duration of action than pyridostigmine and neostigmine methyl sulfate. Administration of atropine is usually unnecessary, but this agent should be readily available, especially for older patients. After intravenous administration muscle strength increases in myasthenic patients within one to three minutes and lasts for five to ten minutes.

A smaller dose of edrophonium is used to differentiate a myasthenic crisis from a cholinergic crisis: An intravenous dose produces a brief remission of symptoms if these are caused by an exacerbation of the illness but further weakens patients suffering from an overdose of medication.

For untoward effects, see the Introduction.

ROUTES, USUAL DOSAGE, AND PREPARATIONS
Intravenous: For diagnosis, *adults*, 2 mg injected within 15 to 30 seconds; if no response occurs within 45 seconds, an additional 8 mg should be given. The test may be repeated after one to two hours (see manufacturer's labeling for details). *Children under 75 lb*, 1 mg; *over 75 lb*, 2 mg. I

no response is observed after 45 seconds, an additional dose of up to 5 mg in children under 75 lb and up to 10 mg in children over 75 lb should be administered.

For differential diagnosis of myasthenic crisis and cholinergic crisis, *adults*, 1 to 2 mg. This test should be undertaken only if facilities for endotracheal intubation and controlled ventilation are immediately available.

Intramuscular: For diagnosis, *infants*, 0.5 mg as a single dose. *Children up to 75 lb*, 2 mg; *over 75 lb*, 5 mg. There is a delay of two to ten minutes before a reaction is noted with this route of administration.

   Tensilon (Roche). Solution 10 mg/ml in 1 and 10 ml containers.

ADRENAL CORTICOSTEROIDS

PREDNISONE

Oral treatment with an adrenal corticosteroid such as prednisone is beneficial in patients with severe myasthenia gravis not controlled by anticholinesterase drugs or thymectomy. The success rate is high, but treatment must be continued indefinitely and the patient must be observed closely for adverse effects.

Adverse reactions usually associated with the prolonged use of steroids may occur and must receive appropriate attention. Alternate-day therapy is preferable in order to minimize reactions. For further discussion, see Chapter 41, Adrenal Corticosteroids.

ROUTE, USUAL DOSAGE, AND PREPARATIONS. *Oral*: Initially, 25 mg daily is given for two days; the dose is increased gradually by 5 mg every two days until an optimal response occurs (usually, 50 to 60 mg daily). An alternate-day program is gradually substituted by adding 10 mg to the first day's dose (60 mg) and subtracting 10 mg from the second day's dose (40 mg) each week until improvement reaches a plateau (ie, the patient experiences weakness on the "off" day) or until 100 mg is given every other day. The dosage then should be reduced very gradually over a period of many months to establish a minimal maintenance dose given on alternate days (usually, 30 to 60 mg). In patients with severe myasthenia gravis who do not respond to 100 mg of prednisone every other day, doses as large as 100 to 200 mg daily, or equivalent doses of longer-acting adrenal corticosteroids such as dexamethasone, may be needed.

The dosage of anticholinesterase drugs should be adjusted as necessary during steroid therapy.

   For preparations, see Chapter 41, Adrenal Corticosteroids.

Selected References

Drachman DB: Myasthenia gravis. *N Engl J Med* 298:136-142, 186-193, 1978.

Fields WS (ed): Myasthenia gravis. *Ann NY Acad Sci* 183:1-386, 1971.

Grob D (ed): Myasthenia gravis. *Ann NY Acad Sci* 274:1-682, 1976.

Havard CWH: Progress in myasthenia gravis. *Br Med J* 2:1008-1011, 1977.

Hofmann WW: Treatment of myasthenia gravis. *Ration Drug Ther* 13:1-8, (Feb) 1979.

Patten BM: Myasthenia gravis: Review of diagnosis and management. *Muscle Nerve* 1:190-205, 1978.

Simpson JA: Myasthenia gravis: Personal view of pathogenesis and mechanism, parts 1 and 2. *Muscle Nerve* 1:45-56, 151-156, 1978

Local Anesthetics | 19

Local anesthetics produce loss of sensation and motor activity in circumscribed areas of the body by reversibly blocking nerve conduction (regional anesthesia). The majority are organic amine bases classified as esters or amides. Agents in both chemical groups usually consist of a secondary or tertiary amine linked through an aliphatic chain to an aromatic moiety. Certain antihistaminic, anticholinergic, and adrenergic agents having a similar configuration also have some local anesthetic action.

Selected references are listed for more information on local anesthetics (Covino and Vassallo, 1976; de Jong, 1977; Dripps et al, 1977; Ralston and Shnider, 1978).

Local anesthetic bases are relatively insoluble in water but are soluble in lipid vehicles (eg, ointments). Salts of local anesthetic bases are water soluble and stable. Under aqueous conditions, the ratio of the nonionized base to the cationic form depends upon the pKa of the compound (range, 7.6 to 9.0) and tissue fluid pH. The nonionized base penetrates the nerve sheath and membrane. After re-equilibration at the internal pH of the axon, the charged cation is quantitatively the principal agonist that produces nerve block.

A current working hypothesis for the site and mechanism of action of local anesthetics is as follows: The cationic form attaches to the internal axoplasmic membrane, probably a phospholipid receptor, to decrease ion flux, particularly sodium. The rate of increase and amplitude of the local action potential are depressed to the degree that depolarization is not sufficient for a propagated action potential. This nondepolarizing or stabilizing block is similar to that induced by curare at the neuromuscular junction. In fact, some local anesthetics have been reported to have neuromuscular blocking effects that may be additive to those produced by tubocurarine-like muscle relaxants. The clinical significance of this finding remains to be established. At least 1 cm of nerve should be exposed to the local anesthetic to ensure blockade because the impulse in myelinated fibers is capable of skipping over two or three nodes.

The nonionized base also blocks nerve conduction at tissue fluid pH, but this action is less prominent. The site appears

285

to be the lipophilic areas of the nerve membrane, and the mechanism is believed to be similar to that of the general anesthetics, which are thought to act through a physicochemical mechanism rather than through specific receptors. After the anesthetic occupies a critical volume fraction of the nerve membrane, expansion and fluidization of the membrane occurs; this interferes with the protein conformational changes necessary for ion flux and depolarization. Topical anesthetics that possess a very low pKa (eg, benzocaine: pKa 3.5) or certain non-nitrogenous local anesthetic alcohols (eg, benzyl alcohol) may produce nerve block almost exclusively via the physicochemical mechanism.

The onset of anesthesia (essentially the rate and degree of penetration into individual nerves) principally depends upon the lipid solubility, molecular size, and quantity of available nonionized form of the local anesthetic. The anesthetic's vasoactive action, the blood flow and pH at the site of injection, and the total volume of the anesthetic solution and its concentration also are important determinants.

Although all local anesthetics act on all parts of a neuron, they are generally applied to the axons of peripheral nerves. Such nerves are generally blocked in sequence according to their size. Thus, small nonmyelinated autonomic C fibers, thinly myelinated sensory delta A fibers (carrying pain, pressure, fine touch, and temperature sensations), and myelinated autonomic preganglionic B fibers are blocked before larger myelinated A fibers carrying visceral sensory proprioception and motor functions. The clinical appearance of sensory or motor loss may vary from this order in larger nerves because of the geographical location of fibers (either near the surface or core of the nerve). The total amount of drug required to block large nerve trunks is greater than that needed for smaller peripheral nerves. The duration of the block depends upon all of the factors listed for onset of anesthesia, as well as upon the extent of protein binding and whether or not a vasoconstrictor is added to the solution.

Ester-type local anesthetics are partly or completely hydrolyzed by plasma cholinesterase and, to a much lesser extent, by hepatic cholinesterase; metabolites are excreted in the urine. An exception is cocaine, 10% to 12% of which is excreted unchanged in the urine. The amides are metabolized in the liver by microsomal enzymes; the small quantity of unchanged amides excreted in urine is not usually relevant in patients with impaired renal function. The metabolism of both the esters and amides may be reduced in patients with hepatic disease.

For most local anesthetics, the perineural concentration necessary to produce block is several hundredfold greater than the tolerable plasma level; therefore, the drug should be injected precisely at the appropriate site to avoid systemic toxicity. In general, the greatest rate of absorption and hence the highest plasma level is achieved by injection into highly vascular sites (eg, head and neck region, intercostal and paracervical blocks), by topical application to respiratory mucous membranes, by use of large volumes or high concentrations, or by use of solutions that do not contain a vasoconstrictor (eg, epinephrine). Plasma levels are relatively unaffected by the speed of injection (except with the intravenous route) or by the age (except the very young and very old) of the patient. Thus, the least volume of the most dilute solution that is effective should be administered.

There is much less experience with the use of local anesthetics in children compared to use of general anesthetics in this age group. Total maximal dosages vary markedly; the amount depends upon the specific nerve block and should be calculated according to the child's age, surface area, or other variables (see the section on Pediatric Patients in Chapter 2).

Solutions of local anesthetics are usually isotonic to avoid edema, local irritation, and inflammation at the site of injection. Solutions prepared by the physician for subarachnoid anesthesia can be varied in baricity to obtain the desired level of anesthesia.

Regional Anesthetic Techniques

Regional (conduction) anesthetic techniques are classified according to the site of application: (1) infiltration (local), including extravascular and intravascular (intravenous regional anesthesia); (2) peripheral nerve block (nerve or field block); (3) central nerve block, including epidural (peridural, extradural, caudal) and subarachnoid (spinal, intrathecal); and (4) surface (topical).

To prevent accidental intravascular injection, needle placement must always be checked by aspiration with a syringe prior to injection of the local anesthetic. In addition, local anesthetics should not be administered unless resuscitative equipment is available: oropharyngeal airways, anesthesia masks, endotracheal tubes, and a laryngoscope. An intravenous infusion should always be started prior to injection of a substantial dose of a local anesthetic.

Current therapy for local anesthetic toxicity has been recently summarized (de Jong, 1978). Apparatus for administering oxygen and artificial ventilation, diazepam, ultrashort- or short-acting barbiturates, neuromuscular blocking agents, vasopressors, intravenous fluids, and any additional drugs and equipment that may be useful for resuscitation should be available.

Infiltration Anesthesia: *Extravascular anesthesia* includes the conventional technique of injecting the anesthetic in the immediate area of surgery. With *intravascular anesthesia*, which is synonymous with *intravenous regional anesthesia*, the entire distal portion of an extremity is anesthetized. A butterfly-type needle is inserted into a distal peripheral vein and secured in place. A pneumatic tourniquet is then applied to the upper arm or leg above the operative site and inflated to a pressure adequate to occlude arterial flow. A dilute solution of local anesthetic is then injected and diffuses from the veins and capillaries to produce an evenly distributed infiltration to all nerves in the occluded limb. Satisfactory anesthesia is obtained within several minutes and is maintained as long as the circulation of the extremity is occluded.

Peripheral Nerve Block Anesthesia: In *field block anesthesia*, the solution is injected close to the nerves around the area to be anesthetized. In *nerve block anesthesia*, a localized perineural injection is made at an access point along the course of a nerve distant from the operative site. More concentrated solutions of drug often are required because these nerves have a sheath and a relatively large diameter.

The drugs most commonly used for infiltration and peripheral nerve block anesthesia include chloroprocaine [Nesacaine], lidocaine [Xylocaine], mepivacaine [Carbocaine], prilocaine [Citanest], and procaine [Novocain]. Bupivacaine [Marcaine] and etidocaine [Duranest] are indicated if a more prolonged block is desired. Tetracaine [Pontocaine] is seldom used because of its high potency and risk of toxicity, even with small injection volumes.

Central Nerve Block Anesthesia: The technique of *epidural anesthesia* is accomplished by injecting a local anesthetic into the epidural space. In lumbar epidural anesthesia, the injection is usually made between the second lumbar and first sacral vertebrae to avoid injury to the spinal cord, which ends at the first lumbar vertebra in 95% of individuals. In caudal anesthesia, the solution is introduced into the caudal canal (an epidural space) through the sacral hiatus. In both techniques, the site of action is believed to be the paravertebral and epidural sections of the spinal nerves and/or the spinal cord rootlets in the subarachnoid space. In general, the number of spinal segments blocked is determined by the site of injection (lumbar or caudal), the position of the patient (fewer segments with sitting), the volume and concentration of solution injected (more segments with high volume or concentration), the age of the patient (more segments in children and the elderly), pregnancy (more segments at term), and extent of arteriosclerosis (more segments if occlusive arterial disease is present). Physiologic changes with epidural anesthesia are more moderate and slower in onset than those that occur with subarachnoid anesthesia. Many physicians believe that a test dose should be administered at least five minutes before the main dose in an attempt to detect an inadvertent intravenous or subarachnoid (spinal) injection. The relatively large dose needed and the great vascularity of the epidural space increase the possibility of systemic toxic reactions. Repeated fractional injections through an in situ catheter (continuous epidural anesthesia) may be used to prolong epidural anesthesia.

The drugs most commonly used for epidural anesthesia are bupivacaine, etidocaine, lidocaine, and mepivacaine; procaine, chloroprocaine [Nesacaine-CE], and prilocaine also can be administered. Piperocaine [Metycaine] is now rarely given for caudal anesthesia. Only single-dose containers should be used to minimize the danger of injecting a solution contaminated by chemicals or bacteria. The use of epinephrine in epidural anesthesia reduces the blood concentration of most local anesthetics.

For *subarachnoid anesthesia*, a local anesthetic is injected into the subarachnoid space, usually between the second lumbar and first sacral vertebrae. The drug is believed to act initially on the nerve roots as they emerge from the spinal cord. The level of anesthesia is determined by the site of injection; specific gravity, volume, and concentration of solution; and position of the patient. The dose should be reduced markedly in advanced pregnancy, and injection should be avoided when the patient is having strong uterine contractions or is bearing down during labor, for an excessively high level of anesthesia may result. Consciousness is preserved at all times unless a total spinal block occurs or profound arterial hypotension develops secondary to the relative sympathetic blockade that is always produced. The duration of anesthesia depends upon the rate at which the drug leaves the nerve tissue. Duration may be increased 50% to 100% by adding epinephrine or phenylephrine to the solution. Repeated fractional injections of solutions (without a vasoconstrictor) through an in situ catheter (continuous spinal anesthesia) also may prolong spinal anesthesia, but the incidence of postspinal headache is increased because of the size of the catheter. The local anesthetic diffuses within the cerebrospinal fluid and is removed primarily by the venous circulation; a small quantity is removed by lymphatic drainage. Enzymatic hydrolysis of the drugs in cerebrospinal fluid is insignificant.

In addition to isobaric solutions of local anesthetics for use in subarachnoid anesthesia, hyperbaric (diluted with dextrose) or hypobaric (diluted with distilled water) solutions also are available to assure that their specific gravity is higher or lower than that of cerebrospinal fluid, respectively. The hypobaric (light) solutions gravitate caudad and the hyperbaric (heavy) solutions gravitate cephalad when the patient is tilted in the head-down position. Tetracaine and lidocaine are most widely used for subarachnoid anesthesia; procaine and dibucaine [Nupercaine] also can be administered. Only single-dose containers should be employed to minimize the danger of injection of a contaminated solution, and only local anesthetics specifically prepared for subarachnoid anesthesia should be used.

The dose of local anesthetics used for subarachnoid anesthesia is too small, even if absorbed, to produce systemic toxicity or to exert any direct depressant effects upon the fetus when given during labor and delivery.

Surface Anesthesia: Cationic forms of local anesthetics do not penetrate intact skin, but unionized (base) forms penetrate to a limited degree. As a result, only certain local anesthetics are appropriate to relieve pruritus, burning, and surface pain on intact skin and the less sensitive mucous membranes (anus and rectum). Cationic and unionized forms penetrate skin that has been abraded. Wounds, ulcers, and burns are treated with preparations that are relatively insoluble in tissue fluids; this generally precludes systemic toxicity if the area of application is not too extensive and administration is not repeated too frequently. Mucous membranes of the nose, mouth, pharynx, larynx, trachea, bronchi, vagina, and urethra are readily anesthetized by both cationic and unionized forms. However, since absorption from these areas is quite rapid, the smallest dose required for adequate analgesia should be administered to minimize the incidence of systemic toxic reactions. The addition of a vasoconstrictor does not generally lessen the incidence of these reactions.

The use of local anesthetics on conjunctival and corneal tissues represents a form of topical application. Benoxinate [Dorsacaine] and proparacaine [Ophthaine] are only used topically on the eye (see Chapter 25, Miscellaneous Ophthalmic Preparations). The ophthalmologic use of cocaine and tetracaine [Pontocaine] is discussed in Chapter 25; however, their evaluations appear in this chapter as well in view of their more widespread local anesthetic use.

Adjuncts for Regional Anesthetics

Vasoconstrictors may be added to solutions for infiltration, peripheral nerve block, epidural, and subarachnoid anesthesia to decrease the rate of absorption. In general, this prolongs the anesthetic effect and reduces the risk of systemic toxic reactions, as well as increases the frequency of complete conduction blocks at low anesthetic concentration. The addition of epinephrine is more appropriate than increasing the concentration to prolong the duration. Epinephrine 1:200,000 is the vasoconstrictor most commonly used for infiltration, nerve block, and epidural anesthesia. Norepinephrine [Levophed], nordefrin [Cobefrin], and phenylephrine [Neo-Synephrine] also are used, but the latter two must be given in higher concentrations and are no more satisfactory. Epinephrine and phenylephrine are most commonly used to prolong subarachnoid anesthesia.

Local anesthetic solutions containing epinephrine should not be used for nerve blocks in areas supplied by end-arteries (eg, digits, ears, nose, penis) because they may cause ischemia, which could progress to gangrene. These solutions also should not be administered in excessive dosage, intravenously, or with inhalation anesthetics that sensitize the heart to catecholamines, since severe ventricular arrhythmias may result. It is undesirable to use solutions containing epinephrine for infiltration and nerve blocks in patients in labor because of the danger of producing vasoconstriction in uterine blood vessels, which may decrease placental circulation or diminish the intensity of uterine contractions and prolong the period of labor. It also is undesirable to use solutions containing epinephrine in patients with severe cardiovascular disease or thyrotoxicosis. The systemic effects of epinephrine may be potentiated in patients receiving tricyclic antidepressants or monoamine oxidase inhibitors.

Cocaine is the only local anesthetic that has a well-documented vasoconstrictor action, although there is some evidence that low concentrations of mepivacaine and lidocaine also possess an inherent vasoconstrictor effect. Moderate to high concentrations of all local anesthetics except cocaine have a vasodilator effect. It is for this reason that patients in whom epinephrine is contraindicated should receive only minimal effective doses of local anesthetics. Epinephrine should not be used in nerve blocks performed to determine the presence or absence of vasospasm.

Hyaluronidase [Alidase, Wydase] has been added to local anesthetics to facilitate their diffusion into tissues during infiltration and nerve block anesthesia. However, because a higher incidence of systemic reactions caused by too rapid absorption of the anesthetic and local irritation and sensitization have been reported with use of this enzyme, its value is seriously questioned and it is now seldom used for this purpose.

Adverse Reactions

Unpredictable adverse reactions (ie, hypersensitivity, including anaphylaxis) are extremely rare. If a patient is hypersensitive to a particular local anesthetic, a drug from a different chemical group should be substituted. Use of a test dose to determine hypersensitivity is not necessarily reliable to predict an allergic response. If rash, urticaria, edema, or other manifestations of allergy develop during use of a topical anesthetic, the drug should be discontinued permanently. To minimize the possibility of a serious allergic reaction, topical preparations should not be applied for prolonged periods except under the continuing supervision of a physician.

Predictable systemic reactions occur when plasma concentrations reach a critical level. Relative overdosage is most frequently observed as a result of inadvertent intravascular injection or rapid absorption from highly vascular areas. The resulting high plasma levels of the local anesthetic may cause alarming, sometimes fatal, systemic reactions that are qualitatively similar for all local anesthetics. However, it is important to note that when absorption is slow, peak plasma levels (and presumably the possibility of severe systemic reactions) may not be observed until approximately 30 to 40 minutes after the drug is injected. Because of accumulation, systemic reactions are more likely to occur after a number of repeated doses during continuous epidural anesthesia unless the amount administered is reduced. Systemic reactions primarily involve the central nervous and cardiovascular systems. Initial manifestations usually involve the central nervous system.

Signs and symptoms of central nervous system toxicity are characterized by uneasiness, perioral paresthesias, tinnitus, tremors, and shivering; convulsions may follow, particularly if the reaction is not treated adequately. If the drug plasma level is high, ventilatory depression progressing to respiratory arrest and coma may develop as a result of generalized central nervous system depression.

The most important and initial treatment should be assuring and maintaining a patent airway and supporting ventilation using oxygen and assisted or controlled respiration as required.

Persistent convulsions may be controlled by the intravenous administration of diazepam [Valium] in 2.5 mg increments or of small increments (50 to 100 mg) of an ultrashort-acting barbiturate (eg, thiopental [Pentothal], thiamylal [Surital], methohexital [Brevital]). If none of these drugs are available, a short-acting barbiturate (eg, secobarbital [Seconal], pentobarbital [Nembutal]) may be given in increments of 25 mg every two to three minutes. The barbiturate should be given in sufficient quantity to control the seizures, but caution must be exercised because overdosage may occur if sufficient time is not allowed for the anticonvulsant action of the individual doses to become apparent. Neuromuscular blocking agents also may be used to terminate muscular manifestations of persistent convulsions, but artificial ventilation is required to support respiration. Usual preoperative doses of barbiturates given for prophylaxis have little or no value in averting central nervous system reactions. However, diazepam has been recommended for prophylaxis of convulsions.

The cardiovascular reaction is the result of depression of myocardial force and impulse conduction and of systemic vasodilatation. It is characterized by bradycardia, hypotension, and heart block that may ultimately progress to cardiac and ventilatory arrest. The onset of cardiovascular symptoms usually occurs after signs of central nervous system toxicity are established. However, rapid inadvertent intravenous injection or profound sympathetic blockade, particularly following some local anesthetics, can cause an abrupt hypotensive episode. Acute circulatory failure is treated with fluids and vasopressors (eg, ephedrine, metaraminol [Aramine], mephentermine [Wyamine], phenylephrine [Neo-Synephrine]) administered intravenously. If ventilatory arrest occurs or asystole is suspected, artificial ventilation and external cardiac massage must be instituted immediately.

The most common local adverse reaction is contact dermatitis, characterized by erythema and pruritus that may progress to vesiculation and oozing. This occurs most commonly in individuals frequently exposed to ester-type local anesthetics (eg, physicians, dentists). Since the amides were introduced, these reactions have become rare.

Systemic symptoms and signs (anxiety, restlessness, tremors, palpitations, tachycardia, anginal pain, dizziness, headache, and hypertension) may be produced by the epinephrine added to local anesthetics for parenteral use. These effects tend to be mild and transient when a 1:200,000 concentration is used.

Local anesthetics diffuse readily through the placenta and reports have appeared in the literature of diminished muscle strength and tone and decreased rooting behavior in the infant, although Apgar scores are normal. If used in excessive quantities, particularly in paracervical block, these agents may accumulate and cause fetal bradycardia, expulsion of meconium before birth, and marked central nervous system depression after birth. Bupivacaine [Marcaine] and etidocaine [Duranest] have much lower umbilical vein/maternal vein plasma concentration ratios than alternative agents. This may be related to their high degree of protein binding (94% to 96%); however, it more likely reflects their greater uptake by fetal tissues. Both drugs have high lipid partition coefficients and are absorbed by fetal

tissues in greater amounts than lidocaine. In neurobehavioral tests administered to infants a few hours after birth, bupivacaine-induced epidural anesthesia was reported to cause less depression than lidocaine or mepivacaine.

INDIVIDUAL EVALUATIONS

Recommendations for selected uses of currently available local anesthetics appear in Tables 1 and 2. Alternative agents within a group or among groups should be considered when allergic, pharmacokinetic, or individual factors require that a different agent be administered. Some topical preparations listed in the evaluations may contain a small quantity of antimicrobial agent as a preservative, but no claim is made for antimicrobial action.

Suggested maximum single doses are

TABLE 1.
LOCAL ANESTHETICS PRINCIPALLY RECOMMENDED FOR INJECTION

Drugs	Infiltration	Nerve Block	Intravenous Regional	Epidural	Subarachnoid	Relative Duration of Action
AMIDES						
Bupivacaine [Marcaine]	+	+	investigational	+	investigational	long
Dibucaine [Nupercaine]	—	—	—	—	+	long
Etidocaine [Duranest]	+	+	—	+	—	long
Lidocaine [Xylocaine]	+	+	+	+	+	intermediate
Mepivacaine [Carbocaine]	+	+	investigational	+	—	intermediate
Prilocaine [Citanest]	+	+	investigational	+	—	intermediate
AMINOBENZOATE ESTERS						
Chloroprocaine [Nesacaine]	+	+	investigational	+	investigational	short
Procaine [Novocain]	+	+	—	+	+	short
Tetracaine [Pontocaine]	—	—	—	+	+	long

TABLE 2.
LOCAL ANESTHETICS PRINCIPALLY RECOMMENDED FOR SURFACE APPLICATION

	EYE	MUCOUS MEMBRANES Oropharynx Laryngotracheal Bronchi	Urethra Vagina Rectum	MUCOCUTANEOUS JUNCTION AND SKIN
AMIDES				
Lidocaine [Xylocaine]	—	—	—	+
Lidocaine Hydrochloride [Xylocaine]	—	+	+	+
Dibucaine [Nupercainal]	—	—	—	+
ESTERS				
Benzoic Acid Esters				
Cocaine Hydrochloride	+	+	+	—
Hexylcaine Hydrochloride [Cyclaine]	—	+	+	—
Piperocaine Hydrochloride [Metycaine]	—	+	+	—
Proparacaine Hydrochloride [Ophthaine]	+	—		
Aminobenzoate Esters				
Benzocaine [Americaine]	—	—	—	+
Benoxinate Hydrochloride [Dorsacaine]	+	—	—	—
Butamben Picrate [Butesin Picrate]	—	—	—	+
Tetracaine Hydrochloride [Pontocaine]	+	+	+	+
MISCELLANEOUS				
Cyclomethycaine Sulfate [Surfacaine]	—	—	+	+
Dimethisoquin Hydrochloride [Quotane]	—	—	—	+
Diperodon Monohydrate [Diothane]	—	—	—	+
Dyclonine Hydrochloride [Dyclone]	—	+	+	+
Pramoxine Hydrochloride [Tronothane]	—	—	+	+

listed in the evaluations for those local anesthetics recommended for injection; however, there is considerable evidence to support the view that these doses may be insufficient for certain types of extensive regional anesthesia and excessive in other clinical situations (Moore et al, 1977; Covino, 1978). Therefore, suggested doses should be viewed only as a guideline. The most common cause of toxic reactions to local anesthetics is still inadvertent intravascular injection of these agents.

BENZOCAINE
[Americaine]

$$H_2N-\text{C}_6H_4-\overset{\text{O}}{\underset{}{\text{C}}}\text{OCH}_2\text{CH}_3$$

Benzocaine is used for surface anesthesia of the skin and mucous membranes. It is one of the most widely used agents for relief of sunburn, pruritus, and minor burns. Ointments containing less than 10% benzocaine or acidic preparations are ineffective on intact or mildly sunburned skin. Since benzocaine is poorly soluble in water and poorly absorbed, it remains in contact with the skin for a long time and thus produces a sustained anesthetic effect with a low incidence of systemic toxic reactions.

The possibility of sensitization should always be considered. Preparations containing benzocaine (usually suppositories) may cause methemoglobinemia in susceptible infants. For additional information on adverse reactions and precautions, see the Introduction.

ROUTE, USUAL DOSAGE, AND PREPARATIONS.
Topical: The appropriate preparation is applied as required.

Drug available generically: Cream 5%; ointment 5%; spray 20%; bulk (crystals, powder).

Americaine Aerosol (Arnar-Stone). Solution containing benzocaine 20% in a water-dispersible base in 20, 60, and 120 ml containers (nonprescription).

Americaine Hemorrhoidal Ointment (Arnar-Stone). Ointment containing benzocaine 20% and benzethonium chloride 0.1% in a water-soluble polyethylene glycol base in 30 g containers (nonprescription).

Americaine Anesthetic Lubricant (Arnar-Stone). Lubricant containing benzocaine 20% and benzethonium chloride 0.1% in a water-soluble base of polyethylene glycol 300 and 4000 in 2.5 and 30 g containers.

Americaine Otic (Arnar-Stone). Liquid containing benzocaine 20% in a water-soluble base of 1% (w/w) glycerin and polyethylene glycol 300 with benzethonium chloride 0.1% in 15 ml containers.

BUPIVACAINE HYDROCHLORIDE
[Marcaine]

This amide, related chemically to mepivacaine, is used for infiltration, nerve block, and epidural anesthesia (Moore et al, 1978); it is currently being investigated for subarachnoid anesthesia. Its most important property is its long duration of action. Bupivacaine is particularly useful when administered by continuous epidural techniques to relieve pain during labor, since the need for supplemental doses, with the attendant risk of excessive plasma levels, is less than with mepivacaine or lidocaine. When the 0.5% solution is used, the interval between doses is usually two to three hours, but occasionally may be three to five hours. The addition of epinephrine 1:200,000 may increase this interval slightly but decreases both umbilical and maternal venous plasma levels. Although bupivacaine may accumulate in the mother during continuous epidural anesthesia, few systemic toxic reactions have been reported. Data on use of bupivacaine in children and elderly or debilitated adults are incomplete.

The potency of bupivacaine is similar to that of etidocaine and tetracaine (ie, four-times greater than that of mepivacaine, lidocaine, and prilocaine). In general, the onset of action is slower and the interval to maximal anesthesia is longer with bupivacaine than with lidocaine. The duration of action is two to three times longer than with mepivacaine and lidocaine; the time usually can be lengthened slightly by adding epinephrine. Some peripheral nerve blocks may last more than 24 hours; neuropathy caused by such prolonged blocks has not been reported.

The systemic toxic reactions produced by bupivacaine are qualitatively similar to those produced by other local anesthetics. However, this agent does not cause methemoglobinemia or fetal depression after use in obstetrical epidural anesthesia. No residual effects have followed inadvertent subarachnoid injection in several patients, including one parturient. For additional information on adverse reactions and precautions, see the Introduction.

ROUTE, USUAL DOSAGE, AND PREPARATIONS. *Injection*: As a general guide, the maximal single dose in healthy *adults* should not exceed 200 mg without epinephrine and 250 mg with epinephrine 1:200,000. This dose should not be repeated at intervals of less than three hours. A maximal total dose of 600 mg (8 mg/kg of body weight) in 24 hours generally should not be exceeded. If the 0.5% solution without epinephrine is used for continuous epidural anesthesia in obstetric patients, the total dose probably should not exceed 320 mg.

Infiltration: Without epinephrine, up to 70 ml of the 0.25% solution; with epinephrine, up to 90 ml of the 0.25% solution.

Intravenous regional: The use of bupivacaine for intravenous regional anesthesia is still considered investigational at this time (Ware, 1979). The recommended dose is 1.5 mg/kg of body weight of the 0.25% solution without epinephrine. Plasma levels are well below the toxic range within four minutes after release of the tourniquet, and the only adverse reaction noted was drowsiness in one patient.

Nerve block: Without epinephrine, up to 70 ml of the 0.25% solution or 35 ml of the 0.5% solution; with epinephrine, up to 90 ml of the 0.25% solution or 45 ml of the 0.5% solution. The 0.5% solution is required to produce a consistent complete motor block of the larger nerves.

Caudal: With or without epinephrine, for obstetrical analgesia and perineal surgery, up to 30 ml of the 0.25% solution; for surgery of the lower extremities, up to 30 ml of the 0.5% solution. A single dose of either the 0.25% or 0.5% solution does not reliably produce motor block and, when used for a continuous technique, supplemental doses of the 0.25% or 0.5% solution are necessary. Only single-dose containers should be used.

Lumbar epidural: With or without epinephrine, for obstetrical analgesia and perineal surgery, up to 20 ml of the 0.25% solution; for obstetrical analgesia and surgery of the lower extremities, up to 20 ml of the 0.5% solution. When used for a continuous technique, supplemental 5- to 10-ml doses of the 0.25% or 0.5% solution are usually adequate to produce excellent sensory analgesia. Motor block, such as that required for abdominal surgery, usually can be obtained by use of up to 30 ml of the 0.75% solution. Repeated use of the 0.75% solution for continuous epidural anesthesia is inadvisable because of the possibility of accumulation. Only single-dose containers should be used.

Drug available generically: Solution 0.5% in 20 ml containers.

Marcaine (Breon). Solution 0.25% in 50 ml single- or multiple-dose containers; solution 0.5% in 30 ml single-dose containers and 50 ml multiple-dose containers; solution 0.75% in 30 ml single-dose containers.

Solutions are prepared with or without epinephrine bitartrate 1:200,000. Solutions that do not contain epinephrine may be autoclaved. Solutions in multiple-dose containers also contain methylparaben.

BUTAMBEN PICRATE
[Butesin Picrate]

Butamben is used on the skin to relieve pruritus and burning. Since it is relatively insoluble in water and thus poorly absorbed, this drug remains in contact with the skin for a prolonged period and produces a sustained anesthetic effect with a low incidence of systemic toxic reactions.

Butamben picrate may cause a rash in sensitive individuals; the incidence is increased because of the picrate component. For additional information on adverse reactions and precautions, see the Introduction.

ROUTE, USUAL DOSAGE, AND PREPARATIONS. *Topical*: The ointment is applied to affected areas as required.

Butesin Picrate (Abbott). Ointment 1% in 30 g containers (nonprescription).

CHLOROPROCAINE HYDROCHLORIDE
[Nesacaine, Nesacaine-CE]

Chloroprocaine, a chlorinated analogue of procaine, is used for infiltration, peripheral nerve block, and epidural anesthesia. The drug is not effective topically and has not been studied sufficiently to be used for subarachnoid anesthesia. Its anesthetic potency is slightly greater than that of procaine, and its duration of action is slightly shorter. Nerve blocks last an average of one hour; the addition of epinephrine 1:200,000 prolongs the duration to as much as two hours.

The systemic toxicity of chloroprocaine is less than that of all other local anesthetics because of its rapid degradation by plasma cholinesterase and short plasma half-life. No evidence of intact drug in the infant's cord blood at delivery after paracervical and epidural blocks has been reported. For additional information on adverse reactions and precautions, see the Introduction.

ROUTE, USUAL DOSAGE, AND PREPARATIONS.
Injection: As a general guide, the maximal single dose is 800 mg (20 mg/kg of body weight) without epinephrine and 1 g with epinephrine 1:200,000. Repeated doses of up to 300 mg without epinephrine and 600 mg with epinephrine 1:200,000 may be given at 50-minute intervals.
Infiltration: Without epinephrine, up to 80 ml of the 1% solution; with epinephrine 1:200,000, 100 ml of the 1% solution.
Peripheral nerve block: The dose of the 1% or 2% solution, with or without epinephrine 1:200,000, depends upon the type of block and intensity and duration of effect needed.
Caudal: Initially, 15 to 25 ml (depending upon the size of the patient) of the 2% or 3% Nesacaine-CE solution. Repeated doses may be given at 40- to 60-minute intervals as required; epinephrine 1:200,000 may be used to prolong the action.

Lumbar epidural: The usual total initial dose, with or without epinephrine 1:200,000, is 15 to 25 ml (approximately 2 to 2.5 ml per nerve segment to be blocked) of the 2% or 3% Nesacaine-CE solution. Supplemental doses of 10 to 20 ml may be given at 40- to 50-minute intervals.
    Nesacaine (Pennwalt). Solution 1% and 2% in 30 ml multiple-dose containers (not for caudal or epidural anesthesia).
    Nesacaine-CE (Pennwalt). Solution 2% and 3% in 30 ml single-dose containers (for caudal or epidural anesthesia; contains no preservative).

COCAINE HYDROCHLORIDE

Cocaine is a naturally occurring alkaloid that produces excellent surface anesthesia and intense vasoconstriction when applied to mucous surfaces. It is not used parenterally. Onset of action is rapid (one minute) and the duration is up to two hours, depending upon the dose and concentration applied. Cocaine is used for surface anesthesia in the ear, nose, and throat and in bronchoscopy; many physicians have concluded that it produces the most complete anesthesia of the upper airway passage possible. The addition of epinephrine not only is unnecessary because it does not delay absorption, but it also may increase the likelihood of arrhythmias and ventricular fibrillation. The moistening of dry cocaine powder with epinephrine solution to form so-called "cocaine mud" for use on the nasal mucosa is particularly dangerous and not recommended.

Toxic symptoms occur frequently because cocaine is absorbed readily after topical application in spite of its vasoconstrictor action and dosage is often not carefully monitored. Central nervous system effects include euphoria and cortical stimulation manifested by excitement and restlessness. Stimulation of the lower motor centers causes tremors, while stimulation of the medullary centers causes hypertension, tachycardia, and tachypnea. Acute poisoning produces marked cortical stimulation manifested by excitement, restlessness, confusion, tremor, hypertension, tachycardia, tachypnea, nausea, vomiting, abdominal pain, exophthalmos, and mydriasis. Stimulation is followed by depression and, finally, by death from ventilatory depression.

Repeated use results in psychic dependence and tolerance; therefore, cocaine is classified as a Schedule II drug under the Controlled Substances Act.

Cocaine exerts an indirect adrenergic effect by interfering with the tissue uptake of circulating catecholamines. This effect potentiates the actions of endogenous and exogenous epinephrine and norepinephrine (levarterenol). Ventricular fibrillation caused by absorption of excessive amounts of cocaine may occur, particularly if a general anesthetic that sensitizes the myocardium to catecholamines is also being administered. For this reason, cocaine should be used with extreme caution, if at all, in patients with hypertension, severe cardiovascular disease, or thyrotoxicosis and in patients taking drugs that also potentiate catecholamines (eg, guanethidine, monoamine oxidase inhibitors). Solutions of cocaine are unstable and deteriorate on standing; boiling and autoclaving cause decomposition.

For additional information on adverse reactions and precautions, see the Introduction.

ROUTE, USUAL DOSAGE, AND PREPARATIONS.
Topical: For the ear, nose, and throat and for bronchoscopy, concentrations of 1% to 4% are used. As a general guide, the maximal single dose is 1 mg/kg of body weight. The lowest concentration and smallest volume possible should be applied. Use of concentrations greater than 4% is not advisable because of the potential for increasing the incidence and severity of systemic toxic reactions.

> Drug available generically: Tablets (soluble) 135 mg. Also supplied in bulk form (crystals, powder).

CYCLOMETHYCAINE SULFATE
[Surfacaine]

Cyclomethycaine is applied topically on the skin and mucous membranes of the rectum, vagina, urethra, and urinary bladder to treat thermal or chemical burns; abrasions; dermatologic conditions characterized by pain, pruritus, and irritability; and in various proctologic, gynecologic, and urologic manipulations. This drug is relatively ineffective in anesthetizing the mucous membranes of the mouth, nose, trachea, bronchi, eye, and ear.

Cyclomethycaine may produce transitory stinging or burning in sensitive patients. The ointment form should not be used on vesicular lesions. For additional information on adverse reactions and precautions, see the Introduction.

ROUTE, USUAL DOSAGE, AND PREPARATIONS.
Topical:

Skin: The 0.5% cream or 1% ointment is applied as required.

Urethra: The 0.75% jelly is used in the untraumatized urethra. The optimal dose is up to 4 ml in women and 10 ml in men.

Anus: The 1% ointment or 0.75% jelly is used for rectal pain.

Vagina, Rectum: The 10 mg suppository relieves pain for up to eight hours; the 1% ointment also may be used.

> *Surfacaine* (Lilly). Cream 0.5% in 30 and 454 g containers (nonprescription); jelly 0.75% with thimerosal 1:10,000 as a preservative in 3.5, 30, and 150 g containers; ointment 1% in 30 and 454 g containers; suppositories 10 mg (nonprescription).

DIBUCAINE
[Nupercainal]

DIBUCAINE HYDROCHLORIDE
[Nupercaine]

Dibucaine is the most potent and one of the most toxic of the long-acting anesthetics when used parenterally. It is 15 to 20 times more potent and 15 times more toxic than procaine when injected. The parenteral dosage form is indicated only for spinal anesthesia. Hyperbaric (heavy), hypobaric (light), and isobaric solutions are available for subarachnoid anesthesia. The onset of action is relatively slow (up to 15 minutes); the duration of spinal anesthesia is three to four hours but can be prolonged to six hours by the addition of epinephrine. The topical dosage form is applied to the skin and rectal mucocutaneous junction for long-acting surface anesthesia. Dibucaine is partially metabolized and a portion is eliminated unchanged.

For adverse reactions and precautions, see the Introduction.

ROUTES, USUAL DOSAGE, AND PREPARATIONS.
Topical:
Skin: The 0.5% cream or 1% ointment is applied as required.
Rectum: The ointment or suppository is used morning and night, preferably following bowel movements.

DIBUCAINE:
Drug available generically: Ointment 1%.
Nupercainal (Ciba). Cream 0.5% in 45 g containers; ointment 1% in 30 and 60 g containers; suppositories 2.5 mg (nonprescription).

Injection:
Subarachnoid: Saddle block (including obstetrical but not involving abdomen), 2.5 to 5 mg (1 to 2 ml of hyperbaric solution); lower extremities, 4 mg (6 ml of hypobaric solution); abdomen, 7.5 to 10 mg (11 to 15 ml of hypobaric solution). For dosage for isobaric subarachnoid anesthesia, see the manufacturer's literature.

DIBUCAINE HYDROCHLORIDE:
Drug available generically in bulk form.
Nupercaine (Ciba). Solution (for spinal anesthesia only) 5 mg (0.25%) with dextrose (5%) 100 mg in 2 ml containers (hyperbaric); 0.667 mg (3.33%) (1:1,500) in 20 ml containers (hypobaric); and 10 mg (0.5%) (1:200) in 2 ml containers (isobaric).

DIMETHISOQUIN HYDROCHLORIDE
[Quotane]

Dimethisoquin is applied topically on the skin and mucocutaneous junctions. for relief of pruritus, irritation, burning, or pain in a variety of dermatoses, including nonspecific pruritus and sunburn. The incidence of sensitization is low. Onset of action is rapid (within a few minutes) and the duration is two to four hours. This drug is not used for injection.

For adverse reactions and precautions, see the Introduction.

ROUTE, USUAL DOSAGE, AND PREPARATIONS.
Topical: Ointment is applied no more than four times daily.
Quotane (Menley & James). Ointment 0.5% with thimerosal 1:50,000 in 30 g containers.

DIPERODON MONOHYDRATE
[Diothane]

Diperodon is used for surface anesthesia on the skin and mucocutaneous junctions. It is as potent as cocaine and has a longer duration of action.

Diperodon may cause burning or stinging and contact allergic reactions. For additional information on adverse reactions and precautions, see the Introduction.

ROUTE, USUAL DOSAGE, AND PREPARATIONS.
Topical: 1% ointment is used.

> **Diothane** (Merrell-National). Ointment 1% preserved with oxyquinoline benzoate 0.1% in 30 g containers (nonprescription).

DYCLONINE HYDROCHLORIDE
[Dyclone]

Dyclonine is used topically to anesthetize mucous membranes prior to endoscopy, to suppress the gag reflex, to relieve the pain of minor burns and gynecologic or proctologic procedures, and in the management of pruritus ani or vulvae. The potency of dyclonine is comparable to that of cocaine. Generally, up to ten minutes are required for onset of action and the duration is up to one hour.

The toxicity of dyclonine is low; however, this drug is contraindicated in cystoscopic procedures following intravenous pyelography because contrast media containing iodine can cause a precipitate to form, and this interferes with visualization. For additional information on adverse reactions and precautions, see the Introduction.

ROUTE, USUAL DOSAGE, AND PREPARATIONS.
Either the 0.5% or the 1% solution may be used for most of the indications described below. When continuous or repetitive application is anticipated, as in some oral or anogenital uses, the 0.5% solution may be preferred to reduce transmucosal absorption and the attendant possibility of cumulative systemic toxicity.
Topical: As a general guide, the maximal single dose is 200 mg.
Skin: 0.5% or 1% solution is applied as required.
Mouth, esophagus, oral endoscopy: For relief of oral pain, 5 to 10 ml of the 0.5% or 1% solution is swabbed, gargled, or sprayed and then expectorated. For esophagoscopy after pharyngeal anesthesia, 10 to 15 ml of the 0.5% solution is swallowed. For relief of esophageal pain, 5 to 15 ml of the 0.5% solution is swallowed.

Bronchoscopy: The tongue is pulled forward and the larynx and trachea are sprayed with 2 ml of the 1% solution every five minutes until the laryngeal reflex is abolished. This usually requires two or three sprayings. Five minutes should be allowed before instrumentation.
Urologic endoscopy: 6 to 30 ml of the 0.5% to 1% solution (usually 10 to 15 ml) is instilled into the urethra and retained for five to ten minutes before instrumentation.
Gynecology: 0.5% or 1% solution is used as a wet compress or spray.
Proctology: A cotton pledget saturated with the 0.5% or 1% solution is applied for relief of pain and discomfort.

> **Dyclone** (Dow). Solution 0.5% and 1% with chlorobutanol 0.1% in 30 ml containers.

ETIDOCAINE HYDROCHLORIDE
[Duranest]

This amide-type local anesthetic has a pKa of 7.7, which is similar to that of lidocaine (7.9); however, like bupivacaine, it is much more highly bound to protein (94%) than lidocaine. Etidocaine has a much higher lipid partition coefficient than either lidocaine or bupivacaine. Onset of action is rapid and the duration of anesthesia is comparable to that with bupivacaine. At equipotent levels of anesthesia, the duration of action of etidocaine is usually at least twice as long as that of lidocaine.

This agent is currently recommended for infiltration, peripheral nerve block, and epidural (but not subarachnoid) anesthesia. A 0.5% concentration is generally adequate for infiltration anesthesia, but the 1% or 1.5% concentration is suggested for epidural anesthesia. Onset of sensory block in epidural anesthesia is rapid (about five minutes), with complete block in 12 minutes. Although etidocaine and bupivacaine elicit seizures at the same plasma concentration level, the decreased rate of absorption, more rapid plasma decay, and increased volume of distribution are probably responsible for the fact that, experimentally, etidocaine is less toxic than bupivacaine after injection of the same dose.

Like other amides, etidocaine is metabolized primarily by the liver and metabolic products are excreted in the urine; little unchanged drug is excreted in the urine.

Etidocaine may cause mild pain on injection. This anesthetic produces a profound motor nerve paralysis after epidural administration; this is desirable for abdominal surgery but may be undesirable during the third stage of labor. Regression of anesthesia following epidural administration of etidocaine is similar to that seen with spinal anesthesia, ie, the patient may experience pain at the operative site while motor block is still profound. For additional information on adverse reactions and precautions, see the Introduction.

ROUTE, USUAL DOSAGE, AND PREPARATIONS.
Injection: The 0.5% solution is recommended for infiltration and peripheral nerve block, although the 1% solution may be more appropriate for certain peripheral nerve blocks if a smaller volume is preferable. Total dose of either the 0.5%, 1%, or 1.5% solution should not exceed 5.5 mg/kg of body weight for solutions with and 4 mg/kg for solutions without epinephrine. The 1% solution is recommended for epidural nerve blocks for various gynecological and obstetrical procedures. The 1.5% solution may be required in intra-abdominal procedures and cesarean sections.

> *Duranest* (Astra). Solution 0.5% in 30 ml single-dose containers; 0.5% with epinephrine 1:200,000 in 30 ml single-dose and with methylparaben in 50 ml multiple-dose containers; 1% with and without epinephrine 1:200,000 in 30 ml single-dose containers; 1.5% with epinephrine 1:200,000 in 20 ml containers. Single-dose containers without epinephrine may be autoclaved.

HEXYLCAINE HYDROCHLORIDE
[Cyclaine]

Hexylcaine is used for surface anesthesia of intact mucous membranes in endoscopy, intubations, and manipulations of the respiratory, upper gastrointestinal, and urinary tracts. Anesthesia is produced in five minutes and lasts approximately 30 minutes. Hexylcaine is not used by injection because of its local and systemic toxicity. Tissue irritation, burning, swelling, and tissue necrosis with slough have been reported after topical or inadvertent parenteral administration. For additional information on adverse reactions and precautions, see the Introduction.

ROUTE, USUAL DOSAGE, AND PREPARATIONS.
Topical: *Adults*, as a general guide, the maximal single dose is 200 mg. A 1% or 2% concentration usually gives adequate anesthesia.
Nose: The area is swabbed, packed, or sprayed with a 0.5% to 5% solution. A concentration of 1% or more may be required for antral puncture.
Bronchoscopy, endotracheal intubation: No more than 10 ml (200 mg) of a 2% solution should be used.
Gastroscopy: The patient should gargle four times with the 1% or 2% solution; the procedure is repeated twice at five-minute intervals. The excess should not be swallowed.
Genitourinary: The dose ordinarily should not exceed 10 ml of the 2% solution.

> *Cyclaine* (Merck Sharp & Dohme). Solution 5% with propylparaben 0.02% and methylparaben 0.15% in 60 ml containers.

LIDOCAINE
[Xylocaine]

LIDOCAINE HYDROCHLORIDE
[Xylocaine Hydrochloride]

This amide is one of the most widely used local anesthetics for infiltration, intravenous regional, nerve block, epidural, and subarachnoid anesthesia; it also is commonly used for topical anesthesia.

Compared to procaine, the action of lidocaine is more rapid in onset, more intense, and of longer duration; lidocaine also is more potent. This anesthetic has excellent powers of diffusion and penetration. It has a local vasodilating action but is usually administered with epinephrine. When used alone, anesthesia after perineural injection lasts 60 to 75 minutes; with epinephrine, anesthesia lasts two hours or more.

When administered by extravascular injection, lidocaine is approximately one and one-half times as toxic as procaine. When given intravenously, lidocaine is twice as toxic as procaine. Rapid absorption of large amounts of lidocaine generally causes convulsions, but central nervous system depression rather than stimulation may occur in some patients. Even therapeutic doses of lidocaine may cause drowsiness, lassitude, and amnesia. Other systemic reactions are similar to those produced by local anesthetics in general. Lidocaine is not irritating and produces relatively little sensitization when used topically. For additional information on adverse reactions and precautions, see the Introduction.

ROUTES, USUAL DOSAGE, AND PREPARATIONS. As a general guide, in healthy *adults*, the maximal single dose for topical use is 300 mg and for injection (excluding subarachnoid) is 300 mg (or 4.5 mg/kg) without epinephrine or 500 mg (or 7 mg/kg) with epinephrine. This dose should not be repeated at intervals of less than two hours. The vascularity of tissue at the site of injection also should be taken into consideration when estimating total dose. In normal *children*, the dose (preferably of the 0.5% or 1% solution) should be reduced according to the type of block and the age and surface area of the child (see Chapter 2).

Topical: The 2% solution is generally recommended for topical anesthesia. The 4% solution is used principally for laryngo-tracheal anesthesia, and it can be used when the lower concentration does not provide adequate anesthesia. The maximal recommended dose is 10 ml of the 2% or 5 ml of the 4% concentration.

Skin: The maximal dose is 35 g of the 2.5% or 5% ointment daily.

Nose and nasopharynx: 1 to 5 ml of a 1% to 4% solution is sprayed or used on cotton applicators, depending upon the procedure.

Pharynx and upper digestive tract: The 2% viscous solution is used. The preparation can be moved around the mouth and pharynx by the cheeks and tongue and then swallowed. The dose should not exceed 15 ml every three hours or 120 ml in 24 hours. The patient should not eat or drink for one hour after application because of the danger of aspiration.

Respiratory tract: 1 to 5 ml of the 4% solution is sprayed or used by applicator or pack to produce anesthesia of the pharynx, larynx, and trachea for laryngoscopy, endotracheal intubation, and bronchoscopy. In addition, 2 to 3 ml of the 4% solution may be injected through the cricothyroid membrane (transtracheal), but a total dose of 5 ml generally should not be exceeded.

Urology: A 2% aqueous solution or 2% jelly may be used. *Men*, prior to catheterization, 5 to 10 ml of the 2% jelly is instilled into the urethra and retained for five to ten minutes. The maximal dose is 30 ml in 12 hours. *Women*, application is the same but the dose is 3 to 5 ml.

Anorectal: The suppositories are used after each bowel movement and before retiring. No more than five suppositories should be used in 24 hours.

LIDOCAINE, LIDOCAINE HYDROCHLORIDE:
Drug available generically: Ointment 5%.
Xylocaine (Astra). Ointment 2.5% in 35 g containers (nonprescription) and 5% in 3.5, 15, and 35 g containers; suppositories 100 mg.
Xylocaine Hydrochloride (Astra). Jelly 2% with methylparaben and propylparaben in 30 ml containers; solution (viscous) 2% in 100 and 450 ml containers; solution 4% in 5 ml sterile containers and with methylparaben in 50 ml containers.

Injection:
Infiltration: Without epinephrine, for extensive procedures, 25 to 60 ml of a 0.5%

solution or 10 to 30 ml of a 1% solution; for minor surgery and relief of pain, 2 to 50 ml of a 0.5% solution. With epinephrine 1:200,000, up to 50 ml of a 1% solution. Maximum single dose should be 7 mg/kg.
Intravenous regional: 40 to 50 ml of a 0.5% solution without epinephrine is used for the arm and approximately 60 ml for the leg.
Nerve block: Without epinephrine, up to 30 ml of a 1% solution or 15 ml of a 2% solution. With epinephrine 1:200,000, up to 50 ml of a 1% or 25 ml of a 2% solution. Retrobulbar block lasting one to one and one-half hours can be accomplished with 4 ml of the 4% solution.
Caudal: Without epinephrine, for obstetrical analgesia, up to 30 ml of the 1% solution; for surgical anesthesia, up to 20 ml of the 1.5% solution. With epinephrine 1:200,000 for surgical anesthesia, up to 30 ml of the 1.5% solution or 25 ml of the 2% solution. Analgesia during labor may be obtained with 20 to 30 ml of a 0.5% solution. Only single-dose containers should be used.
Lumbar epidural: Without epinephrine, for obstetrical analgesia, 8 to 15 ml of the 1% solution; for surgical anesthesia, 15 to 20 ml·of the 1.5% or 10 to 15 ml of the 2% solution. The dose depends on the level of analgesia required but cannot be predicted accurately. With epinephrine 1:200,000, up to 20 ml of the 1%, 1.5%, or 2% solution. Analgesia during labor may be obtained with 8 to 10 ml of a 0.5% solution. Only single-dose containers should be used.
Subarachnoid: The 1.5% and 5% solutions with 7.5% dextrose (hyperbaric) are used for subarachnoid anesthesia. For vaginal delivery, 0.8 or 1 ml (40 or 50 mg) of the 5% solution or 2 ml (30 mg) of the 1.5% solution will provide perineal anesthesia for about one hour; analgesia lasts an additional 40 minutes. For cesarean section, 1.5 ml (75 mg) of the 5% solution may be used. The duration may be prolonged by adding epinephrine.

LIDOCAINE HYDROCHLORIDE:
Drug available generically: Solution 1% and 2% with and without epinephrine, 4% without epinephrine.
Xylocaine (Astra). Solution 0.5% in 50 ml single- and multiple-dose containers and with epinephrine 1:200,000 in 50 ml multiple-dose containers; solution 1% in 2, 5, and 30 ml single- and 20 and 50 ml multiple-dose containers, with epinephrine 1:200,000 in 30 ml single-dose containers, and with epinephrine 1:100,000 in 20 and 50 ml multiple-dose containers; solution 1.5% in 20 ml single-dose containers, with dextrose 7.5% in 2 ml single-dose containers, and with epinephrine 1:200,000 in 30 ml single-dose containers; solution 2% in 2 and 10 ml single- and 20 and 50 ml multiple-dose containers, with epinephrine 1:200,000 in 20 ml single-dose containers, and with epinephrine 1:100,000 in 2 ml single- and 20 and 50 ml multiple-dose containers; solution 4% in 5 and 50 ml multiple-dose containers; solution 5% with dextrose 7.5% in 2 ml single-dose containers. Aqueous solutions without epinephrine can be autoclaved repeatedly if necessary; preparations containing dextrose should not be autoclaved more than once or twice. All multiple-dose containers contain methylparaben 1 mg/ml.

MEPIVACAINE HYDROCHLORIDE
[Carbocaine]

This amide is chemically and pharmacologically related to lidocaine and is indicated for infiltration, nerve block, and epidural anesthesia. Mepivacaine is not effective topically except in large doses and therefore should not be used by this route. The potency of mepivacaine is similar to that of lidocaine. Anesthesia develops in three to five minutes and lasts two to two and one-half hours. Conventional doses of mepivacaine may be used without epinephrine for most purposes. Unless it is contraindicated, epinephrine should be added to reduce plasma levels of mepivacaine with larger doses. Evidence from a randomized, double-blind trial using mepivacaine 1% for obstetrical caudal anesthesia indicates that the addition of epinephrine 1:200,000 may prolong the first stage of labor by approximately 30 minutes and increase the need for augmentation of labor with oxytocics.

The systemic reactions observed with mepivacaine are similar to those produced by other local anesthetics, but the drowsiness, lassitude, and amnesia observed with lidocaine are less with mepivacaine. Therefore, this anesthetic may be desirable for use in outpatient surgery. For additional information on adverse reactions and precautions, see the Introduction.

ROUTE, USUAL DOSAGE, AND PREPARATIONS.
Injection: *Adults*, as a general guide, the doses of mepivacaine are similar to those of lidocaine. The maximal single dose is 7 mg/kg of body weight or 400 mg (550 mg with epinephrine), whichever is less. This dose should not be repeated at intervals of less than 90 minutes, and no more than 1 g should be administered during any 24-hour period. The dosage should be reduced in *children*.
Infiltration: Up to 80 ml of a 0.5% or 40 ml of the 1% solution.
Nerve block: 5 to 20 ml of the 1% or 2% solution.
Epidural: 15 to 30 ml of the 1% solution, 10 to 25 ml of the 1.5% solution, or 10 to 20 ml of the 2% solution. Only single-dose containers should be used.

> *Carbocaine* (Breon). Solution (isotonic) 1% and 2% with methylparaben 0.1% in 50 ml multiple-dose containers; solution (isobaric) 1% and 1.5% (without preservatives) in 30 ml single-dose containers; solution (isobaric) 2% (without preservatives) in 20 ml single-dose containers.

PIPEROCAINE HYDROCHLORIDE
[Metycaine]

Piperocaine is a benzoic acid ester used primarily for surface anesthesia; it is seldom employed for infiltration or peripheral nerve block anesthesia, and it is not used for epidural or subarachnoid anesthesia. Its effects are similar to those of procaine, but piperocaine is more potent, more toxic, and has a faster onset and a somewhat longer duration of action.

For adverse reactions and precautions, see the Introduction.

ROUTES, USUAL DOSAGE, AND PREPARATIONS.
Topical: As a general guide, the maximal single dose is 800 mg of a 1% solution or 1 g of a 0.5% solution.
Nose, larynx: A 2% spray is used for minor procedures, and a 5% or 10% solution is used for removal of polyps and washing antrums.
Stomach and other hollow viscus: No more than 100 ml of a 0.25% solution is instilled.
Urethra: Men, 4 to 8 ml of a 2% to 4% solution is instilled into the urethra and retained for a few minutes, followed by 8 to 16 ml retained for three to ten minutes. *Women*, 15 ml of a 2% to 4% solution is instilled into the bladder; the remaining solution is withdrawn when anesthesia has been established.
Proctoscopy: A 5% solution is commonly used for dilatation and examination, but a 10% or 20% solution may be applied for certain procedures.

> *Metycaine* (Lilly). Powder in 4 oz containers.

Injection:
Infiltration, nerve block: Up to 200 ml of a 0.5% and 80 ml of a 1% solution. The 2% solution also may be used cautiously for nerve block.

> *Metycaine* (Lilly). Powder (for solution) in 120 g containers; solution 2% with chlorobutanol 0.5% in 30 ml containers (infiltration, nerve block).

PRAMOXINE HYDROCHLORIDE
[Tronothane]

Pramoxine is derived from morpholine and, since it is chemically different from ester- or amide-type compounds, may be useful in patients who are sensitive to these classes of drugs. The potency of pramoxine is comparable to that of benzocaine. Onset of action is within three to five minutes.

Pramoxine is applied topically to the skin or mucous membranes to relieve pain caused by minor burns and wounds and to relieve pruritus secondary to dermatoses or hemorrhoids. It also may be used to facilitate sigmoidoscopic examinations and to anesthetize laryngopharyngeal surfaces prior to endotracheal intubation. However, it does not abolish the gag reflex. This anesthetic should not be injected or applied to the nasal mucosa, for it may irritate the tissue, and it should not be used for bronchoscopy or gastroscopy.

For adverse reactions and precautions, see the Introduction.

ROUTE, USUAL DOSAGE, AND PREPARATIONS. *Topical*:
Skin, mucous membranes: The 1% cream or jelly is applied as required, usually every three or four hours. For severe discomfort, preparations may be applied every two or three hours for one or two days; applications should be decreased thereafter to every four hours.
Larynx, trachea: The 1% jelly is used on endotracheal and intragastric tubes.

> *Tronothane* (Abbott). Cream (water-miscible) 1% in 30 g containers; jelly (water-soluble) 1% in 30 g containers (nonprescription).

PRILOCAINE HYDROCHLORIDE
[Citanest]

Prilocaine is similar pharmacologically to mepivacaine and lidocaine and is used for infiltration, intravenous regional, peripheral nerve block, and epidural anesthesia. It is not used topically or for subarachnoid anesthesia. The effectiveness of prilocaine and lidocaine in equivalent dosage is comparable, but the action of prilocaine is slower in onset and of longer duration. Epinephrine will prolong its effect.

Since prilocaine is more rapidly metabolized and excreted and has a larger volume of distribution than lidocaine, it is approximately 40% less toxic. Blood levels are lower after administration of prilocaine for the same reason, and this probably accounts for the reported lack of

psychomotor impairment compared to that occurring after use of bupivacaine, etidocaine, and lidocaine at equianesthetic doses. Therefore, this anesthetic may be desirable for use in outpatient surgery.

Two metabolites of prilocaine, ortho-toluidine and nitroso-toluidine, form methemoglobin. When doses in excess of 600 mg are given, a grayish or slate-blue cyanosis of the lips, mucous membranes, and nail beds may develop, but respiratory and circulatory distress apparently do not occur. Methemoglobinemia also has been observed in neonates whose mothers received prilocaine shortly before delivery. In one clinical study, no signs of inadequate oxygen transport developed in healthy individuals who received 1.2 g of prilocaine. Although methemoglobinemia is readily reversed by the intravenous administration of methylene blue (1 to 2 mg/kg of body weight of a 1% solution injected over a five-minute period), this therapeutic action may cease because of the rapid clearance of methylene blue before conversion of all the methemoglobin to hemoglobin. Prilocaine should not be administered to patients with idiopathic or congenital methemoglobinemia, anemia, or cardiac or ventilatory failure with hypoxia; it should be used with caution for continuous epidural anesthesia since the methemoglobinemic effect of individual doses is additive.

For additional information on adverse reactions and precautions, see the Introduction.

ROUTE, USUAL DOSAGE, AND PREPARATIONS.
Injection: As a general guide, in normal healthy *adults*, the maximal single dose is 600 mg or 8 mg/kg of body weight in a two-hour period or no more than 1.2 g in a four-hour period. A 0.5% to 1% concentration should be used in *children*, and the dose should be reduced appropriately according to the type of block and the age, weight, and height of the child.
Nerve block: Up to 30 ml of the 2% solution or 15 to 20 ml of the 3% solution.
Infiltration: Up to 30 ml of the 1% or 2% solution.
Caudal: 20 to 30 ml of the 1% solution is

adequate for most routine vaginal deliveries. For surgical procedures requiring more profound anesthesia, 20 to 30 ml of the 2% solution or 15 to 20 ml of the 3% solution.

Lumbar epidural: 20 to 30 ml of the 1% or 2% solution or 15 to 20 ml of the 3% solution.

> **Citanest** (Astra). Solution 1% and 2% with and without methylparaben 0.1% in 30 ml single- and multiple-dose containers; solution 3% in 20 ml single-dose containers.

PROCAINE HYDROCHLORIDE
[Novocain]

Procaine was the preferred local anesthetic for injection for many years, but it is now being supplanted by amide local anesthetics and other anesthetics for infiltration, nerve block, and subarachnoid anesthesia. In general, it also has been replaced by more suitable agents for epidural anesthesia because of its slow onset of action and the high incidence of inadequate blocks. Procaine has a slower onset of action than lidocaine and prilocaine; its duration of action is about one hour. It is not applied topically.

Procaine is rapidly metabolized, a factor that accounts for its safety. Much of it is hydrolyzed by plasma cholinesterase; the remainder is metabolized in the liver. The adverse reactions produced by procaine are similar to those of other synthetic local anesthetics. For additional information on adverse reactions and precautions, see the Introduction.

ROUTE, USUAL DOSAGE, AND PREPARATIONS.
Injection: As a general guide, the maximal single dose for *adults* (excluding subarachnoid anesthesia) is 600 mg (10 mg/kg of body weight); epinephrine 1:200,000 should be used with larger doses.
Infiltration: With or without epinephrine 1:200,000, up to 100 ml of a 0.25% or 0.5% solution.
Nerve block: With or without epinephrine

1:200,000, up to 50 ml of the 1% or 25 ml of the 2% solution.
Caudal: The 1% or 2% solution is administered. For continuous caudal anesthesia, initially, 30 ml of a 1.5% solution, with subsequent doses adjusted as required.
Epidural: The 1% or 2% solution is used.
Subarachnoid: The 10% solution diluted with 10% dextrose prepared for subarachnoid anesthesia (hyperbaric) is used. For saddle block (perineum), 0.5 ml of the 10% solution diluted with 0.5 ml of 10% dextrose injection; for lower extremities, 1 ml of the 10% solution diluted with 1 ml of 10% dextrose injection; for level to costal margin, 2 ml of the 10% solution diluted with 1 ml of 10% dextrose injection.

> Drug available generically: Solution 1% and 2%.
> **Novocain** (Breon). Solution 1% in 2 and 6 ml containers and with chlorobutanol 0.25% in 30 ml containers; solution 2% with chlorobutanol 0.25% in 30 ml containers; solution 10% in 2 ml containers (for spinal anesthesia; reautoclaving not recommended).

TETRACAINE HYDROCHLORIDE
[Pontocaine]

Tetracaine is the most widely used drug for subarachnoid anesthesia. It is not recommended for infiltration or peripheral nerve blocks. Tetracaine is approximately ten times more potent and toxic than procaine when injected. The onset of action is slow (approximately five minutes) after injection, but the duration of anesthesia is more than twice as long as that of procaine (two to three hours). Topically, onset of action also develops slowly, and the duration of anesthesia is approximately 45 minutes. Tetracaine is metabolized in the plasma and liver at a slower rate than procaine.

For information on adverse reactions and precautions, see the Introduction.

ROUTES, USUAL DOSAGE, AND PREPARATIONS. As a general guide, the maximal single dose is 50 mg topically and 1.5 mg/kg of body weight by injection (excluding subarachnoid).

Topical:

Skin, anus: The 0.5% ointment or 1% cream is used. No more than 30 g for *adults* or 7.5 g for *children* should be applied in a 24-hour period.

Nose, pharynx: Up to 2 ml of a 1% solution.

Esophageal and laryngeal reflexes: 2 ml of a 1% solution effectively abolishes reflexes in preparation for esophagoscopy, bronchoscopy, and bronchography. These doses should not be exceeded because of the risk of systemic toxicity caused by rapid absorption of the drug.

> Drug available generically: Ointment. Also supplied in bulk form (ointment, powder).
>
> *Pontocaine* (Breon). Cream 1% in 30 g containers (nonprescription); ointment 0.5% in 30 g containers (nonprescription); solution 0.5% in 15 and 60 ml containers and 2% in 30 and 120 ml containers.

Injection:

Infiltration, peripheral nerve block: Tetracaine is not recommended for these procedures now because of its slow onset of action and great systemic toxicity.

Caudal: Up to 30 ml of a 0.15% solution with epinephrine 1:200,000 is used. As anesthesia wears off, subsequent doses of 20 ml may be administered.

Subarachnoid: The 0.2% or 0.3% solutions (hyperbaric) or the 1% solution diluted with an equal volume of 10% dextrose prepared for spinal anesthesia (hyperbaric) is used. For obstetrical saddle block, 2 to 4 mg; for lower extremities and perineal operations, 3 to 6 mg; for most cesarean sections and lower abdominal surgery, 9 to 12 mg; for upper abdominal surgery, 12 to 15 mg. Doses exceeding 15 mg are rarely administered. Epinephrine 1:1,000 (0.1 to 0.3 mg) may be added to prolong the duration of anesthesia by 30% to 50% in the average adult. Epinephrine may prolong the duration of anesthesia excessively in elderly patients.

> *Pontocaine* (Breon). Powder 20 mg; solution 0.2% with dextrose 6% in 2 ml containers, 0.3% with dextrose 6% in 5 ml containers (saddle block, perineal), and 1% in 2 ml containers (subarachnoid).©

Selected References

Covino BG: Systemic toxicity of local anesthetic agents. *Anesth Analg* 57:387-388, 1978.

Covino BG, Vassallo HG: *Local Anesthetics: Mechanisms of Action and Clinical Use.* New York, Grune & Stratton, 1976.

de Jong RH: Toxic effects of local anesthetics. *JAMA* 239:1166-1168, 1978.

de Jong RH: *Local Anesthetics*, ed 2. Springfield, Ill, Charles C Thomas Publisher, 1977.

Dripps RD, et al: *Introduction to Anesthesia: The Principles of Safe Practice*, ed 5. Philadelphia, WB Saunders Co, 1977.

Moore DC, et al: Bupivacaine: Review of 11,080 cases. *Anesth Analg* 57:42-53, 1978.

Moore DC, et al: Factors determining dosages of amide-type local anesthetic drugs. *Anesthesiology* 47:263-268, 1977.

Ralston DH, Shnider SM: Fetal and neonatal effects of regional anesthesia in obstetrics. *Anesthesiology* 48:34-64, 1978.

Ware RJ: Intravenous regional analgesia using bupivacaine: Double blind comparison with lignocaine. *Anaesthesia* 34:231-235, 1979.

General Anesthetics | 20

General anesthetics alter the central nervous system and induce varying degrees of analgesia, depression of consciousness, relaxation of skeletal muscle, and reduction of reflex activity. The ideal general anesthetic should be stable, nonflammable, prompt acting, metabolically inert, and rapidly eliminated. It should provide adequate analgesia and muscular relaxation without producing excitement or adverse effects on vital organs and systems, even during prolonged administration. Recovery of consciousness should occur quickly with no adverse aftereffects or complications. No single agent presently available possesses all of these ideal characteristics.

Currently, general anesthetics are thought to act by fluidizing organized lipid (critical volume hypothesis) in the membranes of nerve cells, which interferes with the normal physiologic functions of the membranes (Kaufman, 1977). This theory is compatible for all general anesthetics and probably also accounts for the action of uncharged lipophilic molecules of local anesthetics and alcohol. Adaptive changes take place in membrane lipid with time and exposure to anesthetics. A corollary to the theory proposes that such adaptive changes result in cross tolerance among alcohol, barbiturates, and general anesthetics.

The classical signs described by Guedel for determining depth of anesthesia are reliable only for ether alone or for ether in combination with nitrous oxide. Anesthetic agents can no longer simply be viewed as producing progressive depression of the central nervous system. Because of the introduction of new and different types of inhalation and intravenous anesthetics, the concept of how anesthetics alter consciousness to prevent response to painful stimuli must be reconsidered. States of altered consciousness correlate reasonably well with electrical activity of the brain; both depression and stimulation can cause functional disorganization of selected brain activities (Winters, 1976). Nitrous oxide, ketamine, and enflurane selectively enhance electrical activity to produce an amnesic and/or cataleptic (dissociative) state which is quite different from that induced by anesthetics that only depress the central nervous system (eg, barbiturates, halothane, isoflurane). Large doses of certain cataleptic agents, such as ketamine and enflurane, can produce convulsions. Diethyl ether can produce anesthesia with characteristics of both stimulation and depression.

Comparative Evaluations

There are two types of general anesthetics, inhalation and intravenous; the arterial concentration required for anesthesia with either type varies with the condition of the patient, the desired depth of anesthesia, and the agent employed. General anesthesia should be undertaken only by individuals who have received adequate training.

Selected references are listed for more detailed information on inhalation anesthetics (Chenoweth, 1972; Collins, 1976; Cohen, 1978), intravenous anesthetics (Dundee and Wyant, 1974; Ghoneim and Korttila, 1977; Hug, 1978; Whitwam, 1978), or both types of anesthetics (Davie, 1977; Clarke and Norman, 1979; Steen and Michenfelder, 1979).

Anesthesia is rarely produced with a single drug, even if preanesthetic medication is not given. Use of inhalation anesthetics is almost always preceded by administration of intravenous induction anesthetics. Short procedures utilizing only an intravenous anesthetic often require supplementation with a muscle relaxant. Thus, most anesthesia represents administration of a number of drugs. The use of certain inhalation and intravenous anesthetics, often in conjunction with narcotic analgesics, neuroleptic drugs, or muscle relaxants, is referred to as combination anesthesia. Special types of combination anesthesia (ie, balanced anesthesia, neuroleptanesthesia) are discussed later in this chapter.

Inhalation Anesthetics: These are gases or volatile liquids (volatility is often expressed as vapor pressure [VP] in torr at 20 C) that vary greatly in their rate of anesthetic induction, potency, and muscle relaxant and analgesic effects. These drugs have an advantage over intravenous agents in that depth of anesthesia can be changed rapidly by varying the inhaled concentration. The rate at which the partial pressure of an inhalation anesthetic in the arterial blood approaches that in the alveoli is largely dependent upon the drug's solubility in blood (the blood gas partition coefficient at 37 C [blood/gas]). When solubility is low, equilibrium is approached rapidly. The clinical potency of these agents is often defined in terms of its MAC: the minimal alveolar concentration necessary to prevent movement in 50% of individuals subjected to a painful stimulus (eg, skin incision).

The anesthetic *gases* are cyclopropane, nitrous oxide, and ethylene. Ethylene has properties similar to those of nitrous oxide but is seldom used because it is flammable (the only such agent that is lighter than air) and has an unpleasant odor.

The *volatile liquids* are ether, halothane [Fluothane], methoxyflurane [Penthrane], enflurane [Ethrane], and the investigational agent, isoflurane [Forane]; all but ether are halogenated compounds. Vinyl ether, chloroform, ethyl chloride, and trichloroethylene have been supplanted by other agents because of their disadvantages (most notably, hepatotoxicity, adverse cardiovascular effects, and, except for chloroform, flammability).

Intravenous Anesthetics: The ultrashort-acting barbiturates, thiopental [Pentothal], methohexital [Brevital], and thiamylal [Surital], are intravenous induction agents that cause rapid loss of consciousness, are not explosive, and provide pleasant induction and recovery. However, they produce little muscle relaxation and frequently do not abolish superficial reflexes. Repeated maintenance doses result in accumulation and prolonged recovery time. Since these agents have little if any analgesic activity, they are seldom used alone except in brief minor procedures.

Ketamine [Ketaject, Ketalar] is a short-acting nonbarbiturate anesthetic that may be given intravenously or intramuscularly. It induces a cataleptic or dissociative state in which the patient appears to be awake but is unconscious and does not respond to pain. Ketamine has been used in various diagnostic procedures; in brief, minor surgical procedures that do not require substantial skeletal muscle relaxation; and in burn patients. It also may be used as an induction agent, especially when cardiovascular or sympathetic depression is undesirable.

Diazepam [Valium] and the investigational drug, flunitrazepam [Rohypnol], are benzodiazepines that are given intravenously for induction. They produce anterograde amnesia that is useful in anesthesia. Diazepam is used alone to produce basal sedation for diagnostic procedures (eg, endoscopy).

An investigational drug, etomidate, has been proposed as a substitute for intravenous barbiturates for induction. It has a shorter duration of action than the barbiturates. The pharmaceutical formulation currently available frequently produces pain on injection.

Adverse Reactions and Precautions

Inhalation Anesthetics: Delirium may develop during induction and recovery despite premedication with a central nervous system depressant and atropine or scopolamine (see Chapter 21, Adjuncts to Anesthesia and Analeptic Drugs). Nausea and vomiting also can occur postoperatively; these untoward effects may or may not be caused by the anesthetic agent alone but are particularly likely to develop following administration of ether and cyclopropane.

Inhalation anesthetics have a direct depressant effect on the myocardium and vascular smooth muscle. The degree of depression varies with different agents and is related to the depth of anesthesia. There is usually little danger of circulatory failure when appropriate concentrations of anesthetic gases or vapors are administered to healthy patients. Halothane [Fluothane], enflurane [Ēthrane], isoflurane [Forane], and methoxyflurane [Penthrane] have pronounced depressant effects on the cardiovascular system, and severe hypotension and circulatory failure may occur with overdosage. Although ether and cyclopropane depress the myocardium by a direct action, cardiac output and arterial pressure are affected minimally because these drugs also stimulate the sympathetic nervous system.

Arrhythmias may develop during administration of any inhalation anesthetic, particularly cyclopropane. Supraventricular arrhythmias are common and usually benign unless they are associated with reduced cardiac output and arterial pressure. Ventricular arrhythmias occur only rarely except in the presence of hypoxia or hypercapnia. Cyclopropane and halothane sensitize the heart to the actions of catecholamines; therefore, administration of epinephrine, norepinephrine [Levophed], or isoproterenol [Isuprel] during anesthesia with these agents may be hazardous, since the combined action of the anesthetic and the catecholamine increases the risk of ventricular arrhythmias. However, cautious use of a limited, nonintravenous dose of epinephrine may be acceptable during administration of halothane.

Ventilatory depression occurs frequently during deeper levels of general anesthesia with inhalation anesthetics, and institution of assisted or controlled ventilation may be necessary. Cyclopropane, halothane, enflurane, isoflurane, and methoxyflurane are most potent in this regard. Although ether has a depressant effect on the respiratory center, ventilation is stimulated during light levels of anesthesia because of reflex effects.

The cause of transient, slight abnormalities in the results of liver function tests is uncertain, but such changes are relatively common after any general anesthetic technique; serious liver damage is relatively rare. Although halothane apparently can cause hepatitis rarely, the diagnosis remains one of exclusion under normal circumstances. The evidence implicating other halogenated compounds (ie, enflurane, methoxyflurane) is not convincing.

Reversible oliguria as a result of reduced renal blood flow and glomerular filtration occurs during general anesthesia. This may be minimized if the patient is adequately hydrated and deep levels of anesthesia are avoided. However, methoxyflurane has produced direct tubular injury with high-output renal failure; therefore, it is contraindicated in patients with impaired renal function and possibly in those receiving other potentially nephrotoxic agents (eg, gentamicin [Garamycin], tetracyclines). Because this complication is dose related and caused by the free fluoride ion produced by metabolism of the drug, methoxyflurane should be administered only in relatively low concentrations for relatively short periods. In comparison to methoxyflurane, enflurane produces substantially less free fluoride ion when metabolized, isoflurane minimal amounts, and halothane essentially none.

Body temperature tends to fall during anesthesia because of exposure, vasodilation, and suppression of thermoregulation. Postoperative shivering is commonly observed after anesthesia with the potent inhalation agents.

Malignant hyperpyrexia is a rare, often fatal, complication of general anesthesia that develops in genetically susceptible individuals and it may have a variable clinical course. Some susceptible families have disturbances of muscle function. The level of blood creatine phosphokinase activity may be elevated but is not a reliable indicator of susceptibility; muscle biopsy for an in vitro contraction test is more reliable. Malignant hyperpyrexia has been associated with many different general anesthetic techniques, and signs of hyper-metabolism (tachycardia, tachypnea) must be recognized early through vigilance and by routine monitoring of temperature during surgery. Hyperpyrexia is treated by eliminating all inhalation agents except oxygen, correcting metabolic and respiratory acidosis, and body cooling (including use of ice packs and cooling blankets and lavage of open body cavities). Therapy also must include supportive measures to combat arrhythmias, hyperkalemia, fluid imbalance, and other problems. The intravenous administration of procaine [Novocain] or procainamide [Pronestyl] (but not of lidocaine [Xylocaine] or mepivacaine [Carbocaine]) may be beneficial, but these drugs must be given slowly (0.5 to 1 mg/kg/min) with extreme caution because of the danger of cardiovascular depression; electrocardiographic monitoring is essential. One experimental study does not support the use of procainamide but recommends dantrolene [Dantrium] (Nelson and Flewellen, 1979). Dantrolene has been reported to prevent or control this syndrome in swine and the results of an early clinical investigation are encouraging (Friesen et al, 1979).

If general anesthesia cannot be avoided in patients susceptible to malignant hyperpyrexia, thiopental, narcotic analgesics, droperidol [Inapsine], and probably ketamine [Ketaject, Ketalar] appear to be safe. The role of nitrous oxide in causing malignant hyperpyrexia is difficult to assess; many anesthesiologists still consider nitrous oxide to be safe for these patients.

Nitrous oxide, ether, enflurane, halothane, isoflurane, and methoxyflurane increase intracranial pressure, but this appears to be of consequence only in patients with intracranial lesions. Since hypocapnia induced by hyperventilation essentially eliminates the increase in intracranial pressure, these agents probably should not be given to patients with intracranial lesions until hyperventilation has been instituted.

Although general anesthetics are teratogenic in animals, they have not been shown to be so in the human fetus; on general principles, they should not be administered during the first trimester of pregnancy unless such use is unavoidable. Neonatal depression can be anticipated if high concentrations of potent inhalation agents are administered for long periods prior to delivery. With the exception of cyclopropane and nitrous oxide, high concentrations of such agents also produce uterine relaxation and may, as a consequence, produce postpartum bleeding; this may be particularly pronounced with halothane, enflurane, and isoflurane.

The dose of nondepolarizing neuromuscular blocking agents (tubocurarine, metocurine [Metubine], pancuronium [Pavulon], and gallamine [Flaxedil]) should be reduced when used with cyclopropane, ether, halothane, enflurane, isoflurane, or methoxyflurane, because these anesthetics potentiate the muscle relaxant effects of the neuromuscular blocking drugs. Cyclopropane and halothane are the least and enflurane and isoflurane the most potent in this regard.

Cyclopropane and ether are flammable and explosive and must be used with appropriate precautions and only in periodically approved areas especially designed to minimize ignition hazards.

Intravenous Anesthetics: Transient hypotension, yawning, coughing, and laryngeal spasm may occur during induction of anesthesia with barbiturates. Hypotension in hypovolemic patients or those with diminished cardiac contractility and undesirably light anesthesia due to rapid elimination of thiopental from the brain can develop. These agents may cause pronounced ventilatory depression and apnea immediately after rapid injection or overdosage. Shivering or excitement and delirium in the presence of pain may be observed during recovery.

The barbiturates may exacerbate acute intermittent porphyria and are contraindicated in patients with this disease. Care should be taken to avoid extravasation or intra-arterial injection of these drugs, for tissue necrosis and gangrene may occur.

See the evaluations for adverse reactions and precautions to be observed with the nonbarbiturate anesthetics.

INHALATION ANESTHETICS

Gases

CYCLOPROPANE

$$H_2C \text{———} CH_2$$
$$\diagdown \diagup$$
$$\underset{H_2}{C}$$

Cyclopropane (blood/gas 0.46, MAC 9.2%) is a pleasant smelling, gaseous anesthetic. It is explosive at all anesthetic concentrations and should be used in a closed system with a carbon dioxide absorber. Its explosiveness is responsible for its relatively rare use. Induction and recovery are rapid. This gas has a wide margin of safety and good analgesic properties and often produces adequate skeletal muscle relaxation except at light planes of anesthesia. Since it potentiates the effects of nondepolarizing neuromuscular blocking agents, the dose of these drugs should be reduced when cyclopropane is the anesthetic (see Chapter 21, Adjuncts to Anesthesia and Analeptic Drugs).

The cardiovascular system usually is not adversely affected during anesthesia, for the drug's direct depressant effect on the myocardium is counteracted by its stimulation of the sympathetic nervous system. Myocardial contractility is usually maintained, the heart rate is unchanged or slightly decreased, peripheral resistance is increased, central venous pressure may rise, and arterial pressure and cardiac output are maintained or moderately elevated. If morphine is given for premedication, cardiac output is diminished and the heart rate may fall.

Cyclopropane increases the irritability of pacemaker and conduction tissues and ventricular arrhythmias can occur, especially if anesthesia is deep or ventilation is inadequate and hypercapnia develops. These reactions are particularly likely to occur and to be severe if a catecholamine or atropine or scopolamine is administered parenterally during anesthesia; if atropine or scopolamine must be given, the initial dose should be 0.08 mg. Severe post-anesthetic hypotension (cyclopropane shock) is observed occasionally.

Ventilation is progressively depressed as anesthesia is deepened, particularly if a narcotic analgesic has been used for pre-medication; therefore, ventilation should be controlled to prevent hypercapnia. Breathholding and laryngeal spasm also may occur under light levels of anesthesia.

Cyclopropane elevates plasma levels of endogenous catecholamines because of increased sympathetic stimulation and re-sultant decreased blood flow to the extremities, kidneys, or liver. This may contribute to reduced urinary output and depleted hepatic glycogen. Moderate ele-vations of blood glucose also occur, possi-bly as a result of sympathetic stimulation. Transient, slight alterations in the results of liver function tests as well as massive he-patic necrosis have been observed.

Although signs of increased bleeding may occur during surgery, this is probably due to accumulation of carbon dioxide re-sulting in increased blood flow to the skin and elevated central venous pressure.

Nausea, vomiting, and headache occur frequently after cyclopropane anesthesia. Emergence is rapid but postanesthetic de-lirium is noted more frequently than after other commonly used inhalation agents, particularly if a narcotic analgesic has not been used for premedication.

ROUTE, USUAL DOSAGE, AND PREPARATIONS. *Inhalation*: For induction, 25% to 50% with oxygen; for maintenance, 10% to 20% with oxygen or intermittent inhalation of higher concentrations with oxygen.

> Drug available generically in sealed orange metal cylinders or chromium-plated cylinders with an orange label.

NITROUS OXIDE

Nitrous oxide (blood/gas 0.47, MAC 101%) is a sweet smelling, nonexplosive gas with low anesthetic potency. It must always be administered with at least 20% oxygen for induction and, preferably, with not less than 34% oxygen for maintenance; induction with 80% nitrous oxide is facili-tated by premedication with a narcotic analgesic or barbiturate.

Nitrous oxide must be supplemented with other agents (thiopental, narcotic analgesics, more potent inhalation agents) to produce surgical anesthesia. It reduces the MAC of other inhalation anesthetics in an additive manner (eg, nitrous oxide 50% reduces the MAC of other inhalation agents by 50%). Since this anesthetic does not provide adequate skeletal muscle re-laxation, a neuromuscular blocking agent also must be given when necessary. Ni-trous oxide has good analgesic properties and is useful as the sole analgesic in brief procedures, in dentistry, and in the second stage of labor. However, it should not be used to produce analgesia or light narcosis for longer than 48 hours (eg, in patients receiving artificial ventilation) because of its tendency to produce leukopenia.

This anesthetic does not appear to have any serious effects on the cardiovascular or ventilatory systems or on the liver, kidneys, or metabolic function, provided that the inhalation mixture contains an adequate concentration of oxygen and ventilation is maintained.

Because nitrous oxide is 35 times more soluble in blood than nitrogen, it diffuses into a closed air-containing cavity faster than nitrogen diffuses out. If the cavity has rigid walls, the pressure within it rises; if the cavity does not have rigid walls, the volume increases. Therefore, nitrous oxide should be used cautiously in the presence of conditions such as air embolism, pneumothorax, pulmonary air cysts, or acute intestinal obstruction and during or after recent pneumoencephalography.

Diffusion hypoxia may develop after discontinuing prolonged anesthesia with nitrous oxide, and it is advisable to admin-ister oxygen briefly during emergence. Recovery is rapid unless large doses of supplementary agents have been used. The incidence of nausea and vomiting is substantially lower after nitrous oxide than after cyclopropane or ether.

Reversible bone marrow depression has occurred following administration of ni-trous oxide for more than three days. It may be fatal if complications develop.

ROUTE, USUAL DOSAGE, AND PREPARATIONS. *Inhalation:* For analgesia, 25% to 50% nitrous oxide with 75% to 50% oxygen. For induction of anesthesia, 80% nitrous oxide with 20% oxygen for two to three minutes. For maintenance, between 66% nitrous oxide with 34% oxygen and 50% nitrous oxide with 50% oxygen, depending upon the condition of the patient and the amount of supplemental agents used.

Drug available generically in sealed blue metal cylinders.

Nonhalogenated Volatile Liquid

ETHER (Ethyl Ether, Diethyl Ether)

This anesthetic (VP 450 torr, blood/gas 12.1, MAC 1.92%) has a pungent, irritating odor and is flammable and explosive. Its flammability and explosiveness account for its current relatively rare use. Because of its high solubility in blood, induction is relatively slow and recovery is prolonged. Induction may be facilitated by concomitant use of nitrous oxide or short-acting intravenous agents. Ether has a wide margin of safety, possesses excellent analgesic properties, and produces profound skeletal muscle relaxation. The depth of anesthesia can be followed by observing the classical signs outlined by Guedel unless supplemental drugs (eg, narcotic analgesics, neuromuscular blocking agents) are used. The skeletal muscle relaxant properties of ether can intensify the action of nondepolarizing neuromuscular blocking agents. Therefore, the dose of these agents should be markedly reduced when ether is the anesthetic (see Chapter 21, Adjuncts to Anesthesia and Analeptic Drugs). Ether also may intensify the neuromuscular blocking action of certain antibiotics (eg, neomycin, polymyxin B).

The cardiovascular system usually is not affected adversely. The drug's direct myocardial depressant effect is usually counteracted by its ability to stimulate the sympathetic nervous system. At moderate levels of anesthesia, heart rate is increased, arterial pressure is maintained, and cardiac output is sustained or elevated. Ether does not sensitize the heart to catecholamines, and ventricular arrhythmias are rare.

Ether dilates the bronchioles and is useful in asthmatic patients; however, it also causes salivation and stimulates bronchial secretions, which may compromise airway patency. Excessive secretions can be minimized by premedication with an anticholinergic drug. Spontaneous ventilation usually remains satisfactory, for ether stimulates the rate of ventilation by reflex mechanisms; this counteracts the central respiratory depressant effect unless extremely deep anesthesia is produced.

Transient effects include reduced urinary output, hyperglycemia, and decreased intestinal tone and motility; transient, slight abnormalities in the results of liver function tests and massive hepatic necrosis have been observed. Postoperative nausea and vomiting occur frequently.

ROUTE, USUAL DOSAGE, AND PREPARATIONS. *Inhalation:* For induction, 10% to 30% ether vapor in oxygen or a nitrous oxide-oxygen mixture is generally required. For maintenance of surgical anesthesia, 5% to 15% is used.

Drug available generically in 0.25, 0.5, 1, and 5 lb airtight, sealed containers lined with copper to prevent oxidation.

Halogenated Volatile Liquids

ENFLURANE
[Ethrane]

$$\begin{array}{ccc} \text{F} & \text{F} & \text{F} \\ | & | & | \\ \text{HCOC} & \text{C} & \text{CH} \\ | & | & | \\ \text{F} & \text{F} & \text{Cl} \end{array}$$

Enflurane (VP 180 torr, blood/gas 1.8, MAC 1.68%) is a pleasant smelling, nonflammable, halogenated ether anesthetic that provides rapid induction with little or no excitement. It appears to provide better muscle relaxation than halothane, but high concentrations may cause cardiovascular depression and central nervous system stimulation; therefore, enflurane is generally given with nitrous oxide. Neuromuscular blocking agents may be used to facilitate muscle relaxation, but the dosage of nondepolarizing drugs must be reduced (see Chapter 21, Adjuncts to Anesthesia and Analeptic Drugs).

The cardiovascular system remains relatively stable. Enflurane has little effect on pulse rate and cardiac rhythm; the arterial pressure, after decreasing moderately following induction, tends to return to near normal upon surgical stimulation and then remains stable. A dose-related depression of the cardiovascular system occurs. Excessive reduction of arterial pressure occurs following maximum reflex compensation and is the best indication of overdosage.

Results of some studies in man suggest that enflurane does not sensitize the heart to catecholamines. Other studies show that enflurane does sensitize the heart, but the dose-response relationships are more variable and unpredictable than those of halothane. A suggested maximum dose of subcutaneous or submucosal (not intravenous) epinephrine is 3 or 4 mcg/kg during enflurane anesthesia. The drug has been used successfully during resection of a pheochromocytoma.

Enflurane is a respiratory depressant. The ventilatory rate remains essentially constant or slightly elevated, but the tidal volume is decreased with a resulting depression of minute volume. Spontaneous ventilation may be sufficient at light levels of anesthesia but, as the depth increases, assisted or controlled ventilation should be employed.

Transient, slight abnormalities in the results of liver function tests similar to those observed after other anesthetic techniques have been noted. There have been several case reports of hepatic damage.

The clinical implications of the biotransformation of enflurane to free fluoride ion require further study. Fluoride ion plasma concentrations are considerably below the toxic threshold of normal individuals but may be hazardous in those with renal disease.

Central nervous system stimulation, manifested by increased electrical activity and seizure-like patterns in the electroencephalogram, is seen as anesthesia deepens. Paroxysms of tonic-clonic or twitching movements have developed in a few patients, usually in association with deep anesthesia and hypocapnia. These can be terminated without sequelae by lightening anesthesia and reducing minute ventilation to reduce hypocapnia or by substituting another anesthetic agent. Patients with recent or remote closed head injuries and children under 3 years with febrile illnesses or pre-existing convulsive disorders should receive the drug with caution.

Recovery is usually rapid and uneventful; shivering due to hypothermia is relatively common, but restlessness, delirium, nausea, and vomiting are rare.

ROUTE, USUAL DOSAGE, AND PREPARATIONS. *Inhalation*: For induction, 2% to 5% vaporized by a flow of oxygen or a nitrous oxide-oxygen mixture. Generally, 1% to 4% is administered for maintenance. A vaporizer calibrated for enflurane or from which a known concentration of the drug can be obtained must be used.

Ēthrane (Ohio Medical Products). Liquid in 125 and 250 ml containers.

HALOTHANE
[Fluothane]

$$CF_3CH{\overset{\underset{\displaystyle |}{Cl}}{\underset{\underset{\displaystyle Br}{|}}{}}}$$

Halothane (VP 243 torr, blood/gas 2.3, MAC 0.77%) is a nonflammable, halogenated hydrocarbon anesthetic that provides relatively rapid induction with little or no excitement. It does not appear to provide adequate analgesia and high concentrations cause circulatory depression; therefore, it is generally given with nitrous oxide. Halothane may not produce adequate muscle relaxation, and concomitant administration of neuromuscular blocking agents is often required. However, since this anesthetic augments the neuromuscular blocking effects of nondepolarizing muscle relaxants, the dose of these blocking agents must be reduced (see Chapter 21, Adjuncts to Anesthesia and Analeptic Drugs).

Halothane diminishes sympathetic activity, augments vagal tone, and depresses the contractility of the heart and vascular smooth muscle. Cardiac output, arterial pressure, and pulse rate are reduced, usually in proportion to the depth of anesthesia. Severe hypotension and circulatory failure may occur with overdosage. Arrhythmias, including nodal rhythm, may be observed during induction or deep anesthesia; ventricular arrhythmias are uncommon unless ventilation is inadequate. Although small doses of epinephrine (1 to 1.5 mcg/kg) may be administered subcutaneously and submucosally with halothane if adequate ventilation is assured, such a combination is potentially hazardous since this anesthetic sensitizes the heart to catecholamines.

Halothane is not irritating to the respiratory tract and depresses pharyngeal and laryngeal reflexes. It dilates the bronchioles and reduces salivation and bronchial secretions; with the possible exception of ether, halothane is preferred to other anesthetics for patients with bronchial asthma. Since it depresses the respiratory center and produces tachypnea, ventilation should be assisted to avoid respiratory acidosis when deep anesthesia is necessary.

Transient, slight abnormalities in the results of liver function tests have been observed after a single administration; the changes are similar to those noted following administration of other anesthetics. Although many cases of liver damage, ranging from mild hepatitis to massive hepatic necrosis, have been reported after such use, the incidence of the latter is no higher than that associated with other general anesthetic techniques. However, there is evidence suggesting that liver damage is more likely to develop following repeated administration of halothane. Controlled data to prove or disprove this hypothesis are not available; however, the development of hepatitis in two anesthesiologists and its recurrence following a short, deliberate challenge with halothane indicate that the drug rarely is capable of producing unpredictable liver damage by an unknown mechanism. Therefore, it is unwise to give halothane to patients in whom acute liver damage developed after previous exposure to this drug. It also may be unwise to give halothane to patients known to have

developed a similar response following exposure to methoxyflurane and possibly to other halogenated anesthetics, although there is little reliable evidence to substantiate this point.

Reversible effects on the kidney (eg, decreased renal blood flow, glomerular filtration rate, and urine volume) have been observed during anesthesia. No appreciable metabolic disturbances have been noted. Oxygen consumption is reduced.

Controlled studies have indicated that low concentrations of halothane may increase uterine hemorrhage when this agent is used during early pregnancy (therapeutic abortion) but not during late pregnancy (cesarean section). High concentrations of halothane relax the uterus and produce considerable uterine hemorrhage.

Recovery from anesthesia is usually rapid and uneventful; shivering is sometimes observed but restlessness, delirium, nausea, and vomiting are uncommon.

ROUTE, USUAL DOSAGE, AND PREPARATIONS. *Inhalation*: For induction, a 1% to 4% concentration vaporized by a flow of oxygen or a nitrous oxide-oxygen mixture. For maintenance, a 0.5% to 2% concentration is given. A vaporizer calibrated for halothane or from which a known concentration of the drug can be obtained must be used.

> Drug available generically: Liquid in 250 ml containers.
> *Fluothane* (Ayerst). Liquid in 125 and 250 ml containers.

ISOFLURANE
[Forane]

$$HC \overset{\displaystyle F}{\underset{\displaystyle F}{|}} - O - CHCF_3 \;\; \underset{\displaystyle Cl}{|}$$

Isoflurane (VP 250 torr, blood/gas 1.38, MAC 1.3%) is a new, nonflammable, halogenated ether anesthetic which is currently being investigated. Although it is quite similar chemically to enflurane, there are many pharmacologic differences between the two drugs.

Isoflurane is less potent than halothane. The alveolar concentration necessary for surgical stage III anesthesia is 2%; this decreases to approximately 1% in patients over 60 years of age. Although this anesthetic has a slight pungent odor, there is good patient acceptance. Induction is smooth with little excitement when premedication is given and nitrous oxide and oxygen are administered concomitantly. The MAC with 50% nitrous oxide is 0.7%. Muscle relaxation is satisfactory for endotracheal intubation. The effects of neuromuscular blocking drugs are markedly potentiated, and the dose of tubocurarine must be reduced by one-third (see Chapter 21, Adjuncts to Anesthesia and Analeptic Drugs).

Little or no cardiovascular depression is observed with assisted respiration, and there is less tendency to develop arrhythmias with or without epinephrine than after use of halothane or enflurane. An equally important advantage over enflurane is the absence of central nervous system stimulation. Respiration is depressed, but the respiratory rate should not be used as an index of ventilation; instead, the dose is correlated with depression of tidal volume or response to elevated pCO_2. Assisted or controlled ventilation is recommended for that reason. Mental alertness is depressed for two to three hours after anesthesia; however, postoperative nausea, vomiting, and excitation are uncommon.

Isoflurane is minimally metabolized; the major metabolites are trifluoroacetic acid and fluoride ion, which occur in the ratio of about 2:1. In one study, serum fluoride ion concentrations were dose related (maximum value, 5.5 micromoles [mcM]/L). In another study, serum fluoride ion concentrations at the end of anesthesia averaged 3.6 mcM/L (maximum, 12 mcM/L). In comparison, methoxyflurane has been reported to produce serum fluoride ion concentrations as high as 200 mcM/L and enflurane as high as 80 mcM/L. Subtle laboratory evidence of defects in renal concentrating ability occur at serum fluoride ion concentrations above 50 mcM/L, and overt damage is observed at concentrations greater than approximately 100 mcM/L. No evidence of renal dysfunction was observed in patients following use of isoflurane; the only abnormality noted was excretion of fluorine-containing substances for several days after surgery.

Because use of this anesthetic has been limited to date, all toxicologic data and possible hypersensitivity reactions have not been determined. Intraocular and intracranial pressure are not adversely affected if adequate ventilation is assured. Unlike enflurane, no central nervous system stimulation is evident with deep anesthesia, and no major alterations in renal or hepatic function have been observed to date. Safety of use of isoflurane during pregnancy and delivery has not been established.

ROUTE, USUAL DOSAGE, AND PREPARATIONS. *Inhalation*: For induction, 3% to 3.5% vaporized in oxygen or in a nitrous oxide-oxygen mixture. Concentrations between 0.5% and 3% are satisfactory for maintenance. An additional 0.5% to 1% is required when isoflurane is given with oxygen alone. A vaporizer accurately calibrated for isoflurane or from which a known concentration can be delivered must be used.

> *Forane* (Ohio Medical Products). Liquid containing no additives or chemical stabilizers in 125 and 250 ml containers (Investigational drug).

METHOXYFLURANE
[Penthrane]

$$\begin{matrix} & Cl & & F & \\ & | & & | & \\ HC & - & C & & OCH_3 \\ & | & & | & \\ & Cl & & F & \end{matrix}$$

Methoxyflurane (VP 22.5 torr, blood/gas 13.0, MAC 0.16%) is a potent halogenated ether anesthetic with a fruity odor. Because of its low vapor pressure and high solubility in blood and certain components of the anesthesia delivery circle (rubber, soda lime), induction may be slow and recovery prolonged unless the carrier gas includes at least 50% nitrous oxide to permit administration of a small dose of this agent. Methoxyflurane provides adequate analgesia and can be used alone in dentistry and in the second stage of labor.

When used as an anesthetic, it should be given with nitrous oxide to achieve a relatively light level of anesthesia, and a neuromuscular blocking agent should be given concurrently to obtain desired muscular relaxation. However, methoxyflurane augments the neuromuscular blocking effects of nondepolarizing muscle relaxants; therefore, the dose of these agents should be markedly reduced (see Chapter 21, Adjuncts to Anesthesia and Analeptic Drugs).

Methoxyflurane depresses the cardiovascular system to approximately the same degree as halothane. The contractility of the heart is reduced, cardiac output and arterial pressure are reduced in proportion to the depth of anesthesia, and the heart rate is relatively unchanged. Arrhythmias are uncommon, even in the presence of hypercapnia. The drug does not appear to sensitize the heart to catecholamines or stimulate the sympathetic nervous system if adequate ventilation is maintained.

Methoxyflurane does not irritate the respiratory tract or increase secretions. Ventilation is only slightly depressed at light levels of anesthesia, but it should be assisted or controlled when deep anesthesia is attained, for tidal volume is diminished.

Transient, slight abnormalities in the results of liver function tests have been observed, and there are a number of anecdotal reports of hepatic damage, including massive hepatic necrosis. It is unwise to administer methoxyflurane to patients who developed acute liver damage after previous exposure to this drug. It also may be unwise to give methoxyflurane to patients known to have responded similarly following exposure to halothane.

Other anesthetics should be used in patients with renal damage, since impaired renal function has been associated with use of methoxyflurane, particularly if administered for long periods. The symptoms are usually those of vasopressin-resistant, high-output renal failure and include output of a large volume of dilute urine; dehydration; weight loss; increased serum osmolality; significantly increased blood sodium, urea nitrogen, and creatinine levels; elevated serum and urine concentrations of inorganic fluoride; and increased excretion of oxalic acid. Most patients recover completely, but some have oliguric renal failure, a few develop chronic renal failure, and, rarely, a patient dies. High-output renal failure is dose related and is almost certainly caused by the free fluoride ion produced by metabolism of the drug; fluoride ion interferes with sodium transport necessary for concentrating urine and also may render the appropriate renal tubules unresponsive to antidiuretic hormone. The degree of nephrotoxicity depends primarily upon the dose (ie, concentration and time or MAC-hours) of methoxyflurane and secondarily upon the degree of metabolism, the presence of enzyme induction, and variations in sensitivity to the fluoride ion. It is important that the presence of a normal arterial pressure should not be taken as an indication that a light level of anesthesia is being maintained, as this may result in a nephrotoxic dose being given. Methoxyflurane should not be administered to patients receiving other potentially nephrotoxic drugs (eg, gentamicin, tetracyclines), because concurrent use of these agents has been associated with irreversible renal failure.

Nausea and vomiting may occur postoperatively.

ROUTE, USUAL DOSAGE, AND PREPARATIONS. *Inhalation:* For analgesia, 0.5% in air. For induction of anesthesia, 1.5% to 3% vaporized by at least a 1:1 mixture of nitrous oxide and oxygen is administered for the shortest possible time. For maintenance, 0.5% or preferably less used with nitrous oxide or neuromuscular blocking agents so that the lowest effective total dosage is given. Since subclinical nephrotoxicity has been detected after the administration of MAC (0.16%) for two and one-half hours, the total dose of methoxyflurane administered should not exceed this MAC-hour limit. This effectively limits the usefulness of this drug to relatively few indications. When methoxyflurane is used to produce anesthesia, a vaporizer calibrated for methoxyflurane or from which a known concentration of the drug can be obtained must be used, and it must be placed outside the anesthesia delivery circle. A draw-over inhaler is acceptable when the drug is used only to produce analgesia. It may be wise to limit the amount of drug used for self-administration during labor to 15 ml.

> *Penthrane* (Abbott). Liquid in 15 and 125 ml containers.

INTRAVENOUS ANESTHETICS

Barbiturates

THIOPENTAL SODIUM
[Pentothal]

This barbiturate is useful to induce general anesthesia, since loss of consciousness occurs within 30 to 60 seconds after intravenous administration. It has poor analgesic properties but once unconsciousness is attained, anesthesia can be maintained with additional small increments or a dilute intravenous infusion can be given as a supplement to nitrous oxide. Depending upon the type of surgery, narcotic analgesics and neuromuscular blocking agents also may be required. Thiopental is not useful as the sole anesthetic agent for procedures lasting longer than 15 minutes because excessive doses are required. This anesthetic is rarely administered rectally for basal sedation or anesthesia, because of its variable absorption from the rectum. Thiopental reduces intracranial pressure.

In most instances, the arterial pressure is only slightly affected by thiopental. However, a reduction in cardiac output and arterial pressure may occur immediately after rapid intravenous injection of enough thiopental to produce deep anesthesia, especially in hypovolemic or poor-risk patients.

Thiopental is a potent ventilatory depressant, and apnea may occur immediately after intravenous injection. The drug also may cause yawning, coughing, and laryngospasm. Rapid redistribution of thiopental out of the brain can result in light anesthesia characterized in part by stimulation of the airway; therefore, it should be used with caution in patients with bronchospasm, upper airway obstruction, or situations in which coughing is undesirable.

Transient, slight alterations in the results of liver function tests similar to those observed following administration of other anesthetics may occur after use of thiopental. The drug decreases urine output but does not cause renal damage. It is contraindicated in patients with acute intermittent porphyria. Anaphylaxis has been reported rarely following injection of thiopental.

Care should be taken to avoid extravasation or intra-arterial injection, for neuritis and skin slough may occur with the former and arteritis, followed by thrombosis and gangrene, with the latter. Damage is reduced when dilute solutions are administered; concentrations greater than 2.5% should not be used. If extravasation or intra-arterial injection does occur, local injection (preferably through the needle used for thiopental) of 1% procaine (10 ml in adults) will dilute and neutralize the thiopental solution and may lessen vascular spasm. Local injection of heparin may reduce thrombosis, and sympathetic block or general anesthesia with halothane may relieve pain and vascular spasm and assist in opening collateral circulation.

Consciousness returns rapidly unless large doses have been given. Vomiting is uncommon during the postoperative period, but shivering occurs often and excitement and delirium may develop in the presence of pain.

ROUTES, USUAL DOSAGE, AND PREPARATIONS. *Intravenous*: The dosage required to induce and maintain anesthesia varies widely and depends upon premedication, body size, physical status, pre-existing disease, and adequacy of the respiratory and circulatory systems. For induction, *adults*, after a 2-ml test dose of a freshly prepared

2.5% solution, 50 or 100 mg is injected intermittently every 30 to 40 seconds until the desired effect has been obtained, or a single injection of 3 to 5 mg/kg of body weight is given. For maintenance, 50 to 100 mg of a 2.5% solution is injected as required. *Children*, a 2.5% solution is injected slowly and intermittently at 30-second intervals. The total dose recommended for induction is 3 to 5 mg/kg in relatively healthy patients. For maintenance, the usual total dose for children weighing 30 to 50 kg is 25 to 50 mg injected intermittently.

> *Pentothal* (Abbott). Powder (for solution) 0.25, 0.5, 1, 5, and 10 g.

Rectal: For basal anesthesia in *children*, 30 mg/kg of body weight in a 40% suspension.

> *Pentothal* (Abbott). Suspension 0.8 g in 2 g containers.

METHOHEXITAL SODIUM
[Brevital Sodium]

Methohexital is a more potent barbiturate and has a shorter duration of action than thiopental, but it has similar uses and adverse effects. Hiccups may occur after rapid intravenous injection.

ROUTE, USUAL DOSAGE, AND PREPARATIONS. *Intravenous*: *Adults*, for induction, after a 2-ml test dose, 5 to 12 ml of a 1% solution injected at the rate of 1 ml every five seconds. For maintenance, 2 to 4 ml of a 1% solution injected as required.

> *Brevital Sodium* (Lilly). Powder (for solution) 0.5, 2.5, and 5 g.

THIAMYLAL SODIUM
[Surital]

The uses and adverse effects of this rapid-acting barbiturate are similar to those of thiopental sodium.

ROUTE, USUAL DOSAGE, AND PREPARATIONS. *Intravenous*: *Adults*, for induction, after a 2-ml test dose of a freshly prepared 2.5% solution, 2 or 4 ml is injected every 30 to 40 seconds until the desired effect is obtained, or a single injection of 3 to 5 mg/kg of body weight is given. For maintenance, 2 to 4 ml of a 2.5% solution is injected as required.

> *Surital* (Parke, Davis). Powder (for solution) 1, 5, and 10 g.

Nonbarbiturates

DIAZEPAM
[Valium]

Diazepam has been used intravenously both as an induction agent and to produce basal sedation for cardioversion and endoscopic and dental procedures. The claims for superiority of diazepam over thiopental for basal sedation are supported by results of some controlled studies. It is less satisfactory as an induction agent than the ultrashort-acting barbiturates because of its somewhat slower onset of action (at least one minute), more prolonged recovery period, and the wide variation in individual response. Sleep and altered consciousness are usually preceded by nystagmus and slurred speech but not excitement.

Intravenous administration of diazepam produces sedation, hypnosis, and anterograde amnesia. These usually are accomplished with only a slight reduction in arterial pressure and mild respiratory depression. However, cardiovascular collapse has been reported in a healthy adult and respiratory arrest has been observed in a healthy elderly patient after intravenous injections of 20 mg and 10 mg, respectively. Respiratory arrest also has been noted after use of the drug during anesthesia, particularly if a narcotic analgesic was included in the premedication. Diazepam should be injected slowly to minimize the risk of cardiovascular and respiratory depression. Despite some preliminary evidence to the contrary, diazepam does not appear to potentiate the effects of neuromuscular blocking agents. Superficial, painless venous thrombosis may develop at the site of injection in 15% of patients.

Although Apgar scores are little affected by use of diazepam for vaginal delivery, hypotonicity and hypoactivity have occurred in infants after doses of 20 to 50 mg were given to the mother.

For other uses, adverse reactions, and precautions, see Chapters 11, Drugs Used for Anxiety and Insomnia; 15, Anticonvulsants; and 17, Drugs Used to Treat Skeletal Muscle Hyperactivity.

ROUTE, USUAL DOSAGE, AND PREPARATIONS. *Intravenous*: Diazepam should not be mixed with intravenous fluids or solutions of other drugs. It is commonly injected through the intravenous tubing with the intravenous fluid flowing rapidly to prevent prolonged exposure of the vein to the solvent. Concurrent use of local or topical anesthetics will improve anesthetic management in some patients (eg, prior to endoscopy). Outpatients must be accompanied home.

For induction of anesthesia, 0.1 to 1 mg/kg of body weight. Although some healthy patients may fall asleep with doses of 0.4 mg/kg of body weight, or even 0.2 mg/kg if a narcotic analgesic is used for premedication, 0.8 to 1 mg/kg is required if sleep is to be assured; poor-risk patients may require only 0.1 to 0.2 mg/kg.

For basal sedation, increments of 2.5 to 5 mg are given at 30-second intervals until the patient falls into a light sleep or nystagmus, ptosis, or slurred speech develops; 5 to 30 mg usually is required.

Valium (Roche). Solution 5 mg/ml in 2 and 10 ml containers.

ETOMIDATE

$$H_3C-\underset{H}{\overset{|}{C}}-\text{(phenyl)}$$
$$CH_3CH_2OC(=O)-\text{(imidazole ring, N)}$$

This investigational nonbarbiturate, nonanalgesic imidazole derivative produces a rapid, smooth induction 20 seconds after injection. Etomidate is rapidly distributed to the brain and highly perfused organs of metabolism (distribution $t_{1/2}$, 2.8 ± 1.6 minutes). It binds principally to serum albumin (76.5%). Hepatic but not plasma hydrolysis of this ester produces its major inactive acid metabolite, which is then eliminated in the urine ($t_{1/2}$, 3.9 ± 1.1 hours).

In comparison to thiopental, initial investigation suggests that etomidate causes less apnea and cardiovascular depression and recovery is more rapid with less residual headache. A small but significant reduction in systolic pressure and an increase in heart rate, particularly after premedication with narcotics, usually are observed. Injection is painful in one-third to one-sixth of patients, even with rapid administration (within 15 seconds). Also, myoclonic muscle movements have been observed in 10% to 65.5% of those receiving etomidate. These involuntary movements may be related partly to the pain on injection, but most are considered to be centrally induced. Premedication with droperidol and fentanyl decreased the incidence of myoclonic activity, but supplemental doses of another general anesthetic may be required in some patients. If halothane is the anesthetic chosen, the amount of halothane administered should be reduced.

If the formulation can be altered to minimize or abolish the pain on injection, etomidate could be a useful intravenous induction agent in patients with compromised cardiovascular status or for outpatient procedures of short duration.

The data are not yet sufficient to predict the prevalence or type of hypersensitivity reactions.

ROUTE, USUAL DOSAGE, AND PREPARATIONS.
Intravenous: *Adults*, 0.3 mg/kg of body weight administered over a period of 15 to 60 seconds. Data are too limited to recommend a dose for *children*.
(Investigational drug)

FLUNITRAZEPAM
[Rohypnol]

This benzodiazepine has approximately ten times the potency of diazepam and has been suggested as a substitute for that drug to induce anesthesia. Although flunitrazepam was thought to have a more rapid onset of action with less individual variation in response than diazepam, well-controlled studies to date reveal no significant differences between the two drugs in onset of anesthesia or effects on heart rate, blood pressure, PaO2, and PaCO2 in patients who have received pentobarbital, morphine, and atropine for premedication. Controlled studies are needed to confirm the clinical impression that flunitrazepam produces greater amnesia than diazepam.

As with diazepam, the doses of flunitrazepam required to produce rapid onset of anesthesia and smooth induction result in postoperative respiratory depression and drowsiness even when surgery exceeds three to four hours. Transient erythema and a lower than expected incidence of nausea and vomiting were the only other adverse reactions noted in the few investigational studies reported to date. For other possible reactions, see the evaluation on Diazepam.

ROUTE, USUAL DOSAGE, AND PREPARATIONS.
Intravenous: *Adults*, a loading dose of 36 to 50 mcg/kg of body weight is administered over a 20- to 40-second period, followed by doses of 10 mcg/kg as needed. *Children*, insufficient data are available to recommend a dose.
Rohypnol. Solution (sterile) (Investigational drug).

KETAMINE HYDROCHLORIDE
[Ketaject, Ketalar]

Ketamine is a nonbarbiturate anesthetic that can be administered intravenously or intramuscularly. It induces a cataleptic state in which the patient may appear to be awake but is dissociated from the environment and does not respond to pain. Ketamine produces a rapid induction of anesthesia even after intramuscular injection. A small dose (0.5 to 1 mg/kg intramuscularly) can be used to calm agitated children and facilitate insertion of an intravenous cannula. Because this anesthetic can be administered intramuscularly, it is particularly useful for repeated anesthesia in burn patients, for diagnostic studies, and for minor surgical procedures in small children; however, adequate training in its use and the availability of resuscitative equipment are mandatory.

Ketamine also may be of value to induce anesthesia, particularly when a barbiturate cannot be used or cardiovascular depression must be avoided; however, it is not satisfactory as the primary agent for abdominal or other major operations because of its inadequate skeletal muscle relaxant action and adverse effects. An anticholinergic drug should be given for premedication to reduce secretions. The concomitant use of diazepam, hydroxyzine, or secobarbital increases ketamine-induced sleep time (from 100 to 140 minutes). Another general anesthetic and a neuromuscular blocking agent can be administered subsequently, if required. Ketamine potentiates the neuromuscular blocking effects of tubocurarine but not of pancuronium or succinylcholine.

Studies on the effects of ketamine on the fetus when this anesthetic is used during delivery indicate that large doses (over 2 mg/kg of body weight) are likely to cause fetal depression. Although smaller doses

(0.25 to 0.5 mg/kg) appear to be safe and can be used for analgesia, caution is advised and, in general, this is not a preferred drug for obstetrical anesthesia.

Psychic disturbances during emergence (unpleasant dreams, irrational behavior, excitement, disorientation, illusions, delirium, hallucinations) are common and occur more frequently in adults (particularly after gynecologic procedures in young women) than in children. Their reported incidence varies between 3% and 50%. One of several techniques can be employed to reduce the incidence of such reactions: (1) Administer droperidol intravenously just prior to induction or thiopental (150 mg) intravenously at the end of anesthesia. (2) Limit the dose to 2 mg/kg and maintain anesthesia with doses of 0.5 to 1 mg/kg. (3) Utilize a low-dose microdrip intravenous infusion. (4) Maintain anesthesia with other agents. Although there is no evidence that psychic disturbances have any residual effect, it may be advisable to avoid ketamine in patients with psychoses.

Muscular rigidity, athetoid motions of the mouth and tongue, swallowing, random movements of the extremities, laryngeal spasm, fasciculations, tremors, and generalized extensor spasm have occurred occasionally; frank convulsions are extremely rare. Although seizure activity has been observed in electroencephalograms, well-controlled studies have not proved that ketamine causes generalized convulsions in epileptics with abnormal electroencephalograms. Ketamine should be given cautiously to patients with convulsive disorders and only when its superiority to other anesthetics is unquestionable.

Ketamine increases cerebrospinal fluid pressure and should be used with extreme caution in patients with evidence of increased intracranial pressure or a space-occupying lesion. It has been suggested that ketamine may not always produce satisfactory analgesia in patients with cerebral cortical disease; the mechanism is unknown.

Although arrhythmias are seldom observed, ketamine usually increases heart rate, cardiac output, and arterial pressure, principally by stimulating the central sympathetic nervous system and inhibiting reuptake of released norepinephrine. Therefore, the drug should be used with care in patients with mild, uncomplicated hypertension and is contraindicated in those with severe coronary artery disease, severe hypertension, or a history of stroke. The cardiovascular stimulant properties of ketamine are blocked by halothane and enflurane, and the direct myocardial depressant action of ketamine becomes evident.

Transient respiratory depression may occur immediately after intravenous administration of anesthetic doses of ketamine, and respiratory arrest has occurred in neonates. Laryngeal reflexes are depressed during anesthesia. A clinical impression exists that the presence of upper airway infection is associated with a higher incidence of laryngospasm after use of ketamine; no controlled studies are available. Aspiration of stomach contents has been reported, and an endotracheal tube should be used if the stomach is full.

Ketamine may increase intraocular pressure slightly; thus, its usefulness for major intraocular surgery is controversial, and it may be wise to avoid this anesthetic in patients with pre-existing elevation of intraocular pressure.

Ketamine may cause vomiting, hypersalivation, lacrimation, shivering, polyneuropathy, and transient dermatologic reactions. There is some evidence that the drug may interact with thyroid medication to produce severe hypertension and tachycardia.

ROUTES, USUAL DOSAGE, AND PREPARATIONS. *Intravenous*: For induction, 2 mg/kg of body weight (range, 1 to 4.5 mg/kg) administered over a period of 60 seconds. For maintenance, one-half of the full induction dose, repeated as necessary. Using the low-dose, microdrip technique, ketamine 0.1% is administered at a rate of 20 ml/min for induction and 10 mg/min for maintenance as required following the administration of nitrous oxide and a muscle relaxant. The total dose required during this technique is only one-third to one-half of the amount employed for bolus administration.

Intramuscular: For induction, 6.5 to 13 mg/kg of body weight. For maintenance, one-half of the full induction dose, repeated as necessary.

> Ketaject (Bristol), Ketalar (Parke, Davis). Solution 10 mg/ml in 20 and 50 ml containers, 50 mg/ml in 10 ml containers, and 100 mg/ml in 5 ml containers.

COMBINATION ANESTHESIA

Balanced Anesthesia

Because of its low potency, nitrous oxide must be supplemented with other agents to produce conditions suitable for surgery. The use of more potent inhalation or intravenous agents to achieve this goal has been discussed. The intravenous use of an ultrashort-acting barbiturate, a narcotic analgesic, a neuromuscular blocking agent, and nitrous oxide to produce general anesthesia is termed "balanced anesthesia." Meperidine [Demerol], morphine, and fentanyl [Sublimaze] appear to be the most widely employed analgesics and, in combination with a barbiturate, supplement the hypnotic and analgesic effects of nitrous oxide.

Meperidine was the first narcotic analgesic used in this manner. Commonly, a narcotic analgesic is included in the premedication and anesthesia is induced with a barbiturate and nitrous oxide; meperidine is then given intravenously in 10- to 25-mg increments over a period of five to ten minutes until adequate analgesia has been produced. The average adult usually requires 50 to 100 mg. Increments of 10 to 25 mg may be required during surgery if the patient shows signs of reacting to painful stimuli (eg, increasing pulse rate and arterial pressure, pupillary dilation, sweating, muscle movement). If used judiciously in this manner and if not given during the last one to two hours of *prolonged* surgery, adequate intraoperative analgesia can be achieved without the need for postoperative ventilatory support. If a neuromuscular blocking agent is used, controlled ventilation is mandatory during surgery. If a neuromuscular blocking agent is not used,

spontaneous ventilation may be satisfactory during short procedures; however, in general, assisted ventilation is advisable.

Morphine has become popular in balanced anesthesia for use in cardiac surgery and poor-risk patients in general. Large intravenous doses (0.5 to 3 mg/kg of body weight) are administered with nitrous oxide. After it was observed that patients about to undergo cardiac surgery appeared to tolerate large doses of morphine well, a study of the hemodynamic effects of 1 mg/kg of morphine was conducted. Results demonstrated that the response was more satisfactory (eg, increased cardiac index, decreased systemic vascular resistance) in patients with aortic valve disease than in nonaffected patients. However, similar studies indicated that these hemodynamic changes were transient and were less marked in patients with coronary artery disease than in those with valvular heart disease and fixed low cardiac output. Such studies also indicated that the administration of either nitrous oxide in concentrations greater than 60% or halothane 0.21% to 0.23% after 1 mg/kg of morphine produces cardiovascular depression (eg, decreased arterial pressure and cardiac index).

Although the use of large doses of morphine in balanced anesthesia currently is believed to be of value for certain patients, it must be emphasized that if large doses of morphine are used alone with 100% oxygen, amnesia may not be achieved, a high proportion of patients may require appropriate management to combat hypertension, and controlled ventilation must be employed postoperatively, at least during the first 12 to 24 hours. In fact, the easy transition from intraoperative to postoperative analgesia and ventilatory support is one of the major advantages of this technique.

Some anesthesiologists administer a narcotic antagonist to overcome the residual effects of the narcotic analgesic at the end of anesthesia. However, this reduces or eliminates postoperative analgesia and sometimes causes an overshoot reaction characterized by increased sympathetic stimulation, which results in dysrhythmias and increased myocardial work. It also can be hazardous if the effect of the narcotic antagonist wears off before that of the analgesic. If a narcotic antagonist is used in this manner, the patient must be observed carefully and additional doses of the antagonist given as necessary. (See Chapter 86, Specific Antidotes.)

The above dosage schedules represent only general guidelines. In practice, the technique of balanced anesthesia remains somewhat empirical: The choice of narcotic analgesic, the dose used, and the frequency of administration differ and must always be individualized for each patient. The adequacy of spontaneous ventilation always must be carefully and objectively evaluated at the termination of balanced anesthesia.

Clinical experience and some controlled data indicate that, in addition to nonflammability, intraoperative cardiovascular depression and increased peripheral resistance generally do not occur; there is an early return of consciousness, and the incidence of postoperative nausea, vomiting, excitement, and pain is reduced with properly administered balanced anesthesia.

Neuroleptanesthesia

Neuroleptanalgesia historically refers to the combination of a narcotic analgesic and droperidol, a neuroleptic (antipsychotic) drug, to produce an altered state of consciousness and awareness. The cataleptic or dissociative anesthetic, ketamine, and the amnesic antianxiety benzodiazepines are now used on occasion as a substitute for droperidol. Diazepam [Valium], ketamine [Ketaject, Ketalar], or droperidol [Inapsine] have been combined with narcotic analgesics, such as meperidine [Demerol], morphine, fentanyl [Sublimaze], or pentazocine [Talwin], in investigational clinical studies. When nitrous oxide is used to supplement these combinations, the descriptive term, neuroleptanesthesia, is employed. A muscle relaxant may be included.

Neuroleptanesthesia can provide satisfactory general anesthesia under many circumstances, but it may be particularly valuable when the patient's cooperation is required during the procedure, for consciousness should return soon after the flow of nitrous oxide is terminated. Neuroleptanalgesia, in which nitrous oxide is not administered and consciousness is not lost, may be of value for diagnostic and therapeutic procedures performed under local anesthesia (eg, cardiac catheterization, repeated burn dressings).

The narcotic analgesic, fentanyl, has been used most commonly with the butyrophenone antipsychotic agent, droperidol, in neuroleptanesthesia. Droperidol and fentanyl are available as single-entity products or in fixed-dose combination [Innovar]. Although the available reports are encouraging, there is much less experience with other combinations.

FENTANYL CITRATE
[Sublimaze]

Fentanyl has pharmacodynamic effects similar to those of meperidine and morphine; however, this drug has little hypnotic activity. On a milligram basis, fentanyl is 50 to 100 times more potent than morphine, which is approximately eight to ten times more potent than meperidine. The analgesia produced by morphine lasts two to three times longer than that of fentanyl and approximately two times longer than that of meperidine. Fentanyl resembles thiopental, however, in that moderate single doses are short acting due to redistribution. Multiple doses or large amounts result in accumulation and prolonged recovery time. Doses of 0.05 to 0.1 mg can be used in place of meperidine in balanced anesthesia and total doses of 0.015 to 0.1 mg/kg of body weight in place of morphine in cardiac surgery and poor-risk patients.

Fentanyl does not cause the moderate to marked vasodilation produced by morphine and meperidine. Fentanyl is used with the butyrophenone, droperidol, in neuroleptanalgesia and with both droperidol and nitrous oxide in neuroleptanesthesia (see the evaluation on Droperidol and Fentanyl).

If a therapeutic intravenous dose of fentanyl is administered rapidly, a generalized increase in muscle tone, including chest wall spasm, may develop; such rigidity also can occur with use of meperidine or morphine but is much less common. The rigidity is due to a central action of fentanyl and results in a marked decrease in thoracic compliance, which impairs the ability of the anesthetist to assist ventilation when respiratory depression is induced by the narcotic analgesic. Rigidity is exacerbated by nitrous oxide; however, it can be relieved or prevented by general anesthesia with thiopental or halothane. It also can be treated by administration of either a neuromuscular blocking agent and institution of controlled ventilation or by use of a narcotic antagonist. Slowing of the heart rate, which is easily reversed by atropine, may occur when fentanyl is given.

For other uses, adverse reactions, and precautions for fentanyl and other opiate and opioid analgesics used in neuroleptanesthesia, see Chapter 6, General Analgesics.

ROUTE, USUAL DOSAGE, AND PREPARATIONS. See the evaluation on Droperidol and Fentanyl Citrate.

> *Sublimaze* (Critikon). Solution 0.05 mg/ml in 2 and 5 ml containers.

DROPERIDOL
[Inapsine]

Droperidol, an antipsychotic butyrophenone, produces an altered state of awareness and marked sedation, little or no amnesia, and has an antiemetic action. It is not an analgesic. Intravenous administration causes a slight, transient fall in arterial pressure secondary to peripheral vasodilation that may be due to block of alpha-adrenergic receptors, direct vasodilatation, or both. There is little change in ventilation and the drug appears to have little effect on the respiratory depressant action of fentanyl. A dose of 10 mg reduces total body oxygen consumption by approximately 25%.

When droperidol was not used previously during the procedure, intravenous administration of 0.075 mg/kg of body weight at the termination of general anesthesia reduces the incidence of postoperative vomiting. However, because this drug may produce untoward effects and the incidence of severe, protracted postoperative vomiting is less than 3%, the prophylactic use of antiemetics should be reserved for procedures in which vomiting could interfere with the results of surgery (eg, intraocular surgery). (See also Chapter 26, Drugs Used in Vertigo, Motion Sickness, and Vomiting.)

Droperidol has a long duration of action (usually 12 to 24 hours) and occasionally produces extrapyramidal reactions (protrusion and uncontrolled movements of the tongue; dysphagia; lateral movements of the head; torticollis; twitching of limbs; restlessness; agitation; and parkinsonian crises) within 24 to 48 hours. Signs and symptoms can be relieved rapidly by diphenhydramine or benztropine (see Chapter 16, Drugs Used in Extrapyramidal Movement Disorders). Anecdotal evidence suggests that droperidol may antagonize the effects of levodopa resulting in reappearance of parkinsonian symptoms. Because of droperidol's prolonged action, central nervous system depressants should be administered in reduced doses and with caution during the early postoperative period.

ROUTE, USUAL DOSAGE, AND PREPARATIONS. See the evaluation on Droperidol and Fentanyl Citrate.

> *Inapsine* (Critikon). Solution 2.5 mg/ml in 2, 5, and 10 ml containers.

DROPERIDOL AND FENTANYL CITRATE
[Innovar]

This fixed-dose combination contains the narcotic analgesic, fentanyl (0.05 mg/ml), and the neuroleptic butyrophenone, droperidol (2.5 mg/ml). It has been used to produce neuroleptanalgesia and neuroleptanesthesia. As with all such combinations, its use is appropriate only when both drugs are to be administered at the same time and in the dosage ratio present in the mixture; otherwise, the two drugs should be administered separately as necessary.

These drugs usually provide satisfactory amnesia and analgesia. Cardiac output is reduced and systemic vascular resistance is increased initially but return to normal as surgery continues; arterial pressure and pulse rate tend to remain stable, but the heart rate may decrease. Ventricular arrhythmias are uncommon unless the sympathetic nervous system is stimulated by accumulation of carbon dioxide due to inadequate ventilation. Profound depression of the ventilatory rate and minute volume and apnea (caused by fentanyl) are to be expected. Apnea may result from central nervous system depression or peripheral muscle rigidity and can be treated by assisted or controlled ventilation. Central nervous system depression usually tends to be transient when only a single or a few repeated doses are given. Muscle rigidity can be overcome by use of neuromuscular blocking agents.

Transient, slight abnormalities in the results of liver function tests similar to those observed after other anesthetic techniques have been observed. Hyperglycemia occurs, but there is no evidence of metabolic acidosis. Pupils are constricted, intraocular tension is unchanged, and cerebrospinal fluid pressure is reduced in patients with and without space-occupying lesions, in contrast to the effect of the volatile agents. Consciousness and spontaneous respiration return rapidly when nitrous oxide and controlled ventilation are stopped if repetitive large doses have not been administered. Postoperative nausea, vomiting, and shivering due to hypothermia may occur,

but restlessness and delirium are uncommon. Extrapyramidal reactions may develop if a large dose of droperidol has been used (see the evaluation on Droperidol).

Droperidol and fentanyl can be administered safely to patients who have previously experienced malignant hyperpyrexia under general anesthesia.

Evidence that the combination reduces laryngeal competence suggests that this mixture should be used to facilitate "awake intubation" only with great caution and in small quantities.

See also the evaluations on Fentanyl Citrate and on Droperidol.

ROUTE, USUAL DOSAGE, AND PREPARATIONS. *Intravenous:* Neuroleptanesthesia can be induced with doses of 1 ml/9 to 15 kg of body weight administered slowly (1 ml every one to two minutes), followed by nitrous oxide and oxygen when drowsiness develops. A small dose of thiopental (100 mg) also may be used to hasten induction. Anesthesia can be maintained with nitrous oxide and with fentanyl alone (usually given in doses of 0.05 to 0.1 mg every 30 to 60 minutes) when clinical signs indicate that anesthesia may be too light (voluntary movements, rapid or irregular ventilation, increasing pulse rate and arterial pressure, lacrimation). Innovar should not be used for maintenance unless the patient specifically requires the pharmacologic effects of both drugs. Neuromuscular blocking agents and controlled ventilation should be utilized as indicated. If the former are not required, assisted ventilation may be adequate if the total dose of fentanyl does not exceed approximately 0.003 mg/kg. A narcotic antagonist can be given to reverse severe respiratory depression but, unless carefully titrated to a satisfactory level of depression, it will antagonize the analgesic effect as well. The patient must be observed carefully after use of the narcotic antagonist in case the effect of the antagonist wears off before that of the fentanyl.

Because droperidol is long lasting and has a relatively slow onset (10 to 15 minutes) and fentanyl has a relatively rapid onset (1 to 2 minutes) but a short duration of action, an alternative technique that avoids the use of Innovar has been described: Induction is started with a single dose of droperidol (0.15 mg/kg), and six to eight minutes later, fentanyl (0.002 to 0.003 mg/kg) is given in increments over a period of six to eight

minutes. Nitrous oxide is started when drowsiness develops and anesthesia is maintained as described above.

Innovar (Critikon). Each milliliter of solution contains fentanyl citrate 0.05 mg and droperidol 2.5 mg in 2 and 5 ml containers.

Selected References

Chenoweth MB (ed): *Modern Inhalation Anesthetics*. New York, Springer-Verlag, 1972.

Clarke RSJ, Norman J (eds): Symposium on anesthetic pharmacology. *Br J Anaesth* 51:577-710, 1979.

Cohen EN: Toxicity of inhalation anesthetic agents. *Br J Anaesth* 50:665-675, 1978.

Collins VJ: *Principles of Anesthesiology*, ed 2. Philadelphia, Lea & Febiger, 1976.

Davie IT: Specific drug interactions in anesthesia. *Anaesthesia* 32:1000-1008, 1977.

Dundee JW, Wyant GM: *Intravenous Anesthesia*. Edinburgh, Churchill Livingstone, 1974.

Friesen CM, et al: Successful use of dantrolene sodium in human malignant hyperthermia syndrome: Case report. *Can Anaesth Soc J* 26:319-321, 1979.

Ghoneim MM, Korttila K: Pharmacokinetics of in-travenous anesthetics: Implications for clinical use. *Clin Pharmacokinet* 2:344-372, 1977.

Hug CC Jr: Pharmacokinetics of drugs administered intravenously. *Anesth Analg* 57:704-723, 1978.

Kaufman RD: Biophysical mechanisms of anesthetic action: Historical perspectives and review of current concepts. *Anesthesiology* 46:49-62, 1977.

Nelson TE, Flewellen EH: Rationale for dantrolene vs procainamide for treatment of malignant hyperthermia. *Anesthesiology* 50:118-122, 1979.

Steen PA, Michenfelder JD: Neurotoxicity of anesthetics. *Anesthesiology* 50:437-453, 1979.

Whitwam JG: Adverse reactions to I.V. induction agents. *Br J Anaesth* 50:677-687, 1978.

Winters WD: Effects of drugs on electrical activity of brain. *Annu Rev Pharmacol Toxicol* 16:413-426, 1976.

Adjuncts to Anesthesia and Analeptic Drugs | 21

A number of drugs commonly used as adjuncts to anesthesia also are given therapeutically for other purposes and are discussed in more detail in other chapters. The agents included in this chapter fall into the following major categories: agents used for premedication; neuromuscular blocking drugs; the therapeutic gases, oxygen and carbon dioxide; miscellaneous adjuncts; and analeptic drugs.

AGENTS USED FOR PREMEDICATION

Anesthesiologist-patient contact plays an important role in the preoperative preparation of the patient. However, most anesthesiologists employ pharmacologic measures in conjunction with the reassurance developed through personal patient contact. Drugs were originally administered prior to induction of diethyl ether anesthesia to sedate the patient, reduce apprehension, facilitate induction, diminish anesthetic dose, inhibit salivary and other airway secretions, and prevent bradycardia. Originally, morphine was used to achieve the first four effects, and either atropine or scopolamine to achieve the last two. However, with the advent of modern anesthetics and general anesthetic techniques, the rationale for the routine use of any of these drugs is being questioned (Conner et al, 1977; Forrest et al, 1977; Mirakhur et al, 1978). They appear to be of limited benefit during induction of anesthesia with modern agents.

During the last several decades, a large number of drugs have been used in place

329

of morphine, and definitive comparative studies on all of them, including the many combinations possible, are clearly impractical. These newer drugs include certain opiate and opioid analgesics, hypnotics, antianxiety drugs, and neuroleptic drugs.

Analgesics: Opium alkaloids and synthetic opioid derivatives have played a dominant, if controversial, role in preanesthetic medication. It is generally agreed that they are of particular value when pain is present preoperatively.

There are few important differences among the individual drugs. When used alone for premedication, euphoria is noted in less than 10% of patients, although most opiate and opioid analgesics produce sedation. However, few reduce apprehension at recommended doses and none produce amnesia, while all may increase the incidence of pre- and postoperative nausea and vomiting. Other adverse effects include dizziness, tachycardia, sweating, and, less commonly, hypotension, restlessness or excitement, and a decreased respiratory response to carbon dioxide.

If scopolamine is given with morphine or meperidine [Demerol], the incidence of sedation and delayed awakening may be increased, while that of apprehension and pre- and postoperative nausea and vomiting may be reduced. The substitution of atropine for scopolamine does not greatly modify these effects. Both of these anticholinergic drugs may contribute further to the palpitations induced by the narcotic analgesics.

The effects of pantopon and pentazocine [Talwin] are similar to those of morphine except that less hypotension and postoperative nausea and vomiting are noted with pentazocine; however, undesirable psychotomimetic effects have been observed in some adults receiving more than 40 mg of pentazocine.

Fentanyl [Sublimaze] produces less sedation than morphine. The incidence of pre- and postoperative nausea and vomiting appears to be lower with this shorter-acting drug.

See also the Table and Chapter 6, General Analgesics.

Barbiturates: In an attempt to circumvent the adverse effects of the opiate and opioid analgesics, secobarbital [Seconal] and pentobarbital [Nembutal] were tried in the hope that they would be satisfactory substitutes. Evidence from controlled studies supported this hypothesis, and many anesthesiologists consider these barbiturates to be the preferred drugs in adults.

The incidence of tachycardia, bradypnea, and intraoperative cardiorespiratory changes was lower after secobarbital than after the narcotic analgesics. Other adverse effects observed less commonly after secobarbital included dizziness, preoperative nausea and vomiting, and delayed awakening. Postoperative restlessness or excitement and pain were more common after secobarbital. Secobarbital was found to reduce apprehension more than morphine and meperidine, but the narcotic analgesics increased sedation more than the barbiturate. Another controlled study revealed that the barbiturates, narcotic analgesics, and antianxiety drugs did not affect apprehension when the response was based on the opinion of the patient rather than the nurse or anesthesiologist (Forrest, 1977).

In children, pentobarbital and scopolamine or pentobarbital and morphine plus either scopolamine or atropine produce greater sedation and ease of induction than atropine alone; the last two combinations, as well as that of morphine and scopolamine, also produce less postoperative excitement or delirium than atropine alone. Comparison of the effects of pentobarbital, morphine, and meperidine in children revealed that morphine most consistently provides tranquility, ease of induction, and decreased postoperative excitement, while pentobarbital was associated with less postoperative vomiting.

See also the Table and Chapter 11, Drugs Used for Anxiety and Insomnia.

Antianxiety Drugs: Many anesthesiologists use benzodiazepines alone in preference to both the opiate and opioid analgesics and the short-acting barbiturates. When given preoperatively, chlordiazepoxide [Librium], diazepam

[Valium], and lorazepam [Ativan] produce anterograde amnesia, which is most marked with lorazepam (Dundee et al, 1977; Dundee et al, 1979). The incidence and intensity of sedation is least with chlordiazepoxide and most with lorazepam at recommended dose levels. The action of these drugs to allay preoperative apprehension is controversial. Either preoperative apprehension is less responsive to doses that produce adequate antianxiety action or refinements in the methodology of assessing apprehension are needed. Excitement, dizziness, tachycardia, hypotension, or pre- or postoperative nausea and vomiting are not characteristic. The onset of action is rapid after parenteral administration, but erratic absorption (except for lorazepam) and persistent pain at intramuscular injection sites may occur. Because of the latter and because benzodiazepines are more predictably absorbed from the gastrointestinal tract, the oral route is preferred, particularly if a longer sedative effect is desirable postoperatively (ie, four to eight hours). Oral medication can be given 90 to 120 minutes before induction when taken with 1 to 2 ounces of water.

In children, these benzodiazepines produce better sedation, fewer nightmares, and possibly better acceptance of the anesthetic face mask; the incidence of postoperative vomiting also is lower than with meperidine.

See also the Table; Chapter 11, Drugs Used for Anxiety and Insomnia; and Chapter 15, Anticonvulsants.

The antianxiety drug, hydroxyzine [Vistaril], is not chemically related to the benzodiazepines. It is not used as a hypnotic and is less effective in moderate to severe anxiety than the benzodiazepines (see Chapter 11). Hydroxyzine has an antiemetic action, which, coupled with its analgesic and sedative effect, is the basis for its use in preanesthetic medication.

Results of a recent controlled study, which compared diazepam and hydroxyzine after intravenous administration to eliminate absorption differences, determined that hydroxyzine was less satisfactory than diazepam in relief of anxiety, sedative and amnesic effects, and patient acceptance (Wender et al, 1977). Use of 150 mg of hydroxyzine did not offer any advantage over a 75-mg dose; the same conclusion was reached in another study (Bellville et al, 1979) when analgesia was compared at these doses. The differences noted between the two drugs may not be as great after intramuscular administration because of the rather erratic absorption of diazepam when it is given by this route.

Hydroxyzine may produce dizziness, dryness of the mouth, drowsiness, chills and shivering, and occasional persistent pain at the injection site. Since the drug potentiates the effects of opiates and barbiturates, it is necessary to reduce the dosage of these interacting drugs to avoid serious adverse reactions.

Neuroleptic Drugs: When used as the sole agent for preanesthetic medication in adults, the butyrophenone, droperidol [Inapsine], given intramuscularly in doses of 5 mg, causes drowsiness significantly more often than 100 mg of secobarbital but less often than 10 mg of either morphine or diazepam. In addition, the incidence of extrapyramidal signs and symptoms (dystonia, akathisia, and oculogyric crises), dysphoria, tachycardia, and hypotension is higher than with a placebo.

Droperidol alone does not always lessen postoperative nausea and vomiting more than a placebo, and the degree of preoperative nausea and vomiting may be similar to that experienced with 10 mg of morphine. A controlled study demonstrated significant pre- and postoperative antiemetic action of droperidol when it is given in combination with meperidine (Tornetta, 1977). When 5 mg of droperidol is added to 0.1 mg of fentanyl (available in this ratio as the fixed-dose combination, Innovar) for premedication, the quality of sedation may be better than that produced by 10 mg of morphine. The incidence of preoperative nausea and vomiting with the combination is low and that of postoperative nausea and vomiting is significantly less than with 10 mg of morphine. In general, in adults, droperidol is less satisfactory for preanesthetic medication alone than when combined with the analgesics.

See the Table and the section on Neuroleptanesthesia in Chapter 20, General Anesthetics.

Controlled studies have been performed comparing the phenothiazine derivatives, chlorpromazine [Thorazine] and promethazine [Phenergan], with meperidine in combination with atropine. Although these compounds and related derivatives provided sedation comparable to that observed with meperidine and atropine and possibly better relief of apprehension, preoperative tachycardia and/or hypotension and restlessness appeared to be greater. A few phenothiazines also produced postoperative dyskinesia. In spite of the less prominent postoperative nausea and vomiting, the usefulness of most of the phenothiazines for premedication is severely curtailed by these adverse effects.

See also Chapter 12, Antipsychotic Drugs.

Anticholinergic Drugs: Atropine, scopolamine, and glycopyrrolate [Robinul] are given before anesthesia to reduce excessive salivary and other airway secretions caused by some inhalation anesthetics and succinylcholine. They are also used to protect against bradycardia, hypotension, and even cardiac arrest induced by succinylcholine, cyclopropane, or certain surgical manipulations (eg, stimulation of the peritoneum, pressure on the eyeball).

Atropine is preferred to scopolamine for preventing reflex bradycardia because it has a more sustained accelerating effect on the heart rate. Usual premedicant doses of atropine (0.6 mg) do not block the cardiac vagal nerves (this requires 1.5 to 2 mg), and the duration of action of an intramuscular dose is usually short (30 minutes). When given in small doses (up to 0.4 mg), scopolamine may slow rather than accelerate heart rate; therefore, this drug is preferred to atropine for premedication when tachycardia must be avoided (eg, in patients with mitral stenosis). Scopolamine is a more potent antisialogogue than atropine. It has a significant sedative effect and may reduce the incidence of postoperative nausea and vomiting. However, scopola-mine also may produce dizziness, delayed awakening, and prolonged postoperative confusion, especially in the elderly. Scopolamine alone is not particularly effective in producing anterograde amnesia compared with lorazepam, but it does produce significant additive amnesia when used with the benzodiazepines or opiate analgesics.

The quaternary ammonium anticholinergic, glycopyrrolate, is used frequently for preanesthetic medication because its action to reduce secretions is more prolonged and its central anticholinergic effect is minimal.

Anticholinergic drugs inhibit heat loss, presumably by suppressing perspiration. Therefore, they should be given cautiously to patients with fever, particularly children, as hyperpyrexia may ensue. Recent evidence suggests that, in hot climates, children free of fever who receive atropine for premedication do not experience a serious rise in body temperature.

If anticholinergic premedication is required in patients predisposed to angle closure, the hazard of inducing acute glaucoma can be minimized by instilling one drop of 1% pilocarpine in each eye. Anticholinergic premedication can be given safely to patients with open-angle glaucoma (80% of glaucoma patients have the open-angle type), particularly if they are being treated with miotics, and to patients who have had a peripheral iridectomy.

Atropine and scopolamine, but not glycopyrrolate, readily cross the blood-brain barrier and can cause confusion, particularly in the elderly. Toxic doses of these drugs cause hallucinations and coma; scopolamine is more potent in this regard. Although scopolamine usually has a pronounced sedative effect, this drug and atropine may cause postoperative excitement (emergence delirium), especially in elderly patients and in those in pain. Physostigmine is the specific antidote for central anticholinergic intoxication (see Chapter 86).

See the Table for dosage.

AGENTS USED FOR PREMEDICATION

Drug	Route	Dosage
ANALGESICS		
Fentanyl Citrate [Sublimaze]	Intramuscular	*Adults,* 0.1 mg.
Morphine Sulfate	Subcutaneous Intramuscular	*Adults,* 10 mg (range, 5 to 20 mg); *children 1 year and over,* 0.1 mg/kg (maximum, 10 mg).
Meperidine Hydrochloride [Demerol Hydrochloride]	Subcutaneous Intramuscular	*Adults,* 100 mg (range, 50 to 150 mg); *children 1 year and over,* 1 mg/kg (maximum, 100 mg).
Pantopon	Subcutaneous Intramuscular	*Adults,* 20 mg.
Pentazocine Lactate [Talwin Lactate]	Subcutaneous Intramuscular	*Adults,* 20 to 40 mg.
BARBITURATES		
Pentobarbital Sodium [Nembutal Sodium]	Intramuscular	*Adults,* 100 to 150 mg (range, 75 to 200 mg); *children 6 months and over,* 2 to 4 mg/kg (maximum, 100 mg).
Secobarbital Sodium [Seconal Sodium]	Intramuscular	*Adults,* 100 to 150 mg (range, 75 to 200 mg); *children 6 months and over,* 2 to 4 mg/kg (maximum, 100 mg).
ANTIANXIETY DRUGS		
Chlordiazepoxide Hydrochloride [Librium]	Intramuscular Oral	*Adults,* 50 to 100 mg.
Diazepam [Valium]	Intramuscular Oral	*Adults,* 10 to 15 mg; *children 2 years and over,* 0.4 mg/kg.
Hydroxyzine Hydrochloride Hydroxyzine Pamoate [Vistaril]	Intramuscular Oral	*Adults,* 25 to 200 mg; *children,* 1 mg/kg.
NEUROLEPTIC DRUGS		
Droperidol [Inapsine]	Intramuscular	*Adults,* 5 mg.
Droperidol and Fentanyl Citrate [Innovar]	Intramuscular	*Adults,* 0.5 to 2 ml (fentanyl 0.05 mg/ml and droperidol 2.5 mg/ml).
ANTICHOLINERGIC DRUGS		
Atropine Sulfate	Intramuscular	*Adults,* 0.6 mg; *newborn infants,* 0.1 mg; *4 to 12 months,* 0.2 mg; *1 to 3 years,* 0.3 mg; *3 to 14 years,* 0.4 mg.
Glycopyrrolate	Intramuscular	*Adults,* 0.002 mg/lb; *children,* 0.002 to 0.004 mg/lb.
Scopolamine Hydrobromide	Intramuscular	*Adults,* 0.4 mg; *infants 4 to 7 months,* 0.1 mg; *7 months to 3 years,* 0.15 mg; *3 to 8 years,* 0.2 mg; *8 to 12 years,* 0.3 mg.

Subcutaneous or intramuscular doses are administered 45 to 60 minutes before anesthesia and oral doses two to four hours before anesthesia. The amounts should be reduced in elderly or debilitated patients.

Drugs may also be given intravenously. They should be given slowly, with caution, ie, titrated to effect. The intravenous doses are generally smaller than those recommended for other parenteral routes.

NEUROMUSCULAR BLOCKING DRUGS

Neuromuscular blocking drugs are used with general anesthetics to provide skeletal muscle relaxation during surgical procedures, particularly abdominal surgery. These agents provide adequate muscle relaxation and surgical exposure and obviate the need for deep general anesthesia and its attendant risks. Neuromuscular blocking drugs are used to facilitate endotracheal intubation, relieve laryngospasm, provide adequate muscle relaxation during brief diagnostic and surgical procedures performed under light general anesthesia, prevent dislocations and fractures during electroconvulsive shock therapy, produce apnea in order to facilitate controlled ventilation during thoracic surgery and neurosurgery, control muscle spasms in tetanus, and facilitate controlled ventilation by eliminating inadequate spontaneous ventilatory efforts in patients with ventilatory failure.

Although use of a neuromuscular blocking agent obviates the need for deep general anesthesia, these drugs have no anesthetic or analgesic properties. Therefore, they should never be used to compensate for inadequate anesthesia. These agents should be administered only by individuals who have received adequate training in the maintenance of artificial ventilation.

Since the neuromuscular blocking agents affect the ventilatory muscles, most anesthesiologists believe that ventilation must be controlled whenever they are used. An objective evaluation of the extent of residual curarization, and thus of the ability of the patient to breathe adequately, maintain an open airway, take a deep breath, and cough, must be conducted upon completion of surgery. For patients who are not sufficiently awake to permit a satisfactory evaluation of ventilatory recovery, a nerve stimulator can be used to estimate residual curarization directly. Strong, well-sustained muscle contractions in response to tetanic stimulation of the motor nerve can be equated with clinical recovery of neuromuscular transmission.

Either muscle membrane nondepolarizing (competitive) or depolarizing types of neuromuscular blocking agents are available. The *nondepolarizing blocking drugs* (tubocurarine, metocurine [Metubine], gallamine [Flaxedil], and pancuronium [Pavulon]) compete with acetylcholine for cholinergic receptor sites on the postjunctional membrane. They also may compete at presynaptic cholinoceptive sites which would decrease the amount of acetylcholine released at postsynaptic sites. They do not possess the transmitter action of acetylcholine and thus paralyze muscle fibers served by the occupied endplates. This competitive block can be antagonized by anticholinesterases such as neostigmine [Prostigmin], pyridostigmine [Mestinon, Regonol], or edrophonium [Tensilon] (Miller, 1976). The anticholinesterases permit acetylcholine to accumulate at the endplate until it displaces the blocking agent from receptor sites and reaches the concentration needed to excite muscle fiber. The degree of effectiveness of anticholinesterases in reversing paralysis depends upon the doses of nondepolarizing blocking agents used, the total amount of acetylcholine being released, and the depth of neuromuscular block (percentage of recovery from block) at the time of reversal. Edrophonium should be used only as a diagnostic agent because of its short duration of action. Pyridostigmine has a slower onset and longer duration of action than neostigmine, but both drugs have similar cardiac muscarinic properties.

The *depolarizing drugs* (succinylcholine [Anectine, Quelicin, Sucostrin, Sux-Cert] and decamethonium [Syncurine]) are believed to act by depolarizing the postsynaptic membrane in a manner similar to the normal neurotransmitter, acetylcholine. This action produces muscle fasciculations that are usually visible. After the initial muscle stimulation, continued occupation of the receptors by these drugs (which dissociate less readily from the receptor than acetylcholine) results in a persistent depolarization (phase I) block and paralysis ensues. This type of neuromuscular block is not antagonized by anticholinesterase drugs; indeed, since anticholinesterase agents inhibit plasma cholinesterase (the enzyme responsible for the primary metabolism of succinylcholine) as well as true cholinesterase, use of these drugs may prolong the phase I block produced by succinylcholine. Decreased receptor sensitivity may occur after a single large dose, repeated administration, or prolonged infusion of the depolarizing agents; this causes a desensitization block (dual, biphasic, antidepolarizing, or phase II block), which is somewhat similar to that produced by the nondepolarizing drugs. The safest treatment of phase II block is maintenance of controlled ventilation until the block reverses spontaneously. Thus, these drugs can produce two types of block with different characteristics, time courses, and responses to antagonists.

The choice between the two classes of neuromuscular blocking drugs is determined by the expected duration of the procedure (succinylcholine has the shortest duration of action), the possibility of interactions between the blocking agent and the general anesthetic or other drugs, and the presence of pathologic conditions that may influence the patient's pharmacokinetic response (Wingard and Cook, 1977). Generally, a single dose of succinylcholine is used for brief procedures and to facilitate endotracheal intubation. For longer surgical procedures and to facilitate controlled ventilation, repeated doses of nondepolarizing agents are used or, less commonly, succinylcholine is administered by continuous infusion. Occasionally, succinylcholine is given in fractional doses with hexafluorenium [Mylaxen], a pseudocholinesterase inhibitor; this drug increases the duration of the block but also may predispose to development of a phase II block.

Prolonged paralysis does not occur with succinylcholine unless the plasma cholinesterase level is low or atypical or magnesium sulfate is being infused. Doses of succinylcholine should be adjusted when plasma cholinesterase levels are low (eg, in those with severe parenchymatous liver disease or malnutrition, after administration of anticholinesterase agents).

Gallamine and decamethonium are excreted unchanged by the kidney and should not be used in patients with severe renal disease. The effect of a specific dose of tubocurarine and, possibly, of pancuronium may be reduced in patients with high plasma globulin levels as a result of liver disease. Since both the liver and kidneys are involved in the degradation and excretion of tubocurarine and pancuronium, these drugs may be given to patients with renal disease; however, the duration of neuromuscular block may be increased in these patients, particularly after large doses. Although reversal of the block at the end of the procedure is usually satisfactory, caution is advised. Approximately 80% of pancuronium and 40% of tubocurarine are eliminated by the kidney. The dosage should be reduced in patients with moderate to severe impairment of renal function.

The main hazard with use of these drugs is inadequate postoperative ventilation. This complication is dangerous only if it is unrecognized, for the residual curarization is reversed after a period of controlled ventilation. Inadequate ventilation is generally caused by overdosage, interactions between the blocking agent and other drugs (including potent inhalation anesthetics and certain antibiotics, such as aminoglycosides, tetracyclines, polymyxins, and lincomycin), or presence of pathologic conditions that influence the patient's response to the neuromuscular blocking drugs.

Tachycardia and a slight increase in arterial pressure follow administration of gallamine and, to a lesser extent, pancuronium, while tubocurarine often reduces arterial pressure and produces bradycardia. Succinylcholine can produce severe arrhythmias.

Tubocurarine and pancuronium are safe for use in patients with penetrating wounds of the eye, while depolarizing drugs are relatively contraindicated (see the evaluation on Succinylcholine Chloride).

Newborn infants are sensitive to nondepolarizing neuromuscular blocking agents. Infants and children appear to be resistant to succinylcholine when it is administered on the basis of milligram per kilogram of body weight.

NONDEPOLARIZING (COMPETITIVE) BLOCKING DRUGS

TUBOCURARINE CHLORIDE

$2Cl^- \cdot 5H_2O$

Tubocurarine (curare) is used to produce muscle relaxation during surgical procedures of moderate or long duration, to reduce the severity of muscle spasms in severe tetanus, to facilitate controlled ventilation, and, occasionally, in the diagnosis of myasthenia gravis (see Chapter 18). A single intravenous dose produces maximum paralysis in three to five minutes, and the clinical effect may persist for more than 60 minutes in some individuals. About 40% of the dose is excreted unchanged by the kidneys over a period of several hours. In general, when repeated doses are used, the amount of each succeeding fraction should be reduced.

Tubocurarine causes flaccid paralysis of all skeletal muscles. The muscles of the eyes are affected first, followed by those of the face, limbs, and trunk; then the intercostal muscles and, finally, the diaphragm become paralyzed. Paralysis of abdominal muscles cannot be achieved without substantial paralysis of the ventilatory muscles. The neuromuscular blocking effect of tubocurarine can be reversed when signs of returning muscle activity begin by intravenous administration of neostigmine methylsulfate 1 to 3 mg or pyridostigmine 5 to 15 mg (for children, neostigmine 0.08 mg/kg of body weight or pyridostigmine 0.4 mg/kg) with atropine 1 to 1.5 mg (for children, 0.018 mg/kg) to antagonize muscarinic actions. In adults, an additional 1 or 2 mg of neostigmine may be used. Edrophonium chloride (10 mg) may be given intravenously as a diagnostic test to determine residual curarization.

Various drugs can potentiate or prolong the action of tubocurarine at the neuromuscular junction. Of the inhalation anesthetics, enflurane and isoflurane cause the greatest potentiation, ether and methoxyflurane somewhat less, and halothane and cyclopropane the least. When tubocurarine is given with enflurane or isoflurane, the dose of the blocking agent should be reduced to one-third to one-half of that used with halothane. Many antibiotics (eg, streptomycin, neomycin, polymyxin B, colistin, kanamycin, viomycin, bacitracin, gentamicin, amikacin, lincomycin, clindamycin) can enhance the neuromuscular block produced by tubocurarine and other nondepolarizing agents. If extremely large doses of these drugs have been used recently in a patient, especially those in renal failure, controlled ventilation may be required postoperatively. Local anesthetics, quinidine, beta-adrenergic blocking agents, magnesium sulfate, and trimethaphan (but not sodium nitroprusside) also have been reported to potentiate the neuromuscular blocking action of tubocurarine.

Respiratory acidosis and hypokalemia enhance and respiratory alkalosis diminishes the blocking effect of tubocurarine. Patients with myasthenia gravis are sensitive to the blocking effects of nondepolarizing agents; therefore, the dose of these drugs should be reduced considerably in these patients.

Tubocurarine may cause hypotension when large doses are given intravenously. This effect tends to be transient and is related directly to the depth of anesthesia; it is due to peripheral vasodilatation which, in turn, is believed to be caused by sympathetic ganglionic block and release of histamine.

This drug has been reported to cause bronchospasm due to the release of histamine. Although this effect is considered by most authorities to be clinically unimportant in normal patients, pancuronium may be preferred in patients with moderate to marked asthma.

Tubocurarine does not readily penetrate the blood-brain barrier; therefore, it is devoid of central nervous system effects when administered in therapeutic doses. However, since use of this agent may increase intracranial pressure secondary to decreased ventilation with resultant hypercarbia and hypoxia, it probably should be given to patients with increased intracranial pressure only after hyperventilation has been instituted. Tubocurarine does not readily cross the placenta in significant quantities and does not affect the tone of the uterus; therefore, it may be used safely in obstetrical anesthesia. However, repeated use of large doses may result in fetal paralysis.

ROUTE, USUAL DOSAGE, AND PREPARATIONS. The required dose varies greatly among patients; a peripheral nerve stimulator may be of value in choosing the appropriate amount. The doses that follow are for use with nitrous oxide as the only inhalation agent. They must be reduced if tubocurarine is used with more potent inhalation agents. The size of subsequent doses depends upon the anticipated duration of the procedure.
Intravenous: Adults and children, initially, 0.2 to 0.4 mg/kg of body weight; subsequent doses, 0.04 to 0.2 mg/kg. *Newborn infants up to 1 month*, initially, 0.3 mg/kg; subsequent doses, 0.15 mg/kg.
    Drug available generically: Solution 3 mg/ml in 10 and 20 ml containers; solution (concentrate for dilution only) 15 mg/ml in 1 ml containers (Abbott).

METOCURINE IODIDE (Dimethyl Tubocurarine Iodide)
[Metubine]

This semisynthetic derivative of tubocurarine is approximately twice as potent as tubocurarine and has a shorter duration of action; in other respects, there is little difference between the two drugs. There is renewed interest in metocurine

because it has less effect on the circulatory system than tubocurarine. It should not be used in patients who are sensitive to iodides.

For uses and adverse reactions, see the evaluation on Tubocurarine Chloride.

ROUTE, USUAL DOSAGE, AND PREPARATIONS. The required dose varies greatly among patients; a peripheral nerve stimulator may be of value in choosing the appropriate amount. The doses that follow are for use with nitrous oxide as the only inhalation agent. They must be reduced if metocurine is used with more potent inhalation agents. The size of subsequent doses depends upon the anticipated duration of the procedure.
Intravenous: Adults, initially, 0.1 to 0.3 mg/kg of body weight; subsequent doses, 0.02 to 0.03 mg/kg.
    Metubine (Lilly). Solution 2 mg/ml in 20 ml containers.

GALLAMINE TRIETHIODIDE
[Flaxedil]

With usual doses, this synthetic agent has a slightly shorter duration of action than tubocurarine; with very large doses, however, its effect may be longer lasting. The actions of gallamine are similar to those of tubocurarine, but this agent blocks the cardiac vagus and may cause sinus tachycardia and, occasionally, hypertension and increased cardiac output. Therefore, it should be used cautiously in patients at risk from increased heart rate. Gallamine may be preferred for use in patients with bradycardia. In contrast to their effects on the action of tubocurarine, respiratory acidosis diminishes and alkalosis enhances the blocking effect of gallamine. Although gallamine crosses the placenta, it has no perceptible effect on newborn infants when usual doses are given for cesarean section and vaginal delivery and the tone of the uterus is not affected. Since gallamine is excreted unchanged solely by the kidneys, other blocking agents should be used in patients with renal damage. A slightly larger dose of neostigmine may be required to reverse the effect of gallamine than with tubocurarine. See also the evaluation on Tubocurarine Chloride.

ROUTE, USUAL DOSAGE, AND PREPARATIONS. The required dose varies greatly among patients; a peripheral nerve stimulator may be of value in choosing the appropriate amount. The doses that follow are for use with nitrous oxide as the only inhalation agent. They must be reduced if gallamine is used with more potent inhalation agents. The size of subsequent doses depends upon the anticipated duration of the procedure.
Intravenous: *Adults*, initially, 1 to 1.5 mg/kg of body weight; subsequent doses, 0.3 to 1.2 mg/kg. *Children*, initially, 2.5 mg/kg; subsequent doses, 0.3 to 1.2 mg/kg. *Newborn infants up to 1 month*, initially, 1.5 mg/kg; subsequent doses, 1 mg/kg.
> *Flaxedil* (Davis & Geck). Solution 20 mg/ml in 10 ml containers and 100 mg/ml in 1 ml containers.

PANCURONIUM BROMIDE
[Pavulon]

The effects and general spectrum of usefulness of pancuronium appear to be similar to those of tubocurarine; however, there are some important differences in actions between the two drugs. Pancuronium is approximately five times more potent than tubocurarine. When compared at doses of 3

mg and 15 mg, respectively, the onset and duration of action of the two drugs are comparable; with larger doses, pancuronium has a longer duration of action. Endotracheal intubation is accomplished with ease in approximately two to three minutes. This drug has several other apparent advantages over tubocurarine: It does not cause hypotension, presumably because it does not have a ganglionic blocking action. Pancuronium rarely, if ever, causes the release of histamine and thus may be preferred for patients with marked bronchospasm. In addition, there is evidence that it may increase heart rate, cardiac output, and arterial pressure, probably because of its vagolytic action and/or stimulation of cardiac adrenergic receptors. Therefore, the drug is indicated when these effects are desired. Pancuronium occasionally produces ventricular extrasystoles. For other adverse reactions, see the evaluation on Tubocurarine Chloride.

Studies indicate that only insignificant quantities of pancuronium enter the fetal blood stream, which suggests that the drug may be used safely in obstetrical anesthesia.

Pancuronium can inhibit plasma cholinesterase and prolong the action of succinylcholine; however, prior administration of small doses of succinylcholine does not prolong the duration of action of pancuronium.

ROUTE, USUAL DOSAGE, AND PREPARATIONS. The required dose varies greatly among patients; a peripheral nerve stimulator may be of value in choosing the appropriate amount. The doses that follow are for use with nitrous oxide as the only inhalation agent. They must be reduced if pancuronium is used with more potent inhalation agents. The size of subsequent doses depends upon the anticipated duration of the procedure.
Intravenous: *Adults*, initially, 0.04 to 0.1 mg/kg of body weight; for intubation, 0.06 to 0.1 mg/kg; subsequently, 0.01 to 0.02 mg/kg, repeated as required (generally every 20 to 40 minutes), appears to maintain satisfactory muscle relaxation. *Children*, dosage same as for adults. *Neonates*

are especially sensitive to nondepolarizing blocking agents such as pancuronium. It is recommended that a test dose of 0.02 mg/kg be given initially to measure responsiveness.

Pavulon (Organon). Solution 1 mg/ml in 10 ml containers and 2 mg/ml in 2 and 5 ml containers.

DEPOLARIZING BLOCKING DRUGS

SUCCINYLCHOLINE CHLORIDE
[Anectine, Quelicin, Sucostrin, Sux-Cert]

$$\left[\begin{array}{c} \overset{O}{\underset{\|}{C}}OCH_2CH_2N^+(CH_3)_3 \\ (CH_2)_2 \\ \underset{\|}{C}OCH_2CH_2N^+(CH_3)_3 \\ O \end{array}\right] 2Cl^-$$

Succinylcholine has a rapid onset (one minute) and short duration of action (five minutes) because of its rapid hydrolysis by plasma cholinesterase. The drug is used primarily to produce relaxation for brief procedures such as endotracheal intubation, relief of laryngospasm, endoscopy, orthopedic manipulation, and electroconvulsive shock therapy. A single dose usually causes transient and visible muscle fasciculations, followed by profound flaccid paralysis of all skeletal muscles. Tachyphylaxis may occur after repeated administration.

Since succinylcholine is almost completely hydrolyzed by plasma cholinesterase, prolonged postoperative apnea can occur in patients with abnormal succinylcholine-resistant plasma cholinesterase activity caused by a genetically determined variant of plasma cholinesterase. The plasma cholinesterase level also can be significantly reduced by exposure to organophosphorus pesticides or topical use of long-acting anticholinesterase agents (eg, echothiophate) for open-angle glaucoma or accommodative esotropia. Nondepolarizing agents should be used in patients who have been receiving long-acting anticholinesterase drugs.

Prolonged postoperative apnea caused by a phase II block also can develop in normal patients receiving increasing or repeated doses. The dose response curve is quite steep for succinylcholine (ie, 1 to 3 mg/kg for phase I block and 3 to 5 mg/kg for phase II block). Because of this, it is helpful to use a peripheral nerve stimulator to monitor the block when succinylcholine is used to provide continuous muscle relaxation. Prolonged postoperative apnea can be avoided if the infusions are interrupted frequently to evaluate the return of neuromuscular function.

The response to succinylcholine also may be prolonged in the presence of hyperkalemia. Since these drugs may produce generalized myotonia in patients with the myotonic syndrome, tubocurarine should be used in these patients. Patients with myasthenia gravis may be resistant to the depolarizing agents and have a predisposition to phase II block.

Succinylcholine has been reported to cause both nodal and ventricular arrhythmias, decreased or increased heart rate, and increased arterial pressure. Nodal arrhythmias, bradycardia, and sinus arrest have occurred after intravenous injection in children or after fractional doses were given intravenously at three- to ten-minute intervals to adults receiving halothane or cyclopropane. These effects usually can be avoided by administering atropine prior to the repeated doses or by using the intramuscular route in children. The complex cardiovascular effects of this blocking agent have been attributed in part to sympathetic ganglionic stimulation.

Severe ventricular arrhythmias and cardiac arrest have followed administration of succinylcholine to patients with severe burns, massive trauma, brain or spinal cord injuries, tetanus, or diffuse lower motoneuron disease. These adverse effects have been attributed to a pronounced increase in plasma potassium levels in patients with severe injuries or neuromuscular disorders that result in inactivity of muscles for two weeks to six months. Therefore, succinylcholine should be avoided if possible in these patients.

Succinylcholine causes a pronounced increase in the intraocular pressure of unanesthetized or lightly anesthetized patients within one minute, but does not elevate intraocular pressure in patients under deep general anesthesia. This ocular hypertensive effect is transient; it occurs during the stage of generalized muscle fasciculations and subsides when the extraocular muscles become paralyzed. Thus, it may be caused by contraction of the extraocular muscles and the orbital smooth muscle. Succinylcholine can be used safely for intraocular surgery if it is administered at least six minutes before the eye is surgically opened. This blocking agent should not be used after the eye has been opened by the surgeon or if the eye is already open at the beginning of anesthesia (eg, penetrating wounds, iris prolapse). Since succinylcholine has only a brief effect on intraocular pressure, it is not contraindicated in patients with open-angle glaucoma or those predisposed to angle closure. In such patients, one or two drops of pilocarpine may be instilled prior to surgery.

Succinylcholine has no effect on the central nervous system when administered in therapeutic doses. It does not cross the placenta in appreciable quantities and may be used safely in obstetrical anesthesia, unless the patient has atypical plasma cholinesterase activity. Reduced maintenance doses may be required if the patient is receiving magnesium sulfate concurrently, for this agent has been reported to potentiate the neuromuscular blockade produced by succinylcholine.

A few cases of severe bronchospasm have been reported when succinylcholine was administered with hexafluorenium; therefore, these agents should not be used concomitantly in patients with bronchial asthma.

Malignant hyperpyrexia is a rare complication of general anesthesia and may have a genetic basis (see Chapter 20, General Anesthetics). In a large proportion of the reported cases, succinylcholine had been used to provide muscle relaxation during anesthesia. In many of these instances, it appeared to be the causative agent since muscle rigidity preceded the increase in body temperature.

Postoperative pain and stiffness in the shoulder and subcostal and back muscles are common after use of succinylcholine; the incidence varies from 10% in patients maintained on bed rest for one day to 70% in ambulatory patients. These symptoms generally appear 12 to 24 hours after administration of the drug and usually last for several hours to a few days; they are believed to be caused by the muscle fasciculations that occur immediately after injection. Increased intragastric pressure also has been observed in some adults. This may predispose to regurgitation. The incidence of pain and stiffness may be reduced by giving tubocurarine (3 mg) or gallamine (20 mg) three minutes prior to succinylcholine; however, the dose of succinylcholine should be increased by approximately 50% to produce an equal degree of relaxation.

ROUTES, USUAL DOSAGE, AND PREPARATIONS. The dose required varies greatly among patients; a peripheral nerve stimulator is helpful in regulating the rate of infusion. *Intravenous*: *Adults*, initially, 0.6 to 1.1 mg/kg of body weight; for continuous infusion, a 0.1% (1 mg/ml) or 0.2% (2 mg/ml) solution is administered at an average rate of 2.5 mg/min (range, 0.5 to 10 mg/min). *Children*, initially, 1.1 mg/kg; subsequent doses, 0.3 to 0.6 mg/kg. *Newborn infants up to 1 month*, initially, 2 mg/kg. Continuous infusion of succinylcholine is considered unsafe in neonates and children. *Intramuscular*: *Children*, 2.2 mg/kg of body weight. For use of succinylcholine with hexafluorenium, see the evaluation on Hexafluorenium Bromide.

Drug available generically: Solution 20 mg/ml in 10 ml containers.

Anectine (Burroughs Wellcome). Powder 500 mg and 1 g; solution 20 mg/ml in 10 ml containers.

Quelicin (Abbott). Solution 20 mg/ml in 10 ml containers; solution (concentrate for dilution only) 50 mg/ml in 10 ml containers and 100 mg/ml in 10 and 20 ml containers.

Sucostrin (Squibb). Solution 20, 50, and 100 mg/ml in 10 ml containers.

Sux-Cert (Travenol). Powder (lyophilized) 500 mg and 1 g.

DECAMETHONIUM BROMIDE
[Syncurine]

$$(CH_3)_3N^+(CH_2)_{10}N^+(CH_3)_3 \cdot 2Br^-$$

This depolarizing neuromuscular blocking agent is rarely used at the present time. Decamethonium has the same mode of action as succinylcholine; however, it is not hydrolyzed by plasma cholinesterase but is excreted unchanged by the kidneys. It has a longer duration of action than succinylcholine: Complete recovery requires about 20 minutes and is either unaffected or delayed by administration of anticholinesterase drugs. Therefore, succinylcholine is preferred for brief procedures and for patients with renal damage, and the nondepolarizing neuromuscular blocking agents are preferred for long procedures.

For indications and adverse reactions of the depolarizing agents, see the Introduction and the evaluation on Succinylcholine Chloride.

ROUTE, USUAL DOSAGE, AND PREPARATIONS. *Intravenous*: *Adults*, 0.03 to 0.06 mg/kg of body weight.
> *Syncurine* (Burroughs Wellcome). Solution 1 mg/ml in 10 ml containers.

Plasma Cholinesterase Inhibitor

HEXAFLUORENIUM BROMIDE
[Mylaxen]

Hexafluorenium is rarely used to prolong the action of succinylcholine. It is primarily a plasma cholinesterase inhibitor that delays the enzymatic hydrolysis of succinylcholine and thus increases the duration and intensity of its action; however, it also has some nondepolarizing activity and has an effect on the postjunctional membrane. The advantages of the combined use of these two agents over the use of fractional doses of succinylcholine alone have not been clearly demonstrated, although hexafluorenium may diminish or prevent the muscle fasciculations and pain often associated with use of succinylcholine alone.

Since the combined use of succinylcholine and hexafluorenium has occasionally caused bronchospasm, these agents should not be given concomitantly to patients with a history of bronchial asthma. Prolonged depolarization due to the combined use of succinylcholine and hexafluorenium almost always leads to a phase II block.

ROUTE, USUAL DOSAGE, AND PREPARATIONS. *Intravenous*: *Adults*, 0.3 to 0.4 mg/kg of body weight of hexafluorenium, followed in two or three minutes by 0.25 mg/kg of succinylcholine, provides relaxation for 15 to 30 minutes. This relaxation may be sustained with doses of 0.15 mg/kg of succinylcholine repeated every 15 to 30 minutes. When the duration of action of succinylcholine becomes less than 12 to 15 minutes, an additional 0.1 to 0.15 mg/kg of hexafluorenium may be given if the procedure is expected to last more than 30 minutes; if relaxation is required for less than 30 minutes, a larger dose of succinylcholine (0.2 to 0.3 mg/kg) may be given.
> *Mylaxen* (Mallinckrodt). Solution 20 mg/ml in 10 ml containers.

THERAPEUTIC GASES

Gases used therapeutically include the general anesthetics (see Chapter 20) and the two gases involved in normal metabolism and respiration, oxygen and carbon dioxide. Of the latter, oxygen has by far the greater therapeutic importance.

OXYGEN

Oxygen has two primary therapeutic uses: to form mixtures with or vaporize inhalation anesthetics and to prevent or relieve hypoxemia and thereby decrease tissue damage and reduce the energy expenditure of the body's compensatory mechanisms until the cause of the hypoxemia can be corrected by other appropriate measures. It is used to oxygenate perfusates for tissues being held in readiness for transplantation and to oxygenate blood during cardiopulmonary bypass. It is sometimes administered to facilitate the elimination of nitrogen or other gas from the tissues or hollow viscera (eg, after pneumoencephalograms and ventriculograms, in intestinal obstruction, in pneumatosis coli). Selection of the technique of administration depends upon the condition being treated, the need for accessibility to the patient, his cooperativeness and oxygen demands, and the anticipated duration of administration.

Approximate inhaled oxygen concentrations attainable with some currently available devices are: short nasal cannula or nasopharyngeal catheter, 24% to 45% with oxygen flow rates of 1 to 6 L/min; pediatric tent or incubator, approximately 40%; face hood, 25% to 50%; loose-fitting plastic mask, 40% to 70% with oxygen flow rates of 5 to 8 L/min; loose-fitting plastic mask with reservoir bag, 60% to 95% with oxygen flow rates of 6 to 10 L/min; and tight-fitting mask and reservoir bag with non-rebreathing valve, 100%. High-flow gas systems that deliver the entire volume of air inspired (eg, the Venturi mask) prevent uncontrolled dilution with air and thus provide specific concentrations of oxygen. In general, devices that permit the admixture of air and oxygen in a fixed ratio offer a distinct advantage over those that deliver only pure gas, particularly when prolonged administration is required. Artificial ventilation with masks or endotracheal or tracheostomy tubes permits delivery of up to 100% oxygen, or the concentration of oxygen delivered can be varied as desired.

Although high concentrations of oxygen may be necessary in life-threatening situations, they should not be used for long periods. When continuous administration is indicated, the lowest possible concentration should be used. Regardless of the concentration provided by the oxygenating system, measuring the oxygen tension of the arterial blood is the only means of monitoring the effectiveness of therapy.

Oxygen also may be administered in hyperbaric chambers at pressures not exceeding three atmospheres. Hyperbaric oxygen appears to be of value to relieve hypoxemia caused by carbon monoxide poisoning and as an adjunct to recompression in decompression sickness. It also appears to be of value when used to supplement antibiotics and other therapeutic measures employed to arrest infection caused by the anaerobic clostridia that produce gas gangrene, and it may augment the effects of therapeutic radiation by making neoplasms more radiosensitive. Definitive evaluation of the effectiveness and practicality of hyperbaric oxygen for these and other conditions must await the results of adequately controlled studies.

ADVERSE REACTIONS AND PRECAUTIONS.

Prolonged administration of high concentrations of oxygen, even at atmospheric pressure, causes pulmonary irritation, most commonly manifested by substernal pain, coughing, and dyspnea. The irritation may be induced at atmospheric pressure by inhalation of 100% oxygen for 3 to 30 hours. Continued administration of high concentrations may cause more severe pulmonary complications (eg, increased physiologic dead space and shunting, decreased vital capacity), which apparently are related to alveolar and pulmonary capillary exudative and proliferative changes (interstitial edema and fibrosis, alveolar exudation and hemorrhage, hyaline membrane formation). This potentially irreversible syndrome is often referred to as "oxygen toxicity," a type of adult respiratory distress syndrome. It does not occur if the inspired tension is below one-half atmosphere (380 mm Hg) and is not clinically important if one atmosphere (760 mm Hg) is inhaled for less than one day. Since the toxicity is a response to inspired oxygen tension, symptoms develop more rapidly under hyperbaric conditions. Although oxygen therapy must not be withheld because of this adverse response, the concentration of oxygen administered should not exceed that required to relieve the hypoxemia, and other measures that might improve oxygenation (eg, positive end-expired pressure, chest physiotherapy) must be employed. Grand mal convulsions may result from administration of oxygen at greater than two and one-half atmospheres; these cease without permanent sequelae upon resumption of air breathing.

When oxygen is required for premature infants, the inspired oxygen concentration should not exceed 40% for any substantial period without measurement of arterial oxygen tension, unless the infant has cyanotic heart disease or the hypoxemia is dangerous. Arterial oxygen tensions above 150 mm Hg may cause retrolental fibroplasia; permanent blindness occurs several months later. The brief periods of administration of 100% oxygen necessary for resuscitation of premature infants impose little risk of retinal injury. Retinal changes do not occur in full-term infants, although these infants are susceptible to the pulmonary complications observed in adults.

Some data suggest that an important early effect of oxygen inhalation is impairment of macrophage function, which may occur with oxygen concentrations below 50%. Although this harmful effect on the pulmonary defense mechanism may be of little consequence to patients with normal lungs, it may be detrimental to those who cannot cough and take adequate deep breaths or whose upper airways have been bypassed by endotracheal or tracheostomy tubes.

When administering oxygen through any type of apparatus, the possibility of carbon dioxide retention must be considered. This may result from rebreathing expired air due to faulty design or malfunction of apparatus or to failure to provide adequate inflow of fresh gas. Patients with chronic obstructive pulmonary disease may be especially susceptible to carbon dioxide retention. In some of these patients, oxygen may correct the hypoxemia but may diminish ventilation by eliminating the reflex hypoxic stimulus mediated mainly via the carotid and aortic chemoreceptors, thus leading to further retention of carbon dioxide. Delirium, disorientation, or coma from carbon dioxide narcosis may result. This may be avoided by carefully adminis-

tering the oxygen via artificial ventilation, monitoring arterial carbon dioxide tension, and continuous electrocardiographic monitoring; serious ventricular arrhythmias can develop if the arterial carbon dioxide tension is reduced rapidly.

Oxygen drawn from cylinders and piping systems is anhydrous and tends to dry the mucous membranes. This causes thickening of natural or pathologic secretions, reduced ciliary function, and discomfort. Such dehydrating effects are accentuated when the gas bypasses the normal moistening area of the nose and pharynx (eg, through an endotracheal or tracheostomy tube or nasopharyngeal catheter). Use of a heated humidifying apparatus or an ultrasonic nebulizer eliminates or reduces these effects, but the former may produce condensation in the delivery tubing and hyperthermia in the patient, and the latter water intoxication in the patient. A simple bubble jar may be sufficient to overcome dehydrating effects if the upper airway is not bypassed.

The intensity of a fire or explosion in oxygen-enriched atmospheres is directly proportional to the concentration of oxygen in the mixture being supplied. The risk of fire is particularly great with oxygen tents. Electrical appliances must never be used in tents or in the areas close to tents. Smoking should be forbidden in areas where oxygen is being administered.

Bacterial contamination of oxygen and humidifying equipment has been reported; in view of this, all reusable parts, including appropriate parts of ventilators, should be properly sterilized.

Oxygen is prepared by fractional distillation of liquid air. Anhydrous in green-coded cylinders (WHO, white-coded) at about 2,000 psi.

CARBON DIOXIDE

Carbon dioxide is of definite therapeutic value in only one situation: It must be added to the oxygen used in certain types of pump oxygenators to maintain the carbon dioxide tension of the blood.

Too often carbon dioxide is used inappropriately when it is of little value and possibly even harmful. Although it often is administered in an attempt to relieve persistent hiccups, it only occasionally produces transient relief. Use of the gas has been suggested to improve circulation in cerebrovascular disorders (eg, following cerebral thrombosis), but it is of doubtful value in these conditions and may be harmful because it elevates intracranial pressure. Carbon dioxide has been used to induce deep breathing and coughing postoperatively in order to avoid atelectasis, but it generally is of little benefit. In addition, carbon dioxide should not be administered in an attempt to resuscitate victims of carbon monoxide poisoning, drowning, electric shock, or asphyxiation or to treat overdosage with central nervous system depressants because the medullary chemoreceptors are depressed and do not respond.

> Carbon dioxide (100%) is supplied in gray-coded cylinders in liquified form at about 750 psi. The pure gas must be mixed with oxygen, and flowmeters and other appropriate apparatus designed to dispense gases should be used. It is also available premixed with oxygen in gray/green-coded cylinders (WHO, gray/white-coded); the most common concentration is 5% carbon dioxide and 95% oxygen. These mixtures are gaseous at room temperature.

MISCELLANEOUS ADJUNCTIVE DRUGS

Agents Used to Produce Peripheral Vasodilation: The ganglionic blocking agent, trimethaphan camsylate [Arfonad], and the direct-acting peripheral vasodilator, sodium nitroprusside [Nipride], may be infused to reduce arterial pressure and thus avoid excessive hemorrhage during neurosurgery, plastic surgery, and cardiovascular and other types of surgery.

Hypotensive anesthesia should be undertaken only by anesthesiologists familiar with the principles of the technique. Intravenous infusion of trimethaphan 0.05% or 0.1% (0.5 or 1 mg/ml) or sodium nitroprusside 0.005% or 0.01% (0.05 or 0.1 mg/ml) in 5% dextrose injection decreases arterial pressure, primarily as the result of a reduction in peripheral vascular resistance. Trimethaphan also may be ad-

ministered repeatedly in intravenous doses of 1 to 5 mg. The main difference between the two drugs is that, whereas there is a fall in cardiac output in some patients with use of trimethaphan, there is either no change or a slight increase in this variable with use of sodium nitroprusside. The latter drug also increases the heart rate and decreases central venous pressure; additionally, early tachyphylaxis normally does not occur and recovery of arterial pressure is rapid (two to six minutes) upon discontinuation of infusion of usual clinical doses. However, progressive, irreversible hypotension has been reported in baboons given four to six times the usual clinical dose of sodium nitroprusside; a similar fatal complication has been reported in one patient. Until additional clinical data become available, great caution should be exercised when increasing doses of sodium nitroprusside are required to maintain the desired level of hypotension. It may be wise to discontinue administration if tachyphylaxis or acidemia develops or when a total dose of 1.5 mg/kg of body weight has been given during anesthesia.

More studies are required to evaluate the comparative usefulness of these two drugs and to investigate the possible hazards of the cyanide and thiocyanate produced by metabolism of sodium nitroprusside (see Chapter 86, Specific Antidotes). Adverse effects (skin rashes, headache, nausea, muscle spasms, psychotic behavior) do not appear to occur after short-term use of sodium nitroprusside. (See also Chapter 38, Antihypertensive Agents.)

Agents Used in Pheochromocytoma: The alpha-adrenergic blocking agents, phenoxybenzamine [Dibenzyline] and phentolamine [Regitine]; the beta-adrenergic blocking agents, propranolol [Inderal] and metoprolol [Lopressor]; and sodium nitroprusside are used in the surgical management of patients with pheochromocytoma. Phenoxybenzamine and propranolol also are used preoperatively, the former to control hypertension and estimate the intravascular volume for volume replacement, and the latter to control sinus tachycardia and frequent premature ventricular contractions. Since the beta-adrenergic blocking agents may increase peripheral vascular resistance significantly as a result of unopposed alpha adrenergic activity, they should not be used alone.

During anesthesia, paroxysms of severe hypertension may be controlled by infusion of sodium nitroprusside, by intravenous injections of 1 to 2 mg of phentolamine, or by infusion of a 0.01% (0.1 mg/ml) solution of phentolamine. Serious ventricular arrhythmias may be controlled by the slow intravenous injection of increments of propranolol (0.5 to 1 mg) up to a total of 3 mg.

If serious hypotension develops after removal of the tumor, the temporary infusion of norepinephrine (levarterenol) 4 mg/500 ml may be indicated (see also Chapter 37, Agents Used to Treat Shock, and Chapter 38, Antihypertensive Agents).

Pressor Agents: Adrenergic stimulating agents can be injected judiciously to elevate arterial pressure and improve blood flow (to vital organs in particular) by producing peripheral vasoconstriction and a positive inotropic effect during anesthesia (see Chapter 37).

ANALEPTIC DRUGS

Analeptics are general central nervous system stimulants; they stimulate respiration, enhance the response to sensory stimulation, and hasten the return of normal reflexes. Studies have demonstrated that analeptics have limited usefulness in the supportive treatment of ventilatory insufficiency or arrest caused by anesthetic agents and certain other drugs that have hypnotic activity. None of these drugs have the high specificity of action of the narcotic antagonists or anticholinesterase agents; therefore, they should not be substituted for these agents when respiratory depression is caused by narcotics or neuromuscular blocking drugs. Analeptics are being investigated for use in ventilatory insufficiency associated with apnea in premature infants, drowning, electrocution, hypoxemia, and carbon monoxide poisoning. They are ineffective for managing ventilatory depression caused by cardiac arrest or overdosage of central nervous system stimulants.

Analeptics act directly on nervous tissue. When ventilation is improved, their site of action is in the brain stem, particularly the medulla and certain analeptics act on the carotid chemoreceptors as well. Reflex activity is improved when the spinal cord is stimulated in addition to the brain stem. Arousal occurs when higher centers are stimulated. Any improvement of cardiovascular reflexes observed is a result of improved central nervous system function rather than direct myocardial stimulation.

Convulsions may occur with increasing doses of any analeptic. Large doses given frequently within a short period may actually produce respiratory depression. The margin between the analeptic and convulsant dose is narrow with the older analeptics (picrotoxin, nikethamide [Coramine], pentylenetetrazol [Metrazol]). The general analeptic agent, doxapram [Dopram], is safer and thus has supplanted the older agents when analeptic therapy is elected to stimulate ventilation; its usefulness in hastening arousal is less established.

The xanthines, caffeine and theophylline, are not recommended for general analeptic use, but they are being investigated in the treatment of apnea in premature infants; most data have been accumulated on theophylline (see the evaluation on Methylxanthines).

Analeptics, particularly caffeine sodium benzoate and the amphetamines, have been promoted for use in overcoming the "hangover" effects that may occur during the arousal period in patients recovering from drug-induced coma. However, their administration for this purpose is neither logical nor advisable.

Physostigmine [Antilirium] is not a general analeptic like doxapram. Its action is related principally to its ability to hasten arousal and the return of normal reflexes rather than to improve ventilation. It is presumably ineffective in nondrug-induced ventilatory depression and does not antagonize the central depression produced by inhalation anesthetics, opiates and opioids, ketamine (Drummond et al, 1979), or barbiturates. However, physostigmine does reverse the adverse central anticholinergic actions of many drugs, and it may arouse individuals depressed by drugs that have little or no central anticholinergic action (eg, droperidol, benzodiazepines). This implies that its arousal action may be unrelated to its cholinergic activity or it is possible that cholinergic activity may be an integral part of the awake-sleep continuum state.

Physostigmine has been effective in shortening the arousal time in postoperative patients who had received anticholinergic drugs, antihistamines, benzodiazepines, and droperidol and in reducing the disorientation and agitation occasionally caused by these agents. Its routine use is not recommended. Physostigmine also has been administered to arouse patients for brief periods during neuroleptanesthesia when their cooperation is required (eg, in certain neurosurgical procedures).

See the evaluation on Physostigmine Salicylate in Chapter 86, Specific Antidotes. The adverse reactions, precautions, and dosage information given in that evaluation are also applicable to its suggested uses as an arousal drug.

INDIVIDUAL EVALUATIONS

DOXAPRAM HYDROCHLORIDE
[Dopram]

Animal studies have demonstrated that this analeptic causes arousal, stimulates ventilation, and increases arterial pressure. Studies in humans with normal central nervous and respiratory systems confirmed that doxapram increased the ventilatory response to carbon dioxide and the minute ventilation (by increasing tidal volume and, to a lesser extent, the ventilatory rate), but they also indicated that the drug increased oxygen uptake. The resultant effects upon arterial blood gases were a reduction in carbon dioxide tension and elevation of pH, oxygen tension, and oxygen saturation. The adverse effects were not serious enough to reduce the rate of administration, although many subjects commented that doxapram elicited an intense desire to breathe deeply.

The availability of other simple tests (eg, evaluation of the ventilatory rate and pattern, ability of the patient to lift his head, results of peripheral nerve stimulation) renders use of doxapram for diagnostic purposes in cases of postanesthetic apnea or hypoventilation of minimal clinical value.

Controlled double-blind studies reveal that doxapram hastens arousal when it is administered during the immediate postoperative period. It is not widely used, perhaps because the clinical usefulness and possible hazards of this action remain unclear.

Because of the effectiveness of controlled ventilation and standard supportive therapy in the treatment of ventilatory failure, doxapram normally should not be used in patients with drug-induced coma or an exacerbation of chronic lung disease. An infusion of doxapram may allow some patients in hypercarbic ventilatory failure to respond satisfactorily to oxygen administration for two hours, but there are no data to indicate that more prolonged infusions are safe and will reduce the ultimate need for controlled ventilation.

Generalized warmth, sweating, dyspnea, restlessness, fasciculations, hyperreflexia, laryngospasm, coughing, breathholding, retching, tachycardia, hypertension, nausea, lightheadedness, headache, tremor, and convulsions may occur, particularly if large doses are given. Agitation and hallucinations are observed rarely. Doxapram is contraindicated in patients with convulsive disorders, hypertension, cerebral edema, hyperthyroidism, or pheochromocytoma and in those taking monoamine oxidase inhibitors or adrenergic agents.

ROUTE, USUAL DOSAGE, AND PREPARATIONS.
Many physicians believe that use of this
drug is inadvisable because of the reasons
stated above. However, other physicians
feel that doxapram may have a place as an
adjunct in the treatment of certain specific
clinical situations. The manufacturer's
suggested dosages are:
Intravenous: *Adults*, for ventilatory
depression following anesthesia, 0.5 to 1
mg/kg of body weight is injected as a single
dose and repeated at five-minute intervals
until a maximum of 2 mg/kg has been
given. Alternatively, 1.5 to 2 mg/kg is infused. The calculated total dose is added to
dextrose 5% or 10% or sodium chloride
injection and administered at an initial rate
of approximately 5 mg/min until a satisfactory response is observed; for maintenance,
an infusion rate of 1 to 3 mg/min is
suggested. The maximal dosage by infusion is 4 mg/kg or 300 mg for adults of
average weight.
To hasten arousal during the recovery
period, 1 to 1.5 mg/kg is injected. The total
amount is given as a single dose or in
divided doses at five-minute intervals.
For drug-induced depression, initially, 0.5
to 1 mg/kg is injected as a single dose. For
maintenance, the injection is repeated or
an infusion is given as above. The maximal
daily dose is 24 mg/kg/day for two days or
until a total dose of 3 g has been given.
Data are not yet available regarding the
drug's use in *children*.

> *Dopram* (Robins). Solution 20 mg/ml with 0.5%
> chlorobutanol in 20 ml containers.

METHYLXANTHINES

The methylxanthines, theophylline and
caffeine, are effective analeptic (re-
spirogenic) drugs in the treatment of primary apnea of prematurity (Higbee and
Bosso, 1979). The disorder is characterized
by periodic breathing and apneic episodes
of greater than 15 seconds accompanied by
cyanosis and bradycardia. These drugs
should be considered only as adjuncts to
nondrug measures (continuous positive
airway pressure, decreased ambient temperature, oxygen, sensory stimulation, and
mechanical support of ventilation, if
needed).

The methylxanthines decrease the frequency of apneic episodes probably
through a central action, because regulari-
zation of breathing is associated with increased alveolar ventilation and increased
respiratory center sensitivity to carbon
dioxide without alteration of lung compliance. No alterations in the PaO_2, pH,
respiratory rate, or blood pressure is necessarily observed, although $PaCO_2$ is usually
decreased when apneic spells are abolished (Davi et al, 1978).

There has been more experience with
the use of theophylline than caffeine. Unlike the adult, theophylline is metabolized
in part to caffeine in the premature infant
(Bory et al, 1979). More investigation is
required to determine if caffeine produced
by the biotransformation of theophylline
may be responsible for part of the latter
agent's action. In any event, it has been
recommended that the total methylxanthine plasma concentration (caffeine plus
theophylline) may need to be assessed in
order to adjust dosage of theophylline appropriately.

The most common adverse reaction of
theophylline is tachycardia; jitteriness is
observed on occasion with caffeine. The
methylxanthines are irritating to the gastrointestinal mucosa. Vomiting and gastrointestinal bleeding have been observed
during therapy; monitoring of bleeding
with hemoccult slides is recommended.
The methylxanthines are potent central
nervous system stimulants and convulsions
have been reported when plasma concentrations are excessive.

The recommended plasma concentration
for theophylline or caffeine is approximately 6 to 13 mcg/ml; adverse reactions
are common if the plasma concentration is
greater than 20 mcg/ml. The clearance of
theophylline and consequently its half-life
is markedly prolonged in the neonate compared to the adult; the clearance of caffeine
is even more impaired. Unfortunately,
there is also a wide variation among premature infants in their ability to clear the
methylxanthines, which makes it mandatory to individualize maintenance dosage.
This is best managed by determining
methylxanthine plasma concentrations if

possible; in any event, if the heart rate is above 180, the dosage should be reduced or therapy discontinued. The clearance of the methylxanthines is reduced in those with liver disease or congestive heart failure, and oral or intravenous maintenance doses must be reduced. See Chapter 32, Drugs Used in Asthma.

A solution of caffeine citrate is administered orally. Either the alcoholic elixir or the nonalcoholic syrup (to minimize gastritis) of theophylline is administered orally. Theophylline is given intravenously as aminophylline.

ROUTES, USUAL DOSAGE, AND PREPARATIONS.

THEOPHYLLINE:

Oral (nasogastric tube): A loading dose of 6 mg/kg of body weight, followed by a maintenance dose of 2 mg/kg is given every 12 hours. Serum levels of theophylline (or theophylline plus caffeine) should be monitored if possible. Generally, 6 to 13 mcg/ml is an effective range of plasma concentration of theophylline, and toxic signs are often noted if the concentration is above 20 mcg/ml. (Complete data are not available to recommend corresponding concentrations for methylxanthine, ie, theophylline and its metabolite, caffeine, but it is anticipated that these concentrations may not be significantly different from recommended concentrations for theophylline alone.) Smaller doses at more frequent intervals may be necessary to maintain a more constant, effective concentration of theophylline without high, possibly toxic, peak concentrations. It may be necessary to increase the daily dose occasionally to maintain therapeutic blood concentrations, because the clearance of theophylline increases with age during the first month of life.

Intravenous: A loading dose of 5.5 mg of theophylline/kg of body weight, (given as aminophylline which contains 85% theophylline), followed by a constant intravenous infusion of 1.1 mg/kg until a plasma theophylline concentration of 6 to 13 mcg/ml is reached.

Rectal (enema): Either the oral or intravenous route of administration is preferred. When a theophylline enema is given, the same dosage schedule recommended for the oral route can be employed. Since absorption after use of suppositories is erratic, this dosage form is not recommended.

See Chapter 32, Drugs Used in Asthma, for a listing of available theophylline products.

CAFFEINE:

Oral (nasogastric tube): A loading dose of 10 mg of caffeine (caffeine citrate contains 50% caffeine)/kg of body weight, followed by maintenance doses of 2.5 mg/kg/day. Serum levels should be monitored if possible. Generally, 6 to 13 mcg/ml is an effective plasma concentration of caffeine. Toxic signs are often observed if the concentration is above 20 mcg/ml.

Drug available generically: Tablets 60 mg, powder.

Selected References

Bellville JW, et al: Analgesic effects of hydroxyzine compared to morphine in man. *J Clin Pharmacol* 19:290-296, 1979.

Bory C, et al: Metabolism of theophylline to caffeine in premature newborn infants. *J Pediatr* 94:988-993, 1979.

Conner JT, et al: Morphine, scopolamine and atropine as intravenous surgical premedicants. *Anesth Analg* 56:606-614, 1977.

Davi MJ, et al: Physiologic changes induced by theophylline in treatment of apnea in preterm infants. *J Pediatr* 92:91-95, 1978.

Drummond JC, et al: Randomized evaluation of reversal of ketamine by physostigmine. *Can Anaesth Soc J* 26:288-295, 1979.

Dundee JW, et al: Comparison of actions of diazepam and lorazepam. *Br J Anaesth* 51:439-445, 1979.

Dundee JW, et al: Studies on drugs given before anesthesia. XXVI. Lorazepam. *Br J Anaesth* 49:1047-1056, 1977.

Forrest WH Jr, et al: Subjective responses to six common preoperative medications. *Anesthesiology* 47:241-247, 1977.

Gunn TR, et al: Sequelae of caffeine treatment in preterm infants with apnea. *J Pediatr* 94:106-109, 1979.

Higbee MD, Bosso JA: Apnea of prematurity. *Drug Intell Clin Pharm* 13:24-29, 1979.

Miller RH: Antagonism of neuromuscular blockade. *Anesthesiology* 44: 318-329, 1976.

Mirakhur RK, et al: Anticholinergic drugs in anesthesia. *Anaesthesia* 33:133-138, 1978.

Tornetta FJ: Comparison of droperidol, diazepam and hydroxyzine hydrochloride as premedication. *Anesth Anal* 56:496-500, 1977.

Wender RH, et al: Comparison of I.V. diazepam and hydroxyzine as surgical premedicants. *Br J Anaesth* 49:907-912, 1977.

Wingard LB, Cook DR: Clinical pharmacokinetics of muscle relaxants. *Clin Pharmacokinet* 2:330-343, 1977.

Agents Used to Treat Glaucoma | 22

MIOTICS

EPINEPHRINE

BETA-ADRENERGIC BLOCKING DRUGS

INVESTIGATIONAL ADRENERGIC AND
ANTIADRENERGIC AGENTS

CARBONIC ANHYDRASE INHIBITORS

OSMOTIC AGENTS

The primary goal in the treatment of glaucoma is to prevent damage to the optic nerve fibers by lowering elevated intraocular pressure. Most forms of glaucoma result from interference with the outflow of aqueous humor from the eye. Aqueous humor is secreted by the cells of the ciliary processes into the posterior chamber where it passes into the anterior chamber through the pupil. The aqueous leaves the eye by flowing through the trabecular meshwork in the anterior chamber angle, entering Schlemm's canal and passing into the venous system; a second pathway is via the ciliary muscle into the suprachoroidal space and then through the sclera. The drugs used in glaucoma therapy reduce intraocular pressure by decreasing resistance to outflow of aqueous humor (miotics and epinephrine), by decreasing aqueous production (carbonic anhydrase inhibitors, epinephrine, beta-adrenergic blocking drugs, and, possibly, some miotics), or by transiently reducing the volume of intraocular fluids (osmotic agents).

In *primary open-angle glaucoma*, which is the most common form, outflow facility is impaired, presumably because of an abnormality in the trabecular meshwork-Schlemm's canal system. This is a chronic,

slowly progressing multifactorial disorder, and symptoms are usually absent until extensive loss of visual field has occurred. Drug therapy is the primary treatment for open-angle glaucoma. Surgery is usually reserved for patients with progressive optic nerve damage and visual field loss despite maximal medical therapy (ie, miotic, epinephrine, beta-blocking drug, and a carbonic anhydrase inhibitor). It is important to measure the intraocular pressure at different times of day, since patients with open-angle glaucoma frequently show marked diurnal variations. Patients with an elevated intraocular pressure but no visual field loss may be observed closely without treatment unless the level of intraocular pressure, age, family history, or the presence of other risk factors (eg, diabetes) suggest that the advantages of therapy outweigh the potential risks.

When glaucomatous cupping and visual field loss appear to occur in the absence of elevated intraocular pressure, the possibility of intermittent increases in pressure should be eliminated by diurnal pressure recordings; low ocular rigidity (which may give falsely low intraocular pressure readings) should be excluded by use of the applanation tonometer, and other causes of

349

optic atrophy (eg, intracranial tumors, ischemic neuropathy) should be ruled out. *Low-tension glaucoma* without intermittent elevation of intraocular pressure is rare. When it occurs, treatment should be directed toward reducing the intraocular pressure to the lowest possible level as in open-angle glaucoma.

Primary angle-closure glaucoma occurs as an acute episode when the lens is unusually far forward and partially blocks the flow of aqueous from the posterior into the anterior chamber. Pressure in the posterior chamber then pushes the peripheral iris into the filtration angle, blocking aqueous outflow and causing a marked, symptomatic rise in intraocular pressure. Eyes predisposed to angle closure have shallow anterior chambers and narrow angles, and dilation of the pupil by drugs, emotional stress, or darkness may precipitate an acute attack of angle closure. Surgical iridectomy to bypass the pupillary block is the definitive treatment for primary angle-closure glaucoma. Laser iridectomy may be used in some cases. Osmotic agents, short-acting miotics, and carbonic anhydrase inhibitors are important in the management of an acute attack. *Long-term* use of these drugs in lieu of surgery should be avoided because permanent iridotrabecular adhesions may form and preclude successful iridectomy. If residual glaucoma is present following surgery, treatment is the same as for open-angle glaucoma.

The *secondary glaucomas* are associated with various ocular diseases, trauma, or the use of certain drugs and may be of the open-angle or closed-angle variety. The primary goal is to control the underlying disease if possible. Drugs used to treat primary open-angle glaucoma are useful in most cases of noninflammatory secondary glaucoma. In glaucoma associated with inflammation, miotics may aggravate the inflammation and increase synechia formation (see Chapter 23, Mydriatics and Cycloplegics).

Congenital glaucoma is essentially a surgical problem. Drugs may be used preoperatively to obtain optimum conditions for surgery and postoperatively to treat residual glaucoma.

For a more detailed discussion, see Chandler and Grant, 1979; Kolker and Hetherington, 1976; Drance, 1975 (A and B); and Wilensky and Podos, 1975.

MIOTICS

Actions and Uses

The miotics are cholinergic drugs that stimulate parasympathetic effector cells directly (parasympathomimetics) or inhibit cholinesterase, the enzyme that destroys acetylcholine (anticholinesterase agents). When applied topically to the eye, these drugs cause constriction of the pupil, contraction of the ciliary muscle, and a fall in intraocular pressure that is associated with decreased resistance to the outflow of aqueous humor.

In chronic open-angle glaucoma, a miotic is the principal and usually the initial drug used. The mechanism by which miotics lower intraocular pressure in open-angle glaucoma is not fully understood but appears to involve opening of the intertrabecular spaces when the ciliary muscle contracts. The resultant reduction in outflow resistance is the desired effect. Miosis and spasm of accommodation are side effects that may interfere with vision and cause discomfort, particularly in younger patients. An optical correction may be indicated for the induced myopia but is often unsatisfactory because of the variability of this condition.

In contrast, the primary beneficial effect of miotics in angle-closure glaucoma results from constriction of the pupil which pulls the iris away from the trabeculum. In some instances, miotics (particularly strong miotics) may favor closure rather than opening of the angle. This paradoxical effect results from increased resistance to the forward flow of aqueous at the pupil (pupillary block) caused by the small pupil, forward movement of the lens associated with ciliary muscle contraction, or a combination of these factors. In some patients who respond unfavorably to miotics, cycloplegics may be effective in opening the angle, but this form of therapy is used mainly in unusual cases under carefully controlled conditions.

Although miotics are useful in many forms of noninflammatory secondary glaucoma, they should be avoided when iritis is present because they may aggravate the inflammatory process. Moreover, iridolenticular synechiae may result from inflammation and are particularly undesirable in the presence of a small pupil.

Short-Acting Miotics: The parasympathomimetic agent, pilocarpine, is the standard drug for initial and maintenance therapy in primary open-angle glaucoma and most other chronic glaucomas. It often provides adequate control of intraocular pressure and, in patients over age 50, is relatively free of undesirable effects. Adequate concentrations should be administered as frequently as necessary to maintain the intraocular pressure at the level required to prevent further damage to the optic disc and progressive loss of visual field. It may be necessary to consider the diurnal variation in pressure. Stronger concentrations may be required in patients with dark irides than in those with light irides, because topically applied miotics are less effective in heavily pigmented eyes.

Pilocarpine is generally better tolerated than other miotics available in the United States. It seldom causes local irritation or systemic effects and hypersensitivity reactions occur infrequently. Carbachol may be substituted if resistance or intolerance develops to pilocarpine or if a slightly stronger or slightly longer-acting drug is needed. The short-acting anticholinesterase drug, physostigmine (eserine), is not well tolerated and is not commonly used today for long-term therapy. Aceclidine, a miotic available in some other countries, appears to cause less spasm of accommodation than other miotics.

Pilocarpine is usually the miotic used for the emergency treatment of acute angle-closure glaucoma. It should not be administered for long periods to avoid or postpone iridectomy because any miotic may tighten the pupil against the lens and block the flow of aqueous. In selected cases, however, especially in elderly patients, pilocarpine may be used for long-term therapy if the pressure is controlled and the angle opens more widely. It may be used after surgical or laser iridectomy if the intraocular pressure remains elevated.

Long-Acting Miotics: Demecarium [Humorsol] and the organophosphorus compounds, isoflurophate [Floropryl] and echothiophate [Echodide, Phospholine], are long-acting, potent cholinesterase inhibitors employed in the treatment of chronic open-angle glaucoma. Because of their cataractogenic properties and other toxicity, these drugs should be reserved for patients refractory to short-acting miotics, epinephrine, beta-blocking drugs, and, possibly, carbonic anhydrase inhibitors. Some authorities now prefer surgery to long-acting miotics if the lens is present. In the absence of the lens, some ophthalmologists feel that these agents may be employed with less hesitation, and they are often used to treat chronic glaucoma in aphakic patients. These agents should not be administered prior to iridectomy in angle-closure glaucoma because they may aggravate angle closure. They also should be avoided in other types of glaucoma caused by unrelieved pupillary block. Long-acting miotics may be used after iridectomy if continued drug therapy is required and weaker miotics are inadequate.

Adverse Reactions and Precautions

Miotics, particularly the strong agents, may cause a variety of untoward reactions as a result of their local effects on ocular structures. Accommodative myopia can be troublesome in younger patients. Pupillary constriction may interfere with vision, particularly in patients with central lens opacities. Other common local effects include twitching of the eyelids, browache, headache, ocular pain, ciliary and conjunctival congestion, and lacrimation. Localized allergy, manifested by conjunctivitis and contact dermatitis, may develop. This complication occurred frequently when physostigmine solutions were used more often.

The development of cataracts may be hastened by treatment with long-acting anticholinesterase agents, particularly in patients over 60 years of age. These cataracts are characterized by the early appearance of anterior subcapsular vacuoles. Although pilocarpine has been reported to be cataractogenic with long-term use, such an association is difficult to prove. Many patients have retained clear lenses after using pilocarpine for several decades.

Cysts may develop at the pupillary margin of the iris, especially in children, when long-acting miotics are administered for prolonged periods. These rounded nodules of the pigmentary epithelium may enlarge sufficiently to interfere with vision. They generally disappear when the drug is discontinued, and their incidence may be reduced if one drop of phenylephrine 2.5% is used in conjunction with the anticholinesterase agent.

Pupillary block, local vascular congestion, and occasional forward movement of the lens induced by the strong miotics may cause a sudden or insidious closure of the angle and an increase in intraocular pressure in eyes with even moderately narrow angles. These drugs are contraindicated prior to iridectomy in angle-closure glaucoma and also should be avoided in secondary glaucomas caused by unrelieved pupillary block (eg, when iritis has caused complete adhesion of the iris to the lens). Occasionally, short-acting miotics have similarly aggravated angle closure in predisposed eyes. Rarely, if either short- or long-acting miotics are administered after operation for angle closure, the anterior chamber may become very shallow and the intraocular pressure may rise due to development of ciliary block (malignant) glaucoma.

When there is an active inflammatory process (eg, in glaucoma secondary to anterior uveitis), miotics usually are of little therapeutic value and may predispose to development of posterior synechiae. Long-acting miotics may increase the frequency of hemorrhage in the wound during ocular surgery. Their use after filtering operations increases the possibility of posterior synechiae formation. If possible, strong miotics should be discontinued several weeks prior to ocular surgery.

Following prolonged (months to years) use of cholinesterase inhibitors, miosis may persist when the drug is discontinued. This complication is associated with a loss of tone of the dilator muscle and the formation of fine posterior synechiae.

Detachment of the retina has been reported in a few patients treated with miotics, particularly the long-acting cholinesterase inhibitors. This complication usually occurs within the first few days after therapy is begun. These drugs should be used with caution in patients with a high risk of retinal detachment (eg, aphakic or myopic patients), and their use should be preceded by examination of the peripheral retina, especially in aphakia.

Topically applied strong miotics, particularly echothiophate [Echodide, Phospholine] and demecarium [Humorsol], may cause systemic effects. Such reactions are rare following routine administration of pilocarpine, carbachol, or the rapidly hydrolyzed anticholinesterase, isoflurophate [Floropryl], but have been seen with excessive treatment. Symptoms of systemic toxicity include hypersalivation, sweating, nausea, vomiting, abdominal pain, diarrhea, bradycardia, hypotension, and bronchospasm. Toxic doses can cause central nervous system effects (ataxia, confusion, convulsions, coma) and muscular paralysis. Death can result from respiratory failure. Severe reactions are more common in adults than in children (Apt and Gaffney, 1976). The most common symptoms of systemic toxicity in children are abdominal cramping and diarrhea; mild rhinorrhea, lacrimation, and upper respiratory congestion also may be observed. Severe toxic reactions are treated with intravenous atropine; pralidoxime may be used concomitantly when required. Pressure at the inner canthus after instillation minimizes drainage into the nose and throat and may reduce the likelihood of systemic reactions.

Drug Interactions: Plasma cholinesterase levels are significantly depressed during topical therapy with long-acting anticholinesterase miotics, and prolonged apnea may develop if succinylcholine is given to patients using these drugs. Long-acting miotics should be discontinued, if possible, two to four weeks prior to administration of succinylcholine. In any event, the anesthesiologist should be informed that the patient has been receiving an anticholinesterase drug. The hydrolysis of procaine is also decreased by topically applied anticholinesterase agents. An adverse interaction between organophosphate miotics and organophosphate insecticides is possible, and these miotics are particularly hazardous in farm workers exposed to insecticides.

There is evidence from animal studies that chronic administration of a long-acting cholinesterase inhibitor may result in prolonged (up to several months) subsensitivity to pilocarpine. It also has been observed that physostigmine may partially block the effects of the long-acting miotics.

Parasympathomimetic Agents

PILOCARPINE HYDROCHLORIDE
[Adsorbocarpine, Isopto Carpine, Pilocar, Pilocel]

PILOCARPINE NITRATE
[P.V. Carpine]

Pilocarpine is the miotic of choice for initial and maintenance therapy in primary open-angle glaucoma and most other chronic glaucomas and (in conjunction with systemically administered ocular hypotensive drugs) for the emergency treatment of acute angle-closure glaucoma. This agent penetrates the eye well. After topical instillation, miosis begins in 15 to 30 minutes and lasts four to eight hours. The maximal reduction of intraocular pressure occurs in two to four hours, which correlates with the maximal decrease in outflow resistance. The effect on intraocular pressure outlasts the effect on outflow facility, which suggests that

pilocarpine also may decrease aqueous production. Therapy is generally started with weaker strengths and the dosage increased gradually. If resistance to pilocarpine develops during long-term therapy, it has been claimed that responsiveness may sometimes be restored by discontinuing pilocarpine and substituting another miotic such as carbachol for a period of time.

Pilocarpine generally is tolerated better than other miotics. Nevertheless, ciliary spasm and miosis may be troublesome initially. Local irritation, allergic reactions, and systemic effects are uncommon. One case of malfunction in the eustachian tube with disturbances in the middle ear has been reported after use of the 4% solution. (See also the section on Adverse Reactions and Precautions.)

ROUTE, USUAL DOSAGE, AND PREPARATIONS.
Topical: In primary open-angle glaucoma and other chronic glaucomas, pilocarpine should be given in an adequate concentration as frequently as required to maintain intraocular pressure at the level necessary to prevent further damage to the optic nerve and progressive loss of visual field. Initially, one drop of a 1% or 2% solution is instilled in each eye every six to eight hours. The concentration and frequency of administration may be adjusted later as needed. Drops are usually instilled four times daily (range, one to six times daily). Concentrations of 4% occasionally may be necessary, especially in patients with heavily pigmented irides or advanced glaucoma. Rarely, concentrations of 6% to 8% may provide still better control. Strong concentrations may have a longer duration of action.

In primary angle-closure glaucoma prior to surgery, initially, drops (usually the 1% or 2% solution) are instilled frequently until the angle opens and the pressure decreases. Occasionally, pilocarpine is unsuccessful in opening the angle. The unaffected eye may be treated every eight hours to avoid a bilateral attack but, despite prophylactic therapy, acute angle-closure glaucoma may develop in the second eye. If prophylactic miotics are used in the second eye, it is necessary to confirm gonioscopically that they do indeed open the angle more widely. Because of the uncertain prevention of angle closure in the second eye with miotic therapy and because miotics occasionally produce angle closure rather than prevent it, many ophthalmologists advise prophylactic iridectomy.

In congenital glaucoma, some surgeons instill one drop of a 2% solution in the affected eye every six hours. The constricted iris serves to protect the lens during surgery.

All preparations are available as ophthalmic solutions.

PILOCARPINE HYDROCHLORIDE:

Drug available generically: Solution 1%, 2%, 3%, 4%, 6%, and 8%.

Adsorbocarpine (Burton, Parsons). Solution (sterile) 1%, 2%, and 4% with hydroxyethylcellulose, povidone, water-soluble polymers, benzalkonium chloride 0.004%, and edetate disodium 0.1% in 15 ml containers.

Isopto Carpine (Alcon). Solution (sterile) 0.25%, 0.5%, 1%, 1.5%, 2%, 3%, 4%, 5%, 6%, 8%, and 10% with hydroxypropyl methylcellulose 0.5%, benzalkonium chloride 0.01%, boric acid, sodium citrate (in 1%, 1.5%, 2%, and 6% concentrations only), citric acid (in 0.25% and 0.5% concentrations only), and sodium chloride (in 0.25%, 0.5%, and 1% concentrations only) in 15 and 30 ml containers.

Pilocar (SMP). Solution (sterile) 1%, 2%, and 4% with benzalkonium chloride, potassium chloride, boric acid, and sodium carbonate in 1 ml containers; solution 0.5%, 1%, 2%, 3%, 4%, and 6% with hydroxypropyl methylcellulose 0.33%, benzalkonium chloride 0.01%, edetate disodium 0.01%, potassium chloride, boric acid, and sodium carbonate in 15 ml containers.

Pilocel (Professional Pharmacal). Solution 0.25%, 0.5%, 3%, and 6% in 15 ml containers; 1% and 4% in 15 and 30 ml containers. All with methylcellulose 0.25% and benzalkonium chloride 0.004%.

Additional trademarks.

Almocarpine (Ayerst), *Pilomiotin* (SMP).

PILOCARPINE NITRATE:

P.V. Carpine Liquifilm (Allergan). Solution 0.5%, 1%, 2%, 3%, 4%, and 6% with polyvinyl alcohol 1.4%, chlorobutanol 0.5%, sodium acetate, sodium chloride, citric acid, menthol, camphor, phenol, and eucalyptol in 15 ml containers.

OCUSERT PILO-20/PILO-40 OCULAR THERAPEUTIC SYSTEM

The Ocusert pilocarpine system is a new drug delivery unit comprised of two outer membranes with a central reservoir of pilocarpine for use in patients with chronic open-angle glaucoma. This oval unit possesses a visible white margin to aid in placement and retrieval. When the Ocusert is placed in the upper or lower cul-de-sac, pilocarpine gradually diffuses across the two outer polymeric layers that serve as rate-controlling membranes. The unit is available in two strengths, Pilo-20 and -40, which correspond roughly to 0.5% or 1% and 2% pilocarpine. The manufacturer's labeling states that these units deliver the drug at a rate of 20 and 40 mcg/hr for one week following an initial six-hour period of more rapid release. Patients inadequately controlled with the Pilo-40 unit may require concomitant use of other antiglaucoma drugs.

The Ocusert System is more expensive than eyedrops, but it may provide better diurnal control of intraocular pressure and improve compliance in unreliable patients. In younger patients, reduced miosis and spasm of accommodation are definite advantages of the Ocusert. However, because these symptoms can be troublesome during the first few hours after insertion of a new unit, the device should be inserted at bedtime. Signs of conjunctival irritation may be noted in some patients, particularly during initial use.

Although the Ocusert System is labeled for replacement every seven days, the duration of action is variable. In a few instances, a single unit was effective for only two to four days. Occasionally, sudden leakage of pilocarpine has produced marked miosis and decreased vision associated with a further fall in intraocular pressure ("burst phenomenon"). Rarely, the Ocusert may migrate onto the cornea, obstructing vision and causing pain. Two cases have been reported in which the device migrated while the patients were driving. Some patients, particularly those with loose lids, have difficulty retaining the Ocusert and may lose it without noting the loss. Since the unit may fall out at night, the patient should be instructed to make sure that it is in place every morning. It is not yet known whether drug resistance will develop more or less frequently with

Ocusert than with eyedrops or if infection will be a problem.

> **Ocusert Pilo-20 Ocular Therapeutic System** (20 mcg/hour for one week), **Ocusert Pilo-40 Ocular Therapeutic System** (40 mcg/hour for one week) (Alza). Ophthalmic sustained-release systems (sterile) in packages of eight individually wrapped units.

CARBACHOL
[Carbacel, Isopto Carbachol]

$$\underset{\substack{|| \\ \text{H}_2\text{NCOCH}_2\text{CH}_2\overset{+}{\text{N}}-\text{CH}_3} \\ \quad\quad\quad\quad\quad \text{CH}_3}{\overset{\text{O}}{}} \quad\underset{\text{CH}_3}{} \quad \text{Cl}^-$$

Carbachol is used in chronic open-angle glaucoma, usually as a replacement for pilocarpine when resistance or intolerance to the latter has developed or if a slightly stronger, slightly longer-acting drug is needed. It also can be used for emergency treatment of acute angle-closure glaucoma, but pilocarpine usually is preferred. Carbachol does not penetrate the eye as well as pilocarpine and is usually prepared with a wetting agent to enhance corneal penetration.

Although carbachol may cause less pupillary constriction than pilocarpine, it may cause more accommodative spasm and headache and may produce slight conjunctival hyperemia. Resistance may develop suddenly. Other local and systemic adverse reactions occur rarely (see the section on Adverse Reactions and Precautions).

ROUTE, USUAL DOSAGE, AND PREPARATIONS. *Topical*: In primary open-angle glaucoma and other chronic glaucomas, carbachol should be given in an adequate concentration as frequently as required to maintain the intraocular pressure at the level necessary to prevent further optic nerve damage and progressive visual field loss. Initially, one drop of a 0.75% to 3% solution is instilled in each eye every eight hours.

In primary angle-closure glaucoma prior to surgery, initially, drops (usually the 1.5% solution) are instilled in the affected eye frequently until the angle opens and the pressure decreases. This form of therapy is not always successful. (For management of the unaffected eye, see the evaluation on Pilocarpine.)

> All preparations are available as ophthalmic solutions.
> Drug available generically: Solution 0.75% and 1.5%.
> **Carbacel** (Professional Pharmacal). Solution (sterile) 0.75%, 1.5%, and 3% with methylcellulose and benzalkonium chloride 1:7,500 or 1:20,000 (3%) in 15 ml containers; 3% concentration also contains boric acid, sodium borate, and sodium chloride.
> **Isopto Carbachol** (Alcon). Solution (sterile) 0.75%, 1.5%, 2.25%, and 3% with hydroxypropyl methylcellulose 1%, benzalkonium chloride 0.005%, boric acid, sodium chloride, and sodium borate in 15 and 30 ml containers.

Short-Acting Anticholinesterase Agents

PHYSOSTIGMINE SULFATE
[Eserine Sulfate]

PHYSOSTIGMINE SALICYLATE
[Isopto Eserine]

Although not currently popular for primary therapy, physostigmine has been used in open-angle glaucoma and occasionally in the emergency treatment of angle-closure glaucoma and accommodative esotropia (overconvergence caused by excessive accommodation). Miosis occurs in about 30 minutes and the effect may last 12 to 36 hours.

Physostigmine often causes hyperemia of the conjunctiva and iris. It is rarely tolerated for prolonged periods because conjunctivitis and allergic reactions occur frequently. Long-term administration can produce follicles in the cul-de-sac. In blacks, reversible depigmentation of the lid margins occasionally is seen after prolonged treatment with physostigmine ointments. See also the section on Adverse Reactions and Precautions.

Solutions are sensitive to light and heat and should not be used if discolored.

Ointments may cause blurred vision and are usually reserved for nighttime use.

ROUTE, USUAL DOSAGE, AND PREPARATIONS. *Topical*: In primary open-angle glaucoma and other chronic glaucomas, one drop of a 0.25% to 1% solution is applied to each eye every four to six hours or, more commonly, the ointment is used at night. The drug should be given in the lowest effective concentration no more frequently than required to maintain the intraocular pressure at the level necessary to prevent further damage to the optic nerve and progressive loss of visual field.

In primary angle-closure glaucoma prior to surgery, one drop of a 0.25% solution is instilled in the affected eye frequently (sometimes alternated with pilocarpine) until the angle opens and the pressure falls. This treatment is not always successful in opening the angle. (For treatment of the unaffected eye, see the evaluation on Pilocarpine.)

> All preparations are available in ophthalmic form.
> PHYSOSTIGMINE SULFATE:
> Drug available under the name Eserine Sulfate: Ointment 0.25%.
> PHYSOSTIGMINE SALICYLATE:
> Drug available generically: Ointment 0.25%; solution 0.5%.
> *Isopto Eserine* (Alcon). Solution (sterile) 0.25% and 0.5% with hydroxypropylmethylcellulose 0.5%, chlorobutanol, sodium bisulfite, sodium chloride, and citric acid in 15 ml containers.

PHYSOSTIGMINE SALICYLATE AND PILOCARPINE HYDROCHLORIDE

Combinations of miotics offer no advantages over a single-entity drug given in adequate dosage. A disadvantage of this combination is the difference in duration of action of the two components. It also has been suggested that their combined effect may be competitive rather than additive or synergistic and that resistance may develop to both components during long-term therapy.

> Preparations are available as ophthalmic solutions.
> *Miocel* (Professional Pharmacal). Solution (sterile) containing physostigmine salicylate 0.125% and pilocarpine hydrochloride 2% with methylcellulose, phenylmercuric borate

1:25,000, sodium bisulfite, boric acid, and sodium carbonate in 5, 15, and 30 ml containers.
Isopto P-ES (Alcon). Solution (sterile) containing physostigmine salicylate 0.25% and pilocarpine hydrochloride 2% with hydroxypropylmethylcellulose 0.5% and chlorobutanol 0.15% in 15 ml containers.

Long-Acting Anticholinesterase Agents

DEMECARIUM BROMIDE
[Humorsol]

ECHOTHIOPHATE IODIDE
[Echodide, Phospholine Iodide]

ISOFLUROPHATE (DFP)
[Floropryl]

These potent, long-acting miotics are used to treat primary open-angle glaucoma and other chronic glaucomas when short-acting miotics and other agents are inadequate. They often are used to treat glaucoma in aphakia. They should be administered in the lowest effective concentration no more frequently than necessary to maintain intraocular pressure at the level required to prevent further damage to the optic nerve and progressive loss of visual field. Maximal reduction of intraocular pressure occurs within 24 hours after a single instillation, and residual effects may persist for days. When instilled once daily for a number of days, a cumulative effect occurs, with a maximal reduction in pressure occurring only after several days of therapy. In addition to their use in glaucoma, the strong miotics have been employed to diagnose and treat accommodative esotropia. By inducing accommodation peripherally, they reduce the amount of convergence associated with a given amount of accommodation, thus reducing the degree of esotropia.

The development of cataracts with long-term administration has limited the usefulness of these agents in glaucoma therapy. Their usefulness in young patients with strabismus also must be balanced against this potential risk. (See also the section on Adverse Reactions and Precautions.)

If a strong miotic is accidentally applied to the normal eye or if overdosage occurs, the cholinesterase reactivator, pralidoxime, may be injected subconjunctivally as an adjunct to parenteral use of atropine to counteract severe miosis and spasm of accommodation (see the following evaluation).

ROUTE, USUAL DOSAGE, AND PREPARATIONS.
DEMECARIUM BROMIDE:
Topical: Initially, one drop of a 0.125% or 0.25% solution may be instilled in each eye every 12 to 48 hours.

Humorsol (Merck Sharp & Dohme). Aqueous solution (ophthalmic, sterile) 0.125% and 0.25% with sodium chloride and benzalkonium chloride 1:5,000 in 5 ml containers.

ECHOTHIOPHATE IODIDE:
Topical: Initially, one drop of a 0.03% to 0.06% solution may be instilled in each eye every 12 to 48 hours. A stronger concentration (0.125%) is often required in highly pigmented eyes.

Echodide (Alcon). Lyophilized powder (sterile) 1.5, 3, 6.25, and 12.5 mg with diluent containing chlorobutanol 0.5%, boric acid, polysorbate 80, sodium hydroxide and/or hydrochloric acid to make 0.03%, 0.06%, 0.125%, or 0.25% solution, respectively.

Phospholine Iodide (Ayerst). Lyophilized powder (sterile) 1.5, 3, 6.25, and 12.5 mg with potassium acetate 40 mg and 5 ml of diluent containing chlorobutanol 0.5%, mannitol 1.2%, boric acid 0.06%, and exsiccated sodium phosphate 0.026% to make 0.03%, 0.06%, 0.125%, and 0.25% solution, respectively; sodium hydroxide or acetic acid also may be added.

ISOFLUROPHATE:
Topical: Initially, a one-quarter inch strip

of ointment is placed in each eye every 12 to 72 hours.

Floropryl (Merck Sharp & Dohme). Ointment (ophthalmic, sterile) 0.025% in polyethylene-mineral oil gel in 3.5 g containers.

Antidote

PRALIDOXIME CHLORIDE
[Protopam Chloride]

This cholinesterase reactivator is given intravenously as an adjunct to atropine in the treatment of systemic poisoning caused by cholinesterase inhibitors (drugs, pesticides, or "nerve gases"). Since it does not readily penetrate the blood-aqueous barrier or cornea, intravenous or topical administration is generally ineffective in counteracting miosis and spasm of accommodation. However, after subconjunctival injection, pralidoxime enters the eye in therapeutic concentrations. It may be administered by this route to reverse ocular side effects if an anticholinesterase agent is accidentally splashed onto the eye or if overdosage occurs. Pralidoxime is more active in counteracting the effects of agents that phosphorylate the enzyme (echothiophate and isoflurophate) than against those that carbamylate it (demecarium). Unless the acetylcholinesterase is dephosphorylated within hours, the enzyme's structure undergoes secondary changes (aging) that render it inactive even though the phosphate group is hydrolyzed off with pralidoxime. In addition, prolonged use of cholinesterase inhibitors may result in fibrotic changes in the iris and produce an immobile pupil and residual miosis after the drug is discontinued.

Local adverse effects reported after subconjunctival injection include a burning sensation, conjunctival hyperemia, subconjunctival hemorrhage, and mild iritis. These reactions are more common with use of concentrations exceeding 5%. Allergic reactions or systemic effects have not been observed.

ROUTE, USUAL DOSAGE, AND PREPARATIONS. *Subconjunctival*: 0.1 to 0.2 ml of a 5% aqueous solution.

> *Protopam Chloride* (Ayerst). Powder (injection) 1 g in 20 ml containers. (Contains no preservative; contents of vial must be discarded after use.)

EPINEPHRINE

EPINEPHRINE BITARTRATE
[Epitrate, Murocoll, Mytrate]

EPINEPHRINE HYDROCHLORIDE
[Epifrin, Glaucon]

EPINEPHRYL BORATE
[Epinal, Eppy]

$$HO \text{---} \bigcirc \text{---} \overset{\overset{H}{|}}{\underset{\underset{OH}{|}}{C}} \text{---} CH_2 \overset{+}{N}H_2CH_3 \quad Cl^-$$

Although the sphincter and ciliary muscles are largely under parasympathetic control, adrenergic receptors have been described in these tissues, primarily beta receptors in the ciliary muscle and both alpha and beta receptors in the sphincter muscle of the iris (Van Alphen, 1976). Stimulation of alpha receptors reduces resistance to outflow of aqueous humor, presumably through an effect on the trabecular meshwork, while stimulation of beta receptors in the ciliary epithelium decreases aqueous production. The dilator muscle of the iris contains mainly alpha receptors. Activation of these receptors causes pupillary dilatation.

When instilled in eyes with primary open-angle glaucoma, the adrenergic drug, epinephrine, induces a prolonged (12 to 24 hours) fall in intraocular pressure and brief constriction of the conjunctival vessels, followed by a more prolonged vasodilation and minimal, brief mydriasis in some patients. The mechanism by which epinephrine lowers intraocular pressure is independent of its mydriatic action and is believed to involve both an increase in outflow facility (caused by stimulation of alpha-adrenergic receptors) and a decrease in production of aqueous humor (beta-adrenergic effect).

Epinephrine is used most commonly to supplement miotic therapy in patients with primary open-angle glaucoma and other chronic glaucomas. Such combined therapy is reported to be more effective in reducing intraocular pressure than either of the two drugs alone. A similar additive effect has been reported with the combined use of epinephrine and a carbonic anhydrase inhibitor. Epinephrine is sometimes used alone for initial treatment of chronic glaucoma, especially in patients who may not tolerate miotic therapy (ie, relatively young patients with active accommodation, patients with cataracts whose vision is reduced by a small pupil). It may be unsatisfactory for prolonged therapy, however, because of the relatively frequent occurrence of conjunctival hyperemia and allergic reactions.

The responsiveness of each individual should be determined before deciding upon long-term epinephrine therapy because of variability in responsiveness and because a paradoxical elevation of intraocular pressure may occur occasionally, even in eyes with open angles. Highly pigmented eyes are relatively resistant to the effects of epinephrine, and stronger concentrations may be required in patients with dark irides than in those with light irides.

ADVERSE REACTIONS AND PRECAUTIONS.

Epinephrine produces browache, headache, blurred vision, ocular irritation, and lacrimation in some patients. With repeated use, the drug may cause reactive hyperemia, allergic conjunctivitis, and contact dermatitis. About 20% or more of patients cannot tolerate prolonged use of this agent because of these reactions. Corneal edema may occur very rarely after long-term administration. Of particular importance in aphakic eyes is the possibility of inducing cystoid macular edema. This complication has been reported to occur in up to 30% of aphakic patients during long-term therapy. Fortunately, the maculopathy is usually reversible if epinephrine is discontinued when visual acuity first begins to decrease. Many ophthalmologists prefer not to use epinephrine in aphakic eyes unless the glaucoma is sufficiently severe to justify the risk.

Topically applied epinephrine can cause pupillary dilation, even when used with miotics. It is contraindicated preoperatively for the treatment of angle-closure glaucoma because it may precipitate an acute attack. When instilled without miotics in patients with open-angle glaucoma, epinephrine rarely may cause a temporary elevation of intraocular pressure upon initial administration. This phenomenon may be associated with release of pigment particles from the iris into the aqueous humor (aqueous floaters). With long-term administration, melanin-like adrenochrome deposits may appear in the bulbar or palpebral conjunctiva, in roughened or edematous areas of the cornea, or in soft contact lenses. Discoloration of solutions indicates that the oxidation product, adrenochrome, has been formed; these solutions should be discarded. Madarosis (loss of eyelashes) rarely has been associated with topical therapy.

Systemic reactions to topically applied epinephrine are rare but potentially include tachycardia, premature ventricular contractions, hypertension, headache, sweating, tremors, and blanching. As with any drug, the lowest effective concentration should be used. Occasionally, the 0.25% strength is effective and the 0.5% strength is frequently sufficient. In several instances, systemic effects have occurred when the drug was applied after conjunctival permeability was increased by tonometry or administration of local anesthetics. Epinephrine should be used with care in patients with arrhythmias, hypertension, hyperthyroidism, recent myocardial infarction, or arteriosclerotic heart disease. It may cause ventricular premature contractions, tachycardia, and fibrillation in patients undergoing general anesthesia with halothane, cyclopropane, or other agents that sensitize the heart to catecholamines.

ROUTE, USUAL DOSAGE, AND PREPARATIONS.
Topical: In primary open-angle glaucoma and other chronic glaucomas, one drop of a 0.25% to 2% solution is instilled in each eye, usually once or twice daily. The stronger concentration may be required in patients with dark irides.

All preparations are available for ophthalmic use.
EPINEPHRINE BITARTRATE:
Epitrate (Ayerst). Aqueous solution (sterile) 2% (equivalent to 1.1% base) with chlorobutanol 0.5%, sodium bisulfite, sodium chloride, poloxamer 188, and edetate disodium in 7.5 ml containers.
Murocoll No. 29½, 29 (Muro). Solution 1.82% (equivalent to 1% base) and 3.64% (equivalent to 2% base) with chlorobutanol, sodium bisulfite, and sodium chloride in 7.5 ml containers.
Mytrate (Professional Pharmacal). Solution (sterile) 1% and 2% with methylcellulose, benzalkonium chloride 1:25,000, sodium bisulfite, and edetate disodium in 15 ml containers.
EPINEPHRINE HYDROCHLORIDE:
Drug available generically: Solution 1:1,000 in 1 ml containers.
Epifrin (Allergan). Solution (sterile) equivalent to 0.25%, 0.5%, 1%, and 2% base with benzalkonium chloride, sodium metabisulfite, and edetate disodium in 5 ml (0.5%, 1%, and 2% concentrations) and 15 ml (all strengths) containers; 0.25% concentration also contains sodium chloride.
Glaucon (Alcon). Solution (sterile) equivalent to 0.5%, 1%, or 2% base with sodium metabisulfite 0.3%, benzalkonium chloride 0.01%, and sodium chloride in 10 ml containers.
EPINEPHRYL BORATE:
Epinal (Alcon). Solution (sterile) equivalent to 0.25%, 0.5%, or 1% base with benzalkonium chloride 0.01%, ascorbic acid, acetylcysteine, boric acid, and sodium carbonate in 7.5 ml containers.
Eppy, Eppy/N (Barnes-Hind). Solution (sterile) 0.5% and 1% (equivalent to 0.5% and 1% levoepinephrine free base, respectively) with sodium bisulfite, oxyquinoline sulfate, and thimerosal in 7.5 ml containers.

EPINEPHRINE BITARTRATE AND PILOCARPINE HYDROCHLORIDE

Mixtures containing pilocarpine and epinephrine are available for use in the treatment of primary open-angle glaucoma. Although these preparations have the advantage of convenience, the usefulness of these fixed combinations is limited because of the difference in duration of action of the two components and problems associated with sensitivity reactions (ie, identifying which component is causing an allergic reaction).

Preparations are available as ophthalmic solutions.

Mixture available generically: Solution containing epinephrine 1% and pilocarpine hydrochloride 4% in 7.5 ml containers.

E-Carpine (Alcon). Solution (sterile) containing epinephrine bitartrate 1% (equivalent to 0.5% base) and pilocarpine hydrochloride 1%, 2%, 3%, 4%, or 6% with hydroxypropyl methylcellulose, polysorbate 80, sodium chloride (in 1% and 2% concentrations only), sodium bisulfite 0.3%, benzalkonium chloride 0.01%, edetate disodium, and sodium hydroxide and/or hydrochloric acid in 15 ml containers.

E-Pilo (SMP). Aqueous solution (sterile) containing epinephrine bitartrate 1% (equivalent to 0.55% base) and pilocarpine hydrochloride 1%, 2%, 3%, 4%, or 6% with mannitol 5%, benzalkonium chloride 0.01%, sodium bisulfite, monobasic and dibasic sodium phosphate, and edetate disodium in 10 ml containers.

P1E1, P2E1, P3E1, P4E1, and P6E1 (Alcon). Solution (sterile) containing epinephrine bitartrate 1% (equivalent to 0.5% base) and pilocarpine hydrochloride 1%, 2%, 3%, 4%, or 6% with benzalkonium chloride 0.01%, methylcellulose, chlorobutanol, polyethylene glycol, edetate disodium, sodium bisulfite, and sodium phosphate anhydrous in 15 ml containers.

BETA-ADRENERGIC BLOCKING DRUGS

Beta-adrenergic blocking drugs represent a new approach to treatment of chronic open-angle glaucoma. Beta receptors are located primarily in the heart, the arteries and arterioles of skeletal muscle, and the bronchi, where they subserve cardiac excitation, vasodilatation, and bronchial relaxation. Beta receptors also have been described in ocular tissue, primarily in the ciliary muscle and, along with alpha receptors, in the sphincter muscle of the iris (Van Alphen, 1976). Beta-blocking drugs combine reversibly with these receptors to block the response to sympathetic nerve stimulation or circulating catecholamines. The various beta-blocking drugs differ in their affinity for cardiac (beta1) and noncardiac (beta2) receptors, and some show local anesthetic and partial agonist activity.

Beta-blocking agents lower intraocular pressure by decreasing the production of aqueous humor. It is not known whether this effect is due to beta blockade because beta receptor stimulants, such as isoproterenol and epinephrine, also have an ocular hypotensive effect. The effect of beta-blocking drugs on intraocular pressure occurs after either topical or systemic administration. The topical route is usually preferred because of a lower incidence of systemic side effects, although oral therapy may be useful when there are additional indications for a beta-blocking drug (eg, systemic hypertension, angina pectoris).

Topical preparations of propranolol, practolol, atenolol, and pindolol have been used abroad to treat chronic glaucoma. Propranolol proved unsuitable for long-term therapy because of its local anesthetic effect, and practolol was withdrawn from the market because of systemic toxicity not seen with any other beta blockers. A short duration of action and the frequent development of tolerance have limited the usefulness of atenolol. Experience with pindolol is still limited. Timolol [Timoptic], a long-acting "nonselective" (ie, acts on both beta1 and beta2 receptors) beta-blocking drug without significant local anesthetic or partial agonist activity, recently became available in the United States for topical ophthalmic use in chronic open-angle glaucoma.

TIMOLOL MALEATE
[Timoptic]

Timolol lowers the intraocular pressure of normal individuals and most patients with primary open-angle glaucoma and some secondary glaucomas. Following topical application of a single dose, pressure is reduced within 20 minutes and the hypotensive effect is still evident after 24 hours. When instilled in only one eye, pressure is also reduced slightly in the contralateral eye, an effect that has been attributed to systemic absorption, a central action, or contamination from rubbing the eyes (Zimmerman and Kaufman, 1977; Radius et al, 1978). Patients with heavily pigmented eyes, who may be less responsive to miotics and epinephrine, apparently have not shown reduced responsiveness to timolol.

Timolol does not alter pupillary diameter or reactivity to light, but it may cause a slight, clinically unimportant decrease in the amplitude of redilation when the light stimulus is removed. Distant visual acuity is not reduced.

In controlled, short-term studies, timolol was as effective as pilocarpine or epinephrine in lowering elevated intraocular pressure and was better tolerated than either reference drug (Boger et al, 1978 A; Moss et al, 1978; Radius et al, 1978). Results of long-term investigations have not been published. Timolol has additive effects with other antiglaucoma drugs in some patients.

Timolol is initially effective in most patients. In those who respond, the ocular hypotensive effect is maximal when treatment is begun but may diminish during the first few days, particularly when the baseline pressure is high (Boger et al, 1978 A and B). Despite this phenomenon, the residual improvement is often maintained during continued therapy. On the other hand, a tendency toward tolerance has occasionally been noted, and escape from adequate pressure control has been observed during long-term therapy. Experience is not yet sufficient to determine whether this will be an important problem.

Like epinephrine, timolol is a suitable alternative to pilocarpine for initial and maintenance therapy in young individuals who cannot tolerate miotics and in older patients with lens opacities. Either of these drugs also may be given with a short-acting miotic when intraocular pressure is not well controlled by the miotic alone. Timolol may be effective in a larger percentage of patients than epinephrine and appears to be less allergenic, but it is more expensive and its long-term efficacy and toxicity are unknown. In certain patients, the choice of drug therapy also may be influenced by potential adverse systemic reactions (eg, arrhythmias with epinephrine, bronchospasm with timolol) or ocular effects (cystoid macular edema in aphakic patients treated with epinephrine).

Patients who are only marginally controlled with concomitant therapy using both a short-acting miotic and epinephrine may benefit from addition of timolol to the regimen. This addition may obviate the need for substituting a long-acting miotic or introducing a carbonic anhydrase inhibitor. In those patients whose intraocular pressure has been brought under control with traditional maximal medical therapy but who cannot tolerate the side effects of the carbonic anhydrase inhibitor, the addition of timolol may permit withdrawal of the carbonic anhydrase inhibitor or a reduction in its dosage. Timolol also should be tried before resorting to surgery in individuals whose pressure is not adequately controlled by traditional maximal medical therapy. The addition of timolol may further lower the intraocular pressure and defer surgery, although some patients who do not respond to the traditional three-drug regimen are relatively resistant to all medication and are not helped by timolol.

ADVERSE REACTIONS AND PRECAUTIONS.

Timolol may cause mild ocular irritation and, rarely, local hypersensitivity reactions and superficial punctate keratopathy. No other adverse local effects have been reported. Since timolol does not cause ciliary muscle spasm or pupillary constriction, it is tolerated better than miotics in young adults with active accommodation and in older patients with cataracts. Presbyopic patients may need a change in eyeglasses after switching from a miotic to timolol because the increased accommodation induced by miotics compensates for presbyopia. An abrupt rise in intraocular pressure may occur when timolol is substituted for existing antiglaucoma medication, and pressure should be checked shortly after the previous drug is discontinued.

Timolol is absorbed into the systemic circulation and may produce side effects related to blockade of cardiac and noncardiac beta receptors. Its effects may be additive with other beta-blocking drugs, and patients who are also receiving a systemically administered beta blocker, such as propranolol, should be observed carefully. Bradycardia is the most common systemic side effect of timolol. A fall in blood pressure also may occur; therefore, pulse rate and blood pressure should be monitored in patients receiving the drug. If the patient is being treated by another physician for a cardiac disorder, the physician should be consulted prior to instituting therapy. Bronchospasm has been reported occasionally and, like other beta blockers, timolol generally should be avoided in patients with a history of asthma or bronchitis. Some of the cardiac and pulmonary side effects of timolol may be additive with those of the anticholinesterase miotics.

The following reactions have occurred with systemically administered beta-blocking drugs and are theoretically possible with timolol: precipitation of heart failure in patients with inadequate cardiac reserve, A-V conduction disturbances, aggravation of peripheral vascular insufficiency, and hypoglycemia. Central nervous system effects are similar to those reported with orally administered propranolol and include fatigue, lethargy, depression, psychic dissociation, and confusion. As with any new drug, the ultimate side effects are unknown; therefore, timolol should be used cautiously, and patients should be observed carefully until long-term usage has established its safety.

ROUTE, USUAL DOSAGE, AND PREPARATIONS.
Topical: In primary open-angle glaucoma and other chronic glaucomas, initially, one drop of the 0.25% solution is applied to each eye twice daily. If a satisfactory response is not obtained, dosage may be increased to one drop of the 0.5% solution in each eye twice daily. Occasionally, once-daily application of the 0.5% solution may be sufficient for maintenance. If the patient is being transferred from another antiglaucoma drug, the previously used medication should not be discontinued until the second day of therapy with timolol and the pressure should be checked to make sure that an abrupt rise has not occurred.

Timoptic (Merck Sharp & Dohme). Solution (ophthalmic) 0.25% and 0.5% in 5 ml containers.

INVESTIGATIONAL ADRENERGIC AND ANTIADRENERGIC AGENTS

Advances in knowledge concerning the role of adrenergic receptors in regulating aqueous production and outflow has stimulated a search for ocular hypotensive drugs that are better tolerated and more effective than epinephrine. Research has focused on the effects of related catecholamines, agents that enhance the effects of epinephrine, and adrenergic blocking drugs (Ross and Drance, 1975; Sears, 1976).

Catecholamines: Epinephrine lowers intraocular pressure by stimulating both alpha and beta receptors. The related amine, isoproterenol, acts primarily on beta receptors and, when applied topically, has an ocular hypotensive effect comparable to that of epinephrine. The usefulness of isoproterenol is limited, however, because of the frequent occurrence of systemic side effects (tachycardia). A newer beta agonist, salbutamol, which selectively stimulates beta2 (noncardiac) receptors, is also effective when applied topically, but it often causes severe hyperemia and local irritation; tolerance may develop during prolonged therapy (Ross and Drance, 1975; Sears, 1976).

Norepinephrine acts primarily on alpha receptors. A stable ophthalmic preparation (the borate salt) is currently under investigation for the treatment of glaucoma. The ocular hypotensive effect of norepinephrine borate 4% appears to be comparable to that of epinephrine borate 1%. Conjunctival hyperemia is the only significant side effect reported. Norepinephrine may prove to be useful in patients who experience allergic reactions to epinephrine (Pollack and Rossi, 1975).

The prodrug, dipivefrin (dipivalyl epinephrine), penetrates the cornea with greater ease than epinephrine and is then converted to epinephrine inside the eye. It has fewer external side effects than epinephrine and causes less adrenochrome formation.

Agents That Enhance the Effects of Epinephrine: Another approach has been to increase the ocular hypotensive effect of epinephrine or norepinephrine by administering agents that prevent the reuptake of catecholamines into sympathetic nerve terminals. Preliminary data suggest that the tricyclic compound, protriptyline, may accomplish this objective when applied topically.

In other studies, an attempt has been made to induce a state of denervation supersensitivity to exogenous epinephrine by long-term topical application of guanethidine, a drug that prevents reuptake and blocks release of catecholamines. Although some investigators found an enhanced response to epinephrine after pretreatment with guanethidine, the usefulness of this approach is limited because superficial punctate lesions in the corneal epithelium and severe hyperemia have occurred in association with guanethidine therapy.

When administered by the subconjunctival route, 6-hydroxydopamine selectively destroys sympathetic nerve terminals in the anterior uvea, thereby increasing the response to catecholamines (denervation supersensitivity). This agent thereby augments the therapeutic response to exogenous catecholamines. Preliminary studies suggest that 6-hydroxydopamine may be useful in glaucoma that cannot be controlled by maximal drug therapy, but repeated injections are necessary because regeneration occurs in two to four months (Ross and Drance, 1975; Kitazawa et al, 1975).

Alpha-Adrenergic Blocking Drugs: Alpha-blocking drugs constrict the pupil by blocking alpha receptors in the dilator muscle of the iris, thereby permitting parasympathetic dominance via the sphincter muscle. They have no significant effect on the ciliary muscle or aqueous outflow system. One such agent, thymoxamine hydrochloride, has been used abroad to reverse the mydriatic effect of phenylephrine without affecting accommodation or intraocular pressure. One drop of a 0.5% solution rapidly reverses the effect of 10% phenylephrine more effectively and safely than does pilocarpine. Thymoxamine also has been used successfully in the emergency treatment of acute angle-closure glaucoma and may be useful diagnostically to distinguish between angle-closure glaucoma and open-angle glaucoma with a narrow angle (Wand and Grant, 1976).

CARBONIC ANHYDRASE INHIBITORS

ACETAZOLAMIDE
[Diamox]

ACETAZOLAMIDE SODIUM
[Diamox Parenteral]

DICHLORPHENAMIDE
[Daranide, Oratrol]

ETHOXZOLAMIDE
[Cardrase, Ethamide]

METHAZOLAMIDE
[Neptazane]

Carbonic anhydrase inhibitors are given systemically to reduce intraocular pressure. These drugs were originally introduced as diuretics, but their effect on intraocular pressure does not depend upon diuresis. They reduce aqueous production and thus lower pressure, possibly by blocking ocular carbonic anhydrase or by inducing systemic acidosis.

Carbonic anhydrase inhibitors are of greatest value for long-term oral therapy in primary open-angle glaucoma and other chronic glaucomas. They are usually added to the regimen when adequate control cannot be obtained with a miotic, epinephrine, and timolol. Many ophthalmologists now prefer to use carbonic anhydrase inhibitors before a strong miotic is substituted for a weak one. Osmotic agents, miotics, and carbonic anhydrase inhibitors (parenteral or oral) are the mainstay in the emergency treatment of acute glaucoma. By reducing aqueous formation, carbonic anhydrase inhibitors decrease pressure behind the iris and thus assist in opening the closed angle. Carbonic anhydrase inhibitors also are used in some secondary glaucomas (eg, glaucomatocyclitic crisis syndrome, alpha chymotrypsin-induced glaucoma, glaucoma secondary to anterior uveitis or trauma) and in the preoperative treatment of congenital glaucoma.

ADVERSE REACTIONS AND PRECAUTIONS.

Carbonic anhydrase inhibitors commonly cause anorexia, weight loss, gastrointestinal disturbances (gastric distress, nausea, vomiting, or diarrhea), weakness, loss of libido, impotence, and what has been described as a "generally miserable feeling" (Grant, 1973). Lethargy and depression are common and often unrecognized until the drug is discontinued and the patient notices a sudden improvement in his emotional state. Many patients cannot tolerate the drugs for prolonged periods because of these adverse effects. Acetazolamide timed-release capsules may be better tolerated than acetazolamide tablets, ethoxzolamide, or dichlorphenamide. Paresthesias are very common, and headache, drowsiness, fatigue, and dizziness also may occur. The malaise syndrome appears to be related to systemic acidosis and some patients have reported alleviation of symptoms with sodium bicarbonate therapy, despite the fact that this treatment had little effect on the serum CO_2-combining power. In infants, failure to thrive should be considered a sign of possible acidosis. Carbonic anhydrase inhibitors increase the risk of salicylate intoxication in patients receiving large doses of aspirin.

Diuresis may be troublesome initially but subsides during continued therapy. The serum potassium level may fall during the first few weeks of treatment but usually returns to normal unless a potassium-wasting diuretic (thiazide, loop diuretic) is being taken concurrently. The hypokalemia is not associated with a clinically significant reduction in total body potassium. While theoretically possible, no serious problems (eg, enhanced digitalis toxicity) have been associated with the initial hypokalemia. Potassium supplements do not alleviate the symptomatic side effects of carbonic anhydrase inhibitors and are no longer given routinely. Carbonic anhydrase inhibitors should, however, be given cautiously to patients at risk from hypokalemia (eg, digitalized patients, those with cirrhosis), those with diseases associated with increased mineralocorticoid activity (eg, primary hyperaldosteronism, Cushing's syndrome), and *especially* those receiving concomitant therapy with potassium-wasting drugs.

Renal colic, hematuria, and oliguria or anuria occur occasionally during prolonged therapy and are usually evidence of ureteral calculus formation. The renal stones are apparently precipitated by a reduction in the urinary excretion of citrate, which decreases the solubility of calcium. More rarely, renal symptoms have occurred early during therapy in the absence of any evidence of urinary calculi. A sulfonamide-like nephropathy may be involved in these cases, and a few patients have died in acute renal failure.

The carbonic anhydrase inhibitors reduce uric acid excretion and increase the blood uric acid level. The hyperuricemia is usually asymptomatic but rarely has led to an exacerbation of gout. Other untoward effects reported include rash and, rarely, drug fever, hirsutism, thrombocytopenia, agranulocytosis, and aplastic anemia. Transient myopia, which has been noted in a few patients, may result from changes in lens hydration. Since carbonic anhydrase inhibitors may have teratogenic effects, these drugs should be avoided during early pregnancy. Carbonic anhydrase inhibitors should be used cautiously in patients with obstructive pulmonary disease because they may precipitate acute respiratory failure.

If carbonic anhydrase inhibitors are employed in angle-closure glaucoma, they should be used only for *short-term* treatment prior to iridectomy. These agents can temporarily reduce intraocular pressure; however, if surgery is delayed and miotic therapy does not completely open the angle, peripheral anterior synechiae may develop. Eventually, the angle may become sufficiently compromised to preclude successful iridectomy.

It has been suggested that the postoperative use of carbonic anhydrase inhibitors may adversely affect the outcome of filtering operations by reducing the size of the resultant drainage bleb and delaying reformation of the anterior chamber.

ROUTES, USUAL DOSAGE, AND PREPARATIONS.
ACETAZOLAMIDE:
Oral: Adults, 250 mg every six hours. *Children*, 10 to 15 mg/kg of body weight daily in divided doses. The timed-release preparation can be given every 12 to 24 hours; although this dosage form may be better tolerated, it may not be as effective as the regular tablets in some patients.

> Drug available generically: Capsules (plain, timed-release) 500 mg; tablets 250 mg.
> *Diamox* (Lederle). Capsules (timed-release) 500 mg; tablets 125 and 250 mg.

ACETAZOLAMIDE SODIUM:
Intravenous, Intramuscular: Adults, initially, 500 mg; the dose may be repeated, if necessary, in two to four hours. *Infants and children*, 5 to 10 mg/kg of body weight every six hours.

> *Diamox [parenteral]* (Lederle). Powder (injection) 500 mg (should be reconstituted with at least 5 ml of sterile water for injection).

DICHLORPHENAMIDE:
Oral: Adults, 50 to 200 mg every six to eight hours.

> *Daranide* (Merck Sharp & Dohme), *Oratrol* (Alcon). Tablets 50 mg.

ETHOXZOLAMIDE:
Oral: Adults, 125 mg every six to eight hours.

> *Cardrase* (Upjohn), *Ethamide* (Allergan). Tablets 125 mg.

METHAZOLAMIDE:
Oral: Adults, 25 to 100 mg every eight hours.

> *Neptazane* (Lederle). Tablets 50 mg.

OSMOTIC AGENTS

Hypertonic solutions of glycerin [Glyrol, Osmōglyn], isosorbide [Ismotic], urea [Urevert, Ureaphil], or mannitol [Osmitrol] are used for the short-term reduction of intraocular pressure and vitreous volume. By increasing blood osmolarity, these agents induce the withdrawal of fluid from the eyeball by an osmotic effect. They cause an immediate, marked fall in intraocular pressure and reduction in vitreous volume and are generally effective even in patients who do not respond to miotics and carbonic anhydrase inhibitors.

In acute angle-closure glaucoma, osmotic agents are used to reduce intraocular pressure rapidly prior to iridectomy. When the pressure elevation is severe, the iris sphincter becomes ischemic and may not respond to miotics unless pressure is initially reduced with an osmotic agent. Osmotic agents also aid in opening of the angle by reducing the volume of the posterior segment of the eye and transiently reducing posterior pressure behind the iris. If the miotic is then effective in opening the angle, the pressure may remain normal even after the osmotic effect has worn off.

In chronic glaucomas, osmotic agents are used only for the pre- and postoperative treatment of patients who require surgery. They also are used pre- and postoperatively in congenital glaucoma, retinal detachment surgery, routine cataract extraction, and keratoplasty and may be of temporary benefit in some secondary glaucomas. Since their action is dependent upon an intact blood-aqueous barrier, they are sometimes ineffective in inflammatory secondary glaucomas.

Mannitol and urea are given intravenously; they are equally effective in reducing intraocular pressure and vitreous volume, but mannitol is more convenient to administer and less toxic. Orally administered glycerin and isosorbide are not as rapidly effective as the intravenous agents, but are often preferred because of their safety and convenience. Ethanol also has an osmotic action and may be given orally to reduce intraocular pressure in an emergency.

See the evaluations for adverse reactions and precautions.

GLYCERIN
[Glyrol, Osmōglyn]

$$CH_2OH$$
$$|$$
$$CHOH$$
$$|$$
$$CH_2OH$$

Orally administered glycerin is used to reduce intraocular pressure and vitreous volume prior to iridectomy and other ocular surgical procedures. Glycerin is safer than the intravenously administered agents, urea and mannitol, but it has a slower onset of action. A maximal reduction in intraocular pressure and vitreous volume occurs about one hour after administration, with a return to the pretreatment level in about five hours. Because it is rapidly metabolized, glycerin produces little diuresis, and routine urinary bladder catheterization for surgery is not required.

Headache, nausea, and vomiting are the most common untoward effects. Diarrhea occurs occasionally. Glycerin may cause hyperglycemia and glycosuria and should be used cautiously in diabetics. Hyperosmolar nonketotic coma is a rare complication. Any of the systemic effects of dehydration that occur with use of the intravenous osmotic agents are potential hazards but are less likely to occur with glycerin.

ROUTE, USUAL DOSAGE, AND PREPARATIONS. *Oral: Adults and children*, 1 to 1.5 g/kg of body weight, usually given as a 50% or 75% solution. The drug may be administered more than once daily, if necessary. Lemon juice or instant coffee may be added to unflavored preparations. Palatability is also enhanced by serving with crushed ice and drinking through a straw, but patients should not be permitted to drink additional water.

> Drug available generically in bulk form (unflavored) and may be diluted.
> *Glyrol* (SMP). Solution (oral) 75%.
> *Osmōglyn* (Alcon). Solution (oral) 50% (600 mg/ml).

ISOSORBIDE
[Ismotic]

Isosorbide is an oral osmotic agent used for the emergency treatment of acute angle-closure glaucoma and other conditions in which a rapid reduction in intraocular pressure and vitreous volume is indicated. It apparently has the same onset and duration of action as glycerin.

Untoward effects are also similar, although isosorbide does not adversely affect blood glucose levels and may cause less nausea and vomiting. Isosorbide produces a more significant diuresis than glycerin and catheterization may be necessary.

ROUTE, USUAL DOSAGE, AND PREPARATIONS. *Oral: Adults*, initially, 1.5 g/kg of body weight. The drug may be given up to four times daily, if indicated. It may be poured over cracked ice to increase palatability.

> *Isosorbide should not be confused with isosorbide dinitrate, an antianginal drug.*
> *Ismotic* (Alcon). Solution (oral) 45%.

MANNITOL
[Osmitrol]

Mannitol is given intravenously to reduce intraocular pressure and vitreous volume prior to iridectomy and other ocular surgical procedures. A maximal reduction in intraocular pressure occurs in 30 to 60 minutes and lasts six to eight hours.

If an intravenous osmotic agent is indicated, mannitol is generally preferred to urea because it is more convenient and less toxic. Impaired renal function is not a contraindication to its use, and it does not cause tissue necrosis if extravasation occurs. Mannitol may be less likely than urea to penetrate the ocular fluids in the presence of inflammation, and in this situation it would be more effective than urea.

Headache, nausea, vomiting, dehydration, and massive diuresis are common untoward effects of mannitol. Urinary bladder catheterization should be considered routinely in patients who are undergoing surgery. Chills, dizziness, and chest pain also have been reported. The drug occasionally has caused agitation, disorientation, and convulsions. Large doses may cause an acute increase in intravascular volume, resulting in congestive heart failure or intracranial hemorrhage. Fatalities have been reported.

ROUTE, USUAL DOSAGE, AND PREPARATIONS.
Intravenous: Adults and children, 0.5 to 2 g/kg of body weight given as a 20% solution is infused over a period of 30 to 60 minutes. Administration may be discontinued when the desired effect has been obtained, even if the full dose has not been given. A total dose of 1 g/kg of body weight is usually sufficient.

> *Mannitol should not be confused with mannitol hexanitrate, an antianginal drug.*
> Drug available generically: Solution 25%.
> *Osmitrol* (Travenol). Solution (injection) 5% in 1,000 ml containers, 10% in 500 and 1,000 ml containers, 15% in 150 and 500 ml containers, and 20% in 250 and 500 ml containers.

UREA FOR INJECTION
[Ureaphil, Urevert]

$$\begin{array}{c} NH_2 \\ | \\ C=O \\ | \\ NH_2 \end{array}$$

Urea is used less commonly than other osmotic agents. Because the eye is permeable to urea, a rebound elevation in intraocular pressure and vitreous volume may occur after the ocular hypotensive effect has terminated (about 8 to 12 hours after administration).

The systemic toxicity of urea is similar to that of mannitol. Urea is irritating to the tissues; it causes pain at the site of infusion and necrosis may result if extravasation occurs. Superficial and deep thrombosis may result if urea is infused into the veins of the lower extremities. This agent should not be used in patients with severely impaired renal function.

Urea is often reconstituted with invert sugar solution. Invert sugar contains fructose, which can cause severe reactions (hypoglycemia, nausea, vomiting, tremors, coma, and convulsions) in patients with hereditary fructose intolerance (aldolase deficiency).

ROUTE, USUAL DOSAGE, AND PREPARATIONS.
Intravenous: Adults, 0.5 to 2 g/kg of body weight given as a 30% solution is administered at a rate of 60 drops/min. *Children,* 0.5 to 1.5 g/kg of a 30% solution is infused over a 30-minute period. The solution should be prepared just prior to use.

> *Ureaphil* (Abbott). Lyophilized powder (injection) 40 g.
> *Urevert* (Travenol). Lyophilized powder (injection) 40 and 90 g with diluent to make a 30% solution with 10% invert sugar.

Selected References

Apt L, Gaffney WL: Toxicity of topical eye medications used in childhood strabismus, in Leopold IH, Burns RP (eds): *Symposium on Ocular Therapy.* New York, John Wiley & Sons, 1976, vol 8, 1-10.

Boger WP III, et al: Clinical trial comparing timolol ophthalmic solution to pilocarpine in open-angle glaucoma. *Am J Ophthalmol* 86:8-18, 1978 A.

Boger WP III, et al: Long-term experience with timolol ophthalmic solution in patients with open-angle glaucoma. *Ophthalmology* 85:259-267, 1978 B.

Chandler PA, Grant WM: *Glaucoma,* ed 2. Philadelphia, Lea & Febiger, in press.

Drance SM: Medical management of early chronic open angle glaucoma, in *Symposium on Glaucoma: Transactions of the New Orleans Academy of Ophthalmology.* St Louis, CV Mosby Co, 1975, 68-80 A.

Drance SM: Low tension glaucoma and its management, in *Symposium on Glaucoma: Transactions of the New Orleans Academy of Ophthalmology.* St Louis, CV Mosby Co, 1975, 257-265 B.

Grant WM: Antiglaucoma drugs: Problems with carbonic anhydrase inhibitors, in Leopold IH (ed): *Symposium on Ocular Therapy.* St Louis, CV Mosby Co, 1973, vol 6, 19-38.

Kitazawa Y, et al: Chemical sympathectomy with 6-hydroxydopamine in treatment of primary open-angle glaucoma. *Am J Ophthalmol* 79:98-103, 1975.

Kolker AE, Hetherington J: *Becker-Shaffer's Diagnosis and Therapy of the Glaucomas,* ed 4. St Louis, CV Mosby Co, 1976.

Moss AP, et al: Comparison of effects of timolol and epinephrine on intraocular pressure. *Am J Ophthalmol* 86:489-495, 1978.

Pollack IP, Rossi H: Norepinephrine in treatment of ocular hypertension and glaucoma. *Arch Ophthalmol* 93:173-177, 1975.

Radius RL, et al: Timolol: New drug for management of chronic simple glaucoma. *Arch Ophthalmol* 96:1003-1008, 1978.

Ross RA, Drance SM: Effects of catecholamines and related drugs on intraocular pressure. *Can J Ophthalmol* 10:162-167, 1975.

Sears ML: Adrenergic therapy of open angle glaucoma, in Leopold IH, Burns RP (eds): *Symposium on Ocular Therapy*. New York, John Wiley & Sons, 1976, vol 8, 67-78.

Van Alphen GWHM: Adrenergic receptors of intraocular muscles of human eye. *Invest Ophthalmol* 15:502-505, 1976.

Wand M, Grant WM: Thymoxamine hydrochloride: Effects on facility of outflow and intraocular pressure. *Invest Ophthalmol* 15:400-403, 1976.

Wilensky JT, Podos SM: Prognostic parameters in primary open angle glaucoma, in *Symposium on Glaucoma: Transactions of the New Orleans Academy of Ophthalmology*. St Louis, CV Mosby Co, 1975, 7-30.

Zimmerman TJ, Kaufman HE: Timolol: New drug for treatment of glaucoma? in Leopold IH, Burns RP (eds): *Symposium on Ocular Therapy*. New York, John Wiley & Sons, 1977, vol 10, 69-76.

Mydriatics and Cycloplegics | 23

Anticholinergic drugs are applied topically to the eye to produce paralysis of accommodation (cycloplegia) and pupillary dilation (mydriasis). These agents are muscarinic antagonists that paralyze the ciliary and iris sphincter muscles, both of which are parasympathetically innervated. They are used primarily as an aid in refraction, internal examination of the eye, and other diagnostic purposes; pre- and postoperatively in intraocular surgery; and in the treatment of anterior uveitis and some secondary glaucomas. The anticholinergic drugs available commercially as ophthalmic preparations include atropine, scopolamine (hyoscine), homatropine hydrobromide, cyclopentolate [Cyclogyl], and tropicamide [Mydriacyl].

Alpha-adrenergic drugs produce mydriasis without cycloplegia. These drugs dilate the pupil by contracting the dilator muscle of the iris. There are two types of alpha-adrenergic agonists: direct-acting, such as phenylephrine [Efricel, Mydfrin, Neo-Synephrine], and indirect-acting, such as hydroxyamphetamine [Paredrine] and cocaine. Hydroxyamphetamine releases intraneuronal stores of norepineph-rine, and cocaine prevents neuronal reuptake of the neurotransmitter. Phenylephrine, the most commonly used adrenergic drug, is useful to produce mydriasis for diagnostic purposes, ocular surgery, and as an adjunct in the treatment of anterior uveitis.

Since adrenergic and anticholinergic drugs act by different mechanisms, wider mydriasis can be obtained by using both. If an anticholinergic agent is not used concomitantly, much of the mydriasis produced by the adrenergic agent may be counteracted by sphincter muscle activity (eg, the light from the ophthalmoscope will evoke iris sphincter contraction).

Diagnostic Uses

Refraction: Both the cycloplegic and mydriatic actions of the anticholinergic drugs are useful in estimating errors of refraction. Paralysis of accommodation reveals latent refractive errors, and dilatation of the pupil facilitates estimation of the refractive error. The presence of mydriasis does not necessarily indicate adequate cycloplegia, as mydriasis generally occurs more rapidly than cycloplegia, persists longer, and can be obtained with a lower drug concentration. Since melanin binds drugs, highly pigmented eyes are relatively resistant to topical cycloplegics and more frequent instillation or use of a stronger solution may be required.

Atropine is the most potent mydriatic-cycloplegic drug in clinical use. It has a slow onset and a very long duration of action; residual cycloplegia may persist for six days or more and mydriasis for weeks in adults. Because of its prolonged action, atropine is not used for refraction in adults, but it is often preferred for children up to five or six years of age, as accommodation is very active and recovery more rapid in the young. Since excessive accommodation may be present in every type of convergent strabismus, atropine is the drug of choice for refraction in all children with this disorder. Scopolamine has a cycloplegic effect comparable to that of atropine. Although its duration of action is somewhat shorter (approximately three days), it is still too long for adult refraction.

The shorter-acting cycloplegics, homatropine, cyclopentolate, and tropicamide, are used for refraction in adults, older children, and, less commonly, in young children. Homatropine has the slowest onset and most prolonged action of these three drugs; residual cycloplegia may persist for 36 to 48 hours. Cyclopentolate induces maximal cycloplegia within 25 to 75 minutes with complete recovery in 6 to 24 hours. Tropicamide is a weaker cycloplegic but its potency and duration of action are sufficient for refraction in adults. Examination must be performed within 20 to 35 minutes or it may be necessary to instill an additional drop. Complete recovery of accommodation occurs two to six hours after administration (Gettes, 1961).

Intraocular Examination: Adrenergic and short-acting anticholinergic drugs are used to dilate the pupil for examination of the intraocular structures (Gambill et al, 1967). Since phenylephrine and hydroxyamphetamine produce mydriasis without cycloplegia, the patient is spared the inconvenience of residual blurring of vision. Cyclopentolate and tropicamide are more effective mydriatics, however, and these agents may be supplemented with an adrenergic drug for maximal mydriasis. Such combined use may be necessary in patients with dark irides. Another short-acting anticholinergic, eucatropine, has a more delayed onset of action than tropicamide or cyclopentolate but has the advantage of producing little or no cycloplegia. Eucatropine is not commercially available as an ophthalmic preparation and may be difficult to obtain in some areas.

Adrenergic and short-acting anticholinergic drugs may be used safely to produce mydriasis for intraocular examination of patients with open-angle glaucoma. Although the anticholinergic drug may increase intraocular pressure in these patients, the rise in pressure is transitory.

If pupillary dilatation is necessary for ophthalmoscopic examination of a patient with potential angle-closure glaucoma, phenylephrine, eucatropine, or hydroxyamphetamine may be used or, for examination of the posterior pole, a wick of cotton moistened with epinephrine 1:1,000 may be placed in the inferior cul-de-sac for three minutes (Shaffer, 1967). Since mydriatic drugs can precipitate an attack of acute angle-closure glaucoma, the patient should be checked after the examination to make certain that the pupil has returned to normal size, the angle is gonioscopically open, and the intraocular pressure is normal.

Provocative Test for Angle-Closure Glaucoma: Not all patients with anatomically narrow filtration angles will develop acute angle-closure glaucoma. Provocative tests are sometimes performed to detect those who might. No available test is highly reliable and all entail some degree of risk. The safest and most physiologic procedures are the dark room test and the prone test, which may be performed simultaneously and do not require instillation of a mydriatic drug (Wand, 1974). In mydriatic provocative testing, a short-acting mydriatic, such as hydroxyamphetamine or eucatropine, is instilled and results are considered positive if a pressure rise of 8 mm

Hg is observed within one hour and the angle is gonioscopically closed at the time of the elevation. Mydriatic provocative tests are more difficult to reverse if results are positive; therefore, only one eye is tested at a time and the patient should be forewarned that surgery may be necessary if the angle remains closed.

Horner's Syndrome: Unilateral Horner's syndrome can be diagnosed with cocaine eyedrops instilled bilaterally. Results of this test are evaluated 30 minutes after instillation of a 10% solution or 60 minutes after instillation of a 5% solution. In a positive test, there is an increase in the difference of the diameters of the two pupils, the abnormal pupil being the smaller one. Once the presence of Horner's syndrome is known, the lesion can be localized by instilling hydroxyamphetamine 1% in each eye. The denervated pupil will dilate if the lesion is preganglionic but not if it is postganglionic.

Uses In Intraocular Surgery

Maximal mydriasis may be desired during intraocular surgery, particularly to facilitate round pupil cataract extraction and to locate the retinal break during retinal detachment operations. Atropine (alone or with phenylephrine) may be instilled preoperatively for this purpose. Pupillary constriction induced by surgical trauma may be mediated by prostaglandins, and there is experimental evidence suggesting that pretreatment with prostaglandin synthetase inhibitors (eg, aspirin, indomethacin) may reduce the miosis.

The pupil is usually dilated daily after intraocular surgery to prevent formation of posterior synechiae (adhesions). Atropine, scopolamine, or a shorter-acting mydriatic may be instilled one to several times daily until slit-lamp examination shows minimal iritis. An alpha-adrenergic agent, such as phenylephrine, may be used as well. If postoperative inflammation is prolonged, continued mydriasis is recommended. For example, after surgery for congenital cataracts, if mydriatics are discontinued be-

fore all cortex is absorbed, posterior synechiae and secondary glaucoma may occur.

Uses in Anterior Uveitis and Secondary Glaucoma

Anticholinergic drugs are applied locally in the nonspecific treatment of anterior uveitis (iritis, iridocyclitis) and in glaucoma secondary to ocular inflammation. Atropine or scopolamine is generally preferred and may be supplemented with phenylephrine for maximal mydriasis. The shorter-acting agents are used in mild inflammatory conditions and may be preferred when the intraocular pressure is elevated. In addition to mydriatic-cycloplegic therapy, corticosteroids are indicated to reduce inflammation and anti-infective agents are given if the uveitis is caused by an ocular infection. Systemic ocular hypotensive drugs (osmotic agents and carbonic anhydrase inhibitors) and topical epinephrine are also administered if the intraocular pressure is elevated.

Anticholinergic drugs have three beneficial actions: They relax the intraocular muscles, reduce abnormal vascular permeability, and dilate the pupil. Although the mechanism is not clear, relaxation of the iris sphincter and ciliary muscles relieves the pain and photophobia associated with anterior uveitis. Cycloplegia is also usually effective in relieving the photophobia associated with corneal disease.

Increased permeability of the blood vessels of the ciliary body and iris allows an outpouring of protein and inflammatory cells into the anterior chamber which may clog the angle and promote the development of adhesions that seal the iris to the trabecular meshwork (peripheral anterior synechiae). By reducing the abnormal vascular permeability, anticholinergic drugs may prevent this complication.

Contact between the inflamed iris and the anterior surface of the lens leads to the formation of adhesions (posterior synechiae) which seal the iris to the lens and prevent passage of aqueous humor from the posterior to the anterior chamber (pupillary block). This causes the iris to bulge forward and close the filtration angle (iris bombé), with a resultant sharp increase in intraocular pressure. Pupillary block also may occur in the absence of the lens (aphakia) when posterior synechiae seal the iris to the bulging vitreous face or lens capsule. Dilation of the pupil prevents the formation of posterior synechiae and may aid in breaking these adhesions once they have formed. In resistant cases, subconjunctival injection of 0.1 ml of a mixture containing equal proportions of cocaine 4%, atropine 1%, and epinephrine 1:1,000 may break the synechiae (Kolker and Hetherington, 1976). Topically applied cocaine 5% has been used to temporarily relieve vitreous herniation in patients unresponsive to intensive mydriatic-cycloplegic therapy (Sears et al, 1972).

Mydriatic-cycloplegic therapy also may be useful in ciliary block (malignant) glaucoma, a rare complication of ophthalmic surgery (usually for angle-closure glaucoma) in which forward displacement of the lens, ciliary processes, and iris flattens the anterior chamber and closes the filtration angle. Increased vitreous pressure and an abnormal slackness in the zonules of the lens are believed to be causative factors. Therapy with atropine (or scopolamine) and phenylephrine promotes re-formation of the anterior chamber and opening of the angle, presumably by increasing tension in the zonules. An osmotic agent and carbonic anhydrase inhibitor are also administered to help reduce pressure from within the vitreous. If drug therapy is successful, the systemic drugs and phenylephrine may be discontinued eventually, but the cycloplegic must be administered indefinitely (Chandler et al, 1968).

Miscellaneous Uses

Cycloplegic drugs also have been used to discourage accommodation in other ocular disorders. In patients with severe functional spasm of accommodation, atropine is sometimes applied daily for three or four weeks to provide a period of accommodative rest. In suppression amblyopia, atropine has been employed to blur vision in the normal eye, thus forcing fixation with the amblyopic eye, particularly when occlusion therapy is not feasible. Atropine is most effective if the fixing eye is severely hypermetropic because cycloplegia causes greater visual impairment in hypermetropes than in myopes or emmetropes. In accommodative esotropia, atropine has occasionally been used to prevent convergence by paralyzing accommodation. This form of therapy is not consistently effective because the blurred vision induced by the cycloplegic may increase accommodative effort and thereby increase the degree of esotropia, especially initially or as the effect of the drug wears off. There is no convincing evidence that the daily use of cycloplegic eyedrops will retard the progression of myopia.

Phenylephrine and other adrenergic drugs (naphazoline, tetrahydrozoline, and ephedrine) are widely used by the laity to constrict the conjunctival blood vessels and to "whiten" the eye. Although severe adverse effects (eg, acute glaucoma) are rare with the weak concentrations contained in decongestant products, rebound hyperemia occurs frequently. The main danger of self-medication with these agents is the possible neglect of symptoms of severe eye disease (eg, iridocyclitis, keratitis).

Adverse Reactions and Precautions

Local Reactions: Mydriatic drugs (anticholinergic and adrenergic) can precipitate an attack of acute angle-closure glaucoma in eyes with anatomically narrow angles. An abrupt rise in intraocular pressure occurs because pupillary dilatation crowds the iris into the filtration angle. Long-acting mydriatics (atropine or scopolamine) should not be used prior to iridectomy in eyes predisposed to angle closure, and shorter-acting mydriatics should be used cautiously, if at all.

TABLE 1.
AGENTS USED FOR REFRACTION

Drug	Dosage (Topical)
Atropine Sulfate [Atropisol, BufOpto Atropine, Isopto Atropine]	*Children:* One drop of 0.125% solution (in infants less than 1 year), 0.25% solution (in children 1 to 5 years and in all children with blue irides), 0.5% solution or ointment (in children over 5 years) or 1% solution or ointment (in children with dark irides) is applied three times daily for three days prior to refraction and once on the morning of refraction.* Administration should be discontinued if systemic effects occur.
Cyclopentolate Hydrochloride [Cyclogyl]	*Adults:* One drop of 1% solution (or 2% in patients with dark irides) is instilled once, or one drop of 0.5% solution is instilled and repeated in five minutes. *Children,* one drop of 1% solution is instilled and repeated in ten minutes.
Homatropine Hydrobromide [Homatrocel, Isopto Homatropine]	*Adults and Children:* One drop of 2% solution is instilled every 10 to 15 minutes for five doses or one drop of 5% solution is instilled and repeated in 15 minutes.
Scopolamine Hydrobromide [Isopto Hyoscine, Murocoll No. 19]	*Children:* One drop of 0.2% solution or ointment or 0.25% solution is applied twice daily for two days before the refraction.*
Tropicamide [Mydriacyl]	*Adults:* One drop of 1% solution is instilled and repeated in five minutes. If the examination cannot be performed within 20-35 minutes, an additional drop must be instilled.

*If ointment is used, it should not be applied for several hours immediately prior to refraction because it will impair the transparency of the cornea and alter the regularity of its refraction.

TABLE 2.
AGENTS USED FOR OPHTHALMOSCOPY

Drug	Dosage (Topical)
Cyclopentolate Hydrochloride [Cyclogyl]	One drop of 0.5% solution (may be supplemented with phenylephrine for wider mydriasis).
Cyclopentolate and Phenylephrine [Cyclomydril]	One drop of solution containing 0.2% cyclopentolate and 1% phenylephrine.
Eucatropine Hydrochloride	One drop of 5% or 10% solution, repeated in 10 to 15 minutes if necessary.
Tropicamide [Mydriacyl]	One drop of 0.5% or 1% solution (may be supplemented with phenylephrine for wider mydriasis). For examination of patients with primary open-angle glaucoma (especially those being treated with miotics), a solution containing equal parts of 0.5% tropicamide and 10% phenylephrine may be used.
Phenylephrine Hydrochloride [Efricel, Mydfrin, Neo-Synephrine Hydrochloride]	One drop of 2.5% solution (may be used cautiously for ophthalmoscopy in patients with narrow angles and shallow anterior chambers).
Hydroxyamphetamine Hydrobromide [Paredrine]	One drop of 1% solution.

Topically applied anticholinergic drugs increase intraocular pressure in about one out of four eyes with mild primary open-angle glaucoma. This response is not caused by closure of the angle but appears to be due to increased resistance to aqueous outflow caused by loss of ciliary muscle tone or to blocking of the trabecular meshwork by pigment liberated from the iris. Short-acting anticholinergic agents are preferred for diagnostic purposes in open-angle glaucoma; atropine and scopolamine should be used cautiously.

When treating inflammation of the anterior segment, posterior synechiae may form if mydriatic drugs are applied for prolonged periods without moving the pupil. If slit-lamp examination shows that synechiae are forming, the mydriatic should be discontinued and a miotic substituted for a brief period. Also, if there are inflammatory exudates in the angle, peripheral anterior synechiae may form while the pupil is dilated; gonioscopy is necessary to determine whether peripheral anterior synechiae have formed. Concurrent corticosteroid therapy minimizes this problem.

Atropine may cause contact dermatitis of the lids and allergic conjunctivitis. Allergic reactions are less common after ocular use of the other anticholinergic agents.

Adrenergic drugs may cause browache, headache, blurred vision, hypersensitivity reactions, pain, and lacrimation. Pigment granules (aqueous floaters) may appear in the anterior chamber several minutes after drug instillation. They disappear within 12 to 24 hours and occur with decreasing frequency when the drug is administered repeatedly. Aqueous floaters occur most commonly in older patients with dark irides. These pigment granules are apparently released from the iris and are derived from degenerated cells in the iris pigment epithelium that rupture when the dilator muscle contracts. This phenomenon (which appears to be harmless) should not be confused with iritis. Release of the pigment is sometimes associated with an increase in intraocular pressure but, if the angle of the anterior chamber is open, this effect is not long lasting and requires no special treatment.

Systemic Reactions: Systemic reactions may occur after ocular instillation of anticholinergic drugs, particularly in children and elderly patients. They are most common after instillation of atropine, scopolamine, or cyclopentolate [Cyclogyl]. Symptoms of systemic toxicity include dryness of the mouth and skin, flushing, fever, rash, thirst, tachycardia, irritability, dizziness, depression, weeping, hyperactivity, ataxia, confusion, somnolence, hallucinations, delirium, and, rarely, convulsions, coma, and death. Cyclopentolate in particular has been associated with a transient, acute psychosis, especially in children but recently also documented in adults. To avoid systemic effects, anticholinergic drugs should be instilled in the lowest effective concentration and no more often than needed to obtain the desired response. The risk of systemic reactions can be reduced by the use of ointments instead of solutions; pressure at the inner canthus after instillation of solutions will minimize drainage into the nose and throat and may reduce the likelihood of systemic reactions. Physostigmine salicylate is an effective antidote (see Chapter 86, Specific Antidotes).

Tachycardia, hypertension, premature ventricular contractions, myocardial infarction, hyperhidrosis, blanching, tremors, agitation, and confusion may occur following ocular instillation of adrenergic drugs. These systemic reactions are most common if a strong concentration (phenylephrine 10%) is instilled repeatedly. Neonates are particularly at risk. Stroke has been reported after adrenergic drugs were injected subconjunctivally or applied with cotton packs.

See also Grant, 1974; Apt and Gaffney, 1976.

For adverse reactions associated with prolonged use of epinephrine, see Chapter 22, Agents Used to Treat Glaucoma.

ANTICHOLINERGIC DRUGS

ATROPINE SULFATE
[Atropisol, BufOpto Atropine, Isopto Atropine]

Atropine is a potent, long-acting mydriatic and cycloplegic that is widely used in ophthalmology. Its effect on accommodation may last six days or longer and mydriasis may persist for 12 days. Atropine is used for pre- and postoperative mydriasis, in anterior uveitis, and in some secondary glaucomas. It is preferred for refraction in children up to the age of five or six years and is the cycloplegic of choice in children with convergent strabismus. Because of its long duration of action, atropine is not useful for refraction in adults.

Acute angle-closure glaucoma may occur if atropine is instilled in eyes with anatomically narrow angles. This agent also may increase intraocular pressure in eyes with open-angle glaucoma. Systemic reactions may occur, particularly in children and elderly patients. Contact dermatitis and allergic conjunctivitis are not uncommon. (Also see the section on Adverse Reactions and Precautions in the Introduction.)

ROUTE, USUAL DOSAGE, AND PREPARATIONS.
Topical: For preoperative mydriasis, one drop of a 1% solution, supplemented with one drop of phenylephrine 10%, is instilled prior to surgery. Some surgeons prefer to instill drops for several days prior to surgery as well.

In anterior segment inflammation, the concentration and frequency of administration are determined by the severity of inflammation and the pupillary response. At-

ropine may be supplemented with phenylephrine for maximal mydriasis. For anterior uveitis or postoperative mydriasis, one drop of a 1% to 2% solution instilled once daily is often adequate. A 0.5% solution or ointment applied one to three times daily is often adequate in children. When slit-lamp examination reveals minimal inflammation, a less potent agent, such as homatropine, may be substituted.

To break posterior synechiae, drops may be instilled more frequently, eg, one drop of a 2% solution (alternately with phenylephrine 10%) every other minute for five applications of each. The risk of toxicity from each drug is increased with increasing dosage.

For ciliary block (malignant) glaucoma, initially, one drop of a 1% or 2% solution and one drop of phenylephrine 10% three or four times daily. For maintenance, one drop of a 1% solution daily or every other day.

For refraction in *children*, see Table 1.

All preparations available in topical ophthalmic forms.

Atropine Sulfate (Allergan). Solution (sterile) 1% and 2% with chlorobutanol 0.5%, boric acid, sodium citrate, hydrochloric acid and/or sodium hydroxide in 15 ml containers; ointment (sterile) 0.5% and 1% with chlorobutanol 0.5%, white petrolatum, mineral oil, and nonionic lanolin derivatives in 3.5 g containers.

Atropine Sulfate Steri-Unit (Alcon). Solution (sterile) 1% without preservatives in 2 ml containers.

Atropisol (SMP). Solution (sterile) 0.5%, 1%, and 2% with benzalkonium chloride 0.005% in 1 ml containers and with edetate disodium 0.01% and benzalkonium chloride 0.01% in 5 ml containers; 1% solution also available in 15 ml size. All sizes also contain potassium chloride, sodium carbonate, and boric acid.

BufOpto Atropine (Professional Pharmacal). Solution (sterile) 0.5% and 1% with methylcellulose, sodium phosphate monobasic and dibasic, sodium chloride, and benzalkonium chloride 1:10,000 in 15 ml containers.

Isopto Atropine (Alcon). Solution (sterile) 0.5%, 1%, and 3% with hydroxypropyl methylcellulose 0.5%, benzalkonium chloride 0.01%, boric acid, sodium hydroxide, and/or hydrochloric acid in 5 and 15 ml (1% concentration only) containers.

Ophthalmic forms of drug also marketed by other manufacturers under generic name: Solution 0.125%, 0.25%, 0.5%, 1%, 2%, and 4%; ointment 0.5%, 1%.

CYCLOPENTOLATE HYDROCHLORIDE
[Cyclogyl]

Cyclopentolate is an effective mydriatic and cycloplegic with a rapid onset and relatively short duration of action. Cycloplegia is maximum 25 to 75 minutes after instillation, and recovery of accommodation is complete in 6 to 24 hours. This drug is used as an aid in refraction and for ophthalmoscopy.

Cyclopentolate has caused systemic reactions in both children and adults. Severe central nervous system disturbances, manifested by ataxia, hallucinations, and grand mal seizures, have occurred in children. Vomiting, abdominal distention, and adynamic ileus developed in a pair of premature twins following instillation of six drops of the 1% solution. One of the twins subsequently died from necrotizing enterocolitis. See also the section on Adverse Reactions and Precautions in the Introduction.

ROUTE, USUAL DOSAGE, AND PREPARATIONS. *Topical*: For refraction, see Table 1. For ophthalmoscopy, see Table 2.

> *Cyclogyl* (Alcon). Solution (ophthalmic, sterile) 0.5% and 1% with boric acid, potassium chloride, sodium carbonate and/or hydrochloric acid, edetate disodium, and benzalkonium chloride 0.01% in 2, 5, and 15 ml containers; 2% with boric acid, edetate disodium, sodium carbonate and/or hydrochloric acid, and benzalkonium chloride 0.01% in 2, 5, and 7.5 ml containers.

CYCLOMYDRIL

Cyclomydril is a combination of cyclopentolate and phenylephrine used to produce maximum mydriasis for examination of the intraocular structures.

See the evaluations on Cyclopentolate Hydrochloride and Phenylephrine Hydrochloride and the section on Adverse Reactions and Precautions in the Introduction.

ROUTE, USUAL DOSAGE, AND PREPARATIONS.

Topical: For ophthalmoscopy, see Table 2.
> *Cyclomydril* (Alcon). Solution (ophthalmic, sterile) containing cyclopentolate hydrochloride 0.2% and phenylephrine hydrochloride 1% with boric acid, edetate disodium, hydrochloric acid and/or sodium carbonate and benzalkonium chloride 0.01% in 2, 5, and 7.5 ml containers.

EUCATROPINE HYDROCHLORIDE

Eucatropine, a weak anticholinergic drug, produces mydriasis for two to four hours with little or no cycloplegia. It is used for ophthalmoscopy and provocative testing for angle-closure glaucoma.

Eucatropine may be difficult to obtain in some areas. Some pharmacies will prepare an ophthalmic solution upon special request but the solution is unstable.

See also the section on Adverse Reactions and Precautions in the Introduction.

ROUTE, USUAL DOSAGE, AND PREPARATIONS. *Topical*: For ophthalmoscopy, see Table 2. As a provocative test for angle-closure glaucoma, two drops of a 5% solution are instilled in one eye. For details, see the discussion on provocative testing in the Introduction. At the conclusion of the provocative test, the patient should be examined to make certain that the pupil has returned to normal size, the angle is gonioscopically open, and the intraocular pressure is normal.

> No commercial preparation available. Compounding necessary for prescription.

HOMATROPINE HYDROBROMIDE
[Homatrocel, Isopto Homatropine]

Homatropine is a mydriatic and cycloplegic used for refraction and treatment of anterior uveitis. Repeated instillation of the 2% solution at ten-minute intervals produces maximal cycloplegia in 60 minutes. Effects may persist for 36 to 48 hours.

See also the section on Adverse Reactions and Precautions in the Introduction.

ROUTE, USUAL DOSAGE, AND PREPARATIONS.
Topical: For refraction, see Table 1. For mild anterior uveitis, one drop of the 2% or 5% solution is instilled two to three times daily. When homatropine is used for continuing therapy after administration of atropine or scopolamine, the drops may be instilled initially one or more times daily, followed by twice weekly administration.

All preparations available as topical ophthalmic solutions.

Homatrocel (Professional Pharmacal). Solution (sterile) 2% and 5% with methylcellulose, benzalkonium chloride 1:15,000, monobasic and dibasic sodium phosphate, and sodium chloride in 15 ml containers.

Homatropine Hydrobromide (Allergan). Solution (sterile) 2% and 5% with chlorobutanol 0.5%, boric acid, and sodium citrate in 15 ml containers.

Homatropine Hydrobromide (SMP). Solution 2% and 5% with benzalkonium chloride in 1 ml sterile containers and 2% and 5% with edetate disodium and benzalkonium chloride in 5 ml containers. All sizes also contain potassium chloride, sodium carbonate, and boric acid.

Isopto Homatropine (Alcon). Solution (sterile) 2% with hydroxypropylmethylcellulose 0.5%, benzalkonium chloride 0.01%, sodium chloride, polysorbate 80, hydrochloric acid and/or sodium hydroxide in 5 and 15 ml containers; 5% with hydroxypropylmethylcellulose 0.5%, benzethonium chloride 0.005%, sodium chloride, sodium hydroxide and/or hydrochloric acid in 5 and 15 ml containers.

Homatropine Hydrobromide Steri-Unit (Alcon). Solution 5% without preservatives in 2 ml containers.

Drug also marketed by other manufacturers under generic name: Powder; solution 1%, 2%.

SCOPOLAMINE HYDROBROMIDE
[Isopto Hyoscine, Murocoll No. 19]

Scopolamine is a potent mydriatic and cycloplegic. In the concentrations used clinically, it has a shorter duration of action than atropine; cycloplegia may persist for three days. Scopolamine rarely causes local allergic reactions and is useful in patients who are allergic to atropine. It is used occasionally for refraction in children but is employed most commonly for postoperative mydriasis, in anterior uveitis, and in some secondary glaucomas.

Scopolamine can cause acute angle-closure glaucoma if it is instilled in eyes with anatomically narrow angles. It also may increase intraocular pressure in eyes with open-angle glaucoma. Systemic reactions may occur, particularly in children and elderly patients (see also the section on Adverse Reactions and Precautions in the Introduction).

ROUTE, USUAL DOSAGE, AND PREPARATIONS.
Topical: In anterior segment inflammation, the concentration and frequency of administration are determined by the severity of inflammation and pupillary response. Scopolamine may be supplemented with phenylephrine for maximal mydriasis. For postoperative mydriasis, one drop of the 0.2% or 0.25% solution instilled once daily is often adequate. For anterior uveitis, one drop of the 0.2% or 0.25% solution or 0.2% ointment is instilled once daily or more frequently in severe inflammation. When slit-lamp examination reveals minimal inflammation, a less potent agent, such as homatropine, may be substituted.
To break posterior synechiae, one drop of a 0.2% solution is instilled every minute for five minutes. One drop of phenylephrine 10% may be instilled every minute for

three applications to enhance the mydriatic effect.

For ciliary block (malignant) glaucoma, initially, one drop of a 0.25% to 0.5% solution and one drop of phenylephrine 10% three or four times daily or more frequently if required. For maintenance, one drop of a 0.25% or 0.3% solution once daily.

For refraction in children, see Table 1.

> All preparations available in topical ophthalmic forms.
> *Isopto Hyoscine* (Alcon). Solution (sterile) 0.25% with hydroxypropylmethylcellulose 0.5%, benzalkonium chloride 0.01%, glacial acetic acid, sodium acetate, and sodium chloride in 5 and 15 ml containers.
> *Murocoll No. 19* (Muro). Solution (sterile) 0.3% in 7.5 ml containers.
> *Scopolamine* [*hydrobromide*] (Allergan). Solution (sterile) 0.25% with benzalkonium chloride, edetate disodium, hydroxypropyl-methylcellulose, sodium acetate, sodium chloride, and sodium hydroxide and/or hydrochloric acid in 2.5 ml containers; ointment (Scopolamine S.O.P.) (sterile) 0.2% with chlorobutanol 0.5%, white petrolatum, mineral oil, and nonionic lanolin derivatives in 3.5 g containers.

TROPICAMIDE
[Mydriacyl]

Tropicamide is an effective mydriatic and cycloplegic with a rapid onset and short duration of action. It is used as an aid in refraction and for ophthalmoscopy and retinal photography. Maximal cycloplegia occurs within 20 to 35 minutes after two drops of the 1% solution are instilled five minutes apart. The duration of action is very brief and complete recovery of accommodation occurs in two to six hours. The 0.5% solution produces maximal pupillary dilatation within 20 to 25 minutes; residual mydriasis persists for about seven hours.

Because of its short duration of action, tropicamide rarely causes systemic reactions. For adverse reactions of anticholinergic drugs, see the section on Adverse Reactions and Precautions in the Introduction.

ROUTE, USUAL DOSAGE, AND PREPARATIONS. *Topical*: For refraction, see Table 1. For ophthalmoscopy and retinal photography, see Table 2.

> *Mydriacyl* (Alcon). Solution (ophthalmic, sterile) 0.5% and 1% with sodium chloride, edetate disodium, hydrochloric acid and/or sodium hydroxide, and benzalkonium chloride 0.01% in 15 ml containers.

ADRENERGIC DRUGS

PHENYLEPHRINE HYDROCHLORIDE
[Efricel, Mydfrin, Neo-Synephrine Hydrochloride]

Phenylephrine is used to produce mydriasis for examination of the intraocular structures, to facilitate ocular surgery, and as an adjunct in the treatment of anterior uveitis, postoperative inflammation, and some secondary glaucomas. It is often used to supplement anticholinergic drugs to achieve maximal mydriasis. After ocular instillation of a 10% solution, maximal mydriasis is obtained in 60 to 90 minutes, and recovery occurs in about six hours. A 2.5% solution has been found to be as effective as a 10% solution for preoperative mydriasis (Smith et al, 1976). For use of phenylephrine to prevent miotic iris cysts, see Chapter 22, Agents Used to Treat Glaucoma.

Local adverse reactions to phenylephrine include transient pain, release of aqueous floaters with a transitory increase in pressure, and occlusion of structurally narrow angles with angle-closure glaucoma. Striking lid retraction may be observed but is of no clinical importance. (See also the section on Adverse Reactions and Precautions in the Introduction.) In patients over 50, rebound miosis has been noted 24 hours after instillation. A diminished mydriatic response was also observed when the drug was instilled again 24 hours later.

Systemic reactions to phenylephrine may occur (tachycardia, hypertension, and, rarely, myocardial infarction), particularly when a strong concentration is instilled repeatedly or is applied by means of a cotton conjunctival pack. A pronounced increase in blood pressure may occur in neonates and elderly patients following instillation of the 10% solution; this complication may be avoided by use of the 2.5% solution. The 10% solution should be used cautiously if at all in patients with hypertension and/or coronary artery disease.

Thymoxamine hydrochloride, an alpha-adrenergic blocking drug, is widely used abroad to reverse the mydriatic effect of phenylephrine. One drop of a 0.5% solution rapidly reverses the effect of one drop of phenylephrine 10% more effectively and safely than does pilocarpine. Thymoxamine is not commercially available in the United States.

ROUTE, USUAL DOSAGE, AND PREPARATIONS. *Topical*: For ophthalmoscopy and retinal photography, see Table 2.

For preoperative mydriasis, two drops of a 2.5% solution every 15 minutes for 90 minutes.

For postoperative mydriasis after iridectomy, one drop of the 10% solution is instilled once or twice daily. Atropine should be substituted if inflammation is severe. After cyclodialysis, one drop of the 10% solution is instilled once daily for three days in conjunction with miotics. For use of phenylephrine to supplement atropine or scopolamine, see the evaluations on these drugs.

All preparations available as topical ophthalmic solutions.
Efricel (Professional Pharmacal). Solution (sterile) 2.5% and 10% with methylcellulose, sodium bisulfite, and benzalkonium chloride 1:10,000 in 15 ml containers.
Mydfrin (Alcon). Solution (sterile) 2.5% with boric acid, sodium bisulfite, edetate disodium, sodium hydroxide and/or hydrochloric acid, and benzalkonium chloride in 5 ml containers.
Neo-Synephrine Hydrochloride (Winthrop). Solution (sterile) 2.5% with sodium phosphate, sodium biphosphate, benzalkonium chloride 1:7,500, boric acid, and phosphoric acid or sodium hydroxide in 15 ml containers; 10% (viscous, nonviscous) with sodium phosphate, sodium biphosphate, benzalkonium chloride 1:10,000, and phosphoric acid or sodium hydroxide in 5 ml containers. Viscous preparation also contains methylcellulose.
Phenylephrine Hydrochloride (SMP). Solution (sterile) 10% with thimerosal 0.01% and sodium bisulfite 0.3% in 1 ml containers or with benzalkonium chloride 0.01% and sodium bisulfite 0.3% in 5 ml containers.
Drug also marketed by other manufacturers under generic name: Solution 10%.

HYDROXYAMPHETAMINE HYDROBROMIDE
[Paredrine]

Hydroxyamphetamine is used to produce mydriasis for ophthalmoscopy and to localize the lesion in Horner's syndrome. It is a weaker mydriatic than phenylephrine, producing maximal mydriasis in 45 to 60 minutes with recovery in about six hours.

See also the section on Adverse Reactions and Precautions in the Introduction.

ROUTE, USUAL DOSAGE, AND PREPARATIONS. *Topical*: For ophthalmoscopy, see Table 2. To localize the lesion in Horner's syndrome, one drop is instilled in each eye. The denervated pupil will dilate if the lesion is preganglionic but not if it is postganglionic.

Paredrine (Smith Kline & French). Solution (ophthalmic) 1% with boric acid 2% and thimerosal 1:50,000 in 15 ml containers.

Selected References

Apt L, Gaffney WL: Toxicity of topical eye medications used in childhood strabismus, in Leopold IH, Burns RP (eds): *Symposium on Ocular Therapy*. New York, John Wiley & Sons, 1976, vol 8, 1-9.

Chandler PA, et al: Malignant glaucoma: Medical and surgical treatment. *Am J Ophthalmol* 66:495-502, 1968.

Gambill HD, et al: Mydriatic effect of four drugs

determined with pupillograph. *Arch Ophthalmol* 77:740-746, 1967.

Gettes BC, Belmont O: Tropicamide: Comparative cycloplegic effects. *Arch Ophthalmol* 66:336-340, 1961.

Grant WM: *Toxicology of the Eye*, ed 2. Springfield, Charles C Thomas Publisher, 1974.

Kolker AE, Hetherington J Jr: *Becker-Shaffer's Diagnosis and Therapy of the Glaucomas*, ed 4. St Louis, CV Mosby Co, 1976.

Sears ML, et al: Drug-induced retraction of vitreous face in aphakia after cataract extraction. *Trans Am Acad Ophthalmol Otolaryngol* 76:498-510, 1972.

Shaffer RN: Problems in use of autonomic drugs in ophthalmology, in Leopold IH (ed): *Ocular Therapy, Complications and Management*. St Louis, CV Mosby Co, 1967, vol 2, 18-23.

Shaffer RN, Hoskins HD: Ciliary block (malignant) glaucoma. *Trans Am Acad Ophthalmol Otolaryngol* 85:215-221, 1978.

Smith RB, et al: Mydriatic effect of phenylephrine. *Eye Ear Nose Throat Mon* 55:133-134, 1976.

Wand M: Provocative tests in angle-closure glaucoma: Brief review with commentary. *Ophthalmic Surg* 5:32-37, 1974.

Ocular Anti-Infective and Anti-Inflammatory Agents | 24

ANTI-INFECTIVE AGENTS

    Antibacterial Agents

    Antifungal Agents

    Antiviral Agents

    Antiseptics and Preservatives

ANTI-INFLAMMATORY AGENTS

STEROID-ANTIBACTERIAL MIXTURES

TOPICAL OPHTHALMIC PREPARATIONS

ANTI-INFECTIVE AGENTS

Anti-infective agents are applied topically in the form of drops or ointments to treat infections of the lids, conjunctiva, and cornea. In severe infections, eyedrops are applied as often as every 15 to 30 minutes or the solution may be administered by continuous corneal lavage. In milder infections, drops or ointments are applied less frequently. Ointments provide a more prolonged effect than solutions with less systemic absorption, but they may interfere with vision when used for daytime medication. Many superficial infections of the conjunctiva and cornea can be treated successfully with topical therapy alone.

Ophthalmologists employ the subconjunctival route in addition to topical application to obtain therapeutic concentrations of antibiotics in the anterior segment of the eye. This route is used to treat serious conditions for which topical therapy alone is insufficient, such as corneal ulcers and anterior intraocular infections. Drugs given subconjunctivally enter the anterior chamber through the corneal limbus and sclera by simple diffusion. By employing the subconjunctival route, drugs which may cause toxic effects when given systemically can be used effectively with less risk of adverse reactions. The injection is repeated every 12 to 24 hours, with the site varied.

Systemic therapy is also used by ophthalmologists to treat severe corneal ulcers and intraocular infections. Since most anti-infective agents do not readily penetrate the eye, large doses must be employed. In treating severe endophthalmitis following injury or surgery, some ophthalmologists inject an anti-infective agent directly into the vitreous humor or anterior chamber to achieve a high intraocular concentration. Since the interior of the eye will not tolerate high concentrations of most drugs, the amount administered must be carefully chosen to give an effective concentration that is not toxic to the retina or other ocular structures.

Antibacterial, antifungal, and antiviral agents commonly used to treat ocular infections are discussed below. Concentrations for topical use may be found in Table 1 and

382

commercially available topical preparations are listed at the end of this chapter. For other routes of administration (systemic, subconjunctival, intracameral) or for more detailed information on the treatment of ocular infections, the reader should consult more specific references; the following are suggested: Ellis, 1977; Havener, 1978; Leopold, 1972; Leopold and Kagan, 1974; Pettit, 1976; and, for pediatric dosage, Apt, 1968. See also the appropriate chapter in Sections XI and XII for adverse reactions to systemically administered anti-infectives and a listing of preparations for systemic use.

Antibacterial Agents

Most bacterial infections of the eyelids or conjunctiva are caused by *Staphylococcus aureus*. Other common causative organisms in infectious conjunctivitis are *Streptococcus pneumoniae, S. pyogenes, Haemophilus influenzae*, and TRIC agent (trachoma and inclusion conjunctivitis). *Pseudomonas* does not usually cause blepharitis or conjunctivitis. Since infections of the lids and conjunctiva are not generally serious clinical problems, intensive treatment is less essential than for

TABLE 1.
ANTI-INFECTIVE AGENTS FOR TOPICAL OPHTHALMIC THERAPY

Drug	Concentration	
	Solution or Suspension	Ointment
ANTIBACTERIAL AGENTS		
Bacitracin	10,000 units/ml	400-500 units/g*†
Cephaloridine	50 mg/ml	
Cephalothin	50 mg/ml	
Chloramphenicol	5 mg/ml*	10 mg/g *†
Colistin Sulfate	5-10 mg/ml	
Erythromycin	5-10 mg/ml	5 mg/g*
Gentamicin Sulfate	3*-10 mg/ml	3 mg/g*
Lincomycin Hydrochloride Monohydrate	50 mg/ml	
Neomycin Sulfate	2.5-5 mg/ml† 30-50 mg/ml	5 mg/g*†
Polymyxin B Sulfate	5,000-10,000 mg/ml† 20,000 units/ml	5,000-10,000 units/g†
Sulfacetamide Sodium	100-300 mg/ml*	100-300 mg/g*
Tetracycline Hydrochloride	5 mg/ml	10 mg/g*
ANTIFUNGAL AGENTS		
Amphotericin B	1.5 mg/ml	
Nystatin	25,000 units/ml	100,000 units/g‡
Natamycin	50 mg/ml*	
ANTIVIRAL AGENTS		
Idoxuridine	1 mg/ml*	5 mg/g*
Vidarabine		10 mg/g*

*Available in this concentration as single-entity ophthalmic product.
†Available in this concentration as combination ophthalmic product.
‡Dermatologic preparation.

See also Ellis, 1977; Pettit, 1976.

other ocular infections. Antibacterial agents will not usually eradicate the microorganisms in chronic bacterial blepharitis or affect the course of a stye. However, frequent lid scrubs with a weak shampoo (such as diluted baby shampoo) may reduce the incidence of recurrent styes that result from chronic bacterial blepharitis. Bacterial conjunctivitis generally has a self-limited course without sequelae, but antibacterial therapy will shorten the course. Chronic conjunctivitis due to trachoma requires treatment to avoid scarring of the tarsal conjunctiva and cornea, but reinfection is common in endemic areas.

The bacteria most frequently isolated from corneal ulcers are *Staphylococcus, Pseudomonas*, and *Streptococcus pneumoniae*. Postoperative bacterial endophthalmitis is usually caused by penicillin-resistant staphylococci, *Staphylococcus epidermis, Streptococcus pneumoniae*, or gram-negative organisms including *Pseudomonas, Escherichia coli*, and *Proteus. Pseudomonas* has become fairly common as the causative organism in both corneal and intraocular infections, and such infections are rapidly progressive and devastating. Since therapy must usually be begun before identification, drugs and combinations that are most useful for initial therapy of bacterial corneal ulcers and endophthalmitis are broad spectrum and are aimed at the most common agents and the highly destructive *Pseudomonas*.

Topical Therapy: In selecting a drug for topical therapy, preference should usually be given to antibacterial agents that are seldom administered systemically and to those that do not readily produce local sensitivity reactions. The choice of these drugs for topical use will avoid possible sensitization to commonly used systemic drugs and will discourage the development of strains of organisms resistant to commonly used agents. Most external bacterial infections can be controlled by proper selection from among these agents or by use of a combination product. Except for self-limited or minor infections, identification of the causative organism by culture and smears should be attempted, and

treatment may be initiated as soon as the specimen is obtained.

Sulfacetamide sodium, bacitracin, gramicidin, neomycin, polymyxin B, and colistin are rarely or never administered systemically and are commercially available for topical use as single-entity preparations or in mixtures. Commercial ophthalmic preparations containing erythromycin, chloramphenicol, gentamicin, or tetracycline are also available. With the exception of neomycin, these agents are not active sensitizers.

Sulfacetamide sodium [Bleph-10, -30, Cetamide, Sodium Sulamyd, Sulfacel-15, Vasosulf] is useful for prophylaxis after corneal injury and for treatment of some forms of acute bacterial conjunctivitis. There is one report of a patient who developed Stevens-Johnson syndrome after topical ophthalmic use of sulfacetamide sodium; this patient had previously experienced a skin reaction after taking an oral sulfonamide.

The antibacterial spectrum of bacitracin [Baciguent] is similar to that of penicillin G. It is preferred to penicillin for topical treatment of gram-positive infections because few strains of organisms are resistant, allergic reactions occur less frequently, and future sensitization to penicillin is avoided. Gramicidin, which is similar in activity to bacitracin, is available only in combination products.

Neomycin [Myciguent] is active against many gram-positive and gram-negative organisms but it readily produces sensitization. In sensitized individuals, allergic conjunctivitis may worsen the signs and symptoms, causing the unwary physician to intensify therapy instead of discontinuing it.

Polymyxin B [Aerosporin] and colistin [Coly-Mycin S] are bactericidal against most gram-negative organisms, including *Pseudomonas aeruginosa, Escherichia coli, Klebsiella pneumoniae*, and *Aerobacter aerogenes*. They are not effective against *Proteus* or gram-positive organisms.

Combinations of bacitracin (or gramicidin), neomycin, and polymyxin B (eg, Mycitracin, Neo-Polycin, Neosporin,

Polyspectrin, Statrol) are widely used in ocular therapy because of their broad spectrum of activity, which includes *Pseudomonas.*

Erythromycin [Ilotycin] is well tolerated and is effective against many gram-positive organisms, including *Streptococcus pneumoniae, S. pyogenes,* and *Moraxella lacunata.* Staphylococci frequently are resistant to this antibiotic.

Chloramphenicol [Antibiopto, Chloromycetin, Chloroptic S.O.P., Econochlor] is a broad spectrum antibiotic which has been widely used for topical therapy because it rarely causes sensitization. It is not as effective as a bacitracin-neomycin-polymyxin B combination, however, and a controlled study failed to reveal a significant effect on the bacterial flora of the normal eye during long-term therapy. Two cases of bone marrow hypoplasia have been associated with the prolonged, uncontrolled use of chloramphenicol eyedrops. Systemic adverse reactions have not occurred after short-term topical ophthalmic use.

The aminoglycoside, gentamicin [Garamycin], is active against a wide variety of gram-negative and gram-positive organisms, and is particularly useful because of its significant activity against *Pseudomonas, Proteus, Klebsiella, E. coli,* and staphylococci. Since occasional strains of *Pseudomonas* are resistant to gentamicin, polymyxin B or colistin should be considered as additional therapy. Although not available commercially as ophthalmic preparations, tobramycin [Nebcin] and carbenicillin [Geopen, Pyopen] have been used topically to treat pseudomonal corneal ulcers.

The most common topical ophthalmic use of tetracycline [Achromycin] is in the treatment of infections caused by TRIC agent (trachoma and inclusion conjunctivitis). In trachoma, tetracycline or a sulfonamide is usually given concomitantly by the systemic route. The World Health Organization suggests a 21-day course of oral tetracyclines in children over 9 years of age in whom dentition is complete. Doxycycline [Vibramycin] is preferred because it need be administered only once daily. Although tetracyclines are not active sensitizers, antibiotics that are rarely used systemically are usually preferred for other external infections.

In addition to these commercial preparations, antibiotic eyedrops may be formulated from parenteral preparations by diluting the parenteral antibiotic with balanced salt solution or artificial tears and adjusting for isotonicity. The solubility and stability of antibiotics prepared in this manner may vary (Osborn et al, 1976).

Because of the danger of sensitization, penicillins should generally not be applied topically except for the treatment of a potentially perforating corneal ulcer that is highly responsive to the drug. Streptomycin also is an active sensitizer and should not be used topically.

See also Ellis, 1977; Havener, 1978; and Pettit, 1976.

Systemic Therapy: Intraocular infections and severe external ocular infections require intensive systemic therapy in addition to local administration. Because of its superior penetration and broad spectrum of activity, chloramphenicol was formerly considered to be the systemic drug of choice for treating intraocular infections. It is used less commonly today because of potential systemic toxicity and the availability of newer effective antibiotics. Ampicillin, dicloxacillin, lincomycin, cephalothin, and cephaloridine provide therapeutic levels in the aqueous humor when given in adequate doses. Many other agents that do not readily penetrate the normal eye will enter the inflamed eye because the blood-aqueous barrier is decreased by injury or inflammation; these include penicillin G, the penicillinase-resistant penicillins (methicillin, nafcillin, and oxacillin), erythromycin, gentamicin, kanamycin, and the polymyxins (polymyxin B and colistin). Some tetracyclines and streptomycin penetrate the eye poorly when given systemically and are, therefore, of limited usefulness in treating intraocular infections. The major use of streptomycin is in conjunction with isoniazid or aminosalicylic acid for the treatment of ocular tuberculosis. The acid-resistant penicillins do not produce sufficiently high blood levels to be useful in ophthalmology. Some of the newer antibiotics, such as the aminoglycoside, amikacin [Amikin], have not yet been studied to determine ocular penetration.

Penicillin G is preferred for treating intraocular infections caused by non-penicillinase-producing staphylococci, streptococci, pneumococci, gonococci, and clostridia. For resistant staphylococci, methicillin [Staphcillin] is the drug of first choice, as it is less protein-bound than nafcillin [Unipen] or oxacillin [Prostaphlin] and, therefore, enters the eye more readily. Other antibiotics used to treat intraocular infections caused by resistant staphylococci include the cephalosporins, clindamycin, gentamicin, tobramycin, and, occasionally, kanamycin.

The broad spectrum penicillins, ampicillin and carbenicillin [Geopen, Pyopen], are effective against many gram-positive and gram-negative organisms, although they are not active against penicillinase-producing staphylococci. Ampicillin readily penetrates the eye and is active against *H. influenzae* and some strains of *E. coli* but is ineffective against *Pseudomonas*. The antibacterial spectrum of carbenicillin is similar to that of ampicillin; however, carbenicillin is more useful in ophthalmology because of its activity against *Pseudomonas*, indole-positive *Proteus*, and some strains of *Enterobacter* that are not susceptible to ampicillin. Gentamicin [Garamycin] is usually given with carbenicillin in ocular pseudomonal infections. Because of their toxicity, polymyxin B [Aerosporin] and colistin [Coly-Mycin M] are used less commonly for systemic therapy than gentamicin and carbenicillin. Since gentamicin is also active against *Proteus, Klebsiella, E. coli*, and resistant staphylococci, it is often used with methicillin for the initial treatment of intraocular infections caused by unidentified organisms.

See also Apt, 1968; Ellis, 1977; Havener, 1978; Leopold, 1972; and Leopold and Kagan, 1974.

Antifungal Agents

Fungal infections of the eye occur most commonly after injury or surgery or when host resistance is decreased by severe systemic disorders (eg, diabetes mellitus), previous corneal disease, or prolonged therapy with immunosuppressive drugs or corticosteroids. The increased incidence of oculomycosis observed in recent years has been attributed to the widespread use of corticosteroids and, possibly, broad spectrum antibiotics.

Over 100 varieties of fungi have been identified as ocular pathogens. The fungi most frequently cultured from mycotic corneal ulcers are *Aspergillus* (usually *A. fumigatus*), *Fusarium* species, or *Candida albicans*. The antifungal drugs available in the United States for treating oculomycosis include nystatin, natamycin (pimaricin), amphotericin B, and flucytosine (see also Jones, 1975 and Lieberman, 1973).

Nystatin [Mycostatin, Nilstat] is used topically and by the subconjunctival route to treat external ocular infections caused by *Candida* or *Aspergillus*. It is of little or no value in other fungal infections. Generally, a suspension (25,000 units/ml) is applied every 15 minutes or the powder may be dusted on the lesion. Alternatively, a dermatologic ointment containing 100,000 units/g may be applied four times daily.

Natamycin (pimaricin) [Myprozine, Natcyn], a highly effective and well tolerated topical agent, has been used successfully to treat a variety of keratomycoses caused by *Fusarium* and *Cephalosporium* species. Because of its broad spectrum of activity, natamycin appears to be the drug of choice for initial antifungal therapy. The suspension is applied every one or two hours. Both natamycin and nystatin penetrate the eye poorly.

Amphotericin B [Fungizone] has significant activity against various fungi, particularly *Candida, Coccidioides, Cryptococcus, Histoplasma, Blastomyces*, and *Sporotrichum*. It is given intravenously to treat fungal endophthalmitis. Intraocular penetration is poor when amphotericin B is administered systemically and large doses must be used, thereby increasing the risk of hepatic and renal toxicity. The patient should be hospitalized if the drug is given systemically. Amphotericin B may also be given by the topical and subconjunctival routes to treat fungal corneal ulcers. It is usually well tolerated when given topically in a concentration of 1.5 mg/ml or by the subconjunctival route in a dose of 1 to 2 mg. Stronger concentrations may cause severe local irritation and, with subconjunctival injection, yellowing of the conjunctiva and formation of nodules. Amphotericin B does not penetrate well when applied topically.

Flucytosine [Ancobon] is a relatively nontoxic antifungal agent that is administered orally. It has not been widely used in ophthalmology but appears to be useful in ocular infections caused by *Candida albicans* or *Cryptococcus neoformans*. Because resistant strains may develop, concomitant administration of amphotericin B has been recommended. Flucytosine also has been used topically (product not available commercially) in a 1% to 1.5% concentration for treatment of mycotic surface infections of the eye. This agent also penetrates the eye poorly when applied topically.

Antiviral Agents

Idoxuridine (IDU) [Dendrid, Herplex, Stoxil] is used topically to treat herpes simplex infections of the lids, conjunctiva, and cornea. It improves the course of acute dendritic keratitis and also may be of value in controlling recurrences if the infection is confined to the epithelium. One drop of the solution is instilled every hour during the day and every two hours at night. Alternatively, the ointment may be applied four or five times daily or as nighttime medication when the solution is used during the day. Treatment should be continued for at least two weeks. Idoxuridine does not penetrate the cornea and has no proved effectiveness in cases of iritis or deep stromal involvement of the cornea. If stromal keratitis is treated with a topical corticosteroid, however, idoxuridine should be given concomitantly to prevent reactivation of the epithelial infection. The drug also has been used to treat vaccinia infections of the eye.

Adverse effects include local irritation (toxic and/or allergic), photophobia, edema of the eyelids and cornea, punctal occlusion, and small punctate defects in the corneal epithelium. This agent may interfere with corneal epithelial regeneration and inhibit stromal healing.

The antimetabolite, vidarabine (adenine arabinoside) [Vira-A], was originally developed as an antineoplastic agent but has been found to be effective for topical treatment of ocular herpes simplex. In previously untreated patients, vidarabine is similar to idoxuridine in efficacy and toxicity. However, there appears to be little cross resistance or cross sensitivity between the two agents, and patients allergic or resistant to idoxuridine may respond to vidarabine. Combined idoxuridine-vidarabine topical therapy is currently under investigation. Studies are also in progress to evaluate the effect of intravenous vidarabine in patients with stromal herpes and iritis.

Idoxuridine and vidarabine are the only antiviral agents that are commercially available in the United States for treating ocular herpes simplex infections. Some promising investigational agents include trifluridine [Viroptic] and interferon. Trifluridine is administered topically to treat herpetic keratitis. It is more soluble than idoxuridine and may be more effective in stromal disease. Human interferon, given topically once or twice daily, may prove to be useful in preventing recurrent attacks of herpes (Kaufman, 1976).

Antiseptics and Preservatives

Before the advent of antibiotics and sulfonamides, ocular infections were treated with a variety of antiseptics and germicides such as silver nitrate, mild silver protein [Argyrol], copper sulfate, zinc sulfate, thimerosal [Merthiolate], merbromin [Mercurochrome], yellow mercuric oxide, ammoniated mercury, nitromersol [Metaphen], acriflavine [Neutroflavine], benzalkonium chloride, boric acid, and iodine. Some of these agents are no longer used to treat ocular disease because of ineffectiveness or local toxicity, but others still have limited ophthalmic use.

Benzalkonium chloride, thimerosal sodium, and chlorobutanol are widely used as preservatives for eyedrops; benzalkonium chloride also is used to enhance the corneal penetration of drugs and to cleanse the skin and irrigate the eye prior to surgery. Preservatives may cause local adverse reactions, most commonly contact dermatitis. When instilled in the rabbit eye in concentrations up to 2%, chlorobutanol and thimerosal have shown no significant cytotoxic effect, but benzalkonium chloride has produced corneal damage following intensive application (three times an hour for six hours) of a 0.05% concentration. Studies are currently in progress to evaluate possible adverse effects on the corneal endothelium of long-term application of benzalkonium chloride. Benzalkonium chloride is most commonly used in ophthalmic preparations in a 0.01% concentration (or 0.004% in combination with EDTA).

Local application of silver nitrate is legally required in most states for prophylaxis of gonorrheal ophthalmia neonatorum. Although silver nitrate may cause severe local irritation, most authorities feel that it has stood the test of time and should continue to be used in a 1% solution (preferably packaged in wax ampuls) as the prophylactic agent of choice. If an alternate agent is required, bacitracin ointment is considered the drug of second choice. Antibiotics commonly used systemically are not recommended for prophylaxis, but may be used for treatment of ophthalmia neonatorum.

Mild silver protein will color conjunctival secretions, thereby aiding in their identification and removal during preoperative cleansing of the eye. Zinc sulfate, usually in combination with phenylephrine, is sometimes used to treat minor ocular irritations but it is a relatively ineffective antiseptic. Boric acid also has little merit as an antiseptic, but is extensively (and ineffectively) used by the laity as an eyewash.

ANTI-INFLAMMATORY AGENTS

Indications and Routes of Administration: Adrenal corticosteroids are used in the treatment of ocular inflammatory disorders to control inflammation and thereby reduce the amount of permanent scarring and prevent visual loss. They are generally more effective in acute than in chronic conditions. Steroid therapy is useful in the treatment of ocular allergic disorders (eg, vernal conjunctivitis, contact dermatitis of the lids and conjunctiva, allergic blepharitis and conjunctivitis), corneal burns, sterile uveal tract inflammation (iritis, iridocyclitis, posterior uveitis), episcleritis, scleritis, and temporal arteritis. Their value has not been clearly established in optic neuritis.

Corticosteroids are useful in treating postoperative iridocyclitis, but the benefits of prophylactic use must be weighed against their potential adverse effects, ie, delayed healing, increased susceptibility to or masking of postoperative infection, and increased incidence of filtering blebs after cataract surgery. They do not significantly reduce the incidence of uveitis or choroidal detachment following retinal detachment surgery.

Corticosteroids generally should be avoided in most ocular infections because the course of the disease may be worsened by weakening of bodily defense mechanisms. Exceptions are herpes zoster infections and Thygeson's superficial punctate keratitis, which may benefit from steroid therapy. Corticosteroids also may be indicated (with appropriate anti-infective therapy) in other ocular infections if vision is seriously threatened by the acute inflammatory response or stromal edema.

Topical corticosteroid therapy is usually effective in controlling inflammations of the lids, conjunctiva, cornea, and anterior sclera. Cortisone (rarely used), cortisol [Hydrocortone, Optef], dexamethasone [Decadron, Maxidex], fluorometholone [FML], medrysone [HMS], and prednisolone are available as drops or ointment for topical ophthalmic use (see Table 2 and list of preparations at end of chapter). Cortisol, medrysone, and weak concentrations of prednisolone (0.125%) are particularly useful for treating superficial inflammatory conditions (eg, allergic conjunctivitis). These agents do not readily penetrate the eye and have relatively weak anti-inflammatory activity; therefore, they rarely increase the intraocular pressure in susceptible individuals. Prednisolone and dexamethasone penetrate the cornea and aqueous following topical administration and are preferred for treating corneal inflammatory disorders and anterior uveitis. Fluorometholone also may be useful in the treatment of anterior segment inflammation, but it may not penetrate the eye as readily as dexamethasone or prednisolone. In the concentrations available in ophthalmic preparations, all three agents may increase the intraocular pressure, but dexamethasone has the most pronounced ocular hypertensive effect.

Ophthalmologists also inject solutions or suspensions of corticosteroids by the subconjunctival route to supplement topical therapy in resistant inflammations; for a more prolonged action, the repository form of methylprednisolone or triamcinolone acetonide is used. Anterior uveitis can sometimes be controlled by topical and subconjunctival therapy, but often steroids or corticotropin also must be given systemically. Inflammatory disorders of the posterior segment of the globe (eg, posterior uveitis, scleritis) usually require both systemic and subconjunctival therapy. Occasionally, steroids are administered by retrobulbar injection to treat posterior segment inflammation. (See also Ellis, 1977.)

Nonsteroidal anti-inflammatory agents have occasionally been used to treat ocular inflammations. An ophthalmic preparation of the antiasthmatic drug, cromolyn, is currently under investigation and appears to be particularly useful for treating vernal blepharoconjunctivitis. Immunosuppressive and antineoplastic agents have been used effectively in some patients with severe inflammatory disorders refractory to steroids, but their usefulness is limited because of their toxicity. There has been considerable recent interest in the role of prostaglandins in ocular inflammation and the effect of agents that inhibit their synthesis or release. Aspirin and indomethacin, which inhibit prostaglandin synthesis,

TABLE 2.
CORTICOSTEROIDS FOR TOPICAL OPHTHALMIC THERAPY

Agent	Concentration	
	Solution or Suspension*	Ointment†
Cortisol	0.2%, 0.5%	
Cortisol Acetate		0.5%, 1.5%
Cortisone Acetate		1.5%
Dexamethasone	0.1%	
Dexamethasone Sodium Phosphate	0.1%	0.05%
Fluorometholone	0.1%	
Medrysone	1%	
Prednisolone Acetate	0.125%, 0.25%	
Prednisolone Sodium Phosphate	0.125% to 1%	0.25%

*Drops are applied every one or two hours until a response is obtained; the frequency is then reduced.
†Ointments are applied three or four times daily or as nighttime medication.
See also Ellis, 1977.

occasionally have been used to treat uveitis and episcleritis with questionable efficacy. A number of newer agents have been developed and some of these may prove to be useful in treating ocular inflammatory disorders (Burns et al, 1976; Leopold, 1974).

Adverse Reactions and Precautions: Topically applied corticosteroids may cause discomfort, burning, and lacrimation; mydriasis, loss of accommodation, and ptosis occasionally follow local use. Although the severe adverse reactions associated with systemic therapy (see Chapter 41) occur only rarely with topical application, corticosteroid eyedrops are absorbed in amounts sufficient to cause partial adrenal suppression in adults and may lead to development of Cushing's syndrome in young children.

Serious local complications are not infrequent. The corticosteroids are potentially toxic agents and never should be used to treat minor disorders or conditions that can be controlled by safer drugs. They always should be given in the lowest effective concentration, and long-term use should be avoided whenever possible. After prolonged use in some chronic conditions, exacerbation of the disease may occur if the corticosteroid is discontinued abruptly; therefore, the interval between applications should be lengthened gradually.

Corticosteroids lower resistance to infection and, by reducing inflammation, can mask the symptoms of serious ocular disease. When used alone or with antibiotics, topical corticosteroids may increase susceptibility to fungal infections, particularly when the corneal epithelium has been damaged by injury, surgery, or infection. These agents also worsen the course of ocular herpes simplex infections. In the initial stages of dendritic keratitis, the nature of the infection may not be recognized without slit-lamp magnification. If corticosteroids or steroid-antibiotic combinations containing inappropriate or ineffective anti-infectives are prescribed, the eye may appear to improve while the infection is spreading; eventually the deeper corneal structures become involved and the cornea may perforate. Other ocular diseases that

may be activated or worsened by the use of corticosteroids are vaccinia and *Pseudomonas* infections, trachoma, and ocular tuberculosis. (See also Havener, 1978.)

Repeated local administration of corticosteroids may increase intraocular pressure by reducing the facility of outflow of aqueous humor. This response is genetically determined and occurs most frequently in patients with primary open-angle glaucoma and in their relatives and is also common in myopes and diabetics. The rise in pressure is not accompanied by pain and the condition usually is reversible if detected before damage to the optic nerve has occurred.

The magnitude of the ocular hypertensive response to steroids is related to concentration, frequency of administration, duration of treatment, the drug used, and individual susceptibility. A rise in pressure has been reported most frequently after administration of a 0.1% concentration of dexamethasone. A clinically significant increase in intraocular pressure is rare with medrysone, fluorometholone, cortisol, or weaker concentrations of more potent steroids (eg, 0.01% dexamethasone). Intraocular pressure should be determined every two months in patients receiving prolonged topical corticosteroid therapy. Long-term administration should be avoided, especially in patients with primary open-angle glaucoma and in their relatives, in myopes, and in diabetics. Increased intraocular pressure is uncommon with systemic therapy. (See also Cantrill et al, 1975 and Podos and Becker, 1972.)

Posterior subcapsular cataracts have developed in some patients during long-term corticosteroid therapy. This complication was first noted in patients receiving large systemic doses but has also been associated with long-term topical use. Very early lens changes may regress when steroids are discontinued but, if the opacities are more distinct, regression is uncommon. Regression is more likely to occur after topical therapy is discontinued than after systemic therapy is stopped.

Topical corticosteroid therapy has rarely been associated with the development of acute anterior uveitis in individuals (primarily blacks) with no history of pre-existing ocular inflammation or infection. This "corticosteroid-induced uveitis" was usually accompanied by a fall in intraocular pressure and, in a few cases, was associated with a mild conjunctival reaction in the untreated eye. No permanent ocular damage was observed.

Topical corticosteroid preparations should be used sparingly in any conditions that cause thinning of the cornea, as perforation may occur.

STEROID-ANTIBACTERIAL MIXTURES

Mixtures containing a corticosteroid in fixed-dose combination with an antibacterial agent are used by ophthalmologists to treat certain conditions in which both anti-inflammatory and anti-infective activity are required. These include marginal keratitis secondary to staphylococcal infection, blepharoconjunctivitis, allergic conjunctivitis with chronic bacterial conjunctivitis, phlyctenular keratoconjunctivitis, and selected cases of postoperative inflammation.

These mixtures are not indicated for the routine treatment of ocular infections or inflammatory disorders. Corticosteroids reduce resistance to infection, and combined therapy may have an adverse effect on the course of ocular disease if the antibacterial agent is not effective against the invading organism, if it is not present in sufficient concentration, or if nonsusceptible organisms (particularly fungi and viruses) are present. In addition, hypersensitivity may develop to the anti-infective agent, and the corticosteroid may mask the allergic response.

TOPICAL OPHTHALMIC PREPARATIONS

Antibacterial Agents

BACITRACIN:
Drug available generically: Ointment 500 units/g in 3.5 g containers.
Baciguent (Upjohn). Ointment (sterile) 500 units/g with white petrolatum, anhydrous lanolin, and mineral oil in 3.5 g containers.

CHLORAMPHENICOL:
Antibiopto (Professional Pharmacal). Ointment (sterile) 1% in mineral oil and polyethylene in 3.5 g containers; solution (sterile) 0.5% with boric acid, sodium borate, and sodium hydroxide in 7.5 ml containers.
Chloromycetin (Parke, Davis). Ointment 1% with mineral oil and polyethylene in 3.5 g containers; powder 25 mg with boric acid, sodium borate, and (if necessary) sodium hydroxide and 15 ml of diluent.
Chloroptic S.O.P. (Allergan). Ointment (sterile) 1% with chlorobutanol 0.5%, white petrolatum, mineral oil, polyoxyl 40 stearate, polyethylene glycol 300, and nonionic lanolin derivatives in 3.5 g containers; solution 0.5% with chlorobutanol 0.5%, polyethylene glycol 300, polyoxyl 40 stearate, and sodium hydroxide or hydrochloric acid in 7.5 ml containers.
Econochlor (Alcon). Ointment (sterile) 1% with mineral oil, anhydrous liquid lanolin, and white petrolatum in 3.5 g containers; solution (sterile) 0.5% with thimerosal 0.01%, hydroxypropyl methylcellulose, boric acid, and sodium borate in 2.5 and 15 ml containers.

COLISTIN SULFATE:
Coly-Mycin S (Professional Pharmacal). Lyophilized powder for solution (sterile) equivalent to 9.6 mg colistin base. [Product distributed to physicians by manufacturer only.]

ERYTHROMYCIN:
Ilotycin (Dista). Ointment (sterile) 0.5% with mineral oil and white petrolatum in ⅛ oz containers.

GENTAMICIN SULFATE:
Garamycin (Schering). Ointment (sterile) equivalent to 3 mg/g of gentamicin with disodium phosphate, monosodium phosphate, sodium chloride, and benzalkonium chloride in ⅛ oz containers; solution (sterile) equivalent to 3 mg/ml of gentamicin with disodium phosphate, monosodium phosphate, sodium chloride, and benzalkonium chloride in 5 ml containers.

NEOMYCIN SULFATE:
Myciguent (Upjohn). Ointment 5 mg/g with anhydrous lanolin, chlorobutanol 0.5%, mineral oil, and white petrolatum in ⅛ oz containers.

SILVER NITRATE:
Drug available generically: Solution 1%.

SULFACETAMIDE SODIUM:
Drug available generically: Ointment 10% in ⅛ oz containers; solution 10% and 30% in 15 ml containers and 15% in 2 ml containers.
Bleph-10, -30 Liquifilm (Allergan). Solution (sterile) 10% or 30% with polyvinyl alcohol 1.4%, polysorbate 80, thimerosal 0.005%, sodium thiosulfate, potassium phosphate monobasic, edetate disodium, sodium phosphate dibasic anhydrous, and hydrochloric acid in 5 (10% solution only) and 15 ml containers.

Cetamide (Alcon). Ointment (sterile) 10% in white petrolatum, anhydrous liquid lanolin, and mineral oil with methylparaben and propylparaben in 3.5 g containers.

Isopto Cetamide (Alcon). Solution (sterile) 15% with hydroxypropyl methylcellulose 0.5%, sodium thiosulfate 0.3%, methylparaben 0.05%, propylparaben 0.01%, and dried sodium phosphate and/or sodium biphosphate in 5 and 15 ml containers.

Sodium Sulamyd (Schering). Ointment (sterile) 10% with methylparaben 0.5 mg, propylparaben 0.1 mg, benzalkonium chloride 0.25 mg, sorbitan monolaurate, and petrolatum in 3.5 g containers; solution (sterile) 10% and 30% with methylcellulose 5 mg (10% solution only), methylparaben 0.5 mg, propylparaben 0.1 mg, sodium thiosulfate 1.5 or 3.1 mg, and sodium dihydrogen phosphate in 5 (10% solution only) and 15 ml containers.

Sulfacel-15 (Professional Pharmacal). Solution (sterile) 15% with methylcellulose, sodium thiosulfate, monobasic and dibasic sodium phosphate, propylene glycol, methylparaben 0.05%, and propylparaben 0.01% in 5 and 15 ml containers.

Vasosulf (SMP). Solution (sterile) containing sodium sulfacetamide 15% and phenylephrine hydrochloride 0.125% with methylparaben, propylparaben, sodium thiosulfate, monobasic and dibasic sodium phosphate, and hydrochloric acid in 5 and 15 ml containers.

SULFISOXAZOLE DIOLAMINE:

Gantrisin (Roche). Ointment (sterile) 4% with white petrolatum, mineral oil, and phenylmercuric acid 1:50,000 in ⅛ oz containers; solution (sterile) 4% with phenylmercuric acid 1:100,000 in 15 ml containers.

TETRACYCLINE HYDROCHLORIDE:

Achromycin (Lederle). Ointment (sterile) 1% with anhydrous lanolin and petrolatum in ⅛ oz containers; suspension in oil (sterile) 1% with light mineral oil and polyethylene resin in 4 ml containers.

Antibacterial Mixtures

Chloromyxin (Parke, Davis). Each gram of ointment (sterile) contains chloramphenicol 1% and polymyxin B as the sulfate 5,000 units with mineral oil and polyethylene in 3.5 g containers.

Mycitracin Ophthalmic Ointment (Upjohn). Each gram of ointment (sterile) contains polymyxin B sulfate 5,000 units, neomycin sulfate 5 mg, and bacitracin 500 units with chlorobutanol 0.5%, anhydrous lanolin, mineral oil, and white petrolatum in ⅛ oz containers.

Neo-Polycin Ophthalmic (Dow). Each gram of ointment (sterile) contains polymyxin B sulfate

10,000 units, neomycin sulfate equivalent to neomycin 3.5 mg, and bacitracin zinc 500 units with chlorobutanol 5 mg, white petrolatum, and mineral oil in ⅛ oz containers; each milliliter of solution (sterile) contains polymyxin B sulfate 5,000 units, neomycin sulfate equivalent to neomycin 1.75 mg, and gramicidin 0.025 mg with thimerosal 0.01 mg, polyoxyalkylene diol, hydrochloric acid, sodium chloride, and alcohol 0.5% in 10 ml containers.

Neosporin (Burroughs Wellcome). Each gram of ointment (sterile) contains polymyxin B sulfate 5,000 units, neomycin sulfate 5 mg (equivalent to 3.5 mg of the base), and bacitracin zinc 400 units with white petrolatum in ⅛ oz containers; each milliliter of solution (sterile) contains polymyxin B sulfate 5,000 units, neomycin sulfate 2.5 mg (equivalent to 1.75 mg of the base), and gramicidin 0.025 mg with alcohol 0.5%, propylene glycol, polyoxyethylene polyoxypropylene compound, sodium chloride, and thimerosal 0.001% in 10 ml containers.

Polyspectrin (Allergan). Each gram of ointment (sterile) contains bacitracin zinc 400 units, polymyxin B sulfate 5,000 units, and neomycin sulfate 5 mg (equivalent to 3.5 mg of the base) with chlorobutanol 0.5%, white petrolatum, and mineral oil in 3.5 g containers; each milliliter of solution (sterile) contains polymyxin B sulfate 5,000 units and neomycin sulfate 0.5% (equivalent to 0.35% of the base) with polyvinyl alcohol 1.4%, thimerosal 1:100,000, propylene glycol, and sodium acetate in 10 ml containers.

Polysporin Ophthalmic Ointment (Burroughs Wellcome). Each gram of ointment (sterile) contains polymyxin B sulfate 10,000 units and bacitracin zinc 500 units with petrolatum base in ⅛ oz containers.

Pyocidin Ophthalmic Ointment (SMP). Each gram of ointment contains polymyxin B sulfate 5,000 units, neomycin sulfate 5 mg (equivalent to 3.5 mg of the base), and bacitracin zinc 400 units with white petrolatum and mineral oil base in ⅛ oz containers.

Statrol (Alcon). Each gram of ointment (sterile) contains neomycin sulfate equivalent to neomycin 3.5 mg and polymyxin B sulfate 6,000 units with methylparaben 0.05%, propylparaben 0.01%, white petrolatum, and anhydrous liquid lanolin in 3.5 g containers; each milliliter of solution (sterile) contains neomycin sulfate (equivalent to 3.5 mg of the base) and polymyxin B sulfate 16,250 units with hydroxypropyl methylcellulose, benzalkonium chloride 0.004%, boric acid, sodium chloride, hydrochloric acid, and/or sodium hydroxide in 5 ml containers.

Terramycin w/Polymyxin B Sulfate (Pfizer). Each gram of ointment (sterile) contains polymyxin B sulfate 10,000 units and oxytetracycline hydrochloride 5 mg with white petrolatum and mineral oil in ⅛ oz containers.

Antifungal Agents

NATAMYCIN:
Myprozine (Lederle). Suspension 5%.
Natcyn (Alcon). Suspension 5% with benzalkonium chloride 0.02% and sodium hydroxide and/or hydrochloric acid in 3.5 g containers.

Antiviral Agents

IDOXURIDINE:
Dendrid (Alcon). Solution 0.1% with benzalkonium chloride 0.004%, phenylmercuric nitrate, and boric acid in 15 ml containers.
Herplex Liquifilm (Allergan). Solution (sterile) 0.1% with polyvinyl alcohol 1.4%, benzalkonium chloride, sodium chloride, edetate disodium, and purified water in 15 ml containers.
Stoxil (Smith Kline & French). Ointment 0.5% in white petrolatum and mineral oil in 4 g containers; solution 0.1% with thimerosal 1:50,000 in 15 ml containers.
VIDARABINE:
Vira-A (Parke, Davis). Ointment (sterile) 3% in 3.5 g containers.

Corticosteroids

CORTISOL:
Drug available generically: Ointment 0.5% in ⅛ oz containers.
Optef Drops (Upjohn). Solution (sterile) 0.2% with chlorobutanol anhydrous 0.5% and tyloxapol in 2.5 ml containers.
CORTISOL ACETATE:
Drug available generically: Ointment 0.5% in 3.5 g containers.
Hydrocortone Acetate (Merck Sharp & Dohme). Ointment (sterile) 1.5% with white petrolatum and mineral oil in 3.5 g containers.
CORTISONE ACETATE:
Drug available generically: Ointment 1.5% in ⅛ oz containers.
DEXAMETHASONE:
Maxidex (Alcon). Suspension (sterile) 0.1% with benzalkonium chloride 0.01%, hydroxypropyl methylcellulose 0.5%, dried sodium phosphate, polysorbate 80, edetate disodium, sodium chloride, and citric acid in 5 and 15 ml containers.
DEXAMETHASONE SODIUM PHOSPHATE:
Drug available generically: Solution 1% in 5 ml containers.
Decadron Phosphate (Merck Sharp & Dohme). Ointment (sterile) 0.05% with white petrolatum and mineral oil in 3.5 g containers; solution (sterile) 0.1% with creatinine, sodium citrate, sodium borate, polysorbate 80, sodium hydroxide, sodium bisulfite 0.32%, phenylethanol 0.25%, and benzalkonium chloride 0.02% in 2.5 and 5 ml containers.

Maxidex (Alcon). Ointment (sterile) 0.05% (dexamethasone sodium equivalent) with mineral oil and white petrolatum in 3.5 g containers.
FLUOROMETHOLONE:
FML (Allergan). Suspension (sterile) 0.1% with polyvinyl alcohol 1.4%, benzalkonium chloride, edetate disodium, sodium chloride, sodium phosphate monobasic monohydrate, sodium phosphate dibasic anhydrous, polysorbate 80, and (if necessary) sodium hydroxide in 5 and 10 ml containers.
MEDRYSONE:
HMS (Allergan). Suspension (sterile) 1% with polyvinyl alcohol 1.4%, benzalkonium chloride, edetate disodium, sodium chloride, potassium chloride, sodium phosphate monobasic monohydrate, sodium phosphate dibasic anhydrous, hydroxypropylmethylcellulose, and (if necessary) sodium hydroxide or hydrochloric acid in 5 and 10 ml containers.
PREDNISOLONE ACETATE:
Econopred, Econopred Plus (Alcon). Suspension (sterile) 0.125% (Econopred) or 1% (Econopred Plus) with hydroxpropyl methylcellulose, dried sodium phosphate, polysorbate 80, benzalkonium chloride 0.01%, edetate disodium, glycerin, and citric acid in 5 and 10 ml containers.
Pred Mild, Pred Forte (Allergan). Suspension (sterile) 0.125% (Mild) or 1% (Forte) with benzalkonium chloride, polysorbate 80, boric acid, sodium citrate, sodium bisulfite, sodium chloride, edetate disodium, and hydroxypropyl methylcellulose in 5 and 10 ml containers.
Predulose (Professional Pharmacal). Suspension (sterile) 0.25% and phenylephrine hydrochloride 0.125% with methylcellulose, methylparaben 0.04%, propylparaben 0.02%, propylene glycol, sodium phosphate monobasic and dibasic, sodium thiosulfate, and polysorbate 80 in 5 ml containers.
PREDNISOLONE SODIUM PHOSPHATE:
Hydeltrasol (Merck Sharp & Dohme). Ointment (sterile) 0.25% (prednisolone phosphate equivalent) with white petrolatum and mineral oil in 3.5 g containers; solution (sterile) equivalent to 0.5% prednisolone phosphate with creatinine, sodium citrate, polysorbate 80, edetate disodium, potassium phosphate, hydrochloric acid, phenylethanol 0.25%, and benzalkonium chloride 0.02% in 5 ml containers.
Inflamase (SMP). Solution (sterile) 0.125% and 1% (Forte) (equivalent to 0.1% and 0.8% prednisolone, respectively) with benzalkonium chloride 0.01%, edetate disodium, monobasic and dibasic sodium phosphate, and sodium chloride in 5 ml containers.
Metreton (Schering). Solution (sterile) 0.5% (prednisolone phosphate equivalent) with disodium edetate, monobasic and dibasic sodium phosphate, tyloxapol, sodium hydroxide, benzalkonium chloride, and phenylethyl alcohol in 5 ml containers.

Corticosteroid-Antibacterial Mixtures

CHLORAMPHENICOL AND STEROID:

Chloromycetin-Hydrocortisone Ophthalmic Liquid (Parke, Davis). Each 5 ml contains chloramphenicol 12.5 mg and cortisol acetate 25 mg with boric acid-sodium borate buffer, cholesterol, methylcellulose, sodium chloride, and benzethonium chloride in 5 ml containers.

Chloroptic-P S.O.P. (Allergan). Ophthalmic ointment (sterile) containing chloramphenicol 1% and prednisolone alcohol 0.5% with chlorobutanol 0.5%, white petrolatum, mineral oil, polyoxyl 40 stearate, polyethylene glycol 300, and nonionic lanolin derivatives in 3.5 g containers.

CHLORAMPHENICOL, POLYMYXIN B, AND STEROID:

Ophthocort (Parke, Davis). Each gram of ophthalmic ointment (sterile) contains chloramphenicol 1%, polymyxin B sulfate 5,000 units, and cortisol acetate 0.5% with mineral oil and polyethylene in 3.5 g containers.

NEOMYCIN AND STEROID:

Cor-Oticin (Maurry). Each milliliter of suspension contains neomycin sulfate 5 mg (equivalent to 3.5 mg of the base) and cortisol acetate 15 mg with polysorbate 80, carboxymethylcellulose, sodium metabisulfite, and chlorobutanol 0.5% in 5 ml containers.

Neo-Cortef Ophthalmic (Upjohn). Each milliliter of suspension (sterile) contains neomycin sulfate 5 mg (equivalent to 3.5 mg of the base) and cortisol acetate 5 or 15 mg with myristyl-gamma-picolinium chloride, sodium citrate, polyethylene glycol 4000, povidone, and sodium hydroxide and/or hydrochloric acid in 2.5 ml (15 mg cortisol acetate only) and 5 ml containers; each gram of ophthalmic ointment (sterile) contains neomycin sulfate 5 mg and cortisol acetate 5 or 15 mg with anhydrous lanolin, mineral oil, white petrolatum, and chlorobutanol 0.5% in ⅛ oz containers.

Neo-Decadron Ophthalmic (Merck Sharp & Dohme). Each gram of ointment (sterile) contains neomycin sulfate (equivalent to 3.5 mg of the base) and dexamethasone sodium phosphate (equivalent to dexamethasone phosphate 0.5 mg) with white petrolatum and mineral oil in 3.5 g containers; each milliliter of solution (sterile) contains neomycin sulfate (equivalent to 3.5 mg of the base) and dexamethasone sodium phosphate (equivalent to dexamethasone phosphate 1 mg) with creatinine, sodium citrate, sodium borate, polysorbate 80, sodium hydroxide, benzalkonium chloride 0.02%, and sodium bisulfite 0.32% in 2.5 and 5 ml containers.

Neo-Delta-Cortef Ophthalmic (Upjohn). Each gram of ointment (sterile) contains neomycin sulfate 5 mg (equivalent to 3.5 mg of the base) and prednisolone acetate 2.5 or 5 mg with anhydrous lanolin, mineral oil, white petro-latum, and chlorobutanol 0.5% in 3.5 g containers; each milliliter of suspension (sterile) contains neomycin sulfate 5 mg (equivalent to 3.5 mg of the base) and prednisolone acetate 2.5 mg with myristyl-gamma-picolinium chloride, sodium citrate, polyethylene glycol 4000, povidone, and sodium hydroxide and/or hydrochloric acid in 5 ml containers.

Neo-Hydeltrasol (Merck Sharp & Dohme). Each gram of ointment (sterile) contains neomycin sulfate equivalent to neomycin 3.5 mg and prednisolone sodium phosphate equivalent to prednisolone phosphate 2.5 mg with white petrolatum and mineral oil in 3.5 g containers; each milliliter of solution (sterile) contains neomycin sulfate equivalent to neomycin 3.5 mg and prednisolone sodium phosphate equivalent to prednisolone phosphate 5 mg with creatinine, sodium citrate, polysorbate 80, edetate disodium, potassium phosphate, hydrochloric acid, and benzalkonium chloride 0.02% in 2.5 and 5 ml containers.

Neo-Medrol Ophthalmic Ointment (Upjohn). Each gram of ointment (sterile) contains neomycin sulfate 5 mg (equivalent to 3.5 mg of the base) and methylprednisolone 1 mg with anhydrous lanolin, mineral oil, white petrolatum, and chlorobutanol 0.5% in 3.5 g containers.

Neosone Ophthalmic Ointment (Upjohn). Each gram of ointment contains neomycin sulfate 5 mg (equivalent to 3.5 mg of the base) and cortisone acetate 15 mg in ⅛ oz containers.

NEOMYCIN, POLYMYXIN B, AND STEROID:

Cortisporin Ophthalmic (Burroughs Wellcome). Each milliliter of suspension (sterile) contains neomycin sulfate 5 mg (equivalent to 3.5 mg of the base), polymyxin B sulfate 10,000 units, and cortisol 10 mg with thimerosal 0.001%, cetyl alcohol, glyceryl monostearate, mineral oil, polyoxyl 40 stearate, and propylene glycol in 5 ml containers; each gram of ointment (sterile) contains neomycin sulfate 5 mg (equivalent to 3.5 mg of the base), polymyxin B sulfate 5,000 units, bacitracin zinc 400 units, and cortisol 10 mg with white petrolatum in ⅛ oz containers.

Maxitrol (Alcon). Each gram of ointment (sterile) contains neomycin sulfate equivalent to 3.5 mg of the base, polymyxin B sulfate 6,000 units, and dexamethasone 0.1% with white petrolatum, anhydrous liquid lanolin, methylparaben, and propylparaben in 3.5 g containers; each milliliter of suspension (sterile) contains neomycin sulfate equivalent to 3.5 mg of the base, polymyxin B sulfate 6,000 units, and dexamethasone 0.1% with hydroxypropyl methylcellulose, sodium chloride, polysorbate 20, hydrochloric acid and/or sodium hydroxide, and benzalkonium chloride 0.004% in 5 ml containers.

SULFACETAMIDE SODIUM AND STEROID:

Blephamide Liquifilm (Allergan). Ophthalmic suspension (sterile) containing sulfacetamide sodium 10% and prednisolone acetate 0.2% with phenylephrine hydrochloride 0.12%, polyvinyl alcohol 1.4%, phenylmercuric nitrate 0.004%, antipyrine 0.1%, polysorbate 80, edetate disodium, sodium phosphate monobasic and dibasic anhydrous, sodium thiosulfate, and hydrochloric acid in 5 and 10 ml containers.

Blephamide S.O.P. (Allergan). Ophthalmic ointment (sterile) containing sodium sulfacetamide 10% and prednisolone acetate 0.2% with phenylmercuric acetate 0.0008%, mineral oil, white petrolatum, and nonionic lanolin derivatives in 3.5 g containers.

Cetapred (Alcon). Each gram of ophthalmic ointment (sterile) contains sulfacetamide sodium 10% and prednisolone acetate 0.25% with white petrolatum, anhydrous liquid lanolin, mineral oil, methylparaben 0.05%, and propylparaben 0.01% in 3.5 g containers.

Isopto Cetapred (Alcon). Ophthalmic suspension (sterile) containing sulfacetamide sodium 10% and prednisolone acetate 0.25% with hydroxypropyl methylcellulose 0.5%, methylparaben 0.05%, propylparaben 0.01%, sodium thiosulfate 0.1%, sodium biphosphate, benzalkonium chloride 0.025%, dried sodium phosphate, polysorbate 80, edetate disodium, and hydrochloric acid and/or sodium hydroxide in 5 and 15 ml containers.

Metimyd (Schering). Each milliliter of suspension (sterile) contains sulfacetamide sodium 100 mg and prednisolone acetate 5 mg with phenylethyl alcohol, benzalkonium chloride 0.25 mg, disodium dihydrogen and hydrogen phosphate, tyloxapol, sodium thiosulfate, and edetate disodium in 5 ml containers; each gram of ointment (sterile) contains sulfacetamide sodium 100 mg and prednisolone acetate 5 mg with white petrolatum, mineral oil, methylparaben 0.5 mg, and propylparaben 0.1 mg in ⅛ oz containers.

Optimyd (Schering). Ophthalmic solution (sterile) containing sulfacetamide sodium 10% and prednisolone sodium phosphate equivalent to prednisolone phosphate 0.5% with sodium thiosulfate, edetate disodium, monobasic and dibasic sodium phosphate, sodium hydroxide, benzalkonium chloride 0.025%, phenylethyl alcohol 0.05%, and tyloxapol in 5 ml containers.

Sulfapred (Professional Pharmacal). Ophthalmic suspension (sterile) containing sulfacetamide sodium 10%, prednisolone acetate 0.25%, and phenylephrine hydrochloride 0.125% with propylene glycol, monobasic and dibasic sodium phosphate, sodium thiosulfate, polysorbate 80, methylcellulose, methylparaben 0.04%, and propylparaben 0.02% in 5 and 15 ml containers.

Vasocidin (SMP). Ophthalmic solution (sterile) containing sulfacetamide sodium 10%, prednisolone sodium phosphate 0.25% (equivalent to prednisolone 0.2%), and phenylephrine hydrochloride 0.125% with methylparaben, propylparaben, sodium thiosulfate, polyoxyethylene polyoxypropylene compound, and polysorbate 80 in 5 and 15 ml containers.

TETRACYCLINE AND STEROID:

Terra-Cortril Eye-Ear Suspension (Pfizer). Each milliliter contains oxytetracycline hydrochloride equivalent to oxytetracycline 5 mg and cortisol acetate 15 mg with mineral oil and aluminum tristearate in 5 ml containers.

Selected References

Drugs for bacterial conjunctivitis. *Med Lett Drugs Ther* 18:70-72, 1976.

Apt L: Pediatric aspects of drug therapy, in Leopold IH (ed): *Symposium on Ocular Therapy*. St Louis, CV Mosby Co, 1968, vol 3, 88-95.

Burns RP, et al: Immunosuppressive therapy in ophthalmology, in Leopold IH, Burns RP (eds): *Symposium on Ocular Therapy*. New York, John Wiley & Sons, 1976, vol 8, 11-15.

Cantrill HL, et al: Comparison of in vitro potency of corticosteroids with ability to raise intraocular pressure. *Am J Ophthalmol* 79:1012-1017, 1975.

Ellis PP: *Ocular Therapeutics and Pharmacology*, ed 5. St Louis, CV Mosby Co, 1977.

Havener WH: *Ocular Pharmacology*, ed 4. St Louis, CV Mosby Co, 1978.

Jones BR: Principles in management of oculomycosis. *Am J Ophthalmol* 79:719-751, 1975.

Kaufman HE: Antiviral agents in ophthalmology, in Leopold IH, Burns RP (eds): *Symposium on Ocular Therapy*. New York, John Wiley & Sons, 1976. vol 9, 33-39.

Leopold IH: Advances in ocular therapy: Noncorticosteroid anti-inflammatory agents. *Am J Ophthalmol* 78:759-773, 1974.

Leopold IH: Problems in use of antibiotics in ophthalmology, in Leopold IH (ed): *Symposium on Ocular Therapy*. St Louis, CV Mosby Co, 1972, vol 5, 113-153.

Leopold IH, Kagan JM: Antimicrobial therapy in ophthalmology, in Kagan BM (ed): *Antimicrobial Therapy*, ed 2. Philadelphia, WB Saunders Co, 1974, 366-377.

Lieberman TW: Systemic antifungal chemotherapy in treatment of intraocular fungal infections, in Leopold IH (ed): *Symposium on Ocular Therapy*. St Louis, CV Mosby Co, 1973, vol 6, 59-73.

Osborn E, et al: Stability of ten antibiotics in artificial tear solutions. *Am J Ophthalmol* 82:775-780, 1976.

Pettit TH: Management of bacterial corneal ulcers, in Leopold IH, Burns RP (eds): *Symposium on Ocular Therapy*. New York, John Wiley & Sons, 1976, vol 8, 57-65.

Podos SM, Becker B: Intraocular pressure effects of diluted and new topical corticosteroids, in Leopold IH (ed): *Symposium on Ocular Therapy*. St Louis, CV Mosby Co, 1972, vol 5, 90-95.

Miscellaneous Ophthalmic Preparations | 25

LOCAL ANESTHETICS

Agents Used for Surface Anesthesia: Benoxinate [Dorsacaine], proparacaine [Alcaine, Ophthaine, Ophthetic], tetracaine [Anacel], and cocaine are applied topically to the eye to anesthetize the cornea and conjunctiva. Surface anesthesia alone provides sufficient analgesia for superficial procedures such as tonometry and removal of foreign bodies and sutures. Topically applied anesthetics also may be used for operations on deeper structures, most commonly as adjuncts to locally injected anesthetics.

These agents all produce adequate corneal anesthesia within one minute after instillation, and the duration of anesthesia can be prolonged, if necessary, by repeated application. The duration of action is approximately 15 minutes for 0.4% benoxinate, 0.5% proparacaine, or 0.5% tetracaine. Cocaine has not been compared with the other topical anesthetics in well-controlled clinical trials, but there is a strong clinical impression that (1) in achieving anesthesia of the conjunctiva, cocaine is considerably more effective and longer acting than any other agent; (2) in anesthetizing the cornea, cocaine has a more prolonged action than the other topical anesthetics, but the intensity of anesthesia is no greater; and (3) cocaine may loosen the corneal epithelium to a greater extent than other anesthetics, thus facilitating debridement or total removal of the surface epithelium.

Topically applied anesthetics cause transient irregularity in the surface of the corneal epithelium that may interfere with visualization of the inside of the eye. Because protective eyelid reflexes are suppressed by topical anesthesia, the corneal epithelium may become dry. Repeated administration may retard healing and cause pitting and sloughing of the corneal epithelium and formation of a yellow-white ring in the corneal stroma around the original disease area (Burns et al, 1977).

395

Cocaine may be more toxic in this respect than other topical anesthetics, although all of these agents can produce severe corneal damage. They should not be used repeatedly except under close medical supervision, and they are especially dangerous if given to the patient for self-medication.

Tetracaine, benoxinate, and cocaine may cause slight pain immediately after instillation, but proparacaine causes little local discomfort. The patient should be warned not to rub the eye. Allergic reactions have been reported more frequently with tetracaine than with the other agents, but this may reflect its more widespread use. Allergy to the preservative also may occur; for this reason, use of a single-dose sterile containers without preservative are preferred (Smith and Everett, 1973). Cocaine dilates the pupil and has precipitated acute angle closure in predisposed eyes. The amount of anesthetic absorbed after topical instillation in the eye is usually not sufficient to cause systemic reactions.

See also Havener, 1978.

ROUTE, USUAL DOSAGE, AND PREPARATIONS. See Table 1.

TABLE 1.
AGENTS USED FOR SURFACE ANESTHESIA

Drug	Dosage (Topical)	Ophthalmic Preparation
Benoxinate Hydrochloride	One or two drops of 0.4% solution instilled before procedure. For deeper anesthesia, one drop instilled at one-minute intervals for two doses.	Dorsacaine (Dorsey). Solution (sterile) 0.4% with sodium chloride and butylparaben in 15 ml containers.
Cocaine Hydrochloride, U.S.P.	One or two drops of 1% to 4% solution instilled before procedure.	No pharmaceutical dosage form available; compounding necessary for prescription.
Proparacaine Hydrochloride	One or two drops of 0.5% solution instilled before procedure. For deeper anesthesia, more frequent instillation required.	Alcaine (Alcon). Solution (sterile) 0.5% with glycerin and benzalkonium chloride in 15 ml containers. Ophthaine (Squibb). Solution (sterile) 0.5% with glycerin, chlorobutanol, benzalkonium chloride, and sodium hydroxide or hydrochloric acid in 15 ml containers. Ophthetic (Allergan). Solution (sterile) 0.5% with glycerin, sodium chloride, and benzalkonium chloride in 15 ml containers.
Tetracaine Hydrochloride	One or two drops of the 0.5% solution instilled before the procedure. For deeper anesthesia, two to four instillations required.	Anacel (Professional Pharmacal). Solution (sterile) 0.5% with methylcellulose, sodium chloride, and benzalkonium chloride in 15 ml containers. Tetracaine Hydrochloride (Alcon). Solution 0.5% with sodium chloride, hydrochloric acid, and benzalkonium chloride in 15 ml containers; Steri-Unit (without preservatives) in 2 ml containers. Tetracaine Hydrochloride (SMP). Solution (sterile) 0.5% with sodium chloride and chlorobutanol in 1 ml containers.

Agents Used for Local Injection: Procaine [Novocain], lidocaine [Xylocaine], mepivacaine [Carbocaine], and bupivacaine [Marcaine] are injected locally to paralyze the orbicularis oculi muscle (facial nerve akinesia) and extraocular muscles (retrobulbar block). These techniques prevent squeezing of the lids and eye movements during intraocular surgery and also provide sensory anesthesia. Epinephrine may be added to the solution to reduce systemic absorption and thereby prolong the action and decrease the toxicity of the anesthetic, but it is usually not required when slowly absorbed agents, such as mepivacaine and bupivacaine, are employed. Hyaluronidase [Alidase, Wydase] enhances diffusion of the anesthetic and

may be particularly useful when added to solutions for retrobulbar injection, because diffusion of the anesthetic may aid in reducing intraocular pressure (see the evaluation on Hyaluronidase).

Procaine, lidocaine, and mepivacaine also may be injected locally to block nerve endings in the immediate area of surgery (infiltration anesthesia). Infiltration anesthesia is indicated for procedures such as minor lid surgery. Subconjunctival infiltration anesthesia is sometimes employed prior to intraocular surgery.

Because it is rapidly metabolized, procaine has a relatively short duration of action and is relatively safe. Lidocaine diffuses more readily than procaine and is more potent, longer acting, and more toxic

TABLE 2.
AGENTS USED FOR LOCAL INJECTION

| Drug | Dosage[1] | | | Preparations[4] |
	Facial Nerve Akinesia[2]	Retrobulbar Block[3]	Infiltration Anesthesia	
Procaine Hydrochloride	4 to 10 ml of 1% to 2% solution	2 to 3 ml of 1% to 2% solution	0.25% to 0.5% solution	Drug available generically with and without epinephrine Novocain (Breon): Solution 1% and 2%
Lidocaine Hydrochloride	4 to 10 ml of 1% to 2% solution	2 to 3 ml of 2% or 4% solution	0.5% solution	Drug available generically with and without epinephrine Xylocaine Hydrochloride (Astra): Solution 0.5%, 1%, 1.5%, and 2% (all with or without epinephrine 1:200,000) and 4% (without epinephrine)
Mepivacaine Hydrochloride	4 to 10 ml of 2% solution	1.5 to 2 ml of 2% solution	1% to 2% solution	Carbocaine Hydrochloride (Breon): Solution 1%, 1.5%, and 2%
Bupivacaine Hydrochloride	5 to 10 ml of 0.5% solution or 5 to 7 ml of 0.75% solution	2 ml of 0.75% solution	—	Drug available generically: Solution 0.5% Marcaine Hydrochloride (Breon): Solution 0.25%, 0.5%, and 0.75% (all with or without epinephrine bitartrate 1;200,000); solutions without epinephrine may be reautoclaved.

[1]*Epinephrine (1:200,000) may be added to prolong the action of the anesthetic. Hyaluronidase may be added to increase diffusion of the anesthetic.*

[2]*Solution is injected in region of terminal branches of facial nerve or around the proximal trunk of the nerve.*

[3]*Solution is injected inside the muscle cone behind the globe. Low pressure may be applied to the eye intermittently for three to five minutes after the injection.*

[4]*For complete product information, see Chapter 19, Local Anesthetics.*

on a milligram for milligram basis. In a comparative study, the duration of near maximal akinesia of the extraocular muscles was measured following retrobulbar block with procaine or lidocaine, each administered with epinephrine (Russell and Guyton, 1954). The duration of action of procaine was 40 minutes and of lidocaine, 90 minutes. The duration of akinesia was reduced, however, when hyaluronidase was added to the solution (procaine, 30 minutes; lidocaine, 60 minutes). Mepivacaine is similar to lidocaine in potency and toxicity, but it may have a longer duration of action. Bupivacaine, which is related structurally to mepivacaine, has the longest duration of action but the onset of anesthesia is variable; a 0.75% solution with hyaluronidase (without epinephrine) has been used successfully in procedures lasting two hours or more (Smith and Linn, 1974).

Allergic reactions are less common with the amide group of local anesthetics (lidocaine, mepivacaine, bupivacaine) than with the ester group (procaine). Transient pain may occur following injection of bupivacaine. The locally injected anesthetics can cause systemic reactions if excessive amounts are absorbed or if the anesthetic is given intravenously. Systemic reactions (eg, tachycardia, hypertension) also may occur if sufficient quantities of epinephrine are absorbed. These reactions are discussed in detail in Chapter 19, Local Anesthetics. See also Ellis, 1976; Havener, 1978.

ROUTES, USUAL DOSAGE, AND PREPARATIONS. See Table 2.

DYES

FLUORESCEIN SODIUM

Fluorescein is an indicator dye that appears yellow-green in normal tear film and bright green in a more alkaline medium such as the aqueous humor. Fluorescence is activated by blue and ultraviolet light. Because it makes the tear fluid visible, fluorescein is applied topically in the fitting of hard contact lenses and is used as an aid in applanation tonometry to delineate the margin of the applanated area. It is also used to detect corneal epithelial defects caused by injury or infection. Defects in the continuity of the tearfilm layer over the cornea can be detected after topical application of fluorescein. Since the intensity of green fluorescence increases when fluorescein is in contact with the aqueous humor, this dye is useful to locate the site of a wound leak in patients with a persistent flat anterior chamber after cataract surgery. Fluorescein also is instilled in the eye to test lacrimal patency; if drainage is normal, the dye will appear in the nasal secretions (Havener, 1978).

In addition to these topical diagnostic uses, fluorescein is given intravenously as an aid in retinal photography. It is useful to evaluate diabetic retinopathy and to detect occlusion or obliteration of retinal vessels, vascular malformations, neovascularization, changes in vascular permeability, ocular tumors, defects in the retinal pigment epithelium, and abnormalities of the iris vasculature (iris angiography), as well as for studies of aqueous humor flow. Measurement of the arm-to-retina circulation time is employed for diagnosis of carotid artery occlusion.

A nondiagnostic use of fluorescein is for irrigation of the eye after injury by an indelible pencil. The aniline dye in these pencils causes edema and necrosis of ocular tissue which may result in loss of vision unless it is detoxified.

The preservatives commonly used in ophthalmic preparations are inactivated by fluorescein, and contaminated fluorescein solutions have been a frequent source of ocular infections, particularly by *Pseudomonas* organisms. These solutions can be sterilized by autoclaving but are easily contaminated by subsequent use. Sterile, single-dose containers and individually packaged filter-paper strips impregnated with fluorescein are safer than multiple-dose containers.

Nausea and vomiting occur occasionally when fluorescein is given intravenously. Pruritus, urticaria, and paresthesias also have been reported. Anaphylactic reactions have occurred only rarely, but facilities to treat these reactions should be available (Stein and Parker, 1971). Acute pulmonary edema is also an uncommon complication of intravenously administered fluorescein.

ROUTES, USUAL DOSAGE, AND PREPARATIONS. *Topical:* To fit hard contact lenses, with the contact lens in place, a fluorescein strip moistened with ophthalmic irrigating solution is lightly touched to the superior conjunctiva or one drop of a 2% solution is applied. The patient should be instructed to blink several times to circulate the dye. Under blue light, areas that lack fluorescein-stained tears appear black, indicating that the contact lens is touching the cornea at those points. Fluorescein should not be used in the fitting of soft contact lenses, because the lens will absorb the dye.

In applanation tonometry, one drop of a 0.25% solution or a fluorescein strip moistened with ophthalmic irrigating solution is applied to the eye immediately before tonometry. A topical anesthetic should be instilled prior to application of fluorescein. Fluress, a combination product containing benoxinate and fluorescein, may be used for simultaneous staining and local anesthesia. Tetracaine generally should be avoided because it may reduce the intensity of fluorescence.

To detect epithelial defects, a fluorescein strip moistened with ophthalmic irrigating solution is used to touch the conjunctiva, or one drop of a 0.5% to 2% solution is placed in the conjunctival sac. To provide contrast between the lesion and surrounding areas, excess dye should be removed by use of an irrigating solution.

To test lacrimal patency, one drop of a 2% solution is instilled in the conjunctival sac. The patient should be instructed to blink at least four times after the dye is instilled. After six minutes, nasal secretions are examined under blue light. If traces of the dye are present in the secretions, the nasolacrimal drainage system is open.

To test for aqueous leak following ocular surgery, one drop of a 2% solution is instilled in the affected eye. Gentle pressure on the globe may be necessary to determine the site of the leak.

As an antidote to poisoning by aniline dyes, following removal of the pencil point, the eye is irrigated with a 2% solution every 10 minutes until a visible precipitate no longer forms. Irrigation is then repeated every 30 minutes for 12 to 24 hours.

All preparations available in ophthalmic forms.

Fluor-I-Strip (Ayerst). Sterile applicators impregnated with fluorescein sodium 9 mg/strip (lint free) with chlorobutanol, polysorbate 80, boric acid, potassium chloride, and sodium carbonate in individual envelopes in boxes containing 200 envelopes.

Fluor-I-Strip A.T. (Ayerst). Sterile applicators impregnated with fluorescein sodium 1 mg/strip (lint-free) with chlorobutanol, polysorbate 80, boric acid, potassium chloride, and sodium carbonate in boxes containing 100 envelopes (2 strips/envelope).

Ful-Glo (Barnes-Hind). Sterile applicators impregnated with fluorescein 0.6 mg/strip in boxes containing 300 individual strips.

Fluoreseptic (Professional Pharmacal). Solution (sterile) 2% with sodium bicarbonate and phenylmercuric borate 1:25,000 in 7.5 and 15 ml containers.

Fluorescein Sodium (Alcon). Solution 2% with phenylmercuric nitrate in 2 ml (sterile) and 15 ml containers.

Fluorescein Sodium (SMP). Solution (sterile) 2% with boric acid, sodium carbonate, potassium chloride, and thimerosal 0.01% in 1 ml containers.

AVAILABLE MIXTURE.

Fluress (Barnes-Hind). Solution (sterile) containing fluorescein sodium 0.25% and benoxinate hydrochloride 0.4% with boric acid isotonic buffer, povidone, and chlorobutanol 1% in 5 ml containers.

Intravenous: Adults, 500 mg (10 ml of a 5% solution or 5 ml of a 10% solution) is injected rapidly into an arm vein. Some investigators believe that better visualization can be attained with 3 ml of a 25% solution (750 mg). The dye should appear in the central retinal artery in 9 to 15 seconds.

Fluorescite (Alcon). Solution 2.5% in 2 ml containers, 5% in 10 ml containers, 10% in 5 ml containers, and 10% in 10 ml syringe with 5 ml of solution.

Funduscein (SMP). Solution 10% in 5 ml containers and 25% in 3 ml containers.

ROSE BENGAL

Rose bengal is a vital stain with a particular affinity for devitalized corneal and conjunctival epithelium. When viewed under the slit-lamp, the stain consists of rose-colored dots; if inflammation or hemorrhage interferes with visibility, a green filter will give the stain a purplish-blue cast. Rose bengal is used to determine the extent of epithelial damage in various conjunctival or corneal disorders. It is particularly useful for diagnosis of keratoconjunctivitis sicca (a disorder of the cornea and conjunctiva caused by tear deficiency) and for the fine differentiation of the margin of corneal ulcers, especially those caused by herpes simplex virus. (See also Havener, 1978.)

Although rose bengal is more irritating to the eye than fluorescein, a local anesthetic is generally not necessary if small amounts are used.

ROUTE, USUAL DOSAGE, AND PREPARATIONS. *Topical*: One drop is instilled in the conjunctival sac.

> *Rose Bengal* (Barnes-Hind). Solution (ophthalmic, sterile) 1% with povidone, sodium borate, sodium chloride, tyloxapol, and thimerosal in 1 ml containers. The 1% solution may be diluted to a 0.1% solution, if desired. (This preparation may not be currently available but will probably be marketed again in the near future.)

ENZYMES

ALPHA CHYMOTRYPSIN
[Catarase, Zolyse]

Alpha chymotrypsin is a proteolytic enzyme used for dissolving the zonules of the lens (zonulolysis) during intracapsular cataract extraction. It is injected behind the iris into the posterior chamber where it acts within one to two minutes and, when zonulolysis is complete, the lens moves forward or assumes a more rounded contour.

Enzymatic zonulolysis is indicated particularly in young adults (over the age of 20), in high myopes, in patients with traumatic cataracts, and after retinal detachment. The zonules of elderly patients are fragile, and alpha chymotrypsin may not be required to facilitate lens extraction. In patients under the age of 20, the lens is firmly attached to the face of the vitreous, and intracapsular extraction can lead to vitreous loss and subsequent retinal detachment; extracapsular extraction is the method of choice in these patients.

A transient increase in intraocular pressure is a common untoward effect of alpha chymotrypsin; if the pressure is very high, ocular pain and corneal edema may occur. Enzyme-induced glaucoma may persist for a week and presumably is caused by the accumulation of zonular fragments in the trabecular meshwork. The use of alpha chymotrypsin also has been associated with wound disruption and loss of the anterior chamber. These complications apparently result from the enzyme-induced glaucoma and can be avoided by postoperative administration of acetazolamide and by the use of multiple corneoscleral sutures.

Alpha chymotrypsin is extremely toxic to the retina and should not be allowed to penetrate into the vitreous, as posterior diffusion could occur. In patients with fluid vitreous, enzymatic zonulolysis can result in loss of the lens posteriorly and, possibly, to entry of alpha chymotrypsin into the vitreous body. Uveitis also has been observed. Systemic reactions have not been reported.

See also Havener, 1978.

ROUTE, USUAL DOSAGE, AND PREPARATIONS. The anterior chamber should be free of blood before use of alpha chymotrypsin, because blood rapidly inactivates the enzyme.

Injection: 0.2 to 0.5 ml of a freshly prepared 1:5,000 or 1:10,000 solution is injected slowly behind the iris into the posterior chamber. To assure uniform zonulolysis, the irrigating tip may be manipulated so that the solution is distributed around the anterior lens equator. After delivery of the lens, the anterior chamber should be irrigated with a small volume (less than 2 ml) of the diluent, sodium chloride injection, or a balanced salt solution. A second application of alpha chymotrypsin may be required if the zonules are resistant.

> *Catarase* (two strengths) (SMP). Two-compartment vial containing lyophilized alpha chymotrypsin 150 or 300 units in the lower compartment and sodium chloride injection 2 ml in the upper compartment.
> *Zolyse* (Alcon). Lyophilized powder (for solution) 750 units with 9 ml of diluent.

HYALURONIDASE
[Alidase, Wydase]

Hyaluronidase promotes diffusion of injected solutions by increasing tissue permeability. It is used in ophthalmic surgical procedures to increase diffusion of locally injected anesthetics (eg, procaine, lidocaine). When hyaluronidase is added to the injection solution, the time required for induction of complete akinesia is reduced (Mindel, 1978), sensory anesthesia is enhanced, and, with retrobulbar injection, hypotony is increased. Hyaluronidase may increase the rate of absorption of the anesthetic and thus reduce its duration of action, but this problem can usually be avoided if epinephrine is added to the injection solution (Ellis, 1976; Havener, 1978).

No adverse effects have been reported following use of hyaluronidase in ophthalmology.

ROUTE, USUAL DOSAGE, AND PREPARATIONS. *Injection*: 125 units are added to each 10 ml of anesthetic solution.

> Drug available generically: Solution 150 N.F. units/ml.
> *Alidase* (Searle). Powder for solution 150 N.F. units.
> *Wydase* (Wyeth). Lyophilized powder 150 and 1,500 N.F. units; solution 150 N.F. units/ml in sterile sodium chloride injection in 1 and 10 ml containers.

INTRAOCULAR MIOTICS

ACETYLCHOLINE CHLORIDE
[Miochol]

$$CH_3COCH_2CH_2\overset{+}{N}(CH_3)_3 \ Cl^-$$

Acetylcholine is the neurohumoral transmitter at numerous sites in the nervous system, including the neuroeffector junction of the sphincter muscle of the iris. When applied topically to the eye, acetylcholine is of no therapeutic value because of poor corneal penetration and rapid hydrolysis by acetylcholinesterase. However, it produces prompt, pronounced miosis when introduced into the anterior chamber and is useful during certain surgical procedures on the anterior segment of the eye. Acetylcholine has a shorter duration of action than other miotics; this is an advantage during ocular surgery, because prolonged miosis can cause severe postoperative pain or predispose to pupillary block. If miosis is desired during the postoperative period, a longer-acting miotic (ie, carbachol, pilocarpine) must be instilled.

Acetylcholine is commonly used to produce miosis after cataract surgery. By increasing the iris surface, it helps protect the vitreous face and facilitates placement of sutures. It also may prevent formation of peripheral anterior synechiae. During peripheral iridectomy, acetylcholine may be introduced into the anterior chamber to permit excision of only peripheral iris tissue and to aid in repositing of the iris. It also is used during penetrating keratoplasty to facilitate suturing of the graft, to protect the lens, and to prevent incarceration of the iris (Rizzuti, 1967; Havener, 1978).

Because it is rapidly inactivated, acetylcholine seldom produces adverse effects. Systemic reactions (hypotension and bradycardia) have occurred rarely; these cardiovascular reactions are potentially dangerous and should be treated with intravenous atropine. No local toxic effects from acetylcholine itself have been reported; however, the hypertonic solution may cause transient lens opacities. In addition, severe ocular complications have occurred when acetylcholine was gas sterilized. These complications included corneal edema, intraocular inflammation, opacity of the anterior lens capsule, retinal toxicity, and optic atrophy. Acetylcholine should not be gas sterilized because the ethylene oxide gas used in the sterilization process may enter through or around the rubber stopper of the two-compartment vial and react chemically with water and/or chloride ion, both of which are present in the pharmaceutical product. Ethylene glycol and/or ethylene chlorhydrin may form, and both are highly toxic to the eye.

ROUTE, USUAL DOSAGE, AND PREPARATIONS.
Intracameral: 0.5 to 2 ml of a freshly prepared 1:100 solution is instilled into the anterior chamber.

> *Miochol* (SMP). Two-compartment vial containing lyophilized acetylcholine chloride 20 mg and mannitol 100 mg in the lower compartment and sterile water 2 ml in the upper compartment.

CARBACHOL
[Miostat]

$$H_2NCOCH_2CH_2\overset{+}{N}(CH_3)_3 \quad Cl^-$$

The parasympathomimetic agent, carbachol, may be preferred to acetylcholine for use during ocular surgery if more prolonged miosis is desired. In contrast to the transient effect of acetylcholine, the miosis induced by carbachol is still evident 15 hours after intracameral injection. Carbachol has not been used as extensively as acetylcholine, but the two drugs are equally effective in producing prompt, complete miosis after cataract extraction (Beasley, 1971). An advantage of carbachol is its stability in solution; unlike acetylcholine, it does not have to be freshly prepared prior to instillation.

No adverse effects have been reported after intraocular use of carbachol.

ROUTE, USUAL DOSAGE, AND PREPARATIONS.
Intracameral: 0.4 to 0.5 ml of a 0.01% solution is instilled into the anterior chamber.

> *Miostat* (Alcon). Solution (sterile, for intraocular use) 0.01% with citric acid monohydrate, sodium chloride, and dried sodium phosphate in 1.5 ml containers.

CHELATING AGENT

EDETATE DISODIUM (EDTA)
[Endrate, Sodium Versenate]

$$Na^+\ ^-OCCH_2 \diagdown \diagup CH_2CO^-\ Na^+$$
$$NCH_2CH_2N$$
$$HOCCH_2 \diagup \diagdown CH_2COH$$

This chelating agent is applied topically to remove corneal calcium deposits that impair vision or, by penetrating the epithelium, cause pain. It dissolves calcium deposits of endogenous origin (eg, band keratopathies and other calcific corneal deposits associated with chronic uveitis, advanced interstitial keratitis, hypercalcemia) and is also useful for emergency management and subsequent treatment of calcium hydroxide burns of the eye (Grant, 1952). Edetate disodium also has been suggested for decontaminating the eye after injury by zinc chloride (Johnstone et al, 1973).

Edetate disodium extracts calcium from the conjunctiva, corneal epithelium, and anterior layers of the stroma but does not affect deposits extending deeper than the level of Bowman's membrane. The removal of superficial calcium deposits should improve vision unless scarring and vascularization have occurred; however, calcium deposits of endogenous origin tend to recur. Edetate disodium does not penetrate the corneal epithelium. Unless the calcium deposit extends to the surface, the epithelium must be completely removed before application of this agent.

Edetate disodium is well tolerated when applied topically. Transient stinging and chemosis may occur. The stronger concentration (1.85%) may cause stromal edema.

ROUTE, USUAL DOSAGE, AND PREPARATIONS.
Topical: For removal of exogenous or endogenous calcium deposits from the anterior layers of the stroma, a local anesthetic should be instilled before the procedure; cocaine is often preferred because it facilitates epithelial removal. The corneal epithelium is then completely removed and the denuded area is irrigated with edetate disodium (0.35% to 1.85% solution) for 15 to 20 minutes. The solution is applied as a corneal bath, under a contact lens, or by iontophoresis. After the procedure, the eye should be irrigated with sodium chloride injection or a balanced salt solution.

For emergency treatment of calcium hydroxide burns, the eye should first be flushed with water as quickly as possible. The eye is then irrigated with a 0.35% to 1.85% solution of edetate disodium for 15 minutes.

For emergency treatment of zinc chloride injury, after flushing with water, the eye may be irrigated with a 1.7% solution for 15 minutes. Treatment may be ineffective if not begun within two minutes after injury.

> No ophthalmic preparation is available. The intravenous solution must be diluted to the desired concentration with isotonic sodium chloride injection.
> *Endrate* (Abbott). Solution (injection) 150 mg/ml in 20 ml containers.
> *Sodium Versenate* (Riker). Aqueous solution (injection) 200 mg/ml in 15 ml containers.

TOPICAL OSMOTIC AGENTS

ANHYDROUS GLYCERIN
[Ophthalgan]

HYPERTONIC SODIUM CHLORIDE
[Adsorbonac, Hypersal, Muro Ointment No. 128, Murocoll No. 4]

These osmotic agents are applied topically to reduce corneal edema. By removing fluid, they produce a temporary clearing of the cornea in the early stages of epithelial edema, but they are not useful in improving visual acuity if scarring of the epithelium or stroma has occurred (Dohlman and Hyndiuk, 1972).

Glycerin is most commonly used prior to ophthalmoscopy or gonioscopy when the cornea is too edematous to permit diagnosis. It is very effective as a dehydrating agent, but instillation is painful and long-term therapy is not well tolerated.

Hypertonic sodium chloride is usually preferred when repeated instillation is indicated. This osmotic agent may be used to reduce corneal edema following cataract extraction, corneal transplantation, or trauma. It also may be beneficial in the early stages of chronic corneal edema associated with Fuchs' endothelial-epithelial dystrophy and other ocular diseases, but is of limited value for long-term therapy because scarring usually occurs with progression of the disease. In treating the bullous keratopathy that may occur in patients with prolonged corneal edema, hypertonic sodium chloride may produce the best results when the patient is also fitted with a hydrophilic bandage lens (Gasset and Kaufman, 1971). The bandage lens provides significant relief of pain in many patients, may improve corneal pathology, and occasionally improves visual acuity. The lens must be carefully sterilized to prevent infection, particularly in eyes with epithelial disease.

ROUTE, USUAL DOSAGE, AND PREPARATIONS.
ANHYDROUS GLYCERIN:
Topical: To facilitate diagnosis, one to three drops are instilled prior to the examination. A topical anesthetic should be instilled before glycerin is applied.

> *Ophthalgan* (Ayerst). Solution (ophthalmic, sterile) with chlorobutanol 0.5% in 7.5 ml containers.

HYPERTONIC SODIUM CHLORIDE:
Topical: For treatment of corneal edema, one or two drops of the hyperosmotic solution are instilled three or four times daily. The ointment may be applied at bedtime. In patients with bullous keratopathy, after application of a hydrophilic bandage lens, a cycloplegic drug should be instilled for several days to prevent ciliary spasm. During this period, topical osmotherapy should be avoided if the eye is painful. After pain has subsided, one or two drops of 5% hypertonic sodium chloride solution are instilled three or four times daily or as

needed to control edema. The frequency of administration may be reduced or the drug discontinued as edema subsides.

All preparations available in topical ophthalmic form.

Adsorbonac (Burton, Parsons). Solution (sterile) 2% and 5% with povidone 1.67% and other water-soluble polymers, thimerosal 0.004%, and edetate disodium 0.1% in 15 ml containers (nonprescription).

Hypersal (American Optical). Solution (sterile) 5% with sodium phosphate monobasic and dibasic, thimerosal 0.002%, and edetate disodium 0.05% in 15 ml containers (nonprescription).

Murocoll No. 4 (Muro). Solution 5% with methylcellulose 4,000 cps 0.9% with methylparaben 0.023% and propylparaben 0.01% in 15 and 30 ml containers.

Muro Ointment No. 128 (Muro). Ointment 5% in a lanolin, liquid petrolatum, and white petrolatum base in ⅛ oz containers.

OPHTHALMIC IRRIGATING SOLUTIONS

Internal Irrigating Solutions: These preparations are administered during intraocular surgery to irrigate the anterior chamber, extraocular muscles, and lacrimal system and to moisten the cornea. Results of in vitro studies have shown that irrigating solutions differ in their ability to preserve corneal endothelial structure and function and to maintain lens clarity. These differences may be of clinical importance, particularly during procedures that involve prolonged intraocular irrigation (eg, pars plana vitrectomy).

In corneal perfusion studies, commonly used irrigating solutions (sterile isotonic saline, lactated Ringer's solution, balanced salt solution) caused corneal swelling and degeneration. Some investigators have found that structure is best preserved if glutathione and adenosine are added to either sodium bicarbonate-Ringer's solution or balanced salt solution (Edelhauser et al, 1975). Others have found that, while bicarbonate is essential to preserve corneal structure, glutathione and adenosine can be safely omitted (McEnerney and Peyman, 1977).

BSS (Alcon). Solution (ophthalmic, sterile) containing sodium chloride 0.49%, potassium chloride 0.75%, calcium chloride 0.048%, magnesium chloride hexahydrate 0.03%, sodium acetate 0.39%, and sodium citrate dihydrate 0.17% in 15 and 500 ml containers.

External Irrigating Solutions: These solutions are used following foreign body removal and administration of fluorescein and other dyes. The boric acid present in some of these solutions may form an insoluble complex with the polyvinyl alcohol contained in some contact lens wetting solutions.

All preparations available in topical ophthalmic forms.

Blinx (Barnes-Hind). Solution (sterile) containing boric acid, sodium borate, and phenylmercuric acetate 0.004% in 30 and 120 ml containers (nonprescription).

Collyrium (Wyeth). Solution containing boric acid, sodium borate, thimerosal (not more than 0.002%), and antipyrine 0.4% in 180 ml containers (nonprescription).

Dacriose (SMP). Solution (sterile) containing sodium carbonate, potassium chloride, benzalkonium chloride 0.01%, and edetate disodium 0.01% in 15, 27, and 118 ml containers (nonprescription).

Eye Stream (Alcon). Solution containing sodium chloride, potassium chloride, calcium chloride, magnesium chloride, sodium citrate, sodium acetate, and benzalkonium chloride 0.013% in 30 and 120 ml containers (nonprescription).

Irigate (Steri-Med). Solution (sterile) containing boric acid, edetate disodium, potassium chloride, and benzalkonium chloride 1:10,000 in 4 oz containers (nonprescription).

Neo-Flo (American Optical). Solution (sterile) containing boric acid, sodium chloride, potassium chloride, sodium carbonate, and benzalkonium chloride 1:15,000 in 118 ml containers (nonprescription).

TEAR SUBSTITUTES AND OTHER POLYMER PREPARATIONS

Artificial tear solutions are used to prevent corneal damage in patients with keratoconjunctivitis sicca, exposure keratitis, neuroparalytic keratitis, and other conditions in which tear flow is reduced. These solutions contain water-soluble polymers (usually cellulose esters or polyvinyl alcohol) which increase the thickness of the precorneal tear film, possibly by dragging water with them as they spread over the ocular surface with each blink (Benedetto et al, 1975). Formulations containing cellulose esters (eg, methylcellulose) are more viscous than those containing polyvinyl alcohol, but retention times are comparable. Preparations employing other polymeric systems (eg, Adsorbotear, Tears Naturale) are retained longer and may be useful in mucus-deficient dry-eye conditions, such as ocular pemphigoid (Lemp et al, 1975). A hypoosmotic agent [Hypotears] may be useful in balancing the hyperosmolarity of tears found in patients with keratoconjunctivitis sicca (Gilbard et al, 1978). Sterile bland ointments (eg, Duratears, Lacri-Lube S.O.P.) may be used as lubricants after foreign body removal and to provide prolonged lubrication at night.

Artificial tears must be used regularly and as frequently as necessary to keep the conjunctiva moist. During warm dry weather, it may be necessary to apply the drops as often as every 15 minutes. Occlusion of the lacrimal puncta by cauterization will help preserve existing lacrimal secretion and prolong retention of artificial tears. A slow-release artificial tear (SR-AT) currently under investigation consists of a pellet that is inserted in the lower conjunctival cul-de-sac where it dissolves slowly.

In addition to their use in artificial tear preparations, cellulose esters and polyvinyl alcohol are incorporated in liquid ophthalmic formulations to prolong the ocular contact time of drugs; they are not as effective in this respect as ointments (Havener, 1978). Water-soluble polymers are also used to moisten hard contact lenses and to protect the cornea during gonioscopy and other procedures.

Ophthalmic polymers are nonirritating to ocular tissue and can be used for prolonged periods without causing damage to the eye. Viscous preparations may cause discomfort if excess solution is allowed to dry on the upper lid.

All preparations are available in ophthalmic form.

METHYLCELLULOSE:

Methopto (Professional Pharmacal). Solution (sterile) 0.25% with benzalkonium chloride 1:25,000 in 15 and 30 ml containers and 0.5% and 1% (Forte) with benzalkonium chloride 1:25,000 in 15 ml containers (nonprescription).

Methulose (American Optical). Solution (sterile) 0.25% with benzalkonium chloride 1:25,000 in 15 and 30 ml containers (nonprescription).

Visculose (American Optical). Solution (sterile) 0.5% or 1% with benzalkonium chloride 1:25,000 in 15 ml containers (nonprescription).

HYDROXYPROPYLMETHYLCELLULOSE:

Goniosol (SMP). Solution (sterile, for gonioscopy) 2.5% with benzalkonium chloride, edetate disodium, boric acid, sodium carbonate, and potassium chloride in 15 ml containers.

Isopto Alkaline (Alcon). Solution (sterile) 1% with benzalkonium chloride 0.01% in 15 ml containers (pH 7.4) (nonprescription).

Isopto Plain (Alcon). Solution 0.5% with benzalkonium chloride 0.01% in 15 ml containers (nonprescription).

Isopto Tears (Alcon). Solution (sterile) 0.5% with benzalkonium chloride 0.01% in 15 and 30 ml containers (nonprescription).

Lacril (Allergan). Solution 0.5% with polysorbate 80, gelatin A, sodium borate, and chlorobutanol 0.5% in 15 ml containers (nonprescription).

Tearisol (SMP). Solution (sterile) 0.5% with boric acid, sodium carbonate, potassium chloride, benzalkonium chloride 0.01%, and edetate disodium 0.1% in 15 ml containers (nonprescription).

Ultra Tears (Alcon). Solution (4,000 cps) 1% with benzalkonium chloride 0.01% in 15 ml containers (nonprescription).

HYDROXYETHYLCELLULOSE:

aqua-FLOW (SMP). Solution (sterile, mildly hypertonic) with sodium bicarbonate, sodium chloride, potassium chloride, edetate trisodium, and benzalkonium chloride in 25 ml containers (nonprescription).

Comfort Drops (Barnes-Hind). Solution (sterile) with edetate disodium 0.02% and benzalkonium chloride 0.005% in 15 ml containers (nonprescription).

Clērz (SMP). Solution (sterile) with poloxamer 407, edetate disodium, and benzalkonium chloride in 25 ml containers (nonprescription).

Lyteers (Barnes-Hind). Solution (sterile) with sodium chloride, potassium chloride, edetate disodium 0.05%, and benzalkonium chloride 0.01% in 15 ml containers (nonprescription).

CARBOXYMETHYLCELLULOSE:

Bro-Lac (Riker). Solution (sterile) with polysorbate 80, glycerin, sodium borate, chlorobutanol 0.1%, methylparaben, propylparaben, menthol, eucalyptol, and phenol in 15 ml containers.

POLYVINYL ALCOHOL:

Liquifilm Tears (Allergan). Solution 1.4% with chlorobutanol 0.5% in 15 and 30 ml containers (nonprescription).

Liquifilm Forte (Allergan). Solution (sterile) 3% with thimerosal 0.002% and edetate disodium in a buffered balanced isotonic solution in 30 ml containers (nonprescription).

Pre-Sert (Allergan). Solution (sterile) 3% with benzalkonium chloride in 15 ml containers (nonprescription).

Total (Allergan). Solution (sterile) with edetate disodium and benzalkonium chloride in 60 and 120 ml containers (nonprescription).

Wetting Solution (Barnes-Hind). Solution (sterile) with edetate disodium 0.02% and benzalkonium chloride 0.004% in 35 and 60 ml containers (nonprescription).

POLYVINYL ALCOHOL AND CELLULOSE ESTER:

Contique Wetting Solution (Alcon). Solution with hydroxypropylmethylcellulose, benzalkonium chloride 0.004%, and edetate disodium 0.025% in 60 ml containers (nonprescription).

hy-FLOW (SMP). Solution (sterile, mildly hypertonic) with potassium chloride, sodium chloride, edetate disodium, and benzalkonium chloride 0.01% in 60 ml containers (nonprescription).

Lensine (SMP). Solution (sterile, mildly hypertonic) 5 in 1 with poloxamer 407, edetate disodium, and benzalkonium chloride in 60 and 120 ml containers (nonprescription).

Lens-Mate (Alcon). Solution with hydroxypropylmethylcellulose, benzalkonium chloride 0.004%, and edetate disodium 0.025% in 60 and 180 ml containers (nonprescription).

Liquifilm Wetting Solution (Allergan). Solution 2% with hydroxypropylmethylcellulose, benzalkonium chloride 1:25,000, edetate disodium, sodium chloride, and potassium chloride in 20 and 60 ml containers (nonprescription).

Neo-Tears (Barnes-Hind). Solution (sterile) containing hydroxyethylcellulose with sodium chloride, potassium chloride, sodium phosphate and sodium biphosphate, polyethylene glycol 300, thimerosal not to exceed 0.004%, and edetate disodium 0.02% in 15 ml containers (nonprescription).

Visalens Wetting Solution (Leeming). Solution (sterile) with hydroxypropylmethylcellulose, edetate disodium 0.1%, sodium chloride, and benzalkonium chloride 0.01% in 60 ml containers (nonprescription).

OTHER POLYMERIC SYSTEMS:

Adapt (Burton, Parsons). Solution (sterile) containing water-soluble BP polymers, hydroxyethylcellulose 0.55%, thimerosal 0.004%, and edetate disodium 0.1% in 15 ml containers (nonprescription).

Adapettes (Burton, Parsons). Solution (sterile) containing water-soluble BP polymers, thimerosal 0.004%, and edetate disodium 0.1% in 15 ml containers (nonprescription).

Adsorbotear (Burton, Parsons). Solution (sterile) containing water-soluble BP polymers, povidone, hydroxyethylcellulose 0.44%, thimerosal 0.004%, and edetate disodium 0.1% in 15 ml containers (nonprescription).

Hypotears (SMP). Solution (sterile, hypotonic) containing lipodin vehicle with the tonicity adjusted to 0.6% with nonionic agents available in 15 and 30 ml containers (nonprescription).

Tears Naturale (Alcon). Solution containing Duosorb water-soluble polymers, benzal-

konium chloride 0.01%, and edetate disodium 0.05% in 15 and 30 ml containers (nonprescription).

STERILE BLAND OINTMENTS:

Duratears (Alcon). Ointment (sterile) with white petrolatum, anhydrous liquid lanolin, mineral oil, methylparaben 0.05%, and propylparaben 0.01% in 3.5 g containers (nonprescription).

Lacri-Lube S.O.P. (Allergan). Ointment (ophthalmic, sterile) with white petrolatum, mineral oil, nonionic lanolin derivatives, and chlorobutanol 0.5% in 3.5 g containers (nonprescription).

ANTIHISTAMINES

Products containing an antihistamine and decongestant are promoted for treatment of ocular allergy. Topically applied antihistamines are relatively ineffective histamine antagonists, and any symptomatic relief obtained from these products is probably due to the local anesthetic properties of the antihistamine and possibly to the vasoconstrictor action of the decongestant. Systemic antihistamines are more effective.

Antihistamines can cause eczematous contact dermatitis following topical use. Individuals sensitized to one antihistamine may show cross sensitivity to other antihistamines or related agents.

These agents may dilate the pupil and, in patients predisposed to angle-closure glaucoma, could precipitate an acute attack.

TOPICAL OPHTHALMIC PREPARATIONS.

Albalon-A (Allergan). Solution (sterile) containing antazoline phosphate 0.5% and naphazoline hydrochloride 0.05% with polyvinyl alcohol 1.4%, benzalkonium chloride 0.004%, edetate disodium, polyvinyl pyrrolidone, sodium chloride, and sodium acetate in 15 ml containers.

Prefrin A (Allergan). Solution containing pyrilamine maleate 0.1% and phenylephrine hydrochloride 0.12% with sodium bisulfite, sodium citrate, boric acid, edetate disodium, benzalkonium chloride, and antipyrine 0.1% in 15 ml containers.

Vernacel (Professional Pharmacal). Solution (sterile) containing pheniramine maleate 0.5%, phenylephrine hydrochloride 0.125%, methylcellulose, and benzalkonium chloride 1:15,000 in 15 ml containers.

Vasocon-A (SMP). Solution (sterile) containing antazoline phosphate 0.5% and naphazoline hydrochloride 0.05% with sodium carbonate, sodium chloride, boric acid, and phenylmercuric acetate 0.002% in 15 ml containers.

Selected References

Beasley H: Miotics in cataract surgery. *Trans Am Ophthal Soc* 69:237-244, 1971.

Benedetto DA, et al: Instilled fluid dynamics and surface chemistry of polymers in preocular tear film. *Invest Ophthalmol* 14:887-902, 1975.

Burns RP, et al: Chronic toxicity of local anesthetics on cornea, in Leopold IH, Burns RP (eds): *Symposium on Ocular Therapy.* New York, John Wiley & Sons, 1977, vol 10, 31-44.

Dohlman CH, Hyndiuk RA: Subclinical and manifest corneal edema after cataract extraction, in Castroviejo R, et al (eds): *Symposium on Cornea: Transactions of the New Orleans Academy of Ophthalmology.* St Louis, CV Mosby Co, 1972, 214-235.

Edelhauser HF, et al: Intraocular irrigating solutions: Their effect on corneal epithelium. *Arch Ophthalmol* 93:648-659, 1975.

Ellis PP: Local anesthetics, in Leopold IH, Burns RP (eds): *Symposium on Ocular Therapy.* New York, John Wiley & Sons, 1976, vol 8, 17-24.

Gasset AR, Kaufman HE: Bandage lenses in treatment of bullous keratopathy. *Am J Ophthalmol* 72:376-380, 1971.

Gilbard JP, et al: Osmolarity of tear microvolumes in keratoconjunctivitis sicca. *Arch Ophthalmol* 96:677-681, 1978.

Grant WM: New treatment for calcific corneal opacities. *Arch Ophthalmol* 48:681-685, 1952.

Havener WH: *Ocular Pharmacology*, ed 4. St Louis, CV Mosby Co, 1978.

Johnstone MA, et al: Experimental zinc chloride ocular injury and treatment with disodium edetate. *Am J Ophthalmol* 76:137-142, 1973.

Lemp MA, et al: Effect of tear substitutes on tear film break-up time. *Invest Ophthalmol* 14:255-258, 1975.

McEnerney JK, Peyman EA: Simplification of glutathione-bicarbonate-ringer solution: Its effect on corneal thickness. *Invest Ophthal Visual Sci* 16:657-660, 1977.

Mindel JS: Value of hyaluronidase in ocular surgical akinesia. *Am J Opthalmol* 85:643-646, 1978.

Rizzuti AB: Acetylcholine in surgery of lens, iris, and cornea. *Am J Ophthalmol* 63:484-487, 1967.

Russell DA, Guyton JS: Retrobulbar injection of lidocaine (Xylocaine) for anesthesia and akinesia. *Am J Ophthalmol* 38:78-84, 1954.

Smith RB, Everett WG: Physiology and pharmacology of local anesthetic agents. *Int Ophthalmol Clin* 13:35-60, 1973.

Smith RB, Linn JG: Retrobulbar injection of bupivacaine (Marcaine) for anesthesia and akinesia. *Invest Ophthalmol* 13:157-158, 1974.

Stein MR, Parker CW: Reactions following intravenous fluorescein. *Am J Ophthalmol* 72:861-868, 1971.

Drugs Used in Vertigo, Motion Sickness, and Vomiting | 26

Vertigo and nausea are only symptoms and vomiting only a sign of altered function; they are not diseases. Rational therapy, which may or may not include drugs, is first and foremost dependent upon accurate diagnosis.

The drugs presented in this chapter are effective in combating (1) vertigo, (2) motion sickness, and (3) the nausea and vomiting associated with pregnancy, the postoperative period, and toxins (metabolic toxins [eg, uremia, carcinomatosis], microbial toxins), radiation sickness, and cytotoxic drugs. The nausea and vomiting induced by other drugs (eg, digitalis, opiates, estrogens, aminophylline, levodopa, iron preparations) is obviated by reducing the dose or changing the preparation or drug.

In general, use of drug therapy for prophylaxis of vomiting is more successful than for treatment, especially that caused by motion sickness, radiation, or chemotherapy. Oral dosage forms are most useful for prophylaxis; suppository and parenteral forms are preferred for treatment.

The pharmacodynamic classification (see the Table) of drugs used in the prevention and treatment of vertigo, motion sickness, and vomiting (ie, anticholinergic, antihistaminic, antidopaminergic, miscellaneous) is more valuable to define anticipated side effects than efficacy in a particular disorder, because numerous drugs in the same pharmacodynamic classes have little or no such activity in these disorders.

Useful drugs include: (1) the anticholinergic agent, scopolamine, which appears to act by reducing the excitability of labyrinth receptors, thus depressing conduction in vestibular cerebellar pathways or preventing recruitment of impulses at the chemoreceptor trigger zone;

(2) antihistamines (buclizine [Bucladin-S], cyclizine [Marezine], dimenhydrinate [Dramamine], diphenhydramine [Benadryl], hydroxyzine [Vistaril], meclizine [Antivert, Bonine], promethazine [Phenergan, Remsed]), which are assumed to affect neural pathways originating in the labyrinth; and (3) antidopaminergic drugs, which include many of the phenothiazines and the butyrophenone, haloperidol [Haldol]; these drugs act primarily upon the chemoreceptor trigger zone and, to a lesser degree, on the vomiting center. Phenothiazines used most commonly for their antiemetic effect include those in the aliphatic group (chlorpromazine [Thorazine], promazine [Sparine], and triflupromazine [Vesprin]) and the piperazine group (fluphenazine [Prolixin], perphenazine [Trilafon], prochlorperazine [Compazine], and thiethylperazine [Torecan]). The piperidine phenothiazines (eg, thioridazine [Mellaril]) are not effective as antiemetics. Although promethazine is an aliphatic phenothiazine, it is classified and used as an antihistamine because it has only weak dopamine antagonist activity, it possesses considerable antihistaminic activity, and, unlike other phenothiazines but like antihistamines, it is effective in vertigo and motion sickness.

Three miscellaneous agents, diphenidol [Vontrol], trimethobenzamide [Tigan], and benzquinamide [Emete-con], also are used as antiemetics. The first is thought to act upon the aural vestibular apparatus and the latter two primarily upon the chemoreceptor trigger zone.

Two investigational antiemetic agents, domperidone and metoclopramide, are similar to the antidopaminergic agents in spectrum of action and potency. They appear to act in part by stimulating upper gastrointestinal motility (but not secretion), which enhances gastric emptying.

In open and controlled studies in adults and children (Fragen and Caldwell, 1978; Dhondt et al, 1978; Reyntjens, 1979), domperidone was shown to be more effective than placebo. It is well absorbed when given intramuscularly, orally, or rectally and is extensively biotransformed by the liver to inactive metabolites that are excreted in the bile. Domperidone has a half-life of approximately eight hours. No serious adverse effects have been reported at this early stage of clinical investigation. The lack of extrapyramidal reactions may be due to the fact that, even with large doses, domperidone has no antipsychotic (neuroleptic) action in animals, presumably because the drug is poorly distributed

AVAILABLE PREPARATIONS AND PRINCIPAL USES
OF ANTIVERTIGO, ANTIMOTION SICKNESS, AND ANTIEMETIC DRUGS

DRUG CLASSIFICATION	AVAILABLE PREPARATIONS				
	Parenteral	Suppository	Oral	Dermal	Vertigo
ANTICHOLINERGIC Scopolamine Hydrobromide Scopolamine [Transderm V] (delivery system Investigational)	+		+	(+)	+

to most of the central nervous system.

Since metoclopramide [Reglan] blocks the chemoreceptor trigger zone, it is not clear to what extent this action and its gastrointestinal stimulating effect (see Chapter 60) contribute to its antiemetic effect. Its parenteral or oral use to control vomiting is considered investigational. Because metoclopramide increases lower esophageal sphincter pressure (Brock-Utne et al, 1978), it is being investigated to reduce the incidence of regurgitation and aspiration of gastric contents in general anesthesia. Like other antidopaminergic agents, metoclopramide is not effective in the prevention of motion sickness. This drug is metabolized by the liver and the first-pass biotransformation varies significantly among patients after oral administration (Bateman et al, 1978; Bateman and Davies, 1979). Its half-life is approximately three hours. The principal adverse effect is sedation; occasional reactions include agitation, irritability, constipation or diarrhea, urticarial maculopapular rash, dryness of the mouth, glossal or periorbital edema, methemoglobinemia, and neck pain and rigidity. Extrapyramidal reactions, deterioration of parkinsonism, and tardive dyskinesia have been noted when large doses (40 to 80 mg daily) were used for many

months or years (Kataria et al, 1978). Dystonic reactions (characterized by seizures, oculogyric crises, opisthotonus, or akathisia) have been noted even with short-term antiemetic use; they were most common in children and young adults.

Animal studies demonstrate that marijuana and its derivatives are effective in controlling vomiting induced by cytotoxic drugs, but the antiemetic action is not related to an antidopaminergic mechanism (Shannon et al, 1978). The active ingredient of marijuana, delta-9-tetrahydrocannabinol (Sallan et al, 1976), and a synthetic derivative, nabilone (Herman et al, 1979), are proposed for continued investigational studies as prophylactic antiemetics against cytotoxic drugs in man.

VERTIGO

True (objective) vertigo is associated with a hallucination of movement (commonly, but not exclusively, rotational). It can be produced by any lesion or process affecting the brain, the eighth cranial nerve, or the labyrinthine system. Common causes of chronic episodic or unremitting true vertigo include cerebral ischemia, cerebral atrophy, vestibular or labyrinthine

PRINCIPAL USES						COMMENTS
Motion Sickness	Pregnancy	Postoperative Vomiting	Toxins* Radiation Sickness	Cytotoxic Drugs		
+ (+)						Side effects markedly limit the use of scopolamine in vertigo, especially the chronic types. Side effects also limit the routine use of this most effective agent in the prevention of motion sickness; however, a Transdermal Therapeutic System (TTS) of delivery may obviate this problem and prolong effectiveness. Data to recommend TTS-Scopolamine for other antivertigo-antiemetic indications are incomplete. Other anticholinergic drugs are less effective.

DRUG CLASSIFICATION	AVAILABLE PREPARATIONS				
	Parenteral	Suppository	Oral	Dermal	Vertigo
ANTIHISTAMINIC					
Buclizine Hydrochloride [Bucladin-S]			+		±
Cyclizine Hydrochloride [Marezine]			+		+
Cyclizine Lactate [Marezine]	+				+
Dimenhydrinate [Dramamine]	+	+	+		+
Diphenhydramine Hydrochloride [Benadryl]	+		+		+
Hydroxyzine Hydrochloride [Vistaril]	+				±
Hydroxyzine Pamoate [Vistaril]			+		±
Meclizine Hydrochloride [Antivert, Bonine]			+		+
Promethazine Hydrochloride [Phenergan, Remsed]	+	+	+		+
ANTIDOPAMINERGIC					
Aliphatic Phenothiazines					
Chlorpromazine		+			
Chlorpromazine Hydrochloride [Thorazine]	+		+		
Promazine Hydrochloride [Sparine]	+		+		
Triflupromazine Hydrochloride [Vesprin]	+		+		
Piperazine Phenothiazines					
Fluphenazine Hydrochloride [Prolixin]	+		+		
Perphenazine [Trilafon]	+		+		
Prochlorperazine		+			
Prochlorperazine Edisylate	+		+		
Prochlorperazine Maleate [Compazine]			+		
Thiethylperazine Malate	+				
Thiethylperazine Maleate [Torecan]		+	+		
Butyrophenone					
Haloperidol [Haldol]	+		+		

PRINCIPAL USES					COMMENTS
Motion Sickness	Pregnancy	Postoperative Vomiting	Toxins* Radiation Sickness	Cytotoxic Drugs	
+					Buclizine and hydroxyzine are classified as possibly effective in the treatment of vertigo, Cyclizine, dimenhydrinate, diphenhydramine, hydroxyzine, andmeclizine are effective in the prevention of mild to moderate motion sickness and vertigo; these agents are effective in the prevention of vomiting of pregnancy *if* drug therapy is indicated; however, hydroxyzine is not recommended because its safe use in pregnancy has not been established. Chemically, promethazine is an aliphatic phenothiazine; however, its antiemetic and toxic actions are more similar to drugs in this class. It is the most effective antihistamine in the prevention or treatment of vomiting associated with moderate to severe vertigo, motion sickness, and, *if* indicated, hyperemesis gravidarum. Although promethazine and hydroxyzine are effective in mild to moderate postoperative vomiting, they are less effective than the antidopaminergic drugs. In any event, they should not be used routinely for postoperative vomiting.
+	+				
+	+				
+	+				
+	+				
+					
+		+			
+				+	
+	+	+		+	
		+		+	These agents are not recommended for the prevention of vertigo or motion sickness. They may be considered in the treatment of vomiting associated with these conditions or hyperemesis gravidarum, especially if a trial with promethazine is inadequate. The antidopaminergic drugs are most useful in the treatment of moderate to severe postoperative vomiting or that induced by radiation and cytotoxic drugs. Their use should be considered only adjunctive in pancreatitis and metabolic disorders (eg, uremia, carcinomatosis) along with gastric or intestinal decompression and intravenous electrolyte and nutrition therapy. The choice of an antidopaminergic agent is also based on adverse effects. Aliphatic phenothiazines tend to produce more autonomic adverse effects (anticholinergic and alpha-antiadrenergic), while piperazine phenothiazines, haloperidol, and metoclopramide tend to produce more adverse extrapyramidal reactions. Domperidone distributes poorly to the brain and no adverse extrapyramidal effects have been noted. Although metoclopramide is approved for use in single intravenous doses to stimulate gastric emptying and intestinal transit, its use in the treatment of vomiting is investigational.
		+		+	
		+		+	

DRUG CLASSIFICATION	AVAILABLE PREPARATIONS				
	Parenteral	Suppository	Oral	Dermal	Vertigo
ANTIDOPAMINERGIC					
Metoclopramide (investigational) [Reglan]					
Domperidone (investigational)					
MISCELLANEOUS					
Benzquinamide Hydrochloride [Emete-con]	+				
Diphenidol Hydrochloride [Vontrol]	+		+		+
Trimethobenzamide Hydrochloride [Tigan]	+	+	+		
Nabilone (investigational)					

*Toxins include metabolic toxins (eg, uremia, carcinomatosis) and other exogenous toxins (eg, microbial, chemicals

neuronitis, benign positional vertigo, and Meniere's disease; it also may be associated with migraine headaches or hearing loss. Nausea and vomiting are not always present, although they are more likely to be associated with true rather than subjective vertigo. The diagnosis (Turner, 1975) and management (Jackson et al, 1976) of true vertigo, including drug selection if indicated, are dependent upon the etiology, rapidity of onset, and character (episodic or unremitting) of the disorder.

The dizziness of *subjective vertigo* is characterized mainly by the presyncopal feeling of lightheadedness, fainting, or altered consciousness, sometimes associated with a vague sensation of motion described as being within the head. Subjective vertigo may be associated with disorders that result in inadequate blood supply to the cochlea and/or vestibular apparatus (eg,

severe anemia, heart block, hypersensitive carotid sinus syndrome, sick sinus syndrome, transient ischemic attack, stroke, trauma). The latter three disorders also may cause true vertigo, depending upon the location of the impaired area. In addition, subjective vertigo may be associated with psychiatric disturbances, especially when hyperventilation is present.

Drug-induced vertigo occurs most frequently after use of agents that damage the eighth nerve (eg, aminoglycoside antibiotics, ethacrynic acid, furosemide) or produce orthostatic hypotension (eg, antihypertensive agents, phenothiazines).

Drug Therapy: Side effects markedly limit the use of scopolamine in vertigo, especially the chronic types. The antihistaminic group of drugs is often beneficial in *true vertigo* (see the Table). Although these drugs are generally satisfactory, se-

PRINCIPAL USES				COMMENTS
Motion Sickness	Pregnancy	Postoperative Vomiting	Toxins* Radiation Sickness Cytotoxic Drugs	
		(+)	(+)	
			(+)	
		+		None of these agents are indicated for prevention or treatment of nausea and vomiting associated with motion sickness. Diphenidol is used for chronic vertigo, but only in closely supervised outpatients or inpatients. Benzquinamide is at least as effective as the antidopaminergic drugs but overall experience is less and data are insufficient to justify its use in children. Trimethobenzamide is less effective than the antidopaminergic drugs in the prevention or treatment of toxin-induced or postoperative vomiting. Nabilone, a synthetic derivative of delta-9-tetrahydrocannibinol, is being investigated for the prevention of vomiting due to cytotoxic drugs; data in man are incomplete.
		+	+	
		+	+	
			(+)	

vere vomiting associated with vertigo may require the use of antidopaminergic agents or diphenidol. Use of diphenidol generally is limited to hospitalized patients or closely supervised outpatients, because of the potential severity of its adverse effects. Sedatives also may be required (see Chapter 11).

The management program for Meniere's disease, a form of episodic true vertigo usually accompanied by ear symptoms and probably caused by excess endolymphatic fluid, includes a low-salt diet, diuretics, and antivertigo-antiemetic drugs. Since papaverine, histamine, and betazole have been shown to increase cochlear blood flow experimentally (Suga and Snow, 1969), these and other vasodilators (eg, cyclandelate [Cyclospasmol], nicotinic acid, nylidrin [Arlidin]) also have been employed in Meniere's disease. These drugs are occasionally used in sudden-onset hearing loss with vertigo, benign positional vertigo, and disorders in which endolymphatic hydrops or a localized vasospastic condition is suspected rather than atherosclerosis. Well-controlled clinical studies are difficult to conduct because of the spontaneous exacerbations and remissions that occur, and the efficacy of the vasodilators is based principally on the clinical judgment of authorities in the field (Rubin, 1973; Roydhouse, 1974). See the evaluations in Chapter 36, Agents Used in Peripheral Vascular Disorders, for dosage.

Betahistine hydrochloride [Serc], an orally effective histamine derivative, is used as an investigational agent in Meniere's disease. One controlled crossover study of 22 patients with Meniere's disease demonstrated a significant improvement in vertigo, tinnitus, and deafness after use of betahistine compared to placebo (Frew and Menon, 1976); however, follow-up was limited to six months after 32 weeks of treatment, and no other vasodilator was used as a positive control. No adverse reactions were noted, and no statistically significant differences in heart rate or blood pressure were noted between placebo and betahistine, which was given as four 8-mg tablets daily (two at 8 a.m. and one each at 2 p.m. and 8 p.m.). If parenteral vasodilator therapy is required, histamine diphosphate or papaverine is used initially (Jackson et al, 1976). Histamine solution containing 2.5 mg in 250 ml is given after a meal at a rate of 16 to 60 drops/min; flushing of the skin is desirable, but blood pressure should not be allowed to fall more than 10 to 15 mm Hg. The dosage of papaverine also is adjusted to the same end points at a rate of 0.5 mg/kg/min intravenously.

Antivertigo drugs usually play less of a role in the treatment of *subjective vertigo* than management of the underlying disorder. In drug-induced vertigo, withdrawing the offending drug or reducing the dose is preferred to administering labyrinthine suppressants.

If the vertigo is severe enough to produce intolerable anxiety or severe depression, patients may benefit from the use of antianxiety agents or antidepressants (see Chapters 11 and 13, respectively).

MOTION SICKNESS

The principal subjective components of the motion sickness syndrome are malaise and nausea rather than vertigo (Wood, 1979). One-third of the population is highly susceptible and even may experience excessive salivation and vomiting under only mildly rough conditions of travel; another third will require moderately rough conditions of travel to exhibit the same signs and symptoms, while the remainder will become sick only under extreme conditions of motion (eg, storms at sea, aerobatics). Tolerance develops within two to three days providing the intensity of the stimulus does not increase. Use of drugs for prophylaxis one to two hours before travel is more effective than for treatment.

Drug Therapy: Although scopolamine is one of the most effective agents for prevention of motion sickness, its use is limited because of untoward effects (primarily drowsiness, dryness of the mouth, and blurring of vision). Nevertheless, because of its efficacy and short duration of action, scopolamine may be especially useful for severe motion sickness of brief duration when only a few small doses are required. Repeated doses may have a cumulative effect. A recently introduced adhesive unit containing scopolamine [Transderm-V] for placement behind the ear delivers sufficient scopolamine transdermally to combat motion sickness while obviating most of the side effects and prolonging the effectiveness of scopolamine.

The antihistamine drugs are less effective than scopolamine but produce fewer adverse effects. Buclizine, cyclizine, dimenhydrinate, diphenhydramine, hydroxyzine, and promethazine are effective in mild to moderate motion sickness; their duration of action ranges from four to six hours, while the action of meclizine is claimed to persist for 24 hours. Promethazine is the most effective antihistamine for the prophylaxis of moderate to severe motion sickness, although considerable sedation may be produced. It is especially effective when combined with ephedrine. Promethazine also usually is effective in the treatment of vomiting associated with motion sickness. A more potent antidopaminergic antiemetic drug may be required for intractable cases; however, these drugs are relatively ineffective in the prophylaxis of motion sickness.

VOMITING

Emesis is a complex reflex that is coordinated by the vomiting center in the medulla. Stimuli are relayed to this center from peripheral areas (eg, gastric mucosa, peritoneum, joints, tendons). Major sensory stimuli also arise within the central nervous system itself (ie, cerebral cortex, otic vestibular apparatus) and are transmitted through the chemoreceptor trigger zone sensory nucleus (CTZ) in the medulla to the vomiting center. The efferent arc is completed by excitatory impulses transmitted to the salivary glands and the muscles of the diaphragm, anterior abdominal wall, gastric antrum, and duodenum. Inhibitory impulses to the muscles of the gastric fundus, gastroesophageal sphincter, and esophagus arrive simultaneously.

Nausea and vomiting may be symptoms of serious organic disturbances of almost any of the viscera of the chest or abdomen or may be produced by infections, drugs, radiation, painful or noxious stimuli, metabolic and emotional disturbances, exposure to unfamiliar environmental forces, audiovisual-proprioceptive sensory mismatch phenomena (eg, air or ship travel, amusement rides, prolonged car or train travel, exposure to large gravitational forces), or vertigo. Whenever possible, the underlying cause should be determined and corrected. The use of antiemetics is justified only when no alternative therapy exists and the benefits outweigh the risks of adverse reactions or of masking more serious underlying conditions.

Drug Therapy: These drugs should not be used to treat *vomiting during pregnancy* unless absolutely necessary. Generally, less than 1% of pregnant patients have sufficiently severe nausea and vomiting to necessitate antiemetic drug therapy. Nondrug therapy (eg, alteration of diet and time of eating, rest) should always be tried before prescribing antiemetic drugs. If an antiemetic is indicated, cyclizine, dimenhydrinate, diphenhydramine, or meclizine is often used initially. If vomiting persists so that maternal nutrition is compromised, use of promethazine or an antidopaminergic drug (see the Table) may be considered. Pyridoxine hydrochloride (vitamin B₆) is ineffective in these patients (see Chapter 52, Vitamins and Minerals).

Administration of antiemetics to prevent *postoperative vomiting* is justified only in a few clinical situations: when vomiting would endanger the results of surgery (eg, intraocular or intracranial operations); when debilitated patients at risk of dehy-

dration or electrolyte imbalance must undergo surgery (it is unlikely that the fluid and electrolyte loss associated with ordinary postoperative vomiting would reach serious proportions in low-risk patients adequately prepared for surgery); or when labyrinthine function is stimulated, which occurs with almost all ear surgery; usually promethazine, prochlorperazine, or benzquinamide is administered for the latter condition. In other situations, the *routine* use of antiemetics postoperatively is unwarranted because less than 3% of individuals require such therapy. Although promethazine, hydroxyzine, and trimethobenzamide may be adequate for moderate postoperative vomiting, the antidopaminergic agents and benzquinamide are more effective and may be required for the management of severe vomiting.

Some physicians use promethazine or hydroxyzine for premedication in patients with a history of nausea and vomiting after use of a general anesthetic.

The established efficacy of an antiemetic drug in *toxin-, radiation-, and cytotoxic drug-induced vomiting* does not reflect the frequency of use in any of these situations. For example, the self-limited nausea and vomiting associated with acute gastroenteritis may require antiemetics only when a regimen that includes intravenous hydration and nutrition, electrolyte replenishment, rest, and fasting does not satisfactorily improve the patient's condition. Conversely, the prophylactic use of antiemetics to control nausea and vomiting induced by radiation or cytotoxic drugs is often indicated because it makes the therapeutic program more acceptable and improves compliance.

The antidopaminergic drugs are the most effective antiemetics for the management of nausea and vomiting associated with toxins, radiation sickness, and cytotoxic drugs. They are generally the agents of choice, although the risk of toxicity is relatively greater. Since the patient's responsiveness varies considerably in these disorders, an antihistamine-type drug (ie, promethazine, meclizine) may be adequate and may minimize the risk in selected patients. The reported effectiveness of trimethobenzamide is quite variable; it should be used with caution in pregnant patients, since only limited data are available.

Adverse Reactions and Precautions

Caution is required with use of all antiemetics because they may mask the symptoms of organic disease (eg, gastrointestinal or central nervous system disorders) or the toxic effects of other drugs. Drowsiness is the most common untoward effect and may account for some of the antiemetic action. Individuals whose activities require alertness, such 'as those operating vehicles or machinery, should use antiemetics with great caution. Some of these drugs may potentiate the actions of other central nervous system depressants.

Anticholinergic and Antihistaminic Drugs: Drowsiness is the most common untoward effect of these drugs; anticholinergic side effects also may be anticipated, even with the antihistamines. Promethazine [Phenergan, Remsed] is relatively free of the extrapyramidal reactions observed with the phenothiazines and the butyrophenone, haloperidol [Haldol].

Buclizine [Bucladin-S], cyclizine [Marezine], hydroxyzine [Vistaril], and meclizine [Antivert, Bonine] are teratogenic in animals when given in very large doses. The possibility that these drugs may be hazardous to the human fetus has not been completely excluded. However, large drug surveillance programs have not demonstrated that birth defects occur in the dosage ranges employed clinically. (See the discussion on Use of Drugs During Pregnancy in Chapter 2.)

Antidopaminergic Drugs: Phenothiazines in the piperazine group (fluphenazine [Prolixin], perphenazine [Trilafon], prochlorperazine [Compazine], and thiethylperazine [Torecan]) are less likely to cause drowsiness, orthostatic hypotension, dryness of the mouth, and nasal congestion than those in the aliphatic group (chlorpromazine [Thorazine], promazine [Sparine], and triflupromazine [Vesprin]). Cholestatic jaundice, granulocytopenia, ur-

ticaria, dermatitis, thrombocytopenia, leukopenia, agranulocytosis, purpura, pancytopenia, and gastroenteritis have occurred after use of all phenothiazines; less common reactions include galactorrhea, photosensitivity, and edema of the extremities. The incidence of these reactions is quite low when these drugs are used as antiemetics, since the duration of administration is short and the dosage relatively small.

Extrapyramidal reactions, including dystonia, parkinsonian syndrome, akathisia, and dysarthria, have been associated with use of all phenothiazines and haloperidol [Haldol]. The incidence of these reactions is higher with phenothiazines in the piperazine group than with those in the aliphatic group.

The extrapyramidal symptoms and signs that may be produced by the antidopaminergic antiemetics or other antiemetics (eg, promethazine [Phenergan, Remsed], trimethobenzamide [Tigan]) may be confused with the central nervous system signs of an undiagnosed primary disease responsible for the vomiting (eg, Reye's syndrome, other encephalopathy). Thus, use of these drugs and other potential hepatotoxins should be avoided in children and adolescents whose signs and symptoms suggest Reye's syndrome.

Phenothiazines are contraindicated in patients with bone marrow depression, pregnant women with pre-eclampsia, or in patients with a history of hypersensitivity to any of the phenothiazines. They should be used with caution in patients with a history of dyskinetic reactions and, since these drugs are detoxified primarily in the liver, in those with moderate to severe hepatic dysfunction.

The action of phenothiazines and haloperidol may be potentiated if other central nervous system depressants are used concomitantly. The sedation may be desirable in some patients (eg, those with malignancies) but undesirable in others. Phenothiazines are contraindicated in patients with symptoms of marked central nervous system depression and/or hypotension. They also may augment the fall in blood pressure when given to patients receiving spinal or epidural anesthesia or adrenergic blocking agents. See also Chapter 12, Antipsychotic Drugs, and the evaluation on Haloperidol.

Miscellaneous Drugs: See the evaluations.

ANTICHOLINERGIC DRUGS

SCOPOLAMINE
[Transderm-V]

SCOPOLAMINE HYDROBROMIDE

Although available evidence indicates that this is one of the most effective agents in the prevention of motion sickness, scopolamine has been largely supplanted by the antihistaminic antiemetics, principally because of its untoward effects. Scopolamine has been incorporated in a novel transdermal delivery system (ie, an adhesive unit) for postauricular placement to obviate untoward side effects. When a 2.5 cm² adhesive unit is applied, scopolamine is released at a uniform rate for 72 hours. This method protects most individuals susceptible to motion sickness. Dryness of the mouth is noted quite frequently and drowsiness occasionally, but cycloplegia is not a problem (Graybiel et al, 1976).

Results of controlled studies in individuals subjected to severe motion indicate that there is a synergistic effect when 0.3 to 0.6 mg of scopolamine is given with 5 to 10 mg of dextroamphetamine, respectively, or when 0.6 mg of scopolamine is given with 25 mg of ephedrine or promethazine (Wood and Graybiel, 1972). The combination of scopolamine with promethazine or ephedrine has the additional advantages of producing fewer untoward effects and little abuse potential (Wood, 1979). The use of these combinations may be relevant only

for intense conditions of motion (eg, storms at sea, aerobatics, severe rotary experimental circumstances) or for individuals who are highly susceptible to moderately rough conditions of motion.

Anticholinergic side effects (blurred vision, mydriasis, dryness of the mouth, decreased or increased pulse rate, drowsiness, amnesia, and fatigue) often are associated with use of scopolamine, especially in large doses. Less frequent but more severe side effects (urinary retention, constipation, and drowsiness) may develop, especially in children and the elderly. A toxic psychosis consisting of excitement, restlessness, hallucinations, or delirium may occur infrequently.

ROUTES, USUAL DOSAGE, AND PREPARATIONS. SCOPOLAMINE HYDROBROMIDE:
Oral, Subcutaneous: *Adults*, 0.6 to 1 mg; *children*, 0.006 mg/kg of body weight.
> Drug available generically: Tablets (hypodermic) 0.4 and 0.6 mg; solution (for injection) 0.4 mg/ml in 0.5 ml containers, 0.3, 0.4, 0.6, and 1 mg/ml in 1 ml containers, and 0.5 mg/ml in 20 ml containers.

SCOPOLAMINE:
Topical: A transdermal therapeutic system is applied to clean dry skin in the postauricular area several hours before antiemetic protection is required. The duration of action is 72 hours. *Adults*, one 2.5 cm² adhesive unit. This system is not suitable for use in *children* because it is not known whether the amount of scopolamine that is released could produce serious adverse effects.
> *Transderm-V* (Ciba). 2.5 cm² adhesive unit (Delivery system investigational).

ANTIHISTAMINIC DRUGS

BUCLIZINE HYDROCHLORIDE
[Bucladin-S]

Buclizine, a piperazine antihistamine, is useful in preventing motion sickness.

Insufficient controlled studies are available for evaluation of its effectiveness in vertigo; therefore, it is classified as only possibly effective in this condition. The duration of action is four to six hours.

Drowsiness, dryness of the mouth, headache, and agitation may occur. See the Introduction for a discussion of the drug's teratogenic effects in animals.

ROUTE, USUAL DOSAGE, AND PREPARATIONS. *Oral*: For motion sickness, *adults*, 50 mg at least one-half hour before departure and four to six hours later, if necessary. The usual dosage for vertigo is 50 mg twice daily.

Bucladin-S (Stuart). Tablets 50 mg.

CYCLIZINE HYDROCHLORIDE
[Marezine]

CYCLIZINE LACTATE
[Marezine]

Cyclizine is useful in preventing and relieving symptoms of motion sickness and vertigo and other symptoms of aural vestibular disorders. The duration of action is about four hours.

Large doses may cause drowsiness and dryness of the mouth. A large-scale study, including pregnant women receiving cyclizine during the first trimester, failed to confirm that the drug had any teratogenic effect with the doses employed clinically (Milkovich and van den Berg, 1976). See the Introduction for a discussion of the drug's teratogenic effects in animals.

ROUTES, USUAL DOSAGE, AND PREPARATIONS. *Oral*: For motion sickness, *adults*, 50 mg one-half hour before departure, then every four to six hours as necessary (maximum, 200 mg daily); *children 6 to 10 years*, 3 mg/kg of body weight divided into three doses during a 24-hour period.

CYCLIZINE HYDROCHLORIDE:
Marezine [*hydrochloride*] (Burroughs Wellcome). Tablets 50 mg.

Intramuscular: 50 mg every four to six hours as necessary.

CYCLIZINE LACTATE:
Marezine [*lactate*] (Burroughs Wellcome). Solution 50 mg/ml in 1 ml containers.

DIMENHYDRINATE
[Dramamine]

This chlorotheophylline salt of diphenhydramine is useful in preventing and treating vertigo, motion sickness, and nausea and vomiting during pregnancy. Its duration of action is four to six hours. Mild drowsiness occurs.

ROUTES, USUAL DOSAGE, AND PREPARATIONS. *Intramuscular*: *Adults*, 50 mg as needed; *children*, 5 mg/kg of body weight divided into four doses during a 24-hour period (maximum, 300 mg/day).

Intravenous: *Adults*, 50 mg diluted in 10 ml of sodium chloride injection administered over a period of two minutes; *children*, no dosage has been established.

Drug available generically: Solution 50 mg/ml in 1 and 10 ml containers.
Dramamine (Searle). Solution 50 mg/ml in 1 and 5 ml containers.
Additional Trademark.
Dramocen (Central).

Oral: *Adults*, 50 to 100 mg every four hours; *children*, 5 mg/kg of body weight divided into four doses during a 24-hour period (maximum, 300 mg/day).

Drug available generically: syrup 12.5 and 50 mg/4 ml; tablets 50 mg.
Dramamine (Searle). Liquid 12.5 mg/4 ml (nonprescription); tablets 50 mg (nonprescription).

Rectal: *Adults*, 100 mg once or twice daily.

Dramamine (Searle). Suppositories 100 mg.

DIPHENHYDRAMINE HYDROCHLORIDE
[Benadryl]

HYDROXYZINE HYDROCHLORIDE
[Vistaril]

HYDROXYZINE PAMOATE
[Vistaril]

This antihistamine is similar to cyclizine in its actions. It is effective in the prevention and treatment of vertigo, motion sickness, or nausea and vomiting occurring during pregnancy. Its duration of action is four to six hours.

The incidence of drowsiness is high. Individuals whose activities require alertness, such as those operating vehicles or machinery, should use diphenhydramine with caution.

ROUTES, USUAL DOSAGE, AND PREPARATIONS. *Intramuscular (deep), Intravenous:* *Adults,* 10 mg initially; if sedation is not severe, the subsequent dose may be increased to 20 to 50 mg every two or three hours (maximum, 400 mg/day).

Intramuscular (deep): Children, 5 mg/kg of body weight divided into four doses during a 24-hour period (maximum, 300 mg/day).

> Drug available generically: Solution 10 mg/ml in 10 and 30 ml containers and 50 mg/ml in 1 and 10 ml containers.
> *Benadryl* (Parke, Davis). Solution (sterile) 10 mg/ml in 10 and 30 ml containers and 50 mg/ml in 1 and 10 ml containers.

Oral: For motion sickness, *adults,* 50 mg one-half hour before departure and 50 mg before each meal; *children,* 5 mg/kg of body weight divided into four doses during a 24-hour period (maximum, 300 mg/day).

> Drug available generically: Capsules 25 and 50 mg; elixir 10 and 12.5 mg/5 ml.
> *Benadryl* (Parke, Davis). Capsules 25 and 50 mg; elixir 12.5 mg/5 ml.

Hydroxyzine is an antianxiety agent, but it also possesses antiemetic and antihistaminic properties. It is useful for the treatment of motion sickness, postoperative nausea and vomiting, and, possibly, vertigo. The duration of action is four to six hours.

The incidence of drowsiness is low. The drug potentiates the central nervous system depressant actions of narcotics and barbiturates; therefore, the doses of these interacting drugs should be reduced by 50% when hydroxyzine is used concurrently. See the Introduction for a discussion on the drug's teratogenic effects in animals.

ROUTES, USUAL DOSAGE, AND PREPARATIONS. *Intramuscular:* For postoperative vomiting, *adults,* 25 to 100 mg; *children,* 1 mg/kg of body weight.

> HYDROXYZINE HYDROCHLORIDE:
> *Vistaril* [*hydrochloride*] (Pfizer). Solution 25 mg/ml in 1 and 10 ml containers and 50 mg/ml in 1, 2, and 10 ml containers.

Oral: *Adults,* 25 to 100 mg three or four times daily; *children under 6 years,* 50 mg divided into four doses during a 24-hour period; *over 6 years,* 50 to 100 mg divided into four doses during a 24-hour period.

> HYDROXYZINE PAMOATE:
> Drug available generically: Capsules, tablets 25, 50, and 100 mg.
> *Vistaril* [*pamoate*] (Pfizer). Capsules 25, 50, and 100 mg; suspension 25 mg/5 ml (strengths expressed in terms of the hydrochloride salt).

MECLIZINE HYDROCHLORIDE
[Antivert, Bonine]

Meclizine is effective in preventing and treating motion sickness. It has a slower onset and longer duration of action (24 hours) than most other antihistamines used for motion sickness. Meclizine also is used to prevent and to treat nausea and vomiting associated with vertigo of vestibular origin (eg, labyrinthitis, Meniere's disease) and occasionally is effective in preventing vomiting associated with radiation sickness.

Drowsiness, blurred vision, dryness of the mouth, and fatigue have occurred following administration of meclizine. See the Introduction for a discussion on the drug's teratogenic effects in animals.

ROUTE, USUAL DOSAGE, AND PREPARATIONS. *Oral: Adults,* for motion sickness, 25 to 50 mg once daily; the initial dose should be taken at least one hour prior to departure. For vertigo and radiation sickness, 25 to 100 mg daily in divided doses, depending upon clinical response. *Children,* dosage has not been established.

> Drug available generically: Tablets 12.5 and 25 mg; tablets (chewable) 25 mg.
> *Antivert* (Roerig). Tablets 12.5 and 25 mg; tablets (chewable) 25 mg.
> *Bonine* (Pfipharmecs). Tablets (chewable) 25 mg (nonprescription).

PROMETHAZINE HYDROCHLORIDE
[Phenergan, Remsed]

Unlike other phenothiazines, promethazine exhibits pronounced antihistaminic activity, is effective in the prevention and treatment of vertigo and motion sickness, and has limited, if any, effect upon vomiting caused by stimulation of the chemoreceptor trigger zone. However, it is effective in postoperative nausea and vomiting. Promethazine is less effective than the antidopaminergic agents in vomiting induced by toxins, radiation sickness, and cytotoxic drugs. The duration of action is four to six hours.

Results of controlled studies in individuals subjected to severe motion indicate that a synergistic antimotion sickness effect occurs when scopolamine is combined with 10 mg of dextroamphetamine or 25 mg of promethazine or ephedrine (see the evaluation on Scopolamine).

The most frequent and prominent side effect of promethazine is sedation. Anticholinergic and antiadrenergic adverse reactions occur infrequently following oral administration (see the Introduction).

In the usual antiemetic dose, promethazine is relatively free of the extrapyramidal stimulation associated with some phenothiazine and butyrophenone derivatives. However, the drug should be avoided in children and adolescents whose symptoms and signs suggest Reye's syndrome (see the Introduction).

ROUTES, USUAL DOSAGE, AND PREPARATIONS. *Intramuscular, Rectal:* For treatment of nausea and vomiting, *adults,* initially, 25 mg, then 12.5 to 25 mg as needed every four to six hours. A dose of 12.5 mg (which is usually effective) should be tried initially in selected high-risk postoperative patients, because hypotension is observed more frequently when the 25-mg dose is given parenterally postoperatively. *Children under 12 years,* the dose should be adjusted on the basis of the age and weight of the patient and severity of the condition; no more than one-half the suggested adult dose should be given.

> Drug available generically: Solution 25 and 50 mg/ml in 1 and 10 ml containers.
> *Phenergan* (Wyeth). Solution 25 and 50 mg/ml in 1 ml containers; suppositories (rectal) 12.5, 25, and 50 mg.

Oral: For motion sickness, *adults,* 25 mg twice daily. Administration one-half to one hour before anticipated travel is most beneficial. *Children*, 12.5 to 25 mg twice daily may be administered.

For treatment of nausea and vomiting, same as intramuscular and rectal dosage.

> Drug available generically: Tablets 12.5, 25, and 50 mg.
> *Phenergan* (Wyeth). Syrup 6.25 and 25 mg/5 ml; tablets 12.5, 25, and 50 mg.
> *Remsed* (Endo). Tablets 50 mg.

ANTIDOPAMINERGIC DRUGS

CHLORPROMAZINE
[Thorazine]

CHLORPROMAZINE HYDROCHLORIDE
[Thorazine]

$$CH_2CH_2CH_2N(CH_3)_2$$

Chlorpromazine is the prototype of the aliphatic phenothiazine compounds. In addition to its antipsychotic action, this compound is effective in the management of postoperative nausea and vomiting and that caused by cytotoxic drugs, radiation sickness, or toxins. It is not useful in preventing vertigo or motion sickness; however, its antiemetic effect may be useful in combating severe vomiting produced by the latter disorders.

Some patients may become drowsy to an undesirable degree; however, tolerance to excessive sedation usually develops after continued use. Chlorpromazine prolongs postanesthesia sleeping time. Serious untoward effects, which may occur after long-term use or administration of large doses, include extrapyramidal reactions, orthostatic hypotension, cholestatic jaundice, and leukopenia. Because of the severity of these adverse reactions, chlorpromazine should be considered only when vomiting cannot be controlled by relatively less toxic antiemetics. Since all phenothiazines have the potential to produce extrapyramidal reactions, the drug should be avoided in children and adolescents whose symptoms and signs suggest Reye's syndrome (see

the Introduction and Chapter 12, Antipsychotic Drugs).

ROUTES, USUAL DOSAGE, AND PREPARATIONS. This drug generally should not be used in *children under 6 months* except when it is potentially lifesaving. The manufacturer's suggested dosages are:

CHLORPROMAZINE:

Rectal: *Adults*, 50 to 100 mg every six to eight hours; *children*, 1 mg/kg of body weight every six to eight hours.

> *Thorazine* (Smith Kline & French). Suppositories 25 and 100 mg.

CHLORPROMAZINE HYDROCHLORIDE:

Intramuscular: *Adults*, initially, 25 mg. If hypotension does not occur, 25 to 50 mg is given every three or four hours until vomiting stops; the drug is then given orally. *Children*, 0.5 mg/kg of body weight every six to eight hours; maximum daily doses, *up to 5 years* (50 lb), 40 mg and *5 to 12 years* (50 to 100 lb), 75 mg.

> Drug available generically: Solution (aqueous) 25 mg/ml in 1, 2, and 10 ml containers.
> *Thorazine* [*hydrochloride*] (Smith Kline & French). Solution (aqueous) 25 mg/ml in 1, 2, and 10 ml containers.

Oral: *Adults*, 10 to 25 mg every four to six hours; *children*, 0.5 mg/kg of body weight every four to six hours. Since all phenothiazines have prolonged half-lives (12 to 20 hours), the oral timed-release preparation has no significant advantage over the ordinary oral dosage forms for most patients.

> Drug available generically: Tablets 4, 10, 25, 50, 100, and 200 mg; liquid (concentrate) 2, 30, and 100 mg/ml; syrup 10 mg/5 ml.
> *Thorazine* [*hydrochloride*] (Smith Kline & French). Capsules (timed-release) 30, 75, 150, and 200 mg; solution (concentrate) 30 and 100 mg/ml; syrup 10 mg/5 ml; tablets 10, 25, 50, 100, and 200 mg.

FLUPHENAZINE HYDROCHLORIDE
[Prolixin]

$$F_3C \quad CH_2CH_2CH_2-N+ \quad +N-CH_2CH_2OH \quad 2\ Cl^-$$

Fluphenazine, a piperazine phenothiazine, is effective in the management of postoperative nausea and vomiting and that caused by toxins, radiation sickness, and cytotoxic drugs. However, it is not useful in preventing vertigo or motion sickness. This phenothiazine has little sedative effect and does not appreciably prolong postanesthesia sleeping time when given preoperatively.

The incidence of extrapyramidal reactions is higher with fluphenazine than with most other phenothiazine compounds. The drug should be avoided in children and adolescents whose symptoms and signs suggest Reye's syndrome (see the Introduction). This drug has little tendency to produce orthostatic hypotension; however, other anticholinergic effects (blurred vision, dryness of the mouth, and urinary retention) have been reported. See also Chapter 12, Antipsychotic Drugs.

ROUTES, USUAL DOSAGE, AND PREPARATIONS. *Intramuscular, Oral*: *Adults*, 1.25 mg repeated at six- to eight-hour intervals if needed; *children*, dosage is reduced (see the table in Chapter 2).

> *Prolixin* (Squibb). Elixir (oral) 2.5 mg/5 ml; tablets (oral) 1, 2.5, 5, and 10 mg; solution (aqueous for injection, sterile) 2.5 mg/ml in 10 ml containers.

HALOPERIDOL
[Haldol]

The antiemetic action of this antidopaminergic butyrophenone is achieved mainly through inhibition of stimuli at the chemoreceptor trigger zone. Haloperidol is comparable in efficacy and scope of uses to that of the piperazine phenothiazines (eg, fluphenazine, perphenazine, prochlorperazine, thiethylperazine). It has been administered to alleviate nausea and vomiting associated with anesthesia and surgery, radiation therapy, use of cytotoxic drugs, and gastrointestinal disorders. As with other antiemetics, haloperidol must be given with great caution in patients with

gastrointestinal disorders to avoid masking the development of life-threatening conditions that may be amenable to surgery. Haloperidol is not effective in the prevention of vertigo or motion sickness. The drug is not recommended for use during pregnancy or in children until more clinical data are available.

The adverse reactions produced by haloperidol closely resemble those observed with use of the piperazine phenothiazines (see the Introduction and Chapter 12, Antipsychotic Drugs), but these occur only rarely with the small doses and short-term therapy used for these indications. Because the drug has the potential to produce extrapyramidal reactions, it should be avoided in children and adolescents whose symptoms and signs suggest Reye's syndrome (see the Introduction). Elderly or debilitated patients may be more sensitive to the drug.

ROUTES, USUAL DOSAGE, AND PREPARATIONS. *Intramuscular*: 1, 2, or 5 mg given every 12 hours as needed.

> *Haldol* (McNeil). Solution 5 mg/ml in 1 and 10 ml containers.

Oral: 1, 2, or 5 mg twice daily.

> *Haldol* (McNeil). Solution (concentrate) 2 mg/ml; tablets 0.5, 1, 2, 5, and 10 mg.

PERPHENAZINE
[Trilafon]

This piperazine phenothiazine is effective in the management of postoperative nausea and vomiting and that caused by toxins, radiation sickness, and cytotoxic drugs. It is not useful in preventing vertigo or motion sickness.

Untoward effects include extrapyramidal reactions, blurred or double vision, nasal congestion, dryness of the mouth, salivation, headache, and, occasionally, drowsiness. The drug should be avoided in children and adolescents whose symptoms and signs suggest Reye's syndrome (see the Introduction and Chapter 12, Antipsychotic Drugs).

ROUTES, USUAL DOSAGE, AND PREPARATIONS.
Intramuscular: *Adults*, 5 or rarely 10 mg.
> *Trilafon* (Schering). Solution 5 mg/ml in 1 ml containers.

Oral: *Adults*, 8 to 24 mg daily in divided doses. Since all phenothiazines have prolonged half-lives (12 to 20 hours), the timed-release preparation has no significant advantage over ordinary oral dosage forms for most patients.
> *Trilafon* (Schering). Solution (concentrate) 16 mg/5 ml; tablets 2, 4, 8, and 16 mg; tablets (timed-release) 8 mg.

PROCHLORPERAZINE
[Compazine]

PROCHLORPERAZINE EDISYLATE
[Compazine]

PROCHLORPERAZINE MALEATE
[Compazine]

Prochlorperazine is effective in the management of postoperative nausea and vomiting and that caused by toxins, radiation sickness, and cytotoxic drugs, especially when minimal sedation is desired. It is not useful in preventing vertigo or motion sickness.

This piperazine phenothiazine frequently causes extrapyramidal reactions. Although these effects are most likely to occur with large doses, signs may appear abruptly in patients taking only moderate doses. The drug should be avoided in children and adolescents whose symptoms and signs suggest Reye's syndrome (see the Introduction). Drowsiness, dizziness, cutaneous reactions, and amenorrhea occur occasionally, and orthostatic hypotension, neutropenia, and cholestasis have been reported rarely. Particular caution is necessary in patients who are sensitive to other phenothiazines, in those with hepatic disease, and in children. Prochlorperazine should not be used in children under 2 years unless it is potentially lifesaving; the drug is contraindicated in children undergoing surgery. See also Chapter 12, Antipsychotic Drugs.

ROUTES, USUAL DOSAGE, AND PREPARATIONS.
PROCHLORPERAZINE:
Rectal: *Adults*, 25 mg twice daily; *children over 10 kg*, 0.4 mg/kg of body weight divided into three or four doses during a 24-hour period.
> *Compazine* (Smith Kline & French). Suppositories 2.5, 5, and 25 mg.

PROCHLORPERAZINE EDISYLATE:
Intramuscular (deep): *Adults*, 5 to 10 mg every three or four hours (maximum, 40 mg daily); *children over 10 kg*, 0.2 mg/kg of body weight.
> *Compazine* [*edisylate*] (Smith Kline & French). Solution (aqueous) 5 mg/ml in 2 and 10 ml containers.

Oral: *Adults*, 5 to 10 mg three or four times daily; *children over 10 kg*, 0.4 mg/kg of body weight divided into three or four doses during a 24-hour period.
> *Compazine* [*edisylate*] (Smith Kline & French). Solution (concentrate) 10 mg/ml; syrup 5 mg/5 ml.

PROCHLORPERAZINE MALEATE:
Oral: Same as oral dosage for edisylate salt. Since all phenothiazines have prolonged half-lives (12 to 20 hours), the timed-release preparation has no significant advantage over ordinary oral dosage forms for most patients.
> *Compazine* [*maleate*] (Smith Kline & French). Capsules (timed-release) 10, 15, 30, and 75 mg; tablets 5 and 10 mg.

PROMAZINE HYDROCHLORIDE
[Sparine]

Promazine, an aliphatic phenothiazine, is effective in the management of postoperative nausea and vomiting and that caused by cytotoxic drugs, radiation sickness, or toxins. However, its use as an antiemetic has been declining gradually.

The incidence of adverse reactions (eg, drowsiness, orthostatic hypotension) is similar to that of the other aliphatic phenothiazines, especially after parenteral administration. The hypotensive action may be detrimental in patients with cardiac or cerebrovascular insufficiency, especially when administered parenterally, and the anticholinergic-like actions may be detrimental in patients with ileus, angle-closure glaucoma, or urinary retention. Like other phenothiazines, promazine may reverse the pressor effect of epinephrine, thereby exacerbating hypotension. Extrapyramidal reactions are infrequent. Although relatively rare, agranulocytosis is reported to occur more frequently than with use of chlorpromazine or prochlorperazine. The drug should be avoided in children and adolescents whose symptoms and signs suggest Reye's syndrome (see the Introduction).

ROUTES, USUAL DOSAGE, AND PREPARATIONS. *Oral: Adults,* 25 to 50 mg; dose may be repeated at four- to six-hour intervals.

> Sparine (Wyeth). Solution (concentrate) 30 and 100 mg/ml; syrup 10 mg/5 ml; tablets 10, 25, 50, 100, and 200 mg.

Intramuscular: Adults, 50 mg.

> Drug available generically: Solution 25 and 50 mg/ml in 1 and 10 ml containers.
> Sparine (Wyeth). Solution 25 and 50 mg/ml in 1, 2, and 10 ml containers.

THIETHYLPERAZINE MALATE
[Torecan]

THIETHYLPERAZINE MALEATE
[Torecan]

Thiethylperazine is used to treat nausea and vomiting associated with the adminis-

tration of general anesthetics, cytotoxic drugs, radiation sickness, and toxins. This piperazine phenothiazine is not useful in preventing vertigo or motion sickness.

Untoward effects occur infrequently and are mild and transitory with usual doses. Adverse reactions noted occasionally include drowsiness, dizziness, dryness of the mouth and nose, tachycardia, and anorexia. Moderate hypotension has occurred occasionally within 30 minutes after administration to patients recovering from general anesthesia. Like other phenothiazine compounds, thiethylperazine may produce extrapyramidal reactions. Symptoms may appear even after a single dose and abate if therapy is discontinued. The drug should be avoided in children and adolescents whose symptoms and signs suggest Reye's syndrome (see the Introduction and Chapter 12, Antipsychotic Drugs).

ROUTES, USUAL DOSAGE, AND PREPARATIONS. *Intramuscular, Oral, Rectal: Adults,* 10 to 30 mg daily.

> THIETHYLPERAZINE MALATE:
> Torecan [malate] (Boehringer Ingelheim). Solution (aqueous for injection) 5 mg/ml in 2 ml containers.
> THIETHYLPERAZINE MALEATE:
> Torecan [maleate] (Boehringer Ingelheim). Tablets 10 mg; suppositories 10 mg.

TRIFLUPROMAZINE HYDROCHLORIDE
[Vesprin]

This aliphatic phenothiazine is effective in the management of postoperative nausea and vomiting and that caused by cytotoxic drugs, radiation sickness, or toxins. It is not useful in preventing vertigo or motion sickness.

Triflupromazine produces less sedation than some other phenothiazines (eg, promazine), but it prolongs the postanesthesia sleeping time. Extrapyramidal reactions have been observed following even single doses of this compound. The drug should be avoided in children and adolescents whose symptoms and signs suggest Reye's syndrome (see the Introduction and Chapter 12, Antipsychotic Drugs).

ROUTES, USUAL DOSAGE, AND PREPARATIONS. This drug should not be used in *children less than 2½ years of age.*
Intramuscular:Adults, 5 to 15 mg, repeated every four hours if necessary (maximum, 60 mg daily); *elderly or debilitated patients,* 2.5 to 15 mg daily; *children,* 0.2 to 0.25 mg/kg of body weight (maximum, 10 mg daily).
Intravenous: Adults, 1 to 3 mg.
  Vesprin (Squibb). Solution 10 mg/ml in 1 and 10 ml containers and 20 mg/ml in 1 ml containers.
Oral: Adults, 20 to 30 mg daily; *children,* 0.2 mg/kg of body weight in three divided doses (maximum, 10 mg daily).
  Vesprin (Squibb). Suspension 50 mg/5 ml; tablets 10, 25, and 50 mg.

MISCELLANEOUS DRUGS

BENZQUINAMIDE HYDROCHLORIDE
[Emete-con]

Benzquinamide is a benzquinoline derivative chemically unrelated to any other antiemetic. Like the antidopaminergic drugs, it apparently inhibits stimuli at the chemoreceptor trigger zone. It appears to be at least as effective as the antidopaminergic drugs in the treatment of postoperative nausea and vomiting.

Results of a few controlled studies suggest that benzquinamide produces fewer serious adverse reactions than the phenothiazines; however, there is still less overall experience with this agent compared to the latter drugs. Drowsiness is noted most frequently. Shivering, chills, and mild anticholinergic reactions also have been reported. Increased cardiac output, blood pressure, and respiratory rate have been noted both experimentally and clinically with use of benzquinamide. Sudden increase in blood pressure and transient arrhythmias have occurred with intravenous administration. Use of benzquinamide in patients with moderate to severe hypertension or severe cardiovascular disease is questionable, particularly if given intravenously. Data are not sufficient to justify use of benzquinamide during pregnancy or in children.

ROUTES, USUAL DOSAGE, AND PREPARATIONS. *Intramuscular* (preferred route): *Adults,* 0.5 to 1 mg/kg of body weight at least 15 minutes prior to administration of antineoplastic drugs or emergence from anesthesia. (The plasma half-life is approximately 40 minutes.) This dose may be repeated in one hour and then every three to four hours as required.
Intravenous: When therapeutic levels are desired in less than 15 minutes, a single dose of 0.2 to 0.4 mg/kg of body weight is given to *adults;* the drug may be diluted in 5% dextrose in water, sodium chloride injection, or lactated Ringer's injection and administered slowly (one to three minutes) or given in an intravenous infusion. Subsequent doses should be given intramuscularly.
  Emete-con (Roerig). Powder equivalent to benzquinamide 50 mg.

DIPHENIDOL HYDROCHLORIDE
[Vontrol]

Diphenidol acts upon the aural vestibular apparatus and is useful in the management of nausea and vomiting associated with toxins, radiation sickness, cytotoxic drugs, and following general anesthesia. In adults, this drug also is effective in the management of labyrinthine-induced vertigo following surgery of the middle and

428

inner ear and Meniere's disease. Its use in the treatment of vertigo in children has not been investigated.

The use of diphenidol is limited to hospitalized or closely supervised outpatients. Therapy should be discontinued if auditory or visual hallucinations, disorientation, or confusion occurs. The benefits of using this agent should be considered carefully and should unquestionably outweigh the substantial risks. The drug occasionally has produced drowsiness, dryness of the mouth, tachycardia, and dizziness. Untoward effects reported rarely include rash, heartburn, headache, nausea, indigestion, blurred vision, malaise, and mild, transient hypotension.

ROUTES, USUAL DOSAGE, AND PREPARATIONS. This drug should not be used in *infants under 6 months of age or weighing less than 12 kg.*
Intramuscular: *Adults*, 20 to 40 mg four times daily; *children*, 3 mg/kg of body weight daily divided into four doses.
Intravenous: *Adults*, 20 mg initially; the dose is repeated in one hour if necessary. Another route should be used if subsequent administration is necessary. No dosage has been established for *children*.
 Vontrol (Smith Kline & French). Solution 20 mg/ml in 2 ml containers.
Oral: *Adults*, 25 to 50 mg four times daily; *children over 6 months or weighing more than 12 kg,* 5 mg/kg of body weight daily divided into four doses.
 Vontrol (Smith Kline & French). Tablets 25 mg.

TRIMETHOBENZAMIDE HYDROCHLORIDE
[Tigan]

This drug has been shown to inhibit stimuli at the chemoreceptor trigger zone in animals, and it has been promoted for use in alleviating nausea and reducing the frequency of vomiting in the immediate postoperative period, in radiation sickness,

and in gastroenteritis. It is not as effective as the phenothiazines postoperatively. Trimethobenzamide has little or no value in the prevention or treatment of vertigo or motion sickness.

In general, the effectiveness of this drug appears to be somewhat unpredictable when given orally. Part of this unreliability may be related to problems of bioavailability; certain reformulations of oral and suppository dosage forms are currently being explored.

With usual doses, the incidence of adverse effects is low; with larger doses, drowsiness, vertigo, diarrhea, and cutaneous hypersensitivity reactions may occur. Extrapyramidal reactions or convulsions also have been noted; the latter occur more often in children, the elderly, or debilitated individuals. This drug should not be used in children with Reye's syndrome or when this diagnosis is suspected, for the extrapyramidal effects may interfere with the diagnosis of this syndrome or the hepatotoxicity produced by trimethobenzamide may unfavorably alter the course of the disease.

Pain at the site of injection and local irritation after rectal administration have been noted.

ROUTES, USUAL DOSAGE, AND PREPARATIONS. *Intramuscular*: *Adults*, 200 mg three or four times daily. To prevent postoperative vomiting, a single dose of 200 mg may be given before or during surgery; this dose may be repeated three hours after termination of anesthesia if needed. This route should not be used in *children*.
 Tigan (Beecham). Solution 100 mg/ml in 2 and 20 ml containers.

Oral: *Adults*, 250 mg three or four times daily; *children*, 15 mg/kg of body weight divided into three or four doses during a 24-hour period.
 Tigan (Beecham). Capsules 100 and 250 mg.

Rectal: *Adults*, 200 mg three or four times daily; *children*, 15 mg/kg of body weight divided into three or four doses during a 24-hour period. This route should not be used in *premature or newborn infants*.
 Tigan (Beecham). Suppositories 100 (pediatric) and 200 mg (with 2% benzocaine).

MIXTURES

Fixed-ratio combinations containing the ingredients noted in the following preparations are available. No controlled studies exist to support the contention that these combinations are as effective, safer, or have any advantage over single-entity preparations. Thus, their use is not recommended.

Bendectin (Merrell-National). Each tablet contains doxylamine succinate 10 mg and pyridoxine hydrochloride 10 mg.
Emetrol (Rorer). Solution containing balanced amounts of levulose, dextrose, and orthophosphoric acid with controlled hydrogen ion concentration (nonprescription).
WANS (Webcon). Each suppository contains pyrilamine maleate 25 mg and pentobarbital sodium 30 mg (pediatric) or pyrilamine maleate 50 mg and pentobarbital sodium 50 or 100 mg.

Selected References

Bateman DN, Davies DS: Pharmacokinetics of metoclopramide. *Lancet* 1:166, 1979.

Bateman DN, et al: Pharmacokinetic and concentration-effect studies with intravenous metoclopramide. *Br J Clin Pharmacol* 6:401-407, 1978.

Brock-Utne JG, et al: Action of commonly used antiemetics on lower oesophageal sphincter. *Br J Anaesth* 50:295-298, 1978.

Dhondt F, et al: Domperidone (R33 812) suppositories: Effective antiemetic agent in diverse pediatric conditions. Multicenter Trial. *Curr Ther Res* 24:912-923, 1978.

Fragen RJ, Caldwell N: New benzimidazole antiemetic, domperidone, for treatment of postoperative nausea and vomiting. *Anesthesiology* 49: 289-290, 1978.

Frew IJC, Menon GN: Betahistine hydrochloride in Meniere's disease. *Postgrad Med J* 52:501-503, 1976.

Graybiel A, et al: Prevention of experimental motion sickness by scopolamine absorbed through skin. *Aviat Space Environ Med* 48:1096-1100, 1976.

Herman TS, et al: Superiority of nabilone over prochlorperazine as antiemetic in patients receiving cancer chemotherapy. *N Engl J Med* 300:1295-1297, 1979.

Jackson RT, et al: Ear, nose and throat diseases, in Avery GS (ed): *Drug Treatment: Principles and Practice of Clinical Pharmacology and Therapeutics*. Littleton, Mass, Publishing Sciences Group, Inc, 1976, 265-274.

Kataria M, et al: Extrapyramidal side-effects of metoclopramide. *Lancet* 2:1254-1255, 1978.

Milkovich I, van den Berg BJ: Evaluation of teratogenicity of certain antinauseant drugs. *Am J Obstet Gynecol* 125:244-248, 1976.

Reyntjens A: Domperidone as antiemetic: Summary of research reports. *Postgrad Med J* 55:50-54, 1979.

Roydhouse N: Vertigo and its treatment. *Drugs* 7:297-309, 1974.

Rubin W: Vestibular suppressant drugs. *Arch Otolaryngol* 97:135-138, 1973.

Sallan SE, et al: Antiemetic effect of delta-9-tetrahydrocannabinol in patients receiving cancer chemotherapy. *N Engl J Med* 293:795-797, 1976.

Shannon HE, et al: Lack of antiemetic effects of delta-9-tetrahydrocannabinol in apomorphine-induced emesis in the dog. *Life Sci* 23:49-54, 1978.

Suga F, Snow JB Jr: Cochlear blood flow in response to vasodilating drugs and some related agents. *Laryngoscope* 79:1956-1979, 1969.

Turner JS Jr: Practical approach to patient with vertigo: Outline of diagnosis and management for nonspecialist. *South Med J* 68:241-245, 1975.

Wood CD: Antimotion sickness and antiemetic drugs. *Drugs* 17:471-479, 1979.

Wood CD, Graybiel A: Theory of antimotion sickness drug mechanisms. *Aerospace Med* 43:249-252, 1972.

Topical Otic Preparations | 27

The products discussed in this chapter are limited to those applied locally in the external ear canal to treat external otitis or to aid in the removal of excess ear wax.

AGENTS USED TO TREAT EXTERNAL OTITIS

External otitis (otitis externa) is an inflammatory condition involving the skin of the external auditory canal. The most common causative factors include trauma from repeated attempts at cleaning or other manipulation of the ear canal by the patient, use of a hearing aid, environmental factors of high temperature and humidity, and frequent exposure to water, eg, while swimming ("swimmer's ear"). Other causative or contributing factors are allergies (eg, hair spray, earrings); chemicals (eg, industrial exposure); coexistent dermatologic conditions (eg, seborrhea, eczema, psoriasis) of the ear canal skin, or scalp; and atrophic changes of the skin associated with aging. External otitis occasionally results from chronic middle ear infection that drains through a perforated tympanic membrane. When any of these factors decrease the natural defenses of the ear canal, such as altering the normal acid pH, breaking the protective layer of the skin, or modifying the protection provided by cerumen, inflammation develops and infection may result. Infections may be localized (furuncle) or generalized (diffuse) involving the entire canal.

The most common signs and symptoms of diffuse external otitis are pruritus, edema, erythema, pain, and purulent discharge; fullness in the ears and hearing loss may occur if the canal is swollen and filled with debris and pus.

The infecting organisms are primarily gram-negative bacilli, such as *Pseudomonas aeruginosa*, *Escherichia coli*, and *Proteus* species. *Staphylococcus aureus* and other endogenous organisms also are commonly isolated. Mixed infections are not unusual. Mycotic infections of the external ear seldom occur alone except in hot, humid environments, and may follow use of some antibiotics (eg, aminoglycosides) and prolonged use of topical steroid preparations. The most common fungi affecting the external ear are *Aspergillus* and *Candida*. *Penicillium* and *Mucor* are involved rarely.

Management of external otitis includes correct differential diagnosis; the determination and elimination of the causative factor(s), if possible; and the use of appropriate medication. It is important that the ear canal be cleaned before application of medication. Care should be taken not to traumatize the skin of the external canal. Gentle mechanical cleansing with suction is usually employed. Irrigation with diluted 70% alcohol, saline, or saline-hydrogen peroxide (1.5%) at room temperature may be effective in patients with impacted debris or cerumen if there are no perforations of the tympanic membrane. If a culture for sensitivity tests is needed, it may be taken prior to or during cleaning. Drugs instilled into the ear usually are dissolved or suspended in a liquid vehicle, but medicated creams or ointments may be used for dry, crusted lesions. Powders also are used frequently for their desiccant properties.

For the treatment of mild pruritus, two or three drops of light mineral (baby) oil instilled into the canal daily or weekly usually controls this symptom. When the ear canal is swollen, a buffered aluminum acetate solution is effective; this preparation has anti-inflammatory, antipruritic, and astringent properties and is nonsensitizing.

A number of preparations are available for treating bacterial infections, and they appear to be equally effective. Aqueous acetic acid solution (2% to 5%) is active against many pathogens associated with otitis externa, particularly *Pseudomonas*; the acidity of the solution inhibits growth of the organism and resistant organisms do not develop. Antibiotics most commonly employed are the polymyxins (polymyxin B and colistin) and neomycin. When external otitis is complicated by severe inflammation or is associated with allergic dermatitis, a combination preparation containing a corticosteroid may be useful.

Systemic antibiotics are necessary only when there is evidence of cellulitis involving the external meatus or auricle or when there are generalized complications. Therapy with appropriate systemic antibiotics (eg, penicillin) can be started initially but may have to be modified after the causative organism has been identified.

Patients who do not respond to the usual treatment for otitis externa, especially those who are diabetic or elderly, require special attention, for they may develop malignant or necrotizing otitis externa.

This infection, caused by *P. aeruginosa*, begins in the soft tissues of the external auditory canal and spreads to the temporal bone. If the patient is not hospitalized and antibiotic therapy (eg, intravenous carbenicillin and gentamicin) is not instituted promptly, complications such as facial nerve palsy, mastoiditis, sigmoid sinus thrombosis, multiple cranial nerve palsies, and death may result.

ANTIBACTERIAL AGENTS

ACETIC ACID PREPARATIONS

Acetic acid solutions (2% to 5%) have antibacterial and antifungal activity, particularly against *Pseudomonas aeruginosa*, *Candida*, and *Aspergillus*. They reduce swelling of the ear canal and relieve other signs and symptoms associated with external otitis. Preparations of aluminum acetate must not be instilled as unbuffered solutions or they will precipitate.

Acetic acid solution is well tolerated, nonsensitizing, and does not produce resistant organisms. If irritation or symptoms of sensitivity to the vehicle occur, the medication should be discontinued.

ROUTE, USUAL DOSAGE, AND PREPARATIONS.
ORLEX OTIC, VŌSOL OTIC SOLUTION:
Topical: *Adults and children*, initially, a cotton wick is inserted into the ear canal, saturated, and kept moist for 24 hours, followed thereafter by removal of the wick and continued instillation of five drops directly into the ear canal three or four times daily.

> *Orlex Otic* (Baylor). Solution (nonaqueous) containing acetic acid 2% and parachlorometaxylenol 0.1% in propylene glycol in 10 ml containers.
> *VōSol Otic Solution* (Wallace). Solution (nonaqueous) containing acetic acid 2% in propylene glycol and propylene glycol diacetate 3% in 15 and 30 ml containers.

OTIC DOMEBORO SOLUTION:
Topical: *Adults and children*, four to six drops instilled every two or three hours.

> *Otic Domeboro Solution* (Dome). Acetic acid 2% in aluminum acetate (modified Burow's) solution in 60 ml containers.

CHLORAMPHENICOL
[Chloromycetin Otic]

This antibacterial agent has a broad spectrum of activity which includes some strains of *Pseudomonas*, *Staphylococcus aureus*, *Escherichia coli*, and *Proteus* species, the principal infecting organisms of external otitis. It is useful topically in the treatment of superficial infections of the external auditory canal caused by these organisms.

Signs of local irritation have been reported in patients sensitive to this preparation. If these occur, the medication should be discontinued. It should be kept in mind that blood dyscrasias have been associated with systemic use of this drug and have been reported after therapy with a topical ophthalmic preparation.

For further information on antibacterial activity and adverse reactions, see Chapter 71.

ROUTE, USUAL DOSAGE, AND PREPARATIONS. *Topical*: *Adults and children*, two or three drops instilled three times daily.

  Chloromycetin Otic (Parke, Davis). Each milliliter of solution contains chloramphenicol 0.5% (5 mg) in propylene glycol.

NEOMYCIN SULFATE
[Otobiotic]

This aminoglycoside antibiotic is effective against *Escherichia*, *Enterobacter aerogenes*, and most species of *Klebsiella*, *Salmonella*, *Shigella*, and *Proteus*; many strains of *Staphylococcus aureus* also are sensitive. It has weak activity against many strains of *Pseudomonas*, which is the most common bacterial isolate in otitis externa. Topical preparations are indicated in the treatment of external otitis caused by susceptible organisms. The contribution of sodium propionate to the antibacterial effectiveness of neomycin in Otobiotic Otic Solution has not been established.

Neomycin is a topical sensitizer, and cutaneous hypersensitivity reactions may result from its use in the ear. If undue irritation or sensitivity develops, treatment should be discontinued. The physician must always be alert for these reactions, since they frequently mimic the disease being treated. Such reactions usually can be recognized because the inflammatory process spreads to the lobule of the ear and the infection does not respond to treatment.

Cross sensitization can occur between neomycin and other aminoglycosides and may prevent the subsequent use of these antibacterial agents. Aminoglycosides are ototoxic when given systemically and, in laboratory animals, ototoxicity has been demonstrated with *topical* application of agents such as gentamicin and neomycin. Therefore, the possibility of ototoxicity should be considered when aminoglycoside otic preparations are used in patients with perforated tympanic membranes.

For further information on antibacterial activity and adverse reactions, see Chapter 74.

ROUTE, USUAL DOSAGE, AND PREPARATIONS. *Topical*: *Adults and children*, several drops instilled three or four times daily. Saturated gauze or a moist cotton wick also may be used.

  Otobiotic (Schering). Each milliliter of solution contains neomycin sulfate 5 mg (equivalent to 3.5 mg neomycin base), sodium propionate 50 mg, glycerin, and isopropyl alcohol (pH, 6).

POLYMYXINS

Polymyxin B and colistin (polymyxin E) are effective against *Pseudomonas aeruginosa* and some other gram-negative organisms, including *Escherichia*, that commonly infect the ear. However, they are not active against other organisms commonly causing external otitis, such as *Proteus* or gram-positive bacteria. Topical preparations are indicated for external otitis caused by susceptible organisms. One preparation [Lidosporin Otic] contains lidocaine for relief of pain; see comments on local anesthetics in the discussion on Otic Analgesics.

Adverse reactions are uncommon, but treatment should be discontinued if irritation or sensitivity occurs.

For further information on antibacterial

activity and adverse reactions, see Chapter 75.

ROUTE, USUAL DOSAGE, AND PREPARATIONS. *Topical: Adults,* three or four drops instilled three or four times daily. *Children,* two or three drops instilled three or four times daily. Alternatively, saturated gauze or a moist cotton wick also may be left in the ear canal for 24 to 48 hours.

> *Aerosporin Otic* (Burroughs Wellcome). Each milliliter of solution contains polymyxin B sulfate 10,000 units, acetic acid 1%, and propylene glycol.
>
> *Lidosporin Otic* (Burroughs Wellcome). Each milliliter of solution contains polymyxin B sulfate 10,000 units, lidocaine hydrochloride 50 mg, and propylene glycol in 10 ml containers.

MIXTURES OF ANTIBACTERIAL AGENTS WITH A CORTICOSTEROID

A number of otic preparations contain polymyxins in combination with neomycin. The proposed rationale for these mixtures is that they have a wide antibacterial spectrum that includes both gram-positive and gram-negative organisms which may be the causative agents in external otitis. Such fixed-ratio mixtures for topical use have reasonable therapeutic value but may cause the adverse reactions associated with each ingredient, eg, hypersensitivity reactions from neomycin (see the above evaluations).

Commonly, preparations contain a corticosteroid in addition to an antibacterial agent, which alleviates inflammation and pruritus, although there is no evidence that the corticosteroid enhances the efficacy of the antibiotics. However, preparations containing a corticosteroid are contraindicated in patients with herpes simplex, vaccinia, and varicella. For further information on actions and adverse reactions of adrenal corticosteroids, see Chapter 41.

ROUTE, USUAL DOSAGE, AND PREPARATIONS. *Topical: Adults,* four drops instilled three or four times daily. *Children,* three drops instilled three or four times daily. The preparations also may be applied on a wick and inserted into the ear canal; the wick should be kept moist and changed every 24 hours.

> *Coly-Mycin S Otic with Neomycin and Hydrocortisone* (Parke, Davis). Each milliliter of suspension contains colistin base activity 3 mg (as the sulfate), neomycin base activity 3.3 mg (as the sulfate), cortisol acetate 10 mg, and acetic acid in 5 and 10 ml containers.
>
> *Cortisporin Otic Solution and Suspension* (Burroughs Wellcome). Each milliliter of solution or suspension contains polymyxin B sulfate 10,000 units, neomycin sulfate 5 mg (equivalent to 3.5 mg neomycin base), and cortisol 10 mg. [The vehicle of the solution is essentially anhydrous; it contains glycerin and a high concentration of propylene glycol; the solution may cause pain in patients with perforated eardrums or open lesions of the skin. The vehicle of the suspension is essentially aqueous; it contains no glycerin and a low concentration of propylene glycol.]
>
> *Orlex H.C. Otic* (Baylor). Solution (nonaqueous) containing acetic acid 2%, cortisol 1%, and parachlorometaxylenol in propylene glycol in 10 ml containers.
>
> *Otic Neo-Cort-Dome* (Dome). Suspension containing neomycin sulfate equivalent to neomycin 0.35%, microdispersed cortisol 1%, acetic acid 2%, and propylene glycol in 10 ml containers.
>
> *Otic Tridesilon* (Dome). Solution containing acetic acid 2%, desonide 0.05%, and propylene glycol in 10 ml containers.
>
> *Otobione* (Schering). Each milliliter of suspension contains neomycin sulfate 5 mg equivalent to neomycin 3.5 mg, polymyxin B sulfate 10,000 units, cortisol 10 mg, povidone, propylene glycol, and glycerin in 5 ml containers.
>
> *Pyocidin-Otic* (Berlex). Each milliliter of solution contains polymyxin B sulfate 10,000 units and cortisol 5 mg in propylene glycol in 10 ml containers.
>
> *VōSol HC* (Wallace). Solution (nonaqueous) containing acetic acid 2% and cortisol 1% in propylene glycol and propylene glycol diacetate 3% in 10 ml containers.

ANTIFUNGAL AGENTS

Mycotic infections in the ear canal occur most commonly in warm climates. Most fungal infections require a warm, moist, dark area and dead tissue for growth. This is particularly true for the superficial skin fungi. The characteristic appearance of the cotton-like surface in different colors, together with a considerable amount of pruritus and desquamation, give this clinical entity a characteristic specificity. The characteristics of either white, black, or bluish color define the different families of fungi. The precise nature of the fungus may be determined by either removal in culture or appearance on a potassium hydroxide-treated slide. Most important in the management of fungal infections is meticulous cleansing of the skin of the ear canal or mastoid cavity. This may be helped considerably by the use of keratolytic agents. After cleansing, an antifungal preparation is instilled into the ear canal. Treatment should be continued for at least one or two weeks after disappearance of clinical symptoms because recurrence is common. When there is a mixed infection of fungus and bacteria, a preparation containing both antifungal and antibacterial agents and a steroid is useful.

Amphotericin B is the most effective antifungal agent; it is active against a variety of fungi, particularly *Candida*. (See also Chapter 80.) Since propylene glycol is dehydrating to fungi, preparations containing this agent may have some antifungal activity. Also, the low pH of some otic preparations is an undesirable medium for growth of many fungi. Other antifungal agents present in some preparations include clioquinol (iodochlorhydroxyquin) and parachlorometaxylenol.

> **Fungizone Lotion** (Squibb). Lotion containing amphotericin B 3% in an aqueous vehicle with propylene glycol in 30 ml containers.
> **Orlex Otic** (Baylor). Solution (nonaqueous) containing acetic acid 2% and parachlorometaxylenol 0.1% in propylene glycol in 10 ml containers.
> **Orlex H.C. Otic** (Baylor). Solution (nonaqueous) containing acetic acid 2%, cortisol 1%, and parachlorometaxylenol in propylene glycol in 10 ml containers.
> **VōSol Otic Solution** (Wallace). Solution (nonaqueous) containing acetic acid 2% in propylene glycol and propylene glycol diacetate 3% in 15 and 30 ml containers.
> **VōSol HC** (Wallace). Solution (nonaqueous) containing acetic acid 2% and cortisol 1% in propylene glycol and propylene glycol diacetate 3% in 10 ml containers.

OTIC ANALGESICS

To relieve the earache that usually accompanies acute external otitis or otitis media when the tympanic membrane is intact, local anesthetics, most commonly benzocaine, have been applied topically in the ear canal. However, since their absorption from the skin or tympanic membrane is inadequate, they are rarely effective and benzocaine may cause hypersensitivity reactions. Therefore, it is preferable to administer systemic analgesics (eg, aspirin) to relieve pain. The following examples of otic analgesic preparations are listed only for information and not to suggest their use:

> **Americaine Otic Drops** (Arnar-Stone). Solution containing benzocaine 20% and benzethonium chloride 0.1% in 15 ml containers.
> **Auralgan Otic Solution** (Ayerst). Each milliliter contains antipyrine 54 mg and benzocaine 14 mg in 15 ml containers.
> **Tympagesic Ear Drops** (Warren-Teed). Solution containing benzocaine 5%, phenylephrine hydrochloride 0.25%, and antipyrine 5% in 13 ml containers.

CERUMENOLYTIC AND CERUMEN-SOFTENING AGENTS

Cerumen or ear wax is produced by the apocrine and sebaceous glands in the outer one-third of the external ear canal. It is hydrophobic nd probably bacteriostatic and fungistatic; thus, it is important in providing a protective coating for the external auditory canal. Normally, the canal is self-cleaning; however, the normal physiologic mechanism for removing cerumen occasionally becomes inefficient and excessive amounts of wax may accumulate. The most frequent causes for breakdown of this mechanism are misguided attempts to remove wax by the patient, lack of moisture or humidity that causes the cerumen to dry, narrow tortuous ear canals, or excessive hair growth in the ear. Even when large amounts accumulate, cerumen rarely causes enough occlusion to decrease hearing acuity substantially or promote infection.

Patients who have chronic difficulty with hard, but not impacted, cerumen may be advised to instill light mineral oil (baby oil), glycerin, or hydrogen peroxide solution into the ear canal occasionally to soften the cerumen and promote normal removal. The majority of mastoid cavities or canals need cleaning occasionally to remove wax and epithelial debris. This can be performed painlessly and efficiently. Three nights before an office visit, the patient is advised to fill the cavity with baby oil and plug the ear at night with cotton which is removed in the morning; this oil treatment may be continued for one to three days. Besides softening the debris, the dead skin separates from the living surface, permitting almost the entire mass to be removed with a #5 and #7 French suction tip. This minimizes the amount of instrumentation and discomfort frequently occurring in patients with large mastoids and old fenestration cavities. In the normal ear canal, rapid removal of wax and debris with a minimum of discomfort is possible. The advantage of this technique is that the oil is inexpensive and nonallergenic. A solution of carbamide peroxide in glycerin is also useful as an aid in the removal of excessive or hardened cerumen. Glycerin acts as a wax-softening agent and the effervesence of the oxygen released from the carbamide peroxide loosens tissue debris, which aids in cleansing the ear canal. Use of an ear bulb syringe to irrigate the canal gently with warm water or normal saline may facilitate removal of the cerumen. The ear canal should be thoroughly dried after treatment, preferably chemically (eg, 70% isopropanol, Orlex Otic Solution, VōSol Otic Solution) rather than mechanically to prevent maceration of the skin.

If external otitis is present in addition to impacted cerumen, it should be treated as discussed above. The instillation of an antibiotic-steroid preparation to reduce inflammation may also aid in softening the wax and facilitate its removal. If cerumen is impacted with little or no inflammation, its removal under direct visualization with a ring curet or another suitable instrument is preferable to irrigation. Extreme care should be taken not to traumatize the canal, since this portion of the ear is very sensitive to instrumentation. If the wax cannot be removed mechanically, a wax-softening or, rarely, a cerumenolytic agent may be used, followed by irrigation. A solution of triethanolamine polypeptide oleate-condensate in propylene glycol is promoted as a cerumenolytic agent. However, clinical studies comparing its efficacy to that of other preparations are conflicting. It must be used with extreme care since it may cause severe contact dermatitis in some patients.

The following preparations are representative of the various types available. They are listed for information only and not to imply their superiority over other similar preparations.

> *Cerumenex Drops* (Purdue Frederick). Solution of triethanolamine polypeptide oleate-condensate 10% in propylene glycol in 8 and 15 ml containers.
>
> *Debrox Drops* (Marion). Solution containing carbamide peroxide 6.5% in glycerin in 15 and 30 ml containers (nonprescription).

Selected References

Establishment of a monograph for OTC topical otics, proposed rules. *Federal Register* 42:63556-63566, (Dec 16) 1977.

Holman JM: The problem ear: *Diagnostic approach*, monograph. Kansas City, Mo, American Academy of Family Physicians, 1978, 6-11.

Keim RJ: Common ear diseases: Recognition and management. *Postgrad Med* 61:72-80, (May) 1977.

McDowall GD: External otitis: Otological problems. *J Laryngol Otol* 88:1-13, 1974.

Tonkin J: Treatment of otitis-externa. *Drugs* 6:261-266, 1973.

Antihistamines | 28

Histamine, an important chemical mediator in allergic reactions, is produced by decarboxylation of the amino acid, histidine, and is stored in secretory granules within mast cells and basophils, as well as at other tissue sites. In sensitized individuals, antigen-antibody (IgE) reactions cause the discharge of histamine and other autacoids into adjacent tissues without mast cell disruption, which elicits smooth muscle contraction and increases vascular permeability. Other autacoids released include eosinophil chemotactic factor of anaphylaxis (ECF-A) and slow-reacting substances of anaphylaxis (SRS-A). The latter is released from basophils during antigen-antibody reactions and causes slow contraction of tracheobronchial smooth muscle.

Histamine also is released by the direct action of many drugs or substances (eg, dyes, alkaloids, venoms, quaternary ammonium compounds) in individuals not previously sensitized. Following intravenous injection, these agents rapidly deplete histamine from mast cells and produce an immediate anaphylactoid reaction. The effects are relatively transient because histamine diffuses quickly and is metabolized rapidly.

Efforts to treat histamine-mediated responses are directed toward preventing the release of histamine or reducing the amount in order to minimize peripheral effects. Antihistamines are structurally related to histamine and, by occupying the same cellular receptor sites on target organs, competitively antagonize some of its actions. To be effective, the receptor site must be accessible to the antihistamine and the drug must remain in high concentrations at the site; to achieve the latter, continuous administration may be necessary.

Antihistamines antagonize some of the pharmacologic effects of histamine but do not affect antibody production, antigen-antibody interactions, release of histamine, or the actions of other autacoids (eg, ECF-A, SRS-A). There are two types of histamine receptors, and antihistamines can be divided into two categories on this basis: conventional antihistamines (H_1 blocking agents) used in allergic disorders and H_2 blocking agents which antagonize gastrointestinal histamine receptors. This chapter describes only the traditional H_1 blocking antihistamines; H_2 blocking agents, which are useful for treating peptic ulcer, are discussed in Chapter 57, Agents Used in Acid Peptic Disorders.

Like histamine, antihistamines contain an ethylamine chain or ring structure, and H_1 receptor inhibitors are classified according to the group which connects to the ethylamine (ie, ethanolamine, ethylenediamine, alkylamine, piperazine, phenothiazine). In addition, there is a miscellaneous group of drugs with antihistaminic activity that cannot be classified in this manner.

Those antihistamines that have been extensively studied appear to be metabolized in the liver and excreted within 24 hours, chiefly by the kidney. Following oral administration, effects are apparent within 15 to 30 minutes, are maximal within one hour, and persist for four to six hours. Some antihistamines have a significantly longer duration of action. More immediate action is produced by intramuscular or intravenous injection, but rapid intravenous administration may cause hypotension. The action of timed-release preparations may persist for 8 to 12 hours. Although bioequivalence has been demonstrated for some timed-release preparations, others may be less effective than conventional dosage forms because effective blood levels are not attained.

Pharmacologic Actions

Antihistamines prevent rather than reverse the effects of histamine by competing with it for receptor sites. By counteracting the effect of histamine, they give palliative relief of allergic symptoms but are not as potent or as prompt acting as adrenergic antagonists of allergic reactions, such as epinephrine.

The antihistamines show some blocking activity against other amines and have a wide variety of pharmacologic actions, some of which are useful clinically. Because they are structurally similar to atropine, all antihistamines produce atropine-like peripheral and central anticholinergic effects. Depending upon the compound, dosage, and sensitivity of the patient, antihistamines may stimulate or depress the central nervous system. Although these drugs may induce convulsions, they also have anticonvulsant activity but are not used clinically for this purpose. Some antihistamines have antiemetic properties, some suppress vertigo and tremor, and most have local anesthetic activity. The anesthesia induced may be as potent as that produced by procaine, but antihistamines are of limited use for this

purpose because of their local irritant action.

Indications

Antihistamines are used primarily to treat allergic symptoms produced by the release of histamine (eg, increased capillary permeability and edema, pruritus, smooth muscle contraction, urticaria). They generally are more effective in acute rather than chronic reactions. Antihistamines control symptoms but are not curative. Thus, their use for long periods should be supplemented, as appropriate, by other measures such as avoidance of allergens or hyposensitization (immunotherapy).

Because of the wide variability in host response, individualization of dosage is necessary. Drugs from different classes of antihistamines may have to be tried to determine the optimal agent for a particular patient. The optimum dose generally is slightly less than that amount causing incapacitating drowsiness.

Upper Respiratory Disorders: The antihistamines are most effective in the management of hay fever (seasonal allergic rhinitis); 70% to 95% of patients experience some relief of symptoms (sneezing, rhinorrhea, and, to a lesser extent, nasal airway obstruction and conjunctivitis). Long-acting preparations are most beneficial when given at bedtime to control the more severe symptoms that are usually evident in early morning. Therapy should be instituted at the beginning of the hay fever season when pollen counts are still low. If therapy is delayed, the temporary use of an aerosol corticosteroid preparation may be required to control symptoms. Steroids have a direct anti-inflammatory action on cells to reduce capillary dilatation and edema. It is claimed that beclomethasone dipropionate [Vanceril] or dexamethasone sodium phosphate [Decadron Phosphate Turbinaire], synthetic glucocorticoids chemically related to prednisolone, may be used topically with little, if any, systemic absorption. An intranasal dose of beclomethasone (50 mcg) or dexamethasone sodium phosphate (84 mcg) in each nostril four times daily has been used safely in children and adults without suppressing pituitary-adrenal function. However, some data show that systemic absorption, sometimes associated with adrenal suppression, can occur. Furthermore, long-term effects are not known and these drugs should be reserved for trial after traditional treatment has failed (see also Chapter 32, Drugs Used in Asthma).

Antihistamines also are useful in nonseasonal (perennial) allergic rhinitis. They are less consistently effective in vasomotor rhinitis and their value in infectious rhinitis has not been established. The nasal blockage prominent in these forms of the disorder is only minimally responsive to antihistaminic drugs, although the anticholinergic action provides drying effects on the nasal mucosa.

Antihistamines are generally ineffective in the treatment of asthma. They are not bronchodilators and they do not block such mediators as SRS-A that may be more important in inducing acute asthmatic attacks. Cromolyn sodium [Aarane, Intal], which appears to block the release of histamine and other mediators from respiratory mast cells, is effective in many patients for the prevention but not the treatment of asthmatic attacks (see Chapter 32). In patients with both hay fever and asthma, antihistamines can be used to treat the hay fever with little likelihood of aggravating the asthma. Nevertheless, in bronchial allergy, it is possible that antihistamines may aggravate the condition through their drying effect on the bronchial mucosa.

The efficacy of antihistamines in treating the common cold and other respiratory infections is being reviewed. Currently, the evidence indicates that none of the antihistamines prevent colds or shorten the duration of such infection. They may provide slight symptomatic relief of rhinitis through their minimal drying effect on mucous membranes, however. Despite their lack of effectiveness, some antihistamines (particularly chlorpheniramine) are widely used in cold remedies (see Chapter 30).

Dermatologic Conditions: Antihistamines alleviate urticaria and pruritus induced by histamine. They are drugs of choice in acute urticaria but are less effective in the chronic form (except for hydroxyzine [Atarax, Vistaril], which is the agent of choice for chronic urticaria). This potent antihistamine also is the agent of choice for a number of other dermatologic conditions. Cyproheptadine [Periactin] is more effective than other antihistamines in controlling cold urticaria. Among the other indications for use of antihistamines are atopic dermatitis, contact dermatitis, and dermatitis medicamentosa. Antihistamines are sometimes beneficial in treating the pruritus, erythema, and edema of insect bites but are of little value in erythema multiforme and exfoliative dermatitis. Their oral administration, combined with appropriate topical therapy (moist soaks, steroids, emollients), is helpful in reducing the pruritus accompanying fixed drug eruptions and contact dermatitis. Generally, oral administration of antihistamines is preferred. Topical preparations are available to control allergic conjunctivitis but may cause allergic contact dermatitis and may anesthetize the cornea, thereby predisposing to corneal abrasion if the eye is rubbed.

Vascular Disorders: Antihistamines do not affect intracellular mediator release or increase vascular tone. By antagonizing the increase in capillary permeability induced by histamine, antihistamines reduce edema. They may be useful in angioedema, but their use is secondary to that of epinephrine, especially when the site of the edema is life-threatening (ie, larynx). Antihistamines are of no value in hereditary angioedema.

Hypersensitivity Phenomena: Antihistamines are helpful in treating the urticaria and pruritus associated with allergic reactions (eg, penicillin sensitivity, certain food allergies). However, because autacoids other than histamine are involved, antihistamines often are ineffective against the more serious manifestations (ie, hypotension, bronchoconstriction) of antigen-antibody reactions. Epinephrine is the agent of choice for anaphylaxis and other allergic crises, and antihistamines can be used as supplements to control local effects on the skin and mucous membranes. These drugs control urticaria in serum sickness, but they have little effect on arthralgia and fever and do not shorten the course of the reaction.

Antihistamines may ameliorate histamine-induced symptoms (flushing, urticaria, pruritus) associated with mild transfusion reactions not caused by ABO incompatibility or pyrogens, but they do not prevent such reactions. These agents should not be given routinely to patients receiving blood but may be administered prophylactically to those with a history of previous transfusion reactions. Antihistamines should never be added to the blood being transfused.

Miscellaneous Uses: Certain antihistamines, particularly diphenhydramine [Benadryl] and promethazine [Phenergan], are used for their sedative effect and as preoperative medication. In patients with severe pruritus, the dual effects of sedation and histamine inhibition can be particularly helpful. Antihistamines are the principal components of most of the popular over-the-counter preparations promoted as daytime sedatives and sleep aids. The amount of such drugs permitted in nonprescription preparations is generally insufficient to provide effective sedation and tolerance develops quickly. Nevertheless, self-medication with this type of preparation is common and fatalities associated with methapyrilene have been reported. Also, in animals, cancer developed following long-term use of large doses, and methapyrilene was removed from the market.

Antihistamines are ineffective in the treatment of migraine but may be of some use in Meniere's disease and other types of vertigo.

Antihistamines, alone or in combination with corticosteroids, may prevent allergic reactions to contrast media. Diphenhydramine has been employed most commonly for parenteral use and may be administered preferably prior to but also in the intravenous contrast media.

Results of several studies suggest that cyproheptadine [Periactin] accelerates weight gain and stimulates linear growth in children. However, most patients lost weight when the drug was discontinued. Some authorities feel that use of an appetite-stimulant is unnecessary in healthy children, even if they are below average in weight for age or height.

The Table summarizes pertinent information on the individual antihistamines. Piperazine antihistamines (buclizine [Bucladin-S], cyclizine [Marezine], meclizine [Antivert, Bonine]) and the ethanolamine, dimenhydrinate [Dramamine], are used principally for their antiemetic effects and are not included in the Table. Other uses for some drugs in this chapter are discussed in Chapters 11, Drugs Used for Anxiety and Insomnia; 16, Drugs Used in Extrapyramidal Movement Disorders; and 26, Drugs Used in Vertigo, Motion Sickness, and Vomiting.

ANTIHISTAMINES

Drug	Chemical Structure
Ethanolamines	
Diphenhydramine Hydrochloride	

Adverse Reactions and Precautions

The incidence and severity of untoward effects and the dose eliciting the reactions vary with each drug. Adverse reactions may be minimized by determining, through trial and error, which antihistamine a particular patient tolerates best.

The most frequent untoward effect with all antihistamines is sedation. Symptoms include drowsiness, inability to concentrate, dizziness, ataxia, and deep sleep. Among the most potent and highly sedating antihistamines are two ethanolamines (diphenhydramine [Benadryl], doxylamine [Decapryn]) and a phenothiazine (promethazine [Phenergan]). The degree of central nervous system depression caused by other drugs in these chemical subclasses (carbinoxamine [Clistin], methdilazine [Tacaryl], trimeprazine [Temaril]) is lower. The sedative properties of the ethylenediamines are approximately intermediate and those of the alkylamines tend to be relatively low. Sedation is a hazard in ambulatory patients whose activities require mental alertness and motor coordination. In some instances, this effect may disappear after two or three days of therapy. If sedation persists, the dose should be reduced or another antihistamine tried. Alternatively, the antihistamine producing sedation may be beneficial for nighttime use to promote sleep and another type used during the daytime. Alkylamines, which are least sedating and may even stimulate the central nervous system, often are preferred for daytime use.

Hydroxyzine has a broad range of optimal dosage among patients and should be given in increasing doses to the level that is sufficient to control symptoms, especially pruritus, but that does not cause excessive sedation.

Occasionally, the anticholinergic action of an antihistamine may predominate and cause excitation that results in insomnia, tremors, nervousness, irritability, and palpitations. Such effects are more likely to occur in children. Increased sensitivity to antihistamines in patients with focal lesions of the cerebral cortex may result in convulsions. Dryness of the mouth, nose, and throat and thickening of bronchial secretions are frequent untoward effects. Blurred vision, urinary retention, tachycardia, and constipation also may be noted, but these reactions are uncommon unless large doses are used.

Gastrointestinal disturbances (eg, anorexia, nausea, vomiting, epigastric distress) are common, especially with ethylenediamines, and may be reduced by giving the drug with meals.

Rarely, reversible leukopenia, agranulocytosis, hemolytic anemia, or thrombocytopenia have been reported, and the possibility of their occurrence should be considered when prolonged antihistamine therapy is needed. Other rare reactions include disorientation, vertigo, confusion, delirium, acute labyrinthitis, hysteria, neuropathy, fatigue, hyperhidrosis, early menses, headache, paresthesias, premature heart contractions, urinary frequency, and chills.

Usual Dosage	Preparations	Comment
Oral: Adults, 25-50 mg 3 or 4 times daily. *Children under 12 years,* 5 mg/kg in 4 divided doses over a 24-hour period. *Intravenous (preferred), Intramuscular (deep): Adults,* 10-50 mg (maximum, 400 mg daily). *Children,* 5 mg/kg daily in 4 divided doses (maximum, 300 mg daily). *Topical:* Cream applied as needed to affected area.	Generic: Capsules, elixir, syrup, and solution *Benadryl* (Parke, Davis): Capsules 25 and 50 mg Elixir 12.5 mg/5 ml Solution (for injection) 10 mg/ml in 10 and 30 ml containers and 50 mg/ml in 1 and 10 ml containers Powder (for injection) Cream 2% in 1 and 2 oz containers	Most widely used antihistamine for parenteral administration in treatment of anaphylactic and other allergic reactions. May be given with epinephrine but is not a substitute for it. Incidence of drowsiness high. Drug should not be used in premature and newborn infants. Patients hypersensitive to xanthines may also be hypersensitive to this medication. Drug should not be used with ototoxic antibiotics, as the ototoxicity may be masked.

ANTIHISTAMINES

Drug	Chemical Structure

Ethanolamines

Carbinoxamine Maleate

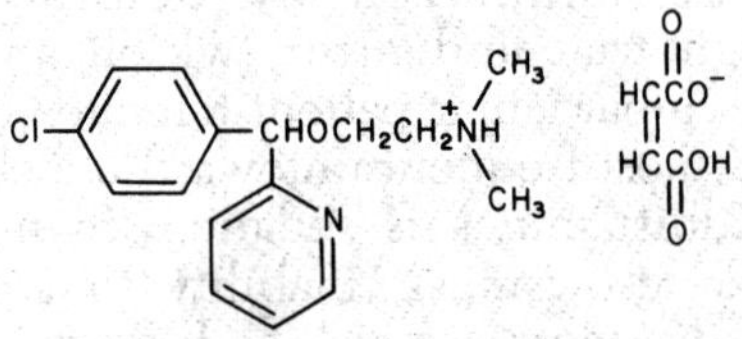

Clemastine Fumarate

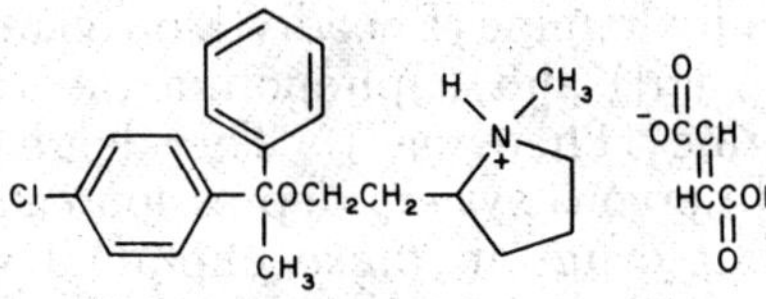

Doxylamine Succinate

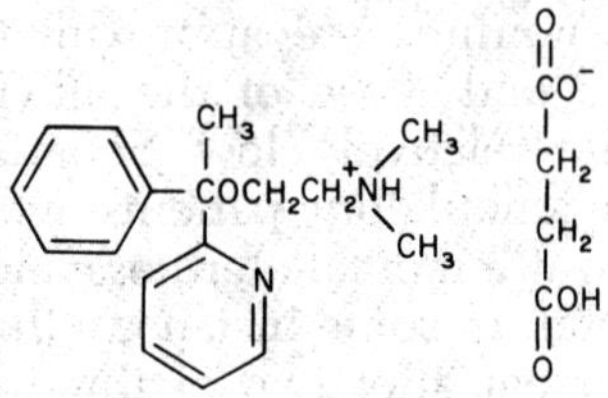

Ethylenediamines

Tripelennamine Citrate

Tripelennamine Hydrochloride

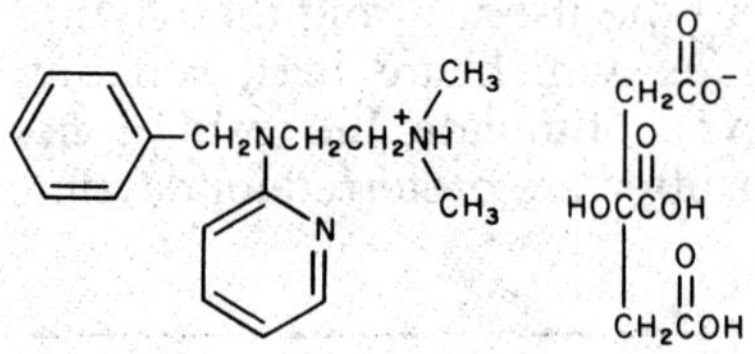

Pyrilamine Maleate

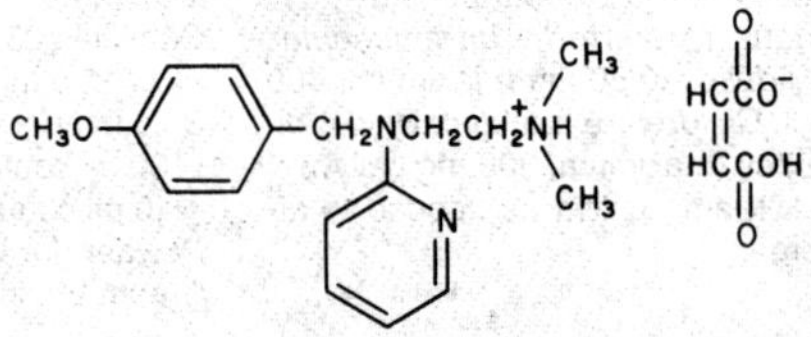

Usual Dosage	Preparations	Comment
Oral: Adults, 12-32 mg daily in divided doses. *Children,* 0.2 mg/kg 3 or 4 times daily.	*Clistin* (McNeil): Elixir 4 mg/5 ml Tablets 4 mg Tablets (timed-release)* 8 and 12 mg	Lowest incidence of drowsiness of the ethanolamines. Anticholinergic effect comparatively weak.
Oral: Adults, 2.68 mg 1 to 3 times daily (maximum, 8.04 mg daily [3 tablets]).	*Tavist* (Dorsey): Tablets 2.68 mg	Drowsiness is the most frequent side effect, but central sedative effects are generally low. Anticholinergic effect very weak.
Oral: Adults, 12.5-25 mg every 4 to 6 hours (maximum, 150 mg daily). *Children, .*2 mg/kg daily divided into 4 to 6 doses (maximum in *children 6-12 years,* 75 mg daily).	*Decapryn* (Merrell-National): Syrup 6.25 mg/5 ml (nonprescription) Tablets 12.5 and 25 mg	Incidence of drowsiness high.
Oral: (Doses expressed in terms of hydrochloride salt.) *Adults,* 25-50 mg every 4 to 6 hours. *Children,* 5 mg/kg/24 hours divided into 4 to 6 doses.	*PBZ Citrate* (Geigy): Elixir 37.5 mg (equivalent to 25 mg of hydrochloride salt)/5 ml	Incidence of sedation lower than with diphenhydramine. Dizziness common.
Oral: Adults, 25-50 mg every 4 to 6 hours (tablets) or 100 mg 2 or 3 times daily (timed-release form); *children,* 5 mg/kg/24 hours in 4 to 6 divided doses (tablets) or, for *children over 5 years,* 50 mg 2 or 3 times daily (timed-release form). *Topical:* Cream or ointment applied as needed.	Generic: Tablets, powder, cream *PBZ-SR* (Geigy): Tablets (timed-release) 100 mg *Pyribenzamine HCl* (Ciba): Tablets 25 and 50 mg Tablets (timed-release)* 50 mg Cream 2% in 1 oz containers Ointment 2% in 1 oz containers	
Oral: Adults, 75-200 mg daily in 3 or 4 divided doses. *Children,* information is inadequate to establish dose.	Generic: Powder (oral) Tablets 25 and 50 mg	Incidence of drowsiness low.

*Bioavailability of drug in timed-release form may be neither uniform nor reliable.

ANTIHISTAMINES

Drug	Chemical Structure

Alkylamines

Chlorpheniramine Maleate

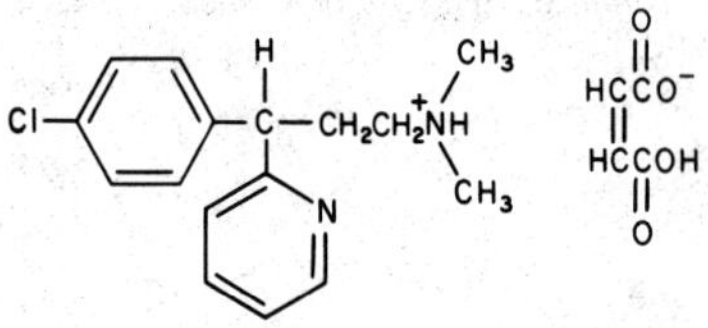

Brompheniramine Maleate

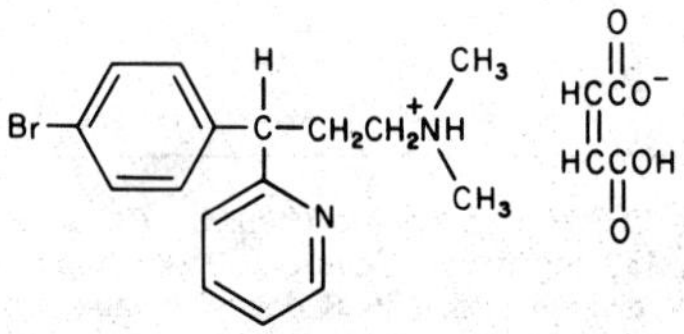

Dexchlorpheniramine Maleate

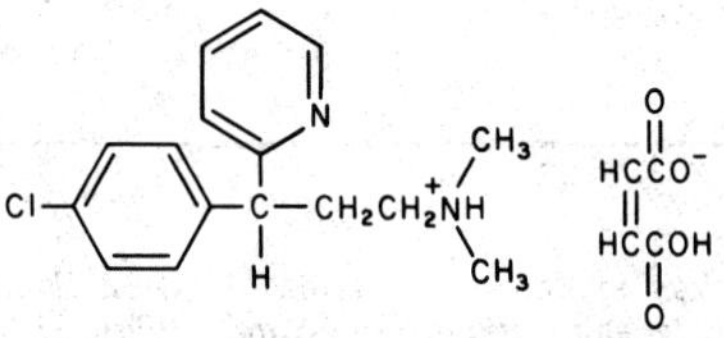

Dimethindene Maleate

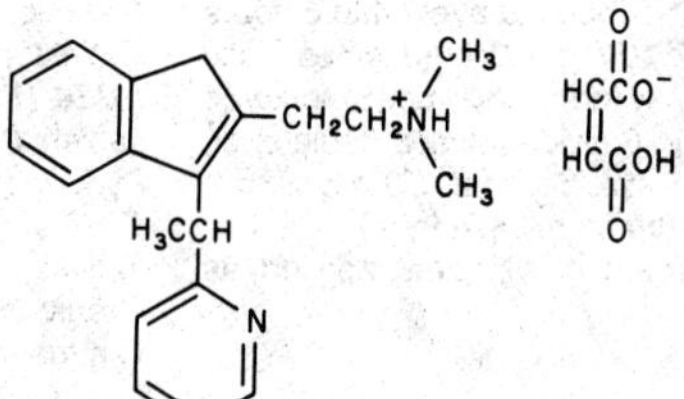

Triprolidine Hydrochloride

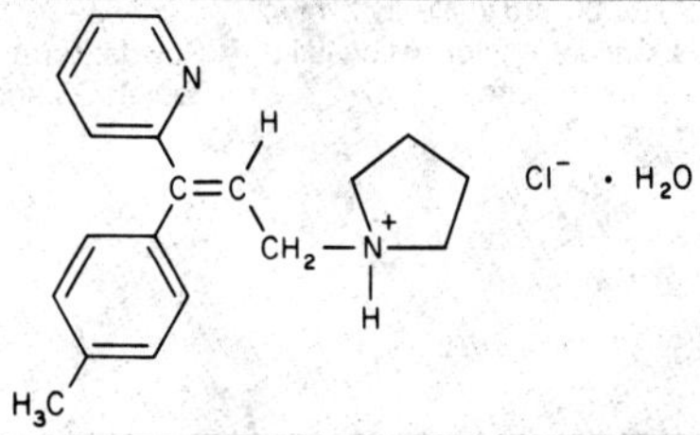

Usual Dosage	Preparations	Comment
Oral: Adults, 2-4 mg 3 or 4 times daily (tablets, syrup) or 8-12 mg 1 to 3 times daily (timed-release form). *Children under 12 years,* 0.35 mg/kg daily divided into 4 doses; *7 years and older,* 8 mg every 12 hours (timed-release form). *Intramuscular, Intravenous, Subcutaneous: Adults,* 5-40 mg (intravenous injection should be made over a period of 1 minute). *Subcutaneous: Children under 12 years,* 0.35 mg/kg daily divided into 4 doses.	Generic: Capsules, tablets, solution *Chlor-Trimeton* (Schering): Syrup 2 mg/5 ml (nonprescription) Tablets 4 mg (nonprescription) Tablets (timed-release) 8 (nonprescription) and 12 mg Solution (for injection) 10 mg/ml in 1 ml containers and 100 mg/ml in 2 ml containers *Histaspan* (USV), *Teldrin* (Smith Kline & French): Capsules (timed-release) 8 and 12 mg	Drowsiness most common reaction, but overall incidence low. Common ingredient in cold remedies.
Oral: Adults, 4 mg every 4 to 6 hours (maximum, 24 mg daily) (tablets, elixir) or 8-12 mg 2 or 3 times daily (timed-release form). *Children 6 to 12 years,* 2 mg every 4 to 6 hours (maximum, 12 mg daily) (tablets, elixir) or 8-12 mg every 12 hours (timed-release form); *2 to 6 years,* 1 mg every 4 to 6 hours (maximum, 6 mg daily) (elixir). *Intramuscular, Intravenous, Subcutaneous: Adults,* 5-20 mg every 6 to 12 hours (maximum, 40 mg daily). *Children under 12 years,* 0.5 mg/kg daily divided into 3 or 4 doses.	Generic: Elixir, tablets, solution *Dimetane* (Robins) (nonprescription): Elixir 2 mg/5 ml Tablets 4 mg Tablets (timed-release)* 8 and 12 mg *Dimetane-Ten* (Robins): Solution (for injection) 10 mg/ml in 1 ml containers *Symptom 3* (Parke, Davis): Liquid 2 mg/5 ml (nonprescription)	Most common reaction is drowsiness.
Oral: Adults, 1 or 2 mg 3 or 4 times daily (tablets, syrup) or 4 or 6 mg 2 times daily and, for resistant cases, 8 mg 2 times daily or 6 mg 3 times daily (timed-release form). *Children under 12 years,* 0.15 mg/kg daily divided into 4 doses.	*Polaramine* (Schering): Syrup 2 mg/5 ml Tablets 2 mg Tablets (timed-release)* 4 and 6 mg	Incidence of reactions low; most common reaction is drowsiness.
Oral: Adults and children over 6 years, 2.5 mg 1 or 2 times daily (timed-release form). *Children under 6 years,* dosage not established.	*Forhistal Maleate* (Ciba): Tablets (timed-release)* 2.5 mg *Triten* (Marion): Tablets (timed-release)* 2.5 mg	Drowsiness occurs frequently.
Oral: Adults, 2.5 mg 3 or 4 times daily. *Children over 6 years,* 1.25 mg 3 or 4 times daily; *under 6 years,* (syrup) 0.3-0.6 mg 3 or 4 times daily, depending on age.	Generic: Syrup, tablets *Actidil* (Burroughs Wellcome): Syrup 1.25 mg/5 ml Tablets 2.5 mg	Incidence of reactions low; most common reaction is drowsiness.

*Bioavailability of drug in timed-release form may be neither uniform nor reliable.

ANTIHISTAMINES

Drug	Chemical Structure

Phenothiazines

Methdilazine

Methdilazine Hydrochloride

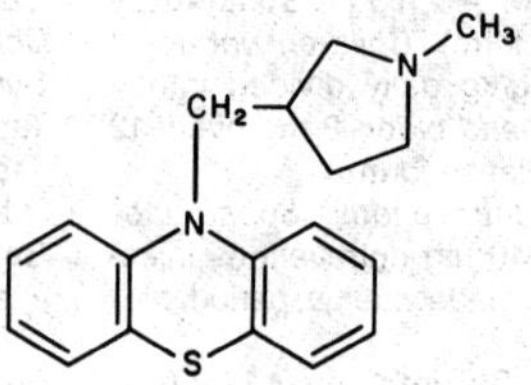

Promethazine Hydrochloride

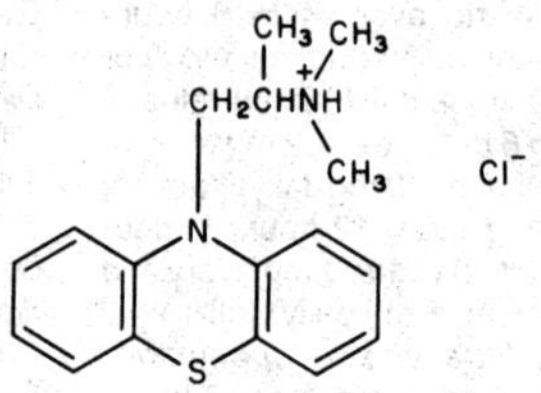

Trimeprazine Tartrate

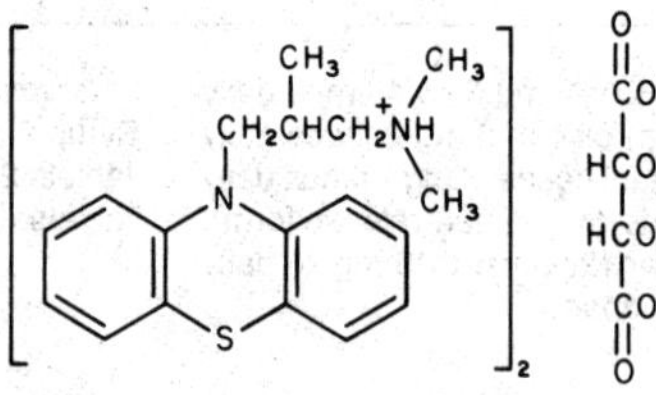

Miscellaneous

Azatadine Maleate

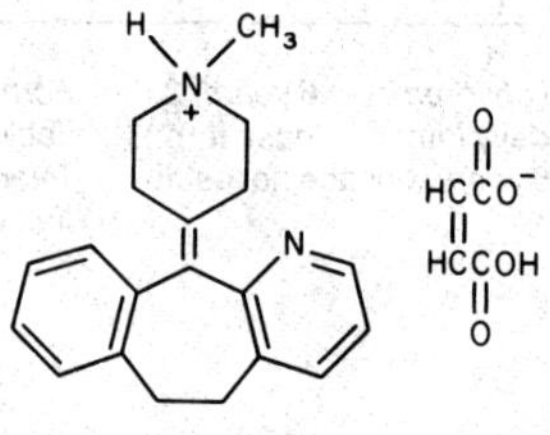

Cyproheptadine Hydrochloride

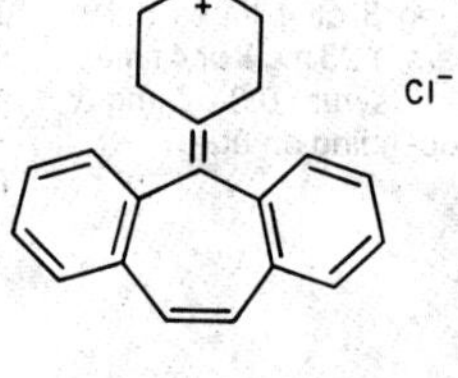

Usual Dosage	Preparations	Comment
Oral: Adults, 16-32 mg daily divided into 2 to 4 doses; *children over 3 years,* 4 mg 2 to 4 times daily.	*Tacaryl* (Westwood): Tablets (chewable) 3.6 mg (equivalent to 4 mg of hydrochloride salt) *Tacaryl Hydrochloride* (Westwood): Syrup 4 mg/5 ml Tablets 8 mg	Used primarily as antipruritic. Drowsiness less prominent than with other phenothiazines used as antihistamines. Most serious adverse reactions of other phenothiazines not reported with methdilazine.
Oral: Adults, 25 mg at bedtime or 12.5 mg 4 times daily; *children,* 25 mg at bedtime or 6.25-12.5 mg 3 times daily. *Rectal, Intramuscular, Intravenous: Adults,* 25 mg repeated in 2 hours if necessary. *Intramuscular: Children,* no more than one-half adult dose.	Generic: Tablets, solution *Phenergan* (Wyeth): Syrup 6.25 and 25 mg/5 ml Tablets 12.5, 25, and 50 mg Suppositories 12.5, 25, and 50 mg Solution (for injection) 25 and 50 mg/ml in 1 ml containers	Pronounced sedative effect limits use in many ambulatory patients. All precautions applicable to phenothiazines should be observed (see Chapter 12). Photosensitization is contraindication to further use.
Oral: Adults, 10 mg daily divided into 4 doses (tablets, syrup) or 2 doses (timed-release form). *Children 6 months to 3 years,* 3.75 mg daily divided into 3 doses; *3 to 12 years,* 7.5 mg daily divided into 3 doses.	*Temaril* (Smith Kline & French): Capsules (timed-release) 5 mg Syrup 2.5 mg/5 ml Tablets 2.5 mg	Used primarily as antipruritic. Drowsiness most common reaction. All precautions applicable to phenothiazines should be observed (see Chapter 12).
Oral: Adults, 1-2 mg twice daily. *Children,* dosage has not been established.	*Optimine* (Schering): Tablets 1 mg	Chemically similar to cyproheptadine. Drowsiness most common side effect.
Oral: Adults, 4-20 mg daily in divided doses. Dosage must be individualized and should not exceed 0.5 mg/kg daily. *Children 2 to 6 years,* 2 mg 2 or 3 times daily (maximum, 12 mg daily); *7 to 14 years,* 4 mg 2 or 3 times daily (maximum, 16 mg daily).	*Periactin Hydrochloride* (Merck Sharp & Dohme): Syrup 2 mg/5 ml Tablets 4 mg	Used to relieve pruritus. Reported to be especially useful in cold urticaria. Drowsiness most common reaction. Weight gain has been reported. Drug should not be used in premature and newborn infants.

*Bioavailability of drug in timed-release form may be neither uniform nor reliable.

ANTIHISTAMINES

Drug	Chemical Structure

Miscellaneous
Hydroxyzine Hydrochloride

Hydroxyzine Pamoate

$$Cl—\text{(ring)}—CH—N^+—\text{(ring)}—^+N—CH_2CH_2OCH_2CH_2OH \quad 2Cl^-$$

Other Antihistamines
Bromodiphenhydramine Hydrochloride
  Ambodryl (Parke, Davis)
Diphenylpyraline Hydrochloride
  Diafen (Riker)
  Hispril (Smith Kline & French)

Although hypersensitivity reactions may develop after oral use of antihistamines, they occur more commonly after topical application. Therefore, with the possible exception of diphenhydramine [Benadryl], these agents should be given orally rather than topically to treat any dermatitis. Sensitization is manifested by urticarial, eczematous, bullous, or petechial lesions, as well as by fixed drug eruptions. In some cases, these eruptions are caused by photosensitization rather than by a primary allergic reaction.

Although diphenhydramine has been used to control drug-induced dyskinesias and to lessen tremor and rigidity in parkinsonism, recent reports suggest that diphenhydramine itself rarely may produce dystonia. This is an idiosyncratic side effect and should not prevent the use of this drug for treatment of dyskinesias.

Since children have less predictable responses to antihistamines (eg, central nervous system stimulation rather than sedation), those 6 to 12 years old should receive approximately one-half the adult dose. Those under 6 should be given antihistamines only under strict medical supervision. These drugs should be prescribed with caution for patients with hepatic or renal dysfunction, prostatic hypertrophy, stenosing peptic ulcer, pyloroduodenal obstruction, bladder neck obstruction, or glaucoma.

Drug Interactions: Patients receiving antihistamines should be warned against the concomitant use of alcoholic beverages or other drugs that depress the central nervous system. They should not be used with drugs that augment their anticholinergic effects (eg, monoamine oxidase inhibitors). Some antihistamines antagonize the effects of antihypertensive drugs such as guanethidine, and control of blood pressure may be lost.

Teratogenicity: Since antihistamines have been used frequently during pregnancy without ill effects, the risk of fetal malformation appears to be very low. However, the risk/benefit ratio should be considered before they are used during the first trimester. Platelet dysfunction has occurred rarely in later stages of pregnancy. Antihistamines may inhibit lactation and may be excreted in breast milk. Since the risk of adverse reactions is higher in infants, use of antihistamines is not recommended in nursing mothers.

Poisoning: Overdosage may be difficult to treat. In children, symptoms resemble atropine poisoning (excitation, convulsions) and, in adults, both depression and stimulation of the central nervous system appear alternately. Cardiorespiratory collapse and death may occur. Mechanical ventilation and supportive care are important, and drugs likely to potentiate the effects of the antihistamines should not be given.

Usual Dosage	Preparations	Comment
Oral: Adults, initially 25 mg 3 times daily, increased if necessary to 100 mg 4 times daily. *Children under 6 years,* 50 mg daily divided into 3-4 doses; *over 6 years,* 50-100 mg daily divided into 3-4 doses.	*Atarax* [hydrochloride] (Roerig): Syrup 10 mg/5 ml Tablets 10, 25, 50, and 100 mg *Vistaril* [pamoate] (Pfizer): Capsules 25, 50, and 100 mg Suspension (oral) equivalent to 25 mg hydrochloride/5 ml	Agent of choice in chronic urticaria and many dermatologic allergies. Drowsiness most common reaction. Contraindicated during early pregnancy.

MIXTURES

Many fixed-ratio combinations containing two or more antihistamines or antihistamines with analgesics, adrenergic agents, adrenal corticosteroids, or antibacterial agents are marketed for use in allergies and other conditions such as the common cold. With the possible exception of antihistamine-adrenergic combinations, in which the adrenergic agent may counteract the drowsiness induced by the antihistamine and augment the drying effect on the nasal mucosa, most such mixtures have an unsound rationale and should not be used. An adequate dose of one ingredient may require the administration of supplementary doses of the other components, thus tending to negate the minor convenience that the combination product appears to offer. In addition, when two or more agents with similar action are combined, the patient is exposed to the possible development of sensitivity to any of them, often without any compensating advantage.

The following are commonly prescribed mixtures containing an antihistamine and an adrenergic agent:

Actifed (Burroughs Wellcome). Each tablet contains triprolidine hydrochloride 2.5 mg and pseudoephedrine hydrochloride 60 mg; each 5 ml of syrup contains triprolidine hydrochloride 1.25 mg and pseudoephedrine hydrochloride 30 mg.

Co-Pyronil (Dista). Each capsule contains pyrrobutamine phosphate 15 mg, methapyrilene hydrochloride 25 mg, and cyclopentamine hydrochloride 12.5 mg; each pediatric capsule and 5 ml of syrup contains pyrrobutamine phosphate 7.5 mg, methapyrilene hydrochloride 12.5 mg, and cyclopentamine hydrochloride 6.25 mg.

Deconamine (Berlex). Each tablet contains chlorpheniramine maleate 4 mg and pseudoephedrine hydrochloride 60 mg; each capsule (timed-release) contains chlorpheniramine maleate 8 mg and pseudoephedrine 120 mg; each 5 ml of elixir contains chlorpheniramine maleate 2 mg and pseudoephedrine hydrochloride 30 mg (alcohol 15%).

Dimetapp (Robins). Each 5 ml of elixir contains brompheniramine maleate 4 mg, phenylephrine hydrochloride 5 mg, and phenylpropanolamine hydrochloride 5 mg (alcohol 2.3%); each tablet (timed-release) contains brompheniramine maleate 12 mg, phenylephrine hydrochloride 15 mg, and phenylpropanolamine hydrochloride 15 mg.

Drixoral (Schering). Each tablet (timed-release) contains dexbrompheniramine maleate 6 mg and pseudoephedrine sulfate 120 mg.

For further information and listings of mixtures containing antihistamines, see Chapters 29, Nasal Decongestants; 30, Cold Remedies; and 31, Agents Used to Treat Cough.

Selected References

Intranasal beclomethasone: Wonder drug or hazard? *Br Med J* 2:1522-1523, 1976.

Ainsworth CA III, et al: A fatality involving methapyrilene. *Clin Toxicol* 11:281-286, 1977.

Church JA, et al: Pharmacotherapy of respiratory allergy. *Drug Ther* 7:33-45, (July) 1977.

Cirillo VJ, et al: Pharmacology and therapeutic use of antihistamines. *J Maine Med Assoc* 67:307-314, 1976.

Cockcroft DW, et al: Beclomethasone dipropionate aerosol in allergic rhinitis. *Can Med Assoc J* 115:523-526, 1976.

Davis WA II: Dyskinesia associated with chronic antihistamine use. *N Engl J Med* 294:113, 1976.

Hermance WE: Antihistamines. *Cutis* 17:1177-1182, 1976.

Krausen AS: Antihistamines: Guidelines and implications. *Ann Otol Rhinol Laryngol* 85:686-691, 1976.

Lavenstein BL, et al: Acute dystonia: An unusual reaction to diphenhydramine. *JAMA* 236:291, 1976.

Levine MI: Perennial rhinitis. *Compr Ther* 4:29-31, (April) 1978.

Pearlman DS: Antihistamines: Pharmacology and clinical use. *Drugs* 12:258-273, 1976.

Nasal Decongestants | 29

The vasomotor integrity of the nasal mucosa depends upon a proper balance between sympathetic and parasympathetic efferent impulses. Activation of the parasympathetic division of the autonomic nervous system produces vasodilatation and increases secretion, while activation of the sympathetic division produces vasoconstriction and decreases secretion. Congestion of the nasal mucosa is usually caused by infection, inflammation, allergy, or emotional upset. Treatment may be directed toward eliciting sympathetic responses or blocking parasympathetic responses.

Adrenergic agents are most commonly used for the symptomatic relief of nasal congestion. They include ephedrine, phenylephrine [Coricidin, Neo-Synephrine, Super Anahist Nasal Spray], phenylpropanolamine [Propadrine], propylhexedrine [Benzedrex], pseudoephedrine [Afrinol, Novafed, Sudafed, Symptom 2], tuaminoheptane [Tuamine], and the imidazolines (naphazoline [Privine], oxymetazoline [Afrin], tetrahydrozoline [Tyzine], and xylometazoline [Neo-Synephrine II, Otrivin, Sinutab Long-Lasting Sinus Spray]). Because they suppress the parasympathetic nervous system, anticholinergic drugs (eg, atropine, glycopyrrolate [Robinul]) occasionally are employed to produce nasal decongestion. Cocaine, which potentiates the actions of norepinephrine, also is used for its nasal decongestant effect in special, restricted circumstances. Adrenal corticosteroids (eg, prednisone, prednisolone) or corticotropin

(ACTH) may be given systemically or certain synthetic steroids (eg, dexamethasone sodium phosphate [Decadron Turbinaire]) may be given topically as aerosols for short periods to counteract inflammation of the nasal mucosa that does not respond to other agents.

The adrenergic nasal decongestants stimulate the alpha (excitatory) adrenergic receptors of vascular smooth muscle, thus constricting dilated arterioles within the nasal mucosa and reducing blood flow in the engorged, edematous area. Opening of obstructed nasal passages improves nasal ventilation and aeration and drainage of the sinuses; this also may relieve headache of sinus origin. The ideal drug exerts an effect on surface vessels as well as on deeper erectile structures.

Antihistamines, which have some antimuscarinic activity, are sometimes combined with an adrenergic agent. Such combinations may be useful in patients with hay fever (pollinosis, seasonal allergic rhinitis), but antihistamines are of little value for relief of nasal congestion in nonseasonal (perennial) allergic rhinitis (see Chapter 28, Antihistamines). There is no justification for including other medications, such as antibiotics, with nasal decongestants (see the section on Mixtures and Chapter 30, Cold Remedies).

Nasal decongestants provide temporary symptomatic relief in acute rhinitis associated with the common cold and other respiratory infections and in hay fever, nonseasonal allergic rhinitis, and other forms of acute and chronic rhinitis and sinusitis. Topical decongestants also are used to facilitate visualization of nasal and nasopharyngeal membranes during diagnostic procedures and to reduce turgescence prior to nasal surgery. Some authorities believe that, by opening obstructed eustachian ostia, the vasoconstrictor action of these drugs may be useful as an adjunct to antibacterial therapy in middle ear infections or as the sole medication in serous otitis media.

Anticholinergic agents are administered before nasal surgery, especially when general anesthesia is to be given. Some patients with severe rhinorrhea and congestion obtain more relief from propantheline [Pro-Banthine] or belladonna alkaloids than from adrenergic agents. Anticholinergic agents also are effective in those with disease that inactivates the sympathetic nerve supply to the nose (eg, Horner's syndrome, adrenocortical insufficiency); adrenergic agents should not be given to these patients. Anticholinergic agents also are useful in laryngectomized individuals who develop boggy rhinitis.

Administration: Most nasal decongestants are applied topically; ephedrine and phenylephrine can be used either topically or orally, and phenylpropanolamine is used only orally. Topical nasal decongestants may not reach all parts of the nasopharyngeal and sinus mucosa, and it has been claimed that systemic therapy with the slower-acting, orally administered preparations is more effective because they ordinarily exert their action on inaccessible parts of the mucous membranes lining the convoluted nasal passages. It also is claimed that more prolonged relief is produced by the systemically acting adrenergic drugs, for topically applied medications tend to be swept away with respiratory tract fluid by the action of the ciliated cells. There is no convincing clinical evidence to support these contentions. Also, systemically administered adrenergic drugs may have undesired effects on tissues other than nasal mucosa.

Topically applied dilute aqueous solutions or inhaled vapors have a more rapid onset of action and are more effective than oral doses of the same drugs because of their immediate and direct contact with the nasal mucosa. Also, the duration of action of some topically applied preparations is comparable to that of the orally administered drugs. However, oral preparations are preferable for prolonged use (more than five days), since the incidence of deleterious effects on the nasal mucosa (eg, rebound congestion, dryness, interference with ciliary action, chronic swelling) increases with prolonged or excessive use of topical agents. (See the section on Adverse Reactions and Precautions.)

Nasal decongestants are used topically in the form of vapors, sprays, or drops; solutions applied by means of wet tampons and nasal packs mechanically injure and remove nasal cilia and are no longer used except for diagnostic or surgical procedures in the office or hospital. For short-term, intermittent use, vaporizers containing the volatile bases of certain nasal decongestants (eg, propylhexedrine) are among the most effective means for reaching the desired areas of the nasal mucosa; they are useful when rapid improvement in ventilation of the nose and eustachian orifices is desired (eg, during airplane descent). Drops instilled on the nasal mucosa usually trickle rapidly over the surface and frequently pass to the hypopharynx, where they are swallowed. Swallowing may be avoided by instilling the drops with the head in the lateral, head-low position. Most plastic spray packs deliver about three drops of finely divided mist over a much larger area of the nasal mucosa than can be reached by an equal volume in drop form. Since the mist is fine, it does not flow readily and is less likely to be swallowed than drops; also, because it is trapped in the upper respiratory tract, the possibility of pulmonary absorption is much less than with vapor.

The following regimen for use of nasal sprays may produce maximal nasal ventilation and opening of the sinus ostia with minimal systemic disturbance: With the patient in the upright position, a spray is delivered into each nostril; three to five minutes later, the nose is thoroughly blown as decongestion begins in the inferior and in part of the middle turbinates. The procedure is then repeated and, if secretions are still being expelled, it may be repeated once more. Congestion of the turbinates high in the nose usually is relieved, providing ventilation of the ostia and drainage of the sinuses. However, since the total doses provided by this procedure are frequently larger than the doses usually recommended for the same time period, untoward adrenergic effects may be more likely to occur when some of these agents are applied in this manner (see the evaluations).

When treating barotitis by producing vasoconstriction in the eustachian tubes, drops should be instilled as follows: The patient lies supine (not hyperextended) with the head turned 15° toward the affected ear. Nasal drops are instilled into the affected side and allowed to run along the floor of the nose and "puddle" at the eustachian orifice which is now the low point. The patient should remain in this position for about five minutes.

Adverse Reactions and Precautions

The topical application of nasal decongestants sometimes causes temporary discomfort such as stinging, burning, or dryness of the mucosa. Inhaled vapors of volatile bases (eg, propylhexedrine [Benzedrex]) particularly may dry the nasal mucosa rapidly and interfere with ciliary action.

Although these agents permit opening of the nasal passages, which improves aeration and drainage of sinuses, a major disadvantage is the occurrence of rebound congestion after the vasoconstrictor action wears off. Because of this, topical nasal decongestants, especially naphazoline [Privine], are often misused. Recurrence or exacerbation of the original discomfort may cause the patient to use the drug more and more frequently, and overdosage with signs of toxicity may result. Irritation from prolonged and continual use produces chronic swelling of the nasal mucosa. Subsequent topical applications reopen the nasal passages only briefly, and the mucosa becomes pale gray or red, boggy, and edematous and is practically identical in

appearance to that seen in nonseasonal allergic rhinitis. This condition usually is alleviated a few days after the medication is discontinued. Generally, topical nasal decongestants should be used only in acute states and for periods not exceeding three to five days.

The orally administered agents generally induce chronic swelling of the nasal mucosa less frequently but are more likely to cause systemic reactions, since their action is not selective for nasal vessels. An oral dose large enough to produce nasal decongestion affects other vascular beds as well, and redistribution of blood flow and cardiac stimulation may occur. Although blood pressure usually is not increased, some patients experience marked hypertension and arrhythmias.

Topical decongestants also may produce systemic reactions, especially in infants and children. Significant absorption may occur from the nasal mucosa or gastrointestinal tract when excess solution trickles down the throat and is swallowed. The proper use of nasal sprays (see previous section) may be the best way to avoid systemic absorption. Use of the spray with the head in the upright position minimizes accumulation, since the medication and secretions drip from the nostril and are not swallowed. For children under six years, it is generally preferable to use drops rather than a spray because of the difficulty of controlling dosage with the latter.

Systemic effects from overdosage of most adrenergic drugs include transient hypertension, nervousness, nausea, dizziness, palpitation, and, occasionally, central nervous system stimulation. Overdoses of tetrahydrozoline [Tyzine] and naphazoline have caused hypertension, bradycardia, drowsiness, and rebound hypotension, and the possibility that such reactions may occur with the other imidazolines (oxymetazoline [Afrin], xylometazoline [Neo-Synephrine II, Otrivin, Sinutab Long-Lasting Sinus Spray]) should be kept in mind. These effects are most commonly seen in children. Severe reactions, characterized by sweating, drowsiness, deep sleep, coma, and even described as "shock-like" with hypotension and bradycardia, have been reported in children following overdosage of naphazoline or tetrahydrozoline. The imidazolines also may cause arrhythmias, presumably because of coronary vasoconstriction. Therefore, the topical nasal decongestants, especially the imidazolines, should be used sparingly and with particular caution in infants, young children, and patients with cardiovascular disease.

Solutions of topical nasal decongestants quickly become contaminated after use and may serve as reservoirs of bacterial and fungal infections. To minimize contamination, the dropper or spray tip should be rinsed in hot water after each use. Patients should be cautioned not to place the dropper in the nostril nor allow more than one person to use the same dropper bottle. The bottle or spray pack should be discarded when the medication is no longer needed. Nasal solutions of many adrenergic agents, especially naphazoline and probably the other imidazolines, should not be used in atomizers having aluminum parts because they interact with this metal.

All adrenergic agents should be given with caution to patients with thyroid disease, hypertension, diabetes mellitus, heart disease, or to those receiving tricyclic antidepressants. Nasal decongestants should not be used in patients receiving monoamine oxidase inhibitors or in those whose sensitivity to even small doses is manifested by insomnia, dizziness, asthenia, tremor, or arrhythmias.

INDIVIDUAL EVALUATIONS

COCAINE

COCAINE HYDROCHLORIDE

Cocaine is a local anesthetic and indirect-acting vasoconstrictor. It is effective when marked decongestion and anesthesia of the nasal mucosa is needed but, because of its abuse potential, it is only rarely used as a nasal decongestant. Its use should be limited to office and surgical procedures. To discourage use of cocaine for illegal purposes, the solution can be strongly tinted with methylene blue or toluidine blue. This provides the added advantages of discouraging mold growth and simplifying identification of pledgets if they are lost in the nose. Cocaine potentiates the effects of norepinephrine, apparently by interfering with its reabsorption by the sympathetic nerve endings and thus prolonging its action locally. Cocaine produces prompt vasoconstriction and temporary paralysis of the cilia. In spite of its local vasoconstrictor action, all mucous membranes may absorb cocaine more rapidly than it can be detoxified and excreted.

Prolonged use causes ischemic damage to the nasal mucosa. Systemic absorption resulting from overdosage causes excitement, chills followed by fever, tachycardia, hypertension, and nervousness. Extreme caution should be observed if epinephrine is added to cocaine because of the risk of inducing a hypertensive episode. For treatment of overdosage or hypersensitivity reactions, see the section on adverse reactions in the chapter on Local Anesthetics. Cocaine is classified as a Schedule II drug under the Controlled Substances Act.

ROUTE, USUAL DOSAGE, AND PREPARATIONS. *Topical*: A 0.5% to 2% solution is applied as a spray or on a tampon. For a more profound effect, a 10% solution is placed on small cotton pledgets and applied to the nasal mucosa. No more than 200 mg should be used in a 70-kg patient over a 30-minute period.

No pharmaceutical dosage form available; compounding by pharmacist necessary.

EPHEDRINE SULFATE

The effects of ephedrine are similar to those of phenylephrine, but the onset of action is slower. This drug is effective topically and orally but is now seldom used because secondary turgescence of the nasal mucosa and tachyphylaxis often occur. Other adverse effects include central nervous system stimulation, transient hypertension, and palpitations. See also the Introduction.

Aqueous solutions are preferred; oily solutions are obsolete and hazardous, especially in children, because of the danger of causing lipid pneumonia. Allergy to ephedrine, which occurs rarely, is a specific contraindication. It also should not be given to patients with heart disease, diabetes, hypertension, or suspected hyperthyroidism.

ROUTES, USUAL DOSAGE, AND PREPARATIONS. *Oral*: *Adults*, 25 to 50 mg every three to four hours; *children*, 3 mg/kg of body weight/24 hours in four to six divided doses.

> Drug available generically: Capsules 25 and 50 mg; syrup 11 and 20 mg/5 ml.

Topical: 1% to 3% solution, generally as drops, applied as needed; drops should be instilled with the head in the lateral, head-low position. The drug also may be applied as a pack or tampon.

> Drug available generically: Solution 3% in 30 ml containers.

EPINEPHRINE HYDROCHLORIDE
[Adrenalin Chloride]

Epinephrine is an effective topical nasal decongestant, but its duration of action is short. It is useful to control epistaxis or to facilitate nasal surgery but is only rarely used today as a nasal decongestant and should be reserved for use by the physician, rather than prescribed for patient self-administration.

Like other topical nasal decongestants, epinephrine frequently causes rebound nasal congestion. Systemic adverse reactions include anxiety, tremor, apprehension, pallor, restlessness, asthenia, dizzi-

ness, throbbing headache, dyspnea, and palpitation. Central nervous system stimulation occurs less frequently than with ephedrine. Adverse effects quickly disappear when the drug is discontinued. It should be used only with extreme caution with cocaine hydrochloride. See also the Introduction.

ROUTE, USUAL DOSAGE, AND PREPARATIONS. *Topical*: 0.1% aqueous solution, instilled as drops or spray, applied as needed (maximum in healthy adults, 1 ml over a 15-minute period). Drops should be instilled with the head in the lateral, head-low position. Some solutions may sting slightly due to the presence of sodium bisulfite added as an antioxidant.

> *Adrenalin Chloride* (Parke, Davis). Solution (aqueous) 0.1% in 30 ml containers.

NAPHAZOLINE HYDROCHLORIDE
[Privine Hydrochloride]

This imidazoline derivative is used topically to relieve local swelling and congestion of nasal mucous membranes.

Adverse reactions include severe rebound congestion, "nose-drop dependence," and irritation and swelling of the nasal mucosa from continued use. Swelling is generally alleviated a few days after the medication is discontinued, but severe withdrawal symptoms requiring hospitalization have been reported following discontinuation of naphazoline after prolonged abuse. Naphazoline also may cause paralysis of the nasal cilia and, occasionally, anosmia. Occasional smarting and sneezing also occur. Other adverse reactions include arrhythmias, probably as a result of coronary vasoconstriction, and transient hypertension, bradycardia, sweating, and drowsiness; rebound hypotension may follow hypertension and bradycardia. Systemic absorption after overdosage has caused deep sleep and, in children, coma.

Because of these effects, naphazoline should be used with particular caution in infants, young children, and patients with cardiovascular disease. The solution should not be used in atomizers containing any parts made of aluminum. See also the Introduction.

ROUTE, USUAL DOSAGE, AND PREPARATIONS. *Topical*: Two drops or two spray inhalations no more often than every three hours (drops) or four to six hours (spray). The drops should be instilled with the head in the lateral, head-low position.

> Drug available generically: Solution 0.05% and 0.1% in 500 ml containers.
> *Privine Hydrochloride* (Ciba). Solution 0.05% in 20 and 473 ml containers; spray 0.05% in 15 ml containers (nonprescription).

OXYMETAZOLINE HYDROCHLORIDE
[Afrin]

Oxymetazoline is an effective topical nasal decongestant that is somewhat longer acting than the other imidazoline derivatives. Subjective clinical evidence indicates that it relieves nasal congestion associated with nonseasonal allergic rhinitis, hay fever, and other forms of acute and chronic rhinitis or sinusitis.

Mild untoward effects that occur with normal use include stinging, burning, and dryness of the nasal mucosa, sneezing, headache, lightheadedness, insomnia, and palpitations. Effects on the central nervous system or blood pressure have not been reported, but presumably overdosage might cause adverse effects similar to those observed with other imidazolines. Rebound congestion, formerly reported only infrequently, has become more common since the drug became a nonprescription item and may be caused by prolonged or excessive use. However, adverse reactions are milder than those elicited by the shorter-acting nasal decongestants. See also the Introduction.

ROUTE, USUAL DOSAGE, AND PREPARATIONS. *Topical*: *Adults and children over 6 years*, two to four drops or two or three squeezes of spray (0.05% concentration) in each nostril in the morning and at bedtime. *Children 2 to 5 years*, two or three drops (0.025% concentration) in each nostril. Some patients may require more frequent administration.

> *Afrin* (Schering). Solution 0.025% (pediatric) and 0.05% in 20 ml dropper containers; spray 0.05% in 15 and 30 ml containers (nonprescription).

PHENYLEPHRINE HYDROCHLORIDE
[Coricidin, Neo-Synephrine Hydrochloride, Super Anahist Nasal Spray]

Phenylephrine is one of the most widely prescribed topical nasal decongestants. Its effects are qualitatively similar to those of epinephrine, but phenylephrine is less potent on a weight basis and has a longer duration of action. Although oral dosage forms are available, this route seldom is effective in producing nasal decongestion at the suggested dosage.

Adverse reactions include all of the untoward effects of ephedrine or epinephrine, except that phenylephrine causes little or no central nervous system stimulation. A concentration of 0.25% is usually effective; stronger concentrations cause chronic swelling of the nasal mucosa within a few days and should probably be used only by (1% concentration) or under the direction of (0.5% concentration) a physician. See also the Introduction.

ROUTE, USUAL DOSAGE, AND PREPARATIONS. *Topical*: *Adults and older children*, several drops of a 0.25% to 1% solution instilled in each nostril as needed with the head in the lateral, head-low position. Administration may be repeated in three or four hours if needed. Alternatively, the nasal spray may be used or a small amount of the jelly may be placed in each nostril and inhaled. *Infants*, the 0.125% solution is used.

Drug available generically: Solution 0.25% and 1% in 500 ml containers.
Coricidin (Schering). Spray 0.5% in 20 ml containers (nonprescription).
Neo-Synephrine Hydrochloride (Winthrop). Solution 0.125% (pediatric) in 30 ml containers, 0.25% and 1% in 30 and 480 ml containers, and 0.5% in 30 ml containers; spray 0.25% and 0.5% in 22.5 ml containers; jelly (water-soluble) 0.5% in 18.75 g containers (nonprescription).
Super Anahist Nasal Spray (Warner-Lambert). Spray 0.25% in 15 ml containers (nonprescription).

PHENYLPROPANOLAMINE HYDROCHLORIDE
[Propadrine Hydrochloride]

Phenylpropanolamine is one of the most frequently used oral nasal decongestants. Its pharmacologic properties are analogous to those of ephedrine. Phenylpropanolamine is approximately equal in potency but usually causes less central nervous system stimulation than ephedrine. See also the Introduction.

ROUTE, USUAL DOSAGE, AND PREPARATIONS.
Oral: *Adults*, 25 mg every three or four hours or 50 mg every six to eight hours. *Children 8 to 12 years*, 20 to 25 mg three times daily.Not recommended for *children under 8 years*.
Drug available generically: Capsules 25 mg; tablets 25, 35, and 50 mg.
Propadrine Hydrochloride (Merck Sharp & Dohme). Capsules 25 and 50 mg; elixir 20 mg/5 ml.

PROPYLHEXEDRINE
[Benzedrex]

Propylhexedrine is used by inhalation for its nasal decongestant effect. It produces considerably less central nervous system stimulation than ephedrine. Because of its wider margin of safety and relative freedom from toxic effects, propyl-

hexedrine may be used in patients in whom an ephedrine-like pressor or stimulant action is undesirable. This nasal decongestant is considered safe for self-medication by adults, but children should not have unsupervised access to an inhaler. The vapors may dry the nasal mucosa and interfere with ciliary action. See also the Introduction.

ROUTE, USUAL DOSAGE, AND PREPARATIONS.
Topical (inhalation): Two inhalations (0.6 to 0.8 mg) in each nostril as needed. The inhaler usually retains its effectiveness for two to three months. If the inhaler is cold, it should be warmed in the hand before use to increase volatility.
Benzedrex (Menley & James). Inhaler 250 mg (nonprescription).

PSEUDOEPHEDRINE HYDROCHLORIDE
[Novafed, Sudafed, Symptom 2]

PSEUDOEPHEDRINE SULFATE
[Afrinol]

Pseudoephedrine is a physiologically active stereoisomer of ephedrine with similar actions, uses, and adverse reactions, although it is not effective in asthma; it may cause less central nervous system stimulation and hypertension. Pseudoephedrine is used in patients with vasomotor rhinitis or those with serous otitis media combined with eustachian tube congestion.

ROUTE, USUAL DOSAGE, AND PREPARATIONS.
Oral: *Adults*, 60 mg three or four times daily. *Children*, 4 mg/kg of body weight daily in four divided doses.
PSEUDOEPHEDRINE HYDROCHLORIDE:
Novafed (Dow). Capsules (timed-release) 120 mg.
Sudafed (Burroughs Wellcome). Syrup 30 mg/5 ml; tablets 30 and 60 mg.
Symptom 2 (Parke, Davis). Liquid 30 mg/5 ml (nonprescription).
PSEUDOEPHEDRINE SULFATE:
Afrinol (Schering). Tablets (timed-release) 120 mg.

TETRAHYDROZOLINE HYDROCHLORIDE
[Tyzine]

This imidazoline derivative is effective topically for temporary relief of nasal congestion.

Adverse effects include hypertension, bradycardia, severe drowsiness accompanied by sweating, rebound hypotension, and arrhythmias, probably as a result of coronary vasoconstriction. Chronic swelling of the nasal mucosa may occur with prolonged use and may persist for a week or more after the medication is discontinued. Coma and hypothermia may occur in children, especially infants. Because of these effects, tetrahydrozoline should be used sparingly, if at all, and with particular caution in infants, young children, and patients with cardiovascular disease. See also the Introduction.

ROUTE, USUAL DOSAGE, AND PREPARATIONS. *Topical: Adults and children 6 years or older,* two to four drops of the 0.1% solution instilled in each nostril no more often than every three hours. *Children 2 to 6 years,* two to three drops of the 0.05% solution instilled in each nostril, with the head in the lateral, head-low position, at intervals of four to six hours. Tetrahydrozoline should be used with extreme caution, if at all, in *infants and children under 6 years* because of the reasons stated above.

Drug available generically: Solution.

Tyzine (Key). Solution 0.05% (pediatric) in 15 ml containers and 0.1% in 15 and 30 ml containers.

TUAMINOHEPTANE SULFATE
[Tuamine Sulfate]

$$CH_3(CH_2)_4CHNH_2$$
$$|$$
$$CH_3$$

Tuaminoheptane is an effective topical nasal decongestant when applied in the form of drops. The vasoconstrictor action of the 1% solution exceeds that of a 1% solution of ephedrine and the duration of effect is longer.

Adverse reactions are the same as those observed with other adrenergic agents. The drug is relatively safe for use in infants and young children. It should be used with caution in patients with cardiovascular disease. See also the Introduction.

ROUTE, USUAL DOSAGE, AND PREPARATIONS. *Topical: Adults and children over 6 years,* four or five drops. *Children 1 to 6 years,* two or three drops. *Infants under 1 year,* one or two drops. The preparation is instilled in each nostril no more than four or five times daily for a maximum of three or four consecutive days.

Tuamine Sulfate (Lilly). Solution 1% in 30 ml containers.

XYLOMETAZOLINE HYDROCHLORIDE
[Neo-Synephrine II, Otrivin Hydrochloride, Sinutab Long-Lasting Sinus Spray]

This imidazoline derivative is effective topically for temporary relief of nasal congestion.

Untoward reactions, which are generally mild and infrequent, include local stinging or burning, sneezing, dryness of the nose, headache, insomnia, drowsiness, palpitations, and chronic swelling of the nasal mucosa with prolonged or excessive use. The solution should not be used in atomizers containing any parts made of aluminum. See also the Introduction.

ROUTE, USUAL DOSAGE, AND PREPARATIONS. *Topical: Adults,* two or three drops of the 0.1% solution or one or two inhalations of the 0.1% nasal spray in each nostril every eight to ten hours. *Children 6 months to 12 years,* two or three drops of the 0.05%

solution in each nostril every four to six hours. *Infants under 6 months*, one drop of the 0.05% solution in each nostril every six hours.

>   *Neo-Synephrine II* (Winthrop). Solution 0.05% (pediatric) and 0.1% in 30 ml containers; spray 0.1% in 15 ml containers.
>   *Otrivin Hydrochloride* (Geigy). Solution 0.05% (pediatric) and 0.1% in 20 ml containers; spray 0.1% in 15 ml containers.
>   *Sinutab Long-Lasting Sinus Spray* (Warner-Lambert). Spray 0.1% in 15 ml containers (nonprescription).

MIXTURES

Mixtures combining a nasal decongestant with one or more additional drugs are available for topical or oral use. Frequently the added drug is an antihistamine, antibiotic, analgesic, glucocorticoid, or a second nasal decongestant. Other compounds occasionally present include atropine or other anticholinergic agents, various wetting compounds, and quaternary ammonium salts.

If nasal decongestion is the therapeutic action desired, there is no good evidence that any of the available mixtures are more effective than a single-entity drug preparation. On the other hand, evidence does exist that the other agents present in the mixture either are detrimental or do not assist the nasal decongestant, and thus simply add cost to the mixture. For example, antihistamines add no beneficial effect to the topical preparations and, even when administered orally, they produce little or no shrinkage of the engorged nasal mucosa, although they may have some effect in ameliorating the symptoms of hay fever. Some added ingredients, particularly the antibiotics, act as sensitizers; in addition, the bacteria present in nasal discharges are simply the normal flora, and an antibiotic may convert these to resistant strains. If headache accompanies the nasal conges-

tion, products containing an analgesic and a decongestant may be useful (see Chapter 30, Cold Remedies).

Topically applied mixtures are used and abused widely by both the medical profession and the lay public. Careful comparative evaluation of these mixtures with single-entity decongestants has not been made; therefore, their use instead of a single-entity drug should be discouraged. The preparation chosen and the total duration of its use must be determined by the physician on the basis of experience and the response of the patient. Since individual tolerance and the tendency toward chronic congestion of the mucosa with prolonged use vary among patients, use of these agents should be regulated on an individual basis. A mixture containing a nasal decongestant cannot be expected to be more effective in relieving nasal congestion than the same quantity of the decongestant drug alone. The following topical mixtures are listed for information only.

For orally administered decongestant mixtures, see Chapter 30, Cold Remedies.

>   *NTZ* (Winthrop). Solution containing phenylephrine hydrochloride 0.5%, thenyldiamine hydrochloride 0.1%, and benzalkonium chloride 1:5,000 (nonprescription).
>   *Triaminicin* (Dorsey). Spray containing phenylpropanolamine hydrochloride 0.75%, phenylephrine hydrochloride 0.25%, pheniramine maleate 0.125%, and pyrilamine maleate 0.125% (nonprescription).

Selected References

Ballenger JJ: *Diseases of the Nose, Throat and Ear*, ed 12. Philadelphia, Lea & Febiger, 1977.

English GM (ed): *Otolaryngology*. Hagerstown, Md, Harper & Row, Publishers, 1976.

Ryan RE, et al: *Synopsis of Ear, Nose, and Throat Diseases*, ed 3. St Louis, CV Mosby Co, 1970.

Saunders WH, Gardier RW: *Pharmacotherapy in Otolaryngology*. St Louis, CV Mosby Co, 1976.

Cold Remedies | 30

Acute infections of the upper respiratory tract have diverse etiologies, including multiple viruses, but symptoms are similar. Most of these viruses are thought to be transmitted by respiratory droplet. However, rhinoviruses may be transmitted from an infected individual to a susceptible one via the hands of each. Because of this and because the virus appears to produce infection when it comes into contact with conjunctival and nasal (but not pharyngeal) mucosa, the incidence of transmission may be reduced by appropriate personal hygiene. By the time the infected person is aware of symptoms, which are presumed to be the result of cellular injury in the host, viral replication is already extensive.

The common cold is one of the most prevalent acute illnesses, but no successful methods to prevent or cure this infection are available. No effective, safe chemotherapeutic agent is presently available because the great variety of pathogenic viruses makes the development of preventive vaccines difficult. Although presently available antiviral agents (eg, amantadine, idoxuridine) are limited in effectiveness against specific viruses, human interferon is nonspecific and is potentially useful in the treatment of the numerous pathogenic viruses attacking man, including cold viruses (see Chapter 81, Antiviral Agents). Controlled studies are required to provide a definitive answer to these possibilities. At present, therefore, treatment must be directed toward relieving symptoms (postnasal drip, nasal congestion, headache,

myalgia, malaise, cough, and, sometimes, fever) until the natural defense and homeostatic mechanisms of the body can restore the patient's health. Failure of symptoms to abate within one week or worsening of symptoms such as headache, fever, cough, grossly purulent nasal discharge, or earache within this period, suggests the possibility that a secondary bacterial infection of the paranasal sinuses, ears, tracheobronchial tree, or lungs may be present. However, administration of an anti-infective agent is indicated only when the infection (bacterial or mycoplasmal) is presumed to be susceptible to the agent and is serious enough to warrant specific treatment.

The common cold is ordinarily benign and self-limited, but it affects virtually all members of society at some time, is sometimes followed by more serious complications, and is responsible for many man-hours of absenteeism from schools and businesses. Even if the infected person is able to maintain his ordinary daily routine, much time will be spent in varying degrees of discomfort. Therefore, drug products that relieve the annoying symptoms provide consolation for the cold sufferer and are worthwhile until specific, effective drugs become available.

Symptomatic Treatment: Because no one therapeutic agent can counteract all symptoms associated with the common cold, many mixtures are formulated that are claimed to relieve discomfort. These mixtures have the principal disadvantage of fixed-dosage combination products: When a therapeutic amount of one agent is given, other drugs in the mixture may be administered at higher or lower levels than are optimally therapeutic. This disadvantage is particularly prominent with some over-the-counter remedies that may have been formulated to satisfy government safety requirements and contain some ingredients in subtherapeutic quantities for some individuals. In addition, some mixtures contain more than one ingredient in a pharmacologic group and each such component is generally present in subtherapeutic quantities. It appears doubtful that a combination of two half-doses, for example, are more effective or even as effective as a full dose of a single ingredient from a given pharmacologic group. On the other hand, if a patient suffers from multiple symptoms, particularly during the early stages of a cold, use of a mixture provides a convenient and possibly less expensive means of relieving symptoms than use of several single-entity products.

Whatever the balance of shortcomings and advantages, cold remedy mixtures are widely used and enjoy a certain amount of endorsement by both the medical profession and the laity. A physician who prescribes a cold remedy should be certain that the ingredients are appropriate for the type and severity of symptoms being treated.

Drugs affording symptomatic relief of the discomforts of colds include nasal decongestants (both topical and oral preparations), analgesics, and antitussives and expectorants (see Chapters 29, Nasal Decongestants; 6, General Analgesics; and 31, Agents Used to Treat Cough).

Nasal decongestants relieve nasal stuffiness in the common cold and also may maintain patency of the eustachian tubes and sinus ostia, thereby inhibiting the development of secondary infections (eg, otitis media, sinusitis). The topical sprays provide the greatest symptomatic relief and have a lower incidence of side effects than systemic preparations except for rebound congestion. Use of topical decongestants should be limited to three to five days days to avoid this side effect, and preference should be given to those preparations that produce minimal rebound. Topical preparations of complex formulations containing decongestants plus other drugs such as antihistamines offer no advantage over the single-entity decongestant (see Chapter 29). Oral formulations are less effective but longer acting than topical preparations.

Side effects with systemic administration are due to the sympathomimetic properties of these drugs and include nervousness, dizziness, and insomnia. At the dosages employed for treatment of colds, the incidence of untoward effects is low. However, caution is advised if drugs with sympathomimetic activity are used in patients with hypertension, ischemic heart disease, or hyperthyroidism; in those taking monoamine oxidase inhibitors; and possibly in those with brittle diabetes in whom increased levels of blood sugar caused by glycogenolysis may present a problem.

Antihistamines also are used, although release of histamine is probably not a significant factor in producing cold symptoms. The effect of these agents in counteracting rhinorrhea is probably due to their anticholinergic properties, and, therefore, is similar to the action of atropine and its derivatives. The efficacy of both types of agents in the common cold is not completely agreed upon. Antihistamines are most useful in colds aggravated by an allergic component. Their drying effect is considered a disadvantage in patients with bronchial asthma or infectious bronchitis in which thinning and liquefaction of bronchial secretions are desirable. For these patients, a preparation without antihistamines should be chosen.

Caffeine is present in some cold preparations, but there is no evidence that it counteracts antihistamine-induced drowsiness. If a decongestant also is present in the formulation, the additional cardiac stimulation provided by caffeine may be undesirable in some patients.

See the Table for a listing of cold remedy products most commonly used.

Since so many cold sufferers are children, it would be useful to have general pediatric dosage guidelines. An FDA Advisory Panel has tentatively recommended

COMPOSITION OF COLD REMEDY PREPARATIONS

Preparation	Decongestant (mg) †	Antihistamine (mg) †	Analgesic (mg) †	Miscellaneous (mg) †
Actifed (Burroughs Wellcome): tablets, syrup	pseudoephedrine HCl 60 mg (tablet), 30 mg (syrup)	triprolidine HCl 2.5 mg (tablet), 1.25 mg (syrup)		sodium benzoate 0.1% methylparaben 0.1%
*Allerest (Pharmacraft): tablets	phenyl-propanolamine HCl 18.7 mg	chlorpheniramine maleate 2 mg		
Comhist LA (Baylor): capsules (timed-release)	phenylephrine HCl 20 mg	phenindamine tartrate 10 mg chlorpheniramine maleate 4 mg		hyoscyamine sulfate 0.1296 mg atropine sulfate 0.0242 mg scopolamine hydrobromide 0.0081 mg
*Contac (Menley & James): capsules (timed-release)	phenyl-propanolamine HCl 50 mg	chlorpheniramine maleate 4 mg		belladonna alkaloids 0.2 mg
*Coricidin (Schering): tablets		chlorpheniramine maleate 0.5, 2 mg	aspirin 80, 325 mg	
*Co-Tylenol (McNeil): tablets	pseudoephedrine HCl 30 mg	chlorpheniramine maleate 2 mg	acetaminophen 325 mg	
Deconamine (Berlex): tablets, elixir, capsules (timed-release)	pseudoephedrine HCl 60 mg (tablet), 30 mg (elixir), 120 mg (capsule)	chlorpheniramine maleate 4 mg (tablet), 2 mg (elixir), 8 mg (capsule)		alcohol 15% (elixir)
Dehist (O'Neal, Jones & Feldman): capsules	phenylephrine HCl 15 mg phenylpropanol-amine HCl 30 mg	chlorpheniramine maleate 8 mg		
*Demazin (Schering): tablets (timed-release), syrup	phenylephrine 10 mg (tablet) phenylephrine HCl 2.5 mg (syrup)	chlorpheniramine maleate 2 mg (tablet), 1 mg (syrup)		alcohol 7.5% (syrup)
Dimetapp (Robins): elixir, tablets (timed-release)	phenylephrine HCl 5 mg (elixir), 15 mg (tablet) phenylpropanol-amine HCl 5 mg (elixir), 15 mg (tablet)	brompheniramine maleate 4 mg (elixir), 12 mg (tablet)		alcohol 2.3% (elixir)
Disophrol (Schering): tablets	pseudoephedrine sulfate 60 mg	dexbrom-pheniramine maleate 2 mg		
*Dristan (Whitehall): capsules (timed-release)	phenylephrine HCl 20 mg	chlorpheniramine maleate 4 mg		

COMPOSITION OF COLD REMEDY PREPARATIONS

Preparation	Decongestant (mg) †	Antihistamine (mg) †	Analgesic (mg) †	Miscellaneous (mg) †
Drixoral (Schering): tablets (timed-release)	pseudoephedrine sulfate 120 mg	dexbrom-pheniramine maleate 6 mg		
Endal (UAD): liquid	phenylpro-panolamine HCl 5 mg phenylephrine HCl 5 mg	chlorpheniramine maleate 2 mg	codeine phosphate 10 mg	guaifenesin 100 mg alcohol 5%
Entex (Baylor): capsules, liquid	phenylephrine HCl 5 mg (capsule, liquid) phenylpro-panolamine HCl 45 mg (capsule), 20 mg (liquid)			guaifenesin 200 mg (capsule), 100 mg (liquid) alcohol 5% (liquid)
*Fiogesic (Sandoz): tablets	phenylpro-panolamine HCl 25 mg	pheniramine maleate 12.5 mg pyrilamine maleate 12.5 mg	calcium carbaspirin 382 mg (equivalent to 300 mg aspirin)	
Hista-Derfule (O'Neal, Jones & Feldman): capsules		chlorpheniramine maleate 2 mg	phenacetin 100 mg salicylamide 130 mg powdered opium 2 mg	atropine sulfate 0.13 mg
Histalet (Reid-Provident): syrup	pseudoephedrine HCl 45 mg	chlorpheniramine maleate 3 mg		
Isoclor (Arnar-Stone): tablets, liquid, capsules (timed-release)	pseudoephedrine HCl 60 mg (tablet), 25 mg (liquid), 120 mg (capsule)	chlorpheniramine maleate 4 mg (tablet), 2 mg (liquid), 8 mg (capsule)		
Naldecon (Bristol): syrup, tablets (timed-release)	phenylpro-panolamine HCl 40 mg (tablet), 20 mg (syrup) phenylephrine HCl 10 mg (tablet), 5 mg (syrup)	phenyltoloxamine citrate 15 mg (tablet), 7.5 mg (syrup) chlorpheniramine maleate 5 mg (tablet), 2.5 mg (syrup)		
Novafed (Dow): capsules (timed-release), *liquid	pseudoephedrine HCl 120 mg (capsule), 30 mg (liquid)			alcohol 7.5% (liquid)
Novafed A (Dow): capsules, (timed-release),*liquid	pseudoephedrine HCl 120 mg (capsule), 30 mg (liquid)	chlorpheniramine maleate 8 mg (capsule), 2 mg (liquid)		alcohol 5% (liquid)

COMPOSITION OF COLD REMEDY PREPARATIONS

Preparation	Decongestant (mg) †	Antihistamine (mg) †	Analgesic (mg) †	Miscellaneous (mg) †
Novahistine Elixir (Dow): elixir	phenylpro-panolamine 18.5 mg	chlorpheniramine maleate 2 mg		alcohol 5%
*Novahistine LP (Dow): tablets	phenylephrine HCl 20 mg	chlorpheniramine maleate 4 mg		
Ornade (Smith Kline & French): capsules (timed-release)	phenylpro-panolamine HCl 50 mg	chlorpheniramine maleate 8 mg		isopropamide iodine equivalent to iso-propamide 2.5 mg
Phenergan Compound (Wyeth): tablets	pseudoephedrine HCl 60 mg	promethazine HCl 6.25 mg	aspirin 600 mg	
Phenergan D (Wyeth): tablets	pseudoephedrine HCl 60 mg	promethazine HCl 6.25 mg		
*Propadrine (Merck Sharp & Dohme): capsules, elixir	phenylpro-panolamine HCl 25, 50 mg (capsule), 20 mg (elixir)			alcohol 16% (elixir)
*Pyrroxate (Upjohn): tablets, capsules		chlorpheniramine maleate 2 mg	phenacetin 150 mg aspirin 210 mg	methoxyphenamine HCl 25 mg caffeine 30 mg
*Rondec (Ross): drops, syrup, tablets	pseudoephedrine HCl 25 mg/ml (drops), 60 mg (syrup, tablet)	carbinoxamine maleate 2 mg/ml (drops), 4 mg (syrup, tablet)		
Rynatan (Mallinckrodt): tablets	phenylephrine tannate 25 mg	chlorpheniramine tannate 8 mg pyrilamine tannate 25 mg		
Singlet (Dow): tablets (timed-release)	phenylephrine HCl 40 mg	chlorpheniramine maleate 8 mg	acetaminophen 500 mg	
Sinubid (Parke, Davis): tablets	phenylpro-panolamine HCl 100 mg	phenyltoloxamine citrate 66 mg	acetaminophen 300 mg phenacetin 300 mg	
*Sinutab (Parke, Davis): tablets	phenylpro-panolamine HCl 25 mg	phenyltoloxamine citrate 22 mg	acetaminophen 325 mg	
*Sudafed (Burroughs Wellcome): tablets, syrup	pseudoephedrine HCl 30, 60 mg (tablets), 30 mg (syrup)			
*Triaminic Syrup (Dorsey): syrup	phenylpro-panolamine HCl 12.5 mg	pheniramine maleate 6.25 mg pyrilamine maleate 6.25 mg		

COMPOSITION OF COLD REMEDY PREPARATIONS

Preparation	Decongestant (mg) †	Antihistamine (mg) †	Analgesic (mg) †	Miscellaneous (mg) †
Triaminic Oral Infant Drops (Dorsey): drops	phenylpro-panolamine HCl 20 mg/ml	pheniramine maleate 10 mg/ml pyrilamine maleate 10 mg/ml		
Triaminic Tablets (Dorsey): tablets (timed-release)	phenylpro-panolamine HCl 50 mg	pheniramine maleate 25 mg pyrilamine maleate 25 mg		

*Nonprescription
†Milligrams in solid dosage form or 5 ml of liquid (except drops)

such dosages for products with a relatively wide margin of safety: for children 6 to 12 years old, one-half the adult dosage; 2 to 6 years, one-fourth the adult dosage; children under 2 years, dosage to be determined by the physician.

Vitamin C: Claims have been made that large doses of vitamin C prevent or cure the common cold. Numerous experiments (some poorly designed or executed) have been performed to determine the relationship between ingestion of megadoses of vitamin C and the occurrence, duration, and severity of cold symptoms. Results and interpretation of these studies have generally been controversial. One series of well-controlled experiments yielded results that were consistently positive, although unspectacular: Vitamin C, taken prophylactically and therapeutically during the symptomatic phase, decreased the number of days spent at home because of disability due to colds by 25% to 30%, but nasal symptoms per se were not relieved (Anderson, 1975). Of interest is the fact that the dosages utilized to attain this effect (500 mg weekly prophylactically; 1 g daily for symptoms) were far below those previously recommended by some promoters of this therapy. Although the body utilizes vitamin C more rapidly during illness, it is not known if this phenomenon serves an important function or is unassociated with repair of the disease process. Therefore, it is not known if maintenance of saturated tissue levels with supplemental doses of vitamin C during illness is beneficial. Any conclusions at this time must be conservative. The effect of vitamin C in decreasing general morbidity during the common cold appears to be minimal, and a population subgroup that is more clearly benefited has yet to be identified. Furthermore, there is insufficient data on the incidence and severity of adverse effects associated with various dosages of vitamin C to be assured that such therapy is entirely without risk.

Selected References

Establishment of a monograph for OTC cold, cough, allergy, bronchodilator and antiasthmatic products. *Federal Register* 41:38312-38424, (Sept 9) 1976.

Anderson TW, et al: Winter illness and vitamin C: Effect of relatively low doses. *Can Med Assoc J* 112:823-826, 1975

Cormier JF, Bryant BG: Cold and allergy products, in *Handbook of Nonprescription Drugs*, ed 5. American Pharmaceutical Association, Washington, DC, 1977, 77-111.

Dykes MHM, Meier P: Ascorbic acid and common cold: Evaluation of its efficacy and toxicity. *JAMA* 231:1073-1079, 1975.

Agents Used to Treat Cough | 31

Cough is a protective physiologic reflex action that clears the respiratory tract of secretions and foreign materials. Although it is a symptom associated with a number of diseases of varied etiology, antitussive therapy is not invariably required. In certain diseases (eg, asthma, chronic bronchitis, cystic fibrosis), coughing maintains an open airway by removing excessive secretions from respiratory passages and, therefore, should not be suppressed indiscriminately.

The most common cause of acute cough in adults and children is a viral upper respiratory infection, "common cold" or "flu." Postnasal drip of mucus stimulates receptors in the pharynx and precipitates cough that is usually transient and self-limiting. Smoking is the most commonly implicated cause of chronic cough. The most common cause of persistent cough in nonsmokers is a chronic postnasal drip, which occurs in association with vasomotor or allergic rhinitis, chronic sinusitis, and obstruction of the nasopharynx by enlarged adenoids.

Other causes of cough include inhalation of allergens or other environmental irritants, aspiration resulting from pharyngeal or gastrointestinal disorders, pulmonary edema, certain infectious diseases, tumors of the trachea or bronchi, and conditions involving the external auditory canal (eg, impacted cerumen, irritation of eardrum by hairs).

Before initiating antitussive therapy, it is important that the cause of the cough should be determined and specific therapy for the underlying disorder employed. The elimination or treatment of the underlying condition often improves the cough. For example, a large percentage of persons who stop smoking report disappearance of or a decrease in coughing; use of antihistamines and/or decongestants improves postnasal drip associated with allergic rhinitis or the common cold, thereby relieving the cough; and bronchodilator therapy may alleviate cough in asthmatic patients or in those in whom bronchospasm follows a viral infection of the lower respiratory tract.

When it is not possible to determine or treat the cause of cough or when coughing does not perform a useful function and may be harmful, symptomatic therapy should be considered. Cough arising from irritation of the pharyngeal mucosa sometimes can be managed temporarily with demulcents (eg, syrups, lozenges) and locally acting sialogogues (eg, hard candy, cough drops). If the cough is nonproductive, an agent that increases the quantity of respiratory tract fluid (expectorant) or decreases its viscosity (mucolytic) may be helpful. Severe nonproductive cough requires treatment with an antitussive. Although antitussive therapy has no direct effect on the underlying disease, it permits rest, facilitates sleep, and reduces the respiratory tract irritation that tends to make cough self-perpetuating.

ANTITUSSIVES

The antitussives are usually classified as centrally or peripherally acting, depending on whether they act on the medullary cough center or at the site of irritation. The centrally acting group includes the opium derivatives (narcotics) (eg, codeine, hydrocodone) and the nonopiate (non-narcotic) agent, dextromethorphan. The peripherally acting group includes agents with local anesthetic or analgesic activities as well as the demulcents. These drugs act on nerve receptors within the respiratory tract. Although local anesthetics applied to the mucous membranes of the respiratory tract suppress cough, their use is impractical for general treatment of cough. The local anesthetic activity of some antitussive agents is claimed to be the basis of their antitussive effect, but this property does not contribute significantly to suppression of cough. The antitussive efficacy of the peripherally acting drugs has not been definitely established.

Because of the difficulties of determining the clinical efficacy of antitussives, reports on the effectiveness of various agents frequently conflict. Most evaluations of single-entity antitussive drugs are based on subjective rather than objective methods, and the placebo effect undoubtedly is an important factor influencing evaluation in subjective studies, particularly in self-limiting conditions. Results of studies on patients with chronic cough may not be applicable to those with acute cough, which improves rapidly and spontaneously, and studies of cough suppression in animals or of experimentally induced cough in man do not adequately predict such activity in pathologic cough treated clinically.

Results of experimental and clinical studies, as well as many years of experience, have shown that codeine is the most useful antitussive in the treatment of acute and chronic cough associated with a wide variety of disease states. The related agent, hydrocodone, is also effective and is more potent than codeine on a milligram basis, but it has a greater dependence liability. All opiate analgesics probably have antitussive activity, although the available evidence of their efficacy is limited. Because they may produce more adverse reactions and have a greater dependence liability than codeine, they are seldom used as general antitussives but are reserved for conditions in which cough is associated with pain, anxiety, and restlessness.

Among the nonopiate agents, dextromethorphan has been shown to be effective in alleviating both experimental and pathologic cough; it has had more extensive study and clinical use than other compounds in this group. In a limited number of studies, benzonatate [Tessalon] appeared to be less effective than codeine. Caramiphen edisylate was found to be effective in some controlled objective studies, but additional studies are needed to establish its efficacy; it is available only in combination products. Although a number of other agents, including noscapine [Tusscapine], levopropoxyphene napsylate [Novrad], pipazethate, chlophedianol [Ulo], and carbetapentane citrate, also have been shown to be effective in some studies, evidence is insufficient to determine their relative efficacy conclusively.

Some antihistamines (eg, diphenhydramine [Benylin]) have been shown to have antitussive activity. The mechanism of this action is not known, but it may be related partly to their sedative effect. Promethazine, a phenothiazine antihistamine, is widely used in combination products for cough, but whether it has a specific antitussive action alone is not known. The antihistamines also have anticholinergic activity, which produces a drying effect on tracheobronchial secretions, an action that may be undesirable in patients who are producing mucus that should be eliminated from the bronchial tree.

EXPECTORANTS AND MUCOLYTICS

Expectorants are used to stimulate the flow of respiratory tract secretions, and mucolytics are used to reduce the viscosity of respiratory tract fluid. Either action allows ciliary motion and coughing to move the loosened material toward the pharynx more easily.

Expectorants: Theoretically, expectorants would be most useful in irritative, nonproductive cough associated with a small amount of secretion. Increasing the amount of secretions facilitates removal of irritants, and it has been claimed that this also may exert a demulcent effect on the irritated airway mucosa, thereby diminishing the tendency to cough. The use of expectorants is based primarily on tradition and the widespread subjective clinical impression that they are effective. Although there is limited experimental evidence to indicate that these drugs affect the amount of respiratory tract fluid secreted, this evidence is unconvincing; thus, the therapeutic efficacy of these agents is doubtful.

Of the many agents used and promoted over the years for their expectorant action, guaifenesin [Robitussin, 2/G] is currently the most widely used. Many experimental and clinical studies have been conducted with this agent and, although the results of some have shown that the drug is effective, other studies have not confirmed these results; thus, conclusive evidence of its efficacy as an expectorant is still lacking.

Of the other commonly used expectorants, the iodides have been reported to be effective when given in adequate dosage in some chronic respiratory diseases, but there is no evidence of their efficacy in acute upper respiratory infection. Use of the iodides is frequently associated with a high incidence of adverse effects, including rashes and even hypothyroidism.

The available evidence on the usefulness of other agents (eg, ammonium chloride, ipecac, guaiacolsulfonate potassium, terpin hydrate) is insufficient to warrant their use as expectorants.

Mucolytics: When secretions are tenacious, the liquefying action of a mucolytic agent may make the secretions easier to eliminate. Acetylcysteine [Mucomyst] reduces the viscosity of some types of mucus, probably by depolymerizing mucopolysaccharides. This agent may be useful in acute or chronic bronchopulmonary diseases and the respiratory complications of cystic fibrosis.

Although the demulcent effect of water may tend to suppress cough produced by upper respiratory tract disorders, the usefulness of hydration is controversial. The oral intake of large amounts of water has been promoted by some clinicians, but it has not been proved conclusively that this has an effect on the volume or viscosity of respiratory tract fluid. The results of some studies have shown that it is not possible by existing means (eg, ultrasonic nebulizer) to deliver enough water by inhalation of aerosols to the lower respiratory tract to affect the secretions.

Adverse Reactions and Precautions

Regardless of the drugs used to treat cough, it should be kept in mind that the primary goal is to treat and eliminate the cause of the cough. Adverse reactions produced by antitussives or expectorants occur infrequently, are generally mild, and usually subside promptly when the drugs are discontinued. Caution is indicated when antitussives are used in sedated or debilitated patients. The cough reflex should not be severely obtunded in patients with productive cough; for example, coughs in infants and children are usually productive. Although serious reactions (eg, depressed respiration, excessive sleepiness) occur only rarely with usual doses of opiate-containing preparations in children under 5 years of age, numerous cases of poisonings and some deaths following ingestion of larger doses have been reported. Therefore, particular care should be taken not to overuse antitussives in this group of patients. Failure to recognize that cough is suppressed by drugs administered after surgery to relieve pain may lead to retention of secretions with bronchial obstruction and atelectasis. Cough and clearing of the respiratory passages are important therapeutically in preventing or reversing the development of atelectasis and pneumonitis. Antitussives should not be used in the acute phase of pertussis or bronchial asthma, as inspissation of mucous plugs may contribute to a fatal outcome.

ANTITUSSIVES

Opiates

CODEINE

CODEINE PHOSPHATE

CODEINE SULFATE

Codeine is considered to be the most useful narcotic antitussive agent and is the drug of choice for treating cough associated with various diseases.

Antitussive doses are generally well tolerated. Nausea, vomiting, constipation, dizziness, palpitations, drowsiness, pruritus, and, rarely, hyperhidrosis and agitation have been reported.

The dependence liability of codeine is considerably less than that of morphine,

although cough syrups containing codeine are misused by drug abusers. Codeine is classified as a Schedule II drug under the Controlled Substances Act. Dependence and ventilatory depression are uncommon because antitussive use is short term and doses are smaller than those given for analgesia. As with other narcotic analgesics, ventilatory depression occurs with overdosage, particularly in children; thus, codeine and codeine-containing preparations should be used with caution in children, especially those under 5 years of age. The depression can be reversed by administering the opiate antagonist, naloxone (see Chapter 86, Specific Antidotes).

ROUTE, USUAL DOSAGE, AND PREPARATIONS. *Oral*: *Adults*, 10 to 20 mg every four to six hours (maximum, 120 mg/24 hrs), as necessary. *Children*, 1 mg/kg of body weight daily divided into four doses (maximum, 60 mg/day). Alternatively, for *children 6 to 12 years*, 5 to 10 mg every four to six hours (maximum, 60 mg/day); *2 to 6 years*, 2.5 to 5 mg every four to six hours (maximum, 30 mg/day).

Base and salts available generically: Powder (base); tablets 30 and 60 mg (phosphate); tablets 15, 30, and 60 mg (sulfate).
See the section on Mixtures for a listing of combination products containing codeine.

HYDROCODONE BITARTRATE
[Codone, Dicodid]

The usefulness of hydrocodone as a narcotic antitussive is similar to that of codeine, and its antitussive potency is approximately three times greater on a milligram basis.

The dependence liability of hydrocodone is greater than that of codeine. This antitussive is classified as a Schedule II drug under the Controlled Substances Act.

The most common adverse reactions are nausea, dizziness, and constipation. Dryness of the pharynx and occasional tightness of the chest have been reported. Other adverse reactions and precautions are the same as those reported for codeine.

ROUTE, USUAL DOSAGE, AND PREPARATIONS. *Oral: Adults*, 5 to 10 mg three or four times daily. *Children*, 0.6 mg/kg of body weight daily in three or four divided doses.

> Drug available generically: Crystals.
> *Codone* (Lemmon), *Dicodid* (Knoll). Tablets 5 mg.
> See the section on Mixtures for a listing of combination products containing hydrocodone.

Nonopiates

DEXTROMETHORPHAN HYDROBROMIDE

Results of clinical studies have shown that dextromethorphan is an effective cough suppressant. Like codeine, its action is mediated centrally by inhibiting incoming cough stimuli. Dextromethorphan is the dextro isomer of the methyl ether of the analgesic, levorphanol but, unlike the latter, it has no dependence liability or analgesic effects.

Adverse reactions are mild and occur infrequently; they include slight drowsiness, nausea, and dizziness. Respiratory depression may occur with very large doses, but no fatalities have been reported.

ROUTE, USUAL DOSAGE, AND PREPARATIONS. *Oral: Adults*, 10 to 20 mg every four hours or 30 mg every six to eight hours (maximum, 120 mg/day). *Children*, 1 mg/kg of body weight daily in three or four divided doses. Alternatively, *children 6 to 12 years*, 5 to 10 mg every four hours or 15 mg every six to eight hours (maximum, 60

mg/24 hrs); *2 to 6 years*, 2.5 to 5 mg every four hours or 7.5 mg every six to eight hours (maximum, 30 mg/day).

> Drug available generically: Powder.
> See the section on Mixtures for a listing of combination products containing dextromethorphan.

DIPHENHYDRAMINE HYDROCHLORIDE
[Benylin]

Experimental and clinical studies have shown that this antihistamine is an effective antitussive but, in comparative studies, it was reported to be less active than codeine.

The most common adverse reaction is drowsiness; patients should be cautioned to avoid driving a motor vehicle or operating heavy machinery while taking the drug. Diphenhydramine also has an undesirable drying effect on a productive cough that may interfere with expectoration by making secretions thicker.

ROUTE, USUAL DOSAGE, AND PREPARATIONS. *Oral: Adults*, 25 mg every four hours (maximum, 100 mg/24 hrs). *Children 2 to 5 years*, 6.25 mg every four hours (maximum, 25 mg/24 hrs); *6 to 12 years*, 12.5 mg every four hours (maximum, 50 mg/24 hrs).

> Drug available generically: Elixir, expectorant, syrup.
> *Benylin* (Parke, Davis). Syrup 12.5 mg/5 ml with alcohol 5%.

BENZONATATE
[Tessalon]

Benzonatate, which is chemically related to the local anesthetic, tetracaine, appears to be less effective than codeine in suppressing cough. It is claimed to exert a peripheral action on the stretch receptors of the respiratory mucosa.

Adverse reactions are mild and include rash, constipation, nasal congestion, slight vertigo, headache, nausea, drowsiness, hypersensitivity reactions, and a vague "chilly" sensation. It has a topical anesthetic effect and produces numbness of the mouth, tongue, and pharynx if the capsules are chewed.

ROUTE, USUAL DOSAGE, AND PREPARATIONS.
Oral: Adults and children over 10 years, 100 mg three to six times daily; *under 10 years,* 8 mg/kg of body weight daily in three to six divided doses.

> *Tessalon* (Endo). Capsules (liquid-filled) 100 mg.

EXPECTORANTS

GUAIFENESIN (Glyceryl Guaiacolate)
[Robitussin, 2/G]

$$OCH_2CHCH_2OH$$
$$OH$$
$$OCH_3$$

Results of subjective clinical studies suggest that the expectorant action of guaifenesin ameliorates dry, unproductive cough; however, results of other studies utilizing objective methods have been conflicting and the reports of beneficial actions have not been confirmed. In experimental studies, guaifenesin increased respiratory tract secretions in animals only when given in doses larger than those used clinically. Thus, the efficacy of this drug has not been conclusively established and, therefore, no dosage information is given.

Nausea and drowsiness may occur rarely. Guaifenesin may produce a false-positive response for urinary 5-hydroxyindoleacetic acid (5-HIAA) and vanillylmandelic acid (VMA).

> Drug available generically under names Guaifenesin and Glyceryl Guaiacolate: Syrup 100 mg/5 ml.

> *Robitussin* (Robins), *2/G* (Dow). Syrup 100 mg/5 ml with alcohol 3.5% (nonprescription). See the section on Mixtures for a listing of combination products containing guaifenesin.

MUCOLYTIC

ACETYLCYSTEINE
[Mucomyst]

$$HSCH_2CHCOH$$
$$O$$
$$NHCCH_3$$
$$O$$

This drug reduces the viscosity of some forms of mucus in vitro. Clinical effectiveness is difficult to assess, but subjective reports and a few controlled studies indicate that acetylcysteine, given by nebulization as an adjunct to other therapy, may be beneficial in reducing the viscosity of abnormal pulmonary secretions in patients with acute or chronic bronchopulmonary diseases or pulmonary complications of cystic fibrosis. The drug also may be instilled directly into the trachea in patients with tracheostomies. This method of administration can be more effective than nebulization. For use of acetylcysteine as an antidote in acetaminophen poisoning, see Chapter 86, Specific Antidotes.

Adverse reactions are uncommon. Production of excessive secretions which require removal by suction (especially when the drug is instilled directly into the trachea) has been reported. For this reason, acetylcysteine should not be used unless suction apparatus is available. Bronchospasm also has been observed, especially in asthmatic patients; it occurs less frequently with the 10% solution than with the 20% concentration. Nausea, vomiting, stomatitis, rhinorrhea, and hemoptysis occur occasionally, and cases of probable sensitization have been reported rarely. Elderly and debilitated patients should be observed closely to avoid aspiration of excessive secretions. Acetylcysteine has an unpleasant odor that may cause gastrointestinal disturbances.

ROUTE, USUAL DOSAGE, AND PREPARATIONS.
Open vials should be covered, refrigerated,
and used within 96 hours.
Inhalation (nebulization): 2 to 20 ml of a
10% solution or 1 to 10 ml of a 20% solution
nebulized into a face mask or mouthpiece
every two to six hours. Since the solution
tends to concentrate, it should be diluted
with sterile water when three-fourths of the
original volume has been used.
Inhalation (instillation): 1 to 2 ml of a
10% to 20% solution instilled into the
trachea by tracheostomy or bronchoscope
as often as every hour.

> *Mucomyst* (Mead Johnson). Solution (sterile)
> 10% and 20% in 4, 10, and 30 ml containers.

MIXTURES

Many antitussive preparations listed in
this section appear to have been formulated primarily for symptomatic treatment
of minor respiratory disorders rather than
for specific relief of cough. In addition to an
antitussive and one or more ingredients
classified as expectorants, most of these
combination products contain one or more
adrenergic agents (bronchodilators or nasal
decongestants) and antihistamines. The effectiveness of these mixtures in comparison to the efficacy of single-entity preparations is not known.

Although it is recognized that it is generally preferable to use single-entity preparations, some patients with cough will have
concurrent symptoms, such as those associated with the common cold, for which
certain combination products may be useful and convenient. If a mixture is selected
for use, it should meet the following
criteria: (1) that not more than three active
ingredients from different pharmacologic
groups be present; (2) that each active
ingredient be present in an effective and
safe concentration and contribute to the
treatment for which the product is indicated; (3) that such products be used only
when multiple symptoms are present concurrently; (4) that the mixture be therapeutically rational for the type and severity of
symptoms being treated; and (5) that the

possible adverse reactions of the components be taken into consideration.

The following list of commonly used
preparations is for information only; inclusion in the list does not indicate approval or
recommendation for use:

Antitussive Mixtures Containing Codeine
(All Schedule V Preparations)

Actifed-C Expectorant (Burroughs Wellcome).
Each 5 ml contains codeine phosphate 10 mg,
guaifenesin 100 mg, pseudoephedrine hydrochloride 30 mg, and triprolidine hydrochloride
2 mg.

Ambenyl Expectorant (Marion). Each 5 ml of
liquid contains codeine sulfate 10 mg, ammonium chloride 80 mg, bromodiphenhydramine hydrochloride 3.75 mg, diphenhydramine hydrochloride 8.75 mg, guaiacolsulfonate potassium 80 mg, menthol 0.5 mg, and
alcohol 5%.

Calcidrine (Abbott). Each 5 ml of syrup contains codeine 8.4 mg, calcium iodide anhydrous
152 mg, and alcohol 6%.

Cerose (Ives). Each 5 ml contains codeine
phosphate 10 mg, pheniramine tartrate 10 mg,
phenylephrine hydrochloride 5 mg, potassium
guaiacolsulfonate 87 mg, sodium citrate 195
mg, citric acid 60 mg, and alcohol 2.5%.

Colrex Compound [sugar free] (Rowell). Each
capsule contains codeine phosphate 16 mg,
acetaminophen 325 mg, phenylephrine hydrochloride 10 mg, and chlorpheniramine maleate
2 mg; each 5 ml of elixir contains codeine
phosphate 8 mg, acetaminophen 120 mg, chlorpheniramine maleate 1 mg, phenylephrine
hydrochloride 5 mg, and alcohol 9.5%.

Dimetane Expectorant-DC (Robins). Each 5
ml contains codeine phosphate 10 mg, brompheniramine maleate 2 mg, guaifenesin 100
mg, phenylephrine hydrochloride 5 mg,
phenylpropanolamine hydrochloride 5 mg, and
alcohol 3.5%.

Histadyl E.C. (Lilly). Each 30 ml of syrup
contains codeine phosphate 60 mg, ammonium
chloride 660 mg, ephedrine hydrochloride 30
mg, methapyrilene fumarate 81 mg, menthol
3.9 mg, and alcohol 5%.

Isoclor Expectorant (Arnar-Stone). Each 5 ml
contains codeine phosphate 10 mg, guaifenesin
100 mg, pseudoephedrine hydrochloride 30
mg, and alcohol 5%.

Novahistine Expectorant (Dow). Each 5 ml
contains codeine phosphate 10 mg, guaifenesin
100 mg, phenylpropanolamine hydrochloride
18.75 mg, and alcohol 7.5%.

Novahistine-DH (Dow). Each 5 ml of liquid
contains codeine phosphate 10 mg, chlor-

pheniramine maleate 2 mg, phenylpropanolamine hydrochloride 18.75 mg, and alcohol 5%.

Nucofed (Beecham). Each capsule or 5 ml of syrup contains codeine phosphate 20 mg and pseudoephedrine hydrochloride 60 mg.

Pediacof (Breon). Each 5 ml of syrup contains codeine phosphate 5 mg, chlorpheniramine maleate 0.75 mg, phenylephrine hydrochloride 2.5 mg, potassium iodide 75 mg, and alcohol 5%.

Phenergan Expectorant W/Codeine (Wyeth). Each 5 ml of expectorant contains codeine phosphate 10 mg, promethazine hydrochloride 5 mg, ipecac fluidextract 0.01 ml, guaiacolsulfonate potassium 44 mg, citric acid anhydrous 60 mg, sodium citrate 197 mg, and alcohol 7%.

Phenergan-VC W/Codeine (Wyeth). Each 5 ml of expectorant contains same formulation as Phenergan W/Codeine plus phenylephrine hydrochloride 5 mg.

Robitussin A-C (Robins). Each 5 ml of syrup contains codeine phosphate 10 mg, guaifenesin 100 mg, and alcohol 3.5%.

Robitussin-DAC (Robins). Each 5 ml of syrup contains codeine phosphate 10 mg, guaifenesin 100 mg, pseudoephedrine hydrochloride 30 mg, and alcohol 1.4%.

Terpin Hydrate and Codeine Elixir (Various Manufacturers). Codeine, glycerin, and terpin hydrate.

Triaminic Expectorant with Codeine (Dorsey). Each 5 ml contains codeine phosphate 10 mg, guaifenesin 100 mg, phenylpropanolamine hydrochloride 12.5 mg, pheniramine maleate 6.25 mg, pyrilamine maleate 6.25 mg, and alcohol 5%.

Tussar-2, Tussar SF [sugar free] (Armour). Each 5 ml of syrup contains codeine phosphate 10 mg, carbetapentane citrate 7.5 mg, chlorpheniramine maleate 2 mg, guaifenesin 50 mg, sodium citrate 130 mg, citric acid 20 mg, and alcohol 5% (Tussar-2) or 12% (Tussar SF).

Tussi-Organidin Expectorant (Wallace). Each 5 ml contains codeine phosphate 10 mg, chlorpheniramine maleate 2 mg, iodinated glycerol 30 mg, and alcohol 15%.

Antitussive Mixtures Containing Hydrocodone (All Schedule III Preparations)

Hycodan (Endo). Each tablet or 5 ml of syrup contains hydrocodone bitartrate 5 mg and homatropine methylbromide 1.5 mg.

Hycomine (Endo). Each 5 ml of syrup or 10 ml of pediatric syrup contains hydrocodone bitartrate 5 mg and phenylpropanolamine hydrochloride 25 mg.

Hycotuss Expectorant (Endo). Each 5 ml contains hydrocodone bitartrate 5 mg, guaifenesin 100 mg, and alcohol 10%.

Triaminic Expectorant DH (Dorsey). Each 5 ml contains hydrocodone bitartrate 1.67 mg, guaifenesin 100 mg, pheniramine maleate 6.25 mg, phenylpropanolamine hydrochloride 12.5 mg, pyrilamine maleate 6.25 mg, and alcohol 5%.

Tussend (Dow). Each tablet or 5 ml of liquid contains hydrocodone bitartrate 5 mg, pseudoephedrine hydrochloride 60 mg, and (in liquid) alcohol 5%.

Tussend Expectorant (Dow). Each 5 ml of liquid contains same formulation as Tussend plus guaifenesin 200 mg and alcohol 12.5%.

Tussionex (Pennwalt). Each capsule, tablet, or 5 ml of suspension contains hydrocodone 5 mg and phenyltoloxamine 10 mg as cationic exchange resin complexes.

Antitussive Mixtures Containing Dextromethorphan

Cerose Compound (Ives). Each capsule contains dextromethorphan hydrobromide 10 mg, chlorpheniramine maleate 2 mg, phenylephrine hydrochloride 7.5 mg, terpin hydrate 64.8 mg, acetaminophen 194 mg, and ascorbic acid 25 mg.

Cheracol D Cough Syrup (Upjohn). Each 5 ml of syrup contains dextromethorphan hydrobromide 10 mg, guaifenesin 15 mg, and alcohol 3% (nonprescription).

Dimacol (Robins). Each capsule or 5 ml of liquid contains dextromethorphan hydrobromide 15 mg, pseudoephedrine hydrochloride 30 mg, guaifenesin 100 mg, and (in liquid) alcohol 4.75% (nonprescription).

Dorcol Pediatric Cough Syrup (Dorsey). Each 5 ml of syrup contains dextromethorphan hydrobromide 7.5 mg, guaifenesin 37.5 mg, phenylpropanolamine hydrochloride 8.75 mg, and alcohol 5% (nonprescription).

Novahistine DMX (Dow). Each 5 ml contains dextromethorphan hydrobromide 10 mg, pseudoephedrine hydrochloride 30 mg, guaifenesin 100 mg, and alcohol 10% (nonprescription).

Phenergan Pediatric Expectorant (Wyeth). Each 5 ml contains dextromethorphan hydrobromide 7.5 mg, promethazine hydrochloride 5 mg, ipecac fluidextract 0.01 ml, guaiacolsulfonate potassium 44 mg, citric acid anhydrous 60 mg, and sodium citrate 197 mg.

Robitussin-CF (Robins). Each 5 ml of liquid contains dextromethorphan hydrobromide 10 mg, guaifenesin 100 mg, phenylpropanolamine hydrochloride 12.5 mg, and alcohol 4.75% (nonprescription).

Robitussin-DM (Robins). Each 5 ml of syrup contains dextromorphan hydrobromide 15 mg, guaifenesin 100 mg, and alcohol 1.4%; each lozenge contains dextromethorphan 7.5 mg and guaifenesin 50 mg (nonprescription).

Rondec-DM (Ross). Each 5 ml of syrup contains dextromethorphan hydrobromide 15 mg, carbinoxamine maleate 4 mg, pseudoephedrine hydrochloride 60 mg, and alcohol less than 0.6%; each milliliter of drops contains dextromethorphan hydrobromide 4 mg, carbinoxamine maleate 2 mg, pseudoephedrine hydrochloride 25 mg, and alcohol less than 0.6%.

Triaminicol Cough Syrup (Dorsey). Each 5 ml contains dextromethorphan hydrobromide 15 mg, ammonium chloride 90 mg, pheniramine maleate 6.25 mg, phenylpropanolamine hydrochloride 12.5 mg, and pyrilamine maleate 6.25 mg (nonprescription).

Trind-DM (Mead Johnson). Each 5 ml of syrup contains dextromethorphan hydrobromide 7.5 mg, phenylephrine hydrochloride 2.5 mg, guaifenesin 50 mg, acetaminophen 120 mg, and alcohol 15% (nonprescription).

Tussagesic (Dorsey). Each 5 ml of suspension contains dextromethorphan hydrobromide 15 mg, acetaminophen 120 mg, pheniramine maleate 6.25 mg, phenylpropanolamine hydrochloride 12.5 mg, pyrilamine maleate 6.25 mg, and terpin hydrate 90 mg; each timed-release tablet contains dextromethorphan hydrobromide 30 mg, acetaminophen 325 mg, pheniramine maleate 12.5 mg, phenylpropanolamine hydrochloride 25 mg, pyrilamine maleate 12.5 mg, and terpin hydrate 180 mg (nonprescription).

Tussi-Organidin DM (Wallace). Each 5 ml of liquid contains dextromethorphan hydrobromide 10 mg, iodinated glycerol 30 mg, chlorpheniramine maleate 2 mg, and alcohol 15%.

Additional Antitussive Mixtures

Conar Expectorant (Beecham). Each 5 ml contains noscapine 15 mg, guaifenesin 100 mg, and phenylephrine hydrochloride 10 mg (nonprescription).

Conar A (Beecham). Each tablet or 10 ml of suspension contains noscapine 15 mg, acetaminophen 300 mg, guaifenesin 100 mg, and phenylephrine hydrochloride 10 mg (nonprescription).

Rynatuss (Mallinckrodt). Each tablet contains carbetapentane tannate 60 mg, chlorpheniramine tannate 5 mg, ephedrine tannate 10 mg, and phenylephrine tannate 10 mg; each 5 ml of pediatric suspension contains carbetapentane tannate 30 mg, chlorpheniramine tannate 4 mg, ephedrine tannate 5 mg, and phenylephrine tannate 5 mg.

Tuss-Ornade (Smith Kline & French). Each timed-release capsule contains caramiphen edisylate 20 mg, chlorpheniramine maleate 8 mg, isopropamide as the iodide 2.5 mg, and phenylpropanolamine hydrochloride 50 mg; each 5 ml of liquid contains caramiphen edisylate 5 mg, chlorpheniramine maleate 2 mg, isopropamide as the iodide 0.75 mg, phenylpropanolamine hydrochloride 15 mg, and alcohol 7.5%.

Mixtures Containing Guaifenesin or Other Expectorants

(See previous lists for other combination products containing guaifenesin.)

Brexin (Savage). Each capsule contains guaifenesin 100 mg, methapyrilene hydrochloride 30 mg, and pseudoephedrine hydrochloride 60 mg.

Dimetane Expectorant (Robins). Each 5 ml contains guaifenesin 100 mg, brompheniramine maleate 2 mg, phenylephrine hydrochloride 5 mg, phenylpropanolamine hydrochloride 5 mg, and alcohol 3.5%.

Phenergan Expectorant (Wyeth). Each 5 ml contains guaiacolsulfonate potassium 44 mg, promethazine hydrochloride 5 mg, ipecac fluidextract 0.01 ml, citric acid anhydrous 60 mg, sodium citrate 197 mg, and alcohol 7%.

Phenergan VC Expectorant (Wyeth). Each 5 ml contains same formulation as Phenergan Expectorant plus phenylephrine hydrochloride 5 mg.

Polaramine Expectorant (Schering). Each 5 ml contains guaifenesin 100 mg, dextrochlorpheniramine maleate 2 mg, pseudoephedrine maleate 20 mg, and alcohol 7.2%.

Robitussin-PE (Robins). Each 5 ml of liquid contains guaifenesin 100 mg, pseudoephedrine hydrochloride 30 mg, and alcohol 1.4% (nonprescription).

Triaminic Expectorant (Dorsey). Each 5 ml contains guaifenesin 100 mg, pheniramine maleate 6.25 mg, phenylpropanolamine hydrochloride 12.5 mg, pyrilamine maleate 6.25 mg, and alcohol 5% (nonprescription).

Trind (Mead Johnson). Each 5 ml of syrup contains guaifenesin 50 mg, acetaminophen 120 mg, phenylephrine hydrochloride 2.5 mg, and alcohol 15% (nonprescription).

Selected References

Report of the FDA Advisory Review Panel on over-the-counter (OTC) cold, cough, allergy, bronchodilator, and antiasthmatic products. *Federal Register* 41:38312-38424, (Sept 9) 1976.

Eddy NB, et al: Codeine and its alternates for pain and cough relief. *Bull WHO* 40:425-454, 639-719, 721-730, 1969.

Irwin RS, et al: Cough. Comprehensive review. *Arch Intern Med* 137:1186-1191, 1977.

Drugs Used in Asthma | 32

Asthma is associated with paroxysms of heightened bronchial muscle activity and inflammatory reactions to allergens and is characterized by episodic, reversible obstruction of the peripheral airways. The bronchospasm, mucosal edema, and mucous plugging of peripheral airways may resolve spontaneously or frequently may respond to drugs that improve pulmonary airflow (adrenergic and xanthine bronchodilators, cromolyn, or anti-inflammatory corticosteroids).

The history, physical examination, radiologic findings, sputum examination, and results of pulmonary function and arterial blood gas studies distinguish asthma from restrictive lung disorders (eg, pleural effusion, respiratory skeletal muscle weakness, thoracic deformity, interstitial pulmonary diseases) and other obstructive lung diseases (eg, chronic obstructive lung diseases [COLD], foreign body, neoplasm) that also limit airflow.

Reversibility of airway obstruction upon use of a bronchodilator and/or corticosteroids during pulmonary function tests helps to distinguish asthma from the poorly reversible or irreversible obstruction present in chronic obstructive lung diseases, such as emphysema, chronic bronchitis, cystic fibrosis, and bronchiectasis. Because these diseases are characterized by cellular loss of elasticity and fibrosis, bronchodilators are ineffective or of limited value if a clinically significant degree of reversible bronchospasm coexists in these diseases. Termination of exposure to environmental pollutants, especially smoking, is much more effective than the use of antiasthmatic drugs in patients with chronic bronchitis and emphysema (Hodgkins et al, 1975).

Therapy to Improve Airflow

The drugs available to improve pulmonary airflow include the adrenergic and theophylline bronchodilators; cromolyn [Intal], which inhibits the release of a number of bronchoconstrictor mediators; and the anti-inflammatory corticosteroids (see the Table).

Parasympathetic stimulation appears to play a significant role in obstructive lung disease. Ipratropium [Atrovent], an investigational anticholinergic drug, is a bronchodilator (Nilsson, 1979) when administered by metered-dose aerosol. Although this form of administration has been associated with minimal systemic side effects, more studies are required to determine potential local adverse effects on sputum viscosity and mucociliary clearance before its final role in the management of asthma can be established.

Oxygen relieves symptoms of hypoxia but does not improve airflow.

DRUGS USED TO IMPROVE PULMONARY AIRFLOW

	AVAILABLE FORMULATIONS			
	Parenteral	Oral Inhalation	Oral	Rectal
Agents Affecting Bronchial Muscle				
BRONCHODILATORS				
Adrenergic Drugs:				
Ephedrine Sulfate			+	
Epinephrine Hydrochloride [Adrenalin Chloride 1:1,000]	+			
Epinephrine (Sustained-Release) [Asmolin, Sus-Phrine]	+			
Epinephrine Hydrochloride [Adrenalin Chloride 1:100, Vaponefrin]		+		
Epinephrine Bitartrate [Medihaler-Epi]		+		
Epinephrine Racemic [microNEFRIN]		+		
Isoproterenol Hydrochloride [Isuprel Hydrochloride 1:100, Isuprel Mistometer, Vapo-Iso]		+		
Isoproterenol Sulfate [Medihaler-Iso, Norisodrine Sulfate]		+		
Isoproterenol Hydrochloride [Isuprel Hydrochloride 1:5,000]	+			
Isoetharine Mesylate [Bronkometer]		+		
Isoetharine Hydrochloride [Bronkosol]		+		
Metaproterenol Sulfate [Alupent, Metaprel]		+	+	
Terbutaline Sulfate [Brethine, Bricanyl]	+		+	
Xanthine Drugs:				
Theophylline			+	+
*Aminophylline	+		+	+
*Oxtriphylline			+	
Dyphylline	+ (intramuscular only)		+	

AVAILABLE FORMULATIONS

	Parenteral	Oral Inhalation	Oral	Rectal
Asthma Prophylactic Drug				
Cromolyn Sodium [Intal]		+		
Anti-Inflammatory Corticosteroids				
Beclomethasone Dipropionate [Beclovent, Vanceril]		+		
Systemic Corticosteroids [see Chapter 41]				
Investigational Drugs				
Adrenergic Drugs:				
Albuterol [Salbutamol]				
Fenoterol [Berotec]				
Anticholinergic Drug:				
Ipratropium [Atrovent]				

Theophylline is the only active bronchodilator ingredient in these formulations.

Adrenergic Drugs: Adrenergic bronchodilator drugs used in the treatment of asthma include ephedrine, epinephrine, isoproterenol [Isuprel, Medihaler-Iso, Norisodrine,Vapo-Iso], isoetharine [Bronkometer, Bronkosol], metaproterenol [Alupent, Metaprel], and terbutaline [Brethine, Bricanyl]. They activate both beta2 and beta1 receptors to varying degrees; activation of beta2 receptors relaxes bronchial smooth muscle by stimulating the production of cyclic adenosine-3,5-monophosphate, and activation of beta1 receptors stimulates the heart.

Ephedrine has a higher affinity for alpha- than beta-adrenergic receptors, and it is a nonselective bronchodilator in that it activates beta2 less than beta1 receptors. It can have a pronounced stimulatory effect on the central nervous system, and its action on the alpha receptors may result in an undesirable increase in peripheral vascular resistance. Ephedrine is available principally in mixtures. The clinical effects of methoxyphenamine [Orthoxine] are similar to those of ephedrine, but the cardiovascular effects of the former are less pronounced. Since other adrenergic agents with greater specificity for beta2 receptors are available (epinephrine, isoproterenol, isoetharine, metaproterenol, and terbutaline), they are preferred to ephedrine and methoxyphenamine in the treatment of asthma.

Metaproterenol and terbutaline are the most selective adrenergic bronchodilators, ie, in doses that produce comparable bronchodilation, they produce less beta1 stimulation than isoproterenol and isoetharine. The investigational drugs, albuterol [Salbutamol] (Leifer and Wittig, 1975; Finkel, 1979) and fenoterol [Berotec] (Heel et al, 1978), are also selective beta2 agonists.

The choice among the adrenergic drugs frequently depends upon the route of administration required, which, in turn, depends upon the desired onset and duration of action. Rapid relief of an acute attack of asthma may be obtained by the subcutaneous injection of epinephrine or terbutaline (terbutaline appears to be at least as effective as epinephrine and is longer acting).

If the attack is less severe, the oral inhalation of isoproterenol, isoetharine, metaproterenol, or terbutaline may be adequate. Metaproterenol produces less cardiac stimulation, is often more effective, and has a longer duration of action than isoproterenol or isoetharine. Because an inhaler containing terbutaline is not available, an aerosol of the solution for injection of this drug is utilized by some physicians as an alternative to metaproterenol.

When a prolonged duration of action is desired for prophylaxis, metaproterenol or terbutaline can be administered orally. A timed-release preparation of an aqueous suspension of epinephrine base is an alternative, but it must be given parenterally. The sublingual preparation of isoproterenol is not always reliably and predictably absorbed; therefore, it has little place in the treatment of asthma.

The concurrent use of aerosolized and oral adrenergic compounds may be needed for better control of wheezing; however, side effects may be more common. Tolerance, refractoriness, and even paradoxical bronchospastic reactions may develop with too frequent administration of epinephrine or isoproterenol. Tolerance is much less of a problem with metaproterenol and terbutaline (Plummer, 1978 B).

Xanthine Drugs: Theophylline is an effective bronchodilator that is especially useful in patients with moderate to severe reversible bronchospasm. In addition to preparations containing anhydrous or monohydrate forms, a number of formulations containing theophylline with solubilizing agents, eg, ethylenediamine (aminophylline), choline (oxtriphylline), monoethanolamine, or sodium glycinate are available. Theophylline is the only active ingredient in all of these preparations. Another xanthine, dyphylline, is not converted to theophylline but is considerably less potent than the latter.

Theophylline formulations are available for intravenous or oral administration but not for inhalation. Some oral preparations are available in a sustained-release form. Rectal suppositories are marketed, but they are erratically absorbed and locally irritating. A rectal retention solution is rapidly and reliably absorbed, although it may cause local irritation.

Asthma Prophylactic Drug: Unlike other drugs in this chapter, cromolyn is used only for prevention of asthma. It is unique in that it inhibits the degranulation and subsequent release of bronchospastic mediators induced by antigen reacting with specific IgE antibody-sensitized mast cell membranes. Asthmatic patients, especially children with extrinsic or exercise-induced asthma, are either partially or completely protected when the drug is inhaled orally prior to antigen exposure or exercise. This effectiveness in extrinsic asthma should not preclude its use in intrinsic asthma, because the absence of allergic factors does not necessarily indicate that the response will be unfavorable. It is emphasized that this drug is not effective for acute attacks of asthma and should not be used to treat status asthmaticus.

Anti-inflammatory Corticosteroids: Corticosteroids are the most potent antiasthmatic drugs available, but their potential systemic adverse reactions are correspondingly greater. Therefore, their longterm use for chronic asthma should be limited to patients who do not respond adequately to other available therapy. In addition to reducing inflammation and edema, corticosteroids potentiate the bronchodilating effect of adrenergic agents. They should be used cautiously or with appropriate antimicrobial therapy when bacterial infection is present.

The short-term use of oral preparations may control severe exacerbations in chronic asthma, although some patients require long-term therapy. Because of the associated hazards of chronic use, alternate-day therapy or inhaled beclomethasone should be employed when long-term corticosteroid treatment is indicated. Although prednisone, prednisolone, and methylprednisolone are appropriate for alternate-day therapy, no single corticosteroid appears to be more effective in asthma than others when equipotent doses are given (see Chapter 41, Adrenal Corticosteroids).

The short-term intravenous administration of large doses may be necessary to alleviate status asthmaticus. Oral therapy can be initiated while the patient is still receiving the steroid intravenously, and relief often can be maintained by the oral preparation while the intravenous dose is gradually decreased. Once status asthmaticus is controlled, an alternate-day schedule with a short-acting corticosteroid should be established if possible and the dosage reduced slowly.

Beclomethasone dipropionate [Beclovent, Vanceril] is available in an aerosol preparation for inhalation in metered doses. This agent exerts a local steroidal effect and, although systemic absorption occurs, beclomethasone is rapidly metabolized and the plasma concentration does not increase significantly if standard doses are not exceeded. Beclomethasone is particularly beneficial in selected individuals with severe, steroid-dependent asthma; in some patients, inhaled beclomethasone can be gradually substituted for oral steroids. The use of an aerosol form of an adrenergic agent just prior to inhalation of beclomethasone may enhance the distribution, and therefore the effectiveness, of the latter and is particularly useful when cough or wheezing occurs with use of beclomethasone.

Drug Selection

A total management program, including drugs and nondrug modalities, is most effective in the treatment of asthma. Drug therapy is much less beneficial if the overall management program is suboptimal. Avoidance of allergens, environmental pulmonary irritants (particularly smoking), cold, infection, and dehydration is important. In addition, reconditioning exercises directed toward developing increased respiratory muscle strength and a more effective cough; patient education, including instruction in postural drainage; and vocational rehabilitation are helpful in both asthma and irreversible chronic obstructive lung disease.

The choice of drug(s) in the treatment of asthma depends primarily upon the severity of the disease (Plummer, 1978 A; Weinberger and Hendeles, 1979). An adrenergic drug (given correctly through a metered-dose inhaler) may be adequate for patients with infrequent episodes of airflow obstruction and may be especially effective prophylactically if the obstruction is related to cold or is induced by exercise.

If wheezing occurs frequently despite numerous inhalations or frequent oral administration of adrenergic drugs, oral theophylline compounds should be added to the regimen temporarily. Such therapy often provides bronchodilation superior to that produced by either type of drug given alone (Wolfe et al, 1978). Theophylline, and possibly the adrenergic drug, may be discontinued when patients with infrequent episodes of asthma have been asymptomatic for a day or two. The continued regular use of theophylline may prolong the remission period in asymptomatic individuals with residual abnormalities of airway function.

More aggressive therapy for long periods is necessary in the chronic asthmatic with more frequent episodes of airway obstruction (Goldstein et al, 1978). In these patients, even milder attacks usually require oral theophylline plus inhalation or oral adrenergic bronchodilators as needed. Cromolyn may be an acceptable alternative to theophylline initially (König, 1978) or in patients who cannot tolerate low doses of theophylline or in whom serum concentrations are difficult to maintain within the recommended range. Although cromolyn is less effective than theophylline, the risk of toxicity also is reduced. Patients who are not adequately controlled on these regimens may respond to a trial of inhaled beclomethasone or alternate-day use of systemic corticosteroids, preferably at the lowest dose necessary for control. Bronchodilator therapy should not be terminated when initiating steroid therapy.

Most physicians administer subcutaneous epinephrine or terbutaline and intravenous theophylline for a sudden, severe attack of asthma, even in patients receiving oral theophylline therapy. If an adrenergic bronchodilator also is being used by inhalation, the frequency of administration may be increased to every two hours as well. A 14- to 21-day course of systemic corticosteroids, with the dose gradually reduced, may be necessary if airflow obstruction cannot be controlled with these drugs. More aggressive therapy, including hospitalization, intravenous fluids, prolonged intravenous aminophylline, steroids, and oxygen, may be necessary. Vigorous therapy must be employed to avoid the use of mechanical ventilation.

Adverse Reactions and Precautions

Adrenergic Drugs: Untoward effects associated with adrenergic bronchodilators involve primarily the cardiovascular, neuromuscular, and central nervous systems. Adrenergic drugs should be administered cautiously to patients with arrhythmias and may be contraindicated in some patients, depending upon the route of administration, dosage, or existence of sensitivity to these drugs. Parenteral or oral inhalation of epinephrine or isoproterenol [Isuprel, Medihaler-Iso, Norisodrine, Vapo-Iso] may cause palpitation, tachycardia, and other disturbances of cardiac rhythm and rate. Although metaproterenol [Alupent, Metaprel] and terbutaline [Brethine, Bricanyl] may cause palpitation and tachycardia, the incidence and severity are less than with epinephrine and isoproterenol, and other disturbances of cardiac rhythm and rate are rare. When adrenergic bronchodilators are used by aerosol inhalation, patients should be observed initially for the development of cardiovascular effects.

Careful instruction of the patient in the proper use of nebulizers, preferably by demonstration and written instructions, is essential whenever these devices are used. There are great variations in response to nebulized agents, and the physician must set firm limits on the frequency of inhalation. With any nebulized preparation, the least number of inhalations of the most dilute solution necessary to obtain relief is the most desirable, because of the danger of tolerance and paradoxical or adverse reactions. Children should be allowed to use handheld nebulizers only under the supervision of a knowledgeable adult.

Rapid absorption of excessive amounts of epinephrine may cause hypertension, headache, and even cerebral hemorrhage. Since hypertension is less likely to occur with isoproterenol and does not occur with metaproterenol, these drugs are preferred for use in hypertensive patients. Indeed, *hypotension* may be observed rarely after the administration of metaproterenol.

Central nervous system stimulation, manifested by nervousness, excitability, and insomnia, is common after oral administration of ephedrine, especially in adults. Sedatives have been used to alleviate these symptoms, but their depressant effect may aggravate the ventilatory problem in patients with respiratory failure. Therefore, sedatives are relatively contraindicated and should be prescribed only with extreme caution for patients with asthma. Rarely, similar stimulation follows the subcutaneous injection of epinephrine and the oral inhalation or sublingual administration of isoproterenol.

Muscle tremor is common with oral use of metaproterenol and terbutaline. A reduction in dose usually eliminates this symptom, although tolerance to this effect develops with prolonged use.

Large doses of adrenergic drugs may cause dizziness, asthenia, lightheadedness, nausea, and vomiting. These reactions are less common after oral inhalation of metaproterenol than after oral inhalation of isoproterenol.

The excessive and prolonged oral inhalation of epinephrine or isoproterenol may cause dryness of the pharyngeal membranes, inflammation of the bronchial mucosa, and, in sensitive individuals, severe, prolonged attacks of asthma. If these preparations are swallowed due to improper administration, they may produce epigastric pain. Refractoriness may develop after repeated use.

Administration of ephedrine may cause urinary retention severe enough to necessitate catheterization in elderly men with prostatic hypertrophy.

Caution should be exercised to avoid hypertension, tachycardia, and increased cardiac oxygen demands when adrenergic bronchodilators are given to patients with hyperthyroidism or ischemic heart disease. Epinephrine may be less effective in the presence of respiratory or metabolic acidosis, and anecdotal evidence suggests that the response to epinephrine is improved if acidemia is corrected by the cautious administration of sodium bicarbonate and/or by improving ventilation. However, it is emphasized that the specific treatment of respiratory acidosis is reduction of arterial carbon dioxide tension by increasing ventilation.

Xanthine Drugs: The most common adverse reactions caused by theophylline and its derivatives are mild gastrointestinal irritation and central nervous system stimulation. Nausea, vomiting, and epigastric pain, generally preceded by headache, often follow the use of excessive doses of theophylline. Theophylline compounds increase gastric acidity and should be used carefully in patients with gastrointestinal ulcers. Prolonged use of suppositories may cause rectal irritation. The rectal absorption of aminophylline suppositories is erratic.

Fatal convulsions occur as a result of excessive plasma concentrations. The dose of theophylline should be reduced if central nervous system stimulation, manifested by irritability, restlessness, and insomnia, occurs. Sedatives should not be given to counteract these effects; instead, the theophylline dosage should be reduced. Agitation, headache, hyperreflexia, fasciculations, fever, hematemesis, clonic and tonic convulsions, and death have occurred following overdosage of theophylline drugs. Rapid intravenous administration of aminophylline has caused severe cardiac arrhythmias and even cardiac arrest.

Miscellaneous Compounds: For adverse reactions produced by the systemically administered corticosteroids, see Chapter 41. Adverse reactions produced by cromolyn and beclomethasone are discussed in the evaluations.

Drug Interactions: Severe hypertension and, rarely, death may occur if ephedrine is administered with a monoamine oxidase inhibitor (isocarboxazid [Marplan], phenelzine [Nardil], tranylcypromine [Parnate]); this is caused by release of excessive amounts of norepinephrine from storage sites. Ephedrine may antagonize the antihypertensive effect of guanethidine [Ismelin]. Adrenergic bronchodilators may be ineffective in patients receiving propranolol [Inderal], or they may antagonize

the action of propranolol, thus exacerbating the condition for which the beta-blocking drug was prescribed. Theophylline is probably the preferred bronchodilator in the rare asthmatic patient for whom propranolol is essential. Caution is advised when barbiturates are administered to asthmatic patients receiving cordicosteroids, for the enzyme-inducing properties of the former may increase the metabolism of the latter. (See also Chapter 5, Drug Interactions and Adverse Drug Reactions.)

BRONCHODILATORS

Adrenergic Drugs

EPINEPHRINE
[Asmolin, Sus-Phrine]

EPINEPHRINE BITARTRATE
[Medihaler-Epi]

EPINEPHRINE HYDROCHLORIDE
[Adrenalin Chloride, Vaponefrin]

EPINEPHRINE RACEMIC
[microNEFRIN]

When given subcutaneously, epinephrine is of value in acute asthmatic attacks. Although its principal therapeutic effect in asthma is bronchodilatation, vasoconstriction and relief of bronchial edema may result in additional improvement in vital capacity. However, the generalized vasoconstriction may increase peripheral vascular resistance. The short duration of action can be prolonged by the cautious subcutaneous administration of the base in aqueous suspension 1:200 [Sus-Phrine].

A nebulized form of epinephrine can be inhaled for both prophylaxis and treatment of bronchospasm, but this is not the preferred drug for oral inhalation. Absorption from the respiratory tract may lead to overdosage and cause adverse effects similar to those observed when epinephrine is administered by other routes. Too frequent inhalation also can irritate the bronchial mucosa.

Adverse reactions due to systemic absorption of epinephrine include symptoms of excessive stimulation of alpha- and beta-sympathetic receptors (anxiety, tremor, palpitation, tachycardia, and headache); these reactions are most common after parenteral administration. Rebound bronchospasm may occur. Excessive doses cause acute hypertension and arrhythmias. The drug generally is contraindicated in patients with hypertension, hyperthyroidism, ischemic heart disease, or cerebrovascular insufficiency. Refractoriness and tolerance may occur after too frequent administration, especially in patients with respiratory or metabolic acidosis. (See also the Introduction.)

ROUTES, USUAL DOSAGE, AND PREPARATIONS. *Subcutaneous*: *Adults*, 0.2 to 0.5 mg (0.2 to 0.5 ml of 1:1,000 solution) every two hours as necessary; *children*, 0.01 mg/kg of body weight every four hours as needed. In severe acute attacks, doses may be repeated every 20 minutes for a maximum of three doses. Alternatively, 0.1 to 0.3 ml of an aqueous suspension of free base 1:200 [Sus-Phrine] for adults (maximum initial dose, 0.1 ml) or 0.01 ml/kg for children (maximum dose, 0.25 ml) may be used when prolonged action is desired. Caution must be exercised, for this preparation is more concentrated than the standard preparation; administration generally should not be repeated within four hours.

EPINEPHRINE:
Drug available generically: Suspension 1:1,000 in 1 and 2 ml containers.
Asmolin (Lincoln). Suspension (aqueous) 1:400 (2.5 mg/ml) in 10 ml containers.
Sus-Phrine (Berlex). Suspension (aqueous) 1:200 (5 mg/ml) in 0.5 and 5 ml containers.

EPINEPHRINE HYDROCHLORIDE:
Drug available generically: Solution 1:1,000 in 1, 10, and 30 ml containers.
Adrenalin Chloride (Parke, Davis). Solution 1;1,000 (1 mg/ml) in 1 and 30 ml containers.

Oral Inhalation: 0.1% to 1% solution or suspension may be inhaled from a nebulizer or metered-dose inhaler as an aerosol and repeated when necessary; however, epinephrine is not a preferred drug for this route of administration.

EPINEPHRINE BITARTRATE:
Medihaler-Epi (Riker). Suspension 7 mg/ml (0.3 mg/measured dose) (nonprescription).
EPINEPHRINE HYDROCHLORIDE:
Adrenalin Chloride (Parke, Davis). Solution 1:100 (10 mg/ml). *Vaponefrin* (Fisons). Solution 2.25% (0.3 mg/metered dose) (nonprescription).
EPINEPHRINE RACEMIC:
microNEFRIN (Bird). Solution 2.25%.

EPHEDRINE SULFATE

The actions of ephedrine are similar to those of epinephrine, but it is not as useful as epinephrine for severe attacks of asthma because its bronchodilator action is weaker. Ephedrine is less effective and no longer acting than adrenergic agents with a greater specificity for beta$_2$ receptors (ie, metaproterenol, terbutaline) in patients who require continuous medication.

Adverse reactions are similar to those caused by epinephrine (see the Introduction and the evaluation on Epinephrine). Central nervous system stimulation, manifested by nervousness, excitability, and insomnia, is common. A sedative is not recommended to reduce these effects; an alternative drug should be chosen instead. An increase in peripheral vascular resistance may result in hypertension. Rarely, a patient may be allergic to ephedrine. Urinary retention may occur in men with prostatic hypertrophy.

ROUTE, USUAL DOSAGE, AND PREPARATIONS. *Oral*: *Adults*, 20 to 50 mg every three to four hours; *children*, 3 mg/kg of body weight every 24 hours in four to six divided doses.
Drug available generically: Capsules 25 and 50 mg; syrup 11 and 20 mg/5 ml.

ISOPROTERENOL HYDROCHLORIDE
[Isuprel Hydrochloride, Vapo-Iso]

ISOPROTERENOL SULFATE
[Medihaler-Iso, Norisodrine Sulfate]

Isoproterenol is effective in preventing and relieving bronchoconstriction. It also relaxes gastrointestinal smooth muscle and skeletal muscle vasculature and increases the rate and force of heart contractions. Its duration of action is similar to that of epinephrine and shorter than that of metaproterenol, and it has less beta2 selectivity than metaproterenol and terbutaline. Oral inhalation is the preferred route of administration for the treatment of asthmatic attacks. Absorption is erratic when isoproterenol is given sublingually. This drug or metaproterenol is preferred to epinephrine for patients with hypertension.

Palpitation, tachycardia and other arrhythmias, hypotension, tremor, headache, and nervousness occur. These side effects are especially frequent with excessive use due to self-medication. Angina has been reported. Excessive inhalation can cause refractory bronchial obstruction and rarely may be followed by sudden death, presumably from arrhythmia. Tolerance and refractoriness may develop with too frequent administration. In sensitive patients, inhalation may cause a severe, prolonged attack of asthma. See also the Introduction.

ROUTES, USUAL DOSAGE, AND PREPARATIONS. *Oral Inhalation: Adults,* one or two deep inhalations from a handheld propellant-operated nebulizer, a preset mechanical nebulizer such as may be found on mechanical ventilators, or an ultrasonic nebulizer. For best results with any of these nebulizers, the breath should be held in full inhalation for a few seconds following a complete exhalation. Administration by metered-dose inhaler is repeated once or twice at five- to ten-minute intervals *if necessary.* This regimen may be repeated at four-hour intervals. If there is evidence of resistance, other medication should be used. *Children,* some physicians believe that a hand-bulb nebulizer is safer, but children can be allowed to use handheld nebulizers if they are supervised by a knowledgeable adult. The dose is 5 to 15 deep inhalations of an aerosol of the 1:200 solution, repeated in 10 to 30 minutes if necessary, or three to seven deep inhalations of the 1:100 dilution. However, some physicians prefer to limit the dose to five inhalations of the 1:200 solution and to avoid use of the 1:100 solution and the 25% concentration [Norisodrine Sulfate].

When an oxygen aerosol nebulizer is used, *adults and children,* up to 0.5 ml of the 1:200 solution or 0.3 ml of the 1:100 solution may be administered with an oxygen flow of 5 to 10 L/min for 15 to 20 minutes, but a dilution of 1:2,000 may be preferable. Dosage with a powder inhalation device is two to four inhalations of normal force and depth only. *If necessary,* the dose may be repeated after five minutes and once more after ten minutes.

ISOPROTERENOL HYDROCHLORIDE:
Drug available generically: Solution 1:200.
Isuprel Mistometer (Breon). Solution 1:400 (2.5 mg/ml) providing 0.125 mg/measured dose.
Isuprel Hydrochloride (Breon). Solution 1:100 (10 mg/ml) and 1:200 (5 mg/ml).
Vapo-Iso (Fisons). Solution 1:200 (5 mg/ml).
ISOPROTERENOL SULFATE:
Medihaler-Iso (Riker). Suspension 2 mg/ml providing 0.075 mg/ measured dose.
Norisodrine Sulfate (Abbott). Powder 10% and 25% in aerosol containers.

Intravenous: This route is used only in intensive care units for children with respiratory failure from asthma and only with great caution. The initial infusion rate is 0.1 mcg/kg/min; the rate is increased by 0.1 mcg/kg/min at 15-minute intervals until a clinical response, a heart rate greater than 180, or an infusion rate of 0.8 mcg/kg/min is achieved.

ISOPROTERENOL HYDROCHLORIDE:
Drug available generically: Solution 1:5,000 in 5 ml containers.
Isuprel Hydrochloride (Breon). Solution 1:5,000 in 1 and 5 ml containers.
Sublingual: Adults, 10 to 15 mg three or four times daily (maximum, 60 mg daily); *children,* 5 to 10 mg three or four times daily (maximum, 30 mg daily). This route is

not preferred because absorption is unpredictable.

ISOPROTERENOL HYDROCHLORIDE:
Isuprel Hydrochloride (Breon). Tablets 10 and 15 mg.

METAPROTERENOL SULFATE
[Alupent, Metaprel]

This drug is primarily a beta2 stimulant and may be administered by oral inhalation or orally; it is absorbed more reliably than isoproterenol by the former route and appears to have little effect on beta1 receptors of the cardiovascular system. The actions, indications, and adverse reactions of metaproterenol are otherwise similar to those of isoproterenol. When inhaled, metaproterenol appears to cause slightly lower peak expiratory flows than inhaled isoproterenol, but its duration of action lasts up to four hours. Patients are less likely to develop tolerance to inhaled metaproterenol than to inhaled isoproterenol. The oral preparation may be more effective than ephedrine. (See also the Introduction.)

ROUTES, USUAL DOSAGE, AND PREPARATIONS.
Oral Inhalation: *Adults and children*, two or three deep inhalations. This may be repeated at four-hour intervals, but the total daily dosage should not exceed 12 inhalations. The manufacturers do not recommend use of this drug in children under 12. In any event, children should be allowed to use handheld nebulizers only under the supervision of a knowledgeable adult.
Alupent (Boehringer Ingelheim), *Metaprel* (Dorsey). Micronized powder 225 mg (0.65 mg/metered dose) in a metered-dose inhaler.
Oral: (Tablets) *Adults*, initially, 10 mg three or four times a day, increased gradually over a period of two to four weeks to 20 mg three or four times daily, if needed. Limited data are available on use of the tablet form in *children*. (Syrup) *Children 6*

to 9 years *(under 60 lb)*, 10 mg three or four times daily; *over 9 years (over 60 lb)*, adult dose.
Alupent (Boehringer Ingelheim), *Metaprel* (Dorsey). Syrup 10 mg/5 ml; tablets 10 and 20 mg.

TERBUTALINE SULFATE
[Brethine, Bricanyl]

This drug is primarily a beta2 stimulant and may be administered subcutaneously or orally. It appears to have little or no effect on beta1 receptors of the cardiovascular system. In general, the subcutaneous preparation resembles that of epinephrine in onset and degree of effect, but some data suggest that equipotent doses of the newer drug are more effective and longer lasting. When administered subcutaneously, the incidence and severity of adverse reactions also resemble those commonly seen with epinephrine when it is administered by this route.

The oral preparation is more effective than the oral forms of metaproterenol and ephedrine, because terbutaline causes higher peak expiratory flows and the action lasts up to eight hours. Although tolerance to terbutaline and other selective beta2 agonists can be demonstrated, it is of considerably less clinical significance than with isoproterenol and ephedrine (Plummer, 1978 B). Oral terbutaline frequently causes tremor but dizziness, nervousness, fatigue, tinnitus, and palpitations are rare. (See also the Introduction.)

ROUTES, USUAL DOSAGE, AND PREPARATIONS.
Subcutaneous: *Adults*, 0.25 mg, repeated in 15 to 30 minutes if necessary; no more than 0.5 mg should be administered in any four-hour period. *Children*, 0.01 mg/kg of body weight (maximum total dose, 0.25 mg). The dose may be repeated once in 30 minutes if necessary but usually is effective for four hours.
Brethine (Geigy), *Bricanyl* (Astra). Solution 1 mg (equivalent to 0.82 mg of free base)/ml in 2 ml containers containing 1 ml of solution.

Oral: *Adults and adolescents*, initially, 2.5 mg three times daily at approximately eight-hour intervals, increased gradually over a period of two to four weeks to 5 mg three times daily, if needed. *Children 12 years and under*, 1.25 to 2.5 mg three times daily at approximately six- to eight-hour intervals, increasing the dose, if needed and tolerated, to a maximum of 5 mg daily.

> *Brethine* (Geigy), *Bricanyl* (Astra). Tablets 2.5 and 5 mg (equivalent to 2.05 and 4.1 mg of free base, respectively).

Xanthine Drugs

THEOPHYLLINE

Except for dyphylline, the action of all other xanthine bronchodilator preparations (theophylline, aminophylline, and oxtriphylline) is dependent upon their content of theophylline. Aminophylline is theophylline (85%) with ethylenediamine (15%), and oxtriphylline is theophylline (64%) with choline (36%), but theophylline is the only active bronchodilator ingredient present. Although aminophylline is too irritating for intramuscular use, it is the only parenteral preparation available and is given intravenously. Oral aminophylline and oxtriphylline preparations offer no advantages over theophylline preparations in most patients.

Moderate or severe reversible bronchospasm almost always requires the use of theophylline. It is an especially effective and safe bronchodilator if care is taken to ensure that the patient is receiving the optimum dose, formulation, and route of administration appropriate for the current status of his disease.

In addition to its bronchodilator effect, theophylline has cardiac positive inotropic, vasodilating, and diuretic actions which also may result from its inhibition of cyclic nucleotide phosphodiesterase activity.

Because theophylline increases cardiac output and decreases peripheral vascular resistance and venous pressure, it is frequently beneficial adjunctively in the treatment of acute pulmonary edema or paroxysmal nocturnal dyspnea due to left-sided heart failure. Theophylline also is useful in the treatment of neonatal apnea because of its central nervous system (medullary) stimulating action (see Chapter 21, Adjuncts to Anesthesia and Analeptic Drugs).

Headache, dizziness, nervousness, nausea, vomiting, and epigastric pain are common, especially after oral administration. These side effects may be related to overdosage. Severe toxic reactions, manifested by arrhythmias, persistent vomiting, agitation, and, sometimes, convulsions that may be fatal, may occur regardless of the route of administration. In children, hematemesis, central nervous system stimulation, diuresis, and fever may be observed. Deaths due to convulsions and shock have been reported following excessive serum concentrations. The danger is particularly great if cough preparations containing theophylline are given concomitantly. Rapid intravenous injection of aminophylline causes arrhythmias, sudden and profound hypotension, and cardiac arrest. Therefore, intravenous injections must be given slowly and cautiously, especially in patients with myocardial ischemia. See also the Introduction.

There are no absolute or relative contraindications to the use of theophylline with other drugs. Smoking and concurrent use of barbiturates increase theophylline elimination, and there is some evidence to suggest that concurrent administration of erythromycin or the presence of an acute infection may have the opposite effect; appropriate dosage adjustments may be necessary. Theophylline is reported to cross the placenta readily (Arwood et al, 1979).

The most important factor in determining theophylline dosage is the theophylline clearance rate of the patient. The rate of clearance varies considerably among individuals (Ginchansky and Weinberger, 1977), and half-lives range from 3 to 13 hours. The average clearance rate is greater in children than in adults. Because of this, children require larger mean mg/kg doses.

The optimal serum theophylline concentration is 10 to 20 mcg/ml. Concentrations above 20 mcg/ml are usually associated with adverse reactions. Levels of 5 to 10 mcg/ml may be adequate in an occasional patient but may be insufficient during times of stress (eg, increased exposure to allergens, infection, excessive exercise).

Absorption of oral theophylline from un-coated tablets and solutions is adequate if tablet disintegration and dissolution are sufficient. Serum theophylline concentrations often fluctuate less with use of selected sustained-release preparations and thus the concentration can be better maintained within a range of 10 to 20 mcg/ml. Sustained-release preparations also may allow maintenance of an effective theophylline serum level in children during eight hours of sleep. However, not all sustained-release preparations have adequate bioavailability or have been evaluated in controlled studies (Bell and Bigley, 1978; Weinberger et al, 1978). Assured bioavailability of the sustained-release product chosen by the physician is essential.

Rectal suppositories are generally irritating and poorly and/or erratically absorbed, in contrast to retention enemas, which are rapidly and completely absorbed.

ROUTES, USUAL DOSAGE, AND PREPARATIONS.
THEOPHYLLINE:
Dosages are expressed as milligrams of *anhydrous theophylline equivalents* per kilogram of ideal body weight for the elixir, syrup, oral solution, oral suspension, tablet, chewable tablet, or capsule forms but not for the sustained-release capsule or tablet preparations (see below). The loading dose should be reduced or eliminated if the patient has received theophylline within 24 hours.
Oral: (*Oral Formulations Except Sustained-Release Tablets*) For an acute attack not requiring parenteral therapy, *adults*, 5 mg/kg initially, followed by a maintenance dose of 3 to 4 mg/kg every six hours to control symptoms. If the initial loading dose is inadequate, an additional

2.5 mg/kg may be given intravenously after one hour, and an intravenous infusion then should be initiated (see the intravenous dosage for aminophylline). The maintenance dose can be increased gradually to 6 mg/kg if necessary to control symptoms. Single doses in excess of 6 mg/kg should not be given until the theophylline serum concentration is determined; effective serum concentrations range between 10 and 20 mcg/ml. The initial maintenance dose should be adjusted for patients in the following categories: Adults who do not smoke and/or are over age 50, 2 to 3 mg/kg; patients with cardiac decompensation or liver disease, 1 to 2 mg/kg. The same dosages and limitations are applicable for *children* except that the maintenance dose is 4 to 5 mg/kg every six hours.

Alternatively, if there is no urgency and laboratory facilities for measurement of serum theophylline concentration are available, the following plan for long-term prophylaxis is recommended to minimize the incidence and severity of side effects and toxic reactions in *children* (Hendeles et al, 1978): Initially, 16 mg/kg or 400 mg/day, whichever is less, is given daily in divided doses. The dose should be increased *if tolerated* in increments of approximately 25% at three-day intervals, and the following limits should not be exceeded: *children less than 9 years*, 24 mg/kg/day; *9 to 12 years*, 20 mg/kg/day; *12 to 16 years*, 18 mg/kg/day; *over 16 years*, 13 mg/kg/day or 900 mg/day, whichever is less. (These limits represent the average therapeutic doses determined for these age groups.) When the maximally tolerated dose or the limits of dose for age are attained, the peak serum theophylline concentration is determined after *assured compliance* for the previous 48 hours. The blood sample should be drawn two hours after the last dose of all oral preparations except sustained-release forms, in which case an interval of four hours is recommended. The final dosage adjustment (expressed as percentage change in total daily dose) is dependent upon the theophylline serum concentration (in mcg/ml). *5 to 7.5*: If the patient is asymptomatic, a drug-free period should be considered. Otherwise, the dose should be increased by 50% (in 25% increments at two-day intervals) and the serum concentration measured again. *8 to 10*: Even if the patient is asymptomatic, increasing the dose by 20% may prevent symptoms during upper respiratory infection (URI) or heavy exposure to an inhalant allergen or vigorous exertion. *11 to 13*: If the patient is asymptomatic, no increase is necessary; if symptoms occur during URI or exercise, the dose should be increased cautiously by 10%. *14 to 20*: If "breakthrough" in asthmatic symptoms occurs at the end of a dosing interval, a sustained-release product is substituted and the serum level measurement is repeated. If side effects occur, the total daily dose is decreased by 10%. *21 to 25*: Even if side effects are absent, the dose is decreased by 10%. *26 to 35*: Even if side effects are absent, the next dose is omitted and the total daily dose is decreased by 30%; measurement of the serum concentration is repeated. *35*: The next two doses are omitted; the subsequent dose is decreased by 50% and the serum concentration is measured again.

Tablets:
Available generically: 100, 200, and 250 mg.
Slo-Phyllin (Dooner) 100 and 200 mg; *Theophyl* (chewable) (Knoll) 100 mg; *Theophyl-225* (Knoll) 225 mg; *Theolair* (Riker) 125 and 250 mg.

Capsules:
Bronkodyl (Breon), *Elixophyllin* (Berlex) 100 and 200 mg: *Somophyllin-T* (Fisons) 100, 200, and 250 mg.

Elixir:
Available generically: 80 mg/15 ml.
Bronkodyl (Breon), *Elixophyllin* (Berlex) 80 mg/15 ml (alcohol 20%).

Oral Solution:
Theolair (Riker) 80 mg/15 ml.

Oral Suspension:
Elixicon (Berlex) 100 mg/5 ml.

Syrup:
Slo-Phyllin-80 (Dooner), *Theoclear 80* (Central), *Theospan* (Laser) 80 mg/15 ml (alcohol 1%, Theospan only).

(Sustained-Release Oral Forms) Adults and children, the recommended initial dose is 4 mg/kg every 8 to 12 hours. If required and *tolerated*, the dose can be gradually increased on the basis of average therapeutic dose levels for age. *Children less than 9 years*, 24 mg/kg/day; *9 to 12*

years, 20 mg/kg/day; *12 to 16 years*, 18 mg/kg/day; *over 16 years*, 13 mg/kg/day or 900 mg/day, whichever is less; the average therapeutic dose for *adults* is 930 mg/24 hours. If required and *tolerated*, these dose limits may be increased gradually, but monitoring of the serum theophylline concentration is recommended (maximum, 20 mcg/ml).

Timed-Release Tablets:
Theo-Dur (Key) 100, 200, and 300 mg; *Theolair-SR* (Riker) 250 and 500 mg; *Sustaire* (Roerig) 100 and 300 mg.

Timed-Release Capsules:
Available generically: 125 and 250 mg.
Slo-Phyllin (Dooner) 60, 125, and 250 mg; *Elixophyllin SR* (Berlex), *Theophyl-SR* (Knoll) 125 and 250 mg.

Rectal: (Retention Unit) Adults and children, 5 mg/kg of ideal body weight no more often than every eight hours; the total daily dose should not exceed the therapeutic dose limits based on age (listed under oral dosage) or a serum theophylline concentration of 20 mcg/ml.

Fleet Theophylline (Fleet) 250 and 500 mg (containing theophylline monoethanolamine 312 and 625 mg, respectively) in 37 ml of aqueous suspension.

(Suppositories) This form is not preferred because of its erratic absorption.

Aqualin (Webcon) 120 and 500 mg.

AMINOPHYLLINE:

Doses are expressed as mg/kg of ideal body weight; theophylline equivalents (mg theophylline = mg aminophylline × 0.85) are given in parentheses for convenience.

Intravenous: Adults and children, for an acute attack, loading dose, 5.6 mg/kg aminophylline (5 mg/kg theophylline) administered slowly at a rate of no more than 25 mg/min. The loading dose should be reduced by 50% if the patient has received theophylline within the previous 24 hours. After the loading dose, the following amounts (mg/kg/hr) are infused for maintenance: *children less than 9 years*, 1 (0.85); *healthy adults who smoke and are younger than 50 years*, 0.9 (0.75); *healthy adults who do not smoke*, 0.45 (0.4); *patients with cardiac decompensation and liver dysfunction*, 0.25 (0.2). The maintenance dose should be reduced if nausea, vomiting, headache, tachycardia, or other toxic effects appear or the serum theophylline concentration exceeds 20 mcg/ml.

> Aminophylline, U.S.P. (Theophylline 85% with Ethylenediamine 15%):
> Solution (intravenous) 25 mg/ml in 10 and 20 ml containers.

Rectal: *(Retention Unit) Adults*, 5 ml (equivalent to 255 mg theophylline) one to three times daily; the total daily dose should not exceed the average therapeutic dose limits based on age (listed under oral administration of theophylline) or a serum theophylline concentration of 20 mcg/ml. *Children*, 5 mg/kg (as theophylline) administered no more often than every six hours; the total daily dose should be based on age and determined as for adults.

> *Somophyllin* (Fisons). Solution 300 mg/5 ml in 3 and 5 oz containers.

(Suppositories) This form is not preferred because of erratic absorption.

> Available generically: 125, 250, 350, 450, and 500 mg.

Oral: Dosage is based on theophylline equivalents.

> Tablets (plain, enteric-coated):
> Available generically: 100 and 200 mg.
> Oral Solution:
> *Somophyllin* (Fisons) 105 mg/5 ml.

OXTRIPHYLLINE (Theophylline 64% with Choline 36%):
Oral: Dosage is based on theophylline equivalents.

> Tablets:
> *Choledyl* (Parke, Davis) 100 and 200 mg.
> Elixir:
> *Choledyl* (Parke, Davis) 100 mg/5 ml (alcohol 20%).

DYPHYLLINE

Dyphylline is a neutral xanthine derivative that is active in its own right; however, it is considerably less potent than theophylline. Dyphylline should not be used with other xanthine preparations, since it does not require conversion to theophylline for bronchodilator activity. The adverse reactions observed are similar to those produced by theophylline.

Compared to theophylline and aminophylline, less pharmacokinetic data are available for suggested initial dosage alterations of dyphylline in various patients (eg, age groups, smokers and nonsmokers, disease states). Dyphylline is rapidly eliminated, principally unchanged, in the urine and has a half-life of two to two and one-half hours (Gisclon et al, 1979). Therefore, theophylline is preferred for use in patients with chronic asthma. Because the therapeutic range of plasma concentrations is not defined, the physician should carefully determine the dosages for any dyphylline product of choice.

Although dyphylline may be given intramuscularly without producing pain because it is a neutral soluble xanthine derivative, the intramuscular route is seldom indicated and is not preferred over intravenous administration of aminophylline. Dyphylline should not be used intravenously.

ROUTES, USUAL DOSAGE, AND PREPARATIONS. The following doses are recommended by the manufacturers.
Intramuscular: *Adults*, 250 to 500 mg every six hours; the dosage should be adjusted individually on the basis of the condition and response of the patient. *Children*, doses have not been established.

> Available generically: Solution 250 mg/ml in 10 ml containers.
> *Dilor* (Savage), *Lufyllin* (Mallinckrodt), *Neothylline* (Lemmon). Solution (for intramuscular use only) 250 mg/ml in 2 and 10 (Dilor only) ml containers.

Oral: *Adults*, 15 mg/kg every six hours; the dosage should be adjusted individually on the basis of the condition and response of the patient. *Children*, doses have not been established.

> Tablets:
> Available generically: 200 mg.
> *Airet* (Baylor), *Dilor* (Savage), *Lufyllin* (Mallinckrodt), *Neothylline* (Lemmon) 200 and 400 mg.
> Elixir:
> *Lufyllin* (Mallinckrodt) 100 mg/15 ml (alcohol 20%).
> Oral Solution:
> *Airet* (Baylor) 100 mg/15 ml (alcohol 10%).

ASTHMA PROPHYLACTIC DRUG

CROMOLYN SODIUM
[Intal]

$$Na^+ \; {}^-OC \quad OCH_2CHCHO_2 \quad CO^-Na^+ \quad OH$$

Unlike other drugs used to treat asthma, cromolyn is used only to prevent attacks of asthma. This drug is ineffective in the treatment of acute attacks of asthma, including status asthmaticus. Cromolyn has no adrenergic, bronchodilator, antihistaminic, or corticosteroid-like actions. Instead it appears to inhibit the degranulation of mast cells and the release of histamine and other spasmogens following immunologic (antigen-IgE antibody) and nonimmunologic (exercise, hyperventilation) stimulation.

Numerous well-controlled clinical trials, including large multicenter studies, have demonstrated conclusively that a large proportion of children with chronic, intractable asthma experience either partial or complete protection after the oral inhalation of cromolyn (Bernstein et al, 1978); a smaller number of adults benefit from prophylactic use of this drug.

Although it is difficult to distinguish between extrinsic (known hypersensitivity to an extrinsic allergen) and intrinsic (no such hypersensitivity known) asthma, the evidence appears to indicate that patients with the former type are more likely to respond to cromolyn than those with the latter type. However, it is not yet possible to predict which specific patients will respond satisfactorily.

The beneficial effects of this drug have been documented by several criteria, including patient preference, evaluation of the incidence and severity of symptoms and signs by patient and physician, the dosage of bronchodilator and corticosteroid drugs required concomitantly, and results of spirometric pulmonary function tests (eg, forced expiration volume in one second). The inhalation of cromolyn shortly before exercise lessens the bronchoconstriction that some asthmatic patients then develop. This effect may be enhanced if the patient is receiving continuous therapy.

Controlled and uncontrolled studies on the long-term use of cromolyn indicate that tolerance usually does not develop and that adults can adjust the dose in a responsible manner. These studies also suggest that children on long-term therapy may demonstrate increased exercise tolerance, reduced school absenteeism, reduced frequency of hospitalization, decreased interference with sleep, reduced need for bronchodilators and corticosteroids, and increased peak expiratory flow rates.

A response to cromolyn is often observed within a few days. Asthmatic patients whose symptoms are not controlled adequately by bronchodilators may be given a trial of cromolyn for three or four weeks. The drug should be used for longer periods only in responsive patients. During the succeeding months, the dose of concomitantly administered bronchodilator and corticosteroid drugs often can be reduced carefully and sometimes these agents can be eliminated, but corticosteroids should *never* be stopped abruptly in asthmatic patients. Although some patients may respond to combined cromolyn, bronchodilator, and corticosteroid therapy, the expense may be prohibitive. If combined therapy is prescribed, the physican must individualize the dose of each drug to obtain maximal benefit with minimal adverse reactions. Although a residual effect may persist for approximately four weeks after cromolyn has been discontinued, patients in whom the dose of corticosteroid had been reduced must be observed carefully for an exacerbation of asthma. If a patient receiving cromolyn has an acute attack, conventional therapy should be instituted immediately.

Approximately 8% of a dose is absorbed into the blood stream (primarily by the lung but also by the gastrointestinal tract). Most of the absorbed drug is excreted unchanged within a few days and none appears to undergo metabolic degradation.

The unabsorbed portion (approximately 80%) is recoverable from the feces. Following inhalation, the maximal plasma level of cromolyn is reached within several minutes, and the plasma half-life is 1 to 1.5 hours. The amount of cromolyn that is absorbed into the blood stream following inhalation of 20 mg does not appear to exert any generalized pharmacologic effects.

Based on the extensive clinical experience that has accumulated in many countries, cromolyn appears to have achieved an unusual record of safety (Settipane et al, 1979). Serious adverse effects (anaphylaxis) have been reported only rarely in man. Urticaria and maculopapular rashes, myositis, and gastroenteritis have occurred rarely but cleared when the drug was withdrawn. Reversible eosinophilic pneumonia has been associated with administration of cromolyn in a few patients. Occasionally, patients have complained of transient coughing, throat irritation, dizziness, nausea, vomiting, hoarseness, and wheezing after oral inhalation. However, since some of these symptoms also developed in patients inhaling a placebo, they may have been caused by the powder rather than by cromolyn. Use of an adrenergic bronchodilator in aerosol form prior to inhalation of cromolyn may be helpful for patients who develop coughing or wheezing following use of this drug.

No alterations in the results of hematologic, urinary, hepatic, or renal function tests, chest roentgenograms, or electrocardiograms have been reported in patients receiving the drug continuously for as long as one year. The small amount of cromolyn that is absorbed is excreted unchanged by the liver and kidneys. The implication of this for patients with impaired function of these organs is unknown, but caution is advised when cromolyn is prescribed in these patients.

The safety of cromolyn during pregnancy has not been established unequivocally, but there are anecdotal observations that no damaging effects on the fetus have occurred. No teratogenic effects have been reported in animals, even after the daily intravenous administration of enormous doses of cromolyn throughout pregnancy.

However, increased fetal resorption and decreased fetal weight were observed with dosages that produced toxic effects in the mother.

ROUTE, USUAL DOSAGE, AND PREPARATIONS. *The physician must ensure that the patient is able to use the inhaler effectively, for its inefficient use will reduce the amount of drug reaching the site of action.*
Oral Inhalation: *Adults and children,* one capsule is punctured in the special inhaler. The patient then inhales through the mouthpiece of the inhaler, thereby spinning and vibrating the capsule and introducing its contents into the stream of inspired air. The patient should remove the spinhaler from his mouth and exhale into the air. This step is repeated until all of the powder is inhaled. Initially, four capsules should be inhaled per day. The number of capsules should then be reduced to the lowest amount that will control symptoms. Since any inhaled particulate matter may produce acute pulmonary airflow obstruction in certain patients with hyperirritable airway, use of an inhaled adrenergic bronchodilator prior to cromolyn may lessen this problem.

> *Intal* (Fisons). Capsules 20 mg. Intal Spinhaler supplied separately.

CORTICOSTEROID

BECLOMETHASONE DIPROPIONATE
[Beclovent, Vanceril Inhaler]

Beclomethasone dipropionate is an esterified chlorinated analogue of betamethasone. This highly potent, lipid-soluble corticosteroid acts locally on the respiratory mucosa. The metered-dose inhaler delivers 42 or 50 mcg/puff. The dosage needed increases with the severity of asthma; two puffs three or four times a day are usually satisfactory in mild asthma, but up to 1 mg/day may be necessary in a patient with severe asthma. Adrenal suppression occurs frequently with daily doses of 2 mg and has been observed in a few adults with 1.6 mg.

Many patients receiving oral prednisone (or an equivalent dose of another steroid), especially those requiring 20 mg or less daily to control asthmatic symptoms, can be transferred to beclomethasone with maintenance of good respiratory function and disappearance of reversible adverse effects caused by systemic administration. Caution must be exercised in the transfer. The weekly decrement in dosage of oral steroid during transfer to beclomethasone therapy should not exceed 2.5 mg prednisone or its equivalent per week. Although early morning cortisol levels should be monitored after slowly withdrawing the systemic steroid, a normal level does not always indicate adequate adrenal reserve. Several asthmatic patients have died during the transfer from oral to inhalation steroid therapy, probably because the degree of adrenal suppression was not appreciated and patients died as a result of adrenal crises. If patients undergo stressful situations (surgery, trauma, respiratory infection, or an exacerbation of severe asthma), a short course of a systemically active steroid in full therapeutic doses is indicated.

Patients receiving beclomethasone aerosol occasionally complain of hoarseness, sore throat, or dryness of the mouth. Patients should receive instructions to gargle with water after inhalation to prevent excessive absorption of the drug. The reported incidence of candidal infection of the oropharynx or larynx has varied considerably but probably is less than 15%. Antifungal therapy usually controls this problem, although in some patients it may be necessary to reduce the dose or discontinue beclomethasone therapy.

ROUTE, USUAL DOSAGE, AND PREPARATIONS.
Oral Inhalation: *Adults*, two to four inhalations three or four times daily. The maximum dose should not exceed 1 mg/day. There are insufficient data to recommend a dosage for *children under 6 years*. For *children 6 to 12 years*, the usual dosage

is one or two inhalations three or four times daily. The maximum dose for children is 800 mcg/day. Use of an adrenergic bronchodilator aerosol one or two minutes before inhalation of the steroid may enhance bronchial distribution of the latter or prevent cough and throat irritation.

Beclovent (Meyer). Aerosol suspension 10 mg (50 mcg/actuation).
Vanceril Inhaler (Schering). Aerosol suspension 10 mg (42 mcg/actuation).

MIXTURES

The following mixtures contain an expectorant or decongestant in addition to one or two bronchodilators. There is no evidence that expectorants are effective in asthma. Iodides are not recommended as expectorants for children and women of childbearing age by the Committee on Drugs of the American Academy of Pediatrics. A decongestant is generally only useful temporarily when asthma is complicated by an acute upper respiratory infection. For these reasons, the use of the following combination products is not advised.

Asbron G (Dorsey). Each tablet or 15 ml of elixir contains theophylline sodium glycinate 300 mg equivalent to 150 mg theophylline and guaifenesin 100 mg.
Brondecon (Parke, Davis). Each tablet or 10 ml of elixir contains oxtriphylline 200 mg and guaifenesin 100 mg (alcohol 20%, elixir).
Dilor-G (Savage). Each tablet or 10 ml of liquid contains dyphylline 200 mg and guaifenesin 200 mg.
Duo-Medihaler (Riker). Each measured dose of aerosol contains isoproterenol hydrochloride 0.16 mg and phenylephrine bitartrate 0.24 mg.
Elixophyllin-KI (Berlex). Each 15 ml of elixir contains theophylline (anhydrous) 80 mg and potassium iodide 130 mg (alcohol 10%).
Lufyllin-GG (Mallinckrodt). Each tablet or 30 ml of elixir contains dyphylline 200 mg and guaifenesin 200 mg (alcohol 17%, elixir).
Norisodrine with Calcium Iodide (Abbott). Each 5 ml of syrup contains isoproterenol sulfate 3 mg and calcium iodide (anhydrous) 150 mg (alcohol 6%).
Quibron (Mead Johnson). Each capsule or 15 ml of elixir contains theophylline (anhydrous) 150 mg and guaifenesin 90 mg.
Theo-Organidin (Wallace). Each 15 ml of elixir contains theophylline (anhydrous) 120 mg and iodinated glycerol 30 mg (alcohol 15%).

Other types of mixtures used in asthma and bronchitis contain a barbiturate or antianxiety agent, one or more bronchodilators, and, in some preparations, an expectorant. Use of such mixtures is inadvisable for the following reasons: The efficacy of barbiturates and antianxiety agents in asthma is not documented; furthermore, any sedative may aggravate ventilatory insufficiency and barbiturates may increase the metabolism of corticosteroids given concomitantly. A combination of two adrenergic drugs is no more effective than an optimum dose of either drug used alone. There is evidence that the concomitant adrenergic and theophylline bronchodilators increase expiratory flows over single agents used separately and, thus, concomitant use of a drug from both classes of bronchodilators may be more efficacious. On the other hand, the adrenergic drugs available in mixtures are those with the least beta2 specificity. The undesirable central nervous system stimulant action of ephedrine may be synergistic with that of theophylline. Adjustment of the initial or maintenance dose of theophylline when correlating clinical effect with theophylline blood level is especially difficult or impossible with fixed-dose combination products. Some physicians elect not to change to single-entity products in chronic asthmatics who have responded satisfactorily for an extended period to one of the following combination products; however, the overall disadvantages of these types of combination products should be considered before initiating therapy in newly diagnosed asthmatics.

Amesec (Lilly). Each capsule or enteric-coated tablet contains aminophylline 130 mg, ephedrine hydrochloride 25 mg, and amobarbital 25 mg.

Amodrine (Searle). Each tablet contains aminophylline 100 mg, racephedrine hydrochloride 25 mg, and phenobarbital 8 mg (nonprescription).

Bronkolixir (Breon). Each 5 ml of elixir contains theophylline 15 mg, ephedrine sulfate 12 mg, phenobarbital 4 mg, and guaifenesin 50 mg (alcohol 19%) (nonprescription).

Bronkotabs (Breon). Each tablet contains theophylline 50 or 100 mg, ephedrine sulfate 12 or 24 mg, phenobarbital 4 or 8 mg, and guaifenesin 50 or 100 mg (nonprescription).

Isuprel Compound (Breon). Each 15 ml of elixir contains isoproterenol hydrochloride 2.5 mg, theophylline 45 mg, ephedrine sulfate 12 mg, phenobarbital 6 mg, and potassium iodide 150 mg (alcohol 19%).

Marax (Roerig). Each tablet contains theophylline 130 mg, ephedrine sulfate 25 mg, and hydroxyzine hydrochloride 10 mg.

Mudrane (Poythress). Each tablet contains aminophylline (anhydrous) 130 mg, ephedrine hydrochloride 16 mg, phenobarbital 8 mg, and potassium iodide 195 mg.

Mudrane GG (Poythress). Each 5 ml of elixir contains theophylline 20 mg, ephedrine hydrochloride 4 mg, phenobarbital 2.5 mg, and guaifenesin 26 mg (alcohol 20%); each tablet contains aminophylline (anhydrous) 130 mg, ephedrine hydrochloride 16 mg, phenobarbital 8 mg, and guaifenesin 100 mg.

Quadrinal (Knoll). Each tablet or 10 ml of suspension contains theophylline calcium salicylate 130 mg (equivalent to 65 mg of theophylline anhydrous), ephedrine hydrochloride 24 mg, phenobarbital 24 mg, and potassium iodide 320 mg.

Quibron Plus (Mead Johnson). Each capsule or 15 ml of elixir contains ephedrine hydrochloride 25 mg, theophylline (anhydrous) 150 mg, butabarbital 20 mg, and guaifenesin 100 mg (alcohol 15%, elixir).

Tedral (Parke, Davis). Each tablet, 10 ml of suspension, or 20 ml of elixir contains theophylline 130 mg, ephedrine hydrochloride 24 mg, and phenobarbital 8 mg (alcohol 15%, elixir) (all forms nonprescription).

Tedral SA (Parke, Davis). Each tablet (timed-release) contains theophylline (anhydrous) 180 mg, ephedrine hydrochloride 48 mg, and phenobarbital 25 mg.

Tedral-25 (Parke, Davis). Each tablet contains theophylline 130 mg, ephedrine hydrochloride 24 mg, and butabarbital 25 mg.

Selected References

Arwood LL, et al: Placental transfer of theophylline: Two case reports. *Pediatrics* 63:844-846, 1979.

Ballin JC: Evaluation of new aerosolized steroid for asthma therapy: Beclomethasone dipropionate (Vanceril inhaler). *JAMA* 236: 2891-2893, 1976.

Bell T, Bigley J: Sustained-release theophylline therapy for chronic childhood asthma. *Pediatrics* 62:352-358, 1978.

Bernstein IL, et al: Therapy with cromolyn sodium. *Ann Intern Med* 89:228-233, 1978.

Finkel MJ: Salbutamol: Lack of evidence of tumor induction in man. *Br Med J* 1:649, 1978.

Ginchansky E, Weinberger M: Relationship of theophylline clearance to oral dosage in children with chronic asthma. *J Pediatr* 91:655-660, 1977.

Gisclon LG, et al: Pharmacokinetics of orally administered dyphylline. *Am J Hosp Pharm* 36:1179-1184, 1979.

Goldstein RS, et al: Severe asthma: Prevention is better than cure. *Drugs* 16:256-267, 1978.

Heel RC, et al: Fenoterol: Review of its pharmacological properties and therapeutic efficacy in asthma. *Drugs* 15:3-32, 1978.

Hendeles L, et al: Guide to oral theophylline therapy for treatment of chronic asthma. *Am J Dis Child* 132:876-880, 1978.

Hodgkins JE, et al: Chronic obstructive airway diseases: Current concepts in diagnosis and comprehensive care. *JAMA* 232:1243-1260, 1975.

König P: Pharmacologic management of childhood asthma. *Adv Asthma Allergy Pulm Dis* 5:2-8, 1978.

Leifer KN, Wittig HJ: Beta-2 sympathomimetic aerosols in treatment of asthma. *Ann Allergy* 35:69-80, 1975.

Nilsson BS (ed): Scandinavian symposium on chronic obstructive airway disease. *Scand J Resp Dis* Suppl 103:105-223, 1979.

Plummer AL: Choosing a drug regimen for obstructive pulmonary disease: 1. Agents to achieve bronchodilatation. 2. Agents other than bronchodilators. *Postgrad Med* 63:36-48, 113-119, (April, May) 1978 A.

Plummer AL: Development of drug tolerance to beta2 adrenergic agents. *Chest* 73(suppl):949-956, (June) 1978 B.

Rangsithienchai P, Newcomb RW: Aminophylline therapy in children: Guidelines for dosage. *J Pediatr* 91:325-330, 1977.

Settipane GA, et al: Adverse reactions to cromolyn. *JAMA* 241:811-813, 1979.

Weinberger M, Hendeles L: Antiasthmatic drugs, in Miller RR, Greenblatt DJ (eds): *Handbook of Drug Therapy*. New York, Elsevier, 1979, 927-951.

Weinberger M, et al: Relation of product formulation to absorption of oral theophylline. *N Engl J Med* 299:852-857, 1978.

Wilson AF, McPhillips JJ: Pharmacological control of asthma. *Annu Rev Pharmacol Toxicol* 18:541-561, 1978.

Wolfe JD, et al: Bronchodilator effects of terbutaline and aminophylline alone and in combination in asthmatic patients. *N Engl J Med* 298:363-367, 1978.

Agents Used to Treat Congestive Heart Failure | 33

The goals in the treatment of congestive heart failure are to increase cardiac output and to relieve pulmonary congestion and peripheral edema. Therapy is directed toward improving one or more of the four determinants of cardiac performance: myocardial contractility, left ventricular filling pressure (preload), systemic vascular resistance (aortic impedance), and heart rate. The principal drugs used are the digitalis glycosides, which increase contractility; diuretics, which reduce preload; and antiarrhythmic agents, which normalize cardiac rate and rhythm (see Chapter 34). Vasodilators reduce aortic impedance and may be useful in selected patients.

DIURETICS

In treating chronic congestive heart failure, the traditional approach has been to initiate therapy with digitalis, a low-sodium diet, and restriction of activities,

with a diuretic given concurrently or added later if symptoms are not adequately controlled. In recent years, the concept that digitalis should be given to all patients with congestive heart failure has been questioned (Cohn, 1974). Reduction of preload with diuretics will often relieve congestive symptoms as effectively as digitalis, particularly when edema is the major manifestation. Diuretics alone are now used frequently for initial therapy of patients with mild congestive heart failure and normal sinus rhythm. They also are useful as adjuncts in the treatment of hypertensive heart failure and acute pulmonary edema resulting from left ventricular failure (see Chapter 39).

DIGITALIS GLYCOSIDES

Digitalis has complex direct and indirect cardiovascular actions that are of value in the treatment of congestive heart failure and most supraventricular tachyar-

497

rhythmias. The beneficial effect of digitalis in congestive heart failure derives from its ability to enhance myocardial contractility. This direct positive inotropic action increases cardiac output and thereby decreases venous pressure, reduces heart size, and slows compensatory *reflex* tachycardia. The consequent improvement in renal hemodynamics promotes diuresis, thus reducing blood volume and relieving edema. The digitalis glycosides also have a mild direct diuretic action that is independent of changes in the glomerular filtration rate and renal blood flow. In patients with congestive heart failure and normal sinus rhythm, the effect of digitalis on resting hemodynamics may be transient, whereas the hemodynamic improvement during exercise is sustained during long-term therapy (Vogel et al, 1977).

The antiarrhythmic actions of digitalis include (1) lengthening of the A-V nodal conduction time and refractory period due to an increase in vagal tone, an antiadrenergic action, and possibly a direct effect; (2) shortening of the atrial muscle refractory period due to enhanced vagal tone; (3) shortening of the ventricular muscle refractory period by a direct action; and (4) enhancement of myocardial contractility.

Uses of Digitalis

The positive inotropic effect of digitalis is useful in most patients with congestive heart failure, but the response to therapy depends upon the underlying etiology and the extent of myocardial damage. Digitalis is most effective in congestive failure associated with coronary artery disease and in hypertensive heart failure that cannot be controlled by antihypertensive therapy. It is of limited usefulness in cor pulmonale or in the high-output failure associated with thyrotoxicosis, chronic anemia, beriberi, or A-V fistulas; in these disorders, effective therapy involves correction of the underlying cause. Glycoside therapy is usually of little value in restoring compensation when congestive heart failure develops in conjunction with chronic constrictive

pericarditis, myocarditis, or mitral stenosis with normal sinus rhythm. In idiopathic hypertrophic subaortic stenosis, digitalis may increase the outflow obstruction and should be avoided unless there is an associated arrhythmia that responds to glycoside therapy.

Opinion is divided on the benefits and potential dangers of glycoside therapy in acute myocardial infarction. Digitalis is not indicated in patients without signs of cardiac decompensation unless a supraventricular tachyarrhythmia is present. Atrial tachyarrhythmias occurring during acute myocardial infarction are often transient but, if they persist, digitalis (or, in emergencies, DC cardioversion) is indicated to slow the ventricular rate. Mild congestive failure is common after myocardial infarction and, if pulmonary congestion develops, a diuretic is often preferred for initial treatment. Digitalis may be administered if heart failure worsens, but therapy should be instituted very cautiously and with small doses to avoid precipitating ventricular arrhythmias. Acute pulmonary edema caused by left ventricular failure represents an immediate threat to life, and glycoside therapy is of secondary importance to more rapidly effective modes of treatment (ie, placing the patient in an upright position; administering morphine, furosemide, and oxygen; applying tourniquets). Vasodilators may be especially helpful in this situation. The treatment of cardiogenic shock is controversial and mortality is high. Digitalis does not appear to be useful for the acute management of this syndrome, but other inotropic agents may be effective (see Chapter 37, Agents Used to Treat Shock). Drug therapy may not always produce an adequate response, however, and cardiac assist systems are often required.

Because it slows A-V conduction and produces a relative degree of A-V block, digitalis is the drug of choice for controlling the ventricular rate in patients with atrial fibrillation, and it may convert the arrhythmia to normal sinus rhythm. Digitalis is less effective in controlling the ventricular response to atrial flutter; in some cases, it may convert flutter to fibrillation (which is easier to control) or to sinus rhythm. Digitalis is also useful in paroxysmal supraventricular tachycardia that does not respond to conventional measures. Sinus tachycardia and supraventricular or ventricular premature beats may respond to digitalis when these arrhythmias are primarily due to congestive heart failure, but sinus tachycardia in the nonfailing heart is *not* altered by digitalis. The indications for use of digitalis in antiarrhythmic therapy are discussed in more detail in Chapter 34.

In patients with heart disease but with no signs of overt failure, digitalis is sometimes given prophylactically prior to cardiac surgery and in other stressful situations (eg, severe illness, pregnancy). There is considerable debate about the merits of prophylactic digitalization, because (1) it is difficult to determine an effective dose in patients who have no signs of congestive heart failure or a supraventricular tachyarrhythmia; (2) if postoperative arrhythmias occur, they may be treated more easily in nondigitalized patients; and (3) if the patient is not receiving digitalis, the drug cannot be implicated as a possible cause of postoperative arrhythmias.

See also Chung, 1971, and Smith, 1973.

Factors Modifying Response to Digitalis Therapy

The response to digitalis is influenced by many factors, including the nature and severity of the underlying heart disease; the patient's age; status of renal function and electrolyte balance; the presence of noncardiac disorders; and the concomitant use of other drugs. Dosage must be individualized, and conditions that predispose to toxicity (eg, hypokalemia, hypercalcemia, hypothyroidism, hypomagnesemia) should be corrected. Impaired renal function (frequently seen in the elderly) necessitates a reduction in digoxin dosage, because this glycoside is excreted largely unchanged in the urine. Digitoxin, on the other hand, is extensively metabolized before excretion and should be used cau-

tiously in patients with hepatic dysfunction.

In the past, digoxin tablets from different manufacturers varied greatly in bioavailability, and a change from one brand to another could result in digitalis intoxication or underdigitalization. Such differences appear to be less of a problem today because of new bioavailability standards (Greenblatt et al, 1976). Antacids, kaolin-pectin preparations, cholestyramine resin, neomycin, and sulfasalazine reduce the bioavailability of digitalis glycosides.

In patients with atrial fibrillation or flutter, the optimal dosage of digitalis is the smallest amount that will control the ventricular rate at rest and during slight exercise. An adequate therapeutic response depends in large measure upon the ability of digitalis to produce a relative degree of A-V block, and larger doses are generally required than for treatment of congestive heart failure. If the ventricular rate is not controlled by nontoxic doses, the addition of propranolol [Inderal] to the regimen may permit a reduction in dose of the glycoside and provide better control of the ventricular response.

It is more difficult to determine proper dosage for patients with congestive heart failure and sinus rhythm. A satisfactory response is manifested by diuresis, weight loss, reduction in pulmonary and systemic venous congestion, decrease in heart size and/or rate, and relief of peripheral edema, fatigue, shortness of breath, and orthopnea. If digitalis is the initial and only therapeutic agent employed, these endpoints are useful as a guide in titrating dosage. However, rest, sodium restriction, and diuretic therapy are also prescribed for most patients with moderately severe heart failure. Since these measures reduce the load on the heart and relieve edema, the relative contribution of digitalis to the therapeutic response often cannot be accurately assessed. If clinical improvement is not satisfactory, the dose of digitalis may be increased cautiously or the diuretic regimen altered.

Patients receiving maintenance therapy with digitalis should be re-evaluated periodically to determine whether dosage should be adjusted or the drug discontinued. This is particularly important in geriatric patients because of the high incidence and severity of toxic reactions in this age group. Many patients with heart failure and/or arrhythmias associated with anemia, beriberi, thyrotoxicosis, or valvular heart disease do not need digitalis after correction of the underlying cause. Heart failure and arrhythmias that occur during the course of acute myocardial infarction also may be transient and may not require long-term glycoside therapy.

All digitalis glycosides possess the same pharmacologic actions, but they vary in potency, onset of action, rate of absorption, and rate and route of excretion. The physician should become thoroughly familiar with one or two preparations (usually digoxin and/or digitoxin) and then restrict his use to those agents. The choice of preparation, dosage, and route of administration depends upon the clinical situation. When prompt action is required (ie, supraventricular tachyarrhythmias with a rapid ventricular rate, acute pulmonary edema due to acute left ventricular failure), a glycoside with a rapid onset of action (digoxin, deslanoside, or ouabain) may be given intravenously. Of these three drugs, ouabain acts most rapidly, but its dosage is the most difficult to regulate for continued digitalization. Digoxin and deslanoside have a comparable onset (10 to 30 minutes) and peak action (two to three hours); digoxin is usually preferred because the oral maintenance dose is easily established after intravenous therapy and because its concentration in the serum can be measured, if necessary.

The orally administered glycosides, digoxin and digitoxin, are used initially when the clinical situation is not sufficiently urgent to require parenteral digitalization and for maintenance after emergency intravenous therapy. Rapid oral digitalization may be suitable for some patients with supraventricular tachyarrhythmias or acute congestive heart failure, although the intravenous route is often preferred. Slower digitalization is indicated in chronic congestive heart failure without acute symptoms and may be accomplished in

two ways: by a loading dose followed by maintenance therapy or, more gradually, by giving the maintenance dose each day and allowing the patient to become fully digitalized over a longer period of time. Digoxin has the advantage of having a relatively short half-life (32 to 48 hours), which makes toxic reactions easier to manage if they occur. Some physicians prefer digitoxin for prolonged therapy because its longer half-life (five to nine days) provides a more sustained therapeutic effect. If digitoxin is substituted for digoxin for maintenance therapy, slow redigitalization may be required because of the difference in duration of action of the two glycosides.

Radioimmunoassay techniques for measuring serum levels of digoxin and digitoxin can be instituted in most hospitals. The serum digitalis concentration can be useful to assess compliance; to detect underdigitalization; to determine whether digitalis has been ingested when this is in doubt; to monitor patients predisposed to toxicity; and to detect problems in absorption caused by gastrointestinal disorders, concomitant use of other drugs, or poor bioavailability (Weintraub, 1977). The value of serum levels in diagnosing toxicity has not been clearly established (Ingelfinger and Goldman, 1976); when used for this purpose, serum levels must be evaluated in conjunction with clinical information, electrocardiographic changes, and results of other laboratory tests. A "therapeutic" serum level for one patient may be excessive or inadequate for another. Infants and children may tolerate higher serum levels than adults.

See also Chung, 1971; Doherty and Kane, 1973; and Doherty et al, 1978.

Adverse Reactions and Precautions

The ratio between the full therapeutic and toxic dose of digitalis is narrow, and results of epidemiologic studies have shown that up to 20% of hospitalized patients receiving digitalis may develop some signs of intoxication. The mortality rate in patients who experience cardiotoxic effects has been estimated to range from 3% to

39%. Digitalis intoxication usually results from too rapid loading, from accumulation of larger than necessary maintenance doses, from prescribing digitalis in doses beyond reasonable limits when it is not likely to be effective, from the presence of conditions that predispose to toxicity, or from intentional or accidental overdose.

In most instances, intoxication can be prevented by evaluating therapy frequently, by decreasing dosage in the presence of factors that tend to cause excessive accumulation (eg, impaired renal function), by correcting conditions that increase toxicity (eg, hypokalemia, alkalosis, hypercalcemia, hypoxia, hypomagnesemia), or by treating underlying diseases (eg, hypothyroidism, anemia, valvular heart disease). When the risk of intoxication is great, use of a short-acting, rapidly eliminated glycoside is advisable. Although intoxication cannot always be avoided by selecting one glycoside over another, certain glycosides may be preferred in patients with fixed disabilities that increase the risk of intoxication (eg, digitoxin for patients with elevated creatinine levels). In homes where young children reside with adults taking digitalis, the medication should be kept safely out of reach.

Quinidine increases serum digoxin levels, possibly by displacing the digoxin from tissue binding sites. This interaction may lead to gastrointestinal disturbances and ventricular arrhythmias, which can be controlled by reducing the dose of digoxin (Leahey et al, 1978). When initiating quinidine therapy in patients receiving digoxin, it may be advisable to monitor serum digoxin levels.

Newborn infants with heart disease, especially premature infants, are particularly susceptible to digitalis intoxication, and frequent electrocardiographic monitoring is essential in these patients. Similarly, special care must be exercised in elderly patients receiving digitalis because their body mass tends to be small and renal clearance is likely to be reduced. In addition, digitalis must be used with great caution in the presence of active heart disease, such as acute myocardial infarction or acute myocarditis. In patients with

acute or unstable chronic atrial fibrillation, digitalis may not normalize the ventricular rate even when the serum concentration exceeds the usual "therapeutic" level. Although these patients may be less sensitive to the toxic effects of digitalis than those with sinus rhythm, it may be preferable to add propranolol to the regimen rather than to increase the dose of digitalis to potentially toxic levels.

Hypokalemia predisposes to digitalis toxicity and even a moderate reduction of the serum potassium concentration can precipitate serious arrhythmias. Hypokalemia is most frequently encountered in patients receiving long-term daily or alternate-day diuretic therapy, for the most widely used and most effective diuretics (ie, thiazides, furosemide) increase the urinary excretion of potassium. A reliable method for maintaining the serum potassium level is to prescribe a potassium-sparing agent (spironolactone [Aldactone] or triamterene [Dyrenium]) along with the potassium-wasting diuretic. Alternatively, potassium chloride supplements may be prescribed; in children, potassium-containing foods may be preferable.

Extracardiac Reactions: The early signs of digitalis intoxication may not be serious, but they serve as a warning that severe cardiac toxicity can result if the drug is not temporarily discontinued or the dosage reduced. Extracardiac manifestations of toxicity include gastrointestinal and neurologic disturbances.

Anorexia, nausea, vomiting, and abdominal pain are the most common gastrointestinal symptoms. Diarrhea occurs rarely. The emetic effect of digitalis is probably of central origin and occurs after either oral or parenteral administration. Digitalis leaf also may cause direct gastric irritation.

Fatigue is the most common neurologic manifestation of toxicity. Other symptoms are depression, drowsiness, weakness, restlessness, nightmares, personality changes, headache, vertigo, confusion, and, rarely, psychotic reactions. Ocular disturbances include blurred vision, photophobia, modified color perception, visions of flashing or flickering lights, scotomata, and amblyopia. These complications may be symptoms of retrobulbar neuritis or they may be caused by an effect of digitalis on the retinal receptor cells.

Gynecomastia and hypersensitivity reactions (urticaria, eosinophilia) occur rarely and generally are not considered to be manifestations of overdosage.

Cardiac Reactions: In a large percentage of patients, a disturbance of cardiac rhythm may be the first evidence of digitalis intoxication. Almost any type of arrhythmia may occur; the most common are multifocal ventricular premature complexes and nonparoxysmal A-V junctional (nodal) tachycardia. The latter dysrhythmia is particularly likely to occur in the presence of pre-existing atrial fibrillation. Other digitalis-induced arrhythmias include sinus irregularities (sinus bradycardia, S-A block, sinus arrest), atrial tachycardia with varying degrees of A-V block, unifocal ventricular premature complexes, accelerated ventricular rhythm, and paroxysmal ventricular tachycardia. A-V dissociation may be induced by a combination of some degree of A-V block plus junctional (or ventricular) tachycardia. A bidirectional tachycardia, recently shown to be ventricular in origin, indicates an advanced stage of digitalis intoxication. Atrial fibrillation or flutter induced by digitalis is very rare. Treatment of digitalis-induced arrhythmias consists of discontinuing glycoside therapy, determining serum potassium levels, and, if indicated, administering potassium chloride and/or antiarrhythmic drugs. (See Chapter 34.)

See also Chung, 1969.

INDIVIDUAL EVALUATIONS

The dosage for all digitalis glycosides should be individualized and titrated in terms of the therapeutic response. The dose needed to increase myocardial contractility is generally smaller than that required to decrease the ventricular response in atrial fibrillation. The dose required to control the ventricular rate during various supraventricular tachyarrhythmias may differ. Generally, a larger amount is required to slow the ven-tricular rate during atrial flutter than during atrial fibrillation, and the ventricular response to atrial flutter is not easily controllable for prolonged periods.

DIGOXIN
[Lanoxin]

$(C_6H_{10}O_3)_3H$
(tridigitoxose)

Digoxin is the most widely used digitalis glycoside. Onset of action is within 5 to 30 minutes after an intravenous dose and within one to two hours after oral administration. The maximal effect is obtained within two to six hours, depending upon the route of administration.

Many cardiologists prefer digoxin to other digitalis glycosides because its rapid onset of action makes it useful in emergency situations; its relatively short duration of action (half-life approximately 32 to 48 hours) makes toxic reactions easier to manage; it can be administered both orally and parenterally, making the maintenance dosage easy to establish after emergency intravenous use; and a liquid preparation is available for oral therapy in infants and children.

Although digoxin is almost completely absorbed when administered in oral solution, tablets from different manufacturers have, in the past, varied in bioavailability. Peak serum levels as well as area under the serum time curve and urinary excretion varied widely with different tablet formulations, and this variation was reflected in the steady-state value. New regulations require all marketed digoxin tablets to conform to a bioavailability standard, and differences among preparations appear to be less of a problem today than in the past (Greenblatt et al, 1976).

Therapeutic serum levels of digoxin generally range from 0.5 to 2.5 ng/ml. (Many commercial digoxin radioimmunoassay kits cannot clearly distinguish digoxin levels between 0 and 0.5 ng/ml. Those with the greatest sensitivity are manufactured by Burroughs Wellcome, Kallestad, and Squibb [Kubasik et al, 1976].) Spironolactone, sex hormones, bile salts, and other digitalis glycosides and metabolites may interfere with results of digoxin assays (Weintraub, 1977).

Digoxin is excreted largely unchanged in the urine. In patients with impaired renal function, dosage must be reduced on the basis of the creatinine clearance, because the half-life of the drug is prolonged when glomerular filtration is impaired.

See the Introduction for a discussion of indications and toxicity.

ROUTES, USUAL DOSAGE, AND PREPARATIONS. The following dosages are given to patients who have not received digitalis for at least two weeks. Smaller loading and maintenance doses should be used in small or elderly patients and in those with impaired renal function, electrolyte disturbances (particularly hypokalemia), or metabolic abnormalities (particularly hypothyroidism).

Oral: *Adults*, the average digitalizing dose is 1 to 1.5 mg. For rapid digitalization, initially, 0.5 to 0.75 mg, followed by 0.25 to 0.5 mg every six to eight hours until full digitalization. For slow digitalization and maintenance, 0.125 to 0.5 mg daily (0.125 to 0.25 mg in the elderly), depending upon lean body weight and renal function as determined by creatinine clearance. The dose should be reduced as renal function decreases. *Institution of maintenance therapy without a loading dose is suitable for many patients with congestive heart failure.* Therapeutic serum levels are achieved after six to seven days of maintenance therapy in patients with normal renal function. Single daily doses are usually satisfactory for maintenance; however, it may be necessary to give the drug in two divided doses to some patients with recurrent supraventricular tachyarrhythmias. For children, the following digitalizing doses are given in divided amounts at

six-hour intervals: *Newborn infants*, 0.03 to 0.05 mg/kg of body weight; *1 month to 2 years*, 0.05 to 0.07 mg/kg; *over 2 years*, 0.03 to 0.05 mg/kg. The daily maintenance dose is approximately 20% to 30% of the digitalizing dose.

Drug available generically: Tablets 0.125, 0.25, and 0.5 mg.

Lanoxin (Burroughs Wellcome). Elixir (pediatric) 0.05 mg/ml; tablets 0.125, 0.25, and 0.5 mg.

Intravenous: *Adults*, the average digitalizing dose is 0.5 to 1 mg. Initially, 0.25 to 0.5 mg, followed by 0.25 mg at four- to six-hour intervals if needed to a total dose of 1 mg. For maintenance, 0.125 to 0.5 mg daily. For children, the following digitalizing doses are given in divided amounts at six-hour intervals: *Newborn infants*, 0.015 to 0.03 mg/kg of body weight; *2 weeks to 2 years*, 0.025 to 0.04 mg/kg; *over 2 years*, 0.015 to 0.03 mg/kg. The daily maintenance dose is approximately 20% to 30% of the digitalizing dose.

Drug available generically: Solution 0.125 mg/ml in 2 ml containers and 0.25 mg/ml in 1 and 2 ml containers.

Lanoxin (Burroughs Wellcome). Solution 0.1 mg/ml in 1 ml containers and 0.25 mg/ml in 2 ml containers.

DIGITOXIN

[Crystodigin, Purodigin]

(tridigitoxose)

Digitoxin is the chief active glycoside in digitalis leaf; 1 mg of digitoxin is therapeutically equivalent to approximately 1 g of digitalis leaf. Although digitoxin is administered less commonly today than formerly, it continues to be useful for maintenance therapy because its long half-life (five to nine days) provides a sustained therapeutic effect even if a dose is missed. This is a particular advantage in patients with recurrent supraventricular tachyarrhythmias.

Digitoxin is almost completely absorbed from the gastrointestinal tract. Equivalent oral or intravenous doses produce essentially the same therapeutic effect, and intravenous administration is generally unnecessary unless the patient is unable to take medication orally. When given orally, the onset of action is one to four hours and the maximal effect is attained in 8 to 12 hours. Therapeutic serum levels range from 15 to 25 ng/ml and no variation in bioavailability has been encountered among different preparations.

Digitoxin is 90% bound to plasma protein. It is extensively metabolized in the liver, excreted in the bile, recycled, and eventually excreted in the urine, 80% as inactive metabolites. Since little of the parent compound is eliminated by renal clearance, the half-life of digitoxin is not increased in patients with impaired renal function, and it may be the glycoside of choice in these patients. Digitoxin should be given with caution and possibly in reduced dosage to patients with hepatic dysfunction. Drugs that increase hepatic microsomal enzyme activity (eg, barbiturates, phenytoin) increase the rate of metabolism of digitoxin and may lower plasma levels.

See the Introduction for a discussion of indications and toxicity.

ROUTES, USUAL DOSAGE, AND PREPARATIONS. The following dosages are given to patients who have not received digitalis for at least two weeks. Smaller loading and maintenance doses should be used in small or elderly patients or in those with electrolyte disturbances (particularly hypokalemia) or metabolic abnormalities (particularly hypothyroidism).

Oral: Adults, for rapid digitalization, initially 0.8 mg, then 0.2 mg every six to eight hours for two or three doses. For slower digitalization, 0.1 to 0.2 mg one to three times daily to a total of approximately 1.2 to 1.8 mg. For maintenance, 0.1 mg daily (range, 0.05 to 0.2 mg). These doses may be given intravenously if the patient cannot take oral medication.

> Drug available generically: Tablets 0.1 and 0.2 mg.
> Crystodigin (Lilly). Tablets 0.05, 0.1, 0.15, and 0.2 mg.

Purodigin (Wyeth). Tablets 0.1, 0.15, and 0.2 mg.

Oral, Intramuscular, Intravenous: For children, the following digitalizing doses are given in three or more divided doses at intervals of six hours or more: Newborn infants, 0.025 mg/kg of body weight; 2 weeks to 1 year, 0.035 to 0.045 mg/kg; 1 to 2 years, 0.04 mg/kg; over 2 years, 0.02 to 0.03 mg/kg. The maintenance dose is approximately 10% of the digitalizing dose.

For oral preparations, see above.

> Drug available generically: Solution 0.2 mg/ml in 1 ml containers.
> Crystodigin (Lilly). Solution 0.2 mg/ml in 1 ml containers.

DIGITALIS LEAF

This preparation contains a mixture of glycosides as active principles and is the least potent digitalis preparation on a weight basis. Its potency is standardized biologically and it is available only for oral use. Digitalis leaf has approximately the same onset, peak effect, duration of action, and route of metabolism as digitoxin; however, since purer, more standardized preparations are preferred, digitalis leaf is used less commonly than digoxin and digitoxin.

Digitalis leaf may cause gastric irritation, but nausea and vomiting are more frequently caused by a central effect. For indications and other adverse reactions, see the Introduction.

ROUTE, USUAL DOSAGE, AND PREPARATIONS. The following dosage is given to patients who have not received digitalis for at least two weeks. Smaller doses should be used in small or elderly patients or in those with electrolyte disturbances (particularly hypokalemia) or metabolic abnormalities (particularly hypothyroidism).

Oral: Adults, the average total digitalizing dose is 1.2 to 1.8 g. The average maintenance dose is 100 mg daily.

> Drug available generically: Capsules, tablets 100 mg.
> SIMILAR DRUGS.
> Digifortis (Parke, Davis), Digiglusin (Lilly).

DESLANOSIDE
[Cedilanid-D]

$(C_6H_{10}O_3)_3 - C_6H_{11}O_5$
(tridigitoxose – glucose)

Deslanoside is derived from lanatoside C. It has essentially the same pharmacologic properties as the natural parent glycoside but is available only for parenteral use. Deslanoside is used intravenously in emergencies, and orally administered glycosides are then substituted for maintenance therapy. The onset of action is 10 to 30 minutes and maximal effects are obtained in two to three hours. Because it may be difficult to transfer a patient from deslanoside to an oral agent, intravenous digoxin is usually preferred.

For a discussion of toxicity, see the Introduction.

ROUTES, USUAL DOSAGE, AND PREPARATIONS. The following dosages are given to patients who have not received digitalis for at least two weeks. Smaller doses should be used in small or elderly patients and in those with impaired renal function, electrolyte disturbances (particularly hypokalemia), or metabolic abnormalities (particularly hypothyroidism).
Intravenous: *Adults*, initially 0.8 mg, then 0.4 mg every two to four hours to a maximum of 2 mg. (The drug may also be given intramuscularly but the intravenous route is preferred for immediate action.)
Intravenous, Intramuscular: For children, the following doses are given in two or three divided portions at three- or four-hour intervals: *Newborn infants*, 0.022 mg/kg of body weight; *2 weeks to 3 years*, 0.025 mg/kg; *over 3 years*, 0.0225 mg/kg.
  Cedilanid-D (Sandoz). Solution 0.2 mg/ml in 2 ml containers.
  Note: This drug is marketed only in a parenteral form. It should not be confused with lanatoside C [Cedilanid], which is used orally.

OUABAIN

$C_6H_{11}O_4$
(rhamnose)

$\cdot\ 8H_2O$

The onset of action of ouabain is three to ten minutes, and maximal effects are obtained within 30 to 60 minutes. Ouabain is metabolized and excreted in the same manner as digoxin (see that evaluation), and its half-life is approximately 21 hours.

Ouabain is administered intravenously in emergencies, and orally administered glycosides are then substituted for maintenance therapy. In fractional doses, ouabain is sometimes used acutely in patients who are already receiving glycoside therapy to determine whether an increase in digitalis dosage would provide further improvement.

Despite its relatively short duration of action, which tends to make toxic manifestations relatively transient, ouabain can easily cause intoxication because of its rapid onset, particularly when a physician is not experienced with its use. For a discussion of toxicity, see the Introduction.

ROUTE, USUAL DOSAGE, AND PREPARATIONS. The following dosages are given to patients who have not received digitalis for at least two weeks. Smaller doses should be used in small or elderly patients and in those with impaired renal function, electrolyte disturbances (particularly hypokalemia), or metabolic abnormalities (particularly hypothyroidism).

Intravenous: *Adults*, initially 0.25 to 0.5 mg, then 0.1 mg every 60 minutes if needed (maximum, 1 mg within a 24-hour period).

  Drug available generically: Solution 0.25 mg/ml in 2 ml containers.

GITALIN
[Gitaligin]

LANATOSIDE C
[Cedilanid]

$(C_6H_{10}O_3)_2 - C_8H_{12}O_4 - C_6H_{11}O_5$
(didigitoxose – acetyldigitoxose – glucose)

These preparations are used less commonly than the other orally administered glycosides, and they have not been studied as extensively as either digoxin or digitoxin. See the Introduction for a discussion of indications and toxicity.

ROUTE, USUAL DOSAGE, AND PREPARATIONS. Following are the manufacturers' recommended dosages for patients who have not received digitalis for at least two weeks. Smaller loading and maintenance doses should be used in small or elderly patients and in those with impaired renal function, electrolyte disturbances (particularly hypokalemia), or metabolic disturbances (particularly hypothyroidism).

GITALIN:

Oral: Adults, for rapid digitalization, initially 2.5 mg, followed by 0.75 mg every six hours to a total dose of approximately 6 mg. For slow digitalization, 1.5 mg daily for four to six days. For maintenance, 0.25 to 1.25 mg daily (average dose, 0.5 mg).
Gitaligin (Schering). Tablets 0.5 mg.

LANATOSIDE C:

Oral: Adults, the average total digitalizing dose is 10 mg given in divided doses over a number of days. For maintenance, 0.5 to 1.5 mg daily.
Cedilanid (Sandoz). Tablets 0.5 mg.
Note: This drug is marketed only in an oral form. It should not be confused with deslanoside [Cedilanid-D], which is used parenterally.

VASODILATORS

Attention has recently been directed toward aortic impedance as an important determinant of left ventricular performance. The reflex increase in sympathetic tone commonly observed in patients with severe heart failure serves to improve myocardial contractility and maintain perfusion of vital organs. On the other hand, cardiac work is increased and cardiac output further reduced because of the elevated systemic vascular resistance. Vasodilator drugs have been used effectively to enhance cardiac performance in selected patients with severe pump failure following acute myocardial infarction (see Chapter 37, Agents Used to Treat Shock) and in those with chronic congestive heart failure refractory to conventional therapy with digitalis and diuretics. By dilating resistance vessels, vasodilators reduce impedance to left ventricular ejection and thus may increase cardiac output in patients with acute or chronic heart failure. Many of these agents also reduce left ventricular filling pressure by increasing venous capacitance, but reduction of aortic impedance is believed to be the major mechanism whereby cardiac performance is improved (Cohn and Franciosa, 1977; Chatterjee and Parmley, 1977; Mason, 1978).

Vasodilators are not indicated for *routine* use. They are beneficial primarily in patients with severe, low-output refractory heart failure due to ischemic heart disease, primary cardiomyopathy, or mitral or aortic insufficiency, and in those with acute myocardial infarction who have pre-existing hypertension or recurrent ischemic pain (Cohn and Franciosa, 1977).

The potent vasodilator, sodium nitroprusside [Nipride], is usually preferred for short-term intravenous therapy. Phentolamine [Regitine], trimethaphan [Arfonad], hexamethonium, and nitroglycerin (intravenous preparation is investigational) also have been used for this purpose. Because it has a balanced dilator action on both the arterial and venous beds, nitroprusside reduces left ventricular filling pressure and increases cardiac output in patients with intractable, low-output chronic congestive heart failure. The increase in stroke volume usually counterbalances the fall in peripheral vascular resistance so that arterial blood pressure is not greatly reduced in these patients. Heart rate is usually not increased and may decrease because of the improved hemodynamics. Nitroprusside appears to be most beneficial in patients with marked pump dysfunction, greatly elevated left ventricular end diastolic pressure, and increased peripheral vascular resistance (Miller et al, 1975). Adrenergic inotropic agents, such as dopamine [Intropin], dobutamine [Dobutrex], and ephedrine, enhance the effectiveness of nitroprusside, and combined inotropic-vasodilator therapy may be particularly useful when congestive heart failure is complicated by

MAJOR VASODILATOR DRUGS USED
TO TREAT REFRACTORY HEART FAILURE

Drug	Actions and Uses	Route of Administration and Doses	Significant Adverse Reactions
Sodium Nitroprusside Nipride (Roche)	Direct-acting vasodilator with balanced effect on arterial and venous beds and little effect on heart rate. Useful for short-term therapy.	*Intravenous:* 15 to 200 mcg/min	Hypotension, increased blood levels of thiocyanate and cyanide*
Phentolamine Mesylate Regitine Mesylate (Ciba)	Alpha-adrenergic blocking drug with predominant effect on arterial bed. Not as useful as nitroprusside because it causes more tachycardia and is expensive.	*Intravenous:* 0.2 to 2 mg/min	Hypotension, tachycardia*
Isosorbide Dinitrate Isordil (Ives) Sorbitrate (Stuart)	Antianginal drug that acts primarily to reduce venous tone; also reduces peripheral vascular resistance and improves coronary blood flow. Oral formulation has relatively long duration of action (4 to 6 hours) and is useful for long-term therapy; chewable formulation has duration of action of approximately 3 hours. Sublingual formulation is less useful because of shorter duration of action.	*Oral:* 20 to 80 mg 3 or 4 times daily	Orthostatic hypotension, headache, dependence (?)†
Nitroglycerin Ointment Nitro-Bid (Marion) Nitrol (Kremers-Urban) Nitrong (Wharton)	Same as isosorbide dinitrate. Hemodynamic effects last up to six hours.	*Topical:* 1.5 to 4 inches	Orthostatic hypotension, headache, dependence (?)†
Hydralazine Hydrochloride Apresoline Hydrochloride (Ciba)	Direct-acting vasodilator that reduces peripheral vascular resistance but has little or no effect on capacitance vessels. May be most useful when given with a nitrate for long-term therapy.	*Oral:* 50 to 75 mg every 6 hours	Tachycardia, headache, fluid retention, SLE syndrome*
Prazosin Hydrochloride Minipress (Pfizer)	Alpha-adrenergic blocking drug with arterial and venous dilator effect. Tolerance has been reported during long-term therapy.	*Oral:* 2 to 7 mg 4 times daily	Orthostatic hypotension, syncopal reactions*

*See also Chapter 38, Antihypertensive Agents.
†See also Chapter 35, Antianginal Agents.

mild or moderate hypotension (Miller et al, 1977). (See also Chapter 37, Agents Used to Treat Shock.)

Several nonparenteral vasodilators are under investigation for long-term therapy. These include isosorbide dinitrate [Isordil, Sorbitrate], nitroglycerin ointment [Nitro-Bid, Nitrol, Nitrong], hydralazine [Apresoline], and prazosin [Minipress]. The nitrates act predominantly to increase venous capacitance, but they also dilate resistance vessels and coronary arteries and arterioles. Although nitrates do not increase cardiac output as effectively as nitroprusside, both oral and chewable isosorbide dinitrate and topical nitroglycerin have produced beneficial hemodynamic effects, relieved symptoms, and improved exercise tolerance in patients refractory to conventional therapy (Franciosa et al, 1978; Hardarson et al, 1977). These agents are generally well tolerated and have a relatively long duration of action; sublingual nitrates are less useful because of their short action.

Hydralazine increases cardiac output by reducing peripheral vascular resistance, but it is not as effective as nitroprusside in reducing left ventricular filling pressure. Combined hydralazine-nitrate therapy reduces both left ventricular filling pressure and aortic impedance as effectively as nitroprusside, while causing only a slight increase in heart rate (Franciosa and Cohn, 1978). The beneficial hemodynamic effect of hydralazine and nitrates (singly or in combination) is sustained during long-term therapy (Massie et al, 1977). The alpha-adrenergic blocking drug, prazosin, has a balanced effect on the arteriolar and venous beds and does not increase heart rate (Miller et al, 1977), but it may not be as effective as hydralazine in increasing cardiac output. There have been reports of tolerance with repeated administration of prazosin, but this has not been a consistent finding.

Since the available vasodilators differ in their hemodynamic effects, therapy can be individualized according to the patient's major symptoms. A nitrate may be most suitable for relieving pulmonary congestion, whereas hydralazine may be more useful when a reduced cardiac output is the primary problem or when mitral regurgitation is present. When it is desirable to reduce left ventricular filling pressure and also elevate cardiac output, prazosin or a combination of hydralazine and a nitrate may be most appropriate. Although vasodilator therapy appears to be an important adjunct in treating severe refractory heart failure, the long-term benefits and possible complications are not yet known. (For specific information on selected vasodilators, see the Table.)

Selected References

Chatterjee K, Parmley WW: Vasodilator treatment for acute and chronic heart failure. *Br Heart J* 39:706-720, 1977.

Chung EK: Current status of digitalis therapy. *Mod Treatment* 8:643-714, 1971.

Chung EK: *Digitalis Intoxication.* Amsterdam, Excerpta Medica, 1969.

Cohn JN: Indications for digitalis therapy: A new look. *JAMA* 229:1911-1914, 1974.

Cohn JN, Franciosa JA: Vasodilator therapy of cardiac failure. *N Engl J Med* 297:27-31, 254-258, 1977.

Doherty JE, et al: Clinical pharmacokinetics of digitalis glycosides. *Prog Cardiovasc Dis* 21:141-158, 1978.

Doherty JE, Kane JJ: Clinical pharmacology and therapeutic use of digitalis glycosides. *Drugs* 6:182-221, 1973.

Franciosa JA, Cohn JN: Hemodynamic responsiveness to short- and long-acting vasodilators in left ventricular failure. *Am J Med* 65:126-133, 1978.

Franciosa JA, et al: Nitrate therapy for congestive heart failure. *JAMA* 240:443-446, 1978.

Greenblatt DJ, et al: Bioavailability of drugs: The digoxin dilemma. *Clin Pharmacokinet* 1:36-51, 1976.

Hardarson T, et al: Prolonged salutary effects of isosorbide dinitrate and nitroglycerin ointment on regional left ventricular function. *Am J Cardiol* 40:90-98, 1977.

Ingelfinger JA, Goldman P: Serum digitalis concentration — Does it diagnose digitalis toxicity? *N Engl J Med* 294:867-870, 1976.

Kubasik NP, et al: Evaluation of sensitivity of commercially available digoxin radioimmunoassay kits. *Chest* 70:217-220, 1976.

Leahey EB Jr, et al: Interaction between quinidine and digoxin. *JAMA* 240:533-534, 1978.

Mason DT: Afterload reduction and cardiac performance: Physiologic basis of systemic vasodilators as a new approach in treatment of congestive heart failure. *Am J Med* 65:106-125, 1978.

Massie B, et al: Hemodynamic advantage of combined administration of hydralazine orally and nitrates nonparenterally on vasodilator therapy of chronic heart failure. *Am J Cardiol* 40:794-801, 1977.

Miller RR, et al: Combined dopamine and nitroprusside therapy in congestive heart failure: Greater augmentation of cardiac performance by addition of inotropic stimulation to afterload reduction. *Circulation* 55:881-884, 1977.

Miller RR, et al: Sustained reduction of cardiac impedance and preload in congestive heart failure with the antihypertensive vasodilator prazosin. *N Engl J Med* 297:303-307, 1977.

Miller RR, et al: Clinical use of sodium nitroprusside in chronic ischemic heart disease: Effects on peripheral vascular resistance and venous tone and on ventricular volume, pump and mechanical performance. *Circulation* 51:328-336, 1975.

Smith TW: Digitalis glycosides. *N Engl J Med* 288:719-722, 942-946, 1973.

Vogel R, et al: Short- and long-term effects of digitalis on resting and posthandgrip hemodynamics in patients with coronary artery disease. *Am J Cardiol* 40:171-176, 1977.

Weintraub M: Interpretation of serum digoxin concentration. *Clin Pharmacokinet* 2:205-219, 1977.

Antiarrhythmic Agents | 34

Cardiac arrhythmias are caused by disorders of electrical impulse formation, by disturbances in impulse conduction, or by a combination of these factors. Disorders of impulse formation occur when the dominant pacemaker function of the sinus node is taken over by specialized cells in the atrium, atrioventricular (A-V) node, or His-Purkinje system, which also possess the property of automaticity (ie, the ability to depolarize spontaneously). This may occur because the normal automaticity of the sinus node is depressed, as in some bradyarrhythmias, or because automaticity in ectopic foci is enhanced, leading to various automatic or re-entrant tachyarrhythmias. Alterations in the rate of impulse formation also may occur when the sinus node is the dominant pacemaker, causing sinus irregularities.

When conductivity is impaired, a normal cardiac impulse entering the affected area may be slowed or blocked (eg, sinus exit block, bundle branch block, varying degrees of A-V block). In special situations with unidirectional block, the nerve impulse may be conducted slowly through adjacent pathways and, in a retrograde fashion, re-enter the normal pathway which has had less time to recover. This establishes a single re-entrant loop or a self-sustaining circus movement that is believed to underlie many tachycardias. Conduction velocity and the duration of the refractory period of cardiac cells are important in determining whether a re-entrant arrhythmia will be perpetuated.

The drugs used to treat tachyarrhythmias and premature complexes reduce automaticity in ectopic foci by depressing spontaneous diastolic depolarization and affect conduction by altering conduction velocity and the duration of the refractory period. Their actions and uses are listed in the Table. Since it is rarely possible to determine the mechanism of a specific tachyarrhythmia or to predict the response to a given drug, it may be necessary to try various drugs, singly or in combination. Although the reported mechanisms of action may suggest logical drug regimens, in practice, the proper choice of drug or drugs is largely empirical.

See also Anderson et al, 1978; Bellet, 1971; Chung, 1977; Dreifus and Likoff, 1973; Mason et al, 1973; Watanabe and Dreifus, 1977; Zipes and Troup, 1978.

ACTIONS AND USES OF ANTIARRHYTHMIC DRUGS

Drug or Class	Actions	Uses
AGENTS USED TO TREAT TACHYARRHYTHMIAS		
Digitalis	Prolongs A-V conduction time and functional refractory period; shortens atrial and ventricular muscle refractory period; enhances myocardial contractility.	Paroxysmal atrial tachycardia; atrial flutter and fibrillation (to control ventricular rate); arrhythmias associated with congestive heart failure.
Quinidine	Depresses automaticity, slows conduction velocity, and increases refractory period duration by both direct and anticholinergic action.	Supraventricular and ventricular tachyarrhythmias, particularly maintenance of sinus rhythm after conversion of atrial flutter and fibrillation and prevention of frequent premature ventricular complexes.
Procainamide	Same as quinidine	Supraventricular and ventricular tachyarrhythmias.
Beta-Adrenergic Blocking Drugs (eg, propranolol)	Block cardiac beta receptors, thereby reducing heart rate and contractility, lengthening A-V conduction time, and suppressing automaticity.	Supraventricular and ventricular tachyarrhythmias, particularly atrial flutter and fibrillation (with digitalis) and arrhythmias associated with increased sympathetic tone or circulating catecholamines.
Disopyramide	Same as quinidine	Ventricular and probably supraventricular tachyarrhythmias.
Lidocaine	Depresses automaticity, reduces refractory period duration, and, in therapeutic doses, does not slow conduction velocity.	Acute control of ventricular tachyarrhythmias and prevention of these arrhythmias after acute myocardial infarction.
Phenytoin	Same as lidocaine	Digitalis-induced arrhythmias.
Bretylium	Prevents release of norepinephrine from sympathetic nerve terminals and acts directly to increase action potential duration.	Refractory ventricular tachyarrhythmias.
Cholinesterase Inhibitors (eg, edrophonium, neostigmine)	Increase parasympathetic activity.	Paroxysmal supraventricular tachycardia.
Vasoconstrictors (eg, phenylephrine, methoxamine)	Increase vagal tone by reflex mechanism.	Paroxysmal supraventricular tachycardia.
*Aprindine	Suppresses automaticity, slows conduction velocity, and lengthens refractory period duration.	Refractory ventricular and supraventricular tachyarrhythmias, particularly arrhythmias associated with Wolff-Parkinson-White syndrome (administered orally and intravenously).
*Tocainide	Similar to lidocaine	Refractory ventricular tachyarrhythmias (administered orally).

ACTIONS AND USES OF ANTIARRHYTHMIC DRUGS

Drug or Class	Actions	Uses
*Mexiletine	Similar to lidocaine.	Refractory ventricular tachyarrhythmias (administered orally and intravenously).
*Verapamil	Interferes with calcium transport across myocardial cell membrane, thereby delaying impulse transmission through A-V node and depressing spontaneous rhythmicity of sinus node.	Supraventricular tachyarrhythmias (administered orally and intravenously).
AGENTS USED TO TREAT BRADYARRHYTHMIAS		
Atropine	Increases sinus rate and A-V conduction velocity.	Sinus bradycardia, sinoatrial arrest, sinoatrial block, type I second-degree A-V block.
Isoproterenol	Increases heart rate and myocardial contractility, enhances automaticity, and increases conduction velocity by stimulating cardiac beta receptors.	Second- or third-degree A-V block, prior to pacing.

Investigational drug.

Sinus Irregularities

Sinus tachycardia is common and usually benign. Generally, the underlying cause (eg, thyrotoxicosis, fever, congestive heart failure) should be determined and corrected rather than treating the sinus tachycardia as a primary disturbance. When therapy is indicated to control symptoms, the beta-adrenergic blocking agent, propranolol [Inderal], may be useful. Propranolol slows a rapid sinus rate resulting from enhanced sympathetic tone or increased levels of circulating catecholamines. Digitalis may control sinus tachycardia associated with congestive heart failure but is not useful when the increased sinus rate is due to other causes.

Sinus bradycardia may require no treatment if cardiac output is adequate. A rate of 50 to 60 beats/minute is usually well tolerated. Marked bradycardia (ie, less than 50 beats/minute) associated with acute myocardial infarction may have serious arrhythmogenic or hemodynamic consequences, and atropine is usually indicated to increase the sinus rate. Temporary pacing may be required in patients who do not respond to atropine. Atropine should not be used routinely in asymptomatic patients because it occasionally precipitates severe ventricular arrhythmias.

Sinoatrial arrest or *sinoatrial block* is sometimes treated with atropine, although drug therapy is only of limited value in these and other sinus disorders (eg, sick sinus syndrome). Sympathomimetic drugs and various antiarrhythmic agents have also been used, but results generally have been disappointing. No drug is available that can reliably increase heart rate on a long-term basis without producing side effects. Permanent pacing is usually preferred for patients with severe symptoms due to sinus node dysfunction.

Supraventricular Tachyarrhythmias

Premature Supraventricular Complexes: Premature atrial or junctional complexes (extrasystoles) are often innocuous and asymptomatic and require no therapy. Propranolol, quinidine, procainamide

[Pronestyl], or disopyramide [Norpace] may be useful in symptomatic patients who do not respond to reassurance. Premature atrial complexes associated with heart failure may respond to digitalization.

Paroxysmal Supraventricular Tachycardia (Without A-V Block): Carotid massage or other measures that increase vagal tone will frequently terminate an acute episode of paroxysmal supraventricular tachycardia. If not effective as the initial approach, vagal maneuvers should be repeated after each pharmacologic intervention. When vagal maneuvers alone are ineffective, administration of an anticholinesterase drug (eg, edrophonium [Tensilon], neostigmine methylsulfate [Prostigmin Methylsulfate]) may terminate the arrhythmia by increasing parasympathetic activity. Occasionally, a vasoconstrictor drug (eg, phenylephrine [Neo-Synephrine], methoxamine [Vasoxyl]) is used to elevate blood pressure rapidly, thereby producing a reflex vagal discharge; however, these drugs may be hazardous in elderly patients and those with hypertension, organic heart disease, hyperthyroidism, or acute myocardial infarction. When normal sinus rhythm cannot be achieved by the preceding measures, digitalis may be administered.

Propranolol is preferred to digitalis in patients with the Wolff-Parkinson-White syndrome because it does not enhance conduction in accessory pathways. Propranolol may be tried in other supraventricular tachycardias refractory to digitalis but should be given cautiously to patients with heart failure. Verapamil, which is currently available only on an investigational basis in the United States, has also been used successfully for acute termination of paroxysmal supraventricular tachycardia. Cardioversion or, rarely, atrial pacing maneuvers may be required in individuals who do not respond to drug therapy. In patients with frequent, symptomatic attacks and a rapid ventricular rate, digitalis, propranolol, quinidine, procainamide, or disopyramide may be administered prophylactically. If prophylactic drug therapy fails to control recurrent severe attacks, the patient should be referred for electrophysiologic testing. Some of these patients will be found to have a surgically correctable accessory atrioventricular pathway.

Digitalis is the drug of choice for terminating paroxysmal supraventricular tachycardia in infants and young children; DC cardioversion may be used in emergencies. Since recurrence is most common during the first year of life, digitalis is usually given for prophylaxis until the infant is 6 to 12 months of age.

Atrial Flutter and Fibrillation: The goal in treating these atrial tachyarrhythmias is to control the ventricular rate and, if possible, restore normal sinus rhythm. The choice of therapy, as with all arrhythmias, depends upon the clinical situation, the condition of the patient, and the ventricular rate. DC cardioversion may be indicated for patients with hypotension, marked heart failure and/or angina, and a very rapid ventricular response; drug therapy may be useful in those who have milder symptoms. Elective cardioversion may not be advisable if the arrhythmia is long-standing, if there is a high risk of thromboembolic complications, or if the patient has a greatly enlarged left atrium, sinus node disease, or a slow ventricular rate.

Digitalis prolongs A-V conduction time and the functional refractory period and is the drug of choice for controlling the ventricular rate. (Digitalis should be avoided, however, when atrial fibrillation or flutter occurs in patients with the Wolff-Parkinson-White syndrome, because it can facilitate conduction in accessory pathways and thus increase the ventricular rate.) In atrial flutter, digitalis may decrease the ventricular response and convert flutter to sinus rhythm or fibrillation; however, the ventricular response to atrial flutter is not easily controllable for any length of time in most patients, and cardioversion is often required. It is easier to decrease the ventricular rate during atrial fibrillation than during flutter. If therapeutic doses of digitalis are not effective, the addition of propranolol to the regimen may permit a reduction in dosage of the glycoside and provide better control of the arrhythmia.

Atrial fibrillation or atrial flutter of recent origin may convert spontaneously to sinus rhythm during digitalization. If fibrillation persists and if conversion to sinus rhythm is indicated, DC cardioversion is the method of choice and is effective in 80% to 90% of patients. Quinidine is the most commonly used antiarrhythmic drug for preventing recurrence of atrial flutter and fibrillation after conversion to sinus rhythm and is generally given in conjunction with digitalis. However, recent reports suggest that quinidine may increase the serum digoxin concentration to potentially toxic levels. Quinidine may be started in maintenance doses 24 to 48 hours prior to cardioversion with the expectation that some cases may revert to sinus rhythm, obviating the need for this procedure. Disopyramide may be used as an alternative agent for this indication.

A-V Conduction Disturbances

First-degree A-V block is usually asymptomatic and does not require therapy. In more severe conduction disturbances, treatment is necessary if the ventricular rate is not sufficient to maintain an adequate cardiac output during rest and exercise or if other arrhythmias accompany the slow ventricular rate. Although atropine may improve A-V conduction in symptomatic patients with Type I (Wenckebach) second-degree A-V block accompanying myocardial infarction, in some cases it may paradoxically increase block by increasing the sinus rate. Type II (Mobitz) second-degree A-V block usually signifies a serious conduction disturbance in the His-Purkinje system and permanent pacing is generally indicated. This conduction abnormality can progress rapidly to third-degree (complete) A-V block, and the resulting sudden reduction in cardiac output may cause syncope and seizures (Stokes-Adams syndrome). Isoproterenol [Isuprel] may be used to maintain heart rate and cardiac output prior to insertion of a pacemaker in these patients. Some individuals with complete A-V block maintain an adequate cardiac output without drug

therapy. Atropine or isoproterenol may improve cardiac output in symptomatic patients, but beneficial effects are usually transient, and these drugs are useful primarily for temporary therapy prior to pacing.

Ventricular Tachyarrhythmias

Premature Ventricular Complexes: Premature ventricular systoles in individuals without underlying heart disease are usually benign. Frequent or complex ventricular ectopy in patients with coronary artery disease may be associated with an increased risk of sudden death (Ruberman et al, 1977). In patients with acute myocardial infarction, treatment is indicated when these arrhythmias cause disturbing symptoms or predispose to ventricular tachycardia and fibrillation. It is currently not known whether antiarrhythmic therapy will prevent sudden death in high-risk patients.

Because it acts rapidly and usually does not depress A-V conduction or myocardial contractility, lidocaine is the drug of choice for immediate control of serious ventricular arrhythmias. If lidocaine is ineffective, procainamide may be tried. Quinidine, procainamide, propranolol, or disopyramide may be used orally for prolonged suppression. Digitalis may be given cautiously when ventricular premature systoles are due to congestive heart failure.

In patients with acute myocardial infarction, frequent premature ventricular complexes may occur in the presence of sinus bradycardia. Atropine (0.5 mg intravenously) may abolish these ectopic beats by increasing the sinus rate, and no other antiarrhythmic agent may be needed.

Ventricular Tachycardia: Ventricular tachycardia usually occurs in the presence of severe cardiac disease and may progress to ventricular fibrillation. Episodes may be paroxysmal or sustained. If the condition is life-threatening or the patient does not respond to drug therapy, DC cardioversion is the method of choice for converting this arrhythmia. The drugs used intravenously to treat an acute attack are, in order of preference, lidocaine, procainamide, and propranolol. In refractory cases, bretylium [Bretylol] may facilitate successful cardioversion. Following conversion, quinidine, procainamide, disopyramide, propranolol, or phenytoin [Dilantin] may be given orally for prophylaxis. Sometimes combinations of antiarrhythmic drugs (eg, quinidine and propranolol) are employed. Special pacing techniques may be effective in some patients who do not respond to these measures.

Ventricular Flutter and Fibrillation: Immediate DC cardioversion is the treatment of choice for ventricular flutter and fibrillation, and after normal cardiac action has been restored, antiarrhythmic drugs are used to prevent recurrence. Usually, lidocaine is infused temporarily; if it is ineffective, procainamide may be tried. Patients refractory to conventional therapy may respond to bretylium. Oral therapy is then instituted with quinidine, procainamide, disopyramide, propranolol, or phenytoin. Long-term therapy with antiarrhythmic drugs is sometimes utilized to prevent sudden cardiac death caused by ventricular fibrillation. The effectiveness of any of these agents in the prophylaxis of sudden cardiac death is not yet proven.

Digitalis-Induced Arrhythmias

The most common arrhythmias produced by digitalis toxicity are multiform premature ventricular complexes, nonparoxysmal A-V junctional (nodal) tachycardia, and paroxysmal atrial tachycardia with block; however, almost any disorder of cardiac rhythm may occur (see Chapter 33, Agents Used to Treat Congestive Heart Failure). Patients with mild symptoms may require no therapy other than temporarily discontinuing digitalis. Additional treatment is necessary in those with more severe disturbances (frequent premature ventricular complexes, supraventricular or ventricular tachyarrhythmias) to prevent the development of ventricular fibrillation. Potassium replacement therapy is indicated if hypokalemia is present, but routine replacement in normokalemic patients is not always advisable because hyperkalemia can intensify A-V block. Electrocardiographic monitoring and frequent determinations of serum potassium levels are essential during replacement therapy.

The drugs most commonly used to treat severe digitalis-induced arrhythmias are lidocaine, phenytoin, and propranolol. Lidocaine is usually preferred. Edetate disodium (EDTA) is rarely used today for this purpose because more effective drugs are available. Antibody fractions against digitalis have been used successfully in severe digitalis intoxication under an investigational protocol. Since digitalis predisposes to postcountershock arrhythmias, DC cardioversion should be avoided unless all other measures have failed and the arrhythmia is life-threatening.

Antiarrhythmic Drug Therapy During and After DC Cardioversion

Lidocaine should be available during DC cardioversion to treat ventricular arrhythmias that may develop. Patients with atrial flutter or fibrillation may require maintenance therapy with quinidine, disopyramide, or procainamide prior to elective cardioversion to prevent immediate postcountershock arrhythmias. These drugs are then administered on a long-term basis to maintain normal sinus rhythm after conversion; however, many patients revert to the abnormal rhythm despite adequate blood levels of the drug. Some patients cannot tolerate prolonged therapy with quinidine or procainamide.

Digitalis predisposes to postcountershock arrhythmias and, until recently, it was the practice to discontinue glycoside therapy before cardioversion. Currently, maintenance doses of digitalis are often continued to reduce the risk of heart failure or recurrence of a rapid ventricular rate. The danger of precipitating severe postcountershock arrhythmias can be reduced if a low energy level is employed initially and the energy level is carefully titrated. If symptoms of digitalis toxicity are present, it may be advisable to administer lidocaine before the countershock. Since quinidine may increase serum digoxin levels, the glycoside probably should be discontinued for 24 to 48 hours prior to cardioversion, if quinidine therapy is begun. Alternatively, quinidine may be omitted before cardioversion.

AGENTS USED TO TREAT TACHYARRHYTHMIAS

DIGITALIS GLYCOSIDES

The digitalis glycosides have complex direct and indirect effects on the heart. The actions that are most important in antiarrhythmic therapy are: (1) lengthening of the A-V nodal conduction time and functional refractory period, which is due to an increase in vagal tone, an antiadrenergic action, and possibly a direct effect; (2) shortening of the atrial muscle refractory period as the result of enhanced vagal tone (although recent evidence suggests that this may not always occur in man); (3) shortening of the ventricular muscle refractory period by a direct action; and (4) enhancement of myocardial contractility.

In atrial fibrillation or flutter, digitalis is the agent of choice to slow the ventricular response to rapid atrial rates; if effective doses are not tolerated, propranolol may be added to the regimen. Digitalis may terminate paroxysmal supraventricular tachycardia after vagal maneuvers have failed and may prevent recurrence; vagal maneuvers may be more effective after digitalization. Sinus tachycardia and supraventricular or ventricular extrasystoles or tachyarrhythmias may respond to digitalis therapy when they are associated with congestive heart failure. Digitalis generally is contraindicated or must be used very cautiously in the presence of A-V block or when treating atrial fibrillation or flutter in patients with the Wolff-Parkinson-White syndrome.

For the treatment of digitalis-induced arrhythmias, see the Introduction. Other adverse effects of the digitalis glycosides are discussed in Chapter 33, Agents Used to Treat Congestive Heart Failure.

Suggested dosages appear in Chapter 33. Since response to the digitalis glycosides varies considerably, these dosages are intended only as a guideline and should be individualized in accordance with the clinical situation. The dose required to slow A-V nodal conduction and prolong the refractory period of the A-V node is generally larger than that needed to increase myocardial contractility. The amount required to control the ventricular rate during various supraventricular tachyarrhythmias also may vary. Generally, a larger dose is required to slow the ventricular rate during atrial flutter than during atrial fibrillation and the ventricular response to atrial flutter is not easily controllable for prolonged periods. Digitalis may be more effective in patients with stable chronic atrial fibrillation than in those whose condition is unstable.

QUINIDINE SULFATE
[Cin-Quin, Quinidex]

QUINIDINE GLUCONATE
[Duraquin, Quinaglute]

QUINIDINE POLYGALACTURONATE
[Cardioquin]

Quinidine has both a direct action on the cell membrane and indirect (anticholinergic) effects. It depresses automaticity, particularly in ectopic sites; retards conduction velocity; and increases the effective refractory period of cardiac cells. Quinidine is useful in both supraventricular and ventricular tachyarrhythmias. Its major uses are to maintain sinus rhythm after conversion of atrial flutter or fibrillation and to prevent frequent premature ventricular complexes or ventricular tachycardia. It is also used prophylactically in patients with paroxysmal supraventricular tachycardia or symptomatic supraventricular premature beats. Administration of a single large oral dose (600 mg of quinidine sulfate) may be useful to determine whether the drug will be effective in controlling ventricular arrhythmias.

Quinidine is usually preferred to procainamide for long-term therapy because the dosage schedule is more convenient and because drug-induced lupus occurs frequently during prolonged therapy with procainamide. In the past, quinidine was often employed to convert atrial tachyarrhythmias to a normal sinus rhythm, but this use has declined in recent years because of the ready availability of cardioversion and the danger of using increasing doses of quinidine for this purpose.

Quinidine sulfate is rapidly absorbed from the gastrointestinal tract whereas the gluconate salt is absorbed more slowly. In a single-dose study in normal subjects, the bioavailability of the sulfate was approximately 80% with peak plasma levels attained in 1.5 hours; the gluconate was approximately 70% bioavailable with peak plasma levels attained in 4 hours (Greenblatt et al, 1977).

Quinidine is 80% to 90% bound to plasma proteins, but protein binding may be decreased in patients with impaired hepatic function. This agent is extensively metabolized in the liver, and some of the metabolites may have antiarrhythmic activity. Approximately 20% of an administered dose appears in the urine as unchanged drug. Plasma concentrations vary according to the assay employed. With the method of Cramer and Isaakson, therapeutic plasma levels range from 2.3 to 5 mcg/ml (Anderson et al, 1978).

The toxic effects of quinidine are generally dose related, but severe reactions may occur after small doses are given to patients who are hypersensitive to the drug. The oral route is preferred because serious cardiovascular reactions are more likely to occur after parenteral (particularly intravenous) administration. Intramuscular injections are painful, increase serum creatine phosphokinase levels, and are erratically and incompletely absorbed (Greenblatt et al, 1977).

Diarrhea, nausea, and vomiting, which may be due to a direct irritant effect, are the most common adverse effects of quinidine. Largely uncontrolled reports suggest that the gluconate and polygalacturonate salts are better tolerated by some patients. If gastrointestinal reactions become severe, procainamide or disopyramide may be substituted. Fever, hepatitis, manifestations of cinchonism (eg, headache, vertigo, palpitations, tinnitus, visual disturbances), blood dyscrasias (hemolytic anemia, thrombocytopenia, agranulocytosis), and dermatologic reactions occur occasionally. (See also Cohen et al, 1977.) Quinidine may unmask or exacerbate myasthenia gravis. There is one report of dementia associated with quinidine therapy.

In patients with atrial flutter or fibrillation, quinidine may increase the ventricular rate, but this complication generally can be avoided by prior and concomitant glycoside therapy (with careful monitoring for digitalis toxicity). Severe hypotension due to peripheral vasodilatation may occur after rapid parenteral administration, and vasopressor amines should be available to treat this complication. Large doses of quinidine may depress myocardial contractility and aggravate or induce heart failure in nondigitalized patients. However, the vasodilator effect may improve the condition of some patients with heart failure. Other manifestations of cardiac toxicity are A-V block, marked prolongation of the Q-T interval, widening of the QRS complex, and ventricular tachyarrhythmias. Quinidine should be used cautiously in patients with partial A-V block and probably should not be used in the presence of high-grade second- or third-degree heart block unless a ventricular pacemaker is in place. Syncopal episodes and sudden death during quinidine therapy may be due to ventricular fibrillation provoked by R-on-T phenomenon, probably as a result of a markedly prolonged Q-T interval. Ventricular arrhythmias, including ventricular tachycardia and fibrillation, may occur at therapeutic or subtherapeutic plasma drug levels and are perhaps the most disconcerting of the adverse effects of quinidine. Some cases of sudden death during quinidine therapy have been attributed to the dislodging of atrial emboli following conversion to sinus rhythm, but there is no convincing evidence that this complication is more common after use of quinidine than after other types of therapy.

Elevated serum digoxin levels (sometimes associated with gastrointestinal disturbances and ventricular arrhythmias) have been noted in patients receiving both quinidine and digitalis. The nature of this interaction is unknown but may reflect displacement of digoxin from tissue binding sites by quinidine. Patients receiving both drugs should be carefully monitored for digitalis toxicity. Phenobarbital and phenytoin reduce the half-life of quinidine, probably by increasing its rate of metabolism. Quinidine should be used cautiously in patients receiving neuromuscular blocking drugs because the effects may be additive.

ROUTES, USUAL DOSAGE, AND PREPARATIONS. Elderly patients and those with congestive heart failure or impaired hepatic or renal function may require a reduction in dosage.

QUINIDINE SULFATE:
Oral: Adults, 200 to 400 mg every six hours. *Children*, 6 mg/kg of body weight every four to six hours.
> Drug available generically: Capsules 180 and 200 mg; tablets 180, 200, and 300 mg.
> *Cin-Quin* (Rowell). Capsules 200 and 300 mg; tablets 100, 200, and 300 mg.
> *Quinidex* (Robins). Tablets (timed-release) 300 mg.

QUINIDINE GLUCONATE:
Oral: Adults, 324 to 972 mg every 8 to 12 hours.
> *Duraquin* (Parke, Davis). Tablets (timed-release) 330 mg.
> *Quinaglute* (Cooper). Tablets (timed-release) 324 mg.

Intramuscular: The oral route is generally preferred, but intramuscular administration may be necessary in severely ill patients; 400 mg is given initially, and this dose may be repeated every four to six hours. In emergencies, administration every two hours (for four or five doses) may be necessary.

Intravenous: This route is rarely indicated and should be employed only in hospitalized patients; 200 to 400 mg in dilute solution may be given very slowly (approximately 10 mg/min). The electrocardiogram and blood pressure should be monitored continuously.
> Drug available generically: Solution 80 mg/ml in 10 ml containers.

QUINIDINE POLYGALACTURONATE:
Oral: The manufacturer's recommended dose for maintenance is: *Adults*, 275 mg two or three times daily.
> *Cardioquin* (Purdue Frederick). Tablets 275 mg (equivalent to 200 mg of quinidine sulfate).

PROCAINAMIDE HYDROCHLORIDE
[Pronestyl]

The electrophysiologic properties and antiarrhythmic actions of procainamide are similar to those of quinidine, and the two agents may be used interchangeably for prophylaxis and maintenance therapy. Quinidine is usually preferred for prolonged oral therapy, however, because of the high incidence of drug-induced lupus associated with long-term administration of procainamide. For intravenous use, procainamide is safer than quinidine and has a more rapid action; given by this route, it is useful in patients with severe ventricular tachyarrhythmias who are unresponsive to lidocaine.

Procainamide is well absorbed after oral administration and bioavailability is approximately 75%. It is 15% bound to plasma proteins. The drug is metabolized in the liver and eliminated by renal excretion of both active drug and metabolites. The major metabolite, N-acetylprocainamide, has antiarrhythmic activity but, in the absence of renal failure, the amount of this metabolite present is probably insufficient to account for much of the antiarrhythmic effect. The rate of acetylation of procainamide is under genetic control and shows a bimodal distribution into slow and fast acetylators. Therapeutic blood levels of procainamide range between 4 and 10 mcg/ml, but severe arrhythmias can occasionally be controlled only at higher levels. Plasma half-life is prolonged in patients with renal insufficiency. Methods available for measuring serum procainamide levels do not measure levels of the active metabolite (Koch-Weser, 1977).

Although procainamide may cause anorexia, nausea, and vomiting, it is better tolerated than quinidine in some patients. Its adverse cardiovascular effects are similar to those of quinidine. The clinical usefulness of procainamide is limited because of a reversible lupus erythematosus-like syndrome which develops in about 30% of patients during prolonged maintenance therapy. An increased titer of antinuclear antibodies develops in about 80% of patients; acetylator status influences the rate, but not the frequency, of antibody development. Other manifestations of hypersensitivity (eg, rash, urticaria, fever, agranulocytosis, pancytopenia) have occurred occasionally. Rarely, mental disturbances (eg, depression, hallucinations, psychosis) have been noted.

ROUTES, USUAL DOSAGE, AND PREPARATIONS. Dosage should be reduced in patients with impaired renal function.
Oral: Adults, 250 to 500 mg every three to four hours. *Children*, 50 mg/kg of body weight daily in four to six divided doses.
> Drug available generically: Capsules 250, 375, and 500 mg; tablets 500 mg.
> *Pronestyl* (Squibb). Capsules and tablets 250, 375, and 500 mg.

Intramuscular: Adults and children, if high blood levels are required immediately, a priming dose double the amount of the oral dose can be given. Usual oral doses then can be given for maintenance.

Intravenous (slow): Adults, 25 to 50 mg/min until the arrhythmia is suppressed (maximum, 1 g). Following the loading dose, for maintenance the drug may be infused at a rate of 2 to 4 mg/min. Blood pressure and the electrocardiogram should be monitored continuously.
> *Pronestyl* (Squibb). Solution 100 mg/ml in 10 ml containers and 500 mg/ml in 2 ml containers.

PROPRANOLOL HYDROCHLORIDE
[Inderal]

The antiarrhythmic effects of propranolol have been attributed to two actions: blockade of cardiac beta-adrenergic receptors and membrane stabilizing activity. Present evidence indicates that the former action is the most important, because the direct membrane effect occurs only at concentrations in excess of those used clinically (Abrams and Davies, 1973). The cardiac effects of beta blockade include a reduction in heart rate and contractility, lengthening of A-V conduction time, and suppression of automaticity. The major indications for use of propranolol as an antiarrhythmic agent are to treat catecholamine-induced arrhythmias, to slow the ventricular response in atrial flutter and fibrillation, and to prevent and convert paroxysmal supraventricular tachycardia and selected ventricular arrhythmias.

Propranolol terminates tachyarrhythmias caused by increased sympathetic tone or an excess of circulating catecholamines. Applications include control of reflex tachycardia induced by vasodilator drugs (hydralazine, nitrates) in antihypertensive and antianginal therapy, suppression of tachyarrhythmias (as an adjunct to alpha-blocking drugs) in pheochromocytoma, and reduction of some of the signs and symptoms of hyperthyroidism (see Chapters 35, 38, and 48).

Because it increases the refractory period of the A-V node and prolongs A-V conduction time, propranolol is often effective in slowing the ventricular rate in patients with atrial fibrillation or flutter who are not adequately controlled by therapeutic doses of digitalis (which should generally be administered initially). This combined therapy represents one of the most important uses of propranolol in the management of arrhythmias. Propranolol may be useful for the short- or long-term treatment of refractory paroxysmal atrial tachycardia, particularly when this arrhythmia is associated with the Wolff-Parkinson-White syndrome. It also may be effective in the treatment of digitalis-induced arrhythmias, but lidocaine or phenytoin is preferred, especially if A-V block is present. Propranolol is usually less effective (although better tolerated) than quinidine or procainamide in suppressing chronic ventricular ectopic activity. It may be useful in recurrent stress-induced ventricular tachycardia. In European studies, long-term therapy with other beta-blocking drugs (practolol, alprenolol) appeared to increase the life expectancy of patients surviving the acute phase of myocardial infarction. A reduction in the incidence of tachyarrhythmias has been suggested, but not established, as the major mechanism. Whether propranolol has a similar action is under investigation.

Significant adverse effects include congestive heart failure, cardiac arrest (in patients with A-V block), and bronchospasm. Although severe bradycardia can occur and requires cessation of therapy, asymptomatic bradycardia (45 to 55 beats/minute) is frequent and should not be cause for stopping the drug. In patients with coronary artery disease, sudden withdrawal of large doses has led to recurrence of unstable angina, ventricular tachycardia, myocardial infarction, and sudden death. For a discussion of the pharmacology and adverse effects of propranolol and other beta-blocking drugs, see Chapter 35, Antianginal Agents.

ROUTES, USUAL DOSAGE, AND PREPARATIONS. *Oral*: When propranolol is administered orally, the degree of beta blockade correlates poorly with dosage; therefore, dosage must be titrated in terms of the therapeutic response. The therapeutic plasma levels for treatment of arrhythmias have not been established. The following dosage is intended only as a guideline: *Adults*, 10 to 80 mg three or four times daily.

Inderal (Ayerst). Tablets 10, 20, 40, and 80 mg.

Intravenous: Adults, 0.1 to 0.15 mg/kg of body weight administered in increments of 0.5 to 0.75 mg every one to two minutes with continuous electrocardiographic and blood pressure monitoring. Smaller doses should be used or the drug avoided if there is a risk of myocardial depression. If excessive bradycardia occurs, 0.5 to 1 mg of atropine should be given intravenously; if myocardial depression is severe, isoproterenol should be given by slow intravenous infusion. The dose of isoproterenol required to reverse the effects of propranolol may be large.

Inderal (Ayerst). Solution 1 mg/ml in 1 ml containers.

DISOPYRAMIDE PHOSPHATE
[Norpace]

The electrophysiologic effects of disopyramide are similar to those of quinidine. It depresses automaticity, retards conduction velocity, and increases the effective refractory period of cardiac cells. Like quinidine, disopyramide has both direct and anticholinergic actions.

Disopyramide has been used successfully to prevent ventricular extrasystoles and ventricular tachycardia and may be effective in suppressing atrial tachyarrhythmias (Heel et al, 1978; Koch-Weser, 1979 B). In comparative (unpublished) studies, both disopyramide and quinidine were effective in preventing ventricular ectopic beats, but there was a slight trend favoring quinidine in the doses used. Both drugs occasionally increased ectopic activity; this complication occurred more frequently with use of disopyramide than with quinidine. One group of investigators reported that disopyramide reduced the incidence of reinfarction and the mortality rate, in addition to suppressing serious arrhythmias, when given prophylactically in the early stages after myocardial infarction; it is generally felt that these conclusions require further documentation.

Disopyramide is well absorbed from the gastrointestinal tract, and peak plasma levels usually are attained within two hours. Therapeutic plasma levels are said to range between 2 and 4 mcg/ml, but others have reported higher ranges for effective acute therapy. Due to unusual protein-binding characteristics, an increase in drug dose results in a less than proportionate increase in *total* drug concentration. However, free (and possibly active) drug concentration does increase in proportion to dose. The mean plasma half-life in patients with normal renal function is 4.5 hours; 80% of an oral dose is excreted in the urine as unchanged drug (52%) and metabolites. The plasma half-life is increased in patients with impaired renal function.

The most common side effects of disopyramide are related to its anticholinergic activity and include dryness of the mouth, blurred vision, constipation, and urinary retention. Rarely, it has precipitated an attack of acute angle-closure glaucoma. Nausea, vomiting, gastric pain, and diarrhea may occur, but these reactions appear to be less common with disopyramide than with quinidine.

Like quinidine, disopyramide may increase the ventricular rate in nondigitalized patients with atrial flutter or fibrillation. It depresses myocardial contractility and may cause heart failure in poorly compensated patients. Therefore, disopyramide should not be used in the presence of poorly compensated or uncompensated congestive heart failure unless the failure is caused by an arrhythmia and proper treatment, including optimal digitalization, has been accomplished. Severe hypotension also has been reported; vasopressor amines should be available to treat this complication. Disopyramide may precipitate or worsen heart block. It should be used cautiously in patients with partial A-V block and probably should not be used in those with high-grade second- or third-degree heart block unless a ventricular pacemaker is in place. Like other antiarrhythmic drugs, disopyramide should be avoided in patients with the sick sinus syndrome because it prolongs sinus recovery time in many of these patients. Disopyramide therapy may cause prolongation of the Q-T interval, widening of the QRS complex, and a prominent U wave; rarely, these electrocardiographic abnormalities may presage ventricular tachycardia, flutter, or fibrillation, sometimes with syncope as the presenting symptom.

Adverse reactions reported rarely include nervousness, dizziness, fatigue, depression, headache, muscle weakness, acute psychosis, hypoglycemia, intrahepatic cholestasis, and dermatologic reactions. The safety of disopyramide in pregnant women and nursing mothers has not been established. In one instance, the drug appeared to initiate uterine contractions.

ROUTE, USUAL DOSAGE, AND PREPARATIONS. *Oral*: *Adults*, 150 mg every six hours. Amounts up to 1.6 g daily have been used occasionally. For patients with renal insufficiency, the manufacturer recommends a maintenance dose of 100 mg every 10 to 30 hours. Patients of small stature or those with hepatic insufficiency, cardiomyopathy, or cardiac decompensation also may require a reduction in dosage.

Norpace (Searle). Capsules 100 and 150 mg (base).

LIDOCAINE HYDROCHLORIDE
[Xylocaine Hydrochloride]

Lidocaine depresses diastolic depolarization and automaticity in the ventricles but has little effect on atrial tissue and, in therapeutic doses, it does not slow conduction velocity. Because it acts rapidly and moderate doses usually do not depress myocardial contractility or A-V conduction, intravenous lidocaine is the drug of choice for immediate suppression of premature ventricular complexes and ventricular tachycardia in acute myocardial infarction.

Since warning arrhythmias may be absent (or undetected) in up to 50% of patients who develop primary ventricular fibrillation after acute myocardial infarction, some authorities have recommended that intravenous lidocaine should be given routinely to all patients with suspected acute myocardial infarction for 24 to 36 hours or until a diagnosis of infarction is excluded (Harrison, 1978). Although this program has been successful in preventing primary ventricular fibrillation, the mortality rate has not been affected. In patients over age 69, the benefits of prophylactic therapy are outweighed by the potential risk (Lie et al, 1974).

Since intravenous therapy may not be practical prior to hospitalization, intramuscular injection of lidocaine has been advocated to suppress ventricular ectopic activity during the prehospital phase of acute myocardial infarction. One group of investigators found that this program improved immediate prognosis (Valentine et al, 1974), but others found no beneficial effects (Lie et al, 1978).

In addition to its use in acute myocardial infarction, lidocaine may control ventricular arrhythmias caused by digitalis toxicity and those occurring during cardiac surgery or cardiac catheterization. Lidocaine usually does not correct supraventricular disturbances and may increase the ventricular rate, particularly in patients also receiving quinidine.

Therapeutic plasma concentrations of lidocaine range from 1.6 to 5 mcg/ml. The drug is extensively metabolized in a single pass through the liver, and plasma levels may be significantly increased and the half-life prolonged in the presence of impaired hepatic blood flow or hepatic disease or after prolonged (more than 24 hours) infusion.

The major adverse effects of lidocaine are attributable to its action on the central nervous system and include drowsiness, paresthesias, muscle twitching, convulsions, coma, and respiratory depression. Large doses may depress myocardial contractility and A-V conduction. Untoward effects are most common in patients with hepatic insufficiency or congestive heart failure, and the dosage should be reduced in patients with these disorders.

ROUTES, USUAL DOSAGE, AND PREPARATIONS. The electrocardiogram and blood pressure should be monitored continuously for patients receiving lidocaine.

Intravenous: *Adults*, for treatment of ventricular arrhythmias, a loading dose of 50 to 100 mg is given over a period of two to three minutes, and this dose may be repeated in five minutes, as necessary (up to 300 mg in a one-hour period). Simultaneously with the loading dose, a 0.1% solution is infused at a rate of 1 to 4 mg/min.

The following regimen has been recommended for prophylaxis after acute myocardial infarction. A loading dose of 200 mg is given as two 100-mg injections ten minutes apart or four 50-mg injections five minutes apart, or 20 mg/min is infused for ten minutes. Some physicians prefer a loading dose of 150 to 175 mg given as a 100-mg injection, followed in ten minutes by the 50- to 75-mg dose. Each bolus should be given slowly. Simultaneously with the loading dose, infusion of a 0.1% solution is started at a rate of 2 to 4 mg/min. The infusion should be continued for 24 to 36 hours following acute myocardial infarction. If symptomatic ventricular arrhythmias occur during infusion, an additional smaller bolus may be given and the infusion rate increased or another antiarrhythmic drug (such as procainamide) may be tried. In patients 70 years and older and those with congestive heart failure, cardiogenic shock, or hepatic disease, the loading dose should be decreased markedly (usually by one-half) and the infusion rate should be reduced to 1 to 2 mg/min. *Children*, 0.5 to 1 mg/kg of body weight every five minutes for a maximum of three doses or a solution containing 5 mg/ml is infused at a rate of 0.03 mg/kg/min.

> *Xylocaine Intravenous Injection for Cardiac Arrhythmias* (Astra). Solution 20 mg/ml in 5 ml containers, 40 mg/ml in 25 and 50 ml single-use containers, and 200 mg/ml in 5 and 10 ml containers.

Intramuscular: *Adults*, 300 mg (3 ml of a 10% solution) injected into the deltoid muscle.

Xylocaine Intramuscular Injection for Cardiac Arrhythmias (Astra). Solution 100 mg/ml in 5 ml containers.

PHENYTOIN
[Dilantin]

PHENYTOIN SODIUM
[Dilantin]

Phenytoin depresses spontaneous depolarization in atrial and ventricular tissues; it usually does not alter intraventricular conduction and may improve (or at least does not slow) A-V conduction. Phenytoin is not a first-line antiarrhythmic drug. Its major indication is to reverse some digitalis-induced arrhythmias (particularly ventricular arrhythmias) but, even for this purpose, lidocaine may be the drug of choice. Phenytoin is usually less effective than other available agents for disorders of cardiac rhythm that are not produced by digitalis.

Effective therapeutic blood levels of phenytoin usually range between 10 and 18 mcg/ml. This drug is extensively metabolized by the liver before excretion. Plasma levels vary widely after administration of a given dose because of individual differences in the rate of metabolism resulting from genetic factors or concurrent administration of drugs that affect microsomal enzyme activity. Therapeutic plasma levels may be difficult to maintain because the drug tends to accumulate at higher doses. Since phenytoin is highly bound to plasma protein, patients with impaired hepatic function or uremia may respond to lower total plasma levels because the free drug concentration is increased.

Fatigue, dizziness, ataxia, nausea, vomiting, pruritus, and rash are common adverse effects. Neurologic side effects are concentration related and progress in severity as the plasma concentration increases. Hepatitis, blood dyscrasias, and pseudolymphoma have occurred rarely. Rapid intravenous administration may cause myocardial depression, bradycardia, hypotension, paradoxical A-V block, and, rarely, cardiac arrest. The drug should not be given faster than 25 to 50 mg/min. Phenytoin can cause a clinically important increase in serum quinidine levels. For other adverse reactions, drug interactions, and precautions, see Chapter 15, Anticonvulsants.

ROUTES, USUAL DOSAGE, AND PREPARATIONS. *Oral*: Large initial doses may be required to achieve an effective plasma level rapidly. *Adults*, 1 g on the first day and 300 to 600 mg on the second and third days. For maintenance, 300 to 400 mg daily in one to four divided doses. *Children*, initially, 10 to 15 mg/kg of body weight in two or three doses over a 24-hour period. For maintenance, 5 to 10 mg/kg daily in two or three divided doses.
PHENYTOIN:
Dilantin (Parke, Davis). Suspension 30 (pediatric) and 125 mg/5 ml; tablets (pediatric) 50 mg.
PHENYTOIN SODIUM:
Drug available generically and under the name Diphenylhydantoin Sodium: Capsules 30 and 100 mg.
Dilantin [*sodium*] (Parke, Davis). Capsules 30 and 100 mg.

Intravenous: This route should be reserved for severely ill patients, and continuous electrocardiographic and blood pressure monitoring is recommended. The infusion rate should not exceed 25 to 50 mg/min. *Adults*, 100 mg every five minutes until the arrhythmia is reversed or toxicity is observed (maximum, 500 mg to 1 g).
PHENYTOIN SODIUM:
Drug available generically: Solution 50 mg/ml in 2 and 5 ml containers.
Dilantin [*sodium*] (Parke, Davis). Powder for solution containing approximately 50 mg/ml when diluted with the special solvent provided in the 100 and 250 mg containers; solution 50 mg/ml in 2 and 5 ml containers.

BRETYLIUM TOSYLATE
[Bretylol]

$$\text{(C}_6\text{H}_4\text{Br)}-\text{CH}_2-\overset{\underset{\displaystyle CH_3}{|}}{\overset{\displaystyle CH_3}{\underset{+}{N}}}-\text{CH}_2\text{CH}_3 \qquad \text{H}_3\text{C}-\text{(C}_6\text{H}_4)-\text{SO}_3^-$$

This quaternary ammonium compound was originally available as an oral preparation for the treatment of hypertension, but it proved unsuitable for long-term therapy because of unpredictable gastrointestinal absorption, troublesome side effects (orthostatic hypotension and parotid pain), and frequent development of tolerance. The parenteral preparation was subsequently found to be useful in antiarrhythmic therapy.

Bretylium has both a direct effect on the cell membrane and an antiadrenergic action. Its major direct effect is an increase in the action potential duration, which is accompanied by prolongation of the refractory period; automaticity is not suppressed nor conduction velocity slowed. Bretylium accumulates in sympathetic ganglia and postganglionic adrenergic neurons where it prevents the release of norepinephrine, thereby inducing a state resembling surgical sympathectomy. It does not antagonize (and may *increase* sensitivity to) the effects of circulating catecholamines. A transient increase in automaticity, heart rate, myocardial contractility, and blood pressure occurs prior to the onset of adrenergic blockade; this effect is caused by the initial release of norepinephrine from sympathetic nerve terminals and can be blocked by propranolol. A temporal dissociation between the antiarrhythmic and antiadrenergic effects of bretylium has been noted (eg, Romhilt et al, 1972), and the antiadrenergic effect can be blocked without blocking the antiarrhythmic action.

Bretylium is used to treat severe refractory ventricular tachyarrhythmias (preferably excluding those associated with digitalis toxicity). Because its onset of action may be delayed and adverse effects may be severe, this drug is usually reserved for patients who have not responded to conventional therapy (ie, DC cardioversion, lidocaine, procainamide, and possibly other antiarrhythmic drugs). Although bretylium has been used successfully to suppress frequent premature ventricular complexes, it is indicated primarily in patients with recurrent refractory ventricular tachycardia or fibrillation. It may terminate these arrhythmias (Bernstein and Koch-Weser, 1972) or facilitate successful cardioversion when previous attempts have failed (Holder et al, 1977). The maximal antiarrhythmic action may not be apparent for 20 minutes to 12 hours after injection. (See also Koch-Weser, 1979 A.)

The initial release of norepinephrine by bretylium may temporarily increase ventricular ectopic activity and elevate blood pressure. These effects may be enhanced if the patient is receiving vasopressor therapy or if the arrhythmia being treated is caused by digitalis toxicity. This initial effect is followed (usually within one hour) by a fall in supine blood pressure, which is the most common and most troublesome adverse effect of bretylium, occurring in up to two-thirds of patients. If the supine systolic pressure falls below 75 mm Hg, dopamine or norepinephrine may be infused, but the blood pressure should be monitored closely because bretylium enhances the pressor effect of catecholamines. Patients with severe aortic stenosis or pulmonary hypertension may not be able to compensate for a fall in peripheral resistance by increasing their cardiac output and, if possible, bretylium should be avoided in these patients. Bretylium may be given if the patient's survival is threatened by the arrhythmia, but the patient should be watched closely and vasoconstrictor amines should be given promptly if hypotension occurs.

Nausea and vomiting may occur, particularly when the drug is given rapidly by the intravenous route; therefore, intravenous infusions in conscious patients should be given slowly over a period of at least eight minutes. Adverse effects reported less commonly include bradycardia, precipitation of anginal attacks, diarrhea, abdominal pain, hiccups, erythematous macular rash, flushing, hyperthermia, sweating, nasal stuffiness, and mild conjunctivitis.

ROUTES, USUAL DOSAGE, AND PREPARATIONS. Blood pressure and the electrocardiogram should be monitored continuously during therapy. Bretylium is eliminated by the kidneys as unchanged drug, and the dosage should be reduced in patients with impaired renal function.

Intravenous: For immediate control of life-threatening ventricular arrhythmias (particularly ventricular fibrillation), *adults*, 5 mg/kg of body weight of undiluted drug given rapidly. Dosage may be increased to 10 mg/kg and repeated at 15- to 30-minute intervals up to a maximal dose of 30 mg/kg.

For immediate control of other ventricular arrhythmias, *adults*, the contents of one ampul should be diluted with at least 50 ml of dextrose injection or sodium chloride injection and infused slowly in a dose of 5 to 10 mg/kg over a period of eight minutes or more; the dose may be repeated in one to two hours.

For maintenance, *adults*, a dilute solution may be infused continuously at a rate of 1 to 2 mg/min or 5 to 10 mg/kg may be given by slow intermittent infusion every six hours.

Intramuscular: *Adults*, 5 to 10 mg/kg of body weight of undiluted drug. The dose may be repeated in one to two hours and thereafter every six to eight hours. The site of injection should be varied and no more than 5 ml should be given in one site.

> **Bretylol** (Arnar-Stone). Solution 50 mg/ml in 10 ml containers.

EDROPHONIUM CHLORIDE
[Tensilon]

Edrophonium is a cholinesterase inhibitor that is used to terminate supraventricular tachycardias that cannot be controlled by vagal maneuvers alone. Because of its rapid onset and brief duration of action, edrophonium is usually preferred to neostigmine for this purpose. In patients with digitalis excess or high degrees of vagal tone, edrophonium may precipitate complete A-V block.

Cholinergic side effects (eg, miosis, sweating, salivation, gastrointestinal disturbances) may occur but are less common with edrophonium than with longer-acting cholinesterase inhibitors.

ROUTE, USUAL DOSAGE, AND PREPARATIONS. *Intravenous*: *Adults*, initially, 5 mg. If this dose is ineffective, an additional 5 to 10 mg may be given. *Children*, 2 mg administered slowly. Administration of edrophonium should be followed by a period of carotid massage.

> **Tensilon** (Roche). Solution 10 mg/ml in 1 and 10 ml containers.

AGENTS USED TO TREAT BRADYARRHYTHMIAS

ISOPROTERENOL HYDROCHLORIDE
[Isuprel Hydrochloride]

This adrenergic drug stimulates beta receptors in the heart, blood vessels, and bronchioles, thereby increasing heart rate and myocardial contractility, enhancing automaticity and conduction velocity, dilating resistance vessels (primarily in skeletal muscle), and causing bronchodilation. It has no significant effect on alpha receptors and therefore lacks the marked pressor effect of norepinephrine or epinephrine.

In patients with second- or third-degree A-V block, isoproterenol is used to maintain adequate heart rate and cardiac output prior to insertion of a pacemaker. It is particularly useful for the emergency treatment of patients with Stokes-Adams seizures and also is indicated for managing severe myocardial depression induced by propranolol.

Isoproterenol may cause tachycardia, extrasystoles, headache, dizziness, flushing, sweating, and tremors. By increasing myocardial oxygen demand, it may precipitate anginal attacks in susceptible individuals. Severe tachyarrhythmias occur occasionally.

ROUTE, USUAL DOSAGE, AND PREPARATIONS. *Intravenous: Adults*, 1 to 2 mg (5 to 10 ml of a 1:5,000 solution), diluted in 500 ml of 5% dextrose injection in water, is infused slowly at a rate of 0.5 to 2 ml/min with continuous monitoring of the electrocardiogram. The rate of infusion is determined by the chronotropic response.

Drug available generically: Solution 1:5,000 in 5 and 10 ml containers.

Isuprel Hydrochloride (Breon). Solution (aqueous) 1:5,000 (0.2 mg/ml) in 1 and 5 ml containers.

ATROPINE SULFATE

Atropine increases heart rate and A-V conduction velocity by blocking effects of the parasympathetic neurotransmitter, acetylcholine. It is used to treat certain reversible bradyarrhythmias that may accompany acute myocardial infarction, particularly marked symptomatic sinus bradycardia. Since a decrease in vagal tone occasionally precipitates severe ventricular arrhythmias, it is current practice not to treat patients who have asymptomatic sinus bradycardia with atropine. Atropine may enhance A-V conduction in Wenckebach Type I second-degree A-V block, but A-V block may be worsened in some patients. This paradoxical effect occurs because small doses of atropine may have little direct effect on the A-V node but nevertheless increase the sinus rate.

Therapeutic doses of atropine cause dryness of the mouth, cycloplegia, and mydriasis. Rarely, systemically administered anticholinergic drugs have induced acute angle-closure glaucoma in predisposed eyes. Large doses of atropine may cause hyperpyrexia, urinary retention, and central nervous system effects (eg, confusion, hallucinations). See also Chapter 21, Adjuncts to Anesthesia and Analeptic Drugs, and Chapter 60, Miscellaneous Gastrointestinal Agents.

ROUTE, USUAL DOSAGE, AND PREPARATIONS. *Intravenous: Adults*, initially, 0.4 to 1 mg every one to two hours as needed; larger doses occasionally may be required (maximum, 2 mg). *Children*, 0.01 to 0.03 mg/kg of body weight.

Drug available generically: Solution 0.3 mg/ml in 30 ml containers; 0.4 mg/ml in 0.5, 1, 20, and 30 ml containers; 0.5 mg/ml in 5 and 30 ml containers; 1 mg/ml in 1 and 10 ml containers; tablets (hypodermic) 0.3, 0.4, and 0.6 mg.

Selected References

Abrams WB, Davies RO: Antiarrhythmic mechanisms of beta-adrenergic blocking agents, in Dreifus LS, Likoff W (eds): *Cardiac Arrhythmias*. New York, Grune & Stratton, 1973, 517-530.

Anderson JL, et al: Antiarrhythmic drugs: Clinical pharmacology and therapeutic uses. *Drugs* 15:271-309, 1978.

Bellet S: *Clinical Disorders of the Heart Beat*, ed 3. Philadelphia, Lea & Febiger, 1971.

Bernstein JG, Koch-Weser J: Effectiveness of bretylium tosylate against refractory ventricular arrhythmias. *Circulation* 45:1024-1034, 1972.

Chung EK: *Principles of Cardiac Arrhythmias*, ed 2. Baltimore, Williams & Wilkins Company, 1977.

Cohen IS, et al: Adverse reactions to quinidine in hospitalized patients: Findings based on data from Boston Collaborative Drug Surveillance Program. *Prog Cardiovasc Dis* 20:151-163, 1977.

Dreifus LS, Likoff W (eds): *Cardiac Arrhythmias*. New York, Grune & Stratton, 1973.

Greenblatt DJ, et al: Pharmacokinetics of quinidine in humans after intravenous, intramuscular and oral administration. *J Pharmacol Exp Ther* 202:365-378, 1977.

Harrison DC: Should lidocaine be administered routinely to all patients after acute myocardial infarction? *Circulation* 58:581-584, 1978.

Heel RC, et al: Disopyramide: Review of its pharmacological properties and therapeutic use in treating cardiac arrhythmias. *Drugs* 15:331-368, 1978.

Holder DA, et al: Experience with bretylium tosylate by a hospital cardiac arrest team. *Circulation* 55:541-544, 1977.

Koch-Weser J: Bretylium. *N Engl J Med* 300:473-477, 1979 A.

Koch-Weser J: Disopyramide. *N Engl J Med* 300:957-961, 1979 B.

Koch-Weser J: Serum procainamide levels as therapeutic guides. *Clin Pharmacokinet* 2:389-402, 1977.

528

Lie KI, et al: Efficacy of lidocaine in preventing primary ventricular fibrillation within 1 hour after a 300 mg intramuscular injection: Double-blind, randomized study of 300 hospitalized patients with acute myocardial infarction. *Am J Cardiol* 42:486-488, 1978.

Lie KI, et al: Lidocaine in prevention of primary ventricular fibrillation. Double-blind randomized study of 212 consecutive patients. *N Engl J Med* 291:1324-1326, 1974.

Mason DT, et al: Antiarrhythmic agents. I. Mechanisms of action and clinical pharmacology. II. Therapeutic considerations. *Drugs* 5:261-291, 292-317, 1973.

Romhilt DW, et al: Evaluation of bretylium tosylate for treatment of premature ventricular contractions. *Circulation* 45:800-807, 1972.

Ruberman W, et al: Ventricular premature beats and mortality after myocardial infarction. *N Engl J Med* 297:750-757, 1977.

Valentine PA, et al: Lidocaine in prevention of sudden death in pre-hospital phase of acute infarction: Double-blind study. *N Engl J Med* 291:1327-1331, 1974.

Watanabe Y, Dreifus LS: *Cardiac Arrhythmias: Electrophysiologic Basis for Clinical Interpretation.* New York, Grune & Stratton, 1977.

Zipes DP, Troup PJ: New antiarrhythmic agents: Amiodarone, aprindine, disopyramide, ethmozin, mexiletine, tocainide, verapamil. *Am J Cardiol* 41:1005-1024, 1978.

Antianginal Agents | 35

The pain of angina pectoris is believed to reflect an imbalance between myocardial oxygen demand and the ability of the diseased coronary arteries to deliver oxygen. The drugs that are useful in antianginal therapy are the sublingually administered nitrates, which are used intermittently to prevent or relieve an acute attack, and the beta-adrenergic blocking agents and oral and topical nitrates, which are administered for long-term prophylaxis. The mechanism by which nitrates and beta-blocking drugs alleviate symptoms is not fully understood but appears to involve hemodynamic changes that reduce the oxygen requirements of the heart. The nitrates also may increase myocardial oxygen supply by their effect on the coronary circulation.

Providing symptomatic relief with antianginal drugs should be part of a general treatment program designed to alleviate symptoms and reduce risk factors that predispose to coronary artery disease (Aronow, 1973; Logue and Robinson, 1972; Paul, 1977; Sostman and Langou, 1978). Cessation of smoking is particularly important, both to avoid the adverse effects of nicotine and carbon monoxide on anginal symptoms and to eliminate one factor which may accelerate atherosclerosis. In obese patients, improvement may occur following weight reduction. Activities or events that precipitate anginal attacks should be recognized and avoided when possible, such as the consumption of heavy meals, undue emotional stress, strenuous unaccustomed exercise (particularly after meals), and exposure to cold air. Many patients benefit

psychologically from a graduated exercise program prescribed according to individual need, and the improvement in physical fitness may enable the patient to exercise without increasing symptoms. Antianxiety drugs may be useful adjunctively in selected patients to reduce the reaction to emotional stress.

Conditions that may aggravate angina (eg, hypertension, arrhythmias, anemia, hyperthyroidism) should be corrected. Reduction of blood pressure in hypertensive patients also reduces myocardial oxygen demand and may alone relieve angina. Congestive heart failure should be treated with digitalis and/or a diuretic. Digitalis is also indicated in patients with a supraventricular tachyarrhythmia and may be useful in those with nocturnal angina. It also counteracts the negative inotropic effect of propranolol in patients with pump dysfunction or left ventricular enlargement.

NITRATES

The nitrates reduce myocardial oxygen requirements through their effects on the systemic circulation. Their systemic actions include (1) a reduction in venous tone, which leads to pooling of blood in peripheral veins, decreased venous return, and reduced ventricular volume and myocardial tension; and (2) a decrease in peripheral vascular resistance, which lowers arterial blood pressure and ventricular outflow resistance. These hemodynamic actions are not always closely correlated with the antianginal effect (Goldstein and Epstein, 1973; Danahy and Aronow, 1977; Lee et al, 1978), and an increase in myocardial blood flow and oxygen supply may play an important role in the therapeutic response. Nitrates dilate coronary arteries and arterioles in normal individuals and also may increase blood flow to ischemic areas. Moreover, by decreasing left ventricular diastolic pressure, they may indirectly decrease coronary collateral resistance, thereby producing a favorable redistribution of myocardial blood flow. There is increasing evidence that coronary artery spasm is the cause of Prinzmetal's variant angina and also may contribute to typical angina.

SUBLINGUAL NITRATES

The sublingually administered nitrates (nitroglycerin, isosorbide dinitrate, and erythrityl tetranitrate) are used intermittently to prevent or relieve acute attacks of angina pectoris (Goldstein et al, 1971; Klaus et al, 1973; Sweatman, 1972; Willis et al, 1976). Because of its more rapid action, long-established efficacy, and low cost, nitroglycerin is the drug of choice among these agents. When taken at the onset of ischemic pain, it usually provides relief within one to three minutes. Since angina of effort frequently subsides spontaneously with cessation of activity, nitroglycerin is most useful when taken shortly before beginning activities that are likely to precipitate an attack. Used in this manner, it prevents the onset of anginal attacks for 20 to 30 minutes and occasionally for up to one hour.

Headache, flushing, and dizziness often are noted early during treatment with nitrates but can be minimized by use of small initial doses. Occasionally, generalized vasodilatation may cause profound hypotension and reflex tachycardia, and the fall in perfusion pressure may worsen anginal symptoms. Because of the pronounced effect of nitrates on capacitance vessels, the therapeutic effect is enhanced but adverse effects also are increased when the patient is in the upright position.

Marked orthostatic hypotension may occur, particularly if doses are repeated within a short period of time, but this frequently can be diminished by reducing the dosage. The patient should be instructed to sit down after taking the tablet.

There is no basis for warnings concerning the use of nitrates in patients with open-angle glaucoma or in those predisposed to angle closure.

ROUTE, USUAL DOSAGE, AND PREPARATIONS.
NITROGLYCERIN:
Sublingual: Adults, initially, 0.15 to 0.3 mg. The dose must be individualized to relieve symptoms with minimal adverse effects. Doses up to 0.6 mg or greater may be required in some patients. If symptoms are not relieved by a single dose, additional doses may be taken at five-minute intervals, but no more than three tablets should be used within a 15-minute period. Nitroglycerin gradually loses potency through volatilization; therefore, the drug must be packaged in glass containers with tightly fitting metal screw caps and with no more than 100-dose units in each container. In addition, it should be dispensed in the original unopened container and closed tightly after each use; nitroglycerin tablets should not be exposed to heat.

Drug available generically: Capsules 0.15, 0.3, 0.4, and 0.6 mg.
Nitrostat (Parke, Davis). Tablets 0.15, 0.3, 0.4, and 0.6 mg.

ISOSORBIDE DINITRATE:
Sublingual: Adults, 2.5 to 5 mg.
Drug available generically: Tablets 2.5 and 5 mg.
Isordil (Ives), *Sorbitrate* (Stuart). Tablets 2.5 and 5 mg.

ERYTHRITYL TETRANITRATE:
Sublingual: Adults, 5 mg.
Cardilate (Burroughs Wellcome). Tablets 5, 10, and 15 mg.

ORAL NITRATES

Orally administered nitrates (isosorbide dinitrate, nitroglycerin, erythrityl tetranitrate, mannitol hexanitrate, pentaerythritol tetranitrate) were developed in an attempt to provide a nitrate preparation with a sufficiently long duration of action for long-term prophylactic use. Controversy concerning the therapeutic value of these agents has revolved around four questions: (1) Are oral nitrates adequately absorbed into the systemic circulation? (2) What dosage is necessary to produce maximal therapeutic effects? (3) Do they produce tolerance and cross-tolerance to sublingual nitrates? (4) Do they induce physiologic dependence?

Doubts about the gastrointestinal absorption of nitrates were generated by experiments in which nitrates injected into the portal vein of rats were degraded by a liver enzyme before reaching the systemic circulation. Subsequent studies in patients with angina demonstrated that, when given orally in adequate dosage, isosorbide dinitrate and nitroglycerin have significant vasodilator activity (usually lasting at least four hours) and improve exercise tolerance. Because they are rapidly metabolized by the liver, doses larger than those usually recommended may be required to achieve therapeutic effects (Abrams, 1978; Danahy et al, 1977; Glancy et al, 1977; Winsor and Berger, 1975). Additional evidence that isosorbide dinitrate and nitroglycerin are absorbed when given orally is provided by numerous studies in which these agents improved cardiac performance for several hours in patients with severe intractable chronic congestive heart failure (see Chapter 33, Agents Used to Treat Congestive Heart Failure). The efficacy of the other oral nitrates in antianginal therapy has not been established, but there are a few studies showing hemodynamic effects in patients with heart failure.

Concern about tolerance and cross-tolerance derived from observations that nitrate headaches usually diminish during long-term therapy and that prolonged administration of oral nitrates attenuates the venodilator response to sublingual nitroglycerin. These hemodynamic changes apparently are not reflected in antianginal activity, since exercise tolerance tests have shown no loss of therapeutic response to isosorbide dinitrate during long-term therapy or evidence of cross-tolerance to sublingual nitroglycerin (Danahy and Aronow, 1977; Lee et al, 1978).

Munitions workers exposed to high levels of nitroglycerin over prolonged periods have developed nitrate dependence. Anginal attacks and, rarely, myocardial infarction and sudden death occurred in some of these workers during periods of withdrawal after prolonged exposure. Nitrate dependence has not been documented in patients receiving oral nitrates. For other adverse effects of nitrates, see the evaluation on Sublingual Nitrates.

ROUTE, USUAL DOSAGE, AND PREPARATIONS. Dosage should be individualized. The patient who does not obtain pain relief from a large dose of sublingual nitroglycerin is unlikely to benefit from oral nitrates.

ISOSORBIDE DINITRATE:

Oral: Adults, 10 to 40 mg four times daily (or three times daily when sustained-release preparations are used). Larger doses (up to 360 mg daily) have been effective in some patients when lower doses have failed.

> Drug available generically: Capsules (timed-release) 40 mg; tablets 5, 10, and 20 mg; tablets (timed-release) 40 mg.
> *Isordil* (Ives). Capsules (timed-release) 40 mg; tablets 5, 10, and 20 mg; tablets (timed-release) 40 mg.
> *Sorbitrate* (Stuart). Tablets 5, 10, and 20 mg.
> Isosorbide dinitrate is also available as a chewable tablet (*Isordil* 10 mg; *Sorbitrate* 5 and 10 mg), but the efficacy of of these preparations in the treatment of angina has not been clearly established.

NITROGLYCERIN:

Oral: Adults, 2.6 or 6.5 mg two or three times daily.

> Drug available generically: Capsules (plain, timed-release) 2.5 and 6.5 mg; tablets 2.5 and 6.5 mg; tablets (timed-release) 2.5 mg.
> *Nitro-Bid* (Marion). Capsules 2.5, 6.5, and 9 mg.
> *Nitroglyn* (Key). Tablets (timed-release) 1.3, 2.6, and 6.5 mg.
> *Nitrong* (Wharton). Tablets (timed-release) 2.6 and 6.5 mg.
> *Nitrospan* (USV). Capsules (timed-release) 2.5 mg.

Information is insufficient to recommend a dosage for the following agents for prophylaxis in angina pectoris:

ERYTHRITYL TETRANITRATE:

> *Cardilate* (Burroughs Wellcome). Tablets 5, 10, and 15 mg; tablets (chewable) 10 mg.

MANNITOL HEXANITRATE:

> Drug available generically: Tablets 30 mg.

PENTAERYTHRITOL TETRANITRATE:

> Drug available generically: Capsules (timed-release) 30 and 80 mg; tablets 10 and 20 mg.

Duotrate (Marion). Capsules (timed-release) 30 and 45 mg.
Pentritol (Armour). Capsules (timed-release) 30 and 60 mg.
Peritrate (Parke, Davis). Tablets 10, 20, and 40 mg; tablets (timed-release) 80 mg.

NITROGLYCERIN OINTMENT 2%
[Nitro-Bid, Nitrol, Nitrong]

Nitroglycerin ointment is well absorbed through the skin and produces hemodynamic effects and improves exercise capacity for at least three hours after topical administration. The antianginal effect is sustained during long-term therapy and cross-tolerance to sublingual nitrates does not occur (Reichek et al, 1974). Although this preparation may be useful as a long-acting antianginal agent, it is not yet known whether toxicity or dependence may prove to be a problem with this route of administration.

Allergic contact dermatitis has rarely been associated with topical nitroglycerin. Precipitation or aggravation of peripheral edema has been reported, but a cause-and-effect relationship has not been established. For other adverse reactions, see the evaluations on Sublingual Nitrates and Oral Nitrates.

ROUTE, USUAL DOSAGE, AND PREPARATIONS.
Topical: The 2% ointment contains 15 mg nitroglycerin per inch. Initially, one-half inch is spread in a thin uniform layer on the chest, back, abdomen, or anterior thighs. This may be increased, if necessary, by one-half inch to the largest amount that does not cause headache. Some patients may require up to 4 or 5 inches.
Nitro-Bid (Marion). Ointment 2% in 20 and 60 g containers.
Nitrol (Kremers-Urban). Ointment 2% in 30 and 60 g containers.
Nitrong (Wharton). Ointment 2% in 60 g containers.

BETA-ADRENERGIC BLOCKING AGENTS

Propranolol [Inderal] and metoprolol [Lopressor] are the only beta-adrenergic blocking drugs that are currently available in the United States. Propranolol has been widely used to treat angina, hypertension, and arrhythmias. Metoprolol has been employed mainly as an antihypertensive agent, and there is not sufficient published data to evaluate its use in angina. A number of other beta-blocking drugs are under investigation.

Beta-adrenergic receptors are located predominantly in the heart, in the arteries and arterioles of skeletal muscle, and in the bronchi, where they subserve cardiac excitation, vasodilatation, and bronchial relaxation. Beta-blocking drugs combine reversibly with these receptors to block the response to sympathetic nerve impulses or circulating catecholamines. Blockade of cardiac (beta₁) receptors reduces heart rate, myocardial contractility, and cardiac output. The atrioventricular (A-V) conduction time is slowed and, at the cellular level, automaticity is suppressed. Blood pressure also is reduced (see Chapter 38, Antihypertensive Agents).

By attenuating the cardiac response to sympathetic stimulation, beta blockade generally reduces myocardial oxygen demand, particularly during exercise, and thereby delays the onset of ischemic pain. The oxygen-sparing action usually overrides other effects that tend to increase myocardial oxygen consumption (ie, prolongation of systolic ejection period, increased ventricular volume) and to decrease myocardial oxygen supply (ie, reduced coronary blood flow, increased coronary vascular resistance).

Blockade of noncardiac (beta₂) receptors increases airway resistance, inhibits catecholamine-induced glycolysis and lipolysis, and inhibits the vasodilating effect of catecholamines on peripheral blood vessels. These noncardiac actions are responsible for some of the adverse effects of beta-blocking drugs (bronchospasm, hypoglycemia, and, possibly, aggravation of peripheral vascular insufficiency).

Beta-blocking agents differ in their relative affinity for beta₁ and beta₂ receptors. Propranolol, nadolol, and timolol are classified as "nonselective" because they block beta receptors equally at all sites. Some beta-blocking drugs (metoprolol, atenolol,

acebutolol, tolamolol) are more cardioselective and may be safer in asthmatics, in
patients prone to develop hypoglycemia,
and in those with peripheral vascular disease. However, cardioselectivity is not absolute and may not be apparent except at
low doses. All beta-blocking drugs should
be used cautiously in patients with these
disorders.

The various beta-blocking drugs also differ in partial agonist properties (intrinsic
sympathomimetic activity) and membrane-
stabilizing (local anesthetic) effects. These
features are not clinically important except
that agents devoid of intrinsic sympathomimetic activity (propranolol, metoprolol, nadolol, sotolol, timolol, tolamolol,
atenolol) may have a broader dose-
response curve than those possessing this
characteristic (oxprenolol, alprenolol, pindolol, acebutolol). Beta-blocking drugs that
readily cross the blood-brain barrier (eg,
propranolol) may cause central nervous
system side effects. Differences in their
effects on plasma renin activity are discussed in Chapter 38.

PROPRANOLOL HYDROCHLORIDE
[Inderal]

Propranolol has provided a significant
advance in the long-term management of
angina pectoris. In addition to its usually
beneficial effect on myocardial oxygen demand, propranolol may increase oxygen
delivery to the marginally perfused
myocardium by shifting the oxygen-
hemoglobin dissociation curve to the right.
During exercise tolerance tests, propranolol usually delays the onset of anginal
symptoms and the appearance of ischemic
electrocardiographic changes. Long-term
administration reduces the frequency of
anginal attacks and decreases nitroglycerin
requirements in many patients (Prichard,
1974). Propranolol may have detrimental

effects, however, in patients with borderline cardiac reserve who rely on
sympathetic stimulation to remain compensated.

Propranolol is usually well tolerated and,
in the absence of specific contraindications, it should be considered for trial in all
patients with frequent attacks of angina.
Sublingual nitrates should be continued, as
needed, to prevent or relieve symptoms,
because propranolol and nitrates reduce
cardiac work by different mechanisms and
may have an additive effect in reducing
myocardial oxygen demand. In addition,
propranolol attenuates the reflex tachycardia induced by the nitrate, while nitrates
tend to counteract the increase in heart size
and prolongation of ventricular systole that
follows beta blockade. The nitrates also
may counteract the tendency of beta-
blocking drugs to decrease coronary blood
flow. This combined regimen is often effective even in patients with severe angina
(Russek, 1974). Although further long-term
documentation is needed, it has been reported that long-term therapy with beta-
blocking drugs may reduce the risk of
myocardial infarction in patients with
coronary artery disease and may prolong
the life of those surviving a prior anterior
infarction (Multicentre International
Study, *Br Med J*, 1975 and 1977;
Fitzgerald, 1976).

In addition to its use in angina, propranolol is effective in the treatment of
hypertension (see Chapter 38), certain arrhythmias (see Chapter 34), and hypertrophic subaortic stenosis.

Propranolol is rapidly and almost completely absorbed from the gastrointestinal
tract, but plasma levels correlate poorly
with dosage. Since it is eliminated mainly
by hepatic metabolism, variability in the
rate of metabolism is believed to account
for most of the individual differences in
bioavailability. Some of the effects of propranolol may be due to a cardioactive
metabolite. It was formerly believed that
doses below 30 mg did not enter the systemic circulation because of hepatic (first
pass) extraction, but it has subsequently
been shown that even smaller doses produce blood levels that, although undetect-

able by conventional fluorometry, can be detected by gas-liquid chromatography (Davies et al, 1978). Attempts to determine therapeutic plasma concentrations have not been consistently effective, largely because of individual differences in sympathetic tone and cardiac reserve.

ADVERSE REACTIONS AND PRECAUTIONS.

Cardiovascular: Propranolol may cause pronounced bradycardia and hypotension, particularly when administered intravenously. It should be used cautiously in patients with extremely low sinus rates. If excessive bradycardia occurs, atropine should be given intravenously or intramuscularly. In the event of severe myocardial depression, isoproterenol should be infused intravenously; because of the competitive nature of beta blockade, large doses may be needed.

Propranolol may precipitate heart failure in patients with inadequate cardiac reserve and should be given with extreme caution to those with frank or borderline congestive heart failure who depend upon sympathetic stimulation to remain compensated. If a beta-blocking drug must be used in such patients, therapy should be initiated with small doses, and digitalis and/or a diuretic should be given concomitantly. Propranolol may cause cardiac arrest in patients with A-V block and is usually contraindicated in the presence of serious A-V conduction disturbances.

Propranolol may precipitate or aggravate Raynaud's phenomenon. It also may exacerbate intermittent claudication and generally should be avoided in patients with chronic occlusive peripheral vascular disease.

Sudden withdrawal of large doses of propranolol has been followed within a two-week period by the recurrence of unstable angina, ventricular tachycardia, fatal myocardial infarction, and sudden death (Harrison and Alderman, 1976). These complications have occurred most frequently in patients with severe angina who were well stabilized on the drug. If it becomes necessary to discontinue propranolol, the dosage should be reduced gradually over a one- to two-week period and the patient should be instructed to restrict physical activity during this time. Most surgeons no longer feel that it is necessary or desirable to discontinue propranolol before coronary bypass surgery.

Respiratory: Propranolol increases airway resistance and may provoke asthmatic attacks. It should be avoided in patients with a history of asthma or bronchitis.

Metabolic: Propranolol should be used cautiously in diabetics because it impairs the sympathetically mediated rebound response to hypoglycemia and may mask hypoglycemic symptoms (sweating and tachycardia). It has produced hypoglycemia in diabetic patients receiving insulin, in patients recovering from anesthesia, in those on dialysis, and in children during periods of restricted food intake. In hypertensive patients, the blood pressure may increase during the hypoglycemic episode. Propranolol has been reported to enhance the effect of thiazides on serum triglyceride and urate levels (see also Chapter 39, Diuretics).

Neurologic: Fatigue and lethargy are the most common central side effects of propranolol. Vivid dreams (with or without insomnia), depression, hallucinations, and paresthesias have been mentioned by several investigators. There is one report of acute organic brain syndrome induced by propranolol.

Miscellaneous: Propranolol may cause nausea, vomiting, diarrhea, and flatulence. Fever, rash, myotonia, cheilostomatitis, Peyronie's disease, thrombocytopenia, and agranulocytosis have occurred rarely. Propranolol crosses the placenta and has caused bradycardia and hypotension in newborn infants whose mothers were receiving the drug. It is also excreted in breast milk.

ROUTE, USUAL DOSAGE, AND PREPARATIONS. When propranolol is administered orally, the therapeutic effect correlates poorly with dosage; therefore, dosage should be titrated in terms of the clinical response. The dosages suggested below are intended only as guidelines.

Oral: Adults, for angina, initially, 10 mg three or four times daily. The dosage may be increased gradually, as needed, to control symptoms. For maintenance, most patients require 160 to 240 mg daily in four divided doses. Rarely, some patients require up to 400 mg daily. Sublingually administered nitrates should be continued, as needed, during therapy with propranolol.

For hypertrophic subaortic stenosis, initially, 20 to 40 mg three or four times daily. Dosage may be increased gradually to control symptoms. A daily maintenance dose of 320 mg or more may be needed.

    Inderal (Ayerst). Tablets 10, 20, 40, and 80 mg.

MISCELLANEOUS AGENT

DIPYRIDAMOLE
  [Persantine]

    Dipyridamole is a potent coronary vasodilator promoted for long-term prophylactic therapy in patients with angina. Double-blind studies have demonstrated that this agent does not significantly decrease the incidence or severity of anginal attacks.

    The adverse effects of dipyridamole include dizziness, headache, syncope, gastrointestinal disturbances, and rash. Rarely, the drug has appeared to aggravate anginal symptoms.

    Because efficacy has not been established, no dosage is suggested.

    Persantine (Boehringer Ingelheim). Tablets 25 mg.

MIXTURES

    These products contain an oral nitrate and a sedative or other drug. Although sedatives are acknowledged to be useful to reduce the reaction to emotional stress in certain patients with angina pectoris, they should be prescribed separately, if needed.

    Equanitrate (Wyeth). Each tablet contains pentaerythritol tetranitrate 10 or 20 mg and meprobamate 200 mg.

    Isordil with Phenobarbital (Ives). Each tablet contains isosorbide dinitrate 10 mg and phenobarbital 15 mg.

    Miltrate (Wallace). Each tablet contains pentaerythritol tetranitrate 10 or 20 mg and meprobamate 200 mg.

    Peritrate with Phenobarbital (Parke, Davis). Each tablet contains pentaerythritol tetranitrate 10 or 20 mg and phenobarbital 15 mg; each timed-release tablet contains pentaerythritol tetranitrate 80 mg and phenobarbital 45 mg.

    Sorbitrate with Phenobarbital (Stuart). Each tablet contains isosorbide dinitrate 10 mg and phenobarbital 15 mg.

Selected References

Improvement in prognosis of myocardial infarction by long-term beta-adrenergic blockade using practolol: Multicentre international study. *Br Med J* 3:735-740, 1975.

Reduction in mortality after myocardial infarction with long-term beta-adrenergic blockade: Multicentre international study. *Br Med J* 2:419-421, 1977.

Abrams J: Usefulness of long-acting nitrates in cardiovascular disease. *Am J Med* 64:183-186, 1978.

Aronow WS: Medical treatment of angina pectoris. IX. Medical management of angina pectoris. *Am Heart J* 85:275-278, 1973.

Danahy DT, Aronow WS: Hemodynamics and antianginal effects of high dose oral isosorbide dinitrate after chronic use. *Circulation* 56:205-212, 1977.

Danahy DT, et al: Sustained hemodynamic and anti-anginal effect of high dose oral isosorbide dinitrate. *Circulation* 55:381-387, 1977.

Davies R, et al: Beta-blockade and blood-levels after low-dose oral propranolol: Hepatic "first-pass" threshold revisited. *Lancet* 1:407-410, 1978.

Fitzgerald JD: Effect of beta-adrenoreceptive antagonists on morbidity and mortality in cardiovascular disease. *Postgrad Med J* 52:770-781, 1976.

Glancy DL, et al: Effect of swallowed isosorbide dinitrate on blood pressure, heart rate and exercise capacity in patients with coronary artery disease. *Am J Med* 62:39-46, 1977.

Goldstein RE, Epstein SE: Nitrates in prophylactic treatment of angina pectoris. *Circulation* 48:917-920, 1973.

Goldstein RE, et al: Clinical and circulatory effects of isosorbide dinitrate: Comparison with nitroglycerin. *Circulation* 43:629-640, 1971.

Harrison DC, Alderman EL: Discontinuation of propranolol therapy: Cause of rebound angina pectoris and acute coronary events. *Chest* 69:1-2, 1976.

Klaus AP, et al: Comparative evaluation of sublingual long-acting nitrates. *Circulation* 48:519-525, 1973.

Lee G, et al: Effects of long-term oral administration of isosorbide dinitrate on antianginal response to nitroglycerin: Absence of nitrate cross-tolerance and self-tolerance shown by exercise testing. *Am J Cardiol* 41:82-87, 1978.

Logue RB, Robinson PH: Medical management of angina pectoris. *Circulation* 46:1132-1145, 1972.

Paul O: Medical management of angina pectoris. *JAMA* 238:1847-1848, 1977.

Prichard BNC: Beta-adrenergic blocking drugs in angina pectoris. *Drugs* 7:55-84, 1974.

Reichek N, et al: Sustained effects of nitroglycerin ointment in patients with angina pectoris. *Circulation* 50:348-352, 1974.

Russek HI: "Natural" history of severe angina pectoris with intensive medical therapy alone: Five-year prospective study of 133 patients. *Chest* 65:46-51, 1974.

Sostman HD, Langou RA: Contemporary medical management of stable angina pectoris. *Am Heart J* 95:775-788, 1978.

Sweatman T: Long-acting hemodynamic effects of isosorbide dinitrate. *Am J Cardiol* 29:475-480, 1972.

Willis WH Jr, et al: Hemodynamic effects of isosorbide dinitrate versus nitroglycerin in patients with unstable angina. *Chest* 69: 15-22, 1976.

Winsor T, Berger HJ: Oral nitroglycerin as prophylactic antianginal drug: Clinical, physiologic, and statistical evidence of efficacy based on three-phase experimental design. *Am Heart J* 90:611-626, 1975.

Agents Used in Peripheral Vascular Disorders | 36

Vasodilator therapy may be beneficial in peripheral arterial disorders such as Raynaud's phenomenon in which blood flow to the skin is markedly reduced by vasoconstriction but there is little or no significant organic involvement. Vasodilators are not useful in chronic occlusive peripheral vascular disorders.

Vasospastic Disorders: The attacks of digital pallor, cyanosis, and rubor that occur in patients with Raynaud's disease (primary Raynaud's phenomenon) are precipitated by exposure to cold and occasionally by emotional stress. These patients have an abnormally small digital capillary blood flow and, when sympathetic tone is increased, the flow is further reduced, probably because of arteriolar constriction (Coffman and Cohen, 1971). Attacks often can be prevented if precipitating factors are avoided; reassurance also may be helpful. In progressive cases that do not respond to these measures, vasodilators may reduce the degree of vasoconstriction and improve digital capillary blood flow (Coffman and Cohen, 1971; Coffman and Davies, 1975; Gifford, 1971; Halperin and Coffman, 1979; Kontos and Wasserman, 1969).

In secondary Raynaud's phenomenon, episodic vasospasm involving the skin of the extremities occurs as a manifestation of collagen disease (especially scleroderma), occlusive arterial disease (arterosclerosis obliterans, thromboembolism, and particularly thromboangiitis obliterans), trauma, ergot toxicity, and a number of other conditions (McGrath and Penny, 1974). Raynaud's phenomenon may be the presenting symptom in some of these disorders, and successful management depends upon identification and treatment of the underlying cause. Vasodilators may improve cutaneous blood flow in some patients but are of marginal value in advanced cases with an obstructive component (Coffman and Cohen, 1971; Coffman and Davies, 1975; Halperin and Coffman, 1979).

Vasodilators are not indicated in the management of acrocyanosis or primary (idiopathic) livedo reticularis, which are benign vasospastic disorders that do not progress significantly.

Chronic Occlusive Peripheral Vascular Disease: Patients with arteriosclerosis obliterans often present with pain during exercise (intermittent claudication) but are asymptomatic at rest, which indicates that skeletal muscle blood flow is not sufficient to meet an increase in metabolic requirements. These patients do not need an increased muscle blood flow during the resting state. Because skeletal muscle circulation is largely under autoregulatory control, vasodilators rarely increase blood flow beyond the level produced by maximal tolerated exercise, and they are ineffective in relieving intermittent claudication (Coffman and Mannick, 1972). Regular exercise to the limits of tolerance may increase walking distance.

Patients with advanced arteriosclerosis obliterans who have rest pain or ischemic skin lesions need an increased blood supply to the skin. No vasodilator consistently increases skin blood flow in the presence of significant organic obstruction (Coffman and Mannick, 1972). By dilating vessels in noninvolved areas, these drugs may actually divert blood from diseased to nondiseased areas and do more harm than good. Avoiding exposure to cold and trauma, cessation of smoking, meticulous foot care, rest, and treatment of major risk factors (diabetes mellitus and hyperlipidemia) are more helpful than vasodilator therapy in these patients (Schatz, 1971). Surgical revascularization, when feasible, is the treatment of choice for patients with severe local ischemia.

Vasodilators are also of no benefit in thromboangiitis obliterans, except possibly in mild cases with considerable peripheral arterial spasm and minimal organic occlusion.

Drug Therapy

Several classes of drugs with vasodilator action have been used to treat peripheral vascular disorders. These agents reduce vascular tone by producing generalized inhibition of sympathetic function, by blocking alpha-adrenergic receptors in the blood vessels of the skin, by directly relaxing vascular smooth muscle, or possibly by stimulating beta-adrenergic receptors in the blood vessels of skeletal muscle. Some

of these drugs are potent hypotensive agents, and care should be taken to avoid a marked fall in blood pressure which may counterbalance the increase in blood flow, particularly in areas supplied by atherosclerotic vessels.

Reserpine [Sandril, Serpasil] dilates blood vessels in the skin by depleting catecholamine stores in sympathetic nerve terminals. It diminishes neurogenic vasoconstriction in Raynaud's disease and other peripheral arterial disorders in which episodes of peripheral ischemia are associated with increased sympathetic activity. Reserpine is inexpensive and is convenient to use because it requires administration only once daily. Other sympathetic depressant drugs, such as guanethidine [Ismelin] and methyldopa [Aldomet], also may be effective in some patients with vasospastic disorders. Since guanethidine does not cause mental depression, it may be particularly useful as an alternative to reserpine in patients with a history of depression.

The alpha-adrenergic blocking agent, phenoxybenzamine [Dibenzyline], acts selectively at alpha receptor sites to block the response to sympathetic nerve impulses or circulating catecholamines. Since alpha receptors are abundant in the resistance vessels of the skin, while skeletal muscle blood flow is largely controlled by local mechanisms, alpha blockade increases blood flow to skin but not to skeletal muscle. Phenoxybenzamine may diminish neurogenic vasoconstriction in primary and secondary Raynaud's phenomenon, although its usefulness is limited by its pronounced side effects.

Tolazoline [Priscoline] directly relaxes vascular smooth muscle, although other actions, including transient alpha blockade, have been demonstrated in animals. Tolazoline has been effective in peripheral arterial disorders associated with significant functional vasoconstriction. It may be of particular value when added to the regimen of patients with severe Raynaud's phenomenon who do not respond to reserpine alone.

Other agents that have a nonspecific relaxant effect on vascular smooth muscle include papaverine, isoxsuprine [Vaso-dilan], cyclandelate [Cyclospasmol], niacin [Nicobid], nicotinyl alcohol [Roniacol], dioxyline [Paveril], and ethaverine [Ethatab, Ethaquin]; they are not potent vasodilators when given orally, and their efficacy in the treatment of peripheral vascular disorders has not been established. The more potent oral or sublingual nitrates are not used for this indication. A 2% nitroglycerin ointment [Nitro-Bid, Nitrol, Nitrong] produces generalized vasodilatation when applied to the skin but has not been promoted for use in peripheral vascular disorders. Some physicians feel that ethyl alcohol is of value, but large amounts (4 oz) are needed to produce vasodilatation. Severe peripheral ischemia caused by ergot poisoning has been successfully treated by continuous infusion of sodium nitroprusside [Nipride], a vasodilator used in hypertensive emergencies (Carliner et al, 1974).

Nylidrin [Arlidin] is usually classified as a beta-receptor stimulant, although animal studies have demonstrated that beta blockade only partially inhibits its vasodilator action. Nylidrin increases muscle blood flow under some circumstances, but it rarely increases calf muscle flow beyond the level produced by exercise to tolerance and is of no value in relieving intermittent claudication. Since nylidrin has no significant effect on blood flow to the skin, it is of no value in vasospastic disorders.

DRUGS THAT REDUCE SYMPATHETIC TONE

RESERPINE
[Sandril, Serpasil]

Reserpine depletes catecholamine stores in sympathetic nerve terminals, thereby reducing adrenergic vasoconstriction in the blood vessels of the skin. When given orally, it may be used for long-term therapy in primary and secondary Raynaud's phenomenon (Coffman and Cohen, 1971; Kontos and Wasserman, 1969). Intra-arterial injection above the site of involvement has been reported to relieve symptoms for variable periods, but one controlled study showed no clearcut benefit over placebo injections (McFadyen et al, 1973); hematemesis has occurred occasionally with this route of administration. Reserpine is not useful in chronic occlusive peripheral vascular disorders.

Nasal stuffiness and bradycardia occur commonly with clinically effective doses of reserpine. More significant adverse effects include lethargy, nightmares, and mental depression, which may be insidious and occasionally is of sufficient severity to require hospitalization or result in suicide. (See also Chapter 38, Antihypertensive Agents.)

ROUTE, USUAL DOSAGE, AND PREPARATIONS. *Oral: Adults*, 0.25 to 1 mg daily.

Drug available generically: Tablets 0.1, 0.25, 0.5, and 1 mg.
Sandril (Lilly). Tablets 0.1 and 0.25 mg.
Serpasil (Ciba). Elixir 0.2 mg/4 ml; tablets 0.1, 0.25, and 1 mg.

GUANETHIDINE SULFATE
[Ismelin Sulfate]

Guanethidine, which interferes with the release of norepinephrine from sympathetic nerve terminals, has been shown to increase finger capillary blood flow in patients with Raynaud's phenomenon (LeRoy et al, 1971). Since guanethidine does not readily cross the blood-brain barrier, mental depression has not been a problem with its use, and it may be a suitable alternative to reserpine for treating vasospastic disorders in patients with a history of depression. It is not useful in chronic occlusive peripheral vascular disorders.

Orthostatic hypotension and hypotension during exercise are common side effects that often limit the clinical usefulness of guanethidine. Other frequent adverse effects are fluid retention, bradycardia, diarrhea, and retrograde ejaculation. See also Chapter 38, Antihypertensive Agents.

ROUTE, USUAL DOSAGE, AND PREPARATIONS.
Oral: *Adults*, 30 to 50 mg daily.
   Ismelin Sulfate (Ciba). Tablets 10 and 25 mg.

METHYLDOPA
   [Aldomet]

Methyldopa is an aromatic amino acid decarboxylase inhibitor that depresses sympathetic nervous system activity through an effect on the central nervous system. It has been used successfully to reduce neurogenic vasoconstriction in some patients with Raynaud's phenomenon (Varadi and Lawrence, 1969). It is not useful in chronic occlusive peripheral vascular disorders.

Drowsiness, dryness of the mouth, and fluid retention are common during methyldopa therapy. Severe reactions (eg, hemolytic anemia, hepatitis) are rare. (See also Chapter 38, Antihypertensive Agents.)

ROUTE, USUAL DOSAGE, AND PREPARATIONS.
Oral: *Adults*, 1 to 2 g daily.
   Aldomet (Merck Sharp & Dohme). Tablets 125, 250, and 500 mg.

PHENOXYBENZAMINE HYDROCHLORIDE
   [Dibenzyline]

Phenoxybenzamine dilates cutaneous blood vessels by blocking alpha-adrenergic receptors and may be used to reduce neurogenic vasoconstriction in primary or secondary Raynaud's phenomenon. Since this drug does not increase skeletal muscle blood flow, it is of no value in chronic occlusive peripheral vascular disease.

When phenoxybenzamine is given in clinically effective doses, orthostatic hypotension and reflex tachycardia occur in most patients. Nasal congestion, gastrointestinal disturbances (nausea, vomiting, diarrhea), and impotence also have been reported.

ROUTE, USUAL DOSAGE, AND PREPARATIONS.
Oral: Only 20% to 30% of an oral dose is absorbed in active form. *Adults*, initially, 10 mg daily; the dose is increased by 10-mg increments at four-day intervals until the desired effect is achieved or adverse effects become intolerable. The usual maintenance dose is 20 to 60 mg daily.
   Dibenzyline (Smith Kline & French). Capsules 10 mg.

DIRECT-ACTING VASODILATORS

TOLAZOLINE HYDROCHLORIDE
   [Priscoline Hydrochloride]

In usual clinical doses, the vasodilator action of tolazoline is probably caused by direct relaxation of vascular smooth muscle, although other actions (alpha blockade, sympathomimetic and cholinergic properties) have been demonstrated in animals. When given orally, tolazoline may be useful in vasospastic disorders, particularly when added to the regimen of patients with severe Raynaud's phenomenon who do not respond to reserpine alone (Coffman and Cohen, 1971). Like all other vasodilators, tolazoline is not useful in conditions in which organic vascular changes are prominent.

Effective doses may cause chilliness, paresthesias of the scalp, and headache. Pronounced tachycardia, anginal pain, arrhythmias, and changes in blood pressure may be observed, but these reactions are less likely to occur with oral than with parenteral administration. Gastrointestinal disturbances (abdominal pain, nausea, vomiting, diarrhea, exacerbation of peptic ulcer) also have been reported.

ROUTE, USUAL DOSAGE, AND PREPARATIONS. *Oral: Adults,* 25 mg four to six times daily. Dosage may be increased, if necessary, up to 50 mg six times daily. Alternatively, 80 mg (in timed-release form) may be given every 12 hours.

> Drug available generically: Tablets 25 mg.
> *Priscoline Hydrochloride* (Ciba). Tablets 25 mg; tablets (timed-release) 80 mg.

PAPAVERINE HYDROCHLORIDE

Papaverine is the prototype of the vasodilators that have a nonspecific relaxant effect on vascular smooth muscle. This drug is promoted for oral therapy in the treatment of various obstructive and vasospastic peripheral vascular diseases, but no objective study has shown it to be effective despite its many years of use.

Adverse reactions include nausea, abdominal discomfort, anorexia, constipation or diarrhea, malaise, drowsiness, vertigo, hyperhidrosis, headache, rash, flushing of the face, and hepatic reactions due to hypersensitivity (jaundice, eosinophilia, altered results of liver function tests).

Because the place of this agent in therapy of peripheral vascular disease has not been established, no dosage is suggested.

> Drug available generically: Capsules (timed-release) 150 mg; tablets 30, 60, 100, and 200 mg.
> **Available Trademarks.**

Cerespan (USV), *Pavabid* (Marion), *Pavacap* (Reid-Provident), *Paverine* (North American), *P-200* (Boots), *Vasal* (Tutag), *Vasospan* (Ulmer) [all timed-release oral forms].

CYCLANDELATE
[Cyclospasmol]

Cyclandelate produces vasodilatation by acting directly on vascular smooth muscle. It is promoted for the treatment of various vasospastic and obstructive peripheral vascular disorders, but its efficacy in these conditions has not been confirmed.

Cyclandelate may cause gastrointestinal disturbances (pyrosis, pain, eructation), flushing, tingling, headache, weakness, and tachycardia.

Because the place of this agent in therapy of peripheral vascular disease has not been established, no dosage is suggested.

> Drug available generically: Capsules, tablets 200 and 400 mg; tablets 200 mg.
> *Cyclospasmol* (Ives). Capsules 200 and 400 mg; tablets 100 mg.

ISOXSUPRINE HYDROCHLORIDE
[Vasodilan]

Isoxsuprine is often classified as a beta-receptor stimulant, although in animal studies its vascular effect is not blocked by propranolol (Manley and Lawson, 1968). Isoxsuprine may increase muscle blood flow in normal individuals but does not significantly affect blood flow to the skin (Coffman, 1968). It does not improve calf muscle blood flow in patients with occlusive vascular disorders and thus is ineffective in relieving intermittent claudication

(Coffman and Mannick, 1972; Zsotér and Baird, 1974). There is also no convincing evidence that isoxsuprine is useful in vasospastic disorders.

Adverse effects include dizziness, hypotension, tachycardia, and, occasionally, severe rash.

Because the place of this agent in therapy of peripheral vascular disease has not been established, no dosage is suggested.

> Drug available generically: Tablets 10 and 20 mg.
> *Vasodilan* (Mead Johnson). Solution (injection) 5 mg/ml in 2 ml containers; tablets 10 and 20 mg.

NIACIN (Nicotinic Acid)
[Nicobid]

NICOTINYL ALCOHOL
[Roniacol]

NICOTINYL ALCOHOL TARTRATE
[Roniacol Tartrate]

The pharmacologic actions of these weak vasodilators are similar; niacin is a metabolic product of nicotinyl alcohol. In clinical doses, these agents act primarily on dermal vessels in the blush area. They have little effect on the vessels of the lower extremities, and there is no convincing evidence that they are of any use in vasospastic disorders or other peripheral vascular disease.

Adverse effects include transient flushing of the face and neck, pruritus, tingling, gastrointestinal disturbances, rash, and urticaria.

Because the place of these agents in therapy of peripheral vascular disease has not been established, no dosage is suggested.

> NIACIN:
> *Nicobid* (Armour). Capsules (timed-release) 125, 250, and 500 mg.
> NICOTINYL ALCOHOL:
> *Roniacol* (Roche). Elixir 50 mg/5 ml.

NICOTINYL ALCOHOL TARTRATE:
> Drug available generically: Tablets 50 mg; tablets (timed-release) 150 mg.
> *Roniacol Tartrate* (Roche). Tablets 50 mg; tablets (timed-release) 150 mg.

BETA-ADRENERGIC STIMULANT

NYLIDRIN HYDROCHLORIDE
[Arlidin]

Nylidrin allegedly improves skeletal muscle blood flow by stimulating beta-adrenergic receptors; however, animal studies suggest that the vasodilator effect may be due in part to a direct action (Manley and Lawson, 1968). When measurements are taken at rest, nylidrin increases calf muscle blood flow in normal individuals and in some patients with arteriosclerosis obliterans. It rarely increases calf flow during exercise, however, and is ineffective in relieving intermittent claudication (Coffman and Mannick, 1972). There is also no convincing evidence that nylidrin is useful in Raynaud's phenomenon.

Adverse effects include dizziness, tachycardia, hypotension, nausea, and vomiting.

Because the place of this agent in therapy of peripheral vascular disease has not been established, no dosage is suggested.

> Drug available generically: Tablets 6 and 12 mg.
> *Arlidin* (USV). Tablets 6 and 12 mg.

Selected References

Carliner NH, et al: Sodium nitroprusside treatment of ergotamine induced peripheral ischemia. *JAMA* 227:308-309, 1974.

Coffman JD: Effect of vasodilator drugs in vasoconstricted normal subjects. *J Clin Pharmacol* 8:302-308, 1968.

Coffman JD, Cohen AS: Total and capillary fingertip blood flow in Raynaud's phenomenon. *N Engl J Med* 285:259-263, 1971.

Coffman JD, Davies WT: Vasospastic diseases: A review. *Prog Cardiovasc Dis* 18:123-146, 1975.

Coffman JD, Mannick JA: Failure of vasodilator drugs in arteriosclerosis obliterans. *Ann Intern Med* 76:35-39, 1972.

Gifford RW Jr: The arteriospastic diseases: Clinical significance and management. *Cardiovasc Clin* 3:127-139, 1971.

Halperin JL, Coffman JD: Pathophysiology of Raynaud's disease. *Arch Intern Med* 139:89-92, 1979.

Kontos HA, Wasserman AJ: Effect of reserpine in Raynaud's phenomenon. *Circulation* 39:259-266, 1969.

LeRoy EC, et al: Skin capillary blood flow in scleroderma. *J Clin Invest* 50:930-939, 1971.

Manley ES, Lawson JW: Effect of beta adrenergic receptor blockade on skeletal muscle vasodilatation produced by isoxsuprine and nylidrin. *Arch Int Pharmacodyn Ther* 175:239-250, 1968.

McFadyen IJ, et al: Intraarterial reserpine administration in Raynaud syndrome. *Arch Intern Med* 132:526-528, 1973.

McGrath MA, Penny R: Mechanisms of Raynaud's phenomenon. *Med J Aust* 2:328-333, 367-375, 1974.

Schatz IW: Medical management of chronic occlusive arterial disease of extremities. *Cardiovasc Clin* 3:94-102, 1971.

Varadi DP, Lawrence AM: Suppression of Raynaud's phenomenon by methyldopa. *Arch Intern Med* 124:13-18, 1969.

Zsotér TT, Baird RJ: Isoxsuprine as oral vasodilator. *Can Med Assoc J* 110:1260-1261, 1974.

Agents Used to Treat Shock | 37

Hypotension does *not* require treatment unless there are signs or symptoms of tissue hypoperfusion. Shock is caused by inadequate tissue perfusion and is often accompanied by increased sympathetic activity. Several of the following signs and symptoms usually are observed in patients in shock: mental obtundation, tachypnea, tachycardia, pallor, cold and clammy skin, oliguria, and metabolic acidosis. Most patients in shock are hypotensive, but the arterial pressure occasionally may be normal, especially in previously hypertensive patients. The goal of therapy is to ensure sufficient blood flow to adequately perfuse vital organs (Moran, 1970; Weil et al, 1975).

In treating the shock patient, a number of hemodynamic, metabolic, and respiratory measurements are employed to detect potentially reversible disturbances and to assess the effectiveness of therapy. Hemodynamic measurements should include continuous electrocardiographic monitoring of cardiac rate and rhythm, intra-arterial pressure (preferably measured directly), and pulmonary artery end-diastolic or pulmonary capillary wedge pressures using a Swan-Ganz flow-directed catheter. The pulmonary artery or wedge pressure gives a more accurate estimate of left ventricular filling pressure, particularly in left ventricular dysfunction, than does measurement of central venous pressure and is particularly useful in evaluating the response to fluid challenge. Cardiac output can be increased in some patients if the wedge pressure is raised to 18 to 20 mm Hg. The system should also include provi-

sions for monitoring arterial blood gases, serum electrolytes and osmolality, skin and core temperature, fluid intake and output, urine osmolality, and plasma colloid osmotic pressure (Weil and Shubin, 1974; Weil et al, 1978). Routine measurement of cardiac output is no longer considered mandatory (Weil and Shubin, 1974; Johnson and Gunnar, 1977) but, as wedge pressure is increased by plasma volume expansion, cardiac output measurement may be useful.

Drug Therapy

Sympathomimetic Amines: When shock is caused by inadequate circulating blood volume, blood or plasma volume expanders should be administered. In normovolemic patients and those unresponsive to adequate plasma volume expansion, sympathomimetic amines may improve perfusion of vital areas until definitive therapy becomes effective or the underlying pathologic state is corrected.

Except in patients with anaphylactic shock or life-threatening hypotension, sympathomimetic amines should not be the initial therapy. They should be used only when volume replacement (if indicated) and treatment of etiologic factors fail to maintain satisfactory circulation. The goal of therapy is to ensure adequate tissue perfusion and not to keep the blood pressure at an arbitrarily set level. The need for and response to a sympathomimetic amine should be assessed on the basis of cerebral and myocardial function, urinary output,

545

and peripheral skin (toe) temperature, together with measurement of arterial blood lactate. The blood lactate is an indirect measure of perfusion failure in that it quantitates the extent of anaerobic metabolism. The rate of infusion must be regulated carefully so that the desired level of blood pressure is not exceeded. Generally, the systolic blood pressure should be maintained between 80 and 90 mm Hg or, in previously hypertensive patients, 30 mm Hg below the usual level.

To be effective, sympathomimetic amines should maintain perfusion of the heart, brain, kidney, and other visceral organs by one or more of the following mechanisms: (1) increasing myocardial contractility, which results in increased cardiac output as long as venous return is adequate; (2) constricting capacitance vessels, thereby preventing venous pooling; and (3) dilating resistance vessels in vital organs without affecting or constricting resistance vessels in nonvital organs.

Sympathomimetic amines mimic the effects of sympathetic nerve stimulation, and their effects vary according to their action on cardiovascular adrenergic receptors. Three distinct receptors have been postulated, alpha-adrenergic, beta-adrenergic, and dopamine receptors, which differ in the type of actions they subserve and in their distribution in the cardiovascular system. Alpha-adrenergic receptors are found in most blood vessels but are most abundant in the resistance vessels of the skin, mucosa, intestine, and kidney. Drugs acting on alpha receptors produce greater vasoconstriction in these vascular beds. Drugs acting on beta-adrenergic receptors increase cardiac contractility and heart rate, accelerate A-V conduction, and may cause vasodilation, primarily in arterioles in skeletal muscles and mesenteric vascular beds. Recent evidence suggests that there are two types of beta-adrenergic receptors: beta$_1$ receptors subserving cardiac stimulation and beta$_2$ receptors subserving bronchial relaxation and vasodilation in peripheral arterioles, particularly in skeletal muscle. Dopamine receptors subserve vasodilation in the renal and mesenteric vascular beds and also have been

described in the coronary and cerebral circulation (Goldberg, 1972; Tarazi, 1974; Weil et al, 1975).

Sympathomimetic amines used in the treatment of shock include the endogenous catecholamines, norepinephrine (levarterenol) [Levophed], epinephrine [Adrenalin], and dopamine [Intropin], and the synthetic compounds, dobutamine [Dobutrex], isoproterenol [Isuprel], and metaraminol [Aramine]. Other sympathomimetic amines are used as pressor agents during anesthesia (ephedrine, mephentermine [Wyamine], methoxamine [Vasoxyl], and phenylephrine [Neo-Synephrine]) (see Chapter 21, Adjuncts to Anesthesia and Analeptic Drugs) or occasionally to treat idiopathic orthostatic hypotension (ephedrine and phenylephrine).

Norepinephrine and dopamine are commonly used as temporary adjunctive measures in the treatment of shock. Norepinephrine stimulates the myocardium and increases cardiac output by acting on beta$_1$ receptors and causes peripheral vasoconstriction by activating alpha receptors. When used in amounts sufficient to raise the arterial pressure to 100 to 110 mm Hg, the inotropic action is predominant; with larger doses, the vasoconstrictor effect becomes more prominent. Cardiac work and myocardial oxygen consumption are increased by norepinephrine, and blood flow may be reduced to all areas except the heart and brain. It is a more potent vasoconstrictor than dopamine.

Dopamine stimulates the heart primarily by a direct action on beta$_1$ receptors in the myocardium and to a lesser extent by releasing norepinephrine from tissue stores. Small doses increase cardiac output without affecting heart rate or blood pressure because of a balance between renal and mesenteric vasodilation (action on dopamine receptors) and vasoconstriction in skeletal muscle vascular beds (action on alpha receptors). Larger doses produce greater vasoconstriction and elevate the blood pressure; the heart rate also may increase.

Metaraminol stimulates the myocardium and causes vasoconstriction, mainly by releasing norepinephrine from adrenergic nerve terminals. The hemodynamic actions and uses of metaraminol are similar to those of norepinephrine, but its duration of action is prolonged and it can be given intravenously or intramuscularly.

Isoproterenol acts on beta₁ receptors in the heart and beta₂ receptors in blood vessels, thereby elevating cardiac output and increasing blood flow, mainly in skeletal muscle. It usually produces pronounced tachycardia through a direct action on the heart and through baroreceptor reflexes. Isoproterenol increases systolic pressure and lowers diastolic pressure; the mean arterial pressure is relatively unchanged. The increase in systolic pressure is caused by its effect on myocardial contractility and cardiac output; the decrease in diastolic pressure is related to arteriolar dilatation and reduction of peripheral vascular resistance. Isoproterenol is used primarily to treat low-output states caused by myocardial failure. Its major disadvantage, particularly in patients with cardiogenic shock, is that it produces a disproportionate increase in myocardial oxygen requirements.

Dobutamine acts primarily on beta₁ receptors and has less pronounced actions on beta₂ and alpha receptors. Moderate doses increase myocardial contractility without greatly increasing heart rate or altering peripheral vascular resistance.

Epinephrine acts on beta₁ receptors in the heart and on both alpha and beta₂ receptors in peripheral blood vessels. Small doses dilate skeletal muscle and mesenteric arterial blood vessels and may decrease blood pressure, but even small amounts constrict cutaneous and renal blood vessels. In large doses, the vasoconstrictor action predominates and blood pressure is increased. Because it dilates constricted bronchioles (by acting on beta₂ receptors) and also raises blood pressure, epinephrine is the drug of choice for treating anaphylactic shock.

Vasodilator Drugs: In recent years, vasodilators have been used in selected patients with severe pump failure following acute myocardial infarction and in other forms of severe left ventricular dysfunction (Cohn and Franciosa, 1977). The rationale for this form of therapy is to improve cardiac performance by reducing peripheral vascular resistance and to limit the extent of ischemic damage by reducing myocardial oxygen demand. Agents that produce both venodilation and arterial dilation (eg, sodium nitroprusside [Nipride], nitrates, alpha-adrenergic blocking agents, ganglionic blocking drugs) are more useful than those with minimal action on veins (eg, hydralazine [Apresoline], diazoxide [Hyperstat]). The intravenously administered direct-acting vasodilators, sodium nitroprusside and nitroglycerin (intravenous preparation not available commercially), are usually preferred. Nonparenteral vasodilators (oral and topical nitrates, prazosin [Minipress], hydralazine) are useful mainly for long-term therapy in patients with severe, refractory chronic congestive heart failure, although sublingual and topical nitrates also have been used after acute myocardial infarction (see Chapter 33, Agents Used to Treat Congestive Heart Failure).

Nitroprusside has a balanced effect on resistance and capacitance vessels and usually does not increase heart rate in patients with left ventricular failure. It may be given with dopamine or dobutamine. Nitroglycerin acts predominantly to reduce venous tone but also dilates resistance vessels. The alpha-adrenergic blocking drug, phentolamine [Regitine], also has been given intravenously to patients with severe heart failure after myocardial infarction, but tachycardia limits its usefulness and it is expensive.

Phentolamine is also used as an adjunct to volume replacement in the treatment of hypovolemic states to estimate the adequacy of volume replacement and to permit administration of a larger volume of fluid without overloading the heart. In the presence of hypovolemia, volume replacement should always precede administration of phentolamine, and fluid should be available in case there is an acute fall in arterial pressure, which indicates inadequate volume replacement. (See Chapter 38, Antihypertensive Agents, for evaluations on Sodium Nitroprusside and Phentolamine.)

Alkalizing Agents: Metabolic acidosis occurring during shock is usually caused by perfusion failure and accumulation of acid metabolites. Measures that improve tissue perfusion generally correct the acidosis, and alkalizing agents are not required unless the arterial blood pH consistently falls below 7.2. In such cases, sodium bicarbonate may be administered cautiously. Therapy for acidosis should be carefully monitored, not only by measuring blood gases but also by monitoring circulatory variables, because overcorrection can be as hazardous as undercorrection. If metabolic alkalosis is produced, there is a danger of further reducing tissue perfusion and precipitating ventricular arrhythmias.

Digitalis and Adrenal Corticosteroids: The use of digitalis glycosides and adrenal corticosteroids in the treatment of shock is controversial. In cardiogenic shock, digitalis (or, in urgent situations, DC cardioversion) is indicated to slow the ventricular rate in patients with atrial flutter or fibrillation; it also may improve left ventricular function if congestive heart failure continues after arterial pressure is established. The rationale for using digitalis in other forms of shock is based on the observation that myocardial function is usually depressed during prolonged shock; its effectiveness in improving myocardial function in this setting is not established.

Adrenal corticosteroids are advocated by some investigators because of experiments demonstrating that these agents stabilize lysosomal membranes and antagonize endotoxin. (See Chapter 41, Adrenal Corticosteroids.) Results of some studies indicate that steroids may be helpful in bacterial shock when given in pharmacologic doses for short periods. There is no convincing evidence that they are useful in other forms of shock.

Clinical Applications

Hypovolemic Shock: Hypovolemic shock may result from external or internal loss of blood, plasma, or water following hemorrhage, trauma, burns, or protracted vomiting or diarrhea. Venous return and cardiac output are reduced and peripheral resistance is usually increased by compensatory mechanisms. Volume replacement is the only effective treatment, and fluid challenge should be guided by measurement of the pulmonary capillary wedge or pulmonary artery end-diastolic pressure. If there is still evidence of perfusion failure, a trial with isoproterenol or phentolamine may be considered. Vasoconstrictors may be necessary in patients who are profoundly hypotensive, but they should not be used for prolonged periods because they may increase ischemic injury by further reducing blood flow through vital organs (Weil et al, 1975).

Cardiogenic Shock: The most common cause of cardiogenic shock is acute myocardial infarction, although myocardial depression also occurs in other forms of shock. The hemodynamic pattern is not always predictable but, in most patients, cardiac output is reduced, pulmonary wedge pressure is elevated, and peripheral resistance is either normal or elevated. Even under the best circumstances, cardiogenic shock is difficult to treat because of extensive myocardial necrosis, and mechanical cardiac assist systems are often required (Gunnar et al, 1976; Kuhn, 1978).

By increasing arterial blood pressure, sympathomimetic amines may improve coronary blood flow and, by stimulating the myocardium, they may increase cardiac output. These agents must be used with caution, however, because they increase myocardial oxygen consumption by a direct effect on myocardial metabolism and by the extra pressure work imposed on the heart. Whether the increased oxygen requirements are met by an adequate increase in coronary blood flow will ultimately depend upon the effect of the amine on the level of blood pressure, especially the diastolic pressure, which determines perfusion through the coronary vessels. In a minority of patients, hypotension in acute myocardial infarction is associated with hypovolemia and a normal or low wedge pressure. These features are most commonly seen in postoperative patients or those who have suffered blood loss. Such patients may benefit from plasma volume expansion, but wedge pressure should be monitored closely.

Because it acts rapidly and is the most potent pressor agent available, norepinephrine (levarterenol) is often preferred for emergency treatment of patients with severe hypotension (da Luz et al, 1976; Kuhn, 1978; Johnson and Gunnar, 1977). Norepinephrine should not be used for prolonged periods because it may cause ischemia of vital organs and depletion of the plasma volume. Dopamine may be useful if adequate perfusion pressure is maintained and the heart rate does not increase too greatly with its use. This drug produces less vasoconstriction than norepinephrine and less vasodilation and tachycardia than isoproterenol; in appropriate doses, it also may increase blood flow to the kidneys and mesentery (Goldberg, 1972). Isoproterenol has been used to treat cardiogenic shock, but its failure to increase coronary perfusion pressure to adequate levels and the tachycardia it produces have greatly restricted its use (Gunnar et al, 1967).

Vasodilator drugs may be useful in selected patients with severe pump failure following acute myocardial infarction (Cohn and Franciosa, 1977; Chatterjee et al, 1976; Chatterjee and Parmley, 1977; Johnson and Gunnar, 1977; Kuhn, 1978). Therapy is initiated with an intravenously infused drug, usually sodium nitroprusside, and, if continued treatment is indicated, a nonparenteral agent, such as sublingual isosorbide dinitrate, may be substituted after about 72 hours. Vasodilators are not indicated for routine use but appear to be most appropriate in patients with pre-existing hypertension or recurrent ischemic pain. If the systolic pressure falls below 100 mm Hg during vasodilator therapy, the drug should be discontinued or its dosage reduced and an inotropic agent, such as dopamine or dobutamine, given concomitantly. While vasodilator therapy has improved short-term prognosis, long-term prognosis remains unfavorable despite continued therapy with oral nitrates. See also Chapter 33, Agents Used to Treat Congestive Heart Failure.

Bacterial Shock: Shock may occur during the course of gram-negative or, less commonly, gram-positive bacterial infections. The severity, hemodynamic changes, and response to therapy vary widely, depending upon the age of the patient, virulence of the bacteria, presence of concurrent disease or other factors (eg, diabetes mellitus, ischemic heart disease, surgery, trauma), and stage of the syndrome. Bacterial shock is associated with a defect in the distribution of blood flow and is currently classified as a distributive form of shock (Weil et al, 1975). In gram-negative bacteremia, the effective blood volume is reduced because of pooling in the venous capacitance bed; peripheral vascular resistance is usually increased. In gram-positive bacteremia, the perfusion deficit may be caused by vascular fluid loss due to increased vascular permeability. Because of increased arteriovenous shunting, peripheral resistance is usually reduced (Weil, 1977).

Bacterial shock requires *immediate intensive antibiotic therapy* and maintenance of an adequate circulating volume. Blood gases should be monitored closely and oxygen should be administered if there is evidence of hypoxemia. Whether sympathomimetic amines should be used adjunctively if volume replacement does not reverse the signs of shock is unsettled. Isoproterenol increases cardiac output if adequate perfusion pressure is maintained and excessive tachycardia does not occur; however, it has the disadvantages of increasing myocardial oxygen requirements and further reducing blood pressure and the potential for precipitating arrhythmias. For these reasons, dopamine is usually preferred. When neither dopamine nor isoproterenol maintains adequate perfusion pressure, norepinephrine may be required for brief periods. These drugs should not be used routinely, because they may intensify perfusion failure and increase myocardial oxygen demands.

Adverse Reactions and Precautions

Therapeutic doses of sympathomimetic amines may cause headache, restlessness, anxiety, weakness, pallor, dizziness, tremor, precordial pain, palpitation, and respiratory distress. Overdosage can induce convulsions, cerebral hemorrhage, and tachyarrhythmias. Excessive cardiac acceleration can reduce cardiac filling time, myocardial efficiency, coronary blood flow, and cardiac output. Since fatal ventricular arrhythmias may be precipitated by sympathomimetic amines that have cardiac excitatory actions, the electrocardiogram should be monitored closely and the drug discontinued or its dosage reduced if an arrhythmia develops. Arrhythmias occur most frequently after administration of large doses of sympathomimetic drugs, during the initial stage of infusion, and in patients with organic heart disease and/or severe shock complicated by extreme hypoxia and electrolyte imbalance. Digitalis therapy also increases the risk of arrhythmias.

Prolonged administration of vasoconstricting sympathomimetic amines may reduce plasma volume because constriction of the postcapillary vessels increases capillary pressure and facilitates transcapillary fluid loss. Renal blood flow and glomerular filtration rate, already decreased by hypotension and compensatory vasoconstriction, may be reduced further by those sympathomimetic amines that constrict the renal vasculature, and severe metabolic acidosis and acute tubular necrosis may develop.

Various pathologic changes have been attributed to prolonged administration of large doses of sympathomimetic amines, particularly norepinephrine. These include edema, hemorrhage, and necrosis of the intestine, liver, and kidneys, as well as focal myocarditis, subpericardial hemorrhage, intravascular platelet aggregation, and local slough and gangrene of fingers or toes. These changes are seen most commonly in patients in severe shock, and it is not certain whether they are caused by drug therapy or by the shock process alone; they apparently develop most frequently in patients with pre-existing vascular disease. Prolonged administration of large doses of sympathomimetic amines produces diffuse necrotic myocardial lesions in experi-

mental animals, and similar lesions have been seen in patients who died after prolonged infusion of norepinephrine (Haft, 1974).

Recurrent hypotension may follow sudden withdrawal of sympathomimetic amines after they have been used for several days or weeks. The fall in arterial blood pressure may be due to generalized loss of vascular tone or exudation of fluid from the vascular space. To avoid this complication, an attempt should be made to discontinue therapy as soon as possible. If there is difficulty in withdrawing the drug, appropriate fluids should be infused and the blood pressure monitored continuously. Measurement of the pulmonary capillary wedge pressure is important for estimating volume loss and as a guide for volume replacement. Use of sympathomimetic amines should not be resumed until the systolic blood pressure falls close to the previous shock level and signs and symptoms of inadequate tissue perfusion are observed. If fluid replacement is unsuccessful, another attempt should be made to discontinue the sympathomimetic amine five or ten minutes later. It may be necessary to repeat this procedure several times.

INDIVIDUAL EVALUATIONS

DOPAMINE HYDROCHLORIDE
[Intropin]

$$HO-\underset{\underset{HO}{\big|}}{\bigcirc}-CH_2CH_2\overset{+}{N}H_3 \quad Cl^-$$

Dopamine exerts a positive inotropic effect due to a direct action on beta-adrenergic receptors and to release of norepinephrine from tissue storage sites. Hemodynamic effects vary with dosage. With low doses (less than 250 mcg/min), cardiac output and renal and mesenteric blood flow increase with little change in heart rate while peripheral resistance decreases. Sodium excretion also is enhanced. With increasing doses, vaso-constriction occurs and arterial pressure rises. With large doses, vasoconstriction predominates and renal blood flow may be reduced; when this occurs, urine output may decrease.

Dopamine is used to treat shock when the marked vasoconstrictor activity of norepinephrine is unnecessary and the vasodilator and cardioaccelerator effects of isoproterenol are undesirable. It is also used to treat acute heart failure following cardiovascular surgery and in severe refractory chronic congestive heart failure (see also Goldberg, 1972). Because of its unique hemodynamic effects, dopamine is often preferred to other sympathomimetic amines for treating patients with impaired renal function. In selected patients, a combination of dopamine and sodium nitroprusside or isoproterenol may produce a greater increase in cardiac output than either drug alone.

Dopamine may cause nausea, vomiting, headache, central nervous system stimulation, tachyarrhythmias, and anginal pain. In cardiogenic shock, the improved hemodynamic status induced by dopamine may be accompanied by an increase in myocardial oxygen consumption (Mueller et al, 1978). Small doses occasionally precipitate a fall in blood pressure due to the vasodilator effect. This can be corrected by increasing the infusion rate.

Polyuria, resulting in volume depletion, has been associated rarely with dopamine therapy in patients with gram-negative bacterial shock. Since dopamine is metabolized by monoamine oxidase, dosage should be reduced to one-tenth the usual amount in patients receiving monoamine oxidase inhibitors. Extravasation of large amounts of dopamine into local tissue may cause ischemic necrosis and slough. If extravasation occurs, the site should be infiltrated with 10 ml of a solution containing 5 to 10 mg of phentolamine using a fine hypodermic needle. Gangrene of fingers and toes after prolonged infusion has been reported. For further information, see the section on Adverse Reactions and Precautions.

ROUTE, USUAL DOSAGE, AND PREPARATIONS.
Intravenous: Adults, the drug is typically prepared as a solution containing 400 or 800 mcg/ml. This can be accomplished by transferring the contents of one ampul to a 250 or 500 ml bottle of sterile sodium chloride injection, 5% dextrose injection, 5% dextrose and 0.45% or 0.9% sodium chloride injection, 5% dextrose in lactated Ringer's solution, or sodium lactate (1/6 Molar) injection. Initially, the diluted solution is infused at a rate of 2 to 5 mcg/kg/min. In more seriously ill patients, an initial infusion rate of 5 mcg/kg/min may be increased gradually (in increments of 5 to 10 mcg/kg/min) to 20 to 50 mcg/kg/min. If larger doses are required, urine output should be checked frequently. When dopamine is discontinued gradually, vasodilation with a decrease in blood pressure may occur when the dose falls below the inotropic level. This complication can usually be avoided if the dosage is not decreased to less than 4 to 5 mcg/kg/min when discontinuing the drug.

Intropin (Arnar-Stone). Solution (aqueous) 40 mg (equivalent to 32.3 mg of the base)/ml in 5 ml containers.

DOBUTAMINE HYDROCHLORIDE
[Dobutrex]

This synthetic catecholamine was developed in a search for new inotropic agents with minimal chronotropic or vascular activity. Dobutamine acts primarily on myocardial beta1 receptors, has less pronounced actions on beta2 and alpha receptors, and does not activate dopamine receptors in the renal and mesenteric vascular beds. Moderate doses increase myocardial contractility without greatly increasing heart rate; large doses increase heart rate and blood pressure may rise. In animal studies, equivalent inotropic doses of dobutamine had less than one-fourth the chronotropic effect of isoproterenol. This difference appeared to be independent of reflex hemodynamic effects and may reflect a relatively selective action on ventricular contractile tissue, with a lesser effect on the S-A node (Tuttle and Mills, 1975).

Dobutamine has been used for short-term therapy to increase the cardiac output of patients with severe chronic congestive heart failure and of those who have undergone cardiac surgery. Experience is still too limited to evaluate its safety and efficacy in patients with acute myocardial infarction.

When used for inotropic support during emergence from cardiac surgery, dobutamine appears to be as effective as isoproterenol in increasing cardiac output. It may cause less tachycardia and fewer arrhythmias than isoproterenol (Tinker et al, 1976), although some investigators have found no significant difference between the two drugs (Kersting et al, 1976).

In patients with severe chronic congestive heart failure, both dobutamine and dopamine increased cardiac output, but dobutamine was more effective in reducing left ventricular filling pressure (Loeb et al, 1977; Stoner et al, 1977) and, in one study, caused less tachycardia (Stoner et al, 1977). When infused in doses producing comparable increases in cardiac output, nitroprusside reduced systemic arterial and wedge pressures more than dobutamine and did not increase heart rate (Berkowitz et al, 1977; Mikulic et al, 1977). Combined therapy with dobutamine and nitroprusside produced a greater increase in cardiac output, a lower wedge pressure, and a greater reduction in systemic and pulmonary vascular resistance than either drug alone (Mikulic et al, 1977).

Dobutamine may occasionally cause nausea, headache, palpitations, anginal pain, and shortness of breath. Tachycardia and hypertension, the most common adverse effects, usually can be controlled by a reduction in dosage. Ventricular arrhythmias may occur but appear to be less common with dobutamine than with isoproterenol. Since dobutamine facilitates A-V conduction, it may increase the ventricular rate in patients with atrial fibrillation.

ROUTE, USUAL DOSAGE, AND PREPARATIONS. Dobutamine is incompatible with alkaline solutions and should not be mixed with sodium bicarbonate injection. It may be reconstituted with sterile water or 5% dextrose injection by adding 10 to 20 ml of diluent to the vial containing 250 mg of dobutamine. This solution can be stored for 48 hours under refrigeration or six hours at room temperature. This solution must be further diluted before infusion to at least 50 ml and should be used within 24 hours.
Intravenous: Adults, the rate of infusion required to increase cardiac output usually ranges from 2.5 to 10 mcg/kg/min. Rarely, infusion rates up to 40 mcg/kg/min may be required.
Dobutrex (Lilly). Powder 250 mg.

EPINEPHRINE HYDROCHLORIDE
[Adrenalin Chloride]

Epinephrine stimulates the heart and large doses constrict capacitance and resistance vessels. In smaller doses, it relaxes resistance vessels in skeletal muscles and the mesenteric vascular bed, and peripheral resistance may decrease. Epinephrine also dilates constricted bronchioles. Because it rapidly relieves laryngeal edema and bronchospasm, epinephrine is the drug of choice for treating anaphylactic shock. Hypoxia should be treated by establishing an airway and administering oxygen. If these measures do not relieve hypotension, fluids should be given to restore the intravascular volume, and a more potent vasoconstrictor, such as norepinephrine, may be infused. Aminophylline, antihistamines, and corticosteroids are administered adjunctively.

For adverse reactions and precautions, see the Introduction.

ROUTES, USUAL DOSAGE, AND PREPARATIONS. *Intramuscular, Subcutaneous, Intravenous: Adults*, initially, 0.5 ml of a 1:1,000 solution injected intramuscularly or sub-cutaneously, followed by 0.25 to 0.5 ml of a 1:10,000 solution given intravenously every 5 to 15 minutes.

Intramuscular: Children, initially, 0.3 ml of a 1:1,000 solution. This dose may be repeated at 15-minute intervals for three or four doses if necessary. In an emergency, the drug may be given intravenously.

> Drug available generically: Solution 1:1,000 in 1 and 30 ml containers and 1:10,000 in 10 ml containers; powder; crystals.
> *Adrenalin Chloride* (Parke, Davis). Solution 1:1,000 (1 mg/ml) in 1 and 30 ml containers.

ISOPROTERENOL HYDROCHLORIDE
[Isuprel Hydrochloride]

This synthetic catecholamine acts exclusively on beta-adrenergic receptors. It stimulates the heart, dilates resistance vessels (primarily those in skeletal muscle), and relaxes bronchial smooth muscle. Isoproterenol is used primarily to treat low-output states caused by myocardial failure, particularly after cardiac surgery, pericardial compression, and bradyarrhythmias (see Chapter 34, Antiarrhythmic Agents). The value of isoproterenol for treatment of hypovolemic and bacterial shock is controversial.

Isoproterenol may cause headache, flushing, hyperhidrosis, tremor, dizziness, nausea, palpitation, and tachycardia. Since arrhythmias may occur, continuous monitoring of cardiac rhythm is advisable during infusion. A major problem, particularly in cardiogenic shock, is that isoproterenol greatly increases myocardial oxygen demand because of its positive inotropic and chronotropic effects; furthermore, perfusion pressure may not increase sufficiently to maintain coronary blood flow, and myocardial ischemia may develop (Gunnar et al, 1967).

ROUTE, USUAL DOSAGE, AND PREPARATIONS. *Intravenous: Adults,* 1 to 2 mg (5 to 10 ml of solution) diluted in 500 to 1,000 ml of 5% dextrose injection and infused at a rate of 0.5 to 5 mcg/min, which may be increased up to 10 mcg/min if necessary.

> Drug available generically: Solution 1:5,000 in 5 and 10 ml containers.
> *Isuprel Hydrochloride* (Breon). Solution 1:5,000 (0.2 mg/ml) in 1 and 5 ml containers.

NOREPINEPHRINE BITARTRATE (Levarterenol Bitartrate)
[Levophed Bitartrate]

This catecholamine has positive inotropic and chronotropic effects and a potent constrictor action on resistance and capacitance vessels. Its marked pressor effect is primarily due to increased peripheral resistance. Despite its direct positive chronotropic effects, it may indirectly reduce heart rate by reflex mechanisms. Norepinephrine has a prompt and reversible action and is used to treat shock when a potent vasoconstrictor is needed to maintain adequate tissue perfusion.

Norepinephrine can cause tissue necrosis at the site of injection. The risk of ischemic injury is reduced if the drug is infused via a catheter in a deeply seated vein and if a small amount of phentolamine is added to the solution. The infusion site should be changed when prolonged administration is necessary. If extravasation occurs, the site should be infiltrated with 10 ml of a solution containing 5 to 10 mg of phentolamine using a fine hypodermic needle. To reduce the incidence of venous thrombosis, heparin may be added to this infusion solution in amounts supplying 100 to 200 units/hour.

For a general discussion of adverse reactions and precautions with sympathomimetic amines, see the Introduction.

ROUTE, USUAL DOSAGE, AND PREPARATIONS.
Intravenous: Adults, 2 to 8 ml of solution is added to 500 ml of 5% dextrose injection and given by continuous infusion at a rate adjusted to maintain a satisfactory perfusion state. *Children*, 1 ml of solution is added to 250 ml of 5% dextrose injection and given by continuous infusion at a rate of 0.5 ml/min.

> *Levophed Bitartrate* (Breon). Solution (aqueous) equivalent to 1 mg of base/ml in 4 ml containers.

METARAMINOL BITARTRATE
[Aramine]

The effects of metaraminol depend largely upon the release of norepinephrine from sympathetic nerve endings. Its hemodynamic effects and uses are similar to those of norepinephrine, except that metaraminol is less potent, has a more gradual onset, and a longer duration of action. In contrast to norepinephrine, it may be given intramuscularly as well as intravenously, as it does not cause tissue necrosis. In addition to its use in shock, metaraminol is used to treat paroxysmal atrial tachycardia, as are other pressor agents.

Theoretically, the effect of metaraminol may be reduced after prolonged administration or with concomitant use of a catecholamine-depleting agent (eg, reserpine, guanethidine). If this complication occurs, metaraminol should be replaced by norepinephrine.

For adverse reactions and precautions, see the Introduction.

ROUTES, USUAL DOSAGE, AND PREPARATIONS.
Intravenous: Adults, 2 to 5 mg as a single injection or 200 to 500 mg diluted in 1 L of 5% dextrose injection and administered by continuous infusion at a rate sufficient to maintain a satisfactory perfusion pressure. *Children*, 0.01 mg/kg of body weight as a single dose; alternatively, a solution containing 1 mg/25 ml in 5% dextrose injection is administered by continuous infusion at a rate sufficient to maintain a satisfactory perfusion state.
Intramuscular: Adults, 5 to 10 mg; *children*, 0.1 mg/kg of body weight.
Subcutaneous: This drug should not be administered by this route because tissue sloughing may occur.

> Drug available generically: Solution 1% in 10 ml containers.
> *Aramine* (Merck Sharp & Dohme). Solution 1% equivalent to 10 mg of base/ml in 1 and 10 ml containers.

Selected References

Berkowitz C, et al: Comparative responses to dobutamine and nitroprusside in patients with chronic low output cardiac failure. *Circulation* 56:918-924, 1977.

Chatterjee K, Parmley WW: Vasodilator treatment for acute and chronic heart failure. *Br Heart J* 39:706-720, 1977.

Chatterjee K, et al: Effects of vasodilator therapy for severe pump failure in acute myocardial infarction on short-term and late prognosis. *Circulation* 53:797-802, 1976.

Cohn JN, Franciosa JA: Vasodilator therapy of cardiac failure. *N Engl J Med* 297:27-31, 254-258, 1977.

da Luz PL, et al: Current concepts on mechanisms and treatment of cardiogenic shock. *Am Heart J* 92:103-113, 1976.

Goldberg LI: Cardiovascular and renal action of dopamine: Potential clinical applications. *Pharmacol Rev* 24:1-29, 1972.

Gunnar RM, et al: Cardiovascular assist devices in cardiogenic shock. *JAMA* 236:1619-1621, 1976.

Gunnar RM, et al: Ineffectiveness of isoproterenol in shock due to acute myocardial infarction. *JAMA* 202:1124-1128, 1967.

Haft JI: Cardiovascular injury induced by sympathetic catecholamines. *Prog Cardiovasc Dis* 17:73-86, 1974.

Johnson SA, Gunnar RM: Treatment of shock in myocardial infarction. *JAMA* 237:2106-2108, 1977.

Kersting F, et al: Comparison of cardiovascular effects of dobutamine and isoprenaline after open heart surgery. *Br Heart J* 38:622-626, 1976.

Kuhn LA: Management of shock following acute myocardial infarction. I. Drug therapy. II. Mechanical circulatory assistance. *Am Heart J* 95:529-534, 789-795, 1978.

Loeb HS, et al: Superiority of dobutamine over dopamine for augmentation of cardiac output in patients with chronic low output cardiac failure. *Circulation* 55:375-381, 1977.

Mikulic E, et al: Comparative hemodynamic effects of inotropic and vasodilator drugs in severe heart failure. *Circulation* 56:528-533, 1977.

Moran NC: Evaluation of pharmacologic basis for therapy of circulatory shock. *Am J Cardiol* 26:570-577, 1970.

Mueller HS, et al: Effect of dopamine on hemodynamics and myocardial metabolism in shock following acute myocardial infarction in man. *Circulation* 57:361-365, 1978.

Stoner JD III, et al: Comparison of dobutamine and dopamine in treatment of severe heart failure. *Br Heart J* 39:536-539, 1977.

Tarazi RC: Sympathomimetic agents in treatment of shock. *Ann Intern Med* 81:364-371, 1974.

Tinker JH, et al: Dobutamine for inotropic support during emergence from cardiopulmonary bypass. *Anesthesiology* 44:281-286, 1976.

Tuttle RR, Mills J: Dobutamine: Development of new catecholamine to selectively increase cardiac contractility. *Circ Res* 36:185-196, 1975.

Weil MH: Current understanding of mechanisms and treatment of circulatory shock caused by bacterial infections. *Ann Clin Res* 9:181-191, 1977.

Weil MH, Shubin H: Monitoring and measurements during shock, in Schumer W, Nyhus LM: *Treatment of Shock: Principles and Practice.* Philadelphia, Lea & Febiger, 1974, 3-22.

Weil MH, et al: Relationship between colloid osmotic pressure and pulmonary artery wedge pressure in patients with acute cardiorespiratory failure. *Am J Med* 64:643-650, 1978.

Weil MH, et al: Treatment of circulatory shock: Use of sympathomimetic and related vasoactive agents. *JAMA* 231:1280-1286, 1975.

Index

Primary headings appear in boldface type and may be drug names (generic and trademark), indications, or adverse reactions. Drug names followed by (M) are mixtures. Boldface page numbers denote individual evaluations.

1

corticosteroids in 634
Eye Infection
  antibacterial agents (systemic) in **384**
  antibacterial agents (topical) in **383**
  antifungal agents in **385**
  antiseptics in **386**
  antiviral agents in **386**
  bacterial 382
  fungal 385
  mixtures in 390
  viral 386
Eye Inflammation
  adrenal corticosteroids in **387**
Eye Stream (M) 404
Eye, Synechia
  mydriatic-induced 374
E-Carpine (M) 360
EDTA (see Edetate Disodium) 902
E.E.S. (erythromycin ethylsuccinate) 1258
E.E.S. 400 (erythyromycin
    ethylsuccinate) 1258
E-Ferol (vitamin E) 826
E-Ferol Succinate (vitamin E) 826
EHDP (see Etidronate Disodium)
E-Ionate P.A. (estradiol cypionate) 675
E-Mycin (erythromycin) 1258
E-Pam (Canada/diazepam)
E-Pilo (M) 360
Factor IX Complex (Human)
  as hemostatic **1107**
Factorate (antihemophilic factor) 1106
Fasciculations
  succinylcholine-induced 340
Fascioliasis
  description 1414
Fasciolopsiasis 1414
Fastin (phentermine hydrochloride) 944
Fat
  in enteral nutrition 857
Febrile Reactions
  transfusion-induced 1094
Fecal Impaction
  sodium polystyrene
    sulfonate-induced 808
Federal Comprehensive Drug Abuse
    Prevention
  and Control Act of 1979 22
Federal Trade Commission 26
Feminone (ethinyl estradiol) 677
Femogen (esterified estrogens) 677
Fenfluramine Hydrochloride
  as anorexiant **942**
Fenicol (Canada/chloramphenicol)
Fenoprofen Calcium
  as analgesic-antipyretic **79**
  in arthritis **95**
Fentanyl Citrate
  in neuroleptanesthesia 324
Feosol (ferrous sulfate) 1056
Feosol Plus (M) 1067
Feostat (ferrous fumarate) 1057

Ferancee (M) 1067
Fergon (ferrous gluconate) 1057
Fermalox (M) 1067
Fero-Folic-500 (M) 1067
Fero-Gradumet (ferrous sulfate) 1056
Fero-Grad-500 (M) 1067
Ferric Subsulfate
  as hemostatic agent 1045
Ferrocholinate
  in iron deficiency anemia **1058**
Ferrolip (ferrocholinate) 1058
Ferrous Fumarate
  in iron deficiency anemia **1057**
Ferrous Gluconate
  in iron deficiency anemia **1057**
Ferrous Sulfate
  in iron deficiency anemia **1056**
Ferro-Sequels (M) 1067
Fersamal (Canada/ferrous fumarate)
Fertility
  physiology 705
Fer-In-Sol (ferrous sulfate) 1056
Festal (M) 1008
Festalan (M) 1008
Fetal Death in Utero
  uterine stimulants in 790
Fever
  anticholinergic agent-induced 991
  antimony-induced 1415
  azathioprine-induced 1127
  flavoxate-induced 613
  immunologic agent-induced 1139
  mercurial agent-induced 603
  oxamniquine-induced 1420
  prostaglandin-induced 793, 795, 796
  quinidine-induced 518
  stibocaptate-induced 1423
  tobramycin-induced 1286
  Intralipid-induced 854
Fibrinolysin with Desoxyribonuclease
    Combined
  as enzymatic debriding agent **1047**
Fibrosis
  bleomycin-induced 1182
  methysergide-induced 127
Filariasis
  description 1413
  diethylcarbamazine in 1416
Filibon preparations (M) 844
Fiogesic (M) 464
Fiorinal with Codeine (M) 84
Fiorinal (M) 84
  in muscle-contraction headache **129**
First Pass Effect
  definition 35
Fissures, Anal
  anorectal preparations in 1006
Flagyl (metronidazole) 970, 1389, 1401
Flavoxate Hydrochloride
  as urinary antispasmodic **612**
Flaxedil (gallamine triethiodide) 337

NOTES

NOTES

NOTES

NOTES

NOTES

NOTES

Antihypertensive Agents | 38

Hypertension is an important risk factor for the development of major cardiovascular complications, including congestive heart failure, coronary heart disease, stroke, and progressive renal failure. There is increasing evidence that salt intake and increasing body weight in acculturated societies are important in the pathogenesis of essential hypertension. This disorder would probably cease to be a major health problem if genetically susceptible individuals would lose excess weight and eliminate salt as a condiment, including elimination of processed foods to which sodium has been added (Freis, 1976). Until this goal is achieved, emphasis must be directed more toward pharmacologic treatment.

Effective reduction of blood pressure reduces the frequency of most complications of hypertension and increases life expectancy. In men with diastolic blood pressures averaging 105 mm Hg or higher, treatment with antihypertensive drugs re-

557

duces the incidence of congestive heart failure, stroke, dissecting aneurysm, and renal failure, but the evidence is less conclusive that such treatment significantly reduces the risk of myocardial infarction. Epidemiologic data indicate that women with similar elevations in blood pressure also should be treated.

There is as yet no conclusive evidence that antihypertensive therapy improves prognosis in patients with mild hypertension (diastolic pressure less than 105 mm Hg), and the decision to initiate active drug therapy in these patients is currently gauged by the presence of major risk factors, including target organ damage, family history of major cardiovascular complications, presence of diabetes mellitus or hyperlipidemia, male sex, black race, age under 50, and cigarette smoking. In the

absence of significant risk factors, patients with early mild hypertension may be managed without drug therapy but should be encouraged to lose weight, exercise regularly, and reduce their sodium intake to 70 mEq daily.

The agents used to treat hypertension are (1) diuretics, (2) drugs that inhibit sympathetic nervous system activity, (3) direct-acting vasodilators, and (4) angiotensin antagonists (see Table 1). The antihypertensive effect of the diuretics is initially due to a reduction in extracellular fluid volume; during long-term therapy, peripheral resistance is decreased. Drugs in the second category act by different mechanisms to reduce sympathetic tone. Their actions, uses, and adverse effects are related to their site(s) of action: central nervous system, autonomic ganglia, post-

TABLE 1. ANTIHYPERTENSIVE AGENTS

DIURETICS	SYMPATHETIC DEPRESSANT DRUGS	DIRECT-ACTING VASODILATORS	ANGIOTENSIN ANTAGONISTS
Thiazide-type	**Centrally Acting Agent**	**Arterial Vasodilators**	**Agents That Block Formation of Angiotensin II**
Bendroflumethiazide	Clonidine	Hydralazine	
Benzthiazide		Minoxidil	Captopril*
Chlorothiazide	**Agents With Both Central**	Diazoxide	Teprotide*
Cyclothiazide	**and Peripheral Actions**		
Hydrochlorothiazide	Rauwolfia Alkaloids	**Arterial and Venous**	**Agent That Blocks Action**
Hydroflumethiazide	Methyldopa	**Vasodilator**	**of Angiotensin II**
Methyclothiazide		Sodium Nitroprusside	Saralasin*
Polythiazide	**Ganglionic Blocking Agents**		
Trichlormethiazide	Trimethaphan		
	Mecamylamine		
Chlorthalidone			
Metolazone	**Agents That Block**		
Quinethazone	**Neuroeffector Transmission**		
	Guanethidine		
Loop			
Furosemide	**Beta-Adrenergic Blocking**		
Ethacrynic Acid	**Drugs**		
	Propranolol		
Potassium-Sparing	Metoprolol		
Spironolactone			
Triamterene	**Alpha-Adrenergic Blocking**		
Amiloride*	**Agents**		
	Prazosin (postsynaptic)		
Uricosuric	Phenoxybenzamine (pre-		
Ticrynafen	and postsynaptic)		
	Phentolamine (pre- and		
	postsynaptic)		

*Investigational

ganglionic nerve endings, and alpha- and beta-adrenergic receptor sites. Vasodilator drugs reduce blood pressure by directly relaxing vascular smooth muscle. Angiotensin antagonists block the formation or the action of the potent endogenous vasoconstrictor, angiotensin II.

The choice of an appropriate drug depends upon the severity of the disease and the patient's response to a therapeutic trial. The following sections present guidelines for therapy in patients with hypertension of varying degrees of severity. (See also Gifford, 1974; Simpson, 1974; Page et al, 1976; Wollam et al, 1977; and reports of the AMA Committee on Hypertension and The Joint National Committee on Detection, Evaluation and Treatment of High Blood Pressure.)

Chronic Hypertension

Prior to beginning life-long treatment, the patient with a mild or moderate elevation in blood pressure should be seen on at least three separate visits to determine whether the elevation is persistent. Therapy should not be delayed in patients with more severe hypertension. The extent of organic changes, particularly those affecting the optic fundi, brain, heart, and kidneys, should be assessed, and baseline measurements of serum or plasma potassium, uric acid, and glucose levels should be obtained. Measurements of plasma renin activity (PRA) and urinary aldosterone level, intravenous urography, renal angiography, and tests for pheochromocytoma are not necessary routinely and should be performed only when specific indications are present. Although patients with high, low, and normal renin levels have been identified and antihypertensive drugs are known to differ in their effects on PRA (diuretics and vasodilators cause an increase and sympathetic depressant drugs a decrease), "renin profiling" generally is not considered to be a useful guide to therapy (Kaplan, 1977).

The goal of antihypertensive therapy is to reduce the blood pressure to normal or to the lowest level tolerated. A diastolic pressure of 90 mm Hg usually can be achieved without prohibitive untoward effects. Because of differences in responsiveness, the regimen must be individualized, and it may be necessary to try various drugs or combinations until the optimal effect is obtained. Effective doses may vary considerably from patient to patient. Therapy usually should be initiated with a single drug and, if additional agents are needed, they should be added to the regimen one at a time. In patients who require more than one drug, use of a fixed-dose combination product may improve compliance, but a mixture should be substituted only if it contains nearly the same proportions of drugs found to be optimal by individual dose titration. Combination products may be unsuitable if the components have markedly different durations of action or if one component is potent, produces marked side effects, and/or has a wide range of effective dosage. Mixtures should not be used if hypertension is difficult to control and frequent adjustment in dosage of one of the drugs is necessary (Gifford, 1974).

Mild to Moderate Hypertension: For patients with mild to moderate hypertension (diastolic blood pressure below 115 mm Hg), treatment is usually initiated with a thiazide diuretic. The uricosuric diuretic, ticrynafen [Selacryn], is a useful alternative in patients with symptomatic hyperuricemia. If renal function is severely impaired (creatinine clearance less than 30 ml/min), a loop diuretic (usually furosemide [Lasix]) may be required. A potassium-sparing agent (spironolactone [Aldactone], triamterene [Dyrenium], or the investigational drug, amiloride [Colectril]) may be given with a thiazide or loop diuretic to patients at risk from hypokalemia.

To ensure an optimal therapeutic response, the diuretic should be given daily; alternate-day therapy is not appropriate for the treatment of hypertension. Diuretics control blood pressure in 30% to 60% of patients without additional therapy. When not effective as single agents, they remain useful to counteract sodium retention and enhance the therapeutic effect of other antihypertensive drugs. The response to the diuretic should be observed for at least two, and preferably four, weeks. If further reduction in blood pressure is indicated, an agent that inhibits sympathetic nervous system activity (reserpine, a beta blocker, methyldopa [Aldomet], clonidine [Catapres], or prazosin [Minipress]) may be added.

Reserpine is convenient because it requires administration only once daily. A thiazide-reserpine regimen provides a simple and inexpensive means for long-term control of hypertension and may be more effective than other two-drug regimens (Veterans Administration Cooperative Study on Antihypertensive Agents, 1977; Finnerty et al, 1979). Reserpine has a delayed onset of action; therefore, unless adverse effects occur, the patient should be observed for four to six weeks before other drugs are added. Because of its central nervous system depressant effect, reserpine may be poorly tolerated by elderly patients and those whose work requires mental alertness and judgment. Individuals receiving reserpine should be observed for subtle or obvious symptoms of mental depression, and the drug should be discontinued if such symptoms appear. Subsequent studies have not confirmed earlier reports of a possible association between long-term reserpine therapy and an increased incidence of breast cancer in older women.

The beta-adrenergic blocking agent, propranolol [Inderal], may be useful in many patients who are not adequately controlled by diuretic therapy alone. Because it does not cause generalized inhibition of adrenergic function, propranolol is usually better tolerated than other sympathetic depressant drugs. The antihypertensive action of a newer beta-blocking drug, metoprolol [Lopressor], appears to be comparable to that of propranolol. Beta-blocking drugs may precipitate heart failure in patients with borderline cardiac reserve and bronchospasm in asthmatics.

Methyldopa or clonidine also may be useful as the second drug in the regimen if the diuretic alone fails to reduce pressure. Both drugs cause drowsiness and dryness

of the mouth initially, but these effects usually subside during long-term therapy. Rarely, methyldopa may cause depression, hepatitis, or hemolytic anemia. The most severe adverse effect of clonidine is the withdrawal syndrome, which is manifested by a marked increase in blood pressure (above pretreatment levels) and symptoms similar to pheochromocytoma crisis.

The vasodilator drug, hydralazine [Apresoline], may be added as the third agent to any of the above regimens if the blood pressure has not been reduced adequately. It is better tolerated and more effective when used with other antihypertensive drugs than when used alone. The marked sodium retention that is seen with all vasodilator drugs is counteracted by a diuretic, while a sympathetic depressant drug minimizes reflex tachycardia. Hydralazine may be suitable as the second drug in the regimen for older patients with less active baroreceptor reflexes. A drug-induced lupus syndrome may develop during long-term therapy with large doses of hydralazine.

The alpha-adrenergic blocking agent, prazosin, causes less tachycardia than hydralazine and may be used as the second or third drug in the regimen. Prazosin is well tolerated except for orthostatic hypotension and syncope, which may occur during the initial few days of therapy.

It is not yet known which of the above drugs or combinations is most effective in reducing the cardiovascular complications of hypertension, and studies are currently in progress to determine whether true differences exist. A thiazide-reserpine-hydralazine combination was used in the studies which demonstrated that treatment was more effective in preventing stroke, congestive heart failure, and progressive renal damage than in preventing myocardial infarction (Veterans Administration Cooperative Study Group on Antihypertensive Agents, 1967 and 1970). Results of a less well-designed study from Sweden suggest that treatment with a beta-blocking drug may reduce mortality from coronary artery disease (Berglund, 1978), but these findings have not been confirmed. There is some evidence that long-term therapy with a beta-blocking drug may reduce mortality after acute myocardial infarction.

Severe Hypertension: Many patients with severe hypertension ·(diastolic blood pressure above 115 mm Hg) can be controlled with a combination of a diuretic, propranolol, and hydralazine, and such a regimen is often well tolerated by patients who have experienced disabling side effects with other types of therapy. Minoxidil [Loniten], a potent vasodilator drug, may prove to be more useful than hydralazine in treating severe hypertension. When there are contraindications to use of a beta-blocking drug, methyldopa or clonidine may be substituted. For patients who do not respond to these multiple-drug regimens, guanethidine [Ismelin] may be given with a diuretic or added to a two- or three-drug regimen. The orthostatic hypotension produced by guanethidine may be troublesome, particularly when first arising in the morning and during the hot summer months. The dose must be adjusted carefully with the patient in the standing position and after mild exercise.

Most patients with severe hypertension can be controlled with one of the several regimens described above. The orally administered ganglionic blocking agent, mecamylamine [Inversine], is rarely used today because of its adverse effects in blocking both parasympathetic and sympathetic function. The monoamine oxidase inhibitor, pargyline [Eutonyl], and the combination of pargyline and a thiazide [Eutron] are seldom used because of the potential for serious adverse reactions when foods containing high levels of tyramine are ingested concurrently. Veratrum alkaloids also are obsolete.

Hypertensive Emergencies

An acute, marked elevation in blood pressure is a medical emergency that may necessitate hospitalization and parenteral administration of antihypertensive drugs. The vasodilator drugs, sodium nitroprusside [Nipride] and diazoxide [Hyperstat I.V.], are the agents of choice in most patients requiring parenteral therapy. Sodium nitroprusside is the most potent and consistently effective drug available for treatment of hypertensive emergencies. Used in appropriate doses, it is effective in more than 90% of patients. Because of its favorable hemodynamic effect on left ventricular function, nitroprusside is the drug of choice for managing hypertensive crises associated with acute left ventricular failure. It is also useful in hypertensive crises complicated by cerebral or subarachnoid hemorrhage because of its very rapid onset and short duration of action. Nitroprusside is given by slow intravenous infusion with continuous monitoring in an intensive care unit.

When administered by rapid intravenous injection, diazoxide reduces blood pressure within one to five minutes, but many physicians now prefer to give the drug intermittently in smaller doses to reduce the risk of myocardial and cerebral ischemia. Diazoxide is often useful in acute hypertensive encephalopathy or when there is a life-threatening elevation of blood pressure in patients with malignant hypertension or any form of renal disease. Marked reflex tachycardia may occur; therefore, diazoxide generally is not used to treat severe hypertension in patients with coronary artery disease. Hyperglycemia is also a common side effect, and the drug should be given cautiously to patients with known or suspected diabetes.

The blood pressure also can be reduced within minutes by intravenous administration of the ganglionic blocking drug, trimethaphan [Arfonad]. Dosage must be carefully adjusted and the blood pressure monitored frequently to avoid excessive hypotension. Since the effect is largely postural, it may be necessary to elevate the head of the bed to obtain an adequate response or use the Trendelenburg position to help correct an overresponse. Trimethaphan decreases myocardial contractility and cardiac output and is preferred to vasodilators such as diazoxide or hydralazine for initial control of blood pressure in patients with acute dissecting aortic aneurysm. Because of its rapid onset and short duration of action, it is also useful in hypertensive patients with cerebral or subarachnoid hemorrhage. Tachyphylaxis may occur with prolonged administration.

Hydralazine, given intramuscularly or intravenously, reduces blood pressure rapidly but is not as consistently effective as sodium nitroprusside or diazoxide. It may be useful in patients with acute or chronic glomerulonephritis. Hydralazine also is the most suitable and widely used antihypertensive drug for treating severe pre-eclampsia and eclampsia and may be given with diazepam or magnesium sulfate when convulsions occur. Reserpine and methyldopa (as methyldopate hydrochloride) also are available in parenteral form but are of limited value in hypertensive emergencies because of their slower onset of action and pronounced sedative effect.

The drugs used to treat hypertensive emergencies may cause marked sodium and water retention which makes the patient resistant to therapy. When oral administration is not feasible, a loop diuretic (usually furosemide) is given intravenously to induce rapid diuresis and counteract secondary expansion of the extracellular fluid volume. Loop diuretics are of particular value in hypertensive emergencies associated with acute pulmonary edema or renal failure.

The alpha-adrenergic blocking agents are used for hypertensive crises caused by an excess of circulating catecholamines (ie, pheochromocytoma, interaction between monoamine oxidase inhibitors and sympathomimetic amines, clonidine withdrawal syndrome). After establishment of effective alpha-adrenergic blockade, propranolol is used if cardiac stimulation is excessive.

DIURETICS

Thiazides and Related Compounds

A thiazide or related compound (chlorthalidone, metolazone, quinethazone) usually serves as the cornerstone of the anti-hypertensive regimen: as sole therapy in patients with mild or moderate hypertension or in combination with other antihypertensive drugs in patients who are not controlled by the diuretic alone. These agents reduce the extracellular fluid (ECF) volume by inhibiting sodium chloride reabsorption in the early distal tubules. Peripheral vascular resistance is reduced during long-term therapy. This effect is not caused by a direct vascular action, but appears to result from autoregulatory mechanisms activated by the reduced ECF volume and initial fall in cardiac output (Bennett et al, 1977; Shah et al, 1978).

The thiazides are preferred for initial therapy because they are well tolerated and inexpensive, they reduce both supine and standing blood pressure, and their antihypertensive effect is maintained during long-term administration. When used with sympathetic depressant or vasodilator drugs, the thiazides prevent secondary volume expansion and thereby allow continued responsiveness. Such combined therapy may permit a decrease in dosage of the antihypertensive drug, thus reducing the incidence and severity of adverse reactions.

The thiazides may cause hypokalemia, hyperuricemia, hyperglycemia, and azotemia. (These and other side effects are discussed in detail in Chapter 39, Diuretics.) Mild hypokalemia is generally well tolerated in the healthy ambulatory patient with hypertension and may require correction less commonly than current practice might suggest. Corrective measures are indicated if symptoms occur, if the serum potassium level falls below 3 mEq/L, or if the patient is receiving digitalis. In such patients, a potassium-sparing diuretic or a potassium supplement may be administered with the thiazide.

The various thiazides and related drugs differ primarily in their duration of action. When given in equipotent doses, no clearcut differences in efficacy or toxicity have been demonstrated. The incidence of biochemical disturbances increases with increasing dosage, whereas the antihypertensive effect is not clearly dose related. For this reason, therapy should be initiated with small amounts. Many patients with mild or moderate hypertension can be controlled with doses that induce minimal biochemical changes (Materson et al, 1978; Tweeddale et al, 1977).

ROUTE, USUAL DOSAGE, AND PREPARATIONS.
See Table 2.

Loop Diuretics

The loop diuretics, furosemide and ethacrynic acid, are chemically distinct but have similar pharmacologic actions. Both drugs block active chloride transport in the thick ascending limb of Henle's loop and thereby interfere with the passive reabsorption of sodium. They have a more rapid onset of action and a greater diuretic effect than the thiazides, but there is no evidence of a greater antihypertensive effect. These agents are usually reserved for patients with impaired renal function unless an immediate action is required to control fluid overload. Their proper use requires an understanding of the electrolyte and fluid derangements that they may induce.

FUROSEMIDE
[Lasix]

Furosemide is a potent nonthiazide sulfonamide diuretic that is useful adjunctively in the treatment of hypertensive crises, particularly in patients with acute pulmonary edema or renal failure. When given intravenously, furosemide causes rapid diuresis and reduces the plasma volume, thereby enhancing the therapeutic response to other antihypertensive agents. This drug is usually preferred to ethacrynic acid because it has a broader dose-response curve, is less ototoxic, produces fewer gastrointestinal disturbances, is more convenient for intravenous use, and may be

less likely to cause alkalosis. When given orally, furosemide is often effective in hypertensive patients with impaired renal function.

Overzealous therapy can cause dehydration, hypotension, and marked hypokalemia and hypochloremic alkalosis. Like the thiazides, furosemide can cause prerenal azotemia, hyperuricemia, and hyperglycemia. Transient deafness has occurred following rapid administration to azotemic or uremic patients. Permanent deafness has occurred rarely. For other adverse effects, see Chapter 39, Diuretics.

ROUTES, USUAL DOSAGE, AND PREPARATIONS.
Intravenous: For hypertensive crises, *adults* with normal renal function, 40 to 80 mg administered over a period of one to two minutes. When the glomerular filtration rate is markedly reduced, larger doses may be required. An oral diuretic should be substituted for parenteral therapy as soon as practical.
   Lasix (Hoechst-Roussel). Solution 10 mg/ml in 2 and 10 ml containers.
Oral: *Adults*, initially, 40 mg twice daily. If an adequate response is not obtained, dosage may be increased gradually. Patients with renal insufficiency occasionally may require doses as large as 640 mg daily.
   Lasix (Hoechst-Roussel). Solution (oral) 10 mg/ml; tablets 20, 40, and 80 mg.

ETHACRYNATE SODIUM
[Sodium Edecrin]

ETHACRYNIC ACID
[Edecrin]

Ethacrynate sodium is given intravenously and is useful as an adjunct in the treatment of hypertensive crises. Ethacrynic acid may be given orally to hypertensive patients with impaired renal function.

Adverse effects are similar to those observed with furosemide, except that ethacrynic acid may be more ototoxic than

TABLE 2. THIAZIDES AND RELATED AGENTS

Drug	Usual Oral Dosage for Hypertension*	Preparations
Chlorothiazide	*Adults*, initially, 250 to 500 mg once or twice daily. *Children*, 20 mg/kg daily in 2 divided doses.	*Generic:* Tablets 250 and 500 mg. *Diuril* (Merck Sharp & Dohme): Tablets 250 and 500 mg. Suspension 250 mg/5 ml
Hydrochlorothiazide	*Adults*, initially, 25 to 50 mg once or twice daily; *children*, 2 mg/kg daily in 2 divided doses.	*Generic:* Tablets 25, 50 and 100 mg. *Esidrix* (Ciba), *HydroDiuril* (Merck Sharp & Dohme): Tablets 25, 50 and 100 mg. *Oretic* (Abbott): Tablets 25 and 50 mg.
Bendroflumethiazide	*Adults*, initially, 5 to 10 mg daily; for maintenance, 2.5 to 10 mg daily. *Children*, initially, 0.1 mg/kg daily in 1 or 2 doses; for maintenance, 0.05 to 0.3 mg/kg daily in 1 or 2 doses.	*Naturetin* (Squibb): Tablets 2.5, 5 and 10 mg.
Benzthiazide	*Adults*, initially, 25 to 50 mg twice daily. *Children*, 1 to 4 mg/kg daily in 3 doses.	*Generic:* Tablets 50 mg. *Aquatag* (Tutag): Tablets 25 and 50 mg. *Exna* (Robins): Tablets 50 mg.
Cyclothiazide	*Adults*, initially, 2 mg once daily. *Children*, 0.02 to 0.04 mg/kg once daily.	*Anhydron* (Lilly): Tablets 2 mg.
Hydroflumethiazide	*Adults*, initially, 50 to 100 mg once daily. *Children*, 1 mg/kg once daily.	*Diucardin* (Ayerst), *Saluron* (Bristol): Tablets 50 mg.
Methyclothiazide	*Adults*, initially, 5 to 10 mg once daily. *Children*, 0.05 to 0.2 mg/kg once daily.	*Aquatensen* (Mallinckrodt): Tablets 5 mg. *Enduron* (Abbott): Tablets 2.5 and 5 mg.
Polythiazide	*Adults*, initially, 1 to 4 mg daily. *Children*, initially, 0.02 to 0.08 mg/kg daily.	*Renese* (Pfizer): Tablets 1, 2 and 4 mg.
Trichlormethiazide	*Adults*, initially, 2 or 4 mg once daily. *Children*, 0.07 mg/kg once daily or in divided doses.	*Generic:* Tablets 2 and 4 mg. *Metahydrin* (Merrell-National), *Naqua* (Schering): Tablets 2 and 4 mg.
Chlorthalidone	*Adults*, initially, 25 mg daily. May be increased to 50 or 100 mg daily.	*Hygroton* (USV): Tablets 25, 50 and 100 mg.
Metolazone	*Adults*, initially, 2.5 to 5 mg daily.	*Diulo* (Searle), *Zaroxolyn* (Pennwalt): Tablets 2.5, 5 and 10 mg.
Quinethazone	*Adults*, initially, 50 mg once or twice daily.	*Hydromox* (Lederle): Tablets 50 mg.

Initial dosage subsequently increased or decreased according to patient's response.

furosemide but is less likely to cause hyperglycemia. See also Chapter 39, Diuretics.

ROUTES, USUAL DOSAGE, AND PREPARATIONS. *Intravenous*: *Adults,* 50 mg or 0.5 to 1 mg/kg of body weight as a single dose; if a second dose is required, it should be injected at another site to avoid thrombophlebitis. An oral diuretic should be substituted for parenteral therapy as soon as practical.

> ETHACRYNATE SODIUM:
> *Sodium Edecrin* (Merck Sharp & Dohme). Powder equivalent to 50 mg ethacrynic acid.

Oral: *Adults,* 100 to 200 mg daily in divided doses.

> ETHACRYNIC ACID:
> *Edecrin* (Merck Sharp & Dohme). Tablets 25 and 50 mg.

Potassium-Sparing Diuretics

Spironolactone, triamterene, and amiloride (investigational drug) promote sodium excretion while conserving potassium. Spironolactone is an aldosterone antagonist, while triamterene and amiloride act directly at the distal exchange sites in the renal tubules. Their major use in the treatment of hypertension is in conjunction with the thiazide diuretics in patients who are at risk from hypokalemia. Such combined therapy reduces potassium excretion, minimizes alkalosis, and may provide better control of hypertension.

SPIRONOLACTONE
[Aldactone]

SPIRONOLACTONE AND HYDROCHLOROTHIAZIDE
[Aldactazide]

In some patients, spironolactone has proven to be equivalent to the thiazides in antihypertensive activity, but it is most effective when given with a thiazide to minimize hypokalemia and enhance the antihypertensive action.

Careful monitoring of the serum potassium level is necessary during therapy with spironolactone because hyperkalemia may occur despite concomitant thiazide therapy. Precipitating factors are impairment of renal function and/or a high potassium intake (dietary, supplements, salt substitutes). Doses greater than 50 mg daily often cause gynecomastia in men. Menstrual irregularities have been reported in women. For a more detailed discussion of actions, uses, and adverse effects, see Chapter 39, Diuretics.

ROUTE, USUAL DOSAGE, AND PREPARATIONS.
SPIRONOLACTONE:
Oral: *Adults,* initially, 50 to 100 mg daily in two divided doses. The dosage should then be adjusted in accordance with the response of the patient as determined by measurements of blood pressure and serum electrolyte levels.

> *Aldactone* (Searle). Tablets 25 mg.

SPIRONOLACTONE AND HYDROCHLOROTHIAZIDE:
Oral: *Adults,* initially, two to four tablets daily. The dosage should then be adjusted in accordance with the response of the patient.

> *Aldactazide* (Searle). Each tablet contains spironolactone 25 mg and hydrochlorothiazide 25 mg.

TRIAMTERENE
[Dyrenium]

TRIAMTERENE AND HYDROCHLOROTHIAZIDE
[Dyazide]

Triamterene is most effective when given with a thiazide to minimize hypokalemia and enhance the antihypertensive response. Triamterene is not a potent antihypertensive drug and is not useful as the sole therapy.

Like spironolactone, triamterene may cause hyperkalemia and the same precautions should be observed. For a more detailed discussion of actions, uses, and adverse effects, see Chapter 39, Diuretics.

ROUTE, USUAL DOSAGE, AND PREPARATIONS.
TRIAMTERENE:
Oral: *Adults*, initially, 100 mg twice daily after meals (maximum, 300 mg daily). The dosage should be adjusted in accordance with the response of the patient as determined by measurements of blood pressure and serum electrolyte levels.

> *Dyrenium* (Smith Kline & French). Capsules 50 and 100 mg.

TRIAMTERENE AND HYDROCHLOROTHIAZIDE:
Oral: *Adults*, initially, one or two capsules twice daily. The dosage should then be adjusted in accordance with the response of the patient.

> *Dyazide* (Smith Kline & French). Each capsule contains triamterene 50 mg and hydrochlorothiazide 25 mg.

Uricosuric Diuretic

TICRYNAFEN
[Selacryn]

Although structurally related to ethacrynic acid, ticrynafen inhibits sodium chloride reabsorption at a site in the nephron similar to that of the thiazides (early distal tubules). Ticrynafen is unique among currently available diuretics in its effect on the renal handling of urate. By inhibiting urate reabsorption at both pre- and postsecretory sites in the proximal tubules, it increases urate excretion and reduces serum

uric acid levels. Because of this action, ticrynafen is the diuretic of choice for hypertensive patients who have a history of gout. Asymptomatic hyperuricemia is *not* an indication to change from a thiazide to ticrynafen.

In comparative studies, ticrynafen (250 to 500 mg) was as effective as hydrochlorothiazide (50 to 100 mg) in reducing the blood pressure of patients with mild to moderate hypertension who were not receiving any other antihypertensive medication. Serum uric acid levels of patients in the ticrynafen groups were significantly reduced from control values, whereas these levels were increased in those receiving the thiazide (Nemati et al, 1977; de Carvalho et al, 1978). The effect of ticrynafen is also comparable to that of hydrochlorothiazide in patients receiving concomitant therapy with nondiuretic antihypertensive drugs. For use in cardiac edema, see Chapter 39, Diuretics.

Like the thiazides, ticrynafen may cause hypokalemia, hyperglycemia, and azotemia. If treatment is necessary to correct hypokalemia, potassium supplements are preferred, because marked elevations in BUN and serum creatinine levels have occurred when triamterene or amiloride was given concomitantly. The combined use of ticrynafen and spironolactone should probably also be avoided.

Like other uricosuric agents, ticrynafen may precipitate acute attacks of gout in susceptible patients, especially during the early months of therapy. For this reason, it is advisable to prescribe prophylactic doses of colchicine if a gouty episode has occurred. The diuretic effect of ticrynafen may reduce the risk of urinary tract obstruction from excessive uricosuria during the first few days of therapy; the risk can be further reduced if fluid intake is increased for three days before and three days after instituting therapy. It also may be advisable to alkalize the urine during this period. Other diuretics should be discontinued for three days before beginning therapy with ticrynafen.

Ticrynafen potentiates the effect of oral anticoagulants, and anticoagulant dosage should be reduced one-quarter or one-half of the maintenance dose and prothrombin time monitored until the patient is stabilized. For other adverse effects and interactions, see Chapter 39.

ADDENDUM: There have been several recent reports of acute renal failure in patients receiving ticrynafen (Selacryn [Smith Kline & French]). Several deaths from hepatic toxicity have also been reported, and the drug was voluntarily removed from the market in January, 1980.

SYMPATHETIC DEPRESSANT DRUGS

Centrally Acting Agent

CLONIDINE HYDROCHLORIDE
[Catapres]

The hypotensive effect of clonidine is associated with a decrease in heart rate and a fall in cardiac output. Peripheral resistance may or may not be reduced during long-term therapy. Clonidine reduces blood pressure by a central action; it inhibits sympathetic outflow from the brain by activating alpha receptors in the vasomotor center of the medulla which may be located on the baroreceptor reflex pathway. The reduction in heart rate is due, in part, to an increase in vagal tone.

Clonidine, administered with a diuretic, is useful in treating all degrees of hypertension. It may be particularly effective in patients with moderately severe hypertension who are not adequately controlled with other regimens or who cannot tolerate other sympathetic depressant drugs. Substituting clonidine for methyldopa is not likely to be helpful, however, if the patient's primary complaints are drowsiness and dryness of the mouth, for these side effects also occur frequently with clonidine.

Clonidine is readily absorbed after oral administration and peak plasma levels are attained within three to five hours. Approximately 60% of an oral dose is excreted in the urine, largely as unidentified metabolites.

The most common adverse effects are drowsiness, dryness of the mouth, and constipation. Orthostatic symptoms occur occasionally. All of these reactions may decrease in severity during long-term therapy. Depression and impotence occur occasionally, and pseudo-obstruction of the large bowel has been reported rarely. By increasing vagal tone, clonidine may potentiate the effect of digitalis in prolonging A-V conduction.

A pronounced withdrawal reaction with rebound hypertension may develop within 12 to 48 hours if clonidine is discontinued abruptly. Initially, the patient may experience restlessness, insomnia, irritability, tremors, and tachycardia, which may be followed by headache, increased salivation, abdominal pain, nausea, and an abrupt rebound increase in blood pressure (higher than pretreatment levels). Some patients may develop symptoms without a marked elevation in blood pressure. The withdrawal syndrome, which resembles the hypertensive crisis seen in pheochromocytoma, is associated with increased plasma and urinary catecholamine levels; however, it is not closely related to a decline in the plasma concentration of clonidine. The likelihood of a withdrawal reaction has been reported by some to be increased if the daily dose exceeds 1.2 mg; however, others have consistently observed rebound hypertension at lower doses.

Because of the danger of a withdrawal reaction, clonidine should not be prescribed for patients who are not reliable in taking medication. All patients receiving clonidine should be warned of the risk of rapid withdrawal and should be instructed to have an adequate supply of the drug available at all times. Withdrawal reactions usually can be controlled by reinstituting clonidine therapy or by substituting a combination of an alpha- and beta-blocking agent. A beta blocker should not be used alone, because it may potentiate the rebound increase in blood pressure. For a planned withdrawal, a reaction usually can be avoided if the dosage is decreased gradually over a period of one week or more; however, rebound phenomena have occurred occasionally during gradual withdrawal. If it is necessary to discontinue clonidine prior to emergency surgery, therapy should be reinstituted in the postoperative period as soon as practical. If this is not possible, rebound hypertension usually can be controlled by phentolamine mesylate (5 to 10 mg intravenously at five-minute intervals to a total dose of 20 to 30 mg), and tachycardia can be controlled by propranolol (1 to 3 mg intravenously administered cautiously over a period of three to five minutes). Sodium nitroprusside also is often effective in treating rebound hypertension associated with clonidine withdrawal.

A marked increase in blood pressure also has been observed following gross overdosage with clonidine. This paradoxical response apparently reflects activation of vasoconstrictor alpha receptors in the peripheral circulation.

Although no serious adverse effects on the eye have been reported, periodic ophthalmologic examinations may be advisable during long-term therapy. This recommendation is based on evidence that clonidine accumulates in the choroid of the eye, caused retinal degeneration in rats, and produced abnormalities in one test of retinal function (electro-oculogram) in man.

ROUTE, USUAL DOSAGE, AND PREPARATIONS. Dosage must be carefully titrated to provide an optimal therapeutic response with minimal side effects. Prior and concomitant administration of an oral diuretic is recommended to enhance the therapeutic response.

Oral: *Adults*, initially, 0.1 mg two or three times daily. Dosage may be increased gradually in increments of 0.1 or 0.2 mg. For maintenance, the usual daily dose ranges from 0.2 to 0.8 mg. Doses larger than 2.4 mg daily are rarely required.

Catapres (Boehringer Ingelheim). Tablets 0.1 and 0.2 mg.

AVAILABLE MIXTURE.

Clonidine and Chlorthalidone: Successful regulation of blood pressure with clonidine requires careful titration of dosage, and an adjustment in dose may be required during the course of continuous therapy. For these reasons, the fixed-dose combination of Combipres may be unsuitable for many patients.

Combipres (Boehringer Ingelheim). Each tablet contains clonidine hydrochloride 0.1 or 0.2 mg and chlorthalidone 15 mg.

Agents With Both Central and Peripheral Actions

RAUWOLFIA ALKALOIDS

Reserpine is regarded as the prototype of the rauwolfia alkaloids and is the most commonly used drug in this group. The antihypertensive effect of reserpine has been attributed to its ability to deplete catecholamine stores in sympathetic nerve terminals and in the central nervous system. Reserpine decreases peripheral vascular resistance and reduces heart rate and cardiac output. The usual oral doses only partially inhibit reflex tonic constrictor impulses to the capacitance vessels and orthostatic hypotension occurs only rarely.

Reserpine is used orally to treat mild or moderate hypertension. When given alone, it is not a potent antihypertensive agent. It is most beneficial when used with a thiazide in patients who are not adequately controlled by the diuretic alone. In comparative studies, a thiazide-reserpine combination was effective in a larger percentage of patients (88% to 100%) than a thiazide-propranolol or thiazide-methyldopa regimen (Veterans Administration Cooperative Study Group on Antihypertensive Agents, 1977; Finnerty et al, 1979). When the desired hypotensive effect is not achieved with a thiazide and reserpine, hydralazine may be added.

Reserpine is rarely used today by the intramuscular route to treat hypertensive crises because the hypotensive effect is delayed for two or three hours, occasional patients develop severe hypotension with repeated doses, and its marked sedative effect may interfere with evaluation of mental status.

Nasal congestion and bradycardia are common with therapeutic doses of reserpine. Sodium and water retention may occur if a diuretic is not given concomitantly. Other adverse effects include diarrhea, lethargy, nightmares, and mental depression that occasionally has been sufficiently severe to require hospitalization or result in suicide. Depression can occur with any amount but is most common with older high-dosage regimens (0.5 to 1 mg or more daily). The rauwolfia alkaloids should not be given to patients with a history of depression and, if depressive symptoms appear, the drug should be discontinued. Barbiturates enhance the central nervous system depressant effects of rauwolfia alkaloids.

An association between long-term reserpine therapy and an increased incidence of breast cancer in hypertensive women over the age of 50 was reported in three retrospective studies. Several subsequent investigations have shown no relationship between use of rauwolfia alkaloids and breast cancer, and the burden of evidence is now against any such association.

Reserpine may increase gastric acid secretion and should be used cautiously in patients with a history of peptic ulcer. If symptoms suggest recurrence of the ulcer, the drug should be discontinued. Because rauwolfia alkaloids increase gastrointestinal tone and motility, they should not be given to patients with a history of ulcerative colitis.

Severe hypotension has occurred occasionally when reserpine was administered repeatedly by the parenteral route for treatment of hypertensive crises. If position change does not relieve the hypotension, norepinephrine (levarterenol) may be given intravenously; vasopressors that act in part by liberating norepinephrine may be less effective, since norepinephrine stores are depleted by the rauwolfia alkaloids.

When given parenterally for treating eclampsia, reserpine passes through the placental circulation and may cause drowsiness, nasal congestion, cyanosis, and anorexia in the newborn infant.

Because rauwolfia alkaloids lower the convulsive threshold, they should be used cautiously in patients with epilepsy. Large doses may cause extrapyramidal reactions.

ROUTES, USUAL DOSAGE, AND PREPARATIONS. The rauwolfia alkaloids have a slow onset and prolonged duration of action. Adjustments in dosage should not be made more frequently than every 7 to 14 days. Concomitant administration of a diuretic is recommended to enhance the therapeutic response.

RESERPINE:

Oral: For chronic hypertension, *adults*, initially, 0.25 mg daily for one week; for maintenance, 0.1 to 0.25 mg daily. *Children*, 0.1 to 0.25 mg daily.

> Drug available generically: Tablets 0.1, 0.25, 0.5, and 1 mg.
> *Reserpoid* (Upjohn). Tablets 0.25 mg.
> *Sandril* (Lilly). Tablets 0.1 and 0.25 mg.
> *Serpasil* (Ciba). Elixir 0.2 mg/4 ml; tablets 0.1, 0.25, and 1 mg.

Intramuscular: For hypertensive crisis, *adults*, initially, 0.5 to 1 mg; if there is little or no fall in blood pressure within three hours, 2 to 4 mg is given at 3- to 12-hour intervals until pressure falls to the desired level. *Children weighing less than 36 kg*, initially, 0.02 mg/kg of body weight; if there is little or no fall in blood pressure within four to six hours, 0.04 mg/kg is given at four- to six-hour intervals. *Children over 36 kg*, initially, 0.5 to 1 mg with subsequent doses adjusted according to response.

> *Sandril* (Lilly). Solution 2.5 mg/ml in 10 ml containers.
> *Serpasil* (Ciba). Solution 2.5 mg/ml in 2 and 10 ml containers.

OTHER RAUWOLFIA ALKALOIDS:

> Rauwolfia Serpentina:
> Drug available generically: Tablets 50 and 100 mg.
> *Raudixin* (Squibb). Tablets 50 and 100 mg.
> Alseroxylon:
> *Rauwiloid* (Riker). Tablets 2 mg.
> Deserpidine:
> *Harmonyl* (Abbott). Tablets 0.1 and 0.25 mg.
> Rescinnamine:
> *Moderil* (Pfizer). Tablets 0.25 and 0.5 mg.

AVAILABLE MIXTURES.

Rauwolfia Alkaloid and An Oral Diuretic: The following orally administered combination products are convenient for patients who require both a thiazide and a rauwolfia alkaloid. Dosage depends upon the requirements of the patient as determined by prior use of the components separately.

> *Diupres-250, -500* (Merck Sharp & Dohme). Each tablet contains chlorothiazide 250 or 500 mg and reserpine 0.125 mg.
>
> *Diutensen-R* (Mallinckrodt). Each tablet contains methyclothiazide 2.5 mg and reserpine 0.1 mg.
>
> *Enduronyl* (Abbott). Each tablet contains methyclothiazide 5 mg and deserpidine 0.25 or 0.5 (Forte) mg.
>
> *Hydromox R* (Lederle). Each tablet contains quinethazone 50 mg and reserpine 0.125 mg.
>
> *Hydropres-25, -50* (Merck Sharp & Dohme). Each tablet contains hydrochlorothiazide 25 or 50 mg and reserpine 0.125 mg.
>
> *Metatensin* (Merrell-National). Each tablet contains trichlormethiazide 2 or 4 mg and reserpine 0.1 mg.
>
> *Naquival* (Schering). Each tablet contains trichlormethiazide 4 mg and reserpine 0.1 mg.
>
> *Oreticyl* (Abbott). Each tablet contains hydrochlorothiazide 25 mg and deserpidine 0.125 mg (Oreticyl 25); hydrochlorothiazide 50 mg and deserpidine 0.125 mg (Oreticyl 50); or hydrochlorothiazide 25 mg and deserpidine 0.25 mg (Oreticyl Forte).
>
> *Rauzide* (Squibb). Each tablet contains bendroflumethiazide 4 mg and rauwolfia serpentina 50 mg.
>
> *Regroton* (USV). Each tablet contains chlorthalidone 25 mg and reserpine 0.125 mg (Demi-Regroton) or chlorthalidone 50 mg and reserpine 0.25 mg.
>
> *Renese-R* (Pfizer). Each tablet contains polythiazide 2 mg and reserpine 0.25 mg.
>
> *Salutensin* (Bristol). Each tablet contains hydroflumethiazide 25 mg and reserpine 0.125 mg (Demi-Salutensin) or hydroflumethiazide 50 mg and reserpine 0.125 mg.
>
> *Serpasil-Esidrix No. 1, No. 2* (Ciba). Each tablet contains hydrochlorothiazide 25 mg (No. 1) or 50 mg (No. 2) and reserpine 0.1 mg.

METHYLDOPA
[Aldomet]

METHYLDOPATE HYDROCHLORIDE
[Aldomet Ester Hydrochloride]

Methyldopa is an aromatic amino acid decarboxylase inhibitor that depresses sympathetic nervous system activity through an effect on the central nervous system. It decreases total peripheral resistance, heart rate, and cardiac output. Both supine and standing blood pressures are reduced. The action of methyldopa is believed to be associated with its metabolism to alpha-methylnorepinephrine. This metabolite presumably lowers blood pressure by activating inhibitory alpha-adrenergic receptors in the central nervous system, thereby reducing sympathetic outflow. Methyldopa also may decrease plasma renin activity, but there is no correlation between this effect and its hypotensive action.

Methyldopa is useful in the treatment of all degrees of hypertension. A thiazide diuretic should be given concomitantly to enhance the antihypertensive effect and prevent the development of drug resistance. If the desired hypotensive effect is not achieved with the thiazide and methyldopa, hydralazine may be added. Methyldopate hydrochloride is used only rarely to treat hypertensive crises because of its erratic onset of action. In addition, the sedative effect may interfere with evaluation of mental status.

Following oral administration, 50% or less of a dose is absorbed from the gastrointestinal tract and neither dosage nor plasma levels correlate with the therapeutic response. Methyldopa is eliminated by renal excretion of active drug or conjugates. In the presence of renal insufficiency, delayed excretion may result in drug accumulation. The pharmacokinetics of the active metabolites have not been studied.

Methyldopa is generally well tolerated. Drowsiness, which usually subsides with continued therapy, is the most common adverse effect. A reversible reduction in mental acuity has been observed in some patients. Mental depression may occur but is less common with this agent than with reserpine. Dryness of the mouth, nasal congestion, nausea, vomiting, diarrhea, and impotence also may occur. Methyldopa occasionally produces symptomatic orthostatic hypotension, and the patient should be informed of this possibility. Sodium and water retention may occur if methyldopa is administered without a diuretic, and this may lead to development of drug resistance (pseudotolerance). A reversible malabsorption syndrome associated with histologic abnormality of the small bowel also has been reported.

With prolonged treatment, a positive Coombs' test has been noted in about 20% of patients. Hemolytic anemia occurs only rarely and is generally reversible when the drug is discontinued, but the Coombs' test may remain positive for several months. Since the great majority of patients with a positive Coombs' test do not develop hemolytic anemia, a positive test is not a contraindication to continued use of the drug.

Alterations in the results of liver function tests (increased serum glutamic oxaloacetic transaminase and alkaline phosphatase levels) have been noted during the first 6 to 12 weeks of treatment. These abnormalities may be accompanied by fever and malaise and are indicative of hepatitis. The hepatitis is usually mild and reversible following discontinuation of methyldopa but, in a few instances, re-exposure to the drug caused fatal hepatic necrosis. Drug fever may occur in some patients without hepatic involvement.

Uncommon adverse effects include reversible leukopenia, thrombocytopenia, retroperitoneal fibrosis, lichenoid reactions, and myocarditis. Hypertensive reactions have been reported rarely after withdrawal of methyldopa or as a result of an interaction with intravenous propranolol or (in patients also receiving a beta blocker) with phenylpropanolamine. Methyldopa produces false elevations of urinary catecholamines when measured by the fluorescent technique and thus may interfere with the diagnosis of pheochromocytoma. Methyldopa may interfere with measurement of serum creatinine (alkaline picrate method), uric acid (phosphotungstate method), and SGOT (colorimetric methods).

Methyldopa crosses the placenta but no adverse effects have been reported when it was used to treat hypertension during pregnancy.

ROUTES, USUAL DOSAGE, AND PREPARATIONS.
Oral: Dosage must be carefully titrated to provide an optimal therapeutic response with minimal side effects, and a diuretic should be given concomitantly to enhance the therapeutic response. For chronic hypertension, *adults*, initially, 250 mg at bedtime; this may be increased to 250 mg twice daily after one week. Daily dosage then may be increased gradually until the blood pressure is controlled or a total daily dose of 2 g is reached. If the patient complains of drowsiness, a larger dose may be given at bedtime than in the morning. It has been suggested that the total daily dose may be administered effectively once daily in some patients; however, further study is warranted. *Children*, initially, 10 mg/kg of body weight daily divided into two to four doses. The daily dosage is then increased or decreased at two-day or longer intervals according to response (maximum, 65 mg/kg daily).

METHYLDOPA:
Aldomet (Merck Sharp & Dohme). Tablets 125, 250, and 500 mg.

Intravenous: *Adults*, 250 to 500 mg every six to eight hours if necessary (maximum, 500 mg every six hours). *Children*, 20 to 40 mg/kg of body weight daily divided into four doses. After the blood pressure has been controlled, oral medication should be substituted.

METHYLDOPATE HYDROCHLORIDE:
Aldomet Ester Hydrochloride (Merck Sharp & Dohme). Solution 250 mg/ml in 5 ml containers.

AVAILABLE MIXTURES.

Methyldopa and a Thiazide: Successful regulation of blood pressure with methyldopa requires careful adjustment of dosage, and the effective dose may vary between 500 mg and 2 g daily. For this reason, fixed-dose combinations containing methyldopa and a thiazide may be unsuitable for many patients.

Aldoclor-150, *-250* (Merck Sharp & Dohme). Each tablet contains methyldopa 250 mg and chlorothiazide 150 or 250 mg.

Aldoril-15, *-25* (Merck Sharp & Dohme). Each tablet contains methyldopa 250 mg and hydrochlorothiazide 15 or 25 mg.

Aldoril D30, *D50* (Merck Sharp & Dohme). Each tablet contains methyldopa 500 mg and hydrochlorothiazide 30 or 50 mg.

Ganglionic Blocking Agents

Ganglionic blocking agents act on autonomic ganglia to inhibit both sympathetic and parasympathetic function. Oral preparations (mecamylamine) are rarely used today because of their untoward effects: severe orthostatic hypotension (due to blockade of sympathetic ganglia) and adynamic ileus and urinary retention (due to blockade of parasympathetic ganglia). Intravenous preparations are still useful occasionally for treating hypertensive emergencies.

TRIMETHAPHAN CAMSYLATE
[Arfonad]

This short-acting ganglionic blocking drug is administered intravenously in hypertensive crises. It has been particularly useful for the initial control of blood pressure in patients with acute dissecting aortic aneurysm. Trimethaphan also is used to produce controlled hypotension for short periods during neurosurgery and some cardiovascular operations in order to avoid excessive blood loss.

Continuous infusion is necessary to maintain the antihypertensive effect. The blood pressure should be monitored frequently while the rate of administration is established initially and every five minutes thereafter. Because they produce marked orthostatic hypotension, the effect of ganglionic blocking agents is enhanced by tilting the head of the bed. If the blood pressure fails to decrease sufficiently with the patient in the supine position, the head of the bed should be elevated.

Trimethaphan may cause urinary retention and orthostatic hypotension. Adynamic ileus is usually not a problem unless the period of infusion exceeds 48 hours. Because prolonged treatment may be associated with sodium and water retention, pseudotolerance can be expected if a diuretic is not given concomitantly. Other adverse effects include anorexia, nausea, vomiting, dryness of the mouth, mydriasis, and cycloplegia.

ROUTE, USUAL DOSAGE, AND PREPARATIONS. *Intravenous*: *Adults,* a 0.1% solution (1 mg/ml) in 5% dextrose injection is continuously infused at a rate determined by the patient's response. The infusion may be started at a rate of 0.5 to 1 mg/min and increased gradually until the blood pressure falls 20 mm Hg or more. After several minutes, the rate can be increased again until the desired level is achieved. While stabilizing the blood pressure with trimethaphan, oral therapy with other antihypertensive drugs should be instituted.

Arfonad (Roche). Solution 50 mg/ml in 10 ml containers.

Agent That Blocks Neuroeffector Transmission

GUANETHIDINE SULFATE
[Ismelin]

This potent antihypertensive agent reduces blood pressure by interfering with the release of norepinephrine from sympathetic nerve terminals. The hypotensive effect is due to both a reduction in cardiac output (resulting from reduced venous return and negative chronotropic and inotropic effects) and a fall in total peripheral vascular resistance. Guanethidine has a marked effect on venous tone, and pronounced orthostatic effects occur frequently. Renal blood flow and glomerular filtration rate may be reduced in the acute treatment phase. Although there are no studies of the long-term effects of guanethidine on renal hemodynamics, chronic therapy is not usually associated with clinically significant changes in renal function.

Guanethidine is usually reserved for patients with severe hypertension who do not respond to other regimens. An oral diuretic should be given concomitantly to prevent sodium and water retention and enhance the antihypertensive response. If side effects are excessive, the dosage may be maintained at the tolerated level and hydralazine or methyldopa added to the regimen. Since guanethidine does not readily cross the blood-brain barrier and central nervous system side effects are, therefore, not a problem, it has been advocated by some for treating selected patients with less severe hypertension who do not respond to a diuretic alone.

Guanethidine is incompletely absorbed and less than 30% of an oral dose enters the systemic circulation. It is eliminated by the renal excretion of unchanged drug and metabolites.

Orthostatic hypotension and post-exercise hypotension are to be anticipated with use of guanethidine, and the patient should be warned of the possible occurrence of these reactions. During initial therapy and whenever dosage is increased, the blood pressure should be measured with the patient in the supine and standing positions and after mild exercise. Orthostatic hypotension may be minimized by cautioning the patient to arise slowly from the recumbent or seated position. Additional measures, such as elevating the head of the bed, are also sometimes helpful. Other common adverse effects are sodium retention (if a diuretic is not given concomitantly), bradycardia, diarrhea, and retrograde ejaculation.

Guanethidine should not be used in patients with pheochromocytoma, since severe hypertension may occur, possibly because of increased sensitivity of the adrenergic receptors to endogenous catecholamines. The response to exogenous catecholamines also may be enhanced. Sympathomimetic agents, such as amphetamines and ephedrine, as well as the tricyclic antidepressants, methylphenidate, cocaine, and, to a lesser extent, chlorpromazine may antagonize the antihypertensive effect of guanethidine.

ROUTE, USUAL DOSAGE, AND PREPARATIONS. Guanethidine has a very broad dose-response curve and dosage should be titrated carefully to provide the desired therapeutic effect with minimal untoward effects. Prior and concomitant administration of a diuretic is recommended to enhance the therapeutic response. Because of guanethidine's long half-life, the maximal effect may not be observed for 7 to 14 days. Effects may persist for seven to ten days or more after withdrawal.

Oral: *Adults*, for ambulatory patients, initially, 10 to 12.5 mg once daily. The dosage may be increased by increments of 10 to 12.5 mg every seven days to 100 mg. If necessary, dosage can be increased by 25-mg increments to a maximum of 300 mg daily; however, daily doses above 100 mg are rarely required because of the availability of newer drugs with fewer side effects. In hospitalized patients, treatment may be initiated with higher doses, eg, 25 to 50 mg daily. *Children*, initially, 0.2 mg/kg of body weight daily, increased by the same amount every seven to ten days if required.

Ismelin (Ciba). Tablets 10 and 25 mg.

AVAILABLE MIXTURE.

Guanethidine and a Thiazide: Guanethidine is particularly unsuitable for incorporation in a fixed-dose product because it is potent, produces marked side effects, and has a wide range of effective dosage. Successful regulation of blood pressure with guanethidine requires careful titration of dosage; the effective dose may range between 10 and 300 mg daily (although doses above 100 mg daily are rarely necessary). In addition, dosage adjustment is often required during the course of continuous therapy. These considerations make use of this fixed-dose combination impractical and undesirable.

Esimil (Ciba). Each tablet contains guanethidine monosulfate 10 mg (equivalent to 8.4 mg guanethidine sulfate) and hydrochlorothiazide 25 mg.

Beta-Adrenergic Blocking Drugs

Propranolol [Inderal] and metoprolol [Lopressor] are the only beta-adrenergic blocking drugs presently available in the United States, but a number of others are currently under investigation. The pharmacology of some of these drugs is discussed in Chapter 35, Antianginal Agents. Another drug under investigation is labetolol, which has both alpha- and beta-blocking properties.

Beta-adrenergic receptors are located primarily in the heart, the arteries and arterioles of skeletal muscle, and the bronchi, where they subserve cardiac excitation, vasodilatation, and bronchial relaxation. Beta-adrenergic blocking agents combine reversibly with these receptors to block the response to sympathetic nerve impulses or circulating catecholamines. Blockade of cardiac (beta1) receptors reduces heart rate and myocardial contractility, thus decreasing cardiac output. The atrioventricular (A-V) conduction time is slowed and automaticity is suppressed at the cellular level.

Beta-blocking drugs reduce both supine and standing blood pressure during long-term therapy without producing orthostatic hypotension. Suggested mechanisms for the antihypertensive action include reduced cardiac output, circulatory adjustments to a chronic reduction in cardiac output, or an effect on adrenergic receptors in the central nervous system. Inhibition of renin release also has been suggested as a possible mechanism, but the evidence is not convincing. There is little or no correlation between the antihypertensive effect of beta-blocking drugs and changes in plasma renin activity, particularly in patients receiving diuretics (Bravo et al, 1975) and/or vasodilators.

Some of the adverse effects of beta-blocking drugs are caused by blockade of noncardiac (beta2) receptors. These include bronchospasm, hypoglycemia, and, possibly, aggravation of peripheral vascular insufficiency. Propranolol is "nonselective" because it blocks beta receptors equally at all sites, whereas metoprolol is classified as "relatively cardioselective."

Since cardioselectivity is not absolute and may not be apparent except at low doses, this property is of limited clinical importance. Various beta blockers also differ in their partial agonist activity (both propranolol and metoprolol have none) and membrane stabilizing action (more pronounced with propranolol than with metoprolol), but these characteristics do not influence safety or efficacy (Davidson et al, 1976). (See also Chapter 35.)

PROPRANOLOL HYDROCHLORIDE
[Inderal]

Propranolol is useful in the treatment of all degrees of hypertension. It is not consistently effective when used alone, but a thiazide diuretic administered concomitantly enhances the antihypertensive response. In a large-scale study on patients with mild hypertension, adequate control of blood pressure was achieved in 52% of patients taking propranolol alone, whereas 81% of those receiving propranolol and a thiazide showed a satisfactory response. The thiazide-propranolol regimen was only slightly less effective than the standard regimen of a thiazide and reserpine (Veterans Administration Cooperative Study Group on Antihypertensive Agents, 1977).

Whether administered alone or with a diuretic, the dosage of propranolol must be carefully titrated, and maximal effects may not be evident for several weeks. The addition of hydralazine permits use of a lower dose of propranolol and further enhances the therapeutic response. In the study mentioned above, combined therapy with a thiazide, propranolol, and hydralazine was effective in 92% of patients with mild hypertension. This diuretic-beta blocker-vasodilator regimen is particularly useful in patients with moderate to severe hypertension and is usually well tolerated by those who have experienced disabling side effects with other forms of therapy (Zacest et al, 1972).

Propranolol also may be administered with an alpha-adrenergic blocking agent for the preoperative management of patients with pheochromocytoma and for prolonged treatment of patients who are not suitable candidates for surgery. In this setting, it is used to protect the heart from the positive inotropic and chronotropic effects of the high level of circulating catecholamines. Propranolol should not be used in patients with pheochromocytoma without first administering adequate doses of an alpha-blocking drug because, if used alone, it may increase blood pressure.

Propranolol is almost completely absorbed from the gastrointestinal tract, but plasma levels correlate poorly with dosage. Individual variability in the rate of hepatic metabolism appears to account for most of the differences in bioavailability (see also Chapter 35).

Because it does not cause orthostatic or postexercise hypotension, propranolol is usually better tolerated than antihypertensive drugs that cause generalized inhibition of sympathetic function. It should be given with great caution, however, to patients with inadequate cardiac reserve because it may precipitate congestive heart failure. Concomitant diuretic therapy may reduce this risk, but it is usually advisable to prescribe digitalis also. Propranolol depresses A-V conduction and may cause A-V dissociation and even cardiac arrest in patients with A-V block. It is generally contraindicated in the presence of severe A-V conduction disturbances.

In patients with severe or unstable angina, sudden withdrawal of large doses of propranolol has been followed by recurrence of unstable angina, ventricular tachycardia, fatal myocardial infarction, and sudden death. If it becomes necessary to discontinue therapy, the dosage should be reduced gradually over a one- to two-week period.

Propranolol increases airway resistance and may provoke asthmatic attacks in patients with a history of asthma or bronchitis. It may precipitate or aggravate peripheral vascular insufficiency. This agent may also mask some of the warning symptoms of hypoglycemia and may prolong the duration of hypoglycemia in diabetics receiving insulin, in patients recovering from anesthesia, in those on dialysis, and in children during periods of restricted food intake. In hypertensive patients, blood pressure may increase during hypoglycemic episodes. For these reasons, beta-blocking drugs should be given cautiously, if at all, to insulin-dependent diabetics. Beta-blocking agents have been reported to have an additive effect on the elevations in serum triglyceride and urate levels induced by thiazides. Other adverse effects include gastrointestinal disturbances, fatigue, lethargy, vivid dreams, insomnia, and other central nervous system effects. The actions, uses, and adverse effects of propranolol are discussed in more detail in Chapter 35, Antianginal Agents. See also Chapter 34, Antiarrhythmic Agents.

ROUTE, USUAL DOSAGE, AND PREPARATIONS. *Oral*: For chronic hypertension, dosage must be titrated on the basis of the therapeutic response, because the effective dose varies widely and plasma levels are not closely correlated with antihypertensive response. *Adults*, initially, 40 mg twice daily with a thiazide diuretic. If the desired response is not obtained, the dosage should be increased to 80 mg twice daily. Further increments may be added, if needed, to a maximum of 640 mg daily. If control is not adequate with twice daily administration, the drug should be given three times daily. If larger daily doses are required, it is generally more practical and effective to add hydralazine to the regimen rather than to continue to increase the dose of propranolol. The daily dose of propranolol usually need not exceed 320 mg when it is given with a diuretic and hydralazine. For pheochromocytoma, there is wide variability in treatment requirements and the dosage must be individualized.

Inderal (Ayerst). Tablets 10, 20, 40, and 80 mg.
AVAILABLE MIXTURE.
Propranolol and a Thiazide: This product recently became available and time has not permitted a thorough evaluation of efficacy.

Inderide (Ayerst). Each tablet contains propranolol hydrochloride 40 or 80 mg and hydrochlorothiazide 25 mg.

METOPROLOL TARTRATE
[Lopressor]

$$CH_3OCH_2CH_2 - \!\!\!\bigcirc\!\!\! - OCH_2CHCH_2\overset{+}{N}H_2CH \overset{CH_3}{\underset{CH_3}{\diagup}} \quad C_4H_6O_6$$
$$\underset{OH}{\vert}$$

Metoprolol is useful in treating mild to moderate hypertension. Its antihypertensive effect appears to be comparable to that of propranolol and other beta-blocking drugs (Davidson et al, 1976). As with other antihypertensive drugs, metoprolol generally should be given with a diuretic. Metoprolol will probably also prove useful as part of a three-drug regimen in patients with severe hypertension, but there is currently little published information on such use.

Metoprolol is well absorbed after oral administration, but plasma levels vary widely because of individual differences in hepatic metabolism. Metoprolol is excreted by the kidney, largely as inactive metabolites.

The adverse effects of metoprolol that are secondary to cardiac beta blockade are identical to those produced by propranolol and other beta blockers and the same precautions apply. (See the evaluation on Propranolol Hydrochloride.) Despite its relative cardioselectivity, clinically effective doses of metoprolol may increase airway resistance in asthmatic patients, although to a lesser extent than propranolol. It should be used cautiously in patients with obstructive airway disease and a beta2 agonist should be given to reduce the risk of bronchospasm. Metoprolol also may potentiate the hypoglycemic effect of insulin and delay the return to normoglycemia and may aggravate peripheral vascular insufficiency. Other adverse reactions include gastrointestinal disturbances, fatigue, dizziness, headache, nightmares, insomnia, and depression.

ROUTE, USUAL DOSAGE, AND PREPARATIONS.
Oral: The effective dose varies widely and must be titrated on the basis of the therapeutic response. Plasma levels do not correlate with the antihypertensive response and are not useful as a guide to therapy. *Adults*, initially, 50 mg twice daily with a thiazide diuretic. If the desired response is not obtained, the dosage may be increased gradually. The daily maintenance dose ranges from 100 to 450 mg. The drug should be given three times daily if control is not adequate with twice daily administration.

Lopressor (Geigy). Tablets 50 and 100 mg.

Alpha-Adrenergic Blocking Agents

Alpha-adrenergic receptors are located primarily in the resistance vessels of the skin, mucosa, intestine, and kidney, where they subserve vasoconstriction. Alpha-adrenergic blocking agents block these receptors and thereby lower peripheral vascular resistance and decrease blood pressure. Phenoxybenzamine and phentolamine block both pre- and postsynaptic alpha-adrenergic receptors, whereas prazosin acts by selective blockade of postsynaptic alpha receptors.

PRAZOSIN HYDROCHLORIDE
[Minipress]

$$CH_3O \qquad CH_3O \qquad NH_2 \qquad N - C \qquad Cl^-$$

Prazosin reduces peripheral vascular resistance by postsynaptic alpha blockade. Prazosin dilates both arterioles and veins and, in addition to its use in hypertension, it has been employed as an adjunct in the treatment of severe refractory congestive heart failure (see Chapter 33). Although prazosin decreases both supine and standing blood pressures, the hypotensive effect is most pronounced when the patient is standing, and marked orthostatic hypotension and syncope may occur with the first dose. Prazosin has little effect on the resting heart rate measured when the patient is in the supine or sitting position; the heart rate increases slightly when the patient is upright and during exercise. Plasma renin activity is not increased.

Since prazosin usually does not cause significant tachycardia, it may be considered for use with a diuretic in selected patients as a component of a two-drug regimen. It also may be a suitable alternative to hydralazine in a three-drug regimen, but may be less effective than hydralazine. The development of drug resistance has been noted in some patients during treatment of congestive heart failure. It is not yet known whether this will be a factor in the long-term control of hypertension.

Prazosin is well absorbed by the gastrointestinal tract, but there is considerable individual variation in plasma levels and no clear correlation between plasma level and therapeutic response. Increased plasma levels have been reported in patients with renal insufficiency, but this has not been a consistent finding.

Marked orthostatic hypotension may occur at the onset of treatment but usually disappears with continued therapy. Reports of syncopal episodes occurring within 30 to 90 minutes following the initial dose led to introduction of the term, "first dose phenomenon." Manifestations include dizziness, headache, palpitations, sweating, weakness, lassitude, blurred vision, nausea, and diarrhea. Marked tachycardia has been noted occasionally and chest pain (without ECG changes) has occurred rarely. In a few patients, the reaction has been characterized by sudden collapse with loss of consciousness which, in some instances, persisted for an hour.

Since symptomatic orthostatic hypotension appears to be more common with an initial 2-mg dose, the first few doses should not exceed 1 mg and should be taken at bedtime. Patients receiving diuretics and/or on a low-sodium diet appear to be particularly susceptible. Those who have experienced the first-dose reaction may tolerate subsequent doses despite the fact that plasma prazosin levels are considerably higher after several days of treatment than after the initial dose. Reactions similar to the first-dose phenomenon have occurred occasionally following a rapid increase in dosage, after addition of another antihypertensive drug to the regimen of patients receiving large doses of prazosin, or during combined therapy with small doses of prazosin and a beta-blocking drug.

Prazosin may cause fluid retention and edema if a diuretic is not given concomitantly. Dryness of the mouth and nasal congestion have been reported. Adverse effects rarely associated with prazosin therapy include urinary frequency, impotence, febrile polyarthritis, and dermatologic reactions.

ROUTE, USUAL DOSAGE, AND PREPARATIONS. As with all antihypertensive drugs, prior and concomitant diuretic therapy is recommended to enhance the therapeutic response. Rapid increases in dosage should be avoided.

Oral: *Adults*, to minimize the danger of a syncopal reaction, the first few doses should not exceed 1 mg and should be given at bedtime. The patient should be instructed to remain in bed for at least three hours. Thereafter, 1 mg may be given two times daily and increased to three times daily later. For maintenance, the dose may be increased gradually to 20 mg daily. (The manufacturer's literature states that a few patients may benefit from further increases up to 40 mg daily.) Prazosin should be added cautiously to the regimen of patients receiving a beta-blocking drug or other sympathetic depressants. When administered with a diuretic and a beta blocker, relatively small doses may be sufficient for maintenance.

Minipress (Pfizer). Capsules 1, 2, and 5 mg.

PHENOXYBENZAMINE HYDROCHLORIDE
[Dibenzyline]

PHENTOLAMINE
[Regitine]

Phenoxybenzamine and phentolamine are used to treat hypertensive states caused by an excess of circulating catecholamines, but they are not useful in essential hypertension. These agents are administered orally for the preoperative management of patients with pheochromocytoma and for long-term treatment of those who are not suitable candidates for surgery. Phenoxybenzamine is preferred because it provides more sustained control of blood pressure. The beta-adrenergic blocking agent, propranolol, should be used concomitantly to prevent excessive cardiac stimulation.

Phentolamine mesylate is given intravenously immediately prior to surgery for pheochromocytoma and during surgical manipulation of the tumor. It has been administered intravenously for diagnosis of pheochromocytoma, but measurement of urinary catecholamines and their metabolites is now the established diagnostic method of choice. The mesylate salt also is used to treat hypertensive crises caused by interaction between monoamine oxidase inhibitors and sympathomimetic amines and in the clonidine withdrawal syndrome.

Reflex tachycardia and orthostatic hypotension are the most common untoward effects of the alpha-adrenergic blocking agents. When these agents are given orally, nasal congestion and gastrointestinal disturbances (nausea, vomiting, diarrhea) may occur.

ROUTES, USUAL DOSAGE, AND PREPARATIONS.
PHENOXYBENZAMINE HYDROCHLORIDE:
Oral: For pheochromocytoma, there is wide variability in treatment requirements and the dose must be individualized.
> *Dibenzyline* (Smith Kline & French). Capsules 10 mg.

PHENTOLAMINE HYDROCHLORIDE:
Oral: For pheochromocytoma, there is wide variability in treatment requirements and the dose must be individualized.
> *Regitine* [*hydrochloride*] (Ciba). Tablets 50 mg.

PHENTOLAMINE MESYLATE:
Intravenous: To control blood pressure immediately prior to or during surgery for pheochromocytoma, there is wide variability in treatment requirements and the dose must be individualized.

For diagnosis of pheochromocytoma, *adults*, 5 mg dissolved in 1 ml of sterile water; *children*, 1 mg. A fall in blood pressure of more than 35 mm Hg systolic and 25 mm Hg diastolic suggests pheochromocytoma.

For hypertensive crisis due to interaction of a monoamine oxidase inhibitor with sympathomimetic amines, *adults*, 5 to 20 mg.

For clonidine withdrawal syndrome, *adults*, 5 to 10 mg at five-minute intervals to a total dose of 20 to 30 mg.
> *Regitine* [*mesylate*] (Ciba). Powder (lyophilized, for solution) 5 mg.

DIRECT-ACTING VASODILATORS

Arterial Vasodilators

HYDRALAZINE HYDROCHLORIDE
[Apresoline]

Hydralazine reduces blood pressure by directly relaxing arteriolar smooth muscle; it has little effect on veins. Heart rate and cardiac output are increased. The tachycardia induced by hydralazine is greater than would be expected solely on a reflex basis and is poorly correlated with changes in blood pressure. Studies in laboratory animals suggest that the cardiac effects may result from a combination of three actions: (1) a reflex response to the fall in blood pressure; (2) a direct beta-adrenergic action on the heart; and (3) an effect on the central nervous system.

Hydralazine is given orally for the management of chronic hypertension, usually as the third agent when adequate control is not obtained with a diuretic and sympathetic depressant drug. Older patients with less sensitive baroreceptor reflexes may not experience tachycardia. Hydralazine may be an effective second drug for such patients because it does not cause sedation or other central nervous system effects.

Hydralazine can be given parenterally in hypertensive emergencies and may be particularly useful in patients with acute glomerulonephritis or eclampsia. The antihypertensive effect begins within 15 minutes after intravenous administration and lasts three or four hours. However, sodium nitroprusside and diazoxide are preferred for most hypertensive emergencies because of their rapid onset of action, greater hypotensive potency, and more consistent effectiveness.

Hydralazine is well absorbed after oral administration and less than 10% of an oral dose is excreted in the feces. It has a relatively short half-life and is eliminated by the kidney as active drug and metabolites. Acetylation is one of the metabolic pathways for inactivation of the drug. Although fast acetylators have lower plasma levels than slow acetylators, the rate of elimination from the plasma does not differ greatly between the two groups; therefore, other metabolic pathways also may be important.

Like other vasodilators, hydralazine causes sodium and water retention if a diuretic is not given concomitantly. Headache and tachycardia, which are common when hydralazine is given alone or with a diuretic, can be minimized by increasing the dosage gradually. Tachycardia also can be reduced or controlled by prior and concomitant administration of a sympathetic depressant drug, particularly a beta blocker. Hydralazine should not be used alone in patients with coronary artery disease or dissecting aortic aneurysm and is generally considered to be contraindicated as sole therapy in patients with congestive heart failure; however, it has recently been shown that hydralazine improves cardiac performance in some patients with intractable left ventricular failure (see Chapter 33). Gastrointestinal disturbances, flushing, dyspnea on exertion, rash, and, rarely, peripheral neuropathy and blood dyscrasias also may occur.

Prolonged administration of large doses has produced an acute rheumatoid syndrome simulating systemic lupus erythematosus (fever, arthralgia, splenomegaly, edema, and LE cells in the peripheral blood). This adverse reaction is most common in slow acetylators and is dose related, occurring only rarely with daily doses below 200 mg. The effects are generally reversible when the drug is withdrawn.

ROUTES, USUAL DOSAGE, AND PREPARATIONS. *Oral*: For chronic hypertension (usually as the third agent in the regimen), *adults*, initially, 10 to 25 mg two or three times daily. Dosage then may be increased by increments of 10 to 25 mg until the blood pressure is reduced to the desired level. The maximal daily dose is 300 mg, usually given in two or three divided doses. *Children*, initially, 0.75 mg/kg of body weight daily in four divided doses. The dosage may be increased gradually over the next three to four weeks to a maximum of 7.5 mg/kg daily.

> Drug available generically: Tablets 10, 25, and 50 mg.
> *Apresoline* (Ciba). Tablets 10, 25, 50, and 100 mg.

Intravenous (slow), Intramuscular: For hypertensive crises, *adults*, 10 to 20 mg, increased to 40 mg if necessary. The dose should be repeated as required. *Children*, 1.7 to 3.5 mg/kg of body weight daily divided into four to six doses. If given with reserpine, the dose may be reduced to 0.15 mg/kg every 12 to 24 hours. While stabilizing the blood pressure, oral antihypertensive therapy should be instituted.

> *Apresoline* (Ciba). Solution 20 mg/ml in 1 ml containers.

AVAILABLE MIXTURES.
Hydralazine and Other Antihypertensive Agents: The products listed below are indicated only if the dosage ratio meets the optimal requirements of the patient. Because the central nervous system side effects of reserpine are dose related, mixtures

containing this drug may not be suitable for patients requiring large doses of hydralazine. If one of the hydralazine-reserpine mixtures is used, a diuretic should be prescribed separately.

Apresazide (Ciba). Each capsule contains hydralazine hydrochloride 25 mg and hydrochlorothiazide 25 mg (25/25); or hydralazine hydrochloride 50 mg and hydrochlorothiazide 50 mg (50/50); or hydralazine hydrochloride 100 mg and hydrochlorothiazide 50 mg (100/50).

Apresoline-Esidrix (Ciba). Each tablet contains hydralazine hydrochloride 25 mg and hydrochlorothiazide 15 mg.

Dralserp (Lemmon). Each tablet contains hydralazine hydrochloride 25 mg and reserpine 0.1 mg.

Ser-Ap-Es (Ciba). Each tablet contains hydralazine hydrochloride 25 mg, hydrochlorothiazide 15 mg, and reserpine 0.1 mg.

Serpasil-Apresoline No. 1, No. 2 (Ciba). Each No. 1 tablet contains hydralazine hydrochloride 25 mg and reserpine 0.1 mg; each No. 2 tablet contains hydralazine hydrochloride 50 mg and reserpine 0.2 mg.

MINOXIDIL
[Loniten]

Minoxidil acts directly on arterioles to reduce peripheral vascular resistance. It has little or no effect on the venous system. When given alone, minoxidil's hypotensive effect is accompanied by a marked increase in heart rate and cardiac output.

Minoxidil is a more potent vasodilator than hydralazine. It is used to treat severe refractory hypertension and is particularly useful as an alternative to bilateral nephrectomy in patients with advanced renal disease (Limas and Freis, 1973; Mitchell and Pettinger, 1978). Both a diuretic and a beta blocker should be given concomitantly to control fluid retention, prevent tachycardia, and enhance the therapeutic response. Large doses of furosemide, sometimes combined with spironolactone

or a thiazide, may be required to prevent the development of congestive symptoms. Other antihypertensive drugs also may be continued or added as necessary.

In addition to fluid retention and tachycardia, the most common side effect of minoxidil is hypertrichosis. If hypertrichosis develops, it does so most commonly after one or two months of therapy. The hirsutism may be accompanied by darkening of the skin and coarsening of facial features. Nausea, headache, fatigue, and dermatologic reactions also may occur. Transient pericardial effusions have been observed occasionally and may be a manifestation of fluid retention. Pulmonary hypertension has been reported in some patients receiving minoxidil, but this may be related to the disease process rather than to the drug.

ROUTE, USUAL DOSAGE, AND PREPARATIONS. *Oral: Adults*, initially, 2.5 mg twice daily. If an adequate response is not obtained within one week, dosage may be increased to 5 mg twice daily. Further increases (up to 40 mg daily) may be necessary in some patients. *Children*, initially, 0.1 to 0.2 mg/kg of body weight daily in two divided doses. Dosages may be increased if necessary up to 1.4 mg/kg/day. A diuretic and beta blocker should be given concomitantly.

Loniten (Upjohn). Tablets 2.5 and 10 mg.

DIAZOXIDE
[Hyperstat I.V.]

Diazoxide is a nondiuretic thiazide derivative that produces a prompt (one to five minutes) reduction in blood pressure when given by the intravenous route. The hypotensive effect is caused by a direct action on the arterioles; capacitance vessels are not affected. Heart rate and cardiac output are increased.

Diazoxide is effective in most hypertensive emergencies. It is particularly useful in patients with hypertensive encephalopathy, malignant hypertension, and severe hypertension associated with acute or chronic glomerulonephritis; it also has been used successfully in pre-eclampsia and eclampsia. Diazoxide is relatively contraindicated in patients with coronary or cerebral vascular insufficiency in whom a rapid reduction in pressure could precipitate coronary or cerebral ischemia. Because it increases cardiac output and left ventricular ejection velocity, it is unsuitable for the treatment of hypertension associated with dissecting aortic aneurysm.

Oral dosage forms of diazoxide [Proglycem] are used in the management of hypoglycemia caused by hyperinsulinism. Oral therapy has occasionally been employed abroad for prolonged treatment of patients with severe hypertension.

Diazoxide is extensively bound to plasma protein. Since the hypotensive action depends upon a high initial concentration of free drug, there is no correlation between serum levels and therapeutic response. It is eliminated by renal excretion, largely as unchanged drug.

Sodium and water retention, hyperglycemia, and hyperuricemia are the major side effects of diazoxide. Administration of adequate doses of an effective diuretic will prevent fluid overload and may enhance the antihypertensive effect. For this reason, furosemide is usually given intravenously concomitantly or prior to each injection of diazoxide. This program is particularly important during repeated injections of diazoxide to avoid volume expansion and to prevent the development of drug resistance.

The hyperglycemic and hyperuricemic effects of diazoxide (which are enhanced by diuretics) are usually mild and transitory. Diabetic patients may require an adjustment in insulin dosage if repeated injections are necessary. Two cases of hyperglycemic hyperosmolar nonketoacidotic coma have been reported following repeated oral or intravenous administration of diazoxide; in one patient, the hyperosmolar coma was associated with the appearance of transient lens opacities.

Marked hypotension may occur in patients treated with large doses of diazoxide and furosemide, and it has been recommended that patients remain recumbent and be closely monitored for 30 minutes after each injection. Severe hypotension, anginal symptoms, cerebral ischemia, hemiplegia, and myocardial infarction have occurred rarely. Diazoxide also may cause gastrointestinal disturbances (nausea, vomiting, anorexia), headache, flushing, and temporary interruption of labor. Hypersensitivity reactions (rash, leukopenia, fever) are uncommon. Hemolytic episodes have occurred rarely during diazoxide therapy. Extravasation causes severe local pain but tissue sloughing has not been reported.

Reversible extrapyramidal symptoms have developed in some patients during long-term oral therapy, which suggests that diazoxide has some effect on central dopaminergic mechanisms. Increased hair growth is common during long-term oral use of the drug. Alopecia and increased hair growth have been observed in the offspring of women who were given diazoxide orally for pre-eclampsia. Similar reactions have not been reported after intravenous use for brief periods.

ROUTE, USUAL DOSAGE, AND PREPARATIONS. *Intravenous*: *Adults*, 300 mg or 5 mg/kg of body weight; *children*, 5 mg/kg. The drug may be injected rapidly (within 30 seconds) and the injection may be repeated, if required, at intervals of 30 minutes to 24 hours. The arterial pressure can be reduced more gradually in many patients by the intermittent injection of smaller doses (50 to 150 mg at 5- to 15-minute intervals) until adequate blood pressure control is achieved. Intravenous administration of furosemide 30 to 60 minutes prior to each injection of diazoxide will prevent fluid overload and ensure a continuing hypotensive response. While stabilizing the blood pressure with diazoxide, oral therapy with other antihypertensive agents should be instituted.

Hyperstat I.V. (Schering). Solution 15 mg/ml in 20 ml containers.

Arterial and Venous Vasodilator

SODIUM NITROPRUSSIDE
[Nipride]

$$Na_2Fe(CN)_5NO \cdot 2H_2O$$

This potent vasodilator acts directly to relax both resistance and capacitance vessels. Heart rate is usually increased by reflex mechanisms. Cardiac output generally is not increased because of the reduction in venous tone and venous return. By reducing impedance to left ventricular ejection, sodium nitroprusside improves cardiac performance and may increase cardiac output in patients with left ventricular failure.

Nitroprusside is the most rapid acting and consistently effective agent for treating hypertensive emergencies regardless of the cause. It reduces blood pressure immediately, but continuous infusion is necessary to maintain the hypotensive response. Because of its beneficial hemodynamic effects, nitroprusside is the drug of choice in the management of hypertensive crises associated with acute myocardial infarction and left ventricular failure. Its rapid onset and brief duration of action are useful in hypertensive patients with cerebral or subarachnoid hemorrhage. Nitroprusside is also used to induce controlled hypotension during certain surgical procedures (see Chapter 21, Adjuncts to Anesthesia and Analeptic Drugs).

Studies are currently in progress to evaluate the efficacy of nitroprusside in the early stages of acute myocardial infarction. The rationale for this use is to reduce impedance to left ventricular ejection and thereby increase cardiac output, while at the same time reducing cardiac work and myocardial oxygen consumption. Also under investigation is the role of vasodilator therapy in improving cardiac function and hemodynamics in patients with intractable low-output chronic congestive heart failure. (See Chapters 33 and 37.)

Nitroprusside has a very brief half-life. It is converted by erythrocytes to cyanide, which is then transformed to the final metabolite, thiocyanate, by the hepatic enzyme, rhodanese. This reaction requires thiosulfate (which is derived endogenously from the amino acid, cysteine). Thiocyanate is eliminated by renal excretion. Its half-life is four to seven days in patients with normal renal function.

Sodium nitroprusside may cause nausea, vomiting, headache, palpitations, restlessness, and sweating. These symptoms generally are caused by the rapid fall in blood pressure and can be relieved by slowing the infusion rate or temporarily discontinuing the infusion. Manifestations of toxicity include muscle spasms, disorientation, delirium, and psychotic behavior. Hypothyroidism developed in one patient following infusion of 3.9 g over a period of 21 days. These reactions are usually attributed to accumulation of thiocyanate which may occur during prolonged administration, particularly in patients with renal insufficiency. If nitroprusside is infused for more than 72 hours, blood thiocyanate levels should be determined daily; if levels do not exceed 10 mg/dl, it is probably safe to continue administration. High levels of blood cyanide may develop during infusion of large amounts, particularly in patients with inadequate endogenous thiosulfate or with hepatic disease. Several deaths associated with the use of nitroprusside during surgery have been attributed to cyanide poisoning. It also has been suggested that increased blood cyanide levels may be responsible for occasional instances of tachyphylaxis to nitroprusside. The blood cyanide level can be reduced by infusion of sodium thiosulfate or hydroxocobalamin. One case of methemoglobinemia has been reported.

ROUTE, USUAL DOSAGE, AND PREPARATIONS. Before using sodium nitroprusside, it is advisable to review the manufacturer's prescribing information.

Intravenous: Sodium nitroprusside should be used only in an intensive care unit and the blood pressure should be monitored frequently during infusion. The solution should be protected from light and, if used continuously, a fresh solution should be prepared every eight hours.

Adults, 50 mg, dissolved in 250 to 1,000 ml of 5% dextrose injection in water, is infused at a rate of 0.5 to 10 mcg/kg/min. Oral therapy with other antihypertensive drugs should be instituted while the blood pressure is being stabilized with sodium nitroprusside.

    Nipride (Roche). Powder (for solution) 50 mg.

ANGIOTENSIN ANTAGONISTS

    Renin is a proteolytic enzyme that is produced and stored in the kidney. It is released in response to various stimuli, the most important being a reduction in renal perfusion pressure resulting from hemorrhage, dehydration, chronic sodium depletion, or other states in which the effective circulating blood volume is reduced. The secretion of renin is also regulated by sympathetic nervous system activity and humoral factors. In the circulatory system, renin reacts with a substrate formed in the liver to produce angiotensin I. This physiologically inactive prohormone is then hydrolyzed to angiotensin II by a converting enzyme present in highest concentrations in the lung. Angiotensin II acts on receptor sites in vascular smooth muscle, the central nervous system, and the adrenal cortex to constrict arterioles, reduce vagal tone, and induce secretion of aldosterone. These actions result in arteriolar constriction, increased heart rate and cardiac output, and increased reabsorption of sodium and water. The resultant increase in blood pressure then activates a feedback loop that reduces secretion of renin. The renin-angiotensin-aldosterone system does not play an active role in maintaining circulatory homeostasis in the normovolemic, sodium-replete individual but is of major importance in maintaining blood pressure and intravascular volume during sodium deprivation or volume depletion.

    Several compounds currently under investigation compete with angiotensin II for receptor sites in vascular smooth muscle and the adrenal cortex (saralasin) or block the conversion of angiotensin I to angiotensin II by inhibiting the converting enzyme (teprotide and captopril). The converting enzyme inhibitors also block degradation of the vasodilator, bradykinin. The role that bradykinin plays in the hypotensive effect of these agents has not yet been determined.

    Angiotensin antagonists have proved useful in studying the function of the renin-angiotensin-aldosterone system, but their diagnostic and therapeutic potential has not yet been clearly defined. The intravenously administered competitive antagonist, saralasin, has been advocated to detect renovascular hypertension (which is presumably angiotensin dependent), but false-negative results may occur in the sodium-replete patient, whereas false-positive results are not uncommon after sodium depletion. There has been less experience with the converting enzyme inhibitors. Teprotide, given intravenously, may be useful for functional lateralization of renal artery stenosis. Captopril, which is administered orally, may have more general applications (and other pharmacologic actions), because it reduces blood pressure in both essential and renovascular hypertension, regardless of initial plasma renin activity (Gavras et al, 1978).

Selected References

Report of Joint National Committee on detection, evaluation and treatment of high blood pressure: Cooperative study. *JAMA* 237:255-261, 1977.

Bennett WM, et al: Do diuretics have antihypertensive properties independent of natriuresis? *Clin Pharmacol Ther* 22:499-504, 1977.

Berglund G, et al: Coronary heart disease after treatment of hypertension. *Lancet* 1:1-5, 1978.

Bravo EL, et al: Beta-adrenergic blockade in diuretic-treated patients with essential hypertension. *N Engl J Med* 292:66-70, 1975.

Committee on Hypertension, AMA: Drug treatment of ambulatory patients with hypertension. *JAMA* 225:1647-1653, 1973.

Davidson C, et al: Comparison of antihypertensive activity of beta-blocking drugs during chronic treatment. *Br Med J* 2:7-9, 1976.

de Carvalho JGR, et al: Ticrynafen: Novel uricosuric antihypertensive natriuretic agent. *Ann Intern Med* 138:53-57, 1978.

Finnerty FA Jr, et al: Step 2 regimens in hypertension: Assessment. *JAMA* 241:579-581, 1979.

Freis ED: Salt, volume and prevention of hypertension. *Circulation* 53:589-595, 1976.

Gavras H, et al: Antihypertensive effect of oral angiotensin converting-enzyme inhibitor SQ 14225 in man. *N Engl J Med* 298:991-995, 1978.

Gifford RW Jr: Drug combinations as rational antihypertensive therapy. *Arch Intern Med* 133:1053-1057, 1974.

Kaplan NM: Renin profiles: Unfulfilled promises. *JAMA* 238:611-613, 1977.

Limas CJ, Freis ED: Minoxidil in severe hypertension with renal failure: Effect of its addition to conventional antihypertensive drugs. *Am J Cardiol* 31:355-361, 1973.

Materson BJ, et al: Dose response to chlorthalidone in patients with mild hypertension: Efficacy of a lower dose. *Clin Pharmacol Ther* 24:192-198, 1978.

Mitchell HC, Pettinger WA: Long-term treatment of refractory hypertensive patients with minoxidil. *JAMA* 239:2131-2138, 1978.

Nemati M, et al: Clinical study of ticrynafen: New diuretic, antihypertensive, and uricosuric agent. *JAMA* 237:652-657, 1977.

Page LB, et al: Drugs in management of hypertension, parts I, II, and III. *Am Heart J* 91:810-815; 92:114-118, 252-259, 1976.

Shah S, et al: Mechanism of antihypertensive effect of thiazide diuretics. *Am Heart J* 95:611-618, 1978.

Simpson FO: Beta-adrenergic receptor blocking drugs in hypertension. *Drugs* 7:85-105, 1974.

Tweeddale MG, et al: Antihypertensive and biochemical effects of chlorthalidone. *Clin Pharmacol Ther* 22:519-527, 1977.

Veterans Administration Cooperative Study Group on Antihypertensive Agents: Propranolol in treatment of hypertension. *JAMA* 237:2303-2310, 1977.

Veterans Administration Cooperative Study Group on Antihypertensive Agents: Effects of treatment on morbidity in hypertension: Results in patients with diastolic blood pressures averaging 90 through 114 mm Hg. *JAMA* 213:1143-1152, 1970.

Veterans Administration Cooperative Study Group on Antihypertensive Agents: Effects of treatment on morbidity in hypertension: Results in patients with diastolic blood pressures averaging 115 through 129 mm Hg. *JAMA* 202:1028-1034, 1967.

Wollam GL, et al: Antihypertensive drugs: Clinical pharmacology and therapeutic use. *Drugs* 14:420-460, 1977.

Zacest R, et al: Treatment of essential hypertension with combined vasodilation and beta-adrenergic blockade. *N Engl J Med* 286:617-622, 1972.

Diuretics | 39

Diuretics reduce the volume of extracellular fluid and thereby prevent or alleviate edema. They act by enhancing the urinary excretion of salt and water by directly or indirectly impairing sodium chloride reabsorption in the renal tubules. The resultant diuresis is influenced primarily by the site of action of the drug in the nephron and, to a lesser extent, by hormonal regulatory mechanisms that promote the reabsorption of sodium and other ions. The selection and proper use of a diuretic require familiarity with the renal regulation of salt and water balance and with the site and mechanism of action of the different classes of diuretics.

Renal Regulation of Salt and Water Balance: Approximately 180 liters of plasma are filtered through the glomeruli daily and, under normal conditions, over 99% of this protein-free filtrate is subsequently reabsorbed. The largest portion of filtered sodium (60% to 70%) is reabsorbed isosmotically in the proximal tubules. In the early proximal tubules, sodium reabsorption occurs by active transport and is coupled electrogenically to the reabsorption of glucose and amino acids and nonelectrogenically to reabsorption of bicarbonate. The transport of sodium bicarbonate, which is linked to hydrogen ion secretion and depends upon the enzyme, carbonic anhydrase, is important in the regulation of acid-base balance. The outward transport of solute in the early proximal tubules creates an osmotic gradient that causes water to flow out of the tubular lumen into the peritubular capillaries. Since bicarbonate is the principal ion accompanying sodium out of the early proximal tubules, fluid entering the late proximal tubules contains a high concentration of chloride. The reabsorption of salt and water that occurs in the late proximal tubules is primarily driven by active sodium transport, although there is increasing evidence favoring additional passive transport of chloride.

Sodium reabsorption in the proximal tubules is directly related to the glomerular filtration rate, inversely related to extracellular fluid volume, and also may be altered by humoral agents, including parathyroid hormone. Although these and other factors may markedly alter proximal sodium reabsorption, the more distal segments of the nephron possess extensive compensatory potential (Burg, 1976 A; Knox, 1973; Stein and Reineck, 1975). For this reason, agents that inhibit sodium reabsorption in the proximal tubules are relatively ineffective diuretics.

The portion of the glomerular filtrate that is not reabsorbed in the proximal tubules passes into the loop of Henle, which provides the primary driving force for concentration or dilution of the urine. The descending limb is highly permeable to the osmotic flow of water. Since the medullary interstitium contains high concentrations of salt and urea, the tubular fluid becomes hypertonic as it approaches the tip of the loop due to outflow of water down its concentration gradient. Approximately 15% to 20% of the filtered load of sodium is reabsorbed in the ascending limb of Henle's loop, which is relatively impermeable to water. The function of the thin ascending limb is not clearly understood; the transport of salt in this segment may occur by passive reabsorption, active transport, or both. The thick ascending limb reabsorbs chloride by active transport, and sodium follows passively. In the medullary portion, sodium chloride is deposited in the medullary interstitium, creating an increasing concentration of solute from cortex to medulla. The separation of salt and water reabsorption in the ascending limb serves two functions: (1) establishment of a hypertonic medullary interstitium, which provides the osmotic driving force for urinary concentration, and (2) generation of a hypotonic tubular fluid. (See also Burg, 1976 A; DuBose and Kokko, 1977; Kleit et al, 1970; and Jacobson and Kokko, 1976.)

At the end of the loop of Henle, the cells of the tubular wall are in close proximity to the glomerular arterioles (macula densa). The chloride ion concentration of the tubular fluid in this region may be important in a feedback system which adjusts the glomerular filtration rate to the reabsorptive capacity of the nephron. This system may protect the body from volume depletion when the tubular reabsorptive mechanisms fail (Thurau and Boylan, 1976).

In the early distal tubules (cortical diluting segment), the tubular fluid becomes further diluted because of additional reabsorption of sodium chloride through the water-impermeable tubular epithelium. In the late distal tubules and cortical collecting ducts, sodium reabsorption is related to the secretion of potassium and hydrogen ions, a reaction that is partially controlled by the adrenal mineralocorticoid, aldosterone. The amount of ion exchange depends upon several interrelated factors, including the rate of delivery of tubular fluid and electrolytes to the exchange sites, the levels of circulating aldosterone, the acid-base balance of the body, the serum potassium level, the relative concentrations of potassium and hydrogen ions in the tubular cell, the concentrations of reabsorbable and nonreabsorbable anions in the glomerular filtrate, and the state of the extracellular fluid volume (Cannon, 1977). Sodium is also actively reabsorbed in the papillary collecting duct, and alterations in reabsorption at this site may play an important role in the control of salt excretion (Burg, 1976 A).

Reabsorption of sodium in the water-impermeable segments of the tubules generates a hypotonic tubular fluid which, in the absence of ADH, is excreted as dilute urine. If there is a need to conserve body water, ADH is released from the posterior pituitary in response to increased plasma osmolality and/or volume depletion. Under the influence of this hormone, the collecting ducts become more permeable to water, which diffuses into the hypertonic medulla, enters the capillaries, and is returned to the general circulation. This process results in formation of a concentrated urine. ADH also facilitates the diffusion of urea out of the collecting ducts into the medullary interstitium, which contributes to the hypertonicity of the medulla.

Site and Mechanism of Action of Diuretics: All diuretics interfere with the reabsorption of sodium and/or chloride in the renal tubules but, because they act at different sites, each class has distinctive effects on the pattern of electrolyte excretion, on acid-base balance, and on the concentrating and diluting capacity of the kidney.

Carbonic anhydrase inhibitors (eg, acetazolamide [Diamox]) enhance sodium excretion by reducing reabsorption of sodium bicarbonate in the proximal tubules. Sodium chloride reabsorption also is decreased, but excess chloride (with accompanying sodium) is subsequently reabsorbed in the loop of Henle. Thus, predominantly sodium bicarbonate is excreted and the total diuretic effect is minimal. Potassium excretion is increased during initial therapy due to the increased flow rate and sodium concentration, the elevated pH of the tubular fluid, and possibly the presence of nonreabsorbable anion in the distal tubular fluid (which increases electronegativity of the tubular lumen). Hypokalemia is seldom a major finding, because excess hydrogen ions in the extracellular fluid tend to diffuse into the cells, displacing potassium ions which move into the extracellular compartment. After several days of continuous administration of a carbonic anhydrase inhibitor, a mild hyperchloremic acidosis develops; because of this acid-base disturbance, tolerance to the diuretic action occurs.

The osmotic diuretics (eg, mannitol [Osmitrol], urea) are currently believed to produce diuresis by more than one mechanism. Mannitol, the most widely used osmotic diuretic, is filtered at the glomerulus and not reabsorbed by the renal tubules. Because of its osmotic action in the proximal tubules, mannitol prevents the reabsorption of water and thus impairs sodium reabsorption by lowering the concentration of sodium in the tubular fluid. (Expansion of the extracellular fluid volume may play a role in the effect of urea on proximal sodium reabsorption, but such an action has not been clearly established for mannitol.) The major site of action of mannitol is in the loop of Henle where it reduces medullary hypertonicity, possibly by increasing medullary blood flow. As a result of this action, as well as the presence of a nonreabsorbable solute within the tubule, reabsorption of both water and sodium in

the loop is markedly impaired, and a large excess of sodium and water is delivered to the distal tubule. The excess water is not reabsorbed at the distal sites because of the washout of the medullary gradient, and little sodium is reclaimed because the increased rate of flow of tubular fluid overwhelms the capacity of the transport system (Gennari and Kassirer, 1974).

The loop diuretics, furosemide [Lasix] and ethacrynic acid [Edecrin], block the active transport of chloride in both the medullary and cortical portions of the thick ascending limb of Henle's loop, thereby inhibiting the concomitant passive reabsorption of sodium. By this action, the loop diuretics reduce the osmotic gradient in the renal medulla and impair both the concentrating and diluting capacity of the kidney. The thiazides (including the related agents, chlorthalidone, metolazone, and quinethazone) block the reabsorption of sodium chloride in the cortical diluting portion of the early distal tubules and thus interfere with urinary dilution but do not affect the concentrating mechanism. In large doses, the thiazides and furosemide also have slight, clinically unimportant carbonic anhydrase inhibitory activity in the proximal tubules (Burg, 1976 B; Jacobson and Kokko, 1976). The uricosuric diuretic, ticrynafen [Selacryn], acts primarily in the cortical diluting segment of the distal tubules and does not inhibit carbonic anhydrase. Since all of these agents increase the rate of delivery of tubular fluid and electrolytes to the exchange sites in the late distal tubules and early collecting ducts, they may cause significant kaliuresis and decrease the serum potassium level. In addition, plasma volume contraction increases the production of aldosterone via the renin-angiotensin system (secondary hyperaldosteronism). If sufficient sodium is delivered to the exchange sites during a diuresis, the combination of increased sodium delivery and high aldosterone levels increases the loss of potassium and hydrogen ions. These changes may be associated with development of hypokalemia and mild hypochloremic alkalosis, with or without an effective diuresis.

Mercurial diuretics impede active

chloride transport in the cortical and possibly also the medullary portion of the thick ascending limb of Henle's loop. They also may act at other sites in the nephron, including the exchange sites where, under conditions of potassium loading, they may partially depress sodium-potassium exchange. In the usual clinical situation, however, significant urinary loss of potassium may occur following massive diuresis. Hypokalemic hypochloremic alkalosis may develop during continued administration, and the mercurials lose their effectiveness in the presence of this acid-base disturbance. Responsiveness generally can be restored by allowing a larger interval between injections or by administering a source of chloride ion.

The potassium-sparing diuretics, spironolactone [Aldactone], triamterene [Dyrenium], and amiloride (investigational agent) interfere with sodium reabsorption at the distal exchange sites and thereby promote sodium excretion while conserving potassium. Spironolactone is a competitive antagonist of aldosterone, while triamterene and amiloride interfere directly with electrolyte transport. These agents are not potent diuretics when used alone but, when given with a more proximally acting diuretic, they reduce potassium loss, enhance sodium excretion, and minimize alkalosis.

Major Uses of Diuretics

Congestive Heart Failure: The kidney plays an important role in the pathogenesis of congestive heart failure (Cannon, 1977). By reducing the extracellular fluid volume, diuretics reduce preload and relieve pulmonary congestion and peripheral edema. The traditional approach has been to initiate therapy with digitalis, a low-sodium diet, and restriction of activities, with a diuretic given concomitantly or added later if symptoms are not adequately controlled. In recent years, the concept that digitalis should be given to all patients with congestive heart failure has been questioned, and diuretics are used frequently for initial therapy of patients with mild congestive failure and normal sinus rhythm.

Because they are generally well tolerated and rarely cause excessive diuresis, the thiazides are the diuretics of choice for treating chronic congestive heart failure in patients with normal renal function. Ticrynafen may be substituted for the thiazide in patients with symptomatic hyperuricemia. When the glomerular filtration rate is below 30 ml/min, a loop diuretic is indicated. Because hypokalemia may predispose to or accentuate digitalis intoxication, potassium-sparing diuretics are particularly useful when given in conjunction with a thiazide or loop diuretic to digitalized patients.

When cardiac failure is difficult to control with a diuretic and moderate doses of digitalis, the possibility of sodium abuse should be considered. In many patients, refractory cardiac edema can be controlled with digitalis and a thiazide if sodium intake is restricted to 50 to 70 mEq daily (Whight et al, 1974).

Given parenterally, the loop diuretics have largely replaced the mercurials for treatment of acute pulmonary edema. Furosemide is often used for the initial management of patients with pulmonary congestion following acute myocardial infarction. Because the symptoms of pulmonary congestion are often relieved before urinary output is increased, the initial beneficial effect of furosemide may involve a reduction in venous tone.

Hypertension: Diuretics initially lower blood pressure by reducing the plasma volume; during long-term therapy, peripheral resistance is reduced. A thiazide usually serves as the foundation of the antihypertensive regimen: as sole therapy in patients with mild or moderate hypertension or in combination with other antihypertensive drugs in patients who are not controlled by the diuretic alone. Ticrynafen is useful in patients with symptomatic hyperuricemia. The loop diuretics are reserved for patients with markedly impaired renal function unless an immediate action is required (ie, in hypertensive crisis). A potassium-sparing diuretic may be given with a thiazide or loop diuretic when hypokalemia is a problem. (See Chapter 38, Antihypertensive Agents.)

Nephrotic Syndrome: Dietary sodium restriction is important in managing edema associated with the nephrotic syndrome. Some clinicians initiate diuretic therapy with a thiazide, adding spironolactone if needed to control secondary hyperaldosteronism. Nephrotic edema may be more difficult to control than cardiac edema, however, and a satisfactory diuresis often can be obtained only with a loop diuretic, usually given with spironolactone. Vigorous diuresis should be avoided because patients with the nephrotic syndrome have a reduced effective arterial blood volume.

Chronic Renal Failure: The management of patients with chronic renal failure requires careful attention to salt and water balance because these patients cannot readily adapt to a marked deficiency or excess of dietary sodium. A loop diuretic (usually furosemide) is useful to control both edema and hypertension. Because of the risk of excessive sodium depletion, daily use is not advisable, especially when chronic renal failure is associated with tubulointerstitial diseases or other salt-losing nephropathies.

Acute Oliguric Renal Failure: In oliguric patients, mannitol and/or furosemide have been used diagnostically, prophylactically, and therapeutically. These diuretics are useful in differentiating prerenal azotemia from established acute renal failure. They may reduce the risk of developing acute tubular necrosis when administered prior to or immediately after some types of renal insult (eg, during aortic surgery); however, in patients with hypovolemic or bacteremic shock, furosemide may precipitate rather than prevent acute renal failure by further reducing the effective blood volume. Furosemide has been employed in an effort to convert acute oliguric renal failure to the nonoliguric form of this disease. This therapy may reduce the need for dialysis, but there is as yet no conclusive evidence that the underlying pathologic picture is changed (Minuth et al, 1976).

Cirrhosis with Ascites: If cirrhotic edema and ascites do not respond to sodium restriction and bedrest, diuretics may be indicated, but therapy must be initiated very cautiously to avoid electrolyte disturbances (particularly hypokalemia) which may precipitate hepatic coma. Secondary hyperaldosteronism is common and usually severe in cirrhotics. Some patients have been treated successfully with spironolactone alone, but combined therapy with spironolactone and a thiazide appears to be more effective. In very resistant cases, a loop diuretic may be substituted for the thiazide, but extreme care must be taken to avoid electrolyte imbalance and volume depletion. Diuretic therapy is relatively safe in the presence of peripheral edema, but vigorous treatment of ascites may result in acute volume depletion.

Edema of Pregnancy: In the past, thiazide diuretics were often used routinely during pregnancy to relieve edema and prevent pre-eclampsia. More recently, enthusiasm for diuretic therapy and/or sodium restriction in pregnant women has lessened. It is now apparent that dependent or generalized edema develops in up to 80% of normotensive women during uncomplicated pregnancy. The phenomenon is thus physiologic and well tolerated, and attempts to mobilize edema by use of diuretics could conceivably compromise uteroplacental perfusion. Furthermore, even when diuretics relieve the edema, there is no convincing evidence that they prevent pre-eclampsia (Lindheimer and Katz, 1973).

Once pre-eclampsia is present, the role of diuretics is controversial. Some clinicians believe that, by decreasing the sensitivity of vascular receptors to endogenous pressor substances, diuretics may be beneficial. Others feel that diuretic therapy does not influence the course of the disease and (since intravascular volume is decreased in pre-eclampsia) may further impair uteroplacental perfusion. Consideration also should be given to the risk of adverse effects on the newborn, because electrolyte disturbances and thrombocytopenia have been reported in neonates whose mothers were treated with thiazide diuretics.

Idiopathic Edema: This disorder occurs primarily in women and is often attributed to a capillary leak of albumin. Treatment has included avoidance of precipitating causes (eg, prolonged standing), mild salt restriction, diuretic therapy, periods of recumbency in the afternoon, use of elastic stockings, and administration of sympathomimetic amines. While idiopathic edema is a poorly understood condition, it now appears that in many cases there is a strong psychological overlay producing habituation to the use of diuretics with excessive sodium retention for a number of days after the diuretic is withdrawn. Patients with this disorder are often overly concerned about weight and appearance and have taken diuretics for many years. Successful long-term treatment involves complete abstinence from diuretics with eventual re-establishment of normal sodium and water homeostasis (MacGregor et al, 1979).

Brain Edema: Intravenously administered mannitol and urea and the orally administered osmotic agent, glycerin, may be used to reduce intracranial pressure temporarily in neurosurgical patients. Mannitol is usually preferred for short-term intravenous therapy because it has less tendency than urea to produce a rebound effect. The efficacy of long-term maintenance therapy with glycerin has not been established. Glucocorticoids are the most effective agents for prolonged therapy (see Chapter 41, Adrenal Corticosteroids).

Hypercalcemia and Renal Calculi: Furosemide increases the urinary excretion of calcium and is useful (in conjunction with saline infusion) for the emergency treatment of acute hypercalcemia. Thiazides decrease urinary calcium excretion and may increase serum calcium levels and, therefore, should not be used to treat hypercalcemia. Because of these actions, thiazides are administered to prevent recurrence of calcium-containing renal calculi in some forms of hypercalciuria. (See Chapter 54, Agents Affecting Calcium Metabolism.)

Diabetes Insipidus: The thiazides have a paradoxical antidiuretic action in patients with diabetes insipidus. This syndrome results from deficient production of antidiuretic hormone (central diabetes insipidus) or from a defect in the renal tubules that renders them insensitive to the hormone (nephrogenic diabetes insipidus). The thiazides are useful in both forms. (See Chapter 49, Antidiuretic Agents.)

Glaucoma Therapy and Intraocular Surgery: Carbonic anhydrase inhibitors reduce intraocular pressure by decreasing the production of aqueous humor. They are used for the long-term treatment of patients with primary open-angle glaucoma and other chronic glaucomas that cannot be controlled by topical therapy alone. They also are administered for the short-term management of some self-limited secondary glaucomas and in the preoperative treatment of acute angle-closure and congenital glaucoma. The osmotic agents are used to reduce intraocular pressure and vitreous volume rapidly prior to iridectomy and other ocular surgical procedures. They are also of temporary benefit in some secondary glaucomas. (See Chapter 22, Agents Used to Treat Glaucoma.)

THIAZIDES AND RELATED COMPOUNDS

The prototype thiazide, chlorothiazide, was introduced in 1958 and became widely recognized as a reliable, well-tolerated, orally effective diuretic. A number of derivatives and three similarly acting nonthiazide agents (chlorthalidone, quinethazone, metolazone) were developed subsequently. The major difference among the various agents involves duration of action (see the Table).

Thiazide-type diuretics increase the urinary excretion of sodium chloride and water by inhibiting sodium reabsorption in the early distal tubules (cortical diluting segment). They also increase the urinary excretion of potassium, magnesium, and, to a small extent, bicarbonate ions (the latter effect is due to their slight carbonic anhydrase inhibitory action). During long-term therapy, calcium excretion is reduced.

When renal function is normal, the thiazides are the diuretics of choice for maintenance therapy in ambulatory patients with cardiac edema; they may be given with a potassium-sparing diuretic to reduce potassium loss and enhance the therapeutic response. Such combined therapy also may be effective in patients with nephrotic edema or cirrhotic edema and ascites. In addition, thiazides are sometimes used to control edema associated with premenstrual tension and corticosteroid or estrogen therapy. Thiazide-type diuretics are usually ineffective in patients with impaired renal function (glomerular filtration rate less than 30 ml/min) and may cause further deterioration of renal function. Metolazone may be useful in patients with chronic renal failure if given in large doses, which suggests that its site of action may differ in some respects from that of the other thiazide-type diuretics.

ADVERSE REACTIONS AND PRECAUTIONS.

The thiazides may cause dizziness, weakness, fatigue, and leg cramps. In patients receiving prolonged therapy, serum sodium, potassium, chloride, and bicarbonate levels should be determined periodically. The serum potassium level frequently falls during long-term therapy, and the hypokalemia may be associated with a mild hypochloremic alkalosis. Thiazide-induced hypokalemia is not progressive, is rarely pronounced, and is not associated with a clinically important deficiency of total body potassium; the serum potassium level usually ranges between 3 and 3.5 mEq/L. Since a further decrease may occur during episodes of diarrhea, vomiting, or anorexia, patients receiving these diuretics should be instructed to report any such occurrence promptly. In addition, careful consideration should be given to the effect of sodium abuse on the potassium wasting action of diuretics. The volume contraction induced by thiazides increases sodium reabsorption in the early renal tubules, thereby limiting the amount of sodium reaching the distal sites where sodium reabsorption is linked with potassium secretion. A high sodium intake may increase potassium loss by counteracting this sodium-conserving mechanism. Often, patients with lower serum potassium levels

are excreting more than 150 mEq of sodium in the urine.

Digitalized patients and those with cirrhosis are most at risk from hypokalemia. Even a modest decrease in the serum potassium concentration can precipitate serious arrhythmias during digitalis therapy and, in cirrhotic patients, a low serum potassium level may precipitate hepatic coma. Concurrent administration of a potassium-sparing diuretic or potassium supplements may be indicated in these patients. In the healthy, ambulatory patient with hypertension, mild hypokalemia is generally well tolerated and corrective measures are not indicated unless symptoms develop or the serum potassium falls below 3 mEq/L (Kassirer and Harrington, 1977; Kosman, 1974).

Thiazides increase fasting blood glucose levels and decrease glucose tolerance during long-term therapy. The hyperglycemic effect is sometimes attributed to potassium loss; however, concomitant therapy with triamterene does not prevent it (Amery et al, 1978). The effect on glucose tolerance is not clinically important except in patients with pre-existing or subclinical diabetes, who may require an adjustment in dosage of hypoglycemic drugs. In the rare instances in which hyperglycemia is difficult to control, it may be advisable to discontinue the thiazide and substitute a diuretic less likely to cause carbohydrate intolerance (Gifford, 1976). Ethacrynic acid appears to be the best choice. Although the potassium-sparing diuretics are unlikely to decrease glucose tolerance, these agents may cause severe hyperkalemia in diabetics and should be avoided in these patients, particularly when there is associated renal insufficiency.

A reversible elevation of the blood urea nitrogen level may occur during thiazide therapy. This prerenal azotemia is caused by a decrease in renal blood flow and glomerular filtration rate secondary to the reduction of blood volume induced by the diuretic. The thiazides also may directly depress renal blood flow.

Thiazides tend to produce an asymptomatic hyperuricemia, which may be caused by decreased secretion of uric acid

THIAZIDES AND RELATED DIURETICS

Drug	Chemical Structure
THIAZIDES Chlorothiazide	
Chlorothiazide Sodium	
Hydrochlorothiazide	
Bendroflumethiazide	
Benzthiazide	
Cyclothiazide	
Hydroflumethiazide	

*See Chapter 38 for antihypertensive doses.

THIAZIDES AND RELATED DIURETICS

Usual Diuretic Dosage*	Duration of Action (hours)	Preparations

Oral: Adults, 500 mg to 1 g once or twice daily; *children*, 22 mg/kg daily in 2 divided doses; *infants under 6 months*, up to 33 mg/kg daily in 2 divided doses.	6 to 12	*Generic:*
		    Tablets 250 and 500 mg
		Diuril (Merck Sharp & Dohme):
		    Tablets 250 and 500 mg
		    Suspension 250 mg/5 ml

Intravenous: Adults, 500 mg twice daily.	6 to 12	*Diuril Sodium* (Merck Sharp & Dohme): Powder (injection) equivalent to 500 mg chlorothiazide

Oral: Adults, initially, 25 to 200 mg once or twice daily for several days; for maintenance, 25 to 100 mg daily or intermittently. *Children*, 2 mg/kg daily in 2 doses; *infants under 6 months*, up to 3 mg/kg daily in 2 doses.	6 to 12	*Oretic* (Abbott):
		    Tablets 25 and 50 mg
		Generic, Esidrix (Ciba),
		HydroDIURIL (Merck Sharp & Dohme):
		    Tablets 25, 50 and 100 mg

Oral: Adults, initially, 5 mg daily, preferably in the morning; dose may be increased to 20 mg as a single dose or in 2 divided doses. For maintenance, 2.5 to 15 mg once daily or intermittently. *Children*, initially, up to 0.4 mg/kg daily in 2 divided doses. For maintenance, 0.05 to 0.1 mg/kg daily in a single dose.	More than 18	*Naturetin* (Squibb): Tablets 2.5, 5 and 10 mg

Oral: Adults, initially, 50 to 200 mg daily for several days, depending upon patient's response. For maintenance, dosage is reduced gradually to minimum effective amount. *Children*, initially, 1 to 4 mg/kg daily divided into 3 doses, For maintenance, dose is reduced as needed.	12 to 18	*Aquatag* (Tutag):
		    Tablets 25 and 50 mg
		Generic, Exna (Robins):
		    Tablets 50 mg

Oral: Adults, initially, 1 to 2 mg daily, preferably in the morning; for maintenance, 1 mg on alternate days or 2 or 3 times weekly. *Children*, initially, 0.02 to 0.04 mg/kg daily; for maintenance, dose is reduced as needed.	18 to 24	*Anhydron* (Lilly): Tablets 2 mg
Oral: Adults, initially, 50 to 100 ml daily; for maintenance, 25 to 200 mg in divided amounts, depending upon response. *Children*, initially, 1 mg/kg daily; for maintenance, dose is adjusted as needed.	18 to 24	*Diucardin* (Ayerst), *Saluron* (Bristol): Tablets 50 mg

THIAZIDES AND RELATED DIURETICS

Drug	Chemical Structure
Methyclothiazide	
Polythiazide	
Trichlormethiazide	
RELATED COMPOUNDS Chlorthalidone	
Quinethazone	
Metolazone	

by the tubular cells into the lumen of the tubule or increased renal tubular reabsorption of uric acid. Asymptomatic hyperuricemia does not appear to produce any long-term deleterious effects and need not be treated. The development of acute gouty arthritis is rare, except in patients with chronic renal failure or a hereditary predisposition to gout. Patients with a history of gout have traditionally been man-

THIAZIDES AND RELATED DIURETICS

Usual Diuretic Dosage*	Duration of Action (hours)	Preparations
Oral: Adults, initially, 2.5 to 10 mg once daily; same dose range is used for maintenance. *Children*, 0.05 to 0.2 mg/kg daily.	More than 24	*Aquatensen* (Mallinckrodt): Tablets 5 mg *Enduron* (Abbott): Tablets 2.5 and 5 mg
Oral: Adults, initially, 1 to 4 mg daily, depending upon response and severity of the condition; for maintenance, 0.5 to 8 mg daily adjusted for optimal response. *Children*, initially, 0.02 to 0.08 mg/kg daily; for maintenance, dose is adjusted according to response.	24 to 48	*Renese* (Pfizer): Tablets 1, 2 and 4 mg
Oral: Adults, initially, 2 to 4 mg after breakfast daily or twice daily if needed; for maintenance, 1 to 2 mg once daily. *Children*, 0.07 mg/kg daily in single or divided doses.	Up to 24	*Generic, Metahydrin* (Merrell-National), *Naqua* (Schering): Tablets 2 and 4 mg
Oral: Adults, initially, 50 to 100 mg after breakfast daily or 100 mg on alternate days or 3 times weekly; some patients may require 200 mg. Maintenance doses should be adjusted individually. *Children*, 2 mg/kg 3 times weekly; maintenance dose should be adjusted individually.	24 to 72	*Hygroton* (USV): Tablets 25, 50 and 100 mg
Oral: Adults, 50 to 100 mg daily, depending upon response and severity of the condition. Some patients may require as much as 150 or 200 mg on alternate days or 3 times weekly.	18 to 24	*Hydromox* (Lederle): Tablets 50 mg
Oral: Adults, 5 to 20 mg daily, depending upon response and severity of the condition. Doses as large as 150 mg daily may be required in patients with chronic renal failure.	12 to 24	*Diulo* (Searle), *Zaroxolyn* (Pennwalt): Tablets 2.5, 5 and 10 mg

aged by continuing the thiazide and administering colchicine with uricosuric agents (probenecid, sulfinpyrazone) or allopurinol. Treatment now has been simplified by the introduction of the uricosuric diuretic, ticrynafen, which may be substituted for the thiazide in gouty patients. Asymptomatic hyperuricemia is not an indication to substitute ticrynafen for a thiazide.

Elevated serum lipid levels have been noted in some patients during therapy with thiazide-type diuretics (Ames and Hill, 1976). The effect on serum cholesterol has been neither consistent nor pronounced, and the possibility of a hemoconcentration effect has not been completely ruled out. An elevation of serum triglyceride levels has been reported more frequently, with a few patients showing increases of 50% or more over control levels. Predisposing or associated factors have not been clearly defined, but obesity, glucose intolerance, and hyperuricemia have been mentioned. Since the increase in serum lipids appears to occur most commonly in patients with lower baseline levels, the clinical implications are unclear, and the data are conflicting regarding the effect of a lipid-lowering diet. There is no definitive information on what diuretic could be substituted for a thiazide in patients with markedly elevated lipid levels.

Since the thiazides block sodium reabsorption in the diluting segment of the nephron, hyponatremia may occur if water intake is excessive. This complication is usually encountered in markedly edematous patients with severe congestive heart failure, cirrhosis, or the nephrotic syndrome who are refractory to diuretics. The hyponatremia results from the combined effects of a disorder of water excretion and excessive intake of sodium-free solutions. Correction depends upon improving the circulatory status, restricting fluid intake, and temporarily liberalizing salt intake.

Hypercalcemia is a rare complication of thiazide therapy. It is usually associated with latent primary hyperparathyroidism and generally persists when the thiazide is discontinued. Hyperparathyroid surgery will reduce the serum calcium level and may normalize the blood pressure. Thiazides also may induce hypercalcemia (which is usually transient) in hypoparathyroid patients receiving vitamin D, particularly when renal function is impaired.

Blood dyscrasias (leukopenia, aplastic anemia, thrombocytopenic purpura, hemolytic anemia, and agranulocytosis), hypersensitivity reactions (eg, pneumonitis, rash, photosensitivity), and pancreatitis have been reported infrequently in patients receiving thiazides. Necrotizing vasculitis of the skin and kidney has occurred in elderly patients, but its relationship to thiazide therapy is still unproved. Muscle cramps, syncope, and epileptiform movements have been associated with administration of metolazone.

Serious problems can develop if patients on long-term thiazide therapy are treated with lithium. Lithium is eliminated from the body largely by renal excretion. The lithium ion is handled like the sodium ion in the proximal tubules, but not at most other sites in the nephron. Prolonged thiazide therapy contracts the plasma volume and this action increases sodium reabsorption in the proximal tubules. Since the transport systems in the proximal tubules do not distinguish between the lithium and sodium ions, lithium clearance is reduced and the serum lithium concentration may rise to toxic levels. If thiazides are used in patients treated with lithium, the serum lithium level should be monitored closely.

Thiazides displace bilirubin from albumin and should be used cautiously in jaundiced infants. These agents may augment the neuromuscular blocking action of tubocurarine in surgical patients.

Since small bowel lesions consisting of stenosis with or without ulceration have occurred in patients who received potassium chloride in enteric-coated form, these products (which are sometimes available in combination with a thiazide) should not be used.

ROUTES, USUAL DOSAGE, AND PREPARATIONS. See the Table.

LOOP DIURETICS

The loop diuretics, furosemide and ethacrynic acid, are chemically distinct but they have similar pharmacologic actions. Both drugs block active chloride transport in the thick ascending limb of Henle's loop and thereby interfere with the passive reabsorption of sodium. The loop diuretics have a much greater diuretic effect than the thiazides. Unlike the mercurials, they remain effective even in the presence of electrolyte and acid-base disturbances, and their proper use requires an understanding of the electrolyte and fluid derangements that they may induce. These potent agents are usually reserved for patients refractory to thiazide therapy unless an immediate action is required to control fluid overload or the glomerular filtration rate is markedly reduced.

Despite the similar actions of the loop diuretics, there are some essential differences between them. Furosemide is usually preferred because (1) it has a broader dose-response curve; (2) it is less ototoxic; (3) it causes fewer gastrointestinal side effects; (4) it is more convenient for intravenous use; and (5) it may be less likely to cause alkalosis.

FUROSEMIDE
[Lasix]

Furosemide is a potent, short-acting sulfonamide diuretic that is chemically similar to the thiazides. When administered orally, onset of action occurs within one hour and the diuretic effect lasts about six hours; with parenteral administration, the diuretic effect is immediate and persists for about two hours. Furosemide has a very wide dose-response curve, and dosage can be adjusted to produce a graded response. In addition to sodium and chloride, furosemide increases the renal excretion of potassium, magnesium, calcium, and, to a lesser extent, bicarbonate ions.

When administered orally, furosemide is usually effective in patients with cardiac edema who do not respond to the thiazides. It is of particular value in the treatment of edema associated with impaired renal function because it is effective even when

the glomerular filtration rate is greatly reduced. Although some patients with the nephrotic syndrome may respond to less potent diuretics, edema and hypertension in patients with chronic renal failure often can be controlled only with the loop diuretics, and large doses may be required. Furosemide is effective but should be administered very cautiously in the management of resistant cirrhotic edema and ascites; intensive diuretic therapy may not be desirable in these patients, especially if plasma volume is borderline.

Patients with pulmonary edema respond rapidly to intravenous administration of furosemide. This drug is often preferred for the initial management of patients with pulmonary congestion following acute myocardial infarction. Since relief of symptoms may precede the diuretic action, a vascular effect (ie, reduction in venous tone) has been postulated. In patients with pulmonary edema and low blood pressure secondary to acute myocardial infarction, excessive diuresis should be avoided because of the danger of precipitating shock.

In oliguric patients, furosemide (often in conjunction with mannitol) is most useful as a diagnostic test for acute renal failure. It also may prevent the development of acute tubular necrosis. In patients with established acute tubular necrosis, furosemide may possibly reduce the need for dialysis, but a favorable effect on the mortality rate has not been reported.

Because of its extreme potency, therapy with furosemide must be instituted cautiously and dosage should be individualized to avoid excessive diuresis. Overzealous therapy can cause dehydration, hypotension, and marked hypokalemia and hypochloremic alkalosis; therefore, it is advisable to begin therapy with small doses and to increase the dosage gradually if larger amounts are required. During rapid mobilization of edema, serum electrolytes should be monitored closely and prophylactic measures may be indicated to prevent severe hypokalemia.

In patients receiving long-term therapy, serum electrolyte levels should be determined periodically. A potassium-sparing diuretic or potassium supplements may be indicated in digitalized or cirrhotic patients. In addition, all patients receiving furosemide should be instructed to report promptly any events that might cause a further fall in the serum potassium level (diarrhea, vomiting, anorexia). Like the thiazides, furosemide may cause azotemia, hyperuricemia, and hyperglycemia. Dermatologic reactions (urticaria, erythema multiforme, phototoxic blisters), hematologic disturbances (agranulocytosis, anemia, thrombocytopenia), allergic interstitial nephritis, and acute pancreatitis have been reported rarely. Transient deafness has occurred following rapid intravenous administration of large doses of furosemide to azotemic or uremic patients. Permanent deafness has been observed rarely. Additive ototoxic effects might be expected with concomitant administration of aminoglycoside antibiotics, since this interaction has occurred with ethacrynic acid.

It has been reported that patients receiving long-term anticonvulsant therapy may show a diminished natriuretic response to oral furosemide. This interaction has been attributed to decreased intestinal absorption of the diuretic. Although there are no reports of elevated lithium levels during furosemide therapy, such an interaction might be expected.

ROUTES, USUAL DOSAGE, AND PREPARATIONS. *Oral*: For edema, *adults*, initially, 20 to 80 mg as a single dose, preferably in the morning. If an adequate diuretic response is not achieved, the dosage may be increased gradually at intervals of six to eight hours. The effective maintenance dose varies widely and no definite upper limit has been established. The frequency of administration also must be determined individually. One or two large doses achieve higher blood levels and appear to be more effective than small doses administered frequently, especially in patients with renal insufficiency. Furosemide may be administered daily, on alternate days, or for two to four consecutive days per week. In some patients, intermittent therapy may be the most efficient method of mobilizing refractory edema. *Children*, initially, 1 to 2 mg/kg of body weight once

or twice daily. If an adequate response is not obtained, the dosage may be increased gradually in increments of 1 mg/kg/dose. Some children with the nephrotic syndrome may require doses as large as 5 mg/kg.

> *Lasix* (Hoechst-Roussel). Solution (oral) 10 mg/ml; tablets 20, 40, and 80 mg.
> Drug available generically, but these products should be avoided because of questionable bioavailability.

Intravenous: For acute pulmonary edema, the usual initial dose is 40 mg, which may be repeated in 60 to 90 minutes. *Children*, initially, 1 mg/kg of body weight. This dose may be repeated at six-hour intervals if needed. (Furosemide also may be administered intramuscularly, but the intravenous route is usually preferred.) For acute renal failure, *adults*, initially, 40 to 80 mg. The amount may then be increased but the total dose should rarely exceed 500 mg in a 24-hour period. It is important to ascertain that the plasma volume is adequate before furosemide is administered as a diagnostic test. In prerenal azotemia, even large doses may not produce a diuresis without volume replacement. Furosemide should be discontinued if oliguria persists for more than 24 hours after adequate dosage. Careful attention should be directed toward maintenance of adequate hydration in the event of successful diuresis. In the absence of edema or cardiopulmonary overload, total losses should be replaced every two to four hours to maintain adequate plasma volume and renal perfusion.

> *Lasix* (Hoechst-Roussel). Solution 10 mg/ml in 2 and 10 ml containers.

ETHACRYNIC ACID
[Edecrin]

ETHACRYNATE SODIUM
[Sodium Edecrin]

Ethacrynic acid is a potent, short-acting diuretic with an onset and duration of action similar to furosemide. The two drugs have the same therapeutic applications, but furosemide is usually preferred.

The electrolyte and fluid derangements induced by ethacrynic acid are identical to those caused by furosemide, and the same precautions should be observed. Ethacrynic acid also may cause azotemia and hyperuricemia. Hyperglycemia occurs rarely, if at all (Gifford, 1976). Transient deafness has been reported following rapid intravenous administration of large doses of ethacrynic acid, most commonly in azotemic or uremic patients. Permanent deafness has occurred rarely but much more commonly than with furosemide. In patients with normal renal function, additive ototoxic effects developed when small doses of ethacrynic acid were administered with aminoglycoside antibiotics. Elevated lithium levels have not been reported when ethacrynic acid and lithium were used concomitantly, but the possibility of this interaction should be kept in mind. When given orally, ethacrynic acid may cause gastrointestinal disturbances, and gastrointestinal bleeding has been associated with intravenous therapy. Dermatologic reactions, abnormal results of liver function tests, agranulocytosis, and thrombocytopenia have been reported rarely.

Routes, Usual Dosage, and Preparations. *Oral*: For edema, *adults*, initially, 50 to 100 mg daily. If an adequate response is not obtained, the daily dosage may be increased, usually in increments of 25 or 50 mg. For maintenance, the dose and frequency of administration must be determined individually. Patients with refractory edema may require 400 mg daily (usually in two divided doses); in such patients, intermittent therapy may be the most efficient method of mobilizing edema fluid. *Children*, initially, 25 mg daily. Dosage may be increased gradually by increments of 25 mg.

ETHACRYNIC ACID:
Edecrin (Merck Sharp & Dohme). Tablets 25 and 50 mg.

Intravenous: For acute pulmonary edema, *adults*, initially, 50 mg or 0.5 to 1 mg/kg of body weight injected slowly; *children*, initially, 1 mg/kg. These doses may be increased if necessary.

ETHACRYNATE SODIUM:
Sodium Edecrin (Merck Sharp & Dohme). Powder equivalent to 50 mg ethacrynic acid.

POTASSIUM-SPARING DIURETICS

The potassium-sparing diuretics, spironolactone, triamterene, and amiloride (investigational drug), interfere with sodium reabsorption at the distal exchange sites in the renal tubules and thereby promote sodium excretion while conserving potassium. Since only a small fraction of filtered sodium is normally reabsorbed at the distal exchange sites, the potassium-sparing agents are not potent diuretics when used alone. Their major use is in conjunction with the thiazides or loop diuretics. Such combined therapy not only reduces potassium excretion and minimizes alkalosis, but also is often effective in mobilizing refractory edema. Since hypokalemia predisposes to digitalis toxicity, combined therapy is particularly useful in digitalized patients. There is also some evidence from animal studies that the potassium-sparing diuretics may reduce digitalis toxicity by mechanisms that are independent of their effect on potassium excretion (eg, direct cardiac action, enhanced glycoside metabolism).

The potassium-sparing diuretics are better tolerated than potassium supplements and are more reliable in raising the serum potassium level during diuretic therapy. Because they block the renal regulatory mechanisms that control potassium excretion, these agents are often effective in patients who do not respond to potassium supplements. Also for this reason, their dosage may be more difficult to manipulate in accordance with changes in the serum potassium level, and they are more prone to cause hyperkalemia, particularly when renal function is impaired or potassium intake is excessive. Because renal function decreases with age, these drugs should be used cautiously in elderly patients. Many diabetics with mild to moderate renal insufficiency have a deficiency in the renin-angiotensin-aldosterone axis. This defect, in addition to insulin deficiency, makes these patients particularly prone to life-threatening hyperkalemia. For this reason, these diuretics should be avoided in diabetics.

SPIRONOLACTONE
[Aldactone]

SPIRONOLACTONE AND HYDROCHLOROTHIAZIDE
[Aldactazide]

Spironolactone is used in the management of edema associated with chronic congestive heart failure, cirrhosis, and the nephrotic syndrome. It is sometimes used as the sole diuretic agent (particularly in cirrhosis with ascites), but is most effective when given with a thiazide or loop diuretic. Spironolactone is more effective than triamterene. At one time, spironolactone was regarded as a specific diagnostic or therapeutic agent for primary hyperaldosteronism, but it has since been found that the effect of the drug in this disorder is a nonspecific response to volume depletion.

Careful monitoring of the serum potassium level is necessary during therapy with spironolactone because hyperkalemia may occur even when a potassium-wasting diuretic is given concomitantly. Precipitating factors are a high intake of potassium (supplements, salt substitutes, or dietary) and/or impaired renal function. Spironolactone should be used very cautiously, if at all, in patients with a reduced glomerular filtration rate and only if the serum potassium level is monitored closely. The concurrent use of potassium-sparing diuretics and potassium supplements can be hazardous.

Hyponatremia may occur following excessive ingestion of water in patients receiving spironolactone. Doses exceeding 50 mg daily often cause gynecomastia in men, which may be related to binding of canrenone (an active metabolite of spironolactone) to tissue androgen receptors. Decreased libido and impotence also have been reported. Menstrual disturbances may occur in women. Breast cancer has developed in some patients during or after spironolactone therapy, but a cause-and-effect relationship has not been established. Gastrointestinal disturbances occur occasionally and gastric ulceration rarely. Rashes also have been reported. Aspirin has been reported to block the diuretic effect of spironolactone, but this interaction has not occurred consistently and requires confirmation. The possibility of an interaction with lithium should be considered.

ROUTE, USUAL DOSAGE, AND PREPARATIONS.
SPIRONOLACTONE:
Oral: *Adults*, 50 to 100 mg daily, usually given with a thiazide or loop diuretic; *children*, 3.3 mg/kg of body weight daily in divided doses. The onset of action of spironolactone is relatively slow and maximal effects usually do not occur until the third day of therapy. When discontinued, effects diminish gradually over a period of two or three days. Food increases the bioavailability of the active spironolactone metabolite, canrenone.

Aldactone (Searle). Tablets 25 mg.
SPIRONOLACTONE AND
HYDROCHLOROTHIAZIDE:
Oral: *Adults*, one tablet one to four times daily.

Aldactazide (Searle). Each tablet contains spironolactone 25 mg and hydrochlorothiazide 25 mg.

TRIAMTERENE
[Dyrenium]

TRIAMTERENE AND HYDROCHLOROTHIAZIDE
[Dyazide]

Triamterene is used with a thiazide or loop diuretic in the management of edema associated with congestive heart failure, cirrhosis, or the nephrotic syndrome. It has a more rapid onset of action than spironolactone but is less effective.

Like spironolactone, triamterene can cause hyperkalemia and the same precautions should be observed (see the evaluation on Spironolactone). Triamterene may increase blood urea nitrogen and serum uric acid levels. Gastrointestinal disturbances and rashes occur occasionally. Megaloblastic anemia has been reported in cirrhotic patients during therapy with triamterene, but a cause-and-effect relationship has not been definitely established. Triamterene should not be given with ticrynafen because combined therapy may cause marked elevations in serum creatinine and BUN levels. The possibility of an interaction with lithium should be considered.

ROUTE, USUAL DOSAGE, AND PREPARATIONS.
TRIAMTERENE:
Oral: Adults, 100 to 300 mg daily in divided doses, usually given with a thiazide or loop diuretic; *children*, 2 to 4 mg/kg of body weight daily in divided doses.
   Dyrenium (Smith Kline & French). Capsules 50 and 100 mg.
TRIAMTERENE AND HYDROCHLOROTHIAZIDE:
Oral: Adults, one capsule one to four times daily.
   Dyazide (Smith Kline & French). Each capsule contains triamterene 50 mg and hydrochlorothiazide 25 mg.

URICOSURIC DIURETIC

TICRYNAFEN
[Selacryn]

Although it is structurally related to ethacrynic acid, ticrynafen appears to act at a different site in the nephron. Like the thiazides, ticrynafen interferes with dilution of the urine but has little effect on the concentrating mechanism, which suggests that it blocks sodium chloride reabsorption in the cortical diluting segment of the distal tubules (Stote et al, 1976). Its site and/or mechanism of action must differ in some respects from that of the thiazides, however, because it enhances the natriuretic response to maximally effective doses of hydrochlorothiazide in laboratory animals. Ticrynafen also increases the urinary excretion of potassium and magnesium, but it does not affect bicarbonate reabsorption in the proximal tubules. Calcium excretion may be reduced during long-term therapy.

Ticrynafen is unique among currently available oral diuretics in that it reduces serum uric acid levels by inhibiting urate reabsorption at both pre- and postsecretory sites in the proximal tubules. The hypouricemic and uricosuric response occurs both in individuals with hyperuricemia and in those with normal serum uric acid levels. Additive natriuretic effects can be obtained when ticrynafen is given with a thiazide or furosemide without a loss of hypouricemic action.

Ticrynafen is used as a diuretic and antihypertensive agent (see Chapter 38). It also has been employed to reduce elevated serum urate levels in normotensive, nonedematous patients (see Chapter 8, Drugs Used in Gout); however, many experts believe that, since effective nondiuretic agents are available, a uricosuric diuretic is not indicated in these patients.

Ticrynafen (usually in doses of 250 to 500 mg daily) has been effective as sole therapy to relieve the signs and symptoms of chronic congestive heart failure in patients with mild cardiac edema or it has been combined with digitalis, antiarrhythmic, and nondiuretic antihypertensive drugs when indicated. Because of its uricosuric effect, this diuretic is useful in patients with chronic congestive heart failure who have a history of gout and require a diuretic similar to the thiazides in potency. However, hydrochlorothiazide (50 to 100 mg daily) produces a more substantial increase in sodium excretion than ticrynafen (250 to 500 mg daily), at least during the first week of therapy (Smith and Clements, 1979). Ticrynafen is also less effective initially than either a thiazide or spironolactone in enhancing the 24-hour sodium excretion of hypertensive patients but, after a month of therapy, sodium output is similar with all three drugs.

Ticrynafen may cause gastrointestinal disturbances, dizziness, fatigue, and leg cramps. In patients with normal renal function, ticrynafen may produce reversible elevations in BUN and serum creatinine levels which may be slightly greater than the increases produced by the thiazides. It should not be used in patients with impaired renal function or hepatic cirrhosis because it is not consistently effective in these patients and may precipitate azotemia. Since ticrynafen increases urinary potassium excretion, it may cause hypokalemia, sometimes associated with a mild hypochloremic alkalosis. The reduction in the serum potassium level is comparable to that induced by the thiazides and the same precautions apply (see the discussion on the Thiazides). If corrective measures are indicated, potassium supplements are preferred because marked elevations in BUN and serum creatinine levels have occurred when triamterene was given concurrently. Experience with the combined use of ticrynafen and spironolactone is limited but, until further information is available, this combination should also be avoided. Hyperglycemia and glucose intolerance appear to develop as frequently with ticrynafen as with the thiazides. Effects on serum triglycerides are unclear.

Like other uricosuric agents, ticrynafen may precipitate acute attacks of gout in susceptible patients, particularly during the early months of therapy. For this reason, it is advisable to prescribe prophylactic doses of colchicine if a gouty episode has occurred. The diuretic effect of ticrynafen reduces the risk of urinary tract obstruction during the first few days of therapy when excess uric acid is excreted; the risk can can be further reduced if fluid intake is increased for three days before and three days after initiating therapy. It also may be desirable to alkalize the urine during this period. When ticrynafen is substituted for another diuretic, the latter should be discontinued for one to two days before starting ticrynafen, if feasible.

Abnormal results of liver function tests (elevated SGOT and SGPT levels) and jaundice have been reported rarely in patients receiving ticrynafen, but a cause-and-effect relationship has not been established. Pruritus, rash, and urticaria also have occurred in a few patients.

Ticrynafen potentiates the effect of oral anticoagulants; the anticoagulant dosage should be reduced one-quarter or one-half in patients receiving both drugs, and prothrombin times should be monitored closely. Because the excretion of penicillin is reduced by ticrynafen, it may be necessary to adjust the dose of penicillin during concomitant therapy. Salicylates inhibit the uricosuric effect of many uricosuric agents, including ticrynafen. The possiblity of an interaction with lithium should be considered.

ADDENDUM: There have been several recent reports of acute renal failure in patients receiving ticrynafen (Selacryn [Smith Kline & French]). Several deaths from hepatic toxicity have also been reported, and the drug was voluntarily removed from the market in January, 1980.

MERCURIAL COMPOUNDS

Mercurial diuretics block active chloride transport in the thick ascending limb of Henle's loop. Until the advent of the thiazides and loop diuretics, these agents were the mainstay of diuretic therapy. The oral mercurials are no longer marketed, and the parenterally administered compounds have largely been replaced by the more convenient and less toxic loop diuretics.

MERCAPTOMERIN SODIUM
[Thiomerin]

MERETHOXYLLINE PROCAINE
[Dicurin Procaine]

These agents can be given intramuscularly or subcutaneously to produce a prompt diuresis (within one to two hours) in patients with edema caused by congestive heart failure, renal disease, or cirrhosis with ascites. With continuous administration, the patient may become refractory to the diuretic action because of the development of hypokalemic hypochloremic alkalosis. Responsiveness generally can be restored by lengthening the intervals between injections or by administering chloride ion in the form of ammonium chloride (1 to 2 g four times daily concurrently) or *L*-lysine monohydrochloride (10 g four times daily for two to four days prior to the mercurial diuretic). Ammonium chloride should be avoided in patients with liver disease.

The intravenous route should be avoided because rapid intravenous administration of mercurial diuretics may cause ventricular fibrillation. Renal failure and hemorrhagic colitis have occurred following prolonged use in patients with impaired renal function.

In sensitive patients, mercurial compounds can cause gastrointestinal disturbances, vertigo, fever, pruritus, and rash; therefore, small amounts should be given to determine sensitivity before full therapeutic doses are administered. Therapy should be discontinued if severe gastric disturbances, vertigo, fever, cutaneous reactions, or electrolyte imbalances develop.

ROUTES, USUAL DOSAGE, AND PREPARATIONS.
MERCAPTOMERIN SODIUM:

Intramuscular, Subcutaneous: *Adults*, initially no more than 0.5 ml (to determine sensitivity), then 0.2 to 2 ml daily.

   Thiomerin (Wyeth). Solution 125 mg (equivalent to 40 mg of mercury)/ml with edetate disodium 0.1 mg in 2 and 10 ml containers.

MERETHOXYLLINE PROCAINE:

Intramuscular, Subcutaneous: *Adults*, initially no more than 0.5 ml (to determine sensitivity), then 1 to 2 ml daily.

Dicurin Procaine (Lilly). Each milliliter of solution contains merethoxylline procaine 100 mg (equivalent to mercury 39.3 mg and procaine base 45 mg) and theophylline anhydrous 50 mg in 10 ml containers.

OSMOTIC DIURETICS

Mannitol, urea, and glycerin produce a rapid diuresis by inhibiting sodium and water reabsorption in the proximal tubules and in Henle's loop. With the exception of mannitol, the osmotic agents are not useful as diuretics. Their main clinical application is to reduce intraocular pressure and vitreous volume prior to iridectomy and other ocular surgical procedures. They also are used to reduce intracranial pressure pre- and postoperatively in neurosurgical patients. Early reports that urea was useful in terminating or preventing sickle cell crises have not been substantiated by subsequent studies.

Mannitol is usually preferred to urea for intravenous therapy because it is more convenient to use, less irritating, less likely to cause thrombophlebitis, does not cause tissue necrosis following extravasation, and is safer in patients with renal failure. It is also less likely than urea to cause a rebound increase in intracranial pressure in patients with brain edema because it remains in the extracellular fluid compartment where it exerts its osmotic effect.

MANNITOL
[Osmitrol]

$$
\begin{array}{c}
CH_2OH \\
|\\
HOCH \\
|\\
HOCH \\
|\\
HCOH \\
|\\
HCOH \\
|\\
CH_2OH
\end{array}
$$

This osmotic diuretic is administered intravenously, usually with furosemide, to evaluate the oliguric patient and possibly to prevent the development of renal failure following an insult to the kidney. It also is used to reduce intraocular pressure and vitreous volume prior to ocular surgery, to reduce intracranial pressure temporarily in patients with brain edema, and to promote urinary excretion of toxic substances.

Headache, nausea, vomiting, chills, dizziness, polydipsia, lethargy, confusion, and sensations of constriction or pain in the chest have been observed following infusion of mannitol. Fatalities have occurred after large doses. Too rapid administration of large amounts will draw intracellular water into the extracellular space, causing cellular dehydration and overexpansion of the intravascular space with congestive heart failure and pulmonary edema. Hyponatremia is a common problem. Mannitol may increase cerebral blood flow and thus the risk of postoperative bleeding in neurosurgical patients.

ROUTE, USUAL DOSAGE, AND PREPARATIONS. Hypertonic solutions of mannitol should not be added to whole blood for transfusion because increased osmotic pressure will cause crenation and agglutination of red blood cells.

Intravenous: To promote diuresis in oliguric patients, *adults*, 300 to 400 mg/kg of body weight of a 20% or 25% solution may be given as a single dose (often in conjunction with furosemide). *Children*, 750 mg/kg. Doses should not be repeated in patients with persistent oliguria, as this can cause a hyperosmolar state and precipitate congestive heart failure and pulmonary edema due to volume overload.

To reduce intracranial pressure, *adults and children*, 1.5 to 2 g/kg of body weight of a 15%, 20%, or 25% solution infused over a period of 30 to 60 minutes.

To promote urinary excretion of toxic substances, *adults*, a 5% to 25% solution may be infused as long as indicated if the urinary output remains high. The concentration will depend upon the fluid requirement and urinary output. Water and electrolytes should be given intravenously to replace the loss of these substances in urine, sweat, and expired air. If benefits are not observed after 200 g have been infused, the drug should be discontinued. *Children*,

2 g/kg of body weight of a 5% to 10% solution.

Mannitol should not be confused with mannitol hexanitrate, an antianginal drug.

Osmitrol (Travenol). Solution (aqueous) 5% in 1,000 ml containers, 10% in 500 and 1,000 ml containers, 15% in 150 and 500 ml containers, and 20% in 250 and 500 ml containers; 5% (in 0.3% sodium chloride injection) in 1,000 ml containers, and 20% (in 0.45% sodium chloride injection) in 500 ml containers.

Mannitol I.V. (Abbott). Solution 5% and 10% in 1,000 ml containers and 15% and 20% in 500 ml containers.

Mannitol (Cutter). Solution 5% and 10% (in 0.45% sodium chloride injection) in 1,000 ml containers, 15% (in 0.45% sodium chloride injection) in 500 ml containers, 10% in 1,000 ml containers, and 15% and 20% in 500 ml containers.

Mannitol (Merck Sharp & Dohme). Solution 25% in 50 ml containers.

Selected References

Amery A, et al: Glucose intolerance during diuretic therapy. *Lancet* 1:681-683, 1978.

Ames RP, Hill P: Elevation of serum lipids during diuretic therapy of hypertension. *Am J Med* 61:748-757, 1976.

Burg MB: Renal handling of sodium chloride, in Brenner BM, Rector FC Jr (eds): *The Kidney*. Philadelphia, WB Saunders Co, 1976 A, vol 1, 272-298.

Burg MB: Mechanisms of action of diuretic drugs, in Brenner BM, Rector FC Jr (eds): *The Kidney*. Philadelphia, WB Saunders Co, 1976 B, vol 1, 737-762.

Cannon PJ: The kidney in heart failure. *N Engl J Med* 296:26-32, 1977.

DuBose TD, Kokko JP: Renal chloride transport and control of extracellular fluid volume. *Cardiovasc Med* 2:967-981, 1977.

Gennari FJ, Kassirer JP: Osmotic diuresis. *N Engl J Med* 291:714-720, 1974.

Gifford RW Jr: Guide to practical use of diuretics. *JAMA* 235:1890-1893, 1976.

Jacobson HR, Kokko JP: Diuretics: Sites and mechanisms of action. *Annu Rev Pharmacol Toxicol* 16:201-214, 1976.

Kassirer JP, Harrington JT: Diuretics and potassium metabolism: Reassessment of need, effectiveness, and safety of potassium therapy. *Kidney Int* 11:505-515, 1977.

Kleit SA, et al: Diuretic therapy: Current status. *Am Heart J* 79:700-712, 1970.

Knox FG: Role of proximal tubule in regulation of urinary sodium excretion. *Mayo Clin Proc* 48:565-573, 1973.

Kosman ME: Management of potassium problems during long-term diuretic therapy. *JAMA* 230:743-748, 1974.

Lindheimer MD, Katz AI: Sodium and diuretics in pregnancy. *N Engl J Med* 288:891-894, 1973.

MacGregor GA, et al: Is "idiopathic" edema idiopathic? *Lancet* 1: 397-400, 1979.

Minuth AN, et al: Acute renal failure: Study of course and progress of 104 patients and of role of furosemide. *Am J Med Sci* 271:317-324, 1976.

Smith JW, Clements P: Renal function during therapy in patients with congestive cardiac failure: Ticrynafen vs hydrochlorothiazide. *Nephron* 23(suppl):41-45, 1979.

Stein JH, Reineck HJ: Effect of alterations in ex-tracellular fluid volume on segmental sodium transport. *Physiol Rev* 55:127-141, 1975.

Stote RM, et al: Tienilic acid: Potent diuretic-uricosuric agent. *J Pharmacol Clin* (special issue) 19-27, Jan 1976.

Thurau K, Boylan JW: Acute renal success: Unexpected logic of oliguria in acute renal failure. *Am J Med* 61:308-315, 1976.

Whight C, et al: Diuretics, cardiac failure and potassium depletion: Rational approach. *Med J Aust* 2:831-833, 1974.

Agents Used to Treat Urologic Disorders | 40

Drugs that stimulate or inhibit smooth muscle activity are useful in some disorders of the lower urinary tract. The goals of therapy are to prevent renal complications and to improve urinary bladder function of storage and emptying. Urinary bladder dysfunction may manifest as recurrent urinary tract infection, recurrent or persistent urinary retention, or urinary incontinence. It is, therefore, of paramount importance to investigate the patient thoroughly prior to institution of therapy. A complete urologic evaluation should include appropriate urodynamic tests such as cystometry, sphincter electromyography, urethral pressure profilometry, and cystourethroscopy. These tests are also useful to objectively document the efficacy or lack of efficacy of drug therapy.

Physiologic Considerations

The two functions of the bladder, urine storage and expulsion, are accomplished by the coordinated activity of the smooth (involuntary) muscle of the bladder wall (the detrusor muscle), the smooth muscle of the

607

bladder neck and proximal urethra (the "internal sphincter"), and the striated (voluntary) muscle surrounding the posterior urethra (the periurethral striated muscles of the urogenital diaphragm and levator ani which constitute the "external sphincter"). The bladder stores urine by virtue of its property of accommodation and, if the intravesical pressure is not excessive, continence is maintained by the tonicity of the internal sphincter. In males, the internal sphincter also prevents seminal fluid from entering the bladder during ejaculation. The external sphincter maintains urinary continence when there is a sudden increase in intravesical pressure and thus prevents leakage during stress.

When the bladder is full, emptying is initiated by nerve impulses generated in stretch receptors of the bladder wall that are activated by bladder distention. The nerve impulses are relayed through the central nervous system to the pelvic parasympathetic nerves, which activate the detrusor muscle. At the same time, motor activity in the pudendal motor nerves is inhibited, causing relaxation of the periurethral striated muscles of the external sphincter. Volitional control of this spinal (or brainstem) reflex is maintained by excitatory and inhibitory pathways originating in the cerebral cortex which regulate both the detrusor and the periurethral striated muscles (Bradley et al, 1974; Kendall and Karafin, 1974; Lapides and Diokno, 1976).

When the detrusor muscle contracts, the bladder neck opens concurrently because some of the smooth muscle layers in the urethra are continuous with the detrusor. In addition to this passive mechanism (which is dependent upon parasympathetic innervation of the bladder), bladder neck resistance is increased by tonic sympathetic impulses which activate alpha receptors in the internal sphincter. This state of constant sympathetic tonus is suppressed during voiding (Kleeman, 1970; Krane and Olsson, 1973). Although sympathetic tone is of minor importance in normal urinary function, it may be a major element of outlet resistance in pathologic conditions.

Neurogenic Bladder and Sphincter Dysfunction

Neurogenic disorders of the lower urinary tract may be associated with hyper- or hypotonicity of the detrusor muscle or of the internal or external sphincter. These disorders may exist singly or in various combinations with coordinated or uncoordinated bladder-sphincter function. In treating these disorders, drugs are only part of a regimen that also may include a program of frequent, periodic voiding, intermittent self-catheterization, external compression, or measures to induce reflex bladder contractions. Surgical procedures may be indicated if these measures are inadequate (Lapides, 1974; Wein et al, 1976). The agents used to treat neurogenic bladder disorders inhibit (antispasmodics) or enhance (cholinergics) detrusor contractions or increase (alpha-adrenergic agents) or decrease (alpha-adrenergic blocking drugs) internal sphincter tonus. There is no drug available that acts selectively on the external sphincter, but several muscle relaxants are under investigation for treatment of external sphincter spasticity.

Uninhibited Neurogenic Bladder: An organic or functional defect in the corticoregulatory tract frees the bladder from inhibitory control by the higher centers, resulting in uncontrolled contractions of the detrusor muscle during bladder filling, reduced bladder capacity, and symptoms of urinary frequency, urgency, and urge incontinence. Strokes, brain tumors, and demyelinating diseases are the most common causes of uninhibited neurogenic bladder in adults. Moderate fluid restriction and anticholinergic drugs may improve symptoms in some patients.

The uninhibited bladder may occur in children without any detectable signs of neurologic damage and is presumably associated with delayed development of cortical control over the detrusor muscle. It has been suggested that this type of neurogenic bladder may be a common cause of recurrent urinary infection in young girls who presumably develop control over the periurethral striated muscles before achieving control over the detrusor muscle. Antibacterial drugs and institution of a regular voiding schedule are the major therapeutic tools in the management of these children. Anticholinergic drugs are helpful adjuvants to control incontinence and prevent recurrent infections if the uninhibited contractions cannot be prevented by frequent voiding and fluid restriction.

The uninhibited bladder also may be a cause of enuresis (see the section on Enuresis).

Reflex Neurogenic Bladder: Spinal cord lesions above the conus medullaris (which usually are associated with trauma) disrupt voluntary control while sparing the vesical reflex arc. Initially, there is a period of detrusor areflexia caused by loss of facilitatory impulses from the higher centers. During this period, intermittent self-catheterization is the preferred method for preventing bladder overdistention. Following the period of spinal shock, the vesical reflex arc gradually returns and bladder contractions occur in an uncontrolled manner. When reflex activity is established, two types of external sphincter activity may be observed. The activity of the periurethral striated muscle may be coordinated with the uncontrolled reflex contractions. The coordinated system is characterized by involuntary detrusor contractions with concomitant relaxation of the external sphincter. With this mechanism, micturition with complete emptying can be accomplished by techniques that trigger the detrusor reflex. The uncoordinated system is characterized by involuntary detrusor contraction and external sphincter contraction resulting in incomplete bladder emptying, high intravesical pressures, and vesicoureteric reflux. The cholinergic drug, bethanechol [Duvoid, Myotonachol, Urecholine], has been used during the recovery phase of spinal shock to enhance weak detrusor contractions but should not be given unless bladder and external sphincter function are coordinated (Diokno and Koppenhoefer, 1976).

The alpha-adrenergic blocking drug, phenoxybenzamine [Dibenzyline], may be useful in patients with voiding difficulties caused by internal sphincter dysfunction (Krane and Olsson, 1973; Mobley, 1976). Transurethral surgical procedures, such as external sphincterotomy, are indicated when urethral resistance is increased because of excessive or inappropriate activity of the periurethral striated muscle (Lapides, 1974).

Autonomous Neurogenic Bladder: All reflex bladder activity is abolished by extensive lesions involving the vesical reflex arc in the sacral spinal cord. Such lesions, which may be produced by congenital defects, trauma, ischemia, tumors, or a herniated nucleus pulposus, result in loss of voluntary control, absence of bladder contractions, and increased bladder capacity and residual urine with both overflow and stress incontinence. Because the motor outflow to the external sphincter also originates in the sacral spinal cord, the external sphincter is usually flaccid and the bladder can be emptied by external compression. An alpha-adrenergic drug such as ephedrine may be used to increase proximal urethral resistance and thus diminish stress incontinence (Lapides and Diokno, 1976). On the other hand, if residual urine is increased because of functional obstruction of the internal sphincter, phenoxybenzamine may be useful (Mobley, 1976; Krane and Olsson, 1973).

Sensory Paralytic Bladder: Lesions involving the afferent limb of the micturition reflex arc are usually associated with tabes dorsalis or sometimes with diabetes mellitus. Although the patient can initiate micturition voluntarily, voiding occurs infrequently because the sensation of bladder fullness is impaired. If a program of frequent periodic voiding is not instituted, prolonged overdistention will lead to a gradual loss of detrusor muscle tone, followed by infection, deteriorating renal function, and overflow incontinence. When motor power is impaired because of prolonged overdistention, bethanechol may reduce residual urine by enhancing detrusor contractions. If these measures are not effective, intermittent self-catheterization should be instituted or surgical procedures may be necessary (Lapides, 1974).

Motor Paralytic Bladder: Lower motor neuron impairment produces urinary retention. Exteroceptive and proprioceptive sensations are intact. This type of neurogenic bladder may be associated with poliomyelitis (when it is transient), polyradiculoneuritis, trauma, or neoplasm. Since detrusor muscle activity is absent, therapy is directed toward preventing overdistention, usually by means of intermittent self-catheterization. On occasion, the external sphincter may be totally denervated. In such cases, bladder emptying can be accomplished by the Valsalva or Credé maneuver. However, patients with complete sphincter denervation have severe stress incontinence. When the bladder is only partially denervated and sphincter function is coordinated, bethanechol may be used for long-term therapy to improve bladder emptying (Lapides, 1974; Lapides and Diokno, 1976). Phenoxybenzamine may be used adjunctively if residual urine volume is increased because of functional outlet obstruction.

Enuresis

Enuresis is a common childhood disorder which is often associated with a positive family history. Nocturnal enuresis is the most common form, although some children also suffer from urgency, frequency, and urge incontinence during the day. Uninhibited bladder contractions, emotional disturbances, and sleep disorders are among the postulated causes; rarely is there any evidence of an organic cause.

Regardless of the method of management, the condition generally improves as the child matures and no treatment may be indicated. The major methods used in these patients (singly or in combination) are psychotherapy, imipramine [Imavate, SK-Pramine, Tofranil], and waking devices. Imipramine has been the most effective drug for treating nocturnal enuresis, while an antcholinergic agent, such as belladonna tincture, may be more effective in patients with marked daytime symptoms (McKendry and Stewart, 1974).

Stress Incontinence

Stress incontinence is manifested by the involuntary loss of urine following a sudden increase in intra-abdominal pressure as may occur with coughing, sneezing, straining, or physical exercise. It is caused by sphincter incompetence rather than detrusor dysfunction and may be of neurogenic or non-neurogenic origin. Neurogenic stress incontinence results from a lesion in the motor nerves supplying the periurethral striated muscle of the external sphincter. Non-neurogenic stress incontinence is a common disorder of older women, and the etiology is controversial; it may be associated with an abnormally short or narrow urethra or loss of the urethrovesical angle due to weakness of the pelvic floor-supporting mechanisms. Other types of non-neurogenic stress incontinence result from urethral injury, inflammation, scarring, or instrumentation.

Although the striated muscle of the external sphincter cannot be activated by drugs, proximal urethral resistance can be increased by drugs that activate alpha receptors in the smooth muscle of the internal sphincter. For this reason, adrenergic drugs such as ephedrine and phenylpropanolamine have been used to treat stress incontinence.

Interstitial Cystitis

Interstitial cystitis is an uncommon bladder disorder of unknown etiology which occurs more commonly in women than in men. Patients with this disorder have symptoms of urgency and frequency with infrapubic or suprapubic pain which may be diminished by voiding. Submucosal edema and vasodilation are characteristic histologic findings, and cystoscopic examination may reveal glomerulations, reduced bladder capacity, and ulceration (Messing and Stamey, 1978).

Interstitial cystitis has been treated by hydrodilation, surgery, and use of various drugs, including corticosteroids and anticholinergic agents. More recently, dimethyl sulfoxide (DMSO [Rimso-50]) has been found useful in some patients.

AGENTS USED TO TREAT URINARY INCONTINENCE

Three classes of drugs are useful in treating urinary incontinence: (1) antispasmodics, which reduce urgency, frequency, and urge incontinence associated with uninhibited detrusor contractions; (2) tricyclic drugs (particularly imipramine), which sometimes alleviate nocturnal enuresis in children; and (3) alpha-adrenergic drugs (particularly ephedrine), which may lessen stress incontinence associated with partial incompetence of the urinary sphincter.

Drugs are not useful in treating incontinence associated with detrusor hypotonicity (overflow incontinence), except to maintain dryness between catheterizations or to facilitate bladder emptying. Other types of incontinence that do not benefit from drug therapy are those associated with marked incompetence of the urinary sphincter or congenital or acquired abnormalities of the urinary tract (eg, ectopic ureter, urinary fistulas).

Antispasmodics

Anticholinergic drugs block the action of acetylcholine at postganglionic cholinergic sites, thereby increasing bladder capacity by reducing the number of motor impulses reaching the detrusor muscle. The response of the detrusor muscle to parasympathetic stimulation is relatively resistant to cholinergic blockade; therefore, doses that inhibit the urinary bladder can be expected to produce the usual anticholinergic side effects (eg, constipation, dryness of the mouth). A large number of anticholinergic agents are available commercially (see Chapter 60, Miscellaneous Gastrointestinal Agents, for a listing and further discussion of these agents), but there is no convincing evidence that any one is more effective or better tolerated than the others. Both the natural belladonna alkaloids (atropine, belladonna tincture, and hyoscyamine [Cystospaz, Levsin]) and various synthetic substitutes (eg, propantheline [Pro-Banthine]) have been used in urology.

Other urinary antispasmodics (flavoxate [Urispas] and oxybutynin [Ditropan]) relax the detrusor and other smooth muscle by both cholinergic blockade and a direct relaxant effect on muscle fibers.

PROPANTHELINE BROMIDE
[Pro-Banthine]

This quaternary ammonium compound is a synthetic anticholinergic agent with both antimuscarinic (atropine-like) and ganglionic blocking properties. Its therapeutic effects are usually attributed to the antimuscarinic component. Although quaternary ammonium anticholinergics are not as well absorbed orally as the natural belladonna alkaloids, they may have a slightly longer duration of action.

Propantheline is given orally to increase bladder capacity and reduce urinary frequency, urgency, and urge incontinence associated with an uninhibited neurogenic bladder. It has been used more commonly for this purpose than other anticholinergic drugs. In paraplegic patients with lesions above the sacral spinal cord (reflex neurogenic bladder), propantheline may also control reflex detrusor activity and thus preserve continence in the interval between catheterizations (Lapides, 1974).

Because the uncontrolled contractions of a neurogenic bladder are mediated by parasympathetic motor fibers, whereas contractions resulting from localized muscle spasm are not, intravenous propantheline is useful in the differential diagnosis of the small-capacity bladder to confirm the presence or absence of neurogenic vesical dysfunction (Lapides and Diokno, 1976).

The adverse reactions produced by propantheline are common to all anticholinergic drugs. Doses that inhibit detrusor contractions also suppress salivation, interfere with ocular accommodation, dilate the pupil, increase heart rate, and reduce gastrointestinal motility, causing constipation. Quaternary ammonium compounds do not readily cross the blood-brain barrier; therefore, central nervous system effects are rare but, because of their ganglionic blocking properties, large doses can cause orthostatic hypotension and impotence. (See also Chapter 60.)

ROUTES, USUAL DOSAGE, AND PREPARATIONS.
Oral: To improve bladder capacity in patients with uninhibited neurogenic bladder, *adults*, initially, 15 mg every four to six hours; *children*, 7.5 mg every four to six hours.
To maintain continence between catheterizations in patients with reflex neurogenic bladder, *adults*, 15 to 30 mg every four to six hours; *children*, 7.5 to 15 mg every four to six hours.
> Drug available generically: Tablets 7.5 and 15 mg.
> *Pro-Banthine* (Searle). Tablets 15 mg.

Intravenous: For differential diagnosis of the small-capacity bladder, *adults*, 30 mg.
> *Pro-Banthine* (Searle). Powder (for injection) 30 mg.

BELLADONNA TINCTURE

This anticholinergic preparation is used primarily in children who, in addition to nocturnal enuresis, experience urgency, frequency, and urge incontinence during the day (McKendry and Stewart, 1974).

Belladonna produces the usual antimuscarinic side effects on the salivary glands, heart, eye, and gastrointestinal tract; large doses may cause flushing, fever, and marked central nervous system effects (eg, excitement, hallucinations, delirium). (See also Chapter 60.)

ROUTE, USUAL DOSAGE, AND PREPARATIONS.
Oral: *Children over 5 years*, initially, 0.25 to 0.5 ml (10 to 20 drops) three times daily. Dosage may be increased gradually, if necessary, to 1 ml/dose. The dose should be reduced if flushing or other signs of toxicity occur.
> Drug available generically in 4 oz, pint, and gallon containers.

HYOSCYAMINE
[Cystospaz]

HYOSCYAMINE SULFATE
[Cystospaz-M, Levsin]

Hyoscyamine has the same actions and side effects as the other belladonna alkaloids. Its most common use in urology has been to treat bladder spasm associated with infection, inflammation, or use of a retention catheter, although these disorders are less responsive to anticholinergic medication than are neurogenic bladder disorders. Adverse effects are similar to those observed with other anticholinergic agents.

ROUTE, USUAL DOSAGE, AND PREPARATIONS.
Oral: *Adults*, 0.15 to 0.3 mg of the base three or four times daily or 0.375 mg of the sulfate twice daily.
> HYOSCYAMINE:
> *Cystospaz* (Webcon). Tablets 0.15 mg.
> HYOSCYAMINE SULFATE:
> *Cystospaz-M* (Webcon). Capsules (timed-release) 0.375 mg.
> *Levsin* (Kremers-Urban). Capsules (timed-release) 0.375 mg (Levsinex); drops 0.125 mg/ml; elixir 0.125 mg/5 ml; tablets 0.125 and 0.25 mg.

FLAVOXATE HYDROCHLORIDE
[Urispas]

Flavoxate has anticholinergic, local anesthetic, and analgesic properties and also may have a direct relaxant effect on smooth muscle. The relative contribution of each of these characteristics to the anti-spasmodic effect is difficult to appraise. Excretion of the drug in the urine with the resultant local action on the urinary tract may play a role.

Flavoxate has been used to reduce dysuria, nocturia, suprapubic pain, and urinary frequency, urgency, and incontinence associated with cystitis, prostatitis, urethritis, and trigonitis. Despite its mixed actions, flavoxate has not proved to be more effective in these disorders than an anticholinergic drug.

Adverse reactions are relatively uncommon, although the following have been reported: nausea, vomiting, dryness of the mouth, nervousness, vertigo, headache, drowsiness, blurred vision, disturbance in visual accommodation, increased intra-ocular pressure, urticaria and other dermatoses, mental confusion (especially in the elderly), dysuria, tachycardia, fever, eosinophilia, and reversible leukopenia (one case). Some of these reactions resemble anticholinergic effects; therefore, the same precautions and contraindications should apply (see Chapter 60).

ROUTE, USUAL DOSAGE, AND PREPARATIONS. *Oral: Adults,* 100 or 200 mg three or four times daily; the dose may be reduced when symptoms improve. The dosage has not been established for *children under 12 years.*

Urispas (Smith Kline & French). Tablets 100 mg.

OXYBUTYNIN CHLORIDE
[Ditropan]

Oxybutynin has both anticholinergic and direct actions and also may possess mild analgesic properties. In a limited number of clinical trials, oxybutynin increased bladder capacity and improved symptoms of urinary frequency, urgency, and urge incontinence in adults and children with uninhibited bladder contractions and also increased bladder capacity and reduced reflex incontinence in those with reflex neurogenic bladder. It has not been consistently effective in relieving bladder spasm following transurethral surgical procedures.

Adverse reactions reflect this agent's anticholinergic activity. Dryness of the mouth is most common; nausea, blurred vision, flushing, and tachycardia also have been reported. The contraindications to oxybutynin are the same as for other drugs with anticholinergic properties (see Chapter 60).

ROUTE, USUAL DOSAGE, AND PREPARATIONS. *Oral: Adults,* 5 mg two or three times daily (maximum, 20 mg daily). *Children over 5 years,* 5 mg two times daily (maximum, 15 mg daily).

Ditropan (Marion). Tablets 5 mg.

Tricyclic Drugs

IMIPRAMINE HYDROCHLORIDE
[Imavate, SK-Pramine, Tofranil]

IMIPRAMINE PAMOATE
[Tofranil-PM]

Imipramine is sometimes used to treat nocturnal enuresis in children. Improvement may or may not be sustained when the drug is discontinued, as reported rates of cure range from 10% to over 50% (Stewart, 1975; McKendry et al, 1975). The mechanism of action of imipramine in enuresis is unclear. An anticholinergic effect on the detrusor muscle appears unlikely because, in contrast to propantheline, imipramine does not abolish uninhibited contractions (Diokno et al, 1972). Other postulated mechanisms include an adrenergic effect on the internal sphincter or central nervous system, an antidepressant action, or an alteration in sleep patterns (Gualtieri, 1977).

Drowsiness, dryness of the mouth, nausea, vomiting, constipation, blurred vision, restlessness, sleep disturbances, and mood changes are common adverse effects. Overdosage can cause convulsions, coma, and severe cardiovascular reactions, including A-V block and marked hypotension. Withdrawal reactions (nausea, headache, and malaise) have been reported following the drug's abrupt cessation after long-term therapy. (See also Chapter 13, Drugs Used in Affective Disorders.)

ROUTE, USUAL DOSAGE, AND PREPARATIONS.
Oral: *Children*, initially, 10 mg every night for one week or longer if improvement occurs. If there is no improvement after one week, dosage may be increased in weekly increments of 10 mg up to the following maximal doses: 40 mg (5 to 6 years), 50 mg (6 to 8 years), 60 mg (8 to 10 years), 70 mg (10 to 12 years), 75 mg (12 to 14 years). The drug may be administered after dinner or up to one hour before bedtime. Some early nighttime bedwetters may benefit from divided doses given in midafternoon or at bedtime. When optimal effects are obtained, administration is continued for two to three months, and then the dose is gradually reduced over a period of three to four months.

> IMIPRAMINE HYDROCHLORIDE:
> Drug available generically: Tablets 10, 25, and 50 mg.
> *Imavate* (Robins), *SK-Pramine* (Smith Kline & French), *Tofranil* (Geigy). Tablets 10, 25, and 50 mg.
> IMIPRAMINE PAMOATE:
> *Tofranil-PM* (Geigy). Capsules equivalent to 75, 100, 125, and 150 mg of imipramine hydrochloride.

Alpha-Adrenergic Drugs

EPHEDRINE SULFATE

This adrenergic drug, which has both alpha- and beta-stimulating properties, is often preferred to other sympathomimetic agents because it is effective orally, is generally well tolerated, and has a relatively long duration of action. By increasing urethral resistance, ephedrine improves urine storage in patients with mild to moderate stress incontinence of neurogenic or non-neurogenic origin, but it is of little value if the periurethral striated muscle is completely denervated or severely damaged or if there is severe damage to the posterior urethra (Diokno and Taub, 1975).

Since ephedrine increases blood pressure and stimulates the heart, it should be used cautiously in patients with hypertension and other cardiovascular disorders and in those with hyperthyroidism. It also stimulates the central nervous system and may cause insomnia and anxiety.

ROUTE, USUAL DOSAGE, AND PREPARATIONS.
Oral: *Adults*, 25 to 50 mg four times daily. *Children*, 11 to 20 mg four times daily.
> Drug available generically: Capsules 25 and 50 mg; syrup 11 and 20 mg/5 ml.

ORNADE

Because stress incontinence is frequently precipitated by sneezing or coughing, some urologists prefer to treat this disorder with a cold preparation containing an alpha-adrenergic drug combined with an antihistamine and an anticholinergic drug. One such product, Ornade, has been effective in women with mild to moderate symptoms of classic stress incontinence. Results are less satisfactory in men with postprostatectomy incontinence, although a few patients with mild symptoms may improve (Stewart et al, 1976).

Ornade may cause sympathomimetic, antihistaminic, and anticholinergic side effects. Sedation and dryness of the mouth are the most common reactions. If these effects are troublesome, dosage should be reduced or ephedrine should be substituted. Ornade should be used cautiously in patients with hypertension and other cardiovascular disorders and in those with hyperthyroidism.

ROUTE, USUAL DOSAGE, AND PREPARATIONS.
Oral: *Adults*, one capsule twice daily.

Ornade (Smith Kline & French). Capsules (timed-release) containing phenylpropanolamine hydrochloride 50 mg, chlorpheniramine maleate 8 mg, and isopropamide iodide equivalent to isopropamide 2.5 mg.

AGENTS USED TO TREAT URINARY RETENTION

The drugs used to treat urinary retention facilitate bladder emptying by increasing detrusor muscle contractility (cholinergic agents) or by reducing outlet resistance (alpha-adrenergic blocking drugs). Bethanechol [Duvoid, Myotonachol, Urecholine] is the cholinergic agent most commonly recommended for management of the chronic hypotonic bladder and for short-term treatment of postoperative urinary retention in selected patients. The cholinesterase inhibitor, neostigmine methylsulfate [Prostigmin], is also used for the latter purpose. The alpha-adrenergic blocking drug, phenoxybenzamine [Dibenzyline], is used in certain neurogenic bladder disorders to facilitate voiding by relaxing the internal sphincter. It may be used in conjunction with bethanechol.

Cholinergic Drugs

BETHANECHOL CHLORIDE
[Duvoid, Myotonachol, Urecholine]

$$H_2NCOCHCH_2 \overset{+}{N}(CH_3)_3 \quad Cl^-$$
$$\underset{CH_3}{|}$$

Bethanechol is a choline ester that acts directly on effector cells. Its effects are similar to those of acetylcholine but are more prolonged because bethanechol is relatively resistant to hydrolysis by cholinesterase. The actions of bethanechol are primarily muscarinic, and it produces minimal effects on autonomic ganglia in normal individuals. The action on the urinary bladder and gastrointestinal tract is more pronounced than that on the cardiovascular system.

In patients with spinal cord lesions above the vesical reflex arc (S2-3-4) and coordinated bladder-sphincter function, bethanechol is sometimes employed during the recovery phase of spinal shock to enhance weak detrusor contractions (Diokno and Koppenhoefer, 1976). If tolerated, it also may be used for long-term therapy in patients with sensory paralytic bladders or in those with incomplete motor lesions and coordinated sphincter function (Lapides, 1974; Lapides and Diokno, 1976). Bethanechol is used, in conjunction with intermittent self-catheterization, to facilitate bladder emptying in patients with hypotonic neurogenic bladder.

Bethanechol has been advocated as a diagnostic aid to determine the presence or absence of neurogenic vesical dysfunction in the patient with a hypotonic bladder. The response to bladder stretching is measured cystometrically before and after subcutaneous injection of a small dose. Because neurologic lesions that damage the micturition reflex arc induce denervation supersensitivity, the patient with a motor or sensory paralytic bladder or an autonomous neurogenic bladder should demonstrate an exaggerated response to the cholinergic drug, ie, the pressure recorded after administration of bethanechol should be 15 cm or more over the control value (Lapides and Diokno, 1976; Wear, 1974). The validity of this test has been questioned, however, because false-positive results may occur in the presence of uremia, urinary tract infection, and bladder outlet obstruction, and a negative or normal result may occur when the bladder muscle is decompensated or the bladder capacity markedly increased (Wein, 1979).

In addition to its use in neurogenic bladder disorders, bethanechol is used to restore normal micturition in selected patients with acute urinary retention related to surgery or parturition.

Bethanechol may cause flushing, headache, salivation, sweating, nausea, vomiting, diarrhea, and difficulty in accommodation. Some patients cannot tolerate prolonged therapy because of these adverse effects. Bethanechol is contraindicated in patients with bronchial asthma because it may cause bronchospasm. It also may lower blood pressure and generally should be avoided in patients with hypotension, bradycardia, or coronary artery disease. Hyperthyroidism is generally listed as another contraindication. Because it increases gastrointestinal motility, bethanechol should not be given to patients with peptic ulcer and other gastrointestinal lesions or to those with intestinal obstruction.

Bethanechol is contraindicated in the presence of organic urinary tract obstruction. This drug also should be avoided in patients with detrusor-external sphincter dyssynergia, because prolonged therapy has caused bladder trabeculation, diverticula, and vesicoureteral reflux. Although dyssynergia resulting from internal sphincter overactivity may be less common, the possibility of adverse effects in such cases should be considered.

Bethanechol should not be given intravenously or intramuscularly because acute severe muscarinic effects, including acute circulatory failure and cardiac arrest, may result.

ROUTES, USUAL DOSAGE, AND PREPARATIONS. In treating neurogenic bladder disorders, bethanechol may be used in conjunction with surgical or pharmacologic (phenoxybenzamine) measures to reduce outlet obstruction.

Subcutaneous, Oral: For patients with incomplete spinal cord lesions above the reflex arc and voluntary control of the external sphincter, initially, 2.5 to 5 mg subcutaneously every four to six hours. The patient should be catheterized once or twice daily and, when residual urine is less than 50 ml, oral therapy may be substituted (50 mg every six hours) or subcutaneous therapy may be continued (2.5 mg every six hours). This regimen should be continued for at least one week and, if residual urine remains low, the drug may be discontinued following a gradual reduction in dosage. Some patients may require several weeks or months of therapy.

In sensory paralytic bladder and partial motor paralytic bladder with coordinated sphincter function, initially, 7.5 to 10 mg subcutaneously every four hours around the clock. (An initial dose of 5 mg may be advisable in very frail patients.) When residual urine is less than 50 ml for three days, each dose may be reduced by 2.5 mg. If the response is satisfactory, dosage may later be reduced to a minimum of 5 mg every four hours. Oral therapy (50 mg four times daily) may be substituted when complete bladder emptying is achieved over a three-day period. When the sensory paralytic bladder is rehabilitated, therapy may be discontinued, but patients with motor lesions require lifetime treatment.

> Drug available generically: Tablets 5, 10, and 25 mg.
> *Duvoid* (Norwich-Eaton). Tablets 10, 25, and 50 mg.
> *Myotonachol* (Glenwood), *Urecholine* (Merck, Sharp & Dohme). Tablets 5, 10, and 25 mg.
> *Urecholine* (Merck Sharp & Dohme). Solution 5 mg/ml in 1 ml containers.

Oral: For patients with complete lesions above the reflex arc and coordinated bladder and sphincter function, initially, 25 mg is given every six hours. Dosage may be increased or decreased depending upon the response, and the drug should be discontinued when reflex voiding is established.

> Drug available generically: Tablets 5, 10, 25, and 50 mg.
> *Duvoid* (Norwich-Eaton). Tablets 10, 25, and 50 mg.
> *Myotonachol* (Glenwood), *Urecholine* (Merck Sharp & Dohme). Tablets 5, 10, and 25 mg.

Subcutaneous: For acute postoperative and postpartum urinary retention in selected patients, *adults*, 5 mg (1 ml). If this dose is ineffective, the patient should be catheterized. Bethanechol should not be used unless the patient is alert.

> *Urecholine* (Merck Sharp & Dohme). Solution 5 mg/ml in 1 ml containers.

Alpha-Adrenergic Blocking Agents

PHENOXYBENZAMINE HYDROCHLORIDE
[Dibenzyline]

Obstructive voiding symptoms in patients with neurogenic bladder disorders may be caused by dysfunction of the external or internal sphincter. In the latter case (in which drug therapy may be beneficial), outlet resistance is increased because (1) detrusor contractions are too weak to open the bladder neck; (2) urethral smooth muscle tone is increased as a result of damage to inhibitory pathways; or (3) bladder and sphincter function are not coordinated.

By blocking alpha receptors in the smooth muscle of the bladder neck and proximal urethra, phenoxybenzamine relaxes the internal sphincter. It may improve voiding efficiency in patients with functional outlet obstruction and obviate or delay the need for transurethral surgical procedures. Phenoxybenzamine has been used successfully in patients with reflex, autonomous, and motor paralytic bladders when urinary retention could not be prevented by other methods such as reflex voiding, Crede maneuver, or administration of bethanechol (Kleeman, 1970; Krane and Olsson, 1973; Mobley, 1976). It has no effect on striated muscle and is therefore ineffective in treating urinary retention caused by excessive or inappropriate activity of the external sphincter. Phentolamine has been employed to identify patients who are likely to benefit from long-term phenoxybenzamine therapy (Olsson et al, 1977).

In addition to its use in neurogenic bladder dysfunction, phenoxybenzamine has been employed to treat voiding symptoms in patients with prostatic obstruction who are not suitable candidates for surgery.

The major side effects of phenoxybenzamine, orthostatic hypotension and reflex tachycardia, result from blockade of alpha receptors in the peripheral circulation. Elastic stockings may be useful to counteract the orthostatic hypotension. Other adverse reactions include nasal congestion and gastrointestinal disturbances (nausea, vomiting, diarrhea).

ROUTE, USUAL DOSAGE, AND PREPARATIONS. *Oral*: *Adults*, initially, 10 mg once daily. The dosage may be increased if needed in 10-mg increments every three to five days to a maximum of 60 mg daily. Daily doses larger than 10 mg should be evenly divided and given every 8 to 12 hours. During long-term therapy, some patients may require as little as 10 mg two or three times a week. Phenoxybenzamine may be used in conjunction with bethanechol.

Dibenzyline (Smith Kline & French). Capsules 10 mg.

AGENT USED TO TREAT INTERSTITIAL CYSTITIS

DIMETHYL SULFOXIDE (DMSO)
[Rimso-50]

$$\begin{array}{c} CH_3 \\ \diagdown \\ S=O \\ \diagup \\ CH_3 \end{array}$$

After being used for many years as an industrial solvent, DMSO was found to possess a variety of pharmacologic effects when applied topically, including anti-inflammatory, analgesic, bacteriostatic, vasodilatory properties, and a softening effect on collagen. These actions lead to its investigational use in various disorders such as arthritis and scleroderma, but it was later withdrawn from clinical testing because of ocular toxicity in laboratory animals.

DMSO is now available as a 50% solution for direct instillation into the bladder for treatment of interstitial cystitis. It relieves symptoms in most patients and may improve bladder capacity and endoscopic appearance of the bladder. However, some patients do not respond and others may relapse after initial improvement (Shirley et al, 1978).

The major side effect of DMSO, which results from systemic absorption, is a garlic-like taste and odor. No serious adverse effects have occurred after intravesical instillation of the 50% solution, but a stronger concentration (100%) has caused severe, transient chemical cystitis. When applied topically to the skin, it has caused urticaria, gastrointestinal disturbances, headache, photophobia, and transient disturbances in color vision. Lens opacities have occurred in animals but have not been reported in man.

ROUTE, USUAL DOSAGE, AND PREPARATIONS. *Intravesical Instillation:* 50 ml of a 50% solution is instilled slowly by catheter directly into the bladder under local urethral anesthesia. An anticholinergic drug may be given to prevent bladder spasm. Instilla-

tion may be repeated at weekly intervals in patients with severe symptoms or at intervals of three to six months in those with milder symptoms.

Rimso-50 (Research Industries Corporation). Solution 50% in 50 ml containers.

Selected References

Bradley WE, et al: Innervation of detrusor muscle and urethra. *Urol Clin North Am* 1:3-27, 1974.

Diokno AC, Koppenhoefer R: Bethanechol chloride in neurogenic bladder dysfunction. *Urology* 8:455-458, 1976.

Diokno AC, Taub M: Ephedrine in treatment of urinary incontinence. *Urology* 5:624-625, 1975.

Diokno AC, et al: Comparison of action of imipramine (Tofranil) and propantheline (ProBanthine) on detrusor contraction. *J Urol* 107:42-43, 1972.

Gualtieri CT: Imipramine and children: Review and some speculations about mechanism of drug action. *Dis Nerv Syst* 38:368-374, 1977.

Kendall AR, Karafin L: Classification of neurogenic bladder disease. *Urol Clin North Am* 1:37-44, 1974.

Kleeman FJ: Physiology of internal urinary sphincter. *J Urol* 104:549-554, 1970.

Krane RJ, Olsson CA: Phenoxybenzamine in neurogenic bladder dysfunction. I. Theory of micturition; II. Clinical considerations. *J Urol* 110:650-656, 1973.

Lapides J: Neurogenic bladder: Principles of treatment. *Urol Clin North Am* 1:81-97, 1974.

Lapides J, Diokno AC: Urine transport, storage, and micturition, in Lapides J (ed): *Fundamentals of Urology.* Philadelphia, WB Saunders Co, 1976, 190-241.

McKendry JBJ, Stewart DA: Enuresis. *Pediatr Clin North Am* 2:1019-1028, 1974.

McKendry JBJ, et al: Primary enuresis: Relative success of three methods of treatment. *Can Med Assoc J* 113:953-955, 1975.

Messing EM, Stamey TA: Interstitial cystitis. *Urology* 12:381-392, 1978.

Mobley DF: Phenoxybenzamine in management of neurogenic vesicle dysfunction. *J Urol* 116:737-738, 1976.

Olsson CA, et al: Phentolamine test in neurogenic bladder dysfunction. *J Urol* 117:481-485, 1977.

Shirley SW, et al: Dimethyl sulfoxide in treatment of inflammatory genitourinary disorders. *Urology* 11:215-220, 1978.

Stewart BH, et al: Stress incontinence: Conservative therapy with sympathomimetic drugs. *J Urol* 115:558-559, 1976.

Stewart MA: Treatment of bedwetting. *JAMA* 232:281-283, 1975.

Wear JB: Cystometry. *Urol Clin North Am* 1:45-67, 1974.

Wein AJ: Pharmacologic approaches to management of neurogenic bladder dysfunction. *J Contin Educat Urol*, 1979 (in press).

Wein AJ, et al: Management of neurogenic bladder dysfunction in adult. *Urology* 8:432-443, 1976.

Adrenal Corticosteroids | 41

Adrenal corticosteroids are administered either in physiologic doses to correct deficiency or in pharmacologic doses to treat inflammatory conditions, collagen disorders, and certain other diseases. Natural and synthetic glucocorticoids can be divided into glucocorticoids or mineralocorticoids, depending upon their predominant activity. In physiologic amounts, the glucocorticoids have primarily carbohydrate-storing, protein catabolic, and corticotropin-suppressing activities. In pharmacologic doses, they also have anti-inflammatory and anti-immunologic actions. The mineralocorticoids have primarily sodium-retaining and potassium-excreting effects and are used in physiologic amounts for replacement therapy and occasionally in orthostatic hypotension to increase extracellular fluid volume.

Numerous synthetic corticosteroids have been developed by varying the chemical structure of cortisol (hydrocortisone, Compound F). Prednisone and prednisolone were produced by introducing a double bond between carbon atoms 1 and 2 (Δ -1 analogues) of cortisone and cortisol, respectively; this increased their glucocorticoid activity while decreasing their mineralocorticoid effect. Other synthetic preparations have either glucocorticoid (ie, dexamethasone, betamethasone) or mineralocorticoid (desoxycorticosterone acetate and pivalate) activities almost exclusively; most have been synthesized primarily for their glucocorticoid activity and are widely used in nonendocrine diseases.

When considering the therapeutic efficacy of the corticosteroids, it is important to remember that separation of glucocorticoid and mineralocorticoid activity is incomplete. Some agents that are considered to be primarily glucocorticoids (eg, cortisol [hydrocortisone], cortisone, prednisone, prednisolone) possess variable mineralocorticoid activity as well and, therefore, cause sodium retention and potassium depletion when used in pharmacologic amounts. The relative potencies of the corticosteroids are listed in the Table.

Physiology and Pharmacology of Corticosteroids

Secretion: Under basal conditions, the adrenal cortex secretes 15 to 25 mg (12 to 15 mg/M^2) of cortisol and 1.5 to 4 mg of corticosterone, the major natural glucocorticoids, daily. In man, aldosterone is physiologically the most important mineralocorticoid secreted by the adrenal cortex; 30 to 150 mcg is produced daily with the rate of secretion inversely related to dietary sodium intake. Desoxycorticosterone is secreted in approximately the same quantity but has only 3% to 5% of the sodium-retaining activity of aldosterone on an equimolar basis. This compound is of historical interest because it was the first corticosteroid synthesized and made available for clinical use.

RELATIVE POTENCIES OF THE SYSTEMIC CORTICOSTEROIDS

Compound (Or Its Esters)	Approximate Glucocorticoid Potency Compared to Cortisol (mg for mg basis)	Mineralocorticoid Potency	Equivalent Dose
Cortisol (hydrocortisone)	1.0	+ +	20.0 mg
Betamethasone	30	0	0.6 mg
Cortisone	0.8	+ +	25.0 mg
*Desoxycorticosterone	≈0	+ + + +	
Dexamethasone	30	0	0.75 mg
*Fludrocortisone	15	+ + + + +	
Fluprednisolone	10	0	1.5 mg
Meprednisone	5	0	4.0 mg
Methylprednisolone	5	0	4.0 mg
Paramethasone	10	0	2.0 mg
Prednisolone	4	+	5.0 mg
Prednisone	4	+	5.0 mg
Triamcinolone	5	0	4.0 mg

*Used only for mineralocorticoid effect.

The adrenal cortex also secretes androgens, principally dehydroepiandrosterone (DHEA) and smaller amounts of androstenedione and testosterone. The adrenal androgens do not normally exert a strong masculinizing effect; however, in women, they may be responsible for the slight masculinization that sometimes occurs after menopause; sexual hair development; and for support of normal libido. The importance of adrenal androgens in normal pubertal development in both sexes is debated. Physiologically insignificant quantities of estrogens are also secreted by the adrenal cortex. In hyperfunctional secretory states or with certain types of adrenal tumors, overproduction of adrenal androgens or estrogens and their metabolites can produce their typical effects on responsive tissues.

Glucocorticoid steroidogenesis and secretion is stimulated by corticotropin (ACTH), whose action on the adrenal cortex is mediated via cyclic adenosine monophosphate (cAMP). The adrenal cortex does not store appreciable amounts of glucocorticoids; the corticotropin signal results in a tightly coupled dual effect of stimulating steroidogenesis and secretion. The responses occur within one or two minutes and are completed in less than one hour after maximal stimulation.

Corticotropin is produced in basophilic cells of the anterior pituitary gland, and its secretion is stimulated by a putative corticotropin releasing hormone (CRH, corticoliberin), the chemical structure of which is unknown. CRH is synthesized in the hypothalamus and transported to the anterior pituitary gland by the hypophyseal portal blood vessels. Corticotropin secretion is inhibited by a negative feedback effect of glucocorticoids (chiefly cortisol), probably at both the hypothalamus (decreasing CRH secretion) and directly at the anterior pituitary gland.

Stimulation of CRH and, therefore, of corticotropin secretion occurs in response to two types of extrahypothalamic central nervous system signals: The first, basal secretion, is stimulated by neural signals relayed from anterior areas of the brain, including the amygdala, and displays circadian rhythmicity. In individuals maintaining a normal sleep-activity cycle, peak blood levels occur before arising (between 4 and 8 AM), with periodic bursts of secretion superimposed upon the basic pattern during the period of maximum secretion. The corticotropin secretion nadir occurs in the late evening. The second type of neural input occurs in response to stressful stimuli (trauma, anxiety, severe infections, hypoglycemia, surgery) and the signals enter the hypothalamus from both anterior and posterior brain areas, the latter probably arising from the reticular formation. The amount of corticotropin secreted at any time is the result of integration of the negative feedback of circulating glucocorticoids and the neural signals associated with basal secretion and response to stress. Severe stress is the most potent stimulus of corticotropin secretion. It supercedes other influences and can result in a tenfold increase in glucocorticoid secretion, but the levels achieved are below those attainable by administration of corticosteroids.

As with glucocorticoids, there is no appreciable storage of aldosterone in the adrenal cortex, and the rates of synthesis and secretion are essentially equal. Aldosterone secretion is partly controlled by the renin-angiotensin system. Decreased blood volume (sometimes causing orthostatic hypotension) and plasma sodium levels stimulate renin production and, ultimately, aldosterone secretion. Corticotropin usually plays only a minor role but large pharmacologic doses also stimulate secretion of aldosterone. Aldosterone does not exert a negative feedback effect on corticotropin production. Plasma aldosterone secretion displays circadian rhythmicity with maximum levels observed after arising in the morning.

The secretion of adrenal androgens is stimulated by corticotropin. Pituitary gonadotropins only stimulate secretion of gonadal sex steroids. Adrenal sex steroids exert no feedback effect on pituitary corticotropin secretion.

Transport and Metabolism: The major proportion of corticosteroids is transported in the blood, reversibly bound to albumin and corticosteroid-binding globulin (CBG).

It is generally accepted that the unbound hormone is the active form which exerts physiologic effects and is available for metabolism. Natural and some synthetic corticosteroids compete for binding to CBG (eg, dexamethasone is not bound to CBG), with cortisol having the highest and aldosterone the lowest affinity. More than 90% of plasma cortisol is protein bound, over 50% to CBG, while only 50% of circulating aldosterone is protein bound, principally to albumin. The chemical structures of the synthetic corticosteroids interfere with their ability to compete for binding to CBG; therefore, they are only about 70% protein bound, and a larger proportion of free hormone is available to exert a therapeutic effect. This may explain why relatively small doses of some synthetic preparations cause cushingoid effects.

In certain conditions in which total blood corticosteroid levels are elevated or decreased, the negative feedback mechanism maintains normal functional levels of the free fraction. For example, during pregnancy or in patients taking estrogens, CBG concentration and thus total plasma corticosteroid levels are elevated, but the physiologically active unbound portion remains functionally normal. When protein binding is altered (disease- or drug-induced), this effect must be taken into account when interpreting certain adrenal function tests.

Natural corticosteroids have relatively short plasma half-lives, ranging from 30 minutes for aldosterone to 90 minutes for cortisol. The plasma half-lives of the synthetic glucocorticoids are variable and those steroids used clinically all have longer half-lives than cortisol; they range from 90 minutes to over four hours. This variability is due to the effects that altering the chemical structure have on plasma protein and tissue binding and metabolism.

The tissue half-lives determine the duration of biological effectiveness; although they generally correlate positively with plasma half-lives, the relationships are not linear. Tissue half-lives range from 8 to 12 hours for cortisol to about three days for dexamethasone.

Seventy percent or more of endogenous corticosteroid is metabolized in the liver, where physiologically inactive water-soluble conjugates are formed. These are excreted in the urine.

Effects of Corticosteroids in Physiologic Concentrations

Corticosteroids exert seemingly diverse effects on physiologic systems through a mechanism that is gradually being understood and is probably common to all steroid hormones: They influence the cellular production of proteins. The steroid molecule enters cells where it forms complexes with specific receptor proteins in target cells. This steroid-receptor complex enters the nucleus where the transcription of a messenger RNA is influenced (probably through an action of the protein moiety of the complex). The result is control of the nature and rate of manufacture of proteins (eg, enzymes) that are ultimately responsible for carrying out the biological activities of the respective hormone. The time course necessary for corticosteroids to accomplish their biological functions is in the range of hours.

Corticosteroids play important roles in almost all systems of the body. These are summarized below.

Intermediary Metabolism: Glucocorticoids affect carbohydrate, protein, and fat metabolism; in contrast, mineralocorticoids serve no function in this area. In general, the glucocorticoids enhance glucose availability and stimulate protein catabolism and lipolysis. They increase glucose availability by (1) stimulating hepatic gluconeogenesis, whereby amino acids are supplied from extrahepatic protein catabolism, as well as stimulating induction of enzymes (transaminases) involved in gluconeogenesis and amino acid metabolism; as a result of protein catabolic processes, urinary excretion of nitrogen is increased; (2) decreasing glucose utilization (anti-insulin effect); and (3) stimulating glycogen storage, particularly by the liver. Glucocorticoid insufficiency results in glucose being less readily available and causes hypersensitivity to insulin.

The mobilization of fatty acids from adipose tissue is enhanced by glucocorticoids, probably because they facilitate the lipolytic response to cAMP. However, there is no consistent change in blood lipid levels.

Water and Electrolyte Balance: The major effects of corticosteroids on water and electrolyte balance are exerted by mineralocorticoids through their control of the renal excretion of cations. Mineralocorticoids promote reabsorption of small but significant portions of filtered sodium in the distal tubules; 98% of filtered sodium is absorbed by active and passive mechanisms before reaching the distal tubules. The renal excretion of potassium and hydrogen ions is enhanced by mineralocorticoids. As a result of these actions, severe mineralocorticoid deficiency produces excessive sodium loss resulting in a hypoosmotic intracellular compartment, decreased extracellular fluid volume, hyperkalemia, mild acidosis, and, eventually, circulatory and renal failure and death. Mineralocorticoids also stimulate sodium reabsorption across other epithelial tissues (eg, colonic mucosa, exocrine pancreatic ducts, sweat and salivary glands).

Glucocorticoids also are involved in the regulation of water balance. In glucocorticoid deficiency, the glomerular filtration rate decreases and antidiuretic hormone (ADH) concentration increases, resulting in an inability to excrete a water load. Administration of a glucocorticoid restores normal function. The glucocorticoids also affect calcium balance by decreasing intestinal uptake and increasing renal excretion.

Cardiovascular System and Blood: Both glucocorticoids and mineralocorticoids play important roles in supporting normal cardiovascular function. Although the mechanism is poorly understood, glucocorticoids appear to be necessary for the vasoconstrictor action of adrenergic stimuli on small vessels. In the absence of glucocorticoids, there is inadequate vasomotor response, decreased blood pressure, and increased capillary permeability. Mineralocorticoids help maintain normal

blood volume by stimulating sodium retention. In deficiency states, hypotension and cardiovascular collapse may occur as a result of decreased volume and increased blood viscosity.

Glucocorticoids increase hemoglobin, erythrocytes, and polymorphonuclear leukocytes in the blood and elevate the total white blood cell count. In contrast, they decrease eosinophils, basophils, monocytes, and lymphocytes. The observation that daily fluctuations occur in blood eosinophil levels is of historical interest because it led to the discovery of the circadian rhythm of glucocorticoid secretion.

Central Nervous System: In general, the role the corticosteroids play in central nervous system function is poorly defined but, in part, it is secondary to their effects on carbohydrate metabolism, electrolyte balance, and cerebral blood flow. Corticosteroids also influence mood, sleep patterns, and EEG activity. Adrenal insufficiency is associated with changes in mood (irritability and depression) and with greater than usual EEG slow wave activity. Both conditions are relieved by administration of glucocorticoids. Seizure thresholds are lowered by glucocorticoids and elevated by mineralocorticoids. The net effect in adrenalectomized animals is lowering of the threshold (increased excitability) to various seizure-inducing stimuli.

Skeletal Muscle: Corticosteroids are required to maintain normal skeletal muscular strength. The muscular weakness of adrenal insufficiency probably is caused primarily by circulatory incompetence and, to a lesser extent, by disorders of carbohydrate metabolism and electrolyte balance.

Stress: Although the mechanisms involved have never been completely determined, two observations support the probable protective nature of increased glucocorticoid secretion in response to stressful stimuli: (1) Glucocorticoid secretion is immediately and greatly enhanced at the initiation of stress. (2) Patients experiencing severe stressful stimuli (eg, surgery) who are incapable of secreting additional glucocorticoids require exogenous administration of hormones to prevent circulatory collapse.

Two characteristics of severe stress in animals with adrenal insufficiency are hypoglycemia and hypotension. During most stress situations, both adrenal medullary and glucocorticoid secretion are increased, and these hormones have synergistic effects in increasing blood glucose levels and blood pressure. The exact function of the increased glucocorticoid requirement during stress is still incompletely defined.

Effects of Excessive Corticosteroid Secretion

Prolonged adrenal cortical hypersecretion due to abnormal corticotropin levels or adenoma has deleterious effects on the body systems affected by these hormones. Since the manifestations of Cushing's syndrome are almost identical to the side effects of therapy with pharmacologic doses of glucocorticoids in nonendocrine disorders, these are described in the section on Glucocorticoids in Nonendocrine Diseases, Adverse Reactions. The destructive effects of sustained excessive levels of glucocorticoids include osteoporosis, myopathy, skin atrophy and striae, abnormal fat distribution, abnormal glucose tolerance, and growth suppression in children.

Excessive secretion of mineralocorticoids (hyperaldosteronism) affects several body functions. Increased excretion of potassium and hydrogen ions results in hypokalemic alkalosis; this condition tends to reduce the amount of ionized, but not total, calcium in the blood and may result in tetany. Increased renal tubular reabsorption of sodium is associated initially with increased extracellular fluid volume. However, the serum sodium level eventually returns to normal or even low levels because of a renal "escape" phenomenon that may occur during long-term mineralocorticoid therapy. Although skeletal muscle weakness results from adrenal insufficiency as well as excessive levels of glucocorticoid or mineralocorticoid, the latter is caused by neuromuscular disturbance associated with hypokalemia. Hypertension frequently occurs with prolonged hypersecretion of aldosterone associated with normal or increased sodium intake.

Administration

Except where noted, the choice of corticosteroid preparation depends largely on the relative mineralocorticoid/glucocorticoid potency desired, the route of administration preferred, and the duration of action appropriate for the particular indication. Drugs that have similar relative potencies and durations of action generally are considered to be equivalent therapeutically. Factors such as cost, preference for older drugs for which cumulative experience is greater, bioavailability, and use of preparations with less capacity to suppress the hypothalamic-pituitary axis often dictate the choice of preparation.

Oral preparations are used most commonly for replacement therapy or in nonendocrine conditions requiring systemic administration. Parenteral preparations are employed when the patient is unable to take oral medication, for emergency administration, and for critically ill patients.

For nonendocrine disorders, a variety of routes of administration can be utilized. When possible, local rather than systemic administration is preferable so that the therapeutic effects can be concentrated on the diseased tissue. Examples include topical application in inflammatory dermatologic conditions, enemas for ulcerative colitis, topical ophthalmic preparations, intrasynovial injections for inflamed joints, and inhalant administration for asthma. Dosage must be regulated carefully for topical preparations because varying degrees of systemic absorption occur. The percentage of a topically applied dose absorbed depends upon factors such as the tissue involved, injury to the integument (eg, diaper rash with inflammation), the penetrating properties of the preparation, the method of application, and the rate of metabolic breakdown of the product. For example, significant systemic absorption occurs when topical dermatologic preparations are applied under occlusive dressings.

ADRENOCORTICAL REPLACEMENT THERAPY

Adequate corticosteroid secretion is important in the normal function of many systems of the body, and additional levels are required for successful response to stressful stimuli. When corticosteroid production is absent or deficient, replacement hormones must be provided.

Conditions requiring replacement therapy include those associated with destruction of the adrenal glands, inadequate corticotropin stimulation of the adrenal cortex, or impaired corticosteroid secretion caused by congenital defects in steroidogenesis. The goal of therapy is to provide enough exogenous hormone to maintain close to normal function in dependent body systems. The doses of glucocorticoids and mineralocorticoids used for replacement therapy are small compared to the pharmacologic quantities of glucocorticoids employed in treating nonendocrine diseases. In the latter case, these large doses have useful effects (anti-inflammatory and anti-immunological) but produce many adverse actions not encountered with use of physiologic concentrations.

Replacement of both glucocorticoids and mineralocorticoids is necessary in primary adrenocortical insufficiency (Addison's disease). In secondary adrenal insufficiency (caused by deficient corticotropin secretion), mineralocorticoid secretion is usually unaffected so that only a glucocorticoid is required. The nature of corticosteroid replacement in congenital adrenal hyperplasia (CAH) syndromes depends upon the nature of the enzymatic defect and the consequent degree of salt loss or retention.

In replacement therapy for primary or secondary adrenal insufficiency, it is desirable to simulate normal glucocorticoid secretory patterns. Administration of two-thirds of the daily dose in the morning and one-third in the afternoon approximates this pattern satisfactorily. When a mineralocorticoid is needed, it is customarily given once daily. In children with congenital adrenal hyperplasia, not only replacement of cortisol but also suppression of corticotropin secretion is required; for the optimum schedule, see the section on Congenital Adrenal Hyperplasia Syndromes.

Indications for Replacement Therapy

Primary Adrenocortical Insufficiency: Addison's disease is associated with adrenal atrophy which may be idiopathic or related to autoimmune disease or destruction of the cortex by tuberculosis, histoplasmosis, metastatic carcinoma, or hemorrhage. Signs and symptoms include weakness, weight loss, hyperpigmentation, anorexia, nausea, vomiting, hypoglycemia, hypotension, hyponatremia, and hyperkalemia. Since production of both cortisol and aldosterone is deficient, both mineralocorticoid and glucocorticoid replacement are necessary. The goals of therapy are to re-establish strength, weight, normal mental processes, normal blood pressure, and electrolyte balance.

Cortisol or cortisone is preferred for replacement therapy in chronic adrenocortical insufficiency because they possess both glucocorticoid and mineralocorticoid activity. A more potent mineralocorticoid is added to the regimen if orthostatic hypotension continues in spite of replacement therapy and a liberal salt intake. The mineralocorticoid most commonly used for this purpose (the only oral preparation available) is fludrocortisone [Florinef]; desoxycorticosterone (DOC) [Doca, Percorten] also can be used. Neither compound has significant glucocorticoid effects at the doses employed to achieve sodium balance.

Secondary and Tertiary Adrenocortical Insufficiency: *Secondary adrenocortical insufficiency* is caused by inadequate secretion of corticotropin as a result of surgical ablation or pituitary disease or prolonged administration of pharmacologic doses of glucocorticoids (see the section on Glucocorticoids in Nonendocrine Diseases, Precautions).

Tertiary adrenocortical insufficiency is caused by inadequate secretion of CRH (see Chapter 46, Agents Related to Anterior Pituitary and Hypothalamic Function). Both the secondary and tertiary forms have similar symptoms and they cannot presently be distinguished from one another. Mineralocorticoid secretion is generally not impaired, but dilutional hyponatremia may result from glucocorticoid insufficiency. Hyperpigmentation does not occur. Symptoms are those characteristic of glucocorticoid insufficiency, including fasting hypoglycemia, malaise, anorexia, inability to handle stress, and, in severe cases, vomiting.

Replacement therapy is the same for secondary and tertiary adrenal insufficiency. The dosage of glucocorticoid used (most commonly cortisol, cortisone, or prednisone) may be less than that employed for Addison's disease, but must be adjusted on an individual basis.

In panhypopituitarism, which requires replacement of thyroid as well as adrenal hormones, the corticosteroid should be administered alone for a few days until adrenal sufficiency is established. If thyroid hormone is administered first, there is a possibility of precipitating acute adrenal insufficiency.

Congenital Adrenal Hyperplasia Syndromes (CAH): In these syndromes, synthesis of cortisol and sometimes aldosterone is partially or completely interrupted due to an inherited enzyme deficiency. Clinical manifestations vary depending upon the specific enzyme(s) involved but, in all patients, the low cortisol levels cause excessive corticotropin to be secreted by the pituitary (lack of negative feedback) and a type of adrenal hyperplasia results which is distinct from that caused by corticotropin hypersecretion due to other etiologies. Hypersecretion of steroids prior to the enzyme block or production of steroids from an alternate pathway occurs. Therefore, symptoms may be related to either hormone deficiency or excess. For example, in the most common form of CAH (21-hydroxylase deficiency), hypersecretion of corticotropin (in response to low cortisol levels) causes secretion of an abnormally large amount of androgen while the pathways to cortisol and, in severe cases, to aldosterone, are partially blocked. Eventually, cortisol levels may be low to almost normal, depending upon the severity of the block and the resultant degree of stimulation by corticotropin. Androgen excess causes virilization of external genitalia in female infants or hirsutism later in life; in males, it causes precocious sexual development, although the testes remain immature. If the enzymatic defect is severe enough to cause aldosterone deficiency, salt loss also occurs. Other forms of CAH (11-β-hydroxylase and 17-hydroxylase deficiencies) induce hypertension through hypersecretion of desoxycorticosterone, a mineralocorticoid that exerts little effect on blood pressure at normal concentrations.

CAH syndromes are treated in the same manner as other types of adrenocortical insufficiency. Cortisol is replaced and salt is added to the diet (almost all patients with CAH have some degree of salt wasting). In patients with severe salt-losing forms of the syndrome, a mineralocorticoid also is prescribed. However, patients with hypertensive forms of CAH preferably are treated with an intermediate-acting glucocorticoid having minimal mineralocorticoid activity (eg, prednisone). Long-acting preparations (eg, dexamethasone) should be avoided because overdosage can occur and growth may be retarded. The patient should be observed for clinical evidence of adequate treatment (eg, rate of growth and bone maturation, signs of steroid insufficiency or excess). Laboratory tests that assist in determining dosage of the glucocorticoid are measurement of either the urinary excretion of 17-ketosteroids and pregnanetriol or, if available, serum levels of 17-hydroxyprogesterone, testosterone, or corticotropin, all of which are elevated in the untreated patient. In patients with the salt-losing form, careful evaluation of electrolyte concentrations is needed to determine a proper regimen. Mineralocorticoid replacement usually can be discontinued cautiously between the ages of 5 and 7 years. Glucocorticoid therapy must be continued throughout life. Usually, the dosage for the initial treatment of infants is greater than that required for maintenance.

In CAH, the schedule of maintenance therapy is similar to that for adrenal insufficiency (ie, two-thirds of the daily dosage in the morning, one-third in the afternoon). However, some clinicians prefer to administer the largest dose at bedtime, which theoretically provides maximum suppression of early morning corticotropin secretion.

Acute Adrenal Insufficiency (Crisis): Adrenal crisis can result from acute adrenal or pituitary failure (following neurosurgery, head trauma, or hemorrhagic shock), from failure to maintain adrenal replacement therapy, or from failure to provide additional corticosteroids to dependent patients subjected to stress. Symptoms may include fever, hypotension, dehydration, weakness, vomiting, and diarrhea. Crisis can be due to lack of cortisol or, in the classic Addisonian type, to sodium loss (mineralocorticoid deficiency) which results in more marked dehydration. The precise deficiency is difficult to distinguish and, in either case, rapid replacement of sodium, fluids, and glucocorticoids is required. Treatment consists of the intravenous administration of 100 mg of a soluble cortisol ester initially, followed by intravenous infusion of normal saline with dextrose containing additional cortisol. The amount of saline administered in the first 24 hours depends upon the degree of dehydration and is generally less than 5% of ideal body weight. The total dose of cortisol in the same period is 300 to 400 mg. The dose may be reduced gradually to replacement levels over several days.

Precautions

All patients receiving corticosteroid replacement therapy require supplemental doses during periods of stress. The dose must be increased in proportion to the severity of the stress. When mineralocorticoids are also required, the dose is not increased but adequate salt replacement must be assured or acute adrenal insufficiency (Addisonian crisis) may result.

Temporary, excessive doses of glucocorticoid are preferred to inadequate replacement. During mild illness, such as upper respiratory infections, doubling the glucocorticoid maintenance dose usually is sufficient. When oral intake of steroids is not possible for any reason, including vomiting, a parenteral preparation (cortisol, prednisolone phosphate or succinate, or dexamethasone sodium phosphate) can be given intramuscularly. Patients receiving replacement therapy who are undergoing major surgery require larger doses during the immediate pre- and postoperative period. Salt and fluid replacement must be assured. If the postoperative course is uncomplicated, the dose can be reduced gradually over a period of two to five days to the usual amount for replacement.

The patient's understanding of his steroid-dependent status and increased dosage requirement under widely variable conditions of stress is of utmost importance. All such patients should carry an identification card and bracelet indicating their dependence on steroid medication. In addition, care should be taken to assure that an adequate supply of steroids is available at all times for emergencies. This should include a sufficient supply of oral medication and a glucocorticoid preparation suitable for intramuscular injection. An injectable mineralocorticoid also should be available for patients requiring it. Older patients and parents of pediatric patients should be trained to administer these injections.

GLUCOCORTICOIDS IN NONENDOCRINE DISEASES

Corticosteroids having predominantly glucocorticoid activity are used most commonly to treat a wide variety of nonendocrine diseases. Efficacy is related to their anti-inflammatory and anti-immunologic actions. It must be emphasized that these extremely valuable therapeutic effects are not associated with normal physiologic concentrations of hormones, but only become apparent when pharmacologic doses are administered. Thus, patients receiving systemic therapy for nonendocrine disorders are at risk of developing cushingoid side effects, increased susceptibility to infection, and suppression of the hypothalamic-pituitary-adrenal (HPA) axis. Because of these possible complications, it is important to weigh the possible adverse effects against the expected benefits of therapy before initiating corticosteroid therapy.

Guidelines for the judicious use of corticosteroids include: (1) Accurate diagnosis should be made to confirm the presence of a steroid-responsive condition. (2) Corticosteroid therapy should be initiated only after alternative treatment has been ineffective. (3) The dosage should be determined according to the severity of the disease rather than the weight or age of the patient; the smallest dose that controls a specific symptom or sign should be used. The purpose of therapy is to achieve an acceptable degree of palliation but complete remission of symptoms is usually not an appropriate therapeutic goal. (4) Dosage and duration of therapy, particularly with systemic administration, influence the therapeutic response and occurrence of adverse reactions. Systemic administration of a single large dose is virtually without ill effects and may be lifesaving; this justifies use of such therapy in life-threatening emergencies when diagnosis is only tentative (eg, brain edema). Generally, the longer systemic glucocorticoid therapy is continued and the larger the dose, the greater the risk of adverse reactions. (5) When possible, the corticosteroid should be administered locally in order to concentrate therapeutic effects on the diseased tissue. (6) Pharmacologic doses of glucocorticoids should not be stopped abruptly to avoid adrenal crisis during the period of recovery of HPA axis responsiveness.

Anti-inflammatory and Anti-immunologic Effects

The therapeutic usefulness of glucocorticoids in nonendocrine disease states is related to their ability to retard normal inflammatory and immunologic responses. They suppress the inflammatory response whether this is part of a disease process or is the result of mechanical, chemical, or immunologic insult by suppressing circulating lymphocytes and monocytes. Sensitization of lymphocytes is blocked, and cell-mediated hypersensitivity reactions (including graft rejection) are inhibited.

Glucocorticoids probably exert their action at multiple sites. They do not block the interaction of antibodies of sensitized lymphocytes and antigen or the release of histamine or kinins that is initiated by this process. Rather, they block the usual tissue responses to these stimuli. Normally, histamine increases capillary permeability with resultant extravasation of fluid and protein and consequent formation of edema; during an antigen-antibody interaction, migration inhibitory factor (MIF) is released from the lymphocytes involved, which inhibits the mobility of macrophages and causes them to accumulate in the surrounding area. Glucocorticoids help to maintain capillary integrity, prevent the macrophage reaction to MIF, inhibit phagocytosis and digestion of antigens, and, in high tissue concentrations, may stabilize lysosomal membranes, thus preventing the release of hydrolytic enzymes. By inhibiting the inflammatory process at the cellular level, glucocorticoids decrease its superficial manifestations (eg, heat, redness, tenderness).

Precautions

Pharmacologic doses of glucocorticoids may suppress diagnostic signs and symptoms of disease through their anti-inflammatory and anti-immunologic actions. Perforation of a peptic ulcer may occur with minimal discomfort, and septicemia may progress without fever, probably due to an effect on hypothalamic temperature control or suppression of pyrogen production. Degradation of glucocorticoids is markedly increased in patients with hyperthyroidism. Pharmacologic doses of glucocorticoids have been given in some cases of thyrotoxic crisis (thyroid storm) because the compensatory increase in adrenal secretion may be inadequate in this condition.

Infection: Decreased resistance to infection occurs during prolonged treatment with pharmacologic doses of glucocorticoids. The same mechanisms that prevent tissue destruction caused by inflammation are also responsible for increasing the vulnerability of tissues to infectious agents. Glucocorticoid therapy predisposes the body to all types of infection (bacterial, viral, fungal, parasitic) but, in many cases, susceptibility may be due to the underlying disease (eg, systemic lupus erythematosus, leukemia). Fewer infections occur when the dose interval is increased, as in alternate-day therapy.

The body requires greater than normal amounts of glucocorticoids under conditions of stress, including infectious illnesses. Individuals with normal adrenal function secrete larger amounts of corticosteroids during the early phase of most infectious diseases. Those dependent on exogenous steroid therapy (whether for replacement or nonendocrine indications) require larger doses in stressful conditions, since they are unable to secrete adequate additional amounts of endogenous hormone. When infection occurs in patients treated for a prolonged period with pharmacologic amounts of glucocorticoids, a dilemma occurs: Administering the larger doses needed for the nonspecific, stress-related functions of glucocorticoids may further compromise resistance to infection. The usual solution is to provide the additional glucocorticoid required (usually doubling the normal dose for mild illness unless the patient is already taking more than 100 mg of prednisone or equivalent daily) and treat the patient concomitantly with an appropriate antimicrobial agent.

Hypothalamic-Pituitary-Adrenal Axis Suppression: Administration of exogenous glucocorticoids will result in some degree of suppression (negative feedback of glucocorticoid) of the hypothalamic-pituitary-adrenal (HPA) axis which is proportional to the size of the dose and duration of therapy. It must be assumed that

patients with such suppression are unable to secrete normal amounts of hormone or to respond to stress by increasing secretion if they have been receiving pharmacologic doses of exogenous hormones for a long period. The same precautions exercised by patients receiving adrenal replacement therapy, such as carrying a steroid identification card and bracelet and keeping emergency supplies of medication, are also applicable to those receiving these hormones for nonendocrine conditions. (See also the section on Adrenocortical Replacement Therapy, Precautions.)

There is wide individual variation in the dose and duration of treatment required to produce HPA suppression. In general, however, less than 5 mg prednisone daily (or the equivalent) causes little suppression. Doses smaller than 15 mg prednisone daily probably will not depress adrenal responsiveness if the duration of therapy is limited to one or two months, but larger doses or longer courses of therapy at this dosage level may result in profound suppression. Divided doses (three or four daily) are more suppressive than single doses, and steroids administered before bedtime are more suppressive than those given earlier in the day.

Withdrawal: When long-term glucocorticoid therapy for nonendocrine disease is terminated, the dosage should be reduced gradually to prevent rapid exacerbation of symptoms and avoid the possibility of adrenal insufficiency. The latter is of particular concern because of HPA suppression (see above). The adrenal gland begins to regain the ability to respond to corticotropin stimulation at daily doses of 5 to 7.5 mg of prednisone or the equivalent. Dosage reduction may begin by administering a single daily dose in the morning (to minimize suppression of corticotropin), then decreasing the dose by 25% weekly until replacement levels are reached. Therapy can then be eliminated on alternate days for one to two months before the drug is discontinued completely (Dluhy et al, 1975).

Recovery of HPA axis function occurs in two stages: First, normal basal cortisol secretion, which is preceded by elevated corticotropin levels, is usually achieved within several months and indicates recovery of adrenal responsiveness to corticotropin and resumption of the cortisol feedback mechanism. Second, normal corticotropin and cortisol secretory responses to stressful stimuli return. The entire process may occur rapidly or may require up to one year for completion; for this reason, patients who have received systemic glucocorticoid therapy within the past year should be given appropriate doses of steroids during times of stress.

Corticotropin injections have been used to accelerate recovery from adrenal atrophy. This is not useful, however, because HPA axis suppression is prolonged while adrenal secretion is stimulated.

In addition to the problems associated with suppression of the HPA axis, withdrawal of glucocorticoid therapy is frequently accompanied by a syndrome characterized by malaise, fever, myalgia, arthralgia, fatigue, and restlessness which may be mistaken for an exacerbation of the underlying disease, particularly in patients with diseases such as rheumatoid arthritis. To minimize these problems after long-term treatment, the dosage should be reduced gradually in appropriate decrements (ie, with larger dosage, decrements may be larger) (Ehrlich, 1978).

The tendency of some patients to become dependent on glucocorticoids should be noted. This may be particularly prevalent in patients given repeated courses of therapy for recurring symptoms (eg, those with asthma or certain dermatologic conditions). Since rapid relief and, sometimes, euphoria occur when glucocorticoid therapy is initiated, it may be difficult to convince the patient to accept repeated attempts to withdraw medication with its attendant discomforts.

Alternate-Day Therapy

After symptoms are controlled with daily use of glucocorticoids, some chronic diseases respond equally well to administration of intermediate-acting glucocorticoids (prednisone, prednisolone, methylpred-

nisolone) on alternate days. Alternate-day therapy is also effective for the initial treatment of childhood nephrosis. The advantages are less suppression of the HPA axis and a lower incidence of adverse effects. For example, when pharmacologic doses of glucocorticoids are given daily to children, the rate of growth is decreased; when alternate-day therapy is employed, children maintain normal growth patterns.

The alternate-day regimen consists of administering a 48-hour dose of an intermediate-acting glucocorticoid at 7 to 8 AM every other morning. This simulates the natural circadian rhythm of glucocorticoid secretion (early morning peak, evening nadir). Administration of the hormone in the morning results in less suppression of the hypothalamic-pituitary axis. Ideally, the level of *exogenous* hormone is high on the morning of treatment and that of *endogenous* hormone is high on the morning medication is withheld, for the HPA axis is not suppressed on that day. Because of established advantages, alternate-day therapy is preferred for maintenance whenever feasible.

This regimen is reported to be particularly effective in the treatment of asthma, systemic lupus erythematosus, uveitis, and nephrotic syndrome. However, some patients, especially those with rheumatoid arthritis and adults with ulcerative colitis, become symptomatic or experience an exacerbation on the day that glucocorticoids are withheld. They may respond to an increase in dosage. If symptoms persist, a single daily dose may be necessary and is preferred to a divided-dose schedule.

Indications

Allergic Disorders: These agents provide prompt palliation of symptoms in many allergic states, including bronchial asthma; nonseasonal allergic rhinitis; hay fever (pollinosis, seasonal allergic rhinitis); reactions to drugs, serum, and transfusions; and dermatoses with an allergic component. Their use is generally reserved for control of acute episodes; they are not a substitute for conventional measures, such as other medication (eg, theophylline for asthma, antihistamines for hay fever) or avoidance of allergens. In emergencies (eg, anaphylactic reactions, status asthmaticus), glucocorticoids should be employed only as adjuncts to the immediate use of epinephrine, cardiorespiratory support, and, in status asthmaticus, a theophylline derivative. (See also the section on Respiratory Disorders.)

Hematologic Disorders: Most cases of idiopathic and acquired *autoimmune hemolytic anemia* respond to glucocorticoids; they are sometimes the sole therapeutic agents utilized. Glucocorticoids do not reduce hemolysis in *transfusion reactions*, although they may lessen drug-induced hemolysis (eg, that produced by methyldopa). In *erythroblastopenia* (pure erythrocyte aplasia, congenital hypoplastic anemia, Blackfan-Diamond syndrome), small maintenance doses on alternate days may eliminate dependence on transfusion and may be the treatment of choice. Glucocorticoids rarely may produce remissions of variable length in *aplastic anemia*; however, if there is no improvement in cellular production after two months of therapy, further use should be reserved for amelioration of complications. Although they do not shorten the duration of disease, glucocorticoids are useful in the early stages of *thrombocytopenic purpura*, because they may reduce the probability of life-threatening intracranial hemorrhages, possibly by improving capillary integrity. In children, the usefulness of glucocorticoids in acute thrombocytopenic purpura or in increasing platelet counts is not universally accepted. Glucocorticoids are of no proven value in the treatment of acute agranulocytosis.

Because of their lympholytic effects, glucocorticoids are used to treat certain *hematologic malignancies* of lymphoid origin (lymphatic leukemia; lymphomas, including Hodgkin's disease; multiple myeloma). A combination of drugs is usually employed. Prednisone and vincristine produce remissions in about 90% of children with acute *lymphoblastic leukemia* and therapeutic responses occur in about 50% of patients with *chronic lymphocytic leukemia*. These drugs are not effective in the treatment of *chronic myelocytic leukemias*. They may be used to treat complications of lymphoid malignancies such as thrombocytopenia, hemolytic anemia, and hypercalcemia.

Cerebral Edema: The effectiveness of glucocorticoids in the treatment of cerebral edema depends upon the underlying cause. They are most effective when edema is caused by brain tumors, especially metastases and glioblastomas, and are somewhat less effective in that caused by astrocytomas and meningiomas. Edema resulting from brain abscesses responds to glucocorticoid therapy and that produced by closed head injury is least responsive. Glucocorticoids have been used with increasing frequency for brain edema associated with stroke, but opinion is divided on their efficacy. They are also used with mannitol to treat brain edema associated with Reye's syndrome, but this practice is not universal. Dexamethasone is commonly chosen for treatment for this indication because of its low mineralocorticoid activity, since very large doses are employed.

Collagen Disorders: Generally, steroids are most beneficial in these conditions when large doses are given during acute exacerbations; the desirability and effectiveness of long-term maintenance therapy are variable. Various manifestations of *systemic lupus erythematosus* may be controlled by glucocorticoids. Topical preparations may be used if dermatologic symptoms predominate, and systemic therapy is appropriate when nephritis, central nervous system disturbances, and hematologic complications, such as hemolytic anemia or thrombocytopenia, are present. Both clinical symptoms and serologic values (eg, serum complement, anti-DNA antibodies) have been reported to be useful in determining effective dosage, with resultant improvement in survival rates (Urman and Rothfield, 1977). Short-term use of large doses (1 to 2 mg/kg of body weight of prednisone or the equivalent) may be required for remission, particularly when the central nervous system is involved. Fewer exacerbations occur if the dosage is reduced gradually at the rate of 10% of the daily dose per week after the patient's condition stabilizes (Yount et al, 1975). Immunosuppressive agents, such as azathioprine [Imuran] and cyclophosphamide [Cytoxan], have been used in conjunction with glucocorticoid therapy for severe symptoms, but the effectiveness of such combinations compared to the use of steroids alone remains unproved.

Polymyositis and *dermatomyositis* are treated initially with large doses of glucocorticoids; the amount can be decreased gradually after the initial response, but maintenance therapy may be required for years.

Steroids relieve the signs of *polyarteritis nodosa*. They may improve survival during the first year, but survival time after four or five years is not affected.

Polymyalgia rheumatica occurs in older patients (usually over 60 years) and is improved by glucocorticoids. These patients have a high incidence of *temporal arteritis* in which there is a risk of sudden and irreversible blindness. Prompt institution of glucocorticoid therapy (1 mg/kg of prednisone daily or the equivalent) within the first 24 hours after developing symptoms rarely results in recovery of vision. Administration of steroids may prevent involvement of the second eye.

Glucocorticoid therapy in *mixed connective tissue disease* (MCTD) is similar to that for systemic lupus erythematosus. Differential diagnosis of MCTD and systemic scleroderma is essential, however, because glucocorticoids do not improve the vascular lesions or fibrosis produced by the latter.

Dermatologic Diseases: Topical glucocorticoid preparations relieve the signs and symptoms of many *allergic, inflammatory*, and *pruritic dermatoses*. If possible, the causal agents should be identified and eliminated. Severe *sunburn*, nonvenomous *insect bites*, acute self-limiting *eczematous conditions*, and the cutaneous manifestations of some *collagen diseases* (see above), such as systemic lupus erythematosus and dermatomyositis, also may respond to topical therapy.

Intralesional injection of glucocorticoids may be utilized in the treatment of *psoriasis, alopecia areata*, and *keloids*. However, atrophy or sloughing of the skin may occur at the site of injection (see Chapter 61, Dermatologic Preparations), and systemic administration on an alternate-day schedule may be preferable.

Systemic administration of glucocorticoids can be lifesaving in *pemphigus vulgaris*. Initially, massive doses (120 to 300 mg of prednisone or the equivalent daily) are used to control acute exacerbations. Prolonged suppression of symptoms usually requires long-term maintenance therapy (alternate-day therapy is sometimes successful) but, occasionally, spontaneous remissions allow gradual withdrawal of therapy. Other agents (azathioprine, gold salts, methotrexate, cyclophosphamide) are sometimes used instead of glucocorticoids in mild cases; concomitantly to allow use of smaller maintenance doses of glucocorticoids; or to replace glucocorticoids as they are gradually withdrawn in maintenance therapy. The immunofluorescent test for pemphigus can be used to titrate the dose of glucocorticoid to determine the best fully effective long-term dosage.

Gastrointestinal Diseases: Glucocorticoids are used as part of a comprehensive program in the management of *inflammatory bowel disorders* and to induce remission in acute attacks. Local application using enemas, rectal drip, or foam is preferred to systemic therapy, although some absorption (20% to 50%, depending upon the condition of the mucosa) does occur with rectal administration. Sulfasalazine [Azulfidine, S.A.S.-500], phthalylsulfathiazole [Sulfathalidine], or certain other antibiotics also are given while the dose of glucocorticoid is gradually reduced and may be administered for prolonged periods in an attempt to maintain remission. Alternate-day therapy during the period of glucocorticoid withdrawal may be successful but daily therapy must be resumed if symptoms persist. Gradual discontinuation of glucocorticoid therapy is usually possible in patients with ulcerative colitis.

The place of glucocorticoids in the treatment of *Crohn's disease* has not been completely determined, but many patients respond to systemic therapy in the early stages of the disease; acute inflammatory manifestations also are responsive. Long-term therapy appears to be beneficial in some patients. (See Chapter 58, Anti-diarrheal Agents.)

Hypercalcemia: Pharmacologic doses of glucocorticoids are generally effective in the treatment of hypercalcemia due to increased intestinal absorption of calcium, because they antagonize the effects of vitamin D; they are, therefore, effective in hypervitaminosis D, sarcoidosis, adrenal insufficiency, and breast cancer. Glucocorticoids also prevent hypercalcemia in patients with multiple myeloma by decreasing reabsorption of calcium from the bone. They usually are ineffective in hypercalcemia caused by increased levels of parathyroid hormone, either from hyperparathyroidism or neoplasms (lung, renal, pancreatic) that secrete a parathyroid hormone-like substance. (See Chapter 54, Agents Affecting Calcium Metabolism.)

Hepatic Diseases: The effectiveness and safety of glucocorticoids in the treatment of liver disease depend upon the form involved and, sometimes, the condition of the patient. These agents are used in the initial therapy of subacute hepatic necrosis (60 to 100 mg/day of prednisolone) and chronic active hepatitis. Medication is withdrawn gradually when there are signs of maximal improvement; if relapse occurs, more prolonged therapy is required. Concomitant administration of azathioprine (1 to 1.5 mg/kg of body weight) may be helpful and sometimes allows the dosage of glucocorticoid to be reduced.

In alcoholic hepatitis, the beneficial effects of glucocorticoid therapy are probably limited to seriously ill patients, in whom survival rates are enhanced. These agents may be used with prophylactic doses of isoniazid in sarcoidosis when acute inflammatory changes coexist with functional abnormalities as demonstrated by liver biopsy. Glucocorticoids also may be effective in other types of hepatic granulomata,

except those due to infections or neoplasms.

Glucocorticoids may be beneficial in some cases of drug-induced hepatic disorders, but controlled studies on which to base guidelines are lacking. Whether these agents are effective in biliary cirrhosis or infectious mononucleosis has not been adequately demonstrated. They are *not* indicated for the treatment of acute viral hepatitis or inactive postnecrotic cirrhosis.

Some patients with liver disease may have low levels of albumin; since albumin is partially responsible for binding glucocorticoids in the blood, the excessive levels of free (biologically active) hormone that result may require an appropriate adjustment in dosage. When liver function is altered by disease, hepatic metabolism of drugs may be compromised: Normally, prednisone is readily converted to its active form, prednisolone, but this conversion may be partially inhibited in patients with hepatic damage. Therefore, prednisolone is theoretically preferable to prednisone in patients with functional liver damage, although the two preparations can be considered equivalent in other patients (Lesene and Fallon, 1975).

Neuromuscular Disease: Glucocorticoids are usually reserved for patients with severe myasthenia gravis who have not responded to anticholinesterase therapy and thymectomy. Because symptoms may worsen during the first ten days of glucocorticoid therapy, such treatment should be carried out in the hospital where ventilatory support equipment is readily available. Patients can be given 10 mg of prednisolone initially, increased by 10 mg daily to a maintenance dose of 80 to 120 mg daily, or 25 mg can be given initially, increasing the dose to 100 mg given on alternate days (*Drug and Therapeutics Bulletin,* 1977). Treatment may be withdrawn gradually after several months. Glucocorticoid therapy may permit reduction in the dose of anticholinesterase agents and may produce prolonged remission. The mechanism by which steroids are effective in this disease has not been resolved but probably involves suppression of an immunoglobulin that binds to the acetylcholine receptor of the neuromuscular junction.

Glucocorticoids have been used to hasten remission in some cases of acute *multiple sclerosis*; alternate-day therapy has been successful. These agents probably act by reducing the inflammatory response within the developing plaque. In the small number of patients who become dependent on steroids, low-dosage maintenance therapy is useful.

Ocular Disorders: Ocular disorders that respond to glucocorticoid therapy include allergic and inflammatory conditions (eg, vernal conjunctivitis, contact dermatitis of the lids and conjunctiva, allergic blepharitis and conjunctivitis, episcleritis, scleritis, temporal arteritis, sterile uveal tract inflammations). Agents may be administered topically, subconjunctivally, systemically, or by retrobulbar injection, depending upon the disease.

Glucocorticoids are generally contraindicated in ocular infections because, by suppressing the inflammatory response, they may mask progression of the infection. However, if vision is threatened by acute, severe uveitis or stromal edema, steroids may be used cautiously in conjunction with appropriate anti-infective therapy (see also Chapter 24, Ocular Anti-infective and Anti-inflammatory Agents). Glucocorticoids are not useful in degenerative diseases such as cataracts (see the section on Adverse Reactions).

When visual acuity is decreased as a result of progressive exophthalmos in Graves' disease, glucocorticoids may be beneficial; decompression surgery may be avoided in some cases.

Renal Disease: In children with the minimal lesion form of idiopathic nephrotic syndrome (INS), glucocorticoid treatment usually induces a remission. Various regimens are used, including both daily and alternate-day programs; 80% to 90% of children respond to treatment within four to eight weeks, although a three-month course of treatment is usual. Two-thirds of those who respond never experience relapse or do so infrequently (no more than once yearly), in which case they may be given repeated courses of glucocorticoids.

The remaining one-third of those who respond have relapses more frequently (two to four times yearly) and may require more prolonged glucocorticoid therapy, preferably on an alternate-day schedule. A regimen consisting of prednisone with one of the alkylating agents (cyclophosphamide [Cytoxan] or chlorambucil [Leukeran]) may be more successful in maintaining remission in frequently relapsing children than prednisone alone (Bacon and Spencer, 1975; *Br Med J*, 1977). Adults with IMS respond to alternate-day prednisone therapy depending upon the subtype present; in decreasing order of responsiveness these are: minimal change nephrosis, membranous nephropathy, diffuse proliferative nephritis, and focal sclerosis (Bolton et al, 1977).

Respiratory Disorders: Glucocorticoids are used in the emergency treatment of status asthmaticus. Long-term therapy may be necessary in *asthma* if conventional measures fail to suppress symptoms. Inhalation of the locally acting glucocorticoid, beclomethasone [Beclovent, Vanceril], may avoid the adverse effects produced by systemic therapy (see also Chapter 32, Drugs Used in Asthma).

The clinical manifestations and complications of *pulmonary tuberculosis* have been treated with a regimen consisting of glucocorticoids and antimycobacterial agents. Although glucocorticoids are useful in treating pleural and pericardial effusions by suppressing inflammation and the formation of fibrous tissue, their use in pulmonary tuberculosis is generally not encouraged. Initial improvement (eg, weight gain, sense of well-being, clearing of pulmonary infiltrate, more rapid elimination of tubercle bacilli from sputum) may be noted, but results are not significantly altered after several months of combined therapy. Short-term glucocorticoid therapy is useful in treating hypersensitivity reactions to antimycobacterial drugs, however.

Glucocorticoids have palliative effects in *pulmonary sarcoidosis* but apparently have little effect on the development of pulmonary fibrosis or the eventual outcome of the disease.

Aspiration pneumonia with serious impairment of pulmonary function occurs within hours after aspiration of the liquid contents of the stomach. Prompt administration of large doses of glucocorticoids has been recommended to reduce the extent of lung damage and decrease the mortality rate. However, the success of this method has not been confirmed, and it has been suggested that administration of glucocorticoids for this indication may actually increase the risk of gram-negative pneumonia.

The *respiratory distress syndrome* (RDS) in neonates can be prevented by the antenatal administration of glucocorticoids. These agents may induce enzymes that accelerate the production of lung surfactant by type 2 pneumocytes; therapy after the development of RDS does not enhance survival because there is a latent period of up to several days before enzyme induction occurs. Glucocorticoid therapy may be considered in pregnancies of less than 34 weeks' gestation or in more advanced pregnancies when the lecithin:sphingomyelin (L/S) ratio is less than 2, indicating immaturity of the production apparatus for lung surfactant and increased likelihood of developing RDS. During premature labor, a uterine relaxant (eg, intravenous ethyl alcohol) is administered concurrently with the glucocorticoid to delay labor for 24 to 48 hours. This treatment is not indicated for women with severe pre-eclampsia or conditions in which immediate delivery is necessary for survival of mother or infant (ie, abruptio placentae, placenta previa).

Two intramuscular injections of betamethasone [Celestone Soluspan] (12 mg, 24 hours apart) given 24 hours to seven days before premature delivery significantly reduced the incidence of respiratory distress syndrome (Ballard and Ballard, 1976). Dexamethasone [Decadron, Hexadrol] also has been beneficial (Caspi et al, 1976). In one study (Block et al, 1977), it was reported that methylprednisolone [Medrol] was ineffective when compared to betamethasone. It has been suggested that betamethasone is preferable to cortisol, prednisone, or prednisolone because the maternal:fetal ratio is lower, thus allowing administration of a relatively smaller effective dose (Ballard et al, 1975). However, in another study, the effects of intravenous cortisol were observed nine hours earlier than those of intramuscular betamethasone, and it was concluded that the former is preferred when rapid action is necessary (Whitt et al, 1976).

In pregnancies complicated by severe pre-eclampsia, the number of fetal deaths was reported to be increased after glucocorticoid therapy, but no other adverse effects have been observed. Apgar scores and onset of lactation are unaffected, and postpartum fever is not observed more frequently. Although the endogenous cortisol level is suppressed in the neonate for several days, adrenal insufficiency has not been reported. In children followed for four years after treatment, no significant alterations of growth or development have been observed. The possibility that a long latent period or rare adverse effect associated with this treatment may eventually be identified cannot be ignored, however, and continued monitoring of children given this treatment is necessary before this form of therapy can be accepted unequivocally.

Rheumatic Disorders: Corticosteroids are not indicated as initial therapy for rheumatoid arthritis but may be useful adjuncts to nonsteroidal anti-inflammatory agents, rest, and physical therapy. Steroids are used only in the active, reversible phases of disease. Systemic administration usually is unnecessary but, when employed, periodic attempts to withdraw medication should be made; this should be done very gradually to avoid withdrawal symptoms or exacerbation of disease. Alternate-day therapy may not be satisfactory in rheumatoid arthritis because symptoms are more pronounced on the day on which medication is withheld.

When only a few joints are persistently inflamed, occasional intra-articular injection can be employed. There is usually dramatic relief of symptoms initially, but inflammation tends to recur and discomfort is sometimes more intense following cessation of treatment. This route should not be employed if infection in the joint is suspected because steroids may accelerate the course of the infection. (See also Chapter 7, Antiarthritic Drugs.)

Shock: Although glucocorticoids are commonly used to treat shock, they are clearly indicated only for that produced by adrenocortical insufficiency (Addisonian shock). When adrenal response to stress is normal, maximal endogenous levels of adrenal corticosteroids are being secreted. However, pharmacologic doses may be of additional therapeutic benefit. The mechanism by which corticosteroids act in shock is not understood, but probably involves effects on cellular and subcellular membranes with consequent effects on cellular metabolism. Although clinical evidence is limited and equivocal, it appears that glucocorticoids are ineffective in the treatment of cardiogenic, hypovolemic, or traumatic shock but they may be useful in septic shock.

A small percentage of patients with septic shock may suffer from relative adrenal insufficiency and are unable to respond appropriately to the severe stress caused by infection. This may account for the variable results reported after glucocorticoid therapy; such therapy may benefit only those patients with inadequate endogenous supplies of adrenal corticosteroids. On the other hand, pharmacologic doses may be necessary to counteract the detrimental effects of bacterial endotoxins. When corticosteroids are used to treat septic shock, they are usually given for short periods in massive doses and are discontinued when the patient's condition is stabilized.

Adverse Reactions

Corticosteroids have many potential adverse effects which, in most instances, are extensions of their pharmacologic actions. The incidence of adverse reactions correlates with the dose, frequency and route of administration, duration of therapy, the age and condition of the patient, and the underlying disease.

Gastrointestinal Reactions: Glucocorticoids decrease the protection provided by the gastric mucus barrier, interfere with tissue repair, and, in some patients, increase gastric acid and pepsinogen production. There is no universal agreement on whether the steroids per se are responsible for peptic ulcers encountered during therapy. However, glucocorticoid therapy may mask the symptoms of peptic ulcer so that perforation or hemorrhage occurs without antecedent pain, and periodic examination of the stools for occult blood is suggested. Although theoretically useful, there is no evidence that prophylactic administration of antacids prevents ulcer formation. Nevertheless, most physicians prescribe antacids for patients on long-term glucocorticoid therapy.

A review of prospective single- or double-blind studies including data from over 5,000 patients has cast doubt on the degree to which corticosteroid therapy is responsible for the development, reactivation, or perforation and bleeding of peptic ulcers (Conn and Blitzer, 1976). Occurrence of peptic ulcers was not significantly correlated with increased daily dosage, and the incidence of hemorrhage was not higher among patients receiving steroids compared to those given a placebo. However, there was some indication that the frequency of peptic ulcer was increased in patients receiving total doses greater than 1 g of prednisone or the equivalent. Consistent with this finding is the observation that patients with cirrhosis or the nephrotic syndrome have an increased tendency to develop peptic ulcer while receiving corticosteroids. This may be related to their hypoalbuminemic condition with decreased plasma protein-binding of corticosteroid resulting in a higher unbound (biologically active) quantity of circulating steroid, although it also may be associated with their general catabolic state.

Edema: Since glucocorticoids with little or no mineralocorticoid activity are now available, electrolyte imbalance is observed less frequently. Edema is best treated by prevention; dietary restriction of sodium at the inception of steroid therapy is urged. If edema occurs, sodium intake should be sharply reduced initially; if edema persists, the patient should receive a glucocorticoid less likely to produce sodium retention. However, caution is required if large doses of any corticosteroid are given for prolonged periods to patients with cardiovascular or severe renal disease, for even slight fluid retention may be dangerous.

Hypokalemia: Severe hypokalemia may cause asthenia, paralysis, or arrhythmias that may proceed to cardiac arrest. The incidence of hypokalemia is related to the mineralocorticoid activity of a specific glucocorticoid and can be avoided in most patients by dietary restriction of sodium and ingestion of foods rich in potassium (eg, bananas). Potassium-wasting diuretics (eg, thiazides) taken concurrently with corticosteroids may cause further potassium loss. (See also Chapter 51, Replenishers and Regulators of Water and Electrolytes.)

Osteoporosis: This common but infrequently recognized adverse effect is associated with long-term use of large doses of glucocorticoids. In some cases, it is difficult to determine the extent to which the underlying disease or glucocorticoid therapy contributes to the development of osteoporosis. Vertebral compression fractures may occur with little or no trauma. This disease may be observed in children with nephrosis, a condition not normally associated with osteoporosis, when long-term treatment with large doses of glucocorticoids is necessary. On the other hand, the incidence of fractures from generalized osteoporosis is high in patients with rheumatoid arthritis regardless of whether glucocorticoids are used in therapy. It also is more likely to occur in postmenopausal women. Nevertheless, prolonged use of glucocorticoids in these patients should be undertaken only after careful consideration. Whenever the underlying illness permits, the patient should be encouraged to be ambulatory. (See also Chapter 54, Agents Affecting Calcium Metabolism.)

Negative Nitrogen Balance: Negative nitrogen balance is a result of the excessive breakdown of protein caused by glucocorticoids; this may be modified somewhat by administration of anabolic agents and a high-protein diet. However, there is no experimental or clinical evidence to show that anabolic agents protect tissues from atrophy and osteoporosis.

Carbohydrate and Lipid Metabolism: Glucocorticoids aggravate known diabetes and make latent diabetes chemically apparent. Ketosis is not a problem, and the diabetes usually can be controlled with diet or hypoglycemic agents. Serum lipid levels may become elevated in some patients.

Central Nervous System Effects: Large doses of glucocorticoids cause behavioral and personality changes manifested most frequently by euphoria. Other signs include insomnia, increased appetite, nervousness, irritability, and hyperkinesia. Psychotic episodes, including manic-depressive and paranoid states and acute toxic psychoses, have been reported occasionally. Patients sometimes increase dosages because of psychological dependence on these drugs. Cases of glucocorticoid abuse have been reported in which patients took the drug without proper indication. Although the newer synthetic glucocorticoids seem less likely to produce psychoses, the reduced incidence of these disorders may actually be the result of more cautious prescription or lack of recognition of abuse.

Patients with psychoses or convulsive disorders are usually poor candidates for glucocorticoid therapy unless these conditions are caused by systemic lupus erythematosus. Although a history of emotional disorders does not necessarily preclude use of corticosteroids, patients should be observed closely for signs of personality changes or other indications of depression or psychosis.

Growth Suppression: Because growth is suppressed in children receiving long-term, daily, divided-dose glucocorticoid therapy, use of such regimens in children should be restricted to the most urgent indications. Some clinicians think that corticotropin does not inhibit growth to the same extent as glucocorticoids and is, therefore, useful in the long-term treatment of chronic diseases. Further studies are needed to substantiate this, however. Alternate-day glucocorticoid therapy usually avoids or at least minimizes growth suppression.

Myopathy: Development of weakness primarily involves the proximal musculature of the upper and lower extremities and responds to a reduction in dosage. Recovery occurs slowly over a period of months. Although myopathy can occur in patients with pituitary-dependent Cushing's syndrome or after use of any glucocorticoid, it is most frequently associated with use of 9α-fluorinated steroids such as triamcinolone.

Cutaneous Effects: The skin may become thin and shiny or violaceous striae may develop due to rupture of subcutaneous collagen fibers when glucocorticoids are used topically for prolonged periods in intertriginous areas or under occlusive dressings. The long-term topical application of potent fluorinated preparations to the face has been associated with the development of rosacea-like skin eruptions, perioral dermatitis, and acne. Therefore, these agents should be used with caution, if at all, on the face. (See Chapter 61, Dermatologic Preparations.)

Ocular Effects: Topical ocular application of glucocorticoids occasionally results in elevated intraocular pressure caused by decreased outflow facility (open-angle glaucoma). The tendency to develop these symptoms is inherited in a recessive autosomal pattern and occurs most frequently in patients with primary open-angle glaucoma and their relatives, especially homozygous individuals. An exaggerated intraocular pressure response is also common among diabetics and myopes. (See Chapter 24, Ocular Anti-infective and Anti-inflammatory Agents.) Topical glucocorticoids also increase susceptibility to eye infection, especially with fungi and herpes simplex.

Posterior subcapsular cataract formation is associated with prolonged systemic glucocorticoid therapy and appears to be dose related. Children are affected more frequently than adults. This may occur even when alternate-day therapy is employed.

Infections: Reactivation of tuberculosis in patients receiving glucocorticoids is well documented. Therefore, tuberculin skin testing is recommended before the initiation of prolonged, high-dose glucocorticoid therapy since skin sensitivity to tuberculin may be lost during treatment with large daily doses of glucocorticoids. Sensitivity remains unchanged in patients on alternate-day therapy. Patients with positive skin tests may be candidates for appropriate chemotherapy (see Chapter 79, Antimycobacterial Agents).

Host defenses are impaired in patients receiving large doses of glucocorticoids, and this effect increases susceptibility to fungal infections, especially candidosis, pneumocystosis, cryptococcosis, aspergillosis, and sporotrichosis. The incidence and severity of bacterial and viral infections also are increased. Since glucocorticoids tend to mask symptoms, intercurrent infections may become severe before their presence is recognized. Glucocorticoids are especially hazardous when herpes simplex keratitis is present. Early recognition and institution of appropriate treatment are the only safeguards against these serious complications. Cutaneous bacterial or yeast infection is the most common complication of topical glucocorticoid therapy. The infection should be treated with appropriate anti-infective agents, and the glucocorticoid should be discontinued if possible.

Miscellaneous Reactions: Acne, hirsutism, menstrual disorders, facial rounding, development of supraclavicular fat pads, weight gain due to increased appetite, headache, pseudotumor cerebri, hypertension, impotence, hyperhidrosis, flushing, vertigo, asthenia, chronic pancreatitis, intestinal perforation, hepatomegaly, hyperlipidemia, and acceleration of atherosclerosis have been associated with glucocorticoid therapy.

Drug Interactions

The metabolism of corticosteroids is increased by drugs that induce certain hepatic metabolizing enzymes (eg, pheno-barbital, phenytoin [Dilantin], rifampin [Rifadin, Rimactane]). If one of these agents is given concomitantly, an increase in the maintenance dose of corticosteroid may be necessary. Since the half-life of cortisol may be reduced in patients who have been taking other corticosteroids, asthmatic patients who have been maintained on steroids may require larger doses of cortisol for an acute attack.

In a controlled study of asthmatic patients, treatment for three weeks with ephedrine (but not theophylline) resulted in more rapid metabolism of radioactive-labeled dexamethasone. This suggests that larger doses of systemic glucocorticoids may be required if ephedrine is taken concomitantly (Brooks et al, 1977).

Other agents reduce the level of active corticosteroids. Estrogen increases levels of corticosteroid-binding globulin, thereby increasing the bound (inactive) fraction, but this effect is at least balanced by decreased metabolism of corticosteroids. When estrogen therapy is initiated, a reduction in corticosteroid dosage may be required, and increased amounts may be required when estrogen is terminated.

Corticosteroids have a hyperglycemic effect and may increase the requirement for hypoglycemic drugs. The potassium balance should be monitored in patients taking corticosteroids, particularly when amphotericin B and thiazide diuretics are taken concurrently, for such combinations can cause potassium depletion. Corticosteroid administration is associated with greater clearance of salicylates and decreased effectiveness of anticoagulants, and the dosage of these drugs may require adjustment when steroid therapy is initiated or discontinued. Corticosteroids are bound to plasma proteins, including albumin. Since the unbound steroid is the physiologically active fraction, in hypoalbuminemic patients taking pharmacologic doses in whom the normal negative feedback mechanisms are inoperable, dosage should be reduced to avoid high levels of unbound hormone and the possibility of increasing the incidence of adverse reactions.

Effects on Laboratory Tests

Corticosteroids may increase the blood level of glucose, sometimes resulting in diabetes mellitus and glycosuria. This reflects not only elevated blood glucose but a lowered renal threshold for glucose. Potent glucocorticoids (eg, dexamethasone) decrease 17-ketosteroid (17-KS) and 17-hydroxysteroid (17-OHCS) levels in urine due to the negative feedback effect on secretion of endogenous hormones.

Pregnancy and Lactation

Corticosteroids readily cross the placenta. If very large pharmacologic doses must be used during pregnancy, fetal adrenal hypoplasia may occur. The state of adrenal function must be assessed in the neonate and replacement therapy provided if necessary. When the suppressing influence of high levels of exogenous steroids is removed, normal function of the adrenal glands is recovered eventually.

Corticosteroids are found in the breast milk of lactating women receiving systemic therapy with these agents. However, it is probably safe for a lactating mother to nurse her infant even if she is taking low pharmacologic doses of corticosteroids.

INDIVIDUAL EVALUATIONS

Dosage requirements are variable and must be individualized on the basis of the disease being treated and the response of the patient. The maintenance dose is determined by reducing the initial dose by small amounts at appropriate intervals until the lowest quantity that maintains an adequate response is found. The dosage for children also should be determined in this manner rather than on the basis of age or body weight.

BETAMETHASONE
[Celestone]

BETAMETHASONE ACETATE AND BETAMETHASONE SODIUM PHOSPHATE
[Celestone Soluspan]

This synthetic analogue of prednisolone is a stereoisomer of dexamethasone. It is used in inflammatory or allergic conditions and other glucocorticoid-responsive diseases. In anti-inflammatory effect, 0.6 mg of betamethasone is equivalent to 20 mg of cortisol. Betamethasone lacks the mineralocorticoid properties of cortisol and is, therefore, not recommended as sole replacement therapy in primary adrenocortical insufficiency.

The base is given orally. A suspension containing the soluble sodium phosphate ester for rapid onset of action and the slightly soluble acetate ester for sustained effect is used intramuscularly, intra-articularly, and for soft tissue injection.

Undesirable effects are similar to those observed with other glucocorticoids. For specific indications, adverse reactions, and precautions, see the Introduction.

ROUTES, USUAL DOSAGE, AND PREPARATIONS.
Oral: Initially, 0.6 to 7.2 mg daily.
> BETAMETHASONE:
> *Celestone* (Schering). Syrup 0.6 mg/5 ml; tablets 0.6 mg.

Intramuscular: 1 to 2 ml (6 to 12 mg).
Intra-articular: 0.25 to 2 ml (1.5 to 12 mg), depending upon the size of the joint.
Soft Tissue Injection: 0.25 to 1 ml (1.5 to 6 mg), depending upon the size of the affected area.
> BETAMETHASONE ACETATE AND BETAMETHASONE SODIUM PHOSPHATE:
> *Celestone Soluspan* (Schering). Each milliliter of sterile aqueous suspension contains betamethasone acetate 3 mg and betamethasone sodium phosphate 3 mg in 5 ml containers.

CORTISOL
[Cortef, Cortenema, Hydrocortone, Rectoid]

CORTISOL ACETATE
[Cort-Dome, Hydrocortone Acetate]

CORTISOL CYPIONATE
[Cortef Fluid]

CORTISOL SODIUM PHOSPHATE
[Hydrocortone Phosphate]

CORTISOL SODIUM SUCCINATE
[A-hydroCort, Solu-Cortef]

Cortisol (hydrocortisone) is a preferred drug for replacement therapy in chronic adrenocortical insufficiency and salt-losing forms of congenital adrenal hyperplasia syndromes because it has both glucocorticoid and mineralocorticoid activities.

The oral preparations (base and cypionate salt) are used for replacement therapy or in inflammatory conditions. The highly water-soluble forms (sodium phosphate, sodium succinate) are given intravenously or intramuscularly in emergencies, such as acute adrenocortical insufficiency (Addisonian crisis) or acute inflammatory conditions, or to prepare steroid-dependent patients for major surgery. For patients in shock, the intravenous route should be used until the blood pressure is stabilized. Cortisol acetate is only slightly soluble in water; aqueous suspensions are used for intra-articular and soft tissue injection when a long-acting effect is desired. The base and acetate forms are also available in preparations for rectal administration as adjuncts in the treatment of ulcerative colitis.

Because of the drug's mineralocorticoid activity, its administration systemically in inflammatory conditions should be limited to short-term use. Prolonged use for such indications may result in sodium and water retention, hypertension, and hypokalemia; sodium restriction and potassium supplementation may be necessary. The Δ -1 analogues of cortisone and cortisol have less mineralocorticoid activity and are preferred for long-term anti-inflammatory therapy.

See the Introduction for specific indications, adverse reactions, and precautions.

ROUTES, USUAL DOSAGE, AND PREPARATIONS. *Oral*: For chronic adrenocortical insufficiency, 20 to 30 mg daily. The daily dosage may be divided, with two-thirds given in the morning upon arising and one-third in the afternoon, to simulate normal adrenocortical secretion.

For congenital adrenal hyperplasia, 10 to 30 mg daily, or 0.6 mg/kg of body weight daily, or 20 mg/M² daily. The daily dosage may be divided with two-thirds given in the morning and one-third in the late afternoon. Alternatively, dosage is divided with the last dose being largest in order to achieve maximum suppression of the early morning surge of corticotropin secretion.

For anti-inflammatory effects, 20 to 240 mg daily; larger amounts may be given in divided doses.

> CORTISOL:
> Drug available generically: Tablets 10 and 20 mg.
> *Cortef* (Upjohn). Tablets 5, 10, and 20 mg.
> *Hydrocortone* (Merck Sharp & Dohme). Tablets 10 and 20 mg.
> CORTISOL CYPIONATE:
> *Cortef Fluid* (Upjohn). Suspension equivalent to cortisol 10 mg/5 ml.

Intravenous: In emergencies, initially, 100 to 500 mg, repeated if necessary. Larger doses have been suggested for treatment of shock.

Intramuscular: For emergencies when the intravenous route is not feasible, initially, 100 to 250 mg, repeated if necessary.

> CORTISOL SODIUM PHOSPHATE:
> *Hydrocortone Phosphate* (Merck Sharp & Dohme). Solution 50 mg/ml in 2 and 10 ml containers and in 2 ml single-dose disposable syringes.
> CORTISOL SODIUM SUCCINATE:
> Drug available generically: Solution 100 and 250 mg/ml in 2 ml containers.
> *A-hydroCort* (Abbott), *Solu-Cortef* (Upjohn). Powder 100, 250, and 500 mg and 1 g.

Intra-articular: 10 to 50 mg, depending upon the size of the joint.

Soft Tissue Injection: 5 to 75 mg, depending upon the size of the affected area.

> CORTISOL ACETATE:
> Drug available generically: Suspension 25 and 50 mg/ml in 5 and 10 ml containers.
> *Hydrocortone Acetate* (Merck Sharp & Dohme). Suspension (aqueous) 25 and 50 mg/ml in 5 ml containers.

Rectal: (Base) A retention enema containing 100 mg is instilled once or twice daily. The enema is inserted with the patient in the left Sims's position. Since optimal absorption is achieved with prolonged retention, the patient should lie quietly for at least 30 minutes after instillation. Dosage usually is reduced over a period of weeks as improvement occurs. (Acetate) For proctitis, one suppository inserted twice daily (maximum, two suppositories twice daily) for two weeks.

See the manufacturers' literature for complete instructions on rectal administration.

> CORTISOL:
> *Cortenema* (Rowell), *Rectoid* (Pharmacia). Retention enema 100 mg in 60 ml single-dose containers.

> CORTISOL ACETATE:
> Drug available generically: Suppositories 25 mg.
> *Cort-Dome* (Dome). Suppositories 15 and 25 mg.

CORTISONE ACETATE
[Cortone Acetate]

Cortisone acetate was the first synthetic corticosteroid preparation developed in 1948. It is readily converted in the body to cortisol, the naturally occurring active form. It is a preferred drug for replacement therapy in chronic adrenocortical insufficiency and the majority of patients with salt-losing forms of congenital adrenal hyperplasia syndrome, because it has both glucocorticoid and mineralocorticoid effects. In anti-inflammatory effect, 25 mg of cortisone acetate is equivalent to 20 mg of cortisol; the mineralocorticoid activity of the two drugs is approximately equal.

The aqueous suspension for intramuscular injection is particularly useful when absorption by the oral route is precluded (eg, vomiting, diarrhea). Intramuscular administration may not be as effective for acute emergencies because of the delayed onset of action.

Although this drug may be given systemically in pharmacologic doses for short periods to treat inflammatory or allergic disorders that respond to glucocorticoids, the Δ-1 analogues of cortisol or cortisone are preferred because they have little mineralocorticoid activity.

If cortisone is used as an anti-inflammatory agent, sodium and water retention, hypertension, and hypokalemia can occur; sodium restriction and potassium supplementation may be necessary.

See the Introduction for specific indications and precautions.

ROUTES, USUAL DOSAGE, AND PREPARATIONS. *Oral*: For chronic adrenocortical insufficiency, 25 to 37.5 mg daily. The daily dosage may be divided, with two-thirds given in the morning upon arising and one-third in the afternoon, to simulate normal adrenocortical secretion.

For congenital adrenal hyperplasia, 15 to 40 mg/M_2 daily. Daily dosage is divided, with two-thirds given in the morning and one-third in the late afternoon. Alternatively, dosage is divided with the last dose being the largest in order theoretically to achieve maximum suppression of the early morning surge of corticotropin secretion.

For anti-inflammatory effects, initially, 25 to 150 mg daily; the larger amounts may be given in divided doses.

> Drug available generically: Tablets 5, 10, and 25 mg.
> *Cortone Acetate* (Merck Sharp & Dohme). Tablets 25 mg.

Intramuscular: For severe inflammatory disorders, 75 to 300 mg daily.

> Drug available generically: Suspension 25 mg/ml in 10 and 20 ml containers and 50 mg/ml in 10 ml containers.
> *Cortone Acetate* (Merck Sharp & Dohme). Suspension (in sodium chloride) 25 mg/ml in 20 ml containers and 50 mg/ml in 10 ml containers.

DESOXYCORTICOSTERONE ACETATE
[Doca Acetate, Percorten Acetate]

DESOXYCORTICOSTERONE PIVALATE
[Percorten Pivalate]

This mineralocorticoid has almost no glucocorticoid activity and is available for parenteral administration as replacement therapy in chronic primary adrenocortical insufficiency and salt-losing forms of congenital adrenal hyperplasia when the patient is unable to take oral medication. It is administered with appropriate doses of a glucocorticoid such as cortisol.

Adverse reactions result from excessive retention of sodium and water and loss of potassium; they include hypertension, edema, hypokalemia, cardiac enlargement, and congestive heart failure.

ROUTES, USUAL DOSAGE, AND PREPARATIONS. *Intramuscular*: For chronic primary adrenocortical insufficiency, initially, 1 to 5 mg desoxycorticosterone acetate (solution in oil) daily.

For salt-losing congenital adrenal hyperplasia, 1 to 5 mg daily for the first three or four days; thereafter, dosage is adjusted on the basis of clinical response and the serum electrolyte level. After the maintenance dose is determined (usually 1 mg), the aqueous suspension of desoxycorticosterone pivalate may be given at a rate of 1 ml (25 mg) for each milligram of the solution in oil; the calculated dose is administered every four weeks.

> DESOXYCORTICOSTERONE ACETATE:
> Drug available generically: Suspension (aqueous, in oil) 5 mg/ml in 10 ml containers.
> *Doca Acetate* (Organon), *Percorten Acetate* (Ciba). Solution (in sesame oil) 5 mg/ml in 10 ml containers.
> DESOXYCORTICOSTERONE PIVALATE:
> *Percorten Pivalate* (Ciba). Suspension (aqueous) 25 mg/ml in 4 ml containers.

Subcutaneous Implantation: After the patient has been maintained on desoxycorticosterone acetate for at least two to three months, pellet implantation may be substituted. Once every 8 to 12 months, the number of pellets equal to twice the number of milligrams of solution required daily are implanted. Caution should be exercised because hypertension may occur. Signs of overdosage or underdosage can be corrected by varying the salt intake or giving the steroid intramuscularly, if necessary.

DESOXYCORTICOSTERONE ACETATE: *Percorten Acetate* (Ciba). Pellets approximately 125 mg.

DEXAMETHASONE
[Decadron, Hexadrol]

DEXAMETHASONE ACETATE
[Decadron-LA]

DEXAMETHASONE SODIUM PHOSPHATE
[Decadron Phosphate, Hexadrol Phosphate]

Dexamethasone is a fluorinated derivative of prednisolone used primarily in inflammatory or allergic conditions and other diseases responsive to glucocorticoids. In anti-inflammatory effect, 0.75 mg of dexamethasone is equivalent to 20 mg of cortisol. Since the drug almost completely lacks mineralocorticoid activity, it is not recommended for sole replacement therapy in acute or chronic primary adrenocortical insufficiency. Mild diuresis with sodium loss may occur in patients who had been receiving other glucocorticoids.

Dexamethasone acetate is available as a long-acting repository suspension for intramuscular or local injection when oral therapy is not feasible. This preparation is not suitable when an immediate effect or a short duration of action is desired.

Dexamethasone sodium phosphate is available as an aqueous solution for intramuscular or intravenous use in acute illnesses and other emergency situations. The value of intra-articular injection is limited by the short duration of action of this soluble salt. An aerosol preparation is used for inhalation therapy in bronchial asthma, but dosage by this route is difficult to control and overuse by the patient is a danger. Since systemic absorption occurs with this form of administration, patients should be observed carefully for adverse reactions. (See also Chapter 32, Drugs Used in Asthma.)

Side effects are qualitatively similar to those produced by other glucocorticoids. Also, this drug often causes increased appetite with weight gain. See the Introduction for specific indications, adverse reactions, and precautions.

ROUTES, USUAL DOSAGE, AND PREPARATIONS. *Oral*: Initially, 0.75 to 9 mg daily; this amount may be divided into two to four doses.

DEXAMETHASONE:
Drug available generically: Elixir 0.5 mg/5 ml; tablets 0.25, 0.5, 0.75, and 1.5 mg.
Decadron (Merck Sharp & Dohme). Elixir 0.5 mg/5 ml (alcohol 5%); tablets 0.25, 0.5, 0.75, 1.5, and 4 mg.
Hexadrol (Organon). Elixir 0.5 mg/5 ml; tablets 0.5, 0.75, 1.5, and 4 mg.

Intramuscular: (Acetate) As repository, 1 to 2 ml, equivalent to 8 to 16 mg of dexamethasone. Dosage may be repeated at intervals of one to three weeks, if needed. (Sodium Phosphate) In emergencies, 0.5 to 9 mg.

Intra-articular, Soft Tissue Injection: (Sodium Phosphate) 0.2 to 6 mg. This form is recommended for use in conjunction with a less soluble form for longer-acting effect.

(Acetate) For longer-acting effect, alone or in conjunction with dexamethasone sodium phosphate, 0.5 to 2 ml, equivalent to 4 to 16 mg of dexamethasone. Dosage may be repeated at one- to three-week intervals if needed.

DEXAMETHASONE ACETATE:
Drug available generically: Suspension 8 mg/ml in 5 ml containers.

Decadron-LA (Merck Sharp & Dohme). Suspension (sterile, timed-release) equivalent to 8 mg dexamethasone/ml in 1 and 5 ml containers.
DEXAMETHASONE SODIUM PHOSPHATE:
Drug available generically: Solution 4 mg/ml in 1, 5, and 25 ml containers.
Decadron Phosphate (Merck Sharp & Dohme). Solution (sterile) 4 mg/ml in 1 ml disposable syringes and in 1, 5, and 25 ml containers; 24 mg/ml (for intravenous use only) in 5 and 10 ml containers.
Hexadrol Phosphate (Organon). Solution (aqueous) 4 mg/ml in 1 and 5 ml containers and 10 mg/ml in 10 ml containers.

Intravenous: Initially, 0.5 to 9 mg.
DEXAMETHASONE SODIUM PHOSPHATE:
For preparations, see above.

FLUDROCORTISONE ACETATE
[Florinef Acetate]

Fludrocortisone is a halogenated derivative of cortisol. It has very potent mineralocorticoid and moderate glucocorticoid effects and is, therefore, useful for mineralocorticoid replacement therapy in primary chronic adrenocortical insufficiency and salt-losing forms of congenital adrenal hyperplasia syndromes. This drug is the only oral mineralocorticoid available. It is not suitable for use as an anti-inflammatory agent.

Adverse reactions are caused by the drug's mineralocorticoid activity (retention of sodium and water) and include hypertension, edema, hypokalemia, and cardiac hypertrophy. Adverse reactions from glucocorticoid effects are not a problem because of the small doses used. Salt intake must be adjusted to meet individual requirements.

ROUTE, USUAL DOSAGE, AND PREPARATIONS.
Oral: For chronic primary adrenocortical insufficiency, 0.05 to 0.2 mg daily. For salt-losing forms of congenital adrenal hyperplasia, initially, up to 0.5 mg daily; this can be reduced gradually to 0.1 to 0.2 mg daily over several months.
Florinef Acetate (Squibb). Tablets 0.1 mg.

FLUPREDNISOLONE
[Alphadrol]

This synthetic glucocorticoid is a fluorinated derivative of prednisolone. In anti-inflammatory effect, 1.5 mg of fluprednisolone is equivalent to 20 mg of cortisol. It is useful in treating inflammatory and allergic conditions and other diseases that respond to glucocorticoids. Because fluprednisolone does not have appreciable mineralocorticoid activity, it is not recommended as the sole agent for replacement therapy in acute or chronic primary adrenal insufficiency.

Undesirable effects are similar to those observed with other glucocorticoids. See the Introduction for specific indications, adverse reactions, and precautions.

ROUTE, USUAL DOSAGE, AND PREPARATIONS.
Oral: Initially, 2.5 to 30 mg daily.
Alphadrol (Upjohn). Tablets 1.5 mg.

MEPREDNISONE
[Betapar]

Meprednisone is the 16 β-methyl derivative of prednisone. It is used primarily in inflammatory or allergic conditions and other diseases responsive to glucocorticoids. In anti-inflammatory effect, 4 mg of meprednisone is equivalent to 20 mg of cortisol. Because the drug almost completely lacks mineralocorticoid activity, it is not recommended as the sole agent in the treatment of primary adrenal insufficiency.

See the Introduction for specific indications, adverse reactions, and precautions.

ROUTE, USUAL DOSAGE, AND PREPARATIONS.
Oral: In inflammatory conditions, initially, 8 to 60 mg daily.

    Betapar (Parke, Davis). Tablets 4 mg.

METHYLPREDNISOLONE
[Medrol]

METHYLPREDNISOLONE ACETATE
[Depo-Medrol, Medrol]

METHYLPREDNISOLONE SODIUM SUCCINATE
[Solu-Medrol]

This methyl derivative of prednisolone has the same actions and uses as the parent compound. It is used to treat inflammatory and allergic conditions and other diseases that respond to glucocorticoids. In anti-inflammatory effect, 4 mg of methylprednisolone is equivalent to 20 mg of cortisol. Since the drug lacks significant mineralocorticoid activity, it is not recommended as the sole agent in replacement therapy for primary adrenal insufficiency.

The base is used orally and may be obtained by the tablet or in packages of tablets designed for scheduled administration (Dosepak for six days of gradual reduction in dosage and ADT for alternate-day therapy).

Methylprednisolone acetate is relatively insoluble and is administered intramus-

cularly, intra-articularly, or by soft tissue injection for a prolonged effect. It also may be given rectally as an adjunct in the treatment of ulcerative colitis. Methylprednisolone sodium succinate is highly soluble in water and may be used intravenously in emergencies (except acute adrenocortical insufficiency).

See the Introduction for specific indications, adverse reactions, and precautions.

ROUTES, USUAL DOSAGE, AND PREPARATIONS.
Oral: For anti-inflammatory effect, initially, 4 to 48 mg daily.
    METHYLPREDNISOLONE:
    Drug available generically: Tablets 4 mg.
    Medrol (Upjohn). Tablets 2, 4, 8, 16, 24, and 32 mg; tablets 4 mg (Dosepak) and 16 mg (ADT Pak).

Intravenous: For emergencies, 10 to 40 mg initially. Larger doses have been suggested for the treatment of shock.
    METHYLPREDNISOLONE SODIUM SUCCINATE:
    Solu-Medrol (Upjohn). Powder 40, 125, and 500 mg and 1 g.

Intramuscular: (Acetate) For a prolonged effect, 40 to 120 mg administered at appropriate intervals.
(Sodium Succinate) In emergencies, following initial intravenous injection or when the intravenous route is not feasible, 10 to 40 mg.
    METHYLPREDNISOLONE ACETATE:
    Drug available generically: Suspension 20 and 40 mg/ml in 5 ml containers.
    Depo-Medrol (Upjohn). Suspension (sterile, aqueous) 20 mg/ml in 5 ml containers, 40 mg/ml in 1, 5, and 10 ml containers, and 80 mg/ml in 1 and 5 ml containers.
    METHYLPREDNISOLONE SODIUM SUCCINATE:
    Solu-Medrol (Upjohn). Powder 40, 125, and 500 mg and 1 g.

Intra-articular: 4 to 80 mg, depending upon the size of the joint.
Soft Tissue: 4 to 30 mg, depending upon the size of the area.
    METHYLPREDNISOLONE ACETATE:
    Depo-Medrol (Upjohn). See under Intramuscular.

Rectal: A retention enema containing 40 mg is instilled once or twice daily. The enema is inserted with the patient in the left Sims's position. Since optimal absorption is achieved with prolonged retention, the patient should lie quietly for at least 30 minutes after instillation. Dosage usually is reduced over a period of weeks as improvement occurs.

METHYLPREDNISOLONE ACETATE:
Medrol (Upjohn). Retention enema 40 mg/unit in 6-unit packs (Medrol Enpak).

PARAMETHASONE ACETATE
[Haldrone]

This synthetic derivative of prednisolone is used to treat inflammatory or allergic conditions and other diseases that respond to glucocorticoids. It is more potent on a weight basis than the parent compound; in anti-inflammatory effect, 2 mg of paramethasone acetate is approximately equivalent to 20 mg of cortisol. Since the drug has essentially no mineralocorticoid activity, it is not recommended as the sole treatment in primary adrenocortical insufficiency.

Side effects are similar to those observed with other glucocorticoids. See the Introduction for specific indications, adverse reactions, and precautions.

ROUTE, USUAL DOSAGE, AND PREPARATIONS.
Oral: For anti-inflammatory effect, initially, 2 to 24 mg daily.
Haldrone (Lilly). Tablets 1 and 2 mg.

PREDNISOLONE
[Delta-Cortef, Sterane]

PREDNISOLONE ACETATE
[Meticortelone Acetate, Savacort, Steraject-50, Sterane Suspension]

PREDNISOLONE ACETATE AND PREDNISOLONE SODIUM PHOSPHATE
[Soluject]

PREDNISOLONE SODIUM PHOSPHATE
[Hydeltrasol]

PREDNISOLONE TEBUTATE
[Hydeltra-T.B.A.]

Prednisolone, a Δ-1 analogue of cortisol, is one of the most commonly used synthetic glucocorticoids for inflammatory and allergic conditions and other diseases that respond to glucocorticoids. In anti-inflammatory effect, 5 mg of prednisolone is equivalent to 20 mg of cortisol. Because it has little mineralocorticoid activity, prednisolone is not suitable as the sole agent in the treatment of primary adrenal insufficiency.

The base is used orally. The sodium phosphate ester is highly soluble in water and can be injected intravenously in emergencies (except acute adrenal insufficiency) or intramuscularly. The acetate form is an aqueous suspension suitable for intramuscular, intra-articular, or soft tissue injection when a prolonged effect is desired. The tebutate form is an aqueous suspension even less soluble than the acetate form, and therefore provides a longer lasting effect. It is suitable for intra-articular, intralesional (in cystic tumors of an aponeurosis or tendon), and soft tissue injection.

See the Introduction for specific indications, adverse reactions, and precautions.

ROUTES, USUAL DOSAGE, AND PREPARATIONS.
Oral: For inflammatory conditions, initially, 5 to 60 mg daily.
PREDNISOLONE:
Drug available generically: Tablets 1, 2.5, and 5 mg.
Delta-Cortef (Upjohn), *Sterane* (Pfipharmecs). Tablets 5 mg.
Intravenous: For emergencies, initially, 4 to 60 mg.

PREDNISOLONE SODIUM PHOSPHATE:
Drug available generically: Solution 20 mg/ml in 10 ml containers.
Hydeltrasol (Merck Sharp & Dohme). Solution equivalent to prednisolone phosphate 20 mg/ml in 2 and 5 ml containers.

Intramuscular: (Sodium Phosphate) For emergencies, initially, 4 to 60 mg.
(Acetate) For a prolonged effect, 4 to 60 mg.
PREDNISOLONE SODIUM PHOSPHATE:
See under Intravenous.
PREDNISOLONE ACETATE:
Drug available generically: Suspension 25 and 50 mg/ml in 10 ml containers.
Meticortelone Acetate (Schering), *Sterane Suspension* (Pfizer). Suspension (aqueous) 25 mg/ml in 5 ml containers.
Savacort (Savage). Suspension 50 and 100 mg/ml in 10 ml containers.
Steraject-50 (Mayrand). Suspension 50 mg/ml in 10 ml containers.
PREDNISOLONE ACETATE AND PREDNISOLONE SODIUM PHOSPHATE:
Compound available generically: Each milliliter of suspension contains prednisolone acetate 80 mg and prednisolone sodium phosphate 20 mg in 10 ml containers.
Soluject (Mayrand). Each milliliter of suspension contains prednisolone acetate 80 mg and prednisolone sodium phosphate 20 mg in 10 ml containers.

Intra-articular, Soft Tissue Injection: For a more prolonged effect, initially, 4 to 60 mg.
PREDNISOLONE ACETATE:
See under Intramuscular.
PREDNISOLONE TEBUTATE:
Drug available generically: Suspension 20 mg/ml in 10 ml containers.
Hydeltra-T.B.A. (Merck Sharp & Dohme). Suspension 20 mg/ml in 1 and 5 ml containers.

PREDNISONE
[Deltasone, Meticorten, Orasone]

Prednisone, a Δ-1 analogue of cortisol, is available for oral administration and is one of the most commonly used synthetic steroid preparations for the treatment of inflammatory or allergic conditions and other diseases that respond to glucocor-ticoids. It is readily converted in the body to the active compound, prednisolone. In anti-inflammatory effect, 5 mg of prednisone is equivalent to 20 mg of cortisol.

Because it has little mineralocorticoid activity, the drug is not suitable as the sole agent in the treatment of primary adrenocortical insufficiency. However, it can be used for replacement therapy in secondary adrenal insufficiency or, with additional mineralocorticoid therapy, for primary adrenal insufficiency or salt-losing forms of congenital adrenal hyperplasia.

See the Introduction for specific indications, adverse reactions, and precautions.

ROUTE, USUAL DOSAGE, AND PREPARATIONS.
Oral: For inflammatory conditions, initially, 5 to 60 mg. For replacement therapy, 5 to 7.5 mg daily may be given. The daily dosage may be divided with two-thirds given in the morning upon arising and one-third in the afternoon to simulate normal adrenocortical secretion.
For congenital adrenal hyperplasia, *infants*, 2 mg daily, increasing the amount to 5 to 7.5 mg/M2 daily during adolescence, given in two or three divided doses.
Drug available generically: Tablets 1, 2.5, 5, 10, and 20 mg.
Deltasone (Upjohn). Tablets 2.5, 5, 10, 20, and 50 mg.
Meticorten (Schering). Tablets 1 and 5 mg.
Orasone (Rowell). Tablets 1, 5, 10, 20, and 50 mg.

TRIAMCINOLONE
[Aristocort, Kenacort]

TRIAMCINOLONE ACETONIDE
[Kenalog]

TRIAMCINOLONE DIACETATE
[Aristocort Diacetate, Kenacort Diacetate]

TRIAMCINOLONE HEXACETONIDE
[Aristospan]

This drug is a fluorinated derivative of prednisolone and is used to treat inflammatory or allergic conditions and other diseases that respond to glucocorticoids. In anti-inflammatory effect, 4 mg of triamcinolone is equivalent to 20 mg of cortisol. Triamcinolone has less mineralocorticoid effect than prednisolone and is not suitable as the sole agent in replacement therapy for primary adrenal insufficiency.

The base and diacetate ester are given orally. Aqueous suspensions of the acetonide or diacetate forms are injected intramuscularly when oral therapy is not feasible or desirable. The intramuscular depot may supplement or replace initial oral therapy. These suspensions are also injected intra-articularly or into soft tissue and form a depot for sustained activity. Triamcinolone hexacetonide, the least soluble salt, is injected intra-articularly; it may provide relief for three months to more than a year and may reverse synovial thickening.

During the first days of treatment with triamcinolone, mild diuresis with sodium loss may occur whether or not the patient is frankly edematous; conversely, edema may occur in patients with a decreased glomerular filtration rate. Triamcinolone does not increase potassium loss except in very large doses.

Certain adverse reactions are dissimilar to those produced by other glucocorticoids; myopathy is encountered more frequently with triamcinolone, and this agent tends to cause anorexia rather than stimulation of appetite (with resultant weight loss) and sedation and depression rather than euphoria.

See the Introduction for specific indications, other adverse reactions, and precautions.

ROUTES, USUAL DOSAGE, AND PREPARATIONS. *Oral*: For anti-inflammatory effect, initially, 4 to 48 mg daily.

TRIAMCINOLONE:
Drug available generically: Tablets 2, 4, and 8 mg.
Aristocort (Lederle). Tablets 1, 2, 4, 8, and 16 mg.
Kenacort (Squibb). Tablets 1, 2, 4, and 8 mg.

TRIAMCINOLONE DIACETATE:
Aristocort [*diacetate*] (Lederle). Syrup 2 mg/5 ml.
Kenacort Diacetate (Squibb). Syrup 4.85 mg equivalent to triamcinolone 4 mg/5 ml.

Intramuscular: To supplement or replace initial oral therapy, 40 to 80 mg.

TRIAMCINOLONE ACETONIDE:
Kenalog (Squibb). Suspension (aqueous) 40 mg/ml in 1, 5, and 10 ml containers.

TRIAMCINOLONE DIACETATE:
Drug available generically: Suspension 40 mg/ml in 5 ml containers.
Aristocort [*diacetate*] (Lederle). Suspension 40 mg/ml [Forte] in 1 and 5 ml containers.

Intra-articular: (Acetonide) 2.5 to 5 mg for smaller joints; 5 to 15 mg for larger joints. (Diacetate) 5 to 40 mg per injection, depending upon the size of the joint. (Hexacetonide) 2 to 20 mg, depending upon the size of the joint.

TRIAMCINOLONE ACETONIDE:
Kenalog (Squibb). Suspension (sterile, aqueous) 10 mg/ml in 5 ml containers and 40 mg/ml in 1, 5, and 10 ml containers.

TRIAMCINOLONE DIACETATE:
See under Intramuscular.

TRIAMCINOLONE HEXACETONIDE:
Aristospan (Lederle). Suspension (sterile) 20 mg/ml in 1 and 5 ml containers.

MIXTURES FOR SYSTEMIC ADMINISTRATION

Adrenal corticosteroids for systemic use are commonly marketed in fixed combinations with other drugs. In general, such fixed-dose combinations are not recommended. Since prolonged systemic use of these potent drugs can produce serious adverse reactions, it is important to individualize dosage so that the smallest amount that produces satisfactory relief of symptoms is used for the shortest period possible. In addition, dosage may have to be adjusted during periods of stress, and use of an appropriate amount of glucocorticoid may lead to overdosage or underdosage of the other ingredients in the mixture.

The concomitant use of potassium chloride, antibacterial agents, or antifungal agents to prevent or lessen adverse reactions caused by glucocorticoids is sometimes indicated. However, these drugs must be prescribed separately in accordance with individual requirements.

Antacids also are frequently combined in inadequate doses with glucocorticoids. Although the latter agents may increase gastric secretion, they do not do so consistently. If antacids are taken concomitantly, it is possible that they will not neutralize acid adequately, and the adsorbent action of some antacids (eg, aluminum hydroxide) may make the glucocorticoid unavailable. (See also the Introduction and Chapter 57, Agents Used in Acid Peptic Disorders.)

The addition of ascorbic acid to glucocorticoids is not justified. Adrenal ascorbic acid content decreases in rats after the administration of corticotropin; however, this does not occur consistently in other animals. There is no evidence to suggest that this combination is of benefit in man. It has been suggested that pantothenic acid improves the ability to withstand stress, but any benefit from the addition of pantothenic acid to glucocorticoid preparations is unproved.

Many mixtures are formulated for use in rheumatoid arthritis and other chronic corticosteroid-responsive arthritides. These mixtures usually also contain a salicylate or other nonsteroidal anti-inflammatory agent and are designed to be given three or four times daily. Since the regimens used for rheumatoid arthritis and other rheumatic diseases must be individualized and the maintenance doses of the glucocorticoid carefully adjusted and subject to change, fixed-dose combinations are not suitable for use in these conditions. (See also Chapter 7, Antiarthritic Drugs.) The addition of aminobenzoic acid or muscle relaxants to such mixtures offers no therapeutic advantage.

Decadron Phosphate with Xylocaine Injection (Merck Sharp & Dohme). Each milliliter of solution contains dexamethasone sodium phosphate equivalent to dexamethasone phosphate 4 mg and lidocaine hydrochloride 10 mg.
Predisal (Mallard). Each tablet contains prednisolone 0.75 mg, aspirin 325 mg, salicylamide 120 mg, and aluminum hydroxide gel 100 mg.
Savacort-S (Savage). Each milliliter of solution contains prednisolone sodium phosphate equivalent to prednisolone phosphate 20 mg, niacinamide 25 mg, edetate disodium 0.05%, sodium bisulfite 0.1%, and phenol 0.5%.

Stero-Darvon with A.S.A. (Lilly). Each tablet contains paramethasone acetate 0.25 mg, propoxyphene hydrochloride 32 mg, and aspirin 500 mg.

MIXTURES FOR TOPICAL USE

For an evaluation and listing of various topical mixtures containing glucocorticoids, see Chapters 61, Dermatologic Preparations; 24, Ocular Anti-infective and Anti-inflammatory Agents; 27, Topical Otic Preparations; and 60, Miscellaneous Gastrointestinal Agents.

Selected References

Management and diagnosis of children with nephrotic syndrome. *Br Med J* 2:1103-1104, 1977.

Management of myasthenia gravis. *Drug Ther Bull* 15:29-32, 1977.

Bacon GE, Spencer ML: Pediatric uses of steroids, in Azarnoff DL (ed): *Steroid Therapy*. Philadelphia, WB Saunders Co, 1975, 191-208.

Ballard PL, et al: Glucocorticoid levels in maternal and cord serum after prenatal betamethasone therapy to prevent respiratory distress syndrome. *J Clin Invest* 56:1548-1554, 1975.

Ballard RA, Ballard PL: Use of prenatal glucocorticoid therapy to prevent respiratory distress syndrome: Supporting view. *Am J Dis Child* 130:982-987, 1976.

Block MF, et al: Antenatal glucocorticoid therapy for prevention of respiratory distress syndrome in premature infant. *Obstet Gynecol* 50:186-190, 1977.

Bolton WK, et al: Therapy of idiopathic nephrotic syndrome with alternate day steroids. *Am J Med* 62:60-70, 1977.

Brooks SM, et al: Effects of ephedrine and theophylline on dexamethasone metabolism in bronchial asthma. *J Clin Pharmacol* 17:308-318, 1977.

Caspi E, et al: Prevention of respiratory distress syndrome in premature infants by antepartum glucocorticoid therapy. *Br Obstet Gynecol* 83:187-193, 1976.

Conn HO, Blitzer BL: Nonassociation of adrenocorticosteroid therapy and peptic ulcer. *N Engl J Med* 294:473-479, 1976.

Dluhy RG, et al: Pharmacology and chemistry of adrenal glucocorticoids, in Azarnoff DL (ed): *Steroid Therapy*. Philadelphia, WB Saunders Co, 1975, 1-14.

Ehrlich GE: Steroids in rheumatic disease: Caution, low doses, slow withdrawal. *Mod Med* 46:78-88, (Oct 15-30) 1978.

Gifford RH: Corticosteroid therapy for rheumatoid arthritis, in Azarnoff DL (ed): *Steroid Therapy*. Philadelphia, WB Saunders Co, 1975, 78-95.

Lesene HR, Fallon HJ: Treatment of liver disease with corticosteroids, in Azarnoff DL (ed): *Steroid Therapy*. Philadelphia, WB Saunders Co, 1975, 96-110.

Urman JD, Rothfield NF: Corticosteroid treatment in systemic lupus erythematosus: Survival studies. *JAMA* 238:2272-2276, 1977.

Whitt GG, et al: Comparison of two glucocorticoid regimens for acceleration of fetal lung maturation in premature labor. *Am J Obstet Gynecol* 124:479-482, 1976.

Yount WJ, et al: Corticosteroid therapy of collagen vascular disorders, in Azarnoff DL (ed): *Steroid Therapy*. Philadelphia, WB Saunders Co, 1975, 269-286.

Androgens and Anabolic Steroids | 42

Physiology

Androgenic hormones are secreted by the testis, adrenal cortex, and ovary. Testosterone, the most important circulating androgen, is the principal secretory product of the Leydig cells, which are located in the interstitial spaces of the testes. Leydig cell function is controlled by the anterior pituitary, primarily through one of the gonadotropic hormones, luteinizing hormone (LH), which was originally called interstitial cell-stimulating hormone (ICSH). The steroidogenic function of LH is mediated by stimulating the synthesis of cyclic adenosine monophosphate (cAMP). Normal men produce 2.5 to 10 mg of testosterone daily, which yields plasma concentrations of 350 to 1,200 ng/dl. There is diurnal fluctuation of serum testosterone levels with maximum values in the early morning. In some target tissues (prostate, seminal vesicles, skin), testosterone is reduced to the active intracellular androgen, 5-α-dihydrotestosterone, which binds to the specific androgen receptor in these tissues. It has not been determined whether this transformation is essential for hormonal action in other tissues such as the seminiferous epithelium or muscle.

Testosterone acts through a negative feedback mechanism involving the hypothalamus and anterior pituitary to suppress secretion of LH and, to a lesser extent, follicle stimulating hormone (FSH). FSH is important in the initiation of spermatogenesis; a putative peptide elaborated by the Sertoli cells of the seminiferous tubules ("inhibin") also seems to exert an inhibitory effect on release of FSH from the pituitary. Estradiol, secreted by the testis and also produced by the peripheral conversion of testosterone and other androgens, participates in the negative feedback control of LH and FSH secretion in men and may directly suppress secretion of testosterone by the Leydig cells.

Under normal conditions, the adrenal cortex and ovary secrete relatively little testosterone; instead, they primarily secrete androgen precursors, such as 4-androstenedione and dehydroepiandrosterone, that are metabolized to testosterone in most peripheral tissues. At least 50% of the circulating testosterone in normal women is derived from the metabolism of androstenedione and, to a lesser extent, dehydroepiandrosterone. The overall production of testosterone in women averages 0.23 mg daily, which results in normal plasma concentrations of 15 to 65 ng/dl. Certain pathologic conditions of the adrenal cortex or ovaries (eg, hyperplasia, adenoma, carcinoma) markedly increase the production of androgens and their precursors, which may cause precocious puberal development and virilism or amenorrhea in females if the overproduction is great and sustained.

In males, more than two-thirds of the testosterone precursors are secreted by the adrenal cortex. However, since the rate of conversion to testosterone is low, they are not as important functionally as the smaller amount of testosterone produced by the testis. If Leydig cell function is lost or markedly impaired, the amount of androgens produced by the adrenal cortex is inadequate to sustain normal male function (eg, libido, sexual potency, secondary sexual characteristics, muscular strength, endurance).

Approximately 99% of circulating testosterone is bound to protein, primarily to sex hormone-binding globulin (SHBG, testosterone-estradiol binding globulin or TEGB), but a small amount is bound to albumin. As with other steroid hormones, the biologically active portion of plasma testosterone is the free (dialyzable) fraction. The concentration of SHBG is decreased by androgens and elevated by estrogens. Testosterone has a greater binding affinity for SHBG than estrogen. The concentration of SHBG is approximately twice as high in women as in men.

Testosterone is metabolized primarily in the liver and is excreted mainly in the urine as the metabolites, androsterone and etiocholanolone; small amounts of testosterone glucuronide and sulfate also are excreted. About 6% of the original hormone is excreted in the feces. Synthetic testosterone derivatives are metabolized in a similar manner, but more slowly, which results in longer plasma half-lives.

The diagnosis of androgen deficiency in men may be confusing since emotional disturbances can reduce libido and cause impotence. Idiopathic primary Leydig cell failure may occur in middle-aged men but this is rare. Much has been written about a male climacteric with symptoms similar to those associated with the menopause in women. Free plasma testosterone levels tend to decrease and gonadotropin levels increase with advancing age in men, but whether this is related to climacteric symptoms is unknown. Insensitivity of the target tissues to hormonal stimulation may be a normal manifestation of the aging process, and androgen treatment does not usually relieve symptoms and may stimulate prostatic hyperplasia causing urinary obstruction. However, when serum testosterone levels decrease abruptly at any age (eg, following surgical trauma or orchiectomy), vasomotor flushing can occur; this is alleviated by testosterone replacement therapy.

Results of experiments that attempted to correlate serum testosterone levels with certain behavioral patterns in men (ie, homosexuality, aggressive behavior) have been inconsistent. Some studies measured total serum testosterone levels but not the unbound (physiologically active) fraction; they also failed to take into account the diurnal variation in testosterone secretion, thereby tending to obscure any real differences that may have existed. The ratio of free estrogen:testosterone in these individuals has not been investigated. Furthermore, it remains to be determined whether differences in hormone level are the cause, the effect, or are unrelated to behavior. However, there is good evidence in animals that androgens program the brain in fetal or neonatal life and set male patterns of gonadotropic hormone secretion and sexual behavior.

Preparations

Testosterone derivatives are used primarily to develop or maintain secondary sexual characteristics and other physiologic functions, such as anabolism, growth, and muscular development, in androgen-deficient males. Testosterone is commonly administered parenterally as the propionate or as the longer-acting esters, cypionate [Depo-Testosterone, T-Ionate-P.A.] and enanthate [Delatestryl]. The long-acting esters are absorbed slowly from intramuscular sites and thus produce a response lasting two to four weeks. Most clinicians prefer these preparations because of the convenience and satisfactory results achieved. In contrast, the more rapid absorption and metabolism of testosterone propionate necessitates injection two to four times weekly.

Methyltestosterone [Metandren, Oreton Methyl, Testred] and fluoxymesterone [Halotestin] are alkylated in the 17-α position; thus, they are effective orally since they are relatively resistant to inactivation by the liver. They must be given daily and their androgenic potency, milligram-for-milligram, is less than that of the parenteral forms of testosterone. Also, 17-α-alkylated androgens are potentially hepatotoxic (see the section on Adverse Reactions and Precautions).

Testosterone and its derivatives have anabolic and somatic growth effects. Attempts to separate the anabolic from the androgenic effects by modifying the testosterone molecule have resulted in the development of a number of synthetic analogues, termed anabolic steroids. Results of laboratory tests and bioassays in animals indicate that a partial separation of effects has been achieved with these compounds. Since it has been suggested that there are separate receptors for androgenic and anabolic steroids in an androgen target tissue in rats (levator ani muscle, which serves as a bioassay tissue in testing potency of these compounds), eventually it may be possible to achieve an even greater separation of activities.

The synthetic anabolic steroids include ethylestrenol [Maxibolin], methandrostenolone [Dianabol], oxandrolone [Anavar], oxymetholone [Adroyd, Anadrol-50], and stanozolol [Winstrol]; all are oral preparations and are given daily. Nandrolone phenpropionate [Durabolin, Nandrolin] and nandrolone decanoate [Deca-Durabolin] are longer acting and are given intramuscularly. Only the oral preparations are 17-α-alkylated compounds. All of these synthetic compounds are weak androgens, but nitrogen may be retained without significant virilization if patients are observed closely and if intermittent therapy is employed in susceptible individuals. Virilization can occur if larger doses are given for a prolonged period. There is substantial evidence that the enhancement of protein anabolism by these agents is of therapeutic benefit only when there is sufficient intake of calories and protein.

Indications

Hypogonadism can occur in males as a result of primary dysfunction, such as a chromosomal defect (eg, Klinefelter's syndrome), or as a result of disease (eg, myotonic dystrophy) or traumatic injury; it also may be secondary to a deficiency in gonadotropin secretion. Etiologic factors in secondary testicular failure include pituitary tumors, pituitary insufficiency secondary to trauma or hypothalamic lesions, and selective gonadotropin deficiency (hypogonadotropic eunuchoidism). When hypogonadism becomes evident because of delayed puberty, the manifestations are more severe than if androgen deficiency first occurs in adulthood. Androgens are useful to stimulate initial development or to maintain secondary sexual characteristics in adult-onset hypogonadism. The undeveloped eunuch requires more intensive therapy (dosage and duration) than men who achieved normal adulthood before androgen deficiency occurred. Stimulation of puberal development requires long-term androgen replacement and is best achieved by use of a long-acting parenteral preparation (eg, testosterone cypionate or enanthate). Once puberal changes are accomplished, an oral preparation may be substituted (eg, methyltestosterone, fluoxymesterone), although the possible hepatotoxic effects of these drugs must be considered. When treatment of eunuchoidism is postponed until later in adulthood, usual replacement doses of androgens may result in psychic disturbances. Smaller doses of an oral preparation may avoid this problem.

Although testosterone maintains secondary sexual characteristics, gonadotropic hormones also are necessary to stimulate normal spermatogenesis. When infertility is a manifestation of hypogonadism secondary to gonadotropin deficiency, a regimen of clomiphene or menotropins (HMG) plus chorionic gonadotropin (HCG) may be successful (see Chapter 45, Agents Used to Treat Infertility).

Testosterone has been used to treat *infertility* due to idiopathic oligospermia. A "rebound" of spermatogenesis has been reported to follow discontinuation of prolonged therapy using large doses of a long-acting testosterone preparation, but the results of such therapy are equivocal (see Chapter 45).

Delayed puberty occurs in about 2.5% of normal children. In boys, puberty may be considered delayed if there is no testicular enlargement by age 14 or, in both sexes, if puberal changes are not complete five years after their initiation. Bone age is less retarded in those with primary gonadal failure. Constitutional delay of puberty is most common and is often familial, but hypothalamic-pituitary dysfunction and gonadal failure also occur. Patients with constitutional delay of growth and development are likely to present with short stature as well as sexual immaturity. They ultimately develop normally and do not require medical treatment. When reassurance, patience, or psychotherapy is not adequate, stimulation of growth and development of secondary sexual characteristics is indicated to prevent severe psychological trauma to the adolescent. There are currently no laboratory tests that will distinguish constitutional delayed puberty from hypogonadotropic hypogonadism. However, in primary gonadal failure (eg, Klinefelter's syndrome, gonadal dysgenesis), serum gonadotropins are elevated.

Drug therapy should not be attempted until the chronological age of 12 or a bone age of 10 has been attained. The earlier medical treatment is initiated, the greater is the risk of compromising adult height through premature epiphyseal closure. Clinicians differ in their preferences for medical management of delayed puberty but, in most regimens, the steroids are administered for several months, followed by an equal period of time during which the patient is observed but no medication is given. Bone age should be determined carefully by roentgenographic examinations before and at 6- to 12-month intervals during and after treatment. Since bone maturation may be stimulated for six months after therapy is discontinued, steroids should be withdrawn well before the skeletal age reaches the norm for the chronologic age. Three- to six-month courses of therapy at six-month intervals using the lowest effective dose are most satisfactory. Puberal changes initiated during treatment often continue to proceed spontaneously.

HCG may be administered and beneficial effects indicate testicular response to gonadotropic stimulation, thus ruling out primary gonadal failure or end-organ insensitivity. However, treatment with HCG is inconvenient and expensive (see Chapter 46, Agents Related to Anterior Pituitary and Hypothalamic Function). A long-acting parenteral testosterone preparation (eg, testosterone enanthate or cypionate) stimulates growth and maturation. Oral preparations of anabolic steroids also may be utilized. Usual doses produce less virilization and have less tendency to cause premature closure of the epiphyses, but the possibility of hepatotoxicity should be considered when these $17-\alpha$-substituted preparations are used. Although androgenic preparations enhance growth and development of secondary sexual characteristics, they may suppress testicular growth and function during the course of therapy. In contrast, HCG stimulates Leydig cell function and thereby increases production of endogenous androgen.

Experimental evidence suggests that androgens and anabolic steroids support erythropoiesis by stimulating renal production of erythropoietin, as well as by direct, dose-related stimulation of the erythropoietin-sensitive elements in bone marrow. Androgens also increase erythrocytic 2-3 diphosphoglycerate levels, thus decreasing hemoglobin-oxygen affinity and making oxygen more readily available to the tissues. Accordingly, large doses of these agents are used to treat some *refractory anemias* caused by defective production of erythrocytes (eg, aplastic anemia, sideroblastic anemia), hereditary conditions (eg, Fanconi's anemia), or associated with disorders such as myelofibrosis. Androgenic-anabolic agents also may alleviate leukopenia and thrombocytopenia, but these effects require longer treatment and are achieved less consistently. Less than half of those affected respond to these agents, but their use is justified because of the otherwise poor prognosis of some anemias. Three months of treatment may be required to achieve therapeutic goals. Best results in acquired aplastic anemia have been obtained in children and women. Also, therapy is most successful when there is some residual erythropoietic and myelopoietic activity. If there are no signs of improvement after three months of therapy or if the drug loses effectiveness, it should be discontinued. However, other patients become dependent on continuing androgen therapy to support adequate hematopoiesis. Preparations with less androgenic potency are used in children and women to avoid masculinizing effects. Androgenic preparations that do not have a 17-α-alkyl group (eg, testosterone and its derivatives, nandrolone phenpropionate, nandrolone decanoate) may be preferred for prolonged therapy with large doses, since liver dysfunction is rare with their use. (See the section on Adverse Reactions and Precautions.)

Androgenic agents are useful in treating anemia secondary to acute or chronic *renal failure* and are particularly effective in acute renal failure of pregnancy. These agents stimulate production of erythropoietin even in anephric patients, but the response is better if the kidneys remain. Treatment is most successful in patients who are adequately nourished and dialyzed. Drug treatment increases erythrocyte mass and reduces the transfusion requirement. The latter effect is a less compelling basis for androgen therapy than formerly thought, since it has been shown that prior transfusion improves renal transplant survival.

Androgens have been used to treat certain *gynecologic conditions* (eg, uterine hemorrhage, dysmenorrhea, menopausal syndrome, premenstrual mastalgia); however, estrogens and oral progestins are pre-

ferred (see Chapter 43). Androgens should not be given to treat breakthrough bleeding that occurs with estrogen therapy. Small doses of androgens, alone or in mixtures with estrogen, have been used to restore libido, especially in menopausal women. However, since results are equivocal and administration of even small amounts of androgen for prolonged periods may result in masculinization in sensitive women, its use for these purposes is discouraged. Androgen in combination with estrogen [Deladumone] has been given intramuscularly at the time of delivery to suppress postpartum lactation, but hormonal preparations are not satisfactory for this indication and use of estrogen is discouraged because of the risk of thromboembolism (see Chapter 43). If drug therapy is desired to suppress lactation, bromocriptine [Parlodel] is preferred (see Chapter 46, Agents Related to Anterior Pituitary and Hypothalamic Function).

The most common indication for large-dose, long-term androgen therapy in women is in selected cases of advanced or *metastatic breast carcinoma*. Since the dosage required to induce remissions in breast carcinoma is larger than that used for androgen replacement in males, patients should be advised that virilizing side effects will occur. The short-acting preparations (eg, testosterone propionate, methyltestosterone, fluoxymesterone) are preferred initially, since prompt withdrawal is necessary if symptomatic hypercalcemia develops. Various derivatives of testosterone have been reported to induce remissions with fewer virilizing effects, and testolactone [Teslac] is free of androgenic activity (see Chapter 68, Antineoplastic Agents). Androgens are contraindicated in the treatment of male breast cancer.

Anabolic steroids reverse the negative nitrogen and calcium balance associated with high-dose glucocorticoid therapy, but there is no unanimous agreement that this treatment is effective on a long-term basis. Although this use of anabolic steroids is a rational approach to prevent some side effects (eg, muscle wasting and weakness, demineralization of bone) and such usage is common, proof of efficacy is inadequate.

Defective protein metabolism with loss of tissue protein may occur in patients with chronic debilitating illness and in those convalescing from severe infections, surgery, burns, trauma, radiotherapy, or cytotoxic drug therapy. Testosterone or related anabolic steroids decrease or may reverse the negative nitrogen balance, but there is no conclusive evidence that they shorten the period of recovery. Their effectiveness is dependent upon adequate protein and total caloric intake. These agents also seem to provide a feeling of well-being and sometimes stimulate appetite. There are no adequate clinical trials proving efficacy, but their use as adjunctive or supportive therapy in such conditions, particularly in terminal patients, is justified.

Anabolic steroids were found to be ineffective in alleviating the symptoms or altering the progress of *muscular dystrophy*. Masculinizing effects have been a problem when these agents were used for this indication in children.

The use of anabolic steroids to improve athletic performance is unanimously condemned. Not only is this a medically trivial indication, but experimental evidence suggests that steroids do not significantly increase muscle size or strength in healthy young men who are already in good physical condition, and reported weight gains are probably due to fluid retention. Nevertheless, it is believed that many athletes (particularly weight lifters, shot-putters, and discus throwers) regularly ingest anabolic steroids in doses that frequently far exceed those used for other anabolic purposes. Furthermore, adverse effects associated with the use of large doses of 17-α-alkylated preparations commonly include alteration of liver function, reduced serum gonadotropin and testosterone levels, and decreased spermatogenesis.

Adverse Reactions and Precautions

The essentially harmless and reversible untoward effects associated with use of androgens and anabolic steroids include acne and hirsutism. Although the anabolic steroids are less likely to produce these reactions, they too will cause masculinizing effects when taken in sufficient quantities. Obviously, such effects are of greater concern in women and children, and for this reason the less androgenic preparations are preferred in these patients.

When these steroids are used for indications other than androgen deficiency, the most frequent undesirable effect of therapy is virilism. Signs in prepuberal children are pubic hair development, phallic enlargement, and increased frequency of erections in boys and clitoral enlargement in girls. In boys, the risk of priapism exists; any increase in erectile frequency is an indication for discontinuing androgen therapy. In women, hirsutism, deepening of the voice, oily skin, alopecia, acne, clitoral enlargement, stimulation of libido, and menstrual irregularities may occur; voice change and clitoral enlargement are probably irreversible but hirsutism may be reversible. Combined estrogen and androgen therapy does not significantly delay or prevent the onset of virilism.

Anabolic steroids should not be used to stimulate growth in children who are small but otherwise normal and healthy. When they are used, the rate of skeletal maturation may exceed the rate of linear growth and thereby induce premature closure of the epiphyses and may reduce the attainable adult height. The extent to which this complication occurs depends upon the child's bone age, the drug used, dose, and duration of therapy. The decision to administer anabolic steroids to children for a specific growth problem should be made only after careful evaluation.

Androgenic and anabolic steroids with an alkyl group substituted in the alpha position on carbon 17 (ie, methyltestosterone [Metandren, Oreton Methyl, Testred], fluoxymesterone [Halotestin], ethylestrenol [Maxibolin], methandrostenolone [Dianabol], oxandrolone [Anavar], oxymetholone [Adroyd, Anadrol-50], stanozolol [Winstrol]) have produced signs of liver dysfunction. Increased sulfobromophthalein (BSP) retention and serum glutamic oxaloacetic transaminase (SGOT) levels appear to be dose related and are relatively unimportant. Increased serum bilirubin and alkaline phosphatase values indicating excretory dysfunction are rare but important idiosyncratic reactions. Clinical jaundice is unusual and reversible when the drug is discontinued. The histologic findings consist of intrahepatic cholestasis with little or no cellular damage. These drugs, therefore, should be used with caution in patients with pre-existing liver disease. Occasionally, hepatocellular and endothelial malignancies, as well as intrahepatic hemorrhage associated with peliotic hepatitis, have developed in anemic patients treated for long periods with large doses of 17-α-alkylated steroids. Abnormal results of liver function tests do not occur with intramuscular preparations of testosterone and its derivatives, nandrolone phenpropionate [Durabolin, Nandrolin], or nandrolone decanoate [Deca-Durabolin].

Women receiving androgen therapy for disseminated breast carcinoma may develop hypercalcemia. If symptoms occur, the patient should be hydrated and treated with appropriate drugs (see Chapter 54, Agents Affecting Calcium Metabolism) and the androgen should be discontinued.

Salt and fluid retention may occur in some patients. It is usually not serious but can be undesirable in patients with congestive heart failure or in those with a tendency to develop edema from other causes (eg, cirrhosis, hypoproteinemia).

Care should be taken when 17-α-alkylated preparations are used in patients on hemodialysis because these drugs may increase blood fibrinolytic activity. Stomatitis has been reported after use of buccal forms of testosterone.

Androgens and anabolic steroids are usually contraindicated in pregnant women because of possible masculinization of the female fetus. Their use in premature and newborn infants is not recommended, since evidence of beneficial effect is lacking. They also are contraindicated in men with carcinoma of the prostate or breast.

Drug Interactions: Caution is required when 17-α-alkylated androgens are ad-ministered to patients receiving anticoagulants. Methandrostenolone and ethylestrenol increase the potency of coumarin and indandione anticoagulants when these agents are given concomitantly, and thus the risk of hemorrhage is increased (see Chapter 5, Drug Interactions and Adverse Drug Reactions). Therefore, when any androgenic steroid is added to or withdrawn from the regimen of a patient receiving an anticoagulant, more frequent prothrombin determinations and adjustments in dosage of the anticoagulant should be made.

Methandrostenolone may decrease the metabolism of oxyphenbutazone [Oxalid, Tandearil], resulting in a longer, more intense, and unpredictable response to the latter. Thus, it is advisable to avoid the concomitant use of these drugs. The requirement for antidiabetic agents may be decreased when anabolic steroids are taken, because steroids may directly reduce blood sugar levels in diabetics and may inhibit the metabolism of oral hypoglycemic agents.

Effects on Laboratory Tests

Androgens reduce the level of circulating thyroxine-binding globulin, thereby decreasing thyroid hormone levels and increasing triiodothyronine resin uptake. However, the free thyroxine index is unaffected and there is no evidence of thyroid dysfunction. Androgens enhance blood fibrinolytic activity, increase hematocrit and serum haptoglobin levels, and have variable effects on serum cholesterol.

INDIVIDUAL EVALUATIONS

FLUOXYMESTERONE
   [Halotestin]

This short-acting preparation (half-life about 10 hours) is used orally. It is less effective as replacement therapy in androgen-deficient males than the intramuscularly injected long-acting esters of testosterone. Full sexual maturation in patients with prepuberal hypogonadism cannot be achieved easily with fluoxymesterone, but the drug is effective for replacement therapy when hypogonadism begins in adult life or after secondary sexual characteristics have developed following therapy with a parenteral preparation. Fluoxymesterone also can be used for its anabolic properties and for the palliative treatment of certain cases of metastatic breast carcinoma in women.

See the Introduction for information on other indications and adverse reactions.

ROUTE, USUAL DOSAGE, AND PREPARATIONS.
Oral: For androgen deficiency, 10 to 20 mg daily. For metastatic breast carcinoma in *women*, 10 to 30 mg daily in divided doses. To stimulate erythropoiesis, 0.4 to 1 mg/kg of body weight daily. For anabolic effect, *adults*, 4 to 10 mg daily. For growth stimulation in *boys*, 2.5 to 10 mg daily.

Halotestin (Upjohn). Tablets 2, 5, and 10 mg.

METHYLTESTOSTERONE
[Metandren, Oreton Methyl, Testred]

This short-acting preparation (half-life about 2.5 hours) is used orally and buccally. Although absorption is more variable, the bioavailability is greater with buccal administration, probably because the hepatic circulation is bypassed. However, the oral route is more commonly used for convenience. Methyltestosterone is much less effective as replacement therapy in androgen-deficient males than the long-acting esters of testosterone. Although methyltestosterone is ineffective in produc-

ing full sexual maturation in patients with prepuberal hypogonadism, it is effective for replacement therapy when hypogonadism begins in adult life or after secondary sexual characteristics have developed following therapy with a parenteral preparation. Methyltestosterone also can be used for its anabolic properties and for the palliative treatment of certain cases of metastatic breast carcinoma in women.

See the Introduction for information on other indications and adverse reactions.

ROUTES, USUAL DOSAGE, AND PREPARATIONS.
Oral: For androgen deficiency, 10 to 40 mg daily. For growth stimulation in *boys*, 10 to 20 mg daily. For metastatic breast carcinoma in *women*, 50 to 200 mg daily. For anabolic effect, *adults*, 10 to 20 mg daily. Because of marked variation in sensitivity, signs of virilism may occur in women even when less than the virilizing dose cited by the manufacturers (300 mg per month) is given. The dosage must be individualized and the daily amount should be given in divided doses.

Drug available generically: Tablets 10 and 25 mg.
Metandren (Ciba), *Oreton Methyl* (Schering). Tablets 10 and 25 mg.
Testred (ICN). Capsules 10 mg.

Buccal: Adults, one-half of oral dosage (rate of absorption is variable).

Drug available generically: Tablets 10 mg.
Metandren (Ciba). Tablets 5 and 10 mg.
Oreton Methyl (Schering). Tablets 10 mg.

TESTOSTERONE CYPIONATE
[Depo-Testosterone, T-Ionate-P.A.]

TESTOSTERONE ENANTHATE
[Delatestryl]

These long-acting, potent esters of testosterone can maintain a testosterone level within the normal male range for two to four weeks and are given intramuscularly to develop or maintain secondary sexual characteristics and other physiologic functions in androgen-deficient males. They are preferred to other androgens to induce full sexual development in eunuchoidal males when testicular disease has interfered with normal puberal development and to treat postpuberal Leydig cell failure. Peak blood levels are achieved a few days after administration and decline to baseline levels by three or four weeks. Either ester may be used for the palliative treatment of breast carcinoma in women who have responded favorably to initial treatment with short-acting preparations. Some clinicians prefer short-acting preparations for the entire treatment because it is possible to stop therapy quickly if adverse effects occur. These preparations also may be given as anabolic agents.

See the Introduction for information on other indications and adverse reactions.

ROUTE, USUAL DOSAGE, AND PREPARATIONS. *Intramuscular:* For induction of puberty in *boys*, 25 to 50 mg/M²/month closely simulates the first year of puberty; 100 to 150 mg/M²/month simulates normal midpuberty sexual development and growth spurt; and 100 to 200 mg every two weeks produces normal adult male testosterone plasma levels. Larger doses (eg, 200 mg weekly) result in full sexual development in two to three years. For androgen deficiency, 200 to 400 mg every four weeks. For metastatic breast carcinoma in *women*, 200 to 400 mg every two or more weeks. For anabolic effects, *adults*, 200 to 400 mg every four weeks. Because of marked variation in sensitivity, virilism may occur in females even with doses lower than those suggested. Signs of virilism occur frequently in women given more than 150 mg a month.

TESTOSTERONE CYPIONATE:
Drug available generically: Solution 100 mg/ml in 10 and 30 ml containers and 200 mg/ml in 10 ml containers.
Depo-Testosterone (Upjohn). Solution (sterile, in cottonseed oil) 50 mg/ml in 10 ml containers and 100 and 200 mg/ml in 1 and 10 ml containers.
T-Ionate-P.A. (Tutag). Solution (in cottonseed oil) 200 mg/ml in 10 ml containers.

TESTOSTERONE ENANTHATE:
Drug available generically: Solution 100 and 200 mg/ml in 10 ml containers.
Delatestryl (Squibb). Solution (sterile, in sesame oil) 200 mg/ml in 1 and 5 ml containers.

TESTOSTERONE PROPIONATE
[Oreton Propionate]

Testosterone propionate can be used to develop or maintain secondary sexual characteristics and other physiologic functions in androgen-deficient males. This relatively short-acting preparation produces a steady response when used parenterally, but this route is not practical for long-term therapy. In older patients, the prostate gland may be sensitive to androgen and bladder neck obstruction may develop; thus, this complication is more easily corrected if a short-acting preparation is used initially. The buccal route may be used for maintenance therapy, but the rate of absorption is less predictable. Its short duration of action makes testosterone propionate useful initially for the palliative treatment of breast carcinoma in women, because prompt withdrawal of the androgen is necessary if hypercalcemia develops. The propionate ester also may be used parenterally for anabolic purposes.

See the Introduction for other indications and adverse reactions.

ROUTES, USUAL DOSAGE, AND PREPARATIONS. *Intramuscular:* For androgen deficiency, 10 to 25 mg two to four times weekly. For metastatic breast carcinoma in *women*, 50 to 100 mg three times weekly. For anabolic effect, *adults*, 10 to 25 mg daily. Because of marked variation in sensitivity, signs of virilism may occur in women when less than the virilizing dose cited by the manufacturers (300 mg per month) is given.

Drug available generically: Solution 25 and 50 mg/ml in 1, 10, and 30 ml containers and 100 mg/ml in 10 and 30 ml containers.

Buccal: For maintenance therapy in androgen-deficient *males*, 5 to 20 mg daily in divided doses; for postpuberal cryptorchidism with evidence of hypogonadism, 15 mg daily. In *women*, for palliation of androgen-responsive, inoperable breast carcinoma, 200 mg daily. Dosage must be individualized and the daily amount should be given in divided doses.

Oreton Propionate (Schering). Tablets 10 mg.

ANABOLIC STEROIDS

These drugs are weak androgens. When given in proper doses for short periods and with appropriate diet to patients with cachexia or debilitating diseases, they may produce anabolic effects without clinical signs of virilism. The synthetic androgens have been used in patients recovering from surgery, infections, burns, fractures, emaciating diseases, and severe traumatic injuries and in those receiving prolonged corticosteroid therapy. Although evidence of their therapeutic efficacy is inadequate, these steroids may be given as adjunctive therapy.

The anabolic agents stimulate erythropoiesis in some patients with congenital and idiopathic aplastic anemia (see the Introduction). They also have been given to children for the management of certain growth disorders, but their use for this purpose may have irreversible adverse effects (see the section on Adverse Reactions and Precautions). If a physician feels that the possible benefits for a specific growth problem outweigh the risks, consultation with experts to determine the dosage regimen is advisable (see the Table for a list of preparations and suggested dosages).

MIXTURES

Androgen-Estrogen Preparations

Short-term administration of androgen-estrogen mixtures has sometimes been used for postpartum suppression of lacta-

ANABOLIC STEROIDS*

Drug	Chemical Structure	Usual Dosage	Preparations
Ethylestrenol		*Oral: Adults*, 8 to 16 mg daily; for growth stimulation in *children*, 0.1 to 0.2 mg/kg daily.	*Maxibolin* (Organon): Elixir 2 mg/5 ml (alcohol 10%) Tablets 2 mg
Methandrostenolone		*Oral: Adults*, initially, 5 mg daily; for maintenance, 2.5 to 5 mg daily.	*Dianabol* (Ciba): Tablets 2.5 and 5 mg
Nandrolone Decanoate		*Intramuscular (deep): Adults*, 50 to 100 mg every 3 to 4 weeks. *Children 2 to 13 years*, 25 to 50 mg every 3 to 4 weeks. For erythropoiesis, 100 to 200 mg weekly.	*Deca-Durabolin* (Organon): Solution (sterile, in sesame oil) 50 mg/ml in 1 and 2 ml containers and 100 mg/ml in 2 ml containers

*For use of more potent androgens for anabolic indications, see the evaluations.

ANABOLIC STEROIDS*

Drug	Chemical Structure	Usual Dosage	Preparations
Nandrolone Phenpropionate	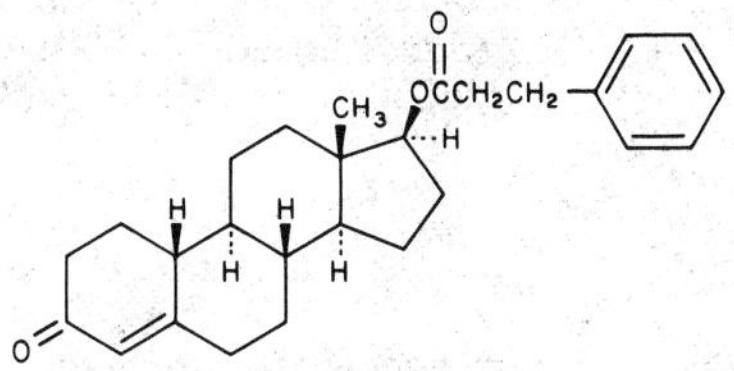	*Intramuscular (deep): Adults*, 25 to 50 mg weekly. *Children 2 to 13 years*, 12.5 to 25 mg every 2 to 4 weeks. For erythropoiesis, up to 100 mg weekly.	*Durabolin* (Organon): Solution (sterile, in sesame oil) 25 mg/ml in 1 and 5 ml containers and 50 mg/ml in 2 ml containers *Nandrolin* (Tutag): Solution 25 mg/ml in 5 ml containers
Oxandrolone	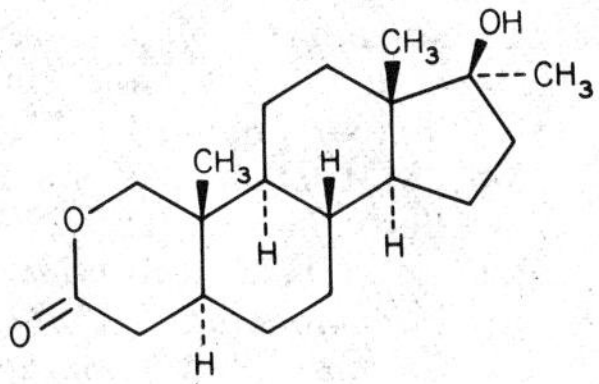	*Oral: Adults*, 2.5 to 10 mg daily. For growth stimulation in *children*, 0.1 mg/kg daily.	*Anavar* (Searle): Tablets 2.5 mg
Oxymetholone	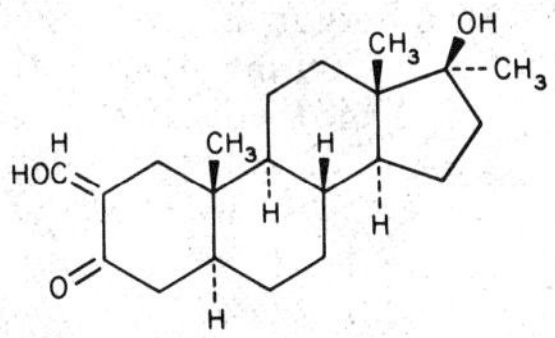	*Oral: Adults*, 5 to 10 mg daily. *Children*, 1.25 to 5 mg daily (depending upon age). For erythropoiesis, *adults and children*, 1 to 5 mg/kg daily (maximum, 100 mg daily).	*Adroyd* (Parke, Davis): Tablets 5 and 10 mg *Anadrol-50* (Syntex): Tablets 50 mg
Stanozolol	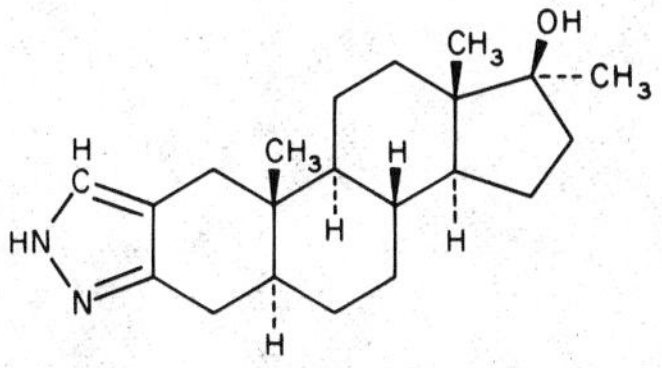	*Oral: Adults*, 6 mg daily. *Children 6 to 12 years*, 2 to 6 mg daily; *under 6 years*, 2 mg daily. These amounts are administered in divided doses before or with meals.	*Winstrol* (Winthrop): Tablets 2 mg

tion. Combined therapy also has been employed empirically to restore libido in postmenopausal women and for a variety of symptoms accompanying aging, but masculinizing effects may occur. There is no evidence that the addition of small amounts of androgen to estrogen is useful to retard symptoms of aging. The use of fixed-dose combinations for any of these problems is irrational.

For postpartum suppression of lactation:

Deladumone OB (Squibb). Each milliliter contains estradiol valerate 8 mg and testosterone enanthate 180 mg in sesame oil.

For menopausal and postmenopausal women:

Deladumone (Squibb). Each milliliter contains estradiol valerate 4 mg and testosterone enanthate 90 mg in sesame oil.

Depo-Testadiol (Upjohn). Each milliliter contains estradiol cypionate 2 mg and testosterone cypionate 50 mg in cottonseed oil.

Di-Genik (Savage). Each milliliter contains estrone 2 mg and testosterone 10 mg (aqueous).
Gynetone (Schering). Each tablet contains ethinyl estradiol 0.02 or 0.04 mg and methyltestosterone 5 or 10 mg.
Premarin with Methyltestosterone (Ayerst). Each tablet contains conjugated estrogens 0.625 or 1.25 mg and methyltestosterone 5 or 10 mg.

Preparations Containing Androgens, Estrogens, And Other Ingredients

Numerous mixtures containing androgens and estrogens combined with vitamins, minerals, progesterone, sedatives, stimulants, and other drugs are available. Many are advocated for use in geriatric patients, but none of these preparations can be considered desirable therapy.

Formatrix (Ayerst). Each tablet contains conjugated estrogens 1.25 mg, methyltestosterone 10 mg, and ascorbic acid 400 mg.
Mediatric (Ayerst). Each tablet or capsule contains conjugated estrogens 0.25 mg, methyltestosterone 2.5 mg, methamphetamine hydrochloride 1 mg, ascorbic acid 100 mg, cyanocobalamin 2.5 mcg, thiamine mononitrate 10 mg, riboflavin 5 mg, niacinamide 50 mg,

pyridoxine hydrochloride 3 mg, pantothenate calcium 20 mg, and ferrous sulfate dried 30 mg.
Mediatric Liquid (Ayerst). Each 15 ml contains conjugated estrogens 0.25 mg, methyltestosterone 2.5 mg, thiamine hydrochloride 5 mg, cyanocobalamin 1.5 mcg, and methamphetamine hydrochloride 1 mg (alcohol 15%).
Os-Cal Mone (Marion). Each tablet contains ethinyl estradiol 5.33 mcg, methyltestosterone 2.67 mg, and calcium carbonate 400 mg.

Selected References

American College of Sports Medicine. Position statement on use and abuse of anabolic-androgenic steroids in sports. *Med Sci Sports* 9:xi-xii, (Winter) 1977.

Karp MM: Diagnosis and treatment of delayed puberty. *Drug Ther* 7:25-33, (June) 1977.

Kochakian CD (ed): *Handbook of Experimental Pharmacology. XLIII. Anabolic-Androgenic Steroids*. New York, Springer-Verlag, 1976.

Root AW, Reiter EO: Evaluation and management of child with delayed pubertal development. *Fertil Steril* 27:745-755, 1976.

Steinberger E: Etiology and pathophysiology of testicular dysfunction in man. *Fertil Steril* 29:481-491, 1978.

Troen P, Nankin H (eds): *The Testis in Normal and Infertile Men*. New York, Raven Press, 1977.

Estrogens and Progestins | 43

Physiology: Estradiol 17-β (hereafter referred to as estradiol) is the major estrogen in premenopausal nonpregnant women. A total of 100 to 600 mcg is secreted daily by the ovary, where androstenedione, an androgen precursor, is converted to testosterone, which in turn is demethylated and aromatized to estrogen. Androstenedione also may be converted to estrone and then to estradiol. Estradiol and estrone (which is about one-half as potent as estradiol) thus are secreted by the ovary, while estriol (a much weaker estrogen) is formed by the peripheral metabolism of ovarian estrogens. Estradiol and estrone may be interconverted in the body. Estrone also is produced by peripheral conversion of androstenedione in a variety of tissues but principally in adipose tissue. In premenopausal women, this accounts for about 25% of the estrone produced; the balance is secreted directly by the ovary. In postmenopausal women, peripheral conversion of androstenedione to estrone is the principal source of estrogen. Although circulating levels of total estrogens decrease and androstenedione levels are about one-half of those in premenopausal women, the daily production of estrone remains similar (about 45 mcg), because of a compensatory increase in the conversion rate of androstenedione. Premenopausally, androstenedione is derived almost equally from ovarian and adrenal secretion, but postmenopausally, the principal source of androstenedione is the adrenal cortex.

Progesterone is produced primarily by direct secretion by the ovary (from the corpus luteum after ovulation) and, to a small extent, by the adrenal cortex. Preovulatory progesterone production is about 3 mg daily; during the luteal phase, 20 to 30 mg is secreted daily. A small quantity of testosterone is produced by the ovary in normal women. About one-half of the testosterone present is derived from peripheral conversion of androstenedione, and the balance is secreted directly by the ovary and adrenal cortex.

Ovarian estrogen (estradiol) is secreted during the follicular and luteal phase of the cycle. In the follicular phase, this hormone is secreted principally by the theca interna (part of this resulting from conversion of progesterone by granulosa cells). During the luteal phase, granulosa cells become vascularized and secrete estrogen as well as progesterone. The increasing preovulatory levels of estrogen act as a positive feedback, modulating the effect of gonadotropin releasing hormone (GnRH) and enhancing the pituitary response to this hormone. This results in a midcycle surge of gonadotropin secretion from the anterior pituitary gland. The high level of luteinizing hormone (LH) is responsible for ovulation of the mature follicle(s). Estrogen and progesterone produced during the luteal phase exert a negative feedback effect on the hypothalamus and anterior pituitary, and gonadotropin secretion during this time is low. In the perimenopausal years, ovulatory cycles decrease in frequency and the production of ovarian steroids by the follicle and corpora lutea becomes less efficient, which may be due to the relative insensitivity of the remaining follicles to gonadotropin effects. After menopause, ovarian secretion of estrogen and progesterone essentially ceases, and circulating estrogen is produced primarily by peripheral conversion of androstenedione.

The placenta produces enormous quantities of estrogens and progesterone during pregnancy resulting in high levels of steroids in the maternal circulation (approximately 130 ng/ml of progesterone, 8 to 13 ng/ml of unconjugated estriol, 7 ng/ml of estrone, and 9.6 ng/ml of estradiol). Since the placenta does not possess the enzyme systems to accomplish this alone, precursors must be supplied for progesterone from the maternal circulation, and for estrogen from the fetal adrenal cortex (the fetoplacental unit for steroid production). The latter relationship is the basis for measuring the maternal urinary excretion of estriol daily to test for fetal well-being in late pregnancy. The functions of the high levels of hormones during pregnancy are not completely understood, but several are probable: Progesterone may suppress the maternal immune response allowing implantation of the blastocyst; it maintains myometrial quiescence and lack of irritability; and it serves as a precursor for formation of fetal adrenal corticosteroids. Estrogen stimulates uteroplacental blood flow.

In nonpregnant women, estrogen and progesterone support physiologic processes which ultimately result in production of an ovum and preparation of the uterine endometrium to support a conceptus. The interaction of steroid hormones and gonadotropins, the influence of steroids on ovum and sperm transport (by affecting motility in the fallopian tubes and quality of cervical mucus), and the steroids' stimulation of growth and glycogen secretion by the endometrial tissue are all directed toward this end.

Estrogen and progesterone stimulate pubertal changes (eg, growth and maturation of uterus and breasts, stimulation and eventual limitation of linear skeletal growth) and later maintain the integrity of responsive tissues (eg, breast, uterus, vaginal and urethral mucosa). These hormones also have widespread effects on various aspects of metabolism (eg, transport protein, electrolyte balance). The reduction of circulating levels of estrogen following menopause often is associated with symptoms referable to these target tissues (eg, atrophic vaginal and urethral irritation).

The cellular mechanism of action of all steroid hormones is similar. Probably most evidence has been obtained with estrogen. This and other steroid hormones cross cell membranes by simple diffusion. The specificity of hormone action (ie, which tissues respond to the hormone) depends upon the presence and concentration of hormone-specific receptors (cytosol proteins). The hormone-receptor complex penetrates the nuclear membrane and binds to nuclear chromatin, which activates selective messenger RNA synthesis. The message undergoes maturation in the nucleus and is transferred to the ribosomes, where enzymes and other proteins are manufactured that carry out the specific cellular function of the hormone.

Estradiol circulates in the blood bound to protein transport carriers. About 80% is bound to sex hormone binding globulin (SHBG), a beta globulin that is also the carrier protein for testosterone; most of the remainder is loosely bound to albumin and about 2% is unbound. Progesterone is bound largely to corticosteroid binding globulin (CBG), which also binds cortisol. Only the relatively small portion of steroid hormone that is unbound is biologically active. The steroids are metabolized to relatively inactive forms in the liver and then excreted in the urine and bile. Estrogens form sulfates and glucuronides, and progesterone is metabolized to a number of products, including pregnanediol. Urine assay for pregnanediol was once widely used to measure progesterone production, but more sensitive, accurate radioimmunoassays and competitive protein binding assays now are widely utilized.

Therapeutic Preparations: Hormones are administered therapeutically to mimic or accentuate the biological effects of endogenous hormones: to supplement inadequate endogenous production (eg, Turner's syndrome, menopause), to correct hormonal imbalance (eg, dysfunctional bleeding), to reverse an abnormal process (eg, hirsutism, endometriosis), and for contraception (see Chapter 44, Contraceptive Agents). Most of the agents used therapeutically are synthetic chemical or naturally occurring analogues of endogenous hormones. Therapy may result in unphysiologic patterns of hormone delivery to the tissues, and certain tissues may have relatively greater exposure to exogenous hormone compared to normal secretory conditions. For example, with the commonly used oral preparations, the hepatic-portal circulation carries a greater concentration of the hormone than under conditions of normal physiologic secretion.

Estrogens, progesterone, and progestins (synthetic compounds possessing progestational activity) are available in a variety of preparations for oral, parenteral, or topical administration. Natural estrogen and progesterone generally are not useful orally because of the poor absorption of the latter and rapid deactivation of estrogen by the liver. An exception is the micronized preparation of estradiol [Estrace] in which particle size is greatly reduced, total surface area is increased, and satisfactory absorption and activity are obtained. Natural estradiol and progesterone are effective when given parenterally. Progesterone also is used as vaginal or rectal suppositories to treat certain infertility cases (see Chapter 45, Agents Used to Treat Infertility).

All natural estrogen products are steroidal, including estradiol (see above) and preparations of conjugated estrogens that are usually prepared from the urine of pregnant mares. Synthetic estrogens may be steroidal or nonsteroidal. The addition of a 17-α ethinyl group to estradiol increases estrogenic potency and enhances oral activity by impeding hepatic degradation. Esters of estradiol (benzoate, cypionate, valerate) in aqueous suspensions or oil for intramuscular injection have more prolonged activity than oral preparations (see the evaluation).

Most nonsteroidal estrogens are related to stilbene in chemical structure. Diethylstilbestrol (DES), a stilbene, was the first to be synthesized and has potent estrogenic activity. Further modifications in structure yielded other nonsteroidal compounds (eg, hexestrol, dienestrol, methallenestril, chlorotrianisene) with varying degrees of estrogenic potency. Clomiphene [Clomid], which is related structurally to chlorotrianisene, possesses both estrogenic and antiestrogenic activity and is used to treat infertility (see Chapter 45).

Synthetic progestins are derived either from modification of the testosterone molecule (norethindrone, norethindrone acetate, and other compounds used only in oral contraceptives), from 17α-hydroxyprogesterone (hydroxyprogesterone caproate, medroxyprogesterone acetate, megestrol acetate), or by changing the position of the C-19 methyl group of progesterone to the α position (dydrogesterone). Depending upon the parent compound and the chemical alterations employed, these agents have varying degrees of progestational, estrogenic, or androgenic potency.

The biological activity of the synthetic estrogens and progestins is similar but not identical to that of the natural compounds. Potency and side effects vary according to the chemical structure or route of administration employed.

Indications

Amenorrhea: Estrogen and progestins are used both to diagnose the etiology of amenorrhea and to treat it, if appropriate. Amenorrhea may be primary or secondary, but generally the same diagnostic approach is employed in either case. A complete medical history and physical examination are necessary to exclude causes outside the reproductive system. Amenorrhea secondary to hyper- or hypofunction of the adrenal cortex or thyroid or to diabetes mellitus may be corrected by treating the primary disorder. Secondary amenorrhea, particularly in adolescents, may result from inadequate nutrition or psychological stress. Other possible causes include a prolactin-secreting pituitary adenoma, abnormal androgen production (see the discussion on Hirsutism), congenital abnormalities (eg, Turner's syndrome), or primary ovarian failure. Hormones are useful to establish the source of the defect (ie, ovary, endometrium, anterior pituitary, hypothalamus). Pregnancy must always be ruled out before exogenous hormones are used.

To test the presence of estrogenic stimulation and ability of the endometrium to respond, intramuscular progesterone in oil (100 or 200 mg) or oral medroxyprogesterone acetate (MPA) (10 mg daily orally for five days) is administered. An oral preparation is often preferred because of the simplicity of administration and the discomfort associated with injection of progesterone. Withdrawal bleeding three to five days after treatment indicates adequate estrogenic stimulation of the endometrium and probable anovulation and suggests either failure of the ovarian follicular apparatus to respond to gonadotropins (high levels of serum gonadotropins support this diagnosis) or inadequate production or abnormal temporal pattern of secretion of gonadotropin (hypothalamic-pituitary-ovarian axis dysfunction). Absence of withdrawal bleeding suggests lack of endogenous estrogen stimulation, obstruction of outflow from the uterus, or ovulation within the last two weeks. If bleeding does not occur, a course of estrogen therapy with the addition of a progestin at the end of the cycle is given.

Ovarian failure may be congenital (eg, Turner's syndrome, presence of Y chromosome, mosaicism) or caused by premature menopausal changes. Replacement therapy should be considered to stimulate development or to maintain secondary sex characteristics and prevent osteoporosis. A progestin is given in addition to estrogen to prevent unopposed endometrial stimulation. Suggested regimens include conjugated estrogens 0.625 (or 1.25 mg if more estrogen is needed) daily for 24 days with oral MPA 10 mg daily during the last seven to ten days of estrogen therapy. Oral contraceptives (OCs) are not used for replacement therapy because they contain pharmacologic, not physiologic, quantities of hormones.) Each cycle can begin on the first of each month for convenience. The adequacy of such therapy can be monitored by the relief of symptoms, the maturational process, the vaginal cornification index, or the level of CBG attained.

If the estrogen-progestin challenge fails to produce withdrawal bleeding, a defect in the outflow tract or endometrium is suggested. The latter may be a result of Asherman's syndrome (uterine synechiae); surgical correction by hysteroscopy and lysis of adhesions is followed by estrogen-progestin therapy designed to rebuild a normal endometrium. Suggested postoperative regimens include (1) conjugated estrogens 5 to 10 mg daily for three weeks plus MPA 10 mg daily during the third week of estrogen therapy, repeated monthly for six months; or (2) conjugated estrogens 5 mg daily for three weeks plus MPA 10 mg daily for the last five days of estrogen therapy, repeated monthly for three cycles.

The treatment of amenorrhea caused by dysfunction of the hypothalamic-pituitary-ovarian (HPO) axis depends upon the goals of the patient. After the presence of a pituitary adenoma is excluded and if the patient desires pregnancy, induction of ovulation may be attempted (see Chapter 45). If the patient does not desire pregnancy, therapy to induce menses may be of psychological benefit but does not necessarily serve a useful physiologic function. However, if the patient has sufficient endogenous estrogen to promote endometrial stimulation, she should be given intermittent progestin therapy to interrupt this steady-state estrogen effect on the endometrium. MPA 10 mg daily for seven to ten days every six to eight weeks will serve this purpose and produce withdrawal bleeding.

Patients with disturbance of the HPO axis may unknowingly experience return of spontaneous cyclicity and therefore may be at risk of pregnancy if they are sexually active. Nonhormonal contraceptives are preferred in these patients, but low-dose OCs are sometimes administered. Although use of these agents will provide contraceptive protection, they may further suppress or alter HPO axis dysfunction.

Dysfunctional Bleeding: Abnormal uterine bleeding may be of organic origin (eg, endometrial cancer, coagulation defects, chronic endometritis, polyps, myomas, complications of pregnancy) or may be dysfunctional, that is, caused by estrogen and progesterone imbalance unassociated with organic pathology. Dysfunctional bleeding is often associated with anovulatory cycles, which are most common in adolescence and the perimenopausal years. This type of cycle produces an estrogen-dominated, fragile, hyperplastic endometrium characterized by periodic profuse bleeding episodes or irregular, possibly chronic, spotting, these abnormalities result from relatively constant, low-level estrogen stimulation which is uninterrupted by progesterone. Dysfunctional bleeding also may be caused by an atrophic endometrium secondary to progestin dominance. A history of combined OC use with a progressively decreasing volume of withdrawal bleeding or progestin-only contraception helps to distinguish the latter type of bleeding. Endometrial biopsy and medical history assist in determining the rationale of drug therapy. Before any hormonal therapy is initiated, pregnancy should be excluded.

If the endometrium is proliferative or hyperplastic, therapy with progesterone (50 to 100 mg in oil intramuscularly) or an oral progestin (5 to 20 mg MPA daily for 5 to 20 days) is useful. The patient with denuded endometrium benefits by administration of a high-potency estrogen-progestin combination or by estrogen alone to build up a structurally stable endometrium (see Chapter 44, Contraceptive Agents, for a listing of oral contraceptive preparations). Conjugated estrogens may be given intravenously initially to control an acute bleeding episode. Suggested oral regimens for initial control or following intravenous estrogen include (1) estrogen plus up to 20 to 30 mg progestin for two days, followed by estrogen plus 10 mg progestin for three days [Enovid 5 or 10], or three Ovral tablets daily for seven to ten days; (2) ethinyl estradiol 50 to 100 mcg plus MPA 10 mg daily for seven to ten days; (3) conjugated estrogens 2.5 to 3.75 mg plus MPA 10 mg daily for seven to ten days or conjugated estrogens 5 mg daily for one week with a progestin added the last five days (MPA 20 mg or norethindrone acetate 10 mg daily).

Bleeding usually is controlled within one to three days, and failure to do so may require curettage. The patient should be prepared for heavy withdrawal bleeding with dysmenorrhea following the above regimens, but the bleeding is usually self-limited. Subsequent cycles are regulated for 6 to 12 months by administering OCs for one year or, if contraception is not required, a progestin alone (MPA 10 mg or norethindrone acetate 5 mg daily for five days) preceding expected withdrawal bleeding can be used during the second six months. The preference of some physicians for long-term nonhormonal contraception in the young anovulatory patient is based on the possibility of suppression of the already compromised HPO feedback control axis (see also the discussion on Amenorrhea).

Hirsutism: The ovary is most often the source of excessive androgen that causes hirsutism (often associated with anovulation), but the adrenal cortex also may be involved. Conditions such as Cushing's syndrome, congenital adrenal hyperplasia, and ovarian or adrenal neoplasms should be considered and treated appropriately if present. Useful diagnostic procedures include determination of 17-ketosteroids (17-KS), 17-hydroxysteroids, serum testosterone, and serum LH levels, usually in that sequence. Increased serum testosterone levels usually are of ovarian origin, and extremely elevated 17-KS suggest an excess of adrenal androgen. If virilism occurs in addition to hirsutism, the likelihood of a tumor as the source of excess androgen is greater.

Alteration of the hormonal milieu may eventually control non-neoplastic (ovarian or adrenal) hirsutism, but up to one year of treatment may be required before effects become apparent because, although suppression of new hair growth can be accomplished, normal levels of androgens maintain hair that is already present. After six months of hormonal therapy, electrolysis is useful to hasten the cosmetic results.

Combination OCs suppress ovarian steroidogenesis secondary to LH inhibition and increase levels of SHBG, which results in decreased levels of free testosterone. Although any preparation may be used, those with low androgenic and progestational activities are preferred (eg, Brevicon, Modicon, Enovid). (See Chapter 44 for table on OC preparations available.) Alternatively, treatment with MPA (oral or depot form) may be attempted if estrogens should be avoided. Since adrenal androgen production is stimulated by ACTH, very low doses of glucocorticoids may suppress excessive androgen secretion of adrenal origin, particularly if given at bedtime. Dexamethasone also may suppress ovarian androgens, possibly by a direct effect on ovarian tissue. However, the usual precautions associated with glucocorticoid administration should be taken if this type of therapy is considered (see Chapter 41, Adrenal Corticosteroids).

Premenstrual Tension and Dysmenorrhea: Prior to menses, some women experience variable manifestations of the premenstrual tension syndrome which may include edema (eg, abdominal bloating, breast tenderness, weight gain), headache, or psychogenic symptoms (eg, irritability, depression). Since the etiology of the syndrome is not clearly understood and may be multifactorial, treatment is often symptomatic (eg, diuretics, antianxiety agents) and is not always effective. Hormonal therapy is not usually employed, but dydrogesterone [Duphaston, Gynorest] is being investigated for use in women who have decreased production of progesterone during the luteal phase. Other therapies are also under study.

Dysmenorrhea may be primary or secondary to other conditions (eg, endometriosis), in which case the specific cause is treated. Primary dysmenorrhea probably occurs as a result of the increased production of prostaglandin (PG) (secondary to progesterone) by the secretory endometrium during the luteal phase. Therefore, agents that inhibit ovulation, steroidogenesis, or prostaglandin production are effective. Mild analgesics often are not effective. Patients who require contraceptive protection as well as relief from dysmenorrhea are sometimes benefited by treatment with OCs. If dysmenorrhea is not relieved with OCs, endometriosis or another organic cause should be considered. Dydrogesterone, a retroprogesterone that does not suppress ovulation, may be useful because it apparently inhibits steroidogenesis and thus reduces the eventual elevation of the prostaglandin level before menses. Finally, potent PG inhibitors (eg, indomethacin, mefenamic acid, flufenamic acid) are being investigated for this indication and appear to be effective. Since they affect PG production throughout the body, further study of the safety of these agents is required before their routine use in dysmenorrhea can be recommended.

Endometriosis: Treatment of endometriosis depends partly on whether or not the patient desires immediate or future pregnancy (see Chapter 45, Agents Used to Treat Infertility). One definitive treatment is surgery; however, various hormonal regimens offer some degree of effectiveness. Since endometrial implants undergo decidualization, necrosis, and reabsorption during pregnancy, induction of a pseudopregnant state by the continuous (noncyclic) administration of combination OCs (eg, Norinyl 2, Ortho-Novum 2, Ovral) for six to nine months may be of benefit. If estrogens are contraindicated, MPA (oral or depot form) may be employed. The depot form may cause amenorrhea over a period of months. Progestin alone produces an atrophic endometrium rather than decidual progression and may be associated with irregular bleeding. Methyltestosterone (10 mg daily) also may relieve symptoms but is not used frequently. Danazol [Danocrine] decreases gonadotropic stimulation of steroid secretion (and consequent growth of the endometrial implants) and does not possess estrogenic or progestational activity. The mild androgenic effect of this agent is responsible for its side effects (eg, weight gain, oily skin and acne, hypoestrogenic symptoms). Although danazol, like all drug therapy, has limited effectiveness and is expensive compared to other drug regimens, it is probably the drug of choice in the treatment of endometriosis when hormonal therapy is indicated (see the evaluation in Chapter 45 for further discussion and dosage information).

Growth Abnormalities: When otherwise normal girls have a predicted adult height (from tables based on present stature and bone age) of greater than six feet and when realization of this growth potential is severely threatening to the child, estrogen therapy is sometimes employed to *suppress the growth rate* and eventual height attained. Estrogens inhibit production of somatomedin and are effective even though growth hormone levels rise concurrently with treatment. Therapy is more effective the earlier it is begun, but this principle has limitations. Treatment initiated at age 8 or 9 may be undesirable because of the psychological impact of the long-term regimen (usually one to two

years) and the pubertal changes, including induced menses, that result from treatment. On the other hand, if therapy is not begun until after the adolescent growth spurt (usually premenarcheal), suppression of growth is not as great. There is usually an initial acceleration of growth before suppression occurs. Once initiated, therapy must be continued until epiphyseal closure occurs or a net stimulation of growth may result.

When estrogen treatment is initiated by bone age of 11 or 12 years (or early to midpuberty), adult height averages 2 to 3 inches less than predicted height. Treatment is most effective when estrogen is taken daily and continuously. However, a progestin is added monthly to induce withdrawal bleeding and thus avoid overstimulation of the endometrium. Dosages given are approximately ten times those used in replacement therapy. Suggested regimens include conjugated estrogens 5 to 10 mg (or the equivalent) daily and continuously, with a progestin (eg, MPA 10 mg, norethindrone 10 mg daily) added for five to seven days each month to induce withdrawal bleeding.

The potential hazards of estrogen therapy must be considered, and the long-term effects of therapy are unknown. The HPO axis apparently is not suppressed, however, since almost all patients experience spontaneous regular menses two to six months after cessation of treatment.

The diagnosis of constitutional *precocious puberty* is likely in girls experiencing pubertal changes before age 8 when ovarian, adrenal, hypothalamic, or pineal tumors have been ruled out. Large doses of the depot form of MPA (400 mg intramuscularly once every three months) effectively suppress gonadotropin secretion. Breast size decreases and menses cease but the rate of linear growth may not be inhibited.

Hypoventilation: Endogenous progesterone stimulates respiration during the luteal phase and pregnancy. MPA administered to normal men has the same effect. This property has proved useful in the treatment of selected patients with the obesity-hypoventilation (pickwickian) syndrome. Patients are predominantly male and demonstrate extreme obesity, hypoventilation (with resultant hypoxemia and hypercapnia), polycythemia, and cor pulmonale. A prominent feature is hypersomnolence caused by multiple nighttime apneic episodes (possibly caused by prolapse of the tongue against the posterior pharynx) that result in sleep deprivation. Life-threatening arrhythmias may occur during apneic episodes. Diagnosis is aided by demonstration of the normalization of blood gases after voluntary hyperventilation. Severe cases may require tracheostomy or treatment with digitalis and diuretics. Milder cases respond to weight reduction, but this method is generally difficult to implement in these patients. Although treatment with MPA does not decrease the number of apneic episodes, blood gases are improved because of the drug's stimulation of alveolar ventilation as well as increased sensitivity of the ventilatory response to hypercapnia and hypoxia. The hematocrit also is reduced. MPA is usually administered sublingually (20 mg three times daily). Oral administration may be equally effective but has not been tested. Some male patients become impotent as a result of therapy.

Cancer: Hormonal ablative therapy (oophorectomy in premenopausal women and adrenalectomy in both premenopausal and postmenopausal women) is employed commonly in *metastatic breast cancer*. Hypophysectomy may further benefit patients who improve with either type of surgery. Demonstration of estrogen receptors in the neoplasm is necessary in selecting patients who will benefit from hormonal treatment (ablative or pharmacologic). Their absence is an excellent predictor of failure, but their presence is not an entirely reliable predictor of success. The longer the interval between mastectomy and the appearance of metastases, the better the likelihood of positive response to endocrine therapy.

Large doses of estrogen may be used in selected patients with metastatic breast cancer ten or more years after menopause. Progestins or androgens also are sometimes employed. The latter appear to be more effective in pre- than in postmenopausal women and when bone metastases occur.

Progestins may benefit up to 40% of patients with metastatic *endometrial carcinoma*. Best results usually are observed in younger patients and those with well differentiated tumors. Large doses produce endometrial atrophy; in addition, tumor nodules may decrease in size and pulmonary metastases may disappear. However, regression or arrest may be only temporary. One to two months of treatment may be necessary before objective response becomes evident. Although response to therapy is not related to site of metastases, undifferentiated tumors or those displaying a papillary growth pattern show poorer response than tumors demonstrating squamous metaplasia.

Hormone-sensitive disseminated *prostatic carcinoma* usually is treated with estrogens and/or bilateral orchiectomy. Hormonal manipulation induces histologic remission of tumor and regression of bone metastases; 80% of patients show improvement which may include decreased gland size with subsequent relief of urinary obstruction, rapid relief of ostealgia, and improvement in well-being. The effect is palliative but may last several years, although survival may not be prolonged. The effectiveness of estrogen therapy is partly due to suppression of LH secretion with resultant suppression of testosterone production and that of castration is due to removal of the primary source of this androgen. Estrogen also may act by directly suppressing the growth of tumor cells and by nonspecific stimulation of the immune response. Undesirable side effects include loss of libido, impotence, gynecomastia, thromboembolic phenomena, and congestive heart failure (due to fluid retention). See also Chapter 68, Antineoplastic Agents.

Other Uses: Although estrogens have been used to treat *habitual* and *threatened abortions* in the past, it is now apparent that such treatment was ineffective. Estrogens now are contraindicated during pregnancy, largely on the basis of the teratogenic effects of diethylstilbestrol (DES) and other estrogens in both female and male offspring (see the section on Metabolic Effects, Adverse Reactions, and Precautions). Progesterone and progestins also have been used for similar indications, and there is some evidence of teratogenicity of the latter agents as well, particularly those with high androgenic potency. In general, progestational agents are not employed during pregnancy, but there are exceptions. Progesterone is used to treat luteal phase dysfunction from ovulation through the early part of pregnancy. Some success has been achieved in preventing premature births in high-risk women by administering hydroxyprogesterone caproate [Delalutin] from the sixteenth week of pregnancy. It should be noted that treatment is initiated after organogenesis has been completed, and thus far no adverse effects have been reported in these fetuses (Johnson et al, 1975) (see Chapter 45, Agents Used to Treat Infertility).

Estrogens, alone or in combination with androgens, have been widely used to prevent *postpartum lactation* and the discomforts associated with its suppression. However, the effectiveness and safety of such therapy are now questioned. In the absence of suckling, lactation will eventually cease without drug treatment. Analgesics may relieve the discomfort accompanying engorgement. There is little difference in the incidence of rebound engorgement or control of lactation between patients treated with hormones and in untreated controls. Furthermore, there is a three- to tenfold increased risk of thromboembolism in patients treated with estrogen. Since bromocriptine [Parlodel] is more promising for suppressing postpartum lactation when drug therapy is deemed desirable, the use of hormonal agents generally is no longer recommended (see Chapter 46, Agents Related to Anterior Pituitary and Hypothalamic Function).

Menopause: The menopause is often accompanied by vasomotor symptoms (ie, hot flushes, sweating) and eventually manifestations of vaginal and urethral atrophy (eg, vaginitis, dyspareunia, urinary frequency) which respond to estrogen therapy. Emotional complaints (eg, irritability, anxiety, depression), insomnia,

fatigability, and headache also sometimes occur. These symptoms, in part, may be secondary to other, particularly vasomotor, disturbances. However, significant improvement in memory and reduction of anxiety have been observed after estrogen therapy in women who did not report vasomotor flushing (Campbell, 1976 B).

Estrogens also may be useful prophylactically and to prevent progression of osteoporosis and must be taken chronically for this purpose but certain risks, including endometrial cancer (see the section on Metabolic Effects, Adverse Reactions, and Precautions), must be considered. Patients taking estrogen therapy should be re-evaluated at 6- to 12-month intervals to confirm the continuing need for medication as well as to monitor status. Blood pressure, breast, and pelvic examinations should be included. Papanicolaou smears should include material from the endocervical canal since this modification improves but does not ensure detection of endometrial cancer.

Osteoporosis sometimes occurs after natural or surgical menopause. It is uncommon in men or black women and it is more prevalent in thin, small-framed women and in women who smoke. About 25% of white women over 60 years of age have vertebral compression fractures. Fractures of the radius and neck of the femur also are common in osteoporotic women. Hip fractures have high associated morbidity and mortality (one-sixth of elderly patients with hip fractures die within three months of injury). Only 25% to 30% of elderly white women do not experience appreciable bone loss. The development of osteoporosis is more closely related to estrogen deficiency than to advancing age per se; estrogens are believed to inhibit bone resorption. The onset of osteoporosis is more rapid after oophorectomy than natural menopause, probably because decline of estrogen levels in the former situation is rapid, whereas the decline is more gradual in natural menopause.

Estrogen replacement therapy is particularly effective in preventing osteoporosis in women with oophorectomy before natural menopause. However, estrogen also retards bone loss after natural menopause. The number of fractures and newly diagnosed cases of osteoporosis is reduced in estrogen-treated women compared to untreated controls. Therapy initiated soon after menopause is more effective than when delayed several years but does not reverse bone changes that have already occurred. The duration of effectiveness in retarding bone loss is not known and there are no firm dosage recommendations. However, it is generally believed that usual menopausal replacement dosages (0.3 to 0.625 mg conjugated estrogens or equivalent) are adequate. Because of the serious consequences of osteoporosis, consideration of long-term estrogen therapy in high-risk or symptomatic women and in those experiencing early hysterectomy (in whom the possibility of endometrial cancer is obviated) is justified. Unfortunately, early diagnostic methods are not routinely available; routine x-ray procedures detect osteoporosis only after considerable bone loss has already occurred. Physical exercise should be encouraged, and adequate intake of vitamin D and calcium should be assured since osteomalacia may be present concurrently in some patients (see also Chapter 54, Agents Affecting Calcium Metabolism).

Preparations and Regimens: The estrogen preparations most commonly used to treat menopausal symptoms in the United States are orally administered conjugated estrogens. Oral administration delivers greater amounts of the hormone to the hepatic circulation than other routes. Other synthetic and natural preparations are also effective, and the superiority of a particular type has not been demonstrated. There have been reports that natural estrogens have fewer undesirable effects on serum lipids and clotting factors, but whether this is true in biologically equivalent amounts and at dosages commonly used in replacement therapy requires further investigation. The route of administration, pattern of delivery (cyclic vs continuous), and dosage may be more important in determining effectiveness and toxicity than the specific compound or preparation.

Topical vaginal estrogen preparations are readily absorbed and produce blood levels approaching those attained after oral ingestion. They are effective for systemic as well as local symptoms and should not be prescribed when use of estrogen is contraindicated. Intramuscular injection is generally inconvenient and therefore seldom appropriate for long-term use. Subdermal implants and long-acting injections may be used but have uncertain rates of absorption, and exposure to the hormone is uninterrupted. If these agents are used when the uterus is *in situ*, periodic administration of progestin may be prescribed.

In general, the goal of menopausal estrogen therapy is to relieve specific responsive symptoms with the lowest effective dosage. Most symptoms can be controlled by conjugated estrogens 0.3 to 0.625 mg or the equivalent given daily and cyclically. Eventual withdrawal of medication is recommended in the absence of continuing symptoms or other indications (ie, prophylaxis or treatment of osteoporosis). For vasomotor symptoms, the dosage can be reduced gradually as symptoms diminish, and therapy may be discontinued eventually.

Estrogen should be administered cyclically when the uterus is intact to avoid uninterrupted stimulation of the endometrium. Medication is administered daily for three weeks followed by one week without treatment or for the first 25 days of each month. The first of the month can be used as the day to initiate each cycle of therapy. If bleeding occurs during the week that treatment is withheld, administration can be resumed before the bleeding ceases. The dose may be decreased to avoid monthly withdrawal bleeding if menopausal symptoms remain controlled. Cyclic therapy is advised even in women who have undergone hysterectomy, since this pattern more closely simulates premenstrual secretion of estrogen and avoids unopposed stimulation of other target tissues.

The practice of adding a progestin to the cyclic regimen of estrogen is gaining favor in the replacement therapy of women with a uterus in place. The progestin (eg, MPA

10 mg) is given daily for the last seven to ten days of estrogen administration. The rationale for this is based on the effects of a progestin on estrogen-primed tissue. Progestin decreases cytoplasmic estrogen receptors, thus inhibiting the ultimate growth-stimulating effect of the hormone. Secretory changes are induced and the endometrial lining regresses, making endometrial conditions unfavorable for the development of hyperplasia.

If long-term estrogen therapy is considered in postmenopausal women, the expected benefits must outweigh the risks and the patient should understand the factors involved and participate in making the decision. More accurate assessment of the risk/benefit ratio would be possible if significant diagnostic improvements permitted early identification of women likely to become osteoporotic and if routine cost-effective methods of endometrial sampling were available to ensure early detection of endometrial pathology.

Metabolic Effects, Adverse Reactions, and Precautions

In general, the side effects of estrogen and progestin therapy are similar to those observed with use of contraceptive hormonal preparations (see Chapter 44, Contraceptive Agents). The dosages prescribed for replacement therapy, the most common noncontraceptive indication for estrogen and progestin treatment, generally are lower than for contraceptive purposes, and hence the associated incidence and intensity of effects would be expected to be lower.

Nausea occurs relatively frequently early in treatment but can be minimized by taking medication with food. This reaction usually disappears with continued treatment, even with the large doses used to treat cancer. Fullness or tenderness of breasts and edema caused by sodium and water retention may occur with estrogen treatment and, if used for replacement therapy, may indicate excessive dosage.

Metabolism: Results of studies suggest that most estrogen replacement therapy does not adversely affect glucose tolerance clinically. Effects on serum lipids are variable; the preponderance of evidence shows that the total cholesterol level is slightly reduced but the triglyceride level is increased. Administration of estrogens is associated with increased levels of high density lipoproteins which are inversely related to the incidence of coronary heart disease. At usual replacement dosages, conjugated estrogens exert minimal effects on protein synthesis. Only slight elevations of CBG levels result. The risk of gallbladder surgery is increased two and one-half times in postmenopausal women treated with estrogen. Changes in hepatic excretory function will result in greater cholesterol saturation in the bile, thus predisposing to gallstone formation. Estrogens should not be given to patients with severe acute liver disease.

When estrogens are administered to patients with breast cancer and bone metastases, hypercalcemia may occur. In such patients, estrogen should be discontinued and the serum calcium level should be reduced by appropriate means.

Cardiovascular System: Although increased levels of some clotting factors have been observed, replacement dosages of estrogen are not associated with an increased risk of thromboembolism. Nevertheless, estrogens generally should not be administered to menopausal patients with thromboembolic disease or a past history of such disease because they are presumably at higher risk. The likelihood of thromboembolic phenomena has been reported to be increased when pharmacologic doses of estrogen are used to treat breast or prostatic cancer. Administration of estrogen to suppress postpartum lactation is associated with a higher incidence of thromboembolism, and this use of estrogen is no longer recommended (see the section on Indications).

Premenopausal women have a lower incidence of coronary heart disease than men of comparable age, but this advantage is lost after the menopause. The possibility that this difference is ascribable to the presence of higher levels of estrogen in premenopausal women and that coronary heart disease may be prevented in men and older women by administration of estrogen has been considered. The incidence of death from myocardial infarction (MI) was increased in men with a history of MI who were treated with pharmacologic doses of conjugated estrogens (5 mg daily). An increased incidence of cardiovascular deaths also has been reported in men receiving DES 5 mg daily for prostatic carcinoma but was not evident at lower dosages. More optimistic data has shown that hypoestrogenic women (from various causes including natural menopause) treated for at least five years with estrogen had fewer new diagnoses of cardiovascular disease and hypertension than untreated women (Hammond et al, 1979 A). In postmenopausal women taking estrogen, the incidence of hypertension generally is not increased, although this may occur in sensitive individuals. However, if hypertension develops or worsens with estrogen therapy, medication should be discontinued. The occurrence of nonfatal MI is not increased, but the associated risk of developing angina pectoris is about doubled (Ryan, 1976; Gordon et al, 1978). Estrogens generally are not administered to patients with migraine headaches.

Teratogenicity: Synthetic progestins should not be administered during pregnancy because of their possible teratogenic potential (see Chapter 44, Contraceptive Agents). Hormonal pregnancy tests are outmoded for this reason and because of the availability of several highly accurate immunological tests of serum or urine HCG concentration.

Although congenital malformations have occurred rarely with 21-carbon compounds (ie, hydroxyprogesterone caproate [Delalutin], progesterone), the incidence is not greater than chance and it is believed that these agents are safe for use in specific appropriate indications during pregnancy. These include prevention of premature birth (hydroxyprogesterone caproate) and treatment of luteal phase dysfunction (progesterone). See the section on Indications and Chapter 45, Agents Used to Treat Infertility.

The administration of any estrogen is contraindicated during pregnancy. The use of synthetic hormones to treat threatened abortion is ineffective and carries the risk of teratogenicity. Administration of DES for this indication during pregnancy is associated with vaginal adenosis and, rarely, adenocarcinoma in female offspring; reproductive tract abnormalities, including infertility, have been observed in male offspring. Although these effects have been associated most freqently with DES, it is not known whether they are specific for nonsteroidal estrogens or whether any estrogenic compound would cause similar aberrations. The high incidence with DES could reflect the widespread use of this agent 20 years ago for prevention of miscarriage. Postpubertal girls whose mothers received DES during pregnancy should be examined yearly for early detection of abnormalities. Management of adenosis is conservative; no treatment is generally given but regular examinations are continued. There is no evidence that adenosis undergoes malignant transformation.

Carcinogenicity: Women should be examined for breast and genital carcinoma before estrogen therapy is instituted and periodically during administration. Therapy should be withdrawn if evidence of estrogen-dependent carcinoma is found or suspected. Available evidence indicates that menopausal estrogen therapy does not increase the risk of developing breast cancer. However, caution is advised in women with a strong family history or in those who are otherwise at increased risk of the disease.

In several studies, an increase in the risk of developing endometrial carcinoma has been reported to be associated with estrogen therapy in postmenopausal women. Generally the risk increases with increasing dosage and duration of use and is higher in women who did *not* have conditions previously identified with a higher risk of endometrial cancer (eg, obesity, diabetes, hypertension). The relative risk varied with the above conditions and among the populations studied from about 4 to 15 times (Antunes et al, 1979). There is some indication that addition of a progestin to cyclic estrogen treatment reduces the risk considerably (Hammond et al, 1979 B).

The putative role of estrogen in endometrial cancer (eg, carcinogen, tumor promoter, growth stimulator) has not been determined, but resolution of this point would not necessarily assist in making therapeutic decisions about estrogen usage. Careful monitoring of patients is always required. Abnormal bleeding requires investigation of endometrial status.

ESTROGENS

Steroidal Estrogens

ESTRADIOL
[Estrace, Progynon]

ESTRADIOL BENZOATE

ESTRADIOL CYPIONATE
[Depo-Estradiol Cypionate, E-Ionate P.A.]

ESTRADIOL VALERATE
[Delestrogen]

Estradiol is the principal and most biologically potent ovarian estrogenic hormone. It is usually injected intramuscularly, but pellets are sometimes implanted subcutaneously (eg, at time of oophorectomy). Oral therapy is generally ineffective because of rapid inactivation following ingestion. However, an oral micronized form of estradiol is effective in relieving menopausal symptoms. With micronization, particle size is reduced, thereby increasing surface area, dissolution, and rate of absorption. The recommended daily dosage for treating menopausal symptoms (1 to 2 mg) is approximately five to ten times the amount of estradiol produced daily by the normal premenopausal ovary. It is not yet known whether long-term therapy with this relatively large quantity of estradiol will have undesirable physiologic effects.

Esters of estradiol are administered intramuscularly in aqueous suspension or oil. Their onset of action is gradual and uncertain and the duration is variable (three or four days to three or four weeks).

See the Introduction for specific indications and adverse reactions. Estrogens used for replacement therapy are frequently given in a regimen with a progestin.

ROUTES, USUAL DOSAGE, AND PREPARATIONS. *Intramuscular*: For replacement therapy, (estradiol benzoate) 0.5 to 1.5 mg two or three times weekly; (estradiol cypionate) 1 to 5 mg weekly for two or three weeks; (estradiol valerate) 10 to 40 mg every one to four weeks.

ESTRADIOL BENZOATE:
Drug available generically: Powder 1 g; solution (in sesame oil, aqueous) 0.5 mg/ml in 30 ml containers.
ESTRADIOL CYPIONATE:
Drug available generically: Solution 5 mg/ml (aqueous) and 2 and 5 mg/ml (in oil) in 10 ml containers.
Depo-Estradiol Cypionate (Upjohn). Solution (in cottonseed oil) 1 mg/ml in 10 ml containers and 5 mg/ml in 5 ml containers.
E-Ionate P.A. (Tutag). Solution (in cottonseed oil) 5 mg/ml in 10 ml containers.
ESTRADIOL VALERATE:
Drug available generically: Powder (for injection) 1 g; solution 10, 20, and 40 mg/ml (aqueous, in oil) in 10 ml containers.
Delestrogen (Squibb). Solution (in sesame oil) 10 mg/ml in 5 ml containers; solution (in castor oil) 20 mg/ml in 1 and 5 ml containers and 40 mg/ml in 5 ml containers.

Oral (micronized): For menopausal symptoms, 1 to 2 mg daily for three weeks, then one week without medication, or daily Monday through Friday with medication withheld on Saturday and Sunday.
ESTRADIOL:
Estrace (Mead Johnson). Tablets (micronized) 1 and 2 mg.

Subcutaneous Implantation: One 25-mg pellet every three to four months or two 25-mg pellets every four to six months.
ESTRADIOL:
Progynon (Schering). Pellets 25 mg.

ESTRONE
[Follestrol, Theelin]

ESTRONE PIPERAZINE SULFATE
[Ogen]

ESTRONE AND ESTRONE POTASSIUM SULFATE
[Theelin R-P]

Estrone is an ovarian estrogenic hormone available in aqueous suspension, solution in oil, and vaginal suppositories. The aqueous mixture of the water-insoluble estrone and the water-soluble potassium salt of the sulfate ester (estrone potassium sulfate) is claimed to have a more prompt effect than insoluble estrone suspensions. The potency of most oral mixtures of estrogenic substances is expressed in terms of the estrone sodium sulfate content.

See the Introduction for specific indications and adverse reactions. Estrogens used for replacement therapy are frequently given in a regimen with a progestin.

ROUTES, USUAL DOSAGE, AND PREPARATIONS.
ESTRONE:
Intramuscular: For menopausal symptoms, 0.1 to 2 mg weekly in single or divided doses. For treatment of prostatic carcinoma, 2 to 4 mg two or three times weekly.

> Drug available generically: Powder (for injection) 1 g; solution 1 mg/ml (in oil) in 10 ml containers, 2 mg/ml (aqueous) in 10 and 30 ml containers, and 5 mg/ml (aqueous) in 10 ml containers.
> *Follestrol* (Bluline). Suspension (aqueous) 2 mg/ml in 10 ml containers.
> *Theelin* (Parke, Davis). Solution (in peanut oil) 1 and 2 mg/ml in 1 and 10 ml containers and 5 mg/ml in 1 and 5 ml containers.

Vaginal: One 0.2-mg suppository is inserted daily.

> *Theelin* (Parke, Davis). Suppositories 0.2 mg.

ESTRONE PIPERAZINE SULFATE:
Oral: For replacement therapy, 0.35 to 1.5 mg daily, cyclically.

> *Ogen* (Abbott). Tablets 0.75, 1.5, 3, and 6 mg (equivalent to estrone sodium sulfate activity 0.625, 1.25, 2.5, and 5 mg, respectively).

ESTRONE AND ESTRONE POTASSIUM SULFATE:
Intramuscular: For replacement therapy, 0.25 to 1 ml one or two times weekly.

> Preparation available generically: Each milliliter of suspension (aqueous) contains estrone 2 mg and estrone potassium sulfate 1 mg in 10 ml containers.
> *Theelin R-P* (Parke, Davis). Each milliliter of solution/suspension contains estrone 2 mg and estrone potassium sulfate 1 mg in 10 ml containers.

CONJUGATED ESTROGENS, U.S.P.
[Premarin]

This is a combination of the sodium salts of the sulfate esters of estrogenic substances, principally estrone and equilin; the esters are similar to the type excreted by pregnant mares. The various preparations contain 50% to 65% estrone sodium sulfate and 20% to 35% equilin sodium sulfate. They are effective orally, parenterally, and topically. There is disagreement about whether the parenteral preparation effectively controls spontaneous capillary bleeding rapidly and reduces capillary bleeding during surgery.

See the Introduction for specific indications and adverse reactions. Estrogens used for replacement therapy are frequently given in a regimen with a progestin.

ROUTES, USUAL DOSAGE, AND PREPARATIONS.
Oral: For menopausal symptoms, 0.3 to 1.25 mg daily, cyclically and a progestin may be added the last seven to ten days. (See also the section on Indications.) Alternatively, estrogen can be given five days a week with two days off medication. A progestin may be added for one week three times a year to prevent unopposed estrogen stimulation.
For replacement therapy in hypogonadism, 0.625 to 1.25 mg daily, cyclically (24 days

with a progestin added during the last five days) (see the section on Indications).

For dysfunctional uterine bleeding due to atrophic endometrium, 2.5 to 5 mg daily in divided doses for a week with a progestin added to the regimen. See also the section on Indications.

For breast carcinoma in women more than five years postmenopausal, 10 mg three times daily for at least three months.

For prostatic carcinoma, 1.25 to 2.5 mg three times daily.

> Drug available generically: Tablets 0.3, 0.625, 1.25, and 2.5 mg.
> *Premarin* (Ayerst). Tablets 0.3, 0.625, 1.25, and 2.5 mg.

Intravenous: For emergency treatment of dysfunctional uterine bleeding, 25 mg initially every four hours for three doses; oral treatment with an estrogen-progestin combination is then initiated. See also the section on Indications.

> *Premarin* (Ayerst). Powder (lyophilized) 25 mg with 5 ml of diluent.

ESTERIFIED ESTROGENS, U.S.P.
[Evex, Menest]

This is a combination of the sodium salts of the sulfate esters of estrogenic substances, principally estrone; the esters are similar to the type excreted by pregnant mares. Preparations of esterified estrogens contain 75% to 85% estrone sodium sulfate and 6.5% to 15% equilin sodium sulfate.

See the Introduction for indications and adverse reactions.

ROUTE, USUAL DOSAGE, AND PREPARATIONS. For dosage, see the evaluation on Conjugated Estrogens.

> *Evex* (Syntex). Tablets 0.625, 1.25, and 2.5 mg.
> *Menest* (Beecham). Tablets 0.3, 0.625, 1.25, and 2.5 mg.

> ADDITIONAL TRADEMARKS.
> *Amnestrogen* (Squibb), *Estratab* (Reid-Provident), *Femogen* (Fellows), *Glyestrin* (Scherer), *Zeste* (Ascher).

OTHER ESTROGENIC SUBSTANCES

Some mixtures of estrogenic substances do not conform to the U.S.P. definitions of conjugated estrogens or esterified estrogens. Most of these preparations combine estrogens of equine origin; some also contain synthetic pure conjugates. Their potency is usually expressed in terms of the sodium estrone sulfate content.

These preparations have the same indications and adverse effects as conjugated or esterified estrogens (see the Introduction and the evaluation on Conjugated Estrogens).

> AVAILABLE TRADEMARKS.
> *Estronol* (Central), *Hormonin No. 1, No. 2* (Carnrick), *Menagen* (Parke, Davis), *Urestrin* (Upjohn).

ETHINYL ESTRADIOL
[Estinyl, Feminone]

This steroid is related to estradiol, the principal ovarian estrogen. It is a potent, orally effective estrogen and is used alone and as a component of some estrogen-progestin oral contraceptive mixtures (see also Chapter 44).

See the Introduction for specific indications and adverse reactions.

ROUTE, USUAL DOSAGE, AND PREPARATIONS. *Oral*: For hypogonadism, 0.05 mg one to three times daily for the first two weeks of an arbitrary cycle, with the addition of a progestin for the last two weeks; for menopausal symptoms, 0.02 or 0.05 mg daily, cyclically; for dysfunctional bleeding, 50 to 100 mcg given with a progestin for seven to ten days (see the section on Indications); for progressive breast carcinoma in selected postmenopausal women, 1 mg three times daily. For prostatic carcinoma, 0.15 to 2 mg daily.

> Drug available generically: Powder 1 g; tablets 0.02 and 0.05 mg.
> *Estinyl* (Schering). Tablets 0.02, 0.05, and 0.5 mg.
> *Feminone* (Upjohn). Tablets 0.05 mg.

Nonsteroidal Estrogens

CHLOROTRIANISENE
[TACE]

Chlorotrianisene is a proestrogen with a long-acting effect; estrogenic activity has been found in adipose tissue up to one month after cessation of therapy. The drug is used most frequently for the palliative treatment of prostatic carcinoma. Its long duration of action makes chlorotrianisene unsuitable for the treatment of menstrual disorders and for replacement when cyclic therapy is desired.

See the Introduction for indications and adverse reactions.

ROUTE, USUAL DOSAGE, AND PREPARATIONS.
Oral: For prostatic carcinoma, 12 to 25 mg daily.
> TACE (Merrell-National). Capsules 12, 25, and 72 mg.

DIENESTROL
[DV]

This nonsteroidal estrogen is related chemically to diethylstilbestrol. It is applied topically to relieve symptoms of hypoestrogenic vaginal atrophy. Dienestrol is contraindicated during pregnancy. See the Introduction and the evaluation on Diethylstilbestrol for indications and adverse reactions.

ROUTE, USUAL DOSAGE, AND PREPARATIONS.
Topical: For atrophic and senile vaginitis, preparation is applied one to two times daily for one to two weeks, then reduced gradually to a maintenance level of one to three times a week.
> Drug available generically: Cream in 78 g containers.
> DV (Merrell-National). Cream 0.01% in 3 oz containers; suppositories 0.7 mg.

DIETHYLSTILBESTROL

DIETHYLSTILBESTROL DIPHOSPHATE
[Stilphostrol]

Diethylstilbestrol (DES) is the most potent nonsteroidal estrogen and has been used extensively. Since the drug is inactivated slowly, it can be given in single daily doses even when large amounts are required. DES is generally believed to cause a greater incidence of nausea than some other estrogen preparations and occasionally causes pigmentation (facies, nipples).

DES is contraindicated in pregnant women, especially during the first 16 weeks, for vaginal adenosis has occurred in 30% to 90% of postpubertal females whose mothers received DES or a closely related congener during pregnancy. Vaginal adenocarcinoma also has been reported rarely. Yearly examination of patients with this history is recommended. Epididymal cysts and impaired fertility have been reported in some postpubertal males whose mothers have a similar history of DES therapy during pregnancy. For contraceptive use of this product, see Chapter 44.

See the Introduction for specific indications and adverse reactions.

ROUTES, USUAL DOSAGE, AND PREPARATIONS.
DIETHYLSTILBESTROL:
Oral: For hypogonadism or replacement therapy, 0.2 to 0.5 mg daily until the desired response is obtained. For breast carcinoma in selected postmenopausal women, initially, 15 mg daily, with the amount increased according to the tolerance of the patient. For prostatic carcinoma, initially, 1 to 3 mg daily; dosage is increased in advanced cases.

Drug available generically: Capsules and tablets (plain, enteric-coated) 0.1, 0.25, 0.5, 1, and 5 mg.

Topical (vaginal): For replacement therapy, a maximum of 7 mg weekly.

Drug available generically: Suppositories 0.1 and 0.5 mg.

DIETHYLSTILBESTROL DIPHOSPHATE:

Intravenous: For prostatic carcinoma, 250 to 500 mg one or two times weekly.

Stilphostrol (Dome). Solution 50 mg/ml in 5 ml containers.

Oral: For prostatic carcinoma, 50 mg three times daily; the dose may be increased to 200 mg or more three times daily.

Stilphostrol (Dome). Tablets 50 mg.

HEXESTROL

This nonsteroidal estrogen is chemically related to diethylstilbestrol. See the Introduction and the evaluation on Diethylstilbestrol for indications and adverse reactions. Hexestrol is contraindicated during pregnancy.

ROUTE, USUAL DOSAGE, AND PREPARATIONS.
Oral: 2 to 3 mg daily until symptoms are controlled, then 0.2 to 1 mg daily.

Drug available generically: Tablets 3 mg.

Estrogens Combined with Other Drugs

ESTROGENS AND ANDROGENS

This type of mixture generally should not be used in women, since administration of androgens for prolonged periods may cause symptoms of masculinization. However, small doses of androgen given with estrogens may decrease stimulation of the breasts and endometrium and enhance libido during the menopause.

See Chapter 33, Androgens and Anabolic Steroids, for a listing of preparations.

ESTROGENS WITH SEDATIVES OR ANTIANXIETY AGENTS

This type of mixture is used to treat menopausal symptoms. Hot flashes and atrophic vaginitis usually respond readily to estrogen therapy alone. However, some patients may have anxiety that cannot be relieved by estrogen therapy. In these patients, mild sedatives or antianxiety agents may be helpful. Therefore, if one of the available combinations contains ingredients appropriate both quantitatively and qualitatively for an individual patient, the use of these mixtures may be acceptable for a *limited* period. Administration of the separate components is preferred, however.

See the Introduction for indications and adverse reactions.

AVAILABLE MIXTURES.
Menrium (Roche). Each tablet contains esterified estrogens 0.2 or 0.4 mg and chlordiazepoxide 5 mg or esterified estrogens 0.4 mg and chlordiazepoxide 10 mg.
Milprem (Wallace). Each tablet contains conjugated estrogens 0.45 mg and meprobamate 200 or 400 mg.
PMB (Ayerst). Each tablet contains conjugated estrogens 0.45 mg and meprobamate 200 or 400 mg.

HORMONE COSMETIC PREPARATIONS

Hormones used topically on the skin are marketed principally as quasi-cosmetic rejuvenating creams. Because of the current FDA restrictions on the concentrations of ovarian hormones permitted in such products, there is little likelihood that they will produce any systemic effects with ordinary use. However, systemic effects have followed *excessive* use of hormone creams. There is some experimental evidence that certain topically applied steroid hormones (both active and inactive biologically) may cause slight histologic thickening in some areas of the epidermis of aged skin. Estrogen can produce a slight increase in dermal thickness, but it is unlikely that this alters facial appearance.

Topical preparations containing physiologic amounts of estrogens or natural progesterone have no effect on human sebaceous glands and oil secretion. There is no scientific evidence that hormone creams are any more effective than simple emollients in relieving dryness of the skin or that hormone creams increase the amount of water that the skin can hold or restore fat to the subcutaneous layer.

Used as directed, topically applied hormones, as presently formulated in cosmetic preparations, appear to be safe.

PROGESTERONE AND PROGESTINS

PROGESTERONE
[Lipo-Lutin]

This natural progestational substance acts on target genital tissues and endocrine glands and also has general systemic effects. Parenteral preparations in oil are used primarily to treat menstrual disorders; responsiveness to progesterone in the target organ depends upon the priming action of estrogen. The drug is ineffective when given orally.

Progesterone is also available in an IUD [Progestasert] (see Chapter 44).

See the Introduction for indications and adverse reactions.

ROUTE, USUAL DOSAGE, AND PREPARATIONS.
Intramuscular: For diagnostic use in amenorrhea, 100 or 200 mg in oil; for dysfunctional uterine bleeding, 50 to 100 mg in oil.

> Drug available generically: Powder (for injection) 5 g; suspension 25 and 50 mg/ml (aqueous) in 10 ml containers and 25, 50, and 100 mg/ml (in oil) in 10 ml containers.
> *Lipo-Lutin* (Parke, Davis). Solution (in peanut oil) 50 mg/ml in 5 ml containers.

DYDROGESTERONE
[Duphaston, Gynorest]

This derivative of retroprogesterone is effective orally. It has no inherent estrogenic activity and no androgenic effects. Priming with estrogen is necessary prior to use. The drug is claimed to be nonthermogenic and does not consistently inhibit ovulation. It is used in other countries to treat premenstrual tension and dysmenorrhea.

See the Introduction for indications and adverse reactions.

ROUTE, USUAL DOSAGE, AND PREPARATIONS.
Oral: For amenorrhea and dysmenorrhea, 10 to 20 mg daily in divided doses for five to ten days prior to the expected menstrual period.

> *Duphaston* (Philips Roxane), *Gynorest* (Mead Johnson). Tablets 5 and 10 mg.

HYDROXYPROGESTERONE CAPROATE
[Delalutin]

This derivative of progesterone is administered parenterally. Its duration of action is about 9 to 17 days. Hydroxyprogesterone has no estrogenic activity. Priming with estrogen is necessary before a response is noted.

See the Introduction for indications and adverse reactions.

ROUTE, USUAL DOSAGE, AND PREPARATIONS.
Intramuscular: For menstrual disorders, 125 to 250 mg per cycle.

> Drug available generically: Solution 125 mg/ml in 10 ml containers and 250 mg/ml in 5 ml containers.
> *Delalutin* (Squibb). Solution (in sesame oil) 125 mg/ml in 2 and 10 ml containers and 250 mg/ml (in castor oil) in 1 and 5 ml containers.

MEDROXYPROGESTERONE ACETATE (MPA)
[Curretab, Depo-Provera, Provera]

This derivative of progesterone is effective both orally and parenterally. The duration of action of the depot preparation is variable and occasionally prolonged and therefore may be undesirable in women desiring pregnancy in the imminent future. The drug has no inherent estrogenic activity. Priming with estrogen is necessary before a response is noted. For use of the parenteral preparation for contraceptive purposes, see Chapter 44.

See the Introduction for indications and adverse reactions.

ROUTES, USUAL DOSAGE, AND PREPARATIONS.
Oral: For amenorrhea and dysfunctional uterine bleeding, 5 to 10 mg daily for five to ten days, depending upon the indication. For endometriosis, 30 mg daily. For menopausal replacement therapy, 10 mg for five to seven days during the third week of estrogen administration (see the section on Indications).

> *Curretab* (Reid-Provident). Tablets 10 mg.
> *Provera* (Upjohn). Tablets 2.5 and 10 mg.

Intramuscular: For endometriosis, 150 mg every three months. For endometrial carcinoma, 400 mg to 1 g weekly initially.

> *Depo-Provera* (Upjohn). Suspension (aqueous) 100 mg/ml in 5 ml containers and 400 mg/ml in 1, 2.5, and 10 ml containers.

MEGESTROL ACETATE
[Megace]

This progestin is used in the palliative treatment of advanced carcinoma of the breast or endometrium. See Chapter 68, Antineoplastic Agents.

ROUTE, USUAL DOSAGE, AND PREPARATIONS.
Oral: For breast carcinoma, 160 mg daily in four divided doses; for endometrial carcinoma, 40 to 320 mg daily in divided doses. At least two months of continuous therapy is considered adequate to determine the efficacy of this agent.

> *Megace* (Mead Johnson). Tablets 20 and 40 mg.

NORETHINDRONE
[Norlutin]

NORETHINDRONE ACETATE
[Norlutate]

This derivative of nortestosterone is a potent oral progestational agent. Its androgenic effects are minor and variable. For therapeutic purposes, the acetate salt is considered to be approximately twice as potent as the base. Norethindrone is also combined with estrogens for many indications, including contraceptive use (see Chapter 44).

See the Introduction for indications and adverse reactions.

ROUTE, USUAL DOSAGE, AND PREPARATIONS.
NORETHINDRONE:
Oral: The manufacturer's recommended

dosage is: For amenorrhea and dysfunctional uterine bleeding, 5 to 20 mg daily, starting with the fifth day of the cycle and ending on the twenty-fifth day; for endometriosis, initially, 10 mg daily for two weeks, increased by increments of 5 mg daily every two weeks until a dose of 30 mg daily is reached, then 30 mg daily for maintenance. See also the section on Indications.

Norlutin (Parke, Davis). Tablets 5 mg.

NORETHINDRONE ACETATE:

Oral: The manufacturer's recommended dosage is: For amenorrhea and dysfunctional uterine bleeding, 2.5 to 10 mg, starting on the fifth day of the cycle and ending on the twenty-fifth day; for endometriosis, initially, 5 mg daily for two weeks, increased by increments of 2.5 mg daily every two weeks until a dose of 15 mg daily is reached, then 15 mg daily for maintenance. See also the section on Indications.

Norlutate (Parke, Davis). Tablets 5 mg.

Selected References

Report of conference on estrogen treatment of the young. *Pediatrics* 62(suppl):1087-1217, (Dec) 1978.

Antunes CMF, et al: Endometrial cancer and estrogen use: Report of large case-control study. *N Engl J Med* 300:9-13, 1979.

Beard RJ (ed): *The Menopause: A Guide to Current Research and Practice*. Baltimore, University Park Press, 1976.

Campbell S (ed): *The Management of the Menopause and Post-Menopausal Years*. Baltimore, University Park Press, 1976 A.

Campbell S: Double blind psychometric studies on effects of natural estrogens on post-menopausal women, in Campbell S (ed): *The Management of the Menopause and Post-Menopausal Years*. Baltimore, University Park Press, 1976 B, 149-172.

Gordon T, et al: Menopause and coronary heart disease. The Framingham Study. *Ann Intern Med* 89:157-161, 1978.

Hammond CB, et al: Effects of long-term estrogen replacement therapy. I. Metabolic effects. *Am J Obstet Gynecol* 133:525-536, 1979 A.

Hammond CB, et al: Effects of long-term estrogen therapy. II. Neoplasia. *Am J Obstet Gynecol* 133:537-547, 1979 B.

Johnson JWC, et al: Efficacy of 17 alpha-hydroxyprogesterone caproate in prevention of premature labor. *N Engl J Med* 293:675-680, 1975.

Mishell DR Jr, Davajan V: *Reproductive Endocrinology, Infertility and Contraception*. Philadelphia, FA Davis Company, 1979.

Ryan KJ: Estrogens and atherosclerosis. *Clin Obstet Gynecol* 19:805-815, 1976.

Speroff L, et al: *Clinical Gynecologic Endocrinology and Infertility*, ed 2. Baltimore, Williams & Wilkins Company, 1978.

Wentz AC: Assessment of estrogen and progestin therapy in gynecology and obstetrics. *Clin Obstet Gynecol* 20:461-482, 1977.

Yen SSC, Jaffe RB (eds): *Reproductive Endocrinology: Physiology, Pathophysiology and Clinical Management*. Philadelphia, WB Saunders Co, 1978.

Contraceptive Agents | 44

Throughout history since man became aware of the relationship between coitus and pregnancy, efforts were made to limit the number of children conceived and to abort unwanted pregnancies. Early attempts, which centered on various vaginal treatments and abortion methods, were ingenious but sometimes crude, dangerous, and often ineffective. Some of the earliest ideas have survived, however, and appear in our culture in the form of condoms, vaginal spermicides, vaginally introduced abortifacients, and a "new" experimental method, a vaginal sponge. The diaphragm used with a spermicide bears resemblance to halved lemons with the acidic juice (spermicide) being expressed from the fruit.

Contraception can be accomplished at any point in the process from gametogenesis in both sexes to endometrial implantation: Combination oral contraceptives (OCs) prevent ovulation (ie, the combination type), and oral agents designed to suppress spermatogenesis are presently being investigated. Sperm are destroyed by vaginal spermicides, but there is no agent available to eliminate ova. Methods used to prevent the union of sperm and ovum utilize timing (eg, natural family planning, "rhythm" using calendar methods), mechanical means (eg, tubal ligation, hysterectomy, vasectomy, condom, diaphragm), or chemical agents (eg, progestins to thicken cervical mucus). Even after fertilization has occurred, pregnancy may be prevented with interceptive ("morning after") methods that alter the uterine environment to prevent nidation (eg, estrogens, OCs, intrauterine devices [IUDs]).

Agents that interfere with the function of the corpus luteum or early function of the placenta are being sought, but a clinically effective luteolytic agent is not yet available. Immunologic approaches are directed toward development of a vaccine to neutralize human chorionic gonadotropin.

Abortion techniques can eliminate an established pregnancy mechanically (eg, suction) or chemically by application of

683

vaginal abortifacients (eg, prostaglandins) or introduction of an intrauterine agent (eg, saline, urea). (See also Chapter 50, Uterine Stimulants and Relaxants.)

CHOICE OF CONTRACEPTIVE

The perfect contraceptive has yet to be designed. The best technique for an individual depends upon factors such as effectiveness and relative safety and the patient's medical history. For example, patients with menorrhagia or dysmenorrhea are benefited by the inhibition of ovulation that occurs with use of combination OCs.

The effectiveness of contraceptive techniques usually is measured by life table methods, which determine the probability of pregnancy with use of a specific contraceptive method within a given time interval. Failure rates also have been expressed by the Pearl index, which is defined as the number of pregnancies/100 woman-years (any product of number of women times years of use that equals 100) of method use. It is important to distinguish between theoretical effectiveness and use effectiveness: The former measures efficacy after consistent correct usage and the latter under actual conditions of use. The higher failure rates shown by the use-effectiveness index may be due to factors such as employing improper technique (barrier methods), forgetting to take pills (OCs), and failing to limit coitus to nonfertile times of the cycle (rhythm). Generally, the theoretical and use-effectiveness rates for IUDs are similar because, once inserted, little further cooperation is required of the patient. However, the use-effectiveness rate may be decreased if the device is inserted improperly, if the patient fails to check IUD strings and is unaware of spontaneous expulsion of the device, or if a medicated device is not replaced at the recommended interval.

Table 1 shows estimates of effectiveness of various contraceptive methods as reported by various sources in the literature. Use of a combination of techniques (eg, diaphragm, condom, vaginal spermicide) enhances the efficacy of any single method and affords protection comparable to OCs. Failure rates for IUDs and diaphragms decline after the first year of use.

The safety of OCs is judged by various measurements of morbidity or mortality. In general, OCs probably cause the widest variety of adverse effects, but complications associated with use of an IUD result in hospitalization more often. Data indicate that use of OCs, IUDs, traditional barrier forms, or first trimester abortion has a lower incidence of mortality than pregnancy that results from failure to use contraception. An exception is use of OCs among women over 40 years of age who smoke; mortality has been calculated to be higher in these patients than with other methods or when no contraception is employed. When noncontraceptive use is excluded, mortality (including that associated with pregnancies resulting from contraceptive failures) is comparable until age 30, when the risk for smokers who take OCs increases. After age

TABLE 1.
ESTIMATES OF CONTRACEPTIVE EFFICACY

Method	Theoretical Effectiveness (Pregnancy Rate per Year)	Use-Effectiveness
Oral Contraceptives (combined regimen)	0.1%	4%—7%
"Minipill" (progestin only)	2.5%	4%
Intrauterine Devices	1%—3%	4%—9%
Vaginal Spermicides	3%	2%—30%
Condoms, Diaphragms	3%	3%—20%
Rhythm	5%	25%—30%
No Contraception	Pregnancy would occur in 80% to 85% of women	

35, the risk of death among nonsmokers taking OCs and those utilizing traditional methods of contraception may be greater than for patients relying on abortion or using IUDs (Tietze, 1977).

Other conditions affecting the choice of contraceptive include the patient's age, attitude toward various methods, frequency of coitus, extent of male participation in contraceptive practice, level of protection desired (ie, absolute versus spacing children), attitude toward contraceptive failure (ie, would response to failure be abortion or unwanted pregnancy), and patient compliance (eg, unreliability in taking OCs or utilizing coitus-related methods favor use of an IUD). Finally, proper instruction in contraceptive capability and use is of utmost importance; methods with a relatively high failure rate (eg, diaphragm) may be very effective (failure rate, 3%) in highly motivated, properly instructed patients.

In women who engage in sporadic sexual activity (eg, teenagers, women without a stable relationship), a barrier, coitus-related method might be more appropriate than OCs; furthermore, compliance with an OC regimen may be lax during periods of abstinence and contraceptive protection would be unreliable. Such patients might be encouraged to plan ahead, to carry contraceptive foam, and to insert a diaphragm prior to a possible sexual encounter.

The risk of pelvic inflammatory disease is higher in women having multiple sexual partners or those with a history of gonorrhea, and contraceptives other than an IUD are preferred in these patients. However, older patients are good candidates for IUDs or barrier methods because the risk of mortality associated with OCs is reported to be increased in this age group. OCs mask menopausal symptoms and contraception may be continued needlessly. Older patients who have completed their families may prefer sterilization (for either the male or female partner) over continuing use of a contraceptive.

Patient preference is paramount when selecting a contraceptive method. A differ-

ence in effectiveness of 1% between two methods may be significant on a population basis, but may be unimportant to a given patient. OCs, IUDs, and barrier methods all are potentially quite effective, and the best choice among them may be the one that the patient feels most comfortable with and which she will use consistently, even though its theoretical effectiveness is not the highest.

VAGINAL SPERMICIDES

Spermicidal agents for topical vaginal application are available in creams, gels, suppositories, foams, and foaming tablets (see Table 2). Most can be obtained without prescription, are easily applied, and, when used correctly (particularly in combination with another method), offer good protection. Some preparations have lower concentrations of active ingredients, and some creams and gels are designed for use only with a diaphragm. Various formulations differ in speed of distribution in the vagina and degree of surface coverage, and some require special applicators. Suppositories are inserted high into the vagina and require a melting time of 10 to 20 minutes for maximum coverage. In general, foams are easy to apply, cover the cervix almost immediately, and are distributed over a larger surface area. Foaming tablets effervesce in the vagina which enhances distribution. Data are unavailable to demonstrate whether these easily spreading preparations are more effective than other formulations.

Vaginal spermicides contain surfactants or acidic agents as active ingredients. They are generally safe, but local irritation (which may be due to the inactive ingredients, especially perfume) may affect either partner. Selection of another product with different components often alleviates the problem. Proper usage of these agents enhances their effectiveness. They should be applied as directed before coitus (from minutes to one hour) and must be reapplied before each ejaculation. Douching should be avoided for six to eight hours

TABLE 2.
VAGINAL SPERMICIDES (Nonprescription)

Product and Manufacturer	Active Ingredient	Other Ingredients
CREAMS		
Anvita (AO Schmidt)	phenylmercuric borate 1:2,000	boric acid, aluminum potassium sulfate, thymol, chlorothymol, aromatics, cocoa butter
Conceptrol (Ortho)	nonoxynol 9 5%	oil-in-water emulsion
Crescent Cream (Milex)	glyceryl ricinoleate 0.36%	sodium lauryl sulfate 0.6%, oxyquinoline sulfate 0.02%
Delfen Cream (Ortho)	nonoxynol 9 5%	oil-in-water emulsion
Immolin Cream-Jel (Schmid)	nonoxynol 1%	methoxypolyoxyethylene glycol 550 laurate 5%, emulsion base
Koromex II Cream (Holland-Rantos)	octoxynol 3%	propylene glycol, stearic acid, sorbitan stearate, poysorbate 60, boric acid, fragrance
Milex Creme (Milex)	glyceryl ricinoleate 0.36%	sodium lauryl sulfate 0.6%, quinoline sulfate 0.02%
Ortho Creme (Ortho)	nonoxynol 9 2%	oil-in-water emulsion
GELS		
Crescent Vaginal Jelly (Milex)	glyceryl ricinoleate 1%	sodium chloride 5%, sodium lauryl sulfate 0.008%, lactic acid
Koromex II and II-A Jelly (Holland-Rantos)	octoxynol 1% (II) nonoxynol 9 2% (IIA)	propylene glycol, cellulose gum, boric acid, sorbitol, simethicone, fragrance
Ortho-Gynol (Ortho)	p-diisobutylphenoxy-polyethoxyethanol 1%	aqueous gel
Ramses "10-Hour" Vaginal Jelly (Schmid)	dodecaethylene-glycol monolaurate 5%	boric acid 1%, ethyl alcohol 5%, jelly base
FOAMS		
Because (Schering)	nonoxynol 9 8%	benzethonium chloride 0.2%, oil-in-water emulsion
Dalkon Foam (Robins)	nonoxynol 9 8%	benzethonium chloride 0.2%, oil-in-water
Delfen Foam (Ortho)	nonoxynol 9 12.5%	oil-in-water foam
Emko (Schering)	nonoxynol 9 8%	benzethonium chloride 0.2%, oil-in-water emulsion
Koromex (Holland-Rantos)	nonoxynol 9 12.5%	propylene glycol, isopropyl alcohol, laureth 4, cetyl alcohol, polyethylene glycol stearate, dichlorodifluoromethane, dichlorotetrafluoroethane, fragrance
SUPPOSITORIES		
Encare Oval Inserts (Norwich-Eaton)	nonoxynol 9	
Semicid (Whitehall)	nonoxynol 9 10%	polyethylene glycol
S'Positive (Jordan-Simner)	nonoxynol 9 10%	hydrogenated vegetable oil fat vehicle

following coitus, since this may dilute the spermicide more effectively than it destroys sperm.

Several vaginal contraceptives are being investigated clinically. In one type, the spermicide is incorporated into squares of water-soluble film resembling plastic wrap. The product can be applied to the erect penis or inserted into the vagina, where it dissolves. A second type, collagen sponges that may contain a spermicide, is designed to be inserted in the vagina and cover the cervix.

INTRAUTERINE DEVICES

Intrauterine devices (IUD) are available in unmedicated and medicated forms. The latter release a hormone (progesterone) or copper ions into the endometrial cavity to enhance the effectiveness of the inert device. Unmedicated devices available in the United States include the Saf-T-Coil and Lippes Loop. Medicated IUDs are the Cu-7 and the Progestasert devices. (See the preparations listing at the end of this section.) Medicated devices combine a design that is easily tolerated by the uterus with a diffusable ingredient that provides greater efficacy than the unmedicated device of the same design. Copper-containing devices must be replaced every three to five years. The Progestasert system requires replacement yearly, but other systems may be developed which permit longer use. In general for inert devices, a greater surface area of the endometrium in contact with the device increases effectiveness, while small size and good conformity with the shape of the uterus results in less discomfort. Efforts to maximize effectiveness and minimize discomfort, bleeding, and expulsion have resulted in the variety of shapes and sizes of IUDs available today.

An IUD often is inserted during menses when the cervical os is dilated and the absence of pregnancy is reasonably assured. However, it may be inserted at any time during the cycle. After a term pregnancy, insertion should be delayed until involution is complete (usually four to eight weeks) to decrease the risk of uterine perforation or spontaneous expulsion. The smaller size of the uterus before an abortion makes it less liable to perforation and involution occurs sooner than after full-term delivery. IUDs usually can be inserted immediately after first trimester abortion.

An IUD may be used as an interceptive measure within three days after unprotected midcycle intercourse. The device may be left in place in women who anticipate a continuing need for contraception if other factors also favor selection of this method. (See also the section on Postcoital Contraceptives.)

Conception is usually not prevented with IUDs, but implantation of the blastocyst is prevented by a combination of effects which alter the biochemical milieu of the endometrium. Leukocytic infiltration occurs soon after insertion of an IUD (a sterile inflammatory reaction that occurs in the endometrial cavity). The serum immunoglobulin level is elevated and this may interfere with the normal immunologic tolerance that allows successful nidation. Sperm transport to the oviducts also may be inhibited.

Medicated IUDs have the additional effects of the active agent. The efficacy of inert models of the medicated devices is unsatisfactory. The addition of copper inhibits synthesis and liquification of endometrial mucus, which may prohibit proper contact between the blastocyst and endometrium. Prostaglandin production is greater with copper than with inert devices, and this probably stimulates the inflammatory reaction. Copper also may have a direct deleterious effect on sperm, since motility is decreased. In addition to enhancing contraceptive efficacy, copper inhibits the growth of gonococci in vitro, but the clinical usefulness of this effect in preventing infection with gonorrhea has not been demonstrated. Copper devices must be replaced every three to five years. Blood copper levels are not measurable by the usual techniques.

With use of the Progestasert device, small quantities (65 mcg daily) of progesterone are continuously released into the endometrial cavity to produce glandular atrophy and a chronic decidual reaction that is unfavorable for implantation. The volume of menstrual blood loss (compared to preinsertion cycles or to cycles in which a copper device was used) also is reported to be decreased, and dysmenorrhea may be reduced compared to non-IUD cycles. The progesterone device presently requires the inconvenience and discomfort of yearly replacement, and spotting may occur throughout the cycle. Normal cyclic function, including ovulation, continues as it does with other IUDs. The amount of progesterone absorbed systemically does not affect carbohydrate or lipid metabolism.

Precautions: Although leukocytic infiltration begins shortly after insertion of an IUD, it is not known exactly when contraceptive protection is assured. Therefore, use of a barrier method for the first one to three months around the time of expected ovulation is sometimes practiced. High fundal placement maximizes efficacy. Partial expulsion may follow low placement, and this is associated with decreased effectiveness and increased risk of infection. When spontaneous expulsion occurs, sometimes undetected by the patient, it is usually within the first six months of use, with the highest incidence in the first month. Insertion of another device is often successful.

The uterus should be carefully sounded before insertion and a device of appropriate size should be used. Insertion into a uterus of less than 6.5 cm may cause discomfort, bleeding, and possibly expulsion. The patient should be examined after the first postinsertion menses to assure proper placement. The presence of the IUD string should be confirmed by the patient after each menses. A missing string requires prompt investigation. If the string is missing, the possibility of pregnancy should first be ruled out (the string can be drawn into the enlarging uterine cavity). Secondly, the presence and location of the device should be confirmed by use of a uterine sound (the string may be found coiled in the endocervical canal); x-ray, ultrasound, or hysterosalpingography may be required.

Perforation of the uterine wall and translocation of the device may occur at insertion or migration might occur at a later time. IUDs also have been reported to become embedded in the endometrium without perforation. Surgery is required if the IUD is found in the peritoneal cavity. This is particularly important when the device contains copper because tenacious adhesions to the omentum may develop.

If pregnancy occurs with an IUD in situ and the patient elects to complete the pregnancy, the risk of spontaneous abortion and midtrimester septic abortion is increased; the rate for the former is up to 50%. If the device can be removed without undue resistance, this should be done whether the pregnancy is to be continued or not. In full-term pregnancies in which the IUD (medicated or inert) is not removed, the incidence of congenital abnormalities is probably not increased.

Reports of deaths from septic abortions in patients wearing Dalkon Shields resulted in the withdrawal of that device from the U.S. market. Evidence suggests that the multifilament tail of this device acted as a wick and carried pathogens into the uterine cavity, which is normally separated from the vaginal flora by the cervical mucus. However, other devices also have been associated with sepsis during pregnancy, and it is possible that any IUD with a string appendage traversing the cervical mucus may have some degree of risk. This would include all IUDs available commercially in the United States. The possibility of infection may be enhanced further if the IUD breaks the endometrial surface. Because of the association of the Dalkon Shield with this serious complication, it usually is recommended that these devices be replaced even in asymptomatic women who are still wearing them.

Adverse Reactions and Contraindications: Insertion of an IUD usually is accompanied by discomfort. A transient vasovagal response (ie, syncope, bradycardia) may occur. Cramping and bleeding are common for up to 24 hours following insertion. Irregular bleeding may be observed during the first few months of use, and menses may begin one or two days earlier and have a more abrupt onset. Dysmenorrhea may be more severe. Caution should be exercised if an IUD is contemplated for a patient with heavy or prolonged menstrual periods, for the total amount of blood lost usually increases. With the Progestasert device, average blood loss actually decreases but spotting may be more of a problem. Allergy to copper has been reported infrequently with use of devices containing copper.

Pregnancies occurring with an IUD in situ are more likely to be ectopic than when other forms of contraception are used. The risk appears to be highest with the Progestasert system (about 16% versus 4% for other IUD users and 0.5% for non-IUD users), but this may be accounted for partially by selection bias of patients who use this device. The incidence of ectopic pregnancy also may increase with the duration of IUD use. The possibility of ectopic pregnancy should be considered when pregnancy occurs with an IUD in situ or when abdominal pain and abnormal bleeding develop. The mechanism of this effect is not completely understood, but it may be that IUDs are more effective in preventing intrauterine than extrauterine (both tubal and ovarian) pregnancy. Women with a history of previous ectopic pregnancy should not use IUDs thereafter.

The incidence of pelvic inflammatory disease (PID) is three to five times greater when IUDs are employed. There is some evidence, which requires confirmation, that the risk is greater among nulligravidous women. If abdominal pain or tenderness, abnormal vaginal discharge, and fever occur, a diagnosis of PID should be considered. If the infection is mild and responds promptly (within one to two days) to antibiotic therapy, the IUD may be left in place. A serious infection requires removal of the device, possibly hospitalization, and prompt, vigorous antibiotic therapy. An IUD should not be inserted in the presence of acute pelvic infection from any cause. Furthermore, women who are at high risk for developing PID (eg, history of PID, multiple sexual partners) are not good candidates for IUD use. The possibility of future infertility caused by PID should be considered before prescribing an IUD for a nulligravid patient who desires children.

IUDs should not be used in pregnant women, in the presence of genital bleeding of unknown etiology, or in patients with suspected or diagnosed uterine carcinoma. Their use generally is not recommended when the uterine cavity is distorted from any cause or in patients with a small uterus or a severely stenotic cervical canal.

Choice of IUD: Comparison of inherent differences in IUD types as they influence event rates (eg, pain, bleeding, expulsions, pregnancy) is difficult for several reasons. Few studies compare several devices in the same population. Factors such as differences in patient populations and proper placement of the device probably are far more important in determining efficacy than characteristics of a particular design. Some generalizations can be made, however, that form a basis for selection of a device in a given patient. In general, because of greater difficulty in tolerating an IUD, young nulligravidous women require a small device; the Cu-7 probably has been used most often in these patients because it is easily inserted and well tolerated. If the patient does not wish to undergo reinsertion of a medicated device or cannot be relied upon to have it replaced when required, a nonmedicated device may be better. The Progestasert may be chosen for patients with a history of heavy menstrual bleeding or a non-IUD form of contraception should be selected.

In the multiparous patient who can tolerate a larger, more rigid device, an inert design is probably the best choice because it avoids the inconvenience of reinsertion. This is particularly convenient for the multiparous patient who desires long-term contraception. Inert devices generally can be left in place until they are no longer needed (at menopause).

PREPARATIONS
NONMEDICATED DEVICES:
Lippes Loop (Ortho). Size A (22.5 mm [for nulliparous]); size B (27.5 mm with reduced radii [for previous pregnancy with uterus less than 3 cm]); size C (30 mm with reduced radii [for use when Loop D cannot be tolerated]); size D (30 mm [for women with one or more children]).

Saf-T-Coil (Schmid). Size 33-S (standard) for multiparous women; size 32-S (intermediate) for primaparous women and those who cannot tolerate standard size; size 25-Nullip (small) for nulliparous women.

MEDICATED DEVICES:

Cu-7 (Searle). 36 mm x 26 mm. Replacement required every three years.

Progestasert (Alza). 36 mm tubular vertical stem containing progesterone 38 mg initially (32 mm horizontal crossarms). Replacement required yearly.

ORAL CONTRACEPTIVES

Oral contraceptives (OCs) contain a synthetic estrogen and progestin or a progestin alone and provide highly effective protection from pregnancy. The most common are mixtures of a synthetic estrogen (ethinyl estradiol or mestranol) and a progestin (norethindrone, norethindrone acetate, norethynodrel, norgestrel, or ethynodiol diacetate). The composition of the OCs and the chemical structures of the steroids appear in Table 3 and the Figure. Ethinyl estradiol, norethindrone, and norethindrone acetate also are available as single-entity drugs for noncontraceptive indications (see Chapter 43, Estrogens and Progestins). Natural steroids are not used because very large doses are required to achieve the desired pharmacologic effect. The addition of a 17 α-ethinyl group enhances the oral activity of the steroids used in OCs by inhibiting hepatic degradation. Combination products are available in "regular" or "low-dose" (ie, less than 50 mcg estrogen) preparations, or in "minipills," which contain only a progestin (norethindrone or norgestrel).

Combination OCs are taken for 21 days of the cycle (usually days 5 through 24), followed by a week of no medication during which withdrawal bleeding occurs. They are available in "memory packets" for each day of the month. Some pills are packaged with 21 active pills and 7 placebos to provide a pill for every day of the month; some preparations contain iron in the nonhormonal pills. Minipills are taken daily and continuously.

Administration of combination OCs may be started two to four weeks after full-term pregnancy. Ovulation is unlikely to have occurred before this time and the danger of thromboembolism following delivery probably is reduced. The risk of thromboembolic phenomena following abortion is not great, but the chance of early ovulation is high; therefore, OCs may be initiated immediately or within one week. Minipills may be started immediately after full-term pregnancy or abortion.

Combination OCs are effective within the first cycle of use if started by the fifth day of the cycle. Some physicians recommend a barrier method for the first month of pill use or until compliance with the regimen is established. Substituting one combined pill formulation for another may be accomplished easily at the initiation of a new cycle or immediately after the last pill of the previous regimen. Contraceptive effectiveness is not interrupted.

Mechanism of Action

Combination OCs inhibit ovulation through a negative feedback effect on the hypothalamus. This results in alteration of the normal pattern of gonadotropin secretion by the anterior pituitary; both follicular phase FSH and the midcycle surge of gonadotropins are inhibited. Changes in the cervical mucus that render it unfavorable to penetration by sperm also augment contraception even if ovulation occurs. In addition, the quality of the endometrium becomes unfavorable to support nidation, and tubal transport may be affected.

Inhibition of ovulation is not a prominent feature of contraception with progestin-only minipills. These agents cause formation of a thick cervical mucus that is relatively impenetrable to sperm and also eventually results in an involuted endometrium.

Choice of Oral Contraceptive

The numerous combination OC preparations on the market (see Table 3) differ in the type and quantity of estrogen and progestin present in the formulation. Their effectiveness is equivalent with certain exceptions. For example, preparations containing the smallest amount of estrogen may be less effective in women taking drugs that enhance the metabolism and thus lower blood levels of the estrogen (see the section on Drug Interactions). In large women, effective drug concentrations may not be achieved with the low-estrogen formulations. Women who miss pills may have a greater risk of failure with low-dose preparations for the same reason.

As a general rule, preparations containing the smallest quantity of hormone consistent with efficacy and tolerable side effects are preferred. This usually means selection of a product containing 50 mcg or less of estrogen that is in the low to intermediate range for estrogen and progestin potency. Estimates of relative hormonal potencies of the various formulations and sensitivity to the hormones employed are other considerations in choosing the most appropriate formulation.

The progestin-only minipill frequently causes menstrual irregularities and is not as widely used (see the section on Adverse Reactions). Although minipills are slightly less effective than the combination regimens, they may be adequate for patients who accept the inconvenience and do not require the most effective protection and in women who should avoid estrogen-containing medications. The following discussion about choice of OC is devoted to combination products.

Relative Potency: There is considerable debate about whether the various formulations available provide real therapeutic alternatives. Attempts have been made to assess the biological activities of the ingredients in order to tailor the OC to the patient's unique hormonal balance. However, numerous considerations complicate interpretation of available data. These include interaction between the estrogen and progestin components and the complexity of biologic activities of some of the synthetic progestins, which possess not only progestational but also estrogenic and androgenic activities. Furthermore, results of the variety of assays available to measure each activity differ, and animal models are not completely analogous to man. Although different assay systems may show significant differences in potency, they may be unimportant at the dosage ranges employed clinically.

The estrogen component of combination OCs marketed in the United States is either ethinyl estradiol or mestranol (3-methylether ethinyl estradiol). Ethinyl estradiol is 50% more potent than mestranol in animal assays, but clearcut differences have not been demonstrated clinically. Comparison of the two hormones in doses of 50 mcg or more reveals that there is little difference in their effects on the reproductive system, including endometrial histology, inhibition of ovulation, and gonadotropin secretion (Goldzieher et al, 1975). Data comparing effects of lower doses of the two estrogens on the reproductive system are not available.

The progestin component of an OC may be one of four derivatives of 19-nortestosterone: norethynodrel, norethindrone, norethindrone acetate, ethynodiol diacetate, or a derivative of gonane, norgestrel. The latter two have the most potent progestational activity; the others possess estrogenic activity as well. Norgestrel has the strongest androgenic and antiestrogenic activity in addition to its prominent progestational effect. Norethynodrel has only progestational and estrogenic activity and no androgenic or antiestrogenic activity. Because of differences in the type and magnitude of potency among the synthetic progestins, comparison of OC formulations on the basis of weight of components alone is meaningless.

A system estimating the relative potencies of OC preparations based on animal and clinical data has been proposed (Dickey, 1978) (see Table 3). The merits of the system are widely argued, but there are no data that unequivocally support or refute its clinical usefulness. However, comparison of commercial products on the basis of their estimated relative hormonal activities provides a rational, though theoretical, approach for selection of an OC preparation.

The relative potencies of OC formulations can be considered in conjunction

TABLE 3.
ORAL CONTRACEPTIVES AVAILABLE IN THE UNITED STATES: CONTENT AND RELATIVE POTENCIES[1]
(Listed within classes according to decreasing estrogenic potency)

Progestin	Mg	Estrogen	Mcg	Trademarks and Manufacturers	Number of Tablets (Active and Inert)[2]	Potency Estimates (0 to +4) Estrogenic	Progestational	Androgenic
PRODUCTS CONTAINING LESS THAN 50 MCG ESTROGEN								
Norethindrone	0.5	Ethinyl estradiol	35	Brevicon (Syntex)	21, 28	+2	+1	+1
Norethindrone	0.5	Ethinyl estradiol	35	Modicon (Ortho)	21, 28	+2	+1	+1
Norethindrone	0.4	Ethinyl estradiol	35	Ovcon-35 (Mead Johnson)	21, 28	+2	+1	+1
Norgestrel	0.3	Ethinyl estradiol	30	Lo/Ovral (Wyeth)	21	+1	+1	+2
Norethindrone Acetate	1.5	Ethinyl estradiol	30	Loestrin 1.5/30 (Parke, Davis)	21, 28 Fe	+1	+3	+3
Norethindrone Acetate	1.0	Ethinyl estradiol	20	Loestrin 1/20 (Parke, Davis)	21, 28 Fe	+1	+2	+2
PRODUCTS CONTAINING 50 MCG ESTROGEN								
Norethindrine	1.0	Ethinyl estradiol	50	Ovcon 50 (Mead Johnson)	21, 28	+2	+2	+2
Norgestrel	0.5	Ethinyl estradiol	50	Ovral (Wyeth)	21, 28	+2	+2	+3
Norethindrone Acetate	1.0	Ethinyl estradiol	50	Norlestrin 1/50 (Parke, Davis)	21, 28, 28 Fe	+2	+2	+2
Norethindrone Acetate	1.0	Ethinyl estradiol	50	Zorane 1/50 (Lederle)	28	+2	+2	+2
Norethindrone	1.0	Mestranol	50	Norinyl 1/50 (Syntex)	21, 28	+2	+2	+2
Norethindrone	1.0	Mestranol	50	Ortho Novum 1/50 (Ortho)	21, 28	+2	+2	+2
Ethynodiol Diacetate	1.0	Ethinyl estradiol	50	Demulen (Searle)	21, 28	+1	+2	+1
Norethindrone Acetate	2.5	Ethinyl estradiol	50	Norlestrin 2.5/50 (Parke, Davis)	21, 28 Fe	+1	+3	+4

PRODUCTS CONTAINING MORE THAN 50 MCG ESTROGEN

Progestin	mg	Estrogen	mcg	Product	Days			
Norethynodrel	9.85	Mestranol	150	Enovid 10 (Searle)[3]	50, 500	+4	+3	0
Norethynodrel	5.0	Mestranol	75	Enovid 5 (Searle)[3]	20	+4	+2	0
Norethynodrel	2.5	Mestranol	100	Enovid E (Searle)	20, 21	+3	+1	0
Ethynodiol Diacetate	1.0	Mestranol	100	Ovulen (Searle)	21, 28	+3	+2	+1
Norethindrone	2.0	Mestranol	100	Norinyl 2 (Syntex)	20	+2	+3	+3
Norethindrone	2.0	Mestranol	100	Ortho Novum 2 (Ortho)	21	+2	+3	+3
Norethindrone	1.0	Mestranol	80	Norinyl 1/80 (Syntex)	21, 28	+2	+2	+2
Norethindrone	1.0	Mestranol	80	Ortho Novum 1/80 (Ortho)	21, 28	+2	+2	+2
Norethindrone	10.0	Mestranol	60	Norinyl 10 (Syntex)[3]	20	N.A.	+4	+4
Norethindrone	10.0	Mestranol	60	Ortho Novum 10 (Ortho)[3]	21	N.A.	+4	+4

PRODUCTS CONTAINING PROGESTIN ONLY
(for continuous administration; all tablets active)

Progestin	mg	Product	Days			
Norethindrone	0.35	Micronor (Ortho)	28	+1	+3	+1
Norethindrone	0.35	Nor Q.D. (Syntex)	42	+1	+3	+1
Norgestrel	0.075	Ovrette (Wyeth)	28	0	+1	+1

[1] Adapted from Dickey, 1978
[2] 20, 21, 50 and 500 –all active; 28 (21 active, 7 inert); 28 Fe (21 active, 7 ferrous fumarate 75 mg)
[3] For noncontraceptive use

ESTROGENS AND PROGESTINS IN ORAL CONTRACEPTIVES

ESTROGENS

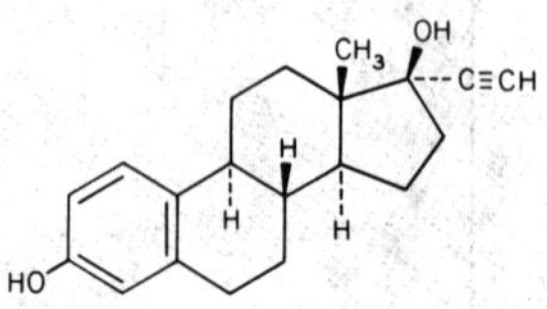

Ethinyl Estradiol

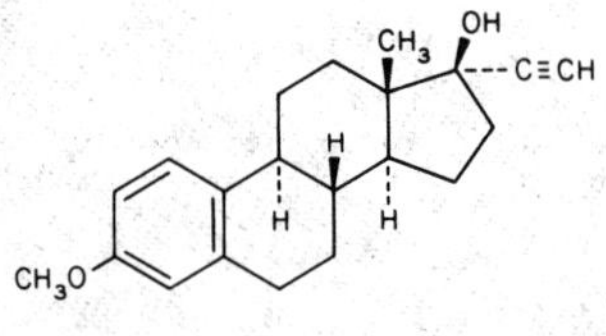

Mestranol

PROGESTINS

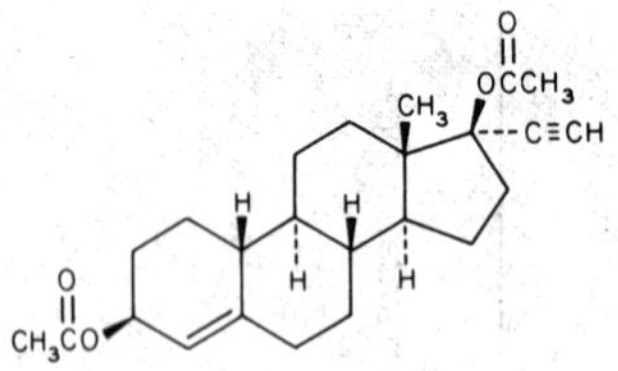

Ethynodiol Diacetate

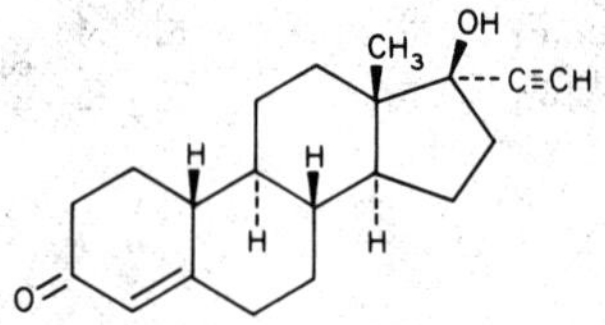

Norethindrone

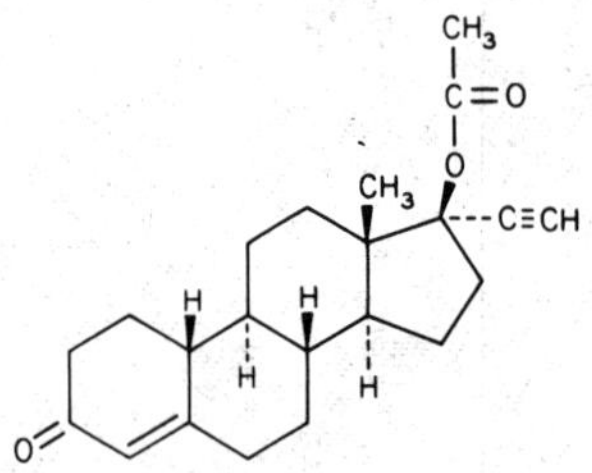

Norethindrone Acetate

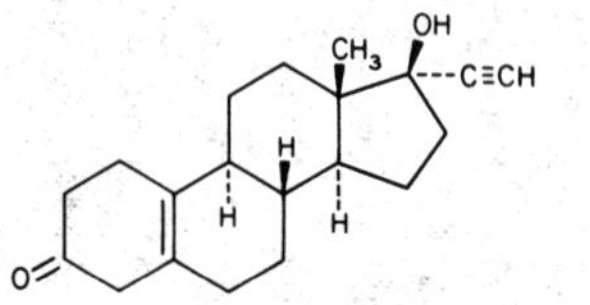

Norethynodrel

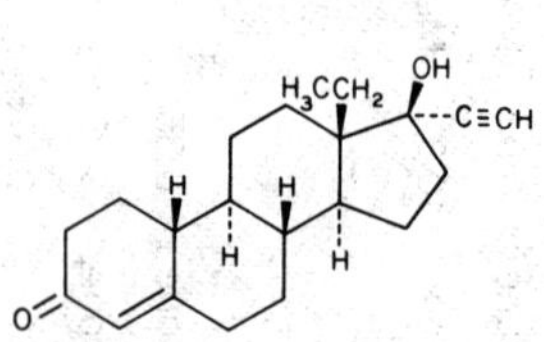

Norgestrel

with the patient's menstrual history or known sensitivities to hormones (eg, response to exogenous administration or pregnancy). Ideally, the preparation chosen would closely mimic the balance of her endogenous hormones or minimize problems she may have with specific hormone sensitivities. For example, a patient with symptoms of estrogen sensitivity (eg, nausea, fluid retention, increased menstrual flow) should be given a preparation with low estrogen content and potency (also, see the section on Adverse Reactions). Those with androgen sensitivity (eg, oily skin and scalp, acne) or progestin sensitivity (eg, depression, noncyclic weight gain) would receive a combination low in androgenic and progestational activities, respectively. Symptoms of estrogen deficiency (eg, vasomotor flushes, atrophic vagina, spotting in the first week of the cycle, no withdrawal bleeding) or progestin deficiency (eg, delayed withdrawal bleeding, heavy flow with clots, spotting in latter part of cycle) might be alleviated by selecting a preparation with an appropriate combination of potencies.

These guidelines can be employed for initial selection or when side effects observed with an initial trial necessitate use of a different product. Most adverse effects caused by OCs are probably due to the high estrogen levels, and adjustments in selection should avoid increasing estrogenic activity if another approach is feasible (ie, change in progestational or androgenic potency). The patient should be encouraged to report unpleasant reactions and be assured that if the problems are not spontaneously resolved, there is a good chance that another preparation will suit her needs adequately.

Precautions

Patients should be warned that the risk of pregnancy is increased if pills are missed during the cycle. If only one or two are omitted, the patient should take an extra pill for one or two days, respectively, following the lapse. A pregnancy test should be performed if menstruation does not occur on time. If three or more pills are omitted, another cycle should be initiated. A barrier method of contraception should be instituted until commencement of the next menses. The risk of pregnancy from missed medication may be greater with use of low-dose estrogen preparations, although clinical evidence is unavailable to support this assumption. Also, the first few pills in the cycle are probably more important in ensuring efficacy than those taken late in the cycle. The minipill is less effective than combined OCs and pregnancies are more likely to occur during the first six months of use. Therefore, a barrier method should be used around the time of expected ovulation, particularly during the first months of use.

Patients taking OCs should be monitored regularly. Biannual blood pressure measurement and annual physical examination including urinalysis, liver palpation, and breast and pelvic examinations should be performed. Patients also should be encouraged to examine their own breasts monthly. Other laboratory tests, such as measurement of serum lipid levels, should be performed when appropriate.

A periodic pill-free interval is not recommended, since it appears to provide no therapeutic advantage and does not enhance the prompt resumption of ovulatory cycles after cessation of OC therapy. Such intervals may, on the other hand, result in noncompliance with the substituted contraceptive and unwanted pregnancies.

Adverse Reactions and Contraindications

Metabolic Effects: The pharmacologic quantities of synthetic hormones that are present in patients taking OC preparations result in numerous metabolic changes. Some of these effects are similar to those experienced during pregnancy when endogenous levels of ovarian steroids are high. These may be minor, tolerable, or temporary but can be potentially serious and even life-threatening. The patient's medical history must be examined carefully to identify possible contraindications.

This is even more compelling with use of OCs than with other drugs, because the majority of patients are healthy before therapy is initiated and alternative contraceptive methods are available.

Most adverse effects associated with OCs are believed to be due to the estrogen component. Although it appears that progestin-only preparations are devoid of the most deleterious effects of the combined preparations, more experience is necessary to determine this with assurance. Likewise, it has not yet been demonstrated that use of low-estrogen preparations produces fewer and less severe adverse effects, but it is reasonable to expect that some untoward effects, just as efficacy, are dose related.

The use of the progestin-only agents has been limited by lack of patient acceptance. The endometrium of the patient taking minipills lacks the structural stability imparted by estrogen, and menstrual irregularities, ranging from intermenstrual spotting to amenorrhea, result. Anxiety about possible pregnancy also is common. When pregnancy occurs during minipill use, there is a higher ectopic/intrauterine ratio than when these agents are not employed.

Common complaints associated with use of combination OC preparations include nausea, sometimes accompanied by vomiting; breast tenderness; and water retention. The nausea is similar to that experienced by some women during early pregnancy and is more common if medication is taken in the early morning or without food. These effects usually occur during the first two or three months of therapy and are relieved after that time.

Effects On Reproductive System: Ovarian size is reduced since large follicles and corpora lutea are absent. Gonadotropic stimulation is diminished and is similar to that occurring in the follicular phase of a normal cycle. Likewise, there is a low rate of endogenous steroid production. Some growth of follicles occurs but is followed by early atresia. Storage of ova and reproductive life span are not increased. The endometrium rapidly progresses from a proliferative to a secretory phase, and glandular atrophy and possibly stromal decidualization then occurs, which accounts for decreased or even absent withdrawal bleeding. Regression of the endometrium after a few cycles may be a factor in short-term, post-treatment amenorrhea. Although breakthrough bleeding and spotting are common in the first few cycles of use (particularly with low-dose preparations), therapeutic intervention with estrogen and/or progestin may be necessary if the bleeding is heavy or prolonged (see Chapter 43, Estrogens and Progestins, for a discussion of dysfunctional bleeding).

Cyclic menses usually resume within two to three months after cessation of OC therapy. Occasional failure of cyclicity after 6 to 12 months has been noted (postpill amenorrhea). If pregnancy is desired, the condition should be treated in the same manner as other cases of secondary amenorrhea; usually clomiphene citrate is utilized (see Chapter 45, Agents Used to Treat Infertility).

The question of whether there is a causal relationship between OC medication and the development of subsequent amenorrhea is unresolved. Most studies report this effect in less than 1% of patients who take OCs. The incidence of spontaneous secondary amenorrhea in women who do not take these agents has not been adequately determined, but it appears to be similar. It does not appear to be related to dosage of either component nor to duration of use. Such amenorrhea is more common in women with previously irregular menstrual cycles, whether or not they have used OCs, and in underweight women. Therefore, this condition may be unrelated to prior OC use. However, some physicians prefer to use another form of contraception in patients with a history of irregular menstrual cycles who desire future pregnancy.

A growing incidence of pituitary microadenomas is being reported. These lesions frequently are associated with amenorrhea (postpill or not) and sometimes galactorrhea. An elevated plasma prolactin level is the most common feature. Although OC use has been considered a possible cause, evidence does not support a significant association. The increased incidence of microadenomas may simply reflect advances in diagnostic technology. However, if amenorrhea persists following OC use and the plasma prolactin level is elevated, appropriate diagnostic procedures and treatment should be undertaken (see also Chapter 45, Agents Used to Treat Infertility).

The quality and quantity of milk produced during lactation may be adversely affected by some OC preparations, especially the older, high-dose formulations. More importantly, the steroids are found in the milk, and their long-range effects on the nursing infant are not known. Nursing mothers should be encouraged to utilize another form of contraception.

Hepatic Effects: There is an increased incidence of *gallbladder disease* and gallstones when OCs are used, which probably is related to increased cholesterol concentrations in bile. Women who had developed jaundice during pregnancy or nulliparous women with a genetic predisposition are at risk of developing cholestatic jaundice during therapy. Results of laboratory tests are similar to those observed in patients with recurrent jaundice of pregnancy (eg, increased bilirubin, alkaline phosphatase, 5-nucleotidase activity; reduced BSP clearance). Biopsies reveal cholestasis and, sometimes, minimal hepatocellular degeneration and necrosis. Upon cessation of OC use, jaundice and pruritus disappear and liver function tests return to normal without residual effects. Patients with this history, as well as those with active liver disease, should not take OCs; those who have recovered from liver disease (eg, hepatitis, mononucleosis) may receive this medication after hepatic function studies are normal for one full year.

Benign hepatic adenomas develop rarely during OC use. Peliosis may accompany adenoma or may be present independently. The case/control estimate of the risk of developing these tumors increases greatly after five years of OC use. However, only about 500 cases have been reported by 1977 and these were not all associated with OCs. The tumors are potentially serious because of the danger of rupture. Although the condition is sometimes accompanied by epigastric pain, the patient may remain asymptomatic until the occurrence of a sudden fatal hemorrhage. Palpation of the liver should be a part of every periodic checkup for patients taking OCs. If a mass is present, appropriate diagnostic procedures should be undertaken. Cessation of OC use is mandatory and spontaneous regression usually occurs.

Carbohydrate, Lipid, and Protein Metabolism: The effect of combination OCs on *carbohydrate metabolism* is complex. Utilization of glucose may be retarded with a compensatory increase in insulin secretion. A peripheral anti-insulin effect of growth hormone may be involved during the first year of use, since OCs increase the pituitary secretion of growth hormone in some patients. After one year, growth hormone secretion appears to return to normal in some individuals. If alterations in glucose tolerance continue, other diabetogenic factors may be responsible. Patients who are diabetic only during pregnancy are particularly vulnerable to developing abnormal glucose tolerance. Also, it is possible that patients who eventually develop diabetes (eg, those with a strong family history of the disease) may become clinically diabetic earlier than without the diabetogenic influence of OCs. Since glucose metabolism may be affected in these patients, other forms of contraception should be encouraged. Adverse effects usually are not observed in controlled diabetic patients; however, their status should be reviewed periodically.

Serum lipids also are affected by OCs. Triglyceride levels rise an average of 50%; there is a smaller increase in low density lipoproteins (LDL) and a variable effect on high density lipoproteins (HDL). The estrogen component of combination OCs causes higher HDL levels, while the progestin component reduces HDL levels. Therefore, the net effect of a given OC preparation depends upon the ratio of hormonal activities. Increased levels of HDL are associated with a lower risk of coronary artery disease, and increased levels of LDL are associated with a higher risk. Periodic measurement of serum triglyceride, HDL, and LDL levels should be performed in women with a strong family history of coronary disease who are taking OCs; if abnormal levels are found (in patients with or without this family history), another form of contraception should be used.

Changes in *serum protein* levels during OC use are qualitatively similar to those that occur during pregnancy, but are generally of less magnitude. Changes in clotting factors (see the discussion on Cardiovascular and Hematologic Effects) occur; alpha-2 globulins (including the renin substrate, angiotensinogen) and beta globulins are increased and serum albumin levels are decreased.

OCs also cause higher levels of circulating corticosteroid-binding globulin (CBG, transcortin), which increases the amount of protein-bound cortisol in peripheral blood. The slight rise in the free (biologically active) cortisol level is probably partly due to the reduced rate of cortisol metabolism. The effect of prolonged elevated cortisol levels is unknown. Pituitary-adrenal response to stress remains normal. The level of thyroxine-binding globulin (TBG) is also greater but, since the concentration of free thyroxine is unchanged, thyroid function is not altered.

Cardiovascular and Hematologic Effects: Intravascular *clot formation* may be enhanced by the presence of larger numbers of platelets or increased platelet adhesiveness, higher levels of blood clotting factors, decreased fibrinolysis, or inflammatory changes in the blood vessel wall. OCs may alter the levels of various clotting factors (increased prothrombin and factors VII, VIII, IX, and X; decreased antithrombin III) and larger numbers of platelets and increased adhesiveness are sometimes observed, although decreases or no change in adhesiveness also have been reported. These changes may or may not be linked causally with the greater risk of thromboembolic phenomena observed among patients taking OCs. The preponderance of data from both prospective and retrospective studies reveals that the relative risk of developing thromboembolic phenomena is approximately 5 to 11 times greater among

women who use OCs. However, although the relative risk of deep vein thrombosis is increased substantially with use of OCs, the actual incidence is low (approximately 80/100,000).

The cardiovascular effects of OCs are believed to be related to the estrogen component. The incidence of deep thrombosis decreased 28% with use of preparations containing 50 mcg estrogen compared to those containing larger amounts (Royal College of General Practitioners Study, 1974), thus demonstrating a probable dose effect for this adverse reaction. Although data are not available to determine if low-dose preparations (less than 50 mcg estrogen) further reduce this incidence, it seems reasonable to assume that this may be the case. Therefore, preparations containing the least amount of estrogen (usually 50 mcg or less) that will provide reliable contraception with a minimum of untoward effects (ie, breakthrough bleeding, spotting) should be utilized.

The incidence of fatal and nonfatal strokes (usually preceded by headaches) is reported to be higher with OC therapy. The reported risk of mortality from general cardiovascular causes, including stroke, malignant hypertension, cardiomyopathy, mesenteric trombosis, and myocardial infarction, is greater among those who have taken the medication for five years or more than among those who have ever used the combination products. The risk of developing one of these cardiovascular problems is enhanced in older women and in those who smoke. The risk of myocardial infarction specifically may be increased slightly in older women taking OCs but is greatly increased in women who also smoke or have one or more additional risk factors (eg, hypertension, obesity, diabetes). Although several estimates have been suggested, the magnitude of the risk cannot be determined accurately on the basis of available information. Cigarette smoking is an important risk factor both quantitatively and qualitatively because it is preventable.

Because of the epidemiologic evidence that use of OCs increases the occurrence of cardiovascular disease, a woman with a history of or active thromboembolic disease, thrombophlebitis, or other serious cardiovascular disease should not take OCs. Moreover, a strong family history of the above indicates caution and close monitoring (ie, glucose and lipid profile annually). In addition, OCs should not be taken within one month before or after surgery or immediately postpartum because of the greater risk of thromboembolism at these times. Women between age 30 and 39 years who have one or more additional risk factors (eg, particularly smoking or hypertension, obesity, diabetes) should consider using another contraceptive measure, and women over 40 with concurrent risk factors also should not take OCs. Since these cardiovascular effects probably develop gradually and are not immediately or completely reversible, substitution of another form of contraception should not be undertaken with such haste that the patient is left unprotected.

Increases in both systolic and diastolic *blood pressure* (1 to 10 mm Hg) have been reported but are usually within the normotensive range. However, the risk of developing hypertension in women who have used OCs for five years is increased two and one-half times. Women who are already hypertensive may experience a further rise in blood pressure with use of OCs. The mechanism of this effect probably involves the renin-angiotensin system. There is an increase in angiotensinogen (renin substrate) levels and impairment of the negative feedback control of renin production; elevated levels of angiotensin, a potent vasoconstrictor, result.

Changes in blood pressure are usually reversible within one to six months after cessation of therapy. One small study showed that, in women using OCs, hypertensive patients had higher blood levels of ethinyl estradiol (ie, the estrogen component of the OC) than normotensive individuals (Ahluwalia et al, 1977). This suggests that any factor that elevates estrogen blood levels (eg, that alters the rate of estrogen metabolism, differences in body weight and resultant volume of distribution) may influence the blood pressure response.

Upon initiation of OC therapy, the blood pressure should be monitored after three months and every 6 to 12 months thereafter. If hypertension develops, another form of contraception should be utilized. Other measures are preferred in women who are already hypertensive, but if OCs are employed, careful monitoring of blood pressure is necessary. Several cases of pulmonary hypertension have been reported in women using OCs, although most of these individuals had predisposing conditions.

OCs have been associated with changes in the pattern of occurrence of migraine headache. Attacks occur frequently during the interval when steroids are not taken or during the first two or three days after resumption of medication. If migraine attacks are first experienced after beginning OC medication or there is an increased frequency or intensity during treatment, therapy should be discontinued since they may be prodromal symptoms of an impending stroke.

Teratogenicity: The teratogenic potential of sex hormones has been studied. Among women who discontinued use of OCs, the risk of spontaneous abortion or congenital abnormalities, including any of the VACTERL anomalies (vertebral, anal, cardiac, tracheal, esophageal, renal, or limb) or Down's syndrome in liveborn infants, was not increased. However, a low incidence of congenital abnormalities, predominantly cardiac, limb reduction, and masculinization of female fetuses, has been noted when progestins (usually not in OC formulations) were taken during early pregnancy. Most abnormalities have been associated with use of hormonal pregnancy tests and progestin therapy for threatened abortion. Most of the abnormalities following ingestion of OCs during early pregnancy involved male infants. These agents should be discontinued if pregnancy is suspected (see the section on Precautions).

Carcinogenicity: Women with a history of fibrocystic disease of the breast are considered to be at higher risk of developing breast cancer than those with no prior benign breast disease. Several studies have shown that the risk of *benign breast disease* is lower in women who use combined OCs but the association may not be causal. These preparations often are not prescribed for women with this history, and this may account for the higher incidence among control subjects. Most studies indicate that the incidence of *breast cancer* is not increased with OC use. One exception was reported after long-term therapy (at least six years) when the risk was increased elevenfold among patients with a history of prior biopsy for benign breast disease. However, this risk was not compared to that in women with a similar history who did not use OCs. Since estrogen can stimulate growth of pre-existing cancerous breast lesions, OCs are contraindicated in women with known or suspected breast carcinoma and caution must be exercised if they are prescribed for patients at high risk of developing breast cancer.

An increased incidence of *endometrial cancer* was observed in women who took the sequential type of OC (compared to those taking combined OCS), and these preparations were subsequently removed from the market in the United States. The incidence of endometrial cancer, carcinoma in situ, or invasive *cervical cancer* was not increased after use of combination OCs. However, since estrogen may stimulate the growth of existing endometrial cancer, OCs should not be prescribed for women with undiagnosed abnormal genital bleeding.

Although the above discussion is optimistic, firm conclusions about the carcinogenicity of OCs are not yet possible because of the long latent period between the administration of a carcinogen and the development of cancer.

Miscellaneous Reactions: Melasma similar to that observed during pregnancy sometimes develops in women who use OCs. Those with dark complexions, excessive exposure to sunlight, or a history of melasma of pregnancy are most likely to exhibit this problem. Decreasing the quantity of estrogen may reduce pigmentation. However, even after cessation of medication, a long time may be required before pigmentation disappears.

Hair loss and changes in hair growth and texture while taking OCs are probably re-

lated to the androgenic potency of the progestin component. Rarely, a male pattern of hair growth may appear on the face and body or recession of temporal hair may occur on the scalp. Other manifestations of androgenicity include oily skin and scalp and acne. A preparation containing a progestin with lower androgenicity or higher estrogen/progestin ratio may be considered. The possibility of androgen-producing ovarian or adrenal pathology should be ruled out. Effects of changes in drug regimen on hair growth may not be apparent for several months.

Some women (most commonly those with previous psychological history) may experience mood changes or develop *depression* while taking OCs. This may be related to associated changes in tryptophan metabolism causing decreased brain serotonin production. Administration of pyridoxine hydrochloride (vitamin B6) is sometimes effective in women with a deficiency of this vitamin.

Alterations in *libido* sometimes occur with OCs. These changes may be in either direction and may be unrelated to hormonal effects (eg, libido may increase because of lack of fear of pregnancy). If decreased libido is a problem, a preparation containing a small amount of estrogen and an androgenic progestin may be helpful.

The use of OCs may be followed by an increase in the diagnosis and frequency of *epileptic seizures*. Women with a history of epilepsy should be encouraged to use another form of contraception.

Changes in blood levels of vitamins and minerals have been observed. Plasma folate, pyridoxine, vitamin B12, carotene, calcium, magnesium, manganese, zinc, and phosphorus levels may decrease while ascorbic acid, vitamin A, iron, and copper levels increase. The clinical significance of these changes is not apparent and decreased levels do not result in deficiency states. Vitamin supplementation is unnecessary in women with adequate diets.

Ocular abnormalities (eg, retinal vascular occlusion, retinal edema, optic neuropathy, retinal vasculitis) have been associated rarely with use of OCs. Symptoms appear during therapy, disappear on withdrawal, and reappear upon resumption of the drugs. OCs should be discontinued if there is an unexplained decrease in vision or other serious symptoms and appropriate diagnostic and therapeutic measures should be taken. Results of controlled studies indicate that OCs probably do not affect *contact lens* tolerance as was earlier thought.

Drug Interactions: OCs may decrease the hypoprothrombinemic response to coumarin anticoagulants, and larger doses of the latter drugs may be required. There have been isolated reports of pregnancies and breakthrough bleeding occurring when OCs were taken with barbiturates, ampicillin, anticonvulsants, and particularly rifampin [Rifadin, Rimactane]. This is probably due to the increased metabolism of estrogen by mixed-function oxidases when these drugs are taken together. In patients taking OCs and pharmacologic amounts of corticosteroids concurrently, the metabolism of the latter is reduced and a reduction in the corticosteroid dosage may be possible. Preliminary reports suggest that doses of tricyclic antidepressants should be reduced when these agents are taken with OCs.

Effects on Laboratory Tests: Reversible sulfobromophthalein (BSP) retention may occur in some women during administration of OCs. The defect is in the transfer of BSP from liver cells to bile; storage is not affected.

Estrogens raise the level of thyroxine-binding globulin (TBG), which increases values for total thyroxine (T4) and decreases values for the T3 resin uptake test.

The free thyroxine index (FTI) and direct measurements of T3 or T4 by radioimmunoassay remain unchanged. Thyroid function test results return to pretreatment levels within two months after discontinuing therapy.

OCs may elevate plasma triglycerides and cause other alterations in lipid levels. Glucose tolerance may be decreased. Serum iron and copper levels may increase due to higher levels of their respective transport proteins, transferrin and ceruloplasmin. OCs may cause a false-positive test for LE cells and/or antinuclear antibodies. Urinary 17-hydroxycorticosteroids may be decreased. See also the section on Adverse Reactions.

POSTCOITAL CONTRACEPTION

When coitus has occurred with no contraceptive protection and pregnancy is not desired, interceptive (ie, at the preimplantation stage) measures may eliminate the unwanted pregnancy and avoid abortion. Postcoital techniques are often referred to as "morning after" contraception. Various estrogen regimens (see Table 4) or IUDs may be used for this purpose.

The most extensive clinical experience and documentation of effectiveness have been obtained with diethylstilbestrol (DES). Large doses are administered within 72 hours after unprotected midcycle sexual exposure. The estrogen may change the sequence of hormonal influences on the fallopian tubes, thereby disturbing the passage of the ovum. Estrogen also may

TABLE 4.
POSTCOITAL CONTRACEPTIVE REGIMENS

Estrogen	Dosage
Diethylstilbestrol	25 mg twice daily for five days
Ethinyl Estradiol	2.5 mg twice daily for five days
Estrone	5 mg three times daily for five days
Conjugated Estrogens	10 mg three times daily for five days
Ethinyl Estradiol and Norgestrel (combination available as Ovral)	100 mcg ethinyl estradiol and 1 mg dl-norgestrel (two Ovral tablets) taken twice 12 hours apart

alter the endometrial milieu and interfere with nidation.

The patient who seeks postcoital contraception should understand that the high-dosage estrogen regimens are to be used infrequently or in emergencies (eg, rape, incest), for the presumed risk of serious side effects after frequently repeated large doses is unacceptable. In addition, nausea and vomiting are routinely a problem. Most of the regimens entail five days of therapy, and the severe nausea that results may require discontinuation of therapy unless an antiemetic is given concurrently. If excessive vomiting occurs, the contraceptive regimen may be ineffective.

Because of the teratogenic potential of estrogens, the possibility of a pre-existing pregnancy must be ruled out before administering a course of postcoital estrogens. DES given during the first trimester of pregnancy is associated with a high incidence of vaginal adenosis and, rarely, adenocarcinoma in female offspring (see Chapter 43, Estrogens and Progestins). Adenosis also has been reported following the use of estrogens other than DES. There is no information on the effects of any estrogen given as an interceptive on a pregnancy that may ensue in the event of contraceptive failure. If a morning-after estrogen fails and pregnancy results, some women will elect abortion simply because the pregnancy is unwanted. However, abortion need not be recommended on the basis of the known teratogenic effects of the estrogen alone. The patient should be provided with a realistic assessment of the risks involved before determining the fate of the pregnancy.

IUDs also are employed as an interceptive method. Although any device may be effective for this indication, most experience has been achieved with the copper-containing devices. They are more easily tolerated in nulliparous women than larger IUDs, which is an advantage in the young population most likely to seek interceptive contraception. The IUD is inserted, preferably within a day, but may be inserted within several days after unprotected intercourse and left in place if continuing contraception is desired.

DEPOT PREPARATIONS

Several long-lasting depot preparations are under clinical investigation for use as contraceptives. These products are usually progestins but may contain both estrogen and a progestin. One such preparation that is widely utilized throughout the world is depot medroxyprogesterone acetate (DMPA) [Depo-Provera]. An intramuscular injection containing 150 mg usually is given every three months, although the effect usually extends beyond the three-month injection interval. The drug is measurable in plasma six to eight months after the last injection. The contraceptive protection provided is as effective as combined OCs.

The major mechanism of action of DMPA is inhibition of ovulation through suppression of the midcycle surge of LH secretion. Other contributing effects include thickening of cervical mucus and development of an atrophic endometrium that cannot support nidation. Gonadotropin suppression is not complete, and there is some follicular development; estrogen production is similar to but slightly lower than that of a normal follicular phase.

Fertility is delayed following use of DMPA for contraception. For this reason, the drug is not recommended for use in young women whose contraceptive needs are to space children. Average time to conception after the last injection is about one year but may be as long as two and one-half years. This may be related to remaining plasma levels of the drug, continuing pituitary suppression after clearance of the progestin, or coincidental pathology. There is considerable variation among women in rate of absorption and metabolism which also could account for the prolonged effect.

Side effects include weight gain, depression, and headache. The most common problems are irregular menstrual cycles and spotting or amenorrhea, and most patients who discontinue therapy do so because of these complaints. If bleeding is a persistent problem that requires correction, hormonal therapy may be attempted (see Chapter 43, Estrogens and Progestins, for a discussion on dysfunctional bleeding). An atrophic endometrium develops progressively, and total amenorrhea occurs frequently 6 to 12 months after therapy is begun. Studies on the effect of DMPA on blood pressure have yielded equivocal results but most often show no effect or decreased blood pressure.

DMPA has glucocorticoid properties, particularly when given in large doses (eg, in treatment of endometrial carcinoma). In contraceptive doses, plasma cortisol levels are sometimes decreased and the response to metyrapone may be diminished, but there is no clinical evidence of adrenal insufficiency.

Glucocorticoids are teratogenic in rabbits and the teratogenic effect of large doses of DMPA in this species is probably related to this activity. DMPA does not appear to have this effect in man. However, administration of progestins during pregnancy is generally not recommended, and there is the possibility of prolonged fetal exposure if a depot preparation is administered during an existing pregnancy or if a rare contraceptive failure occurs.

Large doses of DMPA have caused malignant mammary tumors in beagle dogs, but there is no evidence of similar effect in other test animals (including monkeys) or in women. This appears to be an effect peculiar to the beagle and the appropriateness of the use of this animal model has been questioned. The possibility that there is an increased risk of cervical carcinoma in situ also has been investigated, but firm evidence to either support or reject this relationship does not exist. Endometrial carcinoma was reported in long-term studies of monkeys given 50 times the contraceptive dosage administered to humans.

DMPA may be appropriate for use as a contraceptive in special situations. Its main values lie in its great effectiveness and the need for infrequent administration. The latter property is a drawback in the event of side effects, however. Use of DMPA as a contraceptive remains controversial in this country but is an option for consideration. It seems particularly justified in patients who are unable or unwilling to use other forms of contraception and who are noncompliant in methods requiring cooperation, in women in whom estrogens are contraindicated (eg, those with congenital heart disease, previous thromboembolic disease), and in intellectually or psychologically impaired patients.

Selected References

OCs—Update on usage, safety, and side effects. *Popul Rep* Series A, No. 5, (Jan) 1979.

Oral Contraceptives and Health: Interim Report from the Oral Contraceptive Study of the Royal College of General Practitioners. New York, Pitman Publishing Corporation, 1974.

Ahluwalia BS, et al: Evidence of higher ethynylestradiol blood levels in human hypertensive oral contraceptive users. *Fertil Steril* 28:627-630, 1977.

Beral V, et al: Mortality among oral-contraceptive users. *Lancet* 2:727-731, 1977.

Dickey RP: *Managing Contraceptive Pill Patients.* Aspen, Colo, Creative Infomatics, Inc, 1978.

Goldzieher JW, et al: Comparative studies of ethynyl estrogens used in oral contraceptives I. Endometrial response. II. Antiovulatory potency. III. Effect on plasma gonadotropins. *Am J Obstet Gynecol* 122:615-636, 1975.

Hatcher RA, et al: *Contraceptive Technology 1978-*

1979, ed 9. New York, Irvington Publishers, Inc, 1978.

Keith L, Berger GL: Relationship between congenital defects and use of exogenous progestational contraceptive' hormones during pregnancy: A 20 year review. *Int J Gynaecol Obstet* 15:115-124, 1977.

Mishell DR Jr: Contraception. *Am J Dis Child* 132:912-920, 1978.

Ory HW: Review of association between intrauterine devices and acute pelvic inflammatory disease. *J Reprod Med* 20:200-204, 1978.

Rosenfield A: Oral and intrauterine contraception: 1978 risk assessment. *Am J Obstet Gynecol* 132:92-106, 1978.

Tatum HJ: Clinical aspects of intrauterine contraception: Circumspection 1976. *Fertil Steril* 28:3-28, 1977.

Tietze C: New estimates of mortality associated with fertility control. *Fam Plann Perspect* 9:74-76, 1977.

Agents Used to Treat Infertility | 45

Among couples who desire to have children, 10% to 15% have some form of infertility problem that, in the absence of treatment, will result in a sterile union, and another 10% will have less than the desired number of children. Successful pregnancy is achieved in about one-half of these couples who seek medical attention.

Drug therapy for infertility is effective in some appropriately selected individuals and is directed primarily toward stimulating or enhancing ovulation and facilitating sperm transport in women and stimulating spermatogenesis in men. At this time, pharmacotherapy is more advanced and successful in women than in men. Treatment regimens are continually being refined to fit specific causes of infertility in both sexes.

Couples who embark on a program of treatment for infertility should be selected carefully. In addition to understanding the potential side effects of treatment, the couple should be fully aware of the extended period that may be required. They should be prepared for the anxiety, frustration, and disappointment that may accompany unsuccessful cycles of treatment and realize that these problems are common to many couples in this circumstance. If coitus is evenly spaced two or more times a week, the pattern of sexual activity need not be altered, for under these circumstances sperm capable of fertilization are almost always present in the woman's reproductive tract.

Requirements for Fertility: Fertility depends upon a complex and integrated hormonal milieu as well as the anatomic integrity of the reproductive organs. The responsibility and contribution of the male reproductive system end with the production and delivery of a sufficient number and quality of sperm to effect fertilization. The female role extends beyond that of gamete production to encompass the elegant life support system that nurtures the developing fetus until viability in the external environment is assured.

In both sexes, the physiologic stimulus for gametogenesis emanates from the gonadotropins that are produced and secreted by the anterior pituitary gland. Follicle-stimulating hormone (FSH) and luteinizing hormone (LH) are named for their actions in the female, although they are also necessary for normal reproductive function in the male. In females, LH stimulates androstenedione and testosterone production by the thecal cells of the follicle before ovulation (these hormones are transported to the granulosa cells where aromatization to estradiol takes place) and also stimulates estrogen and progesterone production from the converted granulosa cells of the corpus luteum (CL) after ovulation. FSH stimulates growth of Graafian follicles in the ovary and induces the aromatase enzyme in the granulosa cells.

A surge of LH and FSH secretion occurs at midcycle; at this time, LH stimulates ovulation of the prepared follicle, but the function of FSH is uncertain. Estrogen and progesterone produced by the CL prepare the endometrium for nidation. Progesterone is necessary for support of the uterine lining in the early weeks of pregnancy before the placenta assumes its steroidogenic function. Female infertility can result from any interference in the delicate hormonal integration that results in failure of ovulation, impairs the life and function of the CL, or impedes access of the sperm to the ovum; it also may result from anatomical or physiologic conditions that prevent normal transport of the fertilized ovum through the fallopian tubes or interfere with the ability of the uterus to provide adequate nutrition and support of the fetus.

Although fluctuations in gonadotropin secretion occur in males, there is apparently nothing analagous to the midcycle episodic surge of secretion in females. FSH acts on the Sertoli cells that produce androgen-binding protein (ABP), and LH (originally called ICSH or interstitial cell-stimulating hormone and found to be identical to LH) stimulates production of androgen, principally testosterone, by the Leydig cells. Testosterone maintains libido and potency and has a direct effect on developing germ cells in the seminiferous tubules. ABP is probably responsible for maintaining a greater concentration of testosterone in the tubules than in the serum. Even though the germinal epithelium is able to supply the constant and enormous spermatogenic production rate required for normal function, a compatible epididymal environment (temperature and chemical composition) and a patent duct system are necessary to ensure fertility.

Even in the presence of two perfectly functioning reproductive systems, coitus must occur during a time when the 36-hour fertile life of the sperm and the 24-hour viability of the ovum overlap.

Diagnosis of Infertility: Evaluation of infertility should involve both partners. A detailed description of the procedures used to determine the causes of infertility is beyond the scope of this book. The choice and sequence of tests employed can maximize the amount of information gained and eventually may spare the couple the time and expense of further testing and possibly of inappropriate drug therapy and avoid unwarranted hopefulness. An accurate medical history, including frequency and timing of coitus, may suggest the need for education rather than immediate infertility tests. Other aspects of medical history may pinpoint a likely source of infertility deserving early evaluation (eg, mumps orchitis in the male, pelvic inflammatory disease in the female). Since the male is the sole partner affected in about 40% of infertile couples, or both partners may have impaired reproductive capacity, the simple and inexpensive semen analysis is reasonably the initial diagnostic procedure employed. A postcoital test provides information about both partners (ie, the quality of cervical mucus and semen and their interaction). Patency of the fallopian tubes can be demonstrated by hysterosalpingography. Basal body temperature patterns, measurement of serum progesterone levels, and/or endometrial biopsy provide presumptive evidence of ovulatory function. Optimal timing of tests allows almost complete infertility evaluation in the first cycle (ie, postcoital tests and hysterosalpingogram just before ovulation, endometrial biopsy just before menses, temperature chart throughout cycle). When these diagnostic measures fail to provide an explanation, laparoscopy may reveal a hitherto unsuspected cause (eg, endometriosis, peritubal abnormalities) in up to 40% of women. Usually this procedure is delayed for two to three months after hysterosalpingography because of the increased incidence of pregnancy during this interval.

Drug Therapy: Since FSH and LH are necessary to support both female and male gametogenesis, clomiphene [Clomid], menotropins (HMG) [Pergonal], and human chorionic gonadotropin (HCG) [Antuitrin-S, A.P.L., Follutein, Pregnyl] can be used to treat both female (anovulation) and male infertility secondary to inadequate secretion or abnormal patterns of secretion of these gonadotropic hormones. Clomiphene stimulates while HMG and HCG replace normal gonadotropin secretion.

The effectiveness of clomiphene depends upon the presence of an intact anterior pituitary gland and hypothalamus, because endogenous secretion of gonadotropin is stimulated by this agent. Clomiphene induces ovulation in women and stimulates spermatogenesis in men. Menotropins, a preparation of human menopausal gonadotropins (HMG), contains both FSH and LH activity. It is indicated when the pituitary gland is unable to secrete these hormones in response to stimulation and exogenous gonadotropin must be provided. HCG has the biological activity of LH and stimulates ovulation of prepared follicles (assuming prior stimulation by endogenous FSH or an exogenous agent). It is always used with HMG and, in some instances, after clomiphene.

Agents prescribed to treat other types of infertility include estrogen, oral contraceptives, danazol [Danocrine], and bromocriptine [Parlodel]. In women, estrogen is used to improve the quality of poor cervical mucus that occurs spontaneously or after treatment with clomiphene. Oral contraceptives or danazol are sometimes effective in enhancing fertility impaired by endometriosis. Bromocriptine reduces the secretion of abnormally high levels of prolactin and often normalizes cyclic function and ovulation in women. Gonadotropin-releasing hormone (GnRH) is an investigational drug that directly stimulates the synthesis and secretion of gonadotropins by the anterior pituitary gland. However, treatment of anovulation with this agent currently is impractical, because its short half-life requires frequent administration over the entire period of follicular maturation; therefore, evaluation of its clinical usefulness awaits the development of longer-acting analogues.

FEMALE INFERTILITY

Before instituting drug therapy, possible primary causes of female infertility should be identified and treated if possible. These may be organic (eg, adrenal, thyroid, pituitary disease) or anatomic (eg, obstruction of the fallopian tubes). Those that are amenable to drug therapy include unfavorable cervical mucus, failure of ovulation, luteal phase dysfunction, and endometriosis.

Hostile Cervical Mucus: If copious quantities of the thin, watery cervical mucus characteristic of normal estrogenic stimulation around the time of ovulation are not present and the mucus is instead scant, thick, and opaque, transport of the sperm through the cervix is effectively inhibited. Favorable cervical mucus can be demonstrated by the spinnbarkeit test of viscosity, which is performed by drawing out a strand of cervical mucus between two slides. A strand of 10 to 15 cm indicates cervical mucus favorable to sperm penetration. Test results are valid only in the periovulatory period when the effect of the estrogen peak on the cervical mucus can be seen. However, demonstration of sperm survival by a periovulatory postcoital test is more important, and this may occur sometimes even when the quality of the cervical mucus does not appear to be ideal.

Unfavorable cervical mucus can occur spontaneously or, infrequently, it may be secondary to the antiestrogenic effect of clomiphene, especially with large doses. If poor cervical mucus is associated with failure to ovulate in a clomiphene-treated cycle, a change in drug regimen may be indicated (see below under Clomiphene). If cervical mucus is inadequate in an ovulatory cycle of clomiphene treatment, estrogen supplementation may be indicated. Treatment for spontaneous or clomiphene-associated poor cervical mucus is similar: ethinyl estradiol (0.02 to 0.08 mg daily in divided doses) or an equivalent dosage of conjugated estrogens beginning on day 6 to 8 of the cycle and continuing until day 12 or 13. When used with clomiphene, the estrogen should be given two or three days after the last dose of clomiphene and continued for three days, but the two agents should not be given concurrently because they compete for binding sites and the therapeutic action of clomiphene is blocked. Estrogen should not be given during the luteal phase, when it may be luteolytic, and should not be added to a clomiphene regimen unless the condition of the cervical mucus warrants it. Appropriate antibiotic or other local therapy can be prescribed if the thickened mucus is due to chronic cervicitis. Cervical cryosurgery may be indicated for severe chronic cervical infections.

Anovulation, Oligo-ovulation: Three drugs are presently used to treat ovulation failure: clomiphene citrate (alone or with other agents), HMG, and HCG: the latter two are used in combination. Clomiphene is used to stimulate endogenous secretion of gonadotropins and HMG and HCG to replace inadequate quantities or correct abnormal patterns of gonadotropin secretion that result in failure of ovulation. Dosage regimens vary when ovulatory agents are employed and must be determined on the basis of the expected and actual response to treatment. There may be considerable discrepancy between apparent ovulatory rates and pregnancies achieved. The dosage adequate to stimulate ovulation should not be exceeded unless recurrent anovulation occurs, for once an ovulatory response is attained, the pregnancy rate is not enhanced by increasing the dosage; this only increases the probability of ovarian hyperstimulation. There is no evidence that these drugs improve fertility in normally ovulating women.

Clomiphene:

The ideal patients for clomiphene therapy secrete gonadotropins and estrogen but do not ovulate because of an abnormality in the cycling mechanism that controls gonadotropin secretion. Menstruation is a demonstration that gonadotropin is produced, that the ovary is capable of responding to this stimulus by secretion of estrogen, and that the uterine endometrium is capable of responding to the influence of ovarian steroids. In women with amenorrhea, the presence of a normal endometrium and estrogenic stimulation can be demonstrated by a positive (ie, bleeding within a week) response to a progesterone withdrawal test (preferably one intramuscular injection of progesterone 100 to 200 mg or oral doses of medroxyprogesterone acetate [Provera] 10 mg daily for five days). A negative progesterone withdrawal test and high serum gonadotropins indicate ovarian failure and an unsuitable candidate for clomiphene therapy. Abnormally low levels of gonadotropins suggest pituitary failure and success with clomiphene is also unlikely but may be tried. Women who respond to clomiphene tend to have low to normal FSH levels and normal to high LH levels. The existence of an early pregnancy should be ruled out (using an immunologic assay for HCG) before utilizing a synthetic progestin for the progesterone withdrawal test because of the teratogenic potential of these preparations (see Chapter 43, Estrogens and Progestins). Small doses of clomiphene usually induce ovulation in women with polycystic ovarian disease (high LH and estrogen levels). These women may have associated endometrial hyperplasia, and endometrial carcinoma should be ruled out by biopsy and/or dilatation and curettage (D and C) before induction of ovulation is undertaken.

It is not always necessary to complete the infertility tests before initiating clomiphene therapy. However, pregnancy should be ruled out, a semen analysis performed, and an endometrial biopsy and/or D and C in patients with long-term anovulation should be performed to identify possible endometrial carcinoma. The balance of the diagnosis can proceed during the first treatment cycles as needed.

Clomiphene therapy is usually begun at the lowest dosage (50 mg/day for five days) and is increased in gradual increments until an ovulatory response is obtained. The effective dosage should not be exceeded but may be repeated until pregnancy occurs. (See the evaluation for details on dosage.) Clomiphene is usually administered from day five to ten of a menstrual cycle (spontaneous or induced). To achieve maximum effectiveness, the dosage and duration of treatment is individualized. The patient who fails to ovulate at a given dose and has poor cervical mucus may benefit from a longer duration of therapy rather than an increase in dosage. The appearance of adequate cervical mucus in the absence of ovulation suggests that follicular maturation has occurred but the LH surge has not. In this case, HCG can be administered to replace the LH surge and stimulate ovulation (see below).

Monitoring is necessary during each treatment cycle to evaluate the adequacy of dosage in terms of ovulatory response and the side effects produced. Ovulation is assumed to occur if the basal body temperature is at least 0.5 F higher than during the follicular phase, if an endometrial biopsy in the luteal phase shows a secretory effect, and/or serum progesterone levels during the midluteal phase are consistent with a functioning corpus luteum. When clomiphene therapy is successful, ovulation usually occurs five to ten days after the last dose. Therefore, it is desirable for patients to have intercourse approximately every other day during this period. If ovulation does not occur, the patient should be examined to determine if ovarian enlargement (hyperstimulation) has occurred or if she is pregnant before a subsequent cycle of therapy is begun. In the former case, further treatment is postponed until the ovary regresses to normal size, usually by the following month.

Although the ovulation rate in properly selected patients approaches 70% with use of clomiphene, the pregnancy rate may be only 40%. Several possibilities may explain this discrepancy: First, possibly one-half of clomiphene-treated cycles that are ovulatory result in an inadequate corpus luteum (luteal phase dysfunction) (see below). Second, the antiestrogenic effect of clomiphene may result in thick cervical mucous that is unfavorable to sperm penetration. Third, luteinization of an unruptured follicle may occur; this may cause the presumptive signs of ovulation secondary to progesterone secretion to appear, but the ovum is not available for fertilization.

Menotropins (HMG):

Therapy with HMG is complex and should be undertaken only by a physician with experience in its use and with the patient's full understanding and willingness to cooperate; furthermore, monitoring of the patient during treatment requires the availability of laboratory facilities capable of performing estrogen assays (urinary or serum) and reporting results within 24 hours (preferably less) after sample collection.

Induction of ovulation with HMG is reserved for patients who require exogenous supplementation of gonadotropins in order to achieve pregnancy. Those most likely to respond to therapy are anovulatory and have low gonadotropin and estrogen production. Some patients who are able to produce estrogen but fail to ovulate with clomiphene may respond to HMG. However, patients with polycystic ovarian disease who do not respond to clomiphene and HCG generally should not be given HMG because of their hypersensitivity to this agent. These patients may be candidates for ovarian wedge resection. Patients with evidence of ovarian failure, demonstrated by high levels of serum gonadotropins or the inability of the endometrium to bleed after a progesterone withdrawal test or adequate therapy with estrogen and progesterone (as in Asherman's syndrome of intrauterine synechiae), are not suitable candidates for HMG. Caution should be exercised before HMG is given to a woman with evidence of pituitary tumor. Because of the expense ($15 to $20 per ampul; usually in excess of $300 for drugs in one cycle; cost per conception, $1,000 or more) and the potential for complications (eg, multiple pregnancy, hyperstimulation syndrome), complete infertility testing should be performed prior to initiating HMG treatment to rule out, and treat if possible, other causes of infertility. A course of clomiphene is usually given before beginning HMG therapy, because unpredictably some hypogonadotropic patients will respond.

The goal of therapy with HMG is to replace gonadotropins and stimulate follicular development. The dosage varies widely and should be based upon careful observation of the patient's hormonal profile and response to therapy (see the evaluation for details on dosage). When follicular maturation is optimal (usually after one to two weeks of therapy), ovulation is induced by intramuscular administration of HCG. Since ovulation of properly prepared follicles usually occurs within one day after HCG administration, the couple is instructed to have coitus the evening of the injection and for the next two or three days. Three to five cycles of HMG treatment usually constitute an adequate trial.

Monitoring patient response is crucial to determine that adequate stimulation without ovarian hyperstimulation is provided and to reduce the likelihood of multiple pregnancy. The basal body temperature should be recorded daily. Ideally, the patient also should be examined daily to monitor changes in ovarian size, cervical mucus, and estrogen production, but this may not be necessary during the first several days. Daily examinations and estrogen determinations should be initiated when clinical evidence of improvement is demonstrated (ie, with the spinnbarkeit test), which is a sign of follicular maturation and estrogen production. Follicular maturation occasionally proceeds without the usual clinical signs of estrogen production and, for this reason, estrogen secretion should be measured one week after beginning administration of HMG even if there is no improvement in the quality of cervical mucus. HCG should never be given to induce ovulation unless estrogen production has been measured for the previous 24 hours.

As with use of clomiphene, there is a discrepancy between ovulatory and pregnancy rates with HMG. In properly selected patients, ovulatory rates are close to 100% but pregnancy occurs in only 40% to 70% of treated women. The incidence of multiple gestation is 15% to 30% and up to 75% of these are twins. Spontaneous abortion occurs in about 25% of pregnancies and is more likely with multiple gestations (which are due to ovulation of multiple ova). The incidence of congenital abnormalities with HMG-induced pregnancy is not increased.

Combination Therapy:

In certain patients who fail to respond to standard ovulation induction regimens, various regimens combining the above agents have been employed with variable success. For example, women who apparently ovulate in response to clomiphene but who fail to develop favorable cervical mucus may become pregnant when estrogen is added to the treatment program (see above). It is appropriate to add HCG to a clomiphene regimen in patients who fail to ovulate with clomiphene alone but show evidence of estrogenic stimulation. These patients may be lacking only the LH surge, and HCG replaces this stimulus to ovulation. Other failures with clomiphene may be due to a short luteal phase after ovulation, and this problem also may respond to HCG. (See the evaluation on Clomiphene Citrate for dosages.)

Some candidates for HMG therapy who have some degree of pituitary responsiveness with withdrawal bleeding after administration of progesterone may benefit from the combined actions of clomiphene, HMG, and HCG. The goal of this combination is to achieve partial follicular maturation with clomiphene so that smaller doses of HMG may be used. HCG is employed as usual to stimulate ovulation. Monitoring is the same as with HMG-HCG therapy, and the possibility of ovarian hyperstimulation and multiple gestations also is similar. The rationale for attempting this regimen is based on economic, not physiologic, considerations. The dose of HMG may be reduced by one-half, thus providing financial relief for this costly therapy (see the evaluation on Menotropins for dosage).

Luteal Phase Dysfunction (LPD): Compromise of corpus luteum function, either in the amount of progesterone produced or in the duration of function, can result in infertility or repeated early fetal wastage. It may occur spontaneously or be associated with use of clomiphene. About 4% of infertile women and up to 50% of clomiphene-treated cycles in some women may be affected. The dysfunction is probably caused by gonadotropin deficiency resulting from inadequate FSH stimulation of the follicles prior to ovulation or from failure of adequate support of the corpus luteum by LH (or HCG in early pregnancy). A short luteal phase, more rare than luteal phase defect, can be suspected if the duration of luteal function is subnormal (temperature elevated less than 10 to 12 days) as determined by elevation of the basal temperature which indicates the probable time of ovulation. Diagnosis of luteal phase defect or inadequate luteal phase is more difficult and is not necessarily associated with shortening of the luteal phase. Diagnosis of the latter is based on observation of inadequate secretion of progesterone (determined by serial measurements during the luteal phase) or evidence of abnormal endometrium (determined by biopsy taken within several days before the next expected menses). The results of the biopsy must be more than two days out of phase with the normal histologic appearance for the appropriate stage of the cycle (with reference to the onset of the next menses) (Noyes et al, 1950). Since episodes of luteal dysfunction sometimes occur in women with normal function, drug therapy should be reserved for abnormalities documented in more than one cycle. Efficacy of therapy should be verified by endometrial biopsy during the first treatment cycle.

Pharmacotherapy is directed either toward stimulation of the corpus luteum with HCG or replacement therapy with progesterone. It is important that therapy with the chosen agent be initiated in the cycle of conception and not after the first missed menses. Continuing administration is necessary until steroidogenesis is taken over by the placenta after ten weeks of gestation. There are no comparative data to support recommendation of one mode over another on the basis of efficacy, so the choice is made because of other considerations.

HCG is an effective luteotropic agent, and the initial dose may serve the dual purpose of acting as the ovulatory trigger if ovulation is being induced, as well as supporting the corpus luteum. Less desirable aspects include the necessity of administering the agent parenterally, delay of menses for up to one week if pregnancy does not ensue, and interference of exogenous HCG with the interpretation of a pregnancy test. Rarely, the corpus luteum may be resistant to the normal stimulatory action of HCG and fail to produce progesterone.

Progesterone replacement therapy is effective regardless of the etiology of luteal dysfunction and, unlike HCG, efficacy does not depend upon a secondary response that may fail. Progesterone may be administered daily by intramuscular injection (12.5 mg daily), but this is inconvenient and the injections are painful. Preferably, progesterone suppositories (25 mg twice daily) are inserted vaginally or, less commonly, rectally. Suppositories are not commercially available but may be compounded by a pharmacist (see the evaluation on Progesterone). The route is easily utilized and the dosage is low enough (physiologic) so that menses are not usually delayed more than two days if the patient is not pregnant. Natural progesterone must be used because a synthetic progestin may be luteolytic and/or teratogenic (see also Chapter 43, Estrogens and Progestins).

Endometriosis: Endometriosis is a condition in which endometrial tissue exists in ectopic sites, most frequently the ovaries, the peritoneum of the cul-de-sac, on the uterosacral and round ligaments, the oviducts, and the serosal surface of the uterus. It is characterized by pelvic or lower back pain that is worse during menstruation; dysmenorrhea, particularly if it first appears in the late twenties or thirties and becomes progressively worse; and dyspareunia and/or pain on defecation, particularly during menses. The disease is predominantly one of the childbearing years, for the stimulation of endometrial implants and the associated discomfort depend upon cyclic hormonal stimulation. The ectopic implants respond to the normal cyclic hormonal stimulation similarly to normal endometrium. The pain of endometriosis is probably related to stretching of the peritoneum or other structures that occurs from scarring or as a result of bleeding from the implants during menstruation. However, the degree of pain is not necessarily related to the extent of the disease. Endometriosis may be the single cause of infertility in 10% of infertile women and is a major factor in 25% to 40%. It is a frequent finding upon laparoscopy in those with previously unexplained infertility. Infertility also may result from ovarian or tubal adhesions and, in many cases, may be caused by subtle changes that affect tubal transport of the ovum, although there is no visible cause.

Endometriosis responds to drug therapy or surgery. Surgery is more often curative, but both modes of treatment relieve symptoms and enhance fertility. Surgery is usually indicated if the ovaries are greatly enlarged or if extensive disease is present. Drug therapy is utilized in milder cases or as preparation for surgery. It is difficult to evaluate and compare the effectiveness of surgery and various pharmacotherapeutic regimens because of a lack of understanding of the extent to which the disease interferes with fertility and of the spontaneous pregnancy rate in the presence of endometriosis. Pregnancy rates ranging from 40% to 80% have been reported following conservative surgery (which allows preservation of reproductive function) and probably reflect variation in the severity of the disease.

The drugs used with some degree of success in the treatment of endometriosis include estrogens, progestins, and androgens. Those most widely prescribed currently are combination oral contraceptives, which are taken continuously rather than cyclically for six to nine months; if estrogen should be avoided, a progestin such as medroxyprogesterone acetate [Provera, Depo-Provera] may be used (for dosage, see the evaluation in Chapter 43, Estrogens and Progestins). Breakthrough bleeding is common with progestin alone and, if a depot preparation is used, the return of fertility is delayed. Therapy can be continued for up to nine months and may be repeated later if symptoms recur. The effectiveness of hormonal therapy is secondary to suppression of cyclic changes in the ectopic implant and possibly to direct atrophic effects on the lesions. Oral contraceptive therapy should not be employed in the presence of myomas, since they may stimulate growth. Symptoms may increase initially before improvement is noted, and the usual adverse effects associated with estrogen therapy may occur (see Chapter 43).

The newest drug available for the treatment of endometriosis is an androgen derivative, danazol [Danocrine]. This drug is not primarily estrogenic or progestational but has antigonadotropic and mild androgenic activity. Its use is followed by regression of implants, suppression of symptoms, and by pregnancy in some previously infertile patients. However, no controlled studies are available to compare the effectiveness of danazol with other types of hormonal therapy. As with other forms of drug therapy, lesions tend to reappear after cessation of treatment. The most common side effects include weight gain, oily skin, and acne; decreased breast size and hypoestrogenic symptoms (eg, vasomotor flushes, atrophic vaginitis) also have occurred. Therapy with danazol appears to be more effective than oral contraceptive suppressive therapy, and the continuous administration of oral contraceptives can be avoided. Furthermore, suppression of endometrial implants begins immediately, and potential side effects are less serious than with estrogen-progestin combinations. However, because of the lack of definitive clinical evidence of superiority and the expense of danazol treatment (over $100 monthly for the recommended course of therapy), other hormonal regimes are used commonly.

Prolactinemic Reproductive Dysfunction: Amenorrhea or oligomenorrhea with galactorrhea is usually associated with elevated levels of plasma prolactin. Conversely, hyperprolactinemia also can occur in the absence of galactorrhea and sometimes in women with normal menstrual function. Hyperprolactinemic states are often associated with impaired fertility, whether the patient's condition is a normal physiologic state (postpartum lactation) or is caused by a pathologic condition (eg, pituitary tumor). The etiology of this effect is not completely understood but probably involves central derangement of normal gonadotropin secretion as well as possible peripheral actions that block the gonadotropic effect at the gonad. Both males and females may be affected, but interference with reproductive function is more definitely established in the female.

Bromocriptine [Parlodel] is a dopaminergic agent with many potential clinical uses. Of interest in the treatment of infertility is the ability of this agent to act directly on the dopamine receptors of prolactin-secreting cells in the anterior pituitary, resulting in depressed secretion of prolactin toward normal levels. When used in women with hyperprolactinemic disorders, the decrease in the serum prolactin level is usually followed by normalization of menstrual cycles and return of fertility.

Although bromocriptine restores reproductive function impaired by elevated prolactin levels, caution is advised because excessive prolactin may be produced by a pituitary adenoma. These tumors rarely may expand rapidly during pregnancy with serious consequences (eg, visual impairment, hypopituitarism). Even though the danger of tumor growth is greatest during pregnancy, bromocriptine should not be taken at this time because its safety during gestation and inhibiting effect on tumor cell growth have not been demonstrated. However, there has been no evidence of teratogenicity in patients in whom the drug was inadvertently continued in early pregnancy. Therefore, in women with infertility caused by hyperprolactinemia, every effort should be made to detect the presence of a pituitary macroadenoma or microadenoma (eg, polytomography, pituitary function tests) and most clinicians elect to treat it appropriately (eg, transsphenoidal resection, irradiation) before pregnancy is attempted.

MALE INFERTILITY

Almost one-half of infertility is at least partially due to reproductive dysfunction in the male partner. Whatever the etiology, it is manifested by an effect on the number of sperm produced, their motility or morphology, or the viscosity or volume of the semen. The cause may be an anatomic abnormality, such as varicocele or cryptorchidism, or obstruction of the epididymis due to inflammatory disease (eg, tuberculosis, gonorrhea); genetic (eg, Klinefelter's syndrome); destruction of germinal epithelium (eg, mumps orchitis, irradiation, drugs); environmental (eg, increased scrotal temperature from hot baths, tight underwear); immunologic (eg, sperm antibodies); or acute infection as suggested by leukocytes in the semen. Only a small proportion of male infertility has a recognized endocrinologic basis.

Varicocele is responsible for over one-third of the cases of male infertility and, when surgical correction is appropriate, ligation of the left spermatic vein restores fertility in about 50% of patients (bilateral involvement occurs less often and right varicocele is rare). In men with low sperm count or abnormal semen volume, use of split ejaculates and artificial insemination occasionally achieves pregnancies. HCG (4,000 units twice weekly for ten weeks) has been given empirically to augment the results of surgery in men with varicocele who have low sperm counts (less than 1,000,000/ml) preoperatively. Significant improvement in semen quality may occur about three months after completion of HCG treatment; however, improvement may be preceded by an initial decline in the quality of semen (Dubin and Amelar, 1975).

Few causes of male infertility are amenable to drug therapy. In the past, thyroid and sometimes adrenal supplements were used empirically, but with the sensitive diagnostic endocrine tests available today, such indiscriminate treatment cannot be recommended in the absence of a demonstrated thyroid or adrenal hormone deficiency. Improvement in sperm motility with increased incidence of pregnancies has been reported following low-dose androgen therapy in infertile males with isolated poor sperm motility. Sperm count, morphology, and serum testosterone levels were normal in these subjects (Brown, 1975). In the presence of infection, appropriate antibiotic therapy may be effective. There is no evidence that vitamin supplementation improves male fertility.

Hypothalamic-Pituitary-Gonadal Axis Dysfunction: Hypogonadotropic infertility is uncommon in males. However, in properly selected patients, fertility can be enhanced and pregnancies achieved in one-half of the cases treated. Definitive diagnostic tests include exclusion of infertility of both partners from other causes, measurement of serum concentrations of gonadotropins and testosterone, and testicular biopsy.

Hormonal therapy for male infertility can still be considered experimental, but the long-term administration of small doses of clomiphene [Clomid] appears to be most successful (see the evaluation). As in women, clomiphene stimulates endogenous gonadotropin secretion. Criteria for candidates include serum gonadotropin and testosterone levels usually within the normal range and testicular biopsy indicating presence of all germinal elements although decreased in number (pregerminal hypofertility). Clomiphene usually increases serum testosterone levels and the number and motility of sperm. However, some patients show an early increase in sperm count followed by a decline. Patients with primary germinal hypofertility (increased serum FSH, hyalinization or other evidence of permanent epithelial damage) or postgerminal hypofertility caused by duct obstruction are not candidates for drug therapy (Paulson, 1977).

Although much attention has been given to impairment of female fertility in hyperprolactinemic states, the effects of serum prolactin levels on semen quality have not been studied. Since both men and women require gonadotropic support for gametogenesis, it seems reasonable to expect that the male reproductive system also may be subject to various inhibitions associated with elevated prolactin levels. Galactorrhea sometimes occurs in males with prolactin-secreting tumors, and impotence is often, but not invariably, present. In some men, sperm counts and testosterone levels are increased following normalization of serum prolactin with use of bromocriptine. Hyperprolactinemia may account for refractoriness to gonadotropin in some men whose hormonal profile indicates that they would be successful candidates for clomiphene therapy. In the future, perhaps measurement of serum prolactin will be added to the routine hormonal tests employed in infertile men; identification and treatment of appropriate patients with bromocriptine may improve the pregnancy rates achieved in patients who would otherwise be "failures."

Other hormonal treatment includes the administration of exogenous gonadotropins (HCG or a combination of HCG and HMG). Results have been disappointing and the necessity for repeated intramuscular injections is inconvenient and, particularly when HMG is employed, expensive (in excess of $1,000 for a three-month course of therapy). Unless such regimens eventually produce results superior to those achieved with clomiphene, they probably will be reserved, as in women, for patients refractory to clomiphene. Gonadotropin-releasing hormone (GnRH) also may stimulate the release of gonadotropin from the pituitary, but long-acting analogues must become commercially available before this approach is feasible.

Testosterone rebound therapy has been employed sporadically since its introduction 30 years ago. A depot preparation (testosterone enanthate or cypionate 200 mg injected intramuscularly) is administrated weekly for 12 to 20 weeks. The negative feedback effect of testosterone suppresses pituitary gonadotropic output and azoospermia ensues. Following cessation of therapy, there is sometimes a rebound phenomenon in which the germinal epithelium may recover function and increase sperm production to a level compatible with fertility. The mechanism of action has been ascribed to release of gonadotropin that was stored in the pituitary during the period of testosterone suppression. However, stimulation and support of spermatogenesis probably require a more prolonged period of gonadotropin secretion; furthermore, it is possible that the rebound phenomenon involves increased sensitivity of testicular tissue to the effects of gonadotropin. Success rates with this method are quite variable but do not exceed 40%, and there are several disadvantages: (1) The treatment period is long and, when therapy is successful, the rebound in sperm production is delayed for three to four months after cessation of therapy. (2) In most men, the improvement in sperm production lasts only two to three months. (3) Treatment may be followed by permanent depression of the sperm count (Charny and Gordon, 1978). Because of these problems and the uncertainty of success, the testosterone suppression method is best reserved for patients who do not respond to other therapy and who understand the possible deleterious consequences of the treatment.

INDIVIDUAL EVALUATIONS

CLOMIPHENE CITRATE
[Clomid]

Clomiphene citrate is a nonsteroidal agent related to chlorotrianisene; it is antiestrogenic in humans and mildly estrogenic in laboratory animals. This preparation is a mixture of the cis and trans forms of the compound in approximately a 1:1 ratio. It may stimulate ovulation in anovulatory and oligo-ovulatory women with potentially functional hypothalamic-pituitary-ovarian axes and adequate endogenous estrogens.

Clomiphene decreases the concentration of cytoplasmic receptors in the hypothalamus, producing a low estrogen signal which, in turn, increases the secretion of gonadotropin-releasing hormone (GnRH) and the levels of LH and FSH. Ovarian stimulation results. About one-half of the ingested dose is excreted in five days; traces appear in the feces up to six weeks after administration.

Ovulation occurs in about 70% and pregnancy in up to 40% of properly selected patients. The incidence of multiple pregnancies is about 8% or six times normal but is lower than with HMG. Multiple births are almost always twins; larger multiple gestations have been reported rarely. Spontaneous abortions (mostly early miscarriages) occur in approximately 20% of clomiphene-induced pregnancies, which is only slightly higher than normal.

Clomiphene is administered in incremental dosages until an ovulatory dose is reached. If ovulation is achieved but pregnancy does not occur, the ovulatory dosage should not be exceeded (this may actually decrease the probability of pregnancy) but can be repeated clinically. On the other hand, a dose that has not produced ovulation may be repeated before advancing to the next level, because the patient may not respond identically in different cycles. This conservative approach is not advocated by many physicians, however, especially with lower amounts (50 to 100 mg). Although 75% of clomiphene-induced pregnancies occur in the first three cycles of treatment (and therefore with low doses), a significant number (15%) occur after treatment with doses of 150 to 200 mg.

The addition of other agents (eg, estrogen, HCG, HMG) to the clomiphene regimen may improve the pregnancy rate over that achieved by clomiphene alone. In certain patients, 5,000 to 10,000 IU of HCG may be administered 7 to 10 days after an unsuccessful course of clomiphene to simulate the midcycle LH surge. Other patients refractory to the effects of clomiphene alone may respond to a regimen of clomiphene-HMG-HCG. With this combination, less HMG may be required than if this agent is used alone to stimulate follicular development. (See the sections on Hostile Cervical Mucus and Combination Therapy and the evaluation on Menotropins.)

ADVERSE REACTIONS AND PRECAUTIONS.

Although there is no evidence of an increased incidence of fetal anomalies clinically, these have been observed in offspring of some subprimate animals given clomiphene *during* pregnancy. Since clomiphene is excreted slowly, there is at least theoretical reason for concern about human teratogenicity. Clomiphene should not be administered to pregnant women; there is no indication for clomiphene therapy once conception has been achieved.

The most serious, although rare, adverse reaction of clomiphene is massive cystic enlargement of the ovaries. Maximal enlargement occurs about a week after ovulation and regression is usually spontaneous after several days or weeks. Additional therapy should not be given until the ovaries return to pretreatment size (usually within one month). The patient may then be given a course of a lower dose of clomiphene with the addition of HCG when the cervical mucus appears favorable. Patients should be examined before each course of clomiphene to detect enlarged, hyperstimulated ovaries and to exclude pregnancy.

When clomiphene induces ovulation, luteal phase defect may occur in up to one-half of the cycles in some patients. This can be treated by adding HCG or progesterone to the regimen. (See the discussion on Luteal Phase Dysfunction.)

Blurred vision and scintillating scotomata are dose related and reversible when the drug is discontinued. Objective signs are rarely found, although measurable loss of visual acuity, definable scotomata, and changes in retinal cell function have been reported. The occurrence of vis-

ual abnormalities is considered a contraindication to further use by some physicians, while others continue therapy with lower doses.

Other adverse reactions include hot flashes resembling menopausal vasomotor symptoms (10% to 40%) and, less commonly, nausea, headache, breast engorgement, and abdominal bloating. Symptoms disappear when therapy is stopped. Untoward effects may occur at the lowest dosages in sensitive individuals (see also the Introduction).

Clomiphene is used to stimulate sperm production in certain male patients (see the section on Male Infertility for criteria for patient selection).

ROUTE, USUAL DOSAGE, AND PREPARATIONS. *Oral*: To induce ovulation, initially, 50 mg daily for five days starting on the fifth day of the cycle (spontaneous or induced bleeding) or at any time in patients who have not menstruated recently (provided pregnancy has been ruled out). Lower doses or a shorter duration of treatment is recommended if unusual sensitivity to pituitary gonadotropin is suspected. If ovulation without conception occurs, the same dosage is given cyclically until conception or for six to eight cycles. If ovulation does not occur, the dosage is increased by 50-mg increments in each cycle until 200 mg/day for five days is given.

Alternatively, lower doses can be given for 7 to 10 days (see the section on Female Infertility in the Introduction). If doses of 150 to 200 mg daily for five days fail to stimulate ovulation, if there is evidence of ovulatory failure due to lack of an LH surge, or if there is evidence of a short luteal phase, HCG may be added to the regimen. A dose of 10,000 IU is given by intramuscular injection 12 to 14 days after starting clomiphene or 5,000 IU is given, followed by 5,000 IU five days later.

For oligospermia in selected male patients, 25 mg daily may be given for 25 days, after which the medication is discontinued for five days. This same schedule is followed for 6 to 12 months or until pregnancy is achieved.

Clomid (Merrell-National). Tablets 50 mg.

MENOTROPINS (HMG)
[Pergonal]

Menotropins is a preparation of human menopausal gonadotropin (HMG) which is extracted from the urine of postmenopausal women. FSH and LH activity is present in a 1:1 ratio. Therapeutic effects are usually achieved by combination with HCG or in a clomiphene-HCG regimen. In anovulatory women judged suitable for gonadotropin therapy (see the Introduction), menotropins is given initially in sufficient doses to induce follicular growth and maturation as determined by serial measurements of serum or urinary estrogens. Following follicular maturation, HCG is given to induce ovulation. Induction of ovulation with gonadotropins is difficult and expensive and should be carried out only by physicians with specialized training and experience. Proper administration of menotropins requires individualization of dosage based on the patient's response.

Menotropins has been used experimentally alone or with HCG to treat male infertility. Such treatment is expensive and effective regimens have not been described (see the section on Male Infertility in the Introduction).

Because there is considerable variation in individual response to menotropins, symptoms of ovarian hyperstimulation, which occur in 1% to 2% of patients, may be observed after any dose but are most common after use of large doses. Mild hyperstimulation, evidenced by ovarian enlargement and abdominal discomfort, lasts seven to ten days and requires no treatment. Severe hyperstimulation is life-threatening and hospitalization is required; ovarian enlargement is accompanied by weight gain, ascites, pleural effusion, oliguria, hypotension, and hypercoagulability. Treatment is largely supportive, although ovarian rupture with intraperitoneal hemorrhage often requires surgical intervention.

Multiple gestations are encountered frequently (15% to 20%) in gonadotropin-induced pregnancies and do not appear to be predictable on the basis of the estrogen levels produced. Several treatment cycles may be necessary, but therapy beyond five cycles is not likely to increase the success rate.

ROUTES, USUAL DOSAGE, AND PREPARATIONS. Close monitoring (pelvic examinations and laboratory assessment of estrogen levels) in each treatment cycle is necessary both to increase the pregnancy rate and to reduce the incidence of the hyperstimulation syndrome, which occurs only after HCG has stimulated ovulation. Findings from physical examination are important, but the primary objective measurement of follicular maturation is the level of estrogen secretion. The appearance of cervical mucus and vaginal cytology are helpful but are not sensitive enough to determine the timing of HCG injection. Measurement of 24-hour urinary estrogens or serum estrogen assays may be used for this purpose. If these levels are approximately double the normal value for the preovulatory peak (absolute values may vary among laboratories), HCG should be given within 24 hours. When follicular maturation has reached this stage of active estrogen secretion, the rate of estrogen production can be expected to double daily. Acceptable estrogen levels for HCG-induced ovulation may vary slightly, depending upon the time elapsed between the collection of the sample and HCG administration. If estrogen production is lower than the optimum level, administration of menotropins should be continued. If estrogen production is three to four times greater than the preovulatory level, HCG should not be administered because of the risk of ovarian hyperstimulation. Monitoring is required in each cycle of therapy because the patient's response may vary from cycle to cycle.

MENOTROPINS AND HCG:
Intramuscular: There is no fixed dosage regimen. The goal of therapy is to produce follicular maturation with menotropins in 10 to 15 days and to stimulate ovulation with HCG. The dosage requirement may vary in the same individual and therefore is determined according to the patient's response in each cycle of treatment. Usually patients are initially given one to two ampuls (each containing 75 IU FSH and 75 IU

LH) daily. Dosage may be continued at this level if there is evidence of estrogen production; if such evidence is lacking, the amount may be increased after the first seven days. Occasionally up to six ampuls per day are required to stimulate follicular development. When the patient has reached the appropriate level of estrogen production (see above), HCG is administered to stimulate ovulation (within 24 hours after the last menotropins injection) as a single injection of 10,000 IU, or 5,000 IU is administered followed by 5,000 IU three to five days later. Other variations in the amount and timing of HCG have been employed and are designed not only to provide the ovulatory stimulus but also to support corpus luteum function at a critical stage (particularly if there is evidence of luteal phase deficiency).

MENOTROPINS, CLOMIPHENE, AND HCG:

Oral, Intramuscular: This regimen may be tried in properly selected patients (see the Introduction) to reduce the cost of therapy. Clomiphene administration is started orally on the fifth day of the cycle (spontaneous or induced); 100 mg is given for five to seven days or 200 mg for five days, then two ampuls of menotropins are given intramuscularly each day for four days, followed by one ampul daily for two days. HCG 10,000 IU is given intramuscularly to stimulate ovulation after 24 hours. As with menotropins-HCG therapy, estrogen levels are monitored and serve as a guide for modification of dosage and duration of drug administration.

> *Pergonal* (Serono). Each 2 ml ampul contains 75 IU each of follicle-stimulating hormone (FSH) activity and luteinizing hormone (LH) activity (with 1 ml of sodium chloride solution).

HUMAN CHORIONIC GONADOTROPIN (HCG)
[Antuitrin-S, A.P.L., Follutein, Pregnyl]

Human chorionic gonadotropin (HCG) is a placental hormone extracted from the urine of pregnant women. In most radio-immunoassay systems, there is a cross reaction between HCG and LH; however, substantial differences in the sequence of protein and carbohydrate exist. Biologically, HCG mimics the actions of LH.

HCG is used to treat infertility in both women and men. It serves as a substitute for the LH surge to stimulate ovulation of a prepared follicle when used with clomiphene and/or menotropins. HCG also may be utilized to replace deficient endogenous LH in women with luteal phase dysfunction. The effectiveness of treatment depends upon the ability of the corpus luteum to respond to HCG stimulus (ie, HCG is not effective if the corpus luteum is refractory to stimulation).

HCG, alone or with clomiphene or menotropins, has been used with limited success to restore full spermatogenesis in men who have insufficient gonadotropic stimulation after puberty.

ROUTE, USUAL DOSAGE, AND PREPARATIONS. *Intramuscular*: To stimulate ovulation, see the evaluations on Clomiphene Citrate and Menotropins.

For luteal phase dysfunction, treatment must begin in the cycle of conception; 5,000 IU is injected three days after the elevation in basal body temperature and again three days later, or 2,500 to 5,000 IU is given initially and every two to three days for four injections.

> Drug available generically: Powder 1,000, 5,000, 10,000, and 20,000 units with 10 ml of diluent.
> *Antuitrin-S* (Parke, Davis). Powder 5,000 IU with 10 ml of diluent.
> *A.P.L.* (Ayerst). Powder 5,000, 10,000 and 20,000 USP units with 10 ml of diluent.
> *Follutein* (Squibb). Powder (lyophilized) 10,000 USP units with 10 ml of diluent.
> *Pregnyl* (Organon). Powder 10,000 IU with 10 ml of diluent.

PROGESTERONE
[Lipo-Lutin]

Progesterone is used to treat luteal phase dysfunction when this results in infertility or repeated early spontaneous abortion. This disorder should be documented before progesterone therapy is undertaken. Treatment begins in the cycle of conception and generally continues until placental production of steroids is established or until assay indicates adequate endogenous production of progesterone (8 to 10 weeks). Only progesterone, and not a synthetic progestin, should be administered for this indication.

Progesterone may be administered intramuscularly, which is painful and inconvenient, or in suppository form. Suppositories are not available commercially but may be compounded by a pharmacist using the following formulation: 44 g progesterone powder, 2,096 g polyethylene glycol 400, 1,392 g polyethylene glycol 6,000 (makes 1,760 suppositories containing 25 mg progesterone each). See also the Introduction.

ROUTES, USUAL DOSAGE, AND PREPARATIONS. *Intramuscular*: For support of pregnancy in luteal phase dysfunction, 12.5 mg daily beginning as soon as ovulation can be diagnosed and continuing, if needed, to the eleventh week of gestation.

> Drug available generically: Suspension (aqueous) 25 and 50 mg/ml in 10 ml containers; solution (in oil) 25, 50, and 100 mg/ml in 10 ml containers.
> *Lipo-Lutin* (Parke, Davis). Solution (in peanut oil) 50 mg/ml in 5 ml containers.

Vaginal, Rectal: For support of pregnancy in luteal phase dysfunction, one 25-mg suppository inserted twice daily beginning as soon as ovulation can be diagnosed and continuing, if needed, up to the eleventh week of gestation.

> Not available commercially; see above for preparation of suppositories.

DANAZOL
[Danocrine]

This synthetic derivative of 17α-ethinyl testosterone (ethisterone) is used to treat pelvic endometriosis. This agent does not exhibit estrogenic or progestational properties and its usefulness in endometriosis is probably the result of its antigonadotropic activity. Danazol also may directly inhibit ovarian steroidogenesis. It causes atrophy of endometrial tissue in the uterus and ectopic sites and amenorrhea is usual. Ovulation and menstruation are reestablished promptly on cessation of therapy.

Danazol is indicated for the treatment of endometriosis amenable to hormonal management; it appears to be more effective than estrogen-progestin regimens and is preferable to these preparations, especially when estrogens are contraindicated. Danazol is not indicated when surgery alone is considered the treatment of choice and should not be given to women with underlying abnormal genital bleeding or markedly impaired hepatic, renal, or cardiac function. This agent is more expensive than therapeutically equivalent courses of other medication.

Adverse reactions reported include weight gain, edema, androgenic and anabolic effects (acne, mild hirsutism, oily skin or hair, decrease in breast size), and sequelae of a hypoestrogenic state (flushing, sweating, vaginitis). Danazol should not be administered to pregnant or lactating women.

Its safe use during pregnancy has not been established, although there have been no embryotoxic or teratogenic effects attributable to administration of this agent thus far. In one study, the incidence of second- and third-trimester intrauterine fetal deaths was high (4 of 39 pregnancies) among pregnancies begun within three menstrual cycles after cessation of treatment with danazol. It was postulated that the atrophic effects of the drug on the endometrium may have resulted in inadequate placentation (Dmowski and Cohen, 1978). A cautious approach would be to postpone pregnancy following use of danazol until after the endometrium has recovered normal function as evidenced by a normal menstrual period.

720

ROUTE, USUAL DOSAGE, AND PREPARATIONS.
Oral: For endometriosis, 800 mg daily in
two divided doses for three to nine months,
as necessary. Treatment can be reinstituted
if symptoms recur upon cessation of
therapy.

    Danocrine (Winthrop). Capsules 200 mg.

BROMOCRIPTINE MESYLATE
[Parlodel]

    The clinical usefulness of this
semisynthetic ergot alkaloid is primarily
dependent upon its dopaminergic activity.
Bromocriptine inhibits the secretion of prolactin directly at the anterior pituitary
gland. The drug may be used to correct
female infertility secondary to hyperprolactinemic states (eg, menstrual irregularities
with or without galactorrhea). Impotence or
hypogonadism in males that is associated
with elevated prolactin levels sometimes
responds to bromocriptine. The drug is not
effective in psychogenic impotence or that
caused by conditions other than hyperprolactinemia. Symptoms frequently recur
upon cessation of therapy.

    With the doses employed for reproduc-
tive dysfunction, side effects are generally
not severe. Nausea is most common, but
vomiting, constipation, dizziness, and orthostatic hypotension also occur. These untoward effects can be minimized by taking
the medication with food and by initiating
therapy with small doses and gradually
increasing them to effective levels.

    Bromocriptine suppresses hypersecre-
tion of prolactin caused by a pituitary
adenoma and may even inhibit tumor
growth. However, the drug is not a substitute for surgery or radiation therapy if these
measures are appropriate because of pressure from or growth of the tumor. The
natural course of prolactin-secreting microadenomas (less than 1 cm diameter) is

not clearly understood, but these neoplasms may prove to be relatively common
(asymptomatic microadenomas have been
found during routine autopsies) and without threat of morbidity other than that
associated with their endocrine function.
Bromocriptine should not be used to correct infertility in women until a pituitary
tumor is ruled out and treated if appropriate, since microadenomas occasionally
enlarge greatly during pregnancy.

    Although no teratogenic effects have
been described in humans, cleft lip has
occurred in offspring of rabbits treated with
bromocriptine. Until more evidence of
safety in human pregnancy is obtained, the
drug should be discontinued as soon as
pregnancy is documented.

ROUTE, USUAL DOSAGE, AND PREPARATIONS.
Oral: For amenorrhea-galactorrhea and related conditions, initially, 1.25 to 2.5 mg
once daily, increasing the amount after two
or three days to 2.5 mg twice daily. If
necessary, dosage may be increased by 2.5
mg every two or three days. Other doses
and treatment schedules also have been
employed. Bromocriptine should be taken
with food.

    Parlodel (Sandoz). Tablets 2.5 mg.

Selected References

Amelar RD, et al: *Male Infertility*. Philadelphia, WB
    Saunders Co, 1977.

Behrman SJ, Kistner RW (eds): *Progress in Infertil-
    ity*, ed 2. Boston, Little, Brown and Company,
    1975.

Brown JS: Effect of orally administered androgens
    on sperm motility. *Fertil Steril* 26:305-308,
    1975.

Charny CW, Gordon JA: Testosterone rebound
    therapy: Neglected modality. *Fertil Steril*
    29:64-68, 1978.

Crosignani PG, Mishell DR (eds): *Ovulation in the
    Human*. New York, Academic Press, 1976.

Dmowski WP, Cohen MR: Antigonadotropin
    (danazol) in treatment of endometriosis. *Am J
    Obstet Gynecol* 130:41-48, 1978.

Dubin L, Amelar RD: Varicocelectomy as therapy
    in male infertility: Study of 50 cases. *Fertil
    Steril* 26:217-220, 1975.

Hammond CH, Haney AF: Conservative treatment
    of endometriosis: 1978. *Fertil Steril* 30:497-509,
    1978.

Marshall JR: Induction of ovulation. *Clin Obstet
    Gynecol* 21:147-162, 1978.

Moghissi KS: *Infertility*, monograph. Kansas City, Mo, American Academy of Family Physicians, 1978.

Noyes RW, et al: Dating the endometrial biopsy. *Fertil Steril* 1:3-25, 1950.

Paulson DF: Clomiphene citrate in management of male hypofertility: Predictors for treatment selection. *Fertil Steril* 28:1226-1229, 1977.

Speroff L, et al: *Clinical Gynecologic Endocrinology and Infertility*, ed 2. Baltimore, Williams & Wilkins Company, 1978.

Taymor ML: *Infertility*. New York, Grune and Stratton, 1978.

Agents Related to Anterior Pituitary and Hypothalamic Function | 46

INTRODUCTION

GROWTH HORMONE

THYROID

ADRENAL CORTEX

GONADOTROPINS

PROLACTIN

BETA-LIPOTROPIN

The anterior pituitary gland (adenohypophysis) synthesizes three large polypeptides and three glycoproteins whose hormonal actions in man are well defined, as well as another polypeptide whose function in man is now being elucidated. The more familiar polypeptides include (1) growth hormone (GH, somatotropin), which has growth-promoting and anabolic properties; (2) prolactin (PRL), which is similar in size to GH and plays a primary role in stimulating lactation, is involved in regulating gonadal function and possibly has some additional as yet undefined metabolic actions; and (3) corticotropin (ACTH), which stimulates glucocorticoid secretion by the adrenal cortex. The less understood polypeptide is lipotropic hormone (LPH, lipotropin), which contains within its structure several biologically active hormones, the exact functions of which remain unknown. The glycoprotein hormones are (1) thyrotropin (TSH, thyroid-stimulating hormone), which regulates thyroid gland function and the synthesis and release of thyroid hormones, including thyroxine (T_4) and triiodothyronine (T_3); (2) luteinizing hormone (LH, interstitial cell stimulating hormone or ICSH), which stimulates ovulation, promotes formation of the corpus luteum in the ovary, and is the primary regulator of Leydig cell function in men; and (3) follicle-stimulating hormone (FSH), which stimulates follicular growth and maturation in the ovary and is essential for spermatogenesis.

Because biological activity usually has been found in only a portion of these complex molecules, the potential for synthesizing smaller active compounds than those produced by the anterior pituitary gland is being explored. The amino acid sequence of all anterior pituitary hormones is known, and several have been partly or completely synthesized.

Pituitary hormones can be grouped according to overlapping similarities in chemical structure and biologic function. ACTH and LPH and its derivatives form one group; the larger polypeptides, GH and PRL, form another; and the glycoprotein hormones, LH, FSH, and TSH, form the third group. The glycoprotein hor-

723

mones have alpha (α) and beta (β) subunits, each with carbohydrate and sialic acid moieties. The specificities of these hormones are the result of the unique structure of the β subunits and carbohydrate groups; their α subunits are similar and possibly identical.

Staining characteristics and morphologic characteristics revealed by electron microscopy have shown that histologically distinct cells produce the various anterior pituitary hormones. The two gonadotropins may be secreted by a single type, as are ACTH and LPH; other cells secrete only one hormone.

The synthesis and release of anterior pituitary hormones are largely regulated by factors or hormones synthesized in the hypothalamus and transported to the anterior pituitary via the hypothalamic-hypophyseal portal system. Several of these hypothalamic hormones, which affect the release and/or synthesis of individual hormones by the anterior pituitary, have been identified. Each is named for what was initially postulated to be its biological function, although additional actions may coexist. The tripeptide, thyrotropin-releasing hormone (TRH, protirelin), was named for its role in inducing synthesis and release of thyrotropin, but it is now also known to be a potent stimulator of prolactin synthesis and secretion. Similarly, the decapeptide, gonadotropin-releasing hormone (GnRH, LHRH, gonadorelin), stimulates the synthesis and release of LH and FSH. Prolactin secretion is controlled primarily by prolactin-inhibiting factor (PIF), but a stimulating factor probably also plays a role. Corticotropin-releasing factor (CRF) stimulates ACTH synthesis and secretion. Growth hormone secretion is regulated by a releasing factor (GHRF) and an inhibiting factor (GH-RIH, somatostatin). Some of these factors (TRH, GnRH, somatostatin) have been isolated, purified, and characterized as small polypeptides; they have been synthesized and analogues that mimic their biological activity are under investigation.

Control of the hypothalamic releasing factors and pituitary secretion is complex.

In most instances, there is a negative feedback control mechanism. For instance, hypersecretion or exogenous administration of cortisol decreases CRF release with subsequent reduction of ACTH secretion. In other segments of the hypothalamic-hypophyseal system, a positive feedback mechanism is involved, that is, tropic hormone levels increase with elevations of the target organ hormone. The best example of positive feedback is the elevation of plasma LH levels (midcycle "surge") induced by increasing amounts of plasma estrogen during the late follicular phase of the ovarian cycle. Also, pituitary response to releasing hormones may be modulated by hormones produced by the target organ (eg, thyroid, ovary, testis).

The concepts of negative and positive feedback have limited applicability in explaining some phenomena of hypothalamic-hypophyseal actions, however. The importance of the central nervous system in integrating environmental influences that alter anterior pituitary hormone levels (eg, the diurnal variation in corticotropin levels) has been well documented. Finally, some alterations in pituitary function result from stimuli originating within the central nervous system; the nocturnal elevation of LH secretion during puberty is an example.

GROWTH HORMONE

Several hormones are particularly important in assuring normal growth and development: growth hormone, thyroid hormones, insulin, androgen in boys, and estrogen in girls. Deficient secretion of growth hormone (GH, somatotropin) in childhood may be idiopathic or secondary to systemic disease, traumatic injury, or tumor growth and may involve only GH or other tropic hormones as well. If untreated, hypopituitary dwarfism may result. True GH deficiency as a cause of growth failure is rare and can be treated only by administration of human GH; hormone from animal sources is relatively ineffective. Human GH is purified from pituitaries obtained at necropsy, and one year of therapy requires GH from approximately 100 pituitaries. Thus, the hormone is in very short supply and can be obtained only under special circumstances (see the evaluation on Somatropin). Candidates for treatment must have documented abnormally slow growth rate and GH deficiency as demonstrated by failure of standard stimuli to provoke release of GH.

Human GH is a single-chain polypeptide consisting of 191 amino acid residues with a molecular weight of 22,000. A semisynthetic GH preparation that possesses full biologic potency has been produced in the laboratory. It consists of a noncovalent combination of a natural amino terminal fragment and a synthetic carboxy terminal fragment (Li, 1978). Further research, especially that using recombinant DNA techniques, may eventually result in a fully synthetic active product and a more abundant supply of GH for therapeutic use.

GH has many effects on body systems, including both anti-insulin (eg, increased plasma glucose level) and insulin-like actions (eg, inhibition of fatty acid release, stimulation of amino acid uptake). Some, if not all, of its actions are mediated by a group of intermediate growth factors (somatomedins) elaborated by the liver and, probably, by the kidney and muscles. In certain growth-retarded patients, the ability to produce somatomedin is diminished; these individuals do not respond to GH therapy and, in fact, have high endogenous blood levels of GH.

GH hypersecretion in childhood produces gigantism and, in adulthood, acromegaly. Dopamine stimulates the secretion of GH acutely by a central mechanism in individuals with normal secretory rates, but inhibits secretion at the level of the pituitary in the presence of acromegaly. The dopaminergic agent, bromocriptine [Parlodel], is therefore sometimes effective in the treatment of acromegaly (see the evaluation in the section on Prolactin).

Somatostatin (GH-RIH), a tetradecapeptide, is the first hormone to be synthesized by recombinant DNA techniques. It is found endogenously not only in the hypothalamus, but also in other areas of the central nervous system and in the gastrointestinal system (stomach antrum, small intestine, D cells of pancreatic islets). This hormone inhibits the secretion of GH, TSH, gastrin, glucagon, insulin, and exocrine pancreatic secretions. Research is being directed toward developing long-acting analogues with separate activities that would be useful in the treatment of diabetes, acromegaly, and peptic ulcer.

SOMATROPIN
[Asellacrin]

H-Phe-Pro-Thr-Ile-Pro-Leu-Ser-Arg-Leu-Phe-Asp-Asn-Ala-Met-Leu-Arg-Ala-His-Arg-
Leu-His-Gln-Leu-Ala-Phe-Asp-Thr-Tyr-Gln-Glu-Phe-Glu-Glu-Ala-Tyr-Ile-Pro-Lys-Glu-
Gln-Lys-Tyr-Ser-Phe-Leu-Gln-Asn-Pro-Gln-Thr-Ser-Leu-Cys-Phe-Ser-Glu-Ser-Ile-Pro-
Thr-Pro-Ser-Asn-Arg-Glu-Glu-Thr-Gln-Gln-Lys-Ser-Asn-Leu-Gln-Leu-Leu-Arg-Ile-Ser-
Leu-Leu-Leu-Ile-Gln-Ser-Trp-Leu-Glu-Pro-Val-Gln-Phe-Leu-Arg-Ser-Val-Phe-Ala-Asn-
Ser-Leu-Val-Tyr-Gly-Ala-Ser-Asn-Ser-Asp-Val-Tyr-Asp-Leu-Leu-Lys-Asp-Leu-Glu-Glu-
Gly-Ile-Gln-Thr-Leu-Met-Gly-Arg-Leu-Glu-Asp-Gly-Ser-Pro-Arg-Thr-Gly-Gln-Ile-Phe-
Lys-Gln-Thr-Tyr-Ser-Lys-Phe-Asp-Thr-Asn-Ser-His-Asn-Asp-Asp-Ala-Leu-Leu-Lys-Asn-
Tyr-Gly-Leu-Leu-Tyr-Cys-Phe-Arg-Lys-Asp-Met-Asp-Lys-Val-Glu-Thr-Phe-Leu-Arg-Ile-
Val-Gln-Cys-Arg-Ser-Val-Glu-Gly-Ser-Cys-Gly-Phe-OH

This preparation of growth hormone is extracted from human pituitary glands that are obtained from cadavers, sterilized, and lyophilized. Its potency is determined by bioassay in hypophysectomized rats. The only indication for somatropin (as distinguished from somatotropin, which is endogenous growth hormone) is in growth failure due to deficiency of growth hormone. This agent is not effective in patients with closed epiphyses or in those who are unable to produce somatomedin after stimulation with GH. It also should not be given when there is an enlarging intracranial lesion, unless this has been treated previously.

Somatropin is administered intramuscularly, with the site of injection being rotated. Subcutaneous injection may produce lipoatrophy and enhance formation of neutralizing antibodies. The half-life of somatropin is only 20 minutes, but intracellular effects in target tissues are long-lasting, allowing administration only several times per week. This hormone may be administered to boys in conjunction with androgen to obtain the greatest growth rate in selected cases when a concomitant androgen deficiency exists. Although neutralizing antibodies to GH develop in 30% to 40% of individuals receiving somatropin, GH treatment is effective in more than 95% of the patients. However, the accelerated growth rate gradually decreases and this may be associated with increasing titers of GH antibodies. Therapy usually is continued until epiphyseal closure, until a satisfactory (usually five feet) adult height is attained, or until there is no further response to treatment.

Somatropin is diabetogenic and may cause hyperglycemia and ketosis. Particular caution should be exercised when it is administered to diabetic patients or those with a family history of diabetes. Testing for glycosuria should be performed routinely in all patients. Since growth retardation is a side effect of glucocorticoid therapy and administration of these agents may inhibit the response to somatropin, daily doses larger than 10 to 15 mg/M^2 of cortisol or the equivalent are not recommended for concomitant administration with somatropin.

Because the supply of GH from autopsy pituitaries is extremely small, documentation of the patient's condition must be furnished before somatropin may be obtained. This includes the patient's chronological age, size, growth rate, bone age, and etiology of deficiency. Evidence of GH deficiency should be demonstrated by results from at least two GH stimulation tests (hypoglycemia, oral levodopa, glucagon, intravenous arginine). Somatropin may be obtained after these criteria are satisfied. The cost for a year's supply is approximately $2,400. For information, contact Hoechst-Roussel Pharmaceuticals, Inc., Medical Research Department, Route 202-206 North, Somerville, NJ, 08876, (201) 685-2000. For patients involved in research projects conducted by qualified investigators, a similar preparation of human GH is available without cost from the National Pituitary Agency, 210 W. Fayette St., Baltimore, MD, 21201. Similar

criteria are employed for patient selection.

ROUTE, USUAL DOSAGE, AND PREPARATIONS. *Intramuscular:* Initially, 2 IU three times weekly with a minimum of 48 hours between injections; if growth does not exceed 2.5 cm in a six-month period, dosage may be doubled for six months. If this is ineffective, treatment should be discontinued and the patient re-evaluated.

Asellacrin (Hoechst-Roussel). Powder (sterile, lyophilized) 10 IU with mannitol 40 mg.

THYROID

Normal thyroid function requires an intact hypothalamic-hypophyseal axis and adequate iodine intake. Sensitive and precise methods for measuring circulating thyroid hormone levels (free and bound T$_4$ and T$_3$) are available to augment clinical judgment. The anterior pituitary gland secretes thyrotropin (TSH), a double-chain glycoprotein hormone with about 96 amino acid residues in the α chain and 113 amino acid residues in the β chain; its molecular weight is 28,000. The radioimmunoassay of TSH is used to distinguish between primary (thyroid failure) and secondary (pituitary failure) hypothyroidism. Increased serum TSH levels occur after thyroidectomy or destruction of the thyroid by autoimmune thyroiditis and precede the clinical manifestations of hypothyroidism. On the other hand, when sufficient thyroid hormone is administered to correct hypothyroidism or when high levels of endogenous hormone are present in thyrotoxic states, serum TSH levels are low. (See also Chapter 48, Agents Used to Treat Thyroid Disease.)

Some hypothyroid patients with low serum T$_4$ and normal TSH levels may not have pituitary dysfunction. Some of these patients respond to stimulation with thyrotropin-releasing hormone (TRH) by secreting TSH. This disorder has been referred to as tertiary hypothyroidism, and the defect is thought to be in the hypothalamus, in contrast to secondary hypothyroidism, in which the defect is in the pituitary.

PROTIRELIN (TRH)
[Relefact TRH, Thypinone]

These synthetic preparations of the tripeptide (pyroglutamyl-histidyl-proline amide), thyrotropin-releasing hormone (TRH), are the first hypothalamic-releasing hormones commercially available in the United States. In animals, natural TRH is present in highest concentrations in the hypothalamus, but the majority of the total content is in various other areas of the central nervous system, including the spinal cord and pineal. TRH stimulates both synthesis and release of TSH from the pituitary. Protirelin is used to test pituitary and, indirectly, thyroid function. Thyrotropin (TSH) levels are measured before and 30 minutes after administration of protirelin. Protirelin stimulation may be used adjunctively to distinguish between secondary (pituitary) and tertiary (hypothalamic) thyroid deficiency. If deficiency is due to pituitary failure, approximately 60% of patients do not exhibit stimulation of TSH secretion; if the deficiency is caused by hypothalamic malfunction, a delayed but quantitatively normal or increased elevation of TSH is usually obtained. In suspected hyperthyroidism with borderline serum thyroid hormone levels, a normal TSH response to protirelin stimulation excludes thyrotoxicosis. Protirelin also may be utilized as part of a general pituitary evaluation when central lesions are suspected. Although the TSH response may be used to distinguish primary (high TSH) and secondary (low TSH) hypothyroidism, this is readily accomplished by measurement of the basal serum TSH level. The normal response to protirelin may be slightly higher in women, particularly in the presence of high estrogen levels, and lower in older men.

TRH also is a potent stimulator of prolactin secretion by the anterior pituitary gland and is sometimes included in the diagnostic profile of hyperprolactinemic disorders, although its usefulness is limited. Pituitary tumors that secrete prolactin usually produce high concentrations of serum prolactin with little or no further increase after protirelin stimulation. However a normal increase in the serum prolactin level following use of protirelin in individuals with elevated prolactin levels has been found in a few patients with pituitary adenoma. Demonstration of prolactin response to protirelin confirms a diagnosis of isolated TSH deficiency. A marked elevation of the growth hormone level following use of protirelin is not usually observed in normal individuals, but occurs commonly in patients with acromegaly; this finding may be of diagnostic value in some cases. Protirelin also is used experimentally in the treatment of depression, but opinion is divided on its usefulness for this indication.

ROUTE, USUAL DOSAGE, AND PREPARATIONS.
Intravenous: TSH levels are measured in serum samples taken immediately before and 30 minutes after a bolus injection of 500 mcg. Protirelin is administered over a period of 10 to 15 seconds. (Since thyroid hormones suppress TSH response, thyroid replacement therapy must be stopped for four to five weeks before administration.) The same procedure is followed for measurement of serum prolactin levels. Serum samples are obtained at the time of the expected prolactin peak (15 to 20 minutes after protirelin injection). Prolactin response also is suppressed (but to a lesser extent) in the presence of high levels of thyroid hormone.
  Relefact TRH (Hoechst-Roussel), *Thypinone* (Abbott Diagnostic). Solution 0.5 mg/ml in 1 ml containers.

THYROTROPIN (TSH)
[Thytropar]

Thyrotropin is isolated from bovine anterior pituitary glands. It stimulates iodine uptake and the formation and secretion of thyroid hormones. TSH is used to increase the uptake of therapeutic doses of radioactive iodine in patients with toxic adenomatous goiters or certain types of thyroid carcinoma and to demonstrate the presence of normal thyroid tissue on a scan in patients with toxic nodule. TSH is administered infrequently to assess thyroid function in patients receiving thyroid replacement therapy. Thyroid replacement therapy may be continued prior to and during the testing procedure. TSH also may be used to differentiate primary hypothyroidism from secondary hypothyroidism but, because of the wide availability of radioimmunoassay of serum TSH, it is not commonly used for this purpose today. Following administration of TSH to a hypothyroid patient, serum thyroxine is elevated and thyroidal radioiodine uptake is increased when the defect is in the pituitary; however, patients with mild primary (thyroidal) hypothyroidism also may respond similarly.

This agent can induce symptoms of hyperthyroidism, especially when repeated injections are given; thus, it should be used with caution in patients with cardiovascular disease who might not tolerate the added stress (eg, those with congestive heart failure or coronary artery disease with or without angina). TSH must be administered with caution to patients with primary (adrenal) or secondary (pituitary) adrenocortical hypofunction because of the danger of precipitating adrenocortical insufficiency. These patients should receive replacement corticosteroid therapy before and during administration of TSH.

Minor untoward effects include nausea, vomiting, headache, and urticaria. More serious reactions include hypotension, arrhythmias, and thyroid swelling. A few anaphylactic reactions also have been reported. Repeated injection can give rise to antibody formation that causes falsely elevated values in TSH assays and resistance to subsequent administration of TSH.

ROUTES, USUAL DOSAGE, AND PREPARATIONS. *Intramuscular, Subcutaneous*: To assess thyroid functional capacity, 10 IU is given intramuscularly on three successive days, and a radioactive iodine uptake test is performed on the last day of treatment. A 24-hour uptake of over 10% demonstrates functional thyroid tissue. To increase the uptake of radioactive iodine, 10 IU is given daily for one to three days prior to a therapeutic dose of iodine. There is no indication for use of TSH in the treatment of either secondary or tertiary hypothyroidism.

Thytropar (Armour). Powder (lyophilized) 10 IU of thyrotropic activity with diluent.

ADRENAL CORTEX

Secretion of adrenal corticosteroids, particularly glucocorticoids, depends upon stimulation by corticotropin (adrenocorticotropin, ACTH). Secretion of ACTH, in turn, is modulated by a hypothalamic corticotropin-releasing factor (CRF), as well as by glucocorticoid negative feedback. ACTH is secreted in a circadian pattern: In normal individuals maintaining a day-night schedule, maximal ACTH and cortisol concentrations are present prior to and upon awakening and levels are lowest in the late evening. This periodicity appears to be controlled by the central nervous system. Since the periodicity of plasma corticosteroid concentrations is secondary to that of plasma corticotropin levels, knowledge of the time of day when the blood sample was obtained is important in interpreting measurements of plasma corticotropin or cortisol.

Excessive secretion of ACTH in the presence of intact adrenal cortices causes Cushing's syndrome. The normal set point of the negative feedback mechanisms controlling the pituitary secretion of ACTH is perturbed in such instances. Hypersecretion of ACTH also can occur in the presence of normal functioning of the negative feedback system. This situation occurs in uncontrolled Addison's disease due to lack of glucocorticoid feedback inhibition of ACTH. The skin pigmentation characteristic of Addison's disease may be caused by the intrinsic skin-darkening properties of ACTH.

In hypopituitarism, deficient ACTH secretion markedly reduces the production of glucocorticoids and adrenal androgens, but synthesis of mineralocorticoid is not seriously affected because of continuing stimulation from the renin-angiotensin system. These patients may not experience symptoms under normal circumstances, but acute adrenal insufficiency may develop in the presence of severe stress. Some patients with deficient secretion of ACTH may have a defect in the hypothalamus. Although there is sufficient evidence that there is a hypothalamic corticotropin-releasing factor (CRF), its structure is as yet unknown. CRF stimulation, a key step in diagnosing tertiary hypoadrenocorticism, is therefore not yet possible.

Corticotropin is a straight-chain polypeptide consisting of 39 amino acids. The sequence of the first 24 amino acids is common to man, cattle, pigs, and sheep, but the arrangement of the remaining amino acids (positions 25 to 39) differs from one species to another. These heterologous segments are clinically important, since they may lead to production of antibodies and cause allergic reactions when corticotropin of animal origin is injected into humans. In addition, animal preparations are highly purified but may contain other pituitary proteins or peptides that may be antigenic. Corticotropin sometimes is used diagnostically and, in certain cases, therapeutically (see the evaluation).

Synthetic corticotropin analogues containing subunits of the 39 amino acid polypeptide have been prepared. Cosyntropin [Cortrosyn] contains the first 24 amino acids. The absence of the heterologous part of the molecule greatly decreases the risk of allergic reactions, since the synthetic polypeptide has little immunologic activity in vivo. Cosyntropin is used as a diagnostic agent (see the evaluation).

Various disease states have a characteristic pattern of hormone levels and response to ACTH. In primary adrenal failure, the plasma level of ACTH is elevated and that of cortisol depressed, whereas both are decreased in hypopituitarism. Administration of corticotropin is used to diagnose adrenal insufficiency (ACTH stimulation test). In hypopituitarism, adrenal response to corticotropin is retained, although repeated administration may be necessary to initiate steroidogenesis. In primary adrenal failure, steroid secretion is not stimulated by exogenous ACTH. Direct measurement of plasma ACTH can now be performed by radioimmunoassay. High levels of plasma ACTH indicate primary adrenal insufficiency and low levels indicate that the insufficiency is secondary to pituitary failure.

In adrenocortical hyperfunction (Cushing's syndrome) secondary to adrenocortical hyperplasia, an exaggerated corticosteroid response may be seen following administration of corticotropin. The response is normal or absent when the disease is secondary to a hypersecreting adrenal adenoma, and usually is absent when adrenal carcinoma is the underlying disorder.

CORTICOTROPIN (ACTH)
[Acthar, Cortrophin Gel, Cortrophin-Zinc]

Corticotropin is prepared from animal pituitaries and is bioassayed against a standard preparation. It stimulates the adrenal cortex to secrete cortisol, desoxycorticosterone, androgens, and other steroids. Corticotropin can be used to determine the competency of the hypophyseal-adrenal axis, although the synthetic analogue, cosyntropin, is preferred since the risk of allergic reactions is reduced and it acts more rapidly.

This hormone also may be used to treat glucocorticoid-responsive diseases in patients with functional adrenal glands; however, treatment with corticotropin is less predictable and less convenient and appears to possess no advantages over glucocorticoids in most patients. Some investigators prefer corticotropin to glucocorticoids in patients with ulcerative colitis and multiple sclerosis, but objective evidence of its superiority is lacking. It has been reported that use of corticotropin in children with chronic diseases that respond to long-term glucocorticoid therapy does not inhibit growth to the same extent as glucocorticoids, but these results require confirmation.

Although corticotropin causes adrenal hyperplasia rather than atrophy, prolonged therapy impairs the ability of the hypophyseal-adrenal axis to respond to stress. Its use during the period of withdrawal of glucocorticoids does not hasten the establishment of adrenal responsiveness.

The activity of corticotropin is destroyed by proteolytic enzymes in the gastrointestinal tract; therefore, the drug is administered intramuscularly and, occasionally, subcutaneously or intravenously.

In addition to the adverse effects caused by increased secretion of glucocorticoids, corticotropin also can produce electrolyte disturbances and undesirable androgenic effects in women (acne, hirsutism, amenorrhea). Acute allergic reactions have followed its administration in sensitized patients.

ROUTES, USUAL DOSAGE, AND PREPARATIONS. Since adrenal glands vary in their response to corticotropin, the dosage must be individualized to obtain a satisfactory therapeutic effect with minimal dosage and alteration in metabolism. The gel form delays uptake from tissues, thereby prolonging the hormone's action.

Intramuscular: For therapeutic use, 40 units of aqueous solution daily in four divided doses (10 units every six hours) or 40 units of gel (repository) or aqueous suspension with zinc hydroxide (repository) every 12 to 24 hours. For diagnostic use, 40 to 80 units daily for one to three successive days.

Subcutaneous: For diagnostic use, 40 units of aqueous solution daily in four divided doses (10 units every six hours) or 40 units of gel every 24 to 72 hours.

Intravenous: For diagnostic use, 25 to 40 units of aqueous solution in 500 ml of 5% dextrose or physiologic sodium chloride injection given as a continuous infusion for eight hours once daily or as a continuous 48-hour infusion (40 units every 12 hours).

Drug available generically and as ACTH: Gel (repository) 40 and 80 units/ml in 5 ml containers; powder 25, 40, and 80 units/ml in 5 ml containers (ACTH only).

Acthar (Armour). Powder (lyophilized) 25 and 40 U.S.P. units; gel (repository) 40 and 80 U.S.P. units/ml in 1 and 5 ml containers (H.P. Acthar Gel).

Cortrophin Gel (Organon). (intramuscular, subcutaneous) Gel (repository) 40 U.S.P. units/ml in 1 and 5 ml containers and 80 U.S.P. units/ml in 5 ml containers.

Cortrophin-Zinc (Organon). Suspension (intramuscular) 40 U.S.P. units with 2 mg of zinc/ml in 5 ml containers.

COSYNTROPIN
[Cortrosyn]

Cosyntropin, a synthetic corticotropin analogue, contains amino acids 1-24 of the corticotropin molecule. The absence of most of the antigenic part of the molecule reduces the risk of sensitivity reactions, since synthetic polypeptides containing amino acids 1-24 have little immunologic activity. Cosyntropin is used diagnostically in patients suspected of having adrenal insufficiency and is preferred to corticotropin for this purpose. This preparation is not used therapeutically.

Hypersensitivity reactions are uncommon and the previous occurrence of one is the only contraindication to use of cosyntropin. Caution should be exercised when giving cosyntropin to patients who are hypersensitive to natural corticotropin, but this is not a contraindication to its use.

ROUTES, USUAL DOSAGE, AND PREPARATIONS. *Intramuscular, Intravenous*: For diagnostic use, *adults*, 0.25 mg (equivalent to 25 units of corticotropin); *children 2 years of age or less*, 0.125 mg. Plasma cortisol levels are determined before and 30 or 60 minutes after intramuscular injection; in most patients, a normal response is an approximate doubling of the basal cortisol level. A cortisol level that exceeds 18 mcg/ml 30 minutes after injection of cosyntropin and that shows an increment of at least 10 mcg/dl above the basal level is considered normal. Lack of a normal response indicates adrenal insufficiency of either adrenal or pituitary origin. To distinguish between the two when assay of plasma ACTH is unavailable, cosyntropin 0.25 to 0.75 mg is infused intravenously over a period of four to eight hours. This dosage should be adequate to elicit a response in all patients with functional adrenal cortical tissue. The response can be determined by measuring plasma cortisol levels or urinary excretion of steroids (17-ketosteroids or 17-hydroxysteroids). The diagnosis of hypopituitarism in responsive patients can be confirmed by other tests of pituitary function. Little or no response is obtained in patients with Addison's disease.

Cortrosyn (Organon). Powder (lyophilized) 0.25 mg with mannitol 10 mg in 1 ml containers with 1 ml of diluent.

GONADOTROPINS

Both the ovaries and testes have dual functions: Each produces gametes as well as steroid hormones essential for establishing and maintaining secondary sexual characteristics. The glycoproteins, follicle-stimulating hormone (FSH) and luteinizing hormone (LH), were first named for their most prominent action upon the ovary. Thus, FSH is essential for follicular maturation and LH for the formation and maintenance of the corpus luteum. In logical consequence, FSH enhances estrogen secretion and LH, estrogen and progesterone secretion. In addition, a surge of LH at midcycle serves as the trigger for ovulation. The same glycoprotein molecules also have effects on the testis. LH, once known as interstitial cell stimulating hormone (ICSH) in the male, stimulates the production of testosterone by the Leydig cells and elevates serum estrogen levels in men. Both LH and FSH are essential for spermatogenesis, although FSH appears to be more critical for the final stages.

FSH and LH are secreted by the anterior pituitary gonadotrophs. Both hormones are double-chain glycoproteins. Their α chains have about 95 amino acid residues, while their β chains contain 115. Molecular weights are 29,000 (FSH) and 28,000 (LH). Preparations of human gonadotropins purified from pituitaries obtained at au-topsy are available in limited amounts for investigational use.

Negative feedback is important in regulating gonadotropin production. The high serum LH and FSH levels seen after castration and in gonadal dysgenesis result from lack of negative feedback from gonadal steroids. However, control of gonadotropin secretion is much more complex. In women, the manner in which administration of estradiol affects serum gonadotropin levels depends upon the stage of the ovarian cycle in which it is given. In men, estradiol is probably a more potent suppressant of gonadotropin than testosterone, although it is not as important as testosterone physiologically because levels are low in males. Finally, on the basis of animal experiments and the frequent finding of elevated FSH levels but normal steroid hormone levels in men with azoospermia, many investigators postulate that a feedback substance (often called "inhibin") selectively inhibits FSH secretion and is synthesized in the germinal epithelium of the testis (a similar "follicular inhibin" is probably produced in the ovary).

Some feedback modulation of gonadotropin regulation is to be anticipated, for, at present, there is only one hypothalamic factor known to be of importance in regulating pituitary LH and FSH release. The decapeptide, gonadotropin-releasing hormone (GnRH), releases both LH and FSH; the differential patterns of release of these hormones must be the result of interactions at the level of the anterior pituitary gland unless additional unidentified hypothalamic factors are involved. Synthetic GnRH is available for investigational use only.

Drugs available to treat dysfunction of the hypothalamic-pituitary-gonadal axis include human chorionic gonadotropin (HCG), human menopausal gonadotropin (menotropins, HMG), and clomiphene. These drugs are used almost exclusively to treat infertility in both women and men (see Chapter 45, Agents Used to Treat Infertility). A drug that possesses anti-gonadrotropic activity, danazol, is also available.

DANAZOL
[Danocrine]

Danazol is a synthetic derivative of 17 α-ethinyl testosterone (ethisterone), which has mild androgenic activity. This agent does not exhibit estrogenic or progestational properties, and its clinical usefulness is probably the result of its antigonadotropic activity, manifested as suppression of the midcycle surge of LH and FSH.

Danazol is used to treat endometriosis; it causes atrophy of endometrial tissue in the uterus and ectopic sites and amenorrhea usually results. Ovulation and menstruation are re-established promptly on cessation of therapy. Contraception should be employed after therapy if pregnancy is not desired, since treatment of endometriosis with danazol may restore fertility (see also the evaluation of this drug in Chapter 45, Agents Used to Treat Infertility).

Danazol has been used experimentally as a component of a male oral contraceptive and in the treatment of gynecomastia, menorrhagia, and precocious puberty. It appears to have particular promise as a therapeutic agent in the treatment of benign breast disease, particularly in patients who cannot tolerate other hormonal therapy (Asch and Greenblatt, 1977; Lauersen and Wilson, 1976), and in hereditary angioedema (Gelfand et al, 1976).

Most adverse reactions caused by danazol are related to its weak androgenic and anabolic activity. They include weight gain, edema, acne, oily skin, decreased breast size, hirsutism, and hypoestrogenic symptoms (flushing, sweating, vaginitis) in women. The safety of this drug during pregnancy has not been determined. Danazol is not indicated for patients with markedly impaired hepatic, renal, or cardiac function or in women with underlying abnormal genital bleeding.

ROUTE, USUAL DOSAGE, AND PREPARATIONS. *Oral*: For endometriosis, 800 mg daily in two divided doses, continued for three to nine months as necessary. Treatment can be reinstituted if symptoms recur upon cessation of therapy. For fibrocystic breast disease, 100 to 400 mg daily. For angioedema, 600 mg daily.

Danocrine (Winthrop). Capsules 200 mg.

HUMAN CHORIONIC GONADOTROPIN (HCG)
[Antuitrin-S, A.P.L., Follutein, Pregnyl]

Human chorionic gonadotropin (HCG) is a placental hormone extracted from the urine of pregnant women. Its biological activity is the same as that of LH and it is used clinically as a substitute for human LH, which is available only in small quantities for investigational studies.

HCG is indicated for the medical treatment of cryptorchidism. Since little spontaneous testicular descent occurs after 12 months of age, and progressive and irreversible tubular damage may begin by age 5 in the absence of treatment, drug therapy should preferably be instituted by 2 years of age. Some testicular function may be spared even if treatment is started later in prepuberal boys, but delay until puberty results in inability to produce sperm. Testicular descent occurs in 25% to 30% of those treated for unilateral cryptorchidism; success rates are slightly higher in those with bilateral cryptorchidism. Even if HCG therapy does not induce complete descent, scrotal development is stimulated and surgical correction (orchidopexy) is facilitated. If hormonal therapy is unsuccessful, surgical correction (or removal if this fails) should be performed. Uncorrected cryptorchid testes have a high potential for malignancy, and androgen production may begin to be compromised after age 30 due to fibrosis of testicular tissue.

HCG is sometimes used diagnostically in males with delayed puberty when there is doubt about the steroidogenic ability of the testes to respond to gonadotropin stimulation (see also Chapter 42, Androgens and Anabolic Steroids). It also is used occasionally in hirsute females in an attempt to differentiate the source (ie, ovary or adrenal) of androgen secretion. However, the test is unreliable in females because a lack of androgen secretion after administration of HCG does not exclude an ovarian source and occasionally adrenal androgen production by a tumor may be stimulated by HCG.

Daily injections of HCG have been used in conjunction with a low-calorie diet in weight reduction programs. Results of a controlled double-blind study comparing subjects on such a regimen to those on the same diet but receiving saline instead of HCG demonstrated no difference between the two groups in weight loss, body measurements, hunger appeasement, and various metabolic measurements (Shetty and Kalkhoff, 1977). There is no evidence that HCG causes weight reduction beyond that due to caloric restriction; therefore, it is not indicated in the treatment of obesity.

For use in the treatment of female or male infertility, see the evaluation in Chapter 45, Agents Used to Treat Infertility.

ROUTE, USUAL DOSAGE, AND PREPARATIONS. *Intramuscular*: In cryptorchidism, for minimal sexual development, 5,000 units every other day for four injections; for greater degree of sexual development, 500 units three times per week for three weeks, or, for *boys 10 years or older*, 1,000 units three times per week for three weeks. In males, for diagnosis of responsiveness to gonadotropin stimulation, 2,000 units daily for three days. Blood levels of testosterone are measured at baseline and on the fourth day (day following last injection). An approximate doubling of testosterone levels is normal.

Drug available generically: Powder 1,000, 5,000, 10,000, and 20,000 units with 10 ml of diluent.

Antuitrin-S (Parke, Davis). Powder 5,000 IU with 10 ml of diluent.

A.P.L. (Ayerst). Powder 5,000, 10,000, and 20,000 U.S.P. units with 10 ml of diluent.
Follutein (Squibb), *Pregnyl* (Organon). Powder 10,000 IU with 10 ml of diluent.

PROLACTIN

Although prolactin was known to exist in animals, it was not identified as a separate hormone in humans until 1970. Before then it was thought that lactogenic activity in humans was solely the result of growth hormone (GH) activity. Human prolactin is a linear polypeptide with 198 amino acid residues and a molecular weight of 23,000. Human growth hormone also demonstrates lactogenic activity, and 16% of its amino acid sequence is identical to that of human prolactin.

The only well-defined function of prolactin in humans is to stimulate milk production by the postpartum breast. The function of prolactin in human males is not understood, but it may serve some permissive function in normal reproductive capacity. In lower animals (particularly birds), prolactin is responsible for stimulating parental behavior in males and females.

Although the function of prolactin appears to be quite restricted in humans, secretion is elevated in a wide variety of physiologic circumstances. Increased secretion occurs in both sexes during sleep, exercise, and in response to stress and in women throughout pregnancy, in the postpartum period (even in the absence of suckling), and in association with orgasm. The most effective and specific stimulus to prolactin secretion is suckling. In nonphysiologic states, prolactin secretion also can be elevated in the presence of a prolactin-secreting pituitary adenoma, by drugs (eg, neuroleptics, H_2 antihistamines, antihypertensive agents), and occasionally in those with hypothyroidism, renal or hepatic failure, or anorexia nervosa.

As with other anterior pituitary hormones, secretion of prolactin is subject to control by hypothalamic substances. However, unlike these other hormones, the predominant hypothalamic influence is inhibitory (prolactin-inhibiting factor, PIF). Dopamine inhibits prolactin secretion and may itself be a PIF. Prolactin-releasing factor (PRF) also is involved in regulating production and secretion of this hormone. There is some indirect evidence to suggest that serotonin exhibits prolactin-releasing activity. Thyrotropin-releasing hormone (TRH), which is used to stimulate thyrotropin (TSH) and prolactin secretion diagnostically, is probably not important in the normal regulation of prolactin production. In the absence of normal hypothalamic control (eg, stalk section), hypersecretion of prolactin occurs but secretion of other anterior pituitary hormones is decreased. Large amounts of prolactin are often secreted in patients with tumors of the anterior pituitary gland.

Other than rare cases of isolated prolactin deficiency that prevent normal postpartum lactation, no clinical symptoms have been described from prolactin deficiency. However, hypersecretion is associated with a variety of symptoms of reproductive malfunction that can affect both men and women. Hyperprolactinemic reproductive dysfunction may be manifested in women by amenorrhea, galactorrhea, and infertility. Any or all of these symptoms may occur concomitantly. It is interesting to note that, even during the physiologic hyperprolactinemia associated with lactation, reproductive capacity is partially or wholly compromised. Elevated prolactin levels in men can cause decreased libido and potency and, rarely, galactorrhea.

Options for treatment of hyperprolactinemia are few and are related to the etiology of the condition. Pituitary tumors are usually treated by surgery or irradiation. Bromocriptine [Parlodel], a dopaminergic agent that inhibits prolactin secretion, is sometimes used in conjunction with or in lieu of ablative therapy. This drug may reduce prolactin secretion of any etiology. There is some evidence that tumor growth also may be retarded. Functional hyperprolactinemia unrelated to a known cause may be an early manifestation of a pathologic continuum that may eventually present as a pituitary adenoma.

BROMOCRIPTINE MESYLATE
[Parlodel]

Bromocriptine is a synthetic ergot alkaloid with dopaminergic properties. It is employed in a variety of conditions in which dopaminergic activity is useful (eg, hyperprolactinemic reproductive dysfunctional disorders, suppression of postpartum lactation, acromegaly, Parkinson's disease) (see Chapter 16, Drugs Used to Treat Extrapyramidal Movement Disorders). Bromocriptine acts directly on dopaminergic receptors of pituitary cells. It also may exert a central effect, but this is of lesser importance. There have been several reports (some confirmed radiologically) of regression of prolactin-secreting adenomas in both men and women after treatment with bromocriptine. Bromocriptine lowers elevated prolactin levels from physiologic, pathologic, or iatrogenic (eg, drug ingestion) causes. However, on cessation of therapy, prolactin levels again increase unless the underlying disorder is corrected. When bromocriptine is used to suppress postpartum lactation, discontinuation of medication does not usually result in increased prolactin secretion and continued lactation, however. In this case, once secretion is inhibited and in the absence of the suckling stimulus, the hormonal conditions necessary to reinitiate lactation are no longer present. Bromocriptine also inhibits secretion of prolactin in normal individuals, but the reduction is less pronounced than when the secretory rate is abnormally high.

Severe hyperprolactinemia in women is usually accompanied by oligomenorrhea or amenorrhea. The mechanisms have not been completely elucidated, but it appears that both central and peripheral effects are involved. Elevated prolactin levels may affect hypothalamic mechanisms controlling normal gonadotropin secretion and probably also interfere directly with steroid production by the ovary. Bromocriptine is used to restore fertility in women (see Chapter 45) or to alleviate galactorrhea. If pregnancy is not desired in a sexually active woman being treated with bromocriptine, nonhormonal contraception should be employed throughout the treatment period. If hyperprolactinemia is caused by pituitary adenoma, there is a danger of tumor expansion during pregnancy which may endanger vision or impair the pituitary vascular supply. Bromocriptine usually decreases prolactin secretion even in the presence of a tumor, but this drug is not a substitute for surgery or irradiation if these are indicated.

After six weeks of treatment with bromocriptine, about 75% of women with amenorrhea and galactorrhea experience a resumption of menses or a significant reduction of galactorrhea. Complete cessation of galactorrhea occurs in 60% of women after about three months of treatment, and normalization of menstrual cycles and complete cessation of galactorrhea occur in about 50% of the women treated. Some success has been reported when bromocriptine was given to correct amenorrhea in normoprolactinemic women, but this use requires further study before it can be recommended routinely.

Bromocriptine appears to be a promising drug for use when suppression of postpartum lactation is indicated. Lactation will eventually cease without drug intervention in the absence of suckling, but breast engorgement and pain (which can be relieved by analgesics) are common. Estrogens, alone or with androgen therapy, have been used commonly to prevent lactation and the discomforts associated with its suppression. However, there is an increased risk of thromboembolic phenomena with estrogen, and rebound lactation often occurs after withdrawal of medication. In controlled studies, bromocriptine has been more effective than all other hormonal therapy in preventing breast engorgement, discomfort, and lactation. This drug is also more effective in suppressing established lactation; rebound lactation occurs only infrequently. Further experience is necessary to determine the most effective regimen that will avoid the problem of rebound lactation entirely.

The etiology of premenstrul tension (abdominal distention, mastodynia, edema, headache, depression) is probably multifactorial and is related to alterations in steroid and other hormonal balance. Prolactin has been suggested as a cause of these symptoms, for women with premenstrual tension have higher serum concentrations of prolactin (but within the normal range) throughout the cycle and a greater elevation occurs premenstrually than in women who do not exhibit this syndrome (Halbreich et al, 1976). Bromocriptine has been used experimentally to reduce levels of prolactin in these patients. Although statistically significant relief of symptoms has been reported in some, results have been less favorable in others. However, a causal relationship between prolactin levels and premenstrual tension has not been definitely demonstrated. If bromocriptine does prove to be effective, it is possible that the mechanism may involve a dopaminergic target unrelated to that which inhibits prolactin secretion.

In men with hyperprolactinemia, impotence and decreased libido are common complaints. Several reports suggest that bromocriptine may alleviate these problems coincident with the drug-induced decrease in prolactin secretion; however, therapy has not been uniformly successful. Best results may require both reduction in serum prolactin and treatment of testosterone deficiency if this is not corrected within six months by bromocriptine therapy. There is no reason to expect bromocriptine to be effective in treating impotence due to causes other than hyperprolactinemia. More study is necessary to determine its usefulness in male reproductive dysfunction (see also Chapter 45).

Bromocriptine provides a medical alternative for the treatment of acromegaly, which in the past was treatable only by surgery or irradiation. The drug is used alone or with an ablative procedure, particularly irradiation. Bromocriptine is most effective in mild cases and should not be used as the sole treatment in patients with suprasellar extension of tumor. About 75% of patients show improvement with bromocriptine, but the drug is not curative. If the cause of acromegaly (ie, pituitary tumor) is not eliminated, cessation of drug treatment is followed by resumption of increased secretion of growth hormone (see the section on Growth Hormone).

The response to bromocriptine is prompt; blood levels of GH are decreased within hours and effectiveness of treatment may be assessed within weeks. However, GH levels are not generally reduced to normal. Some patients show clinical improvement without a fall in serum GH levels; the mechanism for this improvement is unknown. Indications of a favorable response may include improvement in results of the glucose tolerance test; reduction of insulin requirements in diabetics, sweating, excretion of hydroxyproline, and incidence of headaches; and improved libido in men. The latter may be due to concomitant inhibition of prolactin secretion (hyperprolactinemia is an occasional feature of acromegaly). Improvements in morphologic features may include softening of facial features, decreased skin and tongue thickness, and decreased hand and foot size. It is difficult to determine the extent of improvements due only to bromocriptine, since many patients are treated surgically or by irradiation before or during treatment with bromocriptine. The effect of bromocriptine on the growth of GH-producing tumors is not known, but regression of early visual defects and evidence of radiologic improvement following therapy have been observed. Although some patients have been treated for acromegaly for one to two years, more experience is necessary to determine the long-term effectiveness and safety of bromocriptine for this indication.

Adverse reactions occur commonly when bromocriptine therapy is initiated. Thereafter, their incidence and severity depend upon the dosage and rate of incremental increases. Common untoward effects include nausea, vomiting, dizziness, and orthostatic hypotension. In acromegalic patients (eg, patients taking larger doses), decreased alcohol tolerance, constipation, dryness of the mouth, and nocturnal leg cramps have been reported. Nausea may be minimized by taking the medication with food. No teratogenic effects have been reported in man, but cleft lip has occurred in offspring of rabbits treated with bromocriptine.

ROUTE, USUAL DOSAGE, AND PREPARATIONS. *Oral*: Initially, 2.5 mg is given in the evening for two or three days. This dose is increased by increments of 2.5 mg on alternate days until the maintenance level is reached. For hyperprolactinemic reproductive functional disorders, 2.5 mg two or three times daily is usually sufficient. For acromegaly, the most common dosages reported are 15 to 20 mg daily in three or four divided doses. Depending upon clinical response, the amount may be increased to 60 mg daily in four divided doses.

Parlodel (Sandoz). Tablets 2.5 mg.

BETA-LIPOTROPIN

Beta-lipotropin (β-LPH) is found in the intermediate (in β animals only, since humans do not have an intermediate lobe) and anterior lobes of the pituitary gland. Unlike other pituitary hormones and biologically active compounds, chemical isolation and identification (91 amino acid residues) preceded description of its function. The hormone was named after demonstration of its lipolytic activity, but this does not appear to be its primary function in the body. In fact, although much has been learned about biologically active peptides that are present within the molecule, β-LPH remains a "hormone in search of a function."

β-LPH contains within its structure the amino acid sequences for β-melanocyte stimulating hormone (β MSH, β-endorphin, and met-enkephalin (methionine enkephalin). Although β MSH is important in control of the synthesis and dispersement of pigment granules in animals, it probably does not exist as a separate hormone in man. Rather, it is generated as an artifactual fragment of β-LPH during pituitary extraction procedures. Melanocyte-stimulating hormone activity in man may be due to the pigmentary properties of ACTH. β-endorphin, in turn, contains within its structure the pentapeptide, met-enkephalin. Both of these peptides exhibit opiate-like activities (analgesia, catatonia, hypothermia) and cross tolerance to morphine, and their effects are blocked by the morphine antagonist, naloxone. The peptides are found within neurons in the central nervous system in areas involved with transmission of pain and expression of anxiety and emotion (limbic system). The neurons that contain β-endorphin and their distribution are distinct from those containing met-enkephalin. Pituitary β-LPH is probably not the source of endorphins found in the central nervous system; these are apparently synthesized in situ.

The synthesis and release of pituitary β-LPH are closely linked to those of ACTH. Both hormones have a common precursor molecule, both are secreted by the same cell, and the secretion of both is controlled in parallel by positive (eg, stress, CRF stimulation) and negative (eg, dexamethasone) feedback mechanisms. The parallelism between ACTH and β-LPH secretion suggests a function related to the generalized stress response. β-endorphin also stimulates the release of growth hormone (GH) and prolactin by the rat pituitary through a central nervous system-mediated mechanism, events that occur in response to stress in some species.

β-LPH may serve as a prohormone, releasing any of its constituent biologically active fragments after cleavage by proteolytic enzymes in the pituitary. The function of pituitary β-LPH may be entirely unrelated to the opiate-like properties of the smaller molecules it contains. However, it seems likely that the central nervous system endorphins are involved in modulating functions responsive to administration of opiates (Snyder, 1977; Way and Glasgow, 1978; Brown and Doe, 1978).

There are presently no drugs derived from β-LPH marketed anywhere in the world. However, it is anticipated that preparations or analogues of this hormone or its derivatives will eventually be useful in the treatment of chronic pain, opiate addiction, and perhaps certain psychiatric conditions. Numerous enkephalin analogues currently are being used investigationally for these purposes.

Selected References

Archer DF: Current concepts of prolactin physiology in normal and abnormal conditions. *Fertil Steril* 28:125-134, 1977.

Asch RH, Greenblatt RB: Use of impeded androgen-danazol in management of benign breast disorders. *Am J Obstet Gynecol* 127:130-134, 1977.

Brown JD, Doe RP: Pituitary pigmentary hormones: Relationship of melanocyte-stimulating hormone to lipotropic hormone. *JAMA* 240:1273-1278, 1978.

Frantz AG: Prolactin. *N Engl J Med* 298:201-207, 1978.

Friesen HG: Growth retardation, in Ezrin C, et al (eds): *Clinical Endocrinology: A Survey of Current Practice.* New York, Appleton-Century-Crofts, 1977, 60-68.

Gelfand JA, et al: Treatment of hereditary angioedema with danazol: Reversal of clinical and biochemical abnormalities. *N Engl J Med* 295:1444-1448, 1976.

Halbreich U, et al: Serum prolactin in women with premenstrual syndrome. *Lancet* 2:654-656, 1976.

Kleinberg DL, et al: Galactorrhea: Study of 235 cases, including 48 with pituitary tumors. *N Engl J Med* 296:589-600, 1977.

Lauersen NH, Wilson KH: Effect of danazol in treatment of chronic cystic mastitis. *Obstet Gynecol* 48:93-98, 1976.

Li CH: Chemical messengers of adenohypophysis from somatotropin to lipotropin. *Perspect Biol Med* 21:447-465, 1978.

Martini L, Besser GM (eds): *Clinical Neuroendocrinology.* New York, Academic Press, 1977.

Neelon FA, Sydnor CF: Assessment of pituitary function. *DM* 24: 1-55, 1978.

Shetty KR, Kalkhoff RK: Human chorionic gonadotropin (HCG): Treatment of obesity. *Arch Intern Med* 137:151-155, 1977.

Snyder SH: The brain's own opiates. *Chem Engineer News* 55:26-35, 1977.

Taylor AL: Hypothalamic hormones: Applications to endocrine diagnosis. *Hosp Formul* 12:865-869, 1977.

Tolis G, Friesen HG: Prolactin and human reproduction. *Can Med Assoc J* 115:709-711, 1976.

Wass JAH, et al: Long-term treatment of acromegaly with bromocriptine. *Br Med J* 1:875-878, 1977.

Watts NB, Keffer JH: *Practical Endocrine Diagnosis,* ed 2. Philadelphia, Lea & Febiger, 1978.

Way LE, Glasgow CE: Endorphins: Possible physiologic roles and therapeutic applications. *Clin Ther* 1:371-386, 1978.

Agents Used to Regulate Blood Glucose | 47

HYPOGLYCEMIC AGENTS

Diabetes mellitus is a disorder with metabolic and vascular components that probably are interrelated. A relative or absolute deficiency of insulin activity is associated with hyperglycemia and altered lipid and protein metabolism. Vascular components consist of accelerated atherosclerosis throughout the body and angiopathy that primarily affects the renal and retinal microcirculation.

Diabetic patients may be classified as either ketoacidosis-prone (juvenile, growth-onset) or ketoacidosis-resistant (nonketotic, adult or maturity-onset). The ketosis-prone patient generally experiences the onset of disease prior to age 20 and is dependent upon exogenous insulin to prevent ketoacidosis. Patients who develop diabetes between 20 and 30 years of age frequently have ketosis-prone insulin-dependent diabetes. Ketosis-resistant patients generally experience the onset of diabetes after age 40, tend to be overweight, and usually do not develop ketoacidosis in the absence of insulin therapy. Hereditary influence (probably multifactorial) is important in both types of diabetes and is predominant in ketosis-resistant patients, whereas environmental factors may be more important in ketosis-prone diabetics. The genetics of diabetes mellitus is complicated and not clearly understood.

Diet therapy is fundamental in the management of both types of diabetes. An appropriate diet that will provide a body weight consonant with height and build, with reasonable adjustments to fit the individual's living habits, should be prescribed initially for both symptomatic and asymptomatic patients.

The goals, strategies, and priorities of diet therapy vary for the different types of diabetes. In the ketosis-prone patient, composition and timing of meals must be constant. Adequate carbohydrate and protein are needed at each meal to accommodate growth and the variable amounts of exercise of the juvenile. Three meals a day plus midmorning, midafternoon, and bedtime snacks may help to modulate the effects of treatment. Hypoglycemia may occur if meals are delayed even 15 to 30 minutes. In the ketosis-resistant, middle-aged, overweight patient, precise timing of meals is of secondary importance, while caloric restriction to achieve ideal body weight is paramount. In both types of diabetes, 0.8 to 1.2 g/kg (lower range for adults, upper range for children and lactating women) of *ideal* body weight usually is provided in protein and the remainder of total calories is divided between carbohydrate and fat, with 30% to 50% in fats (polyunsaturated preferred). Monosaccharides and disaccharides are avoided because they are absorbed rapidly and cause postprandial hyperglycemia; complex carbohydrates, such as starches, are preferred. For special diet considerations in controlled diabetics with hyperlipidemia, see Chapter 55, Agents Used to Treat Hyperlipidemia.

Choice of Hypoglycemic Agent: Ketosis-prone diabetics are insulin-deficient and require administration of exogenous insulin. They do not respond to oral hypoglycemic agents. Insulin also should be used in ketosis-resistant patients with impaired renal or hepatic function and during pregnancy.

Most ketosis-resistant diabetics are obese and tend to have elevated levels of endogenous insulin, but their tissues are resistant to the hormone. There is a negative feedback between insulin levels and the concentration of insulin receptors in target tissues, and tissue responsiveness to insulin is correlated with the concentration of these receptors. The treatment of choice in these patients is dietary restriction and weight reduction, which increases sensitivity to insulin by increasing the concentration of insulin receptors. The use of any hypoglycemic agent has the potential of worsening the problem of insulin resistance (ie, physiologic resistance, nonimmune type). This is because the lipogenic action of insulin, whether provided exogenously or endogenously (eg, stimulated by a sulfonylurea), enhances further weight gain, which then increases insulin resistance. Therefore, weight reduction is the most important aspect of therapy in obese diabetics. An adequate and documented trial of diet therapy alone should be performed before any hypoglycemic agent is prescribed in these patients. If a hypoglycemic agent is then deemed necessary, it should be considered only as a supplement to continuing caloric restriction rather than as a substitute for weight reduction. Successful control of weight and blood glucose levels has been achieved in 80% of patients in a program that utilizes a team approach (physician, nurse, dietitian, patient, person responsible for food preparation) in an extensive and continuing program (Davidson, 1976). However, this success rate may be difficult or impossible to attain in a private practice setting.

Opinions differ on when hypoglycemic therapy should be instituted in ketosis-resistant patients. Some physicians defer medication until symptoms appear or the blood glucose level consistently reaches 200 to 250 mg/dl. The desirability of strict rather than flexible control of the blood glucose concentration depends largely on whether maintaining near normal levels serves a useful function, such as preventing the progression of diabetic complications.

There is strong evidence to support the importance of rigorous control of blood glucose levels. Most experts probably agree that hyperglycemia is a factor in the development of the nephropathy, neuropathy, and retinopathy of diabetes. A casual association between hyperglycemia and macrovascular complications is more tenuous, and the etiology probably involves multiple factors. Observations in animals or man that support the probable causal association of hyperglycemia and diabetic microvascular and neuronal complications include development of glomerular abnormalities in normal kidneys transplanted into diabetic rats; reversal of glomerular pathology in rats after they receive beta cell transplants; and slowing of nerve conduction velocity associated with hyperglycemia which normalizes after insulin treatment. It has been suggested that small reductions (about 45 mg/dl) in blood glucose may not prevent vascular complications in patients with mild ketosis-resistant diabetes (UGDP, 1978). In one study, it was proposed that complications in ketosis-resistant diabetics may be associated with lack of insulin secretory reserve (as judged by deficient insulin secretion after the glucose tolerance test) rather than degree of hyperglycemia (Turkington and Weindling, 1978). There are well recognized metabolic differences between the ketosis-prone and resistant forms of diabetes, and it is possible that the progression of complications also is influenced differently. However, strong evidence will have to be offered to counter the opinion of most observers that the goal of reducing blood glucose concentration is of primary importance. Attempts are usually made to normalize glucose levels if this does not require unreasonable therapeutic demands. However, the acceptable degree of control may be less stringent in patients who remain asymptomatic, those who are uncooperative or unsuccessful with a weight reduction diet, those unresponsive to drug therapy, and in the elderly.

If it is decided that a hypoglycemic agent should be given to the nonketotic diabetic patient, a choice between insulin and an oral sulfonylurea (acetohexamide [Dymelor], chlorpropamide [Diabinese], tolazamide [Tolinase], tolbutamide [Orinase]) must be made. The only biguanide on the United States market, phenformin [DBI, Meltrol], was withdrawn in 1978, although it may be obtained under special circumstances (see the evaluation). The choice between an oral agent and insulin has been complicated by the continuing decade-long controversy over the findings of the University Group Diabetes Program (UGDP) (see references under UGDP at the end of this chapter).

UGDP Study: The UGDP study was initiated to determine whether the development and progression of vascular complications in patients with maturity-onset, noninsulin-dependent, asymptomatic, mild diabetes mellitus could be avoided or mitigated by controlling the blood glucose level. The answer to this question was not provided by the UGDP. The Study was discontinued because of the emerging pattern of a higher incidence of cardiovascular deaths in the groups treated with oral agents. The assumption was widely made that oral antidiabetic drugs had cardiotoxic properties and that they may be inappropriate for use in adult-onset diabetics who commonly already have cardiovascular risk factors. Subsequent to the publication of these results, various aspects of the UGDP Study (eg, study design and interpretation, irrelevance of results obtained from experimental groups that received inappropriate treatment by later therapeutic standards) have been criticized. Compelling arguments have been offered on both sides by recognized authorities (Biometric Society, 1975; Boyden and Bressler, 1979; Feinstein, 1979; Williamson and Kilo, 1979), but the issue of the potential cardiotoxicity of oral hypoglycemic drugs remains unsettled.

Smaller studies that differed substantially in design from the UGDP do not corroborate the finding of increased mortality from cardiovascular disease with long-term use of tolbutamide and phenformin. However, the possibility that tolbutamide has detrimental cardiovascular effects, whether or not they are associated with increased mortality, is consistent with evidence demonstrating this drug's inotropic effect on the myocardium. In addition, a pharmacogenetic study of tolbutamide metabolism demonstrated a ninefold variation in its rate of disappearance from plasma in almost one-fourth of the subjects studied. This appeared to be an inherited autosomal trait. If tolbutamide does have cardiotoxic properties, the pharmacogenetic findings may account for manifestation of this complication in "slow inactivators" (Scott and Poffenbarger, 1978).

It is not possible to state that cardiovascular effects, if present, will be similar for all sulfonylureas. Nevertheless, it seems prudent to consider that these drugs are similar to tolbutamide until proved otherwise, since the four sulfonylureas that reduce blood glucose levels are closely related in structure. The emphasis on the putative cardiotoxicity of the sulfonylureas has diverted attention from other considerations in the choice of hypoglycemic therapy. Generally, insulin is preferred in the younger or middle-aged patient, while oral agents are sometimes chosen for older patients. Insulin also is preferred in lean patients, but oral agents are sometimes effective in obese patients whose hyperglycemia is not controlled by diet alone.

Sulfonylureas are associated with other adverse effects and a large number of significant drug interactions (see the discussion in the section on Oral Hypoglycemic Agents). Furthermore, insulin is more effective in controlling blood glucose on a long-term basis, for the secondary failure rate (after initial control) with the sulfonylureas may be as high as 25% per year. Thus, sulfonylureas have not proved to be superior to insulin, although they are easier and more convenient to administer. The importance of this property cannot be denied, however, especially in debilitated elderly patients who may have difficulty in self-administering insulin injections or even in patients who exhibit strong aversion to insulin therapy unless it is necessary. Therefore, although insulin is probably more effective, the physician must assess other factors that may favor use of an oral agent in selected patients (AMA Advisory Panel on Oral Hypoglycemic Drugs, in press).

INSULINS

The seven forms of insulin available in the United States differ with respect to time of onset and duration of action. They may be divided into rapid-, intermediate-, and long-acting groups (see Table 1). Insulin injection (crystalline zinc insulin, regular insulin) has a rapid onset and short duration of action. Globin zinc, isophane (NPH), and protamine zinc insulins are conjugated with large protein molecules, which delays absorption from subcutane-

ous sites and prolongs their duration of action (the latter two preparations have an isoelectric point at physiologic pH, causing slow solubility of the complexes, which contributes to their long action). The larger particle size and crystalline form of extended insulin zinc suspension (Ultralente insulin) also delays absorption and prolongs its duration of action. Because of its smaller particle size and amorphous structure, prompt insulin zinc suspension (Semilente insulin) is more rapidly absorbed and shorter acting. The combination of 70% Ultralente and 30% Semilente insulin results in insulin zinc suspension (Lente insulin), which has an intermediate duration of action and approximates the general characteristics of isophane insulin. Some clinicians prefer insulins in the Lente series because they do not contain a modifying protein and may be mixed in any proportion to provide necessary dosage adjustments.

Advances in industrial chemistry have continued to improve the stability and purity of insulin. Unbuffered regular insulin with neutral pH (7.4) has been termed Neutral Regular Insulin (NRI). When stored at room temperature, full potency has been retained for almost one year. Chromatographic purification has produced two very highly purified insulins: (1) "single-peak" insulin, which is about 99% insulin plus desamido and arginine insulins, and (2) "single component" or "monocomponent" insulin, which is over 99% pure insulin, free from common contaminants of commercial insulin (proinsulin, other insulin forms and fragments, and certain proteins with molecular weights over 10,000). However, immunogenicity in humans is decreased only with the monospecies porcine preparations. Most patients allergic to insulin can be desensitized to "single-peak" pork insulin. Lipoatrophy or lipodystrophy is corrected in some patients when highly purified insulins are injected directly into the lesions. Dosage reduction has been possible in some patients transferred from mixed beef-pork or monospecies beef to monospecies "single component" pork insulin. Single component insulins are coming into general use in several countries outside the United States. They are less likely to stimulate formation of circulating insulin antibodies and appear to have reduced the frequency of resistance.

Insulin U 100 (100 units/ml) is more concentrated and will replace U 40 and U 80 forms following adequate patient education programs, thus obviating the serious dosage errors produced by using U 40 syringes with U 80 insulin or vice versa. It is expected that the Food and Drug Administration will soon cease certification of other than U 100 insulins, although lots of U 40 and U 80 that are already certified will be available until they are depleted. Syringes that can measure the small volumes of U 100 insulin accurately are now available.

Previously Untreated Patients: An intermediate-acting preparation is chosen for initial treatment of ketoacidosis-prone diabetes. In the absence of ketosis or other acute complications, the initial dose may be 10 to 20 units given before breakfast. Depending upon the symptomatic response, postprandial blood glucose levels, and urine tests, this dose may be increased by increments of up to 10 units weekly until satisfactory control is obtained. Spot urine samples before meals and at bedtime and occasional blood glucose measurements are useful to pinpoint the timing of hyperglycemia.

Best regulation in ketosis-prone diabetics is usually achieved by giving two injections daily, one before breakfast and the other before supper. Increasing the morn-

TABLE 1.
INSULIN PREPARATIONS AVAILABLE IN THE UNITED STATES
(In Order of Duration of Action)

| | | | Hours After Subcutaneous Administration[1] | | |
Action	Preparation	Animal Source	Onset of Action	Interval to Maximal Action	Duration of Action[2]
Rapid	Insulin Injection (regular, crystalline zinc)	Porcine Mixed Bovine-Porcine	<1	2-3	5-7
	Prompt Insulin Zinc Suspension (Semilente)	Bovine Mixed Bovine-Porcine	<1	4-6	12-16
Intermediate	Globin Zinc Insulin Injection (globin)	Mixed Bovine-Porcine	1-2	6-10	12-18
	Isophane Insulin Suspension (NPH)	Mixed Bovine-Porcine	2	8-12	18-24
	Insulin Zinc Suspension (Lente)	Bovine Mixed Bovine-Porcine	2-4	8-12	18-24
Long	Protamine Zinc Insulin Suspension	Mixed Bovine-Porcine	4-6	16-18	36
	Extended Insulin Zinc Suspension (Ultralente)	Bovine Mixed Bovine-Porcine	4-6	16-18	36

[1]*The duration of action is for a single injection. With daily injections, the duration of the longer-acting insulins is longer than indicated.*

[2]*The onset, interval to maximal action, and duration are influenced by such factors as concentration and volume of insulin injected, depth and site of injection, condition of the injection site, possible binding by antibodies, and state of capillary permeability. (Diabetes Mellitus: Diagnosis and Treatment, vol III, American Diabetes Association, 1971.)*

ing dose generally corrects glycosuria occurring before the evening meal or at bedtime; prebreakfast glycosuria that is not a sequel of nocturnal hypoglycemia is often controlled by reducing the size of the bedtime snack and/or giving an additional dose of an intermediate-acting preparation before the evening meal.

Sometimes it is necessary to add regular insulin to the intermediate-acting preparation to control glycosuria before the latter becomes effective. Regular insulin often is added to the prebreakfast dose of the intermediate-acting preparation and given in the same injection to prevent glycosuria before lunch; less commonly, regular insulin is added to the intermediate-acting insulin before the evening meal to prevent overnight fasting glycosuria. Most commonly, the total dosage is divided to provide two-thirds to three-fourths in the morning; this injection can be given 30 to 90 minutes before breakfast. The longer interval is used for the mixture and allows the peak of carbohydrate absorption to coincide more closely with the peak activity of regular insulin.

Dividing the dose is indicated (1) in unstable diabetes that is otherwise difficult to control; (2) in the presence of severe prebreakfast hyperglycemia that cannot be corrected by one dose of insulin daily; and (3) in patients requiring more than 50 units daily. In these patients, dietary carbohydrate is often divided into six or seven feedings.

A between-meal snack containing 15 to 25 g of carbohydrate plus additional protein and fat should be provided at the time of peak action of the insulin preparation being used. All patients given insulin also should have a bedtime snack. These help to prevent hypoglycemic reactions occurring either at night or between meals and, along with regular exercise, permit the patient's insulin requirements to be tailored to his specific needs.

Vigorous exercise is important in the program of diabetic management because it increases utilization of glucose by muscle. The patient may find it helpful to take a small snack before exercise to prevent hypoglycemia.

Complications: Prompt recognition and appropriate management of the complications of insulin therapy are essential for the safety of the patient and the effective control of diabetes mellitus. Patients who have intercurrent illness, emotional stress, or trauma or those hospitalized for major illness may require, at least temporarily, multiple injections of a rapid-acting insulin. Almost invariably, a temporary increase in total requirements will have been created by the complication. The degree of glycosuria and hyperglycemia occurring subsequently determines the timing, type, and amount of insulin needed.

Diabetic ketoacidosis, a potentially life-threatening emergency, requires prompt diagnosis, accurate estimation of severity, and diagnosis and treatment of any precipitating factor, as well as skillful administration of insulin, fluids, and electrolytes (particularly potassium) and prompt treatment of any coexistent condition. This indication is now treated with much smaller doses of insulin than were formerly utilized. Older regimens (100 units subcutaneously, followed by 50 to 100 units every two to four hours) required 200 to 400 units of insulin to control an episode, whereas less than 100 units may be needed using new, low-dose regimens (see the evaluation on Insulin Injection). With low-dose regimens, the blood glucose level decreases at a similar rate and there is less hazard of hypoglycemia and hypokalemia (Alberti, 1977; Heber et al, 1977; Kreisburg, 1978).

Hyperosmolar (nonketotic) coma occurs rarely and may be confused initially with stroke or a severe hypoglycemic reaction. It is observed most commonly in individuals over 60 years of age who may or may not have a history of diabetes. However, it also may occur in younger diabetics. Associated illness is common and the mortality rate is high (40% to 60%). Polydipsia, polyuria, weight loss, rapid onset of coma, severe dehydration, and very high levels of blood glucose are observed. Azotemia and hyperosmolarity are present, but extreme changes in ketone levels are not seen. The insulin requirement is usually less than for diabetic ketoacidosis and more fluid may be needed; 10 or more liters of hypotonic electrolyte solution (eg, half normal saline) may be required during the first 12 to 36 hours of therapy to correct hyperosmolarity.

Pregnancy: The most common form of diabetes in pregnancy is gestational diabetes, in which symptoms are apparent only during pregnancy. These patients commonly have a family history of diabetes and may have a greater propensity to develop overt diabetes later in life. The diabetogenic effects of the hormones produced during pregnancy (eg, human placental lactogen, estrogen, progesterone) increase insulin requirements, while the placenta simultaneously promotes the metabolism of insulin. Symptoms may respond to diet therapy alone but, if a hypoglycemic agent is indicated, insulin is required; an oral agent should not be used.

Diabetic pregnancies are subject to many complications, which are generally related to the severity of the disease. Diabetes is associated with complications *in utero* (eg, anomalies, pre-eclampsia, hydramnios, fetal wastage) and neonatally (eg, prematurity, respiratory distress syndrome, neonatal glycemia). More careful control of blood glucose levels is necessary than in nonpregnant patients, and this may require more frequent injections and/or the combination of short- and intermediate-acting preparations which was formerly unnecessary. Of particular importance is the avoidance of ketoacidosis, which tends to occur in the second or third trimester, since this often causes fetal death.

Insulin requirements generally are unchanged or even decreased slightly during the first trimester but increase during the second and third trimesters. Patients with pre-existing ketosis-prone diabetes may require two to three times their usual dosage during this period. These patients are at risk of developing ketosis and of fetal loss in about the seventh month of pregnancy. During the last month of pregnancy, insulin needs may decrease slightly, but a 50% decrease may indicate placental malfunction and fetal distress.

Delivery of the infant and placenta abruptly ends the diabetogenic stress, and the insulin requirement may decrease precipitously in the first day postpartum to one-half of the prepregnancy level. Thereafter, there is a gradual increase to the usual prepregnancy level of insulin needed.

Adverse Reactions and Precautions

Every diabetic patient taking insulin should carry some form of readily available carbohydrate as well as an identification card containing pertinent information.

Hypoglycemia: This may be observed in any patient receiving insulin. It often occurs near the time of maximal activity of the particular insulin preparation used and at almost the same time of the day or night. Common manifestations are hunger, anxiety, warmth and sweating, tremulousness, weakness, confusion, emotional lability, palpitation, pallor, abnormal behavior, fatigue, paresthesias, and hyperesthesias of the lips, nose, or fingers. In severe hypoglycemia, profound cerebrocortical dysfunction may occur, manifested by convulsions, coma, and death. Autonomic signs and symptoms may develop as a result of the *rate* of decrease in blood glucose, and those of the central nervous system are related to the blood glucose concentration. Therefore, if glucose levels decrease slowly, autonomic symptoms may not precede central nervous system depression. The symptoms of hypoglycemia are quite variable in children: A child may have a voracious appetite, tremors, or simply be faint or easily fatigued. He may appear to be apathetic or sleepy and the parent mistakenly assumes he wishes to sleep longer.

Causes of hypoglycemia are (1) reduction or change in diet (eg, omission or delay of a meal), especially decreased intake of carbohydrate; (2) weight reduction; (3) termination or completion of pregnancy; (4) exercise; (5) alleviation of stress; (6) correction of disorders associated with hyperglycemia or onset of disorders associated with hypoglycemia, including overindulgence in alcohol; and (7) insulin or sulfonylurea overdosage. Hypoglycemia also may be caused by errors in insulin administration (eg, failure to agitate the container before use, improper measurement, improper injection technique) or remission in the diabetic state. (See the section on Hyperglycemic Agents for treatment.) Patient education is an integral part of initiating insulin therapy. Patients should be taught how to recognize an insulin reaction and how to treat it.

Somogyi Effect: Use of unnecessarily large doses may produce this hyperglycemic rebound phenomenon. It results from unrecognized, uncorrected, or overcompensated hypoglycemia with subsequent reactive hyperglycemia; occasionally a test for ketones is positive. This leads to the mistaken idea that there is an increased need for insulin. The larger doses given then perpetuate the cycle and wide fluctuations in the blood glucose level occur. Less commonly recognized manifestations of the Somogyi effect include moderate fasting hyperglycemia, glycosuria, and weight gain. This effect is sometimes encountered in patients with maturity-onset diabetes who are overweight before insulin therapy is started. Treatment of the Somogyi effect consists of reducing the dose of insulin. In juvenile diabetics, reducing the dose by 2 to 6 units may be all that is required, while patients with maturity-onset diabetes may require a 20% to 30% reduction.

Allergic Reactions: Allergic reactions to insulin can be either systemic or local; the latter occur about ten times more frequently than the former, and both forms may be observed in some patients.

Local allergy is manifested by an erythematous, indurated area at the site of injection that develops within a few minutes to hours and may persist for several days. The reaction commonly occurs within the first few days after initiation of insulin treatment, which suggests previous sensitization to beef or pork protein. Local reactions are thought to be caused by noninsulin or large-molecular-weight materials present in some preparations. Local inflammatory responses (which some consider irritant and others allergic) or infection may result from improper cleansing of the skin, contamination of the injection site, use of a sensitizing antiseptic, or accidental intracutaneous rather than subcutaneous injection. These reactions usually subside spontaneously.

Generalized reactions are characterized by urticarial skin eruptions with or without systemic manifestations that may include angioedema, gastrointestinal disturbances (nausea, vomiting, diarrhea), respiratory symptoms (eg, asthma, dyspnea), and, occasionally, hypotension, shock, and death. These reactions have been ascribed to sensitivity to the insulin molecule itself. Patients with a systemic allergy to insulin commonly have a history of (1) intermittent treatment with insulin; (2) allergy to other materials (eg, penicillin); (3) obesity; or (4) increased serum antibody titers to beef insulin. Pork insulin, which is less antigenic than the beef product, is used for desensitization and subsequent treatment.

Desensitization is indicated in patients with symptoms of systemic allergy or persistent local allergy who require insulin. Although desensitization to any insulin preparation usually is possible theoretically, desensitization to a particular batch of single-peak insulin does not consistently confer desensitization to subsequent batches. Fortunately, however, the composition of single component insulin is sufficiently consistent from lot to lot so that desensitization to one batch often confers desensitization to others.

Some patients may be susceptible to lipodystrophy, an atrophy of fat tissue underlying the site of insulin injection. This condition may be due to an immune phenomenon and tends to occur more frequently when less pure insulin preparations are used. It may be minimized by injecting single-peak insulin into the affected lesions. A minority of patients, however, will develop or have no improvement in insulin lipoatrophy when treated with mixed beef-pork single-peak insulin. These patients should be treated with pork single-peak insulin and, if no improvement occurs, with single component pork insulin. In about 85% of patients with lipoatrophy, the injection of single-peak insulin directly into the atrophic areas results in dramatic reappearance of subcutaneous fat and correction of the cosmetic defect. Unless the insulin is injected into areas affected by lipodystrophy every two to four weeks, atrophy may recur.

Lipohypertrophy is an accumulation of subcutaneous fat that sometimes develops at sites of repeated insulin injection and is a normal tissue response to insulin. Regression occurs gradually if the affected sites are not used for injections.

Insulin Resistance: Resistance to insulin may have an immune or nonimmune mechanism. The presence of insulin antibodies is believed to be of significance in the development of the immune type of resistance. Impaired insulin binding at the receptor site has been suggested as a possible cause in obese patients and appears to correct itself with weight loss. Generally the term "resistant" has been applied to patients who require more than 200 units daily for several days or more in the absence of intercurrent complications. In immunologic insulin resistance, changing the species source from beef or mixed beef-pork to pork may reduce hyperglycemia. If this is tried and the patient still requires 300 to 500 units daily, glucocorticoid therapy is indicated. Prednisone (40 to 80 mg daily) is given for one week or until the insulin requirement decreases; therapy should not be continued for more than one month. The glucocorticoid may decrease IgG production or decrease the binding of insulin to the antibody. This condition is best treated with regular (crystalline) insulin because of the increased duration of action associated with IgG binding of insulin. It is advisable to begin glucocorticoid therapy in the hospital or under careful outpatient control because insulin requirements may increase in the initial days of steroid therapy.

Vision Changes: In uncontrolled diabetes, a transient loss of accommodation has been attributed to changes in the physical properties of the lens; this condition is reversed during the early phase of effective management. Alterations in osmotic equilibrium between the lens and vitreous and aqueous fluids may not stabilize for a few weeks after initiating therapy; thus, it is wise to postpone evaluation for new corrective lenses for three to six weeks.

Interactions: Hormones that tend to counteract the hypoglycemic effect of insulin include growth hormone (somatotropin), corticotropin, glucocorticoids, thyroid hormone, estrogens, progestins, and glucagon. Epinephrine inhibits insulin secretion and stimulates glycogenolysis. Excessive levels of these hormones should be considered in assessing insulin therapy. Guanethidine [Ismelin] decreases blood glucose levels and the dosage of insulin may require adjustment when this agent is added to or omitted from the regimen. Hypoglycemia has occurred in diabetics who have taken beta-blocking agents, and these drugs may mask the tachycardia associated with hypoglycemia. The hypoglycemic effect of insulin also may be potentiated by monoamine oxidase inhibitors, anabolic steroids, and fenfluramine [Pondimin].

INDIVIDUAL EVALUATIONS

INSULIN INJECTION (Crystalline Zinc Insulin, Regular Insulin)
[Regular Iletin]

This rapid-acting agent has a short duration of action and is the only insulin preparation that may be given intravenously or intramuscularly as well as subcutaneously (see Table 1). It may be mixed in the same syringe with isophane (NPH) insulin. It also may be combined with insulin zinc suspension (Lente insulin) in any proportion, and the mixture is stable for up to three months when refrigerated. The clinical effect of such mixtures is to provide more flexibility in delivering appropriate amounts of insulin at the time of food intake.

Insulin injection is widely used to supplement intermediate- and long-acting preparations. It is the preparation of choice in unstable diabetes when complications such as infection, shock, or surgical trauma occur. Insulin injection may be administered intravenously in the presence of ketoacidosis or during surgery. Adherence of insulin to infusion equipment is impeded by adding human serum albumin or

5 ml of the patient's whole blood to the infusate.

See the introduction to this section for further information.

ROUTES, USUAL DOSAGE, AND PREPARATIONS. *Subcutaneous*: Dosage must be individualized. As an adjunct to intermediate-acting preparations, 5 to 10 units given in the same syringe (except with globin insulin) before breakfast or the evening meal.

Intravenous: For ketoacidosis, *adults*, 6 to 10 units, followed by 6 to 10 units/hr given by infusion. *Children*, 0.1 unit/kg of body weight/hr (limitation up to the adult dose above) given as a continuous infusion.

Intramuscular: For ketoacidosis when facilities for continuous intravenous infusion are limited, 10 to 20 units, followed by 5 to 10 units hourly.

> *Regular Iletin* (Lilly). Solution (aqueous) 40, 80, and 100 units/ml in 10 ml containers [mixed bovine-porcine source]; 500 units/ml (concentrated) in 20 ml containers [porcine source].
> *Insulin Injection* (Squibb). Solution 40, 80, and 100 units/ml in 10 ml containers [mixed bovine-porcine source].

PROMPT INSULIN ZINC SUSPENSION
[Semilente Iletin, Semilente Insulin]

This preparation is rapid acting (see Table 1) and is used most commonly to supplement intermediate- and long-acting forms when the duration of action of these preparations is not quite appropriate for a specific patient. A mixture composed of prompt insulin zinc suspension 30% and the long-acting extended insulin zinc suspension (Ultralente insulin) 70% has an intermediate duration of action (Lente) (see the evaluation on Insulin Zinc Suspension).

ROUTE, USUAL DOSAGE, AND PREPARATIONS. *Subcutaneous* (should never be given intravenously): No standard dose can be cited. For patients with newly diagnosed mild diabetes, initially, 10 to 20 units given 30 minutes before breakfast. It may be necessary to inject at least two doses daily.

> *Semilente Iletin* (Lilly) [mixed bovine-porcine source], *Semilente*
> *Insulin* (Squibb) [bovine source]. Suspension 40, 80, and 100 units/ml in 10 ml containers.

ISOPHANE INSULIN SUSPENSION
[NPH Iletin, NPH Insulin]

Isophane insulin is an intermediate-acting preparation (see Table 1). Absorption is delayed because the insulin is conjugated with protamine in a protein complex of reduced isoelectric solubility. This preparation contains less protamine than protamine zinc insulin and is useful in all forms of diabetes except the initial treatment of diabetic ketoacidosis or in emergencies. Isophane insulin or insulin zinc suspension is the drug of choice for previously untreated diabetic patients.

Hypoglycemic reactions in mid to late afternoon may be less obvious in onset, more prolonged, and more frequent than with rapid-acting preparations because of the prolonged effect of the dose. See the introduction to this section for additional information on adverse reactions.

ROUTE, USUAL DOSAGE, AND PREPARATIONS. *Subcutaneous* (should never be used intravenously): Dosage must be individualized. Initially, 10 to 20 units or, for obese adults, 30 to 40 units 30 to 60 minutes before breakfast. If needed, the dose may be divided to provide one-third of the daily amount 30 minutes before supper or at bedtime (see the discussion on Previously Untreated Patients).

> *NPH Iletin* (Lilly), *NPH Insulin* (Squibb). Suspension 40, 80, and 100 units/ml in 10 ml containers [mixed bovine-porcine source].

INSULIN ZINC SUSPENSION
[Lente Iletin, Lente Insulin]

This intermediate-acting preparation is a mixture of 30% prompt insulin zinc suspension (Semilente insulin) and 70% extended insulin zinc suspension (Ultralente insulin) (see Table 1). It may be used interchangeably with isophane insulin, and one of these preparations is most frequently the drug of choice for previously untreated diabetics. Insulin zinc suspension is not a suitable substitute for insulin injection (regular insulin) in emergencies because of its delayed onset of action.

Hypoglycemic reactions in mid or late afternoon may be less obvious in onset, more prolonged, and more frequent than with rapid-acting preparations because of the prolonged effect of the dose. Insulins in the Lente series are sometimes preferred because they do not contain a modifying protein and can be mixed in any ratio. See the introduction to this section for additional information on adverse reactions.

Patients receiving isophane insulin may be transferred directly to insulin zinc suspension on a unit-for-unit basis. For the first two or three days, the total amount should be reduced by one-third in patients who previously received regular insulin or by one-half when protamine zinc insulin was the preparation used formerly.

ROUTE, USUAL DOSAGE, AND PREPARATIONS. *Subcutaneous* (should never be given intravenously): See the dosage for Isophane Insulin Suspension.

> *Lente Iletin* (Lilly) [mixed bovine-porcine source], *Lente Insulin* (Squibb) [bovine source]. Suspension 40, 80, and 100 units/ml in 10 ml containers.

GLOBIN ZINC INSULIN INJECTION

This intermediate-acting insulin preparation (see Table 1) contains globin, a protein prepared from beef blood, which delays absorption from the subcutaneous injection site. This preparation was one of the first intermediate-acting insulins but has been superseded by isophane (NPH) insulin or insulin zinc suspension (Lente insulin), because its duration of action is less than 24 hours in some patients. This form is indicated for patients who require more than one daily injection of regular insulin, those whose condition cannot be controlled by other forms of insulin, or those who are sensitive to protamine. It is not recommended for the treatment of diabetic ketoacidosis. Globin insulin should not be mixed in the same syringe with regular insulin because the excess globin delays absorption of the regular insulin component.

Hypoglycemic reactions in mid to late afternoon may be less obvious in onset, more prolonged, and more frequent than with rapid-acting preparations because of the prolonged effect of the dose. See the introduction to this section for information on adverse reactions.

ROUTE, USUAL DOSAGE, AND PREPARATIONS. *Subcutaneous* (should never be given intravenously): See the dosage for Isophane Insulin Suspension.

> *Globin Zinc Insulin Injection* (Squibb). Solution 40, 80, and 100 units/ml in 10 ml containers [mixed bovine-porcine source].

PROTAMINE ZINC INSULIN SUSPENSION
[Protamine, Zinc & Iletin]

This long-acting preparation contains more modifying protein (protamine) and zinc than isophane insulin (see Table 1). Combining regular insulin with protamine zinc insulin is complicated by the conversion of a portion of the unmodified insulin to an insoluble form. In the past, mixtures of the two in ratios of 2 or more to 1 were utilized; however, use of insulin in the Lente series is much more flexible. The protamine form of insulin is best suited for control of mild to moderately severe hyperglycemia in patients with stable diabetes when insulin timing is not critical. Like extended insulin zinc suspension (Ultralente insulin), this form has limited usefulness when given alone; it is usually administered in combination with a shorter-acting preparation. Long-acting preparations are less adaptable than intermediate-acting forms given in divided doses.

Free protamine forms an insoluble complex with prothrombin and may cause lymphedema around the injection site. The long duration of action of protamine zinc insulin may result in recurrent hypoglycemic reactions if the dosage is not properly adjusted. A readily available carbohydrate (eg, orange juice) may be given to prevent such reactions, but the carbohydrate content of the meal following injection may have to be limited to avoid hyperglycemia. Between-meal snacks may be needed and bedtime snacks are essential. The long delay in onset of action makes this form unsuitable for emergencies. See the introduction to this section for additional information on adverse reactions.

ROUTE, USUAL DOSAGE, AND PREPARATIONS. *Subcutaneous* (should never be given intravenously): See the dosage for Isophane Insulin Suspension.

Protamine, Zinc & Iletin (Lilly), **Protamine Zinc Insulin** (Squibb). Suspension 40, 80, and 100 units/ml in 10 ml containers [mixed bovine-porcine source].

EXTENDED INSULIN ZINC SUSPENSION
[Ultralente Iletin, Ultralente Insulin]

The action, indications, and possibility of hypoglycemic reactions for this long-acting preparation are similar to those for protamine zinc insulin. (See Table 1 and the previous evaluation.) Like prompt insulin zinc suspension (Semilente insulin), this form contains no modifying protein to which patients may be sensitive and, like protamine zinc insulin, it has limited usefulness when given alone. It is usually administered in combination with a shorter-acting form. In slightly reduced doses, this preparation may be combined with insulin zinc suspension (Lente insulin) when fasting blood glucose levels are not adequately controlled during the daytime. It is not suitable for use in emergencies because of its delayed onset of action.

ROUTE, USUAL DOSAGE, AND PREPARATIONS. *Subcutaneous* (should never be given intravenously): See the dosage for Isophane Insulin Suspension.

Ultralente Iletin (Lilly) [mixed bovine-porcine source], **Ultralente Insulin** (Squibb) [bovine source]. Suspension 40, 80, and 100 units/ml in 10 ml containers.

ORAL HYPOGLYCEMIC AGENTS

The sulfonylurea compounds (acetohexamide [Dymelor], chlorpropamide [Diabinese], tolazamide [Tolinase], and tolbutamide [Orinase]) reduce the blood glucose level and are given orally to selected patients with diabetes. The biguanide compound, phenformin [DBI, Meltrol], is available in the United States only under special circumstances (see the evaluation). The absorption of all oral hypoglycemic agents is fairly rapid. See Table 2 for the half-lives and duration of action of these agents.

Although the sulfonylureas are sulfonamide derivatives, they have no antibacterial action. They appear to act initially by stimulating the release of endogenous insulin from pancreatic islet tissue and also

TABLE 2.
ORAL HYPOGLYCEMIC AGENTS AVAILABLE IN THE UNITED STATES

Type	Drug	Maximal Effective Dose	Half-Life (Hours)*	Duration (Hours)
Sulfonylurea	Acetohexamide Dymelor (Lilly)	1.5 g	6-8 (includes metabolites)	12-24
	Chlorpropamide Diabinese (Pfizer)	750 mg	30-36	60
	Tolazamide Tolinase (Upjohn)	1 g	7	up to 24
	Tolbutamide Orinase (Upjohn)	3 g	4-6	6-12
Biguanide	Phenformin Hydrochloride DBI (Geigy) Meltrol (USV)	200 mg	3	4-6
	Phenformin Hydrochloride (timed-release) DBI-TD (Geigy) Meltrol (USV)	200 mg	3	8-14

*Biological half-life regarding hypoglycemic potential.

affect the peripheral utilization of insulin. Tolbutamide potentiates the action of insulin on carbohydrate transport across skeletal muscle membrane, inhibits the output of glucose from the intact liver, and increases the number of insulin receptors. Results of some studies suggest that the sulfonylureas are effective for several years, but their long-term action has not been established conclusively.

Acetohexamide, chlorpropamide, tolazamide, and tolbutamide decrease blood glucose levels in nondiabetic as well as in diabetic individuals. Conversely, usual therapeutic doses of phenformin have no hypoglycemic effect in individuals without diabetes, because increased peripheral glucose utilization is exactly compensated by increased hepatic release of glucose.

Ideally, adequate time is allowed for the patient to learn and practice the necessary dietary habits before other modes of therapy are introduced. Failure to emphasize the necessity and principles of continuous dietary management is perhaps the primary shortcoming in the present treatment of diabetes. Mild elevation of blood glucose levels during this initial period is not life-threatening, and administering oral hypoglycemic agents before the principles of dietary therapy are understood is not the wisest course for long-term management. If hyperglycemia and symptomatic glycosuria continue after an appropriate trial with diet alone, it may be necessary to administer insulin or an oral agent.

Oral hypoglycemic agents may be particularly useful in ketosis-resistant patients who are allergic to insulin and unwilling or unable to undergo desensitization or who are otherwise unable or unwilling to inject insulin. These agents are also useful in elderly diabetics with poor vision who live alone and are at risk of developing hypoglycemia from incorrect insulin dosage. However, some patients who develop diabetes in the late 70's and 80's have the ketoacidosis-prone form in which the oral agents are not indicated.

If substitution of an oral agent for insulin is considered, an insulin-free interval must be established to determine whether dietary regulation alone is effective. If moderate to severe ketonuria occurs within 12 to 24 hours after withdrawal of insulin, control cannot be maintained without this agent. Primary failure of control with the oral agents may be considered to have occurred when hyperglycemia is not controlled by the maximal recommended dosage.

Relapse or secondary failure occurs frequently in patients treated with the sulfonylureas. This may be due to progressive decrease in endogenous insulin reserve or to development of resistance to the drugs. Only 6% to 12% of patients remain well controlled for more than six or seven years. It is advisable to discontinue use of these drugs briefly every six months to determine if their continued administration is essential. This test may demonstrate that (1) patients who are well controlled on the combination of diet and oral agents will continue to be well controlled on diet alone, or (2) patients in whom the dosage of the oral agents had been gradually increased in an attempt to control elevated blood glucose levels will be found to have represented secondary failure.

Adverse Reactions and Precautions

Acute toxic effects occurring after the use of oral hypoglycemic agents appear to be relatively rare, but the use of combinations of these drugs increases the risk of untoward reactions.

Hypoglycemic reactions have been reported after use of all four sulfonylureas; although they are rarely severe, some fatalities have occurred. Hypoglycemia also has occurred in nondiabetic individuals who received sulfonylureas for other diseases on an investigational basis. Because of the prolonged action of chlorpropamide [Diabinese], hypoglycemia may persist for several days and repeated administration of dextrose may be necessary; the severity of this reaction fluctuates during such episodes. Hypoglycemic reactions have occurred after one dose of a sulfonylurea, after two or three days of therapy, or after many months of therapy that had previously produced no untoward effects. Hypoglycemia may develop after treatment with a single sulfonylurea, after a change from one oral drug to another, or after an oral drug is substituted for insulin. It may occur in patients who receive an inappropriately large dose of drug, in those who do not eat properly, or in those who fail to metabolize or excrete the drug because of impaired hepatic or renal function. Thus, these agents should not be used in patients with hepatic or renal disease or congestive heart failure who are more vulnerable to the hypoglycemic effects of the sulfonylureas. These factors become even more significant in the elderly, for their counterregulatory mechanisms are diminished; they may be more prone to have insufficient food intake, and hypoglycemia may not be as easy to recognize because it may develop insidiously without acute signs and may be manifested as brain dysfunction and, ultimately, coma. A decreased rate of excretion is most likely to intensify the hypoglycemia produced by chlorpropamide.

Allergic skin reactions (pruritus, erythema, urticaria, and morbilliform or maculopapular rash) have been noted after use of sulfonylureas and phenformin. Most of these effects are transient; if they persist, the drug should be discontinued. Gastrointestinal disturbances (eg, nausea, vomiting, gastritis), which occur most frequently with phenformin and rarely with sulfonylureas, may be troublesome. They are lessened by taking the drug with meals, adjusting the dosage, or substituting timed-release capsules for the tablets. If symptoms persist, the drug should be discontinued at least temporarily.

Water retention and dilutional hyponatremia (inappropriate ADH syndrome) have been associated with administration of chlorpropamide to patients with diabetes mellitus, particularly those with a tendency to retain water (eg, patients with congestive heart failure or hepatic cirrhosis). Tolbutamide rarely causes dilutional hyponatremia. Signs of hyponatremia include serum hypo-osmolarity, continued sodium excretion despite hyponatremia, and an impaired ability to dilute urine and to excrete a water load. Chlorpropamide potentiates endogenous antidiuretic hormone activity at the renal tubular level and augments the hypothalamic-pituitary release of ADH. These abnormalities have been corrected by withdrawing the drugs but have reappeared with readministration (see Chapter 49, Antidiuretic Agents).

Leukopenia; thrombocytopenia; agranulocytosis; aplastic anemia; hemolytic anemia; jaundice from cholestasis, parenchymal changes, or both; and acute intermittent porphyria have been reported rarely after use of the sulfonylureas but not after use of phenformin.

The oral hypoglycemic agents have not yet been shown to have any teratogenic effects in humans, but such effects have been observed after use of large doses in animals. However, these agents are not recommended for use in diabetic women who may become pregnant. Insulin is the drug of choice during pregnancy. Oral agents are not used during pregnancy, principally because their transplacental passage may cause hypoglycemia in the neonate.

The sulfonylureas are contraindicated in *nondiabetic* patients with renal glycosuria, because their hyperresponsiveness to these agents may result in prolonged or fatal hypoglycemia. Except for investigational use, the oral hypoglycemic agents have no place in the treatment of chemical or latent diabetes, subclinical (suspected) diabetes, prediabetes, or in combination with insulin and they are contraindicated in patients with diabetic ketoacidosis.

The possible cardiotoxicity of sulfonylureas is discussed in the section on UGDP Study.

Interactions: Agents that aggravate the diabetic state by increasing blood glucose levels include glucocorticoids, estrogens, and thiazides. The dosage requirements for oral hypoglycemic agents may be increased in those receiving chlorpromazine [Thorazine], thiazides, or phenytoin [Dilantin], since these drugs inhibit the release of endogenous insulin and may cause hyperglycemia.

Drugs that may increase the risk of

hypoglycemia in patients taking the sulfonylureas include insulin, alcohol, phenformin, sulfonamides, propranolol [Inderal], salicylates, phenylbutazone [Azolid, Butazolidin], oxyphenbutazone [Oxalid, Tandearil], dicumarol, chloramphenicol, monoamine oxidase inhibitors, guanethidine [Ismelin], anabolic steroids, fenfluramine [Pondimin], and clofibrate [Atromid-S].

The sulfonylureas, especially chlorpropamide, may decrease tolerance to alcohol; this is manifested by unusual flushing of the skin, particularly of the face and neck, similar to that caused by disulfiram [Antabuse].

SULFONYLUREA COMPOUNDS

ACETOHEXAMIDE
[Dymelor]

Acetohexamide is similar to other oral hypoglycemic agents in the sulfonylurea class. However, since it is the only one with uricosuric properties, some clinicians prefer this agent for diabetic patients with gout. Acetohexamide is hydroxylated in the liver to a metabolite with more pronounced hypoglycemic effects, which prolongs its biological half-life.

The incidence of untoward effects is low and reactions are reversible when acetohexamide is discontinued. Relatively severe hypoglycemic reactions have been observed occasionally in patients given large doses for prolonged periods without close observation. Rarely, hypoglycemic reactions due to hyperresponsiveness have occurred in patients given usual therapeutic doses. Since the active metabolite is excreted by the kidneys, this drug should be avoided in patients with renal dysfunction.

See also the introduction to the section on Oral Hypoglycemic Agents.

ROUTE, USUAL DOSAGE, AND PREPARATIONS. *Oral*: Dosage should be individualized. The usual range is 250 mg to 1.5 g daily; doses in excess of 1.5 g daily should not be used. Most patients receiving 1 g or less per day can be given the full amount once daily; however, the drug should be given in divided doses before the morning and evening meals if 1.5 g is required. Those who have recently discontinued use of a long-acting insulin preparation should be given relatively small initial doses.
Dymelor (Lilly). Tablets 250 and 500 mg.

CHLORPROPAMIDE
[Diabinese]

Chlorpropamide has essentially the same actions, uses, and limitations as the other sulfonylureas. Primary and secondary failures have been reported less frequently with this sulfonylurea. Chlorpropamide is bound to protein in the blood and is excreted by the kidneys without undergoing metabolic degradation. Because of its long half-life, maximal accumulation and effect may not be apparent for one to two weeks, and several weeks may be required for complete elimination of the drug from the body.

Untoward reactions, including intolerance to alcohol, have occurred more frequently with chlorpropamide than with the other sulfonylureas and, in a few older patients, hypoglycemic reactions have been severe. Chlorpropamide-induced water retention can be life-threatening in patients with a tendency to retain water (eg, those with congestive heart failure or hepatic cirrhosis). This drug should not be used in patients with renal insufficiency, because the duration of action is more prolonged. See also the introduction to the section on Oral Hypoglycemic Agents.

ROUTE, USUAL DOSAGE, AND PREPARATIONS. *Oral*: Dosage should be individualized;

the total amount is usually given once daily with breakfast. For *middle-aged patients*, initially, up to 250 mg daily; *older patients*, 100 to 125 mg daily. After five to seven days, the blood glucose level reaches a plateau and the dosage may be increased or decreased by 50 to 125 mg at weekly intervals. The maintenance dose depends upon the response of the patient and the severity of the disease; the usual range is 100 to 500 mg daily (maximum, 750 mg daily). Patients who do not respond adequately to 500 mg daily usually will not respond to larger doses.

Diabinese (Pfizer). Tablets 100 and 250 mg.

TOLAZAMIDE
[Tolinase]

Tolazamide is similar to other oral hypoglycemic agents in the sulfonylurea class. However, this potent agent lacks antidiuretic action and may be especially useful in the treatment of patients with a tendency to retain water. Tolazamide is metabolized in the liver to several substances, some of which have hypoglycemic activity. The metabolites are excreted by the kidney.

Generally, the untoward effects associated with tolazamide are the same as those noted with the other sulfonylureas; the incidence is low and reactions are reversible when tolazamide is discontinued. Hypoglycemia has been reported occasionally.

See also the introduction to the section on Oral Hypoglycemic Agents.

ROUTE, USUAL DOSAGE, AND PREPARATIONS. *Oral*: Dosage should be individualized. Initially, 100 to 250 mg daily is given with breakfast; the amount then is adjusted every four to six days as needed. A single daily dose is effective in most patients; if 500 mg or more is required daily, the drug should be given in two doses. Amounts larger than 1 g daily probably will not improve control.

Tolinase (Upjohn). Tablets 100, 250, and 500 mg.

TOLBUTAMIDE
[Orinase]

Tolbutamide has the same actions, uses, and limitations as other sulfonylurea compounds. This drug is of greatest value in patients who, because of poor general physical status, should receive a short-acting compound. Tolbutamide is carboxylated in the liver to an inactive metabolite.

The toxicity of tolbutamide appears to be low, and reactions are similar to those observed with other sulfonylureas. When chloramphenicol and tolbutamide are given together, the action of tolbutamide is prolonged and hypoglycemia may occur.

See also the introduction to the section on Oral Hypoglycemic Agents.

ROUTE, USUAL DOSAGE, AND PREPARATIONS. *Oral*: Dosage should be individualized. Initially, 500 mg is given twice daily; the dose then is adjusted gradually until the minimal amount adequate for satisfactory control of blood glucose and glycosuria is established. The maintenance dose is 250 mg to 3 g daily. The total daily dose may be taken in the morning or in divided doses throughout the day. Amounts greater than 3 g daily produce no better results than smaller doses. Tolbutamide should be administered for at least five to seven days to determine its effectiveness.

Drug available generically: Tablets 500 mg.
Orinase (Upjohn). Tablets 250 and 500 mg.

TOLBUTAMIDE SODIUM
[Orinase Diagnostic]

In patients with pancreatic islet cell tumor, the blood glucose level drops quickly after intravenous injection of tolbutamide sodium and remains low for three hours. Since other hypoglycemic states usually are not affected, tolbutamide sodium may be used in conjunction with estimates of plasma insulin to rule out this condition. This agent also has been used during ulcer surgery to verify the completeness of vagus nerve section (by measurement of gastric acid secretion after tolbutamide-stimulated insulin release).

Thrombophlebitis has occurred following intravenous injection of tolbutamide sodium in a small percentage of patients (0.8% to 2.4%); no important sequelae have been reported from this reaction.

ROUTE, USUAL DOSAGE, AND PREPARATIONS. *Intravenous* (diagnostic): 1 g.

> *Orinase Diagnostic* (Upjohn). Powder (for diagnostic use only) 1 g (present as 1.081 g tolbutamide sodium).

BIGUANIDE COMPOUND

PHENFORMIN HYDROCHLORIDE
[DBI, Meltrol]

This drug was removed from the general market in the United States by the FDA in 1978 because of the lactic acidosis associated with its use. This complication usually occurs in diabetic patients who are seriously ill with conditions accompanied by hypoxia (eg, cardiac failure, hypotension, liver or kidney disease) or in those who take the drug with alcohol or following the onset of severe anorexia or vomiting and ketosis. However, lactic acidosis also develops in the absence of known predisposing conditions. The mortality rate in these cases is approximately 50%. Probably very few, if any, patients who cannot be managed by other therapeutic measures require phenformin. However, it may be obtained under special circumstances for use in selected patients.

Phenformin is now available only through an Investigational New Drug Application (IND) under conditions set forth by the FDA. These conditions include documentation that the patient is nonketotic and has not responded to diet or diet plus sulfonylureas; sulfonylureas cannot be tolerated because of side effects; the patient has responded to phenformin treatment in the past; there is no contraindication to the use of phenformin; and insulin cannot be taken. Informed consent must be obtained from the patient or guardian. Physicians desiring further information may address their inquiries to: Division of Metabolism and Endocrine Drug Products (HFD-130), Food and Drug Administration, 5600 Fishers Lane, Rockville, Maryland 20857.

Phenformin is not related chemically to the insulins or the sulfonylurea compounds. It does not stimulate insulin secretion from the islet cells but possible mechanisms include inhibition of hepatic glyconeogenesis, decreased intestinal absorption of glucose, and increased anaerobic glycolysis, which increases glucose utilization. Large doses appear to inhibit the conversion of alanine to glucose (glyconeogenesis) and lactate to glucose, whereas small doses enhance glycolysis without inhibiting glyconeogenesis or the conversion of lactate to glucose in vitro. However, it has not been shown with certainty that these effects are responsible for the hypoglycemic action noted with doses used clinically.

Although some physicians believe that the use of phenformin may cause weight loss in the obese, mildly diabetic patient, some double-blind studies have failed to confirm this finding. In addition to inducing anorexia, phenformin may retard the absorption of food. This agent has been shown to inhibit the uptake of glucose in water by isolated, full-thickness human ileum.

Occasionally, patients in whom normal blood glucose concentrations are maintained by phenformin may experience weight loss, asthenia, and "starvation" ketonuria unless insulin also is administered. Phenformin alone rarely causes hypoglycemia, but this has occurred when it was given with another oral hypoglycemic agent.

HYPERGLYCEMIC AGENTS

Hypoglycemic reactions may follow use of many drugs (eg, alcohol, large doses of salicylates or acetaminophen, dicumarol, phenylbutazone [Azolid, Butazolidin], propranolol [Inderal]) but probably are most common after administration of insulin or the sulfonylureas (see the section on Adverse Reactions and Precautions for Oral Hypoglycemic Agents). It is important that the diabetic patient be aware of the earliest manifestations of hypoglycemia so that a readily available carbohydrate (eg, fruit juice, sugar) can be taken immediately. For severe hypoglycemia, 50 to 100 ml of 50% dextrose solution should be administered intravenously; alternatively, glucagon may be given. If there is no response to glucagon, 50% dextrose must be used. In unconscious or stuporous patients, the intravenous administration of 50% dextrose is the treatment of choice, although glucagon may be given subcutaneously before the physician arrives. Upon rousing, carbohydrate may be given orally. Subsequent management of profound hypoglycemic shock depends more upon the patient's clinical status than the blood glucose levels.

Hyperglycemic agents are used to counteract the effects of increased insulin secretion in pathologic states. Diazoxide [Proglycem] blocks insulin secretion and is sometimes given preoperatively for insulinomas. Prolonged therapy may be administered in mild cases of islet cell tumors or when tumors could not be found at surgery. This agent is sometimes used concurrently with streptozocin. The latter is preferred for treating malignant insulinomas because it destroys the beta cells of the islet tissue (see also Chapter 68, Antineoplastic Agents).

Leucine-sensitive hypoglycemia is a familial condition occurring in young children; it usually improves spontaneously by age 3 to 6 years. Overstimulation of insulin secretion is avoided by restricting leucine intake, and hypoglycemic effects are counteracted by supplementing carbohydrate intake and administering diazoxide.

Treatment of idiopathic reactive (functional) hypoglycemia is primarily dietary. Hyperglycemic agents are not indicated in this condition.

INDIVIDUAL EVALUATIONS

DIAZOXIDE
[Proglycem]

This nondiuretic thiazide has primarily hyperglycemic actions when given orally [Proglycem] and antihypertensive effects when given intravenously [Hyperstat]. It produces a prompt, dose-related increase in blood glucose by directly inhibiting insulin secretion and, possibly, by inhibiting peripheral glucose utilization and stimulating hepatic glucose production. Diazoxide is used to counteract hyperinsulinism in conditions such as insulinoma or leucine-sensitive hypoglycemia. The hyperglycemic action is antagonized by alpha-adrenergic blocking agents.

Over 90% of diazoxide is bound to plasma proteins in the blood. The half-life of the oral form is 24 to 36 hours but may be more prolonged after overdosage or in those with impaired renal function. Because of its long half-life, prolonged observation of patients is necessary. Overdosage can cause marked hyperglycemia sometimes associated with ketoacidosis or nonketotic hyperosmolar coma.

Oral diazoxide may potentiate the effects of other antihypertensive drugs, although the effect on blood pressure is not marked when this agent is used alone. Although diazoxide is a thiazide, it causes sodium and water retention, which may necessitate concurrent administration of a diuretic; thiazide diuretics may intensify the drug's hyperglycemic and hyperuricemic effects. Diazoxide also may cause gastrointestinal irritation, thrombocytopenia, and neutropenia. Excessive hair growth of a lanugo type, which occurs most frequently in children, may be associated with its use. Diazoxide is teratogenic in animals (cardiovascular and skeletal deformities) and causes degeneration of fetal beta islet cells.

The safety of this drug in pregnant women has not been established. It is not indicated in the treatment of functional hypoglycemia.

See Chapter 38, Antihypertensive Agents, for other uses of diazoxide.

ROUTE, USUAL DOSAGE, AND PREPARATIONS. *Oral*: *Adults and children*, 3 to 8 mg/kg of body weight daily; *infants*, 8 to 15 mg/kg daily. The drug is given in two or three equally divided doses.

> *Proglycem* (Schering). Capsules 50 and 100 mg; suspension 50 mg/ml.

GLUCAGON

Glucagon is a polypeptide produced by the alpha cells of the pancreas. Like insulin, its normal function appears to be to control the homeostasis of glucose, amino acids, and possibly free fatty acids. However, in contrast to insulin, glucagon has potent glycogenolytic and glyconeogenic activity and these effects form the basis for its clinical usefulness.

Glucagon is given principally to treat severe hypoglycemia in diabetic patients and is often administered by a member of the family at home to a patient with frequent and severe hypoglycemic episodes that cause loss of consciousness. It also has been given to counteract hypoglycemia caused by administration of insulin for shock therapy in psychiatric patients. Glucagon has been used in the diagnosis of insulinomas. It increases the blood glucose concentration by mobilizing hepatic glycogen and thus is effective only when hepatic glycogen is available. Patients with reduced glycogen stores (eg, in the presence of starvation, adrenal insufficiency, chronic hypoglycemia) are unable to respond to glucagon.

Glucagon is effective only when administered parenterally. Its hyperglycemic effect is more gradual than that of dextrose and is of relatively brief duration. After the initial response, blood glucose levels usually fall to normal or hypoglycemic levels in one to one and one-half hours. Therefore, supplementary carbohydrates should be given as soon as possible after the patient responds in order to restore hepatic glycogen and prevent secondary hypoglycemia. This is especially important in juveniles, since their response is less pronounced than that of adults with stable diabetes. If the patient does not respond within 20 minutes, dextrose should be given intravenously to avoid the potential deleterious effects of cerebral hypoglycemia.

Nausea and vomiting have occurred occasionally after injection of glucagon, but these effects also develop with hypoglycemia. Hypersensitivity reactions are possible because the drug is a protein of animal origin.

ROUTES, USUAL DOSAGE, AND PREPARATIONS. *Intramuscular, Intravenous, Subcutaneous*: *Adults*, 0.5 to 1 mg (usually subcutaneously, but intramuscularly or intravenously if desired) every 15 to 20 minutes for two or three doses. (See the manufacturer's literature for directions on preparing the solution.) The manufacturer's literature also contains instructions for the administration of glucagon by the family of the patient; however, the drug should be used only under the direction of the physician. If it is used in such an emergency, the physician should be notified.

> *Glucagon for Injection* (Lilly). Powder (lyophilized) 1 and 10 mg with diluent.

Selected References

Advisory Panel on Oral Hypoglycemic Drugs, AMA. *JAMA* (in press).

Biometric Society Report of Committee for Assessment of Biometric Aspects of Controlled Trials of Hypoglycemic Agents. *JAMA* 231:583-608, 1975.

Drug interactions in diabetics. *Drug Ther Bull* 17:37-40, 1979.

Management of diabetes. *Compr Ther* 4:1-80, (June) 1978.

Alberti KGMM: Low-dose insulin in treatment of diabetic ketoacidosis. *Arch Intern Med* 137:1367-1376, 1977.

Alberti KGMM, Nattrass M: Highly purified insulins. *Diabetologia* 15:77-80, 1978.

Bonar JR: *Diabetes. A Clinical Guide*. Flushing, NY, Medical Examination Publishing Company, Inc, 1977.

Boyden T, Bressler R: Oral hypoglycemic agents. *Adv Intern Med* 24:53-70, 1979.

758

Bressler R (ed): Diabetes symposium: Putting basics into practice. *Drug Ther* 8:22-144, (March) 1978.

Brownlee M: Normoglycemia as a therapeutic goal in insulin-dependent diabetes. *Drug Ther* 8:13-20, (July) 1978.

Carey RM, et al: Diabetes mellitus updated: Standards of quality care in office and hospital practice. *Virginia Med* 105:195-218, 1978.

Davidson JK: Controlling diabetes mellitus with diet therapy.*Postgrad Med* 59:114-122, (Jan) 1976.

Feinstein AR: How good is statistical evidence against oral hypoglycemic agents? *Adv Intern Med* 24:71-95, 1979.

Gabbe SC: Diabetes in pregnancy: Clinical controversies. *Clin Obstet Gynecol* 21:443-453, 1978.

Galloway JA, Bressler R: Insulin treatment in diabetes. *Med Clin North Am* 62:663-680, 1978.

Heber D, et al: Low-dose continuous insulin therapy for diabetic ketoacidosis. Prospective comparison with "conventional" insulin therapy.*Arch Intern Med* 137:1377-1380, 1977.

Kreisburg RA: Diabetic ketoacidosis: New concepts and trends in pathogenesis and treatment. *Ann Intern Med* 88:681-695, 1978.

Lebovitz HE, Feinglos MN: Sulfonylurea drugs: Mechanism of antidiabetic action and therapeutic usefulness. *Diabetes Care* 1:189-198, 1978.

Moss JM, Tucker HST: New trends in management of diabetic ketoacidosis. *Am Fam Physician* 17:111-118, (Feb) 1978.

Owen OE, et al: Managing insulin-dependent diabetic patients. *Postgrad Med* 59:127-134, (Jan) 1976.

Raskin P: Diabetic regulation and its relationship to microangiopathy. *Metabolism* 27:235-252, 1978.

Scott J, Poffenbarger PL: Pharmacogenetics of tolbutamide metabolism in humans. *Diabetes* 28:41-51, 1978.

Shen S-W, Bressler R: Clinical pharmacology of oral antidiabetic agents, parts I and II. *N Engl J Med* 296:493-497, 787-793, 1977.

Tchobroutsky G: Relation of diabetic control to development of microvascular complications. *Diabetologia* 15:143-152, 1978.

Turkington RW, Weindling HK: Insulin secretion in diagnosis of adult-onset diabetes mellitus. *JAMA* 240:833-836, 1978.

University Group Diabetes Program: Effects of hypoglycemic agents on vascular complications in patients with adult-onset diabetes. I. Design, methods, and baseline results. II. Mortality results. *Diabetes* 19(suppl): 747-783, 785-830, 1970. III. Clinical implications of UGDP results. *JAMA* 218:1400-1410, 1971. IV. A preliminary report on phenformin results. *JAMA* 217:777-784, 1971. V. Evaluation of phenformin therapy. *Diabetes* 24(suppl 1):65-184, 1975. VI. Supplementary report on nonfatal events in patients treated with tolbutamide. *Diabetes* 25:1129-1153, 1976. VII. Mortality and selected nonfatal events with insulin treatment.*JAMA* 240:37-42, 1978.

Williamson JR, Kilo C: New evidence that controlling hyperglycemia in diabetes is important. *Res Staff Physician* 25:46-52, (April) 1979.

Agents Used to Treat Thyroid Disease | 48

Thyroid hormones principally affect metabolism, growth, and development, and their most fundamental metabolic actions are calorigenic and protein anabolic effects. The former accelerates the rate of cellular oxidation, thus increasing energy expenditure and heat production. This, in turn, affects the metabolism of vitamins, proteins, carbohydrates, lipids, electrolytes, and water and the activity of hormones and drugs. Their protein anabolic effect is important in many aspects of growth and development.

Physiology: The two metabolically important thyroid hormones are triiodothyronine (T_3, liothyronine) and tetraiodothyronine (T_4, levothyroxine). All of the T_4 and 10% to 20% of the T_3 produced daily are derived from thyroid gland follicular cells where iodide from the blood is concentrated (mostly by an active transport process), oxidized ("activated" iodine), and incorporated into mono- and diiodotyrosine (MIT and DIT). DIT then couples with MIT or another DIT molecule within the thyroglobulin matrix to form T_3 or T_4, respectively. Thyrotropin (thyroid stimulating hormone, TSH) stimulates each step of hormone synthesis.

T_3 and T_4 are stored within thyroglobulin in the follicular lumina of the gland until they are released into the blood. The

759

thyroid stores 10 to 20 times more T_4 than T_3; about 1% of the stored hormone is released daily. After release, thyroglobulin is returned to the epithelial cell by endocytosis and is subsequently hydrolyzed. The T_4 and T_3 thus freed are secreted into the blood stream where they are largely bound to serum protein. T_4 is bound primarily to thyroid hormone-binding globulin (TBG) and to a lesser extent to prealbumin (TBPA) and albumin. T_3 is bound almost entirely to TBG but less firmly than T_4; thus, it has a greater turnover in the circulation. Only the small proportions of free thyroid hormones are biologically active; the ratio of free T_4 to T_3 is usually 10:1. About 75% to 90% of circulating T_3 is formed by monodeiodination of T_4 in peripheral tissues; the rest is secreted directly by the thyroid. Although it has been suggested that T_4 acts only as a precursor or prohormone for T_3, both T_4 and T_3 probably are metabolically active, although T_3 is three to five times more potent calorigenically. The protein-bound hormone serves principally as a reservoir.

Circulating thyroid hormone levels are regulated through a feedback system involving the thyroid, anterior pituitary, and hypothalamus. As the blood levels of free thyroid hormones increase, the secretion of pituitary TSH is inhibited, thereby decreasing thyroid secretion. Conversely, subnormal levels of thyroid hormones increase the release of TSH, which stimulates the secretion of thyroid hormones. The major negative feedback effect on thyroid hormones occurs within the anterior pituitary gland. TSH secretion is activated by hypothalamic thyrotropin-releasing hormone (TRH), but the regulatory mechanisms controlling its synthesis and release have not been clearly elucidated; positive as well as negative feedback systems may be involved. There also is an intrathyroidal autoregulatory system in which increased concentrations of iodide within the thyroid inhibit iodination of tyrosine; iodide also directly inhibits release of hormones from the gland.

In certain conditions, TBG levels may be abnormal, thus altering the total extrathyroidal pool of thyroid hormones. However, in such circumstances (as in normal individuals), the physiologically active free hormone is maintained at a normal level. For example, TBG levels are elevated during pregnancy and reduced during androgen therapy. The increased TBG levels increase the total amount of T_4 and T_3 but not the amount of free T_4 and T_3. These latter biologically active moieties are kept within normal limits, and thyroid function remains normal.

Thyroid hormones are metabolized at different rates; in euthyroid individuals, the half-life of T_4 is about six to seven days and that of T_3 is about one and one-half days. The half-life of T_4 is shortened in hyperthyroid patients (as little as three days) and may be prolonged in hypothyroid patients (up to ten days). Approximately 85% of the hormones are deiodinated in tissues, and the iodine released is available for re-incorporation into new thyroid hormone; the portion that is not reutilized is excreted in the urine. T_4 has two catabolic pathways: The first involves deiodination of T_4 at the 5 position to form the active metabolite, T_3. The second is the deiodination at the 5 position to form an inert metabolite, reverse T_3 (rT_3). The latter is preferentially generated under certain pathologic conditions (eg, starvation, surgery, cirrhosis, renal failure). In the developing fetus and neonate, rT_3 is the major metabolite. The concentrations of the two metabolites in serum assume a reciprocal relationship.

Thyroid hormones increase oxygen utilization by the tissues through mechanisms involving cell nuclei and mitochondria. They bind to nuclear protein (about 85% of iodothyronine specifically bound to nuclei is T_3; 15% is T_4) and stimulate synthesis of messenger RNA with the eventual production of enzymes which carry out the metabolic effects of the hormone. These enzymes increase ADP production and mitochondrial oxygen consumption. Thyroid hormones also directly stimulate mitochondria to further increase oxygen usage.

Thyroid dysfunction, whether characterized by overproduction or underproduction of hormones, has profound effects on many body systems (eg, cardiovascular, gastrointestinal, skeletal, neuromuscular, reproductive). However, effective treatment is available for most thyroid diseases.

Diagnosis: Some thyroid diseases are easily recognized by clinical examination, and extensive laboratory testing is not always necessary. However, a number of thyroid function tests can define the pathophysiologic state more specifically. The *serum T4* determination frequently is used as a screening test; it measures total serum T4 (protein-bound and unbound) by radioimmunoassay (RIA) and is closely correlated with the clinical status of overall thyroid activity. This test is subject to misinterpretation, however, if TBG levels are abnormal. Misinterpretation is avoided with the *free thyroxine index (FTI)* obtained by multiplying the serum T4 concentration by results of a resin T3 uptake test. The *resin T3 uptake test* is *not* a measurement of serum T3 levels, but provides an indirect estimate of serum TBG levels. It is useful only in conjunction with the measurement of total circulating T4 levels. FTI, which is expressed as a unitless number since it is not an expression of a specific quantity of hormone, more accurately reflects the free fraction of total serum T4. This fraction is more closely correlated with the functional state of the thyroid than the total T4 level. It provides essentially the same information about thyroid function as the more expensive *free T4 concentration test (FT4)*, which measures unbound serum T4 by dialysis. The protein-bound iodine (PBI) test is rarely used now but may be of value in determining the amount of serum non-T4 iodoprotein in certain pathologic states (eg, thyroiditis).

The *serum T3* radioimmunoassay test measures the total serum T3 concentration and is useful in detecting certain cases of mild hyperthyroidism since, in this condition, T3 may become elevated earlier and more markedly than T4. However, increased levels of T3 also may be observed in iodine deficiency hypothyroidism or, following radioiodine therapy, the patient

may be euthyroid with depressed serum T4 and elevated T3. The determination of *serum TSH* by radioimmunoassay can assist in distinguishing between primary (thyroidal) and secondary (pituitary) hypothyroidism. In these conditions, serum TSH levels are elevated or undetectable, respectively. Measurement of serum TSH also is useful for assessing patient progress (see the section on Monitoring Therapy).

Dynamic tests of thyroid function also are utilized. Administration of TRH (thyroid-releasing hormone) often can distinguish hypothalamic hypothyroidism (TSH secretion increased) from pituitary hypothyroidism (TSH secretion not increased). In a *thyroid scan*, a small amount of radioactive iodine or technetium is given, and the morphology of the areas of radioactive uptake are outlined; this is useful in determining whether the hyperthyroidism is caused by Graves' disease, thyroid adenoma, or multinodular goiter and in distinguishing between malignant and nonmalignant nodules. The *radioactive iodine uptake test* assists in determining the dosage for radioactive iodide ablation therapy and in differentiating Graves' disease from subacute thyroiditis.

Although mostly employed as research tools, tests are also available to detect abnormal immunoglobulins present in Graves' disease (see the section on Hyperthyroidism). Antibodies against thyroid tissue and thyroglobulin that may be present in certain disease states (ie, Graves' disease, Hashimoto's thyroiditis, primary myxedema) also can be measured. Presence of these antibodies is an indication of an autoimmune process but does not identify the specific disease present.

The most recent thyroid function test to become available is a radioimmunoassay kit for direct measurement of free serum T4 concentrations. It is technically less difficult to perform than the FT4 test, which requires dialysis. It provides direct measurement of serum T4 without the need to correct for differences in TBG levels as in the two-step FTI determination. For detailed descriptions of these and other tests and their interpretation, see specialty texts.

HYPOTHYROIDISM

The prototype of substances used to treat hypothyroidism is Thyroid, U.S.P., which is derived from the desiccated thyroid gland of animals. This product contains not only the active hormonal substances, T_3 and T_4, but also iodotyrosines and other organic materials. Other preparations used are thyroglobulin [Proloid], a substance prepared from animal thyroid glands; synthetic salts of the pure thyroid hormones, T_4 (levothyroxine sodium [Levothroid, Synthroid]) and T_3 (liothyronine sodium [Cytomel]); and a mixture of the synthetic salts of pure thyroid hormones (liotrix [Euthroid, Thyrolar]). All produce similar qualitative metabolic and clinical effects, but they differ in potency and duration of action. The clinical response to 60 mg of Thyroid, U.S.P. is approximately equal to that produced by 60 mg of thyroglobulin, 0.1 mg or less of levothyroxine, 40 mcg of liothyronine, or preparations of liotrix containing either 60 mcg of levothyroxine and 15 mcg of liothyronine or 50 mcg of levothyroxine and 12.5 mcg of liothyronine.

Dosages of thyroid preparations must be established individually. Generally, the initial dose is small, and the amount is increased gradually until an optimal response is produced. The dose required to maintain this response is then given once daily for an indefinite interval. Hypothyroid patients have increased sensitivity to thyroid hormones, and determination of the optimum maintenance dose should be based on apparent clinical status, age, and appropriate laboratory test results (see the section on Monitoring Therapy). Replacement doses for adults are lower (100 to 200 mcg of levothyroxine daily) than those formerly utilized. If a patient is now taking amounts in excess of those recommended, the dosage may be reduced gradually to the minimum required to suppress serum TSH or to maintain normal serum T_4 levels. Initial doses are generally lower in older patients. In children, maintenance levels are relatively higher than in adults, and so-called adult levels for replacement are usually required by adolescents. In general, dosage is *not* related to body mass.

Indications for Therapy: Clinical hypothyroidism is most commonly of thyroidal origin (primary hypothyroidism), occurring either spontaneously without known cause or following destruction of the thyroid gland by radioactive iodine therapy, surgical removal, or autoimmune disease (Hashimoto's thyroiditis, chronic lymphocytic thyroiditis). It also may result from hypopituitarism (secondary) or hypothalamic injury (tertiary) such as tumor or trauma. In children, cretinism results from thyroid hormone deficiency during fetal or early life. It usually is caused by failure of the thyroid to develop normally but may result from TSH or TRH deficiency, genetic defects in hormonogenesis associated with goiter, maternal ingestion of antithyroid drugs, or extreme deficiency of iodine. Juvenile hypothyroidism develops after the neonatal period in children who apparently were previously normal; it is often produced by autoimmune mechanisms, but errors in hormonogenesis also may be causative factors. Hypothyroidism in adults (myxedema) may result from primary atrophy of the gland, chronic lymphocytic thyroiditis, or lack of thyrotropin secretion by the pituitary gland. The manifestations of myxedema may develop gradually over a period of many years. Hypothyroidism also may be drug induced (eg, lithium, antithyroid compounds, cough preparations with high iodine content), and withdrawal of the causative agent, if possible, may cure the condition. If continuing use of these agents is necessary, thyroid replacement therapy may be given concomitantly.

Regardless of the etiology or severity of hypothyroidism, replacement therapy with thyroid hormone is necessary. Improvement is noted in objective signs such as the classic myxedema facies with its round, puffy, sleepy appearance; dry, rough skin and brittle hair; bradycardia; and slightly elevated diastolic blood pressure. Fatigue, somnolence, irritability or apathy, constipation, and intolerance to cold also are relieved, and growth and development resume in children and adolescents. The hyperlipidemia usually associated with hypothyroidism also improves or disappears.

Early diagnosis and adequate treatment are mandatory for the management of *cretinism*. Widespread use of screening programs for congenital hypothyroidism in neonates should ensure the earliest possible detection. Most defects associated with this form of hypothyroidism, including inadequate development of the brain, bones, teeth, and muscles, can be minimized if not avoided when treatment is begun immediately after birth. Appropriate therapy must be established as soon as possible in order to allow the child to attain full potential of physical and mental development. Treatment of affected patients after about three months of age does not reverse all of the mental stigmata that have already occurred, but some of the physical effects are reversible. Hypothyroidism developing after two to three years of age is not associated with mental retardation.

Mild hypothyroidism can be treated initially with one-half the expected maintenance dosage, with full replacement dosage being attained in one month. In *myxedema* (severe hypothyroidism), the increase in dosage is more gradual and up to four to six months of therapy may be required to achieve euthyroidism. Factors that favor conservatism in treatment include coronary artery disease; severe, prolonged thyroid disease; and advanced age of the patient. In elderly patients, particularly those with arterial vascular disease, the maintenance dosage should be lower than in healthy adults. Pituitary insufficiency resulting in adrenal insufficiency must not be treated with thyroid until the adrenal insufficiency has been corrected. In patients with cardiovascular disease, the use of propranolol [Inderal] in conjunction with thyroid replacement therapy has been reported to decrease the risk of arrhythmia and angina and allow greater tolerance of levothyroxine.

Because of its severity, *myxedema coma* should be treated as soon as definitive diagnosis is made. Treatment addresses three sets of needs. First, thyroid hormone

(levothyroxine, liothyronine, or a combination) is replaced by giving relatively large initial oral or intravenous doses, followed by oral therapy after the first day; second, appropriate supportive measures are provided (ventilatory assistance, regulation of fluids and electrolytes, dextrose if hypoglycemic); and third, intravenous corticosteroids may be given because adrenal insufficiency is difficult to rule out immediately.

Thyroid preparations may be beneficial in *simple nonendemic goiter* and in *chronic lymphocytic (Hashimoto's) thyroiditis*. Exogenous thyroid hormones act not only as replacement therapy but also tend to reduce the size of the goiter by suppressing TSH secretion.

Temporary periods of hypothyroidism may occur during the course of the frequently encountered subacute viral thyroiditis. Permanent hypothyroidism rarely results, but symptomatic improvement can be achieved with thyroid replacement during hypothyroid phases of the disease.

Thyroid hormone is used in the management of *carcinoma of the thyroid gland* and has frequently caused a demonstrable regression of metastatic lesions.

Thyroid hormones have been given to treat so-called *metabolic insufficiency* without adequate laboratory documentation that thyroid hormone deficiency exists. Mild hypothyroidism resulting from reduced production of thyroid hormone responds to thyroid hormones, but vague symptoms suggesting hypometabolism (eg, dry skin, fatigue, slight anemia, constipation, apathy) should not be treated indiscriminately with thyroid hormone. Since specific and precise tests of thyroid function are available, administration of thyroid preparations without proper documentation is obsolete.

Since abnormalities of reproductive function (amenorrhea, menorrhagia, dysmenorrhea, premenstrual tension, sterility, habitual abortion, and oligospermia) may be associated with hypothyroidism, questionable logic has led to the use of thyroid preparations in these disorders. There is no evidence that this is beneficial unless the patient is hypothyroid; therefore, thyroid hormones or mixtures containing them should not be used to treat these problems without a specific indication of thyroid deficiency.

Thyroid hormones are frequently used inappropriately to effect weight loss in euthyroid obese individuals. Since it is necessary to induce a state of hyperthyroidism to accomplish this, thyroid hormones or preparations containing them should not be used for this purpose (see Chapter 56, Agents Used in Obesity).

Choice of Preparations: Hypothyroid patients probably can be maintained satisfactorily on any of the thyroid replacement products available. The various preparations have different properties, however, that influence the choice for a given patient. Some patients have been maintained successfully for years on desiccated animal thyroid (Thyroid, U.S.P.) and, for such patients, there is no need to change therapy because newer, purer products are available. Some desiccated thyroid preparations are standardized on the basis of iodine content rather than active thyroid hormone content and may have variable, undefined biological potency. Other desiccated thyroid preparations and thyroglobulin (a purer preparation also made from animal glands) are assayed for biological potency in addition to iodine content. This decreases, but does not eliminate, variability in potency of different batches due to the inherent limitations of the bioassay utilized.

Generally, the preferred thyroid preparation for replacement therapy is synthetic T_4 (levothyroxine sodium). It is also the drug of choice for congenital hypothyroidism (Committee on Drugs, American Academy of Pediatrics, 1978) and enhances assessment of clinical progress (see the section on Monitoring Therapy). Synthetic T_3 (liothyronine sodium) generally is not preferred for maintenance since it is difficult to monitor plasma levels of the hormone, and wider oscillations in plasma concentration are produced. However, because of its short half-life, some physicians prefer liothyronine for initial therapy in myxedema and myxedema coma. Liothy-

ronine also has better absorption characteristics and may be preferred when the reliability of absorption from the gut is in doubt. Preparations containing both T_4 and T_3 in a physiologic ratio (liotrix [Euthroid, Thyrolar]) also are available. They offer no therapeutic advantage over levothyroxine alone, because peripheral conversion of T_4 to T_3 results in normal levels of T_4 and T_3 with administration of levothyroxine alone. However, in the adequately treated patient, the combination products usually produce an FTI in the euthyroid range. In contrast, levothyroxine produces an FTI about 20% above normal, possibly leading to confusion. Further, conversion of T_4 to T_3 is reduced in disease and the importance of this possible variation in T_3 availability is as yet unknown.

Thyroid preparations are ordinarily administered orally. Parenteral preparations are used in emergencies and when oral administration is impossible. The slight difference in cost among the various thyroid replacement products makes this an unimportant consideration in drug selection.

Monitoring Therapy: Assessment of therapy requires the monitoring of clinical signs and symptoms as well as laboratory values. It is important for the physician to understand the difficulties of interpreting thyroid function tests when patients are taking thyroid medication. The clinically optimal serum T_4 levels vary widely, depending upon the preparation used. This is partly due to differences in protein-binding capacity among the various agents. Also, even though standard assay kits are employed, results obtained from different laboratories may vary. It is, therefore, wise to use the services of a single laboratory.

A satisfactory means of monitoring thyroid therapy appears to be by assay of serum TSH, which is a highly specific test. TSH levels begin to decrease within hours after initiating therapy, and normal levels correlate with normal thyroid hormone levels. Elevated levels indicate that the replacement dosage is inadequate. However, the serum TSH measurement is unreliable as the sole indicator of adequate thyroid therapy in congenital hypothyroidism, because levels may remain elevated for months when appropriate or even excessive doses of thyroid hormone are given. In these cases, serum T_4 should be monitored by radioimmunoassay and maintained in the upper half of the normal level for the age of the infant or child (serum FTI also may be used). This ensures sufficient hormone for the growing child between changes in regimen.

Adverse Reactions: If the appropriate amount of thyroid hormone replacement is provided, no adverse reactions occur. However, overdosage of any thyroid preparation causes thyrotoxicosis. Signs and symptoms include tachycardia, palpitations, elevated pulse pressure, angina pectoris, tremor, nervousness, insomnia, headache, change in appetite, vomiting, diarrhea, weight loss, hyperhidrosis, heat intolerance, and fever. The dose of thyroid hormone that produces thyrotoxicosis varies widely from patient to patient.

The American Thyroid Association has reviewed data that suggested that the incidence of breast cancer was increased in women receiving thyroid replacement therapy. They found the evidence tenuous and have recommended that patients with a documented need for thyroid medication continue their therapeutic program (Education Committee, American Thyroid Association, 1977).

Precautions: Since hypothyroid patients may be inclined to discontinue medication when euthyroidism has been attained, it is important to stress their life-long need for thyroid replacement therapy and the necessity of informing any new physician of their condition.

Hypothyroid patients respond rapidly to replacement doses of thyroid hormones and, if the dosage is increased too rapidly in those with underlying arteriosclerosis or myocardial disease, the capacity of the heart to handle the increased metabolic demands of the body may be exceeded. If cardiovascular symptoms appear, the dose must be reduced. On the other hand, for patients with myxedema coma or severe myxedema with bowel obstruction, it may be lifesaving to accept the hazard associated with rapid replacement of thyroid

hormone. The dose for younger patients may be increased to full replacement dosage more rapidly without undue risk.

When hypothyroidism and adrenal insufficiency coexist, as in pituitary insufficiency, adequate amounts of cortisone or cortisol (hydrocortisone) must be given before attempting thyroid replacement therapy, since thyroid hormones increase the metabolic turnover and degradation of adrenocortical hormones and may precipitate acute adrenocortical insufficiency.

Plasma levels of TBG may increase two- to fourfold during pregnancy. This is not a problem in women with an intact pituitary-thyroid axis, because the negative feedback system ensures initial adjustment of production of thyroid hormones; thereafter, hormone turnover is normal and normal levels of unbound hormone are maintained. In pregnant women dependent on thyroid replacement therapy, an increase in the dosage of thyroid may be necessary.

Drug Interactions: Thyroid hormones enhance the effect of oral anticoagulants, and a decrease in anticoagulant dosage may be required if these agents are given concomitantly. Thyroid hormone increases catabolism of vitamin K-dependent clotting factors, and the compensatory increase in synthesis of clotting factors is impaired by the anticoagulant.

Cholestyramine binds orally administered thyroid hormone in the intestine, delaying or preventing absorption. To prevent this interaction, there should be a four- to five-hour interval between administration of cholestyramine and thyroid hormone.

Initiation of thyroid therapy in diabetic patients may increase the requirement for insulin or oral antidiabetic agents, and the initiation of thyroid replacement therapy in digitalized patients may result in an increased requirement for digoxin.

INDIVIDUAL EVALUATIONS

THYROID, U.S.P.

This preparation is the cleaned, dried, powdered thyroid gland of domesticated animals used for food. The U.S.P. standards for all thyroid products from animal sources require that these preparations contain 0.17% to 0.23% iodine by weight in the organic combination peculiar to thyroid tissue. No requirement is included in these standards for metabolic potency, which is a function of the proportions of the metabolically active compounds present. Since the major portion of iodine in thyroid is present in metabolically inert forms (iodide and iodotyrosines), a given preparation may satisfy the U.S.P. assay requirements and yet not contain sufficient amounts of the metabolically active forms (triiodothyronine and tetraiodothyronine) to produce the desired therapeutic effect. In addition, the variable ratios of T_4:T_3 in different animal preparations results in variable serum concentrations of T_4 and T_3. Thyrar (a beef extract) and Armour Thyroid Tablets (a pork extract) employ additional biological assays to help ensure constant potency from batch to batch. However, even this measure is subject to some defined limit of error for the bioassay and, hence, these products, though less variable than preparations assayed on the basis of iodine content alone, are not as uniform as synthetic products. Some of the variations due to tablet texture can be obviated by instructing the patient to chew the tablet.

Thyroid is used most commonly as replacement therapy in hypothyroidism. Other uses include the treatment of simple nonendemic goiter, chronic lymphocytic (Hashimoto's) thyroiditis, and thyrotropin-dependent carcinoma of the thyroid (see the Introduction). It also may be used to prevent the goitrogenic effects of other therapeutic agents (eg, lithium, aminosalicylic acid, some sulfonamide compounds).

ROUTE, USUAL DOSAGE, AND PREPARATIONS. For replacement therapy, the dose of thyroid must be individualized, with the optimal amount determined primarily by clinical response and confirmed by results of laboratory tests. The initial dose is usually small and is increased gradually until a euthyroid state is obtained; the patient is then maintained on this dose.

Oral: For *younger adults*, the common practice has been to give 15 to 30 mg daily initially, increasing this amount by increments of 15 to 30 mg at two-week intervals until the desired response is obtained; however, some authorities start younger patients on nearly full replacement doses. The usual maintenance dose is 60 to 120 mg daily in a single dose. *Older adults*, initially, 7.5 to 30 mg daily; the dose is doubled at six- to eight-week intervals until an optimal response is obtained.

For suppressive therapy, as for replacement therapy, the initial dose for *adults* should be lower than the maintenance dose (eg, 60 mg) and increased as indicated by the response; for maintenance, 90 to 180 mg daily.

> Drug available generically: Capsules 60, 120, 180, 240, and 300 mg; tablets 15, 30, 60, 90, 120, 180, 240, and 300 mg; tablets (chewable) 180 mg; tablets (enteric-coated, timed-release) 30, 60, 120, and 200 mg.
> *Thyrar* (Armour). Tablets (beef extract) 30, 60, and 120 mg.
> *Armour Thyroid Tablets* (Armour). Tablets (pork extract) 15, 30, 60, 90, 120, 200, 240, and 300 mg.

THYROGLOBULIN
[Proloid]

Thyroglobulin is obtained from a purified extract of frozen hog thyroid. It meets the U.S.P. standard for iodine in thyroid and is assayed for biologic activity. On a weight basis, the potency of this preparation is equal to that of thyroid, and the indications, adverse effects, precautions, and doses are the same (see the Introduction and the evaluation on Thyroid).

> Drug available generically: Tablets 60 mg.
> *Proloid* (Parke, Davis). Tablets 16, 32, 65, 100, 130, 200, and 325 mg.

LEVOTHYROXINE SODIUM
[Levothroid, Synthroid]

This preparation is the synthetic sodium salt of the levorotatory isomer of T4 (thyroxine) and has the same indications, adverse reactions, and precautions as thyroid (see the Introduction and the evaluation on Thyroid). Levothyroxine is less completely absorbed from the gastrointestinal tract than liothyronine and has a slower onset of action when given orally. For most indications requiring thyroid replacement, this is the drug of choice. Levothyroxine usually is administered orally, but the intravenous route is used in myxedema coma or when oral administration is impractical.

ROUTES, USUAL DOSAGE, AND PREPARATIONS.
Oral: For mild hypothyroidism, *young and middle-aged adults*, initially, 50 to 100 mcg daily, increased by increments of 50 to 100 mcg at two- to three-week intervals until the desired response is maintained. For severe hypothyroidism, initially, 25 mcg daily, increased by increments of 25 mcg at two-week intervals to 100 mcg daily. Further increases by increments of 50 to 100 mcg may be made at the same intervals until the desired response is maintained. Most patients can be maintained in a full clinical euthyroid state with doses of 100 to 200 mcg daily. *Older adults*, initially, 12.5 to 50 mcg daily for six weeks; this amount is then doubled every six to eight weeks until the desired response is maintained. For otherwise normal *newborn infants*, initially, 25 to 50 mcg daily in a single oral dose (usually, 37.5 mcg is appropriate). *Premature infants less than 2 kg and infants at risk of cardiac failure*, initially, 25 mcg daily. The dose usually can be increased to 50 mcg daily in four to six weeks. *Children over 1 year*, 3 to 5 mcg/kg of body weight daily until the adult dose of about 150 mcg daily is reached in early or midadolescence. The maintenance dose should produce serum T4 and T3 concentrations in the upper half of the normal range for the child's age.
The largest dosage size still available is a 500 mcg tablet. This large quantity of hormone serves no justifiable medical need in the treatment of hypothyroidism, and care should be taken that this tablet is not misprescribed for the 50 mcg size.

Levothroid, (Armour), *Synthroid* (Flint). Tablets 25 mcg (0.025 mg), 50 mcg (0.05 mg,) 100 mcg (0.1 mg), 150 mcg (0.15 mg), 175 mcg (0.175 mg) [Levothroid only], 200 mcg (0.2 mg), and 300 mcg (0.3 mg).

Intravenous: For *newborn infants* unable to take oral medication, 50% to 75% of the oral dose (see above) is given daily. For myxedema coma, *adults*, 200 to 500 mcg of a solution containing 100 mcg/ml; 100 to 300 mcg may be given on the second day if necessary. After the patient's condition is stabilized, the drug is given orally for maintenance.
  Synthroid (Flint). Lyophilized powder (for reconstitution) 500 mcg with mannitol 10 mg.

LIOTHYRONINE SODIUM
[Cytomel]

This drug is the synthetic sodium salt of the levorotatory isomer of T3. Liothyronine has a rapid onset and short duration of action, and monitoring of blood levels is difficult. Because of this, it is not as useful as levothyroxine for maintenance therapy. Liothyronine is sometimes used to initiate therapy in patients with heart disease, although this is not a universal practice. It may be preferred to levothyroxine if intestinal absorption is impaired. Liothyronine may be given intravenously to treat myxedema coma, since its rapid action facilitates the adjustments in dosage often required. (See the Introduction.) Although liothyronine sodium is not available commercially in a form suitable for intravenous use, the manufacturer will supply this form upon request. Alternatively, administration of crushed tablets through a nasogastric tube is sometimes used.

ROUTES, USUAL DOSAGE, AND PREPARATIONS.
Oral: For mild hypothyroidism, *young and middle-aged adults*, initially, 25 mcg daily, increased by increments of 12.5 to 25 mcg at intervals of one to two weeks until the

desired response is maintained. For severe hypothyroidism, initially, 5 mcg daily, increased by increments of 5 to 10 mcg at intervals of one to two weeks until a daily dose of 25 mcg is reached; thereafter, this amount is increased by increments of 12.5 to 25 mcg at one- to two-week intervals until the desired response is maintained. The usual maintenance dose is up to 75 to 100 mcg/day. *Older adults*, initially, 2.5 to 5 mcg daily for three to six weeks; the amount is then doubled every six weeks until the desired response is maintained.

> Drug available generically: Tablets 25 and 50 mcg.
> *Cytomel* (Smith Kline & French). Tablets 5, 25, and 50 mcg.

Intravenous: For myxedema coma, *adults*, 10 to 25 mcg every 8 to 12 hours as necessary. The drug is given orally for maintenance.

> *Cytomel* (Smith Kline & French). Powder (for solution) 114 mcg/ml. Not available commercially; manufacturer will supply kit upon request for use in myxedema coma.

LIOTRIX
[Euthroid, Thyrolar]

Liotrix is a mixture of levothyroxine sodium and liothyronine sodium in a ratio of 4:1, respectively. The indications, adverse reactions, and precautions are the same as those for thyroid (see the Introduction and the evaluation on Thyroid). The mixture is equivalent to but offers no clinical advantage over the use of levothyroxine alone, since peripheral tissue conversion of T_4 to T_3 usually results in a normal physiologic ratio of the two hormones. However, with usual replacement dosages, the serum FTI is more typically normal with this compound.

ROUTE, USUAL DOSAGE, AND PREPARATIONS.
Oral: For hypothyroidism, *young and middle-aged adults*, initially, one tablet daily containing either 30 mcg of levothyroxine sodium and 7.5 mcg of liothyronine sodium [Euthroid] or 25 mcg of levothyroxine sodium and 6.25 mcg of liothyronine sodium [Thyrolar]; depending upon the response, the dose is increased by one tablet every two weeks. For maintenance, tablets that conveniently provide optimal therapy as determined by results of laboratory tests and clinical status are given. The final maintenance dose may be greater in children than in adults. *Older adults*, initially, one-fourth to one-half the amount given to younger adults; the dose is doubled at six- to eight-week intervals until the desired response is maintained.

> *Euthroid* (Parke, Davis). Tablets Euthroid-½, -1, -2, and -3 containing, respectively, 30, 60, 120, and 180 mcg of levothyroxine sodium and 7.5, 15, 30, and 45 mcg of liothyronine sodium. *Thyrolar* (Armour). Tablets Thyrolar-¼, -½, -1, -2, -3, and -5 containing, respectively, 12.5, 25, 50, 100, 150, and 250 mcg of levothyroxine sodium and 3.1, 6.25, 12.5, 25, 37.5, and 62.5 mcg of liothyronine sodium.

HYPERTHYROIDISM

Hyperthyroidism results from the excessive secretion of thyroid hormones and may be caused by Graves' disease, multinodular goiter, thyroiditis, or hyperfunctioning single nodules. In each case, the ratio of T_4:T_3 secreted may vary from normal. If T_3 predominates, T_3 thyrotoxicosis may occur. In this condition, the serum level of T_3 is invariably increased, but the serum level of T_4 may be normal. This disorder appears to be only diagnostically important since, clinically, patients with T_3 thyrotoxicosis have the same symptoms as those with other forms of hyperthyroidism and the treatment is similar.

The cause of Graves' disease, the most common form of hyperthyroidism, has not been elucidated, but evidence suggests that it may be an autoimmune disorder with circulating humoral stimulators acting on the thyroid gland. These immunoglobulins are designated TSI (thyroid stimulating immunoglobulins). They differ from TSH and have been found in the serum of many patients with this disease. They include LATS (long-acting thyroid stimulator), HTSI (human thyroid-stimulating immunoglobulin, formerly LATS-protector), and other immunoglobulins. It is believed that HTSI binds to thyroid membranes, resulting in stimulation of the thyroid gland. However, the precise role of TSI in the pathogenesis of Graves' disease is still uncertain.

The treatment of hyperthyroidism is directed toward reducing the excessive production of thyroid hormones. This can be accomplished by antithyroid drugs (which render the patient euthyroid until a spontaneous remission is achieved) or by radiation or surgery, both of which are more definitive. Since many of the signs and symptoms of hyperthyroidism reflect increased cellular sensitivity to adrenergic stimulation, the beta-adrenergic blocking drug, propranolol [Inderal], also may be used as an adjunct to other methods. Accurate diagnosis is essential before treatment is started, and the choice of therapy depends upon a careful evaluation of each patient.

When ophthalmopathy occurs with hyperthyroidism, some improvement in ocular complications may be noted with effective treatment of hyperthyroidism, but the condition tends to worsen if the patient then becomes hypothyroid. The unpredictability of the ophthalmopathy must be emphasized to the patient. Pretibial myxedema, an uncommon occurrence, usually is observed simultaneously with exophthalmos, and correction of the thyroid state often does not control this disorder. Severe cases of pretibial myxedema or exophthalmos may be relieved by high-dose glucocorticoid therapy.

Heart disease is a common complication of hyperthyroidism, especially in the elderly. If congestive heart failure occurs, it must be treated with conventional methods while control of thyrotoxicosis is initiated. However, digitalis preparations are less effective than usual in these patients unless hyperthyroidism is corrected. Also in the aged, hyperthyroidism may exist without the classical signs and often assumes the picture of "apathetic" hyperthyroidism.

Choice of Therapy

The choice of antithyroid drugs, radiation, or surgery as treatment for hyper-thyroidism is influenced by the patient's age and sex, status of the cardiovascular system and hyperthyroidism, and history of previous management of the disease. Opinions of experts vary regarding preference for radiation or surgery (for definitive therapy) or whether to initiate treatment with antithyroid drugs (propylthiouracil and methimazole). These drugs have been utilized for the initial treatment of Graves' disease in most patients, since spontaneous and, possibly, permanent remission may occur during the course of therapy. However, the rate of remission now appears to be much lower than formerly observed (25% rather than 50%); this may be due to the increased dietary iodine intake in recent years. Because of this lower remission rate, many physicians and patients choose to employ irradiation of the thyroid with radioactive iodine or subtotal thyroidectomy initially; with the latter, control is achieved in the shortest period of time. Nevertheless, antithyroid drugs remain the treatment of choice for children, pregnant women, patients being prepared for surgery, and those with cardiac disease being prepared for radiation therapy. If antithyroid drugs are ineffective in children after two to three years, surgery might be chosen (the risk decreases with increasing age). Surgery may be performed on pregnant women in the second trimester if necessary. Irradiation is used in patients who are poor surgical risks or who have had previous thyroid surgery; the risk of complications is greater if surgery is performed a second time.

Both surgery and radiation therapy carry a long-term potential for the development of hypothyroidism. Surgery is associated with a higher risk of recurrent hyperthyroidism. Although morbidity and mortality are greater with surgery, these are greatly reduced with a surgeon experienced in performing these operations. In general, radiation is a relatively safe procedure, although a brief increase in thyrotoxic manifestations may occur for a few days following I 131 treatment. This may be of consequence in patients with limited cardiac reserve. The chief hazards are thought to be a possible future carcinogenic effect, damage to gametes or a developing fetus (such treatment is contraindicated in pregnancy), and hypothyroidism. However, follow-up studies of patients irradiated with sodium iodide I 131 have shown that there is no increase in the incidence of leukemia or other malignancies, and, since the radiation exposure of the gonads is quite low, the chance of damage to gametes is considered insignificant. Therefore, some physicians advocate abandoning the age limits (ie, only for those over 40 years) formerly used to select patients for radiation therapy. This procedure continues to be contraindicated during pregnancy and, because data are lacking on long-term effects in children, it still seems wise to avoid irradiation in young patients.

Drug Therapy: The principal agents used to suppress the production of thyroid hormone are thioamide derivatives. The drugs used in this country are propylthiouracil (PTU) and methimazole [Tapazole], which have replaced the parent compound, thiouracil, a more toxic agent. They inhibit the incorporation of iodide into thyroglobulin, but usual doses do not inactivate or interfere with the release of thyroid hormone previously formed and stored in the gland. There is no permanent effect upon the thyroid gland. These drugs are used primarily to prepare patients for surgery (thyroid or other) or irradiation or in long-term suppression of hyperthyroid function.

Propylthiouracil is the most commonly used drug in this class, and it appears to offer some therapeutic advantages: propylthiouracil, but not methimazole, decreases the peripheral conversion of T_4 to T_3 and may increase conversion of T_4 to the physiologically inactive rT_3. Methimazole is more potent than propylthiouracil, thus requiring lower dosages, but this is not particularly advantageous because the incidence of adverse effects with the two drugs is similar with therapeutically equivalent doses. Propylthiouracil also may cross the placenta less readily during pregnancy than does methimazole.

The clinical effects of these drugs are not apparent until the stored supply of thyroid hormone has been utilized, and several weeks may elapse before there are signs of decreased thyroid activity. Since patients with severe hyperthyroidism dissipate their stores rapidly, they may respond to therapy more quickly than those with mild hyperthyroidism. It also should be remembered that, as the abnormally high metabolic state is corrected, the half-life of propylthiouracil and methimazole may increase, which would contribute to reduced dosage requirements.

An antithyroid agent sometimes is given with thyroid replacement therapy in order to facilitate maintenance of the euthyroid state. However, clinical status can be determined more accurately by frequent serum T_4 determinations and appropriate reductions in dosage of the antithyroid drug can be prescribed. The implications of combined antithyroid-thyroid therapy in pregnancy are more complex (see below).

Thioamide derivatives have a short half-life (1.5 hours), necessitating frequent administration to maintain therapeutic blood levels. The interval between doses should be no less than eight hours, particularly during initial therapy. Many so-called treatment failures probably result from inadequate frequency of drug administration. If the patient does not respond to therapy at a given dosage level, a shorter dosage interval (eg, four hours) may be tried before the total dose is increased. Adjustment of dosage interval also helps to avoid dose-related side effects. For maintenance, the drug can be administered less frequently; once-a-day dosage sometimes is successful.

If the vascularity and size of the thyroid gland increase during treatment, this may suggest overdosage and indicate a need for a reduction in dose. This is best accomplished by lengthening the interval between doses.

In general, the adverse reactions produced by antithyroid drugs are similar (see the evaluation on Propylthiouracil). Cross sensitivity sometimes occurs between drugs. Since some mild reactions (eg, rash) may disappear spontaneously with continued treatment, some clinicians do not change drugs unless the reaction fails to clear promptly. On the other hand, if a severe reaction necessitates withdrawal of one drug, another may be tried cautiously, although there is an increased risk of recurrence with administration of a related agent.

In Graves' disease, the goal of long-term antithyroid drug therapy is to inhibit hormone synthesis and secretion until spontaneous remission occurs. This takes about six months to one year in responsive patients, although there is considerable variability. Decrease in the size of the gland during therapy increases the likelihood of remission. Remission is not likely in patients with large goiters or in whom relapse has followed previous remissions. If there is doubt about whether a remission has occurred, a TRH challenge test may be performed.

When hyperthyroidism occurs during pregnancy, moderate dosages of propylthiouracil may be given with relative safety but, since this drug crosses the placenta, goiter and hypothyroidism may occur in the neonate. Some physicians have proposed administering a combination of antithyroid drug and thyroid hormone to the mother on the theory that exogenous thyroid hormone will also cross the placenta and may retard the effect of propylthiouracil on the fetus. However, it is now clear that thyroid hormones do not readily cross the placenta. Also, larger doses of antithyroid drug are required to maintain euthyroidism in pregnant women receiving combination therapy (Mestman et al, 1974). Therefore, the more reasonable approach seems to be use of propylthiouracil alone in the lowest effective dosage, erring on the side of slight maternal hyperthyroidism if necessary. This reduces the incidence of prematurity, which is high in untreated hyperthyroidism. Since antithyroid agents are secreted in breast milk, mothers receiving this medication should avoid nursing their infants.

Potentially fatal thyrotoxic crisis (thyroid storm) may occur in hyperthyroid patients who experience trauma or infection or who are not adequately prepared for surgery. It is manifested by irritability or apathy, followed by fever, extreme tachycardia, profound asthenia, possible high-output heart failure, and, finally, syncope and coma. Treatment includes administration of antithyroid medication, iodine, propranolol [Inderal], cortisol, and digitalis glycosides if necessary. Rapid reversal of this potentially dangerous state can be effected by charcoal hemodialysis. Neonatal thyrotoxicosis also occurs, usually in infants of thyrotoxic mothers, presumably caused by placental transfer of maternal LATS or other immunoglobulins. The condition has a high mortality rate and is treated with antithyroid drugs, propranolol, sedation, and digitalization, as well as appropriate supportive measures. This disorder typically resolves within two months and medication can be gradually withdrawn.

Adrenergic blocking agents may be beneficial adjuncts in the initial treatment of hyperthyroidism and in exacerbations of the disease. The beta-blocking agent, propranolol, is most widely used for this purpose and is preferred to reserpine and guanethidine [Ismelin], which produce general sympathetic blockade. Propranolol rapidly controls tachycardia and is, therefore, quite useful as an adjunct to other appropriate therapy for thyroid storm and neonatal thyrotoxicosis. It is used with antithyroid drugs preoperatively (thyroid or other surgery) and in patients with limited tolerance of antithyroid drugs. Investigationally, propranolol has been administered as the sole agent for the preoperative preparation of hyperthyroid patients and for the long-term control of thyrotoxic symptoms. However, this agent probably does not significantly affect total thyroid secretion, and metabolic effects (increased oxygen consumption) remain unaltered. Continued oxygen demand and the negative inotropic effect may produce congestive heart failure. Propranolol may increase uterine irritability during pregnancy.

At one time, iodine was the only substance available for the management of hyperthyroidism. It inhibits the synthesis and release of thyroid hormones and also may suppress trapping of iodide by the thyroid follicular cell membrane. Iodine usually is only partially effective and control often is not sustained (iodine escape). Therefore, its use as an antithyroid drug is now limited to special circumstances: to treat potentially fatal thyrotoxic crisis (thyroid storm) or neonatal thyrotoxicosis and, preoperatively, to decrease the vascularity of the thyroid gland. It should not be given alone.

The observation that some patients receiving lithium for psychiatric disorders developed hypothyroidism led to the trial of this drug in the treatment of hyperthyroidism. In a limited number of patients, lithium ameliorated thyrotoxicosis and decreased circulating thyroid hormone levels, apparently by blocking hormone release. However, this drug frequently causes adverse effects in the therapeutic dosage range. It does not offer any advantage over thiocarbamides for the initial treatment of thyrotoxicosis.

Radiation: Administration of sodium iodide I 131 [Iodotope I-131, Theriodide-131] is effective in the treatment of hyperthyroidism caused by Graves' disease, multinodular goiter, or a single toxic adenoma. Radioactive iodine accumulates in thyroid tissue and partially destroys the gland. A radioactive iodine uptake test should be performed prior to therapy to determine the dosage that will ensure adequate thyroidal accumulation of the radioisotope. A single dose is often sufficient but repeated doses may be required, especially in patients with large nodular goiters. In such patients, the initial dose may be considerably larger than that used in Graves' disease. The release of thyroid hormones may be increased several days after irradiation, which aggravates the thyrotoxic state; thus, it has been recommended that elderly patients or those with severe hyperthyroidism or cardiac disease be treated initially with propylthiouracil or methimazole before radioactive iodine is given. The antithyroid drug must be discontinued two to four days before treatment to avoid interference with uptake of radioactive iodine. Some physicians resume drug therapy after ten days to hasten the return to euthyroidism, although this approach is not accepted by all. If antithyroid medication is administered too soon, the rate of release of I 131 from the gland may be increased, thus decreasing the therapeutic

effect of the irradiation procedure. The therapeutic effect of radioiodine therapy is gradual; two to three months may be required before hormone production is reduced significantly.

Radioactive iodine also is used to treat metastatic thyroid carcinoma. However, this treatment is usually beneficial only when the lesions have an affinity for iodine (papillary and follicular carcinoma).

Hypothyroidism develops frequently after thyroid irradiation. Thyroid insufficiency may become clinically evident only after several years, and up to 50% of patients who are euthyroid after one year may develop hypothyroidism after five years. Long-term follow-up is necessary to identify these patients.

If a young woman elects irradiation, she should be advised to avoid pregnancy during the next year, since retreatment may be required during that time. Radioiodine therapy is contraindicated during pregnancy.

Surgery: When surgery is used to treat hyperthyroidism, propylthiouracil or methimazole should be used initially to induce euthyroidism. Propranolol also may be given with the antithyroid agent to reduce some of the symptoms. About ten days before surgery, iodine (as Strong Iodine Solution, U.S.P. [Lugol's Solution], potassium iodide, or sodium iodide) usually is added to the regimen to promote involution and decrease vascularity of the thyroid gland, thus reducing the tendency toward excessive bleeding during surgery.

Subtotal thyroidectomy controls a high percentage of patients with hyperthyroidism. The principal drawbacks to surgery, in addition to cost and operative morbidity and mortality, are the subsequent complications that can occur (eg, permanent hypothyroidism, hypoparathyroidism, damage to the recurrent laryngeal nerve) and the propensity for recurrence of hyperthyroidism (5% to 20%). If there is a recurrence, radiation or an antithyroid drug is employed instead of a second surgical procedure because of the higher incidence of complications in subsequent operations. An advantage of surgery is that definitive management of the hyperthyroid condition is obtained within three months (including the preoperative preparatory period).

INDIVIDUAL EVALUATIONS

POTASSIUM IODIDE SOLUTION
SODIUM IODIDE
STRONG IODINE SOLUTION

Iodine is commonly administered as Strong Iodine Solution, U.S.P. or Potassium Iodide Solution, U.S.P.; solutions of sodium iodide also are used occasionally. Iodine is given with an antithyroid drug to prepare hyperthyroid patients for thyroidectomy and to treat thyrotoxic crisis or neonatal thyrotoxicosis. It should not be administered alone.

The adverse effects of iodine administration (iodism) usually include the unpleasant (brassy) taste of iodine and burning in the mouth, sore mouth and throat, hypersalivation, painful sialadenitis, acne and other rashes, diarrhea, and productive cough. In patients with nontoxic nodular goiter, iodide administration may be followed by an increase in plasma thyroid hormones and thyrotoxic symptoms (jodbasedow phenomenon).

Acute poisoning is relatively rare but can occur in markedly sensitive individuals; its onset may be immediate or occur several hours after administration. Angioedema with swelling of the larynx may lead to suffocation. There may be manifestations of serum sickness.

Routes, Usual Dosage, and Preparations. *Oral: Adults and children*, to prepare hyperthyroid patients for thyroidectomy, a common practice is to administer Strong Iodine Solution, U.S.P. (2 to 6 drops three times daily) or Potassium Iodide Solution, U.S.P. (5 drops three times daily) for ten days before surgery.

POTASSIUM IODIDE SOLUTION:
Drug available generically: Solution.

SODIUM IODIDE:
Drug available generically: Crystals; granules (bulk).

STRONG IODINE SOLUTION:
Drug available generically: Solution containing iodine 5% and potassium iodide 10%. Also marketed under the name Lugol's Solution.

Intravenous: For treatment of thyrotoxic crisis, 250 to 500 mg of Sodium Iodide, U.S.P. is given daily in addition to an antithyroid drug and propranolol. Other appropriate agents and procedures are described in the introduction to this section.

SODIUM IODIDE:
Drug available generically: Crystals; powder (bulk); solution 100 mg/ml in 10 ml containers.

PROPYLTHIOURACIL

Propylthiouracil (PTU), the prototype of the antithyroid drugs, is used to manage hyperthyroidism, to prepare hyperthyroid patients for thyroidectomy, and to treat thyrotoxic crisis. It also may be given before or after radioactive iodine is used to treat hyperthyroidism. (See also the introduction to this section.) Propylthiouracil inhibits the synthesis of thyroid hormones within the thyroid gland by preventing the iodination of tyrosine in thyroglobulin. Because it also inhibits the conversion of T_4 to T_3, it is preferred to methimazole in elderly patients, in those with cardiac disease, and in the treatment of thyroid storm. Because it probably crosses the placenta less readily than methimazole, it also is preferred for the treatment of pregnant women. The plasma half-life of propylthiouracil is only 1.5 hours; therefore, frequent administration is necessary, especially initially, to achieve maximal clinical effectiveness.

Granulocytopenia and agranulocytosis, which occur rarely, are the most serious adverse reactions and require immediate cessation of therapy and institution of supportive measures. Most cases are observed during the first two months of treatment, and the incidence gradually declines thereafter. Periodic blood cell counts, although helpful in detecting gradual reductions in the leukocyte level, should not be relied upon to detect agranulocytosis because of the rapidity with which this complication can develop. Patients should be instructed to report the occurrence of sore throat or fever immediately, for these symptoms may signal the development of agranulocytosis. Milder leukopenias appear when doses greater than 400 mg/day are used, but discontinuing therapy or reducing the dose is not necessary if blood cell counts are performed periodically and the leukopenia does not become severe.

Pruritus is common; it can be an adverse reaction or can be caused by the disease itself. Rash, commonly urticarial or papular, is observed in approximately 3% of patients; it can be severe but usually is quite mild. Patients occasionally experience nausea, abdominal discomfort, arthralgia, headache, dizziness, paresthesia, loss of taste, and drowsiness.

ROUTE, USUAL DOSAGE, AND PREPARATIONS. *Oral*: For hyperthyroidism, *adults*, initially, 300 to 600 mg daily in divided doses every six to eight hours; some patients may require as much as 1.2 g daily for initial control. These doses are given until the patient is euthyroid. For maintenance, 100 to 300 mg is given daily in three divided doses. *Children 10 years and over*, initially, 150 to 300 mg daily in divided doses every six hours. The usual maintenance dose is 100 to 300 mg daily divided into two doses at 12-hour intervals. *Children 6 to 10 years*, initially, 50 to 150 mg daily in divided doses every six hours. For neonatal thyrotoxicosis, 10 mg/kg of body weight daily in divided doses.

For preoperative preparation of the thyroidectomy patient, the drug is given to *adults and children* in the same doses used for hyperthyroidism until the patient is euthyroid; iodine is then added to the regimen for ten days before surgery.

For thyrotoxic crisis, *adults*, 600 mg to 1.2 g daily in divided doses; the tablets can be taken orally or crushed and delivered by nasogastric tube. The initial dose is followed in a few hours by administration of iodine. (See the evaluation on the iodine salts.)

Drug available generically: Tablets 50 mg.

METHIMAZOLE

[Tapazole]

Methimazole has the same actions and indications as propylthiouracil (see the introduction to this section and the evaluation on Propylthiouracil). It is approximately ten times more potent than propylthiouracil but has no distinct advantage over it. The onset of action, degree of response, and incidence of adverse reactions depend upon dosage. Cross sensitivity to other thioamide derivatives may occur in susceptible patients.

In general, adverse reactions are similar to those caused by propylthiouracil. There is some indication that agranulocytosis occurs less frequently with methimazole but that the overall incidence of adverse reactions is higher; however, these differences have not been established conclusively.

ROUTE, USUAL DOSAGE, AND PREPARATIONS. *Oral: Adults*, initially, 15 to 60 mg in divided doses every six hours until the patient is euthyroid. For maintenance, 10 to 30 mg is given daily in two or three doses. *Children 6 to 10 years*, initially, 0.4 mg/kg of body weight daily in divided doses every six hours.

For preoperative preparation of the thyroidectomy patient, the drug is given to *adults and children* in the same doses used for hyperthyroidism until the patient is euthyroid; iodine is then added to the regimen for ten days before surgery.

For thyrotoxic crisis, *adults*, 60 to 120 mg daily in divided doses; the tablets are taken orally or crushed and delivered by nasogastric tube. The initial dose is followed in a few hours by the dose of iodine (see the evaluation on the iodine salts).

Tapazole (Lilly). Tablets 5 and 10 mg.

SODIUM IODIDE I 131
[Iodotope I-131, Theriodide-131]

This radioactive isotope of iodine accumulates in the thyroid gland where its ionizing beta radiation destroys the functional and regenerative capacities of thyroid cells within weeks. It also emits gamma radiation which contributes relatively little to its biological activity but is useful in providing an accurate means for determining the amount of uptake.

Radioactive iodine is used to treat hyperthyroidism and carcinoma of the thyroid when uptake of the nuclide is sufficient for treatment. Tracer amounts are also used to evaluate thyroid pathology. These procedures are believed to be virtually without hazard if test doses are small (eg, 1 microcurie in infants and small children, 40 microcuries in adults).

Ablative therapy with radioactive iodine may induce temporary but potentially serious thyrotoxic reactions during the first few days or weeks following therapy; these complications are of special significance in patients with severe thyrotoxic heart disease. The area over the thyroid gland may become tender and painful as a result of radiation thyroiditis, but this usually is alleviated by analgesics. Antithyroid drugs should be discontinued two to four days before administration of radioactive iodine.

Permanent hypothyroidism is a common complication of therapy with radioactive iodine. The incidence is about 10% in the first year, with an increase of approximately 2% to 3% each year following treatment. Since follow-up studies of ten years or longer do not reveal any evidence of a plateau, many patients treated with radioactive iodine eventually will develop hypothyroidism and require replacement therapy with thyroid hormones. Long-term observation is needed to avoid the deleterious effects of unrecognized hypothyroidism. However, since many patients cannot be followed adequately after radioiodine therapy, some clinicians recommend the use of replacement doses of thyroid hormones prior to the advent of hypothyroidism in anticipation of this complication.

If greater than 30 millicuries are administered, appropriate precautions for care of the patient and disposal of body wastes should be observed. Sodium iodide I 131 is contraindicated during pregnancy and nursing.

ROUTE, USUAL DOSAGE, AND PREPARATIONS.
Oral: For treatment of suitable patients with Graves' disease and other types of hyperthyroidism, the usual therapeutic dose is that which results in 40 to 100 microcuries being retained per gram of gland at 24 hours. This can be calculated using an estimate of the weight of the gland and the percentage of uptake in a radioactive iodine uptake test. Further refinements of dosage can be determined (DeGroot and Stanbury, 1975). However, the use of a standard dose of radioiodine (4 to 10 millicuries) is sometimes preferred. If initial treatment is not successful, retreatment after three to four months is usually recommended. Larger doses are required for patients with toxic nodular goiter.

For thyroid carcinoma, 50 millicuries for ablation of normal thyroid tissue; 100 to 150 millicuries is the usual subsequent therapeutic dose for metastases.

For the use of radioactive iodine in diagnostic procedures, see specialty texts.

Iodotope I-131 (Squibb). Capsules 6, 7, 8, 9, and 10 millicuries; solution 1 to 200 millicuries.
Theriodide-131 (Abbott). Capsules 1, 3, and 5 millicuries.

PROPRANOLOL HYDROCHLORIDE
[Inderal]

Propranolol suppresses some of the clinical symptoms of hyperthyroidism, particularly tachycardia, and also palpitations, hyperhidrosis, tremors, nervousness, weakness, spasticity, and hyperreflexia. Although it does not significantly affect total thyroid secretion, administration is followed by decreased serum levels of T3 and increased levels of rT3; this is probably due to inhibition of monodeiodination of T4 by propranolol. Propranolol acts peripherally on the effector organs to control manifestations of hyperthyroidism. This beta-adrenergic blocking agent is preferred to reserpine or guanethidine, which act as general adrenergic blocking agents. The main advantage that propranolol provides is its rapid control of thyrotoxic manifestations.

Propranolol is useful in controlling symptoms during the interval before the effect of antithyroid drugs or radioactive iodine is noted; this may be two or three weeks with antithyroid drugs or as long as three months with radiation therapy. Its adjunctive use prior to thyroidectomy and in neonatal thyrotoxicosis hastens the control of symptoms. When administered intravenously, propranolol also is useful as an adjunct in the treatment of thyrotoxic crisis, but this agent must be administered cautiously. If appropriate, the patient should be digitalized to counteract the decreased myocardial contractility produced by propranolol. The combined effect of increased oxygen requirement and decreased heart rate may precipitate heart failure. Propranolol also should be avoided or used very cautiously in patients with asthma or chronic bronchitis. (See also the section on Drug Therapy.) Abrupt withdrawal of propranolol from hypertensive patients may be followed by symptoms of hyperthyroidism due to increased serum levels of T3, but not T4 or total thyroid hormones, which occur simultaneously with decreased blood levels of propranolol.

Propranolol appears to be better tolerated by hyperthyroid than euthyroid patients. For a discussion of adverse reactions and precautions, see the evaluation in Chapter 35, Antianginal Agents.

ROUTES, USUAL DOSAGE, AND PREPARATIONS. **Oral**: 40 to 240 mg daily in divided doses.
    Inderal (Ayerst). Tablets 10, 20, 40, and 80 mg.
Intravenous: A maximum of 5 mg is administered cautiously at a rate of not more than 1 mg/min. The dose may be repeated, if necessary, in four to six hours; the electrocardiogram should be used to monitor the patient.
    Inderal (Ayerst). Solution 1 mg/ml in 1 ml containers.

Selected References

Bolinger RE: Diseases of thyroid gland, in: *Endocrinology: New Directions in Therapy.* Flushing, NY, Medical Examination Publishing Company, 1977, 7-51.

Committee on Drugs, American Academy of Pediatrics: Treatment of congenital hypothyroidism. *Pediatrics* 62:413-417, 1978.

DeGroot LJ, Stanbury JB: *The Thyroid and Its Diseases*, ed 4. New York, John Wiley & Sons, 1975.

Education Committee, American Thyroid Association: ATA statement on breast cancer and thyroid hormone therapy. *J Pediatr* 90:683-684, 1977.

Evered DC: *Diseases of the Thyroid.* New York, John Wiley & Sons, 1976.

Larsen PR: Hyperthyroidism. *DM* 22:3-30, 1976.

Mestman JH, et al: Hyperthyroidism and pregnancy. *Arch Intern Med* 134:434-439, 1974.

Werner SC, Ingbar SH (eds): *The Thyroid*, ed 4. Hagerstown, Md, Harper and Row, Publishers, 1978.

Antidiuretic Agents | 49

Diabetes Insipidus

Diabetes insipidus is a disorder of water metabolism characterized by polyuria, nocturia, low urine osmolality, polydipsia, and hypernatremia. It is caused by a deficiency of antidiuretic hormone (central diabetes insipidus) or by an inability of the kidney to respond to the hormone (nephrogenic diabetes insipidus).

Antidiuretic hormone (ADH) is synthesized in supraventricular and paraventricular nuclei of the hypothalamus. Granules containing ADH and its carrier protein, neurophysin, are transported down axons that terminate in the median eminence and posterior pituitary. The granules are stored in the terminal bulbs, and their contents are released into the circulation in response to a variety of physiologic stimuli, the most important being an increase in plasma osmolality, a decrease in blood volume, and a fall in blood pressure. Antidiuretic hormone, secreted in this fashion, acts on the collecting ducts of the nephron to increase the reabsorption of water and on smooth muscle to increase contractility. The major physiologic function of ADH is to maintain plasma tonicity and effective blood volume (Moses et al,

1976; Schrier and Berl, 1975; Share, 1974).

Central diabetes insipidus may be idiopathic or familial or may be acquired as the result of head trauma, neurosurgery, neoplasms, infection, granulomatous disease, or other conditions that damage the hypothalamus or posterior pituitary. Depending on the location and extent of the lesion, ADH deficiency may be partial or complete and, under certain circumstances (eg, postoperatively), central diabetes insipidus may be transient.

Primary nephrogenic (vasopressin-resistant) diabetes insipidus is a rare hereditary disorder that most frequently affects males. In this disease, the epithelium of the collecting ducts does not respond to ADH, although the hormone may be present in increased amounts. A syndrome resembling nephrogenic diabetes insipidus may accompany thyrotoxicosis, the nephropathies of hypercalcemia, severe potassium depletion, obstructive uropathy, methoxyflurane toxicity, and the distal tubular form of renal tubular acidosis. Certain drugs, particularly lithium carbonate and demeclocycline, produce a reversible nephrogenic diabetes insipidus

(Moses et al, 1976; Schrier and Berl, 1975).

Only the central form of diabetes insipidus is responsive to hormone replacement. This disorder is treated with preparations containing natural or synthetic ADH (vasopressin, lypressin, desmopressin) or with nonhormonal drugs that promote release of endogenous ADH or enhance its peripheral action (eg, clofibrate, chlorpropamide). Posterior pituitary inhalation powder and injection are rarely used today.

Drug Therapy: Aqueous vasopressin [Pitressin], which is administered by the intramuscular or subcutaneous route, is useful for initiating therapy following hypophysectomy, neurosurgery, or head injuries. Vasopressin tannate in oil [Pitressin Tannate] is effective for long-term therapy in severe disease, but the intramuscular injections (which must be given every one to three days) are inconvenient and painful, and large doses may cause cardiovascular and gastrointestinal reactions and water intoxication. Although better tolerated than the obsolete posterior pituitary powder, lypressin nasal spray [Diapid] has a brief duration of action that may result in episodes of abrupt, severe polyuria. A new synthetic vasopressin analogue, desmopressin acetate [DDAVP], which is also administered by the intranasal route, is long-acting, effective, and devoid of pressor activity and is generally regarded as the agent of choice for treating central diabetes insipidus.

The orally administered nonhormonal agents, clofibrate [Atromid-S] and chlorpropamide [Diabinese], which may be given singly or in combination, are useful in mild to moderate central diabetes insipidus but may not be useful in patients with severe disease. Since effective doses of chlorpropamide may cause marked hypoglycemia, the most satisfactory approach is to initiate therapy with clofibrate and, if the response is inadequate, to then add small doses of chlorpropamide. The tricyclic compound, carbamazepine [Tegretol], also has antidiuretic activity, but is of limited usefulness because of its toxicity. Thiazide diuretics also have a paradoxical antidiuretic action in patients with diabetes insipidus. Thiazides are rarely effective alone in the central form of the disease but are the only agents that have proved useful in the management of nephrogenic diabetes insipidus.

Adverse Reactions and Precautions: Patients with diabetes insipidus who have developed a pattern of excessive water drinking must limit their fluid intake when therapy is initiated because water retention with resultant hyponatremia has been observed with all forms of antidiuretic therapy. When the renal excretion of water is impaired and water intake continues, the extracellular fluid volume expands, diluting solutes. An increase in sodium excretion also may contribute to the hyponatremia. Signs and symptoms of water intoxication (ie, headache, nausea and vomiting, confusion, lethargy, coma, convulsions) occur as a result of movement of fluid from the extracellular into the intracellular space with cellular swelling. Water intoxication is most likely to be observed in patients with hypothalamic dysfunction who lack the ability to recognize water requirements, in those receiving hypotonic fluids intravenously, or in infants who cannot voluntarily adjust their water intake. It is uncommon when the thirst mechanism is intact and water intake can be regulated. Water intoxication is managed by water restriction, temporary withdrawal of the antidiuretic agent, and, occasionally, by the use of hypertonic saline with furosemide. For specific adverse reactions, see the evaluations.

Syndrome of Inappropriate Secretion of Antidiuretic Hormone (SIADH)

Under certain conditions, aberrant production or sustained secretion of ADH may occur despite plasma hypotonicity (syndrome of inappropriate secretion of ADH, SIADH). Aberrant production of ADH is observed most commonly in patients with various neoplasms (particularly oat cell carcinoma of the lung) in which the tumor itself produces ADH. SIADH also may be associated with central nervous system lesions, nonmalignant pulmonary disease, pain, trauma, emotional stress, and various drugs, including nicotine, barbiturates, thiazide diuretics, sulfonylurea-type hypoglycemic drugs, and certain psychotherapeutic, analgesic, and antineoplastic agents.

Alcohol inhibits release of ADH from the posterior pituitary but not from neoplasms and has been suggested as a diagnostic test to determine whether SIADH is due to a tumor. In clinical practice, this procedure has not proved to be of value. Several narcotic antagonists have been demonstrated to be capable of inhibiting the release of ADH from the neurohypophysis and may be of value in treating patients with SIADH of central nervous system origin (Miller, 1975; Miller and Moses, 1977). Lithium and demeclocycline interfere with the action of ADH on the renal tubules and have been used occasionally to induce water diuresis in patients with inappropriate ADH secretion (Bartter, 1973; Moses and Miller, 1974; Schrier and Berl, 1975). Demeclocycline is more effective than lithium (Forrest et al, 1978).

ANTIDIURETIC HORMONE PREPARATIONS

VASOPRESSIN INJECTION
[Pitressin]

VASOPRESSIN TANNATE INJECTION
[Pitressin Tannate]

These preparations are used in central diabetes insipidus; they are not effective in the nephrogenic form of the disease. Vasopressin injection (aqueous vasopressin) has been difficult to obtain because of a shortage of animal pituitary glands from which the crude extract is made. It is now available as a synthetic solution, which is expected to ease the shortage. The units used to describe antidiuretic activity are defined by a pressor assay in anesthetized animals; vasopressin contains 20 pressor units and not more than 1 oxytocic unit per milliliter.

The brief (two to eight hours) antidiuretic effect produced by intramuscular or subcutaneous injection makes aqueous vasopressin suitable for precise control of fluid balance when initiating therapy following hypophysectomy, brain surgery, or trauma, and in acutely ill or unconscious patients with central diabetes insipidus. It has been applied topically to the nasal mucous membranes by cotton pledgets, spray, or dropper, but this route is rarely used today because of the availability of lypressin and desmopressin. Aqueous vasopressin also may be given intramuscularly to evaluate the concentrating capacity of the kidneys. It should not be given intravenously except for emergency treatment of bleeding esophageal varices.

Vasopressin tannate in peanut oil suspension has a longer duration of action (24 to 72 hours) and is useful for long-term therapy in patients with moderate to severe central diabetes insipidus. The antidiuretic effect of a single intramuscular dose lasts one to three days in most patients. Because of this long action, accumulation of antidiuretic effect with excessive water retention is more likely to occur with vasopressin tannate than with other preparations (see the Introduction).

Although the official name for ADH, vasopressin, implies primarily vasoconstrictor activity, only doses much larger than those usually given to treat diabetes insipidus will increase blood pressure. Even large doses elevate the blood pressure only slightly (10 to 20 mm Hg) in normal conscious subjects and this is of brief duration.

Vasopressin may cause significant constriction of the coronary arteries. Angina, electrocardiographic evidence of myocardial ischemia, and myocardial infarction have been reported after injection of 20 units of vasopressin; a latent period of several hours may precede chest pain. Patients with ischemic heart disease should be given no more than the minimal dose of vasopressin needed to control polyuria. If cardiac symptoms occur, desmopressin or an oral antidiuretic agent should be used instead of vasopressin to control polyuria.

Large doses of vasopressin (5 to 20 units) stimulate gastrointestinal smooth muscle and may produce nausea, abdominal cramps, diarrhea, and the urge to defecate. These reactions are more common in women than in men. Uterine cramps also may occur after large doses, and menorrhagia has been reported. Allergic reactions are uncommon but have included urticaria, bronchial constriction, and anaphylaxis; alternative therapy should be selected for patients who have experienced these reactions.

Errors in dosage of vasopressin tannate are common because of the separation of the active principle from the oil vehicle. This can be avoided by warming the vial in the hand or under hot water and shaking the warmed vial vigorously until the brown powder is evenly dispersed in the oil. An absolutely dry syringe should be used for injection.

Repeated injections at the same site may cause a severe local inflammatory reaction requiring surgical drainage. For this reason, it is particularly important to vary the site of injection.

ROUTES, USUAL DOSAGE, AND PREPARATIONS.
VASOPRESSIN INJECTION:
Intramuscular, Subcutaneous: *Adults*, 5 to 10 units (0.25 to 0.5 ml) three or four times daily; *children*, 2.5 to 10 units (0.125 to 0.5 ml) three or four times daily.

> *Pitressin* (Parke, Davis). Solution 20 pressor units/ml in 0.5 and 1 ml containers.

VASOPRESSIN TANNATE INJECTION:
Intramuscular: The vial should be warmed and shaken vigorously before administration and a dry syringe should be used for injection. *Adults*, 2.5 to 5 units (0.5 to 1 ml) and *children*, 1.25 to 2.5 units (0.25 to 0.5 ml), as required. These amounts usually are administered every one to three days when the effect of the previous dose has worn off.

> *Pitressin Tannate* (Parke, Davis). Suspension (in peanut oil) 5 pressor units/ml in 1 ml containers.

DESMOPRESSIN ACETATE
[DDAVP]

$$
\begin{array}{c}
\text{S} - \text{CH}_2\text{CH}_2\text{C} - \text{L-Tyr} \\
\mid \qquad\qquad\quad \mid \\
\text{S} \qquad\qquad\quad \text{L-Phe} \qquad\qquad \text{O} \\
\mid \qquad\qquad\quad \mid \qquad\qquad\quad \parallel \\
\text{L-Cys} - \text{L-Asn} - \text{L-Gln} \qquad \text{CH}_3\text{CO}^- \cdot 3\text{H}_2\text{O} \\
\mid \\
\text{L-Pro} - \text{D-Arg} - \text{Gly} - \overset{+}{\text{NH}}_3
\end{array}
$$

Desmopressin was developed in a search for vasopressin analogues with more specific and prolonged antidiuretic effects.

In comparison with the naturally occurring human hormone, arginine vasopressin, the desmopressin molecule has undergone structural alterations that increased the antidiuretic/pressor ratio from 0.9 to 2,000 and prolonged the duration of action from a maximum of 6 to 20 hours. The long action of desmopressin has been attributed to three factors: slow absorption from the nasal mucosa, persistence in the plasma, and enhanced effects on the kidney.

Desmopressin reduces urine volume, increases urine osmolality, and relieves symptoms of polyuria, nocturia, and polydipsia in adults and children with central diabetes insipidus. It has been used successfully in patients with severe, longstanding disease when other antidiuretics were ineffective or were not tolerated and in those with acute, postoperative symptoms. Although vasopressin tannate in oil has a more prolonged action (one to three days), patients who have previously received this injectable preparation have shown no loss of control when desmopressin was substituted. Desmopressin is considerably longer acting and more effective than lypressin nasal spray. After a single dose, the antidiuretic effect persists for 8 to 20 hours, whereas the duration of action of lypressin is only three to four hours (Cobb et al, 1978; Robinson, 1976).

Desmopressin will probably replace the inconvenient and often poorly tolerated vasopressin tannate for long-term management of severe disease. In some cases, it is a suitable substitute for aqueous vasopressin in controlling acute postoperative symptoms; however, a high percentage of pituitary surgery is now done by the transsphenoidal route, necessitating the placement of nasal packing postoperatively and thus precluding the use of intranasal desmopressin. (An intravenous preparation is currently under investigation for this indication.) Since desmopressin is expensive, it may not completely replace other treatment modalities in central diabetes insipidus, although it does offer advantages over both the short-acting lypressin and the less effective (and sometimes more toxic) oral agents. Like all other antidiuretics except the thiazides, desmopressin is not effective in nephrogenic diabetes insipidus.

A transient (one to two days) reduction in the duration of response to desmopressin has been noted occasionally and may be associated with periods of increased physical activity. Rarely, resistance has developed during prolonged therapy (Cobb et al, 1978). Patients in whom resistance develops may benefit from the addition of an oral antidiuretic agent to the regimen. In the presence of upper respiratory tract infection or allergy, the absorption of desmopressin may be impaired with some loss of antidiuretic effect, but substitution of injectable preparations is not usually necessary.

Related to the use of desmopressin in central diabetes insipidus is its application in the evaluation of renal concentrating capacity. When administered following dehydration, desmopressin will induce a further increase in urine osmolality in patients with central diabetes insipidus and little or no increase in those with nephrogenic diabetes insipidus.

Desmopressin is well tolerated. Large doses may cause transient headaches, nausea, and a slight increase in blood pressure; these symptoms disappear if the dosage is reduced. Nasal congestion, mild abdominal cramps, and vulval pain have occurred rarely. Fluid intake should be adjusted during therapy to avoid hyponatremia and water intoxication; this precaution is particularly important in infants and elderly patients. Undertreatment with occasional polyuria is preferable to overtreatment with water intoxication. Although the safety of desmopressin in pregnancy has not been definitely established, the drug has been given without ill effect to two pregnant women.

Route, Usual Dosage, and Preparations. *Topical (intranasal):* Desmopressin is administered intranasally through a flexible calibrated catheter that the patient fills with the appropriate dosage. One end of the catheter is then inserted into the nose, and the patient blows with a swift puff through the other end so that the solution passes deep into the nasal cavity. The drug can be administered to infants, young children, or obtunded patients by attaching the catheter to an air-filled syringe. Therapy should be initiated with a small dose, and the dosage should be adjusted on the basis of changes in urine volume and osmolality and control of nocturia. The usual *adult* dose is 0.1 ml twice daily (range, 0.1 to 0.4 ml daily as a single dose or divided into two or three doses). For *children 3 months to 12 years*, the usual dosage range is 0.05 to 0.3 ml daily as a single dose or divided into two doses.

DDAVP (Ferring). Solution 0.1 mg/ml in 2.5 ml containers.

LYPRESSIN
[Diapid]

Cys—Tyr—Phe—Gln—Asn—Cys—Pro—Lys—Gly—NH$_2$

Lypressin solution contains synthetic lysine-8-vasopressin, a polypeptide similar to arginine-8-vasopressin, the antidiuretic hormone found in the posterior pituitary of man. The lysine analogue occurs in swine and is more stable chemically than arginine-8-vasopressin. It has an activity of 50 posterior pituitary (pressor) units per milliliter.

Lypressin is rapidly absorbed from the nasal mucosa. It is effective as sole therapy in mild to moderate central diabetes insipidus if administered frequently. In more severe disease, treatment may be complicated by episodes of abrupt, severe polyuria as a result of the short action of lypressin. In these patients, desmopressin or vasopressin tannate gives more satisfactory relief. Lypressin is not effective in the nephrogenic form of diabetes insipidus.

No significant local or systemic reactions have been reported, although hypersensitivity, manifested by a positive skin test, occurs rarely. In the presence of edema of the nasal mucosa, as may occur during an upper respiratory tract infection or as a result of allergy, there may be impaired absorption of lypressin with loss of antidiuretic effect.

Route, Usual Dosage, and Preparations. *Topical (intranasal):* One or more sprays in one or both nostrils. The dosage and

782

interval between applications must be determined individually. Each spray delivers approximately 2 posterior pituitary pressor units, but the exact amount depends upon how vigorously the bottle is squeezed. Four sprays in each nostril provide the maximal amount that can be absorbed at one time without waste. Administration three or four times daily usually is necessary. A bottle commonly lasts five to seven days; if it lasts a shorter or longer period, the patient may not be receiving the proper dosage.

> *Diapid* (Sandoz). Solution (spray) 50 pressor units (0.185 mg)/ml in 8 ml containers. [This product has an expiration date of 36 months.]

ORALLY ADMINISTERED AGENTS WITH ANTIDIURETIC ACTIVITY

CLOFIBRATE
[Atromid-S]

$$Cl-\langle\rangle-OC(CH_3)_2-COCH_2CH_3$$

The hypolipidemic agent, clofibrate, has significant antidiuretic action in patients with mild to moderate central diabetes insipidus (Moses et al, 1973). Daily doses of 2 g reduce urine volume by approximately 50% (Thompson et al, 1977). Clofibrate appears to act by increasing the release of ADH from the neurohypophysis; there is no evidence that it enhances the peripheral action of ADH. Although chlorpropamide may be slightly more effective, clofibrate is usually preferred for initial therapy because of the risk of hypoglycemia with the sulfonylurea. If clofibrate alone does not provide an adequate response, some patients may benefit from the addition of small doses of chlorpropamide to the regimen. Like chlorpropamide, clofibrate is less effective in patients with severe central diabetes insipidus and is ineffective in the nephrogenic form of the disease.

Gastrointestinal disturbances (nausea, vomiting, diarrhea, dyspepsia, and flatulence) are the most common side effects of clofibrate. For other adverse effects, see Chapter 55, Agents Used to Treat Hyperlipidemia.

ROUTE, USUAL DOSAGE, AND PREPARATIONS.
Oral: Adults, 1.5 to 2 g daily.
> *Atromid-S* (Ayerst). Capsules 500 mg.

CHLORPROPAMIDE
[Diabinese]

$$Cl-\langle\rangle-SO_2NHCNHCH_2CH_2CH_3$$

The hypoglycemic agent, chlorpropamide, has an antidiuretic action in many patients with central diabetes insipidus. It is most effective in those with less severe disease in whom, presumably, there are small amounts of circulating or releasable ADH (Miller and Moses, 1970). This observation supports the suggestion that chlorpropamide reduces free-water clearance by increasing the sensitivity of the renal tubular epithelium to otherwise inadequate amounts of endogenous ADH and/or by enhancing the release of ADH. Urinary output is decreased approximately 60% with a daily dose of 250 mg. If an adequate therapeutic response is not obtained with chlorpropamide alone, better control often can be achieved when clofibrate or a thiazide is given concomitantly. Chlorpropamide is not effective in patients with nephrogenic diabetes insipidus.

Chlorpropamide reduces fasting blood glucose levels in patients with diabetes insipidus, and significant, symptomatic hypoglycemia is not uncommon (Thompson et al, 1977). This effect can be minimized by reduction of the dose and addition of another oral antidiuretic agent to the regimen. Hypoglycemic reactions are most common in children, in patients with associated anterior pituitary deficiency, and in those with reduced food intake. Patients should be instructed regarding the importance of not missing meals and, since disulfiram-like effects may occur, on the importance of avoiding alcoholic beverages. The effects of long-term chlorpropamide therapy on the beta cells of the normal pancreas are not known (see also Chapter 47, Agents Used to Regulate Blood Glucose).

ROUTE, USUAL DOSAGE, AND PREPARATIONS. *Oral: Adults,* 250 to 500 mg daily; 125 mg daily may be sufficient when another oral antidiuretic agent is given concomitantly.

Diabinese (Pfizer). Tablets 100 and 250 mg.

THIAZIDE DIURETICS

The thiazide diuretics have a paradoxical antidiuretic action in patients with diabetes insipidus (Earley and Orloff, 1962; Lant and Wilson, 1971). The primary use of the thiazides is in patients with nephrogenic diabetes insipidus, in which they are the only effective agents available. In central diabetes insipidus, thiazides are rarely useful as sole therapy but may be used in conjunction with other oral agents, such as chlorpropamide. The mechanism by which

natriuretic agents reduce free-water clearance in diabetes insipidus appears to involve sodium depletion and contraction of the extracellular fluid volume which increases reabsorption of glomerular filtrate in the proximal tubules, thereby reducing delivery of water to the distal diluting segments of the nephron. Thiazides are not effective unless dietary sodium is restricted. The same oral dosage as that used to control edema is given (see Chapter 39, Diuretics).

Thiazide diuretics are generally well tolerated. Mild asymptomatic hypokalemia, which is common during long-term therapy, can be controlled by addition of a potassium-sparing diuretic to the regimen. Thiazides increase serum uric acid levels and may enhance the hyperuricemia observed in some adults with primary nephrogenic diabetes insipidus. For other adverse effects, see Chapter 39.

Selected References

Bartter FC: Syndrome of inappropriate secretion of antidiuretic hormone (SIADH). *DM*, 1-47, Nov 1973.

Cobb WE, et al: Neurogenic diabetes insipidus: Management with dDAVP (1-desamino-8-D arginine vasopressin). *Ann Intern Med* 88:183-188, 1978.

Earley LE, Orloff J: Mechanism of antidiuresis associated with administration of hydrochlorothiazide to patients with vasopressin-resistant diabetes insipidus. *J Clin Invest* 41:1988-1997, 1962.

Forrest JN, et al: Superiority of demeclocycline over lithium in treatment of chronic syndrome of inappropriate secretion of antidiuretic hormone. *N Engl J Med* 298:173-177, 1978.

Lant AF, Wilson GM: Long-term therapy of diabetes insipidus with oral benzothiadiazine and phthalimidine diuretics. *Clin Sci* 40:497-511, 1971.

Miller M: Inhibition of ADH release in the rat by narcotic antagonists. *Neuroendocrinology* 19:241-251, 1975.

Miller M, Moses AM: Clinical states due to alteration of ADH release and action, in Moses AM, Share L (eds): *Neurohypophysis*, Proceedings of the International Conference on the Neurohypophysis. Basel, S Karger, 1977, 153-166.

Miller M, Moses AM: Mechanism of chlorpropamide action in diabetes insipidus. *J Clin Endocrinol Metab* 30:488-496, 1970.

Moses AM, Miller M: Drug-induced dilutional hyponatremia. *N Engl J Med* 291:1234-1239, 1974.

Moses AM, et al: Pathophysiologic and pharmacologic alterations in release and action of ADH. *Metabolism* 25:697-721, 1976.

Moses AM, et al: Clofibrate-induced antidiuresis. *J Clin Invest* 52:535-542, 1973.

Robinson AG: DDAVP in treatment of central diabetes insipidus. *N Engl J Med* 294:507-511, 1976.

Schrier RW, Berl T: Nonosmolar factors affecting renal water excretion. *N Engl J Med* 292:81-88, 141-145, 1975.

Share L: Blood pressure, blood volume, and release of vasopressin in Knobil E, Sawyer WH (eds): *Handbook of Physiology. IV. The Pituitary Gland and Its Neuroendocrine Control*, part 1. Washington, DC, American Physiological Society, 1974, 243-255.

Thompson P, et al: Comparison of clofibrate and chlorpropamide in vasopressin-responsive diabetes insipidus. *Metabolism* 26:749-762, 1977.

Wales JK: Treatment of diabetes insipidus with carbamazepine. *Lancet* 2:948-951, 1975.

Uterine Stimulants and Relaxants | 50

UTERINE STIMULANTS

Oxytocic agents stimulate contraction of the myometrium and are used to induce labor at term, to induce abortion (therapeutic and elective), to prevent or control postpartum or postabortion hemorrhage, and to assess fetal status in high-risk pregnancies. Drugs used clinically include the neurohypophyseal hormone, oxytocin [Pitocin, Syntocinon], the prostaglandins (carboprost tromethamine [Prostin/M15], dinoprost tromethamine [Prostin F₂ alpha], and dinoprostone [Prostin E₂]), hypertonic saline or urea, and the ergot alkaloids, ergonovine [Ergotrate] and methylergonovine [Methergine]. The choice of agent for a specific use is based upon its oxytocic and other pharmacologic properties.

The myometrium is capable of contraction at any time; however, the integrated effects of various factors involved in the physiologic status of uterine smooth muscle result in a state of relative quiescence throughout most of pregnancy. As pregnancy advances, the myometrium becomes sensitive to contractile stimulation. The myometrium, like other smooth muscle, exhibits spontaneous, repetitive action potentials; however, tension is generated only under conditions of synchronized electrical discharge. Noticeable contractions occur weeks before labor begins and are initially weak uncoordinated events involving few muscle fibers, but eventually the strong, synchronous, propagating contractions characteristic of full-term labor begin.

Physiologic and pharmacologic factors favoring contraction include estrogen, prostaglandins, and oxytocin, as well as stretching of muscle fibers; those favoring quiescence include progesterone and beta-adrenergic stimulation. Progesterone production increases throughout most of pregnancy and is generally responsible for maintaining the uterus in a nonexcitable state. Its possible mechanisms of action include hyperpolarization of the muscle cell membrane; limiting conduction of impulses among cells; and increasing binding of calcium to the sarcoplasmic reticulum in the cell, which reduces the cytoplasmic concentration of calcium available for contractile processes. The muscle fibers of the nonpregnant uterus have a resting membrane potential of -40 mv; during pregnancy, the cells are hyperpolarized (-60 mv). In rabbits and possibly in humans, myometrial cells underlying the placenta are hyperpolarized (resistant to stimulation) compared to other areas of the uterus; this may be due to relatively high local concentrations of progesterone produced by the placenta. As pregnancy progresses, the myometrial area under the placenta becomes proportionately smaller and other factors enhancing excitability become dominant. Estrogen production increases throughout pregnancy and may be partly responsible for this shift in dominance, but high estrogen levels are not obligatory for initiation of labor. Hypertrophy of myometrial muscle fibers during pregnancy results in their being stretched, which stimulates smooth muscle activity and results in the muscle fibers approaching resting length (the length at which maximum tension can be generated with contraction). The stretching of these fibers is also associated with the production of endogenous uterine prostaglandins. Apparently, maternal oxytocin does not play an important role in initiating labor at term. However, surges of secretion increase in frequency during the first stage of labor and reach peak levels at the expulsive phase. The function of endogenous oxytocin, therefore, appears to be to stimulate uterine contraction after expulsion of contents.

During the second trimester, uterine muscle is resistant to stimulation. Large doses of prostaglandins can overcome this resistance and are useful to induce labor at this time. Conversely, the myometrium is relatively resistant to the effects of oxytocin at this stage of pregnancy, and this agent is not effective in inducing labor. The difference in myometrial sensitivity to prostaglandins and oxytocin as pregnancy progresses must ultimately be the result of interaction of these agents with cell membrane receptors, effects on transmembrane ionic fluxes, membrane potential, and intracellular calcium concentrations. It has been shown that the ability to inhibit binding of calcium to sarcoplasmic reticulum in the myometrial cell (increasing cytoplasmic calcium available for contraction) increases 10,000 times for oxytocin and only 100 times for prostaglandins during pregnancy. Also, increasing estrogen production during pregnancy may be partly responsible for increased uterine sensitivity to oxytocin with time, since estrogen increases both the number of binding sites and the affinity of uterine oxytocin receptors.

Although the autonomic nervous system probably is not involved in the initiation of labor, uterine contractions can be influenced by autonomic drugs. Beta-adrenergic drugs inhibit uterine contraction, and drugs such as isoxsuprine and ritodrine (not available in the United States) have been used for this purpose. The beta-adrenergic effect is mediated by increased production of cyclic adenosine monophosphate (cAMP). It is not known if changes in cAMP are required for changes in contractility, however.

Indications

Induction of Term Labor: Labor should be induced only when there is a clear medical indication or other compelling reason, such as patients who live in remote areas and are at risk of delivery outside the hospital. Induction of labor is indicated when continuation of pregnancy represents risks to mother or fetus. Premature rupture of the membranes probably is the most common indication. Others include erythroblastosis fetalis, some instances of antepartum bleeding, and placental insufficiency, which may result from diabetes mellitus, pre-eclampsia, or eclampsia. In these situations, induction of labor before term may reduce maternal and neonatal morbidity and mortality. Except for emergencies, fetal maturity should be determined by ascertaining the pregnancy history, determination of uterine growth and size, and noninvasive testing (ie, serial sonography) for fetal size. Amniocentesis can be utilized to obtain amniotic fluid samples (for determination of lecithin/sphingomyelin ratio and creatinine concentration), but this procedure carries some risk to the fetus and continuation of the pregnancy. The L/S ratio should be at least 2 to ensure fetal lung maturity before induction is attempted. Labor also may be induced in prolonged pregnancies, although this practice is not universal; documentation of postmaturity should be assured. Oxytocin may be used to augment certain types of dysfunctional labor (eg, hypotonic myometrial contractions) except for that caused by cephalopelvic disproportion. Premature induction of labor without a clear medical indication is inexcusable.

Intravenous infusion of oxytocin is preferred to induce or augment labor. Small doses stimulate uterine contractility at term, and the pattern of contraction and relaxation of the uterus approximates that of natural labor. Although studies have shown that intravenously administered dinoprost tromethamine (PGF$_2\alpha$) [Prostin F$_2$ alpha] is similarly effective, its superiority over oxytocin has not been demonstrated. Furthermore, dinoprost may produce more adverse effects (gastrointestinal disturbances, decreased vital capacity, greater incidence of uterine hypertonus, and possible deleterious effects on fetal hemodynamics). It has been suggested that these effects are a function of the rate of increase as well as plasma concentrations of the drug per se. At least some reactions might be avoided by slowly increasing the infusion rate and maintaining the dosage level below 20 mcg/min (Fuchs, 1977; Wildemeersch and Schellen, 1976). An oral preparation of dinoprostone (PGE$_2$) may be useful to induce labor and to prepare an unfavorable cervix before induction, but this dosage form is not available commercially in the United States.

In general, induction of labor should not be attempted in cases of cephalopelvic disproportion; malpresentation; complete placenta previa; uterine scar from previous cesarean section, hysterotomy, or myomectomy; unengaged head; and cervical scarring. Extreme caution should be observed in patients with abruptio placentae, partial placenta previa, and uterine overdistension. In women of high parity, labor should be induced only with great caution because of the risk of uterine rupture.

During induced labor, a physician should be immediately available and the mother and fetus should be monitored continuously using electronic methods or clinical observation to determine fetal and maternal pulse rate, maternal blood pressure, and strength of uterine contractility. If uterine hyperstimulation occurs (hypertonus and abnormally frequent contractions), the uterine stimulant should be withdrawn immediately. Fortunately, both oxytocin and prostaglandins (dinoprost and dinoprostone) have very short plasma half-lives.

Other oxytocic agents are not suitable to induce or augment labor. Quinine and quinidine are unreliable in safe doses, and there is considerable danger of producing eighth nerve damage in the infant. The ergot alkaloids and sparteine sulfate, a plant alkaloid with oxytocic properties, are not satisfactory because they are long-acting and produce excessive, unphysiologic uterine contractions with the attendant potential for causing fetal bradycardia; the latter is no longer available in the United States.

Elective Abortion: Elective abortion should be performed as early in pregnancy as possible, since morbidity and mortality increase with the length of gestation. In general, abortions performed in the *first trimester* are accomplished with some form of suction procedure and, if done within four to six weeks after the last menstrual period (menstrual extraction, minisuction, aspiration abortion), require little or no cervical dilation. As the pregnancy progresses in the first trimester, cervical dilation becomes necessary, but oxytocic drugs usually are not required.

When cervical dilation (with or without concomitant administration of uterine stimulants) is required, laminaria tents may be useful. These sticks of surface-sterile seaweed are placed in the cervical canal, usually 4 to 12 hours before the anticipated procedure. As the sticks absorb fluid and expand, the cervix is gradually and painlessly dilated, usually resulting in less cervical damage than with other mechanical dilatation methods. The dose of oxytocic drugs required is often reduced, and the drug-to-abortion time is sometimes decreased.

For elective abortions in the *second trimester*, instillation of hypertonic saline into the amniotic fluid has been widely used. Recently, intra-amniotic administration of urea and use of prostaglandins by various routes have been employed with greater frequency. Some clinicians prefer dilatation and evacuation (D and E), but this is a major procedure for these relatively late abortions. Each method has advantages and disadvantages, and the ultimate choice may depend largely upon the physician's familiarity and skill with a given procedure, as well as upon factors related to the patient's history. A combination of methods may eventually prove to be most advantageous, and many such regimens have been tried. Evaluation of both single and combination methods is complicated by the wide variety of procedures reported and their lack of standardization. Although combination methods have the potential of maximizing therapeutic effectiveness and minimizing the side effects from each agent, they also carry the risk of complications from untried regimens.

Dilation and evacuation is a relatively rapid procedure that eliminates the necessity of undergoing labor, and it can be performed earlier than instillation techniques requiring amniocentesis, thereby reducing the complications associated with abortion later in pregnancy. Several disadvantages of this procedure, all of which increase with the length of gestation, include the necessity of greater skill and experience of the physician than with other methods and the esthetically unpleasant aspects of crushing and manually removing fetal parts and reconstructing them to ensure complete evacuation. Abortions after dilation and evacuation have been reported to have lower total morbidity rates than procedures using intra-amniotic hypertonic saline or prostaglandins (Cates et al, 1977). However, the conclusions of this study require further verification before they can be accepted unequivocally. Patients were not randomized into treatment groups and the general classification of major side effects, which included events from fever for three days to death, was too broad for accurate interpretation of results. Nevertheless, the study did demonstrate the safe utilization of the D and E procedure by skilled physicians for second-trimester abortions, but not necessarily its superiority.

Hypertonic solutions (usually saline 20% or urea 40% to 50%), instilled intra-amniotically, act as chemical poisons on the placenta and fetus and are effective in terminating second-trimester pregnancies. Instillation requires transabdominal amniocentesis and is usually limited to pregnancies of 16 weeks' gestation (from LMP) or longer when the amniotic cavity is adequate in size.

Hypertonic saline is effective in more than 90% of cases, and the mean abortion time is about 36 hours. Complications include inadvertent myometrial or intravascular injection. The latter results in hypernatremia and disseminated intravascular coagulopathy (DIC), which may be fatal. Intravascular injection may be avoided by not injecting saline into bloody amniotic fluid and not using general anesthetics so the patient can report symptoms of hypernatremia promptly. Hypertonic saline should not be used to induce abortion when the ability to handle a sodium load is compromised (eg, in patients with renal or cardiac failure, hypertension).

Although experience with hypertonic urea is not as extensive, it appears to be less effective but safer than hypertonic saline. Inadvertent intravascular injection does not cause serious complications. The mean abortion time is about 43 hours. Urea can produce dehydration, and coagulation defects have been reported. It should not be used in patients with impaired renal or hepatic function.

Prostaglandins are administered by the intra-amniotic or extra-amniotic (extraovular) routes ($PGF_2\alpha$, dinoprost tromethamine), as a vaginal suppository (PGE_2, dinoprostone), or by intramuscular injection (15-methyl $PGF_2\alpha$, carboprost) to induce second-trimester abortions. Intra-amniotic administration is performed, like saline or urea abortion, by transabdominal amniocentesis; extraovular administration is accomplished by placing a catheter through the cervix and instilling the medication between the fetal membranes and the uterine wall. The intra-amniotic route is preferred because systemic absorption is reduced and thus the incidence of adverse effects is decreased. If the uterus is too small for amniocentesis or if this procedure has failed, extraovular administration can be used, but this technique carries the risk of intrauterine infection caused by insertion of the catheter. The incidence of incomplete abortions is generally higher with the extraovular instillation of dinoprost, and both methods produce more incomplete abortions than saline. The incidence of breast engorgement after use of dinoprost was reported to be higher than after saline abortion or suction curettage. However, the prostaglandins do not carry the increased risk of DIC or hypernatremia.

Another prostaglandin abortifacient, dinoprostone (PGE₂), is administered as vaginal suppositories. It has the advantages of being useful over a wide range of gestational ages, is more convenient than intra-amniotic or extraovular methods, and has a high success rate. It also can be used when other abortion methods fail. The newest prostaglandin abortifacient, carboprost, is longer-acting than other available prostaglandins, is easily administered by intramuscular injection, and also can be used over a wide range of gestational ages. It is particularly useful when other methods of abortion have failed (assuming that ectopic pregnancy and absence of pregnancy have been ruled out) and would be preferable to dinoprostone in cases of profuse vaginal bleeding. However, because of the lower incidence of side effects, dinoprost administered intra-amniotically is probably still the preferred prostaglandin for use as the initial agent to induce labor in abortions when the uterus is large enough to perform amniocentesis.

The mean abortion time with prosta-glandins is about 20 hours, considerbly less than after hypertonic saline or urea. Other long-acting analogues of prostaglandins are being used experimentally as abortifacients and are administered by various routes.

All methods of abortion using prostaglandins have the disadvantages of causing a high incidence of adverse effects (nausea, vomiting, diarrhea) and the possibility of delivering a live fetus. Dinoprost and carboprost are more likely to cause bronchospasm in asthmatic patients than dinoprostone, but the incidence of febrile morbidity is significant with the latter agent.

Oxytocin is sometimes used as an adjunct to other abortifacients to stimulate contractions and shorten the abortion time. Caution must be exercised when such combinations are used because effects are often additive and the incidence of adverse effects (DIC, cervical detachments, and uterine rupture) is increased. Also, when larger doses of oxytocin are used, as in second-trimester abortion, the risk of water intoxication is increased. Therefore, the addition of oxytocin to other abortifacient regimens is best utilized for specific indications (eg, prolonged abortion time, prolonged rupture of membranes, incomplete abortion).

Other combination regimens have been used, and one which appears promising is the intra-amniotic administration of hypertonic urea and dinoprost. This regimen has several advantages: The abortion time is short (16 to 17 hours), similar to that after prostaglandins alone; lower doses of dinoprost (5 or 10 mg total) are effective than when this prostaglandin is used alone, thus reducing gastrointestinal reactions; and administration of hypertonic urea prevents the passage of a live fetus (Wellman and Jacobson, 1976; King et al, 1977).

Other Indications for Induction of Labor: Oxytocic agents also are used to stimulate expulsion of hydatidiform moles. Because the presence of a mole increases the risk of pre-eclampsia, uterine hemorrhage, infection, and choriocarcinoma, removal should be effected promptly on diagnosis. Large doses of oxytocin are required for this indication and the attendant risk of water intoxication is increased. Therefore, other methods are preferable (suction or prostaglandins). Intra-amniotic administration of dinoprost is not suitable because of the lack of fetal membranes and amniotic fluid; administration of the relatively large doses required for intra-amniotic administration may result in high concentrations if the amniotic fluid volume is reduced, and this may cause severe systemic reactions. Extraovular administration of dinoprost can be utilized but, because dinoprostone vaginal suppositories are safe and effective, they may prove to be the best method for stimulating molar expulsion. However, a D and C also should be performed to assure complete evacuation.

Fetal death in utero may be followed closely by spontaneous labor but, in some instances, labor may be delayed. Prolonging such pregnancies increases the risk of DIC. Intra-amniotic instillation of saline increases the potential for this risk even further. Large doses of oxytocin are required as discussed above. Extraovular or intra-amniotic dinoprost sometimes is effective; however, the latter route is impractical if resorption of amniotic fluid has occurred. Dinoprostone vaginal suppositories again are a good noninvasive choice. There has not been enough experience with carboprost to judge its usefulness for this indication.

Oxytocin Challenge Test: This is one of several tests of fetal well-being used in certain high-risk obstetrical patients (eg, those with diabetes mellitus, prolonged pregnancy, pre-eclampsia). It is usually performed weekly during late pregnancy and the method is similar to that employed for induction of labor at term. A dilute solution of oxytocin is infused intravenously, and the dose is doubled every 20 minutes until three contractions are observed every ten minutes. A diagnosis of chronic fetal distress (fetal hypoxia, placental insufficiency) may be inferred if there is late deceleration of fetal heart rate (FHR). If the fetus is mature (L/S greater than 2), a positive test serves as one indication for interruption of pregnancy. However, although a negative finding is usually accurate, the results of one-third of those tests that are positive may be false. Therefore, optimal management requires consideration of other factors (estriol excretion patterns, more detailed assessment of FHR patterns) before the decision to terminate pregnancy is made (Braly and Freeman, 1977).

Postpartum Uses: Oxytocin may be used postpartum to produce firm uterine contractions and decrease uterine bleeding (either after term delivery or following abortion). The need for oxytocic stimulation is enhanced if delivery or abortion was performed under general anesthesia, since this usually decreases spontaneous uterine contractility. It may be most convenient to administer oxytocin by slow intravenous infusion in the immediate postpartum period. Rapid intravenous infusion should be avoided because transient hypotension and increased heart rate may occur; these complications could be life-threatening, particularly in patients who have fixed cardiac output or who are hypotensive as a result of hemorrhage.

Ergot alkaloids (ergonovine [Ergotrate], methylergonovine [Methergine]) also can be used postpartum and usually are administered intramuscularly. These drugs are preferred when sustained action is required, since they are effective for several hours. Oral tablets are sometimes given prophylactically for one or two days to patients who have undergone second-trimester abortion. Ergot alkaloids generally should not be given intravenously because of the danger of producing a transient increase in blood pressure, particularly in hypertensive patients. Methylergonovine has less tendency to cause this complication than ergonovine.

Prostaglandins also have been used postpartum experimentally by intramyometrial or intramuscular injection to reduce blood loss and correct uterine atony.

Stimulation of Milk Let-Down Reflex: The suckling infant stimulates sensory receptors around the nipple, which initiate separate neuroendocrine reflexes that release prolactin from the anterior pituitary and oxytocin from the posterior pituitary. Prolactin is important in the initiation and maintenance of milk production, and oxytocin stimulates myoepithelial cells in the mammary gland which causes milk ejection, commonly termed the milk let-down reflex; oxytocin is not galactopoietic. Milk ejection also can be initiated by psychic stimuli (eg, sight of the infant, hearing the infant cry). Occasionally, when failure of the neuroendocrine reflex is thought to be responsible for ineffective breast feeding, intranasal oxytocin may be useful.

Adverse Reactions

All oxytocic agents are potentially dangerous and patients receiving these drugs must be monitored closely. Their injudicious use may cause injury or death of the mother or infant. Hyperstimulation during labor may progress to uterine tetany with marked impairment of uteroplacental blood flow, uterine rupture, cervical laceration, amniotic fluid embolism, or trauma to the infant (eg, hypoxia, intracranial hemorrhage). See also the previous section and evaluations.

OXYTOCIN

OXYTOCIN
[Pitocin, Syntocinon]

```
         NH2
          |
       Cys — Tyr — Ile
          S          |
          |          |
          S          |
          |          |
       Cys — Asn — Gln
          |
       Pro — Leu — Gly — NH2
```

Oxytocin is the drug of choice to induce labor at term and may be given to augment labor in selected patients with uterine dysfunctional inertia. This agent also may be used in inevitable or incomplete abortion after the 20th week of gestation, although prostaglandins stimulate uterine contraction more effectively during the second trimester. Oxytocin may be given postpartum (after term delivery or abortion) to prevent or control hemorrhage and to correct uterine hypotonicity and also is administered as a test of fetal-placental function in high-risk obstetric patients (oxytocin challenge test). For more information, see the section on Indications.

Oxytocin is a cyclic octapeptide which is synthesized in the cells of the paraventricular nucleus in the hypothalamus. It is weakly bound to neurophysin within granules and is transported in this form down the axons of the hypothalamic neurons to the posterior pituitary gland where it is stored. Oxytocin circulates in the blood as the free peptide and has a plasma half-life between one and six minutes. Inactivation occurs principally in the liver and kidneys. Although animal preparations of oxytocin are active in humans, all of the commercial preparations now available are synthetic.

Oxytocin is recommended for intravenous, intramuscular, and nasal administration. For induction of labor, intravenous infusion is preferred because the dosage can be controlled closely and increased gradually while the patient's response is carefully observed. Intramuscular injections are employed to control postpartum bleeding and uterine hypotonus. Nasal application is used to stimulate the milk let-down reflex.

Hypofibrinogenemia and postpartum bleeding have been observed following use of oxytocin during labor, but these conditions are probably related to the underlying obstetrical problem rather than to the drug. Water intoxication with convulsions, which is caused by the inherent antidiuretic effect of oxytocin, is a serious complication that may occur if large doses (40 to 50 milliunits/min) are infused for long periods. However, this complication should not be a problem at the low concentrations employed to induce labor at term. The potential for development of water intoxication (even with the larger doses used when oxytocin is administered as an adjunct to another abortifacient for second-trimester abortion) can be minimized by administering the intravenous infusion in an electrolyte solution (physiologic saline or Ringer's solution) or in a combination of dextrose 5% and a physiologic electrolyte solution instead of dextrose 5% alone.

Injudicious use of oxytocin may result in uterine rupture, anaphylactoid and other allergic reactions, and maternal death. Induced uterine contractility may cause sinus bradycardia, premature ventricular contractions and other arrhythmias in the fetus, and fetal deaths.

Oxytocin should not be used simultaneously by more than one route. If it is given with another oxytocic agent, caution must be exercised to prevent additive myometrial hypertonia. During induction of labor, the state of uterine contractility, fetal pulse, and maternal pulse and blood pressure should be monitored by clinical or electronic devices. Administration should be discontinued immediately if tetany occurs. A physician should be in constant attendance throughout the induction procedure.

Contraindications for induction of labor are cephalopelvic disproportion; malpresentation; and complete placenta previa. Except in unusual circumstances, labor should not be induced in the presence of uterine scar from previous cesarean section or myomectomy; unengaged head; and cervical scarring.

ROUTES, USUAL DOSAGE, AND PREPARATIONS. *Intravenous Infusion:* For induction of labor, a dilute solution (10 milliunits/ml) is administered, preferably with a constant rate infusion pump (counting drops is less reliable). The infusion is begun at the rate of 1 to 2 milliunits/min and may be increased by 1 to 2 milliunits/min every 15 to 30 minutes until an optimal uterine response (three or four contractions of good quality in ten minutes) is obtained. Physiologic saline or Ringer's solution should be used as the diluent, especially if a faster rate of infusion is used. To induce labor at term, 8 to 10 milliunits/min is usually sufficient. As labor progresses, the dosage required to maintain contractions often decreases. For the oxytocin challenge test, initially, 0.5 milliunits/min is given; the rate is doubled every 20 minutes until there are three contractions/ten minutes (the infusion rate should not exceed 20 milliunits/min).

For prevention of postpartum uterine atony and hemorrhage, 20 to 40 milliunits/ml in an electrolyte solution is given at the rate of 40 milliunits/min or a rate sufficient to control uterine atony. The higher concentration assures adequate dosage of drug without excessive fluid.

Intramuscular: To control postpartum bleeding, 3 to 10 units (0.3 to 1 ml).

Drug available generically: Solution 10 units/ml in 1 ml containers.
Pitocin (Parke, Davis). Solution (aqueous) 5 units in 0.5 ml containers and 10 units/ml in 1 and 10 ml containers.
Syntocinon (Sandoz). Solution (aqueous) 10 units in 1 ml containers.

Topical (nasal spray): To promote milk ejection in breast feeding, one spray into one or both nostrils two to three minutes before nursing.

Syntocinon (Sandoz). Nasal spray 40 units (40,000 milliunits/ml) in 2 and 5 ml containers.

ERGOT ALKALOIDS

ERGONOVINE MALEATE
[Ergotrate Maleate]

METHYLERGONOVINE MALEATE
[Methergine]

These drugs are used after delivery of the placenta to produce firm uterine contractions and decrease uterine bleeding. They can be used for the same indications following suction abortion. Both drugs have a rapid onset of action which varies according to the route of administration (intravenous, 40 seconds; intramuscular, 7 to 8 minutes; oral, 10 minutes). Their usefulness is further enhanced by their prolonged duration of action (several hours).

The adverse effects produced by the two drugs are similar but are more severe after intravenous administration; for this reason, the intramuscular and oral routes are preferred. Intravenous injection commonly produces transient hypertension, which is more prominent in patients with chronic hypertension or pre-eclampsia. Hypertensive episodes may be asymptomatic or associated with nausea, vomiting, blurred vision, headaches, and possibly convulsions and death. The intravenous administration of methylergonovine has less tendency to cause hypertension than ergonovine, but neither agent should be given to patients with hypertension.

Ergot alkaloids should not be used in pregnant patients or to induce labor, because they have a long duration of action and stimulate unphysiologic uterine contractions. They also should not be given to those with a history of hypersensitivity to ergot alkaloids. Both drugs should be administered cautiously to patients with puerperal infection or cardiac, hepatic, renal, or obliterative vascular disease.

ROUTES, USUAL DOSAGE, AND PREPARATIONS. *Intramuscular*: To control uterine hemorrhage, 0.2 mg (1 ml); the dose may be repeated in two to four hours if bleeding is severe.
Intravenous: In emergencies when excessive uterine bleeding has occurred, 0.2 mg (1 ml).

> ERGONOVINE MALEATE:
> Drug available generically: Solution 0.2 mg/ml in 1 ml containers.
> *Ergotrate Maleate* (Lilly). Solution 0.2 mg/ml in 1 ml containers.
> METHYLERGONOVINE MALEATE:
> *Methergine* (Sandoz). Solution 0.2 mg/ml in 1 ml containers.

Oral: 0.2 or 0.4 mg two to four times daily, usually for two days.

> ERGONOVINE MALEATE:
> Drug available generically: Tablets 0.2 mg.
> *Ergotrate Maleate* (Lilly). Tablets 0.2 mg.
> METHYLERGONOVINE MALEATE:
> *Methergine* (Sandoz). Tablets 0.2 mg.

PROSTAGLANDINS

CARBOPROST TROMETHAMINE
[Prostin/M15]

Carboprost (15-methyl $PGF_2\alpha$) is a synthetic analogue of the naturally occurring $PGF_2\alpha$. Addition of a methyl group at C-15 produced a compound with a longer duration of biological activity. This agent stimulates uterine contractions that are similar to those observed during term labor. Carboprost is used to induce abortion between the 13th and 20th week of pregnancy.

In clinical studies, the successful abortion rate was 96%, including 78% complete abortions. Mean time to abortion is about 16 hours and the mean total dose required is 2.6 mg, with a total mean blood loss of 140 ml. Length of time to abortion and total dose administered increased with greater gestational age but decreased with greater gravidity or parity. Incomplete abortions or failures usually can be completed by D and C or suction curettage.

The use of carboprost offers several advantages over other prostaglandin abortifacients. Intramuscular injection of this agent is technically less difficult and is devoid of the potential problems inherent in the invasive intra-amniotic or extraovular techniques. Like dinoprostone, carboprost is easily utilized for abortion of pregnancies in the 13th to 15th week and is not contraindicated if rupture of the membranes occurs. An additional advantage of carboprost is that it can be used without the concern that expulsion of vaginal suppositories may occur in the presence of profuse vaginal bleeding. See also the Introduction.

Adverse effects are common but usually are not serious. Vomiting and diarrhea occur in over 60% of patients, and prophylactic and concurrent administration of antiemetic and antidiarrheal agents is recommended. Fever (greater than 2 F) occurs in over 10% of patients, and care must be taken to differentiate drug-induced pyrexia and that due to endometritis.

Carboprost should not be administered to patients who are hypersensitive to the drug or to those with acute pelvic inflammatory disease or active cardiac, pulmonary, renal, or hepatic disease. Patients with a history of asthma; hypertension; cardiovascular, renal, or hepatic disease; anemia; jaundice; diabetes or epilepsy; or those who have had uterine surgery should be given this drug only with caution. Measures should be taken to ensure complete abortion. Although cervical trauma is unusual, the patient should be examined after abortion.

Abortion induced by carboprost may result in delivery of a live fetus. Because of the teratogenic potential of certain prostaglandins in animals, pregnancy should be terminated by another method if induction of abortion fails with carboprost. Carboprost should be administered only by qualified medical personnel in hospitals with intensive care and surgical facilities.

ROUTE, USUAL DOSAGE, AND PREPARATIONS.
Intramuscular: Initially, 250 mcg is administered deep in the muscle. Subsequent doses of 250 mcg should be administered at intervals of one and one-half to three and one-half hours, depending upon the uterine response. Increments in dosage may be increased to 500 mcg if contractility is inadequate after several 250-mcg doses. The total dose administered should not exceed 12 mg.

   Prostin/M15 (Upjohn). Solution (sterile) 250 mcg in 1 ml containers (distribution limited).

DINOPROST TROMETHAMINE
[Prostin F2 alpha]

Dinoprost tromethamine $(PGF_2\alpha)$ stimulates uterine contractility and is usually given intra-amniotically to induce abortion when the size of the uterus is sufficient and there is an adequate amount of amniotic fluid, usually by the 16th week of gestation; it is injected transabdominally into the amniotic sac. From 60% to 100% are complete abortions (ie, complete passage of fetal products without surgical intervention), and the mean abortion time is approximately 20 hours. Dinoprost is transferred slowly across the fetal membranes and acts directly on the myometrium. Although systemic absorption is lowest with this route of administration, low levels of the drug are found in maternal plasma, which accounts for the adverse effects observed.

The extra-amniotic (extraovular) method of administration is not widely used in the United States. This method requires placement of an indwelling catheter between the uterine wall and the fetal membranes. It probably should be reserved for termination of pregnancies between the 13th and 15th weeks when it is technically difficult to utilize the intra-amniotic method or when amniocentesis has failed. The extraovular technique uses much smaller doses than the intra-amniotic method, but the potential for rapid systemic absorption of the drug is probably greater by this route. Incomplete abortion (usually retention of placenta) occurs more frequently with the extraovular technique and the risk of intrauterine infection is greater because of the presence of a transcervical indwelling catheter.

Oxytocin is sometimes employed as an adjunct to prostaglandins to shorten the abortion time. Since effects are additive, the danger of uterine hyperstimulation is greater. There is no universal agreement on the advisability of this practice; if employed, caution should be exercised.

Several other routes of administration and regimens have been used investigationally. Continuous intravenous infusion, intramuscular and subcutaneous administration, and use of oral or intravaginal tablets and solution-soaked tampons have had variable success but generally have been associated with an unacceptable incidence and degree of adverse effects, which are directly related to the circulating level of prostaglandin. Other investigational uses include induction of labor and stimulation of contractions in early rupture of membranes, missed abortion, intrauterine fetal death, and hydatidiform mole.

Cervical or lower uterine laceration or rupture and retention of the placenta and hemorrhage are the most important dangers associated with use of dinoprost for second-trimester abortion. The former hazard is partially avoided by excluding use of the drug in women with a history of cesarean section, previous hysterotomy, uterine fibroids, or cervical stenosis.

Nausea or vomiting occurs in most patients but can be ameliorated or prevented by administration of antiemetics. Breast engorgement and lactation occur more frequently after use of dinoprost than after other methods of abortion such as suction curettage or intra-amniotic administration of saline and oxytocin. Fever, hypotension and syncope, hypertension, headache, and pain and erythema at the site of injection are noted less frequently. Bronchospasm may be observed in asthmatic patients. Grand mal convulsions probably occur only in patients prone to epilepsy. Vasomotor reactions, arrhythmias, atrioventricular conduction disturbances, hyperventilation, paresthesias and hyperesthesias, chest pain, hiccups, and dysuria have been observed after intrauterine administration.

Inadvertent intravenous administration produces immediate bronchospasm, uterine tetanic contraction, and hypotension or hypertension, which could proceed to shock, severe cramping, vomiting, and diarrhea. Since prostaglandins are metabolized rapidly, reactions seldom last longer than 15 to 30 minutes.

ROUTES, USUAL DOSAGE, AND PREPARATIONS. *Intra-amniotic Instillation*: A spinal needle (No. 18 to 22) is used for transabdominal intra-amniotic tap; 1 or more ml of fluid is removed, and 40 mg (8 ml) of dinoprost tromethamine is injected slowly if the amniotic fluid is not bloody. The first milliliter should be injected over a one- to two-minute period to determine sensitivity and to confirm correct needle placement. If there is an absence or minimal degree of response, a second 10- to 20-mg dose is given after six hours.
Extra-amniotic (Extraovular) Instillation: This route is still investigational. A 14 or 16 Foley catheter with a 30-ml balloon is placed into the lower uterine segment posteriorly in the extraovular space. Suggested dosages include (1) 0.5 mg initially, followed by 0.75 mg every two hours until abortion; (2) 0.25 mg initially, fol-

lowed by 0.75 mg in five minutes, 1 mg in 30 minutes, and 1 mg every six hours until abortion; (3) 0.1 mg/ml infused continuously at the rate of 1 mg/hr; or (4) 5 mg bolus injections every two to three hours until a total dose of 15 mg is given.

Prostin F₂ alpha (Upjohn). Solution 5 mg/ml in 4 and 8 ml containers (distribution limited).

DINOPROSTONE
[Prostin E₂]

Dinoprostone (PGE₂) occurs naturally in mammalian tissues, human seminal plasma, and menstrual fluid. It stimulates uterine contractility and is used clinically to induce labor for the expulsion of uterine products in instances of intrauterine fetal death, missed abortion, hydatidiform mole, or elective abortion. This agent also is useful when uterine perforation has occurred at the time of suction curettage but the uterus has not been evacuated. Uterine contractions are qualitatively similar to those that occur during term labor. Prostaglandins stimulate labor at any time of gestation, but it is preferred that elective abortion be performed before the 20th week of pregnancy. Since large doses of oxytocin (with the attending risk of water intoxication) are necessary to induce labor prior to term, prostaglandins are preferred for midtrimester induction of labor.

Like dinoprost, dinoprostone can induce uterine contractions when administered orally, intramuscularly, intravenously, or intra- and extra-amniotically, but use of these routes is still experimental in this country. Because of its short half-life (less than one minute), large amounts are required to maintain effective drug levels when dinoprostone is given systemically (investigational), and this increases the incidence of adverse effects. Drug action is concentrated at the target tissue with localized administration, and this route has the further advantage of being noninvasive. Vaginal application of dinoprostone induces myometrial contractions that empty the uterus in most cases. It also enhances cervical softening, thus often facilitating cervical dilatation if this is necessary for the completion of the evacuation procedure.

Interruption of pregnancy using dinoprostone can be performed before the 16th week of gestation. This is an advantage over intra-amniotic administration of dinoprost because transabdominal amniocentesis is avoided, earlier abortion is associated with fewer complications, and the emotional effect of delaying elective abortion or evacuation of the fetus in instances of intrauterine death is avoided.

The efficacy of the drug can be judged by several criteria, regardless of the specific abortion indication: treatment success (including both complete and incomplete evacuation), time interval from initiating treatment to abortion, and total dosage required. In complete abortion, there is complete expulsion of embryonic and placental tissues; incomplete abortion indicates that surgical intervention is necessary to completely evacuate uterine contents. When used for elective abortion before the 20th week of pregnancy, there is a 92% success rate, including 74% complete abortions. Mean time to abortion is about 17 hours, and the mean dose required is 90 mg; blood loss averages 170 ml throughout the procedure. When dinoprostone is used to stimulate labor in cases of intrauterine fetal death, the success rate is almost 100% (including 95% to 99% complete abortions, depending upon whether the dead fetus has been retained for longer or shorter than three weeks, respectively), the time to abortion is less (11 hours), and total dosage is lower (about 60 mg). However, average blood loss (200 ml) is slightly higher than in elective abortion. This may be accounted for by coagulation defects and hypofibrinogenemia, which are more likely to occur with retention of a dead fetus. For expulsion of benign hydatidiform mole, an average dose of 70 mg is required, and the time to evacuation varies widely (1 to 80 hours), with a mean of 16 hours. Blood loss averages 645 ml and nearly one-half of patients require blood transfusion.

Adverse reactions are common but are not serious. Gastrointestinal disturbances are reported most frequently and are related to contractile effects on smooth muscle. Vomiting occurs in approximately two-thirds and diarrhea in one-half of patients treated. These symptoms can be alleviated by giving antiemetics and antidiarrheal agents and increasing the interval between doses if this is consistent with adequate therapeutic response. Fever (greater than 2 F), frequently with chills, occurs in up to one-half of patients. Differentiation between drug-induced fever and endometritis pyrexia must be made, particularly in intrauterine fetal death in which there is a greater risk of sepsis. Headache and decreased diastolic blood pressure (mean, 29 mm Hg in elective abortion patients) occur in 10% of patients. Blood loss resulting from the procedure may contribute to the reduced blood pressure. Unlike abortion induced by hypertonic saline, there is no risk of hypernatremia and the incidence of DIC is not increased.

Rupture of the membrane is not a contraindication to continuation of dinoprostone as it is for intra- or extra-amniotic administration of prostaglandins. However, profuse vaginal bleeding may cause expulsion of the suppository. Unlike abortion induced by hypertonic saline or urea in which treatment is usually lethal to the fetus, abortions induced by prostaglandins may result in delivery of a live fetus, particularly with increasing gestational age. When dinoprostone is used to stimulate labor in intrauterine fetal death, confirmation of fetal death should be obtained before treatment is initiated. This agent should not be used in the management of fetal death in utero during the third trimester of pregnancy.

As in spontaneous abortion, appropriate measures (eg, suction, curettage) must be taken to complete uterine evacuation if dinoprostone-induced abortion is incomplete. In animal studies, certain prostaglandins have been shown to have teratogenic potential. Therefore, if treatment with dinoprostone fails to abort the fetus, the pregnancy should be terminated by other means.

Dinoprostone should be used cautiously in patients with cervicitis, infected endocervical lesions, or acute vaginitis and in those with a history of asthma; hypertension or hypotension; cardiovascular, renal, or hepatic disease; anemia; jaundice; diabetes; or epilepsy. It should not be given to patients with acute pelvic inflammatory disease or to those hypersensitive to the drug.

The drug should be administered only by qualified medical personnel in hospitals with intensive care and surgical facilities.

ROUTE, USUAL DOSAGE, AND PREPARATIONS. *Vaginal*: Suppositories must be stored at or below -20 C (-4 F) and brought to room temperature just before use. One 20-mg suppository is inserted high in the vagina, and the patient should remain supine for ten minutes following insertion. Subsequent suppositories are inserted at intervals of three to five hours until abortion occurs. Within this interval, administration time is determined by uterine contractility and patient tolerance. If abortion is incomplete, administration of the drug may be continued to completion if the amount of blood loss is not excessive and the adverse reactions are not severe.

Prostin E₂ (Upjohn). Vaginal suppositories 20 mg (distribution limited).

HYPERTONIC SOLUTION

UREA

A hypertonic solution of urea is used as an alternative to hypertonic saline, dinoprost, dinoprostone, or carboprost to induce second-trimester abortions. Like dinoprost, urea is administered by transabdominal amniocentesis. The abortion time is longer (43 versus 36 hours) but the method is probably safer than saline. Oxytocin is sometimes administered after instillation of urea to shorten the abortion time. A solution of urea and dinoprost has been administered intra-amniotically, and the combination appears to reduce abortion time (16 to 17 hours) and decrease adverse effects from either drug because of the smaller doses employed. However, a combination of urea and oxytocin would be preferable to a method utilizing prostaglandins in patients with a history of asthma or epilepsy. See also the section on Indications.

Urea may cause hyponatremia, hypokalemia, or hyperkalemia. It should not be used in patients with severely impaired renal or hepatic function, intracranial bleeding, or dehydration. Patients should be encouraged to drink fluids and should receive intravenous fluid during the procedure in order to enhance excretion of urea. Nausea, vomiting, and headaches also may occur.

ROUTE, USUAL DOSAGE, AND PREPARATIONS. *Intra-amniotic Instillation*: 80 g of urea is reconstituted to a volume of 135 to 200 ml with 5% dextrose solution to make a 40% to 50% solution. Following amniocentesis with a properly placed needle for aspiration of amniotic fluid, the solution is instilled by gravity via a suitably attached administration set connected to the needle.

Sterile Urea (Abbott). Powder (nonpyrogenic) 40 g in 150 ml single-dose containers. The desired diluent can be added directly to the contents.

UTERINE RELAXANTS

Uterine relaxants are used to delay premature labor until term or until the fetus has matured sufficiently for survival. Corticosteroids (which pass transplacentally to the fetus) may be given concurrently to stimulate production of fetal lung surfactant (see also Chapter 41, Adrenal Corticosteroids). Intravenous alcohol has been most widely used to inhibit premature labor, for it has a direct inhibitory effect on the uterine myometrium. Although alcohol inhibits release of oxytocin from the posterior pituitary gland, this does not appear to be the mechanism of its action since oxytocin is only minimally involved, if at all, in the initiation and early stage of labor. Intravenous alcohol causes inebriation and, if general anesthesia is required for delivery, care must be taken to prevent aspiration of gastric contents, since alcohol is a gastric secretagogue.

A variety of beta-adrenergic agents have

been used experimentally to relax the myometrium, including isoxsuprine [Vasodilan], ritodrine, terbutaline [Brethine, Bricanyl], and salbutamol. Isoxsuprine is used to treat peripheral vascular disorders. Although it is more effective in preventing premature labor than bed rest or alcohol, effective doses cause undesirable cardiovascular side effects (maternal hypotension, maternal and fetal tachycardia). These effects do not necessarily preclude use of the drug, but administration should be closely monitored. Terbutaline is used as a bronchodilator; its administration as a uterine relaxant appears promising but is still experimental. Ritodrine is a more specific beta2 adrenergic stimulant (causing uterine and bronchial relaxation) and produces fewer cardiovascular reactions; it increases the maternal heart rate but has no effect on blood pressure. A transient (up to 48 hours) increase in blood glucose and insulin levels occurs and, in some patients, results of the glucose tolerance test are temporarily elevated. This drug is widely used in several foreign countries and is being tested clinically in the United States. Ritodrine is superior to intravenous alcohol, but studies comparing relative efficacies of the various beta-adrenergic agents are lacking.

Beta-adrenergic agents are usually administered intravenously in individualized doses until contractions are inhibited. After discharge from the hospital, the patient is maintained on oral medication until delivery of a mature infant is assured. If premature labor occurs, the intravenous course of therapy may be repeated.

Magnesium sulfate is given to pre-eclamptic patients to prevent convulsions and it also inhibits uterine contractions, probably by a direct effect on myometrial cells. It is administered intravenously and appears to be more effective than alcohol; in some cases, magnesium sulfate can inhibit premature labor for a week. The drug is generally safe but can cause temporary loss of deep tendon reflexes in the mother and may suppress skeletal muscle activity in the neonate. It should not be used in patients with heart disease or seriously impaired renal function.

Prostaglandins probably play a role in stimulating uterine contractions during normal labor, and their concentrations increase in amniotic fluid and serum during active labor. Prostaglandin inhibitors, particularly indomethacin [Indocin], have been used investigationally to delay preterm labor. Although results are promising, no controlled studies have been reported and these drugs produce undesirable side effects. These include nausea, vomiting, dyspepsia, and rash in the mother; additionally, the theoretical possibility of interference with normal fetal to neonatal cardiovascular transformation exists.

In women at high risk of premature delivery (ie, history of premature deliveries or spontaneous abortions), hydroxyprogesterone caproate [Delalutin] has been reported to be more effective than a placebo in maintaining length of pregnancy. The drug was given prophylactically from the 16th to the 37th week of pregnancy or until delivery if this occurred earlier. Isoxsuprine also was administered intravenously to all patients (control and drug group) who were admitted to the hospital for threatened premature labor.

The effectiveness of relaxant agents is enhanced by initiating therapy immediately after contractions begin. If the membranes rupture, treatment should be discontinued because of the danger of infection. The efficacy of treatment is diminished if the cervix is dilated more than 1 to 3 cm at the start of therapy.

Results have been encouraging with use of all of the above agents in preventing or slowing the progress of premature labor. However, more controlled clinical trials are necessary before the risks and benefits can be adequately assessed. Controlled trials are of particular importance for this indication because of the considerable response to placebo alone. Factors in drug selection for a particular patient and guidelines for the most effective regimens have not been delineated. (See references in Caritis et al, 1979 and Niebyl et al, 1978.)

Selected References

Braly P, Freeman RK: Significance of fetal heart rate reactivity with positive oxytocin challenge test. *Obstet Gynecol* 50:689-693, 1977.

Caritis SN, et al: Pharmacologic inhibition of pre-term labor. *Am J Obstet Gynecol* 133:557-578, 1979.

Cates W Jr, et al: Effect of delay and method choice on risk of abortion morbidity. *Fam Plann Perspect* 9:266-273, 1977.

Fuchs A-R: Prostaglandins, in Fuchs F, Klopper A (eds): *Endocrinology of Pregnancy*, ed 2. Hagerstown, Md, Harper & Row Publishers, 1977, 294-326.

Karim SMM, Amy J-J: Interruption of pregnancy with prostaglandins, in Karim SMM (ed): *Prostaglandins and Reproduction*. Baltimore, University Park Press, 1975, 77-148.

Kawada CY: Techniques of second-trimester abortions. *Clin Obstet Gynecol* 20:833-847, 1977.

King TM, et al: Intra-amniotic urea and prostaglandin F$_2\alpha$ for midtrimester abortion: Clinical and laboratory evaluation. *Am J Obstet Gynecol* 129:817-824, 1977.

Neubardt S, Schulman H: *Techniques of Abortion*, ed 2. Boston, Little, Brown and Company, 1977.

Niebyl JR, et al: Pharmacologic inhibition of premature labor. *Obstet Gynecol Survey* 33:507-515, 1978.

Tepperman HM, et al: Drugs affecting myometrial contractility in pregnancy. *Clin Obstet Gynecol* 20:423-445, 1977.

Wellman L, Jacobson A: Intra-amniotic prostaglandin F$_2\alpha$ and urea for midtrimester abortion. *Fertil Steril* 27:1374-1379, 1976.

Wildemeersch DA, Schellen AMCM: Double-blind trial of prostaglandin F$_2\alpha$ and oxytocin in induction of labour. *Curr Med Res Opin* 4:263-266, 1976.

Replenishers and Regulators of Water and Electrolytes | 51

The rational prescription of water and electrolytes requires understanding of the physiology and pathophysiology of fluid and electrolyte balance and the requirements of the patient. In this chapter, the preparations used in fluid and electrolyte therapy are discussed in broad groups according to major indications, and the discussion is limited to general information on therapy for larger children and adults. For more detailed information, the following references are suggested: MacBryde and Blacklow, 1970; Maxwell and Kleeman, 1972; Mudge and Welt, 1975; and Fox and Nahas, 1970. More specialized references (eg, Winters, 1973) should be consulted for information on therapy in infants and smaller children who are much more vulnerable than adults to fluid and electrolyte imbalances.

When drugs are added to parenteral solutions, possible physical, chemical, and pharmacologic incompatibilities should be considered (see Trissel, 1977); some are well known but more subtle incompatibilities also may occur, for example, the inactivation of buffered penicillin G by parenteral solutions containing vitamin B complex with ascorbic acid. Only one drug at a time should be added to an intravenous solution unless it is known that the drugs are compatible. Incompatible drugs should be given separately.

Abnormal States of Hydration

Because of the dynamic interrelationship between solute and fluid volume control, sodium and water depletion may be considered together. Abnormal states of hydration may be characterized by (1) loss of sodium and water in isotonic proportions, (2) loss of water in excess of sodium, (3) loss of sodium in excess of water, and (4) volume excess.

Isotonic loss of sodium and water (volume depletion) may be caused by vomiting, diarrhea, or hemorrhage. Sodium chloride injection 0.9% or balanced isotonic electrolyte solutions may be used to restore the extracellular fluid volume. Actual fluid losses and changes in weight should be measured, and the patient should be observed carefully for signs of water retention. Serum electrolytes should be monitored and electrolytes added to the infusion as indicated. Whole blood is the only complete replacement therapy when volume depletion is caused by hemorrhage (see Chapter 64, Blood, Blood Components, and Blood Substitutes). For a discussion on the treatment of hypovolemic shock, see Chapter 37, Agents Used to Treat Shock.

Loss of water in excess of sodium may result from inadequate water intake (seen primarily in comatose patients or infants given excessively concentrated foods), hyperhidrosis with no water intake, extensive skin damage from burns, or diabetes insipidus. Initially, it is important to correct hypertonicity by providing fluid without electrolytes or with reduced levels of electrolytes; 5% dextrose injection is recommended for this purpose. If more fluid is needed after normal plasma tonicity has been achieved, sodium chloride injection 0.9% may be infused. Electrolyte levels should be monitored closely. For the treatment of diabetes insipidus, see Chapter 49, Antidiuretic Agents.

Loss of sodium in excess of water may occur when the kidneys are unable to conserve sodium appropriately (diuretic therapy, salt-wasting nephropathies, adrenocortical insufficiency), when there is excessive water retention (syndrome of inappropriate secretion of antidiuretic hormone), or when isotonic or hypotonic losses (eg, gastrointestinal losses, excessive sweating) are replaced by water without sufficient salt.

When the serum sodium concentration is moderately reduced and kidney function is normal, administration of sodium chloride 0.9% is the treatment of choice and is often all that is required to expand the extracellular fluid volume and normalize the serum concentration of sodium. In severe hyponatremia, sodium chloride 3% or 5% may be administered cautiously. When the hyponatremia has been corrected, dehydration may have been corrected only partially; sodium chloride injection 0.9% should then be administered.

Hyponatremia due to adrenocortical insufficiency also should be treated with hormone replacement therapy (see Chapter 41, Adrenal Corticosteroids). Hyponatremia associated with inappropriate secretion of antidiuretic hormone is caused by water retention. In most cases, restriction of water intake will correct the imbalance (see Chapter 49).

Volume excess (edema) is observed in patients with congestive heart failure, nephrotic syndrome, or cirrhosis wih ascites. Drugs used to treat edema are discussed in Chapter 33, Agents Used to Treat Congestive Heart Failure, and Chapter 39, Diuretics. Restriction of dietary sodium is important in the management of this imbalance. Water restriction is necessary only when hyponatremia occurs.

Acid-Base Disturbances

Metabolic Acidosis: Metabolic acidosis accompanied by dehydration may be caused by excess production of lactic acid (lactic acidosis) or ketoacids (ketoacidosis), chronic renal failure, a defect in the ability of the kidney to acidify the urine (renal tubular acidosis), intestinal loss of base, or ingestion of certain drugs or toxins (eg, salicylates, ethylene glycol, methanol, paraldehyde). Treatment of the underlying disease usually corrects the acid-base and fluid derangement. If the plasma bicarbonate level falls below 16 mEq/L or the blood pH below 7.25, an alkalizing agent, preferably sodium bicarbonate, should be given. Tromethamine (tris buffer) [Tham-E] is less effective and more expensive than sodium bicarbonate and is rarely used today.

Metabolic Alkalosis: Metabolic alkalosis with dehydration may result from excessive loss of hydrochloric acid because of vomiting in patients with pyloric obstruction or because of gastric suction. Metabolic alkalosis also occurs in certain endocrine disorders (eg, Cushing's syndrome), in cirrhosis, after vigorous or prolonged diuretic or adrenal corticosteroid therapy, and in the posthypercapneic state. Hypokalemia and/or extracellular volume contraction usually accompanies and accentuates metabolic alkalosis; both renal and extrarenal mechanisms are involved in the hypokalemia.

Providing chloride ion, usually as potassium chloride and/or sodium chloride, is essential in all types of metabolic alkalosis, because plasma bicarbonate levels cannot be reduced unless chloride is made available for reabsorption with sodium in the renal tubules. (Other acidifying agents, such as ammonium chloride, or lysine hydrochloride, are not commonly used today; these agents have been administered with mercurial diuretics to correct hypochloremic alkalosis and thereby prevent a reduction in diuretic effect.) Patients with severe metabolic alkalosis refractory to conventional therapy have been treated successfully by direct infusion of a dilute hydrochloric acid solution through a central venous catheter (Abouna et al, 1974). Concentrations of 0.1 N hydrochloric acid (providing 100 mEq hydrochloride per liter) have been used.

Potassium Imbalances

Hypokalemia: Diuretic therapy is the most common cause of hypokalemia today. The hypokalemia is usually mild and well tolerated. Routine replacement therapy is no longer considered necessary except in high-risk patients, such as those receiving digitalis (see Chapter 39, Diuretics). Other causes of hypokalemia include a grossly inadequate dietary intake of potassium, excessive gastrointestinal losses, increased corticosteroid activity (primary hyperaldosteronism, Cushing's syndrome, or corticosteroid thrapy), and potassium-wasting renal disorders (see also Lindeman, 1976).

When oral replacement therapy is indicated, potassium chloride solution is preferred to other salts of potassium because,

if there is an associated alkalosis, the chloride ion is needed to fully correct both the hypokalemia and the alkalosis. Other salts may be used in the rare instances in which hypokalemia is associated with hyperchloremia (eg, renal tubular acidosis), but there is little evidence that any of these preparations is tolerated better than potassium chloride. Since potassium supplements are not retained well in patients receiving diuretics (Down et al, 1972), large doses may be required (Schwartz and Swartz, 1974). Potassium-sparing diuretics are more effective and may be preferred in high-risk patients. (See Chapter 39, Diuretics.)

If correction is indicated in patients unable to take potassium orally, potassium chloride is given intravenously. The electrocardiogram should be checked frequently, because hyperkalemia can be detected more rapidly by changes in the electrocardiogram than by measuring serum potassium levels. An adequate urinary output also must be assured.

Hyperkalemia: Hyperkalemia is usually the result of impaired potassium excretion in patients with decreased renal function and is particularly prevalent in those taking large amounts of potassium or potassium-sparing diuretics. It also may be caused by rapid intravenous administration of potassium-containing solutions or by shift of potassium out of the cells (eg, acidosis, tissue breakdown). (See Whang, 1976, for other causes.)

The measures used for treatment depend upon the degree of hyperkalemia and the severity of its manifestations. In all cases, potassium intake should be discontinued. When the electrocardiogram is distinctly abnormal (eg, absence of P-wave, widening of QRS complex) or the serum potassium rises rapidly to a level above 6.5 mEq/L, the intravenous infusion of an alkaline sodium solution, usually sodium bicarbonate 7.5%, is indicated. Sodium bicarbonate reduces the serum potassium level by causing potassium to shift into cells. In patients with hyponatremia and volume contraction, sodium chloride may be preferred for replacement therapy because it also counteracts the cardiotoxic effect of potassium; a hypertonic solution may be indicated in patients with severe hyponatremia. Intravenous infusion of dextrose plus insulin (15 units) regular insulin for every 50 g of dextrose) also causes a shift of potassium into cells, although less rapidly than sodium bicarbonate. The dextrose and insulin may be given with sodium bicarbonate.

If the patient is not receiving digitalis, it is also advisable to inject calcium gluconate intravenously (5 to 10 ml of a 10% solution over a two-minute period) to overcome the cardiotoxicity of potassium. The electrocardiogram should be monitored constantly. If electrocardiographic abnormalities continue, injections of sodium bicarbonate and calcium gluconate given separately (the latter in doses of 1 g [10 ml]) may be repeated at one- to two-minute intervals. An exchange resin (eg, sodium polystyrene sulfonate [Kayexalate]) should be given orally or rectally to promote gastrointestinal loss of potassium when continued therapy is indicated (Rovner, 1972; Whang, 1976). In oliguric patients, hemodialysis or peritoneal dialysis may be indicated to remove large amounts of potassium from the blood.

Magnesium Imbalances

Hypomagnesemia: Hypomagnesemia may accompany malabsorption, prolonged diarrhea, prolonged intravenous feeding without magnesium, chronic alcoholism, renal tubular damage, and other disorders associated with hypocalcemia or hypokalemia. Magnesium sulfate may be given parenterally for treatment. Magnesium (as the acetate or chloride) also is included as an essential cation in multiple electrolyte solutions to prevent iatrogenic deficiency during routine fluid and electrolyte therapy. It should be administered cautiously if renal function is impaired.

Hypermagnesemia: Most patients can tolerate moderately elevated plasma levels of magnesium, but toxicity may occur with prolonged administration of magnesium (eg, in antacid preparations) in patients with severe renal impairment. In such patients, hypermagnesemia may result in nausea, vomiting, hypotension, and depression of the central nervous system and the neuromuscular junctions. Occasionally, third-degree atrioventricular block and respiratory arrest occur. The administration of calcium salts counteracts the respiratory effects to some extent. Dialysis is indicated in severe hypermagnesemia with coexistent renal insufficiency.

Ammonia Imbalance

Portal systemic encephalopathy is a metabolic disorder of the central nervous system which occurs most commonly as a complication of advanced hepatic cirrhosis. It is usually associated with an elevation in the blood ammonia level due to the entry of portal blood into the systemic circulation through collateral vessels, intrahepatic communications, or surgical shunts. Measures that reduce the blood ammonia level are basic to treatment and prevention of recurrences.

The blood ammonia concentration may be reduced by use of laxatives and enemas, which increase the excretion of ammonia. The formation of ammonia is decreased by restricting dietary protein and preventing gastrointestinal bleeding (a common cause of encephalopathy). The major drugs used to manage portal systemic encephalopathy are neomycin, a poorly absorbed antibiotic that decreases production of ammonia, and lactulose [Cephulac], a synthetic disaccharide that may decrease ammonia production or absorption and/or enhance its excretion (Avery et al, 1972; Schenker et al, 1974). Neomycin may have a more rapid onset of action but lactulose is less toxic and is, therefore, more suitable for prolonged maintenance therapy. In selected patients, a combination of lactulose and neomycin may be more effective than either drug used alone.

AGENTS USED IN ABNORMAL STATES OF HYDRATION

Sodium chloride injection or dextrose injection, in different strengths and combinations, may be used to treat most states of abnormal hydration. Other solutions have been developed for balanced maintenance or replacement of fluid and electrolytes. In addition to sodium and chloride, these solutions provide potassium, magnesium, and bicarbonate precursors such as acetate. A partial list of the available formulations appears in the Table at the end of this chapter.

SODIUM CHLORIDE

SODIUM CHLORIDE INJECTION

Sodium chloride is used to correct extracellular volume depletion. It should be administered orally for replacement therapy whenever possible. A solution containing 3 to 4 g of sodium chloride and 1.5 to 3 g of sodium bicarbonate/L is satisfactory for oral use.

Isotonic sodium chloride injection is a 0.9% solution containing 154 mEq sodium and 154 mEq chloride/L. (In comparison, plasma contains 137 to 147 mEq sodium and 98 to 106 mEq chloride/L.) Concentrations of 0.11% to 0.45% are hypotonic and concentrations of 3% and 5% are hypertonic. The concentration and tonicity of sodium chloride solutions determine their usefulness in different disorders.

Sodium chloride injection 0.9% is infused when sodium and water have been depleted in isotonic proportions. It may be used to maintain effective extracellular fluid volume and a stable circulation during and after surgery in patients with normal cardiovascular and renal function and to postpone the need for blood transfusions by temporarily maintaining plasma volume in emergencies. Hypertonic sodium chloride injection should be reserved for treatment of severe symptomatic hyponatremia and should be used only during the critical phase. Hypotonic solutions generally are given with dextrose for maintenance therapy in patients who are unable to take fluid and nutrients orally for one to three days.

Sodium chloride must be infused with utmost caution, particularly in patients with congestive heart failure, circulatory insufficiency, renal failure, or hypoproteinemia. Signs and symptoms of sodium excess include lethargy, muscle weakness, tremors, seizures, coma, and increased blood urea nitrogen levels. Hypertonic solutions should be given slowly and cautiously in small volumes (200 to 400 ml) because of the danger of hypervolemia due to movement of water from the intracellular to the extracellular compartment. Central venous pressure should be monitored. Overreplacement of extracellular fluid with sodium chloride injection may lead to pulmonary and peripheral edema.

PREPARATIONS.
See Table.

BALANCED ELECTROLYTE INJECTION

RINGER'S LACTATE

The indications for these hypotonic and isotonic electrolyte formulations are similar to those for sodium chloride injection 0.45% and 0.9%. Although these solutions more closely approximate normal extracellular electrolyte concentrations, it may be necessary to add additional electrolytes to meet the specific needs of the patient (eg, to correct acidosis, alkalosis, or deficits of individual electrolytes). These solutions are not indicated to replace blood or plasma expanders when the latter are indicated, except to temporarily maintain the plasma volume in emergencies.

PREPARATIONS.
See Table.

DEXTROSE

DEXTROSE INJECTION

DEXTROSE AND SODIUM CHLORIDE INJECTION

Dextrose is administered intravenously to provide nutriment and water when oral feeding is not feasible. It usually is administered as a 5% aqueous infusion, which is slightly hypotonic compared with blood and provides about 170 calories/L. Dextrose 5% or sodium chloride 0.11% to 0.45% with dextrose 5% in water may be used for intravenous therapy when there has been a loss of water in excess of sodium. Solutions containing 10% dextrose provide more nutriment in less volume, but this concentration may be irritating to the veins. A solution containing 20% to 50% dextrose (often with insulin added) is used to cause potassium to shift into cells. Hypertonic dextrose is infused in a high-flow vein to provide calories in total parenteral nutrition (TPN). (See Chapter 53, Parenteral and Enteral Nutrition.)

The rate of utilization of dextrose varies considerably. As an approximate guide, however, the average maximal rate is 800 mg/kg of body weight/hr (16 ml/kg/hr of 5% injection). If the patient's capacity to utilize dextrose is exceeded, hyperglycemia, glycosuria, and excessive diuresis will occur.

Subcutaneous administration of dextrose is very undesirable because solutions are irritating, temporarily cause leaching of extracellular water and electrolytes, and may distend tissue and lead to necrosis. Dextrose injection should not be used as a diluent for blood because it causes clumping of red blood cells and, possibly, hemolysis.

PREPARATIONS.
DEXTROSE:
Solution 2.5%, 5%, 10%, 20%, 40%, 50%, 60%, and 70% (Abbott, Cutter, McGaw, Travenol); 7.7% (McGaw); 25% (Cutter); 5% with alcohol 5% (Abbott, Cutter, McGaw, Travenol); 5% with alcohol 10% (McGaw).
DEXTROSE AND SODIUM CHLORIDE INJECTION:
See Table.

FRUCTOSE

FRUCTOSE INJECTION

FRUCTOSE AND SODIUM CHLORIDE INJECTION

INVERT SUGAR INJECTION (containing equal parts of dextrose and fructose)

Fructose offers no advantages and some disadvantages over dextrose injection. It may increase serum levels of lactate and urate if given rapidly, and it is considerably more expensive than dextrose. Infusion of fructose has been associated with increased production of uric acid and hyperuricemia. In patients with hereditary fructose intolerance (aldolase deficiency), fructose can cause severe reactions (hypoglycemia, nausea, vomiting, tremors, coma, convulsions) and is contraindicated.

AGENTS USED IN ACID-BASE DISTURBANCES

SODIUM BICARBONATE

Sodium bicarbonate is the drug of choice in the treatment of metabolic acidosis. In acute mild to moderate acidosis, oral treatment is preferable to intravenous therapy; tablets, a 2% to 5% solution, or a solution containing sodium bicarbonate 0.15% to 0.3% and sodium chloride 0.3% to 0.4% may be used. In severe acute acidosis, the drug may be given intravenously. Commercially available bicarbonate solutions are generally hypertonic and require dilution.

Administration of excessive amounts may cause metabolic alkalosis. Sodium bicarbonate should be given cautiously to patients with congestive heart failure or other edematous or sodium-retaining conditions, as well as in those with oliguria or anuria. Sodium bicarbonate should be avoided in patients who have lost large amounts of chloride as a result of vomiting or continuous gastrointestinal suction or in those receiving diuretics known to produce hypochloremic alkalosis.

PREPARATIONS.
See Table.

SODIUM LACTATE

Sodium lactate is metabolized to sodium bicarbonate in the liver and has been used to treat metabolic acidosis. Sodium bicarbonate is preferred for this purpose, however, because the conversion of lactate to bicarbonate may be impaired in severely ill patients and those with hepatic disease.

PREPARATIONS.
See Table.

SODIUM ACETATE

Sodium acetate is often used in total parenteral nutrition as a bicarbonate precursor. Acetate is converted to bicarbonate on almost an equimolar basis. It is readily metabolized outside the liver and its conversion is not impaired in severely ill patients or those with hepatic disease.

PREPARATIONS.
See Table.

AGENTS USED IN POTASSIUM IMBALANCES

POTASSIUM CHLORIDE

Since hypokalemia is usually accompanied by a hypochloremic alkalosis, potassium chloride is the agent of choice for treatment. It is used to counteract the potassium-wasting effect of thiazide and loop diuretics in patients at risk from hypokalemia, such as digitalized or cirrhotic patients (see Chapter 39, Diuretics). In addition, it may be indicated in those with inadequate dietary intake of potassium, excessive gastrointestinal losses, potassium-wasting nephropathy, primary adrenal disease, or in those receiving corticosteroids. Potassium chloride also is used to treat digitalis intoxication and hypokalemic periodic paralysis.

The liquid form of potassium chloride is the preparation of choice for oral therapy. Most commercial preparations contain 10 to 40 mEq of potassium chloride per 15 ml and have been flavored to mask the disagreeable taste. Such preparations *must be diluted* before ingestion to minimize gastric irritation, and administration after meals also is advisable. Slow-release tablets [Slow-K, Kaon-Cl] should be used only when potassium chloride solution is not tolerated.

The intravenous route is indicated in emergencies or when patients cannot take drugs orally. The electrocardiogram and serum potassium concentration should be checked frequently, and adequate urinary output must be assured. Concentrated potassium chloride solutions may cause pain if injected into a small vein.

Uncoated potassium chloride tablets may cause gastric irritation and should not be used. Enteric-coated tablets (sometimes formulated with a thiazide diuretic) also should not be used because they may cause small bowel ulceration and their rate of absorption is undependable. Although slow-release tablets appear to be safer than enteric-coated preparations, they occasionally have caused small bowel lesions, esophageal ulceration and stricture, and perforation of gastric ulcer.

Potassium preparations should be given very cautiously to patients with impaired renal function, for severe hyperkalemia may occur. Potassium supplements are particularly dangerous in patients who are also receiving potassium-sparing diuretics.

ROUTES, USUAL DOSAGE, AND PREPARATIONS.
Oral: Adults, 10 to 15 mEq three or four times daily. Patients receiving diuretics may require 80 to 100 mEq daily.

Drug available generically: Liquid 5%, 10%, and 20%.
AVAILABLE TRADEMARKS
Kay Ciel Elixir and Powder (Berlex), *K-Lor* (Abbott), *Klorvess 10% Liquid* (Dorsey), *K-Lyte/Cl* (Mead Johnson), *Kaochlor, Kaochlor S-F Liquid* (Warren-Teed), *Kato* (Ingram).
SLOW-RELEASE PREPARATIONS.
Slow-K (Ciba). Each tablet contains 600 mg equivalent to 8 mEq potassium chloride in a wax matrix.
Kaon-Cl (Warren-Teed). Each tablet contains 500 mg equivalent to 6.67 mEq potassium chloride in a wax matrix.
AVAILABLE MIXTURES OF POTASSIUM CHLORIDE WITH OTHER POTASSIUM SALTS.
Kaochlor-Eff (Warren-Teed). Effervescent tablets containing potassium chloride, potassium citrate, potassium bicarbonate, and betaine hydrochloride.
Klorvess Effervescent (Dorsey). Tablets containing potassium chloride, potassium bicarbonate, and *L*-lysine monohydrochloride.

Intravenous: Potassium chloride injection must be diluted before infusion. *Adults,* if serum potassium is greater than 2.5 mEq/L, neuromuscular and cardiac abnormalities are minimal, and renal function is not impaired, potassium is given in concentrations usually no greater than 40 mEq/L at a rate not exceeding 10 to 15 mEq/hr. The total dosage usually should not exceed 100 to 300 mEq/day. If the serum potassium level is less than 2 mEq/L in the presence of cardiovascular abnormalities or muscle paralysis, potassium may be given very cautiously in concentrations as high as 60 mEq/L at a rate of up to 40 mEq/hr. Total dosage usually should not exceed 400 mEq/day. Infusions must be regulated carefully on the basis of results of continuous electrocardiographic monitoring and repeated serum and urinary potassium determinations.

> Drug available generically: Solutions of 1.5 to 3.2 mEq/ml are available in 5, 10, 12.5, and 20 ml containers to supply 10 to 40 mEq/container. Also available are mixed large volume parenteral containers of 5% dextrose in water or 0.22% and 0.45% sodium chloride with 10, 20, 30, or 40 mEq of potassium chloride. (See Table.)

POTASSIUM BICARBONATE AND CITRATE
[K-Lyte]

POTASSIUM GLUCONATE
[Kaon]

POTASSIUM TRIPLEX

These preparations are used to treat hypokalemia associated with hyperchloremia (eg, renal tubular acidosis). If they are used in patients with hypokalemic hypochloremic alkalosis, a source of chloride ion must be provided. There is no convincing evidence that any of these products is better tolerated than potassium chloride.

ROUTE, USUAL DOSAGE, AND PREPARATIONS.
POTASSIUM BICARBONATE AND CITRATE:
Oral: *Adults*, one tablet dissolved in 90 to 120 ml of cold water two to four times daily with meals.

> *K-Lyte* (Mead Johnson). Tablets (for solution) containing potassium bicarbonate 2.5 g and citric acid 2.1 g; each tablet supplies 25 mEq of potassium as bicarbonate and citrate.

POTASSIUM GLUCONATE:
Oral: *Adults*, 15 ml of liquid preparation in 1 oz or more of water or fruit juice two or four times daily after meals or two tablets four times a day after meals and at bedtime.

> Drug available generically: Elixir 20 mEq/15 ml.
> *Kaon* (Warren-Teed). Elixir containing 4.68 g (20 mEq elemental potassium)/15 ml with saccharin (alcohol 5%).

POTASSIUM TRIPLEX:
Oral: *Adults*, 5 ml in fruit juice or water three or four times daily after meals.

> *Potassium Triplex* (Lilly). Liquid containing potassium acetate, potassium bicarbonate, and potassium citrate each in 10% concentration; this supplies approximately 15 mEq of elemental potassium/5 ml.

SODIUM POLYSTYRENE SULFONATE
[Kayexalate]

This exchange resin is used occasionally to treat hyperkalemia. It acts by exchanging sodium ion for potassium in the intestine; the potassium-containing resin is then excreted. In clinical use, much of the exchange capacity is utilized for other cations and possibly lipids and proteins; therefore, in vivo exchange of potassium is estimated to be about 0.5 to 1 mEq of potassium per gram of resin. Because its action is not evident for 2 to 24 hours, sodium polystyrene sulfonate is most useful when serum potassium levels are not life-threatening or when other measures have reduced the immediate danger of hyperkalemia.

Adverse reactions include anorexia, nausea, vomiting, hypokalemia, hypocalcemia, and constipation. Serum potassium levels should be determined daily during therapy, and administration should be discontinued or the dose reduced when the level falls to 4 or 5 mEq/L. Sodium polystyrene sulfonate should be used with caution in patients receiving digitalis preparations, since hypokalemia enhances digitalis toxicity. Because fecal impaction may occur when the drug is given orally, a mild laxative (usually sorbital) should be given concomitantly.

Sodium polystyrene sulfonate should be used cautiously in patients requiring salt restriction, since volume overload may occur. Because of this problem, calcium and hydrogen ion exchange resins have been used on an experimental basis, but the former may cause hypercalcemia and the latter acidosis.

ROUTES, USUAL DOSAGE, AND PREPARATIONS.
Oral administration is preferred to rectal use because enemas are not as reliable and often are difficult to recover unless the resin is placed in a dialysis bag.
Oral: *Adults*, 15 g (suspended in 45 to 60 ml of water, syrup, fruit juice, or a soft drink) one to four times daily. The preparation may be given by stomach tube. To prevent constipation, 10 to 20 ml of 70% sorbital is given every two to three hours.
Rectal: *Adults*, 30 to 50 g suspended in 100 ml of aqueous vehicle, such as sorbital, is

given every six hours initially; the frequency of administration may be decreased on succeeding days. The preparation should be retained as long as possible and should be followed by use of a cleansing enema. Some authorities believe that the preferred method of rectal administration is to place the drug in a sealed dialysis bag which is inserted into the rectum.

Kayexalate (Breon). Powder 453.6 g [sodium content: 100 mg/g].

AGENT USED IN HYPOMAGNESEMIA

MAGNESIUM SULFATE INJECTION

Magnesium sulfate is used to treat severe hypomagnesemia, to prevent hypomagnesemia in total parenteral nutrition (TPN), and as a central nervous system depressant in convulsive states, especially in eclampsia, although other effective drugs are available for the latter purpose. When administered orally, it acts as a cathartic. The duration of action of an intramuscular dose is several hours; intravenous doses last only 30 minutes.

Overdosage can cause depression of the central nervous system, respiration, and heart rate. A calcium salt should be available for intravenous injection to counteract the potential hazard of magnesium intoxication. Magnesium sulfate interacts with succinylcholine and possibly other neuromuscular blocking agents. Additive effects may occur if it is administered with barbiturates or other drugs that depress the central nervous system. Magnesium should be given cautiously to patients with impaired renal function and those receiving digitalis. It is contraindicated in patients with heart block.

ROUTES, USUAL DOSAGE, AND PREPARATIONS. *Intramuscular, Intravenous*: *Adults and older children*, for severe hypomagnesemia, 2 to 4 g (4 to 8 ml of 50% solution or 16 to 32 mEq) daily intramuscularly in divided doses; administration is repeated daily until serum levels have returned to normal. If the deficiency is not severe, 1 g (2 ml of 50% solution) can be given once or twice daily. Serum magnesium levels

should serve as a guide to continued dosage. Magnesium sulfate also may be given intravenously in a 10% solution infused at a rate not exceeding 1.5 ml/min. It also may be added to TPN solution (see Chapter 53, Parenteral and Enteral Nutrition).

As an anticonvulsant, 1 g is given either intravenously as a 10% solution or intramuscularly as a 25% to 50% solution. For eclampsia, 4 g of the initial dose (which varies from 8 g for a 100-lb patient to 15 g for a 200-lb patient) is given intravenously with 250 ml of dextrose injection 5% in water; the remainder is given intramuscularly. Dosage for the subsequent 24 hours is based upon the blood level and urinary excretion of magnesium resulting from the initial dose. It will be approximately 65% of the initial dose every six hours. Dosage for subsequent days should be sufficient to replace magnesium excreted in the urine.

Drug available generically: Solution 10%, 12.5%, 25%, and 50%.

AGENTS USED IN HYPERAMMONEMIA

LACTULOSE
[Cephulac]

Lactulose is a poorly absorbed, synthetic disaccharide prepared from lactose. It is not metabolized in the upper intestinal tract, because the small intestine of man contains no disaccharidase capable of splitting it into its component monosaccharides. In the colon, lactulose is degraded by intestinal bacteria into low molecular weight organic acids which decrease the pH of the colonic contents and have an osmotic laxative action. Lactulose reduces blood ammonia levels. It may act by "trapping and dumping" ammonium ion, by serving as a bacterial substrate, or by decreasing colonic transit time, thereby reducing ammonia production.

Lactulose has been used primarily for long-term therapy to prevent recurrences of portal systemic encephalopathy and to improve protein tolerance in patients with advanced hepatic cirrhosis. It reduces the frequency and severity of recurrent episodes in approximately three-fourths of patients and usually permits an increase in protein intake and withdrawal of neomycin. Improvement may be noted within one to three days after beginning therapy, but maximal benefits may not be evident for 10 to 14 days. Lactulose also has been used orally to control acute attacks of encephalopathy, but it has a relatively slow onset of action. Administration by retention enema produces a more rapid (within 12 hours) response; when given by this route, the beneficial effect may be due to the low pH of the solution (Kersh and Rifkin, 1973).

Therapeutic doses of lactulose may cause abdominal distention and discomfort, flatulence, anorexia, nausea, and vomiting. Diarrhea, which indicates overdosage, may produce dehydration, hypernatremia, and prerenal azotemia when fluid intake is severely restricted. Diarrhea also may induce or intensify hypokalemia and thereby decrease the therapeutic response. The diarrhea can be controlled by reducing the dose.

ROUTE, USUAL DOSAGE, AND PREPARATIONS.
Oral: *Adults*, 30 to 45 ml three or four times daily. Dosage should be adjusted every day or two to produce two or three soft stools daily. If lactulose is used for initial therapy of an acute attack of portal systemic encephalopathy, 30 to 45 ml should be given hourly initially; when laxation occurs, the frequency may be reduced to three or four times daily.

Cephulac (Merrell-National). Solution 10 g/15 ml.

NEOMYCIN SULFATE
[Mycifradin Sulfate, Neobiotic]

This aminoglycoside antibiotic is poorly absorbed from the gastrointestinal tract. When given orally, neomycin reduces elevated blood ammonia levels in patients with portal systemic encephalopathy, presumably by destroying some of the intestinal bacteria that generate ammonia. In acute exacerbations, neomycin may act more rapidly than lactulose, but the latter is preferred for long-term therapy because of its lower toxicity.

Diarrhea and malabsorption are the most common adverse effects. Superinfections may result from prolonged use. In patients with inflammatory bowel disease and renal insufficiency, systemic accumulation of neomycin may result in ototoxicity or nephrotoxicity.

ROUTE, USUAL DOSAGE, AND PREPARATIONS.
·*Oral*: *Adults*, initially, 4 to 6 g daily in divided doses; for maintenance, 2 to 3 g daily.

Drug available generically: Tablets 500 mg.
Mycifradin Sulfate (Upjohn). Solution 125 mg/5 ml; tablets 500 mg.
Neobiotic (Pfipharmecs). Tablets 500 mg.

PERITONEAL DIALYSIS SOLUTIONS

Peritoneal dialysis solutions are used to remove excessive body fluid, urea, creatinine, uric acid, serum electrolytes, and toxic ingestions. They are indicated in acute and chronic renal failure, intractable edema, hypercalcemia, hyperkalemia, and poisoning with dialyzable agents. Dialysis solutions containing acetate in place of lactate are recommended for patients prone to lactic acidosis.

Abdominal adhesions may impede peritoneal dialysis by interfering with proper insertion of the catheter and impairing instillation and removal of dialyzing fluid. Peritonitis is not an absolute contraindication; antibiotics may be added to the dialysis solution and also administered systemically. Local edema from subcutaneous infiltration of the dialyzing solution may result if the catheter is incompletely inserted or if leakage around the catheter is not controlled. Adynamic ileus may occur, especially with continuous dialysis; this complication should be managed by gastrointestinal decompression. Both overhydration and hypovolemia should be avoided. Protein loss may occur during prolonged dialysis; therefore, plasma protein levels should be measured frequently. Fluid and electrolyte requirements also must be maintained.

PREPARATIONS.

Dianeal with 1.5% or 4.25% Dextrose (Travenol). Each liter of solution contains approximately 141 mEq sodium, 3.5 mEq calcium, 1.5 mEq magnesium, 101 mEq chloride, 45 mEq lactate, and 15 or 42.5 g dextrose.

Dianeal 137 with 1.5% or 4.25% Dextrose (Travenol) has similar electrolyte concentrations except the sodium content is 132 mEq/L and lactate 35 mEq/L.

Peritoneal Dialysis Solutions (McGaw) have similar electrolyte and dextrose concentrations except for the substitution of acetate for lactate.

Peridial 1½ D and *Peridial 4¼ D* (Cutter) have similar electrolyte concentrations and contain 1.5% or 4.25% dextrose.

Dianeal K with 1.5% Dextrose (Travenol) contains 4 mEq/L of potassium chloride in addition to the ingredients listed for Dianeal except the chloride content is 105 mEq/L.

Dianeal K-141 with 1.5% or 4.25% Dextrose (Travenol) contains 4 mEq/L of potassium chloride in addition to the ingredients of Dianeal 137 except the chloride content is 106 mEq/L.

Inpersol w/1.5% or 4.25% Dextrose (Abbott). Each liter of solution contains 132 mEq sodium, 3.5 mEq calcium, 1.5 mEq magnesium, 35 mEq lactate, 99 mEq chloride, and 1.5 g or 4.25 g dextrose.

Selected References

Abouna GM, et al: Intravenous infusion of hydrochloric acid for treatment of severe metabolic alkalosis. *Surgery* 75:194-202, 1974.

Avery GS, et al: Lactulose: Review of its therapeutic and pharmacological properties with particular reference to ammonia metabolism and its mode of action in portal systemic encephalopathy. *Drugs* 4:7-48, 1972.

Down PF, et al: Fate of potassium supplements in six outpatients receiving long-term diuretics for oedematous disease. *Lancet* 2:721-724, 1972.

Fox CL Jr, Nahas GG (eds): *Body Fluid Replacement in the Surgical Patient*. New York, Grune & Stratton, 1970.

Kersh ES, Rifkin H: Lactulose enemas. *Ann Intern Med* 78:81-84, 1973.

Lindeman RD: Hypokalemia: Causes, consequences and correction. *Am J Med Sci* 272:5-17, 1976.

MacBryde CM, Blacklow RS (eds): *Signs and Symptoms*, ed 5. Philadelphia, JB Lippincott Company, 1970.

Maxwell MH, Kleeman CR (eds): *Clinical Disorders of Fluid and Electrolyte Metabolism*, ed 2. New York, McGraw-Hill Book Co, 1972.

Mudge GH, Welt LG: Agents affecting volume and composition of body fluids, in Goodman LS, Gilman A (eds): *The Pharmacological Basis of Therapeutics*, ed 5. New York, Macmillan Publishing Co, Inc, 1975, 753-781.

Rovner DR: Use of pharmacologic agents in treatment of hypokalemia and hyperkalemia. *Ration Drug Ther* 6:1-6, (Feb) 1972.

Schenker S, et al: Hepatic encephalopathy: Current status. *Gastroenterology* 66:121-151, 1974.

Schwartz AB, Swartz CD: Dosage of potassium chloride elixir to correct thiazide-induced hypokalemia. *JAMA* 230:702-704, 1974.

Trissel LA: *Handbook on Injectable Drugs*. Washington, DC, American Society of Hospital Pharmacists, Inc, 1977.

Whang R: Hyperkalemia: Diagnosis and treatment. *Am J Med Sci* 272:19-29, 1976.

Winters RW (ed): *The Body Fluids in Pediatrics*. Boston, Little, Brown and Company, 1973.

COMMERCIALLY AVAILABLE INTRAVENOUS SOLUTIONS

Generic Name	Manufacturer (Trademark)	Milliequivalents per 1,000 ml							HCO₃ Precursor
		Na+	K+	Ca+	Mg+	NH₄+	Cl−	HPO₄=	
Single Electrolyte Solutions									
Sodium Chloride 0.45%	Abbott	77					77		
	Cutter	77					77		
	McGaw	77					77		
	Travenol	77					77		
Sodium Chloride 0.9%	Abbott	154					154		
	Cutter	154					154		
	McGaw	154					154		
	Travenol	154					154		
Sodium Chloride 3%	Cutter	513					513		
	McGaw	513					513		
	Travenol	513					513		

Generic Name	Manufacturer (Trademark)	Milliequivalents per 1,000 ml							HCO₃ Precursor
		Na+	K+	Ca+	Mg+	NH₄+	Cl−	HPO₄=	HCO₃ Precursor
Single Electrolyte Solutions (continued)									
Sodium Chloride 5%	Abbott	855					855		
	Cutter	855					855		
	McGaw	855					855		
	Travenol	855					855		
Sodium Lactate (M/6) 1.72%	Abbott	167							Lact 167
	Cutter	167							Lact 167
	McGaw	167							Lact 167
	Travenol	167							Lact 167
Sodium Bicarbonate 5%	Abbott	595							595
	McGaw	595							595
	Travenol	595							595
Single Electrolyte Solutions with Dextrose									
Sodium Chloride 0.11% Dextrose 5%	McGaw	19					19		
Sodium Chloride 0.2% Dextrose 5%	Cutter	34					34		
	McGaw	34					34		
	Travenol	34					34		
Sodium Chloride 0.225% Dextrose 5%	Abbott	38.5					38.5		
Sodium Chloride 0.3% Dextrose 3.3%	Cutter	51					51		
Sodium Chloride 0.3% Dextrose 5%	Abbott	51					51		
Sodium Chloride 0.33% Dextrose 5%	McGaw	56					56		
	Travenol	56					56		
Sodium Chloride 0.45% Dextrose 2.5%	Abbott	77					77		
	Cutter	77					77		
	McGaw	77					77		
	Travenol	77					77		
Sodium Chloride 0.45% Dextrose 5%	Abbott	77					77		
	Cutter	77					77		
	McGaw	77					77		
	Travenol	77					77		
Sodium Chloride 0.45% Dextrose 10%	McGaw	77					77		
Sodium Chloride 0.9% Dextrose 2.5%	Cutter	154					154		
	McGaw	154					154		
Sodium Chloride 0.9% Dextrose 5%	Abbott	154					154		
	Cutter	154					154		
	McGaw	154					154		
	Travenol	154					154		

Generic Name	Manufacturer (Trademark)	Milliequivalents per 1,000 ml							HCO₃ Precursor
		Na+	K+	Ca+	Mg+	NH₄+	Cl−	HPO₄=	

Generic Name	Manufacturer (Trademark)	Na+	K+	Ca+	Mg+	NH₄+	Cl−	HPO₄=	HCO₃ Precursor
Single Electrolyte Solutions with Dextrose (continued)									
Sodium Chloride 0.9% Dextrose 10%	Abbott	154					154		
	Cutter	154					154		
	McGaw	154					154		
	Travenol	154					154		
Potassium Chloride 0.7% Dextrose 5%	Abbott		10				10		
Potassium Chloride 0.15% Dextrose 5%	Abbott		20				20		
	Cutter		20				20		
	McGaw (Kadalex L)		20				20		
	Travenol		20				20		
Potassium Chloride 0.2% Dextrose 5%	Abbott		30				30		
	Cutter		27				27		
	McGaw (Kadalex)		27				27		
Potassium Chloride 0.3% Dextrose 5%	Abbott		40				40		
	McGaw (Kadalex M)		40				40		
Multiple Electrolyte Solutions									
Balanced Electrolyte Injection Maintenance Formulas	Travenol (Plasma-Lyte 56)	40	13		3		40		Acet 16
	Cutter (Polysal-M)	40	16	5		3	40		24
Balanced Electrolyte Injection Replacement Formulas	Abbott (Normosol-R, Normosol-R pH 7.4)	140	5		3		98		Acet 27 Gluc 23
	Cutter (Polyonic R-148)	140	5		3		98		Acet 27 Gluc 23
	McGaw (Isolyte S)	140	5		3		98		Acet 27 Gluc 23
	McGaw (Isolyte)	140	10	5	3		103		Acet 44 Citrate 8
	Travenol (Plasma-Lyte 148)	140	5		3		98		Acet 27 Gluc 23
	Cutter (Polysal)	140	10	5	3		103		Acet 55 Lact 8
	Travenol (Plasma-Lyte)	140	10	5	3		103		Acet 47 Lact 8
Lactated Ringer's (Hartmann's Solution)	Abbott	130	4	3			109		Lact 28
	Cutter	130	4	3			109		Lact 28
	McGaw	130	4	3			109		Lact 28
	Travenol	130	4	3			109		Lact 28
Acetated Ringer's	Cutter	130	4	3			109		Acet 28
	McGaw	130	4	3			109		Acet 28
Ringer's Hypotonic	McGaw	103	5	5	3		116		
Ringer's	Abbott	147	4	5			156		
	Cutter	147.5	4	4.5			156		
	McGaw	147	4	4			155		
	Travenol	147.5	4	4.5			156		

	Manufacturer (Trademark)	Milliequivalents per 1,000 ml							HCO₃ Precursor
Generic Name		Na+	K+	Ca+	Mg+	NH₄+	Cl−	HPO₄=	
Multiple Electrolyte Solutions with Dextrose									
Balanced	Abbott (Normosol-M)	40	13		3		40		Acet 16
Electrolyte	Cutter (Polyonic M-56)	40	13		3		40		Acet 16
Maintenance									
Formulas with	Cutter (Polysal-M)	40	16	5	3		40		Acet 12 Lact 12
Dextrose 5%									
	McGaw (Isolyte H)	40	13		3		40		Acet 16
	McGaw (Isolyte R)	40	16	5	3		40		Acet 24
	Travenol (Plasma-Lyte 56)	40	13		3		40		Acet 16
	Travenol (Plasma-Lyte M)	40	16	5	3		40		Acet 12 Lact 12
Balanced Electrolyte Maintenance Formulas with Dextrose 10%	Cutter (Polysal-M)	40	16	5	3		40		Acet 12 Acet 12
Balanced	Abbott (Normosol-R)	140	5		3		98		Acet 27 Gluc 23
Electrolyte									
Replacement	Abbott (Normosol-R/K)	140	30		3		98		Acet 52 Gluc 23
Formulas with									
Dextrose 5%	Cutter (Polyonic R-148)	140	5		3		98		Acet 27 Gluc 23
	Cutter (Polysal)	140	10	5	3		103		Acet 55
	McGaw (Isolyte E)	140	10	5	3		103		Acet 55
	Travenol (Plasma-Lyte 148)	140	5		3		98		Acet 27 Gluc 23
	Travenol (Plasma-Lyte)	140	10	5	3		103		Acet 47
Lactated Ringer's	Abbott	65.5	2	1			54		Lact 14
half-strength	Cutter	65.5	2	1.5			55		Lact 14
with Dextrose	McGaw	65.5	2	1			54		Lact 14
2.5%	Travenol	65.5	2	1.5			55		Lact 14
Lactated Ringer's with Dextrose 2.5%	Cutter	130	4	3			109		Lact 28
Lactated Ringer's	Abbott	130	4	3			109		Lact 28
with Dextrose	Cutter	130	4	3			109		Lact 28
5%	McGaw	130	4	3			109		Lact 28
	Travenol	130	4	3			109		Lact 28
Lactated Ringer's	Cutter	130	4	3			109		Lact 28
with Dextrose 10%	McGaw	130	4	3			109		Lact 28
Acetated Ringer's	Abbott	74	2	2			78		
with Dextrose	Cutter	130	4	3			109		Acet 28
5%	McGaw	130	4	3			109		Acet 28
Ringer's	Cutter	74	2	2			78		
half-strength with Dextrose 2.5%	McGaw	74	2	2			78		

Generic Name	Manufacturer (Trademark)	Na+	K+	Ca+	Mg+	NH₄+	Cl−	HPO₄=	HCO₃ Precursor
Multiple Electrolyte Solutions with Dextrose (continued)									
Ringer's with	Abbott	147	4	4			155		
Dextrose 5%	Cutter	147	4	4.5			155.5		
	McGaw	147	4	4			155		
	Travenol	147.5	4	4.5			156		
Electrolyte No. 2	Abbott (Ionosol B)	57	25			5	49	13	Lact 25
with Dextrose 5%	Cutter	55	23			5	45	12	Lact 26
Electrolyte No. 3 with Dextrose 5%	McGaw (Isolyte G)	63	17			71	150		
Electrolyte No. 3 with Dextrose 10%	Abbott (Ionosol G)	63	17			71	151		
	McGaw (Isolyte G)	63	17			70	150		
Electrolyte No. 48	Abbott (Ionosol MB)	25	20		3		22	3	Lact 23
with Dextrose 5%	Cutter	25	20		3		22	3	Lact 23
	McGaw (Isolyte P)	25	20		3		22	3	Acet 23
	Travenol	25	20		3		24	3	Lact 23
Electrolyte No. 75	Abbott (Ionosol T)	40	35				40	15	Lact 20
with Dextrose 5%	Cutter	40	35				48	15	Lact 20
	McGaw (Isolyte M)	40	35				40	15	Acet 20
	Travenol	40	35				48	15	Lact 20
Potassium Chloride 0.07%, Sodium Chloride 0.225%, Dextrose 5%	Abbott	38.5	10				48.5		
Potassium Chloride 0.15%, Sodium Chloride 0.225%, Dextrose 5%	Abbott	38.5	20				58.5		
Potassium Chloride 0.2%, Sodium Chloride 0.225%, Dextrose 5%	Abbott	38.5	30				68.5		
Potassium Chloride 0.3%, Sodium Chloride 0.225%, Dextrose 5%	Abbott	38.5	40				78.5		
Potassium Chloride 0.07%, Sodium Chloride 0.45%, Dextrose 5%	Abbott	77	10				87		

Generic Name	Manufacturer (Trademark)	Milliequivalents per 1,000 ml								HCO₃ Precursor
		Na+	K+	Ca+	Mg+	NH₄+	Cl−	HPO₄=		

Multiple Electrolyte Solutions with Dextrose (continued)

Generic Name	Manufacturer (Trademark)	Na+	K+	Ca+	Mg+	NH₄+	Cl−	HPO₄=	HCO₃ Precursor
Potassium Chloride 0.15%, Sodium Chloride 0.45%, Dextrose 5%	Abbott	77	20				97		
	Cutter	77	20				97		
Potassium Chloride 0.2%, Sodium Chloride 0.15%, Dextrose 3.5% (Ordway's Solution)	Cutter	26	27				53		
Potassium Chloride 0.2%, Sodium Chloride 0.45%, Dextrose 5%	Abbott	77	30				107		
Potassium Chloride 0.3%, Sodium Chloride 0.45%, Dextrose 5%	Abbott	77	40				117		

Vitamins and Minerals | 52

Vitamins and some minerals are essential for normal metabolism and maintenance of health. Purified forms are available individually or in various combinations. Differentiation should be made between products for prophylactic use as dietary supplements and those suitable only for therapeutic purposes, since both types often are used indiscriminately and inappropriately. Food is the best source of vitamins and minerals, and healthy persons consuming an adequate balanced diet will not benefit from additional vitamins.

There are few valid indications for vitamin or mineral supplementation except to correct deficiency. Massive-dose therapy usually is justified only for patients who cannot utilize these nutrients properly, although such treatment is appropriate in several diseases (see the evaluations). The danger of toxic effects from excessive amounts of vitamin A or D and all minerals,

particularly in infants and children, should be considered.

The Recommended Dietary Allowances (RDA) for vitamins and minerals established by the Food and Nutrition Board of the National Research Council provide authoritative information to assist the physician in evaluating the formulas of multivitamin preparations (see also the section on Mixtures). These allowances (see Table 1) are higher than the minimum requirements necessary to prevent deficiency and are not absolute nutritional standards or recommendations for an ideal diet; instead they represent amounts that will maintain good nutrition in practically all healthy persons. RDA should not be confused with the United States Recommended Daily Allowances (USRDA), which is a simplified table of values established by the Food and Drug Administration for labeling purposes (see Table 2).

The allowances for calories and protein also are shown in Table 1. Requirements for many of the B-complex vitamins are related to caloric intake. Allowances have not been established for all the essential trace elements, but these are supplied by diets containing a variety of foods and normal amounts of protein and calories. To assess nutritional adequacy, the past nutrient intake, clinical symptoms, and biochemical data on blood, tissue, and urinary levels of nutrients, also must be evaluated.

All infants should receive vitamins and minerals to support normal growth and health, either from their diet or by supplementation. Specific requirements of healthy infants for supplementation depend upon the source of nutrients (human or cow's milk or artificial formulas). (See Table 3.)

TABLE 1.
RECOMMENDED DAILY ALLOWANCES (RDA) FOR DIETARY SUPPLEMENTS[1]

	Units of Measurement	Infants 0–6 Months	Infants 6 Months– 1 Year	Children 1 Year– 4 Years
Energy[2]	Kilocalories	Body wt. in Kg × 117	Body wt. in Kg × 108	1,300
Protein[3]	Grams	Body wt. in Kg × 2.2	Body wt. in Kg × 2.0	23
Fat-Soluble Vitamins				
Vitamin A Activity	Retinol equivalent or	420	400	400
	International Units	1,400	2,000	2,000
Vitamin D	International Units	400	400	400
Vitamin E Activity	International Units	4	5	7
Water-Soluble Vitamins[4]				
Ascorbic Acid	Milligrams	35	35	40
Folacin[5]	Micrograms	50	50	100
Niacin	Milligrams	5	8	9
Riboflavin	Milligrams	0.4	0.6	0.8
Thiamin	Milligrams	0.3	0.5	0.7
Vitamin B_6	Milligrams	0.3	0.4	0.6
Vitamin B_{12}	Micrograms	0.3	0.3	1.0
Minerals				
Calcium	Milligrams	360[6]	540[6]	800
Phosphorus	Milligrams	240	400	800
Iodine	Micrograms	35	45	60
Iron	Milligrams	10	15	15
Magnesium	Milligrams	60	70	150
Zinc	Milligrams	3	5	10

Adapted from Report of Food and Nutrition Board, National Academy of Sciences—National Research Council, 8th Revised Edition, 1974.

[1]The allowance levels are intended to cover individual variations among most normal persons living in the United States under usual environmental stress. The recommended allowances can be attained with a variety of common foods that also provide other nutrients for which human requirements have been less well defined.
[2]Energy requirements vary with amount of physical activity. Requirements are increased following illness.
[3]Factors for infants assume protein equivalent to human milk. For proteins not 100% utilized, factors should be increased proportionately.

In some situations (eg, infants and children who are not eating and not developing satisfactorily, those with prolonged diarrhea), it may be advisable to prescribe RDA levels of B-complex vitamin supplements. The most common deficiency in infants and children is of folic acid. Infants who are breast-fed by mothers deficient in folic acid or under the circumstances mentioned above should receive 50 mcg of folacin daily. Healthy growing children consuming an adequate diet do not require vitamin supplements unless adequate quantities of vitamin D-fortified milk or sufficient exposure to sunlight are not supplied; if a supplement is required, 400 IU of vitamin D should be given daily. Similarly, healthy adults require no supplementation except during pregnancy and lactation. The following daily supplements

Children 4 Years– 10 Years	Adults		Pregnancy	Lactation
	Male	Female		
1,800-2,400	2,400-3,000	1,800-2,400	2,400	2,600
30-36	44-56	44-48	74-78	64-68
500-700	1,000	800	1,000	1,200
2,500-3,300	5,000	4,000	5,000	6,000
400	400	400	400	400
10	12-15	12	15	15
40	45	45	60	80
200-300	400	400	800	600
12-16	16-20	12-16	14-18	16-20
1.1-1.2	1.5-1.8	1.1-1.4	1.4-1.7	1.6-1.9
0.9-1.2	1.2-1.5	1.0-1.2	1.3-1.5	1.3-1.5
0.9-1.2	1.6-2.0	1.6-2.0	2.5	2.5
1.5-2.0	3.0	3.0	4.0	4.0
800	800-1,200	800-1,200	1,200	1,200
800	800-1,200	800-1,200	1,200	1,200
80-110	110-150	80-115	125	150
10	10-18	10-18	18+	18
200-250	350-400	300	450	450
10	15	15	20	25

[4]No allowance has been established for pantothenic acid, but it is estimated that a daily intake of 5 to 10 mg is probably adequate for children and adults.

[5]The folacin allowances refer to dietary sources as determined by Lactobacillus casei assay. Pure forms of folacin (eg, folic acid crystalline) may be effective in doses less than 1/4 of the RDA.

[6]Breast-fed infants receive adequate calcium. These allowances apply only to infants fed formulas.

should be prescribed for pregnant women: 400 IU of vitamin D unless a quart of vitamin D-fortified milk is consumed daily, 0.8 mg of folic acid, and 30 mg of elemental iron. It has not been substantiated that elderly persons consuming an adequate diet have higher requirements for vitamins or minerals than other healthy adults.

Circulating coenzymatic compounds derived from folacin, pyridoxine, and ascorbic acid are removed by hemodialysis; therefore, patients being dialyzed should re-ceive compensatory amounts (100% to 300% of the USRDA) of these vitamins. The requirement for other vitamins, with the possible exception of vitamin E, apparently is not increased.

Vitamins and minerals should be administered parenterally only in certain special circumstances (see the discussion on Therapeutic Vitamin Preparations in the section on Mixtures). Mixture with other intravenous medications should be avoided unless this is specified in the

TABLE 2.
U.S. RECOMMENDED DAILY ALLOWANCES (USRDA) FOR DIETARY SUPPLEMENTS DEVELOPED BY FOOD AND DRUG ADMINISTRATION FOR NUTRITION LABELING*

	Units of Measurement	Infants Birth to 12 Months
Protein	Grams	28
Fat-Soluble Vitamins		
Vitamin A	International Units	1,500
Vitamin D	International Units	400
Vitamin E	International Units	5
Water-Soluble Vitamins		
Vitamin C (Ascorbic Acid)	Milligrams	35
Thiamine (Vitamin B_1)	Milligrams	0.5
Riboflavin (Vitamin B_2)	Milligrams	0.6
Vitamin B_6	Milligrams	0.4
Vitamin B_{12}	Micrograms	2
Folic Acid	Milligrams	0.1
Niacin	Milligrams	8
Pantothenic Acid	Milligrams	3
Biotin	Milligrams	0.15
Minerals		
Calcium	Grams	0.6
Iron	Milligrams	15
Phosphorus	Grams	0.5
Iodine	Micrograms	45
Magnesium	Milligrams	70
Zinc	Milligrams	5
Copper	Milligrams	0.6

*These values usually represent the highest allowance for any age group within the broad category and are the amounts judged necessary to maintain health. These specifications replace the generally lower minimum daily requirements which were the amounts necessary to prevent deficiencies.

package insert. (Compatibility data available in most hospitals also should be consulted.)

FAT-SOLUBLE VITAMINS

The fat-soluble vitamins (A, D, E, and K) are absorbed by complex processes that parallel the absorption of fat. Thus, any condition that causes malabsorption of fat (eg, celiac disease, tropical sprue, regional enteritis) may result in deficiency of one or all of these vitamins. Fat-soluble vitamins affect permeability or transport in various cell membranes and act as oxidation-reduction agents, coenzymes, or enzyme inhibitors. They are stored principally in the liver and excreted in the feces. Since these vitamins are metabolized very slowly, overdosage may produce toxic effects.

Children Under 4 Years of Age	Adults and Children 4 or More Years of Age	Pregnant or Lactating Women
65	65	65
2,500	5,000	8,000
400	400	400
10	30	30
40	60	60
0.7	1.5	1.7
0.8	1.7	2.0
0.7	2.0	2.5
3	6	8
0.2	0.4	0.8
9	20	20
5	10	10
0.15	0.3	0.3
0.8	1.0	1.3
10	18	18
0.8	1.0	1.3
70	150	150
200	400	450
8	15	15
1	2	2

VITAMIN A (Retinol)

Vitamin A is essential for growth and bone development in children, for vision (particularly in dim light), and for integrity of mucosal and epithelial surfaces. It includes several active compounds of which retinol is the major naturally occurring form. Precursor carotenoid pigments, especially beta-carotene, may be obtained from green and yellow vegetables, but only about one-third is converted to vitamin A in man. Preformed vitamin A (retinols) is acquired primarily from animal sources (eggs, dairy products, and meat). Dietary fat is necessary for effective absorption of carotene, and protein is required for absorption of retinols. Protein and, possibly, zinc may be required to mobilize vitamin A reserves in the liver.

TABLE 3.
SUPPLEMENTAL NUTRITIONAL REQUIREMENTS FOR FULL-TERM INFANTS

Formula	Supplemental Vitamins and Minerals[1]	Daily Amount[1]
All infants	vitamin K_1	0.5 to 1 mg immediately after birth
	elemental iron	10 to 15 mg 20 mg (premature infants)
	vitamin A[2]	1,500 IU (to 6 months) 2,000 to 2,500 IU (premature [to 6 months])
	vitamin D[2]	400 IU
	ascorbic acid[2]	35 mg
Areas where water supplies are deficient (less than 0.3 ppm)	fluoride	0.25 mg (0.55 mg sodium fluoride)
Additions recommended for special groups fed exclusively the following:		
Cow's milk	copper	0.5 to 1 mg (premature infants)
	folacin	50 mcg (low birth-weight infants)
Breast milk (from mothers with folic acid deficiency)	folacin	50 mcg
Goat's milk	folacin	50 mcg
Artificial or unfortified skim milk[3]	ascorbic acid	50 mg (infants fed high-protein formulas)
	calcium	amount sufficient to maintain calcium:phosphorus ratio of 1.5:1
Formula high in polyunsaturated fat (eg, soybean base)	vitamin E	5 to 7 IU/L of formula

[1]Since cow's milk may be fortified with vitamins A and D and many formulas contain vitamins and minerals, supplemental amounts should be adjusted accordingly.

[2]These supplements are needed in breast-fed infants only if mother's milk is inadequate.

[3]Filled milks, imitation milk, and coffee whiteners are not satisfactory substitutes for whole milk in infant diets.

Human milk supplies sufficient vitamin A for infants unless the maternal diet is grossly inadequate (see Table 3 for infant requirements). Healthy children and adults consuming a well-balanced diet do not require supplementation.

Variable degrees of deficiency occur when the ability to store vitamin A is impaired (eg, in hepatic cirrhosis), when a deficiency of transport protein exists, or when intestinal absorption is impaired. The initial manifestation of hypovitaminosis A is night blindness (nyctalopia) that may progress to xerophthalmia and keratomalacia with corneal perforation and, eventually, blindness. Hyperkeratosis and metaplasia of mucous membranes, which impair local defenses against infection, also may occur.

Vitamin A in excess of normal requirements should not be used for any condition unless deficiency is demonstrable. It is of no value in the prevention or treatment of infections or for renal calculi, hyperthyroidism, anemia, degenerative conditions of the nervous system, sunburn, or cutaneous ulcerative conditions. Prolonged use of large doses to treat acne vulgaris has not been proved beneficial in well-controlled trials and has produced increased intracranial pressure.

Vitamin A toxicity only rarely results from dietary sources; the only sign of carotenemia is yellow discoloration of the skin that disappears when the dietary source is discontinued. The rate of mobilization of vitamin A and the amount required to produce hypervitaminosis A vary considerably. Symptoms of acute intoxication may appear within a few hours after the ingestion of 75,000 to 300,000 IU in infants and at least 2,000,000 IU in adults. In infants, bulging fontanelles, hyperirritability, anorexia, and vomiting may occur; in adults, symptoms include dizziness, severe headache, drowsiness, nausea, vomiting, and erythema with eventual desquamation that persists for several weeks.

When more than 10,000 IU is taken daily, chronic hypervitaminosis A develops within months in children but usually takes several years in adults. Manifestations of chronic intoxication in children include

pseudotumor cerebri, tinnitus, widening of sutures with bulging fontanelles, increased cerebrospinal fluid pressure, lethargy, pruritus, exfoliative dermatitis, angular stomatitis, hyperostosis, metaphyseal cupping, and paronychia. Diplopia and papilledema occur and, in long-standing cases, optic atrophy and blindness may result. Common symptoms in adults are vomiting, skin changes, irritability, headache, hypomenorrhea, and weakness. Psychiatric symptoms may be so prominent that patients have been placed in psychiatric hospitals with a diagnosis of severe depression or schizophrenia. Hepatic dysfunction, often associated with hepatosplenomegaly, may occur, and marked hypercalcemia and ascites have been reported. In children and adults, hypervitaminosis A may cause dryness of the skin and mucous membranes, alopecia, anorexia, brittle nails, myalgia, ostealgia, arthralgia, abdominal pain, splenomegaly, and hypoplastic anemia with leukopenia. Most symptoms disappear when the vitamin is discontinued, but retardation of growth caused by premature epiphyseal closure may occur in children.

ROUTES, USUAL DOSAGE, AND PREPARATIONS. THERAPEUTIC:
Doses larger than 25,000 IU daily should not be prescribed unless the deficiency is severe. The safety of doses exceeding 6,000 IU daily during pregnancy and lactation has not been established. Oral administration is preferred; the intramuscular route may be used for short-term therapy when absorption is grossly impaired, ocular symptoms are prominent, or oral administration is not feasible.

Intramuscular: In severe deficiency, *adults and children over 8 years*, 50,000 to 100,000 IU daily for three days, followed by 50,000 IU daily for two weeks; *1 to 8 years*, 5,000 to 15,000 IU daily for ten days; *infants*, 5,000 to 10,000 IU daily for ten days.

Available generically: Solution 50,000 IU/ml in 10 ml containers and 100,000 IU/ml in 30 ml containers.

Oral: In severe deficiency, *adults and children over 8 years*, 100,000 IU daily for three days, followed by 50,000 IU daily for two weeks and 10,000 to 20,000 IU daily for another two months.

Available generically: Capsules 10,000, 25,000, and 50,000 IU; drops 50,000 IU/ml in 30 ml containers; tablets 10,000 IU.

AVAILABLE TRADEMARKS.

Vitamin A (water-dispersible): *Acon* (Endo), *Aquasol A* (USV); (fat-soluble): *Alphalin* (Lilly).

DIETARY SUPPLEMENTATION OR PROPHYLAXIS: Dosage should be based on the RDA after evaluation of the patient's dietary supply. The diet should be corrected or the dose reduced on the basis of the RDA after a response is obtained.

VITAMIN D

Vitamin D designates several sterols and their metabolites that have antirachitic properties. Ergocalciferol (vitamin D2) derived from yeast and fungal ergosterol sources is the usual active ingredient supplied commercially. Irradiation of the provitamin, 7-dehydrocholesterol, in the skin or irradiation of food produces cholecalciferol (vitamin D3).

Vitamin D is stored mainly in the liver and is excreted slowly. Following absorption, it is hydroxylated in the liver to form 25-hydroxy-vitamin D (25-OHD3). Further hydroxylation occurs in the kidney in response to the need for calcium and phosphorus, and 1,25-dihydroxy-vitamin D (1,25-(OH)2D3) is produced. In conjunction with calcitonin and parathyroid hormone, this most active form of vitamin D regulates calcium and phosphorus metabolism in the intestine, bone, and possibly kidney; it facilitates the intestinal absorption of calcium and also may initiate phosphorus transport, thus increasing serum calcium and phosphorus levels to allow normal mineralization of the skeleton. Paradoxically, vitamin D also mobilizes calcium from bone to maintain proper plasma levels of calcium. It may act in the kidney to suppress parathyroid hormone secretion, thus preventing phosphaturia, and may have a direct action on the proximal tubules to promote phosphorus retention.

While vitamin D is essential, the daily requirement in adults is very small and may be obtained by adequate exposure to sunlight or in the diet. Products containing more than 400 IU should be used only when deficiency is documented. Premature infants and those fed breast milk or unfortified formulas should receive 400 IU daily. Infants and children receiving adequate amounts of vitamin D-fortified food require no supplementation; in fact, use of a supplement can result in overdosage. Members of dark-skinned races inhabiting northern climates have a slightly higher requirement for vitamin D because melanin interferes with irradiation. Pregnant and lactating women may need supplementation if 400 IU daily is not provided in the diet. However, excessive amounts during pregnancy are potentially dangerous to the fetus (eg, they may cause supravalvular aortic stenosis, vascular injury, suppression of parathyroid function with resultant hypocalcemic tetany in the neonate).

Primary nutritional deficiency of vitamin D is rare in the United States. An absolute or relative deficiency may occur secondary to malabsorption syndromes or in patients with inherited or acquired metabolic disorders (eg, hypoparathyroidism, genetic vitamin D-dependent rickets, renal osteodystrophy). Deficiency causes hypocalcemia and hypophosphatemia, which stimulates parathyroid hormone secretion to restore plasma calcium levels at the expense of bone. This causes rickets in infants and children and osteomalacia in adults. When produced by dietary deficiency, these conditions respond rapidly to adequate doses of vitamin D, but treatment of other disorders may depend upon blood levels of calcium, phosphate, and parathyroid hormone as well as the degree of derangement of vitamin D metabolism. See also Chapter 54, Agents Affecting Calcium Metabolism.

In all deficiency states, the dose of vitamin D should be reduced to the RDA after symptoms are relieved and before normal biochemical levels are achieved or bone healing is complete. When bone healing has occurred, the requirement may decrease suddenly and, since its action may persist long after administration is discontinued, hypercalcemia and renal damage may result.

Vitamin D activity may be reduced in those taking anticonvulsants; thus, epileptics being given hydantoins or barbiturates should receive prophylactic doses of vitamin D.

Administration of vitamin D to treat lupus vulgaris is obsolete, and its topical use for other dermatoses is not justified.

Vitamin D is very toxic in large doses. In infants and children, the margin of safety between prophylactic or therapeutic and toxic doses is narrow. Hypercalcemia may develop in some hypersensitive infants at doses very close to 400 IU. In addition, large amounts inadvertently may be ingested by children who consume a great variety of foods fortified with vitamin D. Prolonged hypervitaminosis D in infants causes mental and physical retardation, elfin facies, renal failure, and death. Symptoms of toxicity may occur with doses greater than 1,000 IU daily, and retardation of linear growth has been reported after daily doses of 1,800 IU. Amounts exceeding 50,000 IU daily produce hypercalcemia in normal adults and children. Initial manifestations of toxicity are associated with symptoms of hypercalcemia (eg, weakness, anorexia, vomiting, diarrhea, polydipsia, polyuria). Proteinuria may indicate renal impairment, and prolonged hypercalcemia may result in ectopic soft tissue calcifications (calcinosis universalis). Chronic use of massive doses ultimately results in irreversible renal failure and death.

Vitamin D intoxication usually is reversible if administration is discontinued unless renal impairment is severe. Some patients also require a low-calcium diet, glucocorticoids, and other measures to reduce plasma calcium levels to normal.

ROUTE, USUAL DOSAGE, AND PREPARATIONS.

PROPHYLACTIC:

Oral: Premature or breast-fed infants or those given unfortified formulas, 400 IU daily. *Infants abnormally susceptible to rickets,* up to 30,000 IU daily. In *adults,* based on dietary intake and exposure to sunlight, supplementation may be needed during pregnancy and lactation and in the elderly to assure a daily intake of 400 IU. If doses larger than 400 IU are used for prolonged periods, blood calcium levels and 24-hour urine specimens should be checked frequently. Blood calcium levels should be maintained at 9 to 10 mg/dl.

No single-entity preparations for prophylactic use are available.

See Table 4 for the appropriate mixture according to age and use.

THERAPEUTIC:

See Chapter 54, Agents Affecting Calcium Metabolism.

VITAMIN E (Tocopherol)

Vitamin E refers to a group of fat-soluble substances occurring in plants. Of the several tocopherols, only alpha-tocopherol is considered because it is the most active and abundant, although soybean products contain gamma-tocopherol, which is less potent but may contribute substantially to vitamin E intake.

Vitamin E is considered an essential nutrient, but its biochemical functions are not completely understood; 50% to 80% is absorbed and transported by lipoprotein in essentially the same manner as fats. It is stored in adipose tissue and is thought to stabilize the lipid portions of cell membranes. Vitamin E protects polyunsaturated fatty acids (PUFA) from oxidative deterioration and appears to influence the synthesis of heme, porphyrin, and heme proteins. Other functions attributed to vitamin E are enhancement of vitamin A utilization, inhibition of the oxidative production of prostaglandins, and stimulation of an essential cofactor in steroid metabolism. A number of other substances that occur naturally in foods (eg, selenium, sulfur, amino acids, coenzyme Q) can function as partial substitutes for vitamin E in certain metabolic reactions.

Surveys indicate that adequate amounts of vitamin E are supplied in the usual diet, that human requirements are small, and that the RDA exceeds the actual needs of normal persons. The requirement for vitamin E increases as the intake of PUFA increases. However, foods that supply PUFA (vegetable oils, shortenings, and margarine) also are good sources of vitamin E. Nevertheless, consumption of excessive amounts of PUFA (more than 20 g/day over normal dietary intake) may warrant supplementation with vitamin E, particularly if the PUFA intake is discontinued abruptly, thus producing a relative deficiency of the vitamin. Vitamin E requirements may be increased in people exposed to high-oxygen environments or in those taking therapeutic doses of iron or large doses of thyroid. Skin lesions, hematologic changes, and edema have developed in premature infants receiving formulas high in PUFA and low in vitamin E; recovery followed administration of 37.5 to 75 IU of alpha-tocopherol daily.

Vitamin E therapy should be restricted to deficiency states demonstrable by low serum vitamin E levels and/or increased fragility of red cells to hydrogen peroxide. These may occur in malabsorption syndromes with steatorrhea (eg, celiac disease, tropical sprue, gastrointestinal resections) and other conditions characterized by prolonged malabsorption of fats (eg, cystic fibrosis, hepatic cirrhosis, biliary obstruction, excessive ingestion of mineral oil).

There is no evidence to support the efficacy of vitamin E in the numerous conditions for which it is popularly used. Large doses do not protect against arteriosclerosis, cancer, pulmonary damage from air pollution, or deterioration from aging, and vitamin E is ineffective in inflammatory skin disorders, habitual abortion, heart disease, menopausal syndrome, infertility, peptic ulcer, burns, porphyria, and neuromuscular disorders.

Excessive use of vitamin E may deplete vitamin A stores, although doses of 300 to 400 IU daily may be taken for prolonged periods without adverse effects. However, the long-term use of 400 to 800 IU daily has been reported to produce nausea, muscular weakness, fatigue, headache, and blurred vision in a few patients, and excessively large doses (2,000 to 12,000 IU daily) have been reported to cause gonadal dysfunction, creatinuria, and gastrointestinal upset (Hayes and Hegsted, 1973). Symptoms disappeared within a few weeks when excessive doses were discontinued.

ROUTES, USUAL DOSAGE, AND PREPARATIONS. *Oral, Intramuscular*: *Adults and children*, in suspected deficiency, four to five times the RDA. Commercial formulas for infant feeding that are high in polyunsaturated fats should contain at least 5 IU/L; for low birth-weight or premature infants, the formula should contain 7 IU/L.

Available generically under the names Vitamin E (capsules 30, 50, 100, 200, 600, 800, and 1,000 IU; solution [injection] 100 and 200 mg/ml in 10 ml containers; drops 10 IU/drop in 15 ml containers; tablets [chewable] 100, 250, and 400 IU; wafers 400 IU), Tocopherol (capsules 100, 200, 400, and 1,000 IU), and Tocopheryl (capsules 100, 200, and 400 IU).

Aquasol E (USV). Capsules 30, 100, and 400 IU; drops 50 IU/ml; elixir 33.3 IU/5 ml (alcohol 15%) (nonprescription).

E-Ferol (O'Neal, Jones & Feldman). Capsules 100, 200, 400, and 800 IU (nonprescription); solution (injection) 200 mg/ml in 10 ml containers.

E-Ferol Succinate (O'Neal, Jones & Feldman). Capsules 100, 200, and 400 IU (nonprescription).

Eprolin (Lilly). Capsules 50 and 100 mg (equivalent to 50 and 100 IU vitamin E activity, respectively) (nonprescription).

Viterra E (Pfipharmecs). Capsules 100, 200, 400, and 600 IU (nonprescription).

VITAMIN K

Hypoprothrombinemia due to vitamin K deficiency may occur secondary to malabsorption of fats, prolonged hyperalimentation, or inhibition of intestinal bacterial biosynthesis. Relative deficiency also may result from imbalance of fat-soluble vitamins following excessive doses of one or all of the other fat-soluble vitamins (A, D, E). Newborn infants, especially those who are premature, have low concentrations of vitamin K-dependent clotting factors that decrease for a few days after birth. Small doses (0.5 to 1 mg) of phytonadione administered either intramuscularly or intravenously immediately after birth are advocated for all newborn infants. This dose may be repeated if needed. For a more detailed discussion on the therapeutic and prophylactic uses of vitamin K, see Chapter 65, Hemostatics.

WATER-SOLUBLE VITAMINS

The water-soluble vitamins include ascorbic acid and the B-complex vitamins, thiamine (B_1), riboflavin (B_2), pyridoxine (B_6), niacin (nicotinic acid), pantothenic acid, biotin, B_{12} (cyanocobalamin), and folic acid. Since the last two are used principally to treat deficiency anemias (see Chapter 62), they are discussed only briefly in this chapter.

Water-soluble vitamins are structurally diverse and act as coenzymes or oxidation inhibiting agents. Metabolism is rapid and the excess is excreted in the urine and, except for niacin, overdosage of these vitamins seldom causes toxic effects in individuals with normal renal function.

ASCORBIC ACID
ASCORBATE CALCIUM
ASCORBATE SODIUM

Ascorbic acid (vitamin C) acts as a reducing agent and antioxidant. It is indicated for the prevention and treatment of scurvy. Unlike most mammals, man lacks the enzyme necessary for conversion of gluconate to vitamin C and ascorbic acid must be supplied exogenously. If maternal intake is adequate, breast-fed infants need no additional ascorbic acid; infants fed cow's milk or a milk-free formula require a dietary source or supplement daily (see Table 3). Requirements are increased during periods of physiologic stress (eg, pregnancy, lactation, infections, postoperatively) and in response to increased excretion caused by some drugs (eg, salicylates, atropine, ammonium chloride, tetracycline, barbiturates).

White blood cell-platelet ascorbic acid levels of 20 to 30 mg/dl are adequate; scurvy is evident at levels below 2 mg/dl (Beeson and McDermott, 1975). Nonspecific signs and symptoms of early hypovitaminosis C include malaise, irritability, emotional disturbances, arthralgia, hyperkeratosis of hair follicles, nosebleeds, and petechial hemorrhages. Clinical scurvy occurs after three to five months on an ascorbic acid-free diet; this is rare in the United States but those most susceptible are the elderly or chronically ill, alcoholics, and dietary cultists. Pathology is manifest in most body tissues, especially those of mesodermal origin (ie, collagen, growing bones, teeth, blood vessels). Defective ground substance is formed and scar tissue formation is delayed. Capillary fragility combined with defective calcification of cartilage causes subperiosteal hemorrhages and, eventually, bone resorption and abnormal bone development with defective development of teeth in growing children. Ecchymoses appear and hemorrhages into muscles and joints may occur. A normocytic or macrocytic anemia, which is multifactorial in origin, is common. Rarely, megaloblastic anemia is observed if there is a deficiency of both ascorbic and folic acids. If untreated, convulsions, coma, and death occur.

Vitamin C facilitates wound healing and recovery from extensive burns or severe trauma, and daily doses 300% to 500% higher than the RDA may be useful in patients with such disorders. However, it is of no value in the treatment of pyorrhea and gingival infections not caused by scurvy. The use of massive doses (1 to 15 g/day) for prevention of the common cold has not been supported by objective data (Chalmers, 1975). Doses greater than 1 g/day may cause diarrhea and increase the danger of developing renal calculi, since ascorbic acid is partially metabolized and excreted as oxalate. It increases iron absorption and, thus, large doses may be dangerous in patients with hemochromatosis, thalassemia, or sideroblastic anemia. Mild hemolysis has been reported in patients with erythrocyte G6PD deficiency; in one patient, acute hemolysis resulted in disseminated intravascular coagulation, acute renal failure, and death (Campbell et al, 1975).

For prophylaxis or correction of deficiency, vitamin C may be given as fresh or frozen orange juice (contains approximately 0.5 mg/ml of ascorbic acid). Crystalline ascorbic acid is a suitable alternative; oral administration is preferred, but ascorbate sodium may be given intramuscularly or intravenously.

ROUTES, USUAL DOSAGE, AND PREPARATIONS.
PROPHYLACTIC:
Oral, Intramuscular: For the first few weeks of life, *infants on formula feedings*, 35 mg daily or, if the formula contains two or three times the amount of protein in human milk, 50 mg daily. *Older infants, children, and adults*, at least 2 to 4 oz of orange juice or other source of vitamin C or 30 to 60 mg of crystalline ascorbic acid daily.

THERAPEUTIC:
Oral, Intramuscular, Intravenous: *Adults and children*, the diet should be corrected to supply at least 2 oz of orange juice or other source of vitamin C. For treatment of scurvy, 100 mg three times daily for one week, followed by 100 mg daily for several weeks until tissue saturation is normal. For severe burns, 200 to 500 mg daily until healing has occurred or grafting operations are completed. During periods of increased requirement (eg, infections, trauma), 150 mg daily.

ASCORBIC ACID:
Available generically: Capsules (timed-release) 250 and 500 mg; solution (injection) 100 mg/ml in 5 and 10 ml containers, 200 mg/ml in 5, 10, 20, and 50 ml containers, and 250 mg/ml in 2, 30, and 50 ml containers; syrup 100 mg/5 ml; tablets 25, 50, 100, 250, and 500 mg and 1 g; tablets (chewable) 100, 250, and 500 mg.
Cevi Bid (Geriatric). Capsules (timed-release) 500 mg (nonprescription).
Cecon (Abbott). Drops 100 mg/ml (nonprescription).
Cevalin (Lilly). Solution (intramuscular) 50 mg/ml in 2 ml containers, 100 mg/ml in 10 ml containers, and 500 mg/ml in 1 ml containers; tablets 100, 250, and 500 mg (nonprescription).
Ce-Vi-Sol (Mead Johnson). Drops 35 mg/0.6 ml (nonprescription).
Viterra C (Pfipharmecs). Tablets 250 and 500 mg (nonprescription).
ASCORBATE CALCIUM:
Available only in multivitamin preparations.
ASCORBATE SODIUM:
Available generically: Solution (injection) 100 mg/ml in 10 ml containers.
Cenolate (Abbott). Solution (injection) 500 mg/ml in 1 and 2 ml containers.
C-Ject (Lincoln). Solution (injection) 200 mg/ml in 10 ml containers.
Liqui-Cee (Arnar-Stone). Solution (oral) 1 g/5 ml.

BIOTIN

This member of the B-complex group of vitamins is a coenzyme essential for fatty acid synthesis and other carboxylation reactions. Biotin normally is synthesized by intestinal bacteria, and deficiency can be produced only by prolonged ingestion of large amounts of raw egg white, which contains the inactivating protein, avidin. Because of uncertainty regarding the contribution of intestinal microorganisms, no RDA has been determined. Federal regulations permit inclusion of 0.15 mg of biotin in multivitamin supplements for infants and children and 0.3 mg in supplements for adults.

FOLIC ACID (Folacin)

Folacin is the generic term for several compounds having folic acid activity. Adequate varied diets provide sufficient amounts for normal individuals. Amounts present in human or cow's milk are adequate to fulfill infant requirements, although supplementation may be needed in low-birth-weight infants or those who are breast-fed by mothers with folic acid deficiency (50 mcg daily) or in those with infections or prolonged diarrhea. Folic acid requirements are markedly increased during pregnancy and lactation and deficiency will result in fetal damage.

Except during pregnancy and lactation, folic acid should not be given in therapeutic doses greater than 0.4 mg daily until pernicious anemia has been ruled out. Patients with pernicious anemia receiving more than 0.4 mg of folic acid daily who are inadequately treated with vitamin B_{12} may show reversion of the hematologic parameters to normal, but neurologic manifestations due to vitamin B_{12} deficiency will progress. Doses of folic acid exceeding the RDA should not be included in multivitamin preparations; if therapeutic amounts are necessary, folic acid should be given separately.

For a more detailed discussion of folic acid, see Chapter 62, Agents Used to Treat Deficiency Anemias.

NIACIN (Nicotinic Acid)

NIACINAMIDE (Nicotinamide)

Niacin, including niacinamide and tryptophan, is converted to physiologically active diphosphopyridine nucleotide (DPN or NAD) and triphosphopyridine nucleotide (TPN or NADP). As coenzymes of numerous dehydrogenases, these nucleotides are functional groups of electron transfer agents active in cellular respiration, glycolysis, and lipid synthesis.

Chief dietary sources are proteins of animal origin, yeast, and green vegetables. Bound forms, which are unavailable for conversion to nucleotides, are present in many foods, especially cereals. The conversion of dietary tryptophan to NAD and NADP requires thiamine, riboflavin, and pyridoxine; approximately 60 mg of precursor tryptophan is equivalent to 1 mg of niacin. Thus, the dietary requirement for niacin is influenced by the protein content of the diet. Increased amounts are needed during stress (eg, pregnancy, lactation, prolonged infection, hyperthyroidism, burns).

Primary dietary deficiency is rare in the United States except in areas where corn (which is low in tryptophan) is the main constituent of the diet. Secondary deficiency may occur in those with malabsorption syndromes, in alcoholics, or in dietary cultists. Deficiency causes pellagra, which is characterized by erythematous lesions on areas of the skin exposed to sun, friction, or pressure. As lesions become chronic, pigmentation and hyperkeratinization occur. Diarrhea and abdominal pain are prominent. Early symptoms also include mental depression or apathy, headache, insomnia, atrophy of sebaceous glands and hair follicles, inflammation and atrophy of mucous membranes, angular stomatitis, sialorrhea, and glossitis. As pellagra progresses, psychoses (eg, hallucinations, disorientation) often occur. The condition may be complicated by thiamine deficiency with associated peripheral neuritis. The macrocytic anemia that frequently accompanies pellagra probably is related to concomitant folic acid deficiency. Therefore, treatment of pellagra should include small doses of all B-complex vitamins and a well-balanced diet with adequate protein to provide tryptophan.

Pellagra may be associated with isoniazid therapy (competitive inhibition of niacin incorporation into NAD), carcinoid syndrome (deviation of precursor tryptophan for conversion by tumor to serotonin), Hartnup disease (a genetic disorder characterized by impaired absorption of tryptophan), or cirrhosis (decreased hepatic dehydrogenases leading to decreased niacin activity).

The usefulness of niacin's vasodilating effect is doubtful (see Chapter 36), and the large doses used in psychiatry have not been proved to be efficacious. Although niacin (but not niacinamide) is effective in reducing blood lipid levels, adverse effects may limit its usefulness in some individuals (see Chapter 55, Agents Used to Treat Hyperlipidemia).

Therapeutic doses of niacin may cause pruritus, flushing, headache, paresthesias, nausea, and other symptoms of gastrointestinal irritation. Large doses may activate peptic ulcer, impair glucose tolerance, or produce liver damage and hyperuricemia. These reactions are usually reversible when therapy is stopped. Anaphylaxis has been reported following intravenous administration of niacin.

ROUTES, USUAL DOSAGE, AND PREPARATIONS. *Oral, Intramuscular, Intravenous*: For deficiency, 50 mg three times daily. A preparation containing 5 mg each of thiamine, riboflavin, and pyridoxine should be given daily to treat pellagra. Associated anemia may require the use of iron, folic acid, or B_{12}.

NIACIN:

Available generically and under the name Nicotinic Acid: Capsules (timed-release) 125, 250, 400, and 500 mg; tablets 25, 50, 100, and 500 mg; solution (injection, sodium salt) 10 mg/ml in 10 ml containers and 100 mg/ml in 10 and 30 ml containers; powder (bulk).
Nicobid (Armour). Capsules (timed-release) 125, 250, and 500 mg.

Nico-400 (Marion). Capsules (timed-release) 400 mg.
Nicotinex (Fleming). Elixir 50 mg/5 ml (alcohol 14%) (nonprescription).

NIACINAMIDE:

Available generically and under the name Nicotinamide: Capsules 500 mg; tablets 25, 50, 100, and 500 mg; tablets (buffered) 500 mg; solution (injection) 100 mg/ml in 2, 5, 10, and 30 ml containers.

PANTOTHENIC ACID

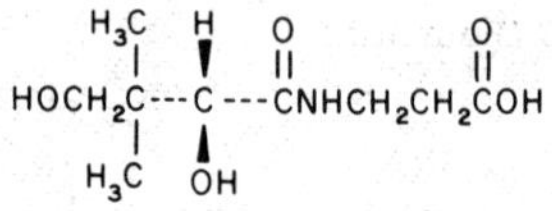

As a precursor of coenzyme A, pantothenic acid is essential in the intermediary metabolism of fats, carbohydrates, and proteins. An RDA has not been established, but a daily intake of 5 to 10 mg is believed to be adequate; a balanced 2,500-calorie daily diet contains about 10 mg.

No cases of spontaneously occurring clinical deficiency have been observed, presumably because pantothenic acid is present in almost all plant and animal tissues. Deficiency is unlikely except in association with other B vitamin deficiencies (eg, pellagra, beriberi, alcoholism), and there is no indication for use of this vitamin alone. Large doses are ineffective in the prevention or treatment of graying hair, adynamic ileus, diabetic neuropathy, or psychiatric states. Pantothenic acid is essentially nontoxic.

ROUTE, USUAL DOSAGE, AND PREPARATIONS. *Oral*: Pantothenic acid is considered suitable for inclusion in multivitamin preparations in amounts of 5 to 10 mg.

See Table 4 for listings.

PYRIDOXINE HYDROCHLORIDE (Vitamin B₆)

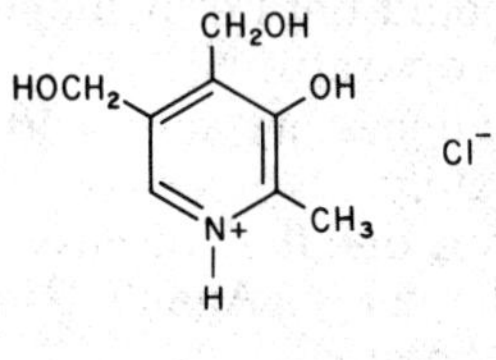

The vitamin B₆ group is composed of three compounds (pyridoxine, pyridoxal, pyridoxamine) that are metabolically and functionally interrelated. These compounds, collectively called pyridoxine, are converted to pyridoxal phosphate, which functions principally in protein and amino acid metabolism (eg, as coenzyme for decarboxylations or transaminations).

The requirement for pyridoxine appears to parallel protein intake and to be increased during pregnancy, lactation, and in some women taking oral contraceptives. Most ordinary diets provide adequate amounts, but artificial formulas for infants should be fortified with pyridoxine.

Dietary deficiency is rare except in combination with other vitamin B-complex deficiencies (eg, in alcoholism, malabsorption syndromes), but inadequate pyridoxine utilization has been implicated in a number of conditions that appear to be genetically determined. For example, infants may exhibit hyperirritability and epileptiform convulsions during the first week of life that promptly respond to administration of pyridoxine. If untreated, pyridoxine-responsive anemia and mental retardation may result. Also, patients with inborn errors of metabolism manifested by homocystinuria or xanthurenic aciduria require large amounts of this vitamin (Mudd, 1971).

Pyridoxine-responsive anemia (usually sideroblastic) is uncommon and may occur in patients without pyridoxine deficiency. It cannot be induced in normal persons either by deficiency in the diet or administration of pyridoxine antagonists. Therefore, a genetic defect is presumed to be the cause (see also Chapter 62, Agents Used to Treat Deficiency Anemias).

Pyridoxine has been reported to improve symptoms such as cheilosis, seborrheic dermatitis, glossitis, and stomatitis that do not respond to thiamine, riboflavin, and niacin. It is also indicated to prevent or treat peripheral neuritis caused by certain drugs (eg, isoniazid, cycloserine, hydralazine, penicillamine) that act as pyridoxine antagonists and/or increase its excretion in the urine. Pyridoxine may be given prophylactically in doses 300% to 500% higher than the RDA during therapy with pyridoxine antagonists.

Pyridoxine supplements should not be given to patients receiving levodopa, because the action of the latter drug is antagonized by pyridoxine. However, this vitamin may be used concurrently in patients receiving a preparation containing both carbidopa and levodopa.

No toxic effects have been reported clinically following intravenous doses of 200 mg or oral doses of 300 mg daily.

ROUTES, USUAL DOSAGE, AND PREPARATIONS. *Oral (preferred), Intramuscular, Intravenous*: In pyridoxine dependency syndromes, *infants*, 2 to 15 mg daily; *adults and children*, 30 to 500 mg daily. For drug-induced peripheral neuritis, *adults and children*, 50 to 200 mg daily. For deficiency, *adults and children*, 10 to 20 mg daily for three weeks, followed by 2 to 5 mg daily in a multivitamin preparation for maintenance.

Available generically: Solution (injection) 50 mg/ml in 10 ml containers and 100 mg/ml in 10 and 30 ml containers; tablets 5, 10, 25, 50, and 100 mg.

Hexa-Betalin (Lilly). Solution (injection) 100 mg/ml in 10 ml containers; tablets 10, 25, and 50 mg.

Hexavibex (Parke, Davis). Solution (injection) 100 mg/ml in 5 ml containers.

RIBOFLAVIN (Vitamin B₂)

Riboflavin functions as the coenzyme for flavin adenine dinucleotide (FAD) and flavin mononucleotide (FMN), which primarily influence hydrogen transport in oxidative enzyme systems (eg, cytochrome C reductase, succinic dehydrogenase, xanthine oxidase). Riboflavin is readily absorbed from the intestine and is distributed to all tissues, but little is stored. A well-balanced diet provides adequate amounts for normal individuals. Requirements parallel carbohydrate intake and are increased during pregnancy and lactation. The requirement also is reported to be increased by prolonged administration of phenothiazines, phenothiazine derivatives, or tricyclic antidepressants.

Ariboflavinosis is characterized by cheilosis, angular stomatitis, glossitis, seborrheic dermatitis of the nose and scrotum, and corneal vascularization (injection and proliferation of capillaries of the limbic plexus). Ocular symptoms include pruritus, burning, blepharospasm, photophobia, and visual impairment. The lesions of the skin and mucous membranes also are noted in other B-complex deficiencies.

Riboflavin deficiency seldom occurs alone; it often is associated with pellagra and other vitamin B-complex deficiency states (eg, alcoholism, malabsorption syndromes). Therefore, ariboflavinosis should be treated with multivitamin B preparations.

There is no acceptable scientific evidence that riboflavin therapy has any effect other than in the treatment or prevention of its deficiency state. No toxic effects have been reported in man.

ROUTE, USUAL DOSAGE, AND PREPARATIONS.
Oral: For deficiency, 5 to 10 mg daily, preferably in a preparation containing the other B-complex vitamins also.

> Available generically: Tablets 5, 10, 25, 60, and 100 mg.
> AVAILABLE TRADEMARK.
> *Hyrye* (O'Neal, Jones & Feldman).

THIAMINE HYDROCHLORIDE (Vitamin B₁)

Thiamine is an essential coenzyme for carbohydrate metabolism. Requirements parallel caloric intake, particularly of carbohydrate.

Thiamine deficiency occurs in the United States, although severe deficiency (beriberi) is relatively rare. Mild deficiency may occur even with apparently adequate diets, especially when energy needs are increased (eg, in hyperthyroidism, during heavy manual labor). Beriberi most commonly occurs in alcoholics, in pregnant women receiving inadequate diets, or in those with malabsorption syndromes, prolonged diarrhea, or hepatic diseases causing defective utilization of thiamine. Beriberi has two principal forms: (1) chronic dry beriberi characterized mainly by polyneuropathy, and (2) acute wet beriberi, in which edema and serous effusions predominate.

Chronic dry beriberi occurs most often in adults and usually is associated with malabsorption or multiple vitamin deficiencies. In chronic alcoholism with associated malnutrition, Wernicke's encephalopathy may develop. The characteristic symptoms (ophthalmoplegia, ataxia, polyneuropathy, mental deterioration) often are accompanied by Korsakoff syndrome (amnestic confabulatory psychosis). This condition is considered a medical emergency and immediate parenteral thiamine therapy is necessary to limit the degree of permanent central nervous system damage.

Wet beriberi is endemic in areas where polished, nonenriched rice forms a large part of the diet. In adults, it may progress from anorexia, muscle weakness, and personality changes to severe circulatory disturbances with edema and high-output heart failure. Severe deficiency in infants may cause death within 24 hours after the onset of symptoms (anorexia, vomiting, convulsions, cyanosis) unless intensive treatment is begun immediately.

There is no evidence that thiamine is of value for anything other than deficiency. Oral administration corrects most uncomplicated deficiencies, but the parenteral route may be utilized in severe, acute situations. In all individuals, the absorptive capacity is restricted and the maximum individual dose absorbed probably is 5 mg.

Thiamine produces no toxic effects when given orally and the excess is excreted rapidly in the urine. Anaphylactoid reactions, a few of which were fatal, have occurred rarely after intravenous administration of large amounts in sensitive patients.

ROUTES, USUAL DOSAGE, AND PREPARATIONS. *Oral, Intramuscular, Intravenous*: For deficiency, 5 to 10 mg three times daily. Larger parenteral doses have been recommended in severe cases, but no satisfactory evidence exists to show that an increased response occurs with doses larger than 30 mg daily. After signs of deficiency have been corrected, the dose should be determined by the RDA as supplied by correction of the diet, if possible, or by a daily supplement. Unless evidence indicates that the deficiency is clearly one of thiamine alone or a therapeutic test is being employed, administration of a vitamin B-complex preparation is preferred.

Available generically: Tablets 5, 10, 25, 50, 100, and 250 mg; solution (injection) 100 mg/ml in 1, 2, 10, and 30 ml containers and 200 mg/ml in 30 ml containers.

AVAILABLE TRADEMARKS.
Betalin S (Lilly), *Bewon* (Wyeth).
SIMILAR PREPARATION.

Thiamine Mononitrate, U.S.P. Used in some multivitamin preparations.

VITAMIN B₁₂ (Cyanocobalamin)

Vitamin B₁₂ is a generic term for several cobalt-containing compounds. As a component of various coenzymes, it is important in the synthesis of nucleic acid, thereby influencing cell maturation and maintenance of the integrity of neuronal

tissue. Animal products are the primary food sources, and dietary deficiencies are rare except in strict vegetarians. Since milk is a relatively good source of vitamin B₁₂, supplementation is unnecessary in infants unless artificial formulas lacking this vitamin are used.

The absorption of vitamin B₁₂ depends upon the presence of sufficient intrinsic factor and calcium ions. Intrinsic factor deficiency causes pernicious anemia, which may be associated with subacute combined degeneration of the spinal cord. Prompt parenteral administration of vitamin B₁₂ prevents progression of neurologic damage. Oral supplements are inadequate for treatment of this disorder; these should be reserved for patients in whom pernicious anemia has been ruled out and they may be necessary during pregnancy and lactation or in vegetarians. Vitamin B₁₂ should be included in B-complex preparations that also include folic acid. See Chapter 62, Agents Used to Treat Deficiency Anemias, for a more detailed discussion of vitamin B₁₂.

ROUTE, USUAL DOSAGE, AND PREPARATIONS. *Oral*: For treatment of dietary deficiency, *adults*, 6 mcg daily; *children*, 3 mcg daily.

No single-entity products available for deficiency. For listing of multivitamin preparations containing vitamin B₁₂, see Table 4.

MINERALS

Many mineral elements function as essential constituents of enzymes and are responsible for regulation of a variety of physiologic functions (eg, maintenance of osmotic pressure, oxygen transport, muscle contraction, central nervous system integrity) and for growth and maintenance of tissues and bones. Some minerals (calcium, phosphorus, sodium, potassium, magnesium, sulfur, and chloride) are present in the body in relatively large amounts, while there are only trace quantities of the others. Trace elements recognized as essential in man are cobalt (as vitamin B₁₂), copper, iodine, iron, and zinc. Since deficiency has been demonstrated in man under special circumstances, chromium and manganese also are thought to be necessary. Because of their presence in human enzyme systems, selenium, molybdenum, nickel, tin, silicon, and arsenic are considered essential. A balanced, varied diet supplies adequate amounts of trace elements, and dietary supplements containing minerals should be used only when evidence of deficiency exists or when demands are known to be increased (eg, during pregnancy and lactation). Unless absorption is impaired, mineral deficiency is uncommon, since most minerals (except zinc) are widely distributed in foods. Also, large quantities of any mineral may interfere with utilization of other elements, and all minerals damage various tissues if present in excessive amounts.

Deficiencies may be created by prolonged total parenteral nutrition. Serum and urine concentrations of trace metals should be monitored every two to four weeks and abnormal levels corrected. The suggested daily intravenous intake of trace minerals for maintenance of adults in stable condition is zinc 2.5 to 4 mg, copper 0.5 to 1.5 mg, chromium 10 to 15 mcg, manganese 0.15 to 0.8 mg, iron (elemental) 1 mg, and iodine 75 mcg. For administration of potassium, magnesium, calcium, and phosphorus, see Chapter 53, Parenteral and Enteral Nutrition. Such therapy should be given routinely to those who would be expected to require supplementation (eg, patients with Crohn's disease, ileal bypass surgery or other resections, malabsorption syndromes). In patients with renal disease or biliary tract obstruction, caution is necessary to avoid excessive dosage.

Minerals Present in Relatively Large Amounts

Calcium: This element is present in the body in greater amounts than any other mineral. Its metabolism and functions are discussed in Chapter 54, Agents Affecting Calcium Metabolism.

An adequate amount of vitamin D is required for efficient absorption of calcium. Quantities of calcium greater than those required to maintain equilibrium have no beneficial effects. Dietary requirements are increased in growing children and during pregnancy and lactation, and infants given artificial formulas or skim milk require supplementation.

Magnesium: Magnesium activates many enzyme systems (alkaline phosphatase, enolases, leucine aminopeptidase) and is an essential cofactor in oxidative phosphorylation, thermoregulation, muscular contractility, and nerve excitability. Deficiency is uncommon in normal individuals eating a varied diet, but the requirement for magnesium parallels the level of protein, calcium, and phosphorus ingested.

Hypomagnesemia causes increased neuronal excitability and neuromuscular transmission; severe deficiency may result in tetany and convulsions. Hypomagnesemia has been observed in alcoholics; in patients with kwashiorkor, infantile tetany, diabetes, malabsorption syndromes, hyper- or hypoparathyroidism, and renal diseases; during diuretic therapy; in burn patients treated with daily saline baths; in patients receiving total parenteral nutrition without adequate magnesium supplements; and postoperatively in some patients.

Hypermagnesemia produces peripheral vasodilatation and loss of tendon reflexes; it has a curare-like effect at the myoneural junction and blocks release of catecholamine from the adrenal glands. Respiratory failure and cardiac arrest occur after very large doses.

For a more detailed discussion of magnesium imbalances, see Chapter 51, Replenishers and Regulators of Water and Electrolytes.

Phosphorus: This mineral is necessary for the utilization of many of the B-complex vitamins. It is present in bones and teeth in amounts nearly equal to those of calcium and is a prominent component of all body tissues. Lipids, proteins, carbohydrates, and various enzymes involved in energy transfer contain phosphorus. A varied diet supplies sufficient phosphorus, but the calcium:phosphorus ratio also is important. If an adequate amount of vitamin D is ingested, diets supplying excess phosphorus in relation to calcium are tolerated. However, neonates fed cow's milk, which has a calcium:phosphorus ratio of 1.2:1 (human milk, 2:1), need dietary manipulation to assure a ratio of at least 1.5:1. Deficiency does not occur in adults unless there is prolonged excessive use of alcohol or antacids, prolonged vomiting, liver disease, and, less commonly, hyperparathyroidism. For further discussion of the therapeutic use of phosphorus, see Chapter 54, Agents Affecting Calcium Metabolism.

Potassium: The differential concentration of potassium (the principal cation of intracellular fluid) and sodium (the principal cation of extracellular fluid) across the cell wall regulates the excitability of the cell, nerve impulse conduction, and body fluid balance and volume. Although deficiency is rare in individuals consuming an adequate diet, hypokalemia may occur in children whose diet lacks protein. Other causes of hypokalemia include prolonged diarrhea, particularly in infants; aldosteronism; inappropriate or inadequate parenteral fluid therapy; and chronic use of adrenal corticosteroids, laxatives, or certain diuretics (eg, thiazides, furosemide). The most serious consequences of hypokalemia are neuromuscular disorders that may progress to areflexic paralysis of the skeleton, gut, and heart.

Hyperkalemia most commonly is caused by impaired renal excretion of potassium, which may occur in patients with adrenocortical insufficiency, acute renal failure, or terminal chronic renal failure or with use of aldosterone antagonists. Severe arrhythmias and conduction defects are the most serious sequelae of hyperkalemia; other manifestations include weakness and paresthesias.

For information on the therapeutic uses of potassium, see Chapters 39, Diuretics; 51, Replenishers and Regulators of Water and Electrolytes; 48, Agents Used to Treat Thyroid Disease; and 80, Antifungal Agents.

Sodium: Sodium helps maintain fluid balance and volume and its concentration in body fluids is under homeostatic control. Imbalances occur only when these mechanisms fail or losses are greater than the compensatory abilities of adaptive mechanisms. Sodium often is added during the processing of food. Many individuals have higher than desirable intakes of sodium, and dietary restriction is recommended in patients with congestive heart failure or hepatic cirrhosis to reduce water retention and in those with hypertension to reduce blood pressure. Hyponatremia is rarely encountered in normal individuals but may occur after prolonged diarrhea or vomiting, particularly in infants; in renal disorders, cystic fibrosis, or adrenocortical insufficiency; or with use of diuretics. Excessive sweating may cause pronounced sodium loss, and replacement therapy should include both water and sodium chloride.

Chloride: Chloride is the most important anion in the maintenance of electrolyte balance. Excessive loss may occur with excessive loss of sodium and, when sodium intake is curtailed, substitution of another source of chloride may be necessary.

Sulfur: Several essential amino acids, thiamine, and biotin contain sulfur. Although this mineral is known to be essential for man, its precise function is not known and no daily requirements have been established.

Trace Elements

Chromium: Trivalent chromium probably acts as a cofactor complex for insulin and thus is necessary for normal glucose utilization. Deficiency has been reported in a few patients receiving total parenteral nutrition for five months to three years. These patients had peripheral neuropathy and/or encephalopathy that was alleviated by administration of 150 mcg of chromium daily. Symptoms included a diabetes-like condition with impaired utilization of glucose. Other patients with similar symptoms of glucose intolerance also had protein-calorie malnutrition. Marginal levels of chromium have been associated with decreased glucose utilization during pregnancy and in the elderly. In these patients, administration of the metal has improved glucose tolerance. However, these findings need further clarification and confirmation.

Supplemental amounts of chromium do not have a hypoglycemic effect in normal individuals or in patients with insulin-dependent diabetes mellitus.

Cobalt: Cobalt is a component of vitamin B12; it has no other known function in normal human nutrition. The daily requirement is easily obtained from a balanced, varied diet. Cobalt salts have been used with dubious success to treat certain types of anemias refractory to other therapy.

Copper: Copper is present in ceruloplasmin (the copper-carrying protein in blood) and is a constituent of several other enzymes (eg, dopamine beta-hydroxylase, cytochrome C oxidase). It is bound to albumin and is an essential component of a number of proteins (eg, erythrocuprein, hepatocuprein). This mineral is thought to act as a catalyst in the storage and release of iron to form hemoglobin. Most unprocessed foods are excellent sources of copper and deficiency is rare. Recently, however, copper deficiency has been reported in malnourished children with anemia and neutropenia; a similar condition has not been observed in adults. Copper supplements should be given during prolonged parenteral or enteral alimentation. In adults, 5 mg of copper sulfate should be given initially, followed by 1.6 mg daily for maintenance; infants and children should receive 0.05 to 0.1 mg/kg of body weight of elemental copper daily. If tolerated, the oral route is preferred but copper also may be used parenterally.

Hypocupremia unrelated to nutritional factors may result from defective ceruloplasmin formation as in the rare genetic disorders, Wilson's disease (hepatolenticular degeneration) or Menkes syndrome (kinky hair disease). Although hypocupremia has been observed in patients with protein-calorie malnutrition, tropical sprue, celiac disease, or the nephrotic syndrome, it is thought to be secondary to disturbances of protein metabolism in which there is loss of copper-protein complexes.

Elevated serum levels of copper occur in various diseases and are produced by some drugs (eg, estrogens, thyroid, corticotropin), but associated abnormalities are rare. For a discussion on the treatment of hypercupremia and excessive tissue accumulation of copper (eg, in Wilson's disease), see the evaluation on Penicillamine in Chapter 86, Specific Antidotes.

Fluoride: Fluoride is incorporated into teeth and decreases the incidence of dental caries, especially in children. The need for fluoride persists throughout life, and there is evidence that it also aids in retention of calcium in bones. However, evidence regarding fluoride supplementation as a means of preventing or alleviating bone diseases such as osteoporosis, especially in older people, remains controversial. (See Chapter 54, Agents Affecting Calcium Metabolism.)

Fluoridation of the water supply (optimum concentration, 0.7 to 1.2 ppm) is the most efficient and economical method of assuring adequate fluoride intake. Dietary supplements should be used only when water supplies contain less than 0.3 ppm (for maximal anticariogenic effects, a daily dose of 0.25 mg of fluoride [0.55 mg sodium fluoride] should be ingested from birth to 2 years of age, 0.5 mg of fluoride [1.1 mg sodium fluoride] from age 2 to 3, and 1 mg [2.2 mg sodium fluoride] from 3 to 16 years) and the dose should be adjusted according to the amount of fluoride in the water. Fluoride supplements are not required when water contains more than 0.7 ppm. Use of fluoride should be discontinued or reviewed if the family moves or when the fluoride content of the water changes.

Chronic toxicity (fluorosis) usually results from prolonged exposure to insecticides or industrial dusts or prolonged use of doses larger than 3 ppm daily. Mottled enamel (dental fluorosis) may occur if teeth are developing, and osteomalacia and osteosclerosis may be induced in older people. Except for orthopedic and supportive measures, there is no treatment for fluorosis; therefore, all efforts should be directed at its prevention.

Reports that persons residing in areas where water supplies are fluoridated have experienced a higher incidence of cancer have been refuted by the American Cancer Institute, which found that some forms of cancer are actually reduced (*J Am Diet Assoc*, 1977).

Iodine: Iodine is an integral part of the thyroid hormones, tetraiodothyronine (thyroxine) and triiodothyronine. Deficiency results in compensatory hyperplasia and hypertrophy of the thyroid gland (endemic goiter). Endemic goiter occurs in areas where the soil is deficient in iodine. This condition was common in many areas before the iodization of table salt but no longer appears to be a problem in the United States, where recent nutrition surveys suggest that iodine intake exceeds the amount necessary to meet human needs. The use of iodized table salt is the most economical and efficient source of iodine supplementation. Iodate in bread and use of iodophores as antiseptic agents by the dairy industry also may contribute iodide to diets, but seafoods are the most reliable food source.

Amounts of 100 to 300 mcg daily are desirable and up to 1 mg daily may be consumed safely. Requirements for iodine are increased in growing children and pregnant or lactating women. However, the prolonged ingestion of large amounts of iodides during pregnancy may result in neonatal thyroid enlargement, hypothyroidism, or cretinism.

Manifestations of acute iodine intoxication are related to the organ systems that incorporate iodine (eg, thyroid gland, salivary apparatus, eye) and include edema, fever, and conjunctivitis. Laryngeal edema resulting in airway obstruction is serious and potentially fatal. Local reactions in the gastrointestinal tract include abdominal pain, vomiting, and diarrhea, sometimes bloody, which may lead to dehydration and shock.

Chronic iodine poisoning (iodism) is more common. There is considerable individual variation in sensitivity to iodine, and some patients may experience inhibition of thyroid activity with subsequent development of hypothyroidism after taking 6 mg or more daily. Hypersensitivity reactions include rash and dermatoses (which appear to be dose related), nausea, edema of the face and eyes, headache, cough, and symptoms of gastric irritation.

For therapeutic use of iodine, see Chapter 48, Agents Used to Treat Thyroid Disease, and Chapter 61, Dermatologic Preparations.

Iron: Ionic iron is an essential component of a number of enzymes necessary for energy transfer and is also present in compounds necessary for oxygen transport and utilization. About 10% of inorganic iron is absorbed when given orally; increased absorption (up to 20%) occurs in iron-deficient individuals. Iron from meat (heme iron) is better absorbed than the primarily nonheme iron from vegetable sources. Requirements are increased in children, adolescents, menstruating women, and during pregnancy and lactation. They are greatest during infancy and, because of the low iron content of milk, formulas should supply 10 to 15 mg of iron daily during the first year of life. Pregnant women cannot obtain sufficient iron from a normal diet unless large amounts of meat are consumed, and this deficit can be corrected only by supplementation (usually 30 mg of elemental iron daily).

Phytates, phosphates, and antacids bind iron as relatively insoluble complexes and thus decrease its absorption; inorganic iron in food also is often bound in these poorly utilized insoluble complexes.

Bleeding associated with gastrointestinal disease (eg, hemorrhoids, peptic ulcer, ulcerative colitis, neoplasms) frequently produces iron deficiency, and malabsorption of iron may occur in tropical sprue or celiac disease, gastrectomy, prolonged diarrhea, or achlorhydria. Deficiency increases the absorption of other elements, which may lead to chronic lead, cobalt, and manganese poisoning. After iron stores in ferritin and hemosiderin are depleted, hemoglobin production is reduced and anemia results. See Chapter 62, Agents Used to Treat Deficiency Anemias.

Excess iron is stored in the liver, kidneys, heart, and other organs, and iron overload can be hazardous, particularly in those with certain diseases (eg, primary and secondary hemochromatosis, porphyria cutanea tarda). Acute iron poisoning is most common in children under 5 years of age. Iron-containing medications should be labeled as hazardous, kept out of reach of children, and packaged in child-proof containers. For treatment of iron poisoning, see Chapter 85, General Antidotes.

Manganese: This element is concentrated in cell mitochondria, mostly in the pituitary gland, liver, pancreas, kidney, and bone. It influences the synthesis of mucopolysaccharides, stimulates hepatic synthesis of cholesterol and fatty acids, and is a cofactor in many enzymes, among them arginase and alkaline phosphatase in the liver. Manganese is abundant in many foods. Deficiency is unknown in humans and an RDA has not been established. Nevertheless, it is advisable to include manganese in a regimen of long-term total parenteral nutrition.

Chronic manganese intoxication is an occupational hazard in mining and industrial areas, although there is no evidence that manganese released into the atmosphere from its many industrial uses is a general hazard to man. In cases of exposure, the onset of parkinsonian symptoms is subtle and may progress unless the exposure ends quickly. Levodopa may relieve rigidity or dystonia.

Molybdenum: This element is an essential constituent of many enzymes. It is easily absorbed and is present in the bones, liver, and kidneys. Human deficiency is unknown and a requirement has not been established.

Selenium: There appears to be a close relationship between vitamin E and selenium, but the latter's function remains obscure. Some evidence suggests it may protect sulfhydryl groups from oxidation. Selenium is depleted in protein-calorie malnutrition, and studies suggest that it may induce weight gain when given to children with kwashiorkor. Little is known of the human requirement and no RDA has been established.

Zinc: This element is a cofactor of enzymes and is essential for cell growth; nucleic acid, carbohydrate, and protein synthesis; and normal utilization of vitamin A. Adequate zinc is provided by a diet containing sufficient animal protein. Its availability in whole grain cereals is unreliable due to the presence of substances such as phytin that interfere with zinc absorption. Diets in which protein is primarily obtained from vegetable sources may supply only marginal amounts of zinc.

The amount of zinc may be insufficient in those with an inadequate diet, in institutionalized patients, or during periods of increased requirement (eg, growing children, pregnancy, lactation), but severe deficiency in this country probably occurs only secondary to malabsorption syndromes. Zinc deficiency with cutaneous manifestations resembling acrodermatitis enteropathica has been reported following long-term parenteral nutrition. Patients receiving intravenous alimentation should receive zinc supplements (2.5 to 4 mg of elemental zinc as the sulfate added to one unit of alimentation solution daily) after about one month of therapy. When enterally administered defined formula diets are the sole source of nutrients, 100% of the USRDA for zinc should be given also.

Symptoms of deficiency include disturbances in taste and smell, anorexia, and suboptimal growth in children. More severe deficiency results in delayed bone maturation, hepatosplenomegaly, hypogonadism, and decreased growth or dwarfism. Other manifestations are hair loss, rashes, multiple cutaneous lesions, glossitis, stomatitis, blepharitis, and paronychia. Gonadal dysfunction in renal disease can be partially corrected in some patients by administering zinc. During dialysis, zinc chloride (400 mcg/L) may be added to the dialysis bath.

Decreased body concentration may occur in patients with acute or chronic infection, myocardial infarction, neoplastic disease, alcoholism with liver disease, and pernicious or sickle cell anemia, while increased concentrations may occur in those with hypertension, hyperthyroidism, polycythemia, and following irradiation. Evidence suggesting that zinc may promote healing of wounds or chronic ulcers is controversial; accelerated healing following zinc administration probably occurs only in those with deficiency.

Miscellaneous Elements: Deficiencies of elements such as nickel, titanium, tin, silicon, aluminum, vanadium, and zirconium have been produced in animals under rigid experimental conditions, but their importance in human nutrition is unknown.

MIXTURES

Clinically apparent vitamin deficiencies are rare in the United States, and subclinical deficiencies are difficult to detect. Excessive use of one or more vitamins may cause relative deficiencies of other essential micronutrients, and large doses of all minerals are toxic. Also, multivitamin preparations used by adequately nourished individuals may exceed nutrient needs by several hundred percent and represent needless expense. Nevertheless, properly formulated multivitamin preparations are useful since clinical vitamin deficiencies are almost always multiple. Such preparations should contain only those ingredients essential for human nutrition in amounts proportional to the RDA. Additional components such as liver, yeast, and wheat germ do not confer any special advantage over the pure chemical ingredients, and inclusion of agents that have no proved value (eg, choline, methionine, lecithin, bioflavonoids, inositol) is unwarranted. The amount of vitamin D in the preparation should not exceed the RDA (400 IU) because of the dangers of hypervitaminosis D. Quantities of folic acid should not exceed the RDA because, although excessive amounts produce a satisfactory hematologic response in pernicious anemia, the neurologic symptoms of this disorder worsen.

Caution is necessary when selecting multivitamin preparations because many manufacturers use the same general trademark for several preparations having very different formulas. *The preparations listed in Table 4 are those considered to have logical formulations when used appropriately. They contain no unwarranted ingredients, inappropriate combinations, or excessive amounts of any individual vitamin or mineral.* Until multivitamin preparations are brought into greater conformity with current nutritional knowledge, the physician should make an effort to prescribe only those having a rational quantitative basis. There seems to be little logic in a formulation containing less than 50% of the RDA for some vitamins and more than 500% of the RDA for other vitamins (particularly the interrelated B vitamins). Dosage should take into account the contribution of the patient's diet, especially vitamins A and D and all minerals.

Supplemental Vitamin Combinations

Prophylactic multivitamin preparations may reasonably contain one-half to one and one-half times the RDA (except that vitamin D should not exceed the RDA) and should be chosen to fit the needs of the individual. These preparations may be useful during periods of increased requirements (eg, pregnancy, lactation), during relatively brief illnesses that cause impaired absorption of nutrients, and in patients who are not eating properly. They should be discontinued after recovery or when correction of the diet has been assured. Preparations containing one and one-half times the RDA may be useful for supplementing therapeutic but nutritionally inadequate diets (eg, in allergy) or when food intake is drastically reduced (eg, in rapid weight reduction programs, during prolonged illness). During pregnancy and lactation, supplemental preparations should reasonably contain folic acid, cyanocobalamin, and iron, for these nutrients probably cannot be supplied adequately by the diet.

Supplemental amounts of a particular vitamin may sometimes be contraindicated. For example, supplementation with vitamin D should be avoided in normal individuals, especially infants and children, who are receiving adequate amounts by exposure to sunlight or in the diet. Pyridoxine may interfere with the effectiveness of levodopa in the treatment of parkinsonism and, therefore, amounts exceeding the RDA should be avoided in these patients.

Therapeutic Multivitamin Preparations

Multivitamin preparations for therapeutic use may contain as much as five times the RDA. If the required dose for a vitamin greatly exceeds the RDA, that vitamin should be given separately. Therapeutic multivitamin preparations should not contain more than the RDA of vitamin D or folic acid. In addition, the intake of vitamin A must be limited in order to avoid hypervitaminosis A.

Therapeutic multivitamin preparations should be labeled as such and prescribed only for the treatment of deficiency states and for supportive therapy in pathologic conditions that markedly increase nutritional requirements (eg, alcoholism, postoperative cachexia). *They should not be used as dietary supplements*, and medical supervision is important when such amounts are administered.

Preparations conforming to the limits stated in this chapter appear in Table 4. The ingredients are listed to enable the physician to select those suitable for particular applications.

Multivitamin preparations for parenteral administration are essential during long-term total parenteral nutrition (TPN) or to treat conditions in which oral intake or absorption of vitamins is inadequate. Current formulations are not satisfactory for use in TPN; none contain all the vitamins and minerals required for a nutritionally complete regimen, nor are all ingredients present in proper amounts.

Guidelines for formulations of vitamins for intravenous use were made by an Expert Panel, Nutrition Advisory Group, AMA Department of Foods and Nutrition in December, 1975. (See Table 5.) It was recommended that a pediatric formulation be prepared for infants and children to age

TABLE 4.
RECOMMENDED MULTIVITAMIN MIXTURES

		Vitamins			
	Category of Use[1]	A (IU)	D (IU)	E (IU)	Ascorbic Acid (mg)
DIETARY SUPPLEMENTS (50% to 150% of USRDA for all ingredients)	(1 tablet unless otherwise noted)				
Adeflor Drops (Upjohn)	I, II (0.6 ml)	2,000	400	—	50
Centrum Tablets (Lederle)	III	5,000	400	30	90
Chocks Multivitamin Tablets (Miles)	III	5,000	400	15	60
With Iron	III	5,000	400	15	60
Dayalets Tablets (Abbott)	III	5,000	400	30	60
With Iron	III	5,000	400	30	60
Dentavite Vitamin Drops with Fluoride (Reid-Provident)	II (1 ml)	3,000	400	5	60
Flintstones Multivitamin Tablets (Miles)	III	5,000	400	15	60
With Iron	III	5,000	400	15	60
Ganatrex Elixir (Merrell-National)	III (3 Tbs)	5,000	400	30	60
Gerilets Tablets (Abbott)	III	5,000	400	45	90
Gevral (Lederle)	III	5,000	—	30	60

10 and an adult formulation be prepared for those age 11 and older. The preparations intended for use during TPN should be incorporated routinely into intravenous feedings daily and should include the fat-soluble vitamins. When parenteral administration is necessary in other conditions, intramuscular injection is usually more satisfactory. For intramuscular use, the same formulation as shown in Table 5 for water-soluble vitamins is recommended *without* the fat-soluble vitamins. Fat-soluble vitamins should be available as single entities in appropriate form for intramuscular administration when needed but are not indicated for routine use except in patients with specific deficiencies.

Ideally, all essential minerals should be included in supplements given during long-term TPN. However, the toxicity of these elements and the difficulty in sol-

ubilizing them for intravenous administration preclude current use of some minerals. The following should be added to intravenous alimentation fluids or given as separate intravenous injections daily: iron, iodine, cobalt (as vitamin B_{12}), zinc, copper, chromium, and manganese. The dosage should be individualized on the basis of the patient's age and clinical and metabolic status. Daily doses suggested for stable adults by the Expert Panel are zinc 2.5 to 4 mg, copper 0.5 to 1.5 mg, chromium 10 to 15 mcg, and manganese 0.15 to 0.8 mg with frequent monitoring of blood levels and adjustment of dosage to meet individual needs. (See also Chapter 53, Parenteral and Enteral Nutrition.) Other clinicians suggest that iron be given in doses of 1 to 5 mg daily and iodine in doses of 70 to 150 mcg daily or appropriate doses may be given once weekly if desired.

| Vitamins | | | | | | Minerals | |
Folic Acid (mcg)	Niacin (mg)	Pyridoxine HCl (mg)	Riboflavin (mg)	Thiamin (mg)	B_{12} (mcg)	Fluoride[2] (mg)	Iron (mg)
—	—	1	—	—	—	0.5	—
400	20	3	2.6	2.25	9	—	27
400	20	2	1.7	1.5	6	—	—
400	20	2	1.7	1.5	6	—	18
400	20	2	1.7	1.5	6	—	—
400	20	2	1.7	1.5	6	—	18
—	8	1	1.2	1	—	0.5	—[3]
400	20	2	1.7	1.5	6	—	—
400	20	2	1.7	1.5	6	—	18
—	20	2	1.7	1.5	6	—	—
400	30	3	2.6	2.25	9	—	27[4]
400	20	2	1.7	1.5	6	—	18

	Category of Use[1]	Vitamins			
		A (IU)	D (IU)	E (IU)	Ascorbic Acid (mg)
Initia Drops with Fluoride (Parke, Davis) (0.6 ml)	II	1,500	200	—	50
Mulvidren Tablets (Stuart)	III	4,000	400	—	75
Mulvidren-F Tablets (Stuart)	III	4,000	400	—	75
Multiple Vitamin Liquid (Abbott) (13.5 ml)	II, III	2,500	400	15	60
One-A-Day Tablets (Miles)	III	5,000	400	15	60
With Iron	III	5,000	400	15	60
Poly-Vi-Flor Chewable (Mead Johnson)	II, III	2,500	400	15	60
With Iron	II, III	2,500	400	15	60
Poly-Vi-Flor Drops (Mead Johnson) (1 ml)	I, II	1,500	400	5	35
With Iron (1 ml)	I, II	1,500	400	5	35
Poly-Vi-Sol Chewable (Mead Johnson)	II, III	2,500	400	15	60
With Iron	II, III	2,500	400	15	60
Poly-Vi-Sol Drops (Mead Johnson) (1 ml)	I, II	1,500	400	5	35
With Iron (1 ml)	I, II	1,500	400	5	35
Stuart Formula Tablets (Stuart)	III	5,000	400	15	60
Tri-Vi-Flor Chewable (Mead Johnson)	II, III	2,500	400	—	60
Tri-Vi-Flor Drops (Mead Johnson) (1 ml)	I, II	1,500	400	—	35
Tri-Vi-Sol Drops (Mead Johnson) (1 ml)	I, II	1,500	400	—	35
With Iron (1 ml)	I, II	1,500	400	—	35
Unicap Capsules, Tablets, and Chewable Tablets (Upjohn)	III	5,000	400	15	60
Unicap plus Iron Tablets (Upjohn)	III	5,000	400	15	60
Unicap M Tablets (Upjohn)	III	5,000	400	15	60
Unicap Senior Tablets (Upjohn)	III	5,000	—	15	60
Vi-Daylin ADC Drops (Ross) (1 ml)	II	1,500	400	—	35
Vi-Daylin ADC w/Fluoride Drops (Ross) (1 ml)	I, II	1,500	400	—	35
Vi-Daylin Chewable (Ross)	II, III	2,500	400	15	60
Vi-Daylin Drops (Ross) (1 ml)	I, II	1,500	400	5	35

	Vitamins					Minerals	
Folic Acid (mcg)	Niacin (mg)	Pyridoxine HCl (mg)	Riboflavin (mg)	Thiamin (mg)	B$_{12}$ (mcg)	Fluoride[2] (mg)	Iron (mg)
—	—	1	—	—	—	0.5	—
—	10	1.2	2.0	2.0	3	—	—[3]
—	10	1.2	2.0	2.0	3	1.0	—[3]
—	13.5	1.05	1.2	1.05	4.5	—	—
400	20	2	1.7	1.5	6	—	—[5]
400	20	2	1.7	1.5	6	—	18
300	13.5	1.05	1.2	1.05	4.5	1	—
300	13.5	1.05	1.2	1.05	4.5	1	12
—	8	0.4	0.6	0.5	2	0.5	—
—	8	0.4	0.6	0.5	—	0.5	10
300	13.5	1.05	1.2	1.05	4.5	—	—
300	13.5	1.05	1.2	1.05	4.5	—	12
—	8	0.4	0.6	0.5	2	—	—
—	8	0.4	0.6	0.5	—	—	10
400	20	2	1.7	1.5	6	—	18[6]
—	—	—	—	—	—	1	—
—	—	—	—	—	—	0.5	—
—	—	—	—	—	—	—	—
—	—	—	—	—	—	—	10
400	20	2	1.7	1.5	6	—	—
400	20	2	1.7	1.5	6	—	18[7]
400	20	2	1.7	1.5	6	—	18[8]
400	14	2	1.7	1.2	6	—	10[9]
—	—	—	—	—	—	—	—
—	—	—	—	—	—	0.25	—
300	13.5	1.05	1.2	1.05	4.5	—	—
—	8	0.4	0.6	0.5	1.5	—	—

		Vitamins			
	Category of Use[1]	A (IU)	D (IU)	E (IU)	Ascorbic Acid (mg)
Vi-Daylin Fluoride Chewable (Ross)	III	2,500	400	15	60
Vi-Daylin Fluoride Drops (Ross)	I, II (1 ml)	1,500	400	5	35
Vi-Daylin/F ADC + Iron Drops (Ross)	I, II (1 ml)	1,500	400	—	35
Vi-Daylin/F + Iron Drops (Ross)	I, II (1 ml)	1,500	400	5	35
Vi-Daylin Liquid (Ross)	II, III (5 ml)	2,500	400	15	60
Vi-Daylin Liquid plus Iron (Ross)	II, III (5 ml)	2,500	400	15	60
Vi-Daylin plus Iron Chewable (Ross)	II, III	2,500	400	15	60
Vi-Daylin plus Iron Drops (Ross)	I, II (1 ml)	1,500	400	5	35
Vi-Daylin plus Iron ADC Drops (Ross)	I, II (1 ml)	1,500	400	—	35
Vigran Adult Tablets (Squibb)	III	5,000	400	30	60
Vi-Magna (Lederle)	III	5,000	400	15	60
Vi-Syneral One-Caps (Fisons)	III	5,000	—	30	60
THERAPEUTIC PREPARATIONS (100% to 500% of USRDA for all ingredients)					
Abdec Baby Drops (Parke, Davis)	I, II (0.6 ml)	5,000	400	—	50
Abdec w/Fluoride Drops (Parke, Davis)	I, II (0.6 ml)	5,000	400	—	50
Fortespan Capsules (Menley & James)	III	10,000	400	—	150
Gevral T (Lederle)	III	5,000	400	45	90
Novacebrin Drops (Lilly)	I, II (0.6 ml)	4,000	400	—	60
PREGNANCY AND LACTATION (contains 0.8 to 1 mg folic acid, 18 to 45 mg elemental iron, at least 4 mcg cyanocobalamin, and more than 50% but less than 300% USRDA of all other vitamins with no inappropriate ingredients. None contain 100% USRDA for calcium and magnesium content is insignificant)					
En-Cebrin F (Lilly)	IV	4,000	400	—	50
Engran-HP (Squibb)	IV (2 tablets)	8,000	400	30	60
Filibon F.A. (Lederle)	IV	8,000	400	30	60
Filibon Forte (Lederle)	IV	8,000	400	45	90

	Vitamins					Minerals	
Folic Acid (mcg)	Niacin (mg)	Pyridoxine HCl (mg)	Riboflavin (mg)	Thiamin (mg)	B$_{12}$ (mcg)	Fluoride[2] (mg)	Iron (mg)
200	13.4	1.28	1.2	1.02	4.5	1	—
—	6	0.4	0.6	0.5	—	0.25	—
—	—	—	—	—	—	0.5	10
—	8	0.4	0.6	0.5	—	0.25	10
—	13.5	1.05	1.2	1.05	4.5	—	—
—	13.5	1.05	1.2	1.05	4.5	—	10
300	13.5	1.05	1.2	1.05	4.5	—	12
—	8	0.4	0.6	0.5	1.5	—	10
—	—	—	—	—	—	—	10
400	20	2	1.7	1.5	6	—	—
400	20	2	1.7	1.5	6	—	—
400	20	2	1.7	1.5	6	—	18
—	10	1	1.2	1	—	—	—[10]
—	10	1	1.2	1	—	0.5	—[11]
—	60	6	6	6	15	—	—[12]
400	30	3	2.6	2.25	9	—	27
—	10	0.8	1	1	—	—	—
1,000	10	2	2	3	5	—	30[13]
800	20	2.5	2	1.7	8	—	18[14]
1,000	20	4	2	1.7	8	—	45
1,000	30	3	2.5	2	12	—	45

		Vitamins			
	Category of Use[1]	A (IU)	D (IU)	E (IU)	Ascorbic Acid (mg)
Filibon OT (Lederle)	IV	8,000	400	30	60
Natabec Rx (Parke, Davis)	IV	4,000	400	—	50
Natalins (Mead Johnson)	IV	8,000	400	30	90

PARENTERAL PREPARATIONS (Each 1 ml of solution, when mixed with diluent, contains between 50% and 500% USRDA for all ingredients. When entire vial is used, the 500% limit is exceeded.)

Folbesyn Injection (Lederle) (2 ml vial + diluent containing the folic acid)	V (1 ml)	—	—	—	150
Solu-B with C (Upjohn) (5 ml vial to be mixed with 5 ml of sterile water for injection)	V (1 ml)	—	—	—	100

[1]Infants less than 1 year; II—children 1 to 4; III—children over 4 and adults; IV—pregnancy and lactation; V—adults only.
[2]All preparations containing fluoride require a prescription.
[3]Plus pantothenic acid 3 mg.
[4]Plus biotin 0.45 mg and pantothenic acid 15 mg.
[5]Plus pantothenic acid 10 mg (preparation without iron only).
[6]Included because vitamin formulation appropriate but mineral formulation provides less than 50% USRDA of calcium, phosphorus, or magnesium.
[7]Plus pantothenic acid 10 mg.
[8]Plus pantothenic acid 10 mg, iodine 150 mcg, copper 2 mg, zinc 15 mg, manganese 1 mg, and potassium 5 mg.

TABLE 5.
SUGGESTED COMPOSITION FOR INTRAVENOUS MULTIVITAMIN FORMULATIONS

Vitamin*	Infants/Children (under 11 yrs)	Adult
Vitamin A (retinol)	2,300.0 IU	3,300.0
Vitamin D†	400.0 IU	200.0
Vitamin E (alpha tocopherol)	7.0 IU	10.0
Vitamin K_1 (phylloquinone)	0.2 mg	—
Ascorbic Acid	80.0 mg	100.0
Folacin	140.0 mcg	400.0
Niacin	17.0 mg	40.0
Riboflavin	1.4 mg	3.6
Thiamin	1.2 mg	3.0
Vitamin B_6 (pyridoxine)	1.0 mg	4.0
Vitamin B_{12} (cyanocobalamin)	1.0 mcg	5.0
Pantothenic acid	5.0 mg	15.0
Biotin	20.0 mcg	60.0

*May be provided in appropriate salt or ester form in equivalent potency.
†As ergocalciferol or cholecalciferol.

Vitamins						Minerals	
Folic Acid (mcg)	Niacin (mg)	Pyridoxine HCl (mg)	Riboflavin (mg)	Thiamin (mg)	B$_{12}$ (mcg)	Fluoride[2] (mg)	Iron (mg)
1,000	20	2.5	2	1.7	8	—	30
1,000	10	3	2	3	5	—	30[15]
800	20	4	2	1.7	8	—	45[16]
500	37.5	7.5	5	5	7.5	—	—[17]
—	50	1	2	2	—	—	—[18]

[9]*Plus iodine 150 mcg, copper 2 mg, zinc 15 mg, and potassium 5 mg.*
[10]*Plus pantothenic acid 5 mg.*
[11]*Plus pantothenic acid 5 mg.*
[12]*Plus pantothenic acid 6 mg.*
[13]*Plus pantothenic acid 5 mg, calcium 250 mg, and other minerals.*
[14]*Plus calcium 650 mg (50% USRDA) and other minerals.*
[15]*Plus calcium 600 mg.*
[16]*Plus calcium 200 mg and other minerals.*
[17]*Plus pantothenic acid 5 mg. Parabens and trolamine added as preservatives.*
[18]*Plus pantothenic acid 10 mg. Parabens added as preservatives.*

Selected References

Diseases of nutrition, in Beeson PB, McDermott W (eds): *Textbook of Medicine*, ed 14. Philadelphia, WB Saunders Co, 1975, 1354, 1375.

National nutrition consortium endorses fluoridation. *J Am Diet Assoc* 70:354, 1977.

Recommended Dietary Allowances, ed 8. National Research Council. Washington, DC, National Academy of Sciences, 1974.

Vitamin E. *Med Lett Drugs Ther* 17:69-70, 1975.

Campbell GD Jr, et al: Ascorbic acid-induced hemolysis in G-6-PD deficiency. *Ann Intern Med* 82:810, 1975.

Chalmers TC: Effects of ascorbic acid on common cold: Evaluation of evidence. *Am J Med* 58:532-536, 1975.

Committee on Nutrition, American Academy of Pediatrics. Fluoride supplementation: Revised dosage schedule. *Pediatrics* 63:150-152, 1979.

DeLuca HF: Vitamin D endocrinology. *Ann Intern Med* 85:367-377, 1976.

Hayes KC, Hegsted DM: Toxicity of vitamins, in *Toxicants Occurring Naturally in Foods*, ed 2. Washington DC, National Academy of Sciences, 1973, 235-253.

Jukes TH: Megavitamin therapy. *JAMA* 233:550-551, 1975.

McIntyre N, Stanley NN: Cardiac beriberi: Two modes of presentation. *Br Med J* 4:567-569, 1971.

Mudd SH: Pyridoxine-responsive genetic disease. *Fed Proc* 30:970-976, 1971.

Reinhold JG: Trace elements--A selective survey. *Clin Chem* 21:476-500, 1975.

Ulmer DD: Trace elements. *N Engl J Med* 297:318-321, 1977.

Underwood EJ: Trace elements, in *Toxicants Occurring Naturally in Foods*, ed 2. Washington DC, National Academy of Sciences, 1973, 43-87.

Starvation and inanition may contribute to morbidity and mortality in critically ill patients. The importance of nutritional support in these and other patients with impaired digestion and absorption or inability to ingest food normally has led to the development of new techniques for supplying nourishment and to the formulation of a wide range of commercial dietary preparations. Diets for oral or tube feeding range from liquified conventional foods through defined formula diets (DFD, elemental diets). In addition, parenteral nutrient solutions are available for peripheral or central intravenous alimentation. Therapy is directed toward maintaining good nutritional status when it exists, establishing positive nitrogen balance and increasing weight in the malnourished, and overcoming the multiple effects of malnutrition.

PARENTERAL NUTRITION

Parenteral nutrition is indicated in patients who are unable to ingest, digest, or absorb nutrients in the alimentary tract. For *short-term* therapy (eg, three to five days) after uncomplicated surgical procedures, a carbohydrate-electrolyte solution may be infused to supply total fluid and electrolyte needs and sufficient calories to reduce protein catabolism. Daily infusion of approximately 150 g carbohydrate maintains brain and red blood cell metabolism and reduces protein catabolism from muscle and viscera. Sodium chloride 0.2% to 0.3% with dextrose injection 5% or 10% is commonly used. (Fructose or invert sugar injection offers no advantage and has some disadvantages over dextrose.) Amino acids have a greater protein-sparing effect than dextrose; however, they usually do not completely prevent negative nitrogen balance following surgery. The higher cost of amino acid solutions relative to potential benefit has prevented their widespread use in place of dextrose for short-term therapy (Craig et al, 1977; Greenberg et al, 1976).

When *prolonged* intravenous feeding is indicated because a serious protein and calorie loss has been identified (eg, in patients with severe gastrointestinal disease or hypermetabolic states; those with anorexia, nausea, and vomiting secondary to cancer chemotherapy) or when relatively short-term therapy (seven to ten days) is required to prepare moderately debilitated patients for surgery, a crystalline amino acid solution [Aminosyn, FreAmine II, Travasol, Veinamine] should be given together with hypertonic carbohydrate, fat emulsions, vitamins, and minerals to provide all known nutrients in amounts needed by the patient (Greene et al, 1977). By providing a source of essential amino acids with adequate calories, loss of lean body mass is prevented or repleted, wound healing may be enhanced, and an impaired immune response is improved. The technique of providing total nutrition by parenteral administration of amino acids in conjunction with dextrose solution (usually 50%) is called total parenteral nutrition (TPN) or intravenous hyperalimentation (IVH) (White et al, 1974; Greene et al, 1977; Fleming et al, 1976). Protein hydrolysate solutions [Amigen, Aminosol, Hyprotigen] also have been used in TPN but are now largely obsolete, having been replaced by crystalline amino acid solutions.

TPN solutions are prepared from commercially available parenteral solutions by mixing 50% dextrose (or 70%, if necessary to reduce volume) with the amino acid solution and adding vitamins, minerals, and trace elements. Because of the possibility of bacterial contamination, TPN solutions are prepared aseptically under a laminar air flow hood, refrigerated, and preferably administered within 24 hours. If infusion is not begun within one hour after preparation, the solution should be stored under refrigeration until the time of use. Darkened or cloudy solutions should not be used. Drugs should not be added to TPN solutions unless compatibility and stability have been established. Drugs often can be given more expeditiously from separate bottles running into the central line when they cannot be administered via a peripheral vein.

Since such TPN solutions are hypertonic, they must be infused into a central vein with a high blood flow to provide rapid dilution. The percutaneous approach to the superior vena cava via the subclavian or jugular vein is preferred, and the solution is generally administered continuously at an even flow rate. Bolus administration may result in hyperglycemia, glycosuria, and an osmotic diuresis with eventual dehydration. Intermittent infusion over 12 to 16 hours may be given with the patient on a "heparin lock" during the remainder of the day. If this is done, it is essential that the hypertonic dextrose solution be gradually tapered for one and one-half hours prior to stopping the infusion.

Adult Needs: The infused osmolar load in TPN may produce diuresis if dextrose is infused in an amount and at a rate that exceeds metabolism. As new tissue is formed, requirements for potassium, magnesium, and phosphate are increased. A high rate of glucose metabolism causes potassium and phosphate to enter cells in increased amounts as TPN is initiated. The average adult patient requires approximately 50 to 80 mEq of sodium and 40 to 60 mEq of potassium daily, but requirements may be greater. Sodium and potassium are generally added to TPN solutions as mixtures of chloride, acetate, or lactate salts to achieve a proper anion/cation ratio and prevent development of acidosis or alkalosis.

Magnesium is necessary in many enzyme systems and is also a major intracellular cation. Hypomagnesemia will develop after eight to ten days of TPN unless magnesium sulfate is added to the infusion daily. Usually 17 to 22 mEq are adequate, but more may be needed in the presence of extensive gastrointestinal fluid loss or renal tubular wasting. Magnesium and potassium should be administered cautiously (with monitoring of serum levels) to patients with impaired renal function.

The amount of calcium gluconate and phosphorus (the latter available commercially as mixtures of sodium or potassium mono- and dibasic phosphate salts) added depends upon the amino acid solution infused. The average adult patient requires 200 to 400 mg of calcium and 200 to 400 mg of phosphorus daily for maintenance, but larger amounts are often needed in the early period of TPN to maintain the serum phosphorus level above 2.5 mg/dl. Trace elements, particularly copper and zinc, should be included when TPN is initiated, especially in malnourished patients, and the levels should be monitored periodically. Manganese and chromium also are desirable during long-term therapy.

The water-soluble B-complex vitamins and ascorbic acid may be depleted rapidly in malnourished patients, and requirements may be increased in stress situations such as severe trauma, major surgery, or serious illness. A parenteral preparation of vitamin B complex with ascorbic acid (eg, Folbesyn, Solu-B with C, Berocca-C) should be added to the intravenous solution together with fat-soluble vitamins on a regular schedule. Because water-soluble vitamins are excreted quickly when given too rapidly, bolus administration should be avoided. Care should be taken to avoid overdosage with vitamins A and D. Folic acid and vitamin B_{12} may be given with multiple vitamins or separately. Vitamin K should be administered separately (2 mg once weekly) if there are no contraindications. See also Chapter 52, Vitamins and Minerals.

Essential fatty acid deficiencies may develop during prolonged TPN. Intravenous fat emulsions [Intralipid, Liposyn] provide a source of essential fatty acids and will prevent or correct the deficiencies when infused in amounts sufficient to provide 3% to 5% of the total caloric input. These preparations have a caloric value of 1.1 calories/ml, and since they are isotonic, they can be administered through a peripheral vein. Intralipid also has been infused peripherally as a major source of calories during prolonged TPN in patients whose daily caloric requirement does not exceed 1,800 calories (Meng and Wilmore, 1976); however, since a fat emulsion should provide no more than 60% of the total caloric input, a central catheter usually is needed for infusion of hypertonic dextrose (Fleming et al, 1976). It has also been suggested that hypermetabolic patients cannot achieve positive nitrogen balance unless their resting metabolic expenditure is covered by glucose. When Intralipid is given with 5% or 10% dextrose via a peripheral vein, a large fluid volume may be required to provide sufficient calories and this may be a disadvantage when volume expansion should be avoided. Fat emulsions may cause hyperlipidemia in patients with impaired fat metabolism. Another disadvantage of these solutions is their high cost compared to 50% dextrose.

Prevention of hyperglycemia and glycosuria is best accomplished by giving dextrose as the main constituent initially, with the caloric content of the formula reduced by about 50%. The caloric content then may be increased gradually by 500 to 1,000 kcal every two days as tolerance is demonstrated. This precaution is particularly important for known diabetics and elderly patients. Fractional urine sugar levels should be determined every six hours. For the initial two to four days or longer, the blood sugar should be monitored until glucose tolerance is demonstrated (usually in two to three days as endogenous insulin production increases). If the blood sugar remains greatly elevated, regular insulin may be given intravenously, starting with 2 units/100 kcal and increasing the amount as indicated. Approximately 50% of insulin will adhere to glass or plastic, but the remainder is stable for 24 hours. Accurate charting of intake and output is essential, together with daily weights. Weight gain of more than 0.5 kg/24 hours may signify fluid retention. If documented, this is treated with diuretics or by sodium and/or fluid restriction.

Red blood cell volume should be restored by transfusion of whole blood or packed cells, and appropriate doses of iron should be given either intramuscularly or intravenously. Moderate and severe hypoalbuminemia should be treated early in the course of TPN by the intravenous administration of 12.5 to 50 g of albumin daily as often as needed to maintain the serum level above 2.5 g/dl. The routine use of albumin should be avoided when there are no albumin losses and the serum level is stable. The serum albumin level will increase by endogenous restoration in most patients receiving TPN if adequate amino acids and calories are given and there is no underlying pathologic condition to prevent formation or increase losses.

Serum electrolytes, blood sugar, and blood urea nitrogen or creatinine levels should be measured three times weekly or more often if the patient is unstable metabolically, and liver function studies, albumin, calcium, SMA 12/60, and serum magnesium once weekly. Additions or deletions to the solutions should be made as necessary to correct any electrolyte or fluid imbalance. The efficacy of nutritional support is most simply determined by weight measurements, assessed against possible edema formation. Other methods include the following: (1) creatinine/height index and upper arm circumference, which reflect the status of muscle protein; (2) serum albumin and transferrin (or total iron-binding capacity) levels, which reflect visceral protein status; (3) lymphocyte count and cell-mediated immunity, which indicate immune competence; (4) triceps skinfold, which estimates fat stores; and (5) nitrogen balance measured directly or by urea nitrogen excretion.

Adverse Reactions and Precautions

In addition to catheter-related mechanical problems, the major complications of TPN are infection and metabolic abnormalities resulting from an excess or deficiency of various nutrients (Fleming et al, 1976). Infection is one of the most serious complications. The cause of an elevated temperature, particularly of the spiking type, during TPN should be investigated immediately. The solution and tubing should be replaced, a fever workup initiated, and cultures taken to determine whether the catheter tip and/or solution are contaminated. If the temperature remains elevated for four to six hours and no other explanation can be found, the catheter may be empirically incriminated as a source of infection and should be removed or replaced.

TPN administration should be discontinued gradually over a period of one to one and one-half hours because the pancreatic insulin response does not necessarily cease once the dextrose infusion is stopped and insulin levels are often elevated during infusion. If TPN must be stopped suddenly, 10% dextrose should be infused peripherally for one to two hours to prevent hypoglycemia. The patient with hypoglycemia following abrupt cessation of TPN usually does not develop symptoms if kept supine. Prior to surgery with general anesthesia, TPN always should be discontinued as indicated above and replaced with dextrose-containing intravenous fluids, for hypoglycemia during anesthesia may be unrecognized and can result in irreversible brain damage or death.

Hyperglycemia, glycosuria, and osmotic diuresis may occur with excessive dextrose infusion. FreAmine I, but not FreAmine II, has caused hyperchloremic acidosis occasionally. Hyperammonemia has been associated with infusion of protein hydrolysates and amino acid solutions. Liver disease in premature infants receiving long-term parenteral nutrition has been attributed to many factors, including essential fatty acid deficiency and protein hydrolysate toxicity; however, this complication has also occurred in infants receiving amino acids and Intralipid (Postuma et al, 1979).

INDIVIDUAL EVALUATIONS

CRYSTALLINE AMINO ACID SOLUTION
[Aminosyn, FreAmine II, Travasol, Veinamine, Nephramine]

Aminosyn, FreAmine II, Travasol, and Veinamine contain a mixture of essential and nonessential amino acids but no peptides. They are indicated for intravenous administration when there is interference with ingestion, digestion, or absorption of protein for long periods or when parenteral supplementation of oral protein intake is required. Free amino acids are utilized more efficiently than the peptides of enzymatic protein hydrolysates, and crystalline amino acid solutions have largely-replaced protein hydrolysates in TPN (Fleming et al, 1976). These amino acid solutions (3.5%) also have been used in place of or with 5% dextrose for short-term therapy in surgical patients, but the high cost has prevented their widespread use for this purpose (Craig et al, 1977; Greenberg et al, 1976). These solutions are useful in place of 5% dextrose in marginally depleted patients with diabetes. Nephramine, a mixture of eight essential amino acids, is used as a component of TPN in patients with serious renal failure who require restriction of nitrogen intake.

Mild thrombophlebitis has occurred rarely during infvsion of amino acid solutions. Flushing, fever, and nausea also have been reported. Because amino acids increase the blood urea nitrogen level more than a protein-free infusion, they should be given cautiously and in restricted amounts to patients with impaired renal function. Since Nephramine contains only the essential amino acids, it is preferred to other amino acid preparations in patients with serious renal failure.

In patients with chronic or acute liver disease, hepatic coma may be precipitated by accumulation of nitrogenous substances in the blood. For this reason, amino acid solutions should be used cautiously in patients with cirrhosis, severe viral hepatitis, and major involvement of the liver by cancer. Amino acid solutions containing significant amounts of sodium should be used cautiously in patients requiring sodium restriction, and those containing potassium should generally be avoided in those with renal failure.

PREPARATIONS.
See Table 1.

PROTEIN HYDROLYSATE INJECTION
[Amigen, Aminosol, Hyprotigen]

Protein hydrolysate solutions may be administered intravenously when there is interference with ingestion, digestion, or absorption of protein for prolonged periods or when parenteral supplementation of oral protein intake is required. These preparations are rarely used today, however, because of the increasing popularity of crystalline amino acid solutions.

Protein hydrolysate solutions contain amino acids and short-chain peptides. Two products are derived from casein [Amigen, Hyprotigen] and one is derived from fibrin [Aminosol]. In most, only about 60% of the

TABLE 1.
AMINO ACID SOLUTIONS

Preparation (Manufacturer)	Milliequivalents Per 1,000 ml			
	Na+	K+	Mg++	C1-
Aminosyn 3.5% (Abbott)	40	18	3	40
Aminosyn 5%, 7%, 10% (Abbott)		5		
Aminosyn with electrolytes 7% (Abbott)	70	66	10	96
FreAmine II 8.5% (McGaw)	10			
Nephramine* 5% (McGaw)	6			
Travasol 5.5% (Travenol)	70	60	10	70
Travasol 8.5% (Travenol)	70	60	10	70
Travasol without electrolytes 5.5% (Travenol)				22
Travasol without electrolytes 8.5% (Travenol)				34
Veinamine 8% (Cutter)	40	30	6	50

*For patients with renal failure.

amino acids are free; the remainder are present as peptides which are probably metabolized in part, but utilization in various disease states is not well documented. The preparations may be modified during manufacture by addition of one or more amino acids so that the final solution has an amino acid content that approximates the requirements for human nutrition. These preparations contain varying quantities of electrolytes.

Adverse reactions to protein hydrolysates, noted most frequently with rapid infusion, include nausea, vomiting, headache, fever, flushing, hypotension, abdominal pain, convulsions, phlebitis and thrombosis, and edema at the site of injection. These reactions are uncommon and when they occur, other causes should be searched for. Protein hydrolysate solutions should be given in restricted amounts to patients with impaired renal function or severe liver disease. Some solutions contain significant amounts of sodium and should be used cautiously in patients on sodium-restricted diets.

PREPARATIONS.

(All amounts given per 1,000 ml.)
Amigen (Baxter). Solution containing casein hydrolysate 5%, sodium 35 mEq, potassium 19 mEq, calcium 5 mEq, magnesium 2 mEq, chloride 20 mEq, and HPO₄ 30 mEq; solution containing casein hydrolysate 10%, sodium 60 mEq, potassium 31 mEq, calcium 10 mEq, magnesium 4 mEq, chloride 44 mEq, and HPO₄ 60 mEq.

Aminosol (Abbott). Solution containing fibrin hydrolysate 5%, sodium 10 mEq, potassium 17 mEq, calcium 1 mEq, magnesium 2.2 mEq, chloride 10.2 mEq, and HPO₄ 10 to 15 mM (P).

Hyprotigen (McGaw). Solution containing casein hydrolysate 5%, sodium 25 mEq, potassium 20 mEq, calcium 5 mEq, magnesium 2 mEq, chloride 18 mEq, and HPO₄ 25 mEq; solution containing casein hydrolysate 10%, sodium 50 mEq, potassium 36 mEq, calcium 10 mEq, magnesium 4 mEq, chloride 36 mEq, and HPO₄ 50 mEq. (Also available as a kit with 40% or 50% dextrose for preparing hyperalimentation fluid.)

INTRALIPID

Intralipid is an intravenous fat emulsion containing 10% soybean oil stabilized with egg yolk phospholipids. The major component fatty acids are linoleic (54%), oleic (26%), palmitic (9%), and linolenic (8%). The total caloric value of Intralipid is 1.1 calories/ml.

Intralipid is used to prevent or correct essential fatty acid deficiencies and to provide calories in high density form during prolonged TPN (Meng and Wilmore, 1976). Since Intralipid is isotonic with plasma, it is suitable for peripheral infusion and, if sufficient calories can be provided by this method, the use of hypertonic (more than 10%) dextrose via a central vein catheter may sometimes be avoided. Weight gain, healing of fistulas, and increased serum protein levels have been observed in some patients during long-term parenteral nutrition using Intralipid as the main nonprotein calorie source. (See also the Introduction.)

Intralipid is thought to be metabolized in the same manner as natural chylomicrons, and a transient increase in plasma triglycerides occurs after infusion. The triglycerides are hydrolyzed to free fatty acids and glycerol by the enzyme, lipoprotein lipase. The free fatty acids either enter the tissues (where they may be oxidized or resynthesized into triglycerides and stored) or circulated in the plasma, bound to albumin. In the liver, circulating free fatty acids are oxidized or converted to very low density lipoproteins that re-enter the blood stream.

In contrast to previously available fat emulsions, Intralipid rarely causes severe adverse reactions. Thrombophlebitis, febrile reactions, vomiting, pain in the chest or back, and hypersensitivity reactions have occurred occasionally.

Hyperlipidemia may occur if Intralipid is infused too rapidly or if it is administered to patients with impaired fat metabolism. Excessive accumulation can be recognized by visual inspection of the plasma, determination of triglyceride concentrations, or measurement of plasma light-scattering activity by nephelometry. This preparation is contraindicated in patients with pathologic hyperlipidemic states.

Newborn infants, particularly those who are premature, small, or acutely ill, may metabolize Intralipid slowly; infusion at a constant rate over a period of 20 to 24 hours may reduce the risk of hyperlipidemia in these patients. Since free fatty acids compete with bilirubin for albumin binding sites, Intralipid may increase the risk of kernicterus in infants with hyperbilirubinemia and may interfere with estimation of serum bilirubin (Andrew et al, 1976). It has also been suggested that the plant sterols present in soybean oil could lead to disturbances in myelin composition of the developing nervous system (Bryan et al, 1976).

The fat particles of Intralipid do not form aggregations, and there appears to be no risk of fat embolism if the recommended infusion technique is followed. After prolonged therapy, there may be a proliferation of Kupfer cells in the liver and deposition of a brown pigment (intravenous fat pigment) throughout the reticuloendothelial system. Hepatomegaly, thrombocytopenia, anemia, transient abnormalities in liver function tests, and decreased pulmonary diffusing capacity have been reported rarely. The "overloading syndrome" (focal seizures, fever, leukocytosis, splenomegaly, and shock) associated with use of earlier fat emulsions is also rare following infusion of Intralipid. Periodic liver function tests and frequent platelet counts should be performed during long-term therapy with this agent.

ROUTE, USUAL DOSAGE, AND PREPARATIONS. Intralipid may be infused via a peripheral or central vein. It should not be mixed with other solutions, and drugs and vitamins should not be added to the infusion bottle. This emulsion may be infused into the same vein as the dextrose-amino acid solution by means of a Y-connector near the infusion site. Filters should not be used for the lipid emulsion. When administered to prevent or correct essential fatty acid deficiency, 3% to 5% of the total caloric input should be provided by Intralipid. When used as a source of calories, Intralipid should comprise no more than 60% of the total caloric input in adults and children and 40% in newborn infants; the remainder should be supplied by dextrose and a source of amino acids.

Intravenous: In *adults*, the initial infusion rate should be no greater than 1 ml/min for 15 to 30 minutes. If no adverse effects occur, the rate may be increased to provide a maximum of 500 ml infused over a period of four hours. On the following day, the dosage may be increased but should not exceed 2.5 g of fat/kg of body weight daily. In *children*, the initial infusion rate is 0.1 ml/min for 10 to 15 minutes which, if tolerated, may be increased to permit infusion of 1 g of fat/kg of body weight in four hours. The daily dose should not exceed 4 of fat/kg.

In *newborn infants*, it has been recommended that Intralipid should be infused at a constant rate over 20 to 24 hours with a maximal daily dose of 2 to 4 g of fat/kg of body weight.

Intralipid (Cutter). Fat emulsion 10% in 500 ml containers.

LIPOSYN

This intravenous fat emulsion contains 10% safflower oil stabilized with egg phospholipids. The major component fatty acids are linoleic (77%), oleic (13%), palmitic (7%), and stearic (2.5%). The total caloric value of Liposyn is 1.1 calories/ml (0.675 calories supplied by linoleic acid).

Liposyn is used to prevent essential fatty acid deficiencies during prolonged TPN. It appears to be comparable to Intralipid in efficacy and safety; however, time has not permitted a detailed evaluation of this new product.

For adverse reactions and precautions, see the evaluation on Intralipid.

ROUTE, USUAL DOSAGE, AND PREPARATIONS. Liposyn may be infused via the same peripheral or central vein as the dextrose/amino acid solution by means of a Y connector. It should not be mixed with other solutions, and drugs and vitamins should not be added to the infusion bottle. Filters should not be used for administration of the emulsion.

Intravenous: For prevention of essential fatty acid deficiencies, the daily requirement is approximately 4% of the caloric intake as linoleate. In *adults*, this can be supplied as 500 ml administered twice weekly. The emulsion is infused initially at a rate of 1 ml/min for 30 minutes. If no adverse effects occur, the rate may be increased but no more than 500 ml should be given over a period of four to six hours. In *children*, the daily dosage ranges from 5 to 10 ml/kg of body weight. The infusion should be started at a rate of 0.1 ml/min for the first 30 minutes. If no adverse effects occur, the rate may be increased but no more than 100 ml should be given per hour.

Liposyn (Abbott). Fat emulsion 10% in 200 and 500 ml containers.

ENTERAL NUTRITION

Total nutritional support can be provided by enteral alimentation in patients with normal or compromised function if (1) the patient's needs can be met by this route, and (2) precautions are taken to assure that aspiration is not likely. Preparations are either nutritionally complete or suitable for use as supplements in specific nutritional deficiencies. Their use may avoid the severe complications of central intravenous alimentation (eg, sepsis) or the possibilities of hemothorax, pneumothorax, and damage to adjacent tissues or pleuritis if fluid gets into the pleural space. Enteral nutrition may be given with peripheral intravenous nutrition to replete malnourished patients when use of either route alone does not provide adequate nutrition.

A conventional balanced diet is the best source of food for people with normal digestion and absorption (see Recommended Dietary Allowances, 1974, for detailed information on requirements of normal individuals). For patients with normal or slightly impaired digestion who are not able to masticate food, oral administration of liquified, finely ground, or blenderized mixtures of conventional food may be satisfactory. Tube feeding of these preparations or commercial products for tube feeding should be reserved for those who cannot or will not consume adequate amounts of food by mouth. Defined formula diets (DFD) often are necessary when there is malab-

sorption or limited intestinal function (eg, patients with anorexia without nausea or vomiting, bowel fistulas, inflammatory bowel disease, or dysphagia secondary to radiation or surgery); for preoperative bowel preparation; or as supplementary feeding when oral intake of regular foods is suboptimal.

Nutritional requirements during illness differ from those of normal, healthy individuals and appear to vary with different diseases. Although many formulations are promoted for use in conditions associated with impaired digestion or absorption, very little basic work has been done to determine the optimum requirements for many of these formulations in disease states or to compare the efficacy of various preparations in a given disease. Formulations with special ingredients (ie, crystalline amino acids) are expensive and are not indicated for patients who have no digestive or absorptive problems.

Dietary Components

The ingredients and nutritional value of enteral alimentation preparations vary greatly. The osmolality as well as the type and amounts of carbohydrates, protein, and fats supplied in a specific formulation may be critical in certain patients. Formulas containing meat, meat products, or whole milk have medium residue; most other formulations provide low residue to enhance excretion.

Carbohydrates: These constitute the major source of calories (40% to 90%) in most formulations; the osmolarity of the formula is greater when carbohydrate is present as simple sugars such as glucose or fructose. The absorptive and digestive capacity of the mucosa should be considered when choosing a carbohydrate source, since most carbohydrates are hydrolyzed and absorbed primarily at the intestinal brush border. If entry into the absorptive mucosa is denied (eg, in disaccharidase deficiency), undigested sugar remains in the intestinal lumen where its osmolality attracts water and bacterial action causes production of acid and gas; osmotic diarrhea ensues. The resulting stimulation of intestinal motility may increase malabsorption of all nutrients and increase the severity of diarrhea.

Lactose intolerance is prevalent in many adolescents and adults, particularly in black, Oriental, or Indian people. It is common in diseases of malabsorption (eg, celiac disease, tropical sprue, regional enteritis) or short bowel syndrome. Formulations containing large amounts of milk or milk products with lactose or those containing large amounts of sucrose or dextrose should be given cautiously to patients likely to have such intolerance. They may be tolerated if given in small amounts or slowly, although use of formulas containing modified starches or glucose oligosaccharides, which have lower osmolality, are preferred. These longer-chain carbohydrates are not sweet but can be mixed with small amounts of sucrose or fructose to satisfy individual preferences. Many of these diets provide amounts of glucose sufficient to cause hyperglycemia and, if used in patients receiving insulin for diabetes, the insulin dosage must be adjusted.

Fat: Fat has a higher caloric density than carbohydrate (9 versus 4 kcal/g), does not increase the osmolarity of the formula as much as simple sugars, and improves palatability when compared to a formula without fat. The amount of fat available in these preparations varies considerably. Most commercially available formulas contain a high percentage of polyunsaturated fat but some have a very low total fat content. Those included most commonly (corn oil, soy oil, safflower oil) are long-chain fats. The triglycerides of all long-chain fats are absorbed rapidly and no one oil has any advantage over others in patients with normal digestion and absorption.

A few formulas contain medium-chain triglycerides (MCT). In some preparations, the amounts of MCT are relatively small compared to the quantity of LCT and the rationale for such mixtures is not apparent. More data are needed to determine whether there is any advantage to the use of various combinations and proportions of MCT and LCT in individuals with normal bowel function. There are ample data to indicate that MCT are absorbed better than LCT in diseases in which (1) there is damage to the endothelium of the intestinal mucosa resulting in inhibition of fat synthesis; (2) the transport of fat from epithelial cells into the lymphatic system is impaired or there is obstruction to lymphatic flow causing impaired fat absorption; or (3) there are decreased amounts of conjugated bile salts. MCT should not be used to correct essential fatty acid (EFA) deficiencies, since such triglycerides do not provide EFAs.

If malabsorption is severe, it is recommended that a low-fat formulation be given initially, and MCT added gradually as tolerated. The ingestion and absorption of large amounts of MCT without carbohydrate may be associated with increased ketone bodies and acidosis. Since elevated levels of shorter-chain fatty acids may be associated with reversible coma in patients with hepatic cirrhosis or portacaval shunts and a tendency to encephalopathy, MCT preparations should be used with caution in these individuals.

Unless the patient has maldigestion and/or malabsorption of fat, formulas with a normal range of fat content are preferred. When a low-fat formulation is used and there is a need for increased calories or a decreased carbohydrate load, the appropriate type and amount of fat should be added if tolerated. To prevent fatty acid deficiency, especially during long-term use, the low-fat formulations should contain some source of linoleic acid; in adults, the amount of EFAs should approximate 1% to 2% and, in children, 2% to 4% of total calories fed.

Protein: Intact proteins from meat, eggs, or milk are present in liquified or blenderized conventional food formulations for oral feeding. Milk, egg white, or soybean proteins; hydrolyzed casein with amino acids; or purified free amino acids are used in formulas for both oral and tube feeding.

Relatively few studies have been performed to determine the digestibility of these proteins in various diseases. Although protein absorption is relatively rapid in the upper jejunum, short-chain oligopeptides (as such or in the form of hydrolyzed protein) appear to be less osmotically active than free amino acids, do not require pancreatic proteolytic enzymes for absorption, and many are absorbed more rapidly than are free amino acids (Adibi, 1977). Dipeptides or tripeptides may be especially useful in patients with a reduced absorptive surface, cystinuria, or Hartnup's disease who are able to absorb dipeptides but not free amino acids. Selection of a formula with the appropriate amount of total nitrogen as protein or amino acids is essential for all patients. However, low-protein formulations are indicated for patients with hepatic encephalopathy or serious renal failure. Increased protein or amino acids (100 g or more/day) are indicated when the nitrogen requirement is increased, as in trauma, burns, or sepsis. The efficient utilization of amino acids is dependent upon adequate caloric intake.

Miscellaneous: Addition of flavorings increases the osmolarity and changes the pH of nutritional supplements. Flavored preparations are preferred by most patients, and physicians and other professional staff should be aware of the taste characteristics of these formulations, since patient preference may be important to acceptance of oral nutrient products. Some oral formulations are best tolerated if kept in an ice bath at the patient's bedside where they may be consumed regularly in small amounts. Initially, hyperosmolar diets should be given at half strength to minimize discomfort induced by increased osmolar load. Diets given by tube should be unflavored, particularly when used in infants.

Water must be made available to satisfy fluid requirements in most patients completely dependent on these formulations, especially when renal concentrating ability is impaired. To prevent dehydration, sufficient water must be given to replace insensible water loss, sweating, urine output, and gastrointestinal losses. Additional electrolytes may be required in patients with some salt-losing nephropathies, burns, or other conditions in which there is excessive electrolyte loss. Some formulas contain inadequate amounts of minerals, particularly zinc and magnesium, and these must be added if enteral alimentation is prolonged. To avoid hypoprothrombinemia, vitamin K also should be included in the preparation if long-term administration is employed.

Indications

Oral feeding of nutritionally complete, blenderized, liquified food is indicated for patients with no special nutritional component requirements and in those with mild to moderate impairment of absorptive surface area or digestive enzyme activities who are capable of digesting intact protein, long-chain fats, or complex branched-chain polysaccharides. If the patient can tolerate oral feeding, such diets are especially useful in those with trauma, malignancies, cachexia, or protein-calorie malnutrition when the gastrointestinal tract is intact.

Some products contain minimally altered foods and others provide nutrients in the form of processed or chemically isolated food derivatives. The palatability of preparations containing intact proteins is much better than those made from hydrolyzed protein or crystalline amino acids, and the former should be used when tolerated. Formulations containing large amounts of milk provide high levels of lactose, calcium, and phosphorus when used in the volumes necessary to meet total nutritional and caloric requirements.

Enteral alimentation is preferred to intravenous alimentation when possible to avoid the septicemia, catheter complications, and high cost associated with intravenous feeding. In one study on burn patients, most of those with major burns (greater than 40% of the body surface area) maintained their weight on an average daily oral intake of 46 kcal/kg with a protein content of 1.6 g/kg (Larkin and Moylan, 1976). Parenteral nutrition has been used to supplement enteral feedings when necessary to assure adequate intake.

Although most complete nutritional supplements are designed for use in a variety of conditions, Lofenalac is indicated only in patients with phenylketonuria. The manufacturer recommends its use in infants and children up to 2 years of age and ingestion of a phenylalanine-free product [Product 3229 (Mead Johnson)] thereafter. The latter permits a wider choice of supplemental foods containing phenylalanine. The phenylalanine concentration of this product is low, and intake should be adjusted to the level necessary to support physical and mental development. Other low-protein foods should be added, as required, to provide calories. Frequent monitoring of blood and urine levels of phenylalanine and tyrosine is essential during prolonged use, with subsequent adjustment of diet as necessary. For children, sufficient Lofenalac and other foods to provide phenylalanine 15 to 30 mg/kg of body weight daily appears to be most beneficial.

MBF, Mull-Soy, Neo-Mull-Soy, Nursoy, Nutramigen, Pregestimil, ProSobee, Similac Isomil, Soyalac, and i-Soyalac are suitable substitutes for cow's milk in individuals with galactosemia, lactose deficiency, allergy to milk protein, milk-induced steatorrhea, or glycogen storage disease. They also are useful in newborn infants with a family history of allergy to cow's milk and as diagnostic agents in determining intolerance to milk. The hypoallergenicity of these products is accomplished by substituting either hydrolyzed casein, soy flour, soy protein isolate, or homogenized beef for the protein in cow's milk. Intolerance to galactose and lactose is avoided by substituting sucrose, maltose, dextrose, dextrins, corn syrup solids, arrowroot starch, or modified tapioca starch. These products usually are administered after diluting to provide 0.67 kcal/ml. They are used in infants, children, and adults in amounts that supply adequate fluid and nutrients.

Tube feeding of conventional liquified food may be necessary when patients are unable to consume food normally (eg, following head or neck surgery, in infants or elderly patients) or have dysphagia. Blenderized formulas of regular foods or meat- or milk-based formulas must be given through larger bore nasogastric tubes, for they do not flow well. DFD or preparations in a highly dispersible form may be given through a finer bore feeding tube directly into the stomach, duodenum, or jejunum.

DFD formulations are indicated for use as adjuncts to or instead of intravenous alimentation in patients with malabsorption syndromes. Many are prepared from chemically isolated food derivatives that may or may not require digestion and may be completely absorbed in the upper small intestine. The degree of absorption is dependent upon the efficiency of the absorptive processes and the amount of normal absorptive surface present.

Use of DFD has been reported to decrease gastric and pancreatic secretions and reduce stool bulk. They have some advantages over standard feedings in patients with the following conditions: (1) Fistulas of the alimentary tract (particularly the lower portion); spontaneous closure of most fistulas has occurred with use of DFD. (2) Pancreatitis complicated by alcoholism or gallstones when oral feeding is not tolerated and sepsis precludes TPN. In chronic pancreatic insufficiency, steatorrhea has been reduced. However, those with pancreatic disorders also may have diabetes, and the additional glucose load imposed by dextrose present in DFD requires adjustment of insulin dosage. (3) Inflammatory bowel disease (eg, Crohn's disease, ulcerative colitis, radiation enteritis); in children with Crohn's disease, excessive diarrhea was controlled and an anabolic response was achieved both pre- and postoperatively (Hartline, 1977). (4) Serious malabsorption and short bowel syndrome; postoperative use, especially as slow drip over many hours, after an initial period of TPN has been reported to stimulate luminal nutrition and encourage intestinal mucosal growth. (5) Gastrointestinal tract neoplasms. DFD has been reported to protect cancer patients from rectal lesions during chemotherapy (Russell, 1975), but more supporting data are needed to confirm this effect. (6) After rectal surgery; the reduced stool bulk may assist healing. (7) For preoperative nutrition in place of clear liquid diets. (8) For individuals with galactosemia, lactose deficiency, allergy to milk protein, glycogen storage disease, and in the diagnosis of food allergy.

As with all oral or enteral feeding, DFD should not be used in patients with total obstruction. They may be given below the site of obstruction (eg, in a gastrostomy with esophageal obstruction or jejunostomy when there is gastric or duodenal obstruction). The nasogastric tube should be placed with care to prevent dislodgement with resulting esophageal reflux and gastric pooling, for this could lead to aspiration and death. These diets are administered through a fine (4F to 8F) nasogastric catheter positioned into the stomach and checked by air insufflation (or by lateral chest x-ray in neonates). Long, fine-bore nasal tubes may be passed into the distal duodenum or upper jejunum with x-ray confirmation of tube placement. The latter two are necessary when gastric retention occurs or intragastric administration is contraindicated. For long-term feeding, surgical placement of an esophagostomy or gastrostomy tube may be necessary. Dosage should be individualized, depending upon the patient's condition, the specific formula administered, and the method of administration. Hyperosmolar formulations should be started at 0.33 to 0.5 kcal/ml given slowly. Jejunal feeding should be initiated at iso-osmolar concentrations (270 to 300 mOsm/L) and gradually increased, if necessary, up to 680 mOsm/L. Use of an automated infusion pump to control the rate of administration and provide continuous feeding is recommended. Absorption and tolerance are improved and the incidence of adverse reactions reduced by slow constant feeding throughout 24 hours rather than repeated bolus feedings (Stephens et al, 1972). This method of administration prevents the dumping syndrome, which occurs when hyperosmolar solutions are introduced rapidly into the small intestine (Kaminski, 1976). The rate should be increased gradually and, if gastric retention, diarrhea, or glycosuria are not encountered, the concentration is increased until the full strength (usually 1 kcal/ml) is given, commonly within 24 to 36 hours. The volume administered is then increased to provide the total caloric input

desired. Patient tolerance generally is reached when 1,800 to 3,500 ml/24 hours is given (maximum dose, about 50 kcal/kg of body weight). If a 1 kcal/ml solution is used, maximum volume in a 70-kg patient is 3,500 ml. These levels can be attained only if hyperglycemia or glycosuria do not occur. Free access to water should be permitted and additional water or electrolyte supplements may be administered if needed.

The DFD commercially available are formulated for adults but can be used in children if the concentration and rate of administration are reduced. In infants, initial concentrations greater than 10% are not tolerated (Stephens et al, 1972). However, if the concentration is increased gradually, strengths of 16% to 18% may be used ultimately. Close monitoring is necessary in infants and children to prevent hyperosmolar dehydration. In one study (Hartline, 1977), a 3 ½ French feeding tube inserted nasogastrically was used with an infusion pump in infants. Initially, 50 ml/kg/day was infused, with the amount increased gradually to 165 ml/kg/day over a period of 40 to 96 hours. Supplemental fluid was provided by peripheral intravenous injection until an adequate enteral volume was tolerated. The concentration was increased from 0.5 cal/ml to 0.67 cal/ml, and 1 to 2 ml of safflower oil (72% linoleic acid) was added daily to provide essential fatty acids. Vitamins A, C, and D and fluoride and iron were also added daily.

All patients should be carefully and frequently monitored for symptoms of malnutrition during therapy. Initially, urine glucose should be checked every six hours and determination of serum glucose, electrolytes, pH, and osmolarity is recommended every two or three days. After the dose is individualized and measurements are stable, the monitoring interval can be gradually increased to once or twice weekly.

Adverse Reactions and Precautions

Most adverse effects are attributable to hypertonicity. Too rapid administration of the more concentrated solutions may produce nausea and delayed gastric emptying (Bury and Jambunathan, 1974), hyperglycemia, and water imbalance (eg, osmotic diuresis secondary to glycosuria). Although administration of additional water or fluid is usually necessary (particularly in children) to prevent dehydration, overhydration also may occur if concurrent intravenous feeding is not decreased to correlate with increased volume from enteral alimentation.

Hyperosmolar dehydration progressing to nonketotic coma results from administration of a high glucose load; this is most likely to occur when preparations containing large amounts of carbohydrate are given both enterally and intravenously. Caution is necessary if these diets are given to patients prone to develop hyperglycemia (eg, those with pancreatitis or diabetes, those taking steroids, adrenergic drugs, or potent diuretics).

Aspiration is always a danger when tube feeding is employed, especially when preparations contain a large amount of fat. Patients should be kept in a semisitting (head of the bed elevated 30°) position during sleep or if they have a poor gag or cough reflex. For elderly patients, infants, or comatose patients, a 30° angle should be maintained. The loss of gag reflex, a tendency to vomit, or presence of significant pulmonary dysfunction are contraindications to bolus feeding through a nasopharyngeal tube and even feeding by slow drip should be undertaken with great caution. Preferably, the tube should be inserted into the duodenum or jejunum or intravenous feeding should be instituted.

Preparations containing large amounts of electrolytes should be given cautiously to patients with cardiovascular, renal, or hepatic disease. All commercial DFD preparations have a substantial sodium content.

Rashes, which have been reported following more than a year of enteral hyperalimentation with diets low in fat, are thought to be caused by fatty acid deficiency.

All dry preparations must be made into solutions and concentrates must be diluted just prior to use, kept refrigerated, and used within 24 hours. Preparations may be kept for extended periods at temperatures below 60 F if dry (see the manufacturers' literature). Once solubilized, they serve as excellent culture media (Russell, 1975).

The enteral route should not be used in patients with intractable vomiting or intestinal obstruction (eg, adynamic ileus, hernia, volvulus). DFD may be administered by constant infusion to patients with chronic diarrhea, but most other enteral preparations should be given with caution.

NUTRITIONALLY COMPLETE FORMULATIONS

These preparations may consist of blenderized conventional foods, liquified preparations of nutrients of varying degrees of complexity, or defined formula diets (DFD) made from purified components. They supply total nutritional support when given in the appropriate concentration and amount (see preceding discussion). Hospital- or home-blenderized formulations tend to have particles too large to pass through small caliber tubes and are more suitable for oral feeding. Commercial formulations are finely dispersed or solubilized and may be fed either orally or through fine-bore tubes, preferably with a pump for close rate control.

Undernourished patients require approximately 3,000 kcal daily to achieve nutritional repletion. The formulation used should provide approximately one and one-half to three times the USRDA for essential nutrients. Patients with burns, trauma, or other hypermetabolic states will require additional protein and calories. Some preparations contain excessive amounts of vitamins and inadequate or excessive amounts of minerals (especially excessive trace elements). Formulas supplying more than 100% of the USRDA/1,000 kcal of vitamin D or large amounts of vitamin A may produce hypervitaminosis when fed in large amounts or for extended periods of time. For discussion of vitamin A and D toxicity, see Chapter 52, Vitamins and Minerals.

See Table 2.

TABLE 2.
COMPLETE NUTRITIONAL PREPARATIONS
(per 1,000 Kcal)[1]

Preparations	Protein (g) Source	Fat (g) Source	Carbohydrate (g) Source	Lactose (g)
Citrotein (Doyle)	60.5 egg white solids	2.6 mono- and diglycerides partially hydrogenated soybean oil	184.2 sucrose 159.1 maltodextrin 25.1	0
Compleat-B (Doyle) [bottles]	40 beef. nonfat dry milk	40 corn oil mono- and diglycerides	120 maltodextrin, fruits, vegetables, hydrolyzed cereal solids 95.6	24.4

Tube feeding only for children over 4 years and adults. Moderate residue; intact protein (containing milk); low cholesterol.

Preparations	Protein (g) Source	Fat (g) Source	Carbohydrate (g) Source	Lactose (g)
Compleat-B (Doyle) [cans]	40 beef, nonfat dry milk	40 corn oil mono- and diglycerides	120 hydrolyzed cereal solids, maltodextrin, fruits, vegetables 95.6	24.4

Tube feeding only for children over 4 years and adults. Moderate residue; intact protein (containing milk); low cholesterol.

Preparations	Protein (g) Source	Fat (g) Source	Carbohydrate (g) Source	Lactose (g)
Ensure (Ross)	35.1 Na & Ca caseinates 30.6 soy protein 4.6	35.1 corn oil	137.2 corn syrup solids 94.7 sucrose 42.5	0

For both oral and tube feeding in children over 4 years and adults. Low residue; intact protein (protein isolates); nutritional analysis of vanilla flavor. \

Preparations	Protein (g) Source	Fat (g) Source	Carbohydrate (g) Source	Lactose (g)
Ensure Osmolite (Ross)	35.1 Na & Ca caseinates 30.8 soy protein 4.4	36.4 MCT 18.2 corn oil 14.6 soy oil 3.6	136.8 glucose oligo- and polysaccharides	0

For both oral and tube feeding in children over 4 years and adults. Low residue; intact protein (protein isolates).

Preparations	Protein (g) Source	Fat (g) Source	Carbohydrate (g) Source	Lactose (g)
Ensure Plus (Ross)	36.6 Na & Ca caseinates 32 soy protein 4.6	35.5 corn oil	133.3 corn syrup solids 103.4 sucrose 29.9	0

For both oral and tube feeding in children over 4 years and adults. Low residue; intact protein (protein isolates).

Preparations	Protein (g) Source	Fat (g) Source	Carbohydrate (g) Source	Lactose (g)
Flexical (Mead Johnson)	22.4 hydrolyzed casein, amino acids	34 soy oil 27.4 MCT 6.6	154 corn syrup solids tapioca starch sugar 100.9 dextrin 48.4 citrate 4.7	0

For both oral and tube feeding in children over 4 years and adults. Low residue; hydrolyzed protein, amino acids.

Preparations	Protein (g) Source	Fat (g) Source	Carbohydrate (g) Source	Lactose (g)
Formula 2 (Cutter)	37.5 nonfat milk, egg yolks, wheat flour, beef	40 corn oil egg yolks beef fat	122.5 sucrose, farina, dextrose, vegetables, orange juice	39.4

For both oral and tube feeding in children over 4 years and adults. Moderate residue; intact protein (containing milk).

Preparations	Protein (g) Source	Fat (g) Source	Carbohydrate (g) Source	Lactose (g)
Isocal (Mead Johnson)	32.5 Na & Ca caseinates, soy protein isolate	42 soy oil 33.6 MCT 8.4	125 corn syrup solids, glucose oligosaccharides	0

For tube feeding only in children over 4 years and adults. Low residue; intact protein (protein isolates).

					Minerals					
Ca (mg)	Cl (mEq)	Cu (mg)	I (mcg)	Fe (mg)	Mg (mg)	Mn (mg)	P (mg)	K (mEq)	Na (mEq)	Zn (mg)
1580	40.2	3.2	237	56.9	632	7.9	1580	26.8	44.8	23.7
625	22.9	1.25	94	11.3	250	2.5	1250	33.6	51.6	9.4
625	22.9	1.25	94	11.3	250	2.5	1250	33.6	51.6	9.4
500	28.2	1	75	9	198	2	500	32.5	30.4	15
500	21.3	1	75	9	198	2	500	21.7	22.2	15
420	29.9	1.1	70.7	9.5	211	1.4	420	32.4	30.7	15.9
600	28.2	1	75	9	200	2.5	500	32	15.2	10
720	53.5	1	75	12.6	100	0.2	560	45.1	26.1	7.5
600	28.2	1	75	9	200	2.5	500	32	21.7	10

TABLE 2. (continued)
COMPLETE NUTRITIONAL PREPARATIONS
(per 1,000 Kcal)[1]

Vitamins (percentage USRDA)
[age group]

A	D	E	C	Folic Acid	Niacin	Riboflavin	Thiamin	B$_6$	B$_{12}$
[children over 4 years and adults]									
158	158	158	592	316	316	316	316	316	316

Citrotein

A	D	E	C	Folic Acid	Niacin	Riboflavin	Thiamin	B$_6$	B$_{12}$
[children over 4 years and adults]									
62.5	62.5	62.5	93.8	62.5	62.5	93.8	93.8	93.8	62.5

Compleat-B [bottles]

A	D	E	C	Folic Acid	Niacin	Riboflavin	Thiamin	B$_6$	B$_{12}$
[children over 4 years and adults]									
62.5	62.5	62.5	93.8	62.5	62.5	93.8	93.8	93.8	62.5

Compleat-B [cans]

A	D	E	C	Folic Acid	Niacin	Riboflavin	Thiamin	B$_6$	B$_{12}$
[children over 4 years and adults]									
50	50	100	250	50	100	100	100	100	100

Ensure

A	D	E	C	Folic Acid	Niacin	Riboflavin	Thiamin	B$_6$	B$_{12}$
[children over 4 years and adults]									
50	50	100	250	50	100	100	100	100	100

Ensure Osmolite

A	D	E	C	Folic Acid	Niacin	Riboflavin	Thiamin	B$_6$	B$_{12}$
[children over 4 years and adults]									
35	35	106	177	35	106	108	117	106	106

Ensure Plus

A	D	E	C	Folic Acid	Niacin	Riboflavin	Thiamin	B$_6$	B$_{12}$
[children over 4 years and adults]									
50	50	75	250	50	125	125	125	125	125

Flexical

A	D	E	C	Folic Acid	Niacin	Riboflavin	Thiamin	B$_6$	B$_{12}$
[children over 4 years and adults]									
50	60	70	65	50	50	50	50	70	50

Formula 2

A	D	E	C	Folic Acid	Niacin	Riboflavin	Thiamin	B$_6$	B$_{12}$
[children over 4 years and adults]									
50	50	125	250	50	125	125	125	125	125

Isocal

Pantothenic Acid	$K_1{}^2$	Volume to Give 1,000 Kcal	mOsm/kg (H_2O)
316	0	1,512 ml	496 (M)[3]
62.5	0	938 ml	405
62.5	0	1,000 ml	390
50	940	943.4 ml	450 (add 15-30 per flavor packet)
50	940	943 ml	300
56	1,060	666.7 ml	600
125	125	1,000 ml	723
47	0	1,000 ml	435-510
125	125	960 ml	350

TABLE 2. (continued)
COMPLETE NUTRITIONAL PREPARATIONS
(per 1,000 Kcal)[1]

Preparations	Protein (g) Source	Fat (g) Source	Carbohydrate (g) Source	Lactose (g)
MBF (Gerber)	43 beef hearts	50 sesame oil	95 cane sugar, tapioca starch	0
For oral feeding only in infants. Moderate residue; intact protein (protein isolates).				
Meritene Liquid (Doyle)	60 concentrated skim milk, Na caseinate	33.3 corn oil, mono- and diglycerides	115 corn syrup solids 37.5 sucrose 20.8	56.7
For both oral and tube feeding in children over 4 years and adults. Low residue; intact protein (containing milk); nutritional analysis is for vanilla flavor.				
Meritene Powder & Whole Milk (Doyle)	65 nonfat dry milk, whole milk	32.5 milk fat	112 corn syrup solids 14.5	97.5
For both oral and tube feeding in children over 4 years and adults. Moderate residue; intact protein (containing milk); nutritional analysis for plain flavor.				
Mull-Soy (Syntex)	48 soy flour	55.5 soy oil	79.5 sucrose fructose	0
For oral feeding only in adults and children 1 year and older. Low residue; intact protein (protein isolates); formula for persons allergic to cow's milk.				
Neo-Mull-Soy (Syntex)	27 soy protein isolate methionine	52.5 soy oil	96 sucrose	0
For oral feeding only in infants. Low residue; intact protein (protein isolates); formula for infants allergic to cow's milk.				
Nursoy (Wyeth)	31 soy protein isolate	53.2 soybean oil, oleo oil, coconut oil, oleic (safflower) oil	102 corn syrup solids sucrose	0
For oral feeding only in infants. Low residue; intact protein (protein isolates); formula for infants allergic to cow's milk.				
Nutramigen (Mead Johnson)	32.5 hydrolyzed casein	39 corn oil	130 sucrose 93.6 tapioca starch 36.4	0
For oral feeding only for all age groups. Low residue; hydrolyzed protein, amino acids; formula for infants allergic to cow's milk.				
Nutri-1000 (Cutter)	37.5 skim milk	55 corn oil	95 sucrose, lactose, corn syrup solids	49.2
For both oral and tube feeding in children over 4 years and adults. Low residue; intact protein (containing milk); nutritional analysis for vanilla flavor.				
Nutri-1000 LF (Cutter)	37.5 casein, soy protein isolates	52.2 corn oil	95.5 corn syrup solids sucrose	0
For both oral and tube feeding in children over 4 years and adults. Low residue; intact protein (containing milk); nutritional analysis for vanilla flavor.				

| | | | | | Minerals | | | | | |
Ca (mg)	Cl (mEq)	Cu (mg)	I (mcg)	Fe (mg)	Mg (mg)	Mn (mg)	P (mg)	K (mEq)	Na (mEq)	Zn (mg)
1500	8.8	0.6	50	21	60	0.3	1000	14.7	11.8	9.5
1250	47	1.7	125	15	333	3.3	1250	42.7	39.8	12.5
2168	58.1	1.8	136	16	361	3.6	1807	71.2	39.3	13.4
1903		0.6	240	12.7	119	4	1269	28.1	66.1	4.8
1269	18	0.6	240	15.9	119	4	952	41.2	26.2	4.8
938	15.4	0.7	101	18.8	102	1.6	656	28	13	5.5
937	19.8	0.9	70	18.7	109	1.6	703	26.8	20.4	6.2
1150	1.7	1	75	9	200	1.3	900	35.9	21.7	7.5
500	26.7	1	75	9	200	1.3	500	35.9	29.5	7.5

TABLE 2. (continued)
COMPLETE NUTRITIONAL PREPARATIONS
(per 1,000 Kcal)[1]

Vitamins (percentage USRDA)
[age group]

A	D	E	C	Folic Acid	Niacin	Riboflavin	Thiamin	B$_6$	B$_{12}$
[infants]									
179	175	180	257	40	138	250	180	325	650

MBF

[children over 4 years and adults]									
83	83	83	125	83	83	125	125	125	83

Meritene Liquid

[children over 4 years and adults]									
90	90	90	135	90	90	135	135	135	120

Meritene Powder & Whole Milk

[infants]									
211	159	318	236	111	179	267	158	158	158

Mull-Soy

[infants]									
211	159	318	236	111	139	267	158	158	156

Neo-Mull-Soy

[infants]									
260	156	282	245	78	185	200	246	150	155

Nursoy

[infants]									
167	156	312	232	156	156	156	156	156	156

Nutramigen

[children over 4 years and adults]									
50	50	50	75	50	50	59	67	50	50

Nutri-1000

[children over 4 years and adults]									
50	50	50	75	50	50	59	67	50	50

Nutri-1000 LF

Pantothenic Acid	K_1^2	Volume to Give 1,000 Kcal	mOsm/kg (H_2O)
100	0	740 ml	136 (1:1 with water) 262 (undiluted)
83	0	1,000 ml	550
90	0	940 ml	690 (M)
133	0	1,500 ml (M)	252
120	135	1,500 ml (M)	275
157	156	1,479 ml (M)	244
156	156	1,478 ml	443
50	0	943 ml	500
50	150	943 ml	380

TABLE 2. (continued)
COMPLETE NUTRITIONAL PREPARATIONS
(per 1,000 Kcal)[1]

Preparations	Protein (g) Source	Fat (g) Source	Carbohydrate (g) Source	Lactose (g)
Osmolite (Ross)	35.1 Na & Ca caseinates, soy protein, isolates	36.4 MCT 18.2 corn oil 14.6 soy oil 3.6	136.8 glucose oligo- & polysaccharides, corn syrup solids	0

For both oral and tube feeding in children over 4 years and adults. Low residue; intact protein (protein isolates).

Portagen (Mead Johnson)	35 Na caseinate	47.7 MCT 41 corn oil 5.5 lecithin 1.3	115 maltodextrin 83.5 sucrose 28.8 corn syrup solids	<0.3

For oral feeding only in children over 4 years and adults. Low residue; intact protein (protein isolates). For patients with impaired fat absorption. Not for patients with abetalipoproteinemia. Use with caution in those with cirrhosis of the liver.

Precision High Nitrogen (Doyle)	41.7 egg white solids	1.2 MCT, hydrogenated soybean oil, mono- and diglycerides	205.7 maltodextrin 193 sucrose 12.7	0

For both oral and tube feeding in children over 4 years and adults. Low residue; intact protein (egg albumin). Do not blenderize. For patients requiring high protein intake (eg, severe burns, infection, major surgery, multiple fractures).

Precision Isotonic (Doyle)	30 egg white solids	31.3 hydrogenated soybean oil, mono- and diglycerides	150 glucose oligosaccharides 112.2 sucrose 37.8	0

For both oral and tube feeding in children over 4 years and adults. Low residue; intact protein (egg albumin); low cholesterol.

Precision LR (Doyle)	23.7 egg white solids	1.4 MCT, hydrogenated soybean oil, mono- and diglycerides	223.2 maltodextrin 208.1 sucrose 15.1	0

For both oral and tube feeding in children over 4 years and adults. Low residue; intact protein (egg albumin); low cholesterol. Do not blenderize. Not for patients with impaired ability to utilize carbohydrates.

Pregestimil (Mead Johnson)	28.5 hydrolyzed casein	40.8 MCT 35.6 corn oil 5.2	137 corn syrup solids 91 tapioca starch 39	0

For oral feeding only in infants. Low residue; hydrolyzed protein, amino acids; formula for infants allergic to cow's milk. For infants and children with dietary intolerances or malnutrition and after intestinal resection or those with cystic fibrosis. For long-term feeding in patients with malabsorption, add 2-3 mEq/kg Na bicarbonate daily to prevent acidosis.

Probana (Mead Johnson)	60 protein milk powder, casein hydrolysate	32 corn oil	118 banana powder dextrose	0

For oral feeding only in infants and children with celiac disease or malabsorption. Low residue; intact protein (containing milk); high protein preparation.

ProSobee (Mead Johnson)	37.5 soy protein isolate L-methionine	50 soy oil	100 sucrose 62 corn syrup solids 38	0

For oral feeding only for all age groups. Low residue; intact protein (protein isolates); for infants allergic to cow's milk.

Soyalac (Loma Linda)	29.8 soy protein isolate	54 soy oil	94.5 corn syrup, soybean lecithin, sucrose	0

For oral feeding only for all age groups. Low residue; intact protein (protein isolates); for infants allergic to cow's milk; cholesterol free.

Minerals

Ca (mg)	Cl (mEq)	Cu (mg)	I (mcg)	Fe (mg)	Mg (mg)	Mn (mg)	P (mg)	K (mEq)	Na (mEq)	Zn (mg)
500	21.3	1	75	9	198	2	500	21.7	22.2	15
951	24.6	1.6	74	19	211	3.2	719	32.4	20.7	9.5
333	32	0.7	50	6	133	1.3	333	22.1	40.6	5
667	30.3	1.3	100	12	267	2.7	667	25.6	34.8	10
526	28.1	1.1	79	9.5	210	2.1	526	20	27.5	7.9
952	24.6	0.9	71	19	111	0.3	634	28.4	20.7	6.3
1718		0.7	102	0	125	3.1	1328	45.9	39.4	0
1171	17.6	0.9	70	18.7	109	1.6	781	28	23.8	7.8
938		1.1	70	23.4	117	1.6	781	29.9	22.5	7.8

TABLE 2. (continued)
COMPLETE NUTRITIONAL PREPARATIONS
(per 1,000 Kcal)[1]

Vitamins (percentage USRDA)
[age group]

A	D	E	C	Folic Acid	Niacin	Riboflavin	Thiamin	B$_6$	B$_{12}$
[children over 4 years and adults]									
50	50	100	250	50	100	100	100	100	100

Osmolite

A	D	E	C	Folic Acid	Niacin	Riboflavin	Thiamin	B$_6$	B$_{12}$
[children over 4 years and adults]									
159	198	106	132	40	106	112	106	106	106

Portagen

A	D	E	C	Folic Acid	Niacin	Riboflavin	Thiamin	B$_6$	B$_{12}$
[children over 4 years and adults]									
33	33	33	50	33	33	50	50	50	33

Precision High Nitrogen

A	D	E	C	Folic Acid	Niacin	Riboflavin	Thiamin	B$_6$	B$_{12}$
[children over 4 years and adults]									
67	67	67	100	67	67	100	100	100	67

Precision Isotonic

A	D	E	C	Folic Acid	Niacin	Riboflavin	Thiamin	B$_6$	B$_{12}$
[children over 4 years and adults]									
53	53	53	79	53	53	79	79	79	53

Precision LR

A	D	E	C	Folic Acid	Niacin	Riboflavin	Thiamin	B$_6$	B$_{12}$
[infants]									
211	159	476	236	159	159	159	159	159	159

Pregestimil

A	D	E	C	Folic Acid	Niacin	Riboflavin	Thiamin	B$_6$	B$_{12}$
[infants]									
521	390	312	232	78	156	267	186	195	195

Probana

A	D	E	C	Folic Acid	Niacin	Riboflavin	Thiamin	B$_6$	B$_{12}$
[infants]									
167	156	438	232	156	156	156	156	156	156

ProSobee

A	D	E	C	Folic Acid	Niacin	Riboflavin	Thiamin	B$_6$	B$_{12}$
[infants]									
208	156	156	268	156	156	156	156	156	156

Soyalac

Pantothenic Acid	K_1^2	Volume to Give 1,000 Kcal	mOsm/kg (H_2O)
50	940	943 ml	300
106	158	1,000 ml (30 cal/fl oz)	357
33	33	950 ml	557 (M)
67	67	1,040 ml	300
53	53	890 ml	505-549
159	159	1,500 ml	590
156	156	1,478 ml(M)	
156	156	1,478 ml	258
156	0	1,479 ml	210

TABLE 2. (continued)
COMPLETE NUTRITIONAL PREPARATIONS
(per 1,000 Kcal)[1]

Preparations	Protein (g) Source	Fat (g) Source	Carbohydrate (g) Source	Lactose (g)
i-Soyalac (Loma Linda)	29.8 soy protein isolates	53.3 soy oil	94.5 tapioca, dextrin, sucrose	0

For both oral and tube feeding for all age groups. Low residue; intact protein (protein isolates); for infants allergic to cow's milk; cholesterol free.

Sustacal Liquid (Mead Johnson)	60.3 skim milk concentrate, Na & Ca caseinates, soy protein isolate 23	23 soy oil	137.8 sucrose 97.2 corn syrup solids 25.4	16.7

For both oral and tube feeding in children over 4 years and adults. Low residue; intact protein (containing milk); vanilla flavor.

Sustacal + Milk (Mead Johnson)	60.3 nonfat dry milk, whole milk	24.4 milk fat	134.4 sucrose 36.2 corn syrup solids 11.8	85.8

For both oral and tube feeding in children over 4 years and adults. Moderate residue; intact protein (containing milk); vanilla flavor.

Sustagen + Water (Mead Johnson)	67.6 nonfat dry milk, whole milk, Na caseinate	10.1 milk fat	191.2 corn syrup solids 104.7 dextrose 9.3	57.3

For both oral and tube feeding in children over 4 years and adults. Moderate residue; intact protein (containing milk). For tube feeding, powder should be diluted to 45 Kcal/fl oz.

Vipep (Cutter)	25 enzymatic digestive fish protein	25 corn oil 5 MCT 20	176 corn syrup solids 147 sucrose 15.5	0

For both oral and tube feeding in children over 4 years and adults. Low residue; hydrolyzed protein, peptides, and amino acids. Add 333 Kcal/flavor packet.

Vital (Ross)	41.7 hydrolyzed soy, meat, whey, free amino acids	10.3 sunflower oil	185 glucose oligo- & polysaccharides	0.5

For both oral and tube feeding in children over 4 years and adults. Low residue; hydrolyzed protein, amino acids; nutritional analysis of banana flavor.

Vivonex HN (Norwich-Eaton)	43.3 crystalline amino acids	0.9 safflower oil	211 glucose oligosaccharides	0

For both oral and tube feeding in children and adults. Low residue; pure crystalline amino acids.

Vivonex Standard (Norwich-Eaton)	20.6 crystalline amino acids	1.5 safflower oil	230 glucose oligosaccharides	0

For both oral and tube feeding in children and adults. Low residue; pure crystalline amino acids.

[1]Most manufacturers cooperated by supplying data and checking the accuracy of the formulations presented. All available published sources were checked but the accuracy of the Mead Johnson products could not be verified.
[2]No USRDA established. Amount (in mcg) present in 1,000 Kcal of preparation.
[3]M = standard dilution.

Precautions:
Provide additional water to meet fluid requirements, especially for patients with limited renal concentrating capacity, fever, dehydration, or those who are comatose.
Postoperative feeding should not be initiated until peristalsis is reinstituted.
Additional iron should be given separately when formulas low in iron are fed.
Those preparations having high concentrations of electrolytes should be used with caution in patients with heart disease or who tend to have edema.

Minerals

Ca (mg)	Cl (mEq)	Cu (mg)	I (mcg)	Fe (mg)	Mg (mg)	Mn (mg)	P (mg)	K (mEq)	Na (mEq)	Zn (mg)
938		1.2	70	23.4	109	1.6	781	23.6	46.6	7.3
1000	43.8	1.9	139	16.7	375	2.8	917	52.6	40.2	13.9
1611	37.6	1.9	139	16.7	375	2.8	1333	64.8	40.2	13.9
2029		1.3	95	11.4	254	3.2	1522	51.9	33.1	12.7
600	47.9	0.9	75	9	200	1.3	600	21.8	32.6	7.5
667	18.8	1.3	100	12	267	1.3	667	29.8	16.7	10
333	52.4	0.7	50	6	133	0.9	333	18	33.5	5
555	51.9	1.1	83	10	222	1.6	555	29.9	37.4	8.3

TABLE 2. (continued)
COMPLETE NUTRITIONAL PREPARATIONS
(per 1,000 Kcal)[1]

Vitamins (percentage USRDA)
[age group]

A	D	E	C	Folic Acid	Niacin	Riboflavin	Thiamin	B₆	B₁₂
208	156	156	268	156	156	156	156	156	156

i-Soyalac

A	D	E	C	Folic Acid	Niacin	Riboflavin	Thiamin	B₆	B₁₂
[children over 4 years and adults]									
100	100	100	100	100	100	100	100	100	100

Sustacal Liquid

A	D	E	C	Folic Acid	Niacin	Riboflavin	Thiamin	B₆	B₁₂
[children over 4 years and adults]									
100	100	100	100	100	100	100	100	100	100

Sustacal + Milk

A	D	E	C	Folic Acid	Niacin	Riboflavin	Thiamin	B₆	B₁₂
[children over 4 years and adults]									
63	63	95	317	63	159	161	161	159	158

Sustagen + Water

A	D	E	C	Folic Acid	Niacin	Riboflavin	Thiamin	B₆	B₁₂
[children over 4 years and adults]									
50	50	50	75	50	50	50	50	50	50

Vipep

A	D	E	C	Folic Acid	Niacin	Riboflavin	Thiamin	B₆	B₁₂
[children over 4 years and adults]									
67	67	67	100	67	67	66	67	67	67

Vital

A	D	E	C	Folic Acid	Niacin	Riboflavin	Thiamin	B₆	B₁₂
[children over 4 years and adults]									
33	33	33	33	34	34	33	34	34	33

Vivonex HN

A	D	E	C	Folic Acid	Niacin	Riboflavin	Thiamin	B₆	B₁₂
[children over 4 years and adults]									
56	56	56	56	50	56	55	55	55	55

Vivonex Standard

Pantothenic Acid	K_1^2	Volume to Give 1,000 Kcal	mOsm/kg (H_2O)
156	0	1,479 ml	280
100	0	1,000 ml	625
100	0		756
159	159	600 ml (50 cal/fl oz)	1334
50	75	1,000 ml	520 (M)
67	1,330	1,000 ml	450 (add 15 to 30/ flavor packet)
33	22	1,000 ml	810 (add 60/flavor packet)
56	37	1,000 ml	550 (add 60/flavor packet)

TABLE 3.
SUPPLEMENTARY NUTRITIONAL PREPARATIONS
(per 1,000 Kcal)[1]

Preparations	Protein (g) Source	Fat (g) Source	Carbohydrate (g) Source	Lactose (g)
Amin-Aid (McGraw)	9.7 essential amino acids	35 soybean oil	162 sucrose, maltodextrin	0
Serum electrolyte concentrations should be monitored. If low electrolyte intake is necessary, dilute with distilled water only. For long-term use, electrolyte and vitamin supplements may be required.				
Cal-Power (General Mills Chemical)	0.27	0	274	0
Casec (Mead Johnson)	237.6 Ca caseinate	5.4	0	0
CHO-Free + Water (Syntex)	47.6 soy protein isolate	92.5 soy oil	1.05	0
Controlyte (Doyle)	trace	48 partially hydrogenated soybean oil	143 maltodextrin	0
Gevral Protein (Lederle)	163.7 Ca caseinate	5.5	74 sucrose	0
Hy-Cal (Beecham)	0.15	0.1	244.7 dextrose	0
Lipomul Oral (Upjohn)	0.1	111.1 corn oil	1.1	0
Lofenalac (Mead Johnson)	32.5 processed casein hydrolysate, amino acids	39 corn oil	130 corn syrup solids, tapioca starch	0
For infants and children up to 2 years. Fed at 50 Kcal/lb or 110 Kcal/kg; provides phenylalanine 9 mg/lb or 20 mg/kg. Other foods must be added to provide adequate caloric intake.				
Lonalac (Mead Johnson)	53 casein	54.7 coconut oil	74.2 lactose	74.2
Patients should be monitored for evidence of sodium deprivation.				
Lytren (Mead Johnson)	0	0	247 corn syrup solids, dextrose	0
Although used as a source of water and electrolytes, this preparation should not be used when fluid loss is severe or in patients with intractable vomiting, adynamic ileus, intestinal obstruction, or impaired renal function. Monitor to prevent excessive intake of electrolyte.				
MCT Oil (Mead Johnson)	0	120.5 medium chain triglycerides of coconut oil	0	0
Use with caution in patients with cirrhosis of the liver or complications such as portacaval shunts or a tendency to encephalopathy.				
Pedialyte (Ross)	0	0	250 dextrose	0

Minerals

Ca (mg)	Cl (mEq)	Cu (mg)	I (mcg)	Fe (mg)	Mg (mg)	Mn (mg)	P (mg)	K (mEq)	Na (mEq)	Zn (mg)
	<3							<3	<3	
1.7							0	11	37	
4320							2160		17.6	
2247	14.9	1.1	396	21	198	6.6	1586	57.5	40.2	7.9
8	0.85	0	0	0	0	0	16	0.2	0.85	0
3767	0	4.2	42	45.1	4.2	4.2	554	3.5	4.6	2.3
4.8	0.7	0	0	0	4.8	0	31.7	0.07	1.5	0
0	0	0	0	0	0	0	0	0.09	2.9	0
952	20.1	0.9	71.4	19	111	1.6	714	26.4	20.7	6.3
1745		0	0	1.6	143	0	1586	48.7	1.7	0
534	100	0	0	0	324	0	0	83.2	83.2	0
									0	0
400	150	0	0	0	245	0	0	100	150	0

TABLE 3. (continued)
SUPPLEMENTARY NUTRITIONAL PREPARATIONS
(per 1,000 Kcal)[1]

Vitamins (percentage USRDA)
[age group]

A	D	E	C	Folic Acid	Niacin	Riboflavin	Thiamin	B$_6$	B$_{12}$
0	0	0	0	0	0	0	0	0	0
Amin-Aid									
0	0	0	0	0	0	0	0	0	0
Cal-Power									
0	0	0	0	0	0	0	0	0	0
Casec									
[infants]									
352	264	528	391	185	231	433	264	264	264
CHO-Free + Water									
0	0	0	0	0	0	0	0	0	0
Controlyte									
[children over 4 years and adults]									
455	569	150	385	0	344	1358	1540	110	152
Gevral Protein									
0	0	0	0	0	0	0	0	0	0
Hy-Cal									
0	0	0	0	0	0	0	0	0	0
Lipomul Oral									
[infants]									
169	159	318	236	159	159	158	158	158	158
Lofenalac									
[children over 4 years and adults]									
30	0	0	0	0	6	159	42	0	0
Lonalac									
0	0	0	0	0	0	0	0	0	0
Lytren									
MCT Oil									
0	0	0	0	0	0	0	0	0	0
Pedialyte									

Pantothenic Acid	K[2]	Volume to Give 1,000 Kcal	mOsm/kg (H$_2$O)	Indications
0	0	215 + 12 oz water	900	Impaired renal function
0	0	444 ml		Source of carbohydrate
0	0	270 g dry weight		Source of protein
220	0	2,500 (M)[3]		Almost carbohydrate-free source of calories
0	0	500 ml (M)	598(M)	Low-protein, low-electrolyte source of calories. Impaired renal or liver function.
231	0	284.8 g dry weight	290-310 (when added to 8 oz whole milk)	Source of protein in low volume
0	0	407	2781	Source of carbohydrate
0	0	166.7 ml		Source of fat
159	159	217 g dry weight or 1,500 ml (20 cal/fl oz)		Phenylketonuria (phenylalanine 173.6 mg)
0	0	223.2 g dry weight or 1,500 ml (20 cal/fl oz)		Milk substitute for sodium-restricted adults
0	0	286 g dry weight or 3,333 ml (M)	290	Source of carbohydrate and electrolytes
				Source of fat when conventional fats are not tolerated
0	0	5,000 ml	370	Source of carbohydrate and electrolytes

TABLE 3. (continued)
SUPPLEMENTARY NUTRITIONAL PREPARATIONS
(per 1,000 Kcal)[1]

Preparations	Protein (g) Source	Fat (g) Source	Carbohydrate (g) Source	Lactose (g)
Polycose (Ross)	0	0	250 glucose polymers of hydrolyzed corn starch	0
Special Formula S-14 (Wyeth)	16 nonfat milk	54.5 oleo oil, coconut oil, oleic (safflower) oil, soy oil	105 lactose	105
Special Formula S-29 (Wyeth)	25 demineralized whey	34 oleo oil, coconut oil, oleic (safflower) oil, soy oil	149.5 lactose	149.5
Special Formula S-44 (Wyeth)	25 demineralized whey	34 oleo oil, coconut oil, oleic (safflower) oil, soy oil	149.5 lactose	149.5

[1]*Most manufacturers cooperated by supplying data and checking the accuracy of the formulations presented. All available published sources were checked, but the accuracy of the Mead Johnson products could not be verified.*
[2]*No USRDA established. Amount (in mcg) present in 1,000 Kcal of preparation.*
[3]*M = standard dilution.*

Minerals

Ca (mg)	Cl (mEq)	Cu (mg)	I (mcg)	Fe (mg)	Mg (mg)	Mn (mg)	P (mg)	K (mEq)	Na (mEq)	Zn (mg)
0	15	0	0	0	0	0	0	0	13.5	0
625	15	0.7	101.5	19	62.5	0.23	469	18	10.2	5.5
203	0.5	0	101.5	19	0	0.23	250	12	0.5	5.5
206	0.5	0	101.5	19	0	0.23	250	12	0.5	5.5

TABLE 3. (continued)
SUPPLEMENTARY NUTRITIONAL PREPARATIONS
(per 1,000 Kcal)[1]

Vitamins (percentage USRDA)
[age group]

A	D	E	C	Folic Acid	Niacin	Riboflavin	Thiamin	B_6	B_{12}
0	0	0	0	0	0	0	0	0	0

Polycose

[children over 4 years and adults]

A	D	E	C	Folic Acid	Niacin	Riboflavin	Thiamin	B_6	B_{12}
78	156	47	143	20	65	88	67	25	25

Special Formula S-14

[children over 4 years and adults]

A	D	E	C	Folic Acid	Niacin	Riboflavin	Thiamin	B_6	B_{12}
78	156	47	143	20	75	88	67	25	25

Special Formula S-29

A	D	E	C	Folic Acid	Niacin	Riboflavin	Thiamin	B_6	B_{12}
0	0	0	0	0	0	0	0	0	0

Special Formula S-44

Pantothenic Acid	K_1^2	Volume to Give 1,000 Kcal	mOsm/kg (H_2O)	Indications
0	0	500 ml	847	Source of oligosaccharides
30	86	1,479 ml	276	For leucine-sensitive hypoglycemia
30	86	1,479 ml	333	For sodium-restricted diet
0	0	1,479 ml	333	For idiopathic hypercalcemia

SPECIALIZED NUTRITIONAL SUPPLEMENTS

Specialized nutritional preparations are designed for use as supplements or as base formulas to which specified components are added as needed for individual requirements. They are not intended for use as the sole source of calories and must be supplemented (eg, with necessary amounts of a nutritionally complete formula or of ordinary foods) to provide essential nutrients. Familiarity with the composition of these formulations is essential, since the products may provide some nutrients in excess of requirements for certain patients. See the discussion on overdosage of vitamins A and D in the previous section.

See Table 3.

TABLE 4.
FORMULAS FOR NORMAL INFANTS
(per 1,000 Kcal)[1,2]

Preparations	Protein (g) Source	Fat (g) Source	Carbohydrate (g) Source	Lactose (g)
Enfamil[1] Enfamil with Iron[2] (Mead Johnson)				
Similac Advance (Ross)	37 cow's milk, soy protein isolate	50 soy oil, corn oil, milk fat	102 lactose, corn syrup solids	23
Similac Concentrate or Ready-to-feed (Ross)	23 nonfat milk	53 coconut oil, soy oil, milk fat	106 lactose	106
Same preparation available with iron 18 mg/1,000 Kcal.				
Similac Isomil [ready-to-use] (Ross)	29 soy protein isolate	53 coconut oil, soy oil	100 corn syrup solids, sucrose	0
Similac PM 60/40 (Ross)	23 Ca & Na caseinate, whey solids (demineralized)	52 coconut oil, corn oil, milk fat	111 lactose	111
Decreased mineral and protein levels for infants with feeding problems.				
Similac Powder (Ross)	23 nonfat milk	53 coconut oil, corn oil	108 lactose	108
SMA (Wyeth)	22 nonfat milk, demineralized whey	53 coconut oil, oleo oil, oleic (safflower) oil, soybean oil	106.5 lactose	106.5

[1]Most manufacturers cooperated by supplying data and checking the accuracy of the formulations presented. All available published sources were checked, but the accuracy of the Mead Johnson products could not be verified.
[2]Levels of intake for thriving infants should approximate 100 Kcal/kg (120 Kcal/kg at birth).
[3]No USRDA established. Amounts (in mcg) present in 1,000 Kcal of preparation.

FORMULAS FOR NORMAL INFANTS

These formulas may be used to provide nutrients for normal premature or full-term bottle-fed infants or as a supplement for breast-fed infants. They have been formulated to provide nutrients in proportions similar to those present in human breast milk. Most formulas are nutritionally complete supplements, although some are deficient in iron content. If the formula contains insufficient iron, supplemental amounts should be given; the American Academy of Pediatrics recommends at least 1 mg iron/100 kcal of formula. Most formulas provide 0.67 kcal/ml and are available as ready-to-feed formulations or as concentrated liquid or powder to be diluted with water.

See Table 4.

Minerals

Ca (mg)	Cl (mEq)	Cu (mg)	I (mcg)	Fe (mg)	Mg (mg)	Mn (mg)	P (mg)	K (mEq)	Na (mEq)	Zn (mg)
812.5	19.4	0.94	102	2.2[1] 18.8[2]	70	1.6	687 (liquid) 625 (powder)	22.1	17	6.25
944	29.6	1.7	111	22	118	0.05	772	40.7	24	11
750	22.1	0.6	147	trace	60	0.05	574	29.4	16.2	7.4
1029	22.1	0.7	221	18	74	0.3	735	26.5	19	7.4
588	19	0.6	62	3.8	62	0.05	294	21.8	10.3	5.9
750	20.2	0.6	147	trace	60	0.05	574	41.2	19.2	7.4
660	15.4	0.7	100	18.8	78	0.23	490	21.1	10	5.5

Selected References

Recommended Dietary Allowances, ed 8. National Research Council, Washington DC, National Academy of Sciences, 1974.

Adibi SA: Oligopeptides as carriers of amino acids for chemically defined diets, in Shils ME (ed): *Defined Formula Diets for Medical Purposes.* Chicago, American Medical Association, 1977, 15-20.

Andrew G, et al: Lipid metabolism in neonate. I. Effects of Intralipid infusion on plasma tri-glyceride and free fatty acid concentrations in neonate. II. Effect of Intralipid on bilirubin binding in vitro and in vivo. *J Pediatr* 88:273-278, 279-284, 1976.

Bryan H, et al: Intralipid: Its rational use in parenteral nutrition of newborn. *Pediatrics* 58:787-790, 1976.

Bury KD, Jambunathan G: Effects of elemental diets on gastric emptying and gastric secretion in man. *Am J Surg* 127:59-64, 1974.

Committee on Nutrition, American Academy of Pediatrics: Commentary on breast-feeding and

TABLE 4. (continued)
FORMULAS FOR NORMAL INFANTS
(per 1,000 Kcal)[1, 2]

Vitamins (percentage USRDA for infants)

A	D	E	C	Folic Acid	Niacin	Riboflavin	Thiamin	B6	B12
167	156	375	232	156	156	156	156	156	156

Enfamil, Enfamil with Iron

A	D	E	C	Folic Acid	Niacin	Riboflavin	Thiamin	B6	B12
296	185	444	263	185	231	278	278	278	231

Similac Advance

A	D	E	C	Folic Acid	Niacin	Riboflavin	Thiamin	B6	B12
245	147	441	231	74	129	245	194	147	110

Similac Concentrate or Ready-to-feed

A	D	E	C	Folic Acid	Niacin	Riboflavin	Thiamin	B6	B12
245	147	441	231	147	165	147	118	147	221

Similac Isomil

A	D	E	C	Folic Acid	Niacin	Riboflavin	Thiamin	B6	B12
245	147	441	231	74	134	245	194	123	110

Similac PM 60/40

A	D	E	C	Folic Acid	Niacin	Riboflavin	Thiamin	B6	B12
245	147	441	231	74	129	245	194	147	110

Similac Powder

A	D	E	C	Folic Acid	Niacin	Riboflavin	Thiamin	B6	B12
260	156	280	246	78	188	267	200	150	80

SMA

[1]Most manufacturers cooperated by supplying data and checking the accuracy of the formulations presented. All available published sources were checked, but the accuracy of the Mead Johnson products could not be verified.
[2]Levels of intake for thriving infants should approximate 100 Kcal/kg (120 Kcal/kg at birth).
[3]No USRDA established. Amounts (in mcg) present in 1,000 Kcal of preparation.

infant formulas, including proposed standards for formulas. *Pediatrics* 57:278-285, 1976.

Craig RP, et al: Intravenous glucose, aminoacids, and fat in postoperative period. Controlled evaluation of each substrate. *Lancet* 2:8-11, 1977.

Department of Foods and Nutrition, AMA: Guidelines for essential trace elements for parenteral use: Statement by expert panel. *JAMA* 241:2051-2054, 1979.

Fleming CR, et al: Total parenteral nutrition. *Mayo Clin Proc* 51:187-199, 1976.

Fomon SJ, et al: Recommendations for feeding normal infants. *Pediatrics* 63:52-59, 1979.

Greenberg GR, et al: Protein-sparing therapy in postoperative patients. Effects of added hypocaloric glucose or lipid. *N Engl J Med* 294:1411-1416, 1976.

Greene HL, et al (eds): *Clinical Nutrition Update. Amino Acids*. Chicago, American Medical Association, 1977.

Hartline JV: Continuous intragastric infusion of elemental diet: Experiences with ten infants having small intestine disease. *Clin Pediatr* 16:1105-1109, 1977.

Heymsfield SB, et al: Enteral hyperalimentation: Alternative to central intravenous hyperalimentation. *Ann Intern Med* 90:63-71, 1979.

Pantothenic Acid	K$_1$[3]	Volume to Give 1,000 Kcal	mOsm/kg (H$_2$O)
156	0	1,478 ml	
247	37	1,850 ml	251
147	44	1,470 ml	290
245	220	1,470 ml	250
147	44	1,470 ml	295
147	44	193.7 g dry weight 1,471 ml	320
103	86	1,479 ml	300

Kaminski MV Jr: Enteral hyperalimentation. *Surg Gynecol Obstet* 143:12-16, 1976.

Kark RM: Liquid formula and chemically defined diets. *J Am Diet Assoc* 64:476-479, 1974.

Larkin JM, Moylan JA: Complete enteral support of thermally injured patients. *Am J Surg* 131:722-724, 1976.

Meng HC, Wilmore DW (eds): *Fat Emulsions in Parenteral Nutrition.* Chicago, American Medical Association, 1976.

Postuma R, et al: Liver disease in infants receiving total parenteral nutrition. *Pediatrics* 63:110-115, 1979.

Russell RI: Progress report elemental diets. *Gut* 16:68-79, 1975.

Shils ME: Guidelines for total parenteral nutrition. *JAMA* 220:1721-1729, 1972.

Shils ME, et al: Liquid formulas for oral and tube feeding. *Clin Bull* 6:151-158, 1976.

Stephens RV, et al: Use of elemental diet in nutritional management of catabolic disease in infants. *Am J Surg* 123:374-379, 1972.

Voitk AJ: Place of elemental diet in clinical nutrition. *Br J Clin Pract* 29:55-62, 1975.

White PL, et al (eds): *Total Parenteral Nutrition.* Acton, Mass, Publishing Sciences Group, Inc, 1974.

Agents Affecting Calcium Metabolism | 54

DISORDERS OF CALCIUM METABOLISM
AND THERAPY

  Hypercalcemia

  Hypocalcemia

  Osteomalacia and Rickets

  Osteoporosis

  Renal Osteodystrophy

  Paget's Disease of Bone

  Nephrolithiasis

INDIVIDUAL EVALUATIONS

  Agents That Increase Calcium Excretion

  Agents That Decrease Calcium Excretion

  Agents That Promote Calcium Uptake by
    Tissues

  Agents That Inhibit Bone Turnover

  Agents That Decrease Gastrointestinal
    Absorption of Calcium

  Calcium Preparations

  Vitamin D Preparations

Calcium homeostasis is maintained by the interaction of intrinsic factors that control the continuous remodeling of bone and regulatory mechanisms that modify calcium absorption, excretion, and exchange. These regulatory mechanisms maintain the concentration of ionized calcium in the extracellular fluid within the narrow range essential for support of important physiologic functions: neuromuscular transmission, muscle cell contraction, blood coagulation, cardiac function, and cell membrane permeability. The metabolic role of calcium has priority over its structural function, and maintenance of calcium ion homeostasis will occur, if necessary, at the expense of bone. Normally, however, homeostasis is maintained largely through regulation of events in the kidney and gastrointestinal tract.

Most of the body calcium is present in skeletal tissue as the phosphate; 2% to 3% is in soft tissue; and 1% is in extracellular fluid where it may be ionized, protein bound, or complexed with various ions (including phosphate, carbonate, citrate, and sulfate). Ionized calcium in the extracellular fluid is in constant equilibrium with a small fraction of skeletal calcium which is available for rapid exchange (approximately 4 g). Maintenance of a normal ionized serum calcium concentration is achieved by the interactions of three homeostatic agents: parathyroid hormone (PTH), vitamin D, and possibly calcitonin (Catt, 1970; Rasmussen and Bordier, 1974).

Under normal conditions, the serum calcium concentration is maintained by a negative feedback mechanism involving ionized serum calcium and PTH secretion. A *fall* in the level of ionized serum calcium stimulates secretion of PTH which, in turn, promotes the renal tubular reabsorption of calcium, decreases the renal reabsorption of phosphate, and increases osteoclastic and osteocytic mobilization of calcium from bone. In addition, PTH acts as a trophic hormone by stimulating the renal synthesis of the vitamin D metabolite, 1,25-dihydroxy-vitamin D_3 [1,25-$(OH)_2D_3$]. The synthesis of this metabolite is also stimulated by a decrease in the serum inorganic phosphate concentration. 1,25-$(OH)_2D_3$ is the major, if not the sole, hormonal regulator of the intestinal absorption of calcium and phosphate and it also acts synergistically with PTH on bone resorption. Although the secretion of calcitonin from parafollicular cells of the thyroid gland is inhibited by a fall in the serum calcium level, the significance of this effect is unclear since a role for this hormone in normal calcium homeostasis is as yet unproven.

A *rise* in the level of ionized serum calcium inhibits the release of PTH and, secondarily, the renal production of 1,25-$(OH)_2D_3$ with effects opposite to those noted above. Hypercalcemia also stimulates secretion of calcitonin. This hormone inhibits mobilization of calcium from bone and increases the renal excretion of calcium, phosphate, sodium, and chloride. In infants and children, calcitonin may serve to modulate postabsorptive hypercalcemia after ingestion of a calcium-containing meal, but no clear role for the hormone has been established in adults. Its long-term effect on the skeleton is to markedly reduce bone remodeling.

Other hormones (eg, glucocorticoids, growth hormone, thyroid hormone, androgens, estrogens) also affect calcium balance and bone metabolism by influencing the secretion and/or action of the primary regulators.

Hypercalcemia

The most common cause of hypercalcemia in adults is neoplastic disease. The etiology appears to involve the synthesis and release by the tumor of parathyroid hormone, prostaglandins, or other substances that stimulate bone resorption in areas of skeletal metastases or that affect both bone turnover and renal excretion of calcium. Hyperparathyroidism, sarcoidosis, hypervitaminosis D, hyperthyroidism, the milk-alkali syndrome, and thiazide therapy are also frequent causes. Less commonly, hypercalcemia may result from hypervitaminosis A, hypothyroidism, acute adrenocortical insufficiency, immobilization, and the syndrome of infantile idiopathic hypercalcemia (Scholz et al, 1972).

The clinical manifestations of hypercalcemia involve many organ systems. Gastrointestinal symptoms are anorexia, nausea, vomiting, constipation, and abdominal pain. Hyperchlorhydria and reduced gastrointestinal motility secondary to the hypercalcemia may account in part for the apparently high incidence of peptic ulcer disease in patients with hyperparathyroidism. Hypercalcemia also affects the central nervous system, causing apathy, depression, poor memory, headaches, drowsiness, and, in severe disease, disorientation, lethargy, syncope, hallucinations, and coma. Muscle weakness and hypotonia, anemia, dysphagia, weight loss, and bone pain also may occur. Renal involvement is manifested by reduced glomerular filtration rate and azotemia with symptoms of polyuria, polydipsia, and dehydration. Calcium may be deposited in various tissues and organs, including the conjunctiva, the cornea (where it produces band keratopathy), and the kidneys (causing potentially irreversible impairment of renal function). Effects on the cardiovascular system include the induction of arrhythmias and hypertension.

The primary objective in treating hypercalcemic disorders is to control the underlying disease. Definitive diagnosis and conservative treatment may be all that is necessary in asymptomatic patients with mild hypercalcemia. Patients with a serum calcium level greater than 12 mg/dl require active treatment, and those with a serum calcium level above 15 mg/dl need intensive and immediate treatment to avoid a hypercalcemic crisis.

The drugs used to treat hypercalcemia lower serum calcium levels (1) by increasing the renal excretion of calcium (saline, loop diuretics, and chelating agents), (2) by promoting calcium uptake by bone and other tissues (phosphates), (3) by inhibiting bone resorption (mithramycin, calcitonin, phosphates, corticosteroids), or (4) by reducing gastrointestinal absorption of calcium (phosphates, glucocorticoids) (Goldsmith, 1972; Newmark and Himathongkam, 1974). The choice of appropriate therapy depends upon the severity of the hypercalcemia, its etiology, and the patient's renal function and response to prior therapy. With any form of treatment, blood calcium levels should be measured frequently so that therapy can be modified as needed.

Because symptomatic patients usually are dehydrated as the result of a combination of vomiting, polyuria, and a reduced sensorium, hydration is the first step in treatment. Intravenous fluids, usually isotonic sodium chloride, are infused and other electrolyte deficits (eg, potassium, magnesium) corrected. In patients with adequate renal and cardiovascular function, the saline infusion may be continued to increase sodium excretion, as volume expansion and natriuresis produce a calcium diuresis. A loop diuretic (furosemide or ethacrynic acid) may be given every one to two hours to enhance this effect and at the same time control overexpansion (Suki et al, 1970). The loop diuretics block active chloride transport in the medullary portion of the thick ascending limb of Henle's loop, thereby interfering with the passive reabsorption of sodium and calcium. (Thiazides should not be used for this purpose because, unlike the loop diuretics, they increase the tubular reabsorption of calcium.) Combined therapy with saline infusion and a loop diuretic reduces the serum calcium level safely and rapidly and is usually preferred for initial management of all hypercalcemic states that require treatment, provided that renal function is not severely impaired. In patients with severe renal insufficiency, hemodialysis and peritoneal dialysis (using calcium-free dialysis fluids) can effectively remove large amounts of calcium.

Because of the effectiveness of the loop diuretics and volume expansion in promoting calciuresis, other methods of increasing calcium excretion are largely obsolete. Since safer agents are available, use of the chelating agent, edetate disodium (EDTA) [Endrate, Sodium Versenate], should be discouraged except possibly in the emergency treatment of refractory cases in which a substantial decrease in ionized calcium is needed within 30 minutes. Sodium sulfate or citrate infusion increases calcium excretion but has no significant advantage over sodium chloride.

Phosphate promotes deposition of calcium in bone and soft tissues and is effective in reducing elevated serum calcium levels regardless of the cause. It is most effective in the presence of hypophosphatemia. Phosphate may be administered intravenously in emergencies but does not act rapidly and is not as effective as saline. Furthermore, the use of intravenous phosphate is potentially dangerous and may lead to sudden, severe hypocalcemia. Excessively rapid infusion can cause acute renal failure. Phosphate should not be used until the serum phosphorus level and status of renal function are determined. The oral route of administration is safer and therefore is preferred. If renal function is normal, oral phosphate can be given daily for prolonged periods without loss of effectiveness. Serum calcium and phosphate levels should be closely monitored to avoid hypocalcemia and hyperphosphatemia. Adequate hydration should be maintained during phosphate administration.

Mithramycin [Mithracin], a cytotoxic agent used principally to treat testicular tumors, reduces elevated serum calcium concentrations, probably by acting directly on bone to inhibit resorption. This drug is particularly useful in treating hypercalcemia associated with advanced neoplastic disease. One-quarter to one-half of the daily antineoplastic dose is given, preferably by intravenous infusion lasting four to eight hours rather than by bolus administration. Toxic manifestations are minimized at this dosage level, although most patients have mild gastrointestinal symptoms, and 10% to 20% may have hemorrhagic complications secondary to platelet deficiency. Transient hepatic and renal impairment also may occur. The onset and duration of action of mithramycin are variable, but most patients who respond will show a significant reduction in serum calcium by the morning after the first infusion. Some authorities believe that, when feasible, the drug should be administered for three or more consecutive days to achieve optimal and long-lasting effects, but others are of the opinion that 48 to 72 hours should elapse between consecutive doses to minimize hematologic reactions. Daily monitoring of the serum calcium level is necessary during therapy.

Calcitonin [Calcimar] is another potentially useful agent for treating any form of hypercalcemia associated with increased bone resorption. Although transient decreases in the serum calcium level of 1 to 3 mg/dl can be achieved safely, calcitonin has not been consistently or continuously effective in the treatment of hypercalcemia (Goldsmith, 1972). Loss of effectiveness may be due in part to the fact that calcitonin lowers serum phosphate levels. Oral phosphate supplements have been used successfully in some patients to restore responsiveness.

Measures that reduce the gastrointestinal absorption of calcium are important in treating hypercalcemia associated with immobilization, the milk-alkali syndrome, sarcoidosis, hyperparathyroidism, vitamin D intoxication, and infantile idiopathic hypercalcemia. The first step in therapy is to reduce the daily intake of calcium. This means alone is effective in the milk-alkali syndrome. The next measure to be employed depends upon the disease state.

Phosphate may be effective when hypophosphatemia and/or elevated serum levels of $1,25\text{-}(OH)_2D_3$ occur, such as in sarcoidosis, hyperparathyroidism, idiopathic hypercalcemia of infancy, and, in some cases, the hypercalcemia of malignancy. A third measure is the use of large doses of glucocorticoids; these agents act in part by inhibiting the intestinal absorption of calcium but also inhibit bone resorption. They are particularly effective in the treatment of vitamin D intoxication but are not useful in treating hyperparathyroidism. Gluocorticoids also may be effective in the treatment of hypercalcemia associated with myeloma, lymphoma, or leukemia. Their mechanism of action in these conditions is probably predominantly through a direct action on the tumor cells and not by an antivitamin D effect. Patients with solid tumors vary in their response to steroids, but those with skeletal metastases usually experience some reduction in serum calcium levels. Since the prolonged use of moderate doses of glucocorticoids may produce serious adverse effects, these drugs should be administered only if other modalities fail and only for short periods (Mundy and Raisz, 1974).

Hypocalcemia

In determining the etiology of a low serum calcium level, it is useful to distinguish between hypocalcemia associated with hyperphosphatemia and that associated with hypophosphatemia. In the former case, the low serum calcium concentration may be caused by PTH deficiency, resistance to PTH (pseudohypoparathyroidism), or advanced renal insufficiency. A low serum calcium level has been encountered occasionally in conditions associated with hypomagnesemia, and it is believed that this is secondary to a combination of decreased PTH release and impaired tissue responsiveness to PTH. Restoration of magnesium stores sometimes corrects this condition (Schneider and Sherwood, 1975). Hypocalcemia with hyperphosphatemia may be seen in patients with leukemia or lymphoma following chemotherapy and rapid tissue lysis with release of large tissue stores of phosphate. If not recognized, the hypocalcemia may lead to death. Rarely, hypocalcemia and hyperphosphatemia in children have been associated with administration of phosphate enemas.

Hypocalcemia with hypophosphatemia is usually indicative of either a deficiency of vitamin D or altered metabolism of this compound (Schneider and Sherwood, 1975). Causes are a simple deficiency of vitamin D, altered vitamin D metabolism, and intestinal malabsorption syndromes. Prolonged administration of anticonvulsant medication (eg, phenytoin [Dilantin], barbiturates) also may induce hypocalcemia and hypophosphatemia secondary to a drug-induced increase in the metabolism of vitamin D. Severe hypocalcemia with hypophosphatemia may occur in patients with hemorrhagic pancreatitis during the acute phase of the disorder; the hypocalcemia may be secondary to extraskeletal deposition of calcium, relative PTH deficiency, and/or calcitonin excess.

Severe alcoholism frequently leads to hypocalcemia secondary to a combination of factors, including deficient intake of calcium, magnesium, and vitamin D, transient malabsorption, and excessive urinary excretion of calcium and magnesium. Rare causes of hypocalcemia are osteoblastic metastases and calcitonin-secreting thyroid tumors (medullary carcinoma).

A low total serum calcium level may be seen secondary to a decrease in the serum albumin concentration but, since the ionized calcium concentration is normal and the bound fraction is inactive, this is not a true hypocalcemia. On the average, 1 g of serum albumin binds approximately 0.8 mg of calcium.

The most prominent symptom attributable to a low ionized serum calcium level in older children and adults is increased neuromuscular excitability that may proceed to tetany. In young children, hypocalcemia is often manifested by convulsions instead of tetany, which may lead to its misdiagnosis as epilepsy. This is a serious error because treatment with anticonvulsants may further decrease the serum calcium concentration. Prolonged hypocal-cemia may be associated with lenticular opacities, calcification of the basal ganglia and choroid plexus, and ectodermal defects involving the nails, skin, and teeth. Abnormal behavior patterns and personality changes may be observed and, in young children, sustained hypocalcemia may result in mental retardation and growth retardation.

Tetany may occur as a result of infused citrate combining with available ionized calcium during exchange transfusions and during massive transfusions with citrated blood, even though the total serum calcium level may not be reduced appreciably.

Most chronic hypocalcemic disorders (excluding primary hypoparathyroidism and those associated with hypomagnesemia) lead to a compensatory increase in the secretion of PTH (secondary hyperparathyroidism) which mobilizes mineral from bone. As a result, the serum calcium level may be raised toward normal at the expense of bone, and there may be skeletal findings of PTH excess.

Regardless of etiology, the initial treatment of severe symptomatic hypocalcemia is the immediate intravenous infusion of a source of rapidly available calcium ions such as calcium gluconate solution 10%. (There is no evidence that parenteral proprietary mixtures of calcium salts have any advantages over single-entity agents.) For maintenance therapy, a calcium salt is given orally (Newmark and Himathongkam, 1974; Schneider and Sherwood, 1975). The calcium content of available salts varies considerably from a high of 40% (calcium carbonate) to a low of 9% (calcium gluconate).

If functional or actual vitamin D deficiency exists, the vitamin is administered after acute hypocalcemic symptoms have been controlled. When the deficiency is severe, there may be a considerable delay before the serum calcium concentration begins to rise. During this period, additional oral and/or intravenous calcium may be required to prevent tetany. Vitamin D is also used to increase serum calcium levels and decrease serum phosphorus levels in hypoparathyroidism and pseudohypoparathyroidism. Its effects on calcium and phosphorus metabolism are similar to those of PTH. Parathyroid injection is rarely used today because its biological activity is uncertain, it may be antigenic, and it is not readily available. In the future, 1,25-$(OH)_2D_3$ (calcitriol [Rocaltrol]) may be the vitamin D agent of choice because of its increased efficacy, biological potency, rapid onset of action, and short duration of action which permits safer therapeutic control.

Osteomalacia and Rickets

Osteomalacia and rickets are disorders in which there is impaired mineralization of bone and accumulation of uncalcified osteoid or cartilage. The osseous changes are usually associated with low serum calcium and phosphorus levels, increased serum alkaline phosphatase level, and signs of secondary hyperparathyroidism. Backache, kyphosis, diffuse bone pain, muscle weakness, waddling gait, bowing of the legs, and fractures of the long bones are the main clinical features of osteomalacia. In children, epiphyseal changes are dominant; delayed bone development, skeletal deformity, and muscle weakness are the principal manifestations.

Vitamin D deficiency (actual or functional), hypophosphatemia, and renal and gastrointestinal disorders are the most common causes of osteomalacia and rickets (Parfitt and Duncan, 1975). Inadequate diet or limited exposure to sunlight contribute to the osteomalacia commonly seen in elderly, bedridden patients and institutionalized patients of all ages. These deficiencies usually respond to physiologic doses of vitamin D, while pharmacologic doses are required in patients with vitamin D-dependent rickets, malabsorption syndromes, and renal disorders.

Osteomalacia in patients with parenchymal or cholestatic liver disease may in part be due to impaired hydroxylation of vitamin D_3 to 25-$(OH)_2D_3$. The low serum levels of 25-OHD_3 observed in patients on long-term anticonvulsant therapy have been attributed to drug-induced stimulation of hepatic microsomal enzymes which presumably accelerates the metabolism of vitamin D_3 to inactive metabolites. For this reason, prophylactic doses of vitamin D may be desirable during prolonged anticonvulsant therapy. Pharmacologic doses are indicated to treat overt bone disease in these patients and in those with impaired hepatic function.

Familial hypophosphatemia (vitamin D-resistant rickets) is an X-linked disorder that usually appears in early infancy; it is characterized by a defect in the renal tubular reabsorption of phosphate and in the synthesis of 1,25-$(OH)_2D_3$. In contrast to other forms of rickets, it usually presents with normocalcemia and no secondary hyperparathyroidism. A nonfamilial (sporadic) form also occurs in adolescents and adults. The severe osseous manifestations of these disorders may benefit from combined therapy with oral phosphate salts (using diarrhea as the dose-limiting factor), large doses of vitamin D, and calcium supplements. Rare instances of hypophosphatemia and osteomalacia associated with benign mesenchymal tumors are corrected when the tumor is excised.

Osteomalacia and/or rickets may occur in patients with renal disorders. In generalized renal disease, this problem is compounded by lack of conversion of vitamin D to 1,25-$(OH)_2D_3$, whereas in pure tubular disorders, the latter aspect is not as prominent. The mineralization defect is usually improved, but not totally corrected, by alkali therapy. The Fanconi syndrome is associated with multiple tubular defects that may contribute to bone demineralization. The treatment of this syndrome is similar to that of familial hypophosphatemia, with alkali therapy also indicated if acidosis is a feature.

For a more detailed discussion of the osteomalacia of chronic renal failure, see the section on Renal Osteodystrophy.

Osteoporosis

Osteoporosis is characterized by a reduction in the total amount of bone tissue with a normal ratio of unmineralized to mineralized matrix. The pathologic process may involve a slightly increased rate of bone resorption without a compensating increase in bone formation, or depressed bone formation with normal resorption. The progressive loss of bone mass is reflected in characteristic clinical manifestations: pain, especially of the spine; loss of height and kyphosis, as vertebral compression and collapse develop; and susceptibility to peripheral fractures. Patients with severe osteoporosis may also show some degree of osteomalacia which contributes to the structural weakness.

Involutional (postmenopausal or senile) osteoporosis, the most common of all metabolic bone disorders, is an important cause of geriatric morbidity. It affects possibly one-fourth of white women over the age of 50, and a smaller but significant number of white males in the same age range. It is uncommon in blacks, but may be as common in orientals as in whites. Other types of osteoporosis include a rare, idiopathic disorder of younger individuals and the secondary forms such as those associated with immobilization or corticosteroid therapy. Although hyperthyroidism is associated with negative calcium balance, it rarely produces sufficient bone loss to cause osteoporosis except in older individuals in whom it may accelerate involutional osteoporosis.

The etiology of involutional osteoporosis is unknown, but genetic factors, sex, hormonal levels, activity, nutrition, and local factors may play a role. Since loss of skeletal mass is a feature of aging, affected individuals may have had a smaller bone mass initially or may have lost bone more rapidly than normal individuals. Race, sex, and body build are believed to be of major importance, as small-framed, fair, thin, fine-skinned women are particularly at risk. Evidence that inactivity is a significant contributory factor comes from studies showing that: (1) the loss of skeletal mass which occurs with aging is proportional to loss of muscle mass; (2) the stress of repeated muscle contraction stimulates bone growth or inhibits resorption; (3) osteoporosis can be induced by prolonged bedrest or immobilization; and (4) bone loss in postmenopausal women can be re-

duced by a regular exercise program.

The association between menopause and osteoporosis and the early onset of bone loss in patients with premature surgical menopause indicate that estrogen deficiency may play a role in the pathogenesis of this disorder. Some investigators have also noted that the incidence of osteoporosis is high in nulliparous women. Dietary causes which have been considered include calcium and vitamin D deficiencies and the excessive consumption of meat and soft drinks (which may increase acid and phosphate loads). Local factors within the bone, such as increase in bone marrow mast cells, also may be involved (Parfitt and Duncan, 1975; Rasmussen and Bordier, 1974; Thomson and Frame, 1976). Possible associations between cigarette smoking, alcohol consumption, and postmenopausal osteoporosis have been noted and merit further study.

Various regimens have been advocated for the prevention or treatment of osteoporosis, but none as yet have provided unequivocal evidence of long-term benefit as evidenced by a substantial reduction in the frequency of fractures. Because calcium intake and/or absorption may be reduced and PTH levels elevated in patients with osteoporosis and because this disorder is said to occur infrequently among patients with hypoparathyroidism, calcium infusion has been suggested as a means of increasing serum calcium levels and suppressing release of PTH. This form of therapy is inconvenient, produces unpleasant side effects, and early reports of efficacy were not confirmed in a later study. Patients with an inadequate dietary intake of calcium should receive oral supplements and vitamin D also may be indicated. Although there is some evidence that bone resorption is decreased by this regimen, skeletal mass is not increased because there is also a secondary decrease in bone formation.

Estrogens reduce the response of bone to PTH, thereby restricting access to skeletal reserves of calcium during reproductive life. Although estrogens have been used for many years to prevent or treat osteoporosis, their role in therapy is still uncertain, and there are no definite guidelines as to who should be treated, at what dosage, and for how long. A decreased rate of bone loss has been reported in some studies, but there is as yet no conclusive evidence that the incidence of fracture is reduced (Heaney, 1976).

Women who have undergone oophorectomy and hysterectomy in the pre- or perimenopausal period are prime candidates for prophylactic therapy, because (1) there is a relationship between early loss of ovarian function and subsequent osteoporosis; (2) estrogen has been effective in preventing bone loss in this group (Lindsay et al, 1976); (3) symptoms of estrogen deficiency (eg, senile vaginitis, vasomotor disturbances) are likely to be present; and (4) these patients are not at risk of developing endometrial carcinoma. Since bone loss is most rapid in the first few years after oophorectomy, therapy should be initiated promptly. Postmenopausal oophorectomy is not associated with rapid loss of bone.

In patients with natural menopause, the indications for replacement therapy are less clearcut, particularly if there are no symptoms of estrogen deficiency. Prospective studies showing a beneficial effect of estrogens have focused on groups composed largely or entirely of oophorectomized women, and the results of these studies may not be directly applicable to women with natural menopause. Until more definitive guidelines become available, the patient's age, race, body build, and muscle mass should be considered in assessing the potential benefits of prophylactic therapy (see Chapter 43, Estrogens and Progestins, for contraindications).

When used to treat older women who have already had spinal compression fractures, estrogen reduces bone resorption, but this effect is partially offset by the secondary decrease in bone formation occurring during long-term therapy. For this reason, estrogen therapy may slow the progression of osteoporosis, but it does not restore skeletal quality to normal (Heaney, 1976; Henneman and Wallach, 1957; Riggs et al, 1972; Thomson and Frame, 1976).

The optimal dose of estrogen has not been determined, but most current recommendations for prophylaxis fall within a range of 0.625 to 1.25 mg of conjugated estrogens or their equivalent given daily, usually in cyclic fashion (Heaney, 1976; Thomson and Frame, 1976). Most authorities feel that cyclic rather than continuous administration is particularly important in women with natural menopause in order to prevent hyperstimulation of the endometrium. Larger doses have sometimes been used for the treatment of established osteoporosis (Riggs et al, 1972). The optimal duration of replacement therapy is not yet known, but estrogens appear to be continually effective for at least eight years. See also Chapter 43.

Results of some population surveys have suggested that an increased fluoride content in drinking water may be associated with a reduced incidence of osteoporosis; others have found no relationship. Fluoride increases bone mass and skeletal density, but large doses cause skeletal fluorosis and osteomalacia and may increase the incidence of fractures in elderly patients. Some investigators believe that normal mineralization will result if supplementary calcium (1 to 2 g daily) and vitamin D (1,000 to 2,000 IU daily) are given with fluoride (40 to 100 mg daily). The safety and efficacy of this regimen remain to be established. Fluoride supplements should never be used in patients with renal insufficiency because toxic levels may accumulate.

There have been reports that progestins, androgens, anabolic steroids, growth hormone, and calcitonin are helpful in osteoporosis, but the place of these agents in therapy is also uncertain. Although inorganic phosphates directly decrease bone resorption and stimulate bone formation, phosphorus supplementation has been found to have the opposite effect upon osteoporotic bone, possibly because of secondary hyperparathyroidism induced during long-term therapy (Goldsmith et al, 1976). Patients treated with etidronate (EHDP) [Didronel] for osteoporosis have developed hyperphosphatemia, secondary hyperparathyroidism, and defective mineralization.

In essence, no drug currently available can restore the 30% to 40% loss of bone mass that occurs in symptomatic osteoporosis. Most of the agents that have been studied are basically inhibitors of bone resorption, with lesser effects on bone formation, and they are probably of greater use in prophylaxis than in restoration of bone mass. Until more potent stimulators of bone formation become available, it may be advisable to work toward the development of precise methods of identifying susceptible individuals and to concentrate effort on detecting early osteoporosis and attempting to prevent further loss. Newer methods of measuring bone mass in vivo (photon beam absorptiometry and total body calcium measurement by neutron activation) offer some hope of detecting osteoporosis prior to the onset of severe symptoms. Routine radiography has unfortunately proved inadequate in this regard.

Renal Osteodystrophy

Osteodystrophy commonly accompanies end-stage renal disease and the resultant uremic syndrome. The disorder in bone metabolism has been attributed to specific hormonal and metabolic responses resulting from a loss of functioning nephrons as well as the accumulation of a variety of uremic toxins. Common symptoms include bone pain, muscle weakness, pathologic fractures, anemia secondary to bone marrow fibrosis, and, in children, skeletal deformity and impaired longitudinal growth. In many patients, the histologic and radiologic manifestations of renal osteodystrophy include some degree of osteomalacia, osteitis fibrosa, and osteosclerosis, while others may present with nearly "pure" osteitis fibrosa or osteomalacia. Hyperphosphatemia and elevated serum alkaline phosphatase levels are common biochemical abnormalities, whereas the serum calcium level may be low, normal, or high depending upon the stage of the disease. Phosphate retention, secondary hyperparathyroidism, impaired vitamin D metabolism, calcium malabsorption, and chronic acidosis are important in the pathogenesis of this disorder (Bricker, 1972; Hosking, 1977; Parfitt and Duncan, 1975).

Osteitis fibrosa, a common lesion in renal osteodystrophy, is caused by severe secondary hyperparathyroidism. The increase in PTH secretion is brought about by a fall in the serum calcium level occurring in response to phosphate retention, impaired vitamin D metabolism, and decreased intestinal calcium absorption. Serum PTH levels also may be elevated because of impaired renal clearance or degradation of the hormone. The increase in parathyroid hormone activity helps to restore homeostasis by decreasing renal phosphate reabsorption and increasing renal calcium retention, but prolonged parathyroid stimulation may eventually lead to hyperparathyroid bone disease with or without hypercalcemia. Although the osseous manifestations of secondary hyperparathyroidism may respond to either medical or surgical therapy, renal osteodystrophy is often accompanied by some degree of osteoporosis which may progress despite treatment.

Osteomalacia is thought to result in large part from a decrease in the renal conversion of vitamin D to its active metabolite, 1,25-$(OH)_2D_3$. Because circulating levels of this metabolite are reduced, the intestinal absorption of calcium is impaired and insufficient calcium is available for mineralization. Serum levels of the major circulating vitamin D metabolite, 25-OHD_3, are variable. This metabolite, which is produced in the liver, is important largely as the precursor of 1,25-$(OH)_2D_3$, but there is increasing evidence that it also may directly affect bone metabolism. Other factors that may contribute to the osteomalacia of chronic renal failure are metabolic acidosis and hypophosphatemia induced by the excessive use of phosphate-binding antacids, depletion during dialysis, low dietary intake, and malabsorption.

An understanding of the pathophysiology of renal osteodystrophy provides a rational approach to therapy. The goals in the prevention and treatment of this disorder are (1) to lower elevated serum phosphate levels by dietary measures and use of phosphate-binding agents, and (2) to improve calcium balance by administering calcium and vitamin D or its active metabolite, calcitriol [Rocaltrol] (1,25-(OH)$_2$D$_3$).

In early renal failure, it may be possible to prevent the development of secondary hyperparathyroidism by progressively reducing phosphate absorption in proportion to the decrease in glomerular filtration rate. This is accomplished by restricting protein and, since it is not practical to limit dietary phosphate to levels below 400 mg daily without producing an intolerable diet, by giving antacids such as aluminum hydroxide, which bind phosphate in the gut and prevent its absorption. Aluminum hydroxide gel is usually given four times daily in doses ranging from 10 to 50 ml. Dosage should be adjusted to maintain serum phosphate levels between 4 and 5 mg/dl because further phosphate depletion may induce or worsen osteomalacia. High levels of aluminum have been found in the brain tissue of uremic patients who died from dialysis encephalopathy, and it has been suggested that the long-term use of aluminum-containing antacids may be a cause of this neurologic syndrome. Aluminum also may contribute to the osteomalacia.

Calcium is administered by high calcium dialysis or by oral supplements. Massive oral doses may be required to ensure absorption of sufficient calcium, but moderate doses (1 to 2 g elemental calcium daily) may be adequate if large doses of vitamin D or dihydrotachysterol [Hytakerol] are given concomitantly. More recently, the active vitamin D metabolite, calcitriol [Rocaltrol] (1,25-(OH)$_2$D$_3$) as well as an investigational analogue, 1-alpha-hydroxy-cholecalciferol (1-α-OHD$_3$), have been used to treat renal osteodystrophy. In small doses, both agents improve calcium absorption, increase serum calcium levels, decrease parathyroid hormone secretion, and improve radiologic and histologic signs of osteitis fibrosa with or without osteomalacia. These compounds have not been consistently effective, however, when osteomalacia alone is the dominant lesion, lending further support to the theory that

impaired renal conversion of vitamin D to its active metabolite is not the only factor involved in the osteomalacic component of renal osteodystrophy.

The serum calcium level should be carefully monitored during therapy with calcium and vitamin D preparations, because severe hypercalcemia may occur and is especially dangerous if there is an associated hyperphosphatemia. Hypercalcemia may be a particular problem following renal transplant.

Paget's Disease of Bone

Paget's disease of bone (osteitis deformans) is a chronic disorder of unknown etiology that occurs primarily in persons over the age of 40. It is characterized by increased bone resorption with formation of structurally abnormal replacement bone. This process is associated with markedly increased vascularity in the affected regions. The rate of progression, degree of disability, and extent of involvement are variable. Patients with mild disease are often asymptomatic and the pagetic lesions may be localized. In about 10% of patients, moderate to severe disease may be present and bone pain and osteoarthritic changes in joints adjacent to affected areas are common. There also may be local or generalized skeletal deformity. Complications include fractures; deafness; neurologic defects resulting from compression of the spinal cord, spinal nerves, and cranial nerves; and, rarely, high-output congestive heart failure and osteogenic sarcoma.

The serum calcium level is normal in ambulatory patients with Paget's disease but may be elevated if the patient is immobilized. When a significant proportion of the skeleton is involved in active Paget's disease, the increased bone turnover is usually reflected by an elevation in serum alkaline phosphatase and urinary hydroxyproline levels.

Asymptomatic patients with only small areas of bone involvement require no treatment, and those with mild pain can often be managed with analgesics and anti-inflammatory agents. In symptomatic patients with more extensive skeletal involvement, agents that inhibit excessive bone turnover are employed to relieve symptoms and possibly to retard progression of the disease. Salmon, porcine, and human calcitonin have been used for this purpose (Mundy and Raisz, 1974). The salmon preparation [Calcimar] has the longest duration of action and is the only form that is currently available commercially.

Serum alkaline phosphatase and urinary hydroxyproline levels are decreased in most patients during calcitonin therapy, and these biochemical changes are usually associated with relief of bone pain. Neurologic symptoms may be relieved and functional capacity increased; improved bone histology and regression of radiologic abnormalities have been reported in a few patients. Calcitonin is generally well tolerated and appears to be safe for long-term therapy, but relapse may occur in some patients after a year or more of treatment.

Diphosphonates inhibit bone resorption and formation and may be useful in treating Paget's disease. Etidronate (EHDP) [Didronel] is the only agent in this group currently available. This agent decreases bone pain, improves the biochemical abnormalities of Paget's disease, and, in contrast to calcitonin, is effective orally. Calcitonin and etidronate have not been compared in controlled clinical trials, however. A major disadvantage of etidronate is that large doses cause defective mineralization.

Nephrolithiasis

One of the most common disorders of calcium metabolism is the formation of kidney stones composed of either calcium oxalate and/or one or more salts of calcium phosphate. The usual presenting complaint is severe colic, but some patients may pass sand or gravel in the urine with little associated discomfort. A number of metabolic states predispose to recurrent renal calculi and/or nephrocalcinosis. These include: (1) hypercalciuria; (2) hyperuricemia and hyperuricosuria; (3) renal tubular acidosis;

(4) recurrent pyelonephritis; and (5) primary hyperparathyroidism.

The pathogenesis of hypercalciuria is not completely understood but at least four possible mechanisms for its occurrence have been described. The first type, absorptive hypercalciuria, is thought to be due to either a primary increase in the renal synthesis of 1,25-$(OH)_2D_3$ or to an increase in the sensitivity of the intestinal calcium transport system to the action of this hormone. The second type, renal hypercalciuria, is ascribed to a primary renal calcium leak with a consequent secondary hyperparathyroidism leading to an increase in 1,25-$(OH)_2D_3$ synthesis and thus to increased intestinal absorption of calcium which is essential to maintain the hypercalciuria. The third is ascribed to a primary renal phosphate leak leading to a reduction of the plasma phosphate level, which in turn acts as a stimulus to 1,25-$(OH)_2D_3$ synthesis, hyperabsorption of calcium, and hypercalciuria. The fourth is primary hyperparathyroidism of either the normocalcemic or hypercalcemic variety (Bordier et al, 1977).

Differential diagnosis can now be made by use of appropriate tests including serum total and ionized calcium, serum phosphate and renal phosphate clearance, plasma parathyroid hormone and/or urinary cyclic AMP, and the response of the patient to an oral calcium tolerance test and an intravenous calcium infusion. A high fluid intake and control of infection are important in treating all patients with hypercalciuria, while dietary measures and thiazide therapy may be useful in some forms. Absorptive hypercalciuria is managed by placing the patient on a moderate calcium intake and instituting treatment with either oral phosphate or thiazides. Renal hypercalciuria should be treated with daily, long-term thiazide therapy. Hypercalciuria secondary to a renal phosphate leak is often associated with osteoporosis. Oral phosphate given in divided doses throughout the day is presently the only adequate therapy. Thiazide administration will correct the hypercalciuria in these patients but probably will not improve the bone disease. Primary hyperparathyroidism should be managed surgically.

Although hyperuricemia and uricosuria may lead to the formation of uric acid calculi, it has recently become evident that these metabolic abnormalities also predispose to the development of recurrent calcium-containing calculi which may contain little or no uric acid. The reason for this association is not completely clear, although there are some data to show that the addition of uric acid to solutions of various calcium salts decreases the solubility of these salts. Of therapeutic importance is the fact that treatment of such individuals with allopurinol often leads to a marked reduction in the recurrence rate of calcium stones.

Nephrolithiasis and/or nephrocalcinosis may occur in patients with renal tubular acidosis. Correction of the acidosis with alkali usually leads to a reduction in calcium excretion and stone formation.

AGENTS THAT INCREASE CALCIUM EXCRETION

FUROSEMIDE
[Lasix]

Furosemide reduces the serum calcium concentration by increasing calcium excretion. This diuretic blocks active chloride transport in the thick ascending limb of Henle's loop, thereby interfering with the passive reabsorption of sodium. Since the calcium ion is handled like the sodium ion in this segment of the nephron, a parallel increase in calcium excretion occurs.

Furosemide is given intravenously in conjunction with saline infusion to reduce the serum calcium level rapidly in the emergency treatment of hypercalcemia. Isotonic sodium chloride should be given

before the diuretic to ensure adequate expansion of the extracellular fluid volume. During diuresis, urinary loss of water and electrolytes (including sodium, potassium, and magnesium) should be carefully measured and replaced. If these measures are not followed, severe fluid and electrolyte disturbances may occur. In addition, volume contraction may increase reabsorption of calcium in the proximal tubules and reduce the therapeutic response.

For adverse effects, see Chapter 39, Diuretics.

ROUTE, USUAL DOSAGE, AND PREPARATIONS. *Intravenous*: *Adults*, in severe cases, 80 to 100 mg every one or two hours until an adequate response is obtained and other therapeutic modalities can be instituted. Smaller doses may be given every two to four hours in less severe cases. *Children*, 25 to 50 mg every four hours.

> *Lasix* (Hoechst-Roussel). Solution 10 mg/ml in 2 and 10 ml containers.

EDETATE DISODIUM (EDTA)
[Endrate, Sodium Versenate]

This chelating agent forms soluble complexes with calcium in the blood which are filtered by the glomeruli and not reabsorbed by the renal tubules. Although edetate disodium is very effective in the treatment of acute hypercalcemia, the nephrotoxic potential of this agent limits its usefulness. Renal tubular damage has resulted from prolonged use or administration of doses larger than 3 g. Other adverse reactions are pain at the site of infusion and hypotension. Marked hypocalcemia may occur if the drug is not diluted sufficiently or if it is administered too rapidly. Because of its potential toxicity, edetate disodium should be used only in dire emergencies when death from hypercalcemic crisis is judged to be imminent. Other therapeutic modalities should be instituted simultaneously so that treatment with this agent will not exceed 48 hours.

An EDTA preparation containing calcium (edetate calcium disodium) designed for use in lead poisoning is already chelated to calcium and is therefore useless in the treatment of hypercalcemia. See also Chapter 86, Specific Antidotes.

ROUTE, USUAL DOSAGE, AND PREPARATIONS. *Intravenous*: *Adults*, for emergency treatment of severe hypercalcemia, 40 mg/kg of body weight infused over a period of four to six hours. The maximal dose is 3 g in 24 hours.

> Drug available generically: Solution 150 mg/ml in 20 ml containers.
> *Endrate* (Abbott). Solution 150 mg/ml in 20 ml containers.
> *Sodium Versenate* (Riker). Solution 200 mg/ml in 15 ml containers.

AGENTS THAT DECREASE CALCIUM EXCRETION

PHOSPHATE SALTS (See the section on Agents That Promote Calcium Uptake by Tissues)

THIAZIDES

Although most diuretics that promote renal sodium loss also increase renal calcium loss, the thiazide diuretics reduce urinary calcium excretion. The mechanism is not clearly understood but appears to involve a dissociation between sodium and calcium reabsorption in the distal tubules. Because of this unique property, these agents have found a secure place in the management of patients with several different forms of hypercalciuria with recurrent renal calculi. Thiazides (in conjunction with a low-sodium diet) have also been recommended as alternatives to vitamin D in the treatment of hypoparathyroidism, but their safety and efficacy in this condition remain to be confirmed. It is unlikely that the thiazides can elevate the serum calcium concentration in patients with severe hypoparathyroidism (eg, serum calcium level less than 7 mg/dl) because

urinary calcium excretion is already minimal in such patients.

The adverse effects that occur with prolonged thiazide therapy are discussed in Chapter 39, Diuretics.

ROUTE, USUAL DOSAGE, AND PREPARATIONS. *Oral*: See Chapter 38, Antihypertensive Agents.

AGENTS THAT PROMOTE CALCIUM UPTAKE BY TISSUES

PHOSPHATE SALTS

Inorganic phosphates (monobasic or dibasic sodium or potassium phosphate) may be used orally in the treatment of mild to moderate hypercalcemia. They are also used for the long-term treatment of patients with hypophosphatemic rickets or osteomalacia and those with certain forms of hypercalciuria and recurrent renal calculi. Phosphates are effective in hypercalcemia regardless of the etiology; the increase in serum phosphorus levels leads to a fall in the serum calcium level. The mechanism is not well understood but may involve all of the following: movement of calcium into cells, decreased bone resorption, increased bone formation, and reduced calcium absorption secondary to a decrease in the renal synthesis of $1,25\text{-(OH)}_2D_3$.

Although intravenous administration is effective, it is dangerous. Hypocalcemia, hypotension, myocardial infarction, tetany, and acute renal failure have occurred following intravenous phosphate therapy, and several deaths have been reported. Ectopic calcification also may occur if phosphate is administered (particularly by the intravenous route) without proper regard for an increase in the serum phosphate concentration. For these reasons, intravenous therapy is rarely justified and should never be the first treatment modality employed. Oral administration is safer, but careful monitoring of serum electrolyte levels and renal function is necessary. Phosphate should not be given to patients with markedly impaired renal function. Nausea, vomiting, and diarrhea may occur after oral administration. Concomitant use of antacids containing aluminum and magnesium should be avoided, because they may bind phosphate and prevent its absorption.

ROUTES, USUAL DOSAGE, AND PREPARATIONS.
Oral: *Adults*, 2 to 4 g of phosphorus daily in divided doses. The sodium-free preparations (K-Phos Original, Neutra-Phos K) should be used in patients on a sodium-restricted diet. Following remission, the dose should be reduced to maintain a normal serum calcium concentration.

> Preparations available generically; compounding necessary for prescription.
> *K-Phos Neutral* (Beach). Each tablet contains phosphorus 250 mg, sodium 298 mg, and potassium 45 mg (nonprescription).
> *K-Phos Alkaline* (Beach). Each tablet contains phosphorus 250 mg, sodium 319 mg, and potassium 90 mg (nonprescription).
> *K-Phos Original (Sodium Free)* (Beach). Each tablet contains phosphorus 114 mg and potassium 144 mg.
> *K-Phos M.F.* (Beach). Each tablet contains phosphorus 126 mg, sodium 67 mg, and potassium 45 mg.
> *K-Phos No. 2* (Beach). Each tablet contains phosphorus 250 mg, sodium 134 mg, and potassium 88 mg.
> *Neutra-Phos* (Willen). Each 75 ml of solution (after reconstitution) or capsule contains phosphorus 250 mg, sodium 7.125 mEq, and potassium 7.125 mEq (nonprescription).
> *Neutra-Phos K* (Willen). Each 75 ml of solution (after reconstitution) or capsule contains phosphorus 250 mg and potassium 14.25 mEq and is sodium free (nonprescription).

Intravenous: *Adults*, 1.5 g of phosphorus infused over a period of six to eight hours. The dose may be repeated daily, but no more than two infusions are usually required.

> Preparations available generically; compounding necessary for prescription.

AGENTS THAT INHIBIT BONE TURNOVER

SALMON CALCITONIN
[Calcimar]

This synthetic polypeptide derived from salmon is used to reduce bone resorption and thereby control symptoms, prevent complications, and possibly halt progression of Paget's disease of bone. It is indicated primarily in symptomatic patients with moderate to severe involvement. In approximately two-thirds of patients, calcitonin reduces the increased levels of serum alkaline phosphatase and urinary hydroxyproline associated with Paget's disease and relieves bone pain. Neurologic deficits resulting from compression of the spinal cord, spinal nerves, or cranial nerves may be relieved and functional capacity increased. If an elevated cardiac output is associated with the pagetic process, calcitonin may reduce cardiac output and relieve congestive symptoms. There have been reports of regression of radiologic abnormalities in some affected bones in a few patients, but it is not yet known whether long-term calcitonin therapy will prevent bony overgrowth and deformities and improve skeletal structure.

After about a year of therapy, a partial loss of effectiveness has been noted in approximately 20% of patients with Paget's disease who initially responded well to calcitonin. The biochemical parameters (serum alkaline phosphatase and urinary hydroxyproline) are affected more often than the symptomatology. In a few cases, loss of response may be related to the formation of neutralizing antibodies to salmon calcitonin, since some patients who developed resistance to this preparation with antibody formation have been successfully treated with human calcitonin. Relapse also may be associated with the development of secondary hyperparathyroidism or the appearance of cellular resistance.

Calcitonin has also been used to treat hypercalcemic states associated with high rates of bone mineral loss, such as hyperparathyroidism, immobilization (particularly in the setting of Paget's disease), and some malignancies. Although initially effective in certain patients, calcitonin is not sufficiently reliable to be a first-line agent in emergencies. In addition, loss of effectiveness may occur after several weeks of use; in some instances, the addition of oral phosphate to the treatment program will restore responsiveness.

Calcitonin is generally well tolerated but may cause nausea, vomiting, diarrhea, facial flushing, and malaise in some patients. Gastrointestinal reactions, which may be due to an increased rate of intestinal fluid secretion, usually diminish with continued therapy. A transient, marked increase in sodium and water excretion has been noted during initial therapy. Soreness and inflammation at the site of injection may occur.

ROUTES, USUAL DOSAGE, AND PREPARATIONS. *Subcutaneous, Intramuscular*: For Paget's disease, *adults*, initially, 50 to 100 MRC units daily or three times a week until a satisfactory clinical or biochemical response is obtained. For maintenance, 50 MRC units three times a week. In patients who relapse, larger doses should be tried but do not consistently improve the clinical response.
Intramuscular: For hypercalcemia, 100 to 400 MRC units once or twice daily.

> Calcimar (Armour). Lyophilized powder 400 MRC units/vial with 4 ml of gelatin as diluent. The final volume should be approximately 0.5 to 1 ml.

ETIDRONATE DISODIUM (EHDP)
[Didronel]

$$\text{Na}^{+-}\text{O} - \underset{\underset{\text{O}}{\overset{\text{OH}}{\overset{|}{\underset{||}{P}}}}{\overset{}{}} - \underset{\underset{\text{CH}_3}{\overset{\text{OH}}{\overset{|}{\underset{|}{C}}}}{\overset{}{}} - \underset{\underset{\text{O}}{\overset{\text{OH}}{\overset{|}{\underset{||}{P}}}}{\overset{}{}} - \text{O}^{-}\text{Na}^{+}$$

This diphosphonate slows the rate of osteoblastic and osteoclastic activity and is used to treat symptomatic patients with moderate to severe Paget's disease of bone. Like calcitonin, etidronate lowers serum alkaline phosphatase and urinary hydroxyproline levels, reduces elevated cardiac output by decreasing bone vascularity, and may improve bone histology and reduce bone pain. One to three months of therapy may be required before there is evidence of biochemical improvement. Although some patients experience a sustained biochemical remission after a single course of therapy, in others the serum alkaline phosphatase and urinary hydroxyproline levels may rise when the

drug is discontinued. When relapse occurs, subsequent courses should be given intermittently because the safety of long-term continuous therapy has not been established. In addition to its use in Paget's disease, etidronate is also given for prevention and treatment of heterotopic ossification due to spinal cord injury.

Etidronate is usually well tolerated, but nausea, vomiting, and diarrhea have been reported, particularly in patients receiving large doses. The serum phosphate level may rise during therapy, presumably because of an increase in the renal reabsorption of phosphate. The hyperphosphatemia is not an indication for discontinuing therapy. Etidronate should be given cautiously to patients with impaired renal function because it is excreted unchanged by the kidney.

Defective bone mineralization is the most serious potential adverse effect of etidronate. Accumulation of unmineralized osteoid is common in patients receiving large doses (10 to 20 mg/kg daily) but also may occur when smaller doses are given for long periods. In some patients, new episodes of incapacitating bone pain and fractures have occurred during a six-month period of treatment with doses of 10 to 20 mg/kg daily but not with lower doses (2.5 to 5 mg/kg daily) (Canfield et al, 1977). Since effects on serum alkaline phosphatase and urinary hydroxyproline are dose related, these biochemical indices cannot be used as the sole guide to therapy. Combined therapy with small doses of etidronate and calcitonin is a promising approach. Some preliminary data suggest that the combined regimen may avoid mineralization defects while providing a more consistent therapeutic response than with calcitonin alone (Hosking et al, 1976).

ROUTE, USUAL DOSAGE, AND PREPARATIONS. *Oral*: *Adults*, for Paget's disease, etidronate should be given as a single daily dose two hours before a meal. Initially, 5 mg/kg of body weight is given daily for a period not to exceed six months. Larger doses should be reserved for use when there is a need for rapid suppression of increased bone turnover or prompt reduction of elevated cardiac output. When doses greater than 10 mg/kg daily are given, the treatment period should not exceed three months; the daily dose should not exceed 20 mg/kg. The drug should be discontinued if bone pain increases or recurs or if fractures develop. Serum alkaline phosphatase and/or urinary hydroxyproline levels should be monitored during and after therapy. Treatment may be initiated again after a drug-free period of at least three months if the biochemical indices approach pretreatment levels.

For heterotopic ossification due to spinal cord injury, initially, 20 mg/kg daily for two weeks, followed by 10 mg/kg daily for ten weeks (total treatment period, 12 weeks).

Didronel (Procter & Gamble). Tablets 200 mg.

MITHRAMYCIN
[Mithracin]

Mithramycin is a cytotoxic antibiotic used primarily to treat testicular neoplasms. It decreases serum calcium levels in both hypercalcemic and normocalcemic individuals, possibly by a direct toxic effect on osteoclasts in bone. Mithramycin is used to treat severe hypercalcemia associated with carcinoma with or without bony metastases and is more effective than glucocorticoids for this purpose. In some patients, a single dose reduces elevated serum calcium levels within 24 hours without producing serious toxic effects; others respond slowly and may require several days of therapy for a satisfactory response. The duration of action may be only a few days but occasionally persists for three weeks or longer, especially if three or more infusions are given. Mithramycin has occasionally been used in Paget's disease, but calcitonin is preferred because it is less toxic.

In addition to anorexia, nausea, and vomiting, mithramycin can produce severe thrombocytopenia which may progress to a hemorrhagic diathesis. Abnormalities in hepatic and renal function tests have also been reported. Although lower doses are used for hypercalcemia than for neoplasms, the same precautions and contraindications apply (see Chapter 68, Antineoplastic Agents). It is also important to monitor serum calcium levels closely.

ROUTE, USUAL DOSAGE, AND PREPARATIONS.
Intravenous: 25 mcg/kg of body weight is given as a single dose by direct injection or preferably added to 5% dextrose in water and infused gradually over a period of four to eight hours. If there is no decline in serum calcium levels by the next morning, 25 mcg/kg may be given daily for two to four days. Additional courses may be given at weekly intervals if the hypercalcemia is not controlled. Alternatively, one to three doses may be given weekly, depending upon the patient's response. The drug should be discontinued after three infusions or sooner when a favorable effect has been achieved.

Mithracin (Dome). Powder (for solution) in vials containing mithramycin 2,500 mcg, mannitol 100 mg, and sufficient disodium phosphate to adjust the pH to 7.

AGENTS THAT DECREASE GASTROINTESTINAL ABSORPTION OF CALCIUM

PHOSPHATE SALTS (See the section on Agents That Promote Calcium Uptake by Tissues)

ADRENAL CORTICOSTEROIDS

Glucocorticoids reduce the intestinal absorption of calcium by antagonizing the action of vitamin D. They are effective in the treatment of hypercalcemia due to hypervitaminosis D, sarcoidosis, and adrenocortical insufficiency. Because of additional direct or indirect effects on bone resorption, they are also useful in some patients with hypercalcemia due to myeloma, leukemia, and lymphoma and in some patients with solid tumors. Large doses of steroids may be necessary initially. The onset of action is variable, but improvement may occur within 24 to 72 hours.

The adverse effects that occur with prolonged glucocorticoid therapy are an important consideration (see Chapter 41, Adrenal Corticosteroids).

ROUTES, USUAL DOSAGE, AND PREPARATIONS.
Intravenous, Intramuscular: Adults, in severe hypercalcemia, parenteral preparations are preferred (cortisol sodium succinate 100 to 500 mg daily or prednisolone sodium phosphate 20 to 100 mg daily); these drugs may be given intramuscularly, intravenously, or, preferably, by intravenous infusion.
Oral: Adults, initially, 40 to 80 mg of prednisone or another glucocorticoid in a therapeutically equivalent dose is given daily in individualized doses until the serum calcium level is satisfactorily controlled. Dosage then is reduced gradually; final dosage is dependent upon the results of serum calcium determinations.

See Chapter 41, Adrenal Corticosteroids, for preparations.

CALCIUM PREPARATIONS

CALCIUM CARBONATE, PRECIPITATED

This orally administered calcium salt (containing 40% calcium) is useful in the treatment of mild hypocalcemia and for maintenance therapy. It is also the preferred calcium salt for calcium supplementation in patients with osteomalacia, rickets, osteoporosis, and renal osteodystrophy. Calcium carbonate is converted in the stomach to soluble calcium salts by interaction with hydrochloric acid. Thus, it is ineffective in patients with achlorhydria.

Hypercalcemia may occur during long-term therapy, particularly in patients who are also receiving vitamin D. Calcium carbonate may cause nausea and gastrointestinal irritation.

ROUTE, USUAL DOSAGE, AND PREPARATIONS.
Oral: Adults, 1 to 2 g three times daily with meals; the preparation is mixed with water or sprinkled on food.

Drug available generically: Antacid preparations containing calcium carbonate are a satisfactory source of this substance.

CALCIUM CHLORIDE

Calcium chloride, which contains 27% calcium, is irritating to the gastrointestinal tract and is rarely given orally. Intravenous calcium chloride is effective in severe hypocalcemia and may increase ionized serum calcium more reliably than other preparations; however, other salts are usually preferred because calcium chloride is more irritating to the veins and subcutaneous tissue, and care must be taken to avoid extravasation. It should never be administered intramuscularly. Hypercalcemia may occur during long-term therapy, particularly in patients who are also receiving vitamin D. Intravenous calcium should be administered cautiously to digitalized patients.

ROUTE, USUAL DOSAGE, AND PREPARATIONS.
Intravenous (slow): Adults, 5 to 10 ml of a 10% solution.

Drug available generically: Solution 10% in 10 ml containers.

CALCIUM GLUCEPTATE

Intravenous administration of calcium gluceptate is effective in the treatment of severe hypocalcemia. A transient tingling sensation and metallic taste may be noted after this route of administration. Calcium gluceptate also may be given intramuscularly to infants and other patients in whom intravenous administration is not feasible; it is well tolerated, although mild local reactions may occur. Intravenous calcium should be administered cautiously to digitalized patients, because calcium enhances the effect of digitalis on the heart and may precipitate arrhythmias.

ROUTES, USUAL DOSAGE, AND PREPARATIONS.
Intravenous: *Adults*, 5 to 20 ml. In *newborn infants*, to prevent hypocalcemia during exchange transfusions, 0.5 ml after every 100 ml of blood exchanged.
Intramuscular: 2 to 5 ml in gluteal region or, in *infants*, in the lateral thigh.

Drug available generically: Solution 220 mg/ml (18 mg/ml of calcium) in 5 ml containers.

CALCIUM GLUCONATE

Calcium gluconate is a source of rapidly available calcium ions; it is administered intravenously and is the treatment of choice in severe hypocalcemia. This agent also is administered orally for mild hypocalcemia and for maintenance therapy. It contains 9% calcium.

The gluconate salt is nonirritating to the veins but may cause nausea and gastrointestinal irritation when given orally. The intramuscular route should not be used because of the large quantity of solution required and the risk of abscess formation. Hypercalcemia may occur during long-term therapy, particularly in patients who are also receiving vitamin D. Intravenous calcium should be administered cautiously to digitalized patients, because calcium enhances the effect of digitalis on the heart and may precipitate arrhythmias.

ROUTES, USUAL DOSAGE, AND PREPARATIONS.
Intravenous: *Adults*, initially, 20 ml of a 10% solution injected slowly, followed by slow infusion of a 0.3% to 0.8% solution (30 to 40 ml of 10% solution in 500 ml to 1 liter of isotonic sodium chloride or 5% dextrose injection) over a period of 3 to 12 hours. *Children*, 500 mg/kg of body weight daily in divided doses.

Drug available generically: Solution 10% in 10 ml containers.

Oral: *Adults*, 15 g daily in divided doses; *children*, 500 mg/kg of body weight daily in divided doses.

Drug available generically: Tablets 450, 500, 600, and 900 mg and 1 g.

CALCIUM LACTATE

This orally administered calcium salt (containing 13% calcium) is readily absorbed and is useful in the treatment of mild hypocalcemia and for maintenance therapy. Hypercalcemia may occur during long-term administration, particularly in patients who are also receiving vitamin D.

ROUTE, USUAL DOSAGE, AND PREPARATIONS.
Oral: *Adults*, 1.5 to 3 g three times daily with meals; *children*, 500 mg/kg of body weight daily in divided doses.

Drug available generically: Tablets 300 and 600 mg.

VITAMIN D PREPARATIONS

Vitamin D is obtained by the ingestion of vitamin D_2 (ergocalciferol) or vitamin D_3 (cholecalciferol) or by ultraviolet irradiation of 7-dehydrocholesterol to vitamin D_3 in the skin. Vitamin D_3 (or D_2) is hydroxylated at the 25 position in the liver to produce 25-hydroxy-vitamin D_3 (or D_2), which is the major metabolite circulating in the plasma. The metabolite is further hydroxylated in the kidney to 1,25-dihydroxy-vitamin D_3 (or D_2), the most active metabolite in initiating intestinal transport of calcium and phosphate and mobilization of mineral from bone. 1,25-dihydroxy-vitamin D_3 ($1,25(OH)_2D_3$) is available commercially as calcitriol [Rocaltrol]. An analogue of this metabolite, 1-α-OHD$_3$, is currently under investigation for treatment of renal osteodystrophy. Another metabolite of vitamin D, 24,25-$(OH)_2D_3$, is formed in the kidney and bone, but its metabolic actions are uncertain.

VITAMIN D

Vitamin D is used as a therapeutic agent in hypoparathyroidism, vitamin D deficiency states (simple deficiency, genetic vitamin D-dependent rickets, malabsorption, impaired renal or hepatic metabolism), and as an adjunct in the management of osteomalacia associated with hypophosphatemia and renal tubular disorders. In parathyroid hormone deficiency, large doses of vitamin D increase serum calcium levels and decrease serum phosphorus levels. This effect on calcium and phosphorus metabolism is similar to that of parathyroid hormone. Large doses of vitamin D may promote phosphaturia, increase mobilization of mineral from bone, and increase intestinal absorption of calcium, phosphate, and magnesium; these effects account for the elevation of serum calcium concentrations. There is a lag between initiation of therapy and the onset of therapeutic effectiveness which can be 10 to 14 days or longer, depending upon the preparation used. Ergocalciferol is employed more commonly than cholecalciferol. Its onset of action is somewhat slower than that of dihydrotachysterol and the duration of effect is more prolonged.

Rickets and osteomalacia caused by dietary deficiency of vitamin D and inadequate exposure to sunlight respond rapidly to physiologic doses of vitamin D, but large doses are required to treat vitamin-D dependent rickets. In malabsorption disorders, effective treatment of the primary cause will usually cure the associated osteomalacia or rickets, but if the condition does not respond to therapy, life-long administration of large doses of vitamin D and calcium may be necessary. Pharmacologic doses are also indicated when overt bone disease is associated with impaired hepatic or renal metabolism of vitamin D. In hypophosphatemic states and renal tubular disorders, large doses of vitamin D may be needed, but correction of hypophosphatemia or acidosis is of primary importance.

The dosage of vitamin D should be regulated by frequent estimation of the serum calcium concentration. Urinary calcium, measured as the amount excreted in 24 hours rather than by a simple Sulkowitch test, can be used as a guide, since the urinary calcium level often rises before the rise in serum calcium.

Vitamin D is potent and potentially harmful, and overdosage can cause gastrointestinal and central nervous system disturbances and soft tissue calcification. The complications affecting the kidneys may be severe and death may result; the possibility of renal damage persists for a considerable period of time after discontinuing the drug. Adverse effects also occasionally result from increased sensitivity in patients not receiving excessively large doses. (See also Chapter 52, Vitamins and Minerals.)

ROUTE, USUAL DOSAGE, AND PREPARATIONS. *Oral*: For hypoparathyroidism, *adults*, initially, 50,000 to 200,000 IU daily as soon as acute tetany is controlled with an intravenous calcium preparation. The maintenance dose is usually 25,000 to 100,000 IU daily. *Children*, 10,000 to 25,000 IU daily.

For osteomalacia and rickets caused by dietary deficiency of vitamin D, *adults*, initially, 1,000 to 2,000 IU daily; for maintenance, 400 IU daily. *Children*, initially, 1,000 to 4,000 IU daily; for maintenance, 400 IU daily.

For genetic vitamin D-dependent rickets, *children*, 5,000 to 50,000 IU daily.

For familial hypophosphatemia (vitamin D-resistant rickets), *children*, 25,000 to 100,000 IU daily in conjunction with a high phosphate intake and calcium supplements.

For sporadic hypophosphatemia, *adults*, 40,000 to 200,000 IU daily in conjunction with a high phosphate intake.

For osteomalacia in malabsorption syndromes, *adults*, 10,000 to 50,000 IU daily. *Children*, 10,000 to 25,000 IU daily.

For osteomalacia in hepatobiliary disease, *adults*, 10,000 to 40,000 IU daily. *Children*, 10,000 to 25,000 IU daily.

For osteomalacia associated with anticonvulsant therapy, *adults and children*, 1,000 IU daily.

For renal osteodystrophy, *adults*, 20,000 to 200,000 IU daily.

For multiple renal tubular defects, *adults,* 40,000 to 100,000 IU daily; *children,* 25,000 to 50,000 IU daily.

ERGOCALCIFEROL (Vitamin D₂):
Drug available generically under names Vitamin D (Capsules 25,000 and 50,000 IU) and Calciferol (Tablets 50,000 IU).
Deltalin (Lilly), *Geltabs* (Upjohn). Capsules 50,000 IU.
Drisdol (Winthrop). Capsules 50,000 IU; solution 8,000 IU/ml.

DIHYDROTACHYSTEROL
[Hytakerol]

This form of vitamin D may act somewhat more rapidly than the D₂ and D₃ forms. In comparison to ergocalciferol, the phosphate diuresis produced by dihydrotachysterol is almost as great, the intestinal absorption of calcium is less, and the serum calcium concentration rises more rapidly. Because its duration of action is shorter, the potential hazards of hypercalcemia are less with dihydrotachysterol than with ergocalciferol. (See the evaluation on Vitamin D.)

Dihydrotachysterol has only weak antirachitic activity (about 1/400 that of vitamin D).

ROUTE, USUAL DOSAGE, AND PREPARATIONS.
Oral: For parathyroid hormone deficiency, *adults,* initially, 0.75 to 2.5 mg daily; specific dosage is determined by frequent estimations of serum calcium levels. For maintenance, 0.25 to 1.75 mg weekly has been given, but larger doses may be required in some patients.
For prevention of renal osteodystrophy, *adults,* initially, 0.1 to 0.25 mg daily. *Children,* initially, 0.01 mg daily. For patients on long-term hemodialysis, *adults,* initially, 0.25 to 0.375 mg daily. Some patients may require doses as large as 1 mg daily.

Drug available generically: Tablets 0.125, 0.2, and 4 mg.
Hytakerol (crystalline) (Winthrop). Capsules 0.125 mg; solution (in oil) 0.25 mg/ml.

CALCITRIOL
[Rocaltrol]

Calcitriol (1,25-dihydroxy-vitamin D₃) is produced in the kidney and is sometimes classified as a renal hormone. It is the most active vitamin D metabolite in initiating the intestinal transport of calcium and phosphate and the mobilization of mineral from bone. Conversion to this active metabolite is enhanced by the presence of parathyroid hormone and/or a decrease in serum inorganic phosphate levels. The major advantages of calcitriol over other vitamin D preparations are (1) its efficacy in patients with renal failure, (2) its rapid onset of action, and (3) its short half-life which makes toxic reactions easier to manage should they occur.

Calcitriol has been used primarily in patients with chronic renal failure on long-term dialysis. In these patients, it is more effective than vitamin D in elevating the serum calcium level and reducing parathyroid hormone secretion (Berl et al, 1978). When renal osteodystrophy is present, calcitriol often relieves bone pain, permits increased physical activity, and may improve bone histology in some patients.

For adverse reactions and precautions, see the evaluation on Vitamin D.

ROUTE, USUAL DOSAGE, AND PREPARATIONS.
Oral: Initially, 0.25 mcg/day. If an adequate response is not obtained, the dosage may be increased by 0.25 mcg/day at two- to four-week intervals. Serum calcium

levels should be measured at least twice weekly and the drug should be discontinued if hypercalcemia occurs. Patients with normal or only slightly reduced serum calcium levels may respond to doses of 0.25 mcg every other day. Most patients undergoing hemodialysis require 0.5 or 1 mcg/day.

Rocaltrol (Roche). Capsules 0.25 and 0.5 mcg.

Selected References

Berl T, et al: 1,25 dihydroxycholecalciferol effects in chronic dialysis: Double-blind controlled study. *Ann Intern Med* 88:774-780, 1978.

Bordier P, et al: On pathogenesis of so-called idiopathic hypercalciuria. *Am J Med* 63:398-409, 1977.

Bricker NS: On pathogenesis of uremic state: Exposition of "trade-off-hypothesis." *N Engl J Med* 286:1093-1099,1972.

Canfield R, et al: Diphosphonate therapy of Paget's disease of bone. *J Clin Endocrinol Metab* 44:96-106, 1977.

Catt KJ: Hormonal control of calcium homeostasis. *Lancet* 2:255-257, 1970.

Goldsmith RS: Treatment of hypercalcemia. *Med Clin North Am* 56:951-960, 1972.

Goldsmith RS, et al: Effects of phosphorus supplementation on serum parathyroid hormone and bone morphology in osteoporosis. *J Clin Endocrinol Metab* 43:523-532, 1976.

Heaney RP: Estrogens and postmenopausal osteoporosis. *Clin Obstet Gynecol* 19:791-803, 1976.

Henneman PH, Wallach S: Review of prolonged use of estrogens and androgens in post-menopausal and senile osteoporosis. *Arch Intern Med* 100:715-723, 1957.

Hosking DJ: Diseases of urinary system: Renal osteodystrophy. *Br Med J* 2:110-112, 1977.

Hosking DJ, et al: Paget's bone disease treated with diphosphonate and calcitonin. *Lancet* 1:615-617, 1976.

Lindsay R, et al: Long-term prevention of postmenopausal osteoporosis by oestrogen. *Lancet* 1:1038-1041, 1976.

Mundy GR, Raisz LG: Drugs for disorders of bone: Pharmacological and clinical considerations. *Drugs* 8:250-289, 1974.

Newmark SR, Himathongkam T: Hypercalcemic and hypocalcemic crises. *JAMA* 230:1438-1439, 1974.

Parfitt AM, Duncan H: Metabolic bone disease affecting the spine, in Rothman RH, Simeone FA (eds): *The Spine.* Philadelphia, WB Saunders Co, 1975, vol 2, 599-720.

Rasmussen H, Bordier P: *The Physiological and Cellular Basis of Bone Disease.* Baltimore, Williams and Wilkins Company, 1974.

Riggs LB, et al: Short- and long-term effects of estrogen and synthetic anabolic hormone in postmenopausal osteoporosis. *J Clin Invest* 51:1659-1663, 1972.

Schneider AB, Sherwood LM: Pathogenesis and management of hypoparathyroidism and other hypocalcemic disorders. *Metabolism* 24:871-898, 1975.

Scholz DA, et al: Diagnostic considerations in hypercalcemic syndromes. *Med Clin North Am* 56:941-950, 1972.

Suki WN, et al: Acute treatment of hypercalcemia with furosemide. *N Engl J Med* 283:836-840, 1970.

Thomson DL, Frame B: Involutional osteopenia: Current concepts. *Ann Intern Med* 85:789-803, 1976.

Agents Used to Treat Hyperlipidemia | 55

The total number of deaths from cardiovascular diseases has declined during the last few years, but the complications of atherosclerosis (eg, coronary heart disease, myocardial infarction, stroke, renal disease) remain major causes of morbidity and mortality in adults, particularly men, in the United States. Although it is recognized that the atherosclerotic process begins in childhood, the pathogenesis of accelerated atherosclerosis is poorly understood.

There are many causes of atherosclerosis. They may be hereditary or acquired and are associated with many biochemical mechanisms. Any factor(s) that contribute to endothelial injury, thickening of the arterial intima, accumulation of connective tissue within the intima, and deposition of lipids or blood constituents may narrow the lumen and decrease blood flow. The potential for developing atherosclerosis is known to be increased by hypertension, cigarette smoking, elevated serum lipid levels, sedentary habits, obesity, and a strong family history of coronary heart disease. These factors are additive, have complex interactions, and have no threshold of abnormality. Those with the greatest predictive value prior to overt events appear to

be hypertension, cigarette smoking, and elevated serum lipid levels, particularly serum cholesterol; inherited hypercholesterolemia may be one of the most important pathogenic determinants of accelerated atherosclerosis. Once heart disease has become clinically manifest, the status and function of the myocardium is more predictive of survival than the presence of risk factors. Nevertheless, the value of reducing risk factors, especially cessation of smoking and control of hypertension, in patients with coronary disease is the only rational approach to therapy at present. Treating hyperlipidemia to reduce the risk of atherosclerosis and delay the onset of complications is based on presumptions derived from epidemiologic data and studies in animals; conclusive validation in man has not yet been accomplished.

Hyperlipidemia, the general term for abnormally elevated concentrations of lipids in the blood, reflects changes in lipoprotein concentrations. Cholesterol, triglycerides, phospholipids, and free fatty acids are insoluble in water; they circulate in plasma as part of protein complexes (lipoproteins) that impart water solubility to the lipid fractions. Lipoproteins are

913

closely interrelated metabolically, but their atherogenicity varies considerably. Thus, diagnosis of hyperlipidemia should be based on determination of specific lipoprotein abnormalities, and therapy should be directed toward correcting the abnormalities of lipoprotein production and distribution, not simply reducing plasma cholesterol and/or triglyceride levels.

Types of Lipoproteins: Because the various lipoproteins differ in electric charge and density, they can be separated by ultracentrifugation or electrophoresis into five major groups:

(1) Chylomicrons, the largest lipoproteins, contain over 90% triglycerides (dietary, exogenous) and less than 5% cholesterol by weight. They are formed by the intestinal mucosa from ingested fats and transported through the lymphatic system to plasma, where they normally are rapidly catabolized by lipoprotein lipase. Triglycerides are hydrolyzed to glycerol and fatty acids, which are utilized by the tissues or re-esterified to triglycerides. Postprandial chylomicronemia subsides about 8 to 12 hours after a meal, and chylomicrons normally are absent in fasting plasma. When present, they form a cream layer on top of cold standing plasma.

(2) Very low density lipoproteins (VLDL, prebeta lipoproteins) contain about 60% triglycerides (endogenous) and 10% to 15% cholesterol. They are synthesized mainly in the liver from precursors such as free fatty acids (FFA). Since FFA and glycerol can be synthesized from carbohydrates, ingestion of large amounts of carbohydrates may cause formation of excessive amounts of VLDL. Triglycerides are degraded rapidly by the same lipases that catabolize chylomicrons. Increased VLDL levels impart turbidity to cold standing plasma and, in the absence of chylomicronemia, this turbidity directly reflects increased levels of triglycerides.

(3) Intermediate density lipoproteins (IDL, beta-VLDL) contain successively less triglyceride and more cholesterol as the catabolic conversion of VLDL to LDL progresses in a continuous process. They represent normal intermediates in the conversion of VLDL to LDL, but normally are not present in large numbers unless further catabolism is blocked to some degree. When excessive amounts are present, IDL may produce some turbidity in cold standing plasma; however, ultracentrifugation usually is necessary to confirm their presence.

(4) Low density lipoproteins (LDL, beta lipoproteins) contain almost 50% cholesterol and less than 5% triglyceride by weight and are derived from the metabolic breakdown of VLDL. Although their exact function and ultimate fate are unknown, they probably are degraded both in the liver and by peripheral cells. LDL carry most of the plasma cholesterol (60% to 75%) and have the highest atherogenic potential. Their concentration in plasma depends upon many factors (eg, dietary cholesterol content, intake of saturated fat, rate of production and removal of LDL and VLDL). LDL are normal constituents of fasting plasma, and cold standing plasma remains clear even when excessive amounts are present because of their relatively small size.

(5) High density lipoproteins (HDL, alpha lipoproteins) may be divided into two subclasses, HDL_2 and HDL_3. Although these differ in molecular weight and density, differences in function have not been established and they are considered collectively as HDL. HDL contain about 20% cholesterol, less than 5% triglyceride, and 50% protein by weight. They appear to be important for triglyceride and cholesterol clearance and for cholesteryl ester metabolism. HDL normally carry 20% to 25% of the cholesterol in blood. With high levels of HDL, the incidence of atherosclerosis and atherosclerotic events is reduced, while with low levels, the incidence, morbidity, and mortality from atherosclerosis are increased. Excessive amounts of HDL may cause a moderate increase in the total plasma cholesterol concentration, and determination of HDL levels and the ratio of HDL to total cholesterol is important in assessing the risk of atherosclerosis in patients with moderate hypercholesterolemia. HDL levels may be elevated in familial hyperalphalipoproteinemia, following exposure to chlori-

TABLE 1.
APOPROTEIN COMPONENTS OF LIPOPROTEINS

	Lipoprotein in which present			
Apoprotein	Chylomicron	VLDL	LDL	HDL
A-I	†	trace		major
A-II	†	trace		major
A-III (see D)				
B	major	major	major	
C-I	major	major		minor
C-II	major	major		minor
C-III*	major	major		minor
D (also called A-III)		minor		minor
E (also called arginine-rich)		major		minor

*Further subdivision of apoprotein C-III according to the number of sialic acid residues present is C-III$_0$, C-III$_1$, C-III$_2$, and C-III$_3$.
†Present, but exact amount not yet determined.

nated hydrocarbon pesticides, and with use of estrogens. HDL normally are present in fasting plasma, but they are even smaller than LDL and cold standing plasma remains clear even when HDL are present in enormous amounts.

Recently, the composition of lipoproteins has been further elucidated to include the protein portion present as part of an envelope enclosing the less soluble lipid portion. These heterogeneous groups of proteins are designated apoproteins. The terminology employed has varied, but in this text the alphabetical system identifying them on the basis of the lipoproteins in which they are usually found will be used (see Table 1). Each of these apoproteins differs in amino acid composition, as well as in immunochemical and biological reactivity.

These protein moieties interact with the lipid complement and affect lipoprotein secretion and degradation. Major functions of the apoproteins are to solubilize and transport plasma lipids. They also have physiologic and/or structural functions. Apoproteins with primarily structural roles are A$_{II}$ in HDL and apo B in chylomicrons, VLDL, and LDL. Apoprotein A$_I$ apparently is bound very loosely to HDL by protein-protein interaction with A$_{II}$ and activates lecithin:cholesterol acyltransferase (LCAT), the enzyme responsible for esterification of plasma cholesterol.

During VLDL metabolism, incremental density changes caused by delipidation result in transfer of apo B to IDL, then to LDL, and defects in apo B structure or function may contribute to increased plasma levels of LDL. During extrahepatic catabolism of chylomicrons or VLDL, C apoproteins are transferred to HDL, transported by HDL, and recycled into newly synthesized VLDL. The C apoproteins also have specific physiologic functions. Apoprotein C$_{II}$ (and possibly C$_I$) activates lipoprotein lipase, the main enzyme responsible for lipolysis of triglycerides. Apoprotein C$_{III}$ appears to inhibit this enzyme activity, which may be further inhibited if large amounts of apoprotein E are present. Since the C apoproteins can be exchanged between HDL, chylomicrons, and VLDL, they may affect the clearance of triglyceride particles. Thus, lipoprotein lipase activity could be decreased by deficiency of the enzyme or by imbalance or deficiency in C apoproteins.

With continuing study of the apoproteins, more complete understanding of both normal and abnormal lipid transport will occur. It is already apparent that apoprotein content and metabolism help explain the interrelationships of the lipoprotein families in normal lipid transport and the mechanisms involved in most forms of hyperlipidemia.

Types of Hyperlipoproteinemia: Five major types of hyperlipoproteinemia have been described, depending on which lipoproteins are abnormally increased. They may be primary (ie, genetically determined, sporadic) or secondary to dietary habits or other diseases. Primary hyperlipoproteinemias differ in their clinical manifestations, prognosis, and response to treatment; often they may be inherited. Secondary hyperlipoproteinemias may be associated with poorly controlled diabetes mellitus, alcoholism, hypothyroidism, obstructive liver disease, nephrotic syndrome, glycogen storage disease, or dysproteinemias (multiple myeloma, macroglobulinemia, lupus erythematosus). Successful treatment of the underlying disease usually corrects the hyperlipoproteinemia. In addition to being associated with atherosclerosis, hyperlipoproteinemia may produce lipid deposits (xanthomas) in the skin and tendons. Hypertriglyceridemia may induce attacks of abdominal pain, hepatosplenomegaly, and pancreatitis.

Lipoprotein patterns (types I to V, see Table 2 and below) do *not* indicate a specific disease mechanism but help to delineate the site of the abnormality in the complex area of lipid transport: Increased concentrations of lipoproteins may result from malfunction in any of the numerous metabolic steps during synthesis, transport, interconversion, or catabolism. Currently, an etiologic diagnosis is not always possible and it is necessary to rely on the lipoprotein patterns, which are purely descriptive. Furthermore, each type of hyperlipoproteinemia is heterogeneous. Although the present classification into types is incomplete, differential diagnosis is important since dietary and drug management vary significantly.

Type I is characterized by massive fasting hyperchylomicronemia induced by a normal dietary intake of fat. It usually is caused by deficiency of a lipoprotein lipase needed for the metabolism of chylomicrons. (One family with absence of apoprotein C$_{II}$ has been reported to have this system complex.) Serum triglycerides are markedly elevated, and the cholesterol/triglyceride ratio is usually less than 0.2:1. Patients with this disorder may be symptomatic before age 10, and colic, recurrent episodes of abdominal pain, eruptive xanthomas, and hepatosplenomegaly often are present in early childhood. Adults may experience episodes of pain that can mimic acute abdominal crises, often accompanied by fever, leukocytosis, anorexia, and vomiting. Acute hemorrhagic pancreatitis is the most severe, often fatal, complication of primary type I hyperlipoproteinemia.

Type II is characterized by elevated levels of LDL, elevated levels of apoprotein B, and normal (IIa) or moderately elevated (IIb) levels of VLDL. In those individuals in whom increased cholesterol intake elevates plasma LDL concentrations, dietary restriction of cholesterol is adequate to control hyperbetalipoproteinemia.

Familial type II hyperlipoproteinemia is manifested clinically in early childhood in homozygous individuals, but clinical symptoms usually do not appear before age 20 in the heterozygote. The most common form of familial type II is thought to be caused by a defect in the cell binding of apoprotein B (LDL) and, hence, in its removal from the plasma. Xanthomas of the tuberous or tendon type occur in both homozygotes and heterozygotes; planar orange-yellow lesions often are evident in homozygotes. In homozygous patients, ischemic heart disease is almost inevitable before age 20; for heterozygotes, the probability is at least 50% by age 50. Since the risk of premature ischemic heart disease appears to be high, early detection is important. If genetically determined type II hyperbetalipoproteinemia is suspected, about one-half of the other family members will be affected; thus, blood relatives should be screened.

Type III is characterized by the accumulation of intermediate forms of lipoproteins, possibly caused by a partial block in the normal metabolic degradation of VLDL to LDL, rapid production of apoprotein B, or increased apoprotein E levels. In some patients, the absence of one isoelectric form of apoprotein E, apo E_{III}, has been reported. Serum cholesterol and triglyceride concentrations are similarly elevated (350 to 800 mg/dl) in this disorder. Palmar planar xanthomas and tuberoeruptive lesions on the elbows, knees, or buttocks may be pathognomonic. Accelerated coronary and peripheral vascular disease frequently occurs in the fourth and fifth decades, and glucose intolerance and hyperuricemia are observed in about 40% of patients with type III.

Type IV is characterized by elevated VLDL levels with resulting hypertriglyceridemia. This genetically diverse disorder may be the most common form of hyperlipoproteinemia. The mechanisms are uncertain, but type IV often is secondary to other diseases or to excessive intake of alcohol or carbohydrates and patients are frequently obese. Ischemic heart disease may occur (although less frequently than in familial type II) during the fourth decade or later in patients with familial type IV hyperlipoproteinemia; there usually are no prior external signs, such as xanthomas. Most of these patients have carbohydrate intolerance and more than 40% have hyperuricemia.

Type V is characterized by accumulation of both VLDL and chylomicrons, probably caused by a defect in the catabolism of both endogenous and exogenous triglycerides. Since all lipoproteins contain some cholesterol, cholesterol concentrations may be elevated if triglyceride levels are very high. This disorder is relatively uncommon, may be genetically heterogeneous, and patients with the familial disorder usually do not become symptomatic until after age 20. These patients have fat and carbohydrate intolerance and usually have hyperuricemia. An association between type V disorder and ischemic heart disease has not been established, but triglyceride levels should be reduced to decrease the incidence of eruptive xanthomas, pancreatitis, and abdominal pain.

Treatment of Hyperlipidemia

There is significant evidence that elevated concentrations of certain plasma lipids are associated with an increased risk of atherosclerosis and its complications. Optimal management includes reduction of plasma lipid levels and elimination of other risk factors, particularly hypertension and smoking. The presence of more than one risk factor, including a familial history of premature atherosclerotic complications, makes active intervention more urgent, especially in younger patients. Many of the important risk factors can and should be diagnosed in children.

Long-term controlled studies have produced some evidence that decreasing blood lipid levels affects morbidity and mortality in patients with established ischemic heart disease who have had at least one myocardial infarction. However, the results are not conclusive, for each of these studies is subject to criticism for various reasons. Furthermore, once atherosclerotic complications have occurred, it is probable that coronary disease is sufficiently advanced and the myocardium damaged so that reducing lipid levels may be ineffective because thrombotic and other factors are functioning. The efficacy of lowering lipid levels in primary prevention of atherosclerosis has not been proved clinically. Nevertheless, it is reasonable to assume that early recognition and application of proper therapy before sequelae have developed may offer the best chance of producing beneficial results.

Type I hyperlipoproteinemia is quite rare, types III and V are uncommon, and types II and IV are relatively common. Since they are often genetically determined and are associated with a high risk of ischemic heart disease (especially types II and IV), family members (particularly children) should be screened for abnormal lipid levels so that treatment can be initiated before irreversible vascular changes have occurred. Unfortunately, manifestations of type IV are uncommon in children.

TABLE 2.
CHARACTERISTICS OF TYPES OF HYPERLIPOPROTEINEMIA*

	Type I Exogenous Hyperlipemia (Hyperchylomicronemia)	Type II a. Hyperbeta-lipoproteinemia (Hypercholesterolemia)	Type II b. Combined Hyperlipidemia (Mixed Hyperlipidemia)
Lipoprotein characteristics of plasma	*Chylomicrons markedly increased* LDL, VLDL, and HDL usually normal or decreased	*LDL increased* VLDL normal Chylomicrons absent	*LDL increased* VLDL increased Chylomicrons absent
Appearance of plasma after standing overnight at 4 C (sample take after 12-14 hr fast)†	*Cream layer on top, clear infranate*	Clear (no cream layer on top)	No cream layer on top, clear to turbid infranate (depending on VLDL level)
Cholesterol: triglyceride ratio	<0.2:1	>1.5:1	Variable
Other laboratory abnormalities	Fat tolerance markedly abnormal PHLA low		
Clinical manifestations	Eruptive xanthomas Hepatosplenomegaly Lipemia retinalis Abdominal pain Pancreatitis	Tendon xanthomas, occasionally associated with polyarthritis Xanthelasma Arcus corneae juvenilis Tuberous xanthomas	
Secondary causes (to be eliminated before treating for hyperlipoproteinemia)	Dysgammaglobulinemia Diabetic acidosis Hypothyroidism	Hypothyroidism Acute intermittent porphyria Obstructive liver disease Macroglobulinemia Multiple myeloma Nephrotic syndrome Excess dietary cholesterol Excess saturated fat in diet	
Incidence	Rare	Common	
Usual age at detection	Early childhood	Infancy or early childhood	
Ischemic heart disease risk	No association	Greatly accelerated	

*VLDL —very low density lipoproteins (pre-β-lipoproteins) represent endogenous triglyceride concentration.
LDL —low density lipoproteins (β-lipoproteins) represent major portions of cholesterol concentration.
HDL —high density lipoproteins (α-lipoproteins) are not included in the chart.
PHLA —post-heparin lipolytic activity represents a group of enzymes necessary for metabolism of triglycerides.
Chylomicrons represent exogenous triglyceride concentration.

Type III Broad Beta Pattern (Dysbetalipoproteinemia)	Type IV Endogenous Hyperlipidemia (Hypertriglyceridemia)	Type V Mixed Hyperlipidemia
Floating β-lipoproteins and VLDL increased Chylomicrons may be present	*VLDL increased* LDL normal (or decreased) Chylomicrons absent	*VLDL increased* Chylomicrons increased LDL normal (or decreased)
Faint cream layer on top, turbid infranate	No cream layer on top, clear to turbid infranate (depending on VLDL level)	Cream layer on top, turbid infranate
Often 1:1, but may vary from 0.3 to 2.0:1	Variable	0.15 to 0.6:1
Carbohydrate sensitivity and glucose tolerance often abnormal Uric acid levels often elevated	Carbohydrate sensitivity and glucose tolerance often abnormal Uric acid levels often elevated	Carbohydrate sensitivity and glucose tolerance usually abnormal Uric acid levels usually elevated Fat tolerance abnormal PHLA sometimes low
Planar xanthomas Tuberoeruptive xanthomas Tendon xanthomas Occasionally, arcus corneae juvenilis Rarely, xanthelasma	Usually none Rarely, eruptive xanthomas	Eruptive xanthomas Abdominal pain Pancreatitis Hepatosplenomegaly Lipemia retinalis Occasionally, tuberoeruptive xanthomas, paresthesias
Hypothyroidism Dysgammaglobulinemia Diabetic acidosis Multiple myeloma	Nephrotic syndrome Juvenile diabetes Multiple myeloma Alcoholism Von Gierke disease (type I glycogenosis) Werner syndrome Use of oral contraceptives or estrogens Obesity Acute metabolic stress	Hypothyroidism Nephrotic syndrome Diabetic acidosis Multiple myeloma Alcoholism Von Gierke disease (type I glycogenosis) Use of oral contraceptives or estrogens
Relatively uncommon	Common	Relatively uncommon
Early adulthood	Adulthood (middle age)	Early adulthood
Peripheral and coronary vascular disease accelerated	Probably accelerated	Data inadequate to determine association

†*Cream layer indicates elevated chylomicron concentration (except in type III, where the large aggregates of β-VLDL form the faint layer); turbid infranate indicates elevated triglycerides (VLDL).*

Therapeutic Guidelines: Rational treatment for hyperlipidemia depends upon definitive differential diagnosis. Proper evaluation also includes complete personal, dietary, and family history; thorough physical examination; and laboratory tests, including carbohydrate tolerance and thyroid, hepatic, and renal function.

Cholesterol and triglyceride analyses are adequate for initial screening, but if above-normal values are found, the lipid transport disorder is not identified. Choles-terol is present in all lipoproteins, and slight to marked hypercholesterolemia may occur when there is an increase in any of the lipoproteins in plasma. After at least one week on a conventional American diet with the patient maintaining a steady weight, cholesterol and triglyceride analyses should be performed on blood samples acquired after a 12- to 14-hour fast. At least three determinations should be obtained at two-week intervals to confirm the diagnosis of hyperlipidemia and estab-

TABLE 3.
GENERAL DIETARY RESTRICTIONS IN TREATMENT OF HYPERLIPOPROTEINEMIAS

	Type I	Type II a	Type II b
General prescription	Low fat Supplement with medium-chain triglycerides High carbohydrate	Low cholesterol Low saturated fat supplemented with unsaturated fat	Low cholesterol Low saturated fat, supplemented with unsaturated fat Weight reduction when necessary Moderate alcohol restriction
Weight reduction	Has little effect	Has little effect	To ideal body weight may be necessary
Calories	Not restricted Patients with high energy requirements may have difficulty maintaining weight	Not restricted	Restricted to maintain ideal body weight
Protein	Not restricted, 15%–20% (50–100 g daily)	Not restricted; 15%–20% (50–100 g daily)	
Fat	Adults, less than 25 g/day; children 6 to 12 years of age, less than 15 g/day. May be either saturated or unsaturated fats. Supplement with medium-chain triglycerides	Not restricted in quantity (40%–45% daily) Low saturated fat (less than 5% of calories) supplemented with unsaturated fat	
Cholesterol	Not restricted	Low. Adults, less than 300 mg daily; children, less than 200 mg daily	
Carbohydrate	Not restricted Substitute carbohydrate for fat	Not restricted	
Alcohol	None allowed	Not restricted	
Remarks	Diet should reduce chylomicrons to normal	Diet should lower LDL 15%–30%	

lish a pretreatment baseline. Office kits are unsatisfactory for these determinations, and analyses of laboratory results preferably should be compared with acceptable standards at regular intervals. If hyperlipidemia is present, examination of the physical appearance of fasting plasma after overnight refrigeration (VLDL and chylomicrons refract light and produce turbidity in hyperlipidemic plasma, but LDL and HDL do not) (see Table 2) identifies the type of hyperlipoproteinemia present in about two-thirds of cases. However, type IIb and mild type IV cannot be differentiated by these tests. Electrophoresis or direct determination of HDL by simple precipitation techniques may be necessary to distinguish between the increased beta lipoprotein of type IIa and increased alpha lipoprotein.

After the type of abnormality has been established, cholesterol and triglyceride determinations are usually adequate for monitoring the effects of diet and drug

Type III	Type IV	Type V
Weight reduction to ideal body weight	Weight reduction to ideal body weight	Weight reduction to ideal body weight
Low cholesterol	Controlled carbohydrate	High protein
Balanced, modified fat and carbohydrate	Modified fat	Moderate fat and carbohydrate reduction
Low alcohol intake	Low alcohol intake	No alcohol intake
To ideal body weight is necessary	To ideal body weight is necessary	To ideal body weight is necessary
Restricted to maintain ideal body weight	Restricted to maintain ideal body weight	Restricted to maintain ideal body weight
Moderate; 18%–21% (75–125 g daily)	Moderate; 18%–21% (75–125 g daily)	High; 21%–24% (90–145 g daily)
Controlled, 35% to 40% daily, with unsaturated fat substituted for a portion of saturated fat	Not restricted except for weight control, and substitution of unsaturated fat for a portion of saturated fat	Restricted to less than 30% daily, with unsaturated fat substituted for a portion of saturated fat
Low. Less than 300 mg daily	Moderate restriction. Less than 500 mg daily	Moderate restriction. Less than 500 mg daily
Controlled to 40% daily	Controlled to 40% daily	Controlled. Less than 50% daily
Restricted to 2 servings daily Substitute for carbohydrate	Restricted to 2 servings daily Substitute for carbohydrate	None allowed

therapy. Since serum triglyceride levels usually increase and serum cholesterol levels decrease immediately after acute myocardial infarction, determination of lipoprotein type should be postponed in these patients until serum lipids have stabilized (usually after two months). Since they complicate interpretation of test results, hypolipidemic drugs, estrogens and contraceptive agents, or steroids should be discontinued, if feasible, at least three weeks prior to diagnostic determinations.

Manipulation of diet is the initial treatment for primary hyperlipoproteinemias. Strong patient motivation is a prerequisite if the prolonged dietary control required is to succeed, and it is usually necessary to be specific about foods that are contraindicated. Foods derived from animal sources should be progressively restricted and vegetable protein substituted, but the amount of polyunsaturated fats need not be increased in many patients. Salt intake should be reduced and convenience and fried foods, especially those prepared in deep fat, should be eliminated. To maintain caloric intake, complex carbohydrates (but not simple sugars) may be increased. See Table 3 for a summary of dietary restrictions correlated to type of hyperlipidemia.

When reduction to ideal body weight is indicated, a standard reducing diet should be prescribed, with the caloric level regulated according to the amount of weight loss necessary. When ideal body weight has been attained or when maximal beneficial effects have been achieved, the appropriate therapeutic diet should then be started.

Some authorities believe that a single diet is appropriate for treating all hyperlipemias (except for the very rare, genetically determined lipoprotein lipase deficiency in type I) and advocate the American Heart Association fat-controlled diet in which saturated fat intake is reduced and polyunsaturated fats and carbohydrates are substituted. However, when polyunsaturated fats are used to replace saturated fats, the P/S ratio probably should not exceed 2:1 until the claims that increased deposition of polyunsaturates in tissues may result in increased cellular damage have been clarified. Recently, a similarly restricted diet has been advocated for all Americans, starting in childhood. However, the Committee on Nutrition of the American Academy of Pediatrics does not advocate dietary changes for *all* children, since current knowledge of the long-term effects of dietary intervention is inadequate to justify widespread alterations.

Maximal effects of diet usually occur within six weeks. Type II heterozygotes rarely attain the normal range of LDL on diet alone and homozygotes never do. Diet therapy may reduce lipids to normal concentrations in types III, IV, and V.

Drugs are indicated only if dietary restrictions, including weight reduction when necessary, are unsuccessful and the risk of atherosclerotic or other complications (eg, pancreatitis, abdominal pain, xanthomas) justifies their use. Dietary regulation must continue during drug therapy, for the effects of diet and drugs are additive. Plasma lipid levels should be determined frequently until they become stable and at gradually increased intervals thereafter. In most instances, the dose should be modified or another drug substituted if lipoprotein levels are not reduced significantly after an adequate trial. Drug therapy must be continuous and lifelong, for plasma lipid levels usually return to pretreatment concentrations if treatment is discontinued. In addition, the patient must be closely monitored indefinitely, since dosage adjustments are required if there are changes in diet or body weight or concomitant medications are used.

Several drugs lower elevated concentrations of plasma cholesterol and triglycerides, but no drug is effective in all types of hyperlipoproteinemia, and their long-term effects have not been established. At present, the agents advocated for treatment of hyperlipidemias are clofibrate [Atromid-S], cholestyramine resin [Questran], colestipol [Colestid], probucol [Lorelco], and niacin (nicotinic acid) [Nicobid, Nico-400, Nicolar]. Dextrothyroxine [Choloxin], neomycin [Mycifradin, Neobiotic], norethindrone [Norlutate], oxandrolone [Anavar], and sitos-terols [Cytellin] are used occasionally. Estrogens are no longer advocated because they increase the incidence of cardiovascular complications. The use of these agents is discussed under the type of hyperlipoproteinemia in which the drugs are effective. Specific indications, untoward reactions, and precautions are discussed in the evaluations.

Several investigational agents have hypolipidemic activity, but further studies of their efficacy and side effects are necessary before use in man can be recommended. Aminosalicylic acid (PAS), a drug used to treat tuberculosis, has potent hypolipidemic action and reduces levels of cholesterol and triglycerides by reducing both LDL and VLDL. However, it is not well tolerated because of gastrointestinal disturbances. A more highly purified aminosalicylic acid preparation (PAS-C) apparently has similar hypolipidemic activity with fewer side effects but rarely may cause hypersensitivity reactions or goiter. Halofenate, a drug structurally similar to clofibrate, reduces VLDL but has caused severe gastrointestinal bleeding. In limited studies, bezafibrate, an analogue of clofibrate, apparently has been shown to have actions similar to those of clofibrate. In several clinical trials, gemfibrozil reduced cholesterol levels, especially in chylomicrons and VLDL, and increased HDL cholesterol levels; triglycerides were decreased in all lipoprotein fractions. Procetofene markedly reduced triglycerides and moderately increased HDL cholesterol in patients with type IV hyperlipoproteinemia and decreased LDL cholesterol in those with type II hyperlipoproteinemia. Several other agents have demonstrated hypolipidemic activity in animal studies but have not been tested in man.

Table 4 summarizes the drug therapy advocated for the treatment of the five major types of hyperlipoproteinemia, listed in order of preference (see also the evaluations). All of these drugs should be discontinued if a patient has an acute myocardial infarction. Drug therapy must be reinstituted cautiously, if at all, during the first month after a myocardial infarction.

Most therapeutic failures are due to inability of the patient to follow the diet and/or take drugs regularly. However, even with ideal therapy, levels of plasma lipids remain elevated in some patients. Many workers are investigating the concomitant use of two hypolipidemic drugs in these individuals. Diet plus cholestyramine and niacin, which act by different mechanisms, has been useful in patients with homozygous type II hyperlipoproteinemia refractory to diet and cholestyramine alone.

When severe hyperlipidemia causes abdominal pain (this occurs fairly often in types I and V), complete fasting for 24 to 48 hours, except for administration of intravenous fluids if necessary, usually relieves the pain and reduces triglyceride levels dramatically. This is the only recommended therapy; no drugs are effective in this acute situation. When pain is relieved, the diet appropriate for the patient's lipid pattern should be started. In type V, high triglyceride concentrations may be further decreased when drugs are added to a dietary regimen to reduce or abolish the frequency of attacks of abdominal pain and/or pancreatitis. Hypertriglyceridemia has been reported to cause neuropathy in a few patients; this condition improved when triglyceride levels were reduced.

A 35% increase in the serum cholesterol level usually occurs during the last trimester of pregnancy and is independent of diet. The use of hypolipidemic drugs during pregnancy is not advocated, because their safety during this period has not been determined.

Other Lipid-Lowering Regimens: Ileal bypass surgery has been used to reduce refractory hypercholesterolemia in patients with type II who are unable or unwilling to take drugs. This surgery may aggravate hyperlipidemia in patients with other types of hyperlipoproteinemia. It should be considered experimental and used with extreme caution. Intermittent plasmapheresis reduces plasma cholesterol levels in patients with homozygous type IIa hyperlipidemia but is considered an experimental procedure at present. Chelation therapy has been advocated by some physicians for treatment of atherosclerosis but has not proved to be effective; data are anecdotal and there is no supporting clinical evidence. Such therapy has no place in the treatment of hyperlipidemia.

Treatment of Hyperlipoproteinemia Types: In familial *type I*, which is rare, and in those secondary states that do not respond to treatment of the underlying dis-

TABLE 4.
DRUG THERAPY IN HYPERLIPOPROTEINEMIA*

Type II

a	b

HETEROZYGOTES:
    Cholestyramine resin (Questran)
        Initial dose: 4 g four times a day.
        Maintenance dose: 4–8 g four times a day, with meals and at bedtime.
        May also give total dose of 16–32 g divided into two or three doses if tolerated.
        LDL levels should decrease 15%–30% over diet alone.
        In IIb, there may be a variable increase in VLDL.
    Alternatively, in Type IIa:
    Colestipol hydrochloride (Colestid)
        Adults: 15–30 g daily divided into 2 to 4 doses, with meals *or*
**Probucol (Lorelco)
        Adults: 500 mg twice daily with morning and evening meal.	

Niacin
    Initial dose 100 mg three times a day.
    Maintenance dose: 1–3 g three times a day, given with meals.
    LDL levels should decrease 15%–35%. VLDL levels should decrease 40% over diet alone.	

Neomycin sulfate (Mycifradin sulfate, Neobiotic)
    Initial dose: 0.5 g/day.
    Maintenance dose: 1–2 g/day.
    LDL levels should decrease 20%–25% over diet alone. Ineffective for lowering VLDL levels.
    Adverse effects limit usefulness.
	Clofibrate (Atromid-S)
	    Dose: 1 g twice daily.
	    LDL levels should decrease 5%–10%. VLDL levels should decrease 35%–50%.

Dextrothyroxine sodium (Choloxin)
    Initial dose: 1 mg/day.
    Maintenance dose: 4–8 mg/day.
    LDL levels should decrease 15%–30% over diet alone.
    Should not be used in patients with organic heart disease or arrhythmias.
	Cholestyramine resin 4 g four times a day and niacin 1–3 g twice a day. The cholestyramine component should decrease LDL 25%–35%: niacin will have some effect on LDL (15%–30%) and should decrease VLDL 35%–50%.

HOMOZYGOTES: Cholestyramine 4–8 g four times a day and niacin 1.2 to 3 g three times a day (with meals). Should be started in childhood before vascular damage becomes too severe.	

*No drug therapy is effective for Type 1.
**Less effective than cholestyramine resin in patients with familial Type IIa disorder.

ease, restriction of dietary fat to 25 g/day or less markedly decreases triglyceride levels, resolves xanthomas, and relieves abdominal pain, although moderate lipemia may persist. At least 1% of total calories should be provided as linoleic acid to meet essential fatty acid requirements and fat-soluble vitamins should be given if not provided in

Type III	Type IV	Type V
Clofibrate (Atromid-S) Initial dose: 0.5–1 g twice a day. Maintenance dose: 1 g twice a day. VLDL levels should decrease 40%–80% over diet alone. Cholelithiasis is a major adverse effect.	Niacin Initial dose: 100 mg three times a day. Maintenance dose: 1–3 g three times a day. Should decrease both LDL and VLDL levels more than 30%. Side effects may limit usefulness.	Niacin Initial dose: 100 mg three times a day. Maintenance dose: 1–3 g three times a day. LDL levels should decrease 30%. VLDL levels should decrease as much as 70% over diet alone. More effective than clofibrate but side effects may limit usefulness.
Niacin Initial dose: 100 mg three times a day. Maintenance dose: 1 g three times a day. Given with meals. VLDL levels should decrease 40%–80% over diet alone.	Clofibrate (Atromid-S) Initial dose: 0.5–1 g twice a day. Maintenance dose: 1 g twice a day. VLDL levels may decrease 10%–50%, but LDL levels may increase more than 50%. Use of clofibrate in type IV requires close supervision.	Clofibrate (Atromid-S) Initial dose: 0.5–1 g twice a day. Maintenance dose: 1 g twice a day. VLDL levels may decrease 10%–50%. Cholelithiasis is a major adverse effect.
		Norethindrone acetate (Norlutate) For use only in women. Initial and maintenance doses 5 mg a day; (premenopausal women should receive the drug 21 days per month to permit regular menses). VLDL levels should decrease 10%–50%.

the diet. The addition of medium-chain triglycerides (MCT), which are transported directly to the liver without requiring chylomicron formation, increases palatability and variety. To supply adequate calories, carbohydrate should be substituted for fat. Alcohol consumption is restricted to prevent abdominal pain. None of the currently available hypolipidemic drugs are effective in type I.

In *type II* hyperlipoproteinemia, the cholesterol intake should be low (less than 300 mg/day) and saturated fat should be restricted in relation to the intake of polyunsaturated fat to give a P/S ratio of approximately 2:1. Weight reduction often is important in type IIb. Drug therapy usually is required in patients with primary familial type II, and cholestyramine resin is the agent of choice. If response is inadequate, niacin may be added to the regimen because its effects are often additive to those of cholestyramine. Colestipol and probucol may be substituted for cholestyramine. The former has the same actions as cholestyramine but is considered an alternate drug because there is less experience with its use; the latter is less effective in patients with familial type II. Niacin also decreases VLDL and thus is especially useful in type IIb; however, adverse effects may limit its usefulness. Dextrothyroxine may reduce LDL concentrations, but it should not be given to patients with arrhythmias or organic heart disease. These complications limit the use of dextrothyroxine, since many patients with type II have latent coronary heart disease. Neomycin sulfate has been used successfully in some patients with type IIa. Clofibrate is only moderately effective in lowering LDL and is often inadequate in familial type IIa, although it may be beneficial in type IIb and nonhereditary type IIa disorders.

Familial homozygous type II is the most malignant form of hyperlipoproteinemia; untreated patients seldom live beyond early adulthood. This form is particularly resistant to therapy, although some success recently has been reported with a combination of diet, cholestyramine, and niacin.

In *type III*, dietary restriction to result in ideal body weight, followed by adherence to a diet low in cholesterol and saturated fat, frequently is the only therapy necessary. In some patients, carbohydrate and alcohol restriction also may be required. If this does not normalize lipid concentrations, concomitant administration of clofibrate usually reduces serum lipids to the normal range and causes xanthomas to regress. Niacin is effective but often is not considered a drug of choice because of the frequency of overt adverse effects. Cholestyramine is not useful in this type of hyperlipoproteinemia and may even worsen it.

Reduction of food intake to achieve ideal body weight is of primary importance in the management of *type IV*, and patients should be maintained on a diet moderately low in carbohydrates and low in alcohol. Excess carbohydrates should be replaced by unsaturated fats and cholesterol should be restricted to less than 500 mg/day. Adherence to this regimen produces complete remission in many patients. The American Heart Association diet does not restrict carbohydrates, and advocates of this regimen suggest that liberal carbohydrate is well tolerated if calories are restricted during weight loss and/or if an isocaloric diet is substituted during subsequent maintenance. Only if the triglyceride concentration remains elevated should cautious use of adjunctive drugs be considered. Although both clofibrate and niacin reduce the VLDL concentration, clofibrate may cause a reciprocal rise in the LDL cholesterol level.

Since most patients with *type V* are overweight, the first step in management is weight reduction. The maintenance diet should be as high in protein and low in fat as is tolerated by the patient; carbohydrate content also should be controlled. Restriction of alcohol consumption often is necessary, especially to prevent abdominal pain. These measures frequently control symptoms and reduce lipid levels. If concomitant drug administration is needed to further decrease these levels, clofibrate may be prescribed but is not uniformly effective. Niacin is more effective but may aggravate hyperglycemia and hyperuricemia. Norethindrone [Norlutate] may be used in women and oxandrolone [Anavar] in men; either may prevent attacks of abdominal pain even though plasma lipids are not normalized.

INDIVIDUAL EVALUATIONS

CHOLESTYRAMINE RESIN
[Questran]

Cholestyramine binds bile acids in the intestine and prevents their reabsorption; the reduced level of bile acids promotes apoprotein B catabolism and increases the rate of conversion of cholesterol to bile acids in the liver. Thus, the major effect of cholestyramine in hyperlipidemia is to increase the rate of LDL removal.

Cholestyramine is the drug of choice for type IIa (hyperbetalipoproteinemia). When used as an adjunct to dietary control, it reduces beta lipoproteins an additional 20% to 25%; 90% of the effect is noted in seven to nine days and maximum effect is apparent within 21 days. In type IIb, usual doses of cholestyramine decrease LDL but may cause further mild elevation of VLDL (triglyceride) in some patients.

In the usual dosage range, cholestyramine is ineffective in hyperprebetalipoproteinemia and is of no benefit in types III, IV, or V hyperlipoproteinemia; in fact, it may aggravate these conditions.

Cholestyramine probably is one of the safest drugs currently available for treatment of hyperlipoproteinemia; because it is not absorbed from the gastrointestinal tract, there are no significant systemic toxic effects. Nevertheless, the large doses required are unpleasant to take. The most frequent untoward effects are bloating, mild nausea, and constipation, which usually subside with continued therapy. One case of intestinal impaction has been reported. Other adverse reactions include epigastric distress and, occasionally, diarrhea. Rarely, vomiting, rash, and irritation of the tongue and perianal region have been reported.

Cholestyramine may interfere with the absorption of fat; associated deficiency of the fat-soluble vitamins A, D, and K may occur and supplementation may be required. Some investigators suggest that folate deficiency occurs during long-term treatment and patients, especially children, should receive 5 mg of folic acid daily, if necessary. Steatorrhea, weight loss, and malabsorption syndrome may be noted with use of doses larger than 30 g daily. For this reason, some investigators consider 24 g daily the maximal dose.

Since cholestyramine may adsorb other drugs given concomitantly (particularly thiazides, thyroid, digitalis, iron, phenylbutazone, antibiotics, barbiturates, and warfarin), these drugs should be given at least one hour before or four hours after cholestyramine. Mild lengthening of the prothrombin time without bleeding has been reported. The dosage of concomitantly administered anticoagulants should be closely monitored.

ROUTE, USUAL DOSAGE, AND PREPARATIONS. *Oral*: Initially, *adults*, 4 g (one packet or one rounded teaspoonful) four times daily with meals and at bedtime. Depending upon the response, this may be increased to 6 g four times daily. A dosage of 24 g daily divided into two or three doses has been shown to be equally effective. The drug should never be swallowed dry because of the hazard of esophageal irritation or blockage. It should be mixed with 4 to 6 oz of a suitable liquid or with pulpy fruit just before ingestion. Although the dosage in *children over 6 years* has not been definitively established, 8 g twice daily with meals, increased to a maximal total daily dose of 24 g, is being given. *Children under 6 years*, dosage has not been established.

Questran (Mead Johnson). Packets (9 g) and powder (378 g) providing 4 g of active drug per packet or 9 g scoop.

CLOFIBRATE
[Atromid-S]

Cl—⟨benzene ring⟩—O—C(CH₃)(CH₃)—COCH₂CH₃ (O)

The mechanism of action of clofibrate is unclear, but this agent may inhibit the hepatic release of lipoproteins (particularly VLDL), interferes with the binding of serum free fatty acids to albumin, increases the excretion of fecal neutral sterols, inhibits cholesterol biosynthesis, and affects the metabolism of some lipoprotein apoproteins. Xanthomas have regressed in patients with type III with reduction of plasma lipid levels. A few studies indicate that clofibrate may accelerate catabolism of VLDL and IDL. Its major effect in hyperlipoproteinemia is to reduce VLDL; in most patients, the hypocholesterolemic effect is moderate.

When used with appropriate dietary regulation, clofibrate is uniformly effective in decreasing IDL (floating beta lipoprotein) levels and is the drug of choice for type III hyperlipoproteinemia; no untoward lipoprotein shift occurs in these patients. Also, dramatic improvement in patients with peripheral vascular disease associated with type III hyperlipoproteinemia has been reported.

This drug also may be effective in reducing VLDL levels in patients with types IV and V abnormalities. However, a reciprocal increase in LDL has been noted in some patients. Cholesterol levels should be monitored in those with type IV or V, and the drug should be discontinued if a significant increase occurs.

Although patients with homozygous type II and heterozygous type IIa usually do not respond satisfactorily to clofibrate, this drug appears to be effective in reducing VLDL levels in some type IIb heterozygotes since the VLDL concentration also is increased. Clofibrate also has been reported to reduce serum fibrinogen levels and may diminish platelet adhesiveness.

Gastrointestinal disturbances (nausea, vomiting, diarrhea, dyspepsia, and flatulence) occur in about 10% of patients taking clofibrate, but these effects are usually transient and disappear with continued therapy. Less frequently, leukopenia, rash, drowsiness, and alopecia areata have been noted. Patients occasionally gain weight.

Clofibrate causes hepatomegaly in animals, but similar changes have not been observed in man. However, elevations in serum transaminase levels, which are reversible when therapy is discontinued, have been noted.

Potentially serious effects on skeletal and cardiac muscle have occurred rarely; creatine phosphokinase levels were increased, sometimes accompanied by frank myositis with asthenia, myalgia, and malaise. Elevated levels may persist when other serum enzymes return to normal and the patient is asymptomatic. In patients with chest pain, increased transaminase and creatine phosphokinase levels caused by clofibrate rather than by myocardial infarction should be considered.

Close supervision of patients on long-term therapy is required. This agent is contraindicated in patients with impaired renal or hepatic function, since delayed detoxification and excretion make the duration of action unpredictable and increased cholelithiasis may result. Clofibrate also is contraindicated during pregnancy and should not be given to nursing mothers, for it may be excreted in milk.

Clofibrate displaces acidic drugs, such as coumarin anticoagulants, phenytoin, and tolbutamide, from binding sites on plasma proteins. The dosage of anticoagulants must be reduced by at least one-half and prothrombin times should be determined frequently, especially during initiation of therapy. SGOT, SGPT, and creatine phosphokinase values should be determined occasionally. A rebound increase in cholesterol and triglyceride concentrations often is observed after clofibrate is discontinued.

The Coronary Drug Project trial of clofibrate for long-term management of men with established ischemic heart disease produced no definitive evidence that this agent reduced total mortality. Furthermore, the incidence of peripheral vascular disease, pulmonary embolism, thrombophlebitis, angina pectoris, increased heart size, arrhythmias, and intermittent claudication was significantly increased. There also was a twofold increase in the incidence of cholelithiasis, and evidence of feminizing effects (decreased libido, breast tenderness) was noted occasionally in these patients. Therefore, clofibrate should not be given indiscriminately to patients who have had a myocardial infarction but generally should be reserved for patients with clofibrate-responsive hyperlipidemia in whom there is substantial risk of ischemic heart disease. The large primary prevention trial of clofibrate conducted in Europe confirms these recommendations (*Br Heart J*, 1978). In this study, there was significant reduction in the incidence of myocardial infarction but a significant increase in total deaths and gastrointestinal problems, especially cholelithiasis. The authors concluded that clofibrate cannot be recommended for all patients with hyperlipidemia. Because of the risks associated with its use, some clinicians suggest it be given only to patients with type III.

Clofibrate is not recommended for use in children, since data are insufficient to determine the drug's safety in this age group.

ROUTE, USUAL DOSAGE, AND PREPARATIONS. *Oral*: *Adults*, 500 mg three or four times daily.

Atromid-S (Ayerst). Capsules 500 mg.

COLESTIPOL HYDROCHLORIDE
[Colestid]

The action and indications for this bile-sequestering agent are similar to those of cholestyramine. Colestipol is odorless and tasteless and, although less experience with its use has accumulated, it may be considered as an alternate to cholestyramine in type IIa patients.

For a discussion of adverse reactions and precautions, see the evaluation on Cholestyramine Resin.

ROUTE, USUAL DOSAGE, AND PREPARATIONS. *Oral*: *Adults*, 15 to 30 g daily (mixed with 4 to 6 oz of suitable liquid) in two to four divided doses with meals. This drug should be given at least one hour before or four hours after other drugs. *Children*, the safety and effectiveness of colestipol has not been established.

Colestid (Upjohn). Powder in 5 g packets and 500 g bottles with scoop providing 5 g/scoop.

CONJUGATED ESTROGENS

ETHINYL ESTRADIOL

Estrogens were used to treat hyperlipidemia after it was found that women have lower serum beta lipoprotein and higher alpha lipoprotein concentrations than men, as well as decreased susceptibility to atherosclerosis and ischemic heart disease until after the menopause. However, estrogens are unsuitable as hypolipidemic agents in men because of their feminizing effects and because they elevate VLDL and triglyceride concentrations. In a long-term trial in men with established ischemic heart disease, their use was discontinued because they increased the incidence of thromboembolism, cardiovascular complications, and mortality from cancer. In women, administration of estrogens may elevate VLDL levels and decrease postheparin lipoprotein lipase activity (PHLA). They also are reported to cause abdominal pain and pancreatitis in women with type V hyperlipoproteinemia.

Although a study in Finland reportedly showed that estrogens reduced LDL concentrations in women with type II hyperlipoproteinemia, these observations require confirmation. At present, estrogens should not be used to treat hyperlipoproteinemia because of the reasons cited above.

See Chapter 43, Estrogens and Progestins, for preparations.

DEXTROTHYROXINE SODIUM
[Choloxin]

Of all the thyroid analogues, dextrothyroxine is reported to have the highest ratio of hypolipidemic/calorigenic activity. The drug effectively reduces LDL by promoting apoprotein B catabolism in both euthyroid and hypothyroid patients. The decrease in serum cholesterol concentrations, which may range from 20% to 50%, is greatest in patients with the highest baseline concentrations. Maximal effects appear in one to two months.

Dextrothyroxine is used in type II hyperbetalipoproteinemia. Since it has no consistent effect on VLDL in the usual dosage range, this drug is seldom useful in patients with types III, IV, or V patterns.

The untoward effects of dextrothyroxine occur frequently, are usually caused by metabolic stimulation, and generally mimic symptoms of hyperthyroidism. Weight loss appears to be the first sign of hypermetabolism. Related effects include nervousness, insomnia, tremors, hyperhidrosis, and menstrual irregularity. Some patients report altered taste sensations, vertigo, and diarrhea during the first six weeks of therapy, but these reactions subside spontaneously. Rash and pruritus may develop in patients who are hypersensitive to iodine. Since this drug increases protein-bound iodine levels, the PBI test cannot be used to measure thyroid function.

In some diabetic patients, prolonged use of dextrothyroxine decreases glucose tolerance, which may necessitate increasing the dose of hypoglycemic agents. Since this drug augments the effect of orally administered anticoagulants, the dose of the latter may require reduction by approximately one-third; prothrombin time determinations should be performed frequently in patients receiving both drugs. Dextrothyroxine should be withdrawn two weeks before elective surgery if use of anticoagulants is contemplated.

Dextrothyroxine should be used judiciously, if at all, in pregnant women and nursing mothers, because its effects on the thyroid gland of the fetus or infant are unknown. The drug also must be given cautiously to patients with hypertension or hepatic or renal disease.

The use of dextrothyroxine in a long-term trial (Coronary Drug Project) in men with established ischemic heart disease was discontinued because of increased mortality in patients with arrhythmias, angina pectoris, or multiple infarctions. Therefore, dextrothyroxine should not be given to patients with pre-existing ischemic heart disease or arrhythmias, especially ventricular premature contractions.

ROUTE, USUAL DOSAGE, AND PREPARATIONS. *Oral: Euthyroid adults*, initially, 1 to 2 mg daily for one month; the daily dose may be increased by increments of 1 to 2 mg at intervals of at least one month until a satisfactory reduction of serum cholesterol has been achieved or a maximal daily dose of 8 mg is reached. In patients receiving digitalis, the maximal dose is 4 mg daily. *Children*, initially, 0.05 mg/kg of body weight daily; this dose may be doubled after one month. The dose is increased by increments of 0.05 mg/kg at monthly intervals until satisfactory reduction of serum cholesterol has been observed or a maximal dose of 4 mg daily has been attained.

Choloxin (Flint). Tablets 1, 2, 4, and 6 mg.

NEOMYCIN SULFATE
[Mycifradin Sulfate, Neobiotic]

Neomycin is only minimally absorbed from the gastrointestinal tract; it reduces the absorption of cholesterol by precipitating it out of micellar solution. Its action is thought to be similar to that of cholestyramine in that it forms insoluble complexes with bile acids, thereby increasing excretion of both bile acids and cholesterol. Small doses given for several years have been reported to lower LDL levels an average of 22% without producing serious adverse effects. Neomycin has variable effects on VLDL. Until additional information on safety and efficacy is available, use of this agent (preferably as an adjunct to clofibrate, 2 g daily) should be reserved for patients with refractory type IIa hyperlipoproteinemia who have a high risk of ischemic heart disease.

Malabsorption syndrome, acute pseudomembranous enterocolitis, nephropathy, and permanent damage to the eighth nerve have occurred after neomycin was given parenterally or in large oral doses. It is claimed that these reactions do not develop with the oral doses used to treat hyperlipidemia. Diarrhea and abdominal cramps, which usually subside spontaneously during continued treatment, have been reported with use of hypolipidemic doses. Neomycin is contraindicated in patients with renal insufficiency, for it may accumulate to toxic levels in these individuals and cause nephrotoxicity and ototoxicity.

Neomycin may potentiate coumarin anticoagulants, and concomitant use requires frequent monitoring of prothrombin time.

For other adverse reactions, see Chapter 74, Aminoglycosides.

ROUTE, USUAL DOSAGE, AND PREPARATIONS. *Oral: Adults*, 0.5 to a maximum of 2 g daily.

> Drug available generically: Tablets 500 mg; powder.
> *Mycifradin Sulfate* (Upjohn). Solution 125 mg (equivalent to 85.7 mg of the base)/5 ml; tablets 500 mg (equivalent to 350 mg of the base).
> *Neobiotic* (Pfipharmecs). Tablets 500 mg.

ALUMINUM NICOTINATE
[Nicalex]

NIACIN (Nicotinic Acid)
[Nicobid, Nico-400, Nicolar]

In contrast to other lipid-lowering agents, studies suggest that niacin reduces the rate of synthesis of LDL and apoprotein B by depressing VLDL synthesis and therefore may be effective in all types of hyperlipoproteinemias except type I. It often is more effective than other drugs in the severe hypertriglyceridemia of type V disease. However, because niacin frequently produces potentially troublesome adverse effects, its usefulness is limited. It is usually well tolerated in patients who respond to doses of 4 g/day or less.

Aluminum nicotinate is hydrolyzed to aluminum hydroxide and niacin in the gastrointestinal tract. In addition to the reactions caused by the niacin component, aluminum hydroxide may decrease the absorption of other drugs, and prolonged use may cause additional adverse effects (see Chapter 57, Agents Used in Acid Peptic Disorders, for adverse reactions of aluminum hydroxide). Therefore, niacin is preferred to aluminum nicotinate for the treatment of hyperlipidemias.

Flushing occurs initially in practically all patients and persists in 10% to 15%. Other common untoward effects are pruritus and gastrointestinal irritation (eg, nausea, vomiting, flatulence, diarrhea). The latter symptoms may subside with continued therapy. Use of small initial doses with gradual increases reduces the severity of these reactions in most patients.

More serious reactions are activation of peptic ulcer, impaired glucose tolerance, hyperuricemia, and liver dysfunction, including cholestatic jaundice. These effects are usually reversible when the drug is discontinued. Many patients with type III, IV, and V already have hyperglycemia and hyperuricemia that may be aggravated by niacin.

Niacin potentiates the effects of ganglionic blocking agents and, when used concomitantly with these drugs in hypertensive patients, it may cause orthostatic hypotension. Toxic amblyopia also has been reported.

The use of niacin in the Coronary Drug Project trial for long-term management of men with established ischemic heart disease produced no definitive evidence that this agent reduced total mortality. It appeared to decrease the incidence of recurrent nonfatal myocardial infarction significantly, but the incidence of atrial fibrillation and other arrhythmias was increased. Therefore, caution must be exercised if niacin is given to patients with established ischemic heart disease.

ROUTE, USUAL DOSAGE, AND PREPARATIONS. *Oral*: *Adults*, initially, 100 mg of niacin three times daily, increased to 2 to 6 g niacin or the equivalent 2.5 to 7.5 g aluminum nicotinate given in three divided doses with or after meals. Doses of niacin as high as 9 to 12 g daily have been used.

ALUMINUM NICOTINATE:
Nicalex (Merrell-National). Tablets 625 mg.
NIACIN:
Drug available generically and under the name Nicotinic Acid: Capsules (timed-release) 125, 250, 400, and 500 mg; tablets 100 and 500 mg.
Nicobid (Armour). Capsules (timed-release) 125, 250, and 500 mg.
Nico-400 (Marion). Capsules (timed-release) 400 mg.
Nicolar (Armour). Tablets 500 mg.

NORETHINDRONE ACETATE
[Norlutate]

Results of recent studies have shown that this progestational agent, when used in conjunction with appropriate diet, decreases levels of VLDL and chylomicrons and decreases levels of HDL and apoprotein A in some women with type V hyperlipoproteinemia. There is a concurrent increase in PHLA and amelioration of abdominal pain or pancreatitis. Noreth-indrone also has been tried in women with types III, IV, or V in whom estrogens or combination oral contraceptives cause undesirable effects (hypertriglyceridemia and decreased PHLA). However, recent studies have shown that progestins may elevate serum cholesterol levels. Therefore, until more experience with its use has accumulated, norethindrone should be reserved for use in women with type V hyperlipoproteinemia who are refractory to established therapy. Its use in men is not advocated because of its estrogenic activity.

For other uses and adverse reactions, see Chapter 43, Estrogens and Progestins.

ROUTE, USUAL DOSAGE, AND PREPARATIONS. *Oral*: *Women*, 5 mg daily. Premenopausal women should receive the drug 21 days per month to permit regular menses.

Norlutate (Parke, Davis). Tablets 5 mg.

OXANDROLONE
[Anavar]

Oxandrolone, an anabolic steroid with weak androgenic properties, is a synthetic derivative of testosterone. It reduces triglycerides (affecting both VLDL and chylomicrons) but has little effect on cholesterol and LDL except that it has caused mild elevations in a few patients. The use of oxandrolone in the treatment of hyperlipidemia is investigational and should be reserved for men with hypertriglyceridemia who are refractory to more conventional agents. It should not be used in women because of its virilizing effect or in children because it may cause disturbances in growth (premature epiphyseal closure) and sexual development.

Since oxandrolone may induce edema, it should be used cautiously in men with cardiac, renal, or hepatic disease and should not be used with adrenal cortico-steroids ·or corticotropin. The dosage of anticoagulants may have to be reduced in patients receiving oxandrolone. For further information on adverse reactions and precautions, see Chapter 42, Androgens and Anabolic Steroids.

ROUTE, USUAL DOSAGE, AND PREPARATIONS.
Oral: Men, 2.5 mg three times daily.
Anavar (Searle). Tablets 2.5 mg.

PROBUCOL
[Lorelco]

$(CH_3)_3C$ $C(CH_3)_3$

CH_3

HO—⬡—S—C—S—⬡—OH

CH_3

$(CH_3)_3C$ $C(CH_3)_3$

The chemical structure of this hypolipidemic agent is unique. It decreases elevated serum cholesterol levels by reducing LDL concentrations but does not reduce serum triglyceride levels appreciably in most patients. The mechanism of the hypocholesterolemic effect is not known. Because the cholesterol precursors, desmosterol and 7-dehydrocholesterol, do not accumulate, it is postulated that probucol blocks one of the early steps in cholesterol biosynthesis but has no effect on the later stages.

Like cholestyramine, this drug appears to be most effective in type IIa hyperlipoproteinemia. There are few data comparing its efficacy with that of other hypolipemic drugs, but results of limited studies indicate that probucol is less effective than cholestyramine in patients with familial type IIa, although it may increase the optimal effect of the diet by an additional 10%. Probucol also may be used with agents that decrease serum triglyceride levels in types IIb,III, and IV when hypercholesterolemia persists.

Absorption is limited, but relatively higher peak blood levels are attained if probucol is administered with meals. Blood levels gradually increase for three or four months with continuous oral administration, after which they remain relatively constant. There is no correlation between blood concentrations and hypocholesterolemic effect.

With prolonged treatment, this fat-soluble agent accumulates slowly in fatty tissues. The major pathway of excretion is through the biliary system into the feces; renal clearance is negligible.

The most common adverse reactions are mild gastrointestinal disturbances (diarrhea, flatulence, abdominal pain, and nausea), which are transient in most patients. Less common reactions include excessive or fetid perspiration, angioedema, headache, dizziness, paresthesias, and eosinophilia. Transient elevations of serum transaminases, alkaline phosphatase, creatine phosphokinase, bilirubin, uric acid, blood urea nitrogen, and blood glucose levels have occurred occasionally.

Clinical experience does not indicate that probucol has an adverse effect on the fetus. Nevertheless, it should not be used in pregnant women, and women of childbearing age should exercise strict birth control measures both during and for six months after therapy is discontinued, since the half-life of this drug in adipose tissue is prolonged. It is not known whether probucol is excreted in human milk, but infants should not be breast-fed while the mother is being treated with probucol.

No interactions have been reported to date between probucol and insulin, oral hypoglycemic agents, or anticoagulants.

ROUTE, USUAL DOSAGE, AND PREPARATIONS.
Oral: Adults, 500 mg with the morning and evening meal. The safety and efficacy of probucol in *children* have not been established. Some investigators have given 250 mg twice daily with meals to children weighing less than 27 kg and 500 mg twice daily with meals to children weighing more than 27 kg.
Lorelco (Dow). Tablets 250 mg.

SITOSTEROLS
[Cytellin]

This mixture of plant sterols has been promoted for the treatment of hyperbetalipoproteinemia. Sitosterols are poorly absorbed and compete with cholesterol for

934

absorption sites in the intestine. They have no effect on elevated VLDL levels, and their effect on LDL is variable. Use is restricted to patients with type IIa hyperlipoproteinemia.

The long-term effects of sitosterols are unknown. Adverse reactions (eg, anorexia, diarrhea, abdominal cramps) occur rarely.

ROUTE, USUAL DOSAGE, AND PREPARATIONS. *Oral: Adults,* 12 to 24 g daily in divided doses taken immediately prior to meals or snacks.

Cytellin (Lilly). Suspension 3 g/15 ml (with alcohol 0.95%).

Selected References

Co-operative trial in primary prevention of ischaemic heart disease using clofibrate: Report from Committee of Principal Investigators. *Br Heart J* 40:1069-1118, 1978.

Ahrens EH Jr: Management of hyperlipidemia: Whether, rather than how. *Ann Intern Med* 85:87-93, 1976.

Berman M, et al: Metabolism of apoB and apoC lipoproteins in man: Kinetic studies in normal and hyperlipoproteinemic subjects. *J Lipid Res* 19:38-56, 1978.

Davignon J: The lipid hypothesis: Pathophysiological basis. *Arch Surg* 113:28-34, 1978.

Day CE: Pharmacologic regulation of serum lipoproteins, in Clarke FH (ed): *Annual Reports in Medicinal Chemistry.* New York, Academic Press, 1978, vol 13, 184-195.

Eder HA, Roheim PS: Plasma lipoproteins and apolipoproteins. *Ann NY Acad Sci* 275:169-179, 1976.

Glueck CJ, Kwiterovich PO Jr: The lipid hypothesis: Genetic basis. *Arch Surg* 113:35-41, 1978.

Glueck CJ, Stein EA: Managing children with hyperlipidemias. *Drug Ther* 8:117-126, (Oct) 1978.

Glueck CJ, et al: Colestipol and cholestyramine resin: Comparative effects in familial type II hyperlipoproteinemia. *JAMA* 222:676-681, 1972.

Gotto AM Jr: Hyperlipidemia: Finding patient at risk. *Mod Med* 46:62-74, (March 30) 1978.

Lees RS, Lees AM: Therapy of hyperlipidemias. *Postgrad Med* 60:99-107, (Sept) 1976.

Levy RI: Effect of hypolipidemic drugs on plasma lipoproteins. *Annu Rev Pharmacol Toxicol* 17:499-510, 1977.

Murphy BF: Probucol (Lorelco) in treatment of hyperlipemia. *JAMA* 238:2537-2538, 1977.

Schaefer EJ, et al: Lipoprotein apoprotein metabolism. *J Lipid Res* 19:667-687, 1978.

Yeshurun D, Gotto AM Jr: Drug treatment of hyperlipidemia. *Am J Med* 60:379-396, 1976.

Agents Used in Obesity | 56

Obesity is often defined as weight more than 25% in excess of "ideal" weight (based on actuarial data on height and body build/weight at various ages); the excess may be as little as 10% in persons with small body build. This condition contributes to morbidity and mortality in a number of diseases (eg, atherosclerotic heart disease, hypertension, stroke, maturity-onset diabetes, gallbladder disease) and can cause emotional damage. It is a serious and ever increasing health problem in the United States; most estimates indicate that 30 to 50 million Americans are overweight.

There are multiple causes of obesity and, whether the cause is physiologic, psychologic, metabolic, or any combination of these, body weight is very resistant to change. Obesity, particularly massive obesity (100% or greater than ideal weight), is a complex condition and treatment must be based upon the patient's personal habits, motivations, and life style. Most authorities agree that the only safe and effective way to lose weight is to consistently eat a balanced diet that supplies fewer calories than the body uses up as energy. Weight reduction is a prolonged procedure, and instruction in sound nutrition is essential.

Research has shown that balanced diets composed of foods familiar to the patient are as conducive to weight loss as those that are high in fat and protein and can be maintained comfortably for extended periods. Balanced diets also are safer than fad diets, modified protein-sparing diets, or total starvation. In general, a daily intake of 1,500 calories for men and 1,000 calories for women induces satisfactory weight loss over an extended period; regimens should include a set of balanced, calorie-restricted choices designed to provide a steady weight loss of approximately one to two pounds per week. Exceptions to these guidelines should be made only under careful supervision by the physician. Diets predesigned for each week, with weekly or biweekly checks and supervision, are desirable, and diet planning should not be left to the patient until adequate training in caloric equivalence has been learned. Excellent calorie guides are available. It is essential that an overweight person makes a permanent change in eating habits if long-term maintenance of weight loss is to be successful. This is usually accomplished by increased intake of foods containing natural fiber and decreased intake of refined carbohydrate foods (eg, sugar, white flour). Fruits, vegetables, and whole grain products with a high proportion of fiber are absorbed more slowly and satisfy hunger longer than the refined carbohydrate equivalent. Proponents claim that new techniques of behavior modification, which are based on the theory that obesity is caused by a learned eating disorder, are more successful than other programs for many patients (Stuart and Davis, 1972).

A discussion of the radical treatment of obesity by means of psychotherapy, starvation regimens in the hospital, plastic surgery, destruction of the hypothalamus, and intestinal bypass surgery is beyond the scope of this presentation.

Drug Therapy

Anorexiants: Anorexiant therapy should be used only as a short-term adjunct in a regimen of weight reduction based on caloric restriction, exercise, and behavior modification. None of the available agents are free of side effects. Anorexiants may suppress the appetite temporarily, which provides psychological support initially. If no significant weight loss occurs during a four- to six-week trial, anorexiant therapy should be discontinued. When weight loss continues during this period, these agents may be given for a total of 12 weeks. Although studies have shown that anorexiants remain effective for periods longer than 12 weeks, it is preferable to use them intermittently to achieve additional weight loss when a weight plateau is reached despite good dietary habits, exercise, and other measures. Furthermore, the prolonged use of these drugs may cause psychic or physical dependence and reinforces a drug habit rather than proper eating habits. The prolonged administration of therapeutic doses or the short-term use of large doses of anorexiants is sometimes followed by a short period of fatigue and mental depression if therapy is discontinued abruptly. Even with short-term use, the average total amount of weight lost remains modest and may not be sustained after the medication is discontinued.

Drugs have no place in the treatment of obesity in children younger than 12. Although data are conflicting, growth impairment has been reported with use of fenfluramine [Pondimin], mazindol [Sanorex], and possibly other anorexiant agents. In some older children and adolescents, short-term use may be helpful temporarily if there is close supervision.

The amphetamines (amphetamine, dextroamphetamine [Dexedrine, Diphylets, Obotan], methamphetamine [Desoxyn]) were the first drugs to be prescribed widely for appetite suppression, and they are still the standard to which newer drugs are compared. Amphetamine, the racemic mixture, is less potent as an appetite suppressant and has a greater effect on the cardiovascular system than dextroamphetamine or methamphetamine. None are advocated for the treatment of obesity because the risk of dependence is great.

The other anorexiant agents (ie, benzphetamine [Didrex], chlorphentermine [Pre-Sate], clortermine [Voranil], diethylpropion [Tenuate, Tepanil], fenfluramine, mazindol, phendimetrazine [Bacarate, Plegine, Statobex], phenmetrazine [Preludin], phentermine hydrochloride [Adipex, Fastin, Tora], phentermine resin [Ionamin]) have some actions similar to those of the amphetamines, although their potency and spectrum of activity vary. These drugs were developed in the hope that they would produce a greater anorexiant effect with fewer untoward reactions than the amphetamines. In spite of differences in their actions and untoward effects, none have been found to be more effective than dextroamphetamine. All presently used anorexiants induce about the same weight loss. Unlike the amphetamines, which have been used for their stimulant effect in other conditions (eg, narcolepsy, hyperkinetic syndrome in children), the other anorexiant agents have been promoted by their manufacturers only for suppression of appetite.

Diethylpropion is effective in some patients and produces few side effects. It is considered to be the safest of the anorexiant drugs for use in patients with mild to moderate hypertension even when myocardial ischemia is present. It should not be used in patients who are tense or nervous unless a mild antianxiety agent (preferably small doses of a benzodiaze-pine) is given concomitantly.

Mazindol is as effective as diethylpro-pion, but the incidence of central nervous system stimulation is greater. Mazindol may increase the heart rate and should be used with caution in patients with severe hypertension or cardiovascular disease. Dextroamphetamine and mazindol cause hyperinsulinemia which improves glucose tolerance, but this effect is probably coun-terbalanced by the increased lipogenesis that also may occur.

Fenfluramine is useful in patients in whom central nervous system stimulant effects are considered undesirable and is the drug of first choice for patients with maturity-onset diabetes who do not have depression. It has been reported to im-prove glucose tolerance in some patients, probably by increasing glucose uptake in muscle or decreasing gastric emptying. However, fenfluramine should not be used to treat glucose intolerance or given to patients with a history of depression, and it should never be discontinued abruptly in any patient.

Phentermine hydrochloride is effective in some patients but is associated with a higher incidence of insomnia than diethyl-propion. Phentermine resin rarely causes insomnia, but both forms may increase blood pressure and produce tachycardia and thus may be considered less preferred agents in patients with hypertension and heart disease. Although benzphetamine, clortermine, and phendimetrazine are ef-fective, all produce a degree of central nervous system stimulation that is unac-ceptable to some patients. Phenmetrazine is as effective as dextroamphetamine but has the same dependence potential and thus is not advocated for use as an anorexiant.

Chlorphentermine is not suitable for use in the treatment of obesity because pulmo-nary complications have been demon-strated in animals and could theoretically occur in man.

Anorexiants stimulate the satiety center in the hypothalamus to decrease appetite, and fenfluramine also decreases activity in the feeding center. The hypothalamic nu-clei (hunger center in the lateral hypo-thalamus with beta-adrenergic receptors, satiety center in the ventromedial nucleus with alpha-adrenergic receptors) also prob-ably are affected by plasma glucose, free fatty acid, and insulin levels. In addition, anorexiant drugs (with the exception of fenfluramine) increase physical activity. They have other metabolic effects involv-ing fat (inhibiting lipogenesis, enhancing lipolysis) and carbohydrate metabolism, but these probably are secondary to loss of weight.

See the Table.

Miscellaneous Drugs: Many drugs not technically classified as anorexiants have been misused in the treatment of over-weight patients, including digitalis, diuret-ics, laxatives, antispasmodics, chorionic gonadotropin, and thyroid. The anorexia produced by digitalis is a symptom of po-tentially fatal intoxication. Thyroid prepa-rations act as anorexiants but may suppress endogenous thyroid secretion and have po-tentially dangerous effects on cardiac func-tion. Diuretics are of little use in decreas-ing adipose tissue, although they cause transient fluid loss. Human chorionic gonadotropin was shown to have no greater effect than a placebo in numerous studies. Laxatives used in doses large enough to produce diarrhea can result in loss of water, but hypokalemia and/or dehydration also may occur after prolonged administration and are potentially fatal. Bulk-producing agents cause gastric distention, inducing a transient sensation of satiety. Methylcel-lulose and water given together relieve hunger briefly but may cause gastrointesti-nal disturbances. Antispasmodics have no effect on body fat or caloric balance. There-fore, use of any of these agents as an aid to weight reduction is unjustified.

Phenylpropanolamine, an adrenergic agent with some stimulant properties, is available without prescription in various proprietary products for weight reduction. It is usually combined with caffeine, and there is no reported evidence of abuse. However, these products are only mini-mally effective.

Adverse Reactions

Most anorexiants are directly or indirectly related to amphetamine and produce central nervous system stimulation. Manifestations include nervousness, irritability, insomnia, decreased sense of fatigue, increased alertness and ability to concentrate, and euphoria. (With usual doses, mazindol does not appear to cause euphoria and fenfluramine has sedative effects; with overdosage, fenfluramine may have stimulant effects.) As the stimulant actions decline, fatigue and depression may occur with most anorexiant agents. Central nervous system effects may be severe enough to require discontinuing the drug.

Sympathetic nervous system effects include dryness of the mouth, blurred vision and mydriasis, dizziness and lightheadedness, tachycardia and palpitations, hypertension, and sweating. Although unpleasant in some patients, these reactions are rarely dangerous.

Nausea, vomiting, and, occasionally, diarrhea or constipation occur. Fenfluramine occasionally may cause severe vomiting and/or diarrhea with abdominal pain.

For additional adverse effects, see the evaluations.

Teratogenicity: Evidence of teratogenicity has not been observed when these agents were taken during pregnancy, although an infant born to a mother who abuses amphetamines may be agitated and have hyperglycemia at birth (see the section on Use of Drugs During Pregnancy in Chapter 2).

Tolerance: Tolerance may occur within 6 to 12 weeks and cross tolerance among the anorexiants is almost universal. Dosage should not be increased to compensate for the loss of anorexiant effect, because larger amounts produce marked restlessness, irritability, and aggressiveness and increase the danger of psychic or physical dependence.

Intoxication and Abuse: Susceptible patients may develop psychic or physical dependence with use of anorexiant agents. Amphetamine, dextroamphetamine, methamphetamine, phenmetrazine, and mixtures containing amphetamine compounds are classified as Schedule II drugs under the Controlled Substances Act. Benzphetamine, chlorphentermine, clortermine, mazindol, and phendimetrazine are classified as Schedule III drugs, and diethylpropion, fenfluramine, and phentermine as Schedule IV drugs. However, abuse of any of these drugs may occur. The risk of dependence is proportional to the stimulant effect in decreasing order: amphetamine, dextroamphetamine (or methamphetamine), phentermine, chlorphentermine, mazindol, diethylpropion, and fenfluramine (Craddock, 1976). See also the section on Controlled Psychotropic Drugs in Chapter 3, Prescription Practices and Regulatory Agencies.

Individuals who abuse an amphetamine frequently inject as much as several grams daily; polyarteritis nodosa (necrotizing angiitis) has been associated with the intravenous administration of large doses of methamphetamine and amphetamine in these individuals. In general, the toxic features of chronic abuse include a distinctive amphetamine psychosis characterized by paranoia, stereotyped behavior, picking at the skin, preoccupation with one's own thoughts, and auditory and visual hallucinations.

Withdrawal of amphetamines or the other anorexiant agents from abusers may unmask symptoms of chronic fatigue (mental depression, asthenia, tremors, and gastrointestinal disturbances) and, in some individuals, the fatigue may be followed by drowsiness and prolonged sleep. Such reactions are now accepted as being a true withdrawal syndrome. Sudden withdrawal of fenfluramine may cause severe depression whether or not the patient has a history of depression.

Acute Overdosage (Poisoning): In general, acute overdosage accentuates the usual pharmacologic effects of excitement, agitation, hypertension, tachycardia, mydriasis, slurred speech, ataxia, tremor, chills, hyperreflexia, tachypnea, fever, headache, and toxic psychoses characterized by auditory and visual hallucinations and paranoid delusions. If these features develop, the drug should be discontinued permanently, sedatives prescribed, and custodial care and psychotherapy employed when needed. In severe cases, overdosage may cause hyperpyrexia, chest pain, acute circulatory failure, convulsions, and coma; death has been reported. Chlorpromazine [Thorazine] or, if an anticholinergic drug has been taken recently, another antipsychotic drug that does not have a prominent anticholinergic action (eg, haloperidol [Haldol]) may be of value in blocking the central nervous system effects. Fenfluramine overdosage appears to have some specific characteristics, including rotary nystagmus and continuous tremor of the lower jaw. Either pronounced drowsiness or agitation may occur.

Precautions

Before prescribing any anorexiant, a patient history is essential to determine whether there is any tendency to abuse drugs, including alcohol, or evidence of pathologic depression. Anorexiants should not be prescribed for these patients since all these drugs have the potential for abuse. The dangers of drug abuse preclude use of amphetamine, dextroamphetamine, methamphetamine, and phenmetrazine except in patients for whom they previously have been found to be effective and who have not experienced side effects.

The use of anorexiants should be closely supervised by the physician and a quantity of drug sufficient only for two weeks prescribed. It is advisable to schedule visits for these intervals, and anorexiants should be given at these subsequent consultations only if the patient has lost weight since the previous visit (unless weight gain is due to premenstrual fluid retention). The physician should personally see the patient at each visit to determine whether euphoria, followed by irritability or depression, is present. If so, continuation of anorexiant therapy is inadvisable.

Interactions: Most anorexiants theoretically release norepinephrine stored in adrenergic neurons and also impair re-entry of hypotensive drugs by blocking the neuronal reuptake of released norepinephrine. However, interference with the action of antihypertensive drugs probably is clinically unimportant when usual doses of anorexiants are given, because their action is offset by the fall in blood pressure which accompanies weight loss. Nevertheless, the blood pressure should be monitored weekly for the first four to six weeks of therapy.

Since anorexiants can precipitate a hypertensive crisis when used with monoamine oxidase inhibitors, they should not be given within 14 days of having taken any monoamine oxidase inhibitor.

Available Anorexiants*

The following agents should be prescribed only as short-term adjuncts (8 to 12 weeks) in the treatment of obesity, and all are capable of producing psychic or, rarely, physical dependence. For effects common to all anorexiant drugs, see the section on Adverse Reactions in the Introduction.

Generally Preferred Anorexiants	Alternative Drugs	Drugs Not Preferred
Diethylpropion (IV)	Clortermine (III)	Amphetamine (II)
Mazindol† (III)	Fenfluramine (IV)	Dextroamphetamine (II)
Phentermine† (IV)		Methamphetamine (II)
		Benzphetamine (III)
		Chlorphentermine (III)
		Phendimetrazine (III)
		Phenmetrazine (II)

* See the evaluations for specific comments.
†Except in patients with severe hypertension or heart disease.

AMPHETAMINES

DEXTROAMPHETAMINE SULFATE
[Dexedrine, Diphylets]

DEXTROAMPHETAMINE TANNATE
[Obotan]

$$\text{(ring)}-CH_2---\underset{\underset{+NH_3}{|}}{\overset{\overset{H}{|}}{C}}---CH_3 \quad \tfrac{1}{2}SO_4^=$$

Dextroamphetamine is a more potent appetite suppressant than amphetamine, and its effect on the cardiovascular system is slightly less pronounced but may still be severe in some individuals. The drug should be stopped immediately if chest pain or arrhythmias occur. Dextroamphetamine causes marked central nervous system stimulation, which may include dystonic movements of the head, neck, and extremities. Severe depression or psychotic reactions may follow prolonged use, and toxic psychoses may occur after large doses.

Because dextroamphetamine may produce euphoria and the danger of dependence is great in susceptible individuals, it is not a preferred drug for use in obesity. It is classified as a Schedule II drug under the Controlled Substances Act.

ROUTE, USUAL DOSAGE, AND PREPARATIONS.
Oral: Adults, 5 to 10 mg three times daily at least one hour before a meal. Alternatively, a timed-release preparation (10 to 15 mg) is taken once daily in the morning.
DEXTROAMPHETAMINE SULFATE:
Drug available generically: Capsules, tablets 10 and 15 mg; capsules (timed-release) 15 mg; powder.
Dexedrine (Smith Kline & French). Capsules (timed-release) 5, 10, and 15 mg; elixir 5 mg/5 ml with alcohol 10%; tablets 5 mg.
Diphylets (Tutag). Capsules (timed-release) 10 and 15 mg.
DEXTROAMPHETAMINE TANNATE:
Obotan (Mallinckrodt). Tablets (timed-release) 17.5 and 26.25 (Forte) (equivalent to 5 and 7.5 mg of base, respectively).

AMPHETAMINE SULFATE

This drug is the racemic form of amphetamine. Because it is less effective as an appetite suppressant and has a more pronounced effect on the cardiovascular system than the dextrorotatory isomer, it is not advocated for use in obesity. Amphetamine is classified as a Schedule II drug under the Controlled Substances Act. The danger of dependence is great in susceptible individuals.

ROUTE, USUAL DOSAGE, AND PREPARATIONS.
Oral: Adults, 5 to 10 mg three times daily at least 30 minutes before each meal.
Drug available generically: Powder; tablets 5 and 10 mg.
AVAILABLE TRADEMARK.
Benzedrine (Smith Kline & French).

METHAMPHETAMINE HYDROCHLORIDE
[Desoxyn]

$$\text{(ring)}-CH_2---\underset{\underset{+NH_2CH_3}{|}}{\overset{\overset{H}{|}}{C}}---CH_3 \quad Cl^-$$

Methamphetamine is essentially equivalent to dextroamphetamine in its effect on the central nervous and cardiovascular systems, as well as in its ability to suppress the appetite. The dangers of dependence are likewise equivalent and methamphetamine is not a preferred drug for use in obesity. It is classified as a Schedule II drug under the Controlled Substances Act.

ROUTE, USUAL DOSAGE, AND PREPARATIONS.
Oral: Adults, 2.5 to 5 mg three times daily 30 to 60 minutes before each meal. Alternatively, a timed-release tablet (10 or 15 mg) is taken once daily in the morning.
Drug available generically under the name Desoxyephedrine Hydrochloride: Tablets 10 mg.
Desoxyn (Abbott). Tablets 2.5 and 5 mg; tablets (timed-release) 5, 10, and 15 mg.

OTHER ANOREXIANT AGENTS

BENZPHETAMINE HYDROCHLORIDE
[Didrex]

$$\text{(ring)}-CH_2CH\underset{\underset{CH_3\ CH_2-(ring)}{|}}{\overset{\overset{CH_3}{+/}}{N}H} \quad Cl^-$$

Benzphetamine is as effective as dextroamphetamine in suppressing the appetite. Although it causes fewer untoward effects than dextroamphetamine, they are similar in character. However, psychotic episodes are rare when recommended doses are used.

Benzphetamine is not a preferred drug for use in obesity because it may produce euphoria and thus there is danger of dependence in susceptible individuals. It is classified as a Schedule III drug under the Controlled Substances Act.

ROUTE, USUAL DOSAGE, AND PREPARATIONS. *Oral*: *Adults*, 25 to 50 mg one to three times daily.
     Didrex (Upjohn). Tablets 25 and 50 mg.

CHLORPHENTERMINE HYDROCHLORIDE
[Pre-Sate]

Chlorphentermine is similar to dextroamphetamine in its ability to suppress appetite. Fewer side effects attributable to central nervous system stimulation have been observed than with the amphetamines, but changes in lung parenchyma of animals have been reported following long-term use of chlorphentermine (Lullman-Rauch and Reil, 1974). Therefore, since pulmonary complications are a possibility in man and other drugs are more effective, chlorphentermine is not considered suitable for use in appetite suppression.

Chlorphentermine is classified as a Schedule III drug under the Controlled Substances Act.
     Drug available generically: Tablets 65 mg.
     Pre-Sate (Parke, Davis). Tablets equivalent to 65 mg of the base.

CLORTERMINE HYDROCHLORIDE
[Voranil]

Clortermine is the ortho-chloro isomer of chlorphentermine hydrochloride, to which it is comparable in suppressing the appetite. There have been no pulmonary changes reported following use of this drug, and it appears to have little effect on blood pressure, pulse, or electrocardiographic readings. Clortermine may be as useful as diethylpropion in some patients who do not have diabetes, severe hypertension, or cardiovascular disease. Nevertheless, the degree of stimulation and/or insomnia is unacceptable to some individuals.

The incidence of psychic or physical dependence is unknown, but the possibility that it may occur remains. The manifestations of chronic intoxication and overdosage with clortermine closely resemble those associated with amphetamines. Clortermine is classified as a Schedule III drug under the Controlled Substances Act.

ROUTE, USUAL DOSAGE, AND PREPARATIONS. *Oral*: *Adults*, 50 mg once daily in midmorning.
     Voranil (USV). Tablets 50 mg.

DIETHYLPROPION HYDROCHLORIDE
[Tenuate, Tepanil]

Diethylpropion is as effective as the amphetamines in suppressing appetite and, although mild restlessness, dryness of the mouth, and constipation are common, the overall incidence of side effects (nervousness, excitability, euphoria, and insomnia) is lower. Psychic and, rarely, physical dependence may occur but are rare despite common worldwide use. No adverse cardiovascular effects have been reported in patients with angina pectoris or hypertension. Therefore, diethylpropion is considered the drug of choice for most patients, particularly those with mild to moderate cardiovascular disease, although fenfluramine is preferred for those who are tense or nervous. Use of this drug in those with severe cardiovascular disease, including marked hypertension, generally is inadvisable.

Diethylpropion is classified as a Schedule IV drug under the Controlled Substances Act.

ROUTE, USUAL DOSAGE, AND PREPARATIONS. *Oral*: *Adults*, 25 mg three times daily one hour before meals. An additional 25 mg may be taken in the evening if needed. Alternatively, one timed-release preparation is taken once daily in midmorning.

> Drug available generically: Tablets 25 mg; capsules, tablets (timed-release) 75 mg.
> *Tenuate* (Merrell-National), *Tepanil* (Riker). Tablets 25 mg; tablets (timed-release) 75 mg.

FENFLURAMINE HYDROCHLORIDE
[Pondimin]

Although this agent is a substituted phenethylamine with some sympathomimetic properties, it differs from other available anorexiants in that it usually depresses rather than stimulates the central nervous system. Its major central nervous system action is through serotonin metabolism rather than norepinephrine and dopamine metabolism. It is comparable to dextroamphetamine in its ability to suppress the appetite, but drowsiness occurs frequently. Therefore, it is useful in patients who are nervous or tense, but it should not be given to those with depression or a history of it or to those who are receiving other central nervous system depressants. The effects in an individual patient are unpredictable.

Fenfluramine does not appear to interfere with the control of hypertension or diabetes mellitus. This drug may increase glucose uptake in muscle and thus improve glucose tolerance. It is considered the anorexiant of choice for patients with maturity-onset diabetes who have not responded to other types of therapy. Fenfluramine also is mildly hypotensive and causes mobilization of fat stores.

Fenfluramine appears to be mildly hallucinogenic in some individuals and has become a drug of abuse in South Africa. Because depth of sleep commonly is decreased, patients may be more aware of vivid dreaming. Sudden withdrawal may lead to depression, sometimes severe. Reinstitution of administration, followed by gradual tapering of the dose, appears to be satisfactory treatment for such patients. Overdosage produces amphetamine-like symptoms plus some specific characteristics (rotary nystagmus, continuous tremor of the lower jaw). Convulsions, coma, and, in a few cases, death have been reported. Ventricular extrasystoles culminating in irreversible ventricular fibrillation have been fatal in several patients. Standard supportive measures are effective in treating most cases of overdosage; forced diuresis with acidification of the urine and/or large doses of diazepam may be helpful in severe cases.

Fenfluramine is classified as a Schedule IV drug under the Controlled Substances Act.

ROUTE, USUAL DOSAGE, AND PREPARATIONS. *Oral*: *Adults*, initially, 20 mg three times daily one hour before meals. Dosage may be increased to 40 mg three times daily one hour before meals.

> *Pondimin* (Robins). Tablets 20 mg.

MAZINDOL
[Sanorex]

Mazindol is an imidazoisoindole. It lacks the phenethylamine structure of the amphetamines and other anorexiant agents. Mazindol's principal effect appears to be blocking of the neuronal uptake of norepinephrine and synaptically released dopamine. However, it is a tricyclic compound and capable of potentiating the effects of catecholamines. Therefore, if concomitant use of pressor amines is necessary, extreme care is needed.

Mazindol is comparable to dextroamphetamine in suppressing the appetite. Although the only cardiovascular action attributed to mazindol is an increase of 10 beats/min in the orthostatic heart rate, use of this drug in patients with severe cardiovascular disease, including marked hypertension, is inadvisable. There is some evidence that the drug may be prescribed safely for patients with stable atherosclerotic heart disease or mild to moderate hypertension. Control of diabetes mellitus does not appear to be adversely affected by mazindol.

Although the incidence of central nervous system stimulation is greater with use of mazindol (eg, insomnia, dizziness, agitation), particularly during the first two weeks of treatment, this anorexiant is as effective as diethylpropion and can be used as an alternate drug of choice for the same patient population.

Mazindol does not appear to produce euphoria; therefore, the abuse potential is low. Otherwise, its stimulant effects are similar to the amphetamines, but the incidence is much lower and they are less severe. There have been no reports of psychic or physical dependence, but the possibility of their occurrence remains. Mazindol is classified as a Schedule III drug under the Controlled Substances Act.

ROUTE, USUAL DOSAGE, AND PREPARATIONS.
Oral: *Adults*, 1 mg daily with the first meal.
Sanorex (Sandoz). Tablets 1 and 2 mg.

PHENDIMETRAZINE TARTRATE
[Bacarate, Plegine, Statobex]

Although cardiovascular effects are infrequent, phendimetrazine is similar to dextroamphetamine both in its ability to suppress the appetite and stimulate the central nervous system. Glossitis, stomatitis, abdominal cramps, headache, and dysuria occasionally occur following its use.

Because it produces euphoria and has abuse potential and because the degree of central nervous stimulation is unacceptable to some patients, phendimetrazine is not considered a preferred anorexiant. It is classified as a Schedule III drug under the Controlled Substances Act.

ROUTE, USUAL DOSAGE, AND PREPARATIONS.
Oral: *Adults*, 35 mg (range, 17.5 to 70 mg) two or three times daily one hour before meals.
Drug available generically: Capsules 35 and 70 mg; tablets 35 mg.
Bacarate (Tutag), *Plegine* (Ayerst). Tablets 35 mg.
Statobex (Lemmon). Capsules, tablets 35 mg.

PHENMETRAZINE HYDROCHLORIDE
[Preludin]

Phenmetrazine is as effective as dextroamphetamine in suppressing the appetite and produces similar untoward effects. The danger of dependence is also comparable to that observed with dextroamphetamine, and psychoses and changes in the electrocardiogram have been reported. Therefore, this agent is not advocated for use in suppression of appetite.

Phenmetrazine is classified as a Schedule II drug under the Controlled Substances Act.

ROUTE, USUAL DOSAGE, AND PREPARATIONS.
Oral: *Adults*, 25 mg two or three times daily one hour before meals. Alternatively, one timed-release tablet once daily in midmorning.
Preludin (Boehringer Ingelheim). Tablets 25 mg; tablets (timed-release) 50 and 75 mg.

PHENTERMINE HYDROCHLORIDE
[Adipex 8, Adipex-P, Fastin, Tora]

PHENTERMINE RESIN
[Ionamin]

Phentermine is available as the hydrochloride salt and as a complex of the base with an ion exchange resin. It is comparable to dextroamphetamine in suppressing the appetite. The incidence and severity of central nervous system effects are less than with dextroamphetamine. Euphoria is rare; therefore, abuse potential is low. However, the degree of stimulation, usually insomnia, is still unacceptable to some patients, although insomnia is rare when phentermine resin is given. Phentermine also can increase blood pressure, produce tachycardia, and commonly causes dryness of the mouth. Therefore, it is considered an alternate drug for some patients, although it may be a drug of choice for many.

Phentermine is classified as a Schedule IV drug under the Controlled Substances Act.

ROUTE, USUAL DOSAGE, AND PREPARATIONS.
PHENTERMINE HYDROCHLORIDE:
Oral: *Adults*, 8 mg three times daily one-half hour before meals or 24 to 30 mg once daily two hours after breakfast.

Drug available generically: Capsules (plain, timed-release) 8, 15, and 30 mg; tablets 8 and 15 mg.
Adipex 8 (Lemmon). Capsules, tablets 8 mg.
Adipex-P (Lemmon). Capsules 30 mg (equivalent to 24 mg of base); tablets 37.5 mg (equivalent to 30 mg of base).
Fastin (Beecham). Capsules 30 mg (equivalent to 24 mg of base).
Tora (Tutag). Tablets 8 mg.

PHENTERMINE RESIN:
Oral: *Adults*, 15 to 30 mg before breakfast or 10 to 14 hours before bedtime. Consistent bioavailability of the resin has been demonstrated.

Ionamin (Pennwalt). Capsules 15 and 30 mg.

MIXTURES

A few mixtures are used in weight control. These include combinations of more than one amphetamine, which may be considered essentially a single-entity drug, and combinations of amphetamines and sedatives. A sedative is present in the formulation to counteract some of the stimulant effects of the anorexiant, but these preparations have the well-recognized disadvantage of a fixed-dosage combination that makes individualization of doses of the constituents in the mixture impossible. All are classified as Schedule II drugs under the Controlled Substances Act.

The following list is supplied for information only.

Biphetamine (Pennwalt). Each timed-release capsule contains resin complexes equivalent to dextroamphetamine 3.75, 6.25, or 10 mg and amphetamine 3.75, 6.25, or 10 mg.
Dexamyl (Smith Kline & French). Each tablet contains dextroamphetamine sulfate 5 mg and amobarbital 32 mg; each timed-release capsule contains dextroamphetamine sulfate 10 or 15 mg and amobarbital 65 or 97 mg.
Eskatrol (Smith Kline & French). Each timed-release capsule contains dextroamphetamine sulfate 15 mg and prochlorperazine maleate 7.5 mg.
Obetrol (Obetrol). Each tablet contains 2.5 or 5 mg each of amphetamine aspartate, amphetamine sulfate, dextroamphetamine saccharate, and dextroamphetamine sulfate.

Selected References

Albrink MJ: Obesity, in Beeson PB, McDermott W (eds): *Textbook of Medicine*, ed 14. Philadelphia, WB Saunders Co, 1975, 1375-1386.
Bray GA: *The Obese Patient*. Philadelphia, WB Saunders Co, 1976, 353-410.
Craddock D: *Obesity and Its Management*, ed 3. Edinburgh, Churchill Livingstone, 1978, 92-109.
Craddock D: Anorectic drugs: Use in general practice. *Drugs* 11:378-393, 1976.
Goldrick RB: Management of obesity. *Drugs* 12:301-304, 1976.
Guggenheim FG: Basic considerations in treatment of obesity. *Med Clin North Am* 61:781-796, 1977.
Hafen BQ (ed): *Overweight and Obesity: Causes, Fallacies, Treatment*. Provo, Utah, Brigham Young University Press, 1975.

Lullman-Rauch R, Reil GH: Chlorphentermine-induced lipidosis-like ultrastructural alterations in lungs and adrenal glands of several species. *Toxicol Appl Pharmacol* 30:408-421, 1974.

Salans LB, Wise JK: Metabolic studies of human obesity. *Med Clin North Am* 54:1533-1542, 1970.

Samuel PD, Burland WL: Drug treatment of obesity, in *Obesity in Perspective*, part 2. Fogarty International Center Series on Preventive Medicine, Washington, DC, US Dept Health, Education and Welfare, 1975, vol 2, 419-428.

Scoville BA: Review of amphetamine-like drugs by Food and Drug Administration: Clinical data and value judgments, in *Obesity in Perspective*, part 2. Fogarty International Center Series on Preventive Medicine, Washington, DC, US Dept Health, Education and Welfare, 1975, vol 2, 441-443.

Stuart RB, Davis B: *Slim Chance in a Fat World*. Champaign, Ill, Research Press Co, 1972.

Sullivan AC, Comai K: Pharmacological treatment of obesity. *Int J Obes* 2:167-189, 1978.

Van Itallie TB, Yang M-U: Current concepts in nutrition: Diet and weight loss. *N Engl J Med* 297:1158-1161, 1977.

Weil WB Jr: Current controversies in childhood obesity. *J Pediatr* 91:175-187, 1977.

Agents Used in Acid Peptic Disorders | 57

When used either separately or together, the recently introduced H₂ receptor antagonists, which inhibit gastric secretion, and the antacids, which neutralize hydrochloric acid, appear to be beneficial in the treatment of acid peptic disorders. Anticholinergic agents also may have a limited effect in selected patients (see Chapter 60, Miscellaneous Gastrointestinal Agents). Other types of adjunctive therapy include physical and emotional rest, cessation of smoking and drinking of alcohol and coffee, and avoidance of potentially ulcerogenic drugs (eg, aspirin and certain other antiinflammatory agents).

The medical treatment of gastric and duodenal ulcer is similar, although the pain associated with gastric ulcer may be more difficult to control. The primary goal of ulcer treatment is to promote healing by neutralizing hydrochloric acid. This is achieved through frequent administration of adequate amounts of antacids and/or by decreasing the secretory activity of the stomach with use of the anticholinergic agents or the more effective H₂ receptor antagonist, cimetidine [Tagamet]. The latter reduces both basal and postprandial secretion in normal subjects and in those with duodenal ulcer. Controlled studies now confirm that adequate ("high-dose") antacid therapy reduces pain initially and then eliminates it and hastens the healing of duodenal ulcer. These findings are in contrast to other studies that concluded that "lower dose" antacids were no more effective than a placebo in relieving pain. There is no evidence that modifying the diet accelerates healing of uncomplicated peptic ulcer.

Carbenoxolone, a triterpenoid licorice derivative which is not available in the United States, has been shown to accelerate the healing of gastric ulcer. Its precise mechanism of action is unknown. However, the adverse effects (eg, hypertension, fluid retention, hypokalemia) encountered with use of carbenoxolone have interfered with the utilization and study of the drug in this country.

Certain alpha2 agonists also inhibit acid secretion, but pressor effects upon the cardiovascular system obviate the usefulness of the presently available compounds. Results with pepsin inhibitors (eg, sulfated polysaccharides, carrageenan) are conflicting. These compounds are not approved for use in man.

Prostaglandins may act as local regulators to stimulate or inhibit acid secretion through their action upon adenyl cyclase. They also may have cytoprotective effects independent of their ability to inhibit acid secretion. Pharmacologic doses of natural prostaglandins and some synthetic analogues inhibit gastric secretion, and, in preliminary studies, long-acting, orally effective prostaglandins with this effect have hastened the healing of duodenal and gastric ulcers. Further investigation must precede widespread acceptance of these agents.

The bismuth salts present in some proprietary mixtures have no significant acid-neutralizing activity, but they are claimed to have antipeptic and demulcent actions which coat and help protect and heal a peptic ulcer. Small controlled studies of an ammoniated bismuth complex [DeNol] demonstrated its effectiveness and lack of toxicity, but larger studies are required to substantiate these findings.

H₂ RECEPTOR ANTAGONISTS

The use of H2 receptor antagonists represents a new means of inhibiting gastric secretion in patients with peptic ulcer and related disorders. The first drug in this class available clinically is cimetidine.

CIMETIDINE
[Tagamet]

CIMETIDINE HYDROCHLORIDE
[Tagamet]

Cimetidine markedly reduces the volume and concentration of acid secreted in the resting state and after stimulation by food, histamine, pentagastrin, insulin, and caffeine. One study in man demonstrated that this agent protected the gastric mucosa from aspirin-induced damage as measured microscopically and by mucosal potential differences. Results of animal studies suggest that chemical erosive gastritis produced by bile salts, alcohol, various antirheumatic drugs, aspirin, and urea may be diminished or prevented by cimetidine. This drug does not appear to exert a clinically significant effect on gastric motility or emptying, on lower esophageal sphincter pressure, or on secretion by the pancreas or gallbladder in man.

Cimetidine has been employed in the treatment of duodenal and gastric ulcer, peptic esophagitis, and upper gastrointestinal bleeding due to acid peptic disorders. Conclusive proof of efficacy is lacking except for its use in duodenal ulcer. It also is effective in the Zollinger-Ellison syndrome and in ulcers associated with systemic mastocytosis and has been tested in the prevention and treatment of stress ulcers associated with burns, severe trauma, and brain and kidney damage. Other proposed uses include reduction of hydrochloric acid secretion to enhance the efficacy of orally administered pancreatic enzymes in patients with pancreatic insufficiency; prevention of alkalosis in patients subjected to prolonged nasogastric aspiration, especially those secreting large amounts of acid; and prevention of the aspiration of acid gastric juice occurring at the time of induction of anesthesia for emergency surgery.

Controlled and uncontrolled studies in hospitalized and outpatients in other countries reveal that when cimetidine was given in a dosage of 0.8 to 2 g daily for six weeks, 70% to 90% of patients with duodenal ulcer and 70% to 100% of patients with gastric ulcer experienced healing; in comparison, beneficial effects were observed in 30% to 70% of the ambulatory control patients and in almost 80% of the hospitalized control patients with duodenal and gastric ulcer. In most instances, these results were confirmed by direct endoscopic visualization.

Early recurrence of both duodenal and gastric ulcer has been reported when cimetidine was discontinued abruptly or used casually by the patient. However, the frequency of recurrences was reduced when a bedtime dose was continued after healing of the crater. Recurrences often are painful but they may be asymptomatic and only discovered when a complication develops or by means of endoscopic visualization.

The possibility of gradually decreasing responsiveness with prolonged use has not been reported and can be determined only with much longer and wider experience. Multicenter, double-blind controlled studies, as well as other studies of different design, are currently being conducted in the United States, and results are similar to those achieved worldwide. An interesting difference between the placebo groups in the United States and European studies has been noted. Healing occurred in a greater percentage of placebo patients in the United States because the antacids used concomitantly were more potent and were given more frequently. By accident of design, it reaffirmed very old clinical observations that frequent adequate doses of antacids are an excellent means of treating peptic ulcer.

Although cimetidine does not increase the tone of the lower esophageal sphincter, it relieves the symptoms caused by gastroesophageal acid reflux by decreasing the output of hydrochloric acid. A few patients with the Zollinger-Ellison syndrome require doses of up to 2.4 g daily to maintain control after many months of therapy; addition of antacids or anticholinergic antispasmodics also helps to re-establish control when hypersecretion recurs.

Adverse effects encountered during short-term trials include diarrhea, dizziness, muscle pain, or rash (which was usually transient). Confusion and more severe central nervous system symptoms have occurred, usually after ingestion of excessive doses, in elderly patients and in those with renal impairment. These symptoms were reversed when the drug was discontinued.

Increased prothrombin time, indicating potentiation of the action of warfarin-like anticoagulants, requires that extra caution be exercised when these drugs are used together. Transformation of cimetidine into an n-nitroso compound in the stomach and its carcinogenic potential are under study.

Drug-related elevations of serum transaminase levels have been noted; no other signs of hepatic dysfunction were observed in these patients. Rarely, unexplained elevations in alkaline phosphatase have been reported. Very slight elevations of creatinine levels without evidence of renal dysfunction occur during treatment. However, interstitial nephritis that clears with discontinuation of the drug has been observed rarely.

The principal route of excretion of cimetidine is through the kidneys; therefore, the dosage must be reduced in patients with impaired renal function. Gastric pH has been maintained at sufficiently high levels to permit candidal overgrowth in the stomach; this may have been the reason for the rare instances of candidal peritonitis found when perforation has occurred in patients receiving cimetidine.

Gynecomastia developed in patients being treated for pathologic hypersecretory states or duodenal ulcer. No endocrine dysfunction has been encountered, but elevated levels of prolactin may be noted in conjunction with the high blood levels encountered occasionally with parenteral administration of cimetidine. Both swelling and nipple tenderness were mild and did not progress after several months of therapy. Decreased sperm counts have been noted in men taking the drug for more than two months.

A few cases of neutropenia and leukopenia have been reported, along with an increased incidence of delayed hypersensitivity reactions after six weeks of treatment; fever and bradycardia and other arrhythmias have occurred, but a direct cause-and-effect relationship is difficult to verify. In animal studies, cimetidine crosses the placenta and is excreted in maternal milk, but dangers associated with pregnancy have not been found. No experience has accumulated in man. Further experience is required before the long-term safety of cimetidine can be established.

For optimal effect, blood levels should be maximal once the stomach has emptied; therefore, cimetidine should be taken with meals. However, since the duration of action is longer than the usual intervals between meals, the patient is protected from the acid stimulating effects of the meal by the previous dose while the current dose of cimetidine is being absorbed. Consequently, if desired, administration may be postponed until the meal is over. The optimal therapeutic interrelationship between cimetidine, antacids, and anticholinergic antispasmodics remains to be established.

ROUTES, USUAL DOSAGE, AND PREPARATIONS. *Oral*: *Adults*, in general, 300 mg is given with or immediately after meals and at bedtime for three to six weeks. Antacids may be taken concomitantly, as needed, to control pain. After endoscopy or x-rays reveal that healing has occurred, once-daily administration at bedtime may be employed to inhibit nocturnal hypersecretion. *Children*, see following parenteral dosages.

CIMETIDINE:
Tagamet (Smith Kline & French). Tablets 300 mg.

Intravenous, Intramuscular: *Adults* (intravenous), 1 to 4 mg/kg/hr is infused or 300 mg is diluted and injected over a two-minute period or infused over a 15- to 20-minute period; (intramuscular) 300 mg is given every six hours. When feasible, the dosage should be adjusted to maintain an intragastric pH greater than 5. Oral administration should be substituted as soon as possible (eg, when signs of bleeding have been absent for 48 hours). For patients with severely impaired renal function, 300 mg twice daily is suggested. *Children*, 20 to 40 mg/kg of body weight daily has been given orally or intravenously in divided doses; however, clinical experience in children is extremely limited, and the benefit/risk ratio should be carefully considered.

CIMETIDINE HYDROCHLORIDE:
Tagamet [*hydrochloride*] (Smith Kline & French). Solution 150 mg/ml in 2 ml containers.

ANTACIDS

The clinically useful antacids are basic salts that react with hydrochloric acid to form neutral, less acidic, or poorly soluble salts. With adequate dosage, antacids increase the pH of the gastric contents to 5 or more, thus inactivating pepsin and facilitating healing of peptic ulcer. Liquid preparations are preferable to tablets because they are generally more effective in neutralizing acid in vivo. Antacids do not provide a beneficial coating on or around the ulcer crater. The precise mechanism whereby symptomatic relief is achieved has not been completely explained.

There is considerable variation in the acid neutralizing effect of different antacids; in vitro differences alone cannot be used to select an antacid. Antacids with a high neutralizing rate are probably more efficacious in vivo, since it is less likely that unconsumed antacid will be lost by gastric emptying. Although comparisons of in vitro acid neutralizing capacity do have some correlation with in vivo effectiveness, the appropriate antacid should be determined individually based upon patient response and acceptance. See the Tables for the acid neutralizing capacity of antacid products; if a generic preparation is to be prescribed, its neutralizing capacity should be known. The dosage of an antacid may be established on the basis of mEq of hydrochloric acid neutralized. In this manner, although the volume may vary, the amount of acid neutralized is the factor of primary importance.

Poorly absorbed antacids are preferred in the treatment of peptic ulcer. Certain highly concentrated aluminum, magnesium, and calcium compounds appear to have a prolonged duration of action and beneficial effects on pH both in vitro and in vivo. Mixtures of aluminum oxide-hydroxide and magnesium oxide-hydroxide or magnesium trisilicate are used most frequently. Calcium carbonate has a greater neutralizing capacity, but its utilization has decreased because of evidence of absorption of calcium and concern created by theoretical considerations regarding acid rebound initiated by increased serum gastrin. All antacids may produce a temporary compensatory increase in the secretion of hydrochloric acid because of their effects on the pH-sensitive antrum and duodenum. Frequent administration during the early painful period maintains acid neutralization and clinically mitigates the effect of acid rebound. The

TABLE 1.
COMPOSITION OF SINGLE-ENTITY ANTACID PREPARATIONS
(per capsule, tablet, or 5 ml)

Product (Manufacturer)	Dosage Form	Acid Neutralizing Capacity OTC Method (mEq)	Al(OH)₃ (mg)	Calcium Carbonate (mg)	Other (mg)	Sodium Content (mg)	(mEq)
*AlternaGEL (Stuart)	Suspension	12	600	—		<2	0.087
Alu-Cap (Riker)	Capsules	11	475	—		<2	<0.1
Alu-Tab (Riker)	Tablets	12	600	—		6	0.26
*Amphojel (Wyeth)	Suspension	6.5	320	—		6.9†	0.30†
	Tablets						
	(0.6 g)	18	600	—		2.8	0.12
	(0.3 g)	9	300	—		1.4	0.06
*Basaljel (Wyeth)	Suspension	14	400**	—		2.4	0.10
	Extra-Strength	22	1,000**	—		23††	1.0††
	Capsules	13	500**	—		2.8	0.12
	Tablets	14	500**	—		2.1	0.09
*Dicarbosil (Arch)	Tablets	9.8	—	500		<3	<0.13
*Robalate (Robins)	Tablets	7			Dihydroxy-aluminum Amino-acetate 500	0.14	
*Rolaids (Warner-Lambert)	Tablets	7.5	—	—	Dihydroxy-aluminum Sodium Carbonate 334	53	2.30
*Titralac (Riker)	Liquid	20	—	1,000		11	0.48
	Tablets	9	—	420		0.3	0.01
*Tums (Lewis-Howe)	Tablets	9.8	—	500		<3.0	<0.130

*Nonprescription
†Maximum allowed per label. Usual value = 6 mg (0.27 mEq).
**Aluminum hydroxide equivalent, present as basic aluminum carbonate.
††Maximum allowed per label. Usual value = 17 mg (0.74 mEq).

clinical significance of any increased acid output associated with use of calcium carbonate is unproved. No comparative studies have demonstrated this agent's lack of efficacy; indeed, in studies conducted 20 and 30 years ago, calcium carbonate was reported to be the most effective antacid and contradictory clinical evidence has not been forthcoming.

Sodium bicarbonate, which is an active ingredient of some proprietary preparations, is very soluble and has an immediate and pronounced neutralizing effect, but the duration of action is extremely brief. This antacid releases large volumes of carbon dioxide in the stomach. Because sodium bicarbonate produces metabolic alkalosis when used excessively or in patients with impaired renal function, it must not be taken for long periods. Sodium bicarbonate should not be used in the routine treatment of peptic ulcer and is contraindicated in patients requiring a low-sodium diet.

Other Uses of Antacids: Antacids are commonly taken to treat functional symptoms such as dyspepsia, heartburn, or so-called acid indigestion. Hypersecretion of hydrochloric acid is not required for the production of these symptoms, which also may occur in patients with achlorhydria. The mechanism whereby antacids relieve these complaints is unclear, and some claim it to be no more than a placebo effect.

Aluminum hydroxide and basic aluminum carbonate [Basaljel] are used to treat renal calculi and to control hyperphosphatemia encountered early in the course of chronic renal failure. The aluminum-magnesium antacids also bind bile salts which reflux into the stomach.

Adverse Reactions and Precautions

The most common adverse reactions associated with prolonged use of antacids are diarrhea and constipation. Magnesium salts cause diarrhea and large frequent doses are not tolerated. Conversely, constipation may occur with large frequent doses of calcium or aluminum preparations; doses of 20 to 40 g of calcium carbonate daily occasionally cause fecal impaction. Disrup-

tion of normal bowel function can be minimized by teaching the patient how to determine the necessary balance of magnesium salts with calcium or aluminum preparations. Very few patients achieve perfect regulation of bowel function with high-dose regimens of the available fixed-ratio mixtures, and further supplementation with laxative or constipating antacids is often required.

By altering gastric and renal pH and thus the ionization of drugs, antacids may interfere with the dissolution, absorption, and excretion of concomitantly used medications. Antacids containing calcium, magnesium, or aluminum interfere with the absorption of tetracycline, digoxin, and quinidine. The slight elevation of urinary pH that is produced by the aluminum-magnesium antacids increases blood levels of quinidine and decreases levels of aspirin as a result of variations in renal excretion. Long-term use of aluminum preparations may produce hypophosphatemic bone resorption. Adverse systemic effects of aluminum and magnesium occur in patients with renal insufficiency; nephrolithiasis has been encountered. (See the evaluations on Aluminum Compounds.)

Almost all antacid gels (aluminum-magnesium oxide, hydroxide, trisilicate) contain enough sodium to preclude their unrestricted use in patients requiring a low-sodium diet. A knowledge of exact amounts of sodium is required when these antacids are prescribed for these patients. (Available information on the sodium content of antacids appears in Tables 1 and 2.)

ALUMINUM COMPOUNDS

ALUMINUM HYDROXIDE GEL
[AlternaGEL, Amphojel]
DRIED ALUMINUM HYDROXIDE GEL
[Alu-Cap, Alu-Tab, Amphojel Tablets]

Aluminum hydroxide is the prototype and the most commonly used aluminum compound. The gel is a poorly soluble antacid-buffer which reacts slowly with hydrochloric acid. It has a low neutralizing capacity; however, the absorptive properties of the gel prolong the duration of action; the rapidity of gastric emptying will thus inversely influence the efficacy of the more slowly reactive preparations. Different preparations of aluminum hydroxide vary in neutralizing potency; solid dosage forms are considered much less effective in vivo. Aluminum hydroxide has demulcent, adsorbent, and astringent properties, but these actions do not contribute to its effect in peptic ulcer.

The toxicity of long-term use of aluminum compounds is not yet fully known; the most common adverse reaction is constipation, which is dose related and thus almost invariably requires combined therapy with a magnesium compound. The astringent action or taste of this agent may produce nausea and vomiting. If phosphate intake is low, patients receiving large doses of this antacid for long periods may develop hypophosphatemia and osteomalacia. Since aluminum hydroxide complexes with the tetracyclines and can interfere with the absorption of excretion of warfarin, digoxin, quinine, and quinidine, the therapeutic effect of these drugs may be affected when antacids are used concomitantly. Adverse central nervous system effects ("dialysis dementia") may occur when aluminum hydroxide is given for prolonged periods to some dialysis patients. Changes in water purification resulting in high levels of aluminum in the water of the dialysis bath have been implicated in some of the cases reported. Neutron activation analysis has demonstrated that the intestinal barrier is permeable to heavy aluminum load and that aluminum may be deposited in bone in those with normal renal function.

ROUTE, USUAL DOSAGE, AND PREPARATIONS.
Oral: The dose and frequency of administration depend upon the disorder being treated, the frequency and severity of pain, and the degree of relief obtained. Although traditional dose recommendations follow, a suggested dosage for duodenal and gastric ulcer is 80 and 40 mEq per dose, respectively. For peptic ulcer, *adults*, 5 to 30 ml of gel. For severe symptoms, 40 ml of gel every 30 minutes may be required; this may be given by continuous intragastric drip after dilution with two to three parts of milk or water. After pain is controlled, this dose may be taken one hour before and one hour after meals and at bedtime. Efficacy of tablet formulations is much less predictable.

Drug available generically: Liquid (gel); tablets 240, 450, and 600 mg (dried gel).
See Table 1 for trademark preparations.

BASIC ALUMINUM CARBONATE GEL
[Basaljel]

DRIED BASIC ALUMINUM CARBONATE GEL
[Basaljel]

This gel reacts slowly with hydrochloric acid but is rarely used today as an antacid. It is prescribed primarily in conjunction with a low-phosphate diet to reduce elevated phosphate levels and demineralization of bones in patients with renal insufficiency and to prevent phosphatic urinary stones.

Generally, patient compliance is difficult, since the quantities required cause upper gastrointestinal discomfort, taste intolerance, and constipation. Serum levels of calcium and phosphorus should be monitored periodically in patients with impaired renal function. As with other amphoteric gels, absorption of tetracycline is prevented when the two drugs are used concomitantly.

ROUTE AND USUAL DOSAGE.
Oral: For phosphatic renal calculi, 10 to 50 ml of suspension or two to six capsules or tablets one hour after meals and at bedtime.
See Table 1 for trademark preparations.

DIHYDROXYALUMINUM AMINOACETATE
[Robalate]

The properties of this agent are similar to those of aluminum hydroxide. In the clinically less effective dried form, dihydroxyaluminum aminoacetate has a greater in vitro neutralizing capacity than dried aluminum hydroxide gel. On an equivalent weight basis, dihydroxyaluminum aminoacetate is as constipating as aluminum hydroxide. Inasmuch as the preparation is available only in tablet form, it is regarded as less effective than the same compound would be if it were available in liquid form.

ROUTE AND USUAL DOSAGE.

Oral: The dose and frequency of administration depend upon the disorder being treated and the degree of relief obtained. A suggested dosage for duodenal and gastric ulcer is 80 and 40 mEq per dose, respectively. The traditional dose recommendation is, *adults*, 500 mg to 2 g four or more times daily.

See Table 1 for trademark preparation.

DIHYDROXYALUMINUM SODIUM CARBONATE
[Rolaids]

This aluminum compound is stated to have properties of both sodium carbonate and aluminum hydroxide; sodium carbonate reacts rapidly while aluminum hydroxide has a more prolonged action. Results of a limited number of studies have shown that this agent is temporarily effective in neutralizing gastric acid; however, there is no convincing comparative study demonstrating its superiority to solid dosage forms of other aluminum compounds. Constipation may occur with large doses.

ROUTE AND USUAL DOSAGE.

Oral: The dose and frequency of administration depend upon the disorder being treated and the degree of relief obtained. A suggested dosage for duodenal and gastric ulcer is 80 and 40 mEq per dose, respectively. The traditional dose recommendation is, *adults*, one or two tablets four or more times daily.

See Table 1 for trademark preparation.

CALCIUM COMPOUNDS

The calcium compound used most commonly as an antacid is calcium carbonate. Tribasic calcium phosphate has been used occasionally, but its neutralizing action is weak and of brief duration; its principal indication is as a source of calcium and phosphate in deficiency states. (See Chapter 54, Agents Affecting Calcium Metabolism.)

CALCIUM CARBONATE
[Dicarbosil, Titralac, Tums]

Calcium carbonate has a rapid onset of action, very high neutralizing capacity, and a relatively prolonged effect. However, its use as an antacid has been abandoned perhaps prematurely by many gastroenterologists because of emphasis on the acid rebound and the elevation in serum gastrin level that occur after single doses. The clinical significance of the gastrin-stimulated acid rebound has not been proved. Sippy and others have shown that the pH of the gastric contents can be maintained above 5.5 by the hourly administration of 2 to 4 g of calcium carbonate. This compound is reconstituted or insoluble calcium soaps or calcium phosphate are formed in the alkaline intestinal milieu; however, significant absorption with resulting hypercalcemia occurs in some patients.

Lack of palatability is a frequent complaint of patients using the hourly regimen for the treatment of active ulcer. Dose-related constipation is common when 20 to 40 g is taken daily; hemorrhoids, painful, bleeding anal fissures, or fecal impaction also may occur. Acute appendicitis has been produced by impacted calcium carbonate fecoliths. Liberation of carbon dioxide in the stomach may cause eructation and flatulence. The constipating effects of this drug can be minimized by substituting sufficient amounts of a magnesium preparation; a mixture of two parts of magnesium oxide to one part of calcium carbonate produces relatively normal stools for many patients. However, if constipation or diarrhea does occur, the ratio of the ingredients must be adjusted.

The milk-alkali (Burnett) syndrome may occur after prolonged administration of calcium carbonate with concomitant use of sodium bicarbonate and/or homogenized milk containing vitamin D. This syndrome is characterized by hypercalcemic alkalosis with normal or elevated phosphorus levels, azotemia, and normal alkaline phosphatase levels. Renal failure and metastatic calcinosis also occur; the urinary excretion of calcium is generally not increased. Conjunctival and episcleral suffusion accompanies the alkalosis, and calcium deposits (manifested by band keratopathy) are noted. Nausea is a common symptom, in part reflecting the hypercalcemia. Symptoms subside gradually following discontinuation of the antacid and/or the milk. Predisposing factors are pre-existing renal dysfunction caused by primary renal disease, hypertension, sarcoidosis, gastrointestinal hemorrhage, and dehydration and electrolyte imbalance due to excessive vomiting or nasogastric aspiration of gastric contents with inadequate intravenous fluid replacement. Magnesium and aluminum salts have not been implicated in this syndrome. The syndrome has become rare as the use of calcium carbonate has declined.

ROUTE, USUAL DOSAGE, AND PREPARATIONS. *Oral*: The dose and frequency of administration depend upon whether an active ulcer or an interval phase is being treated. *Adults*, 1 to 4 g one and three hours after meals and at bedtime; 2 to 4 g every hour may be required to relieve pain. The tablets should be chewed before swallowing. Rarely, a patient may tolerate hourly doses of calcium carbonate alone without becoming constipated.

> Drug available generically: Powder; tablets 600 mg.
> See Table 1 for trademark preparations.

MAGNESIUM COMPOUNDS

The carbonate, hydroxide, oxide, phosphate, and trisilicate salts of magnesium are used as antacids, most commonly in combination with aluminum hydroxide. Magnesium trisilicate reacts slowly in gastric juice, and the stomach may empty before much of the acid is neutralized.

Magnesium salts have a laxative effect; therefore, their correct proportion in combination products will prevent or reduce the constipating effect of aluminum or cal-

cium salts, which reciprocally control the diarrheal effect of magnesium salts. Because large, frequent doses are required for complete control of the pain of active ulcer, most available antacid combinations must be supplemented with additional aluminum or calcium salts to avoid diarrhea. Only very rarely will an ulcer patient tolerate magnesium compounds as the sole antacid for any length of time.

Antacids containing magnesium are not likely to produce serious toxic effects; however, some compounds may cause hypermagnesemia in patients with severely impaired renal function.

MAGNESIUM HYDROXIDE

MAGNESIUM OXIDE

MILK OF MAGNESIA

These antacids have the same properties because magnesium oxide hydrolyzes to the hydroxide in water. They have a high neutralizing capacity with a rapid onset of action. As with all amphoteric antacids, tablets are much less effective than liquid preparations.

For adverse reactions, see the introduction on Magnesium Compounds.

DOSAGE AND PREPARATIONS. Like all antacids used mainly for their laxative properties, the dose and frequency of administration are determined by the number of substitutions for aluminum or calcium salts that result in normal stool consistency.

> MAGNESIUM HYDROXIDE:
> Drug available generically: Powder; tablets 300 and 600 mg.
> MAGNESIUM OXIDE:
> Drug available generically: Capsules 140 mg; tablets 420, 500, and 600 mg; powder available in both heavy and light form (light form suspends more readily in liquid).
> MILK OF MAGNESIA:
> Drug available generically: Suspension (nonprescription).

MAGNESIUM CARBONATE

The effect of magnesium carbonate is similar to that of the hydroxide and oxide salts, but this compound liberates carbon dioxide in the stomach during neutralization. It has a high neutralizing capacity.

For adverse reactions and precautions, see the introduction on Magnesium Compounds.

DOSAGE AND PREPARATIONS.
The dose and frequency of administration depend upon the frequency and intensity of pain and upon bowel function.

Drug available generically: Powder.

MAGNESIUM PHOSPHATE

The action of this alkaline powder is similar to other magnesium preparations. Its neutralizing capacity is less than that of magnesium carbonate but greater than that of magnesium trisilicate.

For adverse reactions and precautions, see the introduction on Magnesium Compounds.

MAGNESIUM TRISILICATE

Magnesium trisilicate is a relatively poor antacid-buffer that reacts slowly with hydrochloric acid to form hydrated silicon dioxide. Thus, its onset of action is delayed

and may not take place if gastric emptying is rapid. It is a common ingredient of many antacid mixtures.

For adverse reactions and precautions, see the introduction on Magnesium Compounds.

Drug available generically: Powder; tablets 450 mg.

MIXTURES

Mixtures of Antacids

Products containing aluminum and/or calcium compounds with magnesium salts, either as mixtures or chemical combinations, are more commonly used in the treatment of peptic ulcer than single-entity antacids. The antacid effect of these combination products usually is the sum of effects of the individual components, but supplemental amounts of aluminum, calcium, or magnesium often are required to reduce constipation or diarrhea when large doses are employed. Newer formulations have been prepared in an attempt to provide a greater neutralizing action.

See Table 2 for product listings.

TABLE 2.
COMPOSITION OF ANTACID MIXTURES
(per capsule, tablet, or 5 ml)

Product (Manufacturer)	Dosage Form	Acid Neutralizing Capacity OTC Method (mEq)	$Al(OH)_3$ (mg)	$Mg(OH)_2$ (mg)	Mg Trisilicate (mg)	Other (mg)	Sodium Content (mg)	Sodium Content (mEq)
*Aludrox (Wyeth)	Suspension	14	307	103	—	—	1.1	0.05
	Tablets	11.5	233	84	—	—	1.6	0.07
Aluscop (O'Neal, Jones & Feldman)	Capsules	12	—	180	—	Dihydroxy-aluminum Amino-acetate 325	NONE	
A-M-T (Wyeth)	Suspension	11	305	—	625	—	11.5§	0.5§
	Tablets	7.5	164	—	250	—	3.5	0.15

TABLE 2.
COMPOSITION OF ANTACID MIXTURES
(per capsule, tablet, or 5 ml)

Product (Manufacturer)	Dosage Form	Acid Neutralizing Capacity OTC Method (mEq)	Active Ingredients				Sodium Content	
			Al(OH)$_3$ (mg)	Mg(OH)$_2$ (mg)	Mg Trisili-cate (mg)	Other (mg)	(mg)	(mEq)
*Camalox (Rorer)						Calcium Carbonate		
	Suspension	18	225	200	—	250	2.5	0.11
	Tablets	18	225	200	—	250	1.5	0.065
Creamalin (Winthrop)	Tablets	12.1	248	75	—	—	<41.0	
*Delcid (Merrell-National)	Liquid	42 .	600	665	—	—	12.2-15	0.53
Escot (Tutag)	Capsules	5	130‡	—	160	Bismuth Aluminate 100	5-6	2.5
Gaviscon (Marion)	Liquid	1.2	53.3	—	13.3	Sodium Alginate	26.8	1.2
	Tablets	0.5	80	—	20	Sodium Alginate	18.4	0.8
*Gelusil (Parke, Davis)	Liquid	11.5	200	200	—	Simethicone 25	0.9	0.039
	Tablets	11.0	200	200	—	Simethicone 25	1.6	0.069
Gelusil-M (Parke, Davis)	Liquid	13.5	300	200	—	Simethicone 25	1.0	0.043
	Tablets	11.0	300	200	—	Simethicone 25	3.0	0.130
Gelusil-II (Parke, Davis)	Liquid	24.0	400	400	—	Simethicone 30	1.3	0.056
	Tablets	20.5	400	400	—	Simethicone 30	2.7	0.117
Glycate (O'Neal, Jones & Feldman)	Tablets	4	—	—	—	Calcium Carbonate 300 Glycine 150	0.112	0.00055
Kolantyl (Merrell-National)	Gel	10.5	150	150	—	—	2.2	0.095
	Wafers	10.8	180	170	—	—	2.0	0.086
*Kudrox (Kremers-Urban)	Suspension	25	540	180	—	Sorbitol	15	0.65
	Tablets	12	400	—	—	Magnesium Carbonate Co-precipi-tate	16	0.7

TABLE 2.
COMPOSITION OF ANTACID MIXTURES
(per capsule, tablet, or 5 ml)

Product (Manufacturer)	Dosage Form	Acid Neutralizing Capacity OTC Method (mEq)	Al(OH)$_3$ (mg)	Mg(OH)$_2$ (mg)	Mg Trisili- cate (mg)	Other (mg)	Sodium (mg)	Content (mEq)
*Maalox (Rorer)	Suspension	13.5	225	200	—	—	2.5	0.11
	Tablets							
	(No. 1)	8.5	200	200	—	—	0.84	0.036
	(No. 2)	18	400	400	—	—	1.80	0.078
*Maalox Plus (Rorer)	Suspension	13.5	225	200	—	Simethicone 25	5.0	0.11
	Tablets	8.5	200	200	—	Simethicone 25	2.6	0.056
Maalox Therapeutic (Rorer)	Suspension	28.3	600	300	—	—	1.25	0.044
*Mylanta (Stuart)	Liquid	12.7	200	200	—	Simethicone 20	0.68	0.03
	Tablets	11.5	200	200	—	Simethicone 20	0.77	0.03
*Mylanta II (Stuart)	Liquid	25.4	400	400	—	Simethicone 30	1.4	0.06
	Tablets	23.0	400	400	—	Simethicone 30	1.3	0.06
Riopan (Robins)	Tablets	2.21	480††	—	—	—	0.3	0.014
	Suspension	2.21	480††	—	—	—	0.3	0.014
*Silain Gel (Robins)	Liquid	15	282†	285	—	Simethicone 25	4.78	0.21
*Simeco (Wyeth)	Suspension	22	300**	300	—	Simethicone 30	6.9-13.8 (usual value 9 mg)	0.3-0.6 (usual value 0.39 mEq)
Tralrnag (O'Neal, Jones & Feldman)	Liquid	11.4	150	150	—	Dihydroxy- aluminum Amino- acetate 200	NONE	
*Trisogel (Lilly)	Liquid	17	150	—	583	—	9.3	0.406
	Capsules	3	97	—	271	—	NONE	
*WinGel (Winthrop)	Liquid	11.6	191	159	—	—	1.97	
	Tablets	12.3	186	160	—	—	1.66	

*Nonprescription.
†Equivalent to dried gel.
**Equivalent to 365 mg dried gel, U.S.P.
‡As a coprecipitate with magnesium carbonate.
§Maximum allowed per label. Usual value = 7.5 mg (0.31 mEq)
††As magaldrate, a complex of aluminum and magnesium hydroxides.

Mixtures of Antacids with Other Ingredients

Several products with antacid and nonantacid ingredients are claimed by their manufacturers to provide additional benefits. The alginic acid in Gaviscon forms a foam that acts as a carrier for antacids. The foam purportedly floats on top of the gastric contents and thus brings the antacids in contact with the mucosa, especially during reflux. The amount of antacids present in the formulation is about one-tenth the usual dose. The antacids do not neutralize the gastric contents but rely more on "local action" to produce their effect. There is no evidence to prove that the effects of Gaviscon are more beneficial than those of conventional antacids, although some studies demonstrate that Gaviscon is at least as effective as other antacids in relieving heartburn. Alginic acid has no demonstrable effect on reflux esophagitis produced by acid peptic or bile reflux. Gaviscon is promoted only for the treatment of heartburn, acid indigestion, and sour stomach.

The simethicone present in some mixtures is claimed to alleviate symptoms of gas; however, its efficacy is doubtful and the rationale for its mechanism of action is dubious (see the evaluation on Simethicone in Chapter 60, Miscellaneous Gastrointestinal Agents). There is no con-vincing evidence of beneficial effects for this apparently safe agent other than those provided by the antacid. The agent has, however, been designated "safe and effec-tive" by the FDA-OTC Antacid and Antiflatulent Review Panel.

The use of these products in the treatment of acid peptic disorders provides no advantage over products containing antacids alone. See Table 2 for product listings.

Selected References

Antacid and antiflatulent products, Part II. *Federal Register* 39:19862-22140, 1974.

Third symposium on histamine H_2-receptor antagonists: Clinical results with cimetidine. *Gastroenterology* 74:338-488, 1978.

Coughlin GP, et al: Effect of tri-potassium di-citrato bismuthate (De-Nol) on healing of chronic duodenal ulcers. *Med J Aust* 1:294-298, 1977.

Gibinski K, et al: Double-blind clinical trial on gastroduodenal ulcer healing with prostaglandin E2 analogues. *Gut* 18:636-639, 1977.

Nagy GS: Evaluation of carbenoxolone sodium in treatment of duodenal ulcer. *Gastroenterology* 74:7-10, 1978.

Peterson WL, et al: Healing of duodenal ulcer with antacid regimen. *N Engl J Med* 297:341-345, 1977.

Smyth RD, et al: Correlation of in vitro and in vivo methodology for evaluation of antacids. *J Pharm Sci* 65:1045-1047, 1976.

Wastell C, Lance, P: *Cimetidine: The Westminister Hospital Symposium 1978.* London, Churchill Livingstone, 1979.

Antidiarrheal Agents | 58

Diarrhea is characterized by excessive fluidity of the stool as manifested by decreased consistency and increased weight (greater than 200 g/day). It is almost always associated with an increased frequency of defecation (more than three times/day) and may be acute or chronic in duration. Causes include infection, intoxication, ischemia, allergy, maldigestion, malabsorption, inflammation, functional disorders, tumors of the bowel, and certain rare extraintestinal hormone-producing neoplasms. The readiness with which diarrhea subsides depends largely upon the underlying cause. Appropriate therapy, if indicated, depends upon proper diagnosis.

Acute severe diarrhea causes water and salt depletion that may lead to dehydration and/or electrolyte imbalance. Even mild chronic diarrhea may produce hypokalemia with profound weakness and malaise. Cramping from intermittent spasm, distention, and borborygmi from swallowed air and gas produced by fermentation occur. The frequency of defecation may cause unbearable discomfort when the number of bowel movements exceeds ten per day. Perianal irritation and hemorrhoids are common in these instances.

Enterotoxigenic *Escherichia coli* and viral infections are probably the most common causes of brief self-limited episodes of diarrhea (24 to 48 hours). No specific treatment is needed except in the aged and infants, in whom dehydration may be life-threatening. In these patients, avoidance of food (with or without intravenous fluid replacement) accompanied by ingestion of a dextrose-electrolyte solution should maintain hydration. For mild cases, antispasmodics, heat applied to the abdomen, and food restriction may be all that is needed to relieve cramps and diarrhea. More vigorous efforts to prevent or reduce the frequency of diarrhea may lengthen the period of morbidity. Alleviation of the symptoms of acute, self-limited diarrhea is optional; when the diarrhea is severe and/or prolonged, hospitalization may be required. Symptomatic treatment of chronic diarrhea may be justified only to provide temporary relief while search for the cause is undertaken. Nutritional status as well as electrolyte balance must be assessed and appropriate replacement therapy given when indicated even prior to a definitive diagnosis.

Patients with disaccharidase deficiencies and gluten-induced enteropathy require diet therapy that is specific. Dietary restriction of fat may ameliorate diarrhea associated with postsurgical vagotomy, hyperthyroidism, lymphangiectasia, and other steatorrheas. Medium-chain triglycerides may serve as an absorbable substitute for fat. Foods high in fiber content (unrefined cereals, fruits, and vegetables) or laxative chemicals should be eliminated whenever diarrhea is present. In absorptive or secretory disorders, temporary intravenous hyperalimentation may be required. Most patients with maldigestive diarrhea caused by pancreatic insufficiency respond to replacement therapy with pancreatic extract, but the associated steatorrhea is not relieved as completely as when replacement therapy is combined with suppression of gastric acid secretion by cimetidine (see Chapter 60, Miscellaneous Gastrointestinal Agents). Dehydration caused by diarrhea associated with abnormal intestinal secretion (eg, in cholera, infantile diarrhea, massive ileal resection) may be treated with oral solutions of dextrose and electrolytes.

Nonspecific Antidiarrheal Agents

The opiates are the most effective and prompt-acting nonspecific antidiarrheal agents. They act by increasing tone and segmenting activity of the large and small intestine, thus providing resistance to transit. Opium tincture and paregoric (camphorated opium tincture) are much more widely used in this country than the purified alkaloids (eg, codeine), which are equally effective in equivalent dosage. Paregoric may be preferable to opium tincture since the dosage of the former is measured by teaspoon while the dosage of the latter is by drops. Because usual oral doses produce neither euphoria nor analgesia, these preparations may be used to treat acute, self-limited diarrhea with little or no risk of addiction. However, physical dependence or addiction may be induced if opiates are used indefinitely to treat chronic diarrhea.

The effectiveness of loperamide [Imodium] and diphenoxylate with atropine [Colonil, Lomotil] is almost the same as that of paregoric. Because these products are available in tablet or capsule form and have little or no abuse potential, they have replaced the opiates as the most widely used, effective, nonspecific antidiarrheal preparations. Both are classified as Schedule V substances under the Controlled Substances Act.

Anticholinergic antispasmodics have been used as antidiarrheal agents, but their primary effect is relief of cramping through reduction of contractile activity. Their effectiveness in the reduction of diarrhea is negligible. There is no conclusive evidence that any drug in this class exerts a selective effect on the gastrointestinal tract, although dicyclomine [Bentyl] has been promoted in such a manner. Sedatives and antispasmodics, when used with specific diet therapy and reassurance, may relieve the cramping and diarrhea or alternating constipation and diarrhea produced by the irritable bowel syndrome.

The use of powders containing bismuth subcarbonate, subgallate, subnitrate, or subsalicylate to treat diarrhea has been empiric. It has been claimed that these salts absorb intraluminal toxins, bacteria, and viruses or provide a protective coating for the mucosa, but the validity of these actions has not been substantiated by appropriate evidence. A controlled study demonstrated the efficacy of bismuth subsalicylate [Pepto-Bismol] in reducing enterotoxigenic E. coli (travelers') diarrhea in Mexico (DuPont et al, 1977). Presumably diarrhea is prevented when the toxin is bound within the lumen and before it can be bound by the receptors of the mucosal cells.

Poorly absorbed powders such as calcium carbonate or the hydrophilic colloids retain fluid to produce a bulkier stool. However, if diarrhea subsides, impaction may follow quickly unless ample oral fluid intake is maintained. The hydrophilic substances (polycarbophil, methylcellulose, and various psyllium seed derivatives) may be effective in the symptomatic treatment of watery diarrhea because of their water and bile salt-binding capacity. The patient may pass fewer and bulkier stools more comfortably. (See also Chapter 59, Laxatives.)

Activated charcoal given to adsorb toxins and infectious agents also has been used empirically in the treatment of diarrhea, but controlled studies to confirm its efficacy for this purpose are lacking. This preparation is used in the treatment of poisoning caused by certain drugs (see Chapter 85, General Antidotes).

Kaolin and other hydrated aluminum silicate clays (eg, activated attapulgite) often are combined with pectin and have been claimed to act as adsorbents and protectants. Adequately controlled clinical studies demonstrating the efficacy of these popular but minimally effective antidiarrheal mixtures have not been published. Recent animal studies suggest that the fluidity of the stool is decreased, but total water loss appears to be unchanged. Small amounts of other ingredients often are present in mixtures of kaolin and pectin, but they too are of unproved efficacy. All of the aforementioned adsorbents may interfere with the absorption of other therapeutic agents.

Viable *Lactobacillus* cultures [Bacid, Lactinex] have been promoted for the treatment of diarrhea caused directly by the toxic action of antibiotics upon the bowel or indirectly by the replacement of normal intestinal flora. There are no convincing well-controlled studies supporting the effectiveness of viable *Lactobacillus* cultures in the treatment of this type of diarrhea.

Two amebicides, clioquinol (iodochlorhydroxyquin) [Entero-Vioform] and iodoquinol (diiodohydroxyquin) [Yodoxin], have been used without proof of efficacy in the prophylaxis of "travelers' diarrhea." Optic atrophy and peripheral neuropathy have occurred in children receiving moderate doses of these and other halogenated hydroxyquinolines for three or more weeks. Transverse myelitis also has been reported in the Far East in adults using clioquinol for six weeks or more. Since amebae cause only a small percentage of the diarrheas encountered while traveling, the indiscriminate use of such potentially toxic agents must be criticized. The risk in no way justifies continued use of these effective amebicides for any other condi-

tion. Manufacturers have voluntarily removed clioquinol from the U.S. market, but iodoquinol continues to be marketed. (See also Chapter 82, Antiprotozoal Agents.)

Antidiarrheal Drugs Having Specific Indications

Drugs used to treat the underlying causes of diarrhea include antibacterial agents (eg, sulfonamides, neomycin [Mycifradin, Neobiotic], chloramphenicol [Chloromycetin, Mychel], ampicillin, vancomycin [Vancocin], tetracyclines), antiprotozoal agents (eg, metronidazole [Flagyl], chloroquine, emetine), adrenal corticosteroids, and certain chelating agents (eg, cholestyramine resin [Questran]). These drugs should be used only when the cause is identified, when there is strong presumptive evidence of such a diagnosis, or when laboratory service for confirmation of a diagnosis is not available. For example, in acute bacterial diarrhea of infancy, appropriate antibacterial therapy may be initiated on the basis of a carefully formed clinical diagnosis when bacteriologic diagnostic service is not immediately available. Nevertheless, the studies should be made since the belated results may still be of vital significance.

Acute, short-term gastroenteritis due to *Salmonella* infections other than typhoid is often self-limited. There is evidence that routine use of antibiotics does not shorten the period of illness and/or may even prolong the excretion of infectious organisms. Antibiotic therapy is advisable in recurrent or severe infections, particularly in patients with associated chronic illness, in infants, or in the elderly. A 10- to 14-day course of chloramphenicol or ampicillin is the treatment of choice for the enteric fevers. If resistant strains emerge, amoxicillin or sulfamethoxazole and trimethoprim [Bactrim, Septra] (three tablets twice the first day, then two tablets twice daily for seven days) has been effective.

Ampicillin (1 g every six hours for five days) is presently the antibiotic of choice in severe acute or chronic *Shigella* infections. The mixture of sulfamethoxazole and trimethoprim has been used for resistant strains. Patients with resistant strains or those who are allergic or do not respond to ampicillin or the sulfonamides may receive a tetracycline (oxytetracycline 250 mg orally every six hours for five days).

When treatment for enteropathogenic or enterotoxigenic infections caused by *Escherichia coli* is necessary, tetracycline (500 mg orally every six hours for three days) shortened the duration of illness and of excretion of the pathogen. Neomycin, doxycycline [Vibramycin], phthalylsulfathiazole [Sulfathalidine], and sulfisoxazole [Gantrisin] have been used prophylactically in travelers' diarrhea. Individual patient reaction to the antibiotic as well as creation of antibiotic-resistant strains warrant careful consideration of benefit versus risk prior to using antibiotics prophylactically. Bismuth subsalicylate [Pepto-Bismol] has also been found to be effective. Lincomycin [Lincocin] or metronidazole [Flagyl] may be of special value in eliminating anaerobic organisms implicated in the blind loop syndrome when tetracycline is not effective. Isolated epidemic outbreaks of diarrhea caused by *Campylobacter, Yersinia,* salt-dependent *Vibrio parahemolyticus*, or the more common pathogens are preferably treated after antibiotic sensitivity is established.

Phthalylsulfathiazole and sulfasalazine [Azulfidine, S.A.S.-500] are adjuncts in the treatment of certain forms of inflammatory bowel disease; however, they are ineffective in the treatment of dysentery. Sulfasalazine is much more widely used than phthalylsulfathiazole, despite the probable higher frequency of adverse effects with its administration. No comparative efficacy or toxicity studies have been performed. Some controlled studies support the use of sulfasalazine in various phases of inflammatory bowel disease. No such studies have been undertaken with the older, poorly absorbed sulfonamide.

See also Chapters 69, Penicillins; 71, Chloramphenicol and Derivatives; 73, Tetracyclines; 74, Aminoglycosides; 75, Polymyxins; 76, Miscellaneous Antibacterial Agents; and 77, Sulfonamides and Related Compounds.

Cholestyramine is of clinical benefit in reducing diarrhea caused by bile salt malabsorption; patients with short bowel and minimal or no steatorrhea (less than 10 g/day) benefit from therapy, whereas those with more severe steatorrhea (more than 15 g daily) are not usually helped; their diarrhea is usually related to the unabsorbed fatty acids that simultaneously increase colonic secretion and reduce colonic absorption of water and electrolytes. Cholestyramine and vancomycin [Vancocin] have been found to be effective in treating a form of diarrhea, called pseudomembranous colitis, that has been observed during or after therapy with many antibiotics. Metronidazole also has been reported to be effective for this type of diarrhea. Evidence implicates the toxin of *Clostridium difficile* as the cause of this potentially fatal condition. It has not been possible to conclude with certainty that pseudomembranous colitis has been observed more frequently with lincomycin [Lincocin] and clindamycin [Cleocin] in man. Elderly, postoperative, or chronically ill debilitated patients receiving antibiotics may be most vulnerable.

Metronidazole (750 mg orally three times daily for ten days) is the drug of choice for acute amebic dysentery. Tetracycline (500 mg four times daily for ten days) is an effective alternative and is combined with amebicides effective against amebic cysts. Metronidazole and quinacrine hydrochloride [Atabrine] are effective in the treatment of giardiasis. (See Chapter 82, Antiprotozoal Agents.)

Propranolol [Inderal], a beta-adrenergic antagonist, has been useful to treat diarrhea accompanying hyperthyroidism. Methysergide [Sansert], a serotonin antagonist, has benefited patients with diarrhea accompanying the carcinoid syndrome. The profuse watery diarrhea observed in patients with pancreatic cholera (Verner Morrison syndrome, secretory diarrhea) produced by metastatic nonbeta cell tumors has been relieved by infusion of streptozocin into the hepatic artery. Indomethacin [Indocin], prednisolone, and nutmeg have been found to be helpful sometimes in controlling the profound diarrhea and other typical symptoms of nonalpha, nonbeta cell pancreatic tumors or medullary carcinomas of the thyroid containing large amounts of prostaglandin E.

Adrenal corticosteroids and corticotropin are used as adjuncts in the treatment of inflammatory bowel disorders and, in enema form, in ulcerative proctitis or proctosigmoiditis. Acute ulcerative colitis and Crohn's disease of the small and/or large intestine respond to oral or parenteral prednisone, prednisolone, dexamethasone, methylprednisolone [Medrol], cortisol (hydrocortisone) [Cortenema, Rectoid], and corticotropin. Triamcinolone and certain other halogenated corticosteroids are not used because they produce rapid profound nitrogen loss in effective dose ranges. Careful judgment and experience are required to minimize the almost inevitable occurrence of adverse reactions which increase with prolonged use. Opinion is divided on whether steroids should be used without concomitant administration of phthalylsulfathiazole or sulfasalazine. Ampicillin or chloramphenicol has been used to treat the severe acute phase of the disease. Discontinuation of treatment is possible in ulcerative colitis, but Crohn's disease may be more resistant to complete withdrawal of steroids. There is no conclusive convincing evidence to support the efficacy of immunosuppressive agents in the treatment of the acute phases of inflammatory bowel disease. Results are conflicting regarding the effectiveness of mercaptopurine [Purinethol] or azathioprine [Imuran] in prolonging remission in Crohn's disease. When effective, these agents may permit reduction in the dosages of steroids if not their complete withdrawal. Adverse effects are common with the use of these drugs.

Adverse Reactions and Precautions

Opiate preparations, loperamide [Imodium], and diphenoxylate with atropine [Colonil, Lomotil] should not be prescribed for long-term unsupervised use because of their small but definite potential for abuse, particularly in dependency-prone individuals. In general, the therapeutic regimens for inflammatory bowel disease need not include an antidiarrheal agent. The factors precipitating ileus or toxic megacolon in the acute phase of the illness, especially when anticholinergic or opiate-like drugs are used, are unclear. Thus, it is questionable whether the risks of precipitating a life-threatening complication justify use of a drug that plays no direct role in recovery. These drugs are better avoided in acute diarrheas caused by antibiotics, poisons, infectious organisms, or exotoxins until mural infection has subsided and/or all toxic material has been eliminated from the gastrointestinal tract which cannot be measured easily.

The more serious untoward effects of the opiates (see Chapter 6, General Analgesics) are not encountered with usual antidiarrheal doses. The opiates, loperamide, and diphenoxylate have the potential for precipitating toxic megacolon in patients with acute colitis caused by amebae, schistosomes, ischemia, or active inflammatory bowel disease. When these agents lessened the cramping and decreased the number of stools in patients with acute infectious diarrhea, sequestration of fluid in dilated loops of bowel has occurred, most often in children and adolescents. Hepatic coma has occurred following use of opiates and opiate-like drugs in patients with severe liver disease, presumably caused by impaired hepatic degradation of the drugs and the increased absorption of ammonia from the colon.

Dryness of the mouth, mydriasis, dizziness, headache, increased intraocular pressure, tachycardia, drowsiness, rash, dysuria, and acute urinary retention may occur after therapeutic doses of anticholinergic antispasmodics. (See also Chapter 60, Miscellaneous Gastrointestinal Agents.)

The adsorbents are quite safe; however, impaction has occurred in infants and elderly debilitated patients. A bizarre, reversible psychosis has been noted among patients employing bismuth subgallate to control the odor of ileostomy discharges. Similar neuropsychiatric reactions have been reported in France in patients using both the subcarbonate and subnitrate salts. Adsorbents are contraindicated in patients with suspected obstructive lesions of the bowel or fever and in children less than 3 years of age. They should not be used for more than two days. Prolonged use also may interfere with the absorption of other therapeutic agents.

Significant amounts of poorly absorbed antibiotics (eg, neomycin, paromomycin [Humatin]) or poorly absorbed sulfonamides (eg, phthalylsulfathiazole [Sulfathalidine]) may be absorbed, particularly in patients with extensive inflammation and ulceration of the bowel. Enough neomycin has been absorbed from the gastrointestinal tract to produce auditory nerve damage; patients with impaired renal function are particularly vulnerable.

The safety of both specific and nonspecific antidiarrheal agents during pregnancy and in infants less than 1 month of age has not been fully determined. Respiratory insufficiency has been reported to be associated with use of diphenoxylate with atropine in infants and young children. Teratogenicity has been observed when sulfonamides were given to rats and mice in doses 7 to 25 times the maximum human therapeutic dose. Sulfasalazine has been reported to cross the placenta and increase the risk of kernicterus.

NONSPECIFIC ANTIDIARRHEAL AGENTS

BISMUTH SUBSALICYLATE
[Pepto-Bismol]

Bismuth subsalicylate has been shown to bind toxins produced by *Vibrio cholerae* and *Esherichia coli*. It also has been suggested that the subsalicylate salt is hydrolyzed by coliforms, liberating salicylic acid which inhibits synthesis of a prostaglandin responsible for intestinal inflammation and hypermotility. In studies performed in Mexico, bismuth subsalicylate reduced travelers' diarrhea.

Use of bismuth may result in impaction in infants and elderly debilitated patients. Grayish-black discoloration of the stool should not be confused with melena.

ROUTE, USUAL DOSAGE, AND PREPARATIONS. *Oral*: *Adults*, 30 ml; *children 3 to 6 years*, 5 ml; *6 to 10 years*, 10 ml; *10 to 14 years*, 20 ml. This dose is repeated every 30 to 60 minutes if needed until eight doses are taken. A dose of 60 ml four times daily has been administered prophylactically for three weeks to young adults.

Drug available generically: Powder.

Pepto-Bismol (Norwich-Eaton). Suspension in 4, 8, 12, and 16 oz containers (nonprescription).

CODEINE PHOSPHATE
CODEINE SULFATE

Codeine is a purified opium alkaloid used for the short-term symptomatic treatment of mild diarrhea. Indications and contraindications are identical to those of the opium extracts, diphenoxylate, and loperamide. The development of dependence is a small but definite risk with prolonged use. Adverse reactions are similar to those produced by other opiates.

ROUTES, USUAL DOSAGE, AND PREPARATIONS. *Oral*: *Adults*, 15 to 60 mg every four to eight hours as needed. Codeine should not be used in *children under 12 years*.

Intramuscular: 15 to 30 mg every two to four hours as needed.

CODEINE PHOSPHATE:
Salt available generically: Solution 30 mg/ml in 1 and 20 ml containers and 60 mg/ml in 1 ml containers; tablets 30 and 60 mg; tablets (hypodermic) 15, 30 and 60 mg; powder.

CODEINE SULFATE:
Salt available generically: Powder; tablets (plain, hypodermic) 15, 30, and 60 mg.

DIPHENOXYLATE HYDROCHLORIDE WITH ATROPINE
[Colonil, Lomotil]

The effectiveness of diphenoxylate in the treatment of diarrhea is comparable to that of the opium derivatives. It apparently limits peristalsis by abolishing the mucosal peristaltic reflex through inhibition of mucosal receptors. It differs from the opiates in that it stimulates segmental contraction while inhibiting longitudinal contraction.

Diphenoxylate hydrochloride with atropine has a minimal potential for producing physical dependence when administered in recommended doses and is classified as a Schedule V substance under the Controlled Substances Act. The presence of atropine helps to prevent abuse and adds the potential for its own unpleasant side effects. The incidence of adverse reactions is relatively low. Untoward effects include abdominal distention, intestinal obstruction, dilation of the colon, rash, drowsiness, dizziness, depression, restlessness, nausea, headache, and blurred vision. Investigationally, large doses (40 to 60 mg) of diphenoxylate have produced a morphine-like euphoria, and toxic doses may cause respiratory depression and coma. Narcotic antagonists are effective antidotes (see Chapter 86, Specific Antidotes). Toxic megacolon or ileus may occur in patients with idiopathic, parasitic, or ischemic colitis. Diphenoxylate may potentiate the actions of barbiturates, opiates, and other central nervous system depressants. It should be used cautiously in patients with liver disease, since hepatic coma has been precipitated in a patient with cirrhosis. Infants and young children may experience respiratory insufficiency with use of this drug.

ROUTE, USUAL DOSAGE, AND PREPARATIONS.
Oral: *Adults*, 5 mg three or four times daily. *Children 8 to 12 years*, 10 mg daily in five divided doses; *5 to 8 years*, 8 mg daily in four divided doses; *2 to 5 years*, 6 mg daily in three divided doses.

> Drug available generically: Tablets containing diphenoxylate hydrochloride 2.5 mg and atropine sulfate 0.025 mg; liquid.
> *Colonil* (Mallinckrodt), *Lomotil* (Searle). Each tablet or 5 ml of liquid contains diphenoxylate hydrochloride 2.5 mg and atropine sulfate 0.025 mg.

LACTOBACILLUS CULTURES
[Bacid, Lactinex]

Bacid is a culture of *Lactobacillus acidophilus*, and Lactinex is a mixed culture of *L. acidophilus* and *L. bulgaricus* (*L. bulgaricus* does not colonize in the colon). These viable cultures are promoted as an aid in restoring normal intestinal flora after administration of antibacterial drugs. No convincing well-controlled studies supporting use of *Lactobacillus* cultures are known to be available.

Because of lack of adequate proof of efficacy, no dosage recommendation is made.

> *Bacid* (Fisons). Capsules containing *Lactobacillus acidophilus* with carboxymethylcellulose sodium 100 mg (nonprescription).
> *Lactinex* (Hynson, Westcott & Dunning). Granules 1 g packet; tablets 250 mg (nonprescription).

LOPERAMIDE HYDROCHLORIDE
[Imodium]

Loperamide is a derivative of haloperidol and structurally resembles meperidine. Its action on the central nervous system has been reduced and separated from its direct action upon intestinal musculature. Inhibition of contraction of both longitudinal and circular muscle fiber has been shown in vitro; however, the exact site of action has not been found. In man, transit time is prolonged, fecal volume reduced, loss of water and electrolytes decreased, while stool viscosity and bulk density are increased.

Open clinical trials as well as double-blind, crossover comparisons with placebo, diphenoxylate, and other opiates have shown that the action of this agent is prompt and prolonged in both acute and chronic diarrheas. However, codeine and the opium extracts are least expensive.

Administration of loperamide has been advocated to reduce the volume of ileostomy effluent and to reduce the frequency of bowel movements and improve the consistency of stools in patients with ulcerative colitis and Crohn's disease. It should not be considered routinely for ileostomy patients. In patients with colectomy performed for ulcerative colitis (in whom, contrasted to those with Crohn's disease, no risk of recurrence exists), loperamide may be of value when dietary measures are insufficient to control the liquidity of the effluent or when renal electrolyte loss is increased and added intestinal loss would be hazardous.

Physical dependence, untoward central nervous system effects, or other significant adverse reactions have not been noted. Loperamide does not potentiate the central nervous system depressant effects of barbiturates or alcohol. Toxic megacolon has occurred. Overdose should be treated with naloxone if morphine-like signs and symptoms of intoxication occur. No serious drug interactions have yet been reported. This agent should be used with caution in the presence of hepatic insufficiency or other conditions in which constipation should be avoided. The danger of perforation exists when the drug is given to patients with bacterial or parasitic infection of the wall of the bowel.

Teratogenicity has not been established. Use in children is not advised since adequate clinical experience has not been accumulated.

ROUTE, USUAL DOSAGE, AND PREPARATIONS. The manufacturer's suggested dosages are: *Oral*: For acute and chronic diarrhea, *adults*, 4 mg followed by 2 mg after each diarrheal stool. Subsequent daily dosage is individualized but is usually 2 to 4 mg once or twice daily. Daily dosage should not exceed 16 mg. Loperamide should be discontinued after 48 hours if no improvement occurs in patients with acute diarrhea. Chronic diarrhea is unlikely to respond if results are not achieved in ten days with doses of 16 mg daily. Use of loperamide in *children under 12 years* is not yet advisable.

Imodium (Ortho). Capsules 2 mg.

OPIUM TINCTURE

Opium tincture is prompt-acting and useful for the treatment of diarrhea. It is less widely used today than paregoric because the latter, despite an unpleasant taste, is more dilute, and teaspoonful doses are more convenient to measure than the dropper quantities of opium tincture prescribed. However, the prescription of the tincture may be smaller in volume and the number of drops adjusted more precisely to the needs of the patient. None of the opiates should be used in diarrhea caused by poisons, toxins, or infectious agents until the material is eliminated from the gastrointestinal tract, and there is no way to be sure when this has been completed.

Effective antidiarrheal doses are not likely to produce euphoria or analgesia because of the relatively small amount needed, but larger doses may produce the undesirable effects of opiates (see Chapter 6, General Analgesics). Opium tincture is classified as a Schedule II drug under the Controlled Substances Act.

ROUTE, USUAL DOSAGE, AND PREPARATIONS. *Oral*: 0.6 ml (range 0.3 to 1 ml) four times daily. The maximal single dose is 1 ml every two to four hours, and not more than 6 ml should be taken in 24 hours.

Drug available generically: Tincture 10% opium containing 10 mg of morphine per milliliter.

PAREGORIC

Paregoric (camphorated opium tincture) is as effective as opium tincture in equivalent doses and provides the convenience of teaspoonful dosage. This preparation should not be used in diarrhea caused by poisons, toxins, or infectious agents until the material is eliminated from the gastrointestinal tract. Paregoric frequently is combined with other antidiarrheal agents of unproven effectiveness, thus exposing the patient to the adverse effects of the other constituents at greater expense and with no additional benefit (see listings under Mixtures).

Adverse effects are rare, but nausea and other gastrointestinal disturbances occur occasionally. Usual oral doses do not produce euphoria or analgesia, but prolonged use has produced physical dependence despite the drug's unappealing taste. Paregoric is classified as a Schedule III drug under the Controlled Substances Act.

ROUTE, USUAL DOSAGE, AND PREPARATIONS. *Oral: Adults*, 5 to 10 ml one to a maximum of four times daily until diarrhea is controlled. *Children*, 0.25 to 0.5 ml/kg of body weight one to a maximum of four times daily. The customary amount per prescription is 1 or 2 ounces.

> Drug available generically: Tincture containing 0.4 mg of morphine/ml. Drug also marketed under the name Camphorated Tincture of Opium.

ANTIDIARRHEAL DRUGS HAVING SPECIFIC INDICATIONS

CHOLESTYRAMINE RESIN
[Questran]

Cholestyramine may be useful in patients with diarrhea caused by increased concentrations of certain bile acids in the colon resulting from defective ileal reabsorption of bile acids or by the presence of colonic flora in the upper small intestine capable of deconjugating bile acids. In patients with extensive ileal resections (short bowel syndrome) or those with postvagotomy diarrhea who are consuming a normal diet, cholestyramine may slightly reduce the fluidity of the diarrhea but may cause increased steatorrhea due to excessive binding of bile salts. In these patients, the concomitant use of small amounts of cholestyramine and a diet low in animal fats supplemented with medium-chain triglycerides and a hydrophilic colloid may control diarrhea while permitting caloric balance. Cholestyramine will bind the toxin of *Clostridium difficile* and thus may be used to treat antibiotic-induced pseudomembranous colitis.

Cholestyramine resin may cause constipation or perianal irritation.

ROUTE, USUAL DOSAGE, AND PREPARATIONS. *Oral: Adults*, initially, 4 g three times daily; for maintenance, 4 g four times daily before meals and at bedtime. In many patients with ileal resection, the maintenance dose can be reduced to 4 g before breakfast or to 2 g before other meals. The preparation is suspended in 120 to 180 ml of water or, when necessary, in pulpy juices, mashed banana, applesauce, gelatin, or cooked cereal. The drug should never be swallowed dry because of the hazard of esophageal irritation or blockage. To reduce the risk of adsorption of thyroid hormones, anticoagulants, digitalis glycosides, and, possibly, other oral medication, cholestyramine resin should be given at least four hours after a dose of other drugs.

> *Questran* (Mead Johnson). Packets (9 g) and powder (378 g) providing 4 g of active drug per packet or 9 g scoop.

CORTISOL (Hydrocortisone)
[Cortenema, Rectoid]

METHYLPREDNISOLONE ACETATE
[Medrol]

Retention enemas containing one of these adrenal corticosteroids are useful in the treatment of nonspecific ulcerative proctitis and ulcerative or Crohn's proctosigmoiditis. They also may be of value in the treatment of irradiation proctitis. Approximately 50% of the steroid is absorbed from noninflamed mucosa, but larger amounts may be absorbed if the mucosa is acutely inflamed. Studies by the manufacturer of Medrol Enpak showed approximately 16% absorption compared to an oral dose. In responsive patients, a beneficial effect is usually noted within 48 hours.

All of the serious toxic reactions accompanying large oral or parenteral doses of adrenal corticosteroids may occur with use of these rectal preparations (see Chapter 41, Adrenal Corticosteroids); the same precautions regarding sodium restriction and anticipation of the metabolic effects of pharmacologic doses of adrenal corticosteroids should be observed.

ROUTE, USUAL DOSAGE, AND PREPARATIONS. *Rectal*: A retention enema containing cortisol 100 mg or methylprednisolone acetate 40 mg is instilled once or twice daily. The enema is inserted with the patient in the left Sims's position. Since optimal absorption is achieved with prolonged retention, the patient should lie quietly for at least 30 minutes after instillation. Dosage usually is reduced over a period of weeks as improvement occurs.

CORTISOL:
Cortenema (Rowell), *Rectoid* (Pharmacia). Retention enema 100 mg in 60 ml disposable single-dose containers.
METHYLPREDNISOLONE ACETATE:
Medrol (Upjohn). Retention enema 40 mg (Medrol Enpak). Preparations also may be prepared by the pharmacist.

METRONIDAZOLE
[Flagyl]

Metronidazole, a trichomonacide and amebicide, is more effective than furazolidone and as effective as quinacrine in the treatment of giardiasis. However, the incidence of untoward effects is lowest with metronidazole. It is bactericidal for anaerobic coliforms and has been used to treat Crohn's disease with uncertain results. More effective results have been obtained in the treatment of anaerobic organisms encountered in variations of the blind loop syndrome.

The drug occasionally causes nausea and, less commonly, diarrhea. Some patients receiving metronidazole experience a disulfiram-type reaction after the ingestion of alcohol or an increase in blood pressure caused by the release of sympathomimetic amines. Reversible distal (usually sensory) polyneuropathy has been noted following completion of longer courses of therapy using larger doses. Mutagenic effects encountered in the laboratory have limited the utilization of metronidazole.

For use of metronidazole in the treatment of amebic dysentery, see Chapter 82, Antiprotozoal Agents.

ROUTE, USUAL DOSAGE, AND PREPARATIONS. *Oral*: For treatment of giardiasis, *adults and children over 30 kg*, 250 mg three times daily; *children 19 to 29 kg*, 250 mg twice daily; *14 to 19 kg*, 125 mg three times daily; *under 14 kg*, 125 mg twice daily. Treatment should be continued for seven days or until stool examinations are negative. For acute amebic dysentery, 750 mg three times daily for ten days.

Flagyl (Searle). Tablets 250 mg.

PHTHALYLSULFATHIAZOLE
[Sulfathalidine]

This drug is hydrolyzed to sulfathiazole in the large intestine; since sulfathiazole is poorly absorbed from the colon, it produces concentrations that inhibit most colonic bacteria. Empirically, phthalylsulfathiazole is beneficial as an adjunct in the long-term management of inflammatory bowel disease (eg, regional enteritis, ulcerative colitis), chronic diverticulitis (but sulfisoxazole is preferred), and the preoperative preparation of patients undergoing bowel surgery. There are no controlled studies establishing efficacy or comparing its usefulness with that of sulfasalazine in these disorders. Phthalylsulfathiazole has been used to treat acute and chronic bacillary dysentery, but sulfadiazine and sulfisoxazole are more effective. The sulfonamides are ineffective against many strains of *Shigella* because of the development of resistance.

Enough sulfathiazole may be absorbed from the colon to produce the usual adverse reactions of the sulfonamides (see Chapter 77). It should not be used in patients with renal insufficiency, urinary or intestinal obstruction, porphyria, sensitivity to other sulfonamides, or glucose-6-phosphate dehydrogenase deficiency. This sulfonamide should be used cautiously during pregnancy.

ROUTE, USUAL DOSAGE, AND PREPARATIONS. *Oral*: *Adults*, 50 to 100 mg/kg of body weight in four or six divided doses. Daily dosage should not exceed 8 g. *Children over 2 years*, 50 mg/kg daily in four or six divided doses.

Drug available generically: Tablets 500 mg.
Sulfathalidine (Merck Sharp & Dohme). Tablets 500 mg.

QUINACRINE HYDROCHLORIDE
[Atabrine Hydrochloride]

This acridine derivative was once widely used for the field prophylaxis of malaria (see Chapter 82, Antiprotozoal Agents). It is as effective as metronidazole in the treatment of giardiasis. Either drug could follow the use of the other in the event of a treatment failure.

Headache and gastrointestinal disturbances occur frequently when the drug is used for giardiasis.

ROUTE, USUAL DOSAGE, AND PREPARATIONS. *Oral*: For giardiasis, *adults*, 100 mg three times daily for five to seven days; *children*, 8 mg/kg of body weight daily divided into three doses for five days.

Atabrine Hydrochloride (Winthrop). Tablets 100 mg.

SULFASALAZINE
[Azulfidine, S.A.S.-500]

Sulfasalazine is partially absorbed in the upper intestine and re-enters the intestine with bile. It is converted to sulfapyridine and 5-aminosalicylic acid by colonic bacteria. Sulfapyridine and its metabolites are absorbed to provide therapeutic blood levels, but 5-aminosalicylic acid is only minimally absorbed. Nevertheless, recent studies suggest that this latter moiety is the active ingredient.

Results of controlled clinical studies suggest that sulfasalazine may prolong remissions in patients with chronic, recurrent idiopathic or granulomatous ulcerative colitis. Its mode of action in ulcerative colitis is unknown, but both beneficial effects and adverse reactions have been thought to be associated with the blood level of sulfapyridine, although increasing evidence suggests that 5-aminosalicylic acid may be responsible for the clinical effect, possibly by inhibiting synthesis of prostaglandins. The degree to which sulfapyridine is acetylated is thought to influence the patient's susceptibility to adverse reactions; those in whom acetylation is slow may require smaller doses and are more likely to develop untoward effects. The effect of sulfasalazine on intestinal flora has not been fully elucidated. It has been suggested that the drug's ability to inhibit anaerobes is a factor in its action in inflammatory bowel disease. This sulfonamide is not effective in the treatment of bacillary dysentery.

Adverse reactions (eg, headache, anorexia, nausea, vomiting, fever, rash, hypersensitivity reactions) are common, especially with daily doses exceeding 2 g. A reduction in dose or discontinuation of therapy may be necessary. Agranulocytosis and other blood dyscrasias, sometimes fatal, have occurred rarely. Both immune and nonimmune hemolytic anemia occur, the latter more commonly in G6PD-deficient patients. Hypersensitivity pneumonitis and a lupus-like syndrome have been reported. The drug should be given cautiously during pregnancy; the potential teratogenicity has not been fully investigated. Kernicterus may occur in newborn infants. Complete blood counts should be performed periodically when long-term drug therapy is undertaken. Crystalluria and nephrolithiasis have been reported. As with use of other early sulfonamides, ample daily fluid intake should be maintained to prevent crystalluria.

ROUTE, USUAL DOSAGE, AND PREPARATIONS. *Oral*: Initially, *adults*, 1 to 4 g daily in four to eight divided doses; *children and infants over 2 months*, 40 to 60 mg/kg of body weight daily in four to eight divided doses. For maintenance, *adults*, up to 2 g daily in four divided doses. To prevent attacks of chronic ulcerative colitis, 3 g may be necessary daily in divided doses. Some patients will not maintain remission with a dose of 2 g daily. *Children*, 30 mg/kg daily in four divided doses. Toxic reactions are common when 8 g daily is administered. The efficacy of enteric-coated tablets in patients with inflammatory bowel disease is not clinically established.

Drug available generically: Tablets 500 mg.
Azulfidine (Pharmacia). Tablets 500 mg; tablets (enteric-coated) 500 mg (Azulfidine-EN).
S.A.S.-500 (Rowell). Tablets (film-coated) 500 mg.

VANCOMYCIN
[Vancocin]

Vancomycin, a bactericidal glycopeptide, is effective in the treatment of staphylococcal enterocolitis. More recently, it has been used successfully against *Clostridium difficile* whose toxin has been shown to be the cause of the antibiotic-associated pseudomembranous colitis. Cholestyramine resin has also been used successfully in this disorder. Studies employing both have shown that vancomycin will control the few cases that do not appear to be responding as promptly as desired. Although this drug is absorbed poorly from the intestine and is usually given intravenously for colitis or enterocolitis, it also may be taken as an oral solution.

Extravasation outside the vein or intramuscular injection produces necrosis. Chills, fever, nausea, rash, and eosinophilia have been encountered. Because of the possible occurrence of ototoxicity and nephrotoxicity, the patient's renal function should be monitored and the drug should not be given concurrently or sequentially with the aminoglycosides. Deafness may progress even when vancomycin is stopped. (See also Chapter 75, Miscellaneous Antibacterial Agents.)

ROUTES, USUAL DOSAGE, AND PREPARATIONS. *Intravenous, Oral*: After dilution with either normal sodium chloride injection or 5% dextrose in water according to instructions provided by the manufacturer, the following dosages are given: *Adults*, 500 mg every 6 hours or 1 g every 12 hours. *Children*, 44 mg/kg of body weight in two or four divided doses. The drug may be stored in the refrigerator for four and seven days for the intravenous and oral forms, respectively.

> *Vancocin Hydrochloride* (Lilly). Powder (injection) 500 mg and (oral) 10 g.

MIXTURES

The use of mixtures containing opiates or poorly absorbed antibacterial agents (often in inadequate dosage) with adsorbents and protectants (most commonly, kaolin and pectin) and antispasmodic agents is unwarranted, since additional benefits beyond those afforded by the single effective agent are questionable, and the patient is subjected to the combined adverse effects of the individual ingredients and the added expense of all of these agents.

The following mixtures are popular with some physicians and the laity. Varying degrees of symptomatic relief may be associated with their use, but their effectiveness in influencing the speed of recovery from diarrhea is questionable. Preparations containing opium are classified as Schedule V substances under the Controlled Substances Act.

> *Bismuth, Pectin, & Paregoric* (Lemmon). Each tablet contains powdered opium 1.2 mg, bismuth subgallate 120 mg, pectin 15 mg, kaolin 120 mg, and zinc phenolsulfonate 15 mg.
> *Corrective Mixture* (Beecham). Each 5 ml of elixir contains zinc sulfocarbolate 10 mg, phenyl salicylate 20 mg, bismuth subsalicylate 80 mg, and pepsin 40 mg with or without paregoric 0.6 ml (nonprescription).
> *Donnagel* (Robins). Each 30 ml of suspension contains kaolin 6 g, pectin 142.8 mg, hyoscyamine sulfate 0.1037 mg, atropine sulfate 0.0194 mg, and scopolamine hydrobromide 0.0065 mg (nonprescription).
> *Donnagel PG* (Robins). Each 30 ml of suspension contains the same formulation as Donnagel plus powdered opium 24 mg.
> *Kaolin Mixture with Pectin*. Suspension; liquid (various manufacturers).
> *Kaopectate* (Upjohn). Each 30 ml of suspension contains kaolin 5.4 g and pectin 120 mg (nonprescription).
> *Kaopectate Concentrate* (Upjohn). Each 30 ml of concentrate contains kaolin 8.1 g and pectin 180 mg (nonprescription).
> *Parepectolin* (Rorer). Each 30 ml of suspension contains opium 15 mg (paregoric equivalent 3.7 ml), pectin 162 mg, and kaolin 5.5 g (nonprescription).
> *Pargel* (Parke, Davis). Each 30 ml of suspension contains kaolin 6 g and pectin 130 mg (nonprescription).
> *Polymagma* (Wyeth). Each tablet contains activated attapulgite 500 mg, pectin 45 mg, and hydrated alumina powder 70 mg (nonprescription).

Selected References

Proposal to establish monographs for OTC laxatives, antidiarrheal, emetic, and antiemetic products, II. Antidiarrheals. *Federal Register* 40:12924-12934, 12942-12943, (March 21) 1975.

Baron JII, et al: Sulphasalazine in asymptomatic Crohn's disease. Multicentre trial. *Gut* 18:69-72, 1977.

Duncombe VM, et al: Double-blind trial of cholestyramine in post-vagotomy diarrhoea. *Gut* 18:531-535, 1977.

DuPont HL, et al: Symptomatic treatment of diarrhea with bismuth subsalicylate among students attending a Mexican university. *Gastroenterology* 73:715-718, 1977.

Kramer P: Effect of antidiarrheal and antimotility drugs on ileal excreta. *Am J Dig Dis* 22:327-332, 1977.

Sack DA, et al: Prophylactic doxycycline for travelers' diarrhea: Results of prospective double-blind study of Peace Corps volunteers in Kenya. *N Engl J Med* 298:758-763, 1978.

Laxatives | 59

Most normally active, healthy people eating a balanced diet have no problem with bowel function. The consistency, frequency, and even the quantity of stool ordinarily can be influenced by eating adequate amounts of high-residue, naturally laxative foods (fruit and vegetables, high-fiber cereals) and drinking an ample amount of liquid. Maintenance of proper toilet habits and regular exercise also are necessary.

Hard dry stools are formed when the frequency of defecation is reduced; increased water reabsorption from the feces in the distal colon or rectum accompanies common constipation. Use of laxatives or inattention to the urge to defecate are among the causes of reduced sensitivity or loss of the rectal defecatory reflex. When some stimulant or saline laxatives are taken, the colon may be evacuated from the ascending colon instead of the usual site, the distal descending or sigmoid colon. After such overemptying, two to five days usually elapse before the normal fecal column can be re-established. Worry regarding the lack of bowel movement during this period provokes repetition of the use of the laxative, and a vicious cycle is established: Spontaneous bowel function is reduced, stronger laxatives in larger doses are used, and the laxative habit becomes fixed. Unfortunately, many people have misconceptions concerning the necessity for daily bowel movements and, because a variety of laxative preparations are available and are advertised aggressively, overuse of laxatives leading to dependence is a problem, especially with stimulant laxatives.

Indications

With few exceptions, there is no justification for prescribing drugs that perpetuate and intensify the condition for which they are used initially. In most instances, laxatives should be used only temporarily, and the agent chosen for treatment of constipation should not overempty the bowel.

Laxatives influence fecal consistency, accelerate the passage of feces through the colon, and facilitate elimination of stool from the rectum. They ease the pain of elimination in patients with an episiotomy wound, painful thrombosed hemorrhoids, anal fissures or perianal abscesses and reduce excessive straining and increased intra-abdominal pressure in those with body wall and diaphragmatic hernias or anorectal stenosis. Patients with aneurysm or other diseases of the cerebral or coronary arterial vessels are spared the brief, potentially hazardous excessive straining during defecation.

Laxatives also are used (1) to relieve constipation during pregnancy or the puerperal period; (2) in geriatric patients with poor eating habits whose abdominal and perineal muscles have lost their tone; (3) in children with congenital or acquired megacolon; (4) in those whose bowel motility has been altered through use of anticholinergic drugs or narcotics; (5) to prevent or decrease colonic absorption of ammonia in patients with hepatic encephalopathy; (6) to prepare the bowel prior to surgery and radiologic, proctoscopic, or colonoscopic procedures; (7) to provide a fresh stool for parasitologic examination; (8) to accelerate excretion of various parasites, including nematodes, after anthelmintic therapy; and (9) to hasten excretion of a poisonous substance in the alimentary tract.

Types of Laxatives

An outmoded classification of laxatives, based upon the consistency of the stool passed and the amount of cramping produced, included: laxatives (mildest), cathartics (stronger), and drastic vegetable purgatives (most irritant). The latter caused violent cramping and watery stool capable of producing hypovolemic shock and hemorrhagic enteritis. Calomel (mercurous chloride), once widely used as a cathartic, produced many deaths from mercury-induced kidney disease. Consequently, use of all of the drastic vegetable purgatives and most of the cathartics has been abandoned.

A classification based on the degree of irritation or stimulation of the bowel includes the following: bulk-forming agents, stimulants, saline cathartics, lubricants, and wetting agents. A more recent classification of laxatives is based on their effect upon intestinal electrolyte transport and the ability of an agent to increase fecal water excretion. As the understanding of mechanisms increases, this last grouping will probably be the surviving classification. When possible, the manner in which increased fecal water excretion is accomplished by the various agents is described. Enemas also are given to empty the rectum and colon.

Bulk-Forming Agents: When taken with adequate amounts of liquid, these agents absorb water and expand, increasing the water content and bulk volume of the stool. Normal peristalsis is stimulated, thereby increasing motility. Bulk-forming agents are generally nonabsorbable and are probably the safest laxatives when adequate quantities of liquids are ingested concomitantly.

The initial response usually occurs in 12 to 24 hours but, in patients who use laxatives chronically, up to three days may be required before the fecal column reaches the rectum. Use of these agents in patients with diverticulosis and the irritable bowel syndrome is increasing. A number of them have been used to improve the consistency of stools in patients with chronic watery diarrhea; anal maceration and discomfort and predefecatory cramps are relieved and the number of evacuations may be reduced, but the water content of the total amount of stool passed is unchanged. An exception may exist with use of bran: Change in the composition of fecal bile acids may enhance water and electrolyte accumulation in the colon. Bulk-forming laxatives may bind bile salts in vivo, and a cholesterol-lowering effect is noted in hypercholesterolemic patients. Claims for the efficacy of bulk-forming preparations in the treatment of obesity have not been substantiated.

Stimulants: The precise mechanism of action for each drug in this group has not been established, but each appears to cause intestinal fluid to accumulate. There is no conclusive evidence that stimulants have a direct mucosal irritant effect; however, morphologic changes of surface epithelium are produced and permeability is increased. Direct stimulation of intramural nerve plexuses has not been proved. Reflex stimulation of peristalsis following stimulation of sensory nerves may partly explain the effect of bisacodyl [Dulcolax] and phenolphthalein, which produce a semifluid or soft stool with little or no colic. Castor oil is hydrolyzed in the upper small intestine to ricinoleic acid, a long-chain fatty acid which stimulates colonic accumulation of water and electrolytes.

The anthraquinone-containing stimulant cathartics (eg, cascara, senna, danthron [Dorbane, Modane]) are widely used and abused. Some of the active glycosides are absorbed in the small intestine, circulated through the portal system and into the general circulation, and excreted in the bile, urine, saliva, colonic mucosa, and in the milk of lactating women. These cathartics usually act within 6 to 12 hours after ingestion. Cascara has the mildest action and produces a soft or formed stool with little or no colic. Danthron, a synthetic compound whose active ingredient is free anthraquinone, has a similar effect. Crude senna also produces a soft or formed stool, but usually there is more muscle contraction with cramping. Rhubarb and aloe are the most potent; since their ingestion almost always results in colic, they should not be used. In view of the availability of wetting agents and bulk-forming laxatives, it is difficult to justify the continued widespread use of stimulant laxatives.

Because of their hyperosmolarity, glycerin suppositories promote defecation by producing tissue dehydration and reflex contraction or act as an irritant to stimulate rectal contraction; they also may lubricate and soften inspissated fecal material. These preparations are safe for temporary use to re-establish proper toilet habits in patients who have lost the rectal reflex. Rectal instillation of hypertonic sorbitol stimulates defecation but appears to have no advantage over glycerin.

Saline Cathartics: These agents include a group of salts, one or both ions of which are poorly and slowly absorbed. A hypertonic solution of such a salt may draw a substantial volume of fluid into the intestinal lumen osmotically and stimulate stretch receptors to increase peristalsis. Release of cholecystokinin-pancreozymin (CCK-PZ) with consequent stimulation of intestinal secretory and motor activity has been proposed as an added mechanism of action of the magnesium salts.

The commonly used salts in this class are magnesium carbonate, oxide, citrate, hydroxide, or sulfate; sodium sulfate or phosphate; and mixed sodium and potassium tartrate. The saline cathartics are used after ingestion of anthelmintics or poisons to hasten the evacuation of worms or toxic materials; certain salts (eg, sodium phosphates oral solution [Fleet's Phospho-Soda]) provide a liquid stool for parasite examination without rupture of trophozoites. Saline cathartics also are given to empty the bowel before various procedures are performed. They usually act within two to six hours.

Lubricants: Mineral oil (liquid petrolatum), olive oil, and cottonseed oil are representatives of this group. However, only mineral oil is indigestible and currently used as a laxative. Its exact mechanism of action is not known but it softens the feces and is used to prevent injury to hemorrhoidal tissue or further irritation of anal fissures and to lessen the strain of evacuation (eg, in patients with hernia or cardiovascular disease).

Wetting Agents: Docusate sodium (dioctyl sodium sulfosuccinate) [Colace], docusate potassium (dioctyl potassium sulfosuccinate) [Kasof], and docusate calcium (dioctyl calcium sulfosuccinate) [Surfak] soften the feces supposedly by lowering surface tension, thus permitting the fecal mass to be penetrated by intestinal fluids. Although this emollient effect may exist, there is evidence that mucosal permeability is increased and water absorption is inhibited in the jejunum and that similar concentrations of docusate sodium inhibit colonic absorption and/or increase intraluminal water and electrolytes. In these respects, the drugs are similar to bile salts, which are anionic detergents. In this manner, they also may be considered as stimulant laxatives. Poloxamer 188 [Magcyl] is similarly promoted, but proof of its efficacy is not as well established. These laxatives are replacing mineral oil when it is important to lessen the strain of defecation.

Miscellaneous Agents: Belladonna tincture may be a useful adjunct in the treatment of constipation-induced cramping associated with irritable colon. Thyroid replacement therapy substantially improves the constipation encountered in patients with hypothyroidism.

Sorbitol and another poorly absorbed sugar, lactulose, are not digested enzymatically but are hydrolyzed in part to lactic, acetic, and pyruvic acids by coliforms and produce an acid pH that may have a mild stimulating effect upon colonic muscle; fluid accumulates in the colon because of the osmotic effect of the acid metabolites of lactulose, and this action may produce loose stools. For use of lactulose to prevent and treat portal systemic encephalopathy, see Chapter 51, Replenishers and Regulators of Water and Electrolytes.

Enemas: Indications for enemas include (1) to assist in the relief of impaction, (2) to empty the rectum and colon for x-ray or endoscopic procedures, and (3) to cleanse the large bowel prior to surgery or delivery. Their regular use also may be helpful in some patients with fecal incontinence or colostomies. Very small enemas occasionally may be substituted for glycerin suppositories to re-establish the rectal reflex in the treatment of constipation. Results are achieved by chemical irritation or distention of the bowel wall with resultant peristalsis and fragmentation, liquefaction, or lubrication of the feces.

Solutions used for enemas include tap water, saline, mineral oil, and hypertonic fluids. Except for administration of adrenal corticosteroids or other agents in distal inflammatory bowel disease, retention enemas are no longer a common mode of administering drugs. The small-volume (4.5 oz) prepackaged lubricant (mineral oil), hypertonic (sorbitol, sodium phosphate-biphosphate), or detergent (docusate potassium) enema kits are convenient and are fairly safe for self-administration.

Numerous complications are associated with either the solution employed or a faulty mode of administration. Most enema solutions produce mucosal irritation, sometimes accompanied by excess mucus in the stool. Early ulcerative proctosigmoiditis is simulated, and patients with this disease may become worse. Peroxide, household detergents, and hypertonic solutions (sodium phosphate-biphosphate) are the most irritating. Thus, if the rectum must be cleansed before proctoscopy, a saline enema is least likely to alter the appearance of the mucosa. If a question regarding the mucosa remains, the examination should be repeated without preparation.

Weakness, excessive perspiration, shock, convulsions, and/or coma may occur as a result of water intoxication and dilutional hyponatremia. This occurs in patients with megacolon given a water enema in the customary volume (500 ml). Children and the elderly are most vulnerable. Tap water or soapsuds enemas have caused weakness and incoordination in elderly patients causing them to fall; fracture of the femur is not uncommon. Convulsions with hypocalcemia have occurred after absorption of large amounts of phosphate by children given enemas with the sodium phosphate-biphosphate-type kit.

Over 250 mEq of potassium has been recorded in the collected output following use of tap water, and serious hypokalemia has occurred. This danger must be anticipated in patients receiving thiazides or more potent congeners as antihypertensive agents or diuretics.

Increased fluid retention follows retention of sodium in patients with congestive heart failure, cirrhosis, or nephrosis. Although use of isotonic sodium chloride solution (one level teaspoon salt/pint of water) is commonly employed in older individuals, a patient's tendency to retain fluid should modify this choice; in studies on sodium phosphate-biphosphate (eg, Fleet's Phospho-Soda) employing a standard unit (4 oz), 36 to 715 mg of radioactive sodium Na 21 has been shown to be absorbed. Small-volume disposable kits containing sorbitol or a wetting agent docusate potassium) may be used instead.

Methemoglobinemia has occurred transiently following a soapsuds enema containing hexachlorophene. Heating this alkaline solution produces an absorbable aromatic amine that, in small quantities, caused the grey cyanosis of methemoglobinemia. Only pure castile soap should be used (20 ml of soap solution to 1 or 1.5 liters of water). Colitis with toxic megacolon, serious serosanguinous fluid loss, anaphylaxis, and rectal gangrene have occurred following use of more concentrated solutions of various soaps. Alkaline soapsuds enemas should be avoided in the presence of portal-systemic encephalopathy, since they increase diffusion of ammonia into the portal circulation.

Rectal abrasion and laceration have been produced by a hard enema tip inserted aggressively. They may sometimes cause bleeding or draining pus. Laceration resulting in perforation may cause ischiorectal abscess. The rectal wall is insensitive above the pectinate line, and thus the patient may be unaware of the injury. Free perforation with fecal peritonitis occurs when the transmural tear is above the peritoneal reflection. Inflamed sigmoidal diverticula are vulnerable to rupture if water pressure is increased even slightly. Syringes should be avoided to prevent high intraluminal pressures. The enema fluid level should be no higher than 18 to 20 inches above the anus, and no more than 750 ml of fluid should be instilled over a 10-minute period. Only soft plastic or rubber tubes with side openings should be inserted. To help prevent damage, the anus should be well lubricated with petroleum jelly or similar preparations.

In view of the above, use of enemas obviously should be confined only to patients in whom they are clearly indicated and when no adequate substitute can be provided.

Adverse Reactions and Precautions

A laxative should never be given to patients with undiagnosed abdominal pain, intestinal obstruction, or fecal impaction. Constipation that reflects a change in bowel habits must be thoroughly investigated.

The continuous use of stimulant laxatives infrequently results in the irritable bowel syndrome or diarrhea that is severe or prolonged enough to cause hyponatremia, hypokalemia, dehydration, hyperaldosteronism, protein-losing gastroenteropathy with hypoalbuminemia, steatorrhea, osteomalacia, and changes in the x-ray appearance of the colon simulating megacolon or ulcerative colitis. It is primarily the stimulant group of laxatives that is abused. A safe rule recommended by some clinicians is that the stimulant should not be used regularly for longer than one week without a laxative-free period to avoid the development of dependence.

Elderly patients prepared for various diagnostic procedures must be watched closely, since weakness, incoordination, and orthostatic hypotension are exaggerated and loss of electrolytes is significant after several copious watery stools. Fractures are not unusual when these patients fall on their way to and from the toilet.

In general, the use of stimulant laxatives should be avoided in children. Some parents give laxatives to their children in the belief that a daily bowel movement is essential; laxative-dependent constipation is created in this manner.

Most anthraquinone-containing stimulants discolor the urine and colonic mucosa (melanosis coli); this is presumed to be innocuous and is reversible. Anthraquinones are excreted in the milk of lactating mothers. Since the need for stimulant laxatives is questionable in these patients, another type of laxative should be prescribed.

Impaction or obstruction may occur if the bulk-forming agents are temporarily arrested in their passage through parts of the alimentary canal. Water is absorbed and the bolus becomes inspissated within the bowel lumen. Thus, any abnormal narrowing of the diameter of the lumen at any level of the gastrointestinal tract represents a hazard to the use of these products. Inspissation does not occur in a normal bowel if bulk laxatives are taken with one or more glasses of water. Allergic reactions (urticaria, nonseasonal rhinitis, dermatitis, and bronchial asthma) may be a serious consequence of the use of plant gums. Digitalis, salicylates, and nitrofurantoin are bound by cellulose. Sodium intake is increased substantially with use of carboxymethylcellulose sodium, which contains approximately 2.7 to 4 mEq sodium/g. Marked fluid retention has been reported when carboxymethylcellulose sodium was used as an anorexiant. A number of these preparations contain significant amounts of dextrose as a dispersing agent; this must be considered when these products are administered to diabetic patients.

Congestive heart failure has been precipitated through indiscriminant use of saline cathartics containing sodium, and coma or death from hyperkalemia and hypermagnesemia has been observed in patients with renal insufficiency who use these drugs. Tetany with hypocalcemia and hyperphosphatemia is also encountered when phosphate salts are used by patients with impaired renal function.

Lipid pneumonia caused by aspiration and syndromes reflecting reduced absorption of the fat-soluble vitamins have occurred after long-term use of mineral oil, and deposits of mineral oil in the liver have been reported. Intestinal absorption is facilitated when mineral oil is taken with a fecal softener.

The calcium and sodium salts of docusate (and probably the potassium salt) are absorbed to some extent in the duodenum and proximal jejunum. Their metabolic fate, the bioavailability of drugs taken with them, and the significance of their absorption are unknown and require further study. Morphologic changes and increased mucosal permeability have been noted in vitro. These potent wetting agents should be prescribed in the smallest effective amounts.

The sodium phosphate-biphosphate preparations (eg, Fleet's Phospho-Soda) and bisacodyl [Dulcolax] may cause sloughing of the surface rectal epithelium. Inflammatory changes after the short-term use of bisacodyl may resemble those seen in mild idiopathic ulcerative proctitis. Se-

cretory doses of ricinoleic acid may produce erosion of villous tips and disorganization of the microvillous surface of the small intestine that results in increased mucosal permeability to molecules as large as 16,000 molecular weight dextran.

BULK-FORMING AGENTS

CARBOXYMETHYLCELLULOSE SODIUM

$$X = H \text{ or } CH_2\overset{O}{\overset{\|}{C}}O^- Na^+$$

METHYLCELLULOSE

These cellulose derivatives are indigestible and nonabsorbable. When mixed with water, a bulky hydrophilic colloid forms which stimulates natural peristalsis and which, upon reaching the colon, becomes part of the stool. These agents have been used to decrease the fluidity of the stools in patients with chronic watery diarrhea. Fluid retention caused by the substantial amounts of sodium in carboxymethylcellulose has occurred after use of this preparation in overweight patients.

ROUTE, USUAL DOSAGE, AND PREPARATIONS. *Oral: Adults*, 4 to 6 g daily; *children over 6 years*, 1 to 1.5 g daily. The drug should be taken with one or two glasses of water and ingested rapidly.

Drugs available generically.

KARAYA GUM (Sterculia Gum)

This indigestible, nonabsorbable vegetable gum contains hydrophilic polysaccharides that act like other bulk-forming laxatives.

Allergic reactions and urticaria have been reported rarely.

ROUTE, USUAL DOSAGE, AND PREPARATIONS. *Oral:* 5 to 10 g daily taken with an adequate amount of fluid.

Drug available generically in bulk form.

PLANTAGO SEED (Psyllium Seed)

PSYLLIUM HYDROPHILIC COLLOID
[Effersyllium, Konsyl, L.A. Formula, Metamucil, Modane Bulk]

The whole or powdered seeds of the three species of *Plantago* or the refined colloid obtained from psyllium seeds are rich in mucilage (a hemicellulose). These preparations increase bulk by imbibing water. They are indigestible and nonabsorbable but may bind bile salts and cholesterol. Choleretic diarrhea caused by vagotomy, small bowel resection, or disease of the terminal ileum may be improved with use of psyllium hydrophilic colloid, but cholestyramine resin is more effective.

Two species of plantago seed (*P. psyllium* and *P. indica*) produce pigmentation of renal tubules in animals, but this effect is not observed with the third species (*P. ovata*). No abnormalities in renal function have been noted in men receiving large doses of the seed for two to seven years.

ROUTE, USUAL DOSAGE, AND PREPARATIONS. PLANTAGO SEED:

Oral: Adults, 2.5 to 30 g daily; *children over 6 years,* 1.25 to 15 g daily. The preparation should be added to a glass of water and ingested rapidly.
    Drug available generically under the name Psyllium Seed.

PSYLLIUM HYDROPHILIC COLLOID:

Oral: Adults, 1 rounded teaspoonful (7 g) or one packet (instant mix) is mixed with a glass of water or other suitable fluid; the liquid is ingested rapidly one to three times daily. A second glass of water enhances the effect.
    Effersyllium (Stuart). Granular powder (instant mix) (nonprescription).
    Konsyl, L.A. Formula (Burton, Parsons). Powder (nonprescription).
    Metamucil (Searle). Powder in effervescent (instant mix; sodium content, 250 mg) and noneffervescent form (nonprescription).
    Modane Bulk (Warren-Teed). Powder (nonprescription).

POLYCARBOPHIL

Polycarbophil, a hydrophilic polyacrylic resin, is indigestible, nonabsorbable, and metabolically inert. It has more water-binding activity than the other bulk-forming agents, absorbing up to 60 times its weight in water. Because of this property, polycarbophil is an effective laxative and antidiarrheal agent. No toxicity has been observed in animal studies.

ROUTE, USUAL DOSAGE, AND PREPARATIONS. *Oral: Adults,* 4 to 6 g daily; *infants up to 2 years,* 0.5 to 1 g daily; *children 2 to 5 years,* 1 to 1.5 g daily; *6 to 12 years,* 1.5 to 3 g daily.
    Drug available generically: Granules.

STIMULANTS

BISACODYL
[Dulcolax]

Bisacodyl produces a soft to formed stool within six hours after ingestion and 15 minutes to one hour after rectal administration. Emptying is sufficient to permit use of this agent to prepare patients for proctoscopic or colonoscopic procedures.

Colic and diarrhea severe enough to cause hypokalemia and muscle weakness have been reported after the occasional use of bisacodyl. Tetany occurs when metabolic alkalosis accompanying the hypokalemia reduces ionized serum calcium levels. The tablets must be swallowed whole to avoid gastric irritation. They should not be taken within one hour after ingestion of milk or antacids in order to prevent premature dissolution of the enteric coating and resultant dyspepsia. The suppository may produce mild smarting or tenesmus, and continued rectal administration may cause proctitis; hence, prolonged use is undesirable.

ROUTES, USUAL DOSAGE, AND PREPARATIONS.
Oral: *Adults*, 10 mg (range, 5 to 15 mg); up to 30 mg may be given to prepare the lower gastrointestinal tract for special procedures. *Children 6 years and older*, 5 mg.

> Drug available generically: Tablets (plain, enteric-coated) 5 mg.
> *Dulcolax* (Boehringer Ingelheim). Tablets (enteric-coated) 5 mg (nonprescription).

Rectal: *Adults and children over 2 years*, 10 mg; *under 2 years*, 5 mg.

> Drug available generically: Suppositories 10 mg.
> *Dulcolax* (Boehringer Ingelheim). Suppositories 10 mg (nonprescription).

CASCARA SAGRADA

Cascara is one of the mildest of the anthraquinone-containing stimulant laxatives. Its effect on the small intestine is insignificant or slight, but it stimulates mass peristalsis in the large intestine. The drug produces a soft or formed stool in six to eight hours with little or no colic when used occasionally in standard doses.

Prolonged use may produce benign pigmentation of the colonic mucosa (melanosis coli) that may regress after cascara sagrada is discontinued. This agent imparts a yellowish-brown color to acid urine and a reddish color to alkaline urine. The active principles of cascara are excreted in the milk of lactating mothers but the amounts are usually insufficient to exert a laxative effect upon the infant. Nevertheless, because many substitutes exist, stimulant laxatives should not be given to lactating mothers.

ROUTE, USUAL DOSAGE, AND PREPARATIONS.
Oral: *Adults*, 200 to 400 mg of extract, 0.5 to 1.5 ml of fluidextract, or 5 ml of aromatic fluidextract.

> Forms available generically: Tablets 300 mg; fluidextract (plain, aromatic), liquid, powder.

CASTOR OIL
CASTOR OIL, AROMATIC
CASTOR OIL, EMULSIFIED
[Neoloid]

Castor oil has been classified as a stimulant because lipolysis in the small intestine liberates ricinoleic acid. This long-chain fatty acid directly stimulates smooth muscle and inhibits the absorption of water and electrolytes resulting in fluid accumulation in vitro, but it is not known whether these changes affect fluid movement or are related to castor oil's laxative effect in vivo.

Castor oil produces one or more copious, watery evacuations two to six hours after ingestion. The colon is emptied so completely that passage of normal stool may be delayed for two days or more. This strong cathartic should not be used to treat common constipation. Since castor oil thoroughly empties gas and feces from the intestines, it is used to prepare patients for radiologic examination. If chilled castor oil is taken with fruit juice or a carbonated beverage is consumed immediately thereafter, tolerance is improved. Neoloid, a mint-flavored emulsion of castor oil, also may be more palatable.

Castor oil causes morphologic changes in the small intestine and increased mucosal permeability. Because of its strong action, the patient experiences more colic and may be more vulnerable to dehydration and electrolyte imbalance.

ROUTE, USUAL DOSAGE, AND PREPARATIONS.
CASTOR OIL; CASTOR OIL, AROMATIC:
Oral: *Adults*, 15 to 60 ml; *children*, 5 to 15 ml; *infants under 2 years*, 1 to 5 ml.

> Forms available generically: Capsules; liquid.

CASTOR OIL, EMULSIFIED:
Oral: *Adults*, 30 to 60 ml; *infants*, 2.5 to 7.5 ml; *children*, dose is adjusted between that used for infants and adults.

> *Neoloid* (Lederle). Liquid 36.4% (nonprescription).

DANTHRON
[Dorbane, Modane]

This synthetic anthraquinone has a mode of action similar to that of other stimulant laxatives (see the Introduction). It produces a soft to semifluid stool in six to eight hours.

Melanosis coli has been reported after prolonged use; this benign pigmentation gradually disappears after the drug is discontinued. Since danthron is excreted in milk, it probably should not be given to lactating mothers. It also imparts a pink color to alkaline urine.

ROUTE, USUAL DOSAGE, AND PREPARATIONS. *Oral*: *Adults*, 75 to 150 mg. Stimulant laxatives should be used sparingly if at all in children. One manufacturer's suggested dosage is: *Children 6 to 12 years*, one-half the adult dose; *1 to 6 years*, one-eighth to one-half the adult dose, depending on age (in liquid dosage form).

 Drug available generically: Tablets 75 mg.
 Dorbane (Riker). Tablets 75 mg (nonprescription).
 Modane (Warren-Teed). Liquid 37.5 mg/5 ml and alcohol 5%; tablets 37.5 (Mild) and 75 mg (nonprescription).

GLYCERIN SUPPOSITORIES

Glycerin suppositories promote fecal evacuation in 15 to 30 minutes by stimulating rectal contraction as a hyperosmotic substance. This preparation also may soften and lubricate inspissated fecal material. It is used temporarily to re-establish proper toilet habits in laxative-dependent patients.

ROUTE, USUAL DOSAGE, AND PREPARATIONS. *Rectal*: *Adults*, 3 g; *children under 6 years*, 1 to 1.5 g.

 Drug available generically.

PHENOLPHTHALEIN

Phenolphthalein (white or yellow) acts primarily on the large intestine to produce a semifluid stool in four to eight hours with little or no colic. An in vitro study has shown that sodium is secreted, which can cause water to accumulate in the ileum. The claim that yellow phenolphthalein is three times more potent than the white form has not been substantiated. The action of a single dose of phenolphthalein may persist for three to four days as a result of its enterohepatic circulation. This stimulant is the active agent in many over-the-counter laxative preparations.

Dermatitis (fixed drug eruptions, pruritus, burning, vesiculation, and residual pigmentation) may occur in hypersensitive patients. Fatal anaphylactic reactions have been reported, but an absolute causal relationship with phenolphthalein has not been established. Nonthrombocytopenic purpura has been reported occasionally, and dehydration from excessive laxative action or electrolyte imbalance after prolonged use occurs infrequently. Phenolphthalein imparts a pink color to alkaline urine or feces.

ROUTE, USUAL DOSAGE, AND PREPARATIONS. *Oral*: *Adults*, 30 to 270 mg daily; *children 6 years and older*, 30 to 60 mg daily; *2 to 5 years*, 15 to 20 mg daily.

 Drug available generically: Powder; tablets, wafers 60 mg.

SENNA WHOLE LEAF PREPARATIONS
SENNOSIDES A AND B
 [Glysennid]
SENNA POD PREPARATIONS
 [Senokot]

The actions and uses of this anthraquinone-type stimulant laxative are similar to those of cascara, but senna is more potent. Defecation occurs 6 to 12 hours after ingestion.

Senna is available as the crude drug (Senna; Senna Fluidextract; Senna Syrup), as crystalline senna glycosides (sennosides A and B [Glysennid]), and as a standardized, purified concentrate from senna pod [Senokot]. The purified preparations are used more commonly than the crude forms and have some different pharmacologic effects; they are claimed to produce colic and loose stools only rarely when used in recommended dosage.

Melanosis coli has not been reported with senna products despite the fact that senna is an anthracene derivative. Crude senna preparations may impart a yellowish-brown color to acid urine and a reddish color to alkaline urine. Senna pod preparations are not excreted in maternal milk.

ROUTES, USUAL DOSAGE, AND PREPARATIONS.

SENNA WHOLE LEAF PREPARATIONS:

Oral: *Adults*, 0.5 to 2 g (senna); 2 ml (senna fluidextract); 8 ml (senna syrup). *Children 6 to 12 years*, one-half adult dose; *2 to 5 years*, one-quarter adult dose; *under 2 years*, one-eighth adult dose.

Drug available generically: Leaves; powder.

SENNOSIDES A AND B:

Oral: *Adults*, one or two tablets before retiring; *children over 10 years*, one or two tablets; *6 to 10 years*, one tablet.

Glysennid (Dorsey). Tablets 12 mg (calcium salt) (nonprescription).

SENNA POD PREPARATIONS:

Oral: (Granules) *Adults*, 1 level teaspoonful to a maximum of 2 level teaspoonsful two times daily; *geriatric, obstetric, or gynecologic patients and children over 27 kg*, dosage reduced by one-half. (Syrup) *Adults*, 2 to 3 teaspoonsful one or two times daily; *geriatric, obstetric, or gynecologic patients*, dosage reduced by one-half; *children 5 to 15 years*, 1 to a maximum of 2 teaspoonsful two times daily; *1 to 5 years*, one-half to a maximum of 1 teaspoonful two times daily; *1 month to 1 year*, one-quarter to a maximum of one-half teaspoonful twice daily. (Tablets) *Adults*, two tablets to a maximum of four tablets two times daily; *geriatric, obstetric, or gynecologic patients and children over 27 kg*, dosage reduced by one-half.

Senokot (Purdue Frederick). Granules, syrup, tablets (nonprescription).

Rectal: *Adults*, one suppository; if necessary, a second suppository may be adminis-tered two hours later. *Children over 27 kg*, one-half suppository.

Senokot (Purdue Frederick). Suppositories (nonprescription).

SALINE CATHARTICS

MAGNESIUM, POTASSIUM, AND SODIUM SALTS

Many different salts having essentially the same actions are used as saline cathartics. They produce a fluid or semifluid evacuation in two to six hours and are most effective if taken with substantial amounts (at least 240 ml) of fluid on an empty stomach. These preparations are given to empty the bowel prior to surgical, radiologic, proctoscopic, or colonoscopic procedures. They also are useful in eliminating parasites and toxic vermifuge after anthelmintic therapy and in removing toxic material in some cases of poisoning. Certain phosphate-biphosphate (phospho-soda) preparations are rendered isotonic in the small intestine. The watery diarrhea produced does not destroy the osmotically sensitive trophozoites of *Entamoeba histolytica* or *Giardia lamblia*. Thus, these preparations are suitable for the collection of fresh stool specimens for parasite examination. The same laxative used as an enema destroys the trophozoites but not the cyst forms of *E. histolytica*.

Magnesium and potassium salts are contraindicated in patients with impaired renal function. The bitter taste of magnesium sulfate may cause nausea, and the magnesium salts should not be used with neomycin. Sodium salts are contraindicated in cardiac patients with edema or evidence of congestive heart failure or in those on a low-sodium diet.

For dosages, see the following Table.

LUBRICANTS

MINERAL OIL (Liquid Petrolatum)

Mineral oil is an indigestible liquid hydrocarbon of limited absorbability. It has been used orally to lessen the strain of evacuation of inspissated stool (eg, in patients with hernia or cardiovascular disease) or rectally to ease the passage of impacted or dried fecal material by softening and lubricating it. The emulsified preparations are claimed to reduce seepage through the anal sphincter and to be more effective than nonemulsified preparations, but conclusive evidence from controlled studies has not been presented. The use of mineral oil has decreased with the advent of the bulk-forming laxatives and wetting agents.

Because prolonged oral use (more than two weeks) coats the mucosa of the small intestine, absorption of fat-soluble vitamins (A, D, E, and K) is reduced. The patient should be warned that lipid pneumonia

may occur if mineral oil is aspirated and that untoward effects such as hepatic infiltration can result from its absorption. Because of this possibility, use of mineral oil with the wetting agents, which may further increase its absorption, is contraindicated. Mineral oil is still used by some surgeons after anorectal surgery, despite the fact that it sometimes causes pruritus ani, and laceration of the area from scratching or rubbing interferes with healing. Droplets of the inert material act as a foreign body in the wound.

ROUTES, USUAL DOSAGE, AND PREPARATIONS. *Oral: Adults,* 15 to 45 ml two times daily; *children over 6 years,* 10 to 15 ml of plain mineral oil at bedtime or 0.25 to 5 ml of the emulsion two times daily.

SALINE CATHARTICS

Preparation	Usual Dose (Adults)[1,2]
Fleet enema (Fleet) (solution containing 16 g sodium biphosphate and 6 g sodium phosphate/dl)	4 oz (rectal only)
Magnesium carbonate	8 g
Magnesium citrate solution (1.55 to 1.9 g/dl magnesium oxide with citric acid anhydrous and potassium bicarbonate for effervescence)	200 ml
Milk of Magnesia (7% to 8.5% magnesium hydroxide suspension)	15 ml
Magnesium oxide	4 g
Magnesium sulfate	10 to 30 g
Phospho-Soda (Fleet) (aqueous solution containing 48 g sodium biphosphate and 18 g sodium phosphate/dl)	10 to 20 ml
Potassium bitartrate	2 g
Potassium phosphate	4 g
Potassium sodium tartrate	5 to 10 g
Sodium phosphate	3.6 to 7.2 g
Sodium phosphate, effervescent, dried	10 g
Sodium phosphate solution	7.5 g
Sodium sulfate	15 g
Seidlitz powders (blue powder paper, sodium bicarbonate 2.5 g and potassium sodium tartrate 7.5 g; white powder paper, tartaric acid 2.2 g)	contents of one blue and one white powder paper mixed in about 60 ml of water.

[1]*Dosage is reduced for children (see table in Chapter 2).*

[2]*Except where indicated, all doses are administered orally. Many manufacturers market their own flavored versions of various saline cathartics, which tend to be more expensive then the generic preparations.*

Rectal: *Adults*, 120 ml; *children over 6 years*, 60 ml.

> Drug available generically.
> AVAILABLE TRADEMARKS.
> *Agoral, Plain* (Parke, Davis), *Fleet Mineral Oil Enema* (Fleet), *Kondremul Plain* (Fisons), *Petrogalar, Plain* (Wyeth) (all nonprescription).

WETTING AGENTS

DOCUSATE CALCIUM (Dioctyl Calcium Sulfosuccinate)
[Surfak]

DOCUSATE POTASSIUM (Dioctyl Potassium Sulfosuccinate)
[Kasof]

DOCUSATE SODIUM (Dioctyl Sodium Sulfosuccinate)
[Colace]

These wetting agents soften the feces and are used to lessen the strain of defecation (eg, in persons with hernia or cardiovascular disease). The drugs are used for constipation produced by delay in rectal emptying. In vitro studies suggest that they lower the surface tension of the stool to permit water and lipids to enter more readily and thus soften the feces. There is, however, no evidence relating this observation to an increase in fecal water excretion. Water absorption may be inhibited in the small and large bowel. Other evidence indicates that they may stimulate secretion of water and electrolytes and alter the microscopic appearance of the epithelium in the colon. These preparations require one to two days or more to exert their full effect, since it may be that long before the softened fecal bolus reaches the rectum.

The potassium salt may be of some benefit in patients requiring sodium restriction. The manufacturer claims that once-a-day dosage is adequate; however, some clinicians believe that twice-daily dosage is more effective.

Wetting agents are often combined with other laxatives with little justification. Their use with mineral oil is contraindicated because they may increase the absorption of the latter. When delay in rectal emptying is the only factor causing constipation, there is no rationale for use of combinations of stimulants and wetting agents.

Diarrhea is the only reported adverse reaction. No serious adverse effects from the use of these agents alone have been reported. However, morphologic damage to the rat intestine has been observed.

ROUTE, USUAL DOSAGE, AND PREPARATIONS.
DOCUSATE CALCIUM, DOCUSATE SODIUM:

Oral: *Adults and children over 12 years*, 50 to 360 mg daily; *2 to 12 years*, 50 to 150 mg daily of the sodium salt. It is suggested that 8 to 10 ounces of water be taken with each dose.

> DOCUSATE CALCIUM:
> *Surfak* (Hoechst-Roussel). Capsules 50 and 240 mg (nonprescription).
> DOCUSATE SODIUM:
> Drug available generically under the name Dioctyl Sodium Sulfocuccinate: Capsules 50, 100, and 250 mg; syrup 20 mg/5 ml; tablets 100 mg.
> *Colace* (Mead Johnson). Capsules 50 and 100 mg; solution for drops 10 mg/ml; syrup 20 mg/5 ml (nonprescription).

DOCUSATE POTASSIUM:
The manufacturer's recommended dosage is:
Oral: *Adults*, 240 mg once daily.

> *Kasof* (Stuart). Capsules 240 mg (nonprescription).

POLOXAMER 188
[Magcyl]

The actions and uses of this oxyalkene polymer are similar to those of docusate calcium and docusate sodium (see the evaluation). Data are insufficient to determine its comparative efficacy as a wetting agent. A three- to five-day period may be required before a laxative effect is noted.

Animal studies suggest that the toxicity of poloxamer 188 is minimal. It should not be administered with mineral oil because absorption of the latter may be increased.

ROUTE, USUAL DOSAGE, AND PREPARATIONS. *Oral: Adults,* 250 mg two or three times daily after meals; 8 ounces of liquid should be taken with each dose.

> *Magcyl* (Elder). Capsules 250 mg (nonprescription).

MIXTURES

There is no satisfactory evidence to prove that laxative mixtures are advantageous. With a knowledge of the mechanism of action of the various laxatives and an understanding of the individual patient's problem, the need for mixtures should be minimized. Too often, constipation caused by delay in passage of fecal material through the colon, delay in evacuating the rectum, or simply insufficient quantity of stool may be converted to a more serious condition if a combination containing a stimulant and bulk-forming agent or a stimulant and wetting agent is used injudiciously. Selecting a single appropriate drug produces the best results. Use of combinations containing wetting agents with stimulants (eg, Dialose Plus, Dorbantyl, Peri-Colace) or lubricants (eg, Milkinol) may increase absorption. Effects upon absorption of other drugs used are unknown and potentially may affect response to other drugs.

The following partial listing of available mixtures is provided only for information; it is not intended to be complete and, in certain instances, represents an unfortunate commentary on the motives that led to the formulation of these products. This listing does not signify a recommendation for use.

Agoral (Parke, Davis). Each 15 ml contains white phenolphthalein 200 mg in an emulsion of 42% mineral oil (nonprescription).

Dialose (Stuart). Each capsule contains docusate sodium 100 mg and carboxymethylcellulose sodium 400 mg (nonprescription).

Dialose Plus (Stuart). Each capsule contains casanthranol 30 mg, docusate sodium 100 mg, and carboxymethylcellulose sodium 400 mg (nonprescription).

Dorbantyl (Riker). Each capsule contains danthron 25 mg and docusate sodium 50 mg; each Forte capsule contains danthron 50 mg and docusate sodium 100 mg (nonprescription).

Doxidan (Hoechst-Roussel). Each capsule contains danthron 50 mg and docusate calcium 60 mg (nonprescription).

Haley's M-O (Winthrop). Liquid emulsion containing milk of magnesia and mineral oil 25% (nonprescription).

Hydrocil (Rowell). Powder containing psyllium mucilloid 40%, karaya gum 10%, and dextrose (nonprescription).

Maltsupex (Wallace). Tablets, liquid, and powder containing malt soup extract and potassium carbonate (liquid, 1.5%; powder, 1.8%) (nonprescription).

Milkinol (Kremers-Urban). Liquid containing docusate sodium and mineral oil (nonprescription).

Peri-Colace (Mead Johnson). Each capsule contains casanthranol 30 mg and docusate sodium 100 mg; each 5 ml of syrup contains casanthranol 10 mg, docusate sodium 20 mg, and alcohol 10% (nonprescription).

Selected References

Dietary fibre. *Lancet* 2:337-338, 1977.

Proposal to establish monographs for OTC laxative, antidiarrheal, emetic, and antiemetic products, I. Laxatives. *Federal Register* 40:12902-12924, 12939-12942, (March 21) 1975.

Binder HJ: Pharmacology of laxatives. *Annu Rev Pharmacol Toxicol* 17:355-367, 1977.

Meisel JL, et al: Human rectal mucosa: Proctoscopic and morphological changes caused by laxatives. *Gastroenterology* 72:1274-1279, 1977.

Phillips SF: A further look at laxatives. *Gastroenterology* 70:464, 1976.

Saunders DR, et al: Effect of bisacodyl on structure and function of rodent and human intestine. *Gastroenterology* 72:849-856, 1977.

Miscellaneous Gastrointestinal Agents | 60

ANTICHOLINERGIC ANTISPASMODICS

Indications: The anticholinergic antispasmodics include the naturally occurring belladonna alkaloids, their derivatives, and numerous synthetic substitutes. These agents are used less frequently in the management of patients with peptic ulcer since the introduction of the H₂ receptor antagonists. There are still instances in which antacids, H₂ receptor antagonists, and anticholinergic agents may be combined: more effective control of nocturnal secretion, of persistent gastric ulcer pain, or of escape from control in Zollinger-Ellison syndrome. Anticholinergic compounds are sometimes given to treat pancreatitis. Pancreatic secretion is stimulated when hydro-chloric acid causes liberation of secretin from the duodenal mucosal epithelium. Inhibition of gastric secretion thus may be of value regardless of any direct inhibition of pancreatic exocrine secretion by anticholinergic drugs. H₂ receptor antagonists may be useful in this condition as well. Anticholinergic compounds also are used to treat certain bradyarrhythmias.

Synthetic antispasmodics, alone or with mild sedatives, are useful as adjuncts in the management of functional bowel disorders (eg, dyspepsia, irritable colon) or mild diarrhea and in the symptomatic control of nonobstructive cramps. These drugs may be effective in symptomatic diffuse esophageal spasm. They are of no value in achalasia, asymptomatic diverticulosis, biliary dyskinesia, and dysmenorrhea. Opinion is divided on their usefulness in regional enteritis and acute ulcerative colitis, probably because it is difficult to determine when the inflammation is severe enough to result in a drug-induced ileus. Toxic megacolon may follow quickly, especially in children and undernourished patients with severe active inflammation.

Actions: The naturally occurring *belladonna alkaloids* are hyoscyamine and scopolamine (hyoscine). Hyoscyamine, the main active alkaloid, racemizes to atropine on extraction. Its antimuscarinic activity is primarily due to the levo isomers, which are 7 to 15 times more potent than racemic mixtures or the dextro forms. There are no qualitative differences in the antimuscarinic effects of atropine and scopolamine. (See Table 1.)

Atropine, the prototype of this group, antagonizes the effect of acetylcholine at peripheral neuroeffector sites. It does not block transmission at the neuromuscular junction of skeletal muscle and has no effect on transmission at autonomic ganglia except when administered in toxic doses. This agent is readily absorbed from the gastrointestinal tract and crosses the blood-brain barrier, where large doses stimulate (presumably by leaving the adrenergic system unopposed) and toxic doses depress the central nervous system.

Atropine reduces both the peristaltic and secretory activity of the entire gastrointestinal system. It reduces the tone of the ureter and urinary bladder and has a slight inhibitory action on the bile ducts and gallbladder. It has little effect upon the myometrium and inhibits bradycardia produced by vagal stimulation. Atropine antagonizes the effects of cholinergic drugs on the gastrointestinal system but is less effective in counteracting the action of these drugs on the urinary bladder. The cholinergic agents, bethanechol [Myotonachol, Urecholine] and neostigmine methylsulfate [Prostigmin], stimulate gastrointestinal smooth muscle. Bethanechol has been shown to be effective in symptomatic esophageal reflux. Tragic consequences can result if these agents are mistakenly used in the treatment of postoperative intestinal atony or adynamic ileus when, in fact, mechanical ileus is present.

The *synthetic anticholinergic agents* (see Table 1) are substituted quaternary ammonium compounds, with the exception of oxyphencyclimine [Daricon], a tertiary amine. Quaternary ammonium compounds are less readily absorbed than tertiary amines when given orally, and there is considerable individual variability in response. These drugs rarely exert an effect on the central nervous system because they do not readily cross the blood-brain barrier. Most of the actions of these synthetic anticholinergics at usual doses are attributable to their antimuscarinic effect.

Adequate doses of anticholinergic antispasmodics relieve pain by inhibiting motility and secretions, and these agents also may have a local anesthetic action. Their use in the treatment of peptic ulcer is based on their ability to block acetylcholine at postganglionic parasympathetic neuroeffector sites in smooth muscle and secretory glands, thus reducing gastric motility and secretion of hydrochloric acid. Although total gastric acid secretion is reduced, the concentration of hydrochloric acid and output of pepsin and mucus are minimally affected. The anticholinergic agents augment the acid-inhibiting action of cimetidine [Tagamet]; however, this property has yet to be fully investigated clinically except in occasional cases of Zollinger-Ellison syndrome in which therapy with cimetidine alone is insufficient. In active ulcer, anticholinergic agents inhibit nighttime secretion. Cimetidine achieves the same result more effectively and with fewer side effects. However, until its long-term effects are better defined, there may be instances in which chronic inhibition may be achieved with less risk using the anticholinergic agents.

Dose requirements vary markedly among patients and may differ from those recommended by the manufacturer. The effective dose of the anticholinergics is determined by increasing the amount to just below that which causes mild adverse effects (eg, dryness of the mouth, blurred vision). However, doses sufficient to inhibit basal secretion generally provoke side effects, and patient compliance may be a problem.

Anticholinergic agents usually are administered orally before meals and at bedtime; timed-release preparations are given less frequently.

A number of *synthetic derivatives of belladonna alkaloids* act mainly but not exclusively as antispasmodics (see Table 2); they relax smooth muscle primarily through a nonspecific direct action on muscle fiber. These agents have little or no antimuscarinic activity and have a minimal effect on gastric secretion.

Adverse Reactions and Precautions: Untoward effects associated with use of anticholinergic agents include dryness of the mouth, anhidrosis, mydriasis, cycloplegia, tachycardia, constipation, dysuria, and acute urinary retention, all of which may appear after administration of therapeutic doses. Dermatologic reactions also may occur. Tolerance to some of these reactions develops with continued use and/or smaller doses, but effectiveness may be reduced. Toxic doses may produce extreme dryness of the mouth accompanied by a burning sensation, dysphagia, thirst, marked photophobia, flushing, fever, leukocytosis, rash, nausea, vomiting, tachycardia, and hypotension or hypertension. Ileus or toxic megacolon has been reported in some patients with severe forms of inflammatory, ischemic, or amebic colitis.

Large doses of the antispasmodics may produce signs of central nervous system stimulation (eg, restlessness, tremor, irritability, delirium, hallucinations). Stimulation may be followed by depression and death from medullary paralysis. Children are more susceptible to the toxic effects of these drugs than adults.

Large doses of the quaternary ammonium compounds may cause ganglionic blockade, as evidenced by orthostatic hypotension and impotence, and toxic doses may cause respiratory arrest as a result of neuromuscular blockade. Since quaternary ammonium compounds do not readily cross the blood-brain barrier, cen-

tral nervous system effects occur only rarely.

Anticholinergic drugs are contraindicated in the treatment of reflux esophagitis because they decrease both esophageal and gastric motility and relax the lower esophageal sphincter; these actions thus promote gastric retention by delaying gastric emptying, which enhances reflux. They should be used with caution in patients with prostatic hypertrophy, pyloric obstruction, obstruction of the bladder neck, and congestive heart failure with tachycardia. The anticholinergic drugs may precipitate an attack of acute glaucoma in patients predisposed to angle closure because of their mydriatic effect. This has occurred occasionally after parenteral administration but only rarely after oral use. Anticholinergic drugs can be given safely to patients with open-angle glaucoma who are being treated with miotics.

Since antacids may interfere with absorption of anticholinergic agents, these drugs should not be taken simultaneously.

Untoward effects reported with some of these drugs include drowsiness, euphoria, dizziness, asthenia, headache, nausea, constipation, diarrhea, hypotension, and rash.

Mixtures Containing Anticholinergic Antispasmodics

Many widely promoted mixtures contain anticholinergic antispasmodics in combination with antianxiety agents, barbiturates, or phenothiazines to facilitate relaxation. Although antispasmodics aid in the relief of symptoms of some functional gastrointestinal disorders, there is no evidence that they directly relieve ulcer pain or hasten healing of an ulcer. Moreover, most combination products do not provide an adequate amount of either anticholinergic agent or sedative. Anticholinergic compounds require greater individualization of dosage than most drugs to be effective. Since the need for adjustments in the dose of the ingredients is seldom parallel, it would be necessary to add or subtract one of the ingredients, eliminating the advantages of the combination. A mixture con-

TABLE 1.
ANTICHOLINERGIC ANTISPASMODICS

Drug	Chemical Structure
BELLADONNA ALKALOIDS Atropine Sulfate	
Belladonna Extract	
Belladonna Leaf	
Belladonna Leaf Fluid- extract	
Belladonna Tincture	
Hyoscyamine Hydrobromide	
Hyoscyamine Sulfate	
MIXTURES OF BELLADONNA ALKALOIDS Bellafoline (total levorotatory alkaloids of belladonna as malates)	
Prydon	

Usual Dosage	**Preparations**
Oral, Subcutaneous: Adults, 0.3 to 1.2 mg every 4 to 6 hours.	Tablets 0.3, 0.4, and 0.6 mg
Subcutaneous: Children, 0.01 mg/kg every 4 to 6 hours.	Solution (for injection) 0.3 mg/ml in 30 ml containers; 0.4 mg/ml in 0.5, 1, 20, and 30 ml containers; 0.5 mg/ml in 5 and 30 ml containers; and 1 mg/ml in 1 and 10 ml containers
	Tablets (hypodermic) 0.3, 0.4, and 0.6 mg
Oral: Adults, 15 mg 3 times daily.	Tablets 15 mg
Oral: Adults, 30 to 200 mg.	No single-entity dosage form available; compounding necessary for prescription.
Oral: Adults, 0.06 ml 3 times daily.	Fluidextract in pint containers
Oral: Adults, 0.6 to 1 ml 3 or 4 times daily. *Children*, 0.03 ml/kg in 3 or 4 divided doses.	Tincture in pint and gallon containers
Oral, Intramuscular, Subcutaneous, Intravenous: Adults, 0.25 mg 3 or 4 times daily.	Powder

Oral: Adults, 0.125 to 0.25 mg every 4 to 6 hours. *Children 2 to 10 years*, one-half above dosage range; *under 2 years*, one-fourth above dosage range.
 	
Intramuscular, Subcutaneous, Intravenous: Adults, 0.25 to 0.5 mg every 4 to 6 hours. When symptoms are controlled, oral medication is substituted. *Children*, dosage not established.
	Anaspaz (Ascher):
	  Tablets 0.125 mg
	Levsin (Kremers-Urban):
	  Drops 0.125 mg/ml
	  Elixir 0.125 mg/5 ml
	  Tablets 0.125 mg
	  Tablets (timed-release) [Levsinex] 0.375 mg
	
	  Solution (for injection) 0.25 mg/ml in 1, 10, and 30 ml containers; 0.5 mg/ml in 1 ml containers

Oral: Adults, 1 or 2 tablets 3 times daily. *Children over 6 years*, ½ to 1 tablet 3 times daily.
Subcutaneous: Adults, 0.5 to 1 ml once or twice daily.
	Bellafoline (Sandoz):
	  Tablets 0.25 mg
	
	  Solution (for injection) 0.5 mg/ml in 1 ml containers

Oral: Adults, 1 capsule every 12 hours.	Prydon (Smith Kline & French): Capsules (timed-release) containing belladonna alkaloids 0.4 or 0.8 mg (hyoscyamine sulfate 0.305 or 0.610 mg, atropine sulfate 0.060 or 0.120 mg, and scopolamine hydrobromide 0.035 or 0.070 mg)

TABLE 1.
ANTICHOLINERGIC ANTISPASMODICS

Drug	Chemical Structure
QUATERNARY AMMONIUM DERIVATIVES OF BELLADONNA ALKALOIDS Homatropine Methylbromide	
Methscopolamine Bromide	
SYNTHETIC SUBSTITUTES Anisotropine Methylbromide	
Diphemanil Methylsulfate	
Glycopyrrolate	

Usual Dosage	Preparations
Oral: Adults, 2.5 to 10 mg 4 times daily. *Children,* 3 to 6 mg 4 times daily (chewable tablets). *Infants,* 0.3 mg dissolved in water 5 or 6 times daily.	Powder

Oral: Adults, 2.5 to 5 mg 4 times daily. *Children,* 0.2 mg/kg daily in 4 doses.
 	
Intramuscular, Subcutaneous: Adults, 0.25 to 1 mg every 6 to 8 hours until acute symptoms are controlled and patient can take oral medication. *Children,* dosage not established.
	Pamine [bromide] (Upjohn):
	  Tablets 2.5 mg
	  Solution (for injection) 1 mg/ml in 1 ml containers
	Drug available generically under the name Scopolamine Methylbromide:
	  Powder

Oral: Adults, 50 mg 3 times daily.	Valpin 50 (Endo): Tablets 50 mg
Oral: Adults, initially, 100 to 200 mg every 4 to 6 hours; for maintenance, 50 or 100 mg every 4 to 6 hours. *Children,* dosage not established.	Prantal (Schering): Tablets 100 mg

Oral: Adults, initially, 1 or 2 mg 3 times daily; for maintenance, 1 mg 2 times daily. *Children,* dosage not established.
 	
Intramuscular, Intravenous, Subcutaneous: Adults, 0.1 or 0.2 mg at 4-hour intervals 3 or 4 times daily. *Children,* dosage not established.
	Robinul (Robins):
	  Tablets 1 and 2 mg (Forte)
	  Solution (for injection) 0.2 mg/ml in 1, 5, and 20 ml containers
	Drug available generically:
	  Tablets 1 and 2 mg

TABLE 1.
ANTICHOLINERGIC ANTISPASMODICS

Drug	Chemical Structure
Mepenzolate Bromide	
Methantheline Bromide	
*Oxyphencyclimine Hydrochloride	
Propantheline Bromide	

*Tertiary amine. All others are quaternary ammonium compounds.

Usual Dosage	Preparations

Oral: Adults, 25 mg 4 times daily. Dosage increased gradually to 50 mg if necessary.	Cantil (Merrell-National):
	    Liquid 25 mg/5 ml
	    Tablets 25 mg

Oral: Adults, initially, 50 to 100 mg every 6 hours; dose reduced to 25 mg for patients who cannot tolerate larger doses. For maintenance, generally one-half initial dose. *Children,* 5 to 10 mg/kg daily in 4 divided doses.	Banthine (Searle): Tablets 50 mg
Oral: Adults, 10 mg twice daily; dose gradually increased to 50 mg if untoward effects do not appear. *Children,* dosage not established	Daricon (Beecham): Tablets 10 mg

Oral: Adults, 15 mg 3 times daily and 30 mg at bedtime, or timed-release preparation given 2 or 3 times daily. *Children,* 1.5 mg/kg daily in 4 divided doses.
 	
Intramuscular, Intravenous: Adults, 30 mg every 6 hours. (Powder dissolved in not less than 10 ml of sodium chloride injection for intravenous administration.)
	Pro-Banthine (Searle):
	    Tablets 7.5 and 15 mg
	    Tablets (timed-release) 30 mg
	    Powder (for injection) 30 mg
	Drug available generically:
	    Tablets 15 mg

TABLE 2.
OTHER SYNTHETIC ANTISPASMODICS

Drug	Chemical Structure

Dicyclomine Hydrochloride

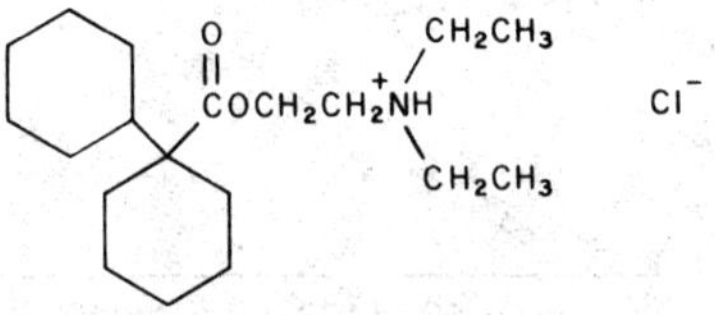

$$\text{(cyclohexyl)}_2 C\text{-}COCH_2CH_2\overset{+}{N}H(CH_2CH_3)_2 \quad Cl^-$$

Methixene Hydrochloride

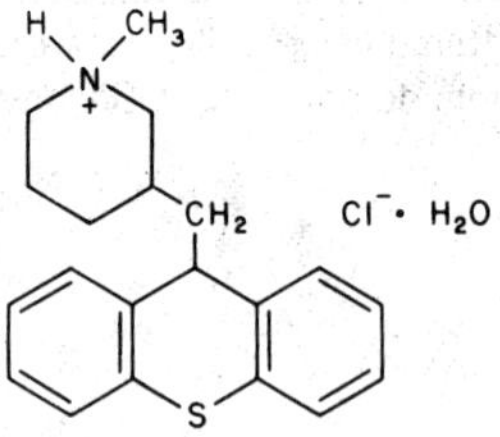

$$\text{(N-methylpiperidinyl)}\text{-}CH_2\text{-}\text{(thioxanthene)} \quad Cl^- \cdot H_2O$$

Thiphenamil Hydrochloride

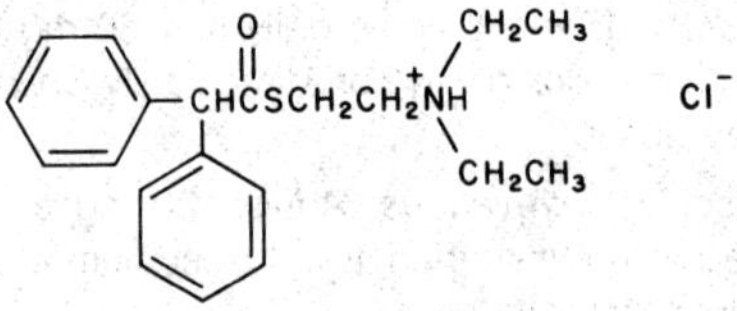

$$(C_6H_5)_2CH\text{-}CSCH_2CH_2\overset{+}{N}H(CH_2CH_3)_2 \quad Cl^-$$

Tridihexethyl Chloride

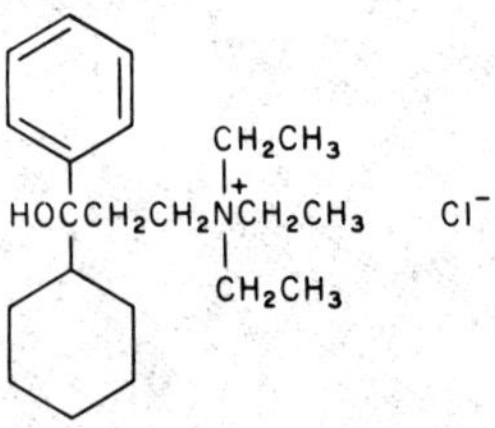

$$HOC(C_6H_5)(\text{cyclohexyl})CH_2CH_2\overset{+}{N}(CH_2CH_3)_3 \quad Cl^-$$

Usual Dosage	Preparations

Oral, Intramuscular: Adults, 10 to 20 mg 3 or 4 times daily. *Children*, 10 mg 3 or 4 times daily. *Infants*, 5 mg 3 or 4 times daily. Solution should not be given intravenously.	Bentyl (Merrell-National):
	  Capsules 10 mg
	  Syrup 10 mg/5 ml
	  Tablets 20 mg
	
	  Solution (for injection) 10 mg/ml in 2 and 10 ml containers
	Dyspas (Savage):
	  Liquid 10 mg/5 ml
	  Tablets 10 and 20 mg
	
	  Solution (for injection) 10 mg/ml in 2 and 10 ml containers
	Drug available generically:
	  Capsules 10 mg
	  Tablets 20 mg
	
	  Solution (for injection) 10 mg/ml in 10 ml containers
	  Syrup

Oral: Adults, 1 mg 3 times daily. Dose increased to 2 mg if necessary. *Children*, dosage not established.	Trest (Dorsey): Tablets 1 mg
Oral: Adults, initially, 400 mg every 4 hours. *Children over 6 years*, 200 mg every 4 hours. Dose given less frequently after symptoms are controlled.	Trocinate (Poythress): Tablets 100 and 400 mg

Oral: Adults, 25 mg 3 times daily before meals and 50 mg at bedtime. Dosage increased to 75 mg 4 times daily if necessary. Alternatively, timed-release preparation given every 12 hours; if necessary, this dose is given every 6 hours.
Subcutaneous, Intravenous, Intramuscular: Adults, 10 to 20 mg every 6 hours.
	Pathilon (Lederle):
	  Capsules (timed-release) 75 mg
	  Tablets 25 mg
	  Solution (for injection) 10 mg/ml in 1 ml containers

taining a phenothiazine is rarely appropriate, because phenothiazines are primarily *antipsychotic* agents and have a potential for serious adverse reactions. For these reasons, these mixtures should be avoided in ulcer therapy and used selectively in functional disorders, in which exact dosage is less critical.

AVAILABLE MIXTURES.

Belap (Lemmon). Each tablet contains belladonna extract 10.8 mg and phenobarbital 16.2 mg; each 5 ml of elixir contains belladonna leaf fluidextract 0.045 mg, phenobarbital 16.2 mg, and alcohol 22%.

Belladenal (Sandoz). Each tablet or timed-release tablet (Belladenal-S) contains levorotatory alkaloids of belladonna as malates 0.25 mg and phenobarbital 50 mg.

Bellergal (Dorsey). Each tablet contains levorotatory alkaloids of belladonna as malates 0.1 mg, ergotamine tartrate 0.3 mg, and phenobarbital 20 mg; each timed-release tablet (Bellergal-S) contains levorotatory alkaloids of belladonna as malates 0.2 mg, ergotamine tartrate 0.6 mg, and phenobarbital 40 mg.

Bentyl W/Phenobarbital (Merrell-National). Each capsule or 5 ml of syrup contains dicyclomine hydrochloride 10 mg, phenobarbital 15 mg, and alcohol 19% (syrup); each tablet contains dicyclomine hydrochloride 20 mg and phenobarbital 15 mg.

Butibel (McNeil). Each tablet or 5 ml of elixir contains belladonna extract 15 mg and butabarbital sodium 15 mg.

Cantil W/Phenobarbital (Merrell-National). Each tablet or 5 ml of liquid (Cantil-PHB) contains mepenzolate bromide 25 mg and phenobarbital 16 mg.

Chardonna-2 (Rorer). Each tablet contains belladonna extract 15 mg and phenobarbital 15 mg.

Combid (Smith Kline & French). Each timed-release capsule contains isopropamide iodide equivalent to isopropamide 5 mg and prochlorperazine maleate 10 mg.

Daricon PB (Beecham). Each tablet contains oxyphencyclimine hydrochloride 5 mg and phenobarbital 15 mg.

Donnatal (Robins). Each capsule, tablet, or 5 ml of elixir contains hyoscyamine sulfate 0.1037 mg, atropine sulfate 0.0194 mg, scopolamine hydrobromide 0.0065 mg, phenobarbital 16.2 mg, and alcohol 23% (elixir); each No. 2 tablet contains same formulation as Donnatal except phenobarbital 32.4 mg; each timed-release tablet contains hyoscyamine sulfate 0.3111 mg, atropine sulfate 0.0582 mg, scopolamine hydrobromide 0.0195 mg, and phenobarbital 48.6 mg.

Donphen (Lemmon). Each tablet contains hyoscyamine sulfate 0.1 mg, atropine sulfate 0.02 mg, scopolamine hydrobromide 6 mcg, and phenobarbital 15 mg.

Enarax (Beecham). Each tablet contains oxyphencyclimine hydrochloride 5 or 10 mg and hydroxyzine hydrochloride 25 mg.

Hybephen (Beecham). Each tablet or 5 ml of elixir contains hyoscyamine sulfate 0.1277 mg, atropine sulfate 0.0233 mg, scopolamine hydrobromide 0.0094 mg, phenobarbital 15 mg, and alcohol 16.5% (elixir).

Kinesed (Stuart). Each chewable tablet contains hyoscyamine sulfate 0.1 mg, atropine sulfate 0.02 mg, scopolamine hydrobromide 0.007 mg, and phenobarbital 16 mg.

Librax (Roche). Each capsule contains clidinium bromide 2.5 mg and chlordiazepoxide hydrochloride 5 mg.

Matropinal (Comatic). Each tablet contains homatropine methylbromide 10 mg and phenobarbital 15 mg; each Forte tablet contains homatropine methylbromide 10 mg and pentobarbital 90 mg; each 5 ml of elixir contains homatropine methylbromide 10 mg, phenobarbital 15 mg, and alcohol 15%; each suppository contains homatropine methylbromide 10 mg and pentobarbital 15 or 90 (Forte) mg.

Milpath (Wallace). Each tablet contains tridihexethyl chloride 25 mg and meprobamate 200 or 400 mg.

Pamine PB (Upjohn). Each tablet contains methscopolamine bromide 2.5 mg and phenobarbital 15 mg.

Pathibamate (Lederle). Each tablet contains tridihexethyl chloride 25 mg and meprobamate 200 or 400 mg.

Pathilon W/Phenobarbital (Lederle). Each tablet contains tridihexethyl chloride 25 mg and phenobarbital 15 mg; each timed-release tablet contains tridihexethyl chloride 75 mg and phenobarbital 45 mg.

Pro-Banthine W/Dartal (Searle). Each tablet contains propantheline bromide 15 mg and thiopropazate hydrochloride 5 mg.

Pro-Banthine W/Phenobarbital (Searle). Each tablet contains propantheline bromide 15 mg and phenobarbital 15 mg.

Robinul-PH (Robins). Each tablet contains glycopyrrolate 1 or 2 mg (Forte) and phenobarbital 16.2 mg.

Valpin 50-PB (Endo). Each tablet contains anisotropine methylbromide 50 mg and phenobarbital 15 mg.

AGENTS USED FOR REPLACEMENT THERAPY

Bile Acids or Salts

The major human bile acids are cholic and deoxycholic acids and chenodeoxycholic acid; the minor bile acids are lithocholic and ursodeoxycholic acids. Cholic acid and chenodeoxycholic acid are present in bile in about equal proportions (30% to 40%); there is usually less deoxycholic acid (10% to 20%). Lithocholic and ursodeoxycholic acids compose less than 5% of the biliary bile acids.

Cholic acid and chenodeoxycholic acid are formed from cholesterol in the liver. Deoxycholic and lithocholic acids result from the dehydroxylating action of anaerobic intestinal bacteria on cholic acid and chenodeoxycholic acid, respectively. Ursodeoxycholic acid is believed to be formed in the liver from the 7-keto derivative of chenodiol, which was previously formed by bacterial hydrogenation in the colon and circulated via the enterohepatic circulation.

Bile acids do not occur as such, but rather as N-glycine or N-taurine conjugates. Lithocholic acid not only is conjugated with glycine or taurine, but also is sulfated at the 3 position. Conjugation increases solubility of bile acids for a given pH, makes the bile acids more resistant to precipitation with calcium, and decreases passive intestinal absorption.

Bile is a concentrated micellar solution. The mixed micelles of bile acids and lecithin facilitate solubility of cholesterol; bile thus serves as the unique excretory pathway for cholesterol in man. Bile is secreted into the intestine during digestion and a mixed micelle with a new composition is formed; it contains predominantly fatty acids and monoglycerides which were formed by the action of lipase and colipase on dietary triglycerides. Bile acids facilitate absorption by enhancing the diffusion of the solubilized fat digestion products through the layer of water that coats the intestinal mucosa. Micellar solubilization of fat-soluble vitamins is essential for their absorption. The bile acids are reabsorbed mainly in the ileum by active transport and return to the liver where they are efficiently extracted and re-excreted in bile. The bile acid pool, that is, the mass of bile acids in the enterohepatic circulation, circulates six to ten times a day. The only input of bile acids into the enterohepatic circulation is by synthesis from cholesterol; the only loss is by fecal excretion.

Many conditions interfere with the enterohepatic circulation of bile acids. The major disturbances are biliary obstruction, interruption caused by bile fistula or ileal disease or resection, and contamination caused by bacterial overgrowth as, for example, in the stagnant loop syndrome. In any of these defects, micelle formation is impaired, causing fat maldigestion and mild to moderate steatorrhea.

At present, there is no satisfactory preparation of conjugated bile acids available for replacement therapy. Commercial ox bile preparations do not provide an adequate amount of conjugated bile acids, since about 4 to 8 g of bile acids are secreted with each meal. In addition, the commercial ox bile preparations induce diarrhea because dihydroxy bile acids cause water and electrolytes to be secreted by the human colon. Thus, use of bile acids in the treatment of vague symptoms attributable to deficiency of bile or intestinal malfunction does not appear justifiable and may cause undesirable side effects.

Bile acids play an important role in solubilizing cholesterol in bile. When bile acid secretion is decreased or cholesterol secretion is increased, bile contains an excess of cholesterol which may precipitate from solution and ultimately lead to the formation of cholesterol gallstones. Relatively large doses of chenodiol (chenodeoxycholic acid) (10 to 15 mg/kg/day) decrease cholesterol secretion in bile; the bile thus becomes desaturated with respect to cholesterol and cholesterol gallstones, if present, will dissolve in a substantial number of patients. Recent work indicates that ursodeoxycholic acid also will induce bile desaturation and dissolve cholesterol gallstones. The long-term place of medical treatment with these drugs versus surgical treatment remains to be established.

No medical treatment of pigment stones or calcium-containing stones has as yet been proposed, since stones ultimately recur when chenodiol is stopped and the cost of drugs for the rest of a patient's life is not small.

INDIVIDUAL EVALUATIONS

CHENODIOL (Chenodeoxycholic Acid)

This bile acid, which is available for investigational use only, increases cholesterol solubility in bile and thus is used to dissolve cholesterol gallstones. Six months to two years of therapy are usually required before an effect is noted. Medical treatment of cholesterol gallstones is most beneficial in patients with early disease in whom irreversible gallbladder damage has not occurred, and the ideal patient has multiple small radiolucent gallstones in a radiologically visualizing gallbladder. Effectiveness may be increased when a low-cholesterol diet is followed. When chenodiol is discontinued, bile becomes supersaturated again and the stones recur in some patients within a year. The newly formed stones may again be dissolved by chenodiol or the patient, if symptomatic, may be referred for a cholecystectomy. Radio-opaque gallstones or cholesterol gallstones containing a calcium surface do not respond to treatment with chenodiol. Efficacy in the treatment of choledocholithiasis has not been established.

To date, the use of chenodiol to dissolve cholesterol gallstones appears to be safe. Mild, transient diarrhea is the only significant adverse reaction observed. Slight elevations in the serum transaminase level occur in some patients, but no evidence of serious liver damage has as yet been reported. Trial of chenodiol during pregnancy has been restricted in the National Cooperative Study.

ROUTE, USUAL DOSAGE, AND PREPARATIONS. *Oral: Adults,* 10 to 15 mg/kg of body weight daily.

(Investigational drug)

DEHYDROCHOLIC ACID
[Decholin, Neocholan]

Dehydrocholic acid, a synthetic derivative of cholic acid, is promoted as a hydrocholeretic that increases bile flow in man. Controlled studies documenting the clinical usefulness of this agent have not been performed. The compound probably has a laxative action, since the dihydroxy bile acids, deoxycholic acid and chenodeoxycholic acid, induce water and electrolyte secretion from the human intestine, but controlled clinical trials are lacking. After absorption, dehydrocholic acid is extensively metabolized by the liver to hydroxyketo acids and ultimately to cholic acid. Therefore, it is likely that the metabolic products formed in the liver are the actual agents that induce water and electrolyte secretion by the human colon. Since the metabolites undergo enterohepatic circulation, it is likely that a laxative effect will not be observed for several days after use of the drug has been initiated.

Drug available generically: Tablets 225 mg.
Decholin (Dome), *Neocholan* (Dow). Tablets 250 mg (nonprescription).
Similar Drug.
KETOCHOLANIC ACID:
Ketochol (Searle). Tablets 250 mg.

Pancreatic Enzymes

Pancreatic enzymes (lipase, protease, and amylase) are extracted from hog pancreas. They are effective as replacement therapy in patients with diseases accompanied by a marked decrease in the secretion of these enzymes (eg, chronic pancreatitis, benign or malignant pancreatic tumors, cystic fibrosis, after pancreatectomy). These enzymes should be used only after the diagnosis of exocrine pancreatic insufficiency has been confirmed. There is no rationale for their use in gastrointestinal disorders unrelated to pancreatic enzyme deficiency or as remedies for dyspepsia or as "digestive aids."

Pancreatin [Panteric, Viokase] and pancrelipase [Cotazym, Ilozyme, Ku-Zyme HP, Pancrease] have largely replaced other pancreatic extracts used clinically. Some preparations are enteric-coated to avoid destruction by gastric pepsin or inactivation by acid pH; however, the coating may partially or completely affect the availability of the enzyme in the duodenum and upper jejunum where it is needed most. Pancrease, a new preparation in which the enzymes are present within small enteric-coated beads, has been shown to resist gastric inactivation. The increase in gastric and duodenal pH induced by cimetidine [Tagamet] more effectively prevents inactivation of pancreatic enzymes by hydrochloric acid than the ingestion of 30 ml of aluminum hydroxide or aluminum-magnesium hydroxide or 2 g of sodium bicarbonate three times daily.

Although allergic reactions to the animal protein in these preparations occur only rarely, allergic rhinitis and bronchospasm have developed as a result of sensitization induced by repeated inhalation of the powder by the patient or by others who handle the granules or tablets. These enzymes should be used cautiously in patients known to be sensitive to pork. However, sensitivity to ingested pork is not always present and does not necessarily develop in those who acquire respiratory symptoms from inhalation of pancreatic powder particles.

A preparation of pancreatin from a bovine source, Beef Viokase, contains 6 N.F. units of lipase activity per milligram. This is equivalent to three times the N.F. strength for pancreatin but provides only about 20% of the lipolytic activity of a porcine product. It does not meet the requirements for Pancreatin, N.F. because beef pancreas is deficient in amylase. This form of Viokase is provided as a service by the manufacturer for the rare patient who is allergic to pork. About three times more of the beef product than the pork product is required to maintain a patient. This preparation is extracted from raw beef pancreas by azeotropic desiccation instead of alcohol extraction.

Dosage should be individualized and should be based on the activity of the lipase, protease, and amylase in each product, not on the weight of the extract. Requirements depend upon the degree of maldigestion and malabsorption, the amount of fat in the diet, and the enzyme activity of each preparation. Preparations of much higher specific activity than those presently available are urgently needed to simplify and facilitate treatment.

The use of bile salts or proteolytic enzymes of plant origin (eg, proteolytic enzymes from *Carica papaya* [Papase]) is of no benefit in the treatment of exocrine pancreatic insufficiency.

INDIVIDUAL EVALUATIONS

PANCREATIN
[Panteric, Viokase]

These preparations are derived from hog pancreas and different products contain varying amounts of amylase, protease, lipase, and other constituents. Preparations containing three or four times the N.F. strength are available and the usual daily doses require 4 to 18 g of the extract.

See the introduction to this section for indications and precautions.

ROUTE, USUAL DOSAGE, AND PREPARATIONS. *Oral*: *Adults*, 4 to 18 g of extract (triple N.F. strength) daily in divided doses at mealtimes, at one- or two-hour intervals throughout the day, or before and within an hour after meals, with an extra dose taken with any food eaten between meals. No apparent advantage is gained from administration of the enzymes at any time other than when food is ingested. *Children*, initially, 300 to 600 mg with each meal. Dosage or frequency of administration may be increased to further reduce steatorrhea if nausea, vomiting, or diarrhea does not occur.

Drug available generically: Capsules 300 mg; powder; tablets 300 mg.

Panteric (Parke, Davis). Capsules 325 mg (three times N.F. strength); tablets (enteric-coated) 325 mg (three times N.F. strength) (nonprescription).

Viokase (VioBin). Powder; each 750 mg (1/3 teaspoon) contains lipase 15,000 N.F. units, protease 75,000 N.F. units, and amylase 112,500 N.F. units. Tablets 325 mg; each tablet contains lipase 6,500 N.F. units, protease 32,000 N.F. units, and amylase 48,000 N.F. units. Other enzymes from whole porcine pancreas are also present.

Beef Viokase (VioBin). Powder: each 1.5 g (2/3 teaspoon) contains amylase 11,500 units, lipase 9,000 units, and protease 75,000 units; each tablet contains not less than amylase 2,500 units, lipase 1,950 units, and protease 16,250 units. Product distributed by manufacturer as a service for those allergic to pork.

PANCRELIPASE
[Cotazym, Ilozyme, Ku-Zyme HP, Pancrease]

The action of pancrelipase, which is derived from hog pancreas, is qualitatively similar to that of other pancreatic enzyme preparations; however, its lipase activity is greater, permitting better control of steatorrhea. (At present, Ilozyme is the most -potent in terms of lipase activity.) Pancrelipase may be more acceptable to patients because of the smaller dosage required. Caution is advised in administering pancrelipase to patients known to be sensitive to pork.

See the Introduction to this section for indications and precautions.

ROUTE, USUAL DOSAGE, AND PREPARATIONS. *Oral: Adults,* 600 to 900 mg (one to three tablets or capsules) before each meal, 900 mg with meals, 600 mg within an hour after meals, and 300 mg with any food eaten between meals. *Children,* 300 to 600 mg taken in the same manner outlined for adults. In severe deficiency, 1 g every waking hour has been given.

Cotazym [porcine source] (Organon). Each capsule (regular, flavored) contains lipase 8,000 N.F. units, protease 30,000 N.F. units, and amylase 30,000 N.F. units; each packet of powder (regular) contains lipase 16,000 N.F. units, protease 60,000 N.F. units, and amylase 60,000 N.F. units; each packet of powder (flavored) contains lipase 40,000 N.F. units, protease

150,000 N.F. units, and amylase 150,000 N.F. units. Also present are other enzymes from whole hog pancreas and calcium carbonate precipitated 25 mg (capsules) or 50 mg (powder).

Ilozyme (Warren-Teed). Each tablet contains lipase 9,600 N.F. units, protease 40,000 N.F. units, and amylase 40,000 N.F. units.

Ku-Zyme HP (Kremers-Urban). Each capsule contains lipase 8,000 N.F. units, protease 30,000 N.F. units, and amylase 30,000 N.F. units.

Pancrease (Johnson & Johnson). Each capsule contains no less than lipase 4,000 N.F. units, protease 25,000 N.F. units, and amylase 20,000 N.F. units in enteric-coated microspheres.

MISCELLANEOUS AGENTS

METOCLOPRAMIDE
[Reglan]

This drug is related closely to procainamide chemically, but it has very little local anesthetic activity and almost no effect on the myocardium. It acts on the muscles of the upper gastrointestinal tract. Metoclopramide may be used in patients with gastric hypotonia, pyloric stenosis or pylorospasm, and spasm of the duodenal bulb who require cine- or still upper gastrointestinal and small intestinal x-ray examination. Duodenal endoscopy, intubation, and biopsy of the jejunum, as well as gastroduodenoscopy for the diagnosis of upper gastrointestinal hemorrhage have been facilitated. Its usefulness in the treatment of reflux esophagitis with and without impaired gastric emptying remains to be established. Clearance of gastric contents prior to and during anesthesia has been demonstrated. Metoclopramide is an effective antiemetic but does not prevent motion sickness (see Chapter 26, Drugs Used in Vertigo, Motion Sickness, and Vomiting).

The exact mechanism of action of metoclopramide in the gastrointestinal tract has not been fully clarified. Gastric, duodenal, and jejunal transit time is accelerated because of increased lower· esophageal sphincter pressure and esophageal body contractions, increased gastric (especially antral) contractions with coordination of antral and duodenal peristalsis, and enhanced pyloric activity and pressure. Effects on the entire small intestine are similar to those observed in the esophagus and stomach. Gastric secretion is not affected. Gallbladder and bile duct pressure is increased, while the sphincter of Oddi is relaxed in the absence of changes in pancreatic secretion. No significant action on colorectal function has been noted. Therapeutic levels of those drugs that are primarily absorbed in the small intestine are achieved more rapidly, because metoclopramide increases the rate of gastric emptying. Metoclopramide also blocks the hypotensive effect of dopamine; its action is blocked by atropine.

When metoclopramide is given in usual therapeutic doses, adverse reactions occur infrequently and are mild, transient, and reversible after the drug is withdrawn. Drowsiness, constipation, diarrhea, urticarial or maculopapular rash, brief episodes of agitation or anxiety, dryness of the mouth, glossal or periorbital edema, and methemoglobinemia have been noted. A hypertensive crisis has been reported when this drug was given to a patient with a pheochromocytoma.

Dystonic extrapyramidal reactions occur infrequently in patients of any age but are more common in infants and children. They are identical to the reactions produced by phenothiazine and butyrophenone drugs. Parkinsonian symptoms occur rarely following administration of therapeutic doses. The drug should not be given with thioxanthene, phenothiazine, or butyrophenone compounds or to patients with extrapyramidal symptoms or epilepsy, although it has been used safely in patients with parkinsonism. Therapy should not be initiated in patients who have received tricyclic antidepressants, adrenergic agents, or monoamine oxidase inhibitors within the previous two weeks. Markedly increased prolactin levels have stimulated lactation, and metoclopramide may be contraindicated in patients with breast cancer who have undergone radiation or chemotherapy. Particular caution should be

employed when metoclopramide is given to infants and young children. Its safety for use during pregnancy has not been established.

ROUTES, USUAL DOSAGE, AND PREPARATIONS. *Intravenous*: To facilitate small bowel intubation or when delayed gastric emptying interferes with x-ray examination of the upper gastrointestinal tract or small bowel, the manufacturer's suggested dose for *adults* is 10 mg (2 ml) injected over a one- to two-minute period. For *children 6 to 14 years*, 2.5 to 5 mg; *children under 6 years*, 0.1 mg/kg of body weight.

Reglan (Robins). Solution 10 mg metoclopramide base (as the monohydrochloride salt) in 2 ml containers.

Oral (investigational): Adults, 10 mg is given 30 minutes before symptoms are likely to occur or before or immediately after meals. *Children and young adults*, a maximum of 0.5 mg/kg of body weight is given daily in three divided doses. *Children under 6 years* should not receive more than 0.1 mg/kg as a single dose.

SIMETHICONE

[Mylicon, Silain]

$$(CH_3)_3Si\left[OSi(CH_3)_2\right]_n CH_3$$

This combination of dimethylpolysiloxanes and silica gel is available as a single-entity product and in mixtures containing antacids, belladonna alkaloids, and/or digestive enzymes. It is promoted to relieve symptoms arising from gaseous distention occurring postoperatively or as a result of aerophagia, but objective evidence from properly constructed and controlled studies to prove that symptoms caused by intestinal gas are benefited by use of this detergent alone or in combination products is not convincing. Simethicone eliminates mucus-embedded bubbles that interfere with visualization during gastroscopy.

No adverse reactions have been reported.

Mylicon (Stuart). Drops 40 mg/0.6 ml; tablets (chewable) 40 and 80 mg (nonprescription).
Silain (Robins). Tablets 50 mg.

SINCALIDE
  [Kinevac]

$$\underset{\begin{array}{c}|\\ \text{Asp}-\text{Tyr}-\text{Met}-\text{Gly}-\text{Trp}-\text{Met}-\text{Asp}-\text{Phe}-\text{NH}_2\end{array}}{\overset{\text{SO}_3\text{H}}{}}$$

This drug is given intravenously for the treatment of postoperative adynamic ileus and has the same spectrum of activities as the endogenous hormone, cholecystekinin. It also has been used diagnostically alone and with other gastrointestinal hormones to evaluate biliary and pancreatic secretions and as a substitute for the fatty meal to stimulate gallbladder contraction during cholecystography. The gallbladder contraction and evacuation of bile is similar to that produced by endogenous cholecystekinin. When injected with secretin, the volume and output of bicarbonate and enzymes are increased. Thus, physiologic and cytologic study of the pancreas is facilitated. Both cholecystekinin and sincalide stimulate intestinal motility while inhibiting gastric emptying.

Before sincalide is used to relieve postoperative ileus, it must be established that no inflammatory disorder (eg, pancreatitis, peritonitis) is present. Its use is contraindicated in the presence of any obstructive lesion of the bowel.

Abdominal cramping and tenesmus are manifestations of the physiologic action of sincalide and often accompany use of this drug. Nausea, dizziness, sweating, and flushing also have been observed. Impaction of stones in the cystic or common bile duct may occur when sincalide is given to patients with cholelithiasis. Complete contraction of the gallbladder does not occur when the drug is given as directed. Sincalide should not be used in pregnant women because it has not been established that the benefits outweigh the potential risk to the fetus. Likewise, the safety of this drug in children is unknown.

Route, Usual Dosage, and Preparations. The powder is reconstituted with 5 ml of sterile water for injection and diluted to 30 ml with sodium chlorde injection prior to administration. It may be kept at room temperature and should be discarded after 24 hours if not used.

Intravenous: The manufacturer's suggested dosage for *adults* is as follows: To stimulate gallbladder contraction, 0.02 mcg/kg of body weight is given over a 30- to 60-second period. A second dose of 0.04 mcg/kg may be administered after 15 minutes if contraction has not occurred. To determine pancreatic function, 0.25 units of secretin/kg is administered intravenously over a period of 60 minutes; 0.02 mcg/kg of sincalide is infused concomitantly (but separately) during the second 30-minute period. To relieve adynamic ileus, 0.04 mcg/kg is administered over a period of 30 to 60 seconds. The same amount or twice this dose may be given every four hours for a total of five doses if a satisfactory response is not obtained.

  Kinevac (Squibb). Powder 5 mcg.

ANORECTAL PREPARATIONS

Hemorrhoids, anal fissures, and cryptitis are common and often are associated with pruritus, bleeding, mucus seepage, and pain, which may become severe, especially during or just after defecation. Of the many available topical preparations, some afford symptomatic relief but none are curative. Most anorectal preparations include protectants or emollients, often in combination with a local anesthetic and, sometimes, a corticosteroid; the latter ingredient is intended to exert an anti-inflammatory effect on acutely inflamed lesions. Some preparations also contain ingredients of questionable value such as belladonna, opium, vitamins, vasoconstrictors, weak antiseptics, and astringents. Convincing data to prove that any one mixture is superior to another in relieving symptoms are lacking. The more bland, simple formulations probably are safer. None effectively controls bleeding.

The local anesthetics commonly incorporated into these preparations include benzocaine, tetracaine, dibucaine, diperodon, dyclonine, lidocaine, and pramoxine. The base forms of local anesthetics afford some degree of relief by penetrating unbroken skin, but salt forms are absorbed only through mucosal or abraded surfaces. In some preparations, the concentration of the base is too low to be effective. Benzocaine, one of the most widely used topical anesthetics, is not absorbed through the skin in concentrations of less than 5% and is poorly soluble in many aqueous vehicles. (See also Chapter 19, Local Anesthetics.)

Untoward systemic effects may result from the absorption of local anesthetics, corticosteroids, or other ingredients from the anal or rectal mucosa or excoriated perianal skin. Symptoms of overdosage are uncommon because of the small quantity of the drugs in the formulation. Hypersensitivity reactions with severe dermatitis may occur after topical application of local anesthetics, antiseptics, and some other drugs present in these preparations. Fatalities have occurred when certain of these products have been ingested by infants.

The suppository is the most common dosage form available. Some products may be applied by introduction of a multiple aperture tip into the anal canal. Thus, the medication is more likely to be applied at the site of the lesion. This overcomes the disadvantage produced when the suppository slips into the rectum to melt. However, the danger of self-inflicted trauma from misdirection of the applicator must be considered. The effectiveness of creams or ointments may be enhanced with intra-anal application up to the distal joint of the rubber-cotted finger.

The preparations listed below are those most commonly prescribed or widely used, but they are not necessarily preferred.

Americaine (Arnar-Stone). Ointment containing benzocaine 20% and benzethonium chloride 0.1%; aerosol containing benzocaine 20%; each suppository contains benzocaine 280 mg, zinc oxide 300 mg, and benzethonium chloride 2.8 mg (nonprescription).

Anusol (Parke, Davis). Each gram of ointment contains pramoxine hydrochloride 10 mg, benzyl benzoate 12 mg, Peruvian balsam 18 mg, and zinc oxide 110 mg; each suppository contains bismuth subgallate 2.25%, bismuth resorcin compound 1.75%, benzyl benzoate 1.2%, Peruvian balsam 1.8%, and zinc oxide 11% (nonprescription).

Anusol-HC (Parke, Davis). Each gram of cream contains bismuth subgallate 22.5 mg, bismuth resorcin compound 17.5 mg, benzyl benzoate 12 mg, Peruvian balsam 18 mg, zinc oxide 110 mg, and cortisol acetate 5 mg; each suppository contains same formulation as Anusol Suppositories plus cortisol acetate 10 mg.

Calmol 4 (Leeming). Each suppository contains cod liver oil, zinc oxide, bismuth subgallate, Peruvian balsam, and theobroma oil (nonprescription).

Corticaine (Meyer). Cream containing dibucaine 0.5% and cortisol 0.5% in a washable base.

Diothane (Merrell-National). Ointment base containing diperodon 1%, petrolatum, propylene glycol, sorbitan sesquioleate, and oxyquinoline benzoate 0.1% (nonprescription).

Preparation H (Whitehall). Ointment containing phenylmercuric nitrate 0.01%, shark liver oil 3%, and live yeast cell derivative (supplying 2,000 units of skin respiratory factor/oz); suppositories containing dilaurate 4.67%, shark liver oil 3%, polyethylene glycol 600 mg, and glycerin 2.5% in theobroma oil and beeswax (nonprescription).

Proctocort Cream (Rowell). Each gram of cream (buffered) contains cortisol 10 mg (1%).

Proctodon (Rowell). Each gram of cream (buffered) contains diperodon hydrochloride 1%, vitamin A palmitate 5,000 units, and vitamin D 1,000 units in a water-miscible base (nonprescription).

Proctofoam HC (Reed & Carnrick). Foam containing pramoxine hydrochloride 1% and cortisol acetate 1% in a mucoadhesive base.

Quotane (Smith Kline & French). Ointment containing dimethisoquin hydrochloride 0.5% preserved with thimerosal 1:50,000 in a water-miscible emulsion base.

Tucks (Parke, Davis). Cream and ointment containing witch hazel 50%; pads containing witch hazel 50%, glycerin 10%, and deionized purified water (nonprescription).

Wyanoid (Wyeth). Ointment containing benzocaine 2%, zinc oxide 5%, boric acid 18%, ephedrine sulfate 0.1%, and Peruvian balsam 1%; each suppository (Wyanoids) contains belladonna extract 15 mg, ephedrine sulfate 3 mg, zinc oxide, boric acid, bismuth oxyiodide, bismuth subcarbonate, and Peruvian balsam in theobroma oil and beeswax (nonprescription).

Wyanoids HC (Wyeth). Each suppository contains belladonna extract 15 mg, ephedrine sulfate 3 mg, zinc oxide 176 mg, boric acid 543 mg, Peruvian balsam 30 mg, bismuth oxyiodide 30 mg, bismuth subcarbonate 146 mg, and cortisol acetate 10 mg in theobroma oil and beeswax.

MIXTURES

The following mixtures containing bile constituents and derivatives, enzymes, sedatives, antispasmodics, cellulase, and other ingredients are marketed for the treatment of many ill-defined gastrointestinal syndromes. There is no scientific rationale or evidence of efficacy to support the use of most of these mixtures. There are no established therapeutic indications for ox bile, pepsin, and hydrochloric acid. Pancreatic enzymes are indicated only when a demonstrated exocrine pancreatic deficiency exists, in which case adequate quantities of the pancreatic enzymes should be prescribed alone. Such other active ingredients of these mixtures deemed necessary (eg, sedatives, antispasmodics) should be prescribed separately and not in combination with useless or inappropriate drugs. For these reasons, use of these mixtures cannot be justified. Examples of commonly used products, which are listed only for information, follow:

Atrocholin (BluLine). Each tablet contains dehydrocholic acid 130 mg and homatropine methylbromide 0.65 mg.

Bilron (Lilly). Each capsule contains bile salts and iron (nonprescription).

Caroid & Bile Salts w/Phenolphthalein (Breon). Each tablet contains digestive ferment from *Carica papaya* 75 mg, desiccated whole bile 70 mg, phenolphthalein 32.4 mg, capsicum 6.48 mg, and cascara sagrada extract 48.6 mg (nonprescription).

Cholan HMB (Pennwalt). Each tablet contains dehydrocholic acid 250 mg, phenobarbital 8 mg, and homatropine methylbromide 2.5 mg.

Cotazym-B (Organon). Each tablet contains pancrelipase 165 mg (lipase 4,000 N.F. units, trypsin 15,000 N.F. units, amylase 15,000 N.F. units, and other pancreatic enzymes), mixed conjugated bile salts 65 mg, and cellulase 2 mg (nonprescription).

Donnazyme (Robins). Each tablet contains pancreatin 300 mg and bile salts 150 mg (in enteric-coated core) and hyoscyamine sulfate 0.0518 mg, atropine sulfate 0.0097 mg, hyoscine hydrobromide 0.0033 mg, phenobarbital 8.1 mg, and pepsin 150 mg (in outer layer).

Entozyme (Robins). Each tablet contains pepsin 250 mg (in outer layer) and pancreatin 300 mg and bile salts 150 mg (in enteric-coated core).

Festal (Hoechst-Roussel). Each enteric-coated tablet contains lipase 10 Willstaetter units (WU), amylase 10 WU, protease 17 WU, hemicellulase 50 mg, and bile constituents 25 mg (nonprescription).

Festalan (Hoechst-Roussel). Each tablet contains lipase 10 Willstaetter units (WU), amylase 10 WU, protease 17 WU, hemicellulase 50 mg, and bile constituents 25 mg (in enteric-coated core); atropine methylnitrate 1 mg (in outer layer).

Phazyme (Reed & Carnrick). Each tablet contains activated simethicone 20 mg (in outer layer) and pancreatin 240 mg and activated simethicone 40 mg (in enteric-coated core) (nonprescription).

Phazyme-PB (Reed & Carnrick). Each tablet contains activated simethicone 20 mg and phenobarbital 15 mg (in outer layer) and pancreatin 240 mg and activated simethicone 40 mg (in enteric-coated core).

Selected References

Antiflatulents, part II. *Federal Register* 39:19862-19877, 1974.

Graham DY: Enzyme replacement therapy of exocrine pancreatic insufficiency in man: Relation between in vitro enzyme activities and in vivo potency in commercial pancreatic extracts. *N Engl J Med* 296:1314-1317, 1977.

Ivey KJ: Anticholinergics: Do they work in peptic ulcer? *Gastroenterology* 68:154-166, 1975.

Ivey KJ: Are anticholinergics of use in irritable colon syndrome? *Gastroenterology* 68:1300-1307, 1975.

Regan PT, et al: Comparative effects of antacids, cimetidine and enteric coating on therapeutic response to oral enzymes in severe pancreatic insufficiency. *N Engl J Med* 297:854-858, 1977.

Schoenfield LJ: Stone dissolution and National Cooperative Gallstone Study. *Am J Dig Dis* 22:1115-1116, 1977.

Dermatologic Preparations | 61

The choice of a topical medication for a cutaneous disorder depends upon the active ingredient(s) and the vehicle. Whereas the choice of active ingredient depends upon a correct diagnosis, the vehicle employed depends upon the character of the skin lesion at the time of treatment. The dermatologic preparations discussed are divided into three main categories: (1) the vehicles available and the criteria for their selection, (2) agents used prophylactically, and (3) agents used therapeutically (see the Outline).

Many dermatologic formulations are available over-the-counter (OTC). The term *Prescription* accompanies those that require it; all others are available over-the-counter. Concentration or dose, vehicle, and container size are listed for prescription drugs but are omitted for most OTC drugs. General guidelines for the amount of topical medication to prescribe once the concentration of the active ingredient(s) and the vehicle have been selected are presented in Table 1. Because of the wide variety of dermatologic compounds used, information on adverse reactions, contraindications, and precautions appear in the introduction for each therapeutic class.

VEHICLES

Criteria to be considered include whether the vehicle has drying or lubricating activity; the manner in which it holds, releases, or assists in the absorption of the active ingredients; and suitability for use on the skin area intended. Liquids (eg, lotions, gels, shampoos, sprays) are convenient for application to hairy areas; emulsified vanishing-type creams are used for intertriginous sites; and ointments may be most suitable for body folds when spread thinly to avoid maceration.

Constituents: The principal constituents of vehicles include liquids (water, hydroalcoholic tinctures, or organic solvents), powders, oils, and ointment bases; pharmaceutic aids often are present as additives.

Liquids have desirable properties in addition to their usefulness as vehicles. Water acts as a vehicle and hydrating agent in wet dressings, lotions, baths, creams, and some ointments. When applied as hot or cold compresses, it increases or decreases skin temperature and macerates the superficial layer of the skin to enhance penetration of active agents. Alcohols are solvents and are used to cool the skin; depending upon the concentration, they may be antiseptic and astringent. Glycerin, a solvent and emollient in lotions, creams, and pastes, is miscible with water and alcohol. Propylene glycol is an excellent solvent and has replaced glycerin as the vehicle in many formulations of topical therapeutic agents, cosmetics, and body and hand lotions. It is hygroscopic and possesses considerable moistening and softening actions. Subjec-

tive irritation (burning and stinging) may limit its use on damaged skin.

Powders increase evaporation, reduce friction and pruritus, and provide a cooling sensation. They are dusted on the skin or are present as a component of lotions and pastes. Examples of U.S.P. powders include zinc oxide, zinc stearate, magnesium stearate, talc, cornstarch, bentonite, titanium dioxide, and precipitated calcium carbonate.

Zinc oxide and talc (mainly hydrous magnesium silicate) are protective and absorb some water when applied as a paste in petrolatum. Zinc oxide mixed with a small amount of ferric oxide has a pink color; this mixture, calamine, is used in shake lotions. Although insoluble in water, bentonite (hydrated aluminum silicate) combines with water to form a gel; it improves the dispersion of zinc oxide and sulfur in oil-in-water mixtures. Titanium dioxide is opaque and is an ingredient of lotions or pastes used as sunscreens. Precipitated calcium carbonate is a fine white powder that is insoluble in alcohol and water; it gives a dry sensation and is more absorbent than talc. Talc may cause severe granulomatous reactions when applied to wounds.

Oils are liquid or semisolid fats of mineral, vegetable, or animal origin. Vegetable and mineral oils are most widely used for

TABLE 1.
AMOUNT OF TOPICAL MEDICATION FOR TREATMENT*

Area Treated	Single Application (g)	Application Three Times Daily For		
		1 week	2 weeks g (oz)	4 weeks
Hands, head, face, anogenital area	2	45 (1.5)	90 (3)	180 (6)
One arm, anterior or posterior trunk	3	60 (2)	120 (4)	240 (8)
One leg	4	90 (3)	180 (6)	360 (12)
Entire Body	30	21 (42) 1¼ (lb)		

*Values given are for cream; double the values for lotion, and add 5% to 10% to the values for ointments.

Adapted from Arndt KA: Manual of Dermatologic Therapeutics with Essentials of Diagnosis, ed 2. Boston, Little, Brown and Company, 1978. Reprinted by permission.

topical therapy. Vegetable oils commonly incorporated in creams and lotions are cottonseed, corn, castor, olive, and peanut. Their emollient effect is similar, but odor, storage stability, and emulsifying capabilities differ.

Mineral oil is a mixture of high-molecular-weight hydrocarbons obtained from petroleum. It is used alone or as an ingredient in lotions, creams, or ointments and, unlike vegetable or animal oils, does not become rancid. Nevertheless, stabilizers (eg, tocopherol, butylhydroxytoluene) are often added. (U.S.P. requires that the stabilizer be identified on the label.) Topically applied mineral oil is relatively free of untoward effects.

Like oils, *ointment bases* are used in various creams and ointments. They include semisolid vegetable and animal fats, petroleum hydrocarbons, and silicones.

Pharmaceutic-aid additives are widely used in topical dermatologic products. When compounding immiscible liquids, dispersing or emulsifying agents provide stability and homogeneity. Glyceryl monostearate, polyethylene glycol derivatives (polyoxyl 40 stearate, polysorbate 80), and sodium lauryl sulfate are used as dispersing agents in lotions, creams, and ointments containing oily ingredients and water. Other widely employed additives include ethylenediamines and cetyl palmitate and related esters that improve the consistency and appearance of creams; stearic acid and stearyl alcohol, which act as lubricants, emollients, or antifoaming agents; and methylcelluose and gum tragacanth, which are inert substances used as suspending agents in ointments and pastes. The parabens (methylparaben and propylparaben), oxyquinoline sulfate, organic quaternary ammonium compounds, hexachlorophene, parachlorometaxylenol, and chlorobutanol frequently are added as antimicrobial preservatives. Most of these agents are innocuous at the low concentrations present; however, the parabens occasionally produce allergic contact dermatitis and sodium lauryl sulfate produces irritation. Many surface agents increase the stratum corneum's permeability not only to medicaments but to noxious agents and

thus may directly or indirectly produce irritation.

Wet Dressings

Wet dressings are indicated for acute inflammation characterized by vesicular eruptions with exudation, oozing (weeping), and crusting. The soft, saturated, tepid dressings should be changed every 5 to 15 minutes for a period of 30 minutes to two hours, depending upon the severity of the inflammation. This process may be repeated three or four times daily.

Water is the most important ingredient in wet dressings. In addition to providing evaporative cooling, it cleanses and helps drain exudates; vasoconstriction resulting from cooling combats the first stage of an acute inflammatory response. These effects are lost if the wet dressing is occluded by wrapping or covering with plastic or rubber. When they are used occlusively, closed wet dressings soften and macerate the skin surface. Aluminum acetate, potassium permanganate, copper and zinc sulfates, acetic acid, or silver nitrate may be added to the water to contribute a mild antibacterial or astringent action.

A 5% aluminum acetate solution, U.S.P. (Burow's solution), diluted 1:10 to 1:40, is commonly used. Potassium permanganate (0.025% to 0.1%) has astringent properties but stains the skin. Tablets should be completely dissolved if placed in a tub of water, because they can produce cutaneous necrosis if the patient inadvertently sits on them. Silver nitrate solution (0.1% to 0.5%) stains the skin but has more antibacterial activity than the other metal salts listed; however, it also permanently stains clothing and linens.

ALUMINUM ACETATE SOLUTION, U.S.P.
ALUMINUM CHLORIDE HEXAHYDRATE, N.F.:
AluWets (Stiefel). Crystals.
ALUMINUM SULFATE AND CALCIUM
ACETATE:
Domeboro (Dome), *Bluboro* (Herbert). Powder.
POTASSIUM PERMANGANATE, U.S.P.
SILVER NITRATE, U.S.P.
ZINC AND COPPER SULFATES AND
CAMPHOR:
Dalbour Powder (Doak), *Dalidome Powder Packets* (Dome).

Lotions

The term lotion (sometimes called "shake lotion") historically refers to a suspension of powder in a liquid medium (most frequently water) that requires shaking before application. The term recently has been extended to include commercial emulsions that are usually of thick, uniform consistency.

Lotions are used for subacute inflammatory lesions after the severe exudative phase is terminated. They provide a protective, drying, cooling effect that is especially useful in intertriginous or widespread eruptions. A basic white "shake lotion" contains zinc oxide, talc, glycerin, and water. Calamine may be added for a flesh tint. Alcohol may be added (to a concentration of 15%) to enhance the drying effect.

Concentrations of 0.25% to 2% menthol, 0.5% to 1.5% phenol, and 1% to 3% camphor in various formulations have an antipruritic action; the latter two agents alter cutaneous nerve transmission, while menthol imparts a cooling sensation. See the evaluation on Phenol in the section on Antiseptics and Disinfectants for precautions. Salicylic acid 1% to 2% and coal tar solution 3% to 10% also have an antipruritic action.

CALAMINE LOTION, U.S.P.
PHENOLATED CALAMINE LOTION, U.S.P.
MENTHOL LOTION WITH PHENOL:
Schamberg's Lotion (C & M Pharmacal).

Gels

Gels used for topical preparations are transparent colloidal dispersions prepared in a solid or semisolid (jelly-like) state. Aqueous, acetone, alcohol, or propylene glycol gels of organic polymers such as agar, gelatin, hydroxypropyl cellulose, methylcellulose, pectin, and polyethylene glycol are primarily used. The gel liquifies on contact with skin and dries to a greaseless nonocclusive film.

The presence of large amounts of water and sometimes other solvents characterize the subclass of gels known as jellies. Jellies are used as vehicles, particularly those applied to the mucous membranes, and serve as lubricants for surgical gloves,

finger cots, catheters, and for sexual intercourse.

A small but significant percentage of patients experience subjective irritation (burning, stinging) or drying after use of gels.

Creams and Ointments

These fluid and semisolid preparations are vehicles for many drugs and are used alone for their emollient and protective properties. Creams and ointments are particularly suitable for the chronic inflammatory stage of skin diseases. Dry, scaling, thickened, pruritic, and lichenified lesions respond to their softening and lubricating properties. Creams and certain ointments can be selected for their ability to hold or attract water to promote skin rehydration; other types of ointments repel water. All creams and ointments are sufficiently occlusive to promote the cutaneous absorption of drugs.

Creams and one class of ointments (*emulsion ointment bases*) consist of emulsions of oil and water. The oils consist of hydrophobic hydrocarbons, animal or vegetable fats, or organic alcohols. Oil-in-water (O/W) emulsions are less greasy and more easily removed (water-washable or vanishing creams) than water-in-oil (W/O) emulsions; however, the latter provide more lubrication and occlusion.

When the amount of oil exceeds that of water by a certain proportion, the emulsion changes from a pourable cream to a semisolid ointment. Although generally true, neither the official nor manufacturers' designation of product as a cream or ointment always correlates with O/W or W/O emulsification type, eg, Cold Cream, U.S.P. (W/O) and Hydrophilic Ointment, U.S.P. (O/W).

Hydrophilic ointment, which contains white petrolatum, stearyl alcohol, sodium lauryl sulfate, and propylene glycol in water with preservatives, is a good vehicle for water-soluble medicaments. It has good esthetic properties and imparts a pleasing sensation. Irritation has been noted, probably due to the emulsifier, sodium lauryl sulfate.

Cold cream, a water-in-mineral oil emulsion containing white wax, cetyl palmitate, and sodium borate, is widely used. It has lubricating qualities, provides some water for hydration of the skin, and imparts a cooling sensation.

The remaining three classes of ointments contain essentially no water. Some are soluble in water or will attract and hold water; others are completely insoluble in water, hold little if any water, or may be water-repellant, depending upon the base used.

Water-absorbent ointment bases are mixtures of oleaginous materials and emulsifying agents. They are insoluble in water but adsorb it, are difficult to wash off, and are oil-in-water emulsion ointment bases when hydrated. Examples include Hydrophilic Petrolatum, U.S.P. and Anhydrous Lanolin, U.S.P. The former is composed of white petrolatum, cholesterol, stearyl alcohol, and white wax and is less greasy and more acceptable cosmetically than petrolatum. Anhydrous lanolin is an oleaginous substance obtained from sheep's wool; it contains less than 0.25% water but is capable of absorbing a considerable amount. It is an ingredient of commercial ointments and some bath oil preparations.

Oleaginous ointment bases (water-repellant) consist of hydrophobic hydrocarbons, hydrogenated vegetable fats, or siloxanes (silicones); some are synthetic mixtures with waxes. They are anhydrous, insoluble in water, and absorb little or no water. They are difficult to wash off, will not dry out, and generally change little during storage (although some fats may become rancid on aging). Oleaginous ointment bases are suitable for use alone or as a vehicle for patients sensitive to other bases and/or their ingredients (emulsifiers, stabilizers, preservatives).

Petrolatum, N.F., the most important agent of this group, is a purified mixture of high-molecular-weight hydrocarbons obtained from petroleum. This ointment is protective and emollient when applied to the skin and is an excellent base or vehicle for topical medicaments. It varies in color (yellow to light amber), composition, and consistency depending upon the petroleum source and manner of preparation.

White Petrolatum, U.S.P., a bleached form of yellow petrolatum, is more esthetically pleasing and, therefore, is the form most commonly used. White Ointment, U.S.P., is white petrolatum with 5% white wax added. This preparation is firmer at room temperature than petrolatum.

Depending upon their degree of polymerization, silicones are available as liquid or semisolid preparations. The latter have the properties of other oleaginous ointment bases, except that they are considerably more water repellent and have a low surface tension, which increases their penetration into skin creases. Silicones are used as aqueous-barrier creams because they are water repellent and provide intimate coverage; however, they do not serve as a barrier for organic compounds that may be contact irritants. The polydimethylsiloxanes (dimethicone) are stable and are neither sensitizing nor irritating.

Water-soluble ointment bases (eg, polyethylene glycol ointment) are greaseless and anhydrous. They absorb water, are water soluble, and are good vehicles for the topical delivery of water-soluble drugs. The oil-in-water emulsion, Hydrophilic Ointment, U.S.P., is soluble in water and can be used similarly.

OIL-IN-WATER EMULSIONS:
Hydrophilic Ointment, U.S.P.
Acid Mantle Cream (Dorsey), *LactiCare Lotion* (Stiefel), *Lubriderm Cream* (Warner/Lambert), *Nivea Cream* (Beiersdorf), *Purpose Dry Skin Cream* (Johnson & Johnson), *Syntex Cream* (Syntex).
WATER-IN-OIL EMULSIONS:
Cold Cream, U.S.P.
Lanolin, U.S.P.
Keri Cream (Westwood), *Eucerin* (Beiersdorf), *Polysorb Hydrate* (Fougera).
WATER-ABSORBENT OINTMENT BASES:
Hydrophilic Petrolatum, U.S.P.
Anhydrous Lanolin, U.S.P.
Aquaphor (Beiersdorf), *Polysorb Anhydrous* (Fougera), *Unibase* (Parke, Davis), *Velvachol* (Texas Pharmacal).
WATER-REPELLANT (OLEAGINOUS) OINTMENT BASES:
Petrolatum, N.F.
White Petrolatum, U.S.P.
White Ointment, U.S.P.
Dimethicone, U.S.P.:
Covicone Cream (Abbott).

WATER-SOLUBLE OINTMENT BASE:
Polyethylene Glycol Ointment, U.S.P.
Carbowax (City Chemical, Doak, Robinson).

Pastes

Simple pastes are made by incorporating a finely divided powder into an ointment base. The resulting mixture protects the skin against external irritants and sunlight. The ointment base is usually petrolatum, and the powder is zinc oxide, talc, starch, bentonite, aluminum oxide, or titanium dioxide. Titanium dioxide has particularly good sunscreen properties. Coloring matter may be added to make the mixture cosmetically acceptable. A paste containing zinc oxide, starch, and white petrolatum in a 1:1:4 ratio, Zinc Oxide Paste. U.S.P. (Lassar's Plain Zinc Paste), is one commonly prescribed protective paste. Starch may act as substrate for some organisms. Pastes generally are poor vehicles for delivering active pharmacologic agents and for inhibiting water evaporation; therefore, they are used only infrequently. They are applied in subacute and chronic dermatoses, particularly in infants, but generally should be avoided in weeping lesions and hairy areas. Pastes protect from friction caused by clothing and bandages.

Soaps, Soap Substitutes, and Shampoos

Ordinary soaps are sodium or potassium salts of fatty acids. These anionic surfactants and cationic detergent cleansers emulsify fats, promoting the removal of foreign particles from the skin. Toilet bars, which exhibit different pH's in solution, are available. Some bar soaps are alkaline (pH 9.5 to 10.5) in solution. Superfatted bar soaps are at the lower end of this range and minimize defatting of the skin. Neutral toilet bars contain synthetic surfactants and have a solution pH of 7.5 or slightly less. Badly irritated skin generally should not be exposed to soaps, detergents, or cleansers other than water.

Medicated soaps are widely available. Some abrasive soaps contain inert alumi-

num oxide, polyethylene, or sodium tetraborate decahydrate particles (see the section on Agents Used in Acne Vulgaris). Antimicrobial soaps may contain antiseptics in sufficient concentration to be effective deodorants or useful as handwashes for health care personnel, preoperatively for preparation of the skin, or for surgical scrubs.

Shampoos are liquid soaps or detergents used to wash the hair and clean the scalp of scales. Most bar soaps can be used similarly. The detergent properties of special shampoos for use on dry, normal, or oily hair are altered, but the same effect can be obtained by applying greater or lesser volumes of regular shampoo. Shampoos also are used as vehicles for applying medication to the scalp for dandruff, seborrheic dermatitis, or psoriasis.

NEUTRAL SOAPS OR SOAP SUBSTITUTES:
Acne-Aid Detergent Soap (Stiefel), *Alpha-Keri* (Westwood), *Caress* (Lever), *Dove* (Lever), *Emulave* (Cooper), *Epi-Clear* (Squibb), *Lowila* (Westwood), *Neutrogena* (Neutrogena), *pHisoDerm* (Winthrop), *Pre-op* (Davis & Geck), *Purpose* (Johnson & Johnson), *Shepard's* (Dermik), *Vel* (Colgate).
SUPERFATTED SOAPS:
Basis (Beiersdorf), *Camay, Coast* (Procter & Gamble), *Derma Lab Soap* (Derma), *Emulave* (Cooper), *Lubriderm Soap* (Warner/Lambert), *Nivea Creme Soap* (Beiersdorf), *Oilatum Soap* (Stiefel).

Baths

Pruritus accompanying acute dermatitis or extensive exanthematous lesions is often alleviated by immersion of the part or the entire body in water. Cooling diminishes pruritus safely and effectively. When baths are used to hydrate the skin, subsequent gentle drying is desirable, followed by use of an emollient to retard water evaporation.

Colloidal substances can be added to baths for their soothing and antipruritic activity. A paste made up of either 2 cups of starch and 4 cups of cold water or 1 cup of oatmeal [Aveeno, Oilated Aveeno] and 2 cups of cold water is added to a tub approximately half-filled with water.

Occasionally it is desirable to add an oil to bath water. Since oils are insoluble in water, emulsifiers are often added to help disperse the oil; the emulsifiers form a milky mixture of microglobules of oil-in-water and a fine film of oil remains on the skin after the bath. These products may be helpful in ichthyosis or pruritic and chronic eczematous dermatosis. Since these surfactant-treated oils impart a pleasing sensation to the skin, they are often used as emollients. Solutions of coal tar oils are available for addition to baths.

MINERAL OIL AND LANOLIN OIL:
Alpha-Keri (Westwood), *Jeri-Bath* (Dermik), *Mellobath* (Beiersdorf).
MINERAL OIL:
Domol (Dome), *Lubath* (Warner/Lambert), *Surfol* (Stiefel).
SESAME SEED OIL:
Neutrogena (Neutrogena).

SUNSCREENS

Individuals with normal skin require only 15 to 20 minutes of exposure to sunlight initially during spring or the early months of summer to produce a perceptible sunburn reaction (minimal erythemal dose, MED). Multiples of this exposure time (dose) can lead to an acute, painful sunburn reaction with blisters. Sun-sensitive patients should minimize direct exposure to sunlight and are able to venture outdoors only at times when solar irradiation is less intense and with as much protection from opaque clothing and accessories as possible. It is better for these individuals to remain indoors between 10 a.m. and 4 p.m., especially during the summer. The variation in sun sensitivity among individuals has led to the following classification of skin types: (1) always burns, never tans; (2) always burns easily, tans minimally; (3) burns moderately, tans gradually; (4) burns minimally, tans well; (5) rarely burns, tans profusely; (6) never burns, deeply pigmented.

Sunscreens help prevent sunburn; these products may be helpful in preventing actinic-induced skin cancer and premature aging of the skin. They are indicated especially in (1) fair-skinned individuals who burn easily (skin types 1 through 3); (2) individuals hypersensitive to sunlight (solar urticaria); (3) patients who are using topical or sytemic medications with photosensitizing or phototoxic properties (eg, thiazides, phenothiazines, sulfonamides, sulfonylureas, psoralens, demeclocycline); (4) medical personnel and patients who may be exposed to ultraviolet bactericidal lamps; and (5) patients with photosensitivity caused by systemic lupus erythematosus or porphyria (especially the erythropoietic form).

Long-range ultraviolet radiation wavelengths of 320 to 400 nm (UVA) tan skin but are relatively weak in the energy required to produce an MED. UV wavelengths of 290 to 320 nm (UVB) cause sunburn, stimulate tanning and require a thousand times less energy than UVA radiation to produce an MED. UV wavelengths of 200 to 290 nm (UVC) do not reach the earth's surface, but artificial sources can emit this radiation. UVC radiation does not stimulate tanning and requires about the same energy as UVA to produce an MED. UVC radiation is an effective germicide. Sunscreen agents vary in their ability to block out UVA, B, or C wavelength radiation.

The Sun Protective Factor (SPF) is the ratio of the amount of energy required to produce the same MED without protection. It has been recommended that each specific sunscreen product be labeled with its SPF number (*Federal Register*, 1978). Five product category designations have been proposed: SPF 2-4, minimal protection from sunburn but permit suntanning; SPF 4-6, moderate protection but permit suntanning; SPF 6-8, extra protection from sunburn and permit limited suntanning; SPF 8-15, maximum protection from sunburn and permit limited suntanning; SPF over 15, most protection from sunburn and permit no suntanning. SPF usually is determined in the laboratory and tends to overestimate the degree of protection.

Chemical sunscreens principally include [UV absorption spectrum in parentheses] para-aminobenzoic acid (280-320) and its esters (280-320), benzophenones (250-360), cinnamates (290-320), salicylates (290-320), and the anthranilides (248-435). Physical sunscreens (zinc oxide, talc, or titanium dioxide) are opaque to all wavelengths of light; these are effective but are cosmetically unappealing. The lack of cosmetic appeal restricts the use of red veterinary petrolatum, which filters out a considerable amount of ultraviolet and visible light and provides partial protection from sunburn in addition to minimizing skin dryness.

Sunscreens exhibit a wide range of effectiveness depending upon the chemical and/or physical agent(s), concentration, and vehicle. Increasing the concentration increases the protection afforded, but concentration and protection are not directly proportional. Both the sunscreen and the vehicle are responsible for the property of substantivity, ie, the ability of the preparation to resist removal during sweating and swimming. Certain esters of para-aminobenzoic acid (PABA) are more substantive than PABA alone (Sayre et al, 1979); creams may be more substantive than alcohol-based formulations. Following initial application, reapplication should be made as directed on the label. Preparations containing less effective sunscreens or lower concentrations of effective agents are marketed for individuals who wish to acquire a tan while avoiding sunburn. These preparations are less suitable for protection of sun-sensitive individuals.

Contact and photocontact sensitization can occur with any of the chemical agents. Individuals sensitive to benzocaine, procaine, paraphenylene diamine, and sulfanilamide should probably avoid para-aminobenzoic acid, and those sensitive to thiazides and other sulfa drugs should avoid PABA esters as well. If patch and photopatch testing facilities can be utilized, definitive determination of sensitivity to these agents is possible. This permits specific recommendations for individual patients and avoids mandating against all related chemicals (Mathias et al, 1978). Highly alcoholic vehicles are not recommended for those with eczematous or otherwise inflamed skin.

Baby oil or mineral oil (with or without iodine), lubricating creams or lotions, cocoa butter, coconut oil, and tanning butters also are available. These preparations provide no protection against sunburn and may induce miliaria and folliculitis; their sole virtue is that they minimize skin dryness.

A number of artificial tanning preparations (bronzers, body gels, face colors) are available to give the skin a tanned appearance without exposure to the sun; these preparations provide no protection against sunburn unless a sunscreen is incorporated in the formulation.

Laboratory methodology is not yet standardized; therefore, the SPF's for the following preparations are estimates (*Medical Letter*, 1979). The lettered designations in parentheses denote the active ingredient(s) and are listed to aid the physician when contact dermatitis is known or anticipated: (a) para-aminobenzoic acid, (b) esters of para-aminobenzoic acid, (c) benzophenones, (d) cinnamates, (e) salicylates, (f) anthranilides, (g) titanium dioxide, (h) zinc oxide, (i) red veterinary petrolatum.

SPF RANGE 10-15 FOR SKIN TYPE 1 (always burns, never tans):
Super Shade 15, Total Eclipse (b,c); *Piz Buin Exclusiv, Extrem Creme* (c,d).
SPF RANGE 6-12 FOR SKIN TYPE 2 (burns easily, tans minimally):
Eclipse (b); *Piz Buin 6* (b,c); *Pabanol, PreSun* (a).
SPF RANGE 4-6 FOR SKIN TYPE 3 (burns moderately, tans gradually):
Pabagel (a); *Pabafilm, Partial Eclipse, Pro-Tan, Sea & Ski 6, Sundown, UVAL* (b); *Solbar* (c); *Sungard* (b,c); *Maxafil* (d,f); *A-Fil* (f,g); *RV Paque* (d,h,i).
SPF RANGE 2-4 FOR SKIN TYPE 4 (burns minimally, tans well):
Coppertone 2 (e); *Sundare and Piz Buin 2* (d); *RVP* (i).

ANTIPERSPIRANTS AND DEODORANTS

Undesirable body odor results from bacterial action on organic constituents of apocrine gland sweat. The more voluminous watery eccrine sweat promotes this process by increasing wetness which favors bacterial growth.

Two classes of nonprescription drugs diminish this phenomenon (*Federal Register*, 1978). Topically applied antiperspirants reduce eccrine, but not apocrine, gland sweat from 20% to 60%, depending upon the drug and method of application; aerosols tend to be least effective. Aluminum chlorohydrate, aluminum zirconium chlorohydrate, aluminum chloride, or buffered aluminum sulfate are the principal active agents present in over-the-counter antiperspirant formulations. They probably interfere with the formation of sweat rather than occlude the ducts. Part of their mechanism of deodorant effect is related to an antibacterial action.

Topically applied antiseptics, usually in the form of antimicrobial bar soaps, represent another approach. This deodorant action should be distinguished from the effect of masking fragrances in cosmetic preparations. The active ingredient is the carbanilide, triclocarban, or the substituted phenol, triclosan. Representative bar soaps include Coast, Dial, Irish Spring, Jergens Clear Complexion Bar, Lifebuoy, Phase III, Safeguard, and Zest. (See the following section on Antiseptics and Disinfectants.)

The most common adverse effects caused by antiperspirant preparations are burning and irritation. Less common reactions include dermatitis and open ulceration. These preparations should be discontinued temporarily at the first sign of irritation, which usually disappears without further complications. Contact sensitization is rare; if patch testing is desirable, the manufacturer should be contacted for appropriate materials, for the final formulation may be inadequate for this purpose.

OTC antiperspirant products are not sufficiently active to treat hyperhidrosis of the palms, soles, and axillae. New prescription products containing aluminum chloride hexahydrate 6.25% [Xerac AC] or 20% [Drysol] in absolute ethyl alcohol appear to be effective in some patients when applied without occlusion or, for greater effectiveness, under plastic occlusion to *dry* axillae; the preparation is used at bedtime and washed off in the morning. The number of treatments required per week depends upon the individual. Considerable irritation has been noted occasionally. Glutaral 2% in a buffered solution (pH 7.5) [Cidex] is available as a nonprescription product and has an anhidrotic effect when applied to the palms and soles but not the axillae. It appears to act by occluding the sweat ducts (see the discussion on Aldehydes in the following section on Antiseptics and Disinfectants).

> **Drysol** (Person & Covey). Aluminum chloride hexahydrate 20% in absolute alcohol in 37.5 ml containers (prescription).
>
> **Xerac AC** (Person & Convey). Aluminum chloride hexahydrate 6.25% in absolute alcohol in 30 ml containers (prescription).

ANTISEPTICS AND DISINFECTANTS

Antiseptics are applied to living tissues either to destroy microorganisms or inhibit their reproduction or metabolic activities. The major prophylactic uses of antiseptics by health care personnel are for surgical hand scrubs, for handwashing to reduce the risk of cross contamination, and preoperatively for preparation of the skin. The laity apply antiseptics as cleansers and protectants to minimize the potential for infection associated with minor cuts, abrasions, burns, or insect bites; antimicrobial-containing soaps also are used to help reduce the number of skin bacteria in order to obtain a deodorant effect. The laity's use of antiseptics as a first-aid measure is of questionable or limited value; they should only be considered at best adjuncts to proper mechanical cleansing (adequate removal of dirt and organic matter by sudsing, emulsification, irrigation, and debridement techniques) and use of protective dressings that assure adequate drainage.

Although the use of antiseptics by health care personnel has been shown to be effective, controversy exists as to which antiseptics are most effective and safe. The FDA's OTC Expert Panel II on Topical Antimicrobial Products is expected to publish a Final Order in 1980 or 1981 formulating guidelines for the role of each antiseptic in each of the prophylactic uses listed above. A Tentative Final Order was published in the *Federal Register* in January, 1978.

The antiseptics most widely employed by health care personnel include ethyl and isopropyl alcohols, cationic surface-active agents (eg, benzalkonium), the biguanide, chlorhexidine, iodine compounds (ie, iodine solution, iodine tincture, iodophors [poloxamer-iodine, povidone-iodine]), and the phenolic compound, hexachlorophene. These antiseptics, except for hexachlorophene, are incorporated into OTC products. Also available are chlorine compounds (eg, sodium hypochlorite; the chlorophor, oxychlorosene); hydrogen peroxide; mercurial compounds (eg, merbromin, nitromersol, phenylmercuric acetate and nitrate, thimerosal); and phenolic compounds (eg, phenol, hexylresorcinol, parachlorometaxylenol).

Silver nitrate is used prophylactically for ophthalmia neonatorum; however, this agent and silver sulfadiazine are used most often in burns. The phenolic compound, triclosan, and the carbanilide, triclocarban, are used principally as components of antimicrobial soaps for deodorant purposes.

Disinfectants are used on inanimate objects to destroy microorganisms and prevent infection. Some disinfectants are used as antiseptics if they can be diluted sufficiently to retain antimicrobial activity but avoid injury to living tissues. The principal disinfectants available are two aldehydes, formaldehyde and glutaral, elemental chlorine, and the phenolic compound, cresol.

Sterilization is the complete and total destruction of all microbial life, including vegetative bacteria, spores, fungi, and viruses. Ethylene oxide is the only chemical available that is approved for sterilization of objects that cannot be heated or sterilized by other physical methods (eg, radiation).

Alcohols: *Ethyl alcohol*, a widely used agent for disinfection of skin, is a good bactericide because it acts rapidly by coagulating protein. The 70% aqueous solution is more effective in reducing the surface tension of bacterial cells than absolute alcohol; the latter precipitates protoplasm at the periphery of the cell and thus tends to retard penetration of the agent.

Isopropyl alcohol has slightly greater bactericidal activity than ethyl alcohol due to its greater depression of surface tension. It rapidly kills vegetative forms of most bacteria when used full strength or as a 70% aqueous solution.

Alcohols are applied to reduce local bacterial flora prior to penetration with needles or other sharp instruments and as a preoperative wash. Their antiseptic action can be enhanced by prior mechanical cleansing of the skin with water and a detergent and gentle rubbing of the skin with sterile gauze while the alcohol is being applied. Ethyl and isopropyl alcohol possess cleansing and lubricant properties and are used as rubefacients and skin conditioners for bedridden patients. Rubbing alcohol contains about 70% (by volume) ethyl alcohol. Alcohol also is applied to cool the skin but it may irritate inflamed or denuded tissue, especially after repeated use. Application of an emollient preparation after an alcohol rub helps alleviate the dry feeling.

Neither ethyl nor isopropyl alcohol are reliable virucidal or fungicidal agents. They are not sporicidal in any concentration; therefore, they are not useful for sterilization of instruments.

Alcohols should not be used to disinfect wounds because they cause tissue irritation, resulting in painful burning and stinging, and they precipitate protein to form a coagulated mass in which bacteria may grow.

ETHYL ALCOHOL:
Alcohol, U.S.P., Diluted Alcohol, U.S.P., Rubbing Alcohol, N.F.
ISOPROPYL ALCOHOL:
Isopropyl Alcohol, N.F.

Aldehydes: *Formaldehyde* is a potent, volatile, wide-spectrum germicide that has been used as a vapor and as a solution in water. The vapor is irritating when inhaled and irritates the skin at concentrations required to produce sufficient antimicrobial activity for antisepsis; therefore, formaldehyde is used principally as a disinfectant in concentrations of 2% to 8%. Formaldehyde has an anhidrotic action when applied to palms and soles, but not axillae.

Glutaral (glutaraldehyde), a potent dialdehyde with a wide range of biocidal activity, is rapidly sporicidal and possesses tuberculocidal activity. A 2% aqueous solution buffered with sodium carbonate 0.3%

to a pH of 7.5 to 8.5 will disinfect and sterilize surgical and endoscopic instruments and plastic and rubber apparatus used for respiratory therapy and anesthesia. Glutaral loses activity within two weeks after preparation because it tends to polymerize in alkaline solution, which is the optimum pH for its germicidal activity. A stabilized alkaline solution formulation with a longer use life is now available (Miner et al, 1977). Like formaldehyde, gluteral has an anhidrotic action when applied to palms and soles, but not axillae.

FORMALDEHYDE SOLUTION, U.S.P.:
Solution containing 37% by weight of formaldehyde with methanol added to prevent polymerization.
GLUTARAL:
Cidex Solution (2% glutaral), *Cidex Formula 7 Long-Life Solution* (2% glutaral) (Arbrook).

Carbanilide: *Triclocarban* is used as an antimicrobial in bar soap; it is antibacterial and antifungal. Tentatively, a concentration limit of 1.5% has been established. Currently, its use is limited to handwashes for health personnel and cleansers for wounds; additional data on substantivity, absorption, distribution, blood levels, excretion, and safety are needed before final guidelines for its use can be established by the FDA Panel II on OTC Topical Antimicrobial Products.

TRICLOCARBAN:
Coast (Procter & Gamble), *Dial* (Armour-Dial), *Jergens Clear Complexion Bar* (Jergens), *Safeguard* (Procter & Gamble), *Zest* (Procter & Gamble).

Cationic Surfactants: Soaps are anionic and organic quaternary ammonium compounds are cationic surface-active agents. Both classes of detergents emulsify sebaceous material which is then removed together with dirt and microbes. The mild desquamating effect of the quaternary ammonium compounds aids this cleansing action. Their antimicrobial properties are limited and thus their usefulness as antiseptics is often less than desired; nevertheless, these compounds are widely used as industrial and home detergents, emulsifiers, and sanitizers. Their antimicrobial action is ascribed to alteration of microbial membrane permeability.

Benzalkonium chloride, the prototype of the organic quaternary ammonium compounds, is active against gram-positive and gram-negative bacteria, some fungi (including yeasts), and certain protozoa (eg, *Trichomonas vaginalis*). Strains of *Pseudomonas aeruginosa* are more resistant and require longer exposure. Aqueous solutions are ineffective against *Mycobacterium tuberculosis*, *Clostridium*, and other spore-forming bacteria and viruses. Benzalkonium chloride may be used preoperatively to diminish the number of organisms on intact skin and mucous membranes and applied to minor lacerations, wounds, and abrasions to limit infection. It is inactivated by organic material, soap, and other anionic substances; therefore, soap should be thoroughly rinsed from the skin with water and alcohol 70% before this agent is applied.

Accidental contact with concentrated solutions can produce corrosive skin lesions with deep necrosis and scarring. Properly diluted solutions are not ordinarily irritating or sensitizing; however, dilute solutions under occlusive dressings, casts, or packs may irritate the skin. Caution is advisable when irrigating body cavities with benzalkonium chloride, for systemic absorption may cause muscle weakness.

The following concentrations are recommended: For use on intact skin, minor wounds, and abrasions, 1:750 (tincture or aqueous solutions); for mucous membranes and broken or diseased skin, 1:2,000 to 1:5,000 (aqueous solution); for storage of instruments, 1:750 to 1:5,000 (aqueous solution). The addition of an antirust agent is recommended to retard corrosion of metallic instruments. Solutions should be checked periodically for contamination by resistant bacteria and spores and replenished frequently to maintain the concentration at an effective bactericidal level.

The quaternary ammonium compounds are inactivated when cotton fabrics, cellulose sponges, certain plastics (particularly polyvinyl chloride), or other porous materials are immersed in the solution, since surface-active agents are absorbed by these materials. For this reason, these agents are of uncertain efficacy in cold sterilization of catheters, flexible endoscopes, or other instruments.

Methylbenzethonium chloride is effective against gram-positive and gram-negative organisms. This cationic surfactant is commonly used as a rinse for diapers and for bed linen and underclothes of incontinent adults to prevent irritant contact dermatitis; articles should be free of soap to avoid inactivation of the antiseptic. It also is applied topically as a dusting powder around genitalia, rectum, thighs, and intertriginous areas for the prevention and treatment of perianal dermatitis, miliaria rubra, and intertrigo. Methylbenzethonium chloride seldom produces irritation.

BENZALKONIUM CHLORIDE:
Drug available generically: Solution, concentrate.
Zephiran (Winthrop). Solution, tincture, tincture spray.
Ionax (Owen). Foam aerosol, scrub paste.
METHYLBENZETHONIUM CHLORIDE:
Diaparene (Glenbrook). Powder, perianal cream, ointment.

Chlorhexidine Gluconate: *Chlorhexidine* is a 1,1' hexamethylene bis[5-*p*-chlorophenyl biguanide]. At pH 5 to 8, it is most effective against gram-positive (10 mg/ml) and gram-negative (50 mg/ml) bacteria and fungi (200 mg/ml) but is sporicidal only at elevated temperatures. High concentrations of nonionic surfactants and serum proteins reduce the bacteriostatic and bactericidal effects of chlorhexidine; however, the drug retains considerable activity even when well diluted. Chlorhexidine is rapid acting, has considerable skin substantivity (residual adherence), a low potential for producing contact sensitivity and photosensitivity with long-term use in man, and is poorly absorbed dermally, even under exaggerated use conditions. The compound is applied as a handwash for health care personnel, as a surgical scrub, and as a wound cleanser in a 4% concentration in a sudsing base formulation. The compound is applied as a preoperative surgical preparation in a 0.5% weight/volume tinted tincture in 70% isopropanol.

Hibiclens, Hibitane Tincture (Stuart).

Chlorine Compounds: *Chlorine* is a potent germicidal agent used to disinfect inanimate objects, water supplies, and swimming pools. It is not recommended for disinfecting medical instruments because of its corrosive properties. The germicidal action is due to the elemental chlorine itself and to the formation of hypochlorous acid in aqueous solution. This effect is decreased by organic matter and an alkaline pH.

Sodium hypochlorite solution is used to disinfect utensils. The undiluted solution contains approximately 5% sodium hypochlorite and is too irritating to tissues for use as an antiseptic except in root canal therapy.

Sodium hypochlorite solution diluted (Modified Dakin's Solution) contains 0.5% sodium hypochlorite adjusted to a neutral pH with sodium bicarbonate. It was once widely used to treat suppurating wounds, but its solvent action on blood clots and its action to delay clotting are disadvantages.

The germicidal chlorophor, *oxychlorosene*, is a mixture of hypochlorous acid and alkylbenzene sulfonates that slowly release the former; the sulfonates appear to enhance the germicidal activity of hypochlorous acid. The sodium salt is used as a topical antiseptic for preoperative preparation of the skin and for wound irrigation in a concentration of 0.4%. Concentrations useful for urologic and ophthalmologic irrigations or applications are 0.1% to 0.2%. The manufacturer states that the compound is nontoxic and nonallergenic in available concentrations.

SODIUM HYPOCHLORITE SOLUTION, N.F.:
Available generically and as household bleach.
DILUTED SODIUM HYPOCHLORITE SOLUTION, N.F.
OXYCHLOROSENE:
Clorpactin XCB (Guardian). Powder (for solution).
OXYCHLOROSENE SODIUM:
Clorpactin WCS-90 (Guardian). Powder (for solution).

Ethylene Oxide: *Ethylene oxide* is readily diffusable, noncorrosive, and biocidal to all organisms at room temperature. This gaseous alkylating agent, widely used as an alternative to heat sterilization of drugs and medical devices, reacts with chloride and water to produce two additional active germicides, ethylene chlorohydrin and ethylene glycol. Ethylene oxide is an alkylating agent and is mutagenic in animals. Controlled studies are in progress to determine the carcinogenic potential of ethylene oxide and ethylene chlorohydrin so that safe residue limits and exposure levels may be established (*Federal Register*, 1978). Special sterilizing chambers are required because the gas must remain in contact with the objects for several hours; it is a pulmonary irritant on inhalation. Ethylene oxide is not used topically as an antiseptic for it is too toxic.

Hydrogen Peroxide: When *hydrogen peroxide* comes into contact with catalase, an enzyme found in blood and most tissue, it is rapidly decomposed into oxygen and water in wounds and on mucous membranes. The liberated oxygen has little bactericidal effect except, possibly, on anaerobes but does debride by loosening masses of infected detritus in wounds. However, the oxygen is released so slowly that use of hydrogen peroxide on intact skin is not recommended.

When diluted with one or more parts of water, hydrogen peroxide is sometimes employed as a mouthwash, but its use to treat stomatitis and gingivitis may irritate the tongue and buccal mucosa. Hydrogen peroxide 3% is often instilled in the external ear to aid in removal of cerumen. It should never be instilled in closed body cavities or abscesses from which the gas has no free egress. Hemiplegia has followed its use to irrigate the pleural cavity; presumably this is caused by the passage of the gas into the vascular system, resulting in cerebral embolism.

Drug available generically: Solution 3%.

Iodine Compounds: Solutions containing elemental iodine or iodophors are antiseptics with a wide spectrum of antimicrobial activity that is fairly persistent. Their activity is reduced by alkaline substances and the presence of organic matter. Iodine can be used to disinfect water when other methods are not available; three drops of tincture of iodine added to one quart of water supposedly kills bacteria and amebae within 15 minutes.

Hypersensitivity reactions may occur after application of any of these compounds. Solutions of iodine are occasionally taken with suicidal intent. The caustic action of elemental iodine affects the gastrointestinal mucosa. Suspensions of starch or protein or solutions of sodium thiosulfate may be used as oral antidotes.

Iodine Solution, U.S.P. contains approximately 2% iodine and 2.4% sodium iodide in water. It is preferred for superficial lacerations to prevent microbial infections, since it is an effective, nonirritating germicide. (Iodine Solution should not be confused with Strong Iodine Solution, U.S.P. [Lugol's solution], which is used to treat thyroid disease.)

Iodine Tincture is a 2% solution of elemental iodine with 2.4% sodium iodide in water and 44% to 50% alcohol. It is preferred to the older 7% iodine tincture for use on the skin and to iodine solution for the decontamination of intact skin prior to intravenous injection or obtaining blood for microbial culture studies. The concentration of alcohol in this 2% tincture is irritating to wounds and does not contribute appreciably to the antibacterial action.

Iodophors are complexes of iodine and organic compounds. The iodophors are divided into two subtypes on the basis of the surfactant nature of the organic compound. *Poloxamer-iodine* is a complex of iodine and the nonionic surfactant copolymer, Pluronic-188. The activity of this preparation is directly related to the availability of free iodine. The second type, *povidone-iodine*, is a complex of iodine and the nonsurfactant polymer, polyvinylpyrrolidone. Free iodine is released slowly from the latter as well. Investigators are seeking to determine if the bound organic iodine moiety has antimicrobial activity in its own right, but present data are insufficient to draw this conclusion.

The iodophors have a broad spectrum of antimicrobial activity. They are used extensively as handwashes for health care personnel; for surgical scrubs; for preparation of the skin prior to surgery, injection, or aspiration; and in the treatment of minor cuts, abrasion, and burns. Povidone-iodine also is used for infected burns and other pyodermas. Development of resistant bacterial strains does not appear to be a potential problem.

Although the iodophors are somewhat less effective than aqueous and alcoholic solutions of elemental iodine, they are usually less irritating; irritation, especially with detergent-containing solutions, does occur occasionally, however. Local hypersensitivity reactions are uncommon. The manufacturer recommends that the rare individual with a history of iodine sensitization should not use the product. Iodophors can be absorbed by starch and the resulting complex is purported to cause serosal adhesions.

None of the following iodine preparations require a prescription.
See also the following section on Anti-infective Agents.
IODINE SOLUTION, U.S.P.
IODINE TINCTURE, U.S.P.
POLOXAMER-IODINE:
Solution, surgical scrub:
Prepodyne (West), *SeptoDyne* (Winthrop).
POVIDONE-IODINE:
Drug available generically: Ointment, solution, surgical scrub, vaginal douche.
Aerosol spray:
Aerodine (Aeroceuticals), *Betadine* (Purdue-Frederick), *Pharmadine* (Sherwood).
Mouthwash and Gargle:
Betadine (Purdue-Frederick), *Isodine* (Blair).
Ointment:
ACU-dyne (Acme United), *Betadine* (Purdue-Frederick), *Isodine* (Blair), *Efodine* (Fougera), *Pharmadine* (Sherwood), *Polydine* (Century).
Skin cleanser:
ACU-dyne (Acme United), *Betadine Liquid, Foam* (Purdue-Frederick), *Isodine* (Blair), *Pharmadine* (Sherwood).
Solution:
ACU-dyne (Acme United), *Betadine* (Purdue-Frederick), *Isodine* (Blair), *Pharmadine* (Sherwood), *Polydine* (Century).
Surgical scrub:
Betadine (Purdue-Frederick), *Mallisol* (Mallard), *Pharmadine* (Sherwood).

Mercurial Compounds: Although organic mercurial compounds are less irritating and toxic than inorganic compounds, they have only weak bacteriostatic activity and are less effective than ethyl alcohol. Except for the phenylmercuric salts, serum and tissue proteins reduce their antimicrobial activity. Skin sensitization is common with their use. Consequently, the antiseptic and disinfectant uses of mercurial compounds are limited.

To avoid systemic absorption of mercury, organic mercurials should not be used on large areas of denuded skin. Acute poisoning with suicidal intent causes gastrointestinal mucosal injury and can cause severe chemical nephrosis with albuminuria, oliguria, azotemia, and irreversible acute renal failure. Dimercaprol is an effective antidote if therapy is begun within four hours (see Chapter 86, Specific Antidotes).

PHENYLMERCURIC NITRATE:
Phe-Mer-Nite (Beecham). Tincture.
THIMEROSAL:
Drug available generically: Solution, tincture.
Merthiolate (Lilly). Aerosol, cream, glycerite, solution, tincture.

Phenolic Compounds: *Phenol* and substituted phenols vary greatly in their antiseptic and disinfectant efficacy and safety. Phenol is bacteriostatic in concentrations of 1:500 to 1:800 and bactericidal and fungicidal in concentrations of 1:50 to 1:100 but is ineffective against spores. At present, phenol is seldom used as an antiseptic or disinfectant. Because it possesses topical local anesthetic activity and has an antipruritic effect at concentrations of 0.5% to 1.5%, its primary use is as a component of numerous topical antipruritic formulations.

Under certain conditions, phenol damages skin which increases the rate of penetration; therefore, its use should be restricted to small areas of skin and occlusive dressings, bandages, or diapers should not be used. Phenol is not recommended for any use on infants under 6 months or for diaper rash in any infant. Phenolic disinfectants have produced epidemics of neonatal hyperbilirubinemia when used to clean bassinets and mattresses in poorly ventilated nurseries. Fatalities have been documented in infants. Since phenol has been implicated as a tumor promoter in concentrations above 5%, controlled studies are under way to determine definitively the potential carcinogenic, mutagenic, and teratogenic activity of this agent in the concentrations used.

Cresol is a mixture of the three methyl isomers of phenol saponified in linseed oil. It is as toxic as phenol but three times more active as a bactericide. Because of its irritating effect on the skin, use of cresol is limited to disinfection. However, neither phenol nor cresol should be used to disinfect rubber, plastic, or fabrics tht may absorb the agent, because burns may result when these come into contact with the skin.

Hexylresorcinol is a more effective bactericide than phenol and is less toxic. It is used in antiseptic mouthwashes and as a skin wound cleanser, but it may be irritating.

Parachlorometaxylenol 2%, a more effective bactericide than phenol, is a component of many OTC mixtures used for acne and seborrhea. More data on skin absorption are needed before its safety can be definitely established.

The short alkyl esters of *p*-hydroxybenzoic acid are known as the *parabens*. Although seldom used as antiseptics, methylparaben and its homologues are commonly included in topical and some parenteral preparations as preservatives. The parabens may sensitize the skin, but the incidence is low.

Hexachlorophene, a chlorinated bisphenol compound with strong bacteriostatic activity, is most effective against gram-positive bacteria, including staphylococci; it has little activity against most gram-negative bacteria or spores. Hexachlorophene is used for handwashing by hospital personnel, as a surgical hand scrub, and for preoperative preparation of the skin.

Although single washings of the skin are no more effective than soap in reducing the number of bacteria, regularly repeated scrubs steadily decrease bacterial flora. Cleansing with alcohol or washing with soap removes the antibacterial residue.

Hexachlorophene may produce irritation, but hypersensitivity reactions are rare. However, since preparations may cause a burning sensation on the skin and in the eyes, suds containing this agent should be rinsed promptly from the eyes with water.

Hexachlorophene is absorbed through intact skin. Since sufficient amounts may be absorbed to produce neurotoxic effects, it should not be applied in the form of compresses and special precautions should be taken to avoid extensive application to broken, denuded, or burned skin. Systemic absorption of hexachlorophene causes symptoms characteristic of cerebral irritability. Hexachlorophene should not be used routinely to bathe infants. When applied to clean small areas of pyoderma in infants, the residue should be rinsed off thoroughly. The drug is available only on prescription.

Triclosan, a 5-chloro-2-(2,4-dichlorophenoxy) phenol, is present as an antimicrobial in bar soaps at concentrations no greater than 1%. Currently, it uses are limited to skin antisepsis and as a wound cleanser and protectant. Since triclosan is not effective against *Pseudomonas*, it cannot be used as a single ingredient in handwashes for health care personnel or surgical hand scrubs or for preoperative preparation. Preparations containing triclosan should not be used in infants under 6 months because the effects of its cumulative absorption through the skin have not been determined.

PHENOL, U.S.P.
SAPONIFIED CRESOL SOLUTION (Lysol)
HEXYLRESORCINOL, N.F.
PARACHLOROMETAXYLENOL, U.S.P.
HEXACHLOROPHENE, U.S.P. (prescription):
Emulsion 3%: *Hexamead-PH* (Spencer Mead) in pt and gal; *pHisoHex* (Winthrop) in 5 oz, pt, and gal; *Soy-Dome Cleanser* (Dome) in 6 oz; *WescoHEX* (West) in 5 oz, pt, and gal.
Emulsion 0.25%:
Septi-Soft (Vestal) in gal.
Sponge 3%:
pHiso Scrub (Winthrop).
Foam 0.23% with 46% alcohol:
Septisol (Vestal) in gal.
TRICLOSAN:
Antimicrobial soaps as *Lifebuoy*, *Phase III*; also with triclocarban as *Irish Spring*.

Silver Compounds: *Silver nitrate* and *silver sulfadiazine* [Silvadene] are the only silver compounds widely used. Colloidal silver preparations (eg, mild silver protein [Argyrol]) are less corrosive, but their disinfecting properties do not equal those of the silver salts because less of the active free silver ion is available; therefore, they are not recommended for such use.

Silver nitrate is strongly bactericidal when applied topically in relatively low concentrations; most microorganisms are rapidly destroyed by a 1:1,000 solution and a 1:10,000 solution is considered to be bacteriostatic.

In many states, instillation of two drops of a 1% solution into the conjunctival sac of newborn infants is required by law to prevent ophthalmia neonatorum. (See Chapter 24, Ocular Anti-infective and Anti-inflammatory Agents.)

Since silver nitrate is an effective germicide and astringent, a 0.1% to 0.5% solution is used on wet dressings but may stain tissue black due to deposition of reduced silver when exposed to sunlight. Occasionally, 0.01% to 0.03% solutions are applied to irrigate the urethra and bladder.

Aqueous solutions containing 0.5% silver nitrate are sometimes applied on dressings for second- and third-degree burns to prevent infections caused by *Pseudomonas aeruginosa*, *Proteus*, and other gram-negative and gram-positive organisms. The most important adverse effect with such use is depletion of sodium and chloride caused by precipitation of insoluble silver chloride; this is particularly likely to occur if silver nitrate is applied to extensive areas over prolonged periods. Silver nitrate stains the skin black; small amounts may be absorbed through the skin after prolonged use, resulting in argyria, a permanent bluish-black discoloration of the skin (only one case of argyria has been reported in association with burn therapy). Pain lasting for one-half to one hour after application of dressings is common if the concentration exceeds 0.5% and is occasionally noted with lower concentrations.

A solid preparation in a pencil-form applicator (toughened silver nitrate) or a cotton pledget dipped in a 10% silver nitrate solution is used to cauterize wounds, fissures, aphthae, and granulomatous tissue.

Silver sulfadiazine is used in burn therapy. See the discussion in the following section on Anti-infective Agents in this chapter and Chapter 77, Sulfonamides and Related Compounds.

SILVER NITRATE, U.S.P.

Drug available generically: Solution (ophthalmic) 1%; ointment; crystals; applicators.

ANTI-INFECTIVE AGENTS

Several antiseptics are used adjunctively with cleansing techniques to treat limited infections associated with minor cuts, abrasions, burns, or insect bites (see the previous section in this chapter). Topically applied antibiotic agents also are beneficial adjunctively, especially in infections in which larger areas are involved or the lesions are more extensive. Other antimicrobial agents, ie, mafenide, nitrofurazone, povidone-iodine 10%, silver sulfadiazine, are principally used for the treatment of infections associated with second- and third-degree burns.

Considerable controversy still exists concerning the precise role of topical application compared to systemic use of antibiotics in moderately severe skin infections. This controversy even extends to treatment of severe burns if adequate facilities are available to minimize contamination and to change wet dressings and perform debridement frequently.

Systemic preparations are available for the treatment of bacterial, fungal, and viral dermatologic infections and infestations such as scabies and pediculosis. See the appropriate chapters in Section XI, Antimicrobial Agents, and Section XII, Antiparasitic Drugs.

Topical Antibiotic Agents

Skin infections (pyodermas) are considered primary or secondary. *Streptococcus pyogenes* and *Staphylococcus aureus* are the most common causative organisms in primary pyodermas (Rosen and Rudolph, 1978). Folliculitis, furuncles, carbuncles, and bullous impetigo are typical of primary staphylococcal pyodermas; nonbullous facial impetigo is usually caused by staphylococci. Ecthyma, cellulitis, erysipelas, and certain types of nonbullous impetigo are generally caused by beta-hemolytic streptococci.

Topical antibiotic therapy, local cleansing, and drainage if indicated are effective in most cases of superficial folliculitis or uncomplicated furunculosis. Deeper lesions associated with surrounding cellulitis and fever or recurrent lesions generally require systemic and possibly topical antibiotic therapy. Systemic administration of a penicillinase-resistant penicillin is employed for staphylococcal impetigo, although erythromycin is preferred by many pediatricians and dermatologists.

Although streptococcal ecthyma responds to topical antibiotic treatment and local cleansing, results are achieved more rapidly with systemic therapy. When the involvement is limited and the patient or family is able to perform gentle debridement of the thick crusts prior to application of the topical antibiotic, systemic antibiotic therapy may not be required (Leyden and Kligman, 1978 B). Systemic administration is almost always indicated in cellulitis, erysipelas, and extensive streptococcal pyoderma; however, aggressive systemic therapy does not significantly reduce the incidence of postpyodermal streptococcal-induced nephritis.

The poorly absorbed topical antibiotics, *bacitracin, gramicidin, neomycin,* and *polymyxin B*, are useful. Neomycin is particularly effective against staphylococci, and streptococci are particularly susceptible to bacitracin. Many gram-negative organisms, except *Proteus* and *Serratia*, are susceptible to polymyxin B, and gramicidin is effective against numerous gram-positive organisms. Since culturing of uncomplicated, limited skin infections is often inappropriate from the standpoint of time and cost and because multiple organisms are commonly associated with a single skin infection, mixtures of the poorly absorbed topical antibiotics are used frequently. Topical erythromycin is also effective and is the drug of choice when contact irritation or sensitivity occurs to the poorly absorbed topical antibiotics; it also is employed in acne vulgaris. Gentamicin is useful occasionally when the causative organism is *Pseudomonas* or other gram-negative species. The development of resistant strains does not appear to be a major problem in outpatient use; however, topical usage is not advised for patients in relatively confined groups (eg, camps, military

units, hospitals) except to treat burns if gentamicin is indicated.

The use of topical tetracycline [Topicycline] and clindamycin is limited almost exclusively to acne therapy (see the section on Agents Used in Acne Vulgaris in this chapter).

The reported incidence of hypersensitivity to a 20% concentration of topically applied neomycin has varied between 3.7% and 60% in individuals with contact dermatitis or chronic dermatoses; the incidence in the general population is about 1% (Prystowsky et al, 1979). Sensitivity to neomycin may extend to other aminoglycoside antibiotics. For more information, see the evaluations on bacitracin and gramicidin (Chapter 76), neomycin (Chapter 74), and polymyxin B (Chapter 75).

Secondary pyodermas appear in conjunction with other skin disorders, such as insect bites, burns, other dermatoses, and pre-existing fungal or viral infections. The most common serious secondary pyodermas are observed in patients with second- or third-degree burns, infectious eczematoid dermatitis, and intertrigo.

BACITRACIN:
Ointment: *Generic, Baciguent* (Upjohn).
ERYTHROMYCIN:
Ointment: *Generic, Ilotycin* (Dista) 1% in 15 and 30 g tubes and 454 g jar (prescription).
GENTAMICIN SULFATE:
Ointment, Cream: *Garamycin* (Schering) 0.1% in 15 g tubes (prescription).
NEOMYCIN:
Cream: *Generic.*
Ointment: *Generic, Myciguent* (Upjohn).
AVAILABLE MIXTURES.
BACITRACIN AND NEOMYCIN:
Ointment: *Generic, Bacimycin* (Merrell-National).
BACITRACIN AND POLYMYXIN B:
Ointment: *Generic, Biotres* (Central), *Polycin* (Dow), *Polysporin* (Burroughs Wellcome).
BACITRACIN, POLYMYXIN B, AND NEOMYCIN:
Aerosol, Powder: *Neosporin* (Burroughs Wellcome) (prescription).
Ointment: *Generic, B.P.N.* (Norwich-Eaton), *Mycitracin* (Upjohn), *Neo-Polycin* (Dow), *Neosporin* (Burroughs Wellcome).
NEOMYCIN AND GRAMICIDIN:
Ointment: *Spectrocin* (Squibb).
NEOMYCIN, GRAMICIDIN, AND POLYMYXIN B:
Cream: *Neosporin-G* (Burroughs Wellcome) (prescription).

Other Topical Antimicrobial Agents

The infected burn wound represents a unique therapeutic problem (Moleski, 1978). Since blood supply to the skin is usually compromised, topical rather than systemic antimicrobial administration is necessary to distribute the compound at the involved site. If invasive infection (bacteremia) is present or anticipated, it may be necessary to institute systemic antibiotic therapy. Gram-negative rods (eg, strains of *Pseudomonas, Klebsiella, Enterobacter, Proteus, Providencia, Serratia*) are most commonly the causative organisms. Streptococcal and staphylococcal strains are observed less commonly; occasionally fungi, especially *Candida albicans*, may be the causative organism.

Silver sulfadiazine and *mafenide* are used most commonly for severe, extensive burns. Silver sulfadiazine does not have the eschar-penetrating power of mafenide; however, it does not possess the potential for producing acid-base disturbance or pain on application that is characteristic of the latter. See the evaluations in Chapter 77, Sulfonamides and Related Compounds.

A 10% solution or 10% ointment of *povidone-iodine* is used extensively for limited pyodermas and burns. Marked systemic absorption of iodine may occur in extensive burns (Lavelle et al, 1975); metabolic acidosis and impairment of renal function occasionally are associated with a high serum iodine concentration; however, these complications may not always be causally related (Blanco and Rothwell, 1976). Until definitive data on absorption and toxicity become available, it is suggested that topical povidone-iodine be used cautiously in extensive burns, particularly when metabolic acidosis and renal impairment are present (Pietsch and Meakins, 1976).

Gentamicin occasionally is used topically for infected severe burns, particularly when the causative organism is *Pseudomonas* or other susceptible gram-negative species. Absorption from limited burn surfaces is clinically insignificant if renal function is adequate. The Council on Drugs of The American Academy of Pediatrics recommends that aminoglycosides not be used on large denuded surfaces because systemic toxicity may ensue; in addition, these agents encourage the growth of resistant organisms in confined populations.

Nitrofurazone is used primarily for burns. It is bactericidal for many gram-positive and gram-negative organisms present in surface infections, but strains of *Pseudomonas* and *Proteus* are often resistant (see also Chapter 78, Urinary Tract Antiseptics). It has been used topically to treat infections of the skin and mucous membranes. As with most topical preparations, severe dermatitis (eg, cutaneous exfoliation) has been reported with this agent; leg ulcer sites are more susceptible to hypersensitivity reactions than normal unabraded skin.

SILVER SULFADIAZINE:
Silvadene (Marion). Cream (water-miscible) 10 mg/g in 50 and 400 g containers or multiple-treatment (3-50 g) packs (prescription).

MAFENIDE ACETATE:
Sulfamylon (Winthrop). Cream 85 mg/g in 2 (56.7 g), 4 (113.4 g), and 14.5 (411 g) oz containers (prescription).

POVIDONE-IODINE:
Drug available generically: Ointment, solution.
Acu-dyne (Acme United). Ointment.
Betadine (Purdue-Frederick). Aerosol foam [Helafoam Solution], aerosol spray, ointment, whirlpool concentrate.
Efodine (Fougera). Ointment.
Pharmadine (Sherwood). Ointment, solution, spray.
Polydine (Century). Ointment.

NITROFURAZONE:
Drug available generically: Ointment, soluble dressing, solution (prescription).
Furacin (Norwich-Eaton). Cream 0.2% in 14, 28, and 368 g containers; powder 0.2% in 14 g containers; soluble dressing 0.2% in 28, 56, 135, and 454 g and 5 lb containers; solution 0.2% in 60 and 473 ml containers (prescription).

ANTI-INFLAMMATORY CORTICOSTEROIDS

Seborrheic dermatitis, atopic dermatitis, lichen simplex chronicus (localized neurodermatitis), pruritus ani, allergic and irritant contact dermatitis (particularly the later phases), and the inflammatory phase of xerosis generally are very responsive to topical corticosteroids of lesser potency (Maibach and Stoughton, 1975). Psoriasis of the face and body folds is responsive, but that affecting the palms, soles, elbows, and knees usually requires more potent topical corticosteroids. The latter also are generally required for discoid lupus erythematosus, necrobiosis lipoidica, lichen planus, pemphigus, granuloma annulare, and pretibial myxedema. If higher concentrations and even occlusion with these more potent corticosteroids are ineffective, intralesional injection may be necessary for acne cysts, hypertrophic lichen planus, and alopecia areata. Intralesional injection is the only method of application of corticosteroids recommended for hypertrophic scars and keloids. Oral or injectable corticosteroids may be required for the acute manifestations of allergic and irritant contact dermatitis.

The mechanism of action of the corticosteroids is related at least in part to their properties of vasoconstriction, suppression of membrane permeability and the immune response, and antimitotic activity. Their vasoconstrictor action decreases extravasation of serum into the skin and inhibits swelling and discomfort. Their lysosomal membrane-stabilizing effect inhibits the release of cytotoxic chemical substances which cause pain and pruritus.

TABLE 2.
DESCENDING ORDER OF POTENCY
OF TOPICAL CORTICOSTEROID PREPARATIONS*

Group	Drug
I	desoximetasone cream 0.25% [Topicort]** fluocinonide cream and ointment 0.05% [Lidex]; gel 0.05% [Topsyn] halcinonide cream 0.1% [Halog]
II	betamethasone benzoate gel 0.025% [Benisone, Uticort] betamethasone dipropionate cream 0.05% [Diprosone] betamethasone valerate ointment and lotion 0.1% [Valisone] triamcinolone acetonide cream 0.5% [Artistocort A, Kenalog]
III	Fluocinolone acetonide ointment 0.025% [Synalar]; cream 0.2% [Synalar HP] flurandrenolide ointment 0.05% [Cordran] triamcinolone acetonide ointment 0.1% [Aristocort, Kenalog]
IV	betamethasone valerate cream 0.1% [Valisone] fluocinolone acetonide cream 0.025% [Synemol] flurandrenolide cream 0.05% [Cordran] hydrocortisone valerate cream 0.2% [Westcort]** triamcinolone acetonide cream 0.1% and 0.025% lotion [Kenalog]
V	desonide cream 0.05% [Tridesilon] flumethasone pivalate cream 0.3% [Locorten]
VI	prednisolone [Meti-Derm] methylprednisolone acetate [Medrol] fluorometholone [Oxylone] dexamethasone [Decadron, Decaderm in Estergel] cortisol (hydrocortisone)

Potency is, at best, an approximation based on vasoconstrictor assays, double blind studies and general clinical observations. No significant difference exists among agents within any given group. Potency is dependent upon the particular corticosteroid, its concentration and the vehicle in that in general, ointment-gel, cream and lotion represent a decreasing order of vehicle effectiveness in enhancing corticosteroid skin penetration.

*Adapted from Maibach HI, Stoughton RB: Topical corticosteroids, in Azarnoff DL (ed): Steroid Therapy, Philadelphia, WB Saunders Co, 1975, 183, and Stoughton RB: Evaluation of new potent steroids, in Frost P, et al (eds): Recent Advances in Dermatopharmacology. New York, Spectrum Publications Inc, 1978, 109. Reprinted by permission.

**These agents were not listed in the original tables. The results of clinical vasoconstrictor assays suggest that diflorasone diacetate cream 0.05% [Florone] belongs in Group I, but clinical use assays are not yet complete.

Suppression of mitotic activity effectively diminishes epidermal hyperplasia, and epidermal and dermal atrophy may result from interference with synthetic pathways. Corticosteroids interfere with lymphokine stimulation which enhances an immune response; therefore, migration of immune-effector substances to a site of inflammation is limited.

In addition to the dermatologic disorder, the selection of a corticosteroid depends primarily upon the drug's inherent potency, concentration, formulation, and application method; the anatomic location of disease; the patient's age; and the expense (Sneddon, 1976). Selected topical corticosteroids are grouped on the basis of potency in Table 2 (Maibach and Stoughton, 1975; Stoughton, 1978). The most potent topical corticosteroids are generally fluorinated compounds. Although the agents in this group may be effective when less potent corticosteroids are inadequate, the risk of adverse reactions is also increased. Consequently, most authorities (Kligman and Kaidbey, 1978) currently recommend that the less potent corticosteroids be administered in conjunction with measures that improve dermal absorption (eg, more frequent application, use of occlusive vehicles or wraps). If more potent steroids are needed for acute conditions in poorly permeable areas, a less potent steroid should be considered for subsequent maintenance therapy, particularly for chronic skin diseases.

The formulation and method of application are not only important in determining the degree of corticosteroid absorption but also are influenced by whether the lesions are wet or dry. See the section on Vehicles for more details. A low-potency steroid may be adequate in permeable areas of skin known to absorb considerably more corticosteroid (eg, scalp, axilla, face, neck, perineal area, genitals); this is particularly true if an occlusive-wrap method of application is employed, for this can increase absorption as much as tenfold. A more potent corticosteroid may be required for less permeable skin regions (eg, palms, soles, back).

Younger individuals, especially infants, and elderly patients with atrophic skin are more susceptible to the effects of topical corticosteroids. Careful monitoring and use of less potent agents (eg, cortisol) are usually indicated.

Expense can be a significant factor. The prototype of this group (cortisol) is available generically; therefore, its cost will generally be less than that of most trademarked higher-potency preparations. However, when not contraindicated, more aggressive therapy with higher-potency, higher-risk corticosteroids may shorten the duration of illness, the number of work days lost, and the incidence of noncompliance in individuals who cannot or will not follow directions (eg, use with occlusive dressings). Therefore, relative expense is best determined by the physician for the individual patient.

Predictable adverse reactions to topically applied corticosteroids are directly related to potency, degree of absorption at the site(s) of application, and the total amount applied (Hill and Rostenberg, 1978; Goette and Odom, 1979). Allergic contact dermatitis is rare compared to the number of prescriptions for topical corticosteroids written; some cases are caused by the vehicle components rather than the corticosteroid. Epidermal and dermal atrophy resulting in thinning of the skin, striae, telangiectasia, and senile-type purpura are most commonly seen in highly absorptive areas (ie, face, neck, axilla, perianal area, genitals). The face, perianal region, or genitals may be affected by a condition termed rebound pustulation that can occur when discontinuing the more potent steroids. Corticosteroids can aggravate existing infections, particularly with occlusive dressings, and they can mask dermatophytoses or scabies infestation (see the section on Corticosteroid-Antibiotic Mixtures).

Systemic toxicity usually is observed only with high-potency corticosteroids when occlusive dressings are employed. It generally does not occur when the total weekly dose does not exceed 30 g in adults or 10 g in small children. If the total weekly dose exceeds 50 g, assessment of hypothalamic-pituitary axis (HPA) function may be indicated. Individuals taking large total doses of high-potency corticosteroids, with or without use of occlusive dressings, should receive supplemental systemic corticosteroid therapy if surgery is necessary. For the signs and symptoms of systemic corticosteroid toxicity, see Chapter 41.

Topical corticosteroids are contraindicated in varicella and vaccinia. Intralesional injection is often valuable in cystic acne, and cortisol may be required temporarily to control an exacerbation of severe erythema and inflammation in acne rosacea and vulgaris.

TOPICAL CORTICOSTEROID PREPARATIONS (Prescription):

CORTISOL (Hydrocortisone):
Drug available generically and as trademarked products. Common forms and concentrations include:
Aeroseb-HC (Herbert). Aerosol spray 0.5% in 58 g containers.
Alphaderm (Norwich-Eaton). Cream 1% in a stabilized carbamide (urea) delivery system in 30 and 100 g containers.
Cetacort (Parke, Davis). Lotion 0.25% in 120 ml containers; 0.5% and 1% in 60 ml containers.
Cort-Dome (Dome). Lotion 0.125% in 240 ml containers, 0.25% in 120 ml containers, and 1% in 15 and 30 ml containers; cream 0.125% in 30 and 120 g containers, 0.25% in 30, 120, and 454 g containers, 0.5% in 15, 30, 120, and 454 g containers, and 1% in 15 and 30 g containers.
Cortef (Upjohn). Ointment 1% and 2.5% in 5 and 20 g containers.
Cortril (Pfipharmecs). Ointment 1% in 15 g containers.
Hytone (Dermik). Cream 0.5% and 1% in 30 and 120 g containers.
Nutracort (Owen). Gel 1% in 15 and 60 g containers.

CORTISOL VALERATE (Hydrocortisone Valerate):
Westcort (Westwood). Cream 0.2% in 15, 45, and 60 g containers.

BETAMETHASONE:
Celestone (Schering). Cream 0.2% in 15 g containers.

BETAMETHASONE BENZOATE:
Benisone (Parke, Davis). Cream and gel 0.025% in 15 and 60 g containers.
Uticort (Parke, Davis). Cream, gel, and ointment 0.025% in 15 and 60 g containers; lotion 0.025% in 15 and 60 ml containers.

BETAMETHASONE DIPROPIONATE:
Diprosone (Schering). Aerosol 0.1% in 85 g containers; cream and ointment 0.05% in 15

and 45 g containers; lotion 0.05% in 20 and 60 ml containers.

BETAMETHASONE VALERATE:
Valisone (Schering). Aerosol 0.15% in 85 g containers; cream 0.1% in 15 and 60 g containers; lotion 0.1% in 20 and 60 ml containers; ointment 0.1% in 5, 15, and 45 g containers.

DESONIDE:
Tridesilon (Dome). Cream 0.05% in 15 and 60 g and 5 lb containers; ointment 0.05% in 15 and 60 g containers.

DESOXIMETASONE:
Topicort (Hoechst-Roussel). Cream 0.25% in 15 and 60 g containers.

DEXAMETHASONE:
Aeroseb-Dex (Herbert). Aerosol 0.01% in 58 g containers.
Decaspray (Merck Sharp & Dohme). Aerosol 10 mg in 25 g pressurized containers.
Decaderm in Estergel (Merck Sharp & Dohme). Gel 0.1% in 15 and 30 g containers.

DEXAMETHASONE PHOSPHATE:
Decadron Phosphate (Merck Sharp & Dohme). Cream 0.1% in 15 and 30 g containers.

DIFLORASONE DIACETATE:
Florone (Upjohn). Cream and ointment 0.05% in 15 and 30 g containers.

FLUMETHASONE PIVALATE:
Locorten (Ciba). Cream 0.03% in 15 and 60 g containers.

FLUOCINOLONE ACETONIDE:
Fluonid (Herbert). Cream 0.01% and 0.025% in 15, 60, and 425 g containers; ointment 0.025% in 15 and 60 g containers; solution 0.01% in 20 and 60 ml containers.
Synalar (Syntex). Cream 0.01% in 15, 45, 60, 120, and 425 g containers and 0.2% (Synalar-HP) in 12 g containers; ointment 0.025% in 15, 60, and 425 g containers; solution 0.01% in 20 and 60 ml containers.
Synemol (Syntex). Cream 0.025% in 15, 30, and 60 g containers.

FLUOCINONIDE:
Topsyn (Syntex). Gel 0.05% in 15, 30, and 60 g containers.
Lidex (Syntex). Cream and ointment 0.05% in 15, 30, and 60 g containers.

FLUOROMETHOLONE:
Oxylone (Upjohn). Cream 0.025% in 15, 60, and 120 g containers.

FLURANDRENOLIDE:
Cordran (Dista). Cream and ointment 0.05% in 15, 30, 60, 225 g containers and 0.025% in 30, 60, and 225 g containers; tape 4 mcg/cm² in 7.5 cm X 60 cm and 7.5 cm X 200 cm rolls; lotion 0.05% in 15 and 60 ml containers.

HALCINONIDE:
Halog (Squibb). Cream 0.1% in 15, 60, and 240 g containers; ointment 0.025% and 0.1% in 15, 60, and 240 g containers; solution 0.1% in 20 and 60 ml containers.

HYDROCORTISONE (See CORTISOL)

METHYLPREDNISOLONE ACETATE:
Medrol Acetate (Upjohn). Ointment 0.25% and 1% in 7.5, 30, and 45 g containers (Medrol Veriderm).

PREDNISOLONE:
Meti-Derm (Schering). Aerosol 0.5% in 150 g containers; cream 0.5% in 10 and 25 g containers.

TRIAMCINOLONE ACETONIDE:
Aristocort (Lederle). Cream 0.025% and 0.1% in 15, 75, and 240 g and 5 lb containers and 0.5% in 15 and 240 g containers; ointment 0.1% in 15, 75, and 240 g and 5 lb containers and 0.5% in 15 and 240 g containers.
Aristocort A (Lederle). Cream 0.1% in 15, 75, and 240 g containers and 0.5% in 15 g containers; ointment 0.1% in 15 and 75 g containers and 0.5% in 15 g containers.
Aristoderm (Lederle). Foam 0.1% in 15 g containers.
Aristogel (Lederle). Gel 0.1% in 15 and 75 g containers.
Kenalog (Squibb). Cream 0.025% in 15, 80, and 240 g and 5.25 lb containers, 0.1% in 15, 60, 80, and 240 g and 5.25 lb containers, and 0.5% in 20 g containers; lotion 0.025% in 60 ml containers and 0.1% in 15 and 60 ml containers; ointment 0.025% in 15, 80, and 240 g containers and 0.1% in 15, 60, 80, and 240 g containers; suspension (spray) 0.147 mg/g in 23 and 63 g containers; Kenalog in Orabase Dental Paste 0.1% for oral application in 5 g containers.

CORTICOSTEROID-ANTIBIOTIC MIXTURES

When a secondary pyoderma is superimposed on a pre-existing dermatitis or an allergic inflammatory dermatitis (eg, eczema) develops in response to a primary pyoderma, the concomitant use of a topical corticosteroid and antibiotic may be indicated. The criteria for selection of parenteral and/or topical antibiotic(s) and a corticosteroid are presented in the preceding sections on Anti-infective Agents and Anti-inflammatory Corticosteroids, respectively.

The appropriateness of simultaneous use of a topical corticosteroid and topical antibiotic is controversial (Leyden and Kligman, 1978 A). Those opposed argue that there is insufficient evidence to show that topical steroid-antibiotic therapy is more effective than the steroid alone in secondary pyodermas, and it carries the additional risk of development of organism re-sistance and allergic contact dermatitis (especially with neomycin). Those in favor point out that well-controlled studies, including quantitative bacteriologic data, show that the combination significantly improves results when therapy is initiated early, is limited to one or two weeks' duration, is avoided in patients with stasic dermatitis or ulcers to decrease the incidence of antibiotic (neomycin) sensitivity, and is chosen on the basis of the area involved (eg, neomycin for glabrous skin infections predominantly caused by *Staphylococcus aureus*, broader spectrum agents for fungal and gram-negative bacteria commonly present in intertriginous areas). Quantitative culturing is also recommended in unresponsive cases.

A listing of representative mixtures containing various corticosteroids and antibiotics follows. Although the concentration of each antimicrobial is not given, the following concentrations are commonly present: neomycin sulfate 0.5%, clioquinol (iodochlorhydroxyquin) 3%, gramicidin 0.025%, polymyxin B sulfate 5,000 to 10,000 units/g, bacitracin 400 to 500 units/g, and nystatin 100,000 units/g.

AVAILABLE MIXTURES
(Prescription):
CORTISOL (Hydrocortisone) AND NEOMYCIN:
Mixture available generically: Ointment containing cortisol 1% and neomycin.
Neo-Cort-Dome (Dome). Cream containing cortisol 0.25%, 0.5%, and 1% and neomycin in 30 and 120 g containers or cortisol 1% and neomycin in 15 g containers.
Neo-Cortef (Upjohn). Cream containing cortisol acetate 1% or 2.5% and neomycin in 20 g containers; lotion containing cortisol acetate 1% and neomycin in 15 ml containers.
CORTISOL AND CLIOQUINOL (iodochlorhydroxyquin) or IODOQUINOL (diiodohydroxyquin):
Mixture available generically: Cream and ointment containing cortisol 0.5% or 1% and clioquinol.
Vioform-Hydrocortisone (Ciba). Cream containing cortisol 0.5% and clioquinol (mild) in 15 and 30 g containers or cortisol 1% and clioquinol in 5 and 20 g containers; lotion containing cortisol 1% and clioquinol in 15 ml containers; ointment containing cortisol 0.5% and clioquinol (mild) in 30 g containers or ointment containing cortisol 1% and clioquinol in 20 g containers.
Vytone (Dermik). Cream containing cortisol 0.5% and iodoquinol in 30 g containers.

CORTISOL, CLIOQUINOL, AND NYSTATIN:
Nystaform-HC (Dome). Ointment containing cortisol 1%, clioquinol, and nystatin in 15 g containers.

CORTISOL, NEOMYCIN, POLYMYXIN B, AND GRAMICIDIN:
Cortisporin (Burroughs Wellcome). Cream containing cortisol acetate 0.5%, neomycin, polymyxin B, and gramicidin in 7.5 g containers.

CORTISOL, NEOMYCIN, POLYMYXIN B, AND BACITRACIN ZINC:
Cortisporin (Burroughs Wellcome). Ointment containing cortisol 1%, neomycin sulfate, polymyxin B sulfate, and bacitracin zinc in 15 g containers.

DEXAMETHASONE AND NEOMYCIN:
NeoDecadron (Merck Sharp & Dohme). Cream containing dexamethasone sodium phosphate 0.1% and neomycin in 15 and 30 g containers; aerosol [NeoDecaspray] containing dexamethasone 10 mg and neomycin sulfate 50 mg in 25 g pressurized containers.

FLUOCINOLONE AND NEOMYCIN:
Neo-Synalar (Syntex). Cream containing fluocinolone acetonide 0.025% and neomycin in 15 and 60 g containers.

FLUOROMETHOLONE AND NEOMYCIN:
Neo-Oxylone (Upjohn). Ointment containing fluorometholone 0.025% and neomycin in 7.5 g containers.

FLURANDRENOLIDE AND NEOMYCIN:
Cordran-N (Dista). Cream and ointment containing flurandrenolide 0.05% and neomycin in 7.5, 15, and 60 g containers.

METHYLPREDNISOLONE AND NEOMYCIN:
Neo-Medrol (Upjohn). Ointment containing methylprednisolone acetate 0.25% or 1% and neomycin in 7.5, 30, and 45 g containers.

PREDNISOLONE AND NEOMYCIN:
MetiDerm w/Neomycin (Schering). Aerosol containing prednisolone 50 mg and neomycin 50 mg in 150 g containers; ointment containing prednisolone 0.5% and neomycin in 10 g containers.
Neo-Delta-Cortef (Upjohn). Ointment containing prednisolone acetate 0.5% and neomycin in 5 and 20 g containers.

TRIAMCINOLONE, NEOMYCIN, GRAMICIDIN, AND NYSTATIN:
Mycolog (Squibb). Cream and ointment containing triamcinolone acetonide 1%, neomycin, gramicidin, and nystatin in 15, 30, 60, and 120 g containers.

AGENTS AFFECTING KERATIN

Several chemicals affect keratin in diverse ways and are useful dermatologic drugs. Urea and propylene glycol hydrate keratin and have a mild keratolytic action that promotes desquamation of the stratum corneum; these actions are sometimes useful in the treatment of dry skin. Both compounds also are used as carriers to improve the penetration of more potent keratolytic agents.

Sulfur and resorcinol have a relatively mild keratolytic action (peeling effect) and also have weak antibacterial and antifungal activity.

Salicylic acid is an effective keratolytic agent in concentrations of 3% to 6%. Concentrations greater than 20% are destructive and are principally employed in the management of verrucae (warts), corns, and callouses.

UREA

Urea, in a suitable cream or ointment vehicle, may soften the skin in ichthyotic and other dry, scaly conditions such as psoriasis or atopic dermatitis. It disrupts the normal hydrogen bonding of keratinic proteins, an effect attributed to its hydrating and keratolytic actions. It has not been established whether the antipruritic effect results from a direct action or from improvement in the skin condition.

Drug available generically: Crystals (bulk).
Aquacare (Herbert). Cream, lotion 2% and 10% (Aquacare/HP).
Aqua Lacten (Herald). Lotion 10%.
Carmol-10 (Syntex). Lotion 10%.
Carmol-20 (Syntex). Cream 20%.
Nutraplus (Owen). Cream, lotion 10%.
U-Lactin (TI-Pharmaceuticals). Lotion 10%.
AVAILABLE MIXTURES.
Carmol-HC (Syntex). Cream containing urea 10% and cortisol 1% in 30 and 120 g containers (prescription).

PROPYLENE GLYCOL

Propylene glycol, a widely used vehicle in dermatologic formulations, is isotonic in 2% concentrations. In concentrations up to 70%, it causes marked hydration and softening of the skin and desquamation of scales, particularly when used under occlusive dressings. Propylene glycol and other hydroalcoholic gels augment the keratolytic action of salicylic acid; this combination may be effective in ichthyosis. Treatment should be limited to no more than 20% of the body surface at any one time to avoid excessive salicylate absorption. The preparation may be applied under occlusive dressing before retiring and washed off in the morning. Nightly therapy is used initially, with the frequency of application reduced when improvement occurs.

Subjective irritation (burning and stinging) occurs, particularly if the skin is damaged. Irritation can occur; this may be especially evident with occlusion. Propylene glycol probably produces allergic contact dermatitis more often than was previously suspected (Fisher, 1978).

> AVAILABLE MIXTURE.
> **Keralyt** (Westwood). Gel containing salicylic acid 6% in a 60% propylene glycol, 20% alcohol vehicle in 30 g containers (prescription).

SULFUR

RESORCINOL

Numerous nonprescription preparations contain sulfur or resorcinol in concentrations of 2% to 10%. They are promoted for the topical treatment of acne vulgaris, dandruff, seborrheic dermatoses, superficial fungal infections, and diaper dermatoses. However, more potent and specific keratolytic, antifungal, and antibacterial agents are available for each of these conditions and should be considered when more than minimal involvement is present.

Nonprescription shampoo mixtures that contain salicylic acid 2% and sulfur 2% to 5% are available for the treatment of seborrheic capitis. Sulfur and/or resorcinol have been combined with one or more active topical ingredients (eg, salicylic acid, coal tar products, anthralin) in nonprescription preparations.

A preparation containing sulfur 3% and salicylic acid 6% in petrolatum is used as an alternative in erythrasma or superficial fungal infections. Because percutaneous penetration and louse resistance to lindane (gamma benzene hexachloride) have been documented, some physicians use sulfur 6% in petrolatum for pediculosis in pregnant women, infants, and young children (see Chapter 84, Scabicides and Pediculicides).

> PRECIPITATED SULFUR, U.S.P.:
> Drug available generically: Powder. Ointments containing sulfur 3% to 15% can be compounded by the pharmacist.
> RESORCINOL:
> Available only as ingredient of mixtures.
> SULFUR AND SALICYLIC ACID:
> **Fostex** (Westwood), **Meted** (Texas), **Rezamid** (Dermik), **Sebaveen** (Cooper), **Sebulex** (Westwood), **Vanseb** (Herbert).

SALICYLIC ACID

Salicylic acid 3% to 6% in an ointment base is a useful keratolytic agent in seborrheic dermatitis, acne, and psoriasis. A 6% concentration in petrolatum is used to thin or remove calluses. This concentration in a gel base with propylene glycol 60% [Keralyt] is particularly effective when applied under occlusive dressings to treat ichthyosis (see the evaluation on Propylene Glycol). Concentrations above 6% are destructive. As a plaster, salicylic acid 40% has been used with variable success in treating warts and corns. Combinations of salicylic acid and lactic acid, each in a concentration of 10% to 20%, in flexible collodion also have been used for the same indications (Bunney et al, 1976).

Salicylic acid is used to treat superficial fungal infections, but more potent antifungal and less keratolytic agents are available. A preparation containing benzoic acid 12% and salicylic acid 6% (Whitfield's ointment) was promoted as an antifungal agent for years. Keratolytic agents may be necessary initially when fungal infections in deeper layers are otherwise inaccessible to the more potent antifungal agents.

This drug is readily absorbed and is slowly excreted in the urine. Thus, salicylic acid should not be applied over large areas or for prolonged periods to avoid salicylism. Caution must be exercised when a 40% plaster is used, particularly on the extremities, in diabetics or patients with peripheral vascular disease, since acute inflammation and ulceration may occur after excessive use. This acid is not effective in a zinc oxide paste (eg, Lassar's Plain Zinc Paste) because it forms zinc salicylate which is pharmacologically inactive. Ointments or lotions containing salicylic acid are odorless and do not stain the skin.

To remove calluses, the ointment is applied at bedtime and washed off in the morning. For the treatment of warts and corns, adhesive plaster is applied to the affected area and changed daily; the skin is washed between treatments. The softened necrotic tissue is then scraped off with an emery board or pared with a scalpel blade or scissors. Plantar warts generally require longer exposures and more frequent debridement. A similar regimen is instituted for most other indications, except that the duration of contact is shortened.

SALICYLIC ACID, U.S.P.:
Drug available generically: Crystals; ointment 25% and 60%; powder.
SALICYLIC ACID COLLODION, U.S.P.;
SALICYLIC ACID PLASTER, U.S.P.:
Numerous commercial products available. Selected concentrations can be compounded by a pharmacist.
AVAILABLE MIXTURES.
Keralyt (Westwood). Gel containing salicylic acid 6% in a 60% propylene glycol, 20% alcohol vehicle in 30 g containers (prescription).
Duofilm (Stiefel), *Salactic Liquifilm* (Pedinol). Flexible collodion containing salicylic acid 16.7% and lactic acid 16.7% in 15 ml containers (prescription).

ANTIDANDRUFF AGENTS

Dandruff and seborrheic dermatitis are associated with an increased rate of maturation and proliferation of epidermal cells, although other characteristics of these disorders, such as type of scale, sebum retention, epidermal hyperplasia, dermal capillary proliferation, areas of involvement, and presence of inflammation, differ considerably.

Dandruff is not considered a pathologic phenomenon; it affects individuals who are at the upper limit of normal variation with respect to rate of turnover of epidermal cells. The excessive scaling (scurf) is most obvious on the scalp and is not accompanied by infection, inflammation, alteration of sebum kinetics, pathologic change, or epidermal hyperplasia. Although dandruff often can be controlled with frequent application of bland shampoos (two to three washings per week), some individuals may require medicated shampoos. Nonprescription shampoos containing sulfur and salicylic acid are beneficial, but preparations containing zinc pyrithione or selenium sulfide are more effective and are required for resistant cases.

Seborrheic dermatitis is an inflammatory scaling disease of the scalp and face; occasionally, the eyelids, upper middle anterior chest, and intertriginous area also are involved. Retention, but not excessive production, of sebum imparts an oily character to the scales; epidermal hyperplasia and an abnormal number of parakeratotic cells are also present. Pruritus is common.

Zinc pyrithione, selenium sulfide, and sulfur-salicylic acid shampoos are effective in seborrheic capitis. Seborrheic blepharitis is treated with preparations containing sulfacetamide and a corticosteroid [Cetapred, Metimyd, Optimyd] or similiar combination preparations containing phenylephrine as well [Blephamide, Sulfapred, Vasocidin] (see Chapter 24, Ocular Anti-infective and Anti-inflammatory Agents). Low- or intermediate-potency topical corticosteroids may be indicated if involvement is widespread, particularly if inflammation is prominent (see the section on Anti-inflammatory Agents).

SELENIUM SULFIDE
[Exsel, Iosel 250, Selsun, Selsun Blue]

Selenium sulfide shampoos are effective in the treatment of dandruff and seborrheic capitis. This agent is used to treat tinea versicolor (see Chapter 80, Antifungal Agents). Selenium sulfide appears to derive its antidandruff effectiveness from its antimitotic activity and its substantivity (ie, residual adherence after shampoo and rinse) to the skin.

Little or no toxicity has been observed when selenium sulfide is applied as directed to normal skin or hair. The drug irritates conjunctival mucosa on contact and should not be applied to large areas of skin with marked dermatitic lesions because it may act as an irritant under such circumstances. The product should not be used when acute inflammation or exudation is present, because absorption may be increased. Allergic contact dermatitis has not been documented.

One or two teaspoonsful are applied and allowed to remain on the scalp for five to ten minutes before being rinsed off thoroughly; the application can be repeated if the involvement is extensive. The preparation may be used one to three times weekly. Contact with the eyes should be avoided.

> Drug available generically: Lotion, shampoo 1% (nonprescription) and 2.5% (prescription); liquid, suspension 2.5% (prescription).
> **Exsel** (Herbert), **Selsun** (Abbott). Lotion 2.5% in 120 ml containers (prescription).
> **Iosel 250** (Owen). Lotion 2.5% in 240 ml containers (prescription).
> **Selsun Blue** (Abbott). Cream 1% (nonprescription).

ZINC PYRITHIONE

Zinc pyrithione shampoos are widely used nonprescription formulations that are effective temporarily in the treatment of dandruff and seborrheic capitis. Zinc pyrithione possesses cytostatic activity in vitro, but this has not been demonstrated in vivo. It is substantive to the skin, allowing continuation of the therapeutic effect after shampooing is completed.

These shampoos have no apparent toxicity when applied as directed to normal skin and hair. One or two teaspoonsful of shampoo are applied and allowed to remain on the scalp for up to five minutes before rinsing off thoroughly; the application is then repeated. Once or twice weekly application is adequate to control dandruff in many individuals. Contact with the eyes should be avoided.

> **Breck One Shampoo** (1%) (Breck), **Danex Shampoo** (1%) (Herbert), **Head and Shoulders Shampoo** (2%) (Procter & Gamble), **Zincon Shampoo** (1%) (Lederle).

CYTOSTATIC AGENTS

Psoriasis is a chronic, dry, scaling papulosquamous disease characterized by acute exacerbations, familial history, and considerable variation in severity; it primarily involves the scalp, elbows, knees, and anogenital areas. Epidermal proliferation is intense; therefore, large numbers of parakeratotic cells are present. Many patients with psoriasis are managed successfully with topical care alone, usually with corticosteroids. The cytostatic agents, tar and anthralin, may be useful in more resistant cases. Tar and anthralin usually restore a normal rate of epidermal cell proliferation and keratinization in psoriasis, other hyperplastic skin disorders, or inflammatory skin disorders, such as eczema. For discussion of photochemotherapy (PUVA) and methotrexate in this disorder, see the sections on Agents Affecting Pigmentation and Cytotoxic Agents, respectively.

ANTHRALIN
[Anthera, Anthra-Derm, Lasan Unguent]

Anthralin was developed as a stable substitute for chrysarobin in the treatment of psoriasis; it reduces the mitotic activity of hyperplastic epidermis. Patients usually are treated with daily tar baths, exposure to ultraviolet light in some cases, and application of anthralin in zinc oxide paste to each

psoriatic plaque overnight, with corticosteroids applied in the daytime. The frequent occurrence of irritation, as well as
the need for specialized care in a supervised setting, has limited the use of this
therapy principally to dermatologists.

Anthralin should be applied only to
quiescent or chronic patches of psoriasis; it
should not be used in the treatment of
acute eruptions or excessively inflamed
areas and should be used with care, if at all,
on the face or intertriginous areas. Contact
with the eyes may cause conjunctivitis.
The drug should be discontinued if sensitivity reactions occur; excessive erythema
of adjacent normal skin may require a reduction in the frequency of application.
Anthralin may stain fabrics and, temporarily, the hair and surrounding skin.

Anthralin therapy usually is withheld
from patients with impaired renal function
because of the possibility of renal irritation
secondary to percutaneous absorption.
However, renal or hepatic toxicity has not
been reported, and short-term toxicologic
studies using both paste and ointment
forms indicate that topical application in
concentrations up to 0.4% does not impair
kidney or liver function.

Anthralin preparations are available in
ointment form. Some preparations also contain 0.2% salicylic acid to minimize staining and act as a preservative. It may be
necessary to add 3% salicylic acid to formulations for thickened lesions on the soles.
The ointment is applied without a dressing
at bedtime and should remain on the lesions for 8 to 12 hours. The next morning,
the ointment is removed and the patient is
treated with a tar bath and ultraviolet light
exposure; a corticosteroid cream may be
applied during the day to control or prevent irritation.

PREPARATIONS (Prescription).
 Drug available generically: Ointment 0.1%,
 0.25%, 0.5%, and 1% in 45 g containers.
 Anthera (Barnes-Hind). Ointment 0.2% with
 salicylic acid 0.2% as preservative in 120 g
 containers.
 Anthra-Derm (Dermik). Ointment in petrolatum 0.1%, 0.25%, 0.5% and 1% in 45 g
 containers.
 Lasan Unguent (Stiefel), Ointment 0.4% with
 salicylic acid as preservative in 120 g containers.

TARS

Tars are used to treat chronic lichenified
and papulosquamous eruptions. Although
they have been largely supplanted by
topical corticosteroid preparations in the
treatment of psoriasis, seborrheic dermatitis, atopic dermatitis, and lichen
simplex chronicus, they are beneficial in
the more severe forms of these disorders.
Coal tar is the most widely used. The
action of tar to suppress hyperplastic skin
in the proliferative disorders may be enhanced by use of ultraviolet light following
removal of the tar from the skin, and a
number of dermatologists use this combination (Goeckerman regimen) for psoriasis.

An important disadvantage of all tar
preparations is their lack of uniformity.
They may be photosensitizing, have an
unpleasant odor, and frequently stain the
skin and hair. They rarely cause allergic
sensitization; juniper tar, birch tar, and
pine tar cause sensitization more frequently and offer no advantage over coal
tar. Inappropriate or excessive use may
aggravate lesions (particularly in spreading
psoriasis) or cause folliculitis. Coal tar has a
tendency to be irritating, although the incidence is minimal in usual concentrations
and appears to be negligible in patients
with psoriasis.

Nonprescription ointment and shampoo
formulations containing tar, sulfur, and
salicylic acid are used if additional
keratolytic action is desired to remove
thick crusts.

Tars incorporated into lotions, creams, or
ointments containing cortisol (hydrocortisone) 0.25% to 1% and iodoquinol
(diiodohydroxyquin) 1% are promoted for
the treatment of infected eczemas and
atopic dermatitis. Controlled studies comparing the efficacy of this regimen to that of
cortisol and the halogenated quinoline
alone are not available.

COAL TAR (Liquor carbonis detergens), U.S.P.:
 Drug available generically: Solution 20%. This
 solution contains an emulsifier, polysorbate 80
 (Tween 80), which forms a fine dispersion
 when 60 ml is added to the bath. The solution
 can be incorporated into creams or ointments
 (2% to 5%) or into tincture of green soap for a
 shampoo (10%).

Bath: *Balnetar* (Westwood) 2.5%, *Lavatar* (Doak) 33.3%, *Polytar Bath* (Stiefel) 25%; *Zetar Emulsion* (Dermik) 30% in 180 ml containers (prescription).
Cream: *Tarbonis* (Reed & Carnrick) 5%.
Emulsion: *Zetar* (Dermik) 30% (prescription).
Gel: *Estar* (Westwood) 5%, *psoriGel* (Owen) 7.5%.
Lotion: *Tar Doak* (Doak) 5% in 180 ml containers.
Ointment: *Supertah* (Purdue-Frederick) 1.25%, *Unquentum Bossi* (Doak) 5%.
Paste: *Tarpaste* (Doak) 5%.
Shampoo: *Pentrax Tar* (Texas Pharmacal) 8.75%, *Polytar* (Stiefel) 1%, *Tersa-Tar* (Doak) 3%, *Zetar* (Dermik) 1%.
Soap: *Packer's Pine Tar* (Cooper) 6%, *Polytar* (Stiefel) 1%.

AVAILABLE MIXTURES.

COAL TAR, SULFUR, AND SALICYLIC ACID:
Ointment: *Pragmatar* (Smith Kline & French). Coal tar 4%, precipitated sulfur 3%, and salicylic acid 3%.
Shampoo: *Sebutone* (Westwood), *Vanseb-T Tar* (Herbert).

CYTOTOXIC AGENTS

Although keratolytic agents are the principal drugs employed in the treatment of verrucae (warts) (see the section on Agents Affecting Keratin), the cytotoxic agents, cantharidin and podophyllin, are used for certain types. Two other cytotoxic agents, fluorouracil and methotrexate, are used to treat actinic keratoses and psoriasis, respectively.

CANTHARIDIN
[Cantharone]

Cantharidin produces intraepidermal vesiculation and resolves various types of warts, especially the periungual variety. It is applied under an occlusive bandage which is removed in 24 hours. The blister that forms will break, crust, and fall off in about ten days.

> *Cantharone* (THEX). Liquid containing cantharidin 0.7% in a vehicle containing acetone, ethyl cellulose, and flexible collodion in 5 ml containers (prescription).

FLUOROURACIL
[Efudex, Fluoroplex]

This cytotoxic drug is used topically to remove multiple premalignant actinic keratoses; curettage or cryotherapy is preferred to treat isolated lesions. Fluorouracil is more effective for keratoses on the face, forehead, bald scalp, and ears. Concentrations of 1% to 2% often are adequate for use on the face and forehead; higher concentrations may produce a severe inflammatory response in these areas. Some physicians prefer to apply a moderate strength (nonfluorinated) topical corticosteroid subsequently to reduce inflammation. Lesions on the hands and arms may require higher concentrations, longer treatment periods, or initial therapy with 0.05% tretinoin [Retin-A] solution or cream. For other uses of fluorouracil, see Chapter 68, Antineoplastic Agents.

Fluorouracil acts selectively against atypical epidermal cells by inhibiting DNA and RNA synthesis. Even lesions that are not clinically visible respond; for this reason, fluorouracil should be applied to the entire affected area. The drug has less effect on normal epidermis unless it is applied under occlusive dressings. The healing process may continue for one to two months after therapy is stopped; restoration of color and texture of the skin is usually satisfactory. Actinic keratoses may recur eventually.

Although the degree of response may be evaluated by limiting the area of initial application, the effectiveness of treatment is related to the duration of therapy and the visible reaction. Pruritus and irritation are the most common adverse reactions and intense burning pain is reported occasionally. Severe reactions can be avoided by careful selection and instruction of patients. Systemic toxic reactions are uncommon after topical use. Before therapy is initiated, the patient should be informed of the inflammatory response, prolonged discoloration of skin, and the accompanying burning sensation.

If there is an excessive inflammatory response on normal skin, treatment should be discontinued. If allergic reactions are not severe, intermittent therapy can be employed every three to seven days to maintain the therapeutic effect. Fluorouracil should not be applied to easily irritated areas (eg, around the eyes, nasolabial folds, wrinkles). Exposure to sunlight during therapy and for one or two months following treatment should be minimized. Allergic reactions occur; the final product may be used for diagnostic patch testing, and intradermal testing sometimes is required.

Commercial preparations provide a choice of concentrations and vehicles. Solutions in propylene glycol are more active than creams containing equivalent concentrations of the drug.

ROUTE, USUAL DOSAGE, AND PREPARATIONS.
Topical: Fluorouracil is applied once or twice daily for two to six weeks until a maximal inflammatory response is obtained; the frequency of application may have to be adjusted in accordance with the intensity of the response.

> *Efudex* (Roche). Cream 5% in 25 g containers; solution 2% and 5% in propylene glycol in 10 ml containers (prescription).
> *Fluoroplex* (Herbert). Cream 1% in 30 g containers; solution 1% in propylene glycol in 30 ml containers (prescription).

METHOTREXATE

Methotrexate is effective when administered orally or parenterally for the symptomatic control of severe, recalcitrant, disabling psoriasis that does not respond adequately to other forms of therapy. Diagnosis must be established by biopsy or after dermatologic consultation. Methotrexate also has some degree of effectiveness in pityriasis rubra pilaris, dermatomyositis, mycosis fungoides, bullous pemphigoid, and pemphigus vulgaris. Since there have been reports that the drug causes bone marrow depression, hepatic cirrhosis and failure, hemorrhagic enteritis, and death, methotrexate must be used cautiously and only by physicians experienced in antimetabolite therapy (Farber et al, 1976; Weinstein, 1977).

Guidelines for the use of methotrexate in the treatment of refractory psoriasis have been published by the Psoriasis Task Force of the National Program for Dermatology (Roenigk, 1972, 1973). The patient should be fully informed of the risks involved and should remain under the close supervision of a physician.

For information on other uses of this drug, see Chapter 68, Antineoplastic Agents.

> *Methotrexate* (Lederle). Tablets 2.5 mg (prescription).

PODOPHYLLIN
[Podoben]

Podophyllin is the active ingredient in podophyllum resin which arrests mitosis in metaphase. A 25% dispersion of podophyllum resin in compound benzoin tincture and alcohol is used principally in the treatment of condyloma acuminatum. Occlusion enhances effectiveness. This preparation should be removed 4 to 12 hours after application. Podophyllin should be applied sparingly on extensive lesions because it can be absorbed and produce psychotoxic confusional states, severe peripheral neuropathy, adynamic ileus, renal damage, leukopenia and thrombocytopenia, and death (Stoehr et al, 1978). Because it is a teratogen, its use during pregnancy is contraindicated. Podophyllin should only rarely be given to the patient for self-administration.

> Drug available generically: Liquid 25% in compound benzoin tincture in 30 ml containers (prescription).
> *Podoben* (Maurry). Podophyllin 25% in compound benzoin tincture 10% and isopropyl alcohol 70% in 5 ml containers (prescription).

AGENTS USED IN ACNE VULGARIS

Acne vulgaris is a disorder of adolescents and young adults which affects the pilosebaceous follicles located on the face, neck, chest, shoulders, and back. It allegedly is caused by an exaggerated response to certain androgenic steroids that results in dilated follicles, increased numbers of normal follicular bacterial flora, increased amounts of follicular sebum and irritant free fatty acids, and alteration in keratinization (Esterly and Furey, 1978). The degree of retentive follicular hyperkeratosis, occlusion, and inflammation determines the therapy required. Mild acne is characterized by oily skin and closed and open comedones; in moderate acne, papules, nodules, pustules, and a variable degree of inflammation and scarring are present. The primary lesions of severe or conglobate acne are inflammatory cysts and abscesses with subsequent pitting or hypertrophic scar formation.

Some acneiform eruptions are induced by occupational chemicals or by drugs, especially corticosteroids, androgens, iodides, bromides, and the androgenic progestins present in some oral contraceptives. Efforts to limit or avoid such drugs, humid environments, and the topical application of occlusive cosmetic oils and greases may be as important in the treatment of acne as the selection and use of drug therapy.

Numerous nonprescription drugs in diverse formulations are available for mild acne. Formulations include bar soap, soap-free cake and liquid cleansers, lotions, gels, and creams. One or more of the following active ingredients are included in each of these preparations: abrasive particles to aid in removal of surface debris (aluminum oxide, sodium tetraborate, polyethylene); keratolytics to promote peeling and comedolysis (sulfur, resorcinol, salicylic acid); astringents to promote drying (zinc oxide, zinc sulfate, sodium thiosulfate); antiseptics, presumably to lessen secondary infection (parachlorometaxylenol, cationic surfactants, povidone-iodine, sodium sulfacetamide, phenol, clioquinol); and various concentrations of alcohol to promote drying.

Some authorities believe that sufficient evidence exists to demonstrate that sulfur is comedogenic (excluding thiosulfate and sulfides); and recommend that sulfur-containing preparations be avoided. A recent study does not support the comedogenicity of sulfur, however (Strauss et al, 1978).

When acne cannot be managed adequately with self-care and nonprescription drugs, aid from the physician is sought. Useful prescription drugs available for topical application include benzoyl peroxide gel, tretinoin, salicylic acid, and topical antibiotics. Prescription drugs for systemic use include antibiotics and isotretinoin (13-*cis*-retinoic acid); the latter is an investigational drug and is not available for general use.

Benzoyl peroxide lotions and creams are nonprescription products, and a 5% or 10% concentration may be used in patients with milder cases of acne who have not previously received any therapy or who have been inadequately treated. Benzoyl peroxide gels are available only by prescription. The gels, particularly those that contain alcohol or acetone, may be required for moderate acne. Tretinoin, an alternate drug, may be more effective. Some physicians employ both drugs: tretinoin for nighttime use and benzoyl peroxide for daytime use.

If inflammation is present and systemic antibiotic therapy is indicated, tetracycline is the drug of choice because of its effectiveness, low toxicity, and low cost. Oral tetracycline, given initially in doses of 250 mg four times daily, may be required for severe inflammation. Optimum response may require four to eight weeks, and prolonged maintenance therapy in daily doses of 250 to 500 mg may be necessary. Acceptable alternative systemic antibiotics include erythromycin or clindamycin. The latter is given orally in doses of 300 to 450 mg/day. Pseudomembranous colitis occurs often enough after oral administration to limit its routine use.

Clindamycin is very effective when applied topically, and pseudomembranous colitis has not been a serious problem with this route (Stoughton, 1979). A topical formulation of clindamycin is not available commercially, but a reasonably stable preparation can be prepared by the pharmacist in a concentration of 1% to 3% in propylene glycol 10% and isopropyl alcohol 50% to 75%. The preparation is applied once or twice a day. Topical erythromycin and tetracycline [Topicycline] are alternatives. However, if bacterial resistance to topical clindamycin or erythromycin is encountered, cross resistance between these antibiotics (but not to oral or topical tetracycline) is usually present. Minocycline [Minocin], in doses of 50 to 200 mg daily, is suggested if resistance develops to all three antibiotics.

The treatment of severe conglobate and cystic acne usually requires dermatologic consultation. More aggressive therapy is employed, eg, larger daily doses of tetracycline (2 g/day) or other appropriate antibiotic therapy if a gram-negative infection is documented; intralesional injection of corticosteroids; hot compresses with sulfurated lime solution (Vlem-Dome); or, in women, oral estrogen therapy. Results with the investigational use of oral isotretinoin have been encouraging. If these results continue to be confirmed and extended, the role of all of the above therapies for severe acne will need re-evaluation.

BENZOYL PEROXIDE

Benzoyl peroxide is of proved efficacy in acne vulgaris. The mechanism of action is probably related to its bacteriostatic activity against *Propionibacterium acnes*, which decreases the amount of irritant free fatty acids in the follicle; this drug also has a keratolytic effect which causes comedolysis. It is available in clear or tinted vehicles in concentrations of 5% to 10%.

Although approximately one-half of a dose of benzoyl peroxide is absorbed after topical application to the forearm of primates (Nacht et al, 1979), systemic toxicity has not been reported in man. Benzoic acid is a major metabolite. Some irritation must be accepted, snce a dose-response relationship exists between efficacy and irritation; local irritation has been severe in some individuals.

Contact sensitivity is observed in 1% to 3% of patients. Benzoyl peroxide is a potent experimental contact sensitizer (delayed hypersensitivity), and a recent study in volunteers revealed that a reaction occurred in 70% of subjects after use of occlusive patches containing either a 5% or 10% concentration. It is assumed that the relative instability, rapid evaporative loss, and dilution in sweat minimize the likelihood of sensitization in clinical use, or that the reported incidence does not reflect the actual incidence. When sensitivity is suspected, patch testing may be performed with a freshly prepared 5% concentration in petrolatum.

ROUTE, USUAL DOSAGE, AND PREPARATIONS. To lessen the possibility of severe irritation, the patient should be carefully instructed to limit the volume of material and frequency of application initially, gradually increasing the amount and duration of contact as tolerance permits.

Topical: The following is a conservative approach and may be modified for individual patients: The formulation is applied for 15 minutes the first evening and then removed with soap and water. The length of the exposure is increased by increments of 15 minutes each evening thereafter until the preparation is tolerated for two hours. The preparation then may be left on overnight and washed off in the morning. An additional application may be necessary in the morning once the level of sensitivity and response is determined. Contact with eyes, eyelids, and mucous membranes should be avoided. There is some evidence that benzoyl peroxide is more readily bioavailable with alcohol-based gels, but the alcohol-based formulations tend to be more drying.

PRESCRIPTION PRODUCTS:

Liquid Cleansers: *Desquam-X Wash* (Westwood). Liquid containing benzoyl peroxide 4% with docusate sodium and sodium lauryl sulfoacetate in 150 ml containers.

Gel (alcohol-based) 5% and 10%: *Generic* in 45 and 120 g containers; *Benzac 5, 10* (Owen) in 60 g containers; *5 Benzagel, 10 Benzagel* (Dermik) in 45 and 90 g containers; *Panoxyl 5, 10* (Stiefel) in 60 and 120 g containers.

Gel (nonalcohol-based) 5% and 10%: *Desquam-X 5, 10* (Westwood), *Persa-Gel* (Texas Pharmacal), *Xerac BP 5, 10* (Person & Covey) in 45 and 90 g containers.

AVAILABLE MIXTURE.

Sulfoxyl (Stiefel). Lotion containing benzoyl peroxide 5% and sulfur 2% (Regular) or benzoyl peroxide 10% and sulfur 5% (Strong) in 30 ml containers.

NONPRESCRIPTION PRODUCTS:

Cream (paraben-free): *Persadox* (5% concentration), *Persadox-HP* (10% concentration) (Texas Pharmacal).

Lotion 5% and 10%: *Generic, Benoxyl 5, 10* (Stiefel), *Loroxide* (5.5% only) (Dermik), *Oxy 5, 10* (Norcliff Thayer), *Persadox* (5% concentration), *Persadox-HP* (10% concentration) (Texas Pharmacal), *Topex* (10% only) (Vicks), *Vanoxide* (5% only) (Dermik).

TRETINOIN
[Retin-A]

This all-*trans* configuration of retinoic (vitamin A) acid is used topically in the treatment of acne vulgaris. It is sometimes effective in keratinizing disorders (eg, lamellar ichthyosis, Darier's disease).

One daily application maintains epidermal sloughing. Tretinoin increases epidermal cell mitosis and cell turnover, and it has been suggested that this increased turnover in the follicular epithelium prevents blocking by keratinous plugs. The process may aggravate acne during the first six weeks of therapy, but good results after three or four months of use are noted in some patients.

Tretinoin is potentially a potent irritant, particularly if used incorrectly; within 48 hours the skin may become red and begin to peel. Once nightly application to dry skin and avoidance of spice/lime aftershave preparations, medicated make-up, and excessive sun or sunlamp exposure will reduce the irritation potential. Tretinoin should be applied to dry skin, eg, not immediately after a shower or washing.

Tretinoin should not be used on eczematous skin. Contact with the corners of the mouth, nose, eyes, or mucous membranes must be minimized. The patient should be instructed to be careful in the concomitant use of other keratolytic preparations (eg, sulfur, resorcinol, salicylic acid, benzoyl peroxide) and abrasive soaps. The number of face washings should be limited, at first, to three a day. The amount and frequency of application should be individualized to minimize irritation while maintaining effective keratolytic action. Tretinoin is available as a gel, a cream, a polyethylene glycol-ethyl alcohol-based solution, or saturated swabs. The latter preparations are generally more irritating.

In the commercially available formulations, tretinoin penetrates the skin slightly, but systemic toxicity has not been observed. Contact sensitization has been noted only rarely. An appropriate patch test concentration for documentation of contact sensitization is 0.1% in petrolatum.

Experimental studies in mice suggest that tretinoin may accelerate the tumorigenic potential of ultraviolet radiation. Until the significance in man is clarified, patients should avoid or minimize sun or sunlamp exposure.

ROUTE, USUAL DOSAGE, AND PREPARATIONS.
Topical: One application nightly to the entire area involved.

> *Retin-A* (Johnson & Johnson). Cream 0.05% and 0.1% in 20 g containers; gel 0.01% in 15 g containers and 0.025% in 15 and 45 g containers; liquid 0.5% in swab form or in 28 ml containers (prescription).

TETRACYCLINE HYDROCHLORIDE
[Topicycline]

This topical preparation of tetracycline is used in the treatment of pustular acne vulgaris. The serum level after continuous twice-daily application is 0.1 mcg/ml or less; this is the lower limit of detection of the analytical method. The effectiveness of topical tetracycline is slightly less than with systemic use. Criteria for precise patient selection have not been established.

No systemic toxicity has been observed. A mild stinging, burning sensation has been noted.

ROUTE, USUAL DOSAGE, AND PREPARATIONS. *Topical*: The powder is dissolved in the diluent and 0.5 to 1 ml of the prepared solution is applied twice daily.

> *Topicycline* (Procter & Gamble). Powder (for reconstitution) with diluent (*n*-decyl methyl sulfoxide and sucrose esters in 40% alcohol) to make 70 ml of solution containing 2.2 mg/ml (prescription).

ISOTRETINOIN (13-*Cis*-Retinoic Acid)

This all-*cis* configuration of retinoic (vitamin A) acid, which is investigational, inhibits the production of sebaceous gland lipid. Complete clearing of conglobate and cystic acne has been observed in 90% of patients after daily oral administration of approximately 1 to 3 mg/kg of body weight for four months (Peck et al, 1979). The drug also appears to act on keratin, because it is effective in the treatment of keratinizing disorders such as lamellar ichthyosis, Darier's disease, and pityriasis rubra pilaris, but it apparently has no direct effect on psoriasis. The keratinizing disorders require more prolonged therapy.

No untoward effects have required discontinuation of therapy, although reversible cheilitis, facial dermatitis, and xerosis occur in almost all patients. Dry nasal mucosa, conjunctivitis, and skin fragility occur in approximately 50% of patients. Inflammation of the urethral meatus was observed in two of eight men treated. Thinning and dryness of the hair persisted in one woman for three months after cessation of therapy. Transient elevations in the sedimentation rate and serum levels of alanine and aspartate transaminases were the only altered laboratory values. Early studies reveal no apparent drug-induced toxicity in the vitamin A target organs (eye, bone, thyroid, central nervous system, and gonads).

Investigational drug (Roche).

AGENTS AFFECTING PIGMENTATION

Hydroquinone and monobenzone are applied topically to treat localized hyperpigmentation. This condition results from increased melanogenesis and is associated with melasma of pregnancy or that induced by oral contraceptives, freckles, and lentigines; it occasionally occurs following skin trauma. Specific systemic therapy is required for diffuse hyperpigmentation disorders (eg, Addison's disease).

Acquired localized disorders of hypopigmentation include vitiligo, which is characterized by a possible immune-mediated loss of melanocytes, or depigmentation resulting from inflammation following bullae, burns, infections, atrophy, or scarring of the skin. Congenital diffuse hypopigmentation and depigmentation (ie, albinism) are distinguished by the presence of melanocytes that do not synthesize melanin. The psoralen compounds, trioxsalen and methoxsalen, may stimulate repigmentation (except in albinism). They are used orally in vitiligo if the process involves less than 40% of the body surface. If the vitiliginous area is less than about 6 cm², topical application of methoxsalen rather than oral administration of these drugs can be considered. If more than 40% of the body surface is affected, it may be easier to lessen the pigmentation of non-vitiliginous areas with monobenzone.

Long-wave ultraviolet light in the A range (320 to 400 nm) is relatively weak in the amount of energy required to produce erythema or pigmentation, but concomitant use of a circulating photosensitizer (eg, psoralen) markedly increases the skin response. This photochemotherapy is termed PUVA (*P*soralen with *UVA* light) and is being used investigationally to treat psoriasis (Roenigk et al, 1979). It is thought to act by causing the formation of psoralen-DNA photo adducts that interfere with the hyperproliferative epidermal cell turnover characteristic of psoriasis. Methoxsalen is used orally in conjunction with controlled exposures to UVA light to optimize the inhibition of epidermal cells and avoid severe burns. Although no serious systemic toxicity has been observed, PUVA therapy increases the incidence of skin cancer and cataracts (Epstein, 1979). The Committee on Drugs of the American Academy of Pediatrics recommends that under no circumstances should children receive such therapy unless it is given by qualified investigators under established investigational new drug protocols. The technique is currently limited to patients who have not responded to conventional treatment regimens (tars, anthralins, steroids, and methotrexate) for psoriasis and who have extensive and active disease.

HYDROQUINONE
[Artra, Eldoquin, Eldopaque]

MONOBENZONE
[Benoquin]

Hydroquinone may decrease cutaneous hyperpigmentation when applied topically to treat various localized disorders such as freckles, lentigenes, and melasma of pregnancy (chloasma gravidarum) or that caused by oral contraceptive drugs. Its effect is usually reversible. Hydroquinone acts by inhibiting tyrosinase in melanocytes, which depresses melanin synthesis; melanin granule movement and melanocyte growth also are inhibited. It is also toxic to melanocytes.

No serious untoward effects have been reported; however, tingling or burning on application and subsequent erythema and inflammation were observed in 8% and 32% of patients, respectively, when a 2% and 5% concentration of hydroquinone was used. Termination of therapy is not required if inflammation occurs, but topical cortisol (hydrocortisone) may be given to alleviate this reaction. Contact with the eyes should be avoided. Allergic contact dermatitis occurs far less frequently than irritation; a 2% concentration of hydroquinone in petrolatum is suitable for patch testing.

For especially resistant cases, a formula composed of 0.1% tretinoin, 5% hydroquinone, and 0.1% dexamethasone in hydrophilic ointment or in equal parts of alcohol and propylene glycol has been recommended (Arndt, 1978). Alternatively, 0.05% tretinoin cream may be applied in the morning, 0.1% betamethasone valerate cream in the afternoon, and 2% hydroquinone cream in the evening (Gano and Garcia, 1979).

Monobenzone is the monobenzyl ether of hydroquinone. Its action is similar to that of hydroquinone except that extensive cytolysis of melanocytes also occurs. Monobenzone causes total, irreversible depigmentation and should be used only to remove the remaining areas of normal pigmentation in patients with disseminated vitiligo. The adverse effects are similar to those caused by hydroquinone, except that the incidence of sensitization is higher.

Monobenzone therapy is often difficult to manage and requires careful patient follow-up; bizarre patterns of hypopigmentation may occur at sites distant from the area of application. Alternative management programs should be considered before monobenzone is tried in the treatment of vitiligo, ie, continuous sunscreen protection, psoralen compounds, masking preparations (eg, Covermark Cream), or staining types of covering cosmetics (eg, Vitadye).

Hydroquinone in concentrations less than 5% has been approved by the FDA as an effective and safe ingredient in nonprescription preparations to lighten limited areas of hyperpigmented skin (*Federal Register*, 1978); monobenzone is available only on prescription.

ROUTE, USUAL DOSAGE, AND PREPARATIONS.
Topical: *Adults and adolescents over 12 years*, the preparation is applied to the involved areas twice daily for six to eight weeks. An opaque sunscreen also should be applied during the day on areas that cannot easily be protected from exposure to the sun to prevent recurrence of hyper-pigmentation.

HYDROQUINONE:
Artra (Plough). Cream 2% in 30, 60, and 120 g containers (nonprescription).
Eldoquin (Elder). Cream 2% or 4% (Forte) in 15 and 30 g containers; lotion 2% in 15 g containers (nonprescription).
Eldopaque (Elder). Ointment 2% in a talc opaque base in 15 g containers (nonprescription).
Eldopaque Forte (Elder). Ointment 4% in a talc opaque base in 15 and 30 g containers.
HCQ Kit (Elder). Eldoquin Forte in 7.5 g tube, Eldopaque Forte in 15 g tube, and Eldecort (with 1% cortisol cream) in 30 g tube (prescription).
AVAILABLE MIXTURE.
Ambi (Nicholas). Cream containing hydroquinone 2% and a para-aminobenzoic acid ester sunscreen (the glyceryl ester of PABA for oily and normal skin in 60 g and the octyldimethyl ester of PABA in 60 and 120 g containers).
MONOBENZONE:
Benoquin (Elder). Ointment 20% in 37.5 g containers (prescription).

TRIOXSALEN
[Trisoralen]

Trioxsalen, a psoralen derivative, is effective in the treatment of vitiligo. Its use to increase tolerance to sunlight in sun-sensitive individuals is potentially dangerous and not always feasible. Tolerance of the skin to ultraviolet light is enhanced by increasing pigmentation and, possibly, by thickening of the stratum corneum; therefore, administration of trioxsalen must be followed, after approximately two hours, by exposure to sunlight or, in expert hands, to long-wave ultraviolet radiation (320 to 400 nm [UVA]) from an artificial light source.

The psoralens are *not* sunscreens. During the first few days of therapy, patients are hypersensitive to sunlight and subject to more severe sunburn than under normal circumstances. Therefore, the dosage and length of exposure to the sun must be controlled closely to prevent injury to the skin, and special sunglasses opaque to UVA and a light-screening lipstick should be used to protect eyes and lips. If over-exposure to sunlight occurs, the patient should remain in a darkened room for eight hours or until cutaneous reactions subside.

Trioxsalen is contraindicated in patients with diseases associated with photosensitivity, such as porphyria (porphyria cutanea tarda and erthropoietic porphyria), discoid or systemic lupus erythematosus, and xeroderma pigmentosum. Other drugs with photosensitizing properties (eg, phenothiazines) should not be given concomitantly.

Extensive clinical experience with short-term administration indicates that trioxsalen has minimal toxicity; gastric discomfort is noted occasionally. See the introduction to this section for references on the possible cataractogenic and carcinogenic actions of the psoralens.

ROUTE, USUAL DOSAGE, AND PREPARATIONS.
Oral: *Adults and children over 12 years*, for large lesions of vitiligo, 0.6 mg/kg of body weight daily is given two hours before exposure to sunlight at noon. The initial exposure is 15 to 20 minutes. As long as erythema develops seven to ten hours after exposure, the patient is maintained on the indicated daily therapy. Once skin tolerance develops and erythema no longer is observed, exposure to sunlight is increased by 15-minute increments and the dose is increased by 10-mg increments to a maximum of 80 mg daily. Repigmentation is usually evident after three to four months of treatment, especially on the face and neck. If no results are obtained after three months of treatment, therapy should be discontinued. To increase tolerance to sunlight, the daily dose usually should not exceed 10 mg. Graduated daily exposures to sunlight should follow two hours later.

The total period of administration should not exceed 14 days.

Trisoralen (Elder). Tablets 5 mg (prescription).

METHOXSALEN
[Oxsoralen]

OCH_3

Methoxsalen is administered topically for the treatment of small vitiliginous lesions. The drug is applied to the affected areas and the patient is then exposed to a long-wave (320 to 400 nm) ultraviolet light source. The procedure should be closely supervised in the physician's office or in appropriate clinical facilities.

The use of oral methoxsalen with specific exposure to controlled long-wave ultraviolet light (PUVA therapy) for the treatment of psoriasis and other skin diseases, such as mycosis fungoides, is still investigational. Methoxsalen may possess cataractogenic and carcinogenic actions (Epstein, 1979).

Topical use can cause acute vesicular cutaneous photosensitization in a large percentage of patients; high concentrations of the drug and overexposure of the treated site to long-wave ultraviolet radiation are the major factors contributing to the development of severe erythema and blistering. Dilution to concentrations of 1:10,000 or 1:1,000 helps avoid excessive reactions.

ROUTES, USUAL DOSAGE, AND PREPARATIONS. *Topical*: Low concentrations are applied daily to the affected area (50 to 200 mcg/in²). The surrounding skin is protected by an opaque sunscreen. After two hours, the treated area is exposed to an artificial long-wave ultraviolet light source for 30 to 60 seconds, the lesions are then washed with soap and water and an opaque sunscreen is applied. Direct sunlight should be avoided. Exposure is increased gradually but should not exceed one-half the minimal erythemal dose.

Oxsoralen (Elder). Lotion 1% in 30 ml containers (prescription). Oxsoralen lotion should never be dispensed directly to the patient.

Oral: *Adults and children over 12 years*, for repigmentation of idiopathic vitiligo, 20 mg/day as a single dose two to four hours before measured periods of ultraviolet exposure that usually is limited to five minutes initially and gradually increased to 30 minutes if required. The risk of severe burn is considerable with methoxsalen. Sun exposure must be limited and sunscreens must be employed. Special sunglasses opaque to UVA should be worn during exposure and the lips protected with a light-screening lipstick (see the manufacturer's literature).

Oxsoralen (Elder). Capsules 10 mg (prescription).

TOPICAL ANESTHETICS

For moderately extensive dermatitic eruptions, the selection of an anti-inflammatory ingredient in an appropriate vehicle will usually relieve pain without resorting to the use of topical local anesthetics. Although of limited value, the incorporation of a local antipruritic agent in the formulation or systemic antipruritic therapy usually provides better relief from itching than a topical local anesthetic. The antipruritic and scabicide, crotamiton [Eurax], is discussed in Chapter 84, Scabicides and Pediculicides.

Topical local anesthetics may be useful in selected disorders affecting mucous membranes, mucocutaneous junctions, and abraded inflamed skin (eg, aphthous stomatitis, oral or anogenital herpes simplex lesions) and for pain caused by cytotoxic therapy for anal and genital warts. They are rarely useful in nonspecific pruritus ani and vulvae. Numerous nonprescription topical mixtures containing a local anesthetic (most commonly, benzocaine) and usually an antiseptic are available for sunburn but they are not usually effective, probably because the concentration of anesthetic is too low and penetration is very poor even in sunburned skin. At least 10% benzocaine, and probably 20%, is necessary for most situations.

Although certain antihistamines have topical local anesthetic activity when applied to mucocutaneous and abraded skin areas, they should not be used topically because of the risk of producing an allergic contact dermatitis. Systemic rather than topical administration of antihistamines is also advisable when these agents are used for pruritus and urticaria.

The selection of a topical local anesthetic is based on the availability of a suitable vehicle (ie, solution, viscous solution, jelly, cream, ointment), the patient's prior history of sensitization, and the desired duration of action. The formulations and container sizes of most available local anesthetics, including a discussion of their adverse reactions, are presented in Chapter 19. For convenience, topical local anesthetic preparations are included below also. Most are available as nonprescription products. They are divided into amide, ester, and miscellaneous (non-amide and nonester) categories for selection in cases of known sensitivity. Dibucaine and dimethisoquin tend to have a longer duration of action (two to four hours).

AMIDE LOCAL ANESTHETICS.

DIBUCAINE:
Drug available generically: Ointment 1%.
Nupercainal (Ciba). Cream 0.5%; ointment 1%; suppositories 0.25%.

LIDOCAINE:
Drug available generically: Ointment 0.025%.
Xylocaine (Astra). Ointment 5% in 3.5, 15, and 35 g containers; solution 2% (viscous) in 100 and 450 ml containers; solution 4% in 50 ml containers (all prescription).
Lida-Mantle (Dome). Cream 3% (prescription).

AMINOBENZOATE ESTER LOCAL ANESTHETICS.

BENZOCAINE:
Drug available generically: Cream, ointment 5%.
Americaine (Arnar-Stone). Aerosol 20% in 20, 60, and 120 g containers; gel lubricant 20% in 2.5 and 30 g containers (prescription); ointment 20% in 3 g and 1 lb containers; suppositories 10%.
Burntame (Buffington). Aerosol 20% in 100 g containers.

BUTAMBEN PICRATE:
Butesin (Abbott). Ointment 1% in 30 g containers.

TETRACAINE HYDROCHLORIDE:
Drug available generically: Ointment, powder.
Pontocaine (Breon). Cream 1%, ointment 5% in 30 g containers.

NON-AMIDE AND NON-AMINOBENZOATE ESTER LOCAL ANESTHETICS.

BENZYL ALCOHOL:
Topic (Syntex). Gel 5% in 60 g containers.

CYCLOMETHYCAINE SULFATE:
Surfacaine (Lilly). Cream 0.5%; ointment 1% in 30 and 454 g containers; suppositories 1%.

DIMETHISOQUIN HYDROCHLORIDE:
Quotane (Smith Kline & French). Ointment 0.5% in 30 g containers.

DIPERODON:
Diothane (Merrell-National). Ointment 1% in 30 g containers.

DYCLONINE HYDROCHLORIDE:
Dyclone (Dow). Solution 0.5% and 1% in 30 g containers (prescription).

PRAMOXINE HYDROCHLORIDE:
Tronothane (Abbott). Cream, jelly 1% in 30 g containers.

CAUSTIC AGENTS

Topically applied caustics are used principally superficially to destroy abnormal epithelium; some are particularly useful in producing hemostasis during limited superficial surgical procedures by coagulating skin proteins (ferric subsulfate).

Bichloracetic acid (Kahlenberg solution), *trichloracetic acid*, and *silver nitrate sticks* are effective cauterants in concentrations of 30% to 50% and are employed to remove warts, although less destructive keratolytic agents usually are preferred. The surrounding normal tissue should be protected with petrolatum and point-application of the cauterant should be done cautiously.

Ferric subsulfate (Monsel's solution) and aluminum chloride solution are effective hemostatic agents but are not used for wart therapy. Excessive or inappropriate use of ferric subsulfate may result in tattoo marks.

ALUMINUM CHLORIDE:
Drug available generically.

BICHLORACETIC ACID:
Drug available generically: Solution (full-strength) 10 ml in a kit with 15 g of petrolatum.

TRICHLORACETIC ACID:
Drug available generically in requested concentration.

FERRIC SUBSULFATE:
Drug available generically.

SILVER NITRATE, TOUGHENED:
Drug available generically: Toughened sticks.

DEBRIDING AGENTS

Topical debriding agents are adjuncts in wound management; the underlying cause (ie, stasis, trauma, inadequate nutrition, infection) must be treated (Nierman, 1978). The use of an appropriate topical antiseptic or antibiotic is advisable to inhibit bacterial growth, and any threatening invasive infection should be treated with systemic antibiotic preparations in addition. Correction of hyperglycemia, uremia, and edema are helpful. It is essential that patients, particularly the elderly who are most likely to develop stasis and decubitus ulcers, receive adequate nutrition; enteral supplementation or total parenteral nutrition may be necessary to resolve resistant ulcers. Bedrest to reduce tissue oxygen demands and frequent changes of position to alleviate pressure ulcers also can be valuable.

Topical debriding enzymes include collagenase [Santyl], the mixture of fibrinolysin with desoxyribonuclease [Elase], streptokinase-streptodornase [Varidase], and sutilains [Travase]. These agents degrade protein, aiding in the removal of necrotic tissue, clotted blood, purulent exudates, or fibrinous accumulations resulting from trauma, inflammation, infected wounds, or ulcers. By promoting the cleansing of a wound, they facilitate healing. Effective enzymatic action depends upon proper wound preparation prior to application (ie, adequate cleansing of the site to remove detritus, providing for subsequent drainage when necessary). Cross hatching of eschar may be necessary to ensure adequate contact of the enzyme with the wound. Insufficient enzymatic action may result from improper storage of the enzyme, use of an inappropriate vehicle, or concomitant administration of other agents that destroy or inhibit the enzyme (eg, heavy metals, antiseptics, hexachlorophene). Failure also may result from drying of the substrate. Persistence of foreign material or sequestra and inaccessible location of pus, as in osteomyelitis of cancellous bone, also reduce enzymatic activity.

Dextranomer [Debrisan] is a hydrophilic cross-linked dextran polymer available in the form of small beads. The mechanism of action of this cleansing agent is novel: It acts by developing powerful suction forces that absorb wound secretions and products so that they will not interfere with wound healing. Its drying action decreases bacterial growth. Its lack of irritation and sensitization is presumably related to its high molecular weight. Dextranomer is expensive, and its final role in wound management has not been fully established.

Benzoyl peroxide is used principally for acne in 5% to 10% concentrations (see the section on Agents Used in Acne Vulgaris in this chapter). A 20% concentration in an oil-in-water emulsion recently has been proposed as an alternative or adjunct to the debriding enzymes in the treatment of dermal ulcers, but this concentration is not available commercially. An ointment is applied to protect normal skin, and benzoyl peroxide is applied to the wound under occlusive dressings. An abdominal pad taped into position over the plastic dressing creates the moist, warm (37 C) environment necessary to promote oxygen release. Dressings are changed every 8 to 12 hours. Use of this drug may be limited by the fact that allergic or primary irritant contact dermatitis occurs in at least 5% of patients.

Enzymes

COLLAGENASE
[Santyl]

Collagenase is an enzyme derived from fermentation of *Clostridium histolyticum*. It has produced a satisfactory response in a large percentage of patients with dermal ulcers from various causes (eg, peripheral vascular disorders, pressure sores); complete debridement usually occurs in 10 to 14 days, followed by granulation and epithelialization with prompt healing. Similar satisfactory results have been obtained in severe burns.

Collagenase is capable of degrading denatured and undenatured collagen, whereas other proteolytic enzymes act only on denatured collagen. For this reason, it has been claimed that this enzyme produces better debridement by acting on collagen fibers at the wound edges which anchor necrotic slough to the base. In vitro studies indicate that collagenase does not act on fat, keratin, fibrin, or muscle. Collagen in healthy tissue or in newly formed granulation tissue is not attacked. Activity is optimal between pH 6 and 8; the enzyme is inactivated at pH 5 or lower and at pH 8.5 or higher, as well as by temperatures above 56 C. It also is inactivated by detergents, benzalkonium chloride, hexachlorophene, nitrofurazone, tincture of iodine, and heavy metals and substances containing them (eg, thimerosal, silver nitrate, aluminum acetate). Several antibiotics (eg, bacitracin, neomycin, polymyxin B) do not interfere with the activity of collagenase.

Adverse reactions are uncommon; slight erythema may develop in surrounding tissue. Irritation may be prevented by applying a protectant (eg, zinc oxide paste, U.S.P. [Lassar's Plain Zinc Paste]) to the surrounding tissue. Enzymatic action can be stopped when desired by application of Aluminum Acetate Solution, U.S.P. (Burow's solution).

ROUTE, USUAL DOSAGE, AND PREPARATIONS. *Topical*: The ointment is applied once daily or more frequently if the dressing becomes soiled. It may be applied directly to deep lesions; for shallow wounds, it can be applied to a sterile gauze pad placed over the wound. Prior to application, the lesion should be cleansed with hydrogen peroxide or Dakin's solution followed by normal saline; antiseptics that inactivate the enzyme should not be used. If such materials have been applied to the lesion, they must be completely removed by washing before collagenase is used. The ointment should be confined to the area of the lesion; surrounding healthy skin can be protected by covering with zinc oxide paste.

Santyl (Knoll). Ointment 250 units/g in white petrolatum in 25 g containers.

FIBRINOLYSIN WITH DESOXYRIBONUCLEASE COMBINED
[Elase]

This preparation is a mixture of fibrinolysin (plasmin) and desoxyribonuclease of bovine origin. The fibrinolysin component acts on the fibrin of blood clots and exudates. It is used topically to remove necrotic debris and exudates from wounds, ulcers, and burns and to irrigate abscess cavities and sinus tracts.

Adverse effects are mild. Local hyperemia may occur. Precautions should be taken to prevent allergic reactions in patients with a history of sensitivity to mercury (from the preservative) or bovine products.

ROUTE, USUAL DOSAGE, AND PREPARATIONS. *Topical: Adults and children*, the ointment or solution is applied at least twice daily until optimal debridement is obtained.

Elase (Parke, Davis). Ointment containing fibrinolysin 10 or 30 units (Loomis) and desoxyribonuclease 6,666 or 20,000 units with thimerosal 0.04 or 0.12 mg in an ointment base containing liquid petrolatum and polyethylene in 10 and 30 g containers; lyophilized powder (for solution) containing fibrinolysin 25 units (Loomis) and desoxyribonuclease 15,000 units (modified Christensen method) with thimerosal 0.1 mg in 30 ml containers.

STREPTOKINASE-STREPTODORNASE
[Varidase]

This preparation is a mixture of enzymes of bacterial origin. Streptokinase (plasminogen activator) rapidly dissolves blood clots and the fibrinous portion of exudates; streptodornase hydrolyzes desoxyribonucleoprotein to liquify the viscous nucleoprotein of dead cells, but it has no effect on living cells. The mixture is injected into cavities or applied topically as a wet dressing. It is used intramuscularly to reduce inflammation and edema, but its effectiveness for this purpose has not been substantiated.

Streptokinase-streptodornase has been most effective when used as a topical debriding agent when purulent exudates, clotted blood, or fibrinous deposits are present as the result of trauma or infection. It is used to supplement surgical debridement and drainage in the treatment of hemothorax, empyema, chronic draining sinuses, osteomyelitis, infected wounds, and ulcers.

Pyrogenic reactions and local irritation are the most common adverse reactions. Streptokinase-streptodornase is contraindicated in the presence of active hemorrhage, acute cellulitis without suppuration, or when there is danger of reopening preexisting bronchopleural fistulas. It should never be given intravenously because of the severe systemic adverse reactions produced by impurities in the preparation.

ROUTES, USUAL DOSAGE, AND PREPARATIONS. *Local*: *Adults and children*, for hemothorax or thoracic empyema, initially, a solution containing streptokinase 200,000 units and streptodornase 50,000 units is injected into one or several sites. For debridement of exudates in small enclosed spaces, the dosage and amount of fluid injected generally depends upon the size of the cavity; provision should be made for drainage of the liquified exudate.

Topical: *Adults and children*, for debridement of exudates, a solution containing 5,000 to 10,000 units of streptokinase/ml is used. The solution should remain in direct contact with the affected area; hence, repeated application is necessary to maintain enzymatic action. For surface lesions of the hands, a jelly containing approximately 5,000 units of streptokinase/g may be placed inside a loose rubber glove which is tied at the wrist.

> *Varidase* (Lederle). Powder (for solution or jelly) containing streptokinase 100,000 units and streptodornase at least 25,000 units with thimerosal 2 mg; preparation containing 15 ml of carboxymethylcellulose gel 4.5% is used for the jelly formulation.

Intramuscular (gluteal): No dosage is cited for the intramuscular use of this mixture to treat inflammation and edema associated with trauma or infection. The manufacturer's suggested dosage is: *Adults*, 0.5 ml of a solution containing streptokinase 5,000 units twice daily.

> *Varidase* (Lederle). Powder containing streptokinase 20,000 units and streptodornase at least 5,000 units with thimerosal 0.2 mg.

SUTILAINS
[Travase]

Sutilains is a sterile preparation of a proteolytic enzyme elaborated by *Bacillus subtilis* in an ointment base. The enzyme is most effective within a pH range of 6.0 to 6.8. It is virtually inactive on viable tissue, but it dissolves and aids in the removal of necrotic tissue. It is used to remove purulent exudate from skin surfaces in second- and third-degree burns. When sutilains has been applied early in the postburn period (first two or three days) on large areas with third-degree burns, some clinicians have noted a high incidence of sepsis; therefore, they recommend using a topical antibiotic (eg, silver sulfadiazine) with the enzyme preparation. In addition, appropriate systemic antibiotic therapy should be initiated. This agent also is used in the management of decubitus ulcers, traumatic and pyogenic wounds, and ulcers secondary to peripheral vascular disease.

Untoward effects are mild and consist of transient pain, paresthesia, hemorrhage, and dermatitis. The drug should be discontinued if bleeding or dermatitis occurs. Although no systemic allergic reactions have been reported in man, immunologic studies have shown that an antibody response may occur.

The concomitant use of detergents or antiseptics (eg, benzalkonium chloride, hexachlorophene, iodine, nitrofurazone) should be avoided because of possible enzyme denaturation. Sutilains should not come into contact with the eyes. If this occurs, the eyes should be rinsed with a copious amount of water (preferably sterile). Use of sutilains is contraindicated in fungating neoplastic lesions; in necrotic areas where bone, tendon, fascia, or cartilage is exposed; or in wounds involving major body cavities or nerve tissue.

ROUTE, USUAL DOSAGE, AND PREPARATIONS. *Topical*: *Adults and children*, after cleansing and irrigating the wounded area, the ointment is applied in a thin layer ¼ to ½ inch beyond the area to be debrided and the site is covered with a loose wet dressing. A wet environment is important for enzymatic action. Application may be repeated three or four times daily. If there is no demonstrable debriding action within 24 to 48 hours, further application is unlikely to have an effect.

> *Travase* (Flint). Ointment containing approximately 82,000 casein units of sutilains/g in a base containing white petrolatum and polyethylene in 14.2 g containers.

Nonenzymatic Agent

DEXTRANOMER
[Debrisan]

Dextranomer is a hydrophilic polymer consisting of a three-dimensional network of cross-linked dextran chains. It is available as beads that are 0.1 to 0.3 mm in diameter; each gram of beads will absorb 4 ml of fluid. Spaces within and between beads are capable of dehydrating suction forces of up to 200 mm Hg. Low-molecular-weight substances less than 1,000 daltons (eg, peptides, bacterial toxins) are absorbed into the beads, and high-molecular-weight substances (eg, proteins such as fibrin and its split products, bacteria, wound detritus) are absorbed into the bead interspaces. Presumably this action creates a more favorable environment for wound healing (Heel et al, 1979). A controlled study demonstrated that dextranomer was more effective than collagenase ointment in the treatment of decubitus ulcers (Parish and Collins, 1979).

Unlike debriding agents (eg, enzymes), dextranomer does not attack collagen or fibrin. It is suggested that large necrotic areas be surgically or enzymatically debrided prior to use of dextranomer. By virtue of its mode of action, dextranomer is indicated only for suppurating lesions. Its ultimate role in the treatment of moist wounds remains to be determined.

Isolated cases of erythema, pain, subjective irritation, and bleeding have been reported, usually associated with dressing changes, although these reactions rarely necessitate discontinuation of dextranomer therapy. Spilling the beads on the floor can make the floor dangerously slippery.

ROUTE, USUAL DOSAGE, AND PREPARATIONS. Dextranomer is indicated only for exudative lesions. The wound is filled with beads to a depth of at least 3 mm. (An area of ulceration 4 cm in diameter will require approximately 4 g of beads.) A light bandage is applied to hold the beads in place. Dextranomer becomes greyish-yellow when saturated and should then be removed by gentle irrigation, although vigorous irrigation may be necessary in some wounds. Dressings are changed once or twice daily, but the frequency depends upon the degree of exudation from the wound.

> *Debrisan* (Pharmacia). Beads in 4, 60, and 120 g containers.

MISCELLANEOUS AGENTS

COLLODION

This mixture of pyroxylin, ether, and alcohol forms a sticky, tenacious film that adheres to the skin upon drying. Flexible collodion contains collodion, camphor 0.2%, and castor oil 0.3%. It is used alone as a protectant from tar in the treatment of psoriasis or from salicylic acid in the treatment of corns, calluses, and warts, and as a vehicle for salicylic and lactic acids.

> COLLODION, U.S.P.:
> Drug available generically: Liquid in 4, 8, and 16 oz containers.
> FLEXIBLE COLLODION, U.S.P.:
> Drug available generically: Liquid in 4, 5, 8, and 16 oz and 2 and 5 gal containers.

DAPSONE
[Avlosulfon]

$$H_2N-\!\!\!\langle\ \rangle\!\!\!-SO_2-\!\!\!\langle\ \rangle\!\!\!-NH_2$$

SULFAPYRIDINE

SULFOXONE SODIUM
[Diasone Sodium]

The sulfonamide, sulfapyridine, formerly was the treatment of choice for dermatitis herpetiformis. The antileprosy sulfone, dapsone, is currently the drug of choice, as it is for leprosy (see Chapter 79, Antimycobacterial Agents). Another antileprosy sulfone, sulfoxone, is available; however, since it is hydrolyzed to dapsone in the intestinal tract, sulfapyridine should be considered the alternative drug when dapsone is not tolerated or is contraindicated.

Dermatitis herpetiformis is a chronic disease characterized by clusters of intensely pruritic papules, urticaria-like lesions, vesicles, and bullae on the extensor surfaces. A gluten-sensitive jejunopathy similar to that found in celiac disease is observed in a sufficient number of these patients so that the jejunopathy and dermatitis are almost considered a single disease. A gluten-free diet reverses the generally asymptomatic jejunal abnormality, but strict adherence to the diet for a number of months is required to reverse the skin lesions. Dapsone usually controls the skin lesions rapidly, and the gluten-free diet usually allows the dose of dapsone to be reduced or eliminated eventually. IgA deposition in dermal papillae, HLA association, gluten sensitivity, and antireticulin antibodies suggest that the disease is an immunologic disorder. An immunosuppressive action of dapsone characterized by inhibition of cytotoxicity induced by the myeloperoxidase-peroxide-halide system also supports that concept (Stendahl et al, 1978).

Daily doses of 150 to 200 mg of dapsone relieve acute dermatologic symptoms within one to three days; however, daily doses of 200 to 300 mg can produce hemolysis, methemoglobinemia, or leukopenia in many patients in less than two weeks. Agranulocytosis is a rare complication. Weekly complete blood counts are recommended during the first month of therapy and every three to four months thereafter. Motor neuropathy, usually manifested by weakness, has been noted and is not always reversible on drug withdrawal.

ROUTE, USUAL DOSAGE, AND PREPARATIONS.
DAPSONE:
Oral: *Adults*, 50 mg three or four times daily.
    Avlosulfon (Ayerst). Tablets 25 and 100 mg.
SULFAPYRIDINE:
Oral: *Adults*, 500 mg to 1 g four times daily. Doses up to 6 g daily have been used.
    Drug available generically: Tablets 500 mg.
SULFOXONE SODIUM:
Oral: *Adults*, 330 mg daily for one week; the dose may then be increased to 660 mg daily. For maintenance, 330 mg daily.
    Diasone Sodium (Abbott). Tablets (enteric-coated) 165 mg.

HYALURONIDASE
[Alidase, Wydase]

This enzyme prepared from bovine testes hydrolyzes intercellular ground substances, thus decreasing the viscosity and barrier action of the latter and enhancing the diffusion and absorption of drugs injected concomitantly. Hyaluronidase has been added to local anesthetics to facilitate their diffusion into tissues during infiltration and nerve block anesthesia. However, because a higher incidence of systemic reactions from too rapid absorption of the anesthetic and local irritation and sensitization have been reported with use of this enzyme, its value is seriously questioned and it is now seldom used. It also is used to facilitate administration of fluids or other drugs (eg, urographic contrast media) by hypodermoclysis. Improved techniques of intravenous administration, particularly in infants and children, have limited the need for this enzyme. It is given occasionally to aid in the resolution of transudates, hematomas, and selected localized edemas.

Hyaluronidase should not be injected into acutely inflamed or cancerous areas because of the danger of spreading infection or cancer. Although sensitivity to hyaluronidase occurs infrequently, skin testing with 0.2 ml prior to use is recommended.

ROUTE, USUAL DOSAGE, AND PREPARATIONS. *Injection*: To increase the absorption of drugs, *adults*, 150 units added to the vehicle containing the drug. For hypodermoclysis, *adults*, 150 units added to each liter of fluid to be administered; *infants and children*, 15 units added to each 100 ml of parenteral fluid. For *children under 3 years*, the maximal volume is 200 ml daily; for *premature or very young infants*, no more than 25 ml/kg of body weight daily. The rate of infusion should not exceed 2 ml/min. To aid in the resorption of transudates, hematomas, and edemas, *adults*, 150 to 1,500 units infiltrated locally. For additional details on administration, see the manufacturers' literature.

Alidase (Searle). Powder (for solution) 150 N.F. units.

Wydase (Wyeth). Lyophilized powder 150 and 1,500 N.F. units; solution 150 N.F. units/ml in sterile sodium chloride injection in 1 and 10 ml containers.

POLYETHYLENE FILM

Polyethylene film is widely used as an occlusive dressing in dermatologic therapy. Occlusion of the skin prevents evaporation of perspiration and enhances penetration of certain medications (eg, adrenal corticosteroids) through the skin. Therefore, polyethylene film is a most useful adjunct in the treatment of psoriasis, some eczemas, and keratodermas.

This form of treatment can cause folliculitis, overgrowth of *Candida*, and other undesirable conditions that result from maceration and heat, especially during hot weather.

Glad Wrap (Union Carbide). Also available in tubular form for occlusion of extremities.

SIMILAR PREPARATION.

Saran Wrap (Dow). Vinylidene polymer plastic.

General References

Handbook of Nonprescription Drugs, ed 6. American Pharmaceutical Association, Washington, DC, 1979.

Arndt KA: *Manual of Dermatologic Therapeutics With Essentials of Diagnosis*, ed 2. Boston, Little, Brown and Company, 1978.

Fitzpatrick TB, et al (eds): *Dermatology in General Medicine*, ed 2. New York, McGraw Hill, 1979.

Marzulli FN, Maibach HI (eds): *Advances in Modern Toxicology: Dermatotoxicology and Pharmacology*. New York, Halstead Press, 1977.

Moschella SL, et al (eds): *Dermatology, Vol I & II*. Philadelphia, WB Saunders Co, 1975.

Selected References

Antiperspirant drug products for over-the-counter human use, proposed rules. *Federal Register* 43:46694-46731, (Oct 10) 1978.

Ethylene oxide, ethylene chlorohydrin, and ethylene glycol, proposed maximum residue limits and maximum levels of exposure. *Federal Register* 43:27474-27483, (June 23) 1978.

OTC topical antimicrobial products, over-the-counter drugs generally recognized as safe, effective and not misbranded, proposed rules. *Federal Register* 43:1210-1249, (Jan 6) 1978.

Skin bleaching products for over-the-counter human use, proposed rules. *Federal Register* 43:51546-51555, (Nov 3) 1978.

Sunscreens. *Med Lett Drugs Ther* 21:46-48, 1979.

Sunscreen drug products for over-the-counter human use, proposed rules. *Federal Register* 43:38206-38269, (Aug 25) 1978.

Blanco C, Rothwell KG: Povidone-iodine and kidney. *Lancet* 1:911, 1976.

Bunney MH, et al: Assessment of methods of treating viral warts by comparative treatment trials based on a standard design. *Br J Dermatol* 94:667-679, 1976.

Epstein JH: Risks and benefits of treatment of psoriasis. *N Engl J Med* 300:852-853, 1979.

Esterly NB, Furey NL: Acne: Current concepts. *Pediatrics* 62:1044-1055, 1978.

Farber EM, et al: Appraisal of current systemic chemotherapy for psoriasis. *Arch Dermatol* 112:1679-1688, 1976.

Fisher AA: Propylene glycol dermatitis. *Cutis* 21:166-178, 1978.

Gano SE, Garcia RL: Topical tretinoin, hydroquinone, and betamethasone valerate in therapy of melasma. *Cutis* 23:239-241, 1979.

Goette DK, Odom RB: Adverse effects of corticosteroids. *Cutis* 23:477-487, 1979.

Heel RC, et al: Dextranomer: A review of its general properties and therapeutic efficacy. *Drugs* 18:89-102, 1979.

Hill CJH, Rostenberg A Jr: Adverse effects from topical steroids. *Cutis* 21:624-628, 1978.

Kligman AM, Kaidbey KH: Hydrocortisone

revisited: Historical and experimental evaluation. *Cutis* 22:232-244, 1978.

Lavelle KJ, et al: Iodine absorption in burn patients treated topically with povidone-iodine. *Clin Pharmacol Ther* 17:355-362, 1975.

Leyden JJ, Kligman AM: Efficacy of steroid-antibiotic combinations. *Drug Ther* 8:114-120, (Feb) 1978 A.

Leyden JJ, Kligman AM: Rationale for topical antibiotics. *Cutis* 22:515-528, 1978 B.

Maibach HI, Stoughton RB: Topical corticosteroids, in Azarnoff DL (ed): *Steroid Therapy*. Philadelphia, WB Saunders Co, 1975, 174-190.

Mathias CGT, et al: Allergic contact photodermatitis to para-aminobenzoic acid. *Arch Dermatol* 114:1665-1666, 1978.

Miner NA, et al: Antimicrobial and other properties of a new stabilized alkaline glutaraldehyde disinfectant/sterilizer. *Am J Hosp Pharm* 34:376-382, 1977.

Moleski RJ: Burn wound: Topical therapy for infection control. *Drug Intell Clin Pharmacy* 12:28-35, 1978.

Nacht S et al: In vitro and in vivo skin penetration and metabolic disposition. *Clin Res* 27:533A, 1979.

Nierman MM: Treatment of dermal and decubitus ulcers. *Drugs* 15:226-230, 1978.

Parish LC, Collins E: Decubitus ulcers: Comparative study. *Cutis* 23: 106-110, 1979.

Peck GL, et al: Prolonged remissions of cystic and conglobate acne with 13-cis-retinoic acid. *N Engl J Med* 300:329-333, 1979.

Pietsch J, Meakins JL: Complications of povidone-iodine absorption in topically treated burn patients. *Lancet* 1:280-282, 1976.

Prystowsky SD, et al: Allergic contact hypersensitivity to nickel, neomycin, ethylenediamine, and benzocaine: Relationships between age, sex, history of exposure, and reactivity to standard patch tests and use tests in a general population. *Arch Dermatol* 115:959-962, 1979.

Roenigk HH Jr, et al: Photochemotherapy for psoriasis: Clinical cooperative study of PUVA-48 and PUVA-64. *Arch Dermatol* 115:576-579, 1979.

Roenigk HH Jr, et al: Methotrexate therapy for psoriasis: Guideline revisions. *Arch Dermatol* 108:35, 1973.

Roenigk HH Jr, et al: Use of methotrexate in psoriasis. *Arch Dermatol* 105:363-365, 1972.

Rosen T, Rudolph AH: Identifying and treating bacterial and fungal infections of skin. *Geriatrics* 33:71-82, (Oct) 1978.

Sayre RM, et al: Performance of six sunscreen formulations on human skin: Comparison. *Arch Dermatol* 115:46-49, 1979.

Sneddon IB: Clinical use of topical corticosteroids. *Drugs* 11:193-199, 1976.

Stendahl O, et al: Inhibition of polymorphonuclear leukocyte cytotoxicity by dapsone: Possible mechanism in treatment of dermatitis herpetiformis. *J Clin Invest* 61:214-220, 1978.

Stoehr GP, et al: Systemic complications of local podophyllin therapy. *Ann Intern Med* 89:362-363, 1978.

Stoughton RB: Topical antibiotics for acne vulgaris: Current usage. *Arch Dermatol* 115:486-489, 1979.

Stoughton RB: Evaluation of new potent steroids, in Frost P, et al (eds): *Recent Advances in Dermatopharmacology*. New York, Spectrum Publications, Inc, 1978, 105-112.

Strauss JS, et al: Reexamination of potential comedogenicity of sulfur. *Arch Dermatol* 114:1340-1342, 1978.

Weinstein GD: Methotrexate. *Ann Intern Med* 86:199-204, 1977.

IRON DEFICIENCY ANEMIAS

  Iron Compounds

MEGALOBLASTIC ANEMIAS

  Vitamin B_{12} Compounds

  Folates

SIDEROBLASTIC AND REFRACTORY ANEMIAS

MIXTURES

Anemia is a common hematologic abnormality that occurs when the hemoglobin concentration of red blood cells is reduced. Differential diagnosis is essential to establish and, if possible, treat the underlying cause. Iron deficiency is present in about one-half of patients with folic acid deficiency and in about one-third of those with vitamin B_{12} deficiency. When the iron deficit is more severe than the vitamin deficiency, diagnosis of the latter may require sophisticated techniques. This chapter discusses the treatment of anemias caused by nutritional deficiency in which replacement of the specific nutrient elicits normal production and maturation of erythrocytes.

In nutritional anemias, impaired production of red cells results from deficiency of substances essential for erythropoiesis, most commonly iron. In the United States, folic acid or vitamin B_{12} deficiency is less common and anemias caused by deficiency of other hematopoietic nutrients are rare. All nutritional deficiencies arise from reduced ingestion, poor absorption, inadequate utilization, increased requirement, or increased excretion. Knowledge of the nutrient sources in food and their metabolism is therefore essential to eliminate the causes of these deficiencies.

IRON DEFICIENCY ANEMIAS

Iron is rigidly conserved; only small amounts are excreted by sloughing of epithelial cells from the skin and gastrointestinal tract, and minute amounts are eliminated in hair, nails, bile, feces, and urine. Homeostasis is maintained by controlled absorption of iron from the gut. However, iron excretion may be increased in patients with proteinuria or iron overload. Iron deficiency often results from acute or chronic blood loss, inadequate intake during periods of accelerated growth in infants and children, or increased demands in pregnant women. In women, menstruation is the most common cause of blood loss and a greater iron intake is required than in men, since blood loss in men occurs only in the presence of disease. When iron replacement therapy is indicated, the source of iron loss must be identified. Neoplastic disease is the causative factor in 2% of adults with iron deficiency anemia. If no obvious source of blood loss exists, occult bleeding is a likely cause and the origin must be sought.

Prophylactic use of iron preparations should be reserved for individuals at high risk of developing iron deficiency, especially pregnant and lactating women, low-birth-weight infants, and infants maintained on unsupplemented milk formulas. Iron supplementation also may be indicated for rapidly growing children consuming diets containing little meat and for adults with chronic blood loss (eg, women with heavy menses, patients with hereditary hemorrhagic telangiectasia).

Iron is widely distributed in the body as a constituent of hemoglobin, myoglobin, and a number of enzymes necessary for energy transfer. It is stored as ferritin or hemosiderin in hepatocytes and in reticuloendothelial cells, especially in the liver, spleen, and bone marrow. Hemoglobin concentration is maintained by mobilization of tissue iron stores if necessary and is reduced only after iron stores are depleted; thus, anemia is not a sensitive indicator of iron depletion. Although hypochromic microcytic red blood cells usually signify iron deficiency, they may be produced by inadequate hemoglobin synthesis from any cause. Early iron depletion produces few recognizable changes in red cell morphology but can be confirmed by decreased or absent bone marrow hemosiderin. Alternatively, if the saturation of serum transferrin is 15% or less and the total iron binding capacity (TIBC) is increased or the serum ferritin level is low (less than 10 to 20 ng/ml), iron deficiency probably is present. If the hemoglobin level and mean corpuscular volume also are low, the most likely diagnosis is iron deficiency anemia (see also Dallman, 1977). Since the diagnosis of iron deficiency usually can be established quickly and easily, the administration of iron compounds may be delayed until appropriate diagnostic procedures to determine the source of iron loss have been completed.

Iron Compounds

Therapeutic doses of iron are used only to treat iron deficiency anemia. Oral administration is the route of choice and, since iron is absorbed more easily in its ferrous form, ferrous salts (sulfate, fumarate, gluconate) are preferred. Ferric salts, including chelated compounds such as ferrocholinate [Chel-Iron, Ferrolip], are absorbed less readily.

Ferrous iron is absorbed through the intestinal mucosa into the blood where it is immediately bound to transferrin and transported to bone marrow. Absorption is most efficient in the duodenum and decreases progressively throughout the intestinal tract. Multiple factors impede or expedite utilization, but hemoglobin synthesis is the primary factor controlling the rate of plasma iron turnover. Iron is conserved through reuse and is only minimally excreted. Storage is principally in liver epithelial cells and consists of reserves from both dietary ingestion and red blood cell destruction, some of which is readily mobilizable for hemoglobin synthesis.

Ferrous sulfate is the standard for other oral iron preparations. Most patients respond to this form and those who do not are unlikely to benefit from any iron salt. Therefore, when ferrous sulfate is well tolerated, there is seldom justification for use of more complex preparations. Some sustained-release and enteric-coated preparations, which are designed to prevent iron release in the stomach where it is irritating and to maximize iron release in the duodenum, transport iron past the sites of maximal absorption and actually reduce the amount available.

Iron is absorbed best when taken between meals but may be taken with food if necessary to reduce intolerance. Gastrointestinal tolerance of any iron preparation depends upon the amount of ionized elemental iron present, not on the form in which it is given. Because the ionized iron content varies greatly among different preparations, calculation of dosage should always be in terms of elemental iron. Despite claims to the contrary, substitution of one form for another when untoward effects develop may not be beneficial if equivalent amounts of elemental iron are given. Adverse reactions often may be lessened by decreasing the size of the individual dose and increasing the number (up to four) of daily doses.

For iron-deficient adults, 50 to 100 mg of elemental iron (one 300-mg ferrous sulfate tablet = 60 mg elemental iron) three times daily has been recommended to replenish body iron stores within six months. However, oral administration of 30 mg of elemental iron three times daily appears to be sufficient to correct most uncomplicated deficiencies rapidly, although iron stores are replenished more slowly. However, tablets or capsules that provide this quantity of elemental iron are not widely available. Ferrous gluconate may be preferred because a 300-mg tablet contains a lower dose of elemental iron (37 mg) than in 300 mg of ferrous sulfate (60 mg) or fumarate (99 mg). Liquid preparations can be used, but this dosage form seldom is popular with adults. Consequently, the usual therapeutic dosage recommendations listed in the individual evaluations follow the traditionally recommended regimens; however, smaller doses are more satisfactory, particularly if gastrointestinal upset becomes a problem. Some clinicians recommend that initially one tablet daily be given with a meal to minimize side effects and increase compliance. If this is tolerated, two, then three or four tablets can be given daily. For most adults, 180 to 200 mg elemental iron daily produces maximum therapeutic effect with minimum adverse effects. Larger doses do not appreciably increase hemoglobin regeneration but do increase side effects (Savin, 1977).

The hematologic response to orally administered iron becomes fully evident after two weeks of therapy. In iron-deficient patients, adequate oral dosage increases hemoglobin production at a rate of 100 to 200 mg/dl of blood daily; a normal value is usually attained in two months unless blood loss continues. Parenteral administration produces a similar increase. To replenish depleted iron stores, oral therapy should be continued for approximately six months after the hemoglobin level has returned to normal. If a satisfactory response is not noted after three weeks of therapy, it is probable that (1) the diagnosis of iron deficiency anemia is incorrect, (2) the dosage regimen is not being followed, (3) blood loss is occurring simultaneously, or (4) complicating factors (eg, defective iron absorption or utilization, infection, chronic disease) are present. If the patient is assimilating iron while blood loss continues, the reticulocyte count may be elevated.

Parenteral iron (iron dextran injection [Imferon]) should be used only after demonstration that bone marrow stores of iron are absent. Iron deficiency need not be corrected rapidly if bleeding has stopped or is known not to be harmful (eg, menorrhagia) and iron metabolism is in positive balance. Because serious reactions are a possibility, parenteral iron should be reserved for patients with a confirmed diagnosis of iron deficiency who cannot tolerate or do not respond to oral administration (eg, continuing loss greater than can be replaced because of limitations to oral absorption) or, most commonly, it is given to noncompliant patients who refuse to take iron orally.

Malabsorption syndromes (eg, tropical sprue, celiac disease, partial gastrectomy) and apparent intolerance to iron usually do not constitute valid reasons for use of parenteral iron preparations. Marked malabsorption of iron is rare and, even in patients with gastric resection, a sufficient amount is absorbed to produce a therapeutic response. Intolerance probably is dose related and may be corrected by reducing the dose.

For a discussion on combination products containing iron, see the section on Mixtures.

Adverse Reactions and Precautions: Iron compounds are contraindicated in patients with primary hemochromatosis and transfusion siderosis. They should not be used to treat hemolytic anemias unless an iron-deficient state also exists, since storage of iron with possible secondary hemochromatosis can result. Iron overload is particularly likely to occur in patients given excessive amounts of parenteral iron, in those taking both oral and parenteral preparations, and in patients with hemoglobinopathies or other refractory anemias erroneously diagnosed as iron deficiency anemia. Iron should not be given to patients receiving repeated blood transfusions, since there is approximately 1 mg of iron/ml of transfused red blood cells. Prolonged administration of therapeutic doses of iron should be avoided except in patients with continued bleeding (including uncorrectable menorrhagia), copious menstrual periods, or repeated pregnancies.

The oral route is preferred because toxic reactions, including hemosiderosis with possible tissue damage, are more likely to occur with parenteral administration that bypasses intestinal regulatory mechanisms. Fever, lymphadenopathy, nausea and vomiting, arthralgias, urticaria, severe toxic dilatation of blood vessels resulting in peripheral vascular failure, and fatal anaphylactic reactions also have occurred after parenteral therapy.

Serious reactions caused by parenteral administration are most likely to occur in patients who also are taking iron orally. Under these conditions, transferrin becomes saturated rapidly and additional iron entering the blood remains unbound; it is this unbound fraction that is responsible for acute toxicity. Hence, *parenteral iron should not be used concomitantly with oral iron preparations*, particularly since the primary indication for parenteral iron therapy is a pre-existing condition that precludes use of oral iron.

Excessive iron storage is rare following oral administration except in patients with increased iron absorption (eg, those with thalassemia, chronic hemolytic states, Laennec's cirrhosis, hemochromatosis, sideroachrestic anemia). Gastrointestinal disturbances, particularly nausea, epigastric pain, diarrhea, or constipation, may occur with oral administration, and pre-existing gastrointestinal diseases (eg, chronic ulcerative colitis, regional enteritis) may be aggravated. Infants and children appear to tolerate therapeutic doses better than adults. Although pregnant women are particularly susceptible to gastrointestinal disturbances, there is no absolute intolerance for orally administered iron. These untoward effects tend to subside with continuation of therapy or ingestion of iron with meals and, if necessary, reduction of the individual dose; most patients tolerate doses below 200 mg of elemental iron in the ferrous form daily.

Brightly coated tablets and flavored syrups are particularly hazardous because they are attractive to children. Parents should be warned that iron is toxic and can be fatal when excessive amounts are ingested by children, and all iron-containing products should be labeled as potentially hazardous if large amounts are ingested. For discussion of iron poisoning, see also the evaluation on Deferoxamine Mesylate in Chapter 86, Specific Antidotes.

ORAL IRON PREPARATIONS

FERROUS SULFATE

[Feosol, Fer-In-Sol, Fero-Gradumet, Mol-Iron]

Ferrous sulfate is the agent of choice for treatment of uncomplicated iron deficiency anemia if the patient can tolerate it. Since conditions for iron absorption are favorable only in the duodenum and upper jejunum, sustained-release or enteric-coated preparations should be used in an effort to decrease gastric irritation only if objective bioavailability data have shown that the preparation is adequately absorbed and the supposed benefits outweigh the disadvantage of added cost. Any iron preparation likely to pass intact beyond the upper gastrointestinal tract is less effective.

Adverse effects are generally dose dependent; in 10% of patients they are severe enough to be intolerable. Gastrointestinal disturbances (usually nausea, bloating, anorexia, pyrosis) are the most frequent reactions noted. This drug is absorbed best when taken between meals, but gastrointestinal symptoms may be minimized by reducing the dose and/or giving it in divided amounts with meals or shortly thereafter. In some patients, administration of one-half the total daily dose at bedtime will improve tolerance. As with other orally administered iron salts, ferrous sulfate may aggravate existing gastrointestinal disease (eg, peptic ulcer, regional enteritis, ulcerative colitis).

Acute severe iron poisoning is uncommon in adults but can occur in children who ingest iron formulations intended for adults. In young children, doses as low as 400 mg of elemental iron are potentially fatal. Initial toxic effects include nausea, vomiting, and shock. Death has resulted from acute circulatory failure, gastric necrosis, and acute hepatic necrosis.

ROUTE, USUAL DOSAGE, AND PREPARATIONS.

Therapeutic:

Oral: *Adults*, initially, 60 mg elemental iron, increased by 30-mg increments to a maximum of 240 mg elemental iron daily in three or four divided doses; *children 6 to 12 years*, 24 to 120 mg elemental iron daily in three or four divided doses (elixir or syrup); *children 1 to 5 years*, 15 to 45 mg elemental iron daily in three or four divided doses; *infants*, a quantity of a pediatric preparation sufficient to provide 10 to 25 mg of elemental iron daily given in three or four divided doses. See also the Introduction to this section.

> Drug available generically: Capsules 150 mg (30 mg elemental iron); tablets (plain, enteric-coated) 192 and 325 mg (39 and 65 mg elemental iron, respectively).
> *Feosol* (Menley & James). Capsules (timed-release) 250 mg (50 mg elemental iron); elixir 220 mg (44 mg elemental iron)/5 ml (alcohol 5%); tablets 325 mg (65 mg elemental iron) (nonprescription).
> *Fer-In-Sol* (Mead Johnson). Capsules 190 mg (equivalent to 60 mg elemental iron); drops 75 mg (15 mg elemental iron)/0.6 ml; syrup 90 mg (18 mg elemental iron)/5 ml (nonprescription).
> *Fero-Gradumet* (Abbott). Tablets (timed-release) 525 mg (105 mg elemental iron) (nonprescription).
> *Mol-Iron* (Schering). Capsules (timed-release) 390 mg (78 mg elemental iron); liquid 195 mg (39 mg elemental iron)/4 ml (alcohol 4.75%); tablets 195 mg (39 mg elemental iron) (nonprescription).

Prophylactic (supplementation):

Oral: *Women of childbearing age, adolescents, and children*, 18 mg of elemental iron daily; *pregnant and lactating women*, 25 mg of elemental iron daily; *men and postmenopausal women*, 10 mg of elemental iron daily. *Low-birth-weight infants and infants with low iron stores*, initially, 2 mg/kg of body weight daily of elemental iron gradually decreasing to approximately 1 mg/kg daily; *normal infants*, 10 to 15 mg of elemental iron daily during the first year. Since many infant formulas contain iron, the amount in the formula should be considered when determining whether supplementation is necessary. Mixtures containing iron usually are given for prophylaxis. (See the section on Mixtures and Chapter 52, Vitamins and Minerals.)

FERROUS FUMARATE
[Feostat, Ircon, Toleron]

FERROUS GLUCONATE
[Fergon]

These compounds are as effective as ferrous sulfate in iron deficiency anemia and are claimed to be less irritating when administered in equal amounts because ionic iron in ferrous sulfate is probably released more quickly. However, equal amounts of *ionic iron*, regardless of the source, are equally irritating to the stomach and intestinal mucosa.

Gastrointestinal disturbances are usually mild and can be minimized by reducing the individual dose and taking the drug shortly after meals. Like ferrous sulfate, ferrous fumarate or gluconate may aggravate existing gastrointestinal disease (eg, regional enteritis, ulcerative colitis). Overdosage has caused acute severe iron poisoning, especially in children.

ROUTE, USUAL DOSAGE, AND PREPARATIONS.
FERROUS FUMARATE:

Therapeutic:

Oral: Adults, 100 to 400 mg (approximately 33 to 133 mg elemental iron) daily in one to four doses; *children 6 to 12 years*, 100 to 300 mg (33 to 100 mg elemental iron) daily in one to four teaspoon doses (suspension); *children 1 to 5 years*, initially, a quantity of a pediatric preparation sufficient to provide 15 mg of elemental iron (12 drops or ½ teaspoon), gradually increased to a maximum of 45 mg elemental iron daily, if necessary, in three or four divided doses; *infants*, 10 to 20 mg elemental iron daily (5 to 16 drops) divided into two to four doses. See also the Introduction to this section.

Prophylactic:

Same as for Ferrous Sulfate.

> Drug available generically: Tablets 195 and 325 mg (64 and 107 mg elemental iron, respectively).
> *Feostat* (O'Neal, Jones & Feldman). Drops 45 mg (15 mg elemental iron)/0.6 ml; suspension 100 mg (33.3 mg elemental iron)/5 ml; tablets (chewable) 150 mg (33.3 mg elemental iron) (nonprescription).
> *Ircon* (Key). Tablets 200 mg (66 mg elemental iron) (nonprescription).
> *Toleron* (Mallinckrodt). Suspension 100 mg (33 mg elemental iron)/5 ml; tablets 200 mg (66 mg elemental iron) (nonprescription).

FERROUS GLUCONATE:

Therapeutic:

Oral: Adults, 320 to 640 mg (38 to 77 mg elemental iron) three times daily. *Children*, 100 to 300 mg (12 to 36 mg elemental iron) three times daily. *Infants*, initially, 120 mg (30 drops of elixir equivalent to 15 mg elemental iron); this amount may be increased gradually to 300 mg (36 mg elemental iron) daily. See also the Introduction to this section.

Prophylactic:

Same as for Ferrous Sulfate.

> Drug available generically: Tablets 300 mg (38 mg elemental iron).
> *Fergon* (Breon). Capsules 435 mg (52.2 mg elemental iron); elixir 300 mg (36 mg elemental iron)/5 ml; tablets 320 mg (38.4 mg elemental iron) (nonprescription).

FERROCHOLINATE
[Chel-Iron, Ferrolip]

IRON-POLYSACCHARIDE COMPLEX
[Niferex]

These ferric iron preparations are not preferred because they are not as well absorbed as the soluble ferrous salt preparations.

Mild gastrointestinal disturbances are the most common adverse effects. Although these complexes appear to be less toxic on a weight basis than the ferrous salts, this is simply a reflection of the smaller quantity of ionic iron reaching the stomach and intestinal mucosa. It is probable that equal quantities of ionic iron from ferrocholinate or iron-polysaccharide complex and the ferrous salts would be equally toxic. The danger of severe iron poisoning still exists, particularly in children. Like other iron preparations, ferrocholinate or iron-polysaccharide complex may aggravate gastrointestinal disease.

ROUTE, USUAL DOSAGE, AND PREPARATIONS.

Oral: Adults, to correct iron deficiency anemia, 330 to 660 mg (40 to 80 mg elemental iron) three times daily; *children*, 1.5 to 2 mg of elemental iron/kg of body weight daily. *Infants*, for prophylaxis, 1 to 1.5 mg of elemental iron/kg daily. See also the Introduction to this section.

(All strengths expressed in terms of elemental iron)

> FERROCHOLINATE:
> *Chel-Iron* (Kinney). Drops (pediatric) 25 mg/ml; liquid 50 mg/5 ml; tablets 40 mg (nonprescription).
> *Ferrolip* (Flint). Syrup 50 mg/5 ml; tablets 40 mg (nonprescription).
> IRON-POLYSACCHARIDE COMPLEX:
> *Niferex* (Central). Capsules 150 mg; elixir 100 mg/5 ml; tablets 50 mg (nonprescription).

PARENTERAL IRON PREPARATION

IRON DEXTRAN INJECTION
[Imferon]

Iron dextran injection should be used only after iron deficiency anemia has been confirmed by diagnostic tests (eg, demonstration that bone marrow stores of iron are absent). This drug is indicated when oral therapy has failed or may further irritate gastrointestinal disease (eg, regional enteritis, ulcerative colitis), when a patient is unwilling or unable to take iron orally (eg, psychiatric, pediatric, or geriatric patients), when iron loss exceeds the amount absorbable from oral ferrous sulfate (more than 500 to 1,000 ml of blood per week [McCurdy, 1977]), when immediate replacement is necessary (eg, severe anemia in late pregnancy), and when it is suspected that a patient is incapable of compliance or that an infant will not receive iron at home.

The parenterally administered iron dextran complex is dissociated by the reticuloendothelial cells to make the iron biologically available; a small proportion may remain complexed for three or four months, particularly after intramuscular injection.

Serious toxic effects (eg, anaphylactic shock, acute circulatory failure, cardiac arrest) have occurred after administration of iron dextran injection. Because the rate of administration can be controlled with intravenous use, which decreases the risk of anaphylaxis compared to intramuscular injection, the former route is preferred. It is recommended that a small test dose be given initially to detect sensitivity. An appropriate injectable form of epinephrine and emergency resuscitative equipment should be readily available, since severe anaphylactic reactions have occurred with doses as small as 0.01 ml. Intramuscular injection can cause painful irritation and skin discoloration that may last for months; divided doses given by deep intramuscular injection (Z-track technique) should be used to minimize this. Although data are not conclusive, development of sarcomas has been reported at the site of in-

tramuscular injection. Iron dextran injection also may cause urticaria, arthralgia, headache, fever, nausea, vomiting, and regional lymphadenopathy. *Parenteral and oral iron preparations should not be used concomitantly.*

ROUTES, USUAL DOSAGE, AND PREPARATIONS. (All dosages expressed in terms of elemental iron)
The response of the patient should be closely followed as an index to the effectiveness of therapy. The dose of iron needed for parenteral therapy is calculated by a number of formulas, one of which is as follows:

$$0.3 \times \text{body weight (lb)} \times$$
$$(100 - \frac{\text{patient's Hg (g/dl)} \times 100)}{14.8} =$$
$$\text{total mg of iron}$$

The value computed by this formula represents a satisfactory replacement dose for iron dextran injection in terms of elemental iron needed to restore blood hemoglobin levels to normal and replenish iron stores. An adult who is not bleeding should receive no more than 3 g as a total parenteral dose. Five to ten times as much may be given orally since iron-deficient persons absorb only about 20% of a normal dose. As they are treated and deficiency is lessened, the amount absorbed decreases to about 10% of the ingested dose. Once determined, the total estimated dose should not be exceeded. If the hemoglobin response is insufficient, other causes of the persisting anemia must be sought. See also the manufacturer's literature.

Intravenous (preferred route): Adults and children, following an initial test dose of 0.5 ml (25 mg), a daily injection of undiluted iron dextran injection may be given in doses no larger than 100 mg a day at a rate not exceeding 50 mg (1 ml)/min. If large doses are indicated, total dose infusion therapy is preferred. Most authorities believe that infusion of the total calculated amount as a single dose is the safer method of administering iron dextran solution to the nonbleeding adult. After dilution with 500 to 1,000 ml of physiologic saline, an initial few ml should be infused slowly. (Use of 5% dextrose in water as the diluent has been associated with development of phlebitis.) After 10 to 15 minutes, the diluted solution may be administered at a rate of 60 drops/min over a period of approximately ten hours.

Intramuscular (deep): If no adverse reaction occurs following a test dose of 25 mg, after 24 hours the following amounts should be administered in divided doses until the total calculated amount is given (maximum, 3 g in nonbleeding adults): *Adults over 50 kg*, up to 250 mg daily. *Small adults and children weighing 9 to 50 kg*, no more than 100 mg daily. *Infants 4.5 to 9 kg*, no more than 50 mg daily; *under 4.5 kg*, no more than 25 mg daily. All injections should be made in the upper outer buttocks using a Z-track technique. Experiments using iron dextran injection radioisotope indicate that approximately 30% of an intramuscular dose remains at the site of injection for more than 30 days.

> Drug available generically: Solution 10 and 50 mg/ml of elemental iron in 10 ml containers.
> *Imferon* (Merrell-National). Solution equivalent to 50 mg of elemental iron/ml in 2 and 5 ml containers (intramuscular, intravenous) and 10 ml containers (intramuscular).

MEGALOBLASTIC ANEMIAS

Since both folic acid and vitamin B_{12} are essential cofactors for DNA synthesis, a deficiency of either causes defective cell division which inhibits normal reproduction of proliferating cells, including hematopoietic cells. The erythroblast nucleus cannot accumulate sufficient DNA to permit cell division (maturation arrest), resulting in large cells in both bone marrow and blood (Beeson and McDermott, 1975). Leukopenia and thrombocytopenia also may be present. The rate of erythrocyte destruction is increased in megaloblastic anemia, which may indicate an accompanying hemolytic process. In other proliferating cells, particularly in the alimentary tract, defective DNA synthesis results in secondary atrophy of epithelial cells in the tongue, stomach, and small intestine. This contributes to the deficiency, since reduced absorption of dietary folic acid and/or vitamin B_{12} may accompany any malabsorptive disorder of the small intestine. However, in pernicious anemia, the cause of vitamin B_{12} deficiency is deficiency or absence of gastric intrinsic factor. The primary defect is a permanent gastric atrophy in which parietal cells fail to secrete intrinsic factor necessary for the absorption of vitamin B_{12}. Maximal absorption of folic acid occurs primarily in the upper one-third of the small intestine and of vitamin B_{12} in the lower one-half of the ileum.

Folate deficiency is more common because folate stores in the body are depleted rapidly, whereas body stores of vitamin B_{12} may last several years. However, in pernicious anemia or following gastric resection, the diminished or absent gastric intrinsic factor causes relatively rapid depletion of vitamin B_{12} because absorption (and thus reabsorption from bile) of vitamin B_{12} is reduced. Most megaloblastic anemias are due to nutritional deficiency of folic acid, vitamin B_{12}, or both. However, malabsorption (eg, in tropical sprue, celiac disease), impaired utilization, or increased losses caused by other diseases, chronic infection, or concomitant use of some drugs may either result in or increase the severity of anemia. Existing anemias also may be aggravated by conditions that increase the requirements for vitamin B_{12}, folate, or both (eg, hemolytic anemias, pregnancy), and anemias may be altered by relative quantities of other agents in the body (eg, pyridoxine, nucleic acids, amino acids, iron). Thus, specific therapy for megaloblastic anemias depends upon accurate diagnosis.

Although hematologic findings produced by folic acid or vitamin B_{12} deficiency frequently are identical and a pharmacologic dose of one may overcome, at least temporarily, the metabolic blockade in hematopoiesis produced by a deficiency of the other, vitamin B_{12} and folic acid are not interchangeable therapeutic agents. The neurologic damage resulting from vitamin B_{12} deficiency will progress and become irreversible unless this vitamin is given promptly. Only rarely is therapy necessary prior to etiologic diagnosis. However, when severe thrombocytopenia associated with bleeding, severe leukopenia associated with infection, severe anemia, marked neurologic damage, or other serious complication makes immediate therapy necessary, both vitamin B12 (100 mcg) and folic acid (15 mg) are given intramuscularly, followed by daily oral administration of folic acid (5 mg) and intramuscular injection of vitamin B12 (100 mcg) for one week (Goodman and Gilman, 1975).

The vitamin B12 or folate deficiency anemias usually respond so rapidly to specific therapy that transfusion of red cell concentrate is indicated only when severe anemia is associated with impending or actual cardiac failure. In these patients, the cautious administration of red blood cell concentrate (up to several units) may produce rapid and dramatic relief. Since the risk of transmitting hepatitis increases with the number of units administered, the dose should be kept as low as practical. A loop diuretic (eg, furosemide 40 mg) should be given (usually when blood is withdrawn for crossmatch) before the blood transfusion is begun. Transfusion in severely anemic patients may cause rapid mobilization of water and produce pulmonary edema disproportionate to the amount being transfused.

Vitamin B12 Compounds

Vitamin B12 is the general name for several cobalt-containing compounds (cobalamins). These are synthesized by microorganisms ingested from soil and water by higher animals and made available to humans through consumption of meat and dairy products. Plants do not provide vitamin B12 and strict vegetarians may develop a cobalamin deficiency. However, deficiency may not appear for several years, since most vitamin B12 is reabsorbed in the enterohepatic circulation and depletion of body stores is gradual. In

these individuals, oral administration of 1 to 2 mcg of vitamin B12 daily will maintain normal hematologic status. In pernicious anemia, the lack of intrinsic factor reduces the absorption of vitamin B12 and deficiency occurs within two to five years. Subnormal intestinal absorption of vitamin B12 is nearly always present in tropical sprue, celiac disease, regional enteritis, and other malabsorption syndromes or following gastric resection. In all patients with defective absorption, only parenteral administration of vitamin B12 is effective.

The average diet supplies about 5 to 15 mcg/day of vitamin B12 in a protein-bound form that is available for absorption after normal digestion. Vitamin B12 is bound to intrinsic factor during transit through the stomach; separation occurs in the terminal ileum in the presence of calcium, and vitamin B12 enters the mucosal cell for absorption. It is then transported by specific B12 binding proteins, transcobalamin I and II. Transcobalamin II is the delivery protein for vitamin B12 in the same sense that transferrin is the delivery protein for iron. In addition, a small amount (approximately 1% to 3% of the total amount ingested) is absorbed by simple diffusion, but this mechanism is significant only with large doses.

The most widely known form of the vitamin B12 group, cyanocobalamin, has hematopoietic activity apparently identical to that of the antianemia factor in purified liver extract. It is clinically effective in the treatment of vitamin B12 deficiency states but has no proven therapeutic value (except as a placebo) in any of the nonhematologic conditions for which it has been used (eg, acute viral hepatitis, trigeminal neuralgia and various other neuropathies, multiple sclerosis, delayed growth, poor appetite, certain dermatologic and psychiatric disorders, allergies, amblyopia, aging, sterility, thyrotoxicosis, malnutrition).

Hydroxocobalamin [alphaREDISOL] is closely related chemically to cyanocobalamin and has equivalent hematopoietic activity. This agent is more highly bound to blood proteins than cyanocobalamin and thus is retained in the body a little longer.

However, because of the dosages generally used, this is not an important clinical consideration and hydroxocobalamin apparently has no advantage over cyanocobalamin. Furthermore, some patients treated with hydroxocobalamin may develop antibodies to the complex of hydroxocobalamin and transcobalamin II. Massive doses of hydroxocobalamin have been used as an antidote to cyanide poisoning and are alleged to be of value in treating tobacco amblyopia.

Preparations of liver for injection provide a source of vitamin B_{12} activity but are outmoded and should no longer be used.

The oral administration of cyanocobalamin should be reserved only for treating *nutritional* vitamin B_{12} deficiency. (See also Chapter 52, Vitamins and Minerals.) Parenteral therapy is universally preferred for pernicious anemia or in patients with other forms of defective absorption (eg, tropical sprue, celiac disease, regional enteritis, gastric resection), because oral therapy generally does not provide a reliable therapeutic response. Although patients receiving oral cyanocobalamin-intrinsic factor combinations respond initially, they frequently become refractory to treatment after a variable period of time.

The treatment of choice for vitamin B_{12} deficiency caused by defective absorption is the intramuscular or deep subcutaneous injection of crystalline cyanocobalamin or hydroxocobalamin solutions. It has been estimated that the total cyanocobalamin deficit in a patient with pernicious anemia is approximately 4,000 to 5,000 mcg. Demonstrable neurologic damage from pernicious anemia that is not reversed after 12 to 18 months of adequate therapy must be considered irreversible.

Vitamin B_{12}-deficient patients respond dramatically to therapy with cyanocobalamin or hydroxocobalamin. Normoblastic hematopoiesis is evident within 48 to 72 hours following intramuscular injection. However, *the patient with pernicious anemia or permanent defective absorption must understand that regular injections of vitamin B_{12} are essential for the rest of his life to prevent development of irreversible neurologic damage.*

INDIVIDUAL EVALUATIONS

CYANOCOBALAMIN

HYDROXOCOBALAMIN
[alphaREDISOL]

The primary established clinical uses of these drugs are to treat confirmed deficiency of vitamin B_{12} and to perform Schilling's test for pernicious anemia or malabsorption. A third occasional use is in suspected cases of pernicious anemia when the patient refuses bone marrow examination, Schilling's test is not available, and serum analysis of vitamin B_{12} content is not completed before therapy is begun.

Hydroxocobalamin has a somewhat longer duration of action than cyanocobalamin. However, antibodies may develop to the complex of hydroxocobalamin and transcobalamin II. No serious toxicity has been reported following use of either preparation. Allergic reactions to impurities in the preparation occur rarely. Injection causes little or no pain, and no adverse local effects have been reported.

ROUTES, USUAL DOSAGE, AND PREPARATIONS. *Intramuscular, Subcutaneous (deep)*: The following regimen is usually recommended: For treatment of uncomplicated pernicious anemia or defective absorption of vitamin B_{12}, *adults*, 30 to 50 mcg daily for five to ten days, followed by 100 to 200 mcg monthly until remission is complete; thereafter, 100 mcg every four weeks will maintain remission. *Children*, a total of

1,000 to 5,000 mcg given in divided doses of 100 mcg each over a period of two or more weeks. Thereafter, 50 to 100 mcg every four weeks will maintain remission. Some authorities now believe that multiple injections and daily office visits are unnecessary because single monthly injections of 1,000 mcg appear to be equally effective. For patients with demonstrable neurologic damage, 1,000 mcg may be given once weekly for several months, then once or twice monthly for another year.

CYANOCOBALAMIN:
Drug available generically: Solution (injection) 100 and 1,000 mcg/ml in 1, 10, and 30 ml containers.
Available Trademarks.
Betalin 12 Crystalline (Lilly), *Redisol Injectable* (Merck Sharp & Dohme), *Rubramin PC* (Squibb), *Sytobex* (Parke, Davis).
HYDROXOCOBALAMIN:
Drug available generically: Solution 1,000 mcg/ml in 10 and 30 ml containers.
alphaREDISOL (Merck Sharp & Dohme). Solution 1,000 mcg/ml in 10 ml containers (intramuscular only).

Oral: This route should be used only to treat dietary vitamin B_{12} deficiency. *Adults and children*, 1 mcg daily; *infants up to 1 year*, 0.3 mcg daily.

For oral preparations, see the section on Mixtures in Chapter 52, Vitamins and Minerals. No single-entity preparations are available in a 1-mcg concentration.

VITAMIN B_{12} WITH INTRINSIC FACTOR CONCENTRATE
[Biopar Forte]

This oral preparation is a mixture of vitamin B_{12} and dried stomach or duodenum from hogs or other food animals. Hematopoietic activity is measured in oral units of activity, 1 oral unit being equivalent to not more than 15 mcg of cyanocobalamin. Since no more than approximately 1% of the administered dose is absorbed, this is a costly method of treatment. Furthermore, this preparation is useless in those with functional or structural intestinal disease, allergic sensitization from hog or other animal protein may occur, and many patients develop refractoriness after varying periods of treatment. Therefore, this preparation should be used only in patients whose primary lesion is caused by lack of secretion of adequate intrinsic factor and who refuse parenteral therapy.

Biopar Forte (Armour). Tablets ½ N.F. unit with cobalamin concentrate 25 mcg.

LIVER INJECTION
[Pernaemon]

The crude soluble vitamin B_{12} activity of liver is available as a single-entity preparation and in vitamin mixtures for injection. Because crystalline cyanocobalamin for injection is superior to all liver preparations, the latter should no longer be used.

Adverse reactions include local hypersensitivity, allergy, anaphylactic reactions, and brownish discoloration of the skin at the injection site.

No dosage regimen is given since use of liver injection is now obsolete.

Drug available generically: Solution 2 mcg/ml (crude) and 10 and 20 mcg/ml (refined) in 10 and 30 ml containers.
Pernaemon (Organon). Solution (injection) vitamin B_{12} activity equivalent to 20 mcg/ml in 10 ml containers.

Folates

Folic acid is widely distributed in nature as a conjugate (usually, heptoglutamate) with one or more molecules of glutamic acid. These forms, called folates, are present in nearly all food stuffs. They are destroyed by prolonged cooking and other types of food processing.

Synthetic folic acid [Folvite], administered orally, is almost completely absorbed even in the presence of the malabsorption caused by tropical sprue, whereas naturally occurring folates must be reduced to mono- and diglutamates by conjugases in the gut before they can be efficiently absorbed from the proximal small intestine. Folates are transported and stored principally as 5-methylhydrofolate, and conversion to the metabolically active form, tetrahydrofolate, may be vitamin B_{12}-dependent.

Folic acid alleviates the megaloblastic anemias that occur during pregnancy, infancy, and in most cases of tropical sprue or celiac disease. Folates also are used to treat hematologic diseases in which there is a fast turnover of red cells (hemolytic disease), especially in children with thalassemia major and in older patients with myelofibrosis and myeloid metaplasia. In these patients, prophylactic daily doses are given routinely; this regimen may reduce the need for transfusions.

Severely ill hospitalized patients may develop subclinical folate deficiency if they are maintained on unsupplemented intravenous fluids. Even in the absence of overt megaloblastic anemia, these individuals have reduced bone marrow reserves that may limit production of granulocytes, platelets, and red cells. Supplementation with folic acid may be beneficial in these patients.

Folic acid and the folates may correct the anemia of pernicious anemia and other types of vitamin B_{12} deficiency but should not be used in these cases (unless adequate concomitant doses of vitamin B_{12} are given) because they neither arrest nor prevent the progression of neurologic damage. Their indiscriminate prophylactic use may mask symptoms and the anemia of pernicious anemia and make diagnosis difficult. Before folic acid is given, serum and red cell folic acid concentrations should be measured to confirm deficiency. If the microbiologic method of assay (*Lactobacillus casei* or *Streptococcus faecalis*) is used, false low values may result if the patient is taking antibiotics.

The minimal adult requirement for folic acid is estimated to be 50 mcg daily (400 mcg for total folacin). The average store of folate in adults is approximately 7.5 mg. Since the free folate content in the average daily diet in the United States is 200 to 300 mcg, dietary sources are generally adequate. When folate deficiency anemia is of dietary origin, correction of the diet is preferred over supplemental medication. The addition of one fresh uncooked fruit or vegetable or glass of fruit juice to the patient's diet each day often constitutes adequate dietary correction. However, during pregnancy and lactation, a daily prophylactic dose should be given routinely to meet the increased demands. Larger doses may be indicated in women with marked absorption defects. Folate-deficient patients generally respond rapidly to folic acid; reticulocytosis generally begins in two to five days.

The sodium salt of folic acid (folate sodium) may be given by intramuscular, intravenous, or deep subcutaneous injection. Parenteral administration has no advantage over the oral route, but it may be preferred when the deficiency is known to be caused by malabsorption or when this drug is included as a constituent of hyperalimentation infusion.

Individuals taking certain anticonvulsant, antimalarial, or contraceptive drugs may develop folic acid deficiency; long-term use of analgesics or steroids to treat chronic diseases (eg, rheumatoid arthritis) also may increase folate requirements. The mechanisms causing the deficiency are not completely understood but include reduction of folic acid absorption by some anticonvulsants and inhibition of dihydrofolate reductase by some antimalarial agents that block the reduction of folic acid to its metabolically active form. Although folic acid deficiency can be corrected by withdrawing the offending drug, this is not always possible. Supplementing the diet with folic acid may overcome the deficiency when the mechanism is not enzyme inhibition. If supplemental folic acid fails to correct the deficiency or if dihydrofolate reductase deficiency is present (eg, in severe hepatic damage; after administration of the folate antagonists, pyrimethamine, trimethoprim, or triamterene), leucovorin calcium (folinate calcium) should be tried. This agent is already in the reduced state and, therefore, is beyond the metabolic step that requires dihydrofolate reductase. Folinic acid also has been employed as an antagonist to methotrexate.

INDIVIDUAL EVALUATIONS
FOLIC ACID
[Folvite]

FOLATE SODIUM
[Folvite Solution]

These agents are specific for the correction of folic acid deficiency. They should never be used as the sole agent to treat pernicious anemia or other vitamin B_{12} deficiency states, for their use in patients with pernicious anemia leads to diagnostic difficulty, and irreversible neurologic damage may occur if vitamin B_{12} is not given promptly.

Oral administration is preferred. Although most patients with malabsorption cannot absorb food folates, they are able to absorb folic acid given orally. Parenteral administration is not advocated but may be necessary in some individuals (eg, patients receiving parenteral or enteral alimentation). Doses greater than 0.1 mg should not be used unless anemia due to vitamin B_{12} deficiency has been ruled out or is being adequately treated with a cobalamin. Daily doses greater than 1 mg do not enhance the hematologic effect, and most of the excess is excreted unchanged in the urine.

Except for one questionable report of an allergic reaction, folic acid is essentially nontoxic in man. There is evidence that the anticonvulsant action of phenytoin is antagonized by folic acid. A patient whose epilepsy is completely controlled by phenytoin may require increased doses to prevent convulsions if folic acid is given.

ROUTES, USUAL DOSAGE, AND PREPARATIONS.
Therapeutic:
Intramuscular, Intravenous, Subcutaneous (deep): *Adults and children*, 0.5 to 1 mg daily for most deficiencies. When clinical symptoms subside and blood tests become normal, a maintenance dose of 0.1 to 0.25 mg daily should be given.
Oral: *Adults and children*, up to 1 mg daily. Although the manufacturers' recommended oral replacement dose of folic acid is 0.25 to 1 mg daily, 0.1 mg produces an adequate hematologic response in patients with uncomplicated folate deficiency.
Prophylactic:
Oral: *Adults and children*, during periods of increased demand (eg, hemolytic disease, alcoholism, infection), 0.5 to 1 mg daily. *During pregnancy*, 0.8 mg daily; *during lactation*, 0.6 mg daily; *low-birth-weight infants and those fed goat milk formulas*, 0.05 mg daily.

For preparations, see the section on mixtures in Chapter 52, Vitamins and Minerals, and the section on infant formulas in Chapter 53, Parenteral and Enteral Nutrition.

FOLIC ACID:
Drug available generically: Tablets 0.1, 0.4, 0.8, and 1 mg.
Folvite (Lederle). Tablets 1 mg.
FOLATE SODIUM:
Folvite Solution (Lederle). Solution (injection) equivalent to folic acid 5 mg/ml in 10 ml containers.

FOLINATE CALCIUM
[Leucovorin Calcium]

Folinic acid (citrovorum factor) is 5-formyl tetrahydrofolic acid, a metabolically active reduced form of folic acid. It is useful to treat overdosage of antagonists to folate (antifols). Although folinic acid also may be administered to treat megaloblastic anemias when oral therapy is not feasible, folic acid is much less expensive and is preferred.

Antifols inactivate dihydrofolate reductase, thus blocking folate metabolism; administration of folic acid will not alleviate the resulting deficiency since no enzyme is available to permit its conversion to a metabolically active form. Folinic acid is beyond the step blocked by the antifols and therapy with this normal metabolite is effective in these patients. Also, when given promptly, folinic acid appears to protect normal tissues from the toxic effects of large doses of methotrexate. In patients with pneumocystosis or toxoplasmosis treated with antifols (eg, pyrimethamine), injections of folinic acid prevent significant bone marrow toxicity without interfering with drug action.

ROUTE, USUAL DOSAGE, AND PREPARATIONS.
Intramuscular: *Adults and children*, for megaloblastic anemia, no more than 1 mg daily; for overdosage of folic acid antagonists, an amount equal to the weight of the antagonist administered within one hour if possible (usually ineffective if delayed more than four hours). To counteract the effects of methotrexate in the treatment of neoplastic disease, 6 to 9 mg every four to six hours. To prevent toxicity during

treatment of toxoplasmosis or pneumocystosis, 3 to 6 mg three times daily.

> *Leucovorin Calcium* (Lederle). Powder for injection (cryodesiccated) 50 mg; solution (injection) 3 mg/ml (folinic acid) in 1 ml containers.

SIDEROBLASTIC AND REFRACTORY ANEMIAS

Sideroblastic anemias are characterized by erythroblasts in the bone marrow that contain a perinuclear ring of stainable iron granules (ring sideroblasts) which represent an accumulation of nonheme iron. Hemoglobin synthesis is defective in that iron is not incorporated into porphyrin to form heme. Causes vary, but alcoholism is most common. In most patients, the anemia is alleviated by abstinence from alcohol and administration of folic acid, but alcoholic patients in whom formation of pyridoxal phosphate is impaired also should be given pyridoxine (50 mg daily for two to four weeks). If the anemia responds to pyridoxine, treatment should be continued indefinitely to prevent relapse, because response to retreatment with pyridoxine is less successful once relapse has occurred.

Since pyridoxal phosphate functions as a coenzyme in porphyrin synthesis, deficiency of pyridoxine or administration of drugs that antagonize its action (eg, isoniazid, chloramphenicol, cycloserine, immunosuppressive agents, lead) also may cause sideroblastic anemias. Some rare, genetically determined disorders (eg, hyperirritability and convulsions in infants, homocystinuria) may be accompanied by anemia that is responsive to pyridoxine or pyridoxal phosphate. Although there is no dietary deficiency of pyridoxine in these and other familial sideroblastic anemias, hemoglobin concentrations improve in some patients following doses of 100 to 300 mg daily; therefore, pyridoxine therapy may be tried in patients with refractory anemias of familial incidence or characterized by siderosis. However, hemoglobin levels remain subnormal and morphologic abnormalities of the red blood cells persist. (One patient with pyridoxine-responsive anemia also responded to crude liver extract or *l*-tryptophan [Horrigan, 1973].)

Androgenic steroids and cobalt have been used to treat some types of anemia refractory to other therapy. Testosterone or cobalt sometimes stimulates erythropoiesis, and cobaltous chloride (60 to 150 mg daily) or large doses of androgens have been used to treat refractory anemias caused by defective production of erythrocytes. Although not all patients benefit from such therapy and the results usually are not dramatic, aplastic and refractory myelophthisic anemias (anemias associated with space-occupying lesions of the bone marrow, such as myelofibrosis) may respond to the extent that fewer transfusions are needed. In some instances, remission has been induced and sustained (see also Chapter 42, Androgens and Anabolic Steroids). Cobalt is a potentially toxic metal; it may cause severe adverse effects, its uses are limited, and it should be given only under the direction of an expert in clinical hematology.

MIXTURES

Deficiency anemias must be properly diagnosed before therapy is initiated. Once a diagnosis has been established, the condition generally responds rapidly to a specific single-entity drug unless there are multiple deficiencies.

Except in nutritional anemias resulting from very poor diets for which use of a multiple vitamin supplement may be considered rational therapy, use of mixtures for treating anemias is strongly discouraged. Combination therapy is indicated when it can be clearly demonstrated that one type of deficiency anemia is superimposed upon another. Even under these circumstances, however, use of the specific agents required is all that is needed to treat the anemias adequately. Avoidance of mixtures not only is better therapy, but may be an absolute necessity because the preferred routes of administration for two therapeutic agents are different. For example, anemia caused by deficiencies of iron and vitamin B_{12} require both agents for treatment. However, the oral route is preferred for iron and the parenteral route for vitamin B_{12}. In pernicious anemia, oral therapy with vitamin B12 is practically useless, even when the preparation contains intrinsic factor.

Mixtures are an added expense when a completely adequate and less expensive regimen is available. For example, although a combination tablet containing an iron salt and a large dose of ascorbic acid may constitute acceptable therapy in the patient having difficulty absorbing iron (ascorbic acid enhances iron absorption), ingestion of one 300-mg ferrous sulfate tablet represents a more than sufficient dose of iron despite poor absorption. Also, large amounts (about 7 mg/1 mg of iron) of ascorbic acid are needed and gastrointestinal side effects are increased. The supplemental vitamins or minerals present in many iron preparations in no way improve the therapeutic effect of the iron. They are not necessary unless other specific deficiencies also are present. Mixtures of iron with folic acid, cyanocobalamin, and pyridoxine generally should not be used, although a combination of folic acid and iron may be a reasonable prophylactic supplement during pregnancy. There is no scientific basis for the inclusion of trace metals (eg, copper, molybdenum, cobalt) in any preparation used to treat anemia.

Hundreds of mixtures are available, but their use for the treatment of anemia should be avoided. They contain almost every imaginable combination of two or more of the following compounds or groups of compounds: iron salts, all the vitamins including folic acid and cyanocobalamin, all the trace minerals, liver extract, and intrinsic factor. A partial listing of some of the more widely used preparations is provided below. For a discussion of the multiple vitamin and vitamin with mineral preparations used in treating deficiency states not related to anemia, see Chapter 52, Vitamins and Minerals.

Baltron (Tutag). Each milliliter of solution contains peptonized iron 29.5 mg, folic acid 1 mg, liver injection (equivalent to vitamin B12) 2.5 mcg, and procaine hydrochloride 1%.

Chromagen Capsules (Savage). Each gel capsule contains ferrous fumarate 200 mg, cyanocobalamin 10 mcg, ascorbic acid 250 mg, and desiccated stomach substance 100 mg.

C-Ron (Rowell). Each tablet contains ferrous fumarate 200 mg (equivalent to 66 mg elemental iron) and ascorbic acid 100 mg or 600 mg (Forte).

Feosol Plus (Menley & James). Each capsule contains ferrous sulfate dried 200 mg (equivalent to ferrous sulfate 325 mg, elemental iron 65 mg), vitamin B12 activity equivalent 5 mcg, folic acid 0.4 mg, thiamine hydrochloride 2 mg, riboflavin 2 mg, pyridoxine hydrochloride 2 mg, ascorbic acid 50 mg, and niacin 20 mg.

Ferancee (Stuart). Each chewable tablet contains ferrous fumarate 200 mg (equivalent to elemental iron 67 mg), ascorbic acid 49 mg, and sodium ascorbate 114 mg (nonprescription).

Fermalox (Rorer). Each tablet contains ferrous sulfate 200 mg and magnesium-aluminum hydroxide 200 mg (nonprescription).

Fero-Folic-500 (Abbott). Each timed-release tablet contains ferrous sulfate 525 mg (equivalent to elemental iron 105 mg), folic acid 800 mcg, and sodium ascorbate 500 mg.

Fero-Grad-500 (Abbott). Each timed-release tablet contains ferrous sulfate 525 mg (equivalent to elemental iron 105 mg) and sodium ascorbate 500 mg (nonprescription).

Ferro-Sequels (Lederle). Each timed-release capsule contains ferrous fumarate 150 mg (equivalent to elemental iron 50 mg) and docusate sodium 100 mg (nonprescription).

Heptuna Plus (Roerig). Each capsule contains ferrous sulfate 311 mg (equivalent to elemental iron 100 mg), undefatted desiccated liver 50 mg, vitamin B12 cobalamin concentrate 5 mcg, intrinsic factor concentrate 25 mg, ascorbic acid 150 mg, thiamine mononitrate 3.1 mg, riboflavin 2 mg, pyridoxine hydrochloride 1.6 mg, niacinamide 15 mg, pantothenate calcium 0.9 mg, copper 1 mg, molybdenum 0.2 mg, calcium 37.4 mg, iodine 0.05 mg, manganese 0.033 mg, magnesium 2 mg, phosphorus 29 mg, and potassium 1.6 mg.

Iberet (Abbott). Each timed-release tablet or 20 ml of liquid contains ferrous sulfate 525 mg (equivalent to elemental iron 105 mg), cyanocobalamin 25 mcg, ascorbic acid 150 mg, thiamine mononitrate 6 mg, riboflavin 6 mg, niacinamide 30 mg, pyridoxine hydrochloride 5 mg, and calcium pantothenate 10 mg (tablet) or dexpanthenol 10 mg (liquid) (nonprescription).

Iberet-500 (Abbott). Each timed-release tablet or 20 ml of liquid contains same formulation as Iberet except ascorbic acid 500 mg (nonprescription).

Iberet-Folic-500 (Abbott). Each timed-release tablet contains same formulation as Iberet-500 plus folic acid 800 mcg.

Iberol (Abbott). Each tablet contains ferrous sulfate 525 mg (equivalent to elemental iron 105 mg), cyanocobalamin 12.5 mcg, ascorbic acid 75 mg, thiamine mononitrate 3 mg, riboflavin 3 mg, niacinamide 15 mg, pyridoxine hydrochloride 1.5 mg, and pantothenate calcium 3 mg (nonprescription).

Iron with Vitamin C (Squibb). Each tablet contains elemental iron 50 mg as stabilized ferrous carbonate and ascorbic acid 25 mg as sodium ascorbate (nonprescription).

Libco 12 (Bluline). Each milliliter of solution contains liver injection 2 mcg, vitamin B_{12} crystalline 15 mcg, iron peptonate 23 mg, thiamine 10 mg riboflavin 0.5 mg, pyridoxine hydrochloride 1 mg, calcium pantothenate 1 mg, and niacin 10 mg.

Pronemia (Lederle). Each capsule contains vitamin B_{12} (as cobalamin concentrate) 15 mcg, intrinsic factor concentrate 75 mg, ferrous fumarate 350 mg (equivalent to elemental iron 115 mg), ascorbic acid 150 mg, and folic acid 1 mg.

Simron (Merrell-National). Each capsule contains ferrous gluconate (equivalent to elemental iron 10 mg) and polysorbate 20 400 mg (nonprescription).

Simron Plus (Merrell-National). Each capsule contains ferrous gluconate (equivalent to elemental iron 10 mg), folic acid 0.1 mg, cyanocobalamin (vitamin B_{12} activity 3.33 mcg), ascorbic acid 50 mg, pyridoxine hydrochloride 1 mg, and polysorbate 20 400 mg (nonprescription).

Stuartinic (Stuart). Each tablet contains ferrous fumarate 300 mg (equivalent to elemental iron 100 mg), ascorbic acid 300 mg, sodium ascorbate 225 mg, cyanocobalamin 25 mcg, thiamine mononitrate 6 mg, riboflavin 6 mg, pyridoxine hydrochloride 1 mg, niacinamide 20 mg, and pantothenate calcium 10 mg (nonprescription).

Tabron (Parke, Davis). Each tablet contains ferrous fumarate (equivalent to 100 mg elemental iron), ascorbic acid 500 mg, thiamine mononitrate 6 mg, riboflavin 6 mg, pyridoxine hydrochloride 5 mg, cyanocobalamin 25 mcg, folic acid 1 mg, niacinamide 30 mg, calcium pantothenate 10 mg, vitamin E 30 IU, and docusate sodium 50 mg.

Theragran Hematinic (Squibb). Each tablet contains ferrous carbonate (equivalent to elemental iron 66.7 mg), cyanocobalamin 50 mcg, folic acid 0.33 mg, ascorbic acid 100 mg, thiamine mononitrate 3.3 mg, riboflavin 3.3 mg, niacinamide 33.3 mg, pyridoxine hydrochloride 3.3 mg, vitamin A acetate 8,333 units, ergocalciferol 133 units, vitamin E 5 IU, pantothenate calcium 11.7 mg, copper sulfate 0.67 mg, and magnesium carbonate 41.7 mg.

TriHEMIC 600 (Lederle). Each tablet contains ferrous fumarate 350 mg (equivalent to elemental iron 115 mg), cyanocobalamin 25 mcg, intrinsic factor concentrate 75 mg, folic acid 1 mg, ascorbic acid 600 mg, vitamin E 30 IU, and docusate sodium 50 mg.

Trinsicon (Dista). Each capsule contains vitamin B_{12} activity (from liver-stomach concentrate containing intrinsic factor and cobalamin concentrate) 15 mcg, ferrous fumarate (equivalent to elemental iron 110 mg), folic acid 0.5 mg, and ascorbic acid 75 mg.

Vitron-C (Fisons). Each chewable tablet contains ferrous fumarate 200 mg (equivalent to elemental iron 66 mg) and ascorbic acid 125 mg (nonprescription).

Selected References

Adams EB: Nutritional anaemias. *Br J Clin Pract* 22:501-504, 1968.

Baker SJ, DeMaeyer EM: Nutritional anemia: Its understanding and control with special reference to work of World Health Organization. *Am J Clin Nutr* 32:368-417, 1979.

Beal RW: Hematinics: I. Patho-physiological and clinical aspects. II. Clinical pharmacological and therapeutic aspects. *Drugs* 2:190-206, 207-221, 1971.

Beeson PB, McDermott W (eds): *Textbook of Medicine*, ed 14. Philadelphia, WB Saunders Co, 1975.

Bryan JA II: Use and abuse of hematinics. *Am Fam Physician* 7:120-128, (June) 1973.

Charlton RW, Bothwell TH: Iron deficiency anemia. *Semin Hematol* 7:67-85, 1970.

Crosby WH: Iron and anemia. *DM* 1-72, Jan 1966.

Dallman PR: New approaches to screening for iron deficiency. *J Pediatr* 90:678-681, 1977.

Das KC, et al: Unmasking covert folate deficiency in iron-deficient subjects with neutrophil hypersegmentation: dU suppression tests on lymphocytes and bone marrow. *Br J Haematol* 39:357-375, 1978.

Erbe RW: Inborn errors of folate metabolism. *N Engl J Med* 293:753-757, 807-812, 1975.

Goodman LS, Gilman A (eds): *The Pharmacological Basis of Therapeutics*, ed 5. New York, Macmillan Publishing Co, Inc, 1975.

Herbert V, et al: Nutritional anemias overview; megaloblastic anemia, in Gordon AS, et al (eds): *The Year in Hematology, 1977*. New York, Plenum Press, 1977.

Horrigan DL: Pyridoxine-responsive anemia: Influence of tryptophan on pyridoxine responsiveness. *Blood* 42:187-193, 1973.

Leavell BS, Thorup OA Jr: *Fundamentals of Clinical Hematology*, ed 4. Philadelphia, WB Saunders Co, 1976.

Matthews JRD, Casey TP: Treatment of common anaemias. *Drugs* 6:244-254, 1973.

McCurdy PR: Microcytic hypochromic anemias. *Postgrad Med* 61:147-151, (June) 1977.

Provisor AJ: Childhood anemia. *Am Fam Physician* 14:124-134, (Oct) 1976.

Savin MA: Practical approach to treatment of iron deficiency. *Ration Drug Ther* 11:1-6, (Sept) 1977.

Streiff RR: Folic acid deficiency anemia. *Semin Hematol* 7:23-39, 1970.

Sullivan LW: Vitamin B_{12} metabolism and megaloblastic anemia. *Semin Hematol* 7:6-22, 1970.

Toskes PP, Deren JJ: Vitamin B_{12} absorption and malabsorption. *Gastroenterology* 65:662-683, 1973.

Wintrobe MM: *Clinical Hematology*, ed 7. Philadelphia, Lea & Febiger, 1974.

Anticoagulants and Thrombolytics | 63

Thromboembolic disorders are a significant cause of morbidity and mortality. Venous thromboembolism occurs as a complication of other diseases. Documented risk factors include trauma, surgery, cancer, diabetes, smoking, heart failure, previous episodes of thromboembolism, varicose veins, obesity, pregnancy, and immobilization following strokes, paraplegia, or heart attacks. Arterial thromboembolism is common in patients with rheumatic heart disease or disorders affecting the coronary, cerebral (intra- and extracranial), or peripheral arteries. The use of estrogen-containing oral contraceptives is associated with a small but definite risk of thrombosis. Therefore, physicians should become familiar with the major factors of thrombogenesis, the mechanisms of coagulation, and the pharmacology of drugs used for prophylaxis or therapy.

Mechanisms of Blood Coagulation: Some knowledge of the complexities of blood coagulation is particularly useful in evaluating the therapeutic effects of anticoagulants and interpreting the laboratory tests required to control therapy (see the figure).

Prothrombin (factor II) is converted to thrombin (factor IIa) in two separate pathways. In the extrinsic system, tissue thromboplastin or tissue factor (factor III), a large lipoprotein complex not normally found in the blood, reacts with factor VII and directly activates factor X to factor Xa in the presence of calcium (factor IV). Thrombin is formed subsequently by the prothrombin-converting activity developed by a complex of factor Xa, factor V, and calcium ions adsorbed on phospholipid micelles of platelets. Only factor Xa is responsible for the proteolytic cleavage of thrombin, but the other factors accelerate the conversion. Thrombin initiates actual coagulation by removing two peptides from each of the alpha (fibrinopeptides A) and beta (fibrinopeptides B) chains; a specific arginyl-glycine bond is cleaved in each. The removal of these peptides from fibrinogen (factor I) leads to spontaneous gelation of fibrin monomers (factor Ia), which are then stabilized only by noncovalent forces and may still be dispersed. The gel is stabilized by cross linkage when covalent bonds are formed by a transglutaminase (factor XIIIa), making fibrin resistant to the action of proteolytic enzymes (eg, plasmin).

In the intrinsic system, all the factors necessary for blood coagulation are present in circulating blood. Despite this, it takes several minutes for whole blood to clot, in contrast to the extrinsic system in which the time-consuming early reactions are bypassed and clotting occurs in seconds. An example of the latter in the test tube is the Quick one-stage prothrombin time test. Coagulation through the intrinsic system is initiated by the conversion of Hageman factor (factor XII) into the activated form, factor XIIa, by contact with a foreign surface (eg, glass tube, subendothelial collagen of a disrupted blood vessel). Upon activation, factor XII undergoes a conformation change accompanied by enzymatic activity but there is no change in the molecular weight. Activated factor XII converts prekallikrein to kallikrein which, by a feedback mechanism, rapidly converts more factor XII to the activated form. This reaction involves the proteolytic cleavage of factor XII to release a fragment with enzymatic activity that does not require calcium ions; it not only activates factor XI but also has been implicated in the formation of plasminogen activator. In a purified system, an additional plasma protein (a high-molecular-weight kininogen) is required for activation of factor XI by factor XIIa. In the presence of calcium ions, the resulting factor XIa transforms factor IX to an active serine protease, factor IXa. Factor X is then activated by a complex of factor IXa, factor VIII (antihemophilic globulin), and calcium ions adsorbed onto platelet phospholipid surface. The rest of the coagulation sequence is identical to that of the extrinsic system. This complicated and repetitive pattern of blood coagulation acts as a biologic amplifier in which a severalfold gain of activity is achieved at each stage. The chain reaction sequence is mandatory, since a gradual generation of thrombin with slow conversion of fibrinogen to fibrin is hemostatically ineffective as isolated platelet aggregates and fibrin threads are washed away by the blood stream. Inactive zymogens are converted to activated forms by limited proteolysis. They participate at various stages of coagulation as a serine protease, for each has a serine residue in the enzymatic active site. Only factors V and VIII apparently do not play proteolytic roles in blood coagulation but, in the presence of calcium ions, they form complexes with other activated coagulation factors as described above.

Antithrombin III (AT III), formerly known as heparin cofactor, is the principal physiologic inhibitor of thrombin (factor IIa) and other activated clotting factors (serine proteases). Normal levels of AT III and binding to activated coagulation factors appear to be necessary to maintain blood fluidity and prevent thrombosis. A few families have been reported to have hereditary AT III deficiency resulting in recurrent venous thromboembolism. Subnormal levels may occur following surgery or estrogen therapy or in disseminated intravascular coagulation, hepatic cirrhosis, nephrotic syndrome, and, frequently, acute thrombosis.

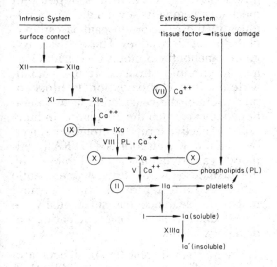

The four factors circled are coumarin-sensitive and vitamin-K dependent.

Mechanisms of Thrombus Formation: After blood vessels are damaged, coagulation is initiated when formed elements of blood and coagulation factors are exposed to extravascular tissues. The extrinsic pathway is activated by tissue thromboplastin (from fibroblasts and damaged endothelial cells), which accelerates the aggregation of platelets at the injured surface and results in the immediate formation of an unstable plug. The intrinsic pathway is activated simultaneously by contact between the collagen of the damaged area and factor XII, and coagulation is accelerated by phospholipid from platelet surfaces. Thrombin is generated which then converts fibrinogen to fibrin (see the figure); fibrin stabilizes platelet aggregates at the site of injury. The hemostatic plug is largely extravascular and is digested slowly by leukocytes and plasma fibrinolysis. Meanwhile, its surface becomes covered with endothelium.

Thrombus formation is similar to the process of hemostasis but occurs intravascularly. Venous thrombi frequently are caused by hypercoagulability rather than as a result of intimal damage and usually develop in regions of slow or disturbed blood flow (eg, valve pockets of deep leg veins). Small deposits of platelets become interspersed with fibrin and extend in the direction of the blood flow. As the thrombus grows, a red tail (mainly fibrin interspersed with red cells) forms; this frequently occludes the vein or may separate and migrate as an embolus.

In contrast, arterial thrombi have a greater platelet component and are called white thrombi. They develop at sites of vascular narrowing or irregularity in areas of rapid blood flow. Platelets aggregate on the surface of damaged vessels or prostheses and become interspersed with fibrin but do not cause occlusion as readily as venous thrombi. They tend to remain fixed and act as a focus for further accumulation of platelet-fibrin layers. The resulting mass interferes with blood flow and causes infarctions or may embolize.

Therapy: Some agents that interfere with the ability of platelets to initiate or perpetuate thrombus formation (ie, aspirin, dipyridamole [Persantine], sulfinpyrazone [Anturane]) are being studied. However, their efficacy and specific indications for this use are controversial. Dextrans inhibit platelet adhesiveness and help prevent vascular stasis through effects on blood flow. Rheomacrodex, a low-molecular-weight dextran (LMD) preparation, has been approved for prophylactic use in patients undergoing surgery who are at high risk of developing thromboembolic complications. However, such preparations have not been shown to be more useful than oral anticoagulants or heparin in patients undergoing general surgery but appear to be beneficial in those having hip surgery. For information on adverse reactions and precautions, see the evaluation on Dextran in Chapter 64, Blood, Blood

Components, and Blood Substitutes. Oral anticoagulants and heparin inhibit fibrin formation and are used prophylactically to reduce the incidence of venous thromboembolism. Once a thrombus has occurred, anticoagulants are given to prevent further growth and diminish the likelihood of embolization, but these agents do not alter the size of the original thrombus or limit subsequent vascular damage. Streptokinase [Streptase] and urokinase [Abbokinase] dissolve existing fresh thrombi and emboli by diffusing into clots to activate trapped plasminogen. Anticoagulants are then given to prevent recurrence.

Surgical interruption of veins may prevent pulmonary embolization, but benefits may last for only a few weeks because of the rapid enlargement of collateral veins. Surgical intervention is considered only when anticoagulants cannot be used.

ANTICOAGULANTS

The anticoagulants used therapeutically are heparin, the coumarin derivatives (dicumarol, phenprocoumon [Liquamar], warfarin sodium [Coumadin, Panwarfin], and warfarin potassium [Athrombin-K]), and the indandione derivatives (anisindione [Miradon] and phenindione [Hedulin]).

Heparin accelerates the formation of complexes involving antithrombin III (a normal plasma alpha 2 globulin) and several coagulation proteases, primarily thrombin and factor Xa. Biochemical data suggest that the primary prophylactic effect of heparin may be mediated by the anti-Xa mechanism rather than by inactivation of thrombin. Commercial preparations are a mixture of low- and high-molecular-weight fractions. The low-molecular-weight fraction (less than 6,000) has potent anti-Xa activity and moderate antithrombin properties; the reverse is true for the high-molecular-weight fraction (more than 25,000). Heparin is metabolized mainly in the liver and is excreted by the kidneys. Up to 50% may be eliminated unchanged, particularly when large doses are injected.

The duration of action is dose dependent: Intravenous doses of 100, 200, and 400 units/kg of body weight have half-lives of 56, 96, and 152 minutes, respectively.

The coumarin and indandione derivatives are administered orally. Warfarin sodium also can be given intravenously or intramuscularly, but parenteral administration has no advantage except in patients who should not or cannot take drugs orally. These compounds block the biosynthesis of factors II, VII, IX, and X by an antivitamin K action. A vitamin K-dependent mechanism converts several glutamate residues in these factors to gamma carboxyglutamic acid residue. These dicarboxyl groups anchor the proteins via calcium ions to phospholipid surfaces. If the vitamin K-dependent carboxylation is blocked, precursors of the coagulation factors mentioned above reach the circulation in functionally inactive forms (as proteins induced by vitamin K antagonists [PIVKAs]). Although carboxylation may be inhibited by the first dose of the drug, a therapeutic effect is not achieved until normal metabolic clearance has substantially reduced the levels of these circulating endogenous factors.

The mechanism of action of all coumarin and indandione anticoagulants is identical. Although the development of individual peak effects is variable, any of these drugs can maintain the therapeutic response established by another. Both abnormal resistance and increased sensitivity to their anticoagulant action have been reported. The oral anticoagulants are metabolized in the liver, and their metabolic products are excreted mainly by the kidneys.

The selection of an oral anticoagulant for use in a given situation is influenced both by individual and class characteristics. The indandiones occasionally produce serious cutaneous, hematologic, renal, and hepatic toxic effects and, therefore, the coumarins are usually preferred. In addition, phenindione (plasma half-life, approximately five hours) may have too short a duration of action to establish good clinical control, but the rapid return of prothrombin activity when the dose is reduced or the drug discontinued may be advantageous. Conversely, anisindione (plasma half-life, three to five days) is so long-acting that it may be hazardous if hemorrhage occurs, but maintenance therapy can be better controlled and alternate-day therapy may be feasible.

The dosage of dicumarol is somewhat difficult to control because this drug is incompletely absorbed and has a dose-dependent half-life of one to four days. Phenprocoumon has a long plasma half-life (approximately six and one-half days) that can be dangerous in the presence of hemorrhage. Therefore, warfarin is probably the oral anticoagulant of choice for many clinical situations. It is rapidly and completely absorbed and has a half-life of two and one-half days. Because cumulative effects may occur, the dose of all anticoagulants must be individualized to produce effective therapeutic levels with minimal complications.

The manufacturers' dosage recommendations for the orally administered anticoagulants reflect the custom of giving a large loading dose, followed by an immediate or gradual tapering off to the maintenance dose. The final amount then is adjusted according to prothrombin test responses. However, many authorities feel that the loading dose technique should be discarded in favor of a uniform daily dose slightly larger than the currently recommended maintenance dose, with the final amount determined by the results of prothrombin tests. Using this regimen, warfarin 15 mg/day produces prothrombin activity of less than 35% only a few days later than when a loading dose is used. Avoiding a loading dose minimizes the danger of hemorrhage, particularly at the inception of treatment, in patients with diminished tolerance or unusual sensitivity to the anticoagulant (eg, those who have recently undergone major surgery; elderly, malnourished, or debilitated patients; those with infections, liver disease, or congestive heart failure).

Indications: Whether administration of heparin or an orally administered drug is most appropriate depends upon the purpose of therapy. Heparin is the drug of choice for initial therapy when the risk of thrombosis is high. However, it must be administered parenterally. The coumarins or indandiones may be preferred after the effects of heparin have been established and when long-term oral anticoagulant therapy is indicated.

It is important to have some understanding of the pathophysiologic process in relation to hemostatic defects (see also Chapter 65, Hemostatics). Disseminated intravascular coagulation (DIC) results when there is excessive activation of the blood coagulation process along with excessive activation of the natural balancing mechanisms that counteract coagulation. Continuous coagulation may coat the vascular system with fibrin, which often occludes small vessels, and imperils adequate perfusion of vital organs. As long as acute DIC persists (unless initial levels are abnormally high or losses are rapidly compensated by synthesis), the concentrations of several normal clotting factors (prothrombin, fibrinogen, factor V, factor VIII) decrease in the circulation, as do platelets that aggregate on the fibrin masses. (Because clotting factors and platelets are being "consumed," this condition occasionally is termed "consumptive coagulopathy.") Hemorrhage can be spontaeous or occur following needle puncture, in surgical wounds, or with other trauma.

Conditions that activate the coagulation system and thereby precipitate DIC include the following: (1) Excessive activation of intrinsic system (massive endothelial damage, deposition and depletion of platelets) caused by sepsis, endotoxin shock, antigen-antibody complexes, and hemolytic-uremic syndrome. (2) Excessive activation of extrinsic system (introduction of tissue factor into the system) produced by transplant rejection, neoplasms, obstetrical accidents (eg, amniotic fluid embolism, retention of dead fetus), massive tissue injury (especially brain), snakebites, and hemolytic transfusion reaction. (3) Decreased hepatic clearance of activated clotting factors (circulatory collapse) caused by hepatic failure, pulmonary embolism, congestive heart failure, and giant hemangiomas.

Extreme caution is required when treating DIC; continuous laboratory monitoring and the assistance of an experienced hematologist are essential. The primary aims are to reverse the underlying pathology and maintain supportive therapy. Transfusion of platelet concentrates may be instituted if thrombocytopenia is severe; however, replacement of clotting factors may accelerate DIC. Heparin is the drug of choice if the diagnosis of DIC is unequivocal and the patient can be carefully monitored clinically and with appropriate laboratory tests. It is given as an intravenous injection (every four hours) or by continuous infusion (adults, 50 to 100 units/kg of body weight; children, 25 to 50 units/kg). If there is no improvement after four to eight hours, the drug should be discontinued. Aminocaproic acid, in conjunction with heparin, has been used to prevent thrombus formation when the fibrinolytic system is active. If bleeding becomes more severe, antifibrinolytic drugs are not useful in most patients and may even be dangerous. Protamine should not be given to these patients even though hemorrhage persists, since complete coagulation of the circulating blood may result.

Heparin reduces fibrin formation by inhibiting several earlier steps in the intrinsic coagulation cascade. One major clinical use is to help maintain extracorporeal circulation during open heart surgery and renal hemodialysis. It also is given when immediate hypocoagulability is required, as in the treatment of massive deep venous thrombosis or pulmonary infarction. For these purposes, regular doses of heparin generally are administered intravenously. The efficacy of small doses (minidoses) given subcutaneously for prophylaxis of venous thromboembolism is well documented. This regimen prevents pulmonary embolism in patients over 40 years of age who have undergone abdominal-thoracic surgery under general anesthesia lasting longer than 30 minutes. No information is available on the safety of this procedure when spinal or epidural anesthesia is employed, and this regimen has not proved to be efficacious in patients who have had prostatic or orthopedic surgery. Also, it should not be used in patients undergoing ocular surgery and is inadequate for those experiencing an active thrombotic process. There are inconclusive data suggesting that small doses of heparin may reduce the incidence of postoperative acute myocardial infarction. No observations are available as yet on heparin's effect on the incidence of mural thrombi or systemic embolism. Clinically significant bleeding occurs more frequently with larger than usual doses but seldom is a problem except in elderly women. Bleeding also is increased when aspirin and small doses of heparin are given concurrently.

It is too early to make recommendations for the inhalation of aerosol preparations of heparin. Prolonged subcutaneous self-administration of heparin is feasible (ie, by pregnant patients with prosthetic heart valves or a history of major thromboembolism).

Oral anticoagulants are generally used for long-term prophylaxis. Despite the lack of stringently controlled trials, many clinicians prescribe oral anticoagulants when mitral valve disease is associated with atrial fibrillation, even if surgical correction of the valve abnormality has been attempted or no embolism is present in the cerebral or limb arteries. Anticoagulants often are given and have been claimed to reduce the incidence of systemic embolism after cardioversion in patients with chronic atrial fibrillation. Controlled clinical trials have shown that these drugs decrease the incidence of thromboembolism in patients with prosthetic heart valves; this effect is enhanced significantly with concomitant use of either dipyridamole [Persantine] (0.45 g daily) or aspirin (1 to 3 g daily). The latter two drugs used alone do not appear to offer the desired protection. However, combined use of an oral anticoagulant and aspirin may be hazardous, because the risk of bleeding is increased. No sound clinical study has been published demonstrating that oral anticoagulants can prevent the occlusion of an aortocoronary bypass.

Studies on the use of oral anticoagulants in patients with peripheral artery disease or after bypass surgery of a limb artery have been uncontrolled or limited to small numbers, but the results suggest that the preventive role of anticoagulants in peripheral vascular disease is probably minimal.

The indications for use of anticoagulants in patients with cerebrovascular insufficiency are restricted to those with transient ischemic attacks (TIA). These agents are beneficial during the first few months of treatment but do not alter mortality. Their prolonged use for more than one year during a trial at the Mayo Clinic was shown to be associated with a significant risk of intracranial hemorrhage. Morbidity and mortality are reduced in patients with recurrent cerebral embolization if anticoagulants are given after the diagnosis is established unequivocally. Anticoagulants are absolutely contraindicated after cerebral hemorrhage and have no place in the treatment of thrombotic cerebral infarction, since hypocoagulation may predispose to hemorrhage in infarcted tissue. Therapy for prevention of recurrences should not be started until several days after a recent cerebral embolism.

Monitoring Therapy: Hypocoagulation induced by heparin or oral anticoagulants must be sufficiently intensive to be effective and to maintain the sharp equilibrium between the desired antithrombotic protection and actual bleeding. This requires not only careful calculation of the dose but also multiple control sampling and reliable laboratory testing. Present evidence indicates that, when small doses of heparin are given subcutaneously to prevent venous embolism, repeated blood sampling is unnecessary even in most high-risk patients. Laboratory monitoring may be required when regular-dose heparin therapy is administered either by intermittent intravenous injection (usually at four-hour intervals) or continuous intravenous infusion.

Authorities have recommended the use of various tests: whole blood clotting time (Lee-White clotting time test), partial thromboplastin time (PTT), or activated partial thromboplastin time (APTT). The latter test is most widely accepted. Experimental thrombosis is prevented in laboratory animals at values one and one-half to

two times normal (60 to 80 seconds if the control value is 40 seconds).

The Quick one-stage prothrombin test or a modification is commonly used to regulate the dosage of oral anticoagulants. This test may be regarded as a means of estimating the combined activity of the complex of prothrombin, factor V, factor VII, factor X, and, to a minor extent, of fibrinogen. Prothrombin, factor VII, and factor X are depressed when anticoagulants are given orally. (Factor IX is vitamin K-dependent and coumarin-sensitive but is not measured by any one-stage prothrombin test.) Since the depression of each of these factors is not additive and each has a markedly different half-life, the factor depressed most quickly and profoundly (usually factor VII) acts as the determinant of a routine prothrombin time determination during the first few days of therapy. During prolonged therapy, factor X ultimately shows the lowest activity in the steady state.

With usual oral anticoagulant doses, the Quick one-stage prothrombin time has a value one and one-half to two times greater than the control when expressed in seconds, or 20% to 30% when expressed as a percentage of normal prothrombin activity interpolated from a standard sodium chloride dilution curve. The prothrombin and proconvertin (P and P) test or the Thrombotest may be used, but they have no advantage over the one-stage prothrombin time for determining the adequacy of oral anticoagulant dosage. The usual therapeutic range for the P and P test is 15% to 20% of the normal control value; for the Thrombotest, the optimum therapeutic range is between 5% and 10%. In terms of prothrombin activity as assessed by various brands of tissue thromboplastins, this is equivalent to 10% to 25% (lower limit) and 18% to 35% (upper limit).

To adjust the dose of oral anticoagulants, prothrombin time should be determined three times during the first week, twice the second week, and weekly thereafter until the maintenance dose is established. The maintenance dose should be re-evaluated monthly and more frequently in those with impaired liver function, congestive heart failure, or frequent diarrhea; when the vitamin K content of the diet is drastically changed; or when new drugs are added to or withdrawn from the regimen. (See also Chapter 5, Drug Interactions and Adverse Drug Reactions.)

Caution must be exercised when interpreting the results of the one-stage prothrombin time test in a patient receiving both full-dose heparin therapy and an oral anticoagulant. Heparin prolongs the one-stage prothrombin time, and the estimated therapeutic doses of the oral anticoagulant may be insufficient to maintain the clinical effect when heparin is discontinued. To circumvent this problem, the effect of the coumarin may be measured with the P and P test of Owren or the Thrombotest, which utilizes a plasma sample diluted tenfold so that the amount of heparin present interferes less with measurement of the coumarin effect.

Treatment of Overdosage of Anticoagulants: The action of heparin can be antagonized by the intravenous administration of protamine sulfate, but there are hazards associated with use of this compound (see Chapter 86, Specific Antidotes). The anticoagulant effect of coumarin and indandione derivatives can be overcome by administration of phytonadione (vitamin K_1), but effects are not apparent for four to eight hours. When anticoagulant therapy is then resumed, larger doses than usual may be required initially. If the effects of the oral anticoagulants must be counteracted quickly, fresh or frozen single-donor human plasma or whole blood may be used; three units of plasma usually correct prothrombin time. However, these products may produce hepatitis and hypervolemia.

Adverse Reactions

Hemorrhage is a hazard of treatment with any anticoagulant and is the main complication of therapy, but the frequency and severity can be minimized by careful management. The incidence of bleeding varies according to the intensity of hypocoagulation, the duration of anticoagulant administration, the compliance of the patient, the reliability of laboratory tests, and the occurrence of drug interactions. When the contraindications are carefully observed, hemorrhage rarely occurs spontaneously because of hypocoagulability alone. Gastrointestinal or urinary tract bleeding may indicate an occult lesion. Cerebral or adrenal hemorrhage, corpus luteum hemorrhage and rupture in women, subdural hematoma, intestinal submucosal hemorrhage with adynamic ileus or colitis, acute hemorrhagic pancreatitis, and cutaneous hemorrhagic necrosis are some of the possible serious hemorrhagic complications. The incidence of hemopericardium after myocardial infarction is greater in patients receiving anticoagulants.

Fever, urticaria, and anaphylaxis occur occasionally after administration of heparin, and myalgia, bone pain, and osteoporosis may be noted with prolonged use. Alopecia or a burning sensation of the feet develops rarely; thrombocytopenia also may be induced by heparin, even with low-dose regimens. Local capillary rupture with subsequent ecchymoses in the area of injection must be anticipated. This has occurred after both subcutaneous and intramuscular injection but is more likely after the latter. Therefore, the intramuscular route should not be used.

Severe, sometimes fatal, hepatic, renal, hematologic, and cutaneous reactions have developed in some patients receiving phenindione [Hedulin] (see the evaluation). Although these effects have not been reported with the other indandione derivatives, all drugs in this group must be considered potentially toxic because of their chemical similarity.

Patients should be advised that the indandione derivatives may discolor alkaline urine orange which may be mistaken for hematuria. The color disappears if the urine is acidified.

The coumarin compounds have been given for prolonged periods without signs of toxicity. Occasional adverse reactions include gastrointestinal disturbances (especially diarrhea), elevated transaminase levels, urticaria, dermatitis, leukopenia, and alopecia. These reactions have not been observed with all coumarin drugs (eg, leukopenia has not been reported with warfarin). Necrotic lesions that are not the result of hemorrhage also have developed, usually at sites rich in fat tissue such as the breasts, abdomen, buttocks, thighs, and calves. Rarely, similar cutaneous lesions are seen.

Precautions

Severe factor IX deficiency has been reported when heparin and the coumarins are used concomitantly. If major hemorrhagic complications occur, all anticoagulants should be discontinued immediately. Bleeding episodes of any kind indicate the need for immediate reappraisal of the patient's condition.

Contraindications to the use of anticoagulants are active ulcerative disease of the gastrointestinal tract, hemorrhagic blood dyscrasias, severe liver or kidney disease, open ulcerative wounds, cerebrovascular hemorrhage, malignant hypertension, and recent surgery of the eye or spinal cord. Anticoagulants should be used with caution in the presence of mild liver or kidney disease, hypertension, alcoholism, subacute bacterial endocarditis, drainage tubes in any orifice, a history of gastrointestinal ulcers, and in those with an occupation that may be hazardous. Other factors that may constitute contraindications to use of anticoagulant drugs are unwillingness or inability of the patient to understand therapy, absence of a reliable laboratory for performance of monitoring tests, or serious risk of drug interactions. Patients receiving anticoagulant therapy have experienced adverse effects when they have undertaken certain fad diets low in vitamin K_1 (eg, when grapefruit are consumed as essentially the only nutritional item). Prolonged therapy in outpatients should never be prescribed unless the patient or someone living with him can assume responsibility for his competent care.

Any woman of childbearing age or one who becomes pregnant while receiving anticoagulants should be informed of the risks associated with their use and possible termination of the pregnancy should be considered. Since orally administered anticoagulants cross the placenta and have been associated with birth defects, small self-administered doses of heparin are preferred. If use of oral anticoagulants is necessary, they should be discontinued after the thirty-seventh week since there is also a risk of hemorrhage in the fetus, particularly during labor.

The indandiones should be discontinued promptly if fever or rash develops. Because severe adverse effects occur in a small percentage of patients, it is recommended that this group of agents be reserved for those who cannot tolerate the coumarins.

The maintenance dose of the orally administered anticoagulants may require adjustment in the presence of conditions that interfere with their actions (eg, the concomitant administration of certain drugs, coexistence of some diseases, change in diet). Thus, careful supervision and use of the one-stage prothrombin time test are mandatory in such instances.

Interactions: Although many drugs affect the action of oral anticoagulants in laboratory animals, a much smaller number have been *clearly* demonstrated to produce such effects in man. Drugs shown to significantly prolong or intensify the action of oral anticoagulants clinically include sulfinpyrazone [Anturane], phenylbutazone [Azolid, Butazolidin], oxyphenbutazone [Oxalid, Tandearil], disulfiram [Antabuse], oral hypoglycemics, clofibrate [Atromid-S], thyroid drugs, anabolic steroids, chloramphenicol, tricyclic antidepressants, quinidine, long-acting sulfonamides, and chloral hydrate or triclofos [Triclos]. The barbiturates, glutethimide [Doriden], and rifampin [Rifadin, Rimactane] are the primary drugs that *diminish* the response, although carbamazepine [Tegretol], oral contraceptives, diuretics, allopurinol [Zyloprim], antacids, laxatives, narcotic analgesics, cholestyramine resin [Questran] and other bile acid sequestrants, griseofulvin [Fulvicin P/G, Fulvicin-U/F, Grifulvin V, Grisactin, Gris-PEG], and anticholinergic drugs also have been implicated. Dicumarol may cause tolbutamide [Orinase] and phenytoin to accumulate in the body. Therefore, doses of these drugs should be reduced when they are given with coumarins or an indandione derivative can be substituted. Two families have been shown to have abnormal resistance to the effects of all orally administered anticoagulant drugs; the resistance was transmitted as a single autosomal dominant trait. See also Chapter 5, Drug Interactions and Adverse Drug Reactions.

HEPARIN

HEPARIN SODIUM

Endogenous heparin, a sulfated mucopolysaccharide, is chemically heterogeneous. It is synthesized in mast cells and is particularly abundant in the lungs. Its physiologic function is not fully understood, but the sudden release of heparin into the blood following anaphylactic shock indicates that it may play a role in immunologic reactions. Since the distribution of heparin in tissues was shown to correspond to the distribution of mast cells within the same tissues, it has commonly been assumed that an injection has the same effect as release of heparin from the mast cells. However, evidence now indicates that disposal within the body is different for endogenous than for exogenously administered heparin.

Commercially prepared heparin consists of straight chain anionic polysaccharides of variable molecular weight (usually 7,000 to 40,000). Heparin prepared from different tissues also appears to vary: More protamine is required to neutralize a unit of beef lung heparin than porcine mucosal heparin, and the forms are significantly different in plasma lipolytic activity, antifactor Xa activity, and activated partial thromboplastin time ratio (APPT is twice as high for porcine mucosal heparin). Heparin is the only anticoagulant commonly used parenterally (warfarin may also be given intramuscularly or intravenously) and is the drug of choice when a rapid effect is desired. Its anticoagulant action apparently plays no significant role in maintaining the normal fluidity of blood.

Heparin binds to the lysine residue of the antithrombin III (AT III) molecule, resulting in a complex with greater affinity for serine proteases than AT III alone. Thus, heparin functions as an anticoagulant by accelerating AT III neutralization of activated clotting factors. Small amounts of heparin with AT III inactivate factor Xa and prevent development of a hypercoagulable state by preventing conversion of prothrombin to thrombin. Larger amounts of heparin with AT III inhibit coagulation by inactivating thrombin and earlier clotting factors, thus preventing conversion of fibrinogen to fibrin. Heparin also inactivates fibrin stabilizing factor and prevents formation of a stable fibrin clot.

The major clinical application of heparin is to help maintain extracorporeal circulation during open heart surgery and renal hemodialysis. It also is given when immediate hypocoagulability is required, such as in the treatment of massive deep venous thrombosis or pulmonary infarction. When heparin is used in the management of pulmonary embolism, it may partially alleviate the bronchoconstriction produced by the embolism. It can be used in place of sodium citrate as an anticoagulant for donor blood during cardiovascular surgery.

Heparin reduces postprandial lipemia by activating lipoprotein lipase and has a slight antihistaminic effect. Because of these actions, it has been claimed that heparin also may be useful as a hypolipidemic or anti-inflammatory agent, but there is no evidence that it is beneficial for such purposes by any route of administration. Heparin interferes with complement and antigen-antibody interactions and depresses aldosterone production, but these effects have no clinical application.

There is evidence that the subcutaneous prophylactic administration of low doses of heparin significantly diminishes massive postoperative pulmonary embolism in patients over the age of 40 (see the Introduction). It is ineffective after thrombosis has developed.

The routine use of low-dose heparin therapy for patients younger than 40 years undergoing general surgery is not advocated, for the risk of hemorrhage and wound complications may exceed the risk of embolization for many of these patients. Heparin should be reserved for those in whom the risk of thromboembolism is high.

Because of its immediate onset of action, heparin often is given with an oral anticoagulant until the desired in vitro depression of clotting factor activity is reached. Administration probably should be continued for 24 to 48 hours after satisfactory depression of prothrombin complex activity is achieved. Since significant quantities of circulating heparin decrease prothrombin time, prothrombin time determinations should be made just before administering the next dose of heparin or, with concomitant administration of an oral anticoagulant, the P and P test of Owren may be substituted. (See the Introduction.)

Full-dose heparin may be administered by intermittent subcutaneous or intravenous injection, by continuous intravenous drip, or by use of a constant infusion pump. This agent is inactive orally. The intravenous route is preferred; in man, continuous infusion and intermittent injection appear to be equally effective in preventing thromboembolism. With full therapeutic doses, the onset of anticoagulant effect is immediate following an intravenous bolus injection and occurs approximately 20 to 30 minutes after subcutaneous injection. When the continuous infusion method is used, the two- to three-hour delay in anticoagulant effect may be avoided by injecting 5,000 units of heparin directly into the tubing when the infusion has been started. The intramuscular route should not be used because of the likelihood of producing tissue irritation, local bleeding, or hematoma; in addition, absorption is unpredictable after intramuscular administration.

Intravenous or subcutaneous injection seldom produces serious adverse reactions such as hemorrhage, anaphylaxis, or myalgia (see the Introduction), although there may be irregular and unpredictable absorp-tion, hematoma formation, and apparent cumulative effects with multiple doses when the subcutaneous route is used. Osteoporosis may occur if doses larger than 20,000 units/day are given for longer than six months. Thrombocytopenia has been observed after administration of porcine mucosal or beef lung heparin preparations; the mechanism of this reaction is obscure.

ROUTES, USUAL DOSAGE, AND PREPARATIONS. The dosage of heparin should be prescribed in units rather than milligrams. The U.S.P. standard for minimal potency is 120 units/mg of dry material derived from lung tissue and 140 units/mg of dry material derived from other sources. The potency of commercial preparations ranges from 140 to 190 units/mg. Thus, doses expressed in milligrams have no practical therapeutic meaning, since 100 mg of heparin may represent between 12,000 and 19,000 units of effect. Also, the U.S.P. unit is approximately 10% greater than the international unit (IU) and the difference should be taken into account when heparin is prescribed.

Intravenous Infusion: *Adults*, initially 5,000 units into the tubing after infusion is started, then 20,000 to 30,000 units daily at an initial rate of 0.5 unit/kg/min in 5% dextrose injection or isotonic sodium chloride injection. The rate is subsequently adjusted according to the results of clotting time tests. *Children*, 50 units/kg initially, followed by 100 units/kg every four hours. An intravenous drip system or an infusion pump can be used to control the dosage. Although the infusion pump is the most accurate of the two methods, the pump must be monitored carefully since it will continue to force fluid extravascularly if the needle is accidentally dislodged, whereas an extravasating intravenous drip will usually stop within a reasonable period of time.

Intravenous (Intermittent): *Adults*, 5,000 units initially, followed by 5,000 to 10,000 units every four to six hours. For disseminated intravascular coagulation (DIC), *adults*, 50 to 100 units/kg of body weight, and *children*, 25 to 50 units/kg every four hours.

Subcutaneous: For low-dose prophylaxis, *adults*, 5,000 units two hours before surgery and every 6 to 12 hours thereafter until the patient is discharged from the hospital. For usual full-dose effects, *adults*, 10,000 to 12,000 units every 8 hours or 14,000 to 20,000 units every 12 hours. Different sites, a small needle (#27), and the smallest volume possible should be used to prevent the development of a massive hematoma.

Intramuscular: This route should not be used.

> Drug available generically: Solution 100, 1,000, 2,500, 3,000, 4,000, 5,000, 6,000, 7,500, 10,000, 20,000, and 40,000 units/ml.
>
> AVAILABLE TRADEMARKS.
> *Hepathrom* (Fellows Testagar), *Heprinar* (Armour), *Lipo-Hepin* (Riker), *Liquaemin Sodium* (Organon), *Panheprin* (Abbott).

COUMARIN DERIVATIVES

DICUMAROL

Dicumarol has the same actions and uses as other oral anticoagulants and can usually maintain the effect established by other anticoagulants. It is long-acting and, in the usual dosage range, three to five days are required for peak action to develop. Once hypoprothrombinemia is established, the action persists for two to ten days following discontinuation of therapy. Dicumarol is incompletely absorbed from the gastrointestinal tract and has a dose-dependent plasma half-life; therapy is therefore somewhat difficult to control. Thus, frequent monitoring is usually indicated and, if overdosage occurs, it can be counteracted by administering phytonadione (vitamin K_1).

Dicumarol frequently causes flatulence and diarrhea. For other adverse reactions, precautions, and general class characteristics of the coumarin compounds, see the Introduction and the evaluation on Warfarin.

ROUTE, USUAL DOSAGE, AND PREPARATIONS.
Oral: *Adults*, 200 to 300 mg on the first day, followed by 25 to 200 mg daily using prothrombin time determinations as a guide. Frequent dosage adjustments may be necessary during the first 7 to 14 days of therapy. Prothrombin time should be determined daily during this period and dosage adjusted to maintain prothrombin activity at approximately 25% of normal. The maintenance dose is 25 to 150 mg daily, depending upon the results of these determinations.

> Drug available generically: Capsules 25 and 50 mg; tablets 25, 50, and 100 mg.

PHENPROCOUMON
[Liquamar]

The actions and uses of this long-acting agent are qualitatively similar to those of other coumarin derivatives. The onset of peak action is 48 to 72 hours after administration of the initial dose; recovery may take up to seven days after the last dose is given. Phenprocoumon usually will maintain the anticoagulant effect established by other anticoagulants. Phytonadione (vitamin K_1) counteracts overdosage.

For adverse reactions, precautions, and general class characteristics of coumarin compounds, see the Introduction and the evaluation on Warfarin.

ROUTE, USUAL DOSAGE, AND PREPARATIONS.
Oral: *Adults*, 24 mg on the first day. Maintenance dosage is individualized on the basis of prothrombin time determinations and varies between 0.75 and 6 mg; the exact amount may have to be adjusted to within 0.5 mg.

> *Liquamar* (Organon). Tablets 3 mg.

WARFARIN POTASSIUM
[Athrombin-K]

WARFARIN SODIUM
[Coumadin, Panwarfin]

Warfarin is the drug of choice when an oral anticoagulant is desired. Like other coumarin compounds, warfarin depresses prothrombin activity. It is readily absorbed from the gastrointestinal tract and may be used orally, intramuscularly, and intravenously, although parenteral routes offer no advantage over oral administration except in those in whom oral therapy cannot be used. Warfarin is intermediate-acting; a peak effect is achieved in 36 to 72 hours and the effect lasts two to five days.

As with all anticoagulants, hemorrhagic complications may occur during therapy. If bleeding occurs, the drug should be discontinued immediately and phytonadione (vitamin K_1) (a single dose of 1 to 5 mg for mild bleeding and 2.5 to 10 mg intravenously for severe bleeding with additional doses at four-hour intervals, as necessary) may be administered to counteract the anticoagulant effect if indicated; its peak effect usually occurs within four to eight hours following oral administration (see also Chapter 65, Hemostatics). Administration of vitamin K_1, particularly in doses above 2.5 mg, results in rebound hypercoagulability and resistance to oral anticoagulants may ensue. If hemorrhage is severe, concomitant administration of whole blood or single-donor plasma may be necessary.

Untoward reactions, which occur infrequently with coumarin derivatives, include dermatitis; necrosis of the breast, buttocks, thighs, abdomen, calves, and skin; purple toes syndrome; alopecia; gastrointestinal irritation; urticaria; and elevated transaminase levels. Unlike other coumarin derivatives, leukopenia has not been noted with warfarin. See also the Introduction and Chapter 5, Drug Interactions and Adverse Drug Reactions.

ROUTES, USUAL DOSAGE, AND PREPARATIONS. *Oral, Intramuscular, Intravenous*: 10 to 15 mg daily until the prothrombin time is within the therapeutic range. If a loading dose is used, 40 to 60 mg is given initially for adults of average weight and 20 to 30 mg for elderly or debilitated patients. With either regimen, the maintenance dose is 2 to 10 mg daily. Prothrombin time should be determined before the initial dose is given and every day thereafter until the response is stabilized. After a steady state is achieved, prothrombin time should be determined at regular intervals (see the Introduction).

WARFARIN POTASSIUM:
Athrombin-K (Purdue Frederick). Tablets 5 and 10 mg.
WARFARIN SODIUM:
Coumadin (Endo). Tablets 2, 2.5, 5, 7.5, and 10 mg; powder (lyophilized, for injection) 50 mg with 2 ml of diluent. *Panwarfin* (Abbott). Tablets 2, 2.5, 5, 7.5, and 10 mg.

INDANDIONE DERIVATIVES

All indandiones are potentially dangerous and should be reserved for use in patients who cannot tolerate the coumarin drugs. Blood dyscrasias and hepatic, renal, and cutaneous toxicity have occurred during phenindione therapy. Some of these reactions have been fatal. Similar reactions may be possible with other agents in this class. If serious adverse effects occur with any of the indandiones, therapy should be discontinued promptly. Patients receiving these compounds should be instructed to report prodromal symptoms such as marked fatigue, chills, fever, and sore throat.

ANISINDIONE
[Miradon]

This long-acting agent is chemically related to phenindione and has actions and uses similar to those of the other oral anticoagulants. For general class characteristics, adverse effects, and precautions for indandione compounds, see the Introduction and the evaluation on Phenindione. After the initial dose, the peak effect is reached in 48 to 72 hours, and coagulation factors gradually return to normal 24 to 72 hours after the drug is discontinued. Phytonadione (vitamin K₁), fresh whole blood, or single-donor plasma counteracts the effect of anisindione, but blood or plasma should be administered only if hemorrhagic complications are severe.

Dermatitis is the only untoward reaction consistently associated with anisindione therapy. However, since other indandione derivatives have produced serious adverse effects (eg, agranulocytosis, jaundice, nephropathy), anisindione has the potential to cause serious reactions. The drug should be discontinued promptly if fever or rash appears, for these reactions may signal the onset of a more severe complication. Like other indandione derivatives, anisindione occasionally discolors alkaline urine orange; this can be differentiated from hematuria by its disappearance on acidification of the urine. The patient should be advised of this possible occurrence.

ROUTE, USUAL DOSAGE, AND PREPARATIONS.
Oral: *Adults*, 300 mg on the first day, 200 mg on the second day, and 100 mg on the third day. The maintenance dose ranges from 25 to 250 mg daily; the amount administered should be that which maintains prothrombin time determinations at two to two and one-half times the normal value.
   Miradon (Schering). Tablets 50 mg.

PHENINDIONE
[Hedulin]

This short-acting indandione derivative is similar in actions and uses to the couma-

rins. Therapeutic levels are usually attained in 18 to 24 hours, and prothrombin time returns to normal 24 to 48 hours after the drug is discontinued. As with other oral anticoagulants, both resistance and sensitivity to its anticoagulant effect have been reported. Phytonadione (vitamin K₁), fresh whole blood, or single-donor plasma will counteract the anticoagulant action of phenindione, but blood or plasma should be used only if hemorrhagic complications are severe (see the Introduction).

Agranulocytosis, leukopenia, leukocytosis, jaundice, hepatitis, nephropathy with acute tubular necrosis, severe exfoliative dermatitis, albuminuria, massive generalized edema, and, rarely, red cell aplasia have been reported with use of phenindione. Some of these effects have been fatal. Phenindione should be discontinued if evidence of hypersensitivity, leukopenia, or agranulocytosis appears. Patients should be instructed to report prodromal symptoms such as marked fatigue, chills, fever, and sore throat.

Phenindione may discolor the urine orange or red, and patients should be so advised to avoid a false impression of hematuria.

ROUTE, USUAL DOSAGE, AND PREPARATIONS.
Oral: *Adults*, 300 mg initially as a single dose or in two equally divided doses in the morning and at bedtime, followed by 200 mg on the second day, and 100 mg daily thereafter until a relatively stable prothrombin depression is achieved. The usual maintenance dose is 50 to 150 mg daily in two equally divided doses in the morning and at bedtime. Prothrombin time should be determined prior to treatment and then daily until an effective maintenance dose is established. Thereafter, determinations should be made at regular intervals (eg, every 7 to 14 days).
   Hedulin (Merrell-National). Tablets 50 mg.

MIXTURES

There is no rationale for using a mixture containing two oral anticoagulants or an anticoagulant with other classes of drugs.

Nevertheless, such mixtures are available commercially and are generally proposed for treating hyperlipidemias or inflammation. They usually contain heparin and some may be taken sublingually as well as by injection. At best, use of the injectable preparations can only be classified as experimental, since heparin has no proved hypolipidemic or anti-inflammatory properties. The sublingual preparations are to be universally condemned because heparin is ineffective by this route. See also Chapter 55, Agents Used to Treat Hyperlipidemia.

THROMBOLYTIC AGENTS

Anticoagulants prevent the extension and propagation of existing thrombi. When a thrombus obstructs an artery or vein, the impeded circulation often is restored by the normal physiologic process, which requires time. Thrombolytic agents are capable of dissolving existing thrombi and emboli by proteolysis of their supporting fibrin network, and they are used when rapid dissolution of the occlusion is required to preserve organ and limb function (arterial occlusion) or valve function (venous occlusion). Anticoagulants are then given to prevent recurrence.

Mechanisms of Thrombolysis: The proteolytic system consists of three main components: the proenzyme, plasminogen; plasminogen activators, the most important of which probably originates in the endothelial cells; and natural inhibitors, which rapidly neutralize plasmin or interfere with the activation of plasminogen.

There is a striking analogy between the coagulation and fibrinolytic systems in which thrombin and plasmin are the key enzymes acting on fibrinogen and fibrin, respectively. Plasmin is formed from its inactive precursor in the circulation (plasminogen) and is capable of hydrolyzing a number of other proteins besides fibrin, including fibrinogen, prothrombin, factors V and VIII, the first component of complement, and prekallikrein. However, in vivo, the main target of plasmin is fibrin because, under normal circumstances, natural inhibitors in the blood limit the action of plasmin to the appropriate substrate and prevent the massive proteolysis and fibrinolysis that would occur if plasmin were allowed to circulate freely. Since inhibitors predominate, free fibrinolytic activity is not normally found in blood. Nevertheless, the fibrinolytic system is very responsive to activation.

Plasminogen is present in human plasma in concentrations of 10 to 15 mg/dl. Analogous to the coagulation system, its activation involves limited proteolytic cleavage of the zymogen molecule. Plasminogen is a single chain protein with multiple molecular isoelectric forms. The most acidic are probably identical to native circulating plasminogen and have an NH_2-terminal glutamic residue (Glu-plasminogen). The more basic forms have an NH_2-terminal lysine residue (Lys-plasminogen), which probably represent partially autocatalytic degraded forms of plasminogen. Plasminogen binds to fibrin via lysine-binding sites which are also responsible for the interaction with lysine and related amino acids (epsilon-aminocaproic acid, 6-aminohexanoic acid). Glu-plasminogen has a weak affinity for fibrin, whereas Lys-plasminogen has a strong affinity. The interaction of the fast-acting and physiologically most important plasmin inhibitor from human plasma, alpha$_2$-antiplasmin, also is mediated via interaction with the lysine-binding sites of plasmin.

The plasminogen molecule appears to be composed of three parts: (1) a small segment or N-terminal, which is released during the formation of Lys-plasminogen; (2) a central region of five triple disulfide loops (heavy chain or A chain of plasmin), which contains the lysine-binding sites of plasminogen; and (3) a C-terminal containing the serine and histidine residues essential for enzyme activity (light chain of plasmin).

Plasminogen activation in blood occurs either by intrinsic pathways, in which plasminogen activator is formed from one or more precursor proteins in plasma, or by extrinsic pathways, in which activators originate from the vascular wall or tissues such as uterus, lung, or heart.

In intrinsic plasminogen activation, two pathways are factor XII-dependent and the third pathway is independent of this factor. In one factor XII-dependent pathway, factor XII and a complex of high-molecular-weight kinogen (Fitzgerald factor) and prekallikrein (kallikreinogen or Fletcher factor) undergo limited proteolysis during contact with a negative surface. Three activation products result: factor XIIa in the form of a surface-bound inactive fragment and a soluble fragment containing the active site; bradykinin; and a soluble complex of kinin-free high-molecular-weight kinogen with kallikrein. Kallikrein then becomes the plasminogen activator. The other factor XII-dependent intrinsic pathway requires the presence of kallikrein as a cofactor of a poorly defined proactivator. About 50% of the total intrinsic activation occurs in the factor-XII independent pathway. In this novel proactivation system, factor XII is activated by polysaccharide sulfates.

Several activators exert an effect in extrinsic plasminogen activation. One humoral activator functions primarily to maintain vascular patency and is present in the endothelial cells of small veins, surface epithelial cells, erythrocytes, and leukocytes. It is released slowly into the circulation and low blood levels usually are present. A variety of stimuli can cause mobilization and discharge of this activator from the cells. Other activators are present in widely different concentrations in tissues, particularly uterus, prostate, and adrenal glands, but are usually absent in the liver. Release of these tissue activators probably is related to tissue repair and wound healing. However, free plasmin is not normally detectable in blood, probably because inhibitor capacity exceeds activation potential.

In all systems studied, activation of plasminogen is accomplished by cleavage of a specific arginyl-valyl bond in the central portion of either Glu-or Lys-plasminogen. Meizoplasmin, a 2-chain disulfide-linked molecule is formed. Secondarily, cleavage by autodigestion of one or more lysyl bonds in the amino terminus of Glu-plasminogen or in the heavy chain of Glu-plasmin causes release of N-terminal peptide. The cleavage of two disulfide bonds in plasmin produces a heavy chain and the light chain that contains the active site of the enzyme.

Therapy: Although several techniques for initiating thrombolysis have been investigated, the only currently practical means is by activation of the fibrinolytic systems with streptokinase [Streptase] or urokinase [Abbokinase]. Both are proteins that convert plasminogen to plasmin, resulting in digestion of fibrin and lysis of blood clots. In addition to their thrombolytic activity, urokinase and streptokinase decrease plasma viscosity and erythrocyte aggregation.

Indications: Use of urokinase or streptokinase appears to be the current treatment of choice to dissolve most *acute massive and severe life-threatening pulmonary emboli* (ie, emboli large enough to occlude two-thirds or more of the main branches of the pulmonary artery or the equivalent in other pulmonary blood supply that cause acute right side heart failure with or without shock, dyspnea, and progressive deterioration). Patients with an unstable hemodynamic condition because of major residual circulatory obstruction who survive for 24 to 48 hours after the initial episode may be considered candidates for this treatment. Although immediate mortality is high and thrombolytic treatment is urgent, these drugs should be used only after pulmonary embolism is confirmed by arteriography. Urokinase or streptokinase can dissolve a major portion of the acute embolus and decrease pulmonary hypertension, improve perfusion of the pulmonary capillary bed, and correct other hemodynamic disturbances. However, morbidity and mortality have not been reduced and surgical embolectomy may be preferred in selected cases. Furthermore, thrombolytic agents are useful only within five days after embolism has occurred.

In patients with *deep venous thrombosis*, these drugs should be used only within 72 hours after clinical symptoms result from recent extensive thrombi in calf or more proximal veins. Approximately two-thirds of thrombi can be dissolved. Older thrombi become increasingly resistant to lysis. Beneficial effects include reduction of edema, induration, and pain and preservation of valvular function. Venous thrombectomy or thrombolytic drug treatment may be indicated in patients with recent occlusive iliofemoral thrombosis, but thrombectomy is more often associated with postphlebetic syndrome due to valve damage and chronic venous insufficiency.

Local instillation of streptokinase into *occluded arteriovenous cannulae* in patients on chronic renal dialysis has successfully salvaged most occluded cannulae and avoided surgical intervention. This treatment should be used following failure of conventional mechanical measures.

In *acute thromboembolism of peripheral arteries*, embolectomy using a Fogarty balloon catheter is preferred if the artery is normal. In arteries with major atheromatous changes, thrombolytic therapy may be effective if the occlusion is less than 72 hours old. However, restoration of circulation also depends on the location of the occlusion, the amount of collateral circulation, and the extent of irreversible tissue damage.

Thrombolytic agents are not indicated for superficial thrombophlebitis; thrombolysis is considered only if the thrombus extends into the femoral vein.

Thrombolytic agents have been useful in some patients with recent (less than 12 hours) myocardial infarction, severe angina pectoris, chronic arterial occlusions of limb arteries, renal artery thrombosis, retinal artery or vein occlusion, and impending renal cortical necrosis. However, more data are needed before thrombolytics can be recommended for these types of thrombotic disorders.

Monitoring Therapy: The thrombin clotting time of plasma is sensitive to decreased fibrinogen levels and increased levels of fibrinogen degradation products. Regimens using standard doses of streptokinase or urokinase usually do not require laboratory testing, but close clinical observation is essential and the thrombin clotting time is useful to determine whether thrombolytic activity is present.

Adverse Reactions

Bleeding is the most common and major complication of thrombolytic therapy. Major bleeding is no more common than following full-dose heparin therapy, but bruising and oozing of blood at sites of needle puncture, invasive procedures, trauma, or recent wounds are more likely. Streptokinase and urokinase impair hemostatic mechanisms by increasing fibrinolytic activity. Also, fibrin(ogen) degradation products may interfere with platelet function and impede fibrin polymerization. Proteolysis of plasma proteins other than fibrin is induced, including splitting of the C-terminal end of the A chains of fibrinogen; these no longer cross link and are more sensitive to plasmin digestion.

A moderate reduction in the hematocrit level not related to clinical bleeding occurs in 20% to 30% of patients receiving thrombolytic drugs.

If bleeding from an invasive site is not serious, local pressure is usually sufficient, and thrombolytic therapy may be continued under close supervision. If serious spontaneous bleeding occurs, treatment should be discontinued and plasma volume expanders used to replace the deficit. If blood loss has been extensive, administration of red blood cells or whole blood may be necessary. For rapid reversal of the fibrinolytic state, fibrinolysis inhibitors, such as epsilon-aminocaproic acid (100 mg/kg of body weight), can be given by slow intravenous injection. See the evaluation on Aminocaproic Acid in Chapter 65, Hemostatics.

Streptokinase acts as a foreign protein and rarely produces antigenic (eg, chills, bronchospasm, rash, malaise) or anaphylactoid reactions. Minor allergic reactions can be avoided if the initial dose is given slowly over a period of about 30 minutes. If allergic reactions are severe, streptokinase should be discontinued and cortisone (40 to 80 mg) may be given intravenously. In hypersensitive individuals, premedication with glucocorticoids (eg, prednisolone 25 mg or equivalent) or chlorpheniramine given intravenously may prevent reactions. Since urokinase occurs naturally in urine or is derived from embryonic human kidney cells, it is not antigenic.

Precautions and Contraindications

Selection of patients for thrombolytic drug therapy should be based on careful assessment of clinical status and patient history, and the potential benefits should be weighed against the risk of bleeding. Intramuscular injections, invasive procedures, and unnecessary handling of the patient should be avoided during thrombolytic therapy.

The primary contraindications for treatment with streptokinase or urokinase are the same as those for anticoagulants. These include manifest or recent hemorrhage, pre-existing hemorrhagic diathesis, conditions with a latent risk of local hemorrhage (eg, gastrointestinal ulceration), and severe hypertension. Use of thrombolytic agents also is contraindicated in patients with serious kidney or liver disease who have a tendency to bleed. The risk of inducing cerebral hemorrhage precludes their use after a recent stroke. Thrombolytics should not be used within ten days following surgical procedures, delivery, kidney or liver biopsy, or lumbar puncture or when there is a suspicion of dissecting aneurysm, visceral carcinoma, active tuberculosis with cavitation of recent onset, subacute bacterial endocarditis, predisposition to allergy, or systemic infection. These agents are contraindicated during the first 18 weeks of pregnancy because the fetus and its membranes are attached to the uterus mainly by fibrin rather than cellular tissue, and there is a risk of premature separation of the placenta. Spontaneous bleeding from internal sites not accessible to control by pressure may occur in patients with abnormalities in platelet count, prothrombin value, partial thromboplastin time, or bleeding time. Therefore, the condition of these patients should be carefully assessed before initiating thrombolytic treatment.

INDIVIDUAL EVALUATIONS

STREPTOKINASE
[Streptase]

Streptokinase, a nonenzymatic protein (molecular weight 47,000 daltons), is a catabolic product secreted by Group C beta-hemolytic streptococci. Although it is antigenic, commercial products are so highly purified that pyrogenic or allergic side effects are rarely serious. Most individuals have some sensitivity from previous streptococcal infections, and a delayed reaction manifested by fever occurs in about one-third of patients given streptokinase. The immune antibodies present in an individual inactivate streptokinase and dosage must be adjusted in each patient to overcome this effect. When the resistance level to streptokinase is in excess of 1,000,000 IU, this agent is probably inactive and should not be used. Similarly, high antibody titers that occur during or immediately following streptococcal infections or in patients recently treated with streptokinase rule out further use of this agent for three to six months.

Streptokinase activates plasminogen in a complex manner: It combines with plasminogen in a 1:1 stoichiometric complex to produce a conformational alteration in plasminogen. The plasminogen thus activated then converts the complex to plasmin-streptokinase from which the streptokinase is fragmented into lower molecular weight products.

Streptokinase has a "fast" half-life of approximately 11 to 13 minutes (due to the action of antibodies) and a "slow" half-life of 83 minutes in the absence of antibodies. Activity ceases within a short period after therapy is discontinued. See the Introduction to this section for information on mechanism of action, indications, adverse reactions, and precautions.

ROUTES, USUAL DOSAGE, AND PREPARATIONS. *Intravenous*: *Adults*, initially, a loading dose of 250,000 IU (maximum, 500,000 IU) of reconstituted solution is infused over a period of 30 minutes, followed by 100,000 IU/hr (usually for no longer than 72 hours). After thrombolytic treatment is discontinued, heparin is given by continuous infusion in a dose that prolongs the activated partial thromboplastin time by 20 to 30 seconds. An oral anticoagulant may be substituted later, if warranted.

Intra-arterial: For local perfusion of an occluded vessel, *adults*, the same dosage as for intravenous use. No advantage for this route of administration has been demonstrated. For local instillation into occluded arteriovenous cannulae after pulling and flushing have been ineffective, 250,000 IU over a period of 30 minutes, followed by clamping of the cannula for two hours. Cannula contents are than aspirated and the cannula is flushed with normal saline and reconnected.

Powder should be reconstituted with isotonic sodium chloride injection or 5% dextrose for injection and used within 24 hours after preparation.
Streptase (Hoechst-Roussel). Powder (lyophilized) 100,000, 250,000, and 750,000 IU. It should be stored at 15 to 30 C.

UROKINASE
[Abbokinase]

Urokinase is an enzyme isolated from human urine or tissue cultures of human kidneys. Two molecular forms exist: S_1, the most active form, has a molecular weight of $34,500 \pm 2,000$ daltons. The S_2 form has a molecular weight of 54,000 daltons. The S_1 form probably represents a breakdown product of urokinase formed during purification procedures; its amino acid sequence is very similar to the B-chain of thrombin and plasmin. Unlike streptokinase, urokinase is a direct activator of plasminogen. It can be purified to a high degree but may be contaminated with thromboplastin, which may cause variable but transient hypercoagulation; low doses may induce platelet aggregation. However, urokinase is nonantigenic and does not cause the allergic reactions encountered with use of streptokinase. It may be used if streptokinase resistance is high or if patients need a second course of treatment.

See the Introduction to this section for information on mechanism of action, indications, adverse reactions, and precautions.

ROUTE, USUAL DOSAGE, AND PREPARATIONS.
Intravenous: *Adults*, 4,400 IU/kg of body weight given over a period of ten minutes, followed by continuous infusion of 4,400 IU/kg/hr for 12 to 24 hours. As with streptokinase, its use should be followed by administration of heparin and later, use of oral anticoagulants.

Abbokinase (Abbott). Powder (lyophilized) containing 250,000 IU with mannitol 25 mg and sodium chloride 45 mg. The material should be reconstituted only with sterile water for injection and used immediately. Any unused portion of the reconstituted material should be discarded. The powder should be stored at 2 to 8 C.

Selected References

Breckenridge A: Oral anticoagulant drugs: Pharmacokinetic aspects. *Semin Hematol* 15:19-26, 1978.

Brozovic M: Oral anticoagulants in clinical practice. *Semin Hematol* 15:27-34, 1978.

Deykin D: Heparin therapy: Regimens and management. *Drugs* 13:46-51, 1977.

Didisheim P, Fuster V: Actions and clinical status of platelet-suppressive agents. *Semin Hematol* 15:55-72, 1978.

Nussbaum M, Moschos CB: Anticoagulants and anticoagulation. *Med Clin North Am* 60:855-869, 1976.

O'Reilly RA: Pharmacodynamics of the oral anticoagulant drugs, in Spaet TH (ed): *Progress in Hemostasis and Thrombosis*, vol 2. New York, Grune & Stratton Inc, 1974, 175-213.

Sherry S: Streptokinase: Use it to lyse clots. *Mod Med* 46:93-98, (May 30-June 15) 1978.

Sherry S: Setting thrombolysis in action. *Drug Ther* 7:23-26, (Aug) 1977.

Thomas DP: Heparin in prophylaxis and treatment of venous thromboembolism. *Semin Hematol* 15:1-17, 1978.

Verstraete M: Biochemical and clinical aspects of thrombolysis. *Semin Hematol* 15:35-54, 1978.

Verstraete M: Are agents affecting platelet functions clinically useful? *Am J Med* 61:897-914, 1976.

Verstraete M, Verwilghen R: Haematological disorders, in Avery GS (ed): *Drug Treatment: Principles and Practice of Clinical Pharmacology*. Acton, Mass, Publishing Sciences Group Inc, 1976, 661-716.

Weiss HJ: Antiplatelet therapy. *N Engl J Med* 298:1403-1406, 1978.

Weiss HJ: Platelet physiology and abnormalities of platelet function. *N Engl J Med* 293:531-541, 1975.

Wessler S: Anticoagulant dilemma: Prescription for its resolution. *Am J Med Sci* 274:106-117, 1977.

Blood, Blood Components, and Blood Substitutes | 64

In order to use blood and its components properly, the physician must know what preparations are available, the effects that can be achieved by administering these preparations, and the properties of fresh and stored blood. In addition, *a blood transfusion should not be given unless the risk/benefit ratio is favorable*. Hepatitis viruses and other infectious diseases (eg, cytomegalovirus, malaria, toxoplasmosis, syphilis) may be transmitted during transfusion of blood or blood components. Plasma fractions that have not been heated at 60 C for ten hours carry a high risk of transmitting hepatitis, except for gamma globulin, which has a very low risk. The administration of incompatible red cells may produce severe and occasionally fatal transfusion reactions.

With the development of techniques to separate freshly donated blood into component preparations under aseptic conditions, the routine use of whole blood has become obsolete except for acute massive blood loss. With few exceptions, component transfusion is superior. It allows administration of that portion of blood required without unnecessarily burdening the circulation; minimizes exposure to sensitizing agents, potentially toxic salts, and metabolites; and maximizes donor utilization, since as many as five patients may benefit from a single blood donation.

Whole Blood or Red Blood Cell Transfusion: When a blood transfusion is considered essential, there is much the physician can do to reduce the risk of untoward effects. Whole blood may be preferred when most of the blood volume is lost or exchanged within a few hours, as in major surgical or medical catastrophes. However, if increasing the oxygen-carrying capacity is the sole aim of transfusion, packed red blood cells (red cell concentrate) should be used. Approximately 70% to 80% of all red cell transfusions can be given in the form of red cell concentrate. Administration of a red cell concentrate with a hematocrit of 70% to 80% reduces the danger of hypervolemia and associated congestive heart failure and, if the plasma is separated just prior to transfusion, also reduces the amount of sodium, potassium, and ammonium ions. The risks of transfusing group O blood to patients of other blood groups during dire emergencies also are decreased because of the low concentrations of anti-A and anti-B alloantibodies in red cell concentrate. Most blood banks now routinely stock packed red cells. If packed in a closed sterile system, their shelf life is the same as that of whole blood. However, if the hermetic seal is broken to separate the plasma, shelf life is reduced to 24 hours. Requirements for crossmatching and method of administration are the same as for whole blood.

Frozen red blood cells are now prepared in a number of blood centers. The high cost of preparation and storage, the time required to thaw and wash the cells (to remove cryoprotective agent) before they can be transfused, and the limited post-thaw shelf life (24 hours) preclude their use for routine transfusions. The risk of bacterial contamination during preparation, storage, thawing, and washing also may be somewhat greater than for the collection and storage of red blood cells or whole blood. Frozen red cells contain very little cellular debris from leukocytes or platelets and usually can be transfused without causing adverse effects in patients with febrile nonhemolytic transfusion reactions produced by antileukocyte antibodies. However, saline-washed red cells may be just as satisfactory for this purpose and thawed, deglycerolized red cells can be reserved for patients who continue to have reactions to washed cells. Frozen red blood cells of rare types can be prepared for either autologous or homologous transfusion. Hemolytic disease in the newborn infant caused by maternal antibodies against high-incidence antigens can be treated with frozen red blood cells obtained from the mother during early pregnancy. Frozen red blood cells formerly were thought to be advantageous for patients scheduled for organ transplants. Most data now suggest that survival of renal transplants is decreased in patients who have received only frozen red blood cells. Prior transfusion of whole blood is preferred, for this has been shown to enhance homograft survival. Claims that the use of frozen red cells reduces the risk of post-transfusion hepatitis have not been confirmed, and animal studies indicate that this may not be the case.

Platelet Transfusion: Thrombocytopenia can develop when there is decreased platelet production or increased platelet destruction, and dilutional thrombocytopenia can develop following massive transfusion of stored blood. Spontaneous bleeding usually does not occur unless the platelet count is less than 20,000/microliter; a level greater than this is desirable but cannot always be achieved in patients with leukemia and other malignancies who are undergoing intensive chemotherapy. Patients with aplastic anemia and some other conditions characterized by prolonged suppression of bone marrow function may not exhibit hemorrhagic manifestations in the presence of low but stable platelet counts of 10,000 to 20,000/microliter, and they do not require maintenance platelet transfusion unless hemorrhage intervenes. During surgery and the postoperative period, it is advisable to maintain the platelet count above 50,000/microliter. Platelet transfusions are indicated for severe thrombocytopenia with active or imminent bleeding, especially in patients whose thrombocytopenia is a consequence of decreased platelet production. Platelet transfusions are less likely to be effective in conditions associated with increased platelet destruction but can be lifesaving in specific situations. Patients with splenomegaly may require large doses of platelets because of splenic pooling of the transfused cells.

Viable platelets act in hemostasis by aggregating into plugs that seal small openings in blood vessels, but platelet-aggregation capacity is lost rapidly upon storage. The proper temperature for platelet storage is controversial. Originally, it appeared that storage at 4 C reduced in vivo recovery and lifespan when compared to storage at room temperature (20 to 24 C), but the former had more immediate hemostatic effectiveness. When platelets are stored at room temperature, the increased acidity which develops from accumulation of lactic acid must be buffered by using a larger volume of suspending plasma (50 to 70 ml), and gentle agitation during storage is essential. Under such conditions, platelets can be kept for up to 72 hours at room temperature and survive longer in vivo than those kept at 4 C. The potential risk of bacterial contamination with storage at room temperature has not been a significant problem and most blood banks are now storing platelets at 20 to 24 C. However, platelets preserved at 4 C appear to be effective if transfused within 24 hours. At either temperature, the sooner platelets are administered after donation, the better the in vivo platelet recovery. Prolonged preservation by freezing in a cryoprotective agent has been accomplished but currently is not practical for routine transfusions. Cryopreserved platelets obtained during remission in patients with hematologic malignancies are effective in treating hemorrhages that occur during subsequent relapse.

Plateletpheresis is a process in which platelets are separated from donated blood, and the plasma and red cells are returned to the donor. With this technique, two to four platelet concentrates may be obtained manually from one donor. If special equipment (continuous or intermittent flow centrifugation) is employed, the equivalent of ten platelet concentrates can be obtained from one donor in a single session.

Platelets from one unit of blood can increase the platelet count of an adult weighing 70 kg by approximately 5,000/microliter. To elevate the platelet count by 35,000/microliter, one unit of platelet concentrate must be transfused for each 10 kg of body weight. The presence of autologous antibodies, histocompatibility, and/or platelet alloantibodies impairs the usefulness of platelet transfusions. Platelet responsiveness also is decreased in the presence of sepsis, fever, active bleeding, disseminated intravascular coagulation, and splenomegaly.

Refractoriness to repeated administration of random donor platelets often occurs within two months after onset of therapy in patients with normal immune mechanisms, and is common even in immunologically compromised patients. This usually results from development of antibodies directed against histocompatibility antigens (HLA) or, less frequently, against specific platelet antigens. Resedimenting platelet preparations to minimize white cell contamination delays the development of refractoriness. HLA-matched platelets may provide more satisfactory survival of platelets once immunization has developed. The ideal donor, an HLA-matched sibling, can provide long-term platelet support, but use of platelets from an HLA-identical sibling is contraindicated for patients in whom marrow transplantation from that sibling is contemplated. Large suppliers of platelets have developed computer-based lists of HLA-typed donors for rapid matching to individual thrombocytopenic patients who are refractory to random donor platelets.

Granulocyte Transfusion: Severe thrombocytopenia and leukopenia caused by marrow hypoplasia frequently result from aggressive antineoplastic chemotherapy, but platelet transfusion has significantly decreased mortality from thrombocytopenic hemorrhage. As a result, infections, particularly those caused by gram-negative organisms, rather than hemorrhage are now the leading cause of death in patients with bone marrow failure. The incidence of infection increases as the granulocyte count falls below 1,000/microliter. Although antibiotics have been helpful, the patient remains at serious risk until remission is achieved and marrow function returns.

It was only after technology for obtaining granulocytes by continuous or intermittent flow centrifugation was developed that granulocyte transfusion became practical. With mechanical leukapheresis, a single donor can provide 1 to 4 X 10^{10} granulocytes in two to three hours. Although this quantity is only about 10% of the normal daily granulocyte production, it appears to be sufficient to combat infection in the recipient. White cell transfusions are beneficial in combating sepsis if the following critera are fulfilled: (1) the patient's granulocyte count is less than 500/microliter, (2) there is proved bacterial or fungal infection, and (3) granulocytes are administered in courses of at least three to four consecutive days in conjunction with appropriate antibiotics.

Plasma Transfusion: Plasma, the cell-free portion of anticoagulated blood, contains the major blood proteins, albumin and globulin, and the various clotting factors.

The use of fresh or fresh frozen single-donor plasma generally should be reserved for patients who require correction of clotting factor abnormalities, because some clotting factors decrease in activity during storage. Factor VIII deficiency can be treated by replacement of the specific factor (see Chapter 65, Hemostatics), but fresh frozen plasma is useful for treating factor IX deficiency as well as multiple deficiencies of coagulation factors. It may be useful adjunctively to control bleeding associated with oral anticoagulant or massive transfusion therapy. Plasma also can be used for its oncotic pressure effect in maintaining circulating blood volume (see the following section).

Single-donor plasma carries the same risk of transmitting hepatitis as a single unit of whole blood and contains anti-A and anti-B isoagglutinins if not from an AB donor. Because of the great risk of transmitting viral hepatitis, pooled plasma is no longer licensed by the Food and Drug Administration.

Plasma Volume Expanders: If temporary maintenance of blood volume is the sole therapeutic objective, plasma volume expanders can be used instead of whole blood or plasma. Albumin (human) [Albuminar, Albumisol, Albuspan, Albutein, Buminate, Plasbumin] and plasma protein fraction (PPF) [Plasmanate, Plasma-Plex, Plasmatein, Protenate] are processed from plasma liquid (normal human plasma) and are indicated in the emergency treatment of shock or to correct hypoproteinemia. However, since serious hypotension has occurred following use of some lots of PPF, this product should be used with caution. These preparations are sterile-filtered and heated for ten hours at 60 C, eliminating the danger of transmitting hepatitis.

Plasma substitutes (eg, dextran 70 [Macrodex], dextran 75 [Gentran-75], hetastarch [Volex]) support circulation during hypovolemic states. They can be given to restore blood volume after hemorrhage when whole blood is not available, to correct the oligemia of burn shock, or to maintain colloidal osmotic pressure temporarily in emergencies or during certain types of cardiovascular surgery. They are not substitutes for blood components in the treatment of anemia or hypoproteinemia. Dextran 40 [Gentran-40, LMD, Rheomacrodex] solutions may be used as adjuncts in the treatment of shock, but the effects are of shorter duration than those of higher molecular weight dextran. Most physicians now believe that hypovolemia and hemoconcentration can be treated by temporary replacement with a balanced electrolyte solution (in amounts two or three times the estimated blood loss). Sodium chloride and Ringer's and dextrose injections also can be used, but their effects last only two hours or less. (See Chapter 51, Replenishers and Regulators of Water and Electrolytes.)

A detailed discussion of transfusion procedures is beyond the scope of this book. The interested reader is referred to a publication of the AMA, *General Principles of Blood Transfusion,* for more complete information.

Rho(D) Immune Globulin: This sterile gamma globulin preparation is obtained by fractionating the plasma of human donors who are nonreactive for hepatitis B surface antigen and who have high titers of antibodies to Rho(D). It is used primarily to prevent active immunization against Rho(D) in the Rho(D)-negative, D^u-negative mother who has delivered an Rho(D)-positive or D^u-positive infant or abortus. It also is given when the Rh status of the abortus is unknown, in tubal pregnancy, following amniocentesis, and to prevent alloimmunization when Rho(D)-positive blood is given accidentally to an Rho(D)-negative recipient. In order to be effective, the dose must be in proportion to the volume of blood infused. A single vial (300 mcg) is considered adequate to prevent sensitization from exposure to about 15 ml of packed cells or 30 ml of whole blood. When fetal-maternal hemorrhage is more severe, the amount of fetal blood in the maternal circulation can be estimated by the acid elution test of Kleihauer which detects fetal hemoglobin. Adverse effects occur infrequently and are mild. Rho(D) immune globulin does not appear to transmit serum hepatitis. (See the evaluation in Chapter 66, Immunomodulators.)

Immune Globulins: These specially prepared concentrates of globulins do not transmit hepatitis. The preparations protect against hepatitis A if administered prior to or within two weeks after exposure. They may provide some protection against non-A, non-B transfusion hepatitis if administered before the blood is given. Also, some preparations with high antibody titers provide postexposure prophylaxis against hepatitis B, pertussis, rabies, and tetanus (see the evaluation in this chapter and in Chapter 67, Vaccines and Antiserums).

Adverse Reactions and Precautions

Viral Hepatitis: This is the most common serious adverse reaction associated with transfusion therapy and may occur after the use of whole blood, packed red cells, plasma, platelets, granulocytes, cryoprecipitated antihemophilic factor, antihemophilic and prothrombin complex concentrates, or fibrinogen. Since there is no practical method for rendering these blood products free of hepatitis virus, components prepared from the blood of volunteer donors should be used whenever possible and all blood *must* be screened by sensitive tests for hepatitis antigens.

Hepatitis B surface antigen (HBsAg) is specific for hepatitis B virus. Mandatory testing of blood donors is required by the Bureau of Biologics of the Food and Drug Administration, the American Red Cross, and the American Association of Blood Banks. A positive test or a history of hepatitis precludes the use of that donor. Currently, only the solid phase radioimmunoassay and reversed passive hemagglutination tests are approved for use in screening. A complete list of licensed products acceptable for use in testing can be obtained from the Bureau of Biologics, Division of Blood and Blood Products, Bethesda, Maryland, 20014.

The exclusion of HBsAg-positive donors has reduced the incidence of post-transfusion hepatitis. However, even the most sensitive test for HBsAg (radioimmunoassay) is not entirely satisfactory, because hepatitis B virus causes only 10% to 30% of post-transfusion hepatitis. The remaining 70% to 90% is caused by agent(s) tentatively designated non-A, non-B for which no tests are available. Type A (infectious) hepatitis has not been reported to be transmitted by blood transfusion.

Based on current procedures, the precise incidence of post-transfusion hepatitis appears to be grossly underestimated; the incidence can only be determined if blood recipients are followed prospectively and periodic measurements of serum aminotransferases are done. Two large-scale prospective studies indicate that approximately 7% to 10% of patients receiving multiple transfusions develop hepatitis. Most are subclinical and anicteric, but even icteric cases seldom are reported to the institution providing the blood. Despite the benign course of the acute phase of anicteric hepatitis, it predisposes the patient to chronic liver disease and may lead to the carrier state. In general, although type B hepatitis tends to be more severe acutely, non-A, non-B hepatitis may progress more readily to chronic liver disease, particularly chronic active hepatitis. The development of a serologic test to detect the agent(s) responsible for non-A, non-B hepatitis prior to transfusion remains a major goal which, if achieved, should lead to a further reduction in post-transfusion hepatitis.

Hypersensitivity Reactions: Donor blood is directly responsible for allergic responses in 1% to 3% of patients receiving transfusions. Fortunately, most of these reactions (eg, urticarial rashes, generalized pruritus) are mild and transitory. However, severe effects (eg, bronchospasm) occur occasionally and rarely cause death. Antihistamines may control milder reactions, but epinephrine, norepinephrine (levarterenol) [Levophed], or corticosteroids may be necessary to control serious ones. Patients with IgA deficiency may be sensitized by even a single blood transfusion and experience an anaphylactic reaction if another transfusion containing IgA is given. Such patients require blood products from IgA-deficient donors or saline-washed or thawed, deglycerolized red cells.

Febrile Reactions: These reactions are characterized by temperatures that may exceed 39.4 to 40 C (103 to 104 F) and usually occur within 15 minutes after transfusion is begun, although they may be observed two hours or more after completion of the transfusion. Febrile reactions are frequently associated with chills, headache, and malaise. When fever develops, the transfusion should be stopped and the cause investigated, since increased temperature may be an early manifestation of a more serious problem, especially hemolytic transfusion reaction or bacterial contamination. However, most febrile reactions are of unknown cause or are attributable to antibodies directed against HLA or other antigens located on granulocytes and platelets. Repetition of these febrile, nonhemolytic reactions can be prevented by administering leukocyte-poor preparations, including saline-washed red cells, red cells filtered to remove granulocytes, and thawed, deglycerolized red blood cells.

Hemolysis: This potentially fatal complication of blood transfusion results from the administration of incompatible blood, usually caused by clerical error (eg, mislabeling of specimens, misidentification of recipients). Only rarely does it result from technical errors in blood typing and crossmatching. The injection of as little as 10 to 50 ml of incompatible blood may cause flushing, nausea, hypotension, tachycardia, restlessness, dyspnea, chills, fever, headache, substernal and/or flank pain, and vomiting. Hemoglobinemia and hemoglobinuria occur, often followed by oliguria and acute renal failure. A hemorrhagic diathesis, with thrombocytopenia and spontaneous bleeding, is observed occasionally and may be caused by disseminated intravascular coagulation (DIC). Rarely, shock and death occur shortly after initiating the transfusion. If a hemolytic reaction is suspected, the transfusion must be stopped immediately. Prompt intravenous administration of a suitable osmotic diuretic (mannitol) or furosemide [Lasix] may help prevent acute renal failure. The transfusion service should be consulted immediately.

Delayed hemolytic transfusion reactions sometimes occur in patients who do not have serologically detectable antibodies at the time of transfusion but later develop an increased antibody titer. This type of reaction may mimic autoimmune hemolytic anemia and a direct antiglobulin test may be positive.

Reactions from Contaminated Products: Administration of whole blood, blood components, or plasma contaminated with bacteria or bacterial endotoxins is a rare cause of catastrophic transfusion reactions. A severe reaction, manifested by nausea and vomiting, chills, fever, profound shock with marked cutaneous erythema (red shock), coma, convulsions, and, frequently, death, may occur after the injection of the first 50 to 100 ml of a product contaminated by gram-negative bacilli. Treatment should include the management of shock and the administration of a broad spectrum antibiotic, followed by use of the most specific antibiotic for the organism once it has been identified and sensitivity tests performed. Systemically administered corticosteroids are useful adjuncts to lessen the severity of the reactions.

Hypervolemia: Hypervolemia can be a serious consequence of transfusions with whole blood, plasma, or plasma substitutes, particularly in the elderly, the very young, and patients with pulmonary or cardiac disease. The use of packed red cells greatly reduces but does not eliminate this hazard. Hematocrit determinations, commonly used as guides for transfusion therapy, are inadequate to detect hypervolemia. The monitoring of central venous or pulmonary wedge pressure is useful in detecting overexpansion of the blood volume. When serious hypervolemia occurs, prompt intravenous administration of a suitable diuretic (eg, furosemide) and/or phlebotomy may be indicated.

Immunization: The recipient of transfusions may become immunized to one or a combination of red blood cell, white blood cell, platelet, and protein antigens. Although this complication is in itself not symptom-producing or life-threatening, it may make red cell compatibility testing more difficult or provoke hemolytic or nonhemolytic transfusion reactions when subsequent transfusions are necessary.

BLOOD AND BLOOD COMPONENTS

WHOLE BLOOD

Whole blood is drawn from a selected donor under rigid aseptic conditions and the ABO and Rh types are identified. Citrate ion (usually as a citrate-phosphate-dextrose mixture, CPD) is used as the anticoagulant. Following crossmatching, blood is administered through a recipient set with a filter. Whole blood is stored between 1 and 6 C, with the temperature held within a 2 C range, except during shipment when the temperature may vary from 1 to 10 C. The expiration date is not later than 21 days after the blood is drawn if a CPD formulation is used. Use of the new anticoagulant-preservative, CPD-adenine (CPDA-1), extends the expiration date from 21 to 35 days. Units on which the hermetic seal is broken are outdated within 24 hours.

Heparinized whole blood contains all the normal constituents of whole blood, but coagulation has been prevented by collection in heparin solution instead of CPD. Occasionally, this product is used for priming pump oxygenators during cardiac surgery, but CPD whole blood less than five days old, modified by the addition of heparin and calcium chloride immediately prior to use, is equally satisfactory. Heparinized whole blood is contraindicated for routine transfusions.

The routine use of whole blood is wasteful, may produce hypervolemia, provides excessive ions or metabolites that could be deleterious in some patients, and results in administration of undesirable alloantibodies. Whole blood transfusion should be reserved for cases of massive bleeding (greater than 20% of the blood volume) that might occur during surgery or following severe trauma or when the need for oxygen-carrying capacity is combined with a need for volume expansion. In all other instances, packed red cells (alone, with electrolyte solutions, or with an indicated specific component) should be utilized. (See also the Introduction.)

ROUTE AND USUAL DOSAGE.
Intravenous: One unit (450 ± 45 ml with 63 ml of CPD or CPDA-1), repeated as indicated. It is administered through a standard filter, and other medications should not be added.

MODIFIED WHOLE BLOOD

Modified whole human blood is prepared in a closed system of containers. Plasma is removed from a fresh unit of whole blood and platelets are separated by centrifugation or antihemophilic factor is removed by cryoprecipitation. The remaining plasma is then reintroduced into the original blood container. The resulting product should not be used to promote or maintain coagulation nor should it be used for exchange transfusions. Otherwise, uses, side effects, hazards, dosage, storage, and dating period are the same as for whole blood.

RED CELL CONCENTRATE (Human Red Blood Cells)

These concentrates are prepared by removing most of the plasma from whole blood at any time during the dating period; the ABO and Rh types are identified, and the hematocrit of the final product usually is between 70% and 80%. Unfrozen red cell concentrate should be stored at 1 to 6 C, with the temperature maintained within a 2 C range. Frozen red blood cells are stored at -65 C or colder. The expiration date for unfrozen cells is not later than that of the whole blood from which it was derived or 24 hours after the hermetic seal is broken. The expiration date for frozen cells is three years, but units have demonstrated adequate in vivo recovery after storage for more than ten years. Once the unit has been thawed and deglycerolized or saline-washed, it is outdated in 24 hours.

Red cell concentrate provides the same hemoglobin content and oxygen-carrying capacity as the whole blood from which it was derived. It is the transfusion product of choice for patients requiring an increased red cell mass (except those with massive hemorrhage who also require volume and coagulation factor replacement).

For adverse reactions and precautions, see the Introduction.

ROUTE AND USUAL DOSAGE.
Intravenous: One unit usually elevates the venous hematocrit approximately 3% in a 70-kg recipient.

PLASMA, FRESH FROZEN (SINGLE DONOR)

This preparation is the liquid portion of a single unit of citrated (CPD, CPDA-1) whole blood that has been separated from the cells within four hours and frozen within six hours after collection from the donor. It may be stored at -18 C or lower for up to one year after the date of collection. The unit is thawed in a waterbath at 37 C with gentle agitation to facilitate thawing and must be used shortly after thawing. Fresh frozen plasma is indicated for treatment of patients with labile plasma coagulation factor deficiencies (ie, factors V and VIII, although antihemophilic factor preparations [cryoprecipitate and concentrates] are preferred for factor VIII deficiencies). This preparation also is indicated to treat factor IX and multiple coagulation factor deficiencies.

ROUTE AND USUAL DOSAGE.
Intravenous: Dosage is determined by clinical response and, when possible, by laboratory assays of appropriate coagulation factors. The preparation administered should be ABO-compatible with the recipient.

PLASMA LIQUID (SINGLE DONOR)

This preparation is the liquid portion of a single unit of citrated (CPD, CPDA-1) whole blood processed no later than 26 days after the collection date of the blood. It may be stored at 1 to 6 C for no more than 26 days after the date of collection of the whole blood. This material may be used as a plasma volume expander and occasionally is used as a source of stable clotting factors (eg, II, VII, IX, X), although commercial concentrates are available that provide in 10 ml the activity equivalent to 250 ml of plasma liquid.

ROUTE AND USUAL DOSAGE.
Intravenous: Dosage is determined by clinical response and, when possible, by laboratory assays of appropriate coagulation factors. The preparation administered should be ABO-compatible with the recipient.

PLATELET CONCENTRATE

Platelet concentrate is prepared by centrifugation of citrated (CPD) whole blood at 20 to 24 C within four hours after collection. An average unit contains more than 5.5 X 10^{10} platelets, and multiple units may be obtained from one donor by platelet-pheresis. The dating period should be no longer than 72 hours after collection from the donor. Platelet concentrates may be stored at either 20 to 24 C or 1 to 6 C (see the Introduction). Those preserved at room temperature must be gently and continuously agitated during storage. Ordinarily, ABO-compatible platelets are used but, when unavailable, platelets from non-ABO-compatible donors may be administered if the preparations are not grossly contaminated with red cells. If necessary, some of the noncompatible plasma may be removed just prior to administration. For indications, see the Introduction.

ROUTE AND USUAL DOSAGE.
Intravenous: Units must be administered through a 170 micron filter (*microfilters must not be used*) within four hours after the hermetic seal is broken. Initially, 1 unit/10 kg of body weight may be given. In patients without platelet antibodies, splenomegaly, sepsis, or disseminated intravascular coagulation, this dose should increase the platelet count by approximately 35,000/microliter. See also the section on platelet transfusion in the Introduction.

ALBUMIN HUMAN (Normal Human Serum Albumin)

[Albuminar, Albumisol, Albuspan, Albutein, Buminate, Plasbumin]

This sterile plasma protein preparation contains at least 96% albumin and is obtained by fractionating blood plasma that is nonreactive for hepatitis B surface antigen (HBsAg). It is sterile filtered and heated for ten hours at 60 C. The heat treatment apparently removes the hazard of viral hepatitis.

Albumin is used to restore the colloidal osmotic pressure of the plasma in hypovolemic states (eg, burns, hemorrhage, surgical procedures, premature birth). It binds bilirubin and has been used as an adjunct in exchange transfusion when treating hyperbilirubinemia, most frequently in association with hemolytic disease in the newborn. It has been given for treating nephrosis and hepatic cirrhosis, but most authorities consider these uses to be questionable and of temporary benefit at best.

Because albumin is a constituent of human blood, it usually can be given with relative safety, although chills, fever, urticaria, and variable effects on blood pressure, pulse, and respiration have been noted following its administration. This preparation does not interfere with normal coagulation mechanisms nor does it promote clotting. It is contraindicated in patients with heart failure, and large amounts should not be given to those with low cardiac reserve, severe anemia, or with no albumin deficiency in order to avoid hypervolemia and possible congestive heart failure. Albumin should not be administered if the solution is turbid or contains sediment.

Albumin preparations contain sodium caprylate and acetyltryptophanate as stabilizers. Unopened stabilized preparations can be stored for approximately three years at temperatures not exceeding 37 C. All albumin preparations should be used promptly once opened.

ROUTE, USUAL DOSAGE, AND PREPARATIONS.
Intravenous: Dosage should be determined by monitoring the pulmonary artery or wedge pressure or the central venous pressure during administration to avoid hypervolemia. No more than 250 g/48 hr should be given. When more than this amount is necessary, the patient should receive whole blood or plasma rather than additional albumin. The 5% solution is given undiluted, usually at a rate of 2 to 4 ml/min. The 25% solution can be administered undiluted or it can be diluted with sterile, nonpyrogenic sodium chloride injection or 5% dextrose injection. (In the presence of edema, the 25% concentrate preferably is given undiluted, although 5% dextrose injection may be used if dilution is necessary.) Albumin must be administered slowly (1 ml/min) to patients with low cardiac reserve to prevent rapid expansion of plasma volume and possible pulmonary

edema. In shock caused by diminished plasma volume, it may be given as rapidly as desired, preferably diluted (an approximately isotonic solution can be prepared by diluting each 20 ml of 25% solution to a volume of 100 ml).

For shock, *adults and children*, 25 g initially, repeated in 15 to 30 minutes if necessary. Whole blood may be required if the patient is hemorrhaging.

For burns, the extent of burn determines the amount and duration of administration. The dose should be sufficient to correct decreased plasma volume and hemoconcentration. Initially, either 500 ml of 5% solution or 1 ml/lb of body weight of 25% solution has been used in addition to other electrolyte solutions administered.

For nonemergency treatment of *children*, 6.25 to 12.5 g may be given.

> Drug available generically: Solution 5% in 50 ml containers and in 250 and 500 ml containers with intravenous administration set; 25% in 20 ml containers and in 50 and 100 ml containers with intravenous administration set. Use of 4% and 20% solutions is permitted according to the Code of Federal Regulations. These concentrations are not manufactured in the United States, but licensure and sale of 4% and 20% solutions manufactured in foreign countries is authorized.
> *Albuminar-5, Albuminar-25* (Armour), *Albumisol* (Merck Sharp & Dohme), *Albuspan* (Parke, Davis), *Buminate* (Hyland), *Plasbumin-5, Plasbumin-25* (Cutter). Solution (aqueous) 5% in 50 ml containers (Plasbumin-5 only) and 250 and 500 ml containers with intravenous administration sets; solution (aqueous) 25% in 50 ml containers (Albumisol, Albuspan) and 20, 50, and 100 ml containers (Albuminar 25, Buminate, Plasbumin-25). The 50 and 100 ml containers are supplied with intravenous administration sets.
> *Albutein* (Alpha Therapeutic). Solution (aqueous) 25% in 50 and 100 ml containers. Supplied with intravenous administration sets.

PLASMA PROTEIN FRACTION (Human Plasma Protein Fraction)

[Plasmanate, Plasma-Plex, Plasmatein, Protenate]

Plasma protein fraction (PPF), a 5% solution of stabilized human plasma proteins (at least 83% albumin, no more than 17% globulin, and no more than 1% of total protein as gamma globulin) in sodium chloride injection, is used to treat hypovolemic shock and to provide protein in patients with hypoproteinemia. It also is effective for the initial treatment of shock in infants and small children with dehydration, hemoconcentration, and electrolyte deficiency caused by diarrhea. Plasma protein fraction does not provide labile clotting factors and should not be given to correct coagulation defects.

Nausea, vomiting, and hypotension have occurred. A number of cases of serious hypotension have been reported in surgical patients following transfusion of plasma protein fraction. Contamination of some lots of the fractions with factor XII (Hageman factor) fragments has been implicated as the cause of prekallikrein activation that has resulted in bradykinin-induced peripheral vasodilatation. All patients, especially those with normal or increased circulatory volume, should be carefully observed for signs of hypervolemia (eg, pulmonary edema) or cardiac failure. Acute viral hepatitis or hypersensitivity reactions have not been reported. Solutions should not be mixed with or administered through the same sets as other intravenous fluids; this does not preclude concomitant administration of other fluids through another vein.

ROUTE, USUAL DOSAGE, AND PREPARATIONS. *Intravenous*: The following amounts will serve as guides; the total amount administered must be adjusted to meet the needs of each patient. *Adults*, for hypoproteinemia, 1 to 1.5 L of solution containing 50 to 75 g of protein infused at a rate of 5 to 8 ml/min, repeated as necessary. Because of the hypotensive reactions associated with its use, plasma protein fraction should be infused slowly. It probably should not be given to treat hypovolemic shock or when rapid intravenous infusion is necessary. *Infants and young children*, for dehydration, 33 ml/kg of body weight infused at a rate of 5 to 10 ml/min.

> Drug available generically: Solution 5% in 50 ml containers and in 250 and 500 ml containers with intravenous administration set.
> *Plasmanate* (Cutter). Solution 5% in 50, 250, and 500 ml containers.
> *Plasma-Plex* (Armour), *Plasmatein* (Alpha Therapeutic), *Protenate* (Hyland). Solution 5% in 250 and 500 ml containers.

IMMUNE GLOBULIN
[Gammagee, H-BIG, Hep-B-Gammagee]

Immune globulin is a sterile concentrated solution of globulins prepared from large pools of normal human plasma of either venous or placental origin by a special fractionation process involving a series of controlled precipitations with cold ethanol (Cohn process). Gamma globulin preparations manufactured in this manner do not transmit hepatitis. This agent protects against the clinical manifestations of hepatitis A when administered before or within two weeks after exposure. It may provide some protection against non-A, non-B transfusion hepatitis, particularly if administered prior to blood transfusion. Immune globulin prevents or modifies rubeola, rubella, and varicella and is used to treat immunoglobulin (IgG) deficiency diseases. Special preparations with high antibody titers provide postexposure prophylaxis against hepatitis B (Hepatitis B Immune Globulin), pertussis, rabies, and tetanus (see the evaluations in Chapter 67, Vaccines and Antiserums).

ROUTE, USUAL DOSAGE, AND PREPARATIONS.
Intramuscular: Dosage varies with the indication. Intramuscular injections are not advocated for patients with bleeding disorders.

> *Gammagee* (Merck Sharp & Dohme) (for hepatitis A). Solution (sterile) containing 16.5 ± 1.5% protein in 2 and 10 ml containers.
> *H-BIG* (Abbott) (for hepatitis B). Solution (sterile) in 3, 4, and 5 ml containers.
> *Hep-B-Gammagee* (Merck Sharp & Dohme) (for hepatitis B). Solution (sterile) in 5 ml containers.

BLOOD SUBSTITUTES

DEXTRAN 40
[Gentran-40, LMD, Rheomacrodex]

DEXTRAN 70
[Macrodex]

DEXTRAN 75
[Gentran-75]

Dextran is a water-soluble glucose polymer biosynthesized by the action of *Leuconostoc mesenteroides* on sucrose. The high molecular weight product thus obtained is further treated by partial acid hydrolysis and differential fractionation to yield finished products of lower and more uniform molecular weight. Dextran 70 and 75 have mean molecular weights of 70,000 and 75,000, respectively. Because they remain in the intravascular space for about 12 hours, these dextran preparations may be used as plasma volume expanders in the treatment of shock or to increase filling pressure. They also may be used to correct the oligemia of burn shock or to maintain colloidal osmotic pressure temporarily during certain types of cardiovascular surgery. Low molecular weight dextran (dextran 40) has a mean molecular weight of approximately 40,000 and a duration of effect lasting two to four hours; it is used as a priming fluid (alone or as an additive) for pump-oxygenators during extracorporeal circulation and as an adjunct in the treatment of shock or impending shock. More recently, dextran 40 preparations have been used to prevent venous thrombosis and thromboembolism (see Chapter 63, Anticoagulants and Thrombolytics).

Hypersensitivity reactions (rash, pruritus, nasal congestion, dyspnea, chest tightness, and mild hypotension) are the primary untoward effects observed. The incidence is very low and reactions generally are mild when adequately hydrolyzed and refined preparations are used. Low molecular weight dextran has considerably less antigenic potential than the higher molecular weight products. Nevertheless, urticaria, angioedema, bronchospasm, and anaphylactic reactions have occurred with both types of preparations. Patients also may develop nausea, vomiting, and, occasionally, acute hypotension. Discontinuation of therapy usually relieves the milder reactions. More serious adverse effects may require the immediate subcutaneous administration of 1:1,000 epinephrine (0.3 to 0.5 ml), followed if necessary by intravenous injection of 0.5 ml diluted with 10 ml of sodium chloride injection. This treatment may be supplemented by the administration of an antihistamine, steroids, and other supportive measures to counteract shock and hypotension. Equipment for emergency resuscitation should be readily available. Because death from anaphylactic reactions has occurred after intravenous administration of as little as 10 ml of dextran 75 solution, the blood pressure should be monitored and the patient observed closely during at least the first 30 minutes of infusion of any dextran preparation.

Increased bleeding time caused by interference with platelet function occurs in a substantial number of patients receiving dextran, especially when the higher molecular weight products are used and the dose exceeds 1 to 1.5 L. This reaction may not appear for six to nine hours following infusion of dextran. Bleeding may occur, especially if there is a pre-existing coagulation defect. Since the renal threshold for dextran is at a molecular weight of about 55,000, more dextran 40 than dextran 70 or 75 is filtered by the glomerulus. In patients with adequate urine flow, dextran has little effect on urine viscosity. However, when urine flow is diminished, dextran can markedly increase urine viscosity and specific gravity that may lead to acute tubular failure, usually associated with dehydration or shock.

Any dextran preparation may induce rouleaux formation and hence interferes with crossmatching techniques; therefore, if blood is to be administered subsequently, the crossmatch specimen should be drawn prior to dextran infusion. Dextran also may interfere with certain tests of renal and hepatic function.

Because of these reactions and the availability of alternative methods of treatment, clinical usage of dextran has declined. The potential hazards must be considered before dextran is selected in lieu of safer (although more expensive) products such as albumin.

Dextran is contraindicated in patients with known hypersensitivity, severe congestive heart failure, renal failure, hypervolemic conditions, or severe bleeding disorders. It should be used with caution in patients with chronic liver disease, impaired renal function, or those likely to develop pulmonary edema or congestive heart failure.

Dextran may precipitate from solution on storage. It can be redissolved by heating in a water bath for a short period of time at the minimal temperature required to effect solution.

ROUTE, USUAL DOSAGE, AND PREPARATIONS.
DEXTRAN 40:
Intravenous: *Adults and children*, for shock, 10 to 20 ml/kg of body weight of 10% solution added to the infusion circuit. The first 500 ml should be infused rapidly with the remaining dose given more slowly. Monitoring of the central venous pressure is strongly recommended as a guide to determine dosage. The total daily dose should not exceed 20 ml/kg. If therapy is continued for more than 24 hours, the total daily dose should not exceed 10 ml/kg. Therapy should not be continued for more than five days.

> *Dextran 40* (Cutter, McGaw), *Gentran-40* (Travenol), *LMD* (Abbott), *Rheomacrodex* (Pharmacia). Solution 10% in 0.9% sodium chloride solution or 5% dextrose in 500 ml containers.

DEXTRAN 70, DEXTRAN 75:
Intravenous: *Adults and children*, 500 to 1,000 ml of 6% solution may be infused at a rate of 20 to 40 ml/min. The total dosage should not exceed 20 ml/kg of body weight during the first 24 hours.

DEXTRAN 70:
Dextran 70 (Cutter, McGaw). Solution 6% in 0.9% sodium chloride solution in 250 and 500 ml containers.
Macrodex (Pharmacia). Solution 6% in 0.9% sodium chloride solution or 5% dextrose in water in 500 ml containers.

DEXTRAN 75:
Dextran 75 (Abbott). Solution 6% in 0.9% sodium chloride solution (Dextran 6%-S) or in 5% dextrose solution (Dextran in D5-W) in 500 ml containers.
Gentran-75 (Travenol). Solution 6% in 0.9% sodium chloride solution in 500 ml containers.

SIMILAR PREPARATION.
6% Gentran 75 in 10% Travert (Travenol). Solution containing dextran 6% with invert sugar 10% in water in 500 ml containers. This preparation, as well as the dextran 75 in dextrose preparation listed above, may be used in patients in whom sodium restriction is indicated.

HETASTARCH
[Volex]

Hetastarch (hydroxyethyl starch, HES, hespan) is an artificial colloid with an average molecular weight of approximately 450,000 and a mean molecular weight of approximately 70,000 (polymer units range from 10,000 to 1,000,000). It is used to expand plasma volume in the emergency treatment of shock or impending shock caused by hemorrhage. It also can be used to correct the oligemia of burn or septic shock and to help maintain blood volume during certain types of surgery (eg, cardiovascular surgery). It is not a substitute for blood.

A 6% solution of hetastarch has approximately the same osmotic properties as human albumin at physiologic concentration. Following intravenous infusion, plasma volume is expanded slightly in excess of the actual volume of hetastarch given. This effect is observed for 24 to 36 hours after infusion. Molecules with a weight of 50,000 or less are readily excreted by the kidneys; 40% of a given dose is eliminated within 24 hours. Heavier molecules are degraded enzymatically by amylase, primarily in the blood stream, and eliminated over a period of two to three weeks.

Nausea, vomiting, mild febrile reactions, chills, pruritus, and urticaria have occurred. Excessive amounts decrease the hematocrit, dilute plasma proteins, and interfere with the normal coagulation mechanism. Thus, hetastarch is contraindicated in patients with severe bleeding disorders. Because it is excreted relatively slowly, primarily by the kidneys, hypervolemia is a potential danger, particularly in patients with impaired renal function. Accordingly, this agent is contraindicated in patients with severe congestive heart failure and renal failure with oliguria or anuria.

No teratogenic effects were demonstrated during studies in mice, but extrapolation of animal data to humans may not be applicable and the risk/benefit potential must be carefully considered before this drug is used in pregnant women. Similarly, no data are available on the use of hetastarch in children.

Studies comparing hetastarch and other plasma expanders (eg, dextran) are limited. One study in England indicated that hetastarch and dextran 70 were similarly useful, but hetastarch had less potential to induce anaphylaxis or coagulation abnormalities. The primary use of hetastarch at present, however, is as a sedimenting agent in the preparation of granulocytes by leukapheresis.

ROUTE, USUAL DOSAGE, AND PREPARATIONS.
Intravenous: *Adults*, 500 to 1,000 ml/24 hours (maximum dose, 1,500 ml), depending upon the amount of blood lost and the hemoconcentration. The maximum infusion rate is 20 ml/kg/hr. Slower rates are indicated when treating burn or septic shock.

   Volex (Arnar-Stone). Solution 6% in 0.9% sodium chloride solution in 500 ml containers.

Selected References

Code of Federal Regulations, section 21, parts 600-1299. Supt of Documents, US Government Printing Office, Washington, DC, 20402.

Dextran and postoperative thromboembolism. *Drug Ther Bull* 13:41-43, 1975.

Hepatitis B immune globulin (human). *Med Lett Drugs Ther* 20:9-10, 1978.

Aach RD: Viral hepatitis-A to e. *Med Clin North Am* 62:59-70, 1978.

Adamkin DH: New uses for exchange transfusion. *Pediatr Clin North Am* 24:599-604, 1977.

Aisner J: Platelet transfusion therapy. *Med Clin North Am* 61:1133-1145, 1977.

Alter HJ, et al: Transmission of hepatitis B ,virus infection by transfusion of frozen-deglycerolized red blood cells. *N Engl J Med* 298:637-642, 1978.

Brzica SM Jr, et al: Blood transfusion for patient who is difficult to transfuse. *Mayo Clin Proc* 52:160-162, 1977.

Brzica SM Jr, et al: Autologous blood transfusion. *Mayo Clin Proc* 51:723-737, 1976.

Czaja AJ, Summerskill WHJ: Chronic hepatitis: To treat or not to treat? *Med Clin North Am* 62:71-85, 1978.

Feinstone SM, Purcell RH: Non-A, non-B hepatitis. *Annu Rev Med* 29:359-366, 1978.

Grady GF: Transfusions and hepatitis: Update in '78. *N Engl J Med* 298:1413-1415, 1978.

Greenwalt TJ (ed): *General Principles of Blood Transfusion*. Chicago, American Medical Association, 1977.

Hoofnagle JH, et al: Type B hepatitis after transfusion with blood containing antibody to hepatitis B core antigen. *N Engl J Med* 298:1379-1383, 1978.

Johnston DG: Blood transfusion: Use and abuse of blood components. *West J Med* 128:390-398, 1978.

Keren DF, Grindon AJ: Blood components instead of blood. *Drug Ther* 6:36-44, (April) 1976.

McCredie KB: Platelet and granulocyte transfusion therapy. *Postgrad Med* 62:151-153, (Aug) 1977.

McCurdy PR: Blood component therapy: Giving what the patient needs. *Postgrad Med* 62:143-147, (Aug) 1977.

Prince AM: Use of hepatitis B immune globulin: Reassessment needed. *N Engl J Med* 299:198-199, 1978.

Ring J, Messmer K: Incidence and severity of anaphylactoid reactions to colloid volume substitutes. *Lancet* 1:466-469, 1977.

Schiffer CA: Principles of granulocyte transfusion therapy. *Med Clin North Am* 61:1119-1131, 1977.

Sherlock S: Clinical aspects of viral hepatitis. *J R Soc Med* 971:430-432, 1978.

Tullis JL: Albumin. 1. Background and use, 2. Guidelines for clinical use. *JAMA* 237:355-363, 460-463, 1977.

Hemostatics | 65

An understanding of blood clotting and fibrinolytic mechanisms is essential in determining the etiology of bleeding and the appropriate hemostatic agent for correction. If bleeding is the result of a specific hereditary deficiency (eg, antihemophilic factor activity), diagnosis and treatment may be relatively simple. Conversely, multiple acquired deficiencies can be difficult to diagnose and may respond poorly to treatment. Four tests of hemostasis that usually provide adequate data for diagnosis are platelet count, bleeding time, one-stage prothrombin time, and activated partial thromboplastin time.

Most hemostatic agents are administered systemically to overcome specific coagulation defects, while others are applied locally to control surface bleeding and capillary oozing. Those prepared as concentrates from human blood for replacement of specific factors include an-tihemophilic factor (factor VIII, AHF) [Factorate, Hemofil, Humafac, Koāte, Profilate], cryoprecipitated antihemophilic factor (human), and factor IX complex (plasma thromboplastin component) [Konȳne, Proplex]. [Fibrinogen is no longer marketed. Cryoprecipitated antihemophilic factor (human) provides adequate fibrinogen and is much less likely to cause hepatitis than fibrinogen.] Other systemic hemostatics used to augment coagulation factor synthesis include vitamin K preparations (phytonadione [AquaMEPHYTON, Konakion, Mephyton], menadione, menadione sodium bisulfite [Hykinone], menadiol sodium diphosphate [Synkayvite]). Aminocaproic acid [Amicar] inhibits the fibrinolytic mechanism. Although estrogens are claimed to control postoperative bleeding when given intravenously, current evidence does not substantiate this effect. The locally applied, absorbable hemostatics that assist in fibrin formation include absorbable gelatin film [Gelfilm], absorbable gelatin sponge [Gelfoam], oxidized cellulose [Oxycel, Surgicel], microfibrillar collagen hemostat [Avitene], and thrombin (bovine source).

HEMOSTATIC AGENTS IN HEMOPHILIA

Before plasma concentrates became available, bleeding associated with classical hemophilia (hemophilia A, factor VIII deficiency) was treated with frequent infusions of large volumes of plasma or, rarely, whole blood. However, this therapy caused hypervolemia and could not provide adequate plasma levels of factor VIII (antihemophilic factor, AHF) during severe hemorrhage. The development of concentrated AHF preparations has virtually eliminated the need to use other products. However, fresh frozen plasma is the only therapy advocated before diagnosis of clotting factor deficiency is established, since both factor VIII and factor IX deficiencies have identical clinical manifestations.

The degree of bleeding resulting from congenital deficiency of factor VIII activity can be highly variable. In some instances, bleeding may be minor or absent and there may be no family history of a bleeding disorder. Definitive diagnosis must be established by a specific assay of plasma for factor VIII activity.

Cryoprecipitated antihemophilic factor (human) obtained from single donor plasma is the only product recommended for patients with hemophilia A. The plasma is frozen rapidly and thawed slowly to yield a solution rich in AHF and fibrinogen. However, the amount of AHF varies, which is the major disadvantage with its use. It also contains more fibrinogen and other materials that may enhance the sensitizing potential. Cryoprecipitated preparations represent more efficient use of community blood resources, since they can be inexpensively prepared in the blood bank laboratory of most hospitals and stored in the freezer until needed for infu-

sion. Furthermore, the material remaining in the plasma can be used to process other component products.

Commercially available AHF concentrates are prepared by a variety of techniques: precipitation by glycine or polyethylene glycol, alcohol, or a combination of the above with subsequent lyophilization. Their use is preferred by some clinicians because they are stable; easy to handle, store, and administer; and contain a standardized amount of AHF. The disadvantages are the expense and the potentially greater risk of hepatitis, since AHF concentrates are prepared from pooled plasma.

Replacement therapy is required in hemophiliacs with active bleeding, whether spontaneous or traumatic, or before surgery. Since the in vivo survival time of these products is brief, the hemostatic should be given just prior to surgery. Correction of a previously abnormal in vitro coagulation time should be monitored carefully. About 10% of patients with hemophilia A develop an immunoglobulin inhibitor which inactivates the infused AHF. The anamnestic response to administration of AHF in these patients complicates correction of the bleeding problem. Assay for this inhibitor should be performed in all hemophiliacs prior to transfusion, especially before surgery. Rarely, this inhibitor may develop in healthy individuals, elderly patients, postpartum women, and patients with systemic lupus erythematosus. For patients with high titers of antihemophilic antibody (most patients treated aggressively have high titers), activated concentrates of vitamin K-dependent clotting factors (eg, factor IX complex) have been used experimentally to bypass the inhibitor.

Each of the many schedules for the use of AHF concentrates is based upon the severity of the bleeding diathesis. Most of the factor VIII transfused remains in the intravascular space, and its biological half-life is approximately 12 hours. In hemophilia A, a factor VIII level that is 5% of normal usually is sufficient to prevent spontaneous bleeding. Control of bleeding in a confined area, such as a joint, requires levels 15% to 20% of normal activity. For effective hemostasis during and after major surgery, a plasma AHF level at least 50% of normal activity must be maintained for several days.

In selected patients under close medical supervision, AHF products may be used for home therapy to reduce cost and allow a more normal life. Also, prompt therapy at home as soon as bleeding occurs may help prevent serious complications. However, most therapeutic programs still have a high failure rate as is evident from the incidence of new or progressive arthropathy. Therefore, prophylaxis in children aged 3 to 8 should be considered. This age group often does not report hemorrhagic episodes promptly, and the consequent bone damage may progress rapidly.

von Willebrand's disease is a hereditary disorder characterized by a deficiency of factor VIII and a prolonged bleeding time; a plasma factor (ristocetin cofactor) responsible for platelet adhesion and capillary stability also may be defective in these patients. Bleeding from mucous membranes is the principal manifestation. Cryoprecipitated antihemophilic factor (human) is the agent of choice for therapy because the von Willebrand factor usually is removed during processing of commercial AHF preparations. Fresh frozen plasma also may be used. Smaller amounts of material are needed than for hemophilia A, because infusion of AHF into these patients increases endogenous factor VIII activity.

Desmopressin [DDAVP] is being investigated for use in hemophilia; this drug markedly increases factor VIII activity in patients with moderate or mild hemophilia and von Willebrand's disease. In patients with these bleeding disorders, doses of 0.3 to 0.5 mcg/kg given before and soon after dental surgery prevented abnormal bleeding. Furthermore, cholecystectomy, thoracotomy, and tonsillectomy were carried out successfully when 0.4 to 0.5 mcg/kg was given every 24 hours as necessary. Desmopressin causes few adverse effects and carries no risk of transmitting hepatitis. Thus, it may be a promising adjunct to plasma concentrates in the management of some patients with hemophilia and von Willebrand's disease.

Hemophilia B (plasma thromboplastin component deficiency, Christmas disease) is similar clinically to hemophilia A but is caused by a functional factor IX deficiency. The mainstay for treatment of hemophilia B is plasma, either fresh frozen or the portion remaining after removal of cryoprecipitate. AHF concentrates are not effective.

Stable, dried, purified preparations of factor IX complex [Konȳne, Proplex] are now available commercially. However, because patients with mild hemophilia B require treatment only infrequently, some physicians use plasma to avoid the risk of hepatitis. Factors II, VII, and X (the other vitamin K-dependent factors) have similar adsorption properties and also are purified in the process. Factor IX complex has been successful in treating deficiency of any of the factors in the complex (eg, congenital deficiency, anticoagulant-induced vitamin K deficiency) but the risk of hepatitis is high. Circulating anticoagulants directed against factor IX are rare in patients with hereditary hemophilia B, but a few patients with lupus erythematosus appear to have an acquired inhibitor of factor IX. Thus, when bleeding is encountered in patients with lupus erythematosus, it is imperative that the presence of an inhibitor and its identity be established prior to treatment.

Hereditary deficiency of plasma thromboplastin antecedent (PTA, factor XI) is a rare, usually mild, autosomally inherited disorder that requires transfusion therapy for hemorrhagic episodes. Since this factor is stable in stored plasma, small amounts of plasma are effective. Other hereditary hemorrhagic disorders related to clotting factor deficiencies are exceedingly rare and a specialized text should be consulted for details of their treatment.

Adverse Reactions and Precautions

Viral hepatitis is the most common adverse effect encountered with administration of concentrated preparations of antihemophilic factor (AHF). Screening of

1106

donors for hepatitis B surface antigen (HBsAg) has decreased the risk of transmitting type B hepatitis. Manufacturers of highly purified, dried AHF products made from pooled plasma screen each unit for HBsAg and eliminate those that are positive but, unfortunately, this screening does not guarantee that the preparations will not transmit hepatitis. The risk of transmitting type B hepatitis with use of cryoprecipitated AHF is the same as that with single units of whole blood. Recent studies suggest that the cumulative risk over long periods of frequent use is probably the same as for the commercial products. Nevertheless, the cryoprecipitate prepared from single donor plasma is recommended for use in those not requiring frequent treatment and for young patients. Factor IX complex [Konȳne, Proplex], like the other factors derived from human plasma, also may transmit viral hepatitis. The use of immune globulin (gamma globulin) to attenuate hepatitis virus is ineffective, and intramuscular injections are dangerous in any patient with a bleeding disorder.

All preparations of factor IX complex, even those with heparin added, carry a significant potential for producing thrombotic complications. To reduce this risk, the smallest effective dose should be given and plasma should be used to control mild bleeding. Intravascular thrombosis has occurred frequently in surgical patients who received large doses. These complications have been particularly severe in patients with underlying liver disease.

Hemolytic anemia may occur when AHF fractions are given to individuals with group A, B, or AB red blood cell antigens, because anti-A or anti-B antibodies may be present in the precipitated fraction. The anemia is mild in most cases and usually abates after administration of AHF is discontinued. Patients with hemolysis should be treated with transfusion of cryoprecipitate from type-matched or type O donors.

AHF preparations may cause marked hyperfibrinogenemia (occasionally tenfold above normal) that interferes with the results of several laboratory tests. Although the increase may not be clinically significant, it has been implicated as a cause of

hemolytic anemia, as a stimulus to fibrinolysis, and as a cause of an increased bleeding tendency due to platelet malfunction. Transient proteinuria with deposits of fibrin and fibrinogen in the kidneys also has been associated with this hyperfibrinogenemia.

INDIVIDUAL EVALUATIONS

ANTIHEMOPHILIC FACTOR
[Factorate, Hemofil, Humafac, Kōate, Profilate]

Antihemophilic factor (factor VIII, AHF) products are prepared commercially as stable, dried, concentrated materials. AHF also can be cryoprecipitated from fresh plasma. The dried preparations contain relatively small amounts of fibrinogen and other plasma proteins. The cryoprecipitated product contains a higher percentage of non-AHF plasma factors than the dried material. The dried preparations may be stored up to four weeks (Kōate may be kept for six months) at room temperature and for longer periods at 2 to 8 C. The cryoprecipitated product must be kept frozen. The normal half-life of AHF in the body is biphasic. There is a short phase (t½, 4 to 8 hours) consistent with equilibrium within the extravascular space and a longer, second phase (t½, 12 to 15 hours) consistent with biodegradation of AHF.

All AHF preparations can be used to treat patients with hemophilia A (factor VIII deficiency) and with acquired factor VIII inhibitors. Commercially prepared AHF products cannot be used to treat von Willebrand's disease because the ristocetin cofactor necessary for platelet adhesion, which is missing in patients with the disease, is removed during the manufacturing process. Cryoprecipitated AHF contains ristocetin cofactor and is suitable for treatment of these patients.

Both dried and cryoprecipitated AHF preparations can be administered rapidly without producing significant adverse effects; neither causes hypervolemic reactions. Since the dried forms are prepared from large pools of fresh human plasma, they may cause acute viral hepatitis even when screened for HBsAg. Although this danger is lessened with the cryoprecipitated material, the prevalence of antibodies to hepatitis B surface antigen (anti-HBs) is similar in patients with hemophilia who require intensive therapy over prolonged periods, regardless of the type of AHF preparation used. Nevertheless, hemophiliacs who require treatment infrequently should receive the single donor products to reduce risk of exposure to hepatitis virus. AHF preparations also contain small amounts of groups A and B isohemagglutinins. When large amounts are given to patients with blood groups A, B, or AB, hemolysis can result. Rarely, chills or mild fever occurs shortly after administration of AHF.

Cryoprecipitated AHF should be thawed in a water bath at 37 C, kept at room temperature after thawing, and used within six hours.

ROUTE, USUAL DOSAGE, AND PREPARATIONS.
Intravenous: A circulating AHF level 20% to 30% of normal usually controls hemarthrosis in patients with hemophilia. Usually, a single dose of 15 to 20 units/kg of body weight achieves hemostasis and, allowing for equilibration and degradation, maintains sufficient levels for healing. For mild bleeding into muscles or soft tissues in noncritical areas, a single dose (usually 10 units/kg) is usually sufficient to achieve the necessary circulating AHF level of 15% to 20% of normal. For surgery, a blood level at least 50% of normal is necessary preoperatively for effective hemostasis; postoperatively, it is desirable to have a circulating level 20% to 25% of normal for seven to ten days. For retroperitoneal, retropharyngeal, or central nervous system bleeding; gross hematuria; severe trauma; or spontaneous bleeding into a body cavity or joint requiring aspiration, hospitalization is required and hemostasis achieved as in surgical patients (50% of normal activity for several days). Bleeding recurs if treatment is discontinued prematurely. Various formulas are available to estimate dosage, and details appear in the manufacturers' literature. Based on experimental evidence, approximately 5 units/kg of body weight produce an increase of about 10%. Regardless of the therapeutic guide, factor VIII assays usually should be performed at frequent intervals, if proper techniques for these determinations are available, to be certain that an adequate level of factor VIII has been reached and is being maintained. These determinations may be imperative when using cryoprecipitated AHF, because there is no uniformity in the concentration of AHF from one plasma donor to the next. If adequate levels are not attained or if hemorrhage is not controlled with adequate dosage, a test for factor VIII inhibitors also should be performed.

Preparation available generically: 250, 500, and 1,000 units.
Factorate (Armour), *Hemofil* (Hyland), *Humafac* (Parke, Davis), *Koāte* (Cutter), *Profilate* (Alpha Therapeutics). Each bottle is labeled with the number of units it contains (200 to 1,000 units/bottle). One unit is the antihemophilic factor activity present in 1 ml of average, normal, human plasma pooled from at least ten donors and tested within three hours after collection. These materials must be reconstituted with sterile water to a volume dependent upon final container assay of potency and dosage/ml desired.
Cryoprecipitated Antihemophilic Factor (Human) can be prepared by the hospital blood bank as a by-product of blood banking. This product cannot be standardized, but each bag usually contains between 60 and 125 units.

FACTOR IX COMPLEX (HUMAN)
[Konȳne, Proplex]

Factor IX complex (plasma thromboplastin component) concentrates are stable, dried, purified plasma fractions containing coagulation factors II, VII, IX, and X, as well as a relatively small amount of other plasma proteins. Products are alleged to be free of thrombin, thromboplastin-like activity, anticomplement activity, and depressor activity. Konȳne contains no heparin, whereas heparin is added to Proplex to help prevent the possible formation of thrombin after the manufacturing process (eg, increased temperature during storage). As anti-A and anti-B agglutinins are present at clinically insignificant levels, factor IX complex (human) may be used safely without typing or crossmatching. Hypervolemic reactions do not occur because of the concentrated nature of these products and the small amount of fluid needed for administration.

Most of these dried preparations must be refrigerated at 2 to 8 C (Konȳne may be stored for up to one month at temperatures below 37 C); freezing should be avoided to prevent breakage of the bottle of diluent. Although factor IX complex (human) is stable after reconstitution for at least 12 hours at room temperature, it should be administered promptly. It is diluted with sterile water for injection and the concentration must not exceed 50 units/ml. The biological half-life of factor IX is biphasic with a short first phase (four to six hours) consistent with equilibration within the extravascular space and a longer second phase (22.5 hours) consistent with biodegradation.

Factor IX complex (human) is used to treat hemophilia B (Christmas disease) or when one or more of the factors contained in this preparation is required to prevent hemorrhage. It should be used in newborn infants only when life-threatening hemorrhagic disease is caused by proven deficiency of factor II, VII, IX, or X. Factor IX complex also may be useful in those patients with factor VIII deficiency who develop an inhibitor, presumably because it supplies activated coagulation factors that are involved in the coagulation mechanism beyond the steps where factor VIII is needed.

Because of the substantial risk of inducing hepatitis with administration of factor IX complex concentrates, these products should never be used in nonhemophiliacs (ie, patients with anticoagulant-induced deficiency of vitamin K-dependent coagulation factors). These patients should receive fresh or fresh frozen plasma.

Many cases of factor IX-induced thromboembolic disease have been reported, particularly after use of Konȳne. Pretesting of individual vials of Konȳne for the presence of activated procoagulants may be indicated. Konȳne is contraindicated in patients with liver disease when there is any suspicion of intravascular coagulation or fibrinolysis.

Transient fever, chills, headache, flushing, or tingling can occur shortly after administration of factor IX complex, particularly if the injection is given rapidly. Since serious hypersensitivity reactions (eg, anaphylactic shock) have been reported following injection of Konȳne, a test dose should be administered before the full dose is given.

ROUTE, USUAL DOSAGE, AND PREPARATIONS. *Intravenous:* The amount of factor IX complex (human) required depends upon the patient and the nature of the deficiency. Coagulation assays performed prior to therapy and at reasonable intervals during treatment are the best guide to appropriate dosage. Each unit contains the factor IX activity of 1 ml of normal fresh plasma; 1 unit/kg of body weight increases factor IX activity 1.5%. Overdosage should be avoided because the long postinfusion half-life of factors II and X can cause unnecessarily high levels of these factors. Specific dosage is similar to the lowest dose employed in factor VIII deficiency (see the evaluation on Antihemophilic Factor). A factor IX level 25% to 30% of normal should be maintained at all times during the healing phase following surgery.

> Each package contains factor IX 500 units and a bottle of sterile water for injection.
> Preparation available generically: 500 units.
> *Konȳne* (Cutter). Contains equal quantities of factors II, IX, and X and a small amount of factor VII (heparin is not present). Preparation should be reconstituted with 20 ml of sterile water for injection.
> *Proplex* (Hyland). Assayed amounts of factors II, VII, IX, and X stated on bottle. Also contains 1 unit of heparin/ml of reconstituted material. Preparation should be reconstituted with 30 ml of sterile water for injection.

HEMOSTATIC AGENTS IN HYPOFIBRINOGENEMIA

Fibrinolysis is an aseptic enzymatic liquefaction of fibrin. In the nonpathologic state, there are checks and balances in the fibrinolytic system. Bleeding episodes associated with hereditary hypofibrinogenemia are generally mild. However, in severe liver disease, a common cause of hypofibrinogenemia, hepatocellular damage results in decreased ability of the liver to remove plasminogen activators from the circulation and decreased synthesis of coagulation factors. In this and other conditions that predispose the individual to pathologic fibrinolysis (eg, stress, postoperative and obstetric complications, neoplastic disease), the deficiencies in fibrinogen and other clotting factors that occur can result in a severe hemorrhagic diathesis. In these acute conditions, administration of fibrinogen may not only have no effect on hemostasis but, by increasing the available substrate, may increase the levels of fibrinogen degradation products and aggravate intravascular clotting. Since most episodes of acquired fibrinolytic bleeding are secondary to intravascular coagulation, an accurate diagnosis must precede the use of fibrinogen-containing materials.

The manufacture of fibrinogen preparations in the United States has been discontinued. These preparations were only rarely indicated and carried a great risk for transmission of hepatitis. If fibrinogen is required, either cryoprecipitated antihemophilic factor (human) or, in patients with increased levels of plasminogen, aminocaproic acid may be given. Aminocaproic acid should not be used in patients with DIC or in those who are thrombosis-prone (see the evaluation).

INDIVIDUAL EVALUATION

AMINOCAPROIC ACID
[Amicar]

$$H_2NCH_2(CH_2)_3CH_2\overset{\overset{\displaystyle O}{\|}}{C}OH$$

Aminocaproic acid may help control serious hemorrhage associated with excessive fibrinolysis due to increased plasminogen (profibrinolysin) activation. This monoamino carboxylic acid is a potent competitive inhibitor of plasminogen activators. It also inhibits plasmin (fibrinoly-

sin) to a lesser degree. Therefore, aminocaproic acid prevents formation of the excessive plasmin responsible for the destruction of fibrinogen, fibrin, and other important clotting components. Since this drug inhibits the dissolution of clots, it may interfere with normal mechanisms for maintaining the patency of blood vessels, particularly in thrombosis-prone patients. Before this hemostatic is used, it is important to understand the role of the fibrinolytic system in maintaining the patency and integrity of the vascular system, the laboratory procedures used to determine coagulation defects, and the mechanism of action of aminocaproic acid.

A pathologic fibrinolytic state may be suspected in patients with a predisposing clinical condition when results of laboratory tests suggest increased fibrinolytic activity, prolonged thrombin and prothrombin times, hypofibrinogenemia, or decreased plasminogen levels. However, these conditions and some of the laboratory findings usually are associated with diffuse intravascular coagulation (DIC). If aminocaproic acid is given to patients with DIC, it may cause serious or even fatal thrombus formation. For this reason, most experts do not use aminocaproic acid to treat "fibrinolytic" hemorrhage unless there is definitive proof that DIC is not the underlying cause. If confusion exists, the following criteria may determine whether DIC or primary fibrinolysis is occurring: In DIC, the platelet count is reduced, the protamine paracoagulation test is positive, and euglobulin clot lysis is normal. In primary fibrinolysis, the platelet count is normal, the protamine paracoagulation test is negative, and euglobulin clot lysis is reduced.

Aminocaproic acid is well absorbed orally and also can be given intravenously. This drug is excreted rapidly in the urine, largely unchanged, and peak plasma levels are obtained about two hours after a single oral dose.

Aminocaproic acid is concentrated in the urine and inhibits the plasminogen activator, urokinase. It is useful in surgical and nonsurgical hematuria arising from the the bladder, prostate, or urethra. In patients undergoing transurethral and suprapubic prostatectomy, a statistically significant reduction of postoperative hematuria has been demonstrated. However, use of aminocaproic acid should be restricted to patients who are seriously threatened by hemorrhage and for whom a correctable cause of bleeding from the prostatic bed has been excluded. Aminocaproic acid also has been used by some neurosurgeons prior to and during surgery for ruptured intracranial aneurysms.

Plasminogen activators such as streptokinase and urokinase are used to treat thromboembolic disorders. Since aminocaproic acid counteracts their thrombolytic effect, it may have some usefulness as an antidote.

Aminocaproic acid does not control hemorrhage caused by thrombocytopenia or most other coagulation defects, although it has been very useful in hemophiliacs prior to and following tooth extraction and for other traumatic bleeding in the mouth. When multiple hemostatic defects exist, other therapeutic measures (eg, administration of fresh frozen plasma, cryoprecipitated antihemophilic factor, or vitamin K) may be required. Since the drug does not control bleeding caused by loss of vascular integrity, valuable time may be lost if it is used in patients with post-tonsillectomy bleeding, gastrointestinal hemorrhage from ulcers or ruptured esophageal varices, hemoptysis due to bronchiectasis, open surgical wounds, or functional uterine bleeding.

The untoward effects of aminocaproic acid include pruritus, erythema, rash, hypotension, dyspepsia, nausea, diarrhea, inhibition of ejaculation, conjunctival erythema, and nasal congestion. The most serious effect is generalized thrombosis, and patients receiving this drug should be tested to evaluate the hemostatic mechanisms in order to prevent the development of a hypercoagulable state.

Cardiac and hepatic necroses were found at postmortem examination in one patient who received therapeutic doses of the drug. Subendocardial hemorrhages and myocardial depression have been associated with administration of aminocaproic acid in several animal species. The drug may transiently alter protein metabolism by inhibiting the utilization of lysine.

Teratogenic studies in animals have produced variable results, but no significant abnormalities have been noted in humans. Nevertheless, the drug should not be used during the first and second trimester unless absolutely essential. It may be administered during the last trimester if specifically indicated and if the potential benefit outweighs the possible hazards to the mother and fetus.

When aminocaproic acid is given during surgery, care must be taken to free the bladder of blood clots, since the drug accumulates in these clots and inhibits their physiologic dissolution.

ROUTES, USUAL DOSAGE, AND PREPARATIONS. Further evidence is needed to determine the safety of prolonged use of aminocaproic acid in the following doses.
Intravenous, Oral: Adults, initially, 5 to 6 g orally or by slow intravenous infusion, then 1 g at hourly intervals or 6 g every six hours if renal function is normal (maximum, 30 g/24 hours). This dosage produces effective therapeutic plasma levels of approximately 13 mg/dl. Smaller doses should be used in patients with renal disease or oliguria. *Children,* 100 mg/kg of body weight every six hours for six days.

When aminocaproic acid is administered intravenously, it should be diluted with sodium chloride injection, 5% dextrose injection, or Ringer's injection. The drug should not be used undiluted or injected rapidly. The patient's condition should be re-evaluated after eight hours of continuous therapy.

Amicar (Lederle). Solution (injection) 250 mg/ml in 20 ml containers; syrup 1.25 g/5 ml; tablets 500 mg.

VITAMIN K

Vitamin K potentiates carboxylation of glutamic acid in the fragment one portion of prothrombin and, by analogy, presumably performs the same function for factors VII, IX, and X. This transformation is responsible for development of the clot-promoting properties of these factors. If a deficiency of vitamin K occurs, the blood level of these procoagulant factors decreases and a hemorrhagic disorder develops.

The vitamin K compounds are fat-soluble naphthoquinones. Phytonadione (vitamin K₁) occurs in a variety of foods and vitamin K₂ is produced by bacteria in the gastrointestinal tract; phytonadione also is prepared synthetically, as is menadione (vitamin K₃).

The daily requirement for vitamin K has not been established in normal individuals but is estimated to be 1 to 5 mcg/kg of body weight for infants and 0.03 mcg/kg for adults. Dietary sources usually satisfy these requirements. It is unlikely that adults, even those with inadequate diets, will develop a deficiency on the basis of dietary deficiency alone. Vitamin K accumulates in the liver, spleen, and lungs, but significant amounts are not stored in the body for long periods.

The K vitamins, except for the water-soluble salts of menadione (menadione sodium bisulfite, menadiol sodium diphosphate), are absorbed from the gastrointestinal tract only in the presence of adequate quantities of bile salts and pancreatic lipase. The natural, fat-soluble vitamin K₁ (phytonadione) is more effective and is preferred for treatment of hypoprothrombinemia, particularly for control of oral anticoagulant-induced bleeding, during the last weeks of pregnancy, or for hemorrhagic disease of the newborn. The water-soluble salts of menadione are useful for treatment of hypoprothrombinemias secondary to conditions limiting absorption or synthesis of vitamin K. None of the vitamin K preparations counteract the anticoagulant effects of heparin.

Intravenous administration should be used during emergencies, but other routes of administration may provide more prolonged action. Phytonadione and the water-soluble salts of menadione can be given orally and by all parenteral routes; menadione is most commonly given orally.

If proper therapy is to be instituted in cases of apparent vitamin K deficiency, it is important to differentiate between true deficiency and defective synthesis of vitamin K-dependent clotting factors. For example, in liver disease with severe cellular damage (eg, cirrhosis, hepatitis, hemochromatosis, porphyria cutanea tarda, Wilson's disease), the vitamin K-dependent clotting factors and factor V may be significantly reduced despite the presence of adequate vitamin K and vitamin K therapy is ineffective.

Patients receiving long-term intravenous feeding may develop vitamin K deficiency, and supplementation with vitamin K should be routine in these patients. Debilitated patients who may have experienced long periods of inadequate diet also develop vitamin K deficiency rapidly when placed on a regimen of parenteral feeding, especially if oral antibiotics are given concomitantly. Uptake of vitamin K is diminished during prolonged oral antibiotic therapy, cleansing of the bowel prior to colonic surgery, or when a malabsorption syndrome exists (eg, pancreatic insufficiency, dysentery, celiac disease, intestinal fistula, blind loop syndrome). In young infants, vitamin K deficiency may result from acute diarrhea, even of short duration. An existing deficiency of vitamin K may be accentuated by alteration of intestinal flora during treatment of bacterial diarrhea.

When insufficient absorption of vitamin K is caused by biliary disease (obstructive jaundice, atresia, fistulas), the prothrombin time gradually increases. If hepatic cell damage also is present, hypoprothrombinemia and the associated deficiency of other vitamin K-dependent factors may become even more severe. Patients with hereditary hypoprothrombinemia or hereditary deficiency of factors VII, IX, or X do not respond to vitamin K therapy.

Inhibition of vitamin K activity in the liver produced by the coumarin derivatives is one of the most common causes of iatrogenic hypocoagulability in man. Coagulation factor levels often are decreased in patients being treated with these drugs, especially if salicylates or phenylbutazone [Azolid, Butazolidin] are being given concomitantly (see also Chapter 63, Anticoagulants and Thrombolytics, and Chapter 5, Drug Interactions and Adverse Drug Reactions). A single oral dose of phytonadione often corrects the defect. However, if severe bleeding occurs, the anticoagulant may have to be discontinued and intravenous vitamin K therapy initiated. Because the response to vitamin K does not develop for 4 to 24 hours, concomitant transfusion of fresh frozen plasma is essential if the hemorrhage is life-threatening. Plasma often restores prothrombin time to therapeutic levels and may be the only therapy necessary for a life-threatening bleeding state. However, the prothrombin time should be measured frequently to monitor the effects of the oral anticoagulant and natural decay of the clotting factors in the transfused plasma. Adults usually require two to three units of plasma. Stored plasma can be used, since the clotting factors are relatively stable. Patients with impaired cardiac reserve must be observed closely for the development of congestive heart failure.

In vitamin K deficiency caused by poor nutrition or malabsorption, a single loading dose of phytonadione frequently stops bleeding within a few hours, and additional doses replenish vitamin K stores in the body. If an absorptive defect cannot be localized, small parenteral doses should be given at regular intervals until the defect is corrected.

The prothrombin level in newborn infants is substantially lower than that in adults, but this may not be reflected in prothrombin time determinations. Prothrombin time often is prolonged in infants at birth and may increase during the next two to four days if vitamin K is not available. Spontaneous hemorrhage caused by deficiency of vitamin K-dependent clotting factors is unlikely after the sixth day, particularly if cow's milk is used for feeding. The enzyme systems that synthesize these factors may not be fully developed at birth, and administration of vitamin K usually does not increase levels in infants to the same extent as in adults. Other conditions that may contribute to defective hepatic synthesis of vitamin K-dependent clotting factors in neonates are a lack of vitamin K-producing bacteria in the gastrointestinal tract (which decreases vitamin K absorption), reduced stores of vitamin K, and maternal drug ingestion (eg, oral anticoagulants, salicylates). If anticonvulsants (phenobarbital, phenytoin) are taken during the third trimester, severe hemorrhagic disease may occur in the newborn infant. In many of these infants, bleeding manifestations can be prevented by administration of phytonadione (vitamin K_1) to the mother before delivery and to the infant immediately after birth.

In pregnant women with vitamin K deficiency or in those who have undergone prolonged labor, the administration of vitamin K 12 to 24 hours before delivery may prevent hemorrhagic disease in the neonate. More commonly, 1 mg is administered to the infant during the first 24 hours after birth. Because large doses of menadione or its salts may cause kernicterus due to hemolysis, phytonadione is the only acceptable preparation for this purpose. Kernicterus has not been reported with use of this agent, and small doses do not hemolyze red cells deficient in glucose-6-phosphate dehydrogenase. In small premature infants with immature liver function or infants with hepatocellular disease, administration of phytonadione may not prevent bleeding and plasma may be required.

The one-stage prothrombin time test is used routinely to monitor vitamin K deficiency. The prothrombin and proconvertin (P and P) test of Owren also is used and is more sensitive, but results are often unreliable in the newborn.

Adverse Reactions

Adverse reactions are observed only rarely in adults after oral administration of vitamin K. Serious reactions, including fatalities, have occurred during and immediately following intravenous injection, even when solutions are dilute and infused slowly. These reactions resemble hypersensitivity or anaphylaxis and may be associated with shock, respiratory arrest, or both. They may occur in some patients receiving vitamin K for the first time.

Therefore, the intravenous route should be used only when other routes are not feasible or the potential risk is considered justified. Other parenteral routes also may be hazardous.

When vitamin K is used to treat hemorrhagic diseases in infants, it can significantly increase hemolysis and the plasma levels of unbound bilirubin, resulting in kernicterus, hemolytic anemia, and hemoglobinuria; however, hyperbilirubinemia has been observed only rarely after use of phytonadione, and this drug has not yet been implicated in causing kernicterus. The hemolytic potential of vitamin K is greatest in infants with relatively low levels of glucose-6-phosphate dehydrogenase (G6PD) but also is observed in adults with this deficiency. Plasma levels of free bilirubin may be increased in premature infants if the mother has received large doses of menadione sodium bisulfite [Hykinone], although moderate doses are relatively safe and often necessary.

Patients with liver disease should not be given repeated large doses of vitamin K if the response to initial administration is unsatisfactory. Patients receiving large doses of vitamin K (25 to 50 mg) may be resistant to coumarin drugs given later, making effective anticoagulant therapy difficult until the vitamin is sufficiently metabolized and excreted.

INDIVIDUAL EVALUATIONS

PHYTONADIONE (Vitamin K₁)

[AquaMEPHYTON, Konakion, Mephyton]

Phytonadione is used either prophylactically or during bleeding episodes to reverse the hypoprothrombinemia produced by oral anticoagulants; it does not combat hemorrhage caused by overdosage of heparin. This preparation also is used to prevent or treat hemorrhagic disease in neonates and hypoprothrombinemia caused by poor nutrition, inadequate absorption of vitamin K, inadequate synthesis of vitamin K in the gastrointestinal tract, the toxic action of certain drugs (eg, salicylates, phenylbutazone) given with the anticoagulants, and hepatic disease. Phytonadione has a more prompt, potent, and prolonged effect than the vitamin K analogues. In contrast to menadione-type drugs, it does not hemolyze red cells in patients who are deficient in glucose-6-phosphate dehydrogenase (G6PD) and is generally safe for use in newborn infants if recommended doses are not exceeded.

This drug is usually administered orally, subcutaneously, or intramuscularly, although the latter may increase the prothrombin time and cause hemorrhage at the site of injection. In emergencies caused by overdosage of coumarin or indandione anticoagulants, transfusions of plasma are essential; slow intravenous injection of phytonadione (not exceeding 1 mg/min) also may be indicated. Since control of hypoprothrombinemia re-exposes the patient to the same hazards of intravascular clotting that existed prior to anticoagulant therapy, the dosage of phytonadione should be as low as possible, prothrombin times should be checked frequently, and heparin should be readily available, for this drug's anticoagulant effect is not impaired by large amounts of phytonadione.

Intravenous injection of phytonadione can cause flushing of the face, hyperhidrosis, a feeling of chest constriction, cyanosis, acute peripheral vascular failure, shock, and hypersensitivity or anaphylactic-type reactions. Fatalities have occurred (see the Introduction to this section). The subcutaneous and intramuscular routes are less reliable than intravenous administration and may cause delayed nodule formation and pain at the site of injection; intramuscular injection may produce bleeding. Parenteral administration in neonates can significantly increase plasma levels of unbound bilirubin and cause hemolytic anemia and hemoglobinuria. These reactions are less likely to occur with use of phytonadione than with the water-soluble analogues (menadiol sodium diphosphate, menadione sodium bisulfite). Kernicterus has not yet been reported.

ROUTES, USUAL DOSAGE, AND PREPARATIONS.
Oral, Subcutaneous, Intramuscular: For hypoprothrombinemic states, *adults and children*, 2.5 to 25 mg; rarely, doses as large as 50 mg may be needed.

> *Mephyton* (Merck Sharp & Dohme). Tablets 5 mg.
> For parenteral preparations, see below.

Intravenous, Intramuscular, Subcutaneous: For prophylaxis of hemorrhagic disease in the newborn, 0.5 to 1 mg immediately after birth; although less desirable, 1 to 5 mg may be given to the mother 12 to 24 hours before delivery. For treatment of hemorrhagic disease in the newborn, 1 mg intramuscularly or subcutaneously. If no improvement occurs within six hours, the condition of the infant should be re-evaluated. Whenever possible, the subcutaneous or intramuscular route is preferred.

Intravenous: For hemorrhage caused by overdosage of oral anticoagulants, *adults and children*, 2.5 to 10 mg. The preparation should be diluted with 5% dextrose or sodium chloride injection and given at a rate not exceeding 1 mg/min, usually by infusion.

> *AquaMEPHYTON* (Merck Sharp & Dohme). Solution 2 mg/ml in 0.5 ml containers and 10 mg/ml in 1, 2.5, and 5 ml containers.
> *Konakion* (Roche). Solution (intramuscular) 2 mg/ml in 0.5 ml containers and 10 mg/ml in 1 and 2.5 ml containers.

MENADIONE (Vitamin K₃)

Menadione has the same actions and uses as phytonadione, although it is not as pharmacologically active on a weight basis (see the evaluation on Phytonadione). This preparation is practically insoluble in water and is most frequently used orally; the presence of bile salts is necessary for intestinal absorption.

The incidence of adverse reactions is low when usual therapeutic doses are used, and reactions are similar to those produced by phytonadione. In addition, menadione hemolyzes red blood cells in patients with glucose-6-phosphate dehydrogenase (G6PD) deficiency, as well as in newborn (especially premature) infants. Therefore, it probably should not be given to newborn infants or to women during the last few weeks of pregnancy.

ROUTES, USUAL DOSAGE, AND PREPARATIONS.
Oral, Intramuscular: 2 to 10 mg daily.

> Drug available generically; Solution (injection) 25 mg/ml in 10 ml containers; tablets 5 mg.

MENADIOL SODIUM DIPHOSPHATE
[Synkayvite]

MENADIONE SODIUM BISULFITE
[Hykinone]

These water-soluble salts of menadione have actions similar to phytonadione (see the evaluation) but, unlike phytonadione, should not be given for the prevention and treatment of hemorrhagic disease in the newborn or for the treatment of hypoprothrombinemia caused by overdosage of oral anticoagulants. Concomitant administration of bile salts is not necessary for intestinal absorption, and their use is not recommended in patients with obstructive jaundice or biliary fistula.

Adverse reactions are similar to those produced by phytonadione, but the incidence is low when usual therapeutic doses are used. Nevertheless, parenteral forms of vitamin K-related compounds should only be used when there is a definite indication for them, since these routes (particularly intramuscular injection) may cause serious toxicity. Like menadione, these salts hemolyze red blood cells in patients with glucose-6-phosphate dehydrogenase (G6PD) deficiency, as well as in newborn (especially premature) infants. Therefore, they probably should not be given to newborn infants or to women during the last few weeks of pregnancy.

ROUTES, USUAL DOSAGE, AND PREPARATIONS.
MENADIOL SODIUM DIPHOSPHATE:
Oral, Subcutaneous, Intramuscular, Intravenous: *Adults*, for secondary hypoprothrombinemia, 5 to 15 mg once or twice daily; *children*, 5 to 10 mg once or twice daily. Doses may be repeated if prothrombin levels do not return to normal.

> *Synkayvite* (Roche). Solution (injection) 5 and 10 mg/ml in 1 ml containers and 37.5 mg/ml in 2 ml containers; tablets 5 mg.

MENADIONE SODIUM BISULFITE:
Subcutaneous, Intramuscular, Intravenous: 2.5 to 10 mg daily, depending upon the route and indications for use. Larger doses may be needed in patients with severe vitamin K deficiency. Intravenous administration produces the most rapid response, but effects may be more long lasting when the other routes are used.

> *Hykinone* (Abbott). Solution 5 and 10 mg/ml in 1 ml containers.

LOCAL ABSORBABLE HEMOSTATICS

The local absorbable hemostatics are absorbable gelatin sponge [Gelfoam], oxidized cellulose [Oxycel, Surgicel], microfibrillar collagen hemostat [Avitene], and thrombin. Absorbable gelatin film [Gelfilm] is not a hemostatic but is used in surgery as an absorbable implant. These agents may help control surface bleeding and capillary oozing and tend to be fairly innocuous. However, if infection is present at the site of application, they may interfere with healing.

INDIVIDUAL EVALUATIONS

ABSORBABLE GELATIN SPONGE
[Gelfoam]

This sterile, gelatin-base surgical sponge is applied locally to help control both capillary oozing and frank hemorrhage. Highly vascular areas that are difficult to suture are primary sites. This preparation is insoluble in water and is usually moistened with sterile sodium chloride or thrombin solution before application (a compressed form is available specifically for dry application).

Since this preparation is absorbable, it may be left in place following closure of a surgical wound. When it is packed into cavities or closed tissue spaces, care should be exercised to avoid overpacking because, as the material absorbs fluid, it expands and may press on neighboring structures. The preparation is absorbed in four to six weeks without causing excessive scar tissue formation or cellular reaction.

ROUTE, USUAL DOSAGE, AND PREPARATIONS.
Topical (in wound or at operative site): The minimal amount required to cover the area and control hemorrhage should be applied.

> *Gelfoam* (Upjohn). Blocks 20 x 60 x 3 mm and 20 x 60 x 7 mm (general and neurologic surgery), 80 x 62.5 x 10 mm and 80 x 125 x 10 mm (general surgery), 80 x 250 x 10 mm (packing for cavities or dead spaces); pleated surgical packs 40 x 2 cm (general packing and filling), 40 x 6 cm (gynecologic and rectal surgery), 10 x 20 x 7 mm and 20 x 20 x 7 mm (dental packing blocks); compressed blocks 125 x 80 mm (dry applications); powder 1 g (sterile) and 10 g (nonsterile [oral]); prostatectomy cones 13 and 18 cm in diameter.

ABSORBABLE GELATIN FILM
[Gelfilm]

This sterile, thin film is used in neurologic and thoracic surgery for nonhemostatic purposes to repair defects in the dura and pleural membranes. It is also used in ocular surgery. Depending upon the site and size of implant, eight days to six months are required for absorption.

ROUTE, USUAL DOSAGE, AND PREPARATIONS.
Topical (in operative site): The minimal amount required to cover the area should be applied.

> *Gelfilm* (Upjohn). Film 25 x 50 mm (ophthalmic) and 100 x 125 mm.

OXIDIZED CELLULOSE
[Oxycel]

OXIDIZED REGENERATED CELLULOSE
[Surgicel]

These celluloses are absorbable fabrics prepared by the controlled oxidation of cellulose or regenerated cellulose. The gauze does not enter into the normal physiologic clotting mechanism but, when exposed to blood, expands and is converted to a reddish-brown or black gelatinous mass that forms an artificial clot. The rate of absorption depends upon the size of the implant, the adequacy of blood supply to the area, and the degree of chemical degradation of the material. Two to seven days are usually required, but complete absorption of large amounts of blood-soaked material may take six weeks or longer. Under optimal conditions, absorption from a body cavity occurs without cellular reaction or fibrosis.

Oxidized cellulose or oxidized regenerated cellulose is useful in surgical procedures to control moderate bleeding when suturing or ligation is technically impractical or ineffective. Such situations include control of capillary, venous, or small arterial hemorrhage encountered in biliary tract surgery; partial hepatectomy; resections or injuries of the pancreas, spleen, or kidneys; bowel resections; amputations; resections of the breast, thyroid, or prostate; oral surgery and exodontia; and certain types of neurologic and otolaryngologic surgery.

These products should not be used for permanent packing or implantation in fractures because they interfere with bone regeneration and can cause cyst formation. They are less effective on surfaces treated by chemical cautery. The Oxycel brand should not be used as a surface dressing except for immediate control of hemorrhage, since it inhibits epithelialization; silver nitrate or other corrosive chemicals should not be applied prior to its use. The hemostatic action of these celluloses is not enhanced by other hemostatic agents (thrombin is destroyed by the low pH of this material).

ROUTE, USUAL DOSAGE, AND PREPARATIONS.
Topical (in wound or at operative site): The minimal amount required to control hemorrhage should be used to facilitate absorption. It should be placed on the bleeding site or held firmly until hemostasis is obtained.

> OXIDIZED CELLULOSE:
> *Oxycel* (Parke, Davis). Pads (gauze type) 3 x 3 inch 8 ply; pledgets (cotton type) 2 x 1 x 1 inch; strips (gauze type) 5 x ½ inch 4 ply, 18 x 2 inch 4 ply, 36 x ½ inch 4 ply.
> OXIDIZED REGENERATED CELLULOSE:
> *Surgicel* (Surgikos). Knitted fabric strips ½ x 2, 2 x 3, 4 x 8, and 2 x 14 inches.

MICROFIBRILLAR COLLAGEN HEMOSTAT
[Avitene]

This water-insoluble powder is prepared from purified bovine corium collagen. When applied directly onto the bleeding surface, it attracts and entraps platelets to initiate aggregation and formation of the platelet plug and a natural clot results. Microfibrillar collagen hemostat is assimilated within seven weeks, leaving very little residue. No systemic allergic reactions or beef antibody responses have been reported. Although weak positive reactions to bovine serum albumin have occurred occasionally, no clinically significant elicitation of antibodies of the IgE class has been demonstrated following use of this product.

Microfibrillar collagen hemostat is indicated as an adjunct during surgical procedures when ligature and/or cautery are ineffective or impractical. However, it should not be used instead of ligation or resection to control large vessel bleeding in surgery, nor is it intended to control routine surgical bleeding. Microfibrillar collagen hemostat is beneficial in diffuse capillary bleeding (eg, from friable tissues or highly vascular organs) and has been effective in controlling hepatic bleeding, such as that following cholecystectomy, lacerations, biopsy, or resections of hepatic tumors and following splenic tears or superficial splenic injuries. It is also used on skin graft donor sites, around vascular anastomoses where only minimal suturing is possible, and to control oozing from cancellous bone. However, this material should not be used on bone surfaces to which prosthetic materials are to be attached with methylmethacrylate adhesives. It appears to retain its effectiveness in heparinized patients and also may be useful in patients with moderate thrombocytopenia but not in those with clinical thrombasthenia or systemic coagulation disorders.

Microfibrillar collagen hemostat adheres to tissue surfaces to form a firm, flexible film; since it also will adhere to any moist surface (eg, gloves, instruments), dry, smooth, sterile forceps should be used for handling. Surfaces to be treated should first be compressed with dry sponges and then covered with microfibrillar collagen hemostat; moderate pressure with a dry sterile sponge should then be exerted. Pressure for one minute may control superficial capillary bleeding, but three to five minutes or more may be needed when high-pressure leaks from artery suture holes or other pronounced bleeding is encountered. If oozing is not controlled, additional microfibrillar collagen hemostat may be used. However, only the amount needed to produce hemostasis should be used and excess material should be removed by teasing or irrigating. This usually can be done without a recurrence of bleeding.

Since it is a foreign protein, microfibrillar collagen hemostat may exacerbate infection, abscess formation, wound dehiscence, mediastinitis, and adhesion formation. By sealing the surface, it may conceal deep hemorrhage or hematoma in penetrating wounds. Use of this hemostatic agent is contraindicated for skin closure, for healing of the wound edges is deterred. However, this preparation does not interfere with epidermal or bone healing.

Microfibrillar collagen hemostat must be kept dry, since moisture impairs its hemostatic capacity. It is inactivated by autoclaving and should not be resterilized. Sterility is not guaranteed once the container is opened; therefore, any unused portion should be discarded. Care should be taken to avoid spillage on nonbleeding surfaces, particularly in abdominal or thoracic viscera.

Information is insufficient to determine its teratogenic potential, and this preparation should be used with caution in pregnant women.

ROUTE, USUAL DOSAGE, AND PREPARATIONS. *Topical*: For capillary bleeding, 1 g is usually sufficient for a 50 cm² area. Thicker coverage is required for more pronounced bleeding. To control oozing from cancellous bone, the preparation should be firmly packed into the spongy bone surface and compressed for 5 to 10 minutes.

> *Avitene* (Avicon). Microfibrillar collagen hemostat (sterile) in 1 and 5 g jars contained in a sealed can. (Distributed by Alcon Laboratories.)

THROMBIN

This sterile plasma protein substance is prepared from bovine prothrombin and is used topically to control capillary oozing in operative procedures. It also has been used successfully to shorten the duration of bleeding from puncture sites in heparinized patients (eg, after hemodialysis). Thrombin is capable of clotting whole blood, plasma, or a solution of fibrinogen without the addition of other substances; it also may be combined with gelatin sponge but should not be used to moisten microfibrillar collagen hemostat. Thrombin alone does not control arterial bleeding.

When applied to denuded tissue, thrombin is rapidly neutralized by antithrombins, and its activity is reduced as a result of absorption on fibrin. There is little danger of thrombin being absorbed into the vascular system.

Thrombin has been instilled into the stomach in an effort to hasten hemostasis in ulcerative disease, but its action is limited because of its rapid transit through the stomach. In addition, thrombin becomes inactive below pH 5.

This compound is stable as a dry powder if stored between 2 and 8 C. In solution, it begins to lose activity within eight hours at room temperature or within 48 hours if refrigerated. It should never be injected, particularly intravenously, for there is danger of thrombosis and death within a few minutes. Since antigenic reactions have occurred in animals, an allergic phenomenon is a remote possibility.

ROUTE, USUAL DOSAGE, AND PREPARATIONS. *Topical* (in wound or at operative site): Thrombin is dusted on as a powder, applied as a solution by flooding or spraying the site, or combined with a suitable sponge matrix (eg, absorbable gelatin sponge).

> *Thrombin, Topical* (Parke, Davis). Powder 1,000, 5,000, and 10,000 unit containers. The 5,000 unit package also contains a 5 ml container of sterile isotonic sodium choride diluent with phemerol 0.02 mg/ml as a preservative.

Selected References

Aledort LM: The Management of Hemophilia: Manual available without charge from the National Hemophilia Foundation, 25 W 39th St, New York, NY, 10018.

Aledort LM: Hematologic management and surgery in hemophilia. *Mt Sinai J Med* 44:371-373, 1977.

Aledort LM: Methods of care, products available, complications of therapy. *Mt Sinai J Med* 44:332-338, 1977.

Aledort LM: Factor IX and thrombosis. *Scand J Haematol* 30(suppl):40-42, 1977.

Aledort LM (ed): Recent advances in hemophilia. *Ann NY Acad Sci* 240:1-426, 1975.

Blatt PM, et al: Antihemophilic factor concentrate therapy in von Willebrand disease. *JAMA* 236:2770-2772, 1976.

Bloom AL, Peake IR: Molecular genetics of factor VIII and its disorders. *Semin Hematol* 14:319-339, 1977.

Fratantoni JC: New concepts in treating hemophilia. *Drug Ther (Hosp)* 2:35-46, (June) 1977.

Girolani A, et al: Immunological investigation of hemophilia B with tentative classification of the disease into five variants. *Vox Sang* 32:230-238, 1977.

Gralnick HR, et al: von Willebrand's disease. Combined qualitative and quantitative abnormalities. *N Engl J Med* 296:1024-1030, 1977.

Green D, Chediak JR: von Willebrand's disease: Current concepts. *Am J Med* 62:315-318, 1977.

Hilgartner MW: Management of hemophilia: Routine and crises. *Drug Ther* 8:141-154, (Feb) 1978.

Hilgartner MW, Sergis E: Current therapy for hemophiliacs: Home care and therapeutic complications. *Mt Sinai J Med* 44:316-331, 1977.

Honig GR: Koagulation vitamin deficiencies. *Drug Ther* 5:108-114, (March) 1975.

Houghie C: Hemophilia: Diseases and patient. *Drug Ther* 5:61-70, (July) 1975.

Hruby MA: Bleeding disorders in children. *Compr Ther* 3:26-34, (Sept) 1977.

Kelly P, Penner JA: Antihemophilic factor inhibitors: Management with prothrombin complex concentrates. *JAMA* 236:2061-2064, 1976.

Mannuci PM: Side effects of antihemophilic concentrates. *Scand J Haematol* 30(suppl):1-5, 1977.

Mannuci PM, et al: 1-Deamino-8-D-arginine vasopressin: New pharmacological approach to management of hemophilia and von Willebrand's disease. *Lancet* 1:869-872, 1977.

Ménache' D: Report of task force on clinical use of factor IX concentrates. *Thromb Haemostas* 35:748-750, 1976.

Ratnoff OD: Antihemophilic factor (factor VIII). *Ann Intern Med* 88:403-409, 1978.

Seeff LB, Hoofnagle J: Chronic hepatitis in hemophilia. *Ann Intern Med* 86:818-820, 1977.

Seeler RA: Vitamin K revisited. *Postgrad Med* 55:179-180, (March) 1974.

Telfer MC, Chediak J: Factor VIII-related disorders and their relationship to pregnancy. *J Reprod Med* 19:211-222, 1977.

Yorke AJ, Mant MJ: Factor VII deficiency and surgery: Is preoperative replacement therapy necessary? *JAMA* 238:424-425, 1977.

Immunomodulators | 66

Once the concept that an immunologic response could be a "double-edged sword" became apparent (for example, the benefit of immunization with viral vaccines contrasted to the detrimental immunologic responses in allergic asthma), diverse clinical applications of the discipline ensued. The province of clinical immunology has paralleled the rapid expansion of basic immunologic knowledge and now embraces the clinical considerations and the care of all the multiple aspects of immune responses as they affect man. Many patients having diseases with immunologic overtones are now considered candidates for immunotherapy.

Perhaps more dramatically than in any other area of drug therapy, the clinical use of agents that affect immune responses has preceded, in large part, an experimental basis for rational use. The relative lack of controlled human trials and less than desirable in vivo and in vitro pharmacologic studies are further complicated by rapidly changing concepts and an increasing awareness of the complexity of human immunologic responses. Much of what seemed thoroughly credible two or three years ago is, at least for the present, no longer tenable.

THE IMMUNE RESPONSE

The hallmark of vertebrate immunologic responses is a two-component system; this is most easily demonstrated in birds, in which two independent and anatomically delineated lymphoid organs exist. The effects of an immunologic response are mediated by the production of specifically modified serum antibodies or by specifically altered, sensitized cells with the capacity to recognize and react with the initiating antigen. Although the two-component concept is too simplistic, it provides an operational approach to understanding immunologic disease.

Cellular Mediators of Immune Response: The progenitors of lymphoid cells appear within fetal liver and primary lymphoid organs during the first two months of gestation. In concert with lymphoid precursor migration, the epithelial framework of the thymus, spleen, and lymph nodes is developing. The thymic stroma appears to be crucial in providing the proper environment for prothymic lymphocytes that have migrated there. An essential component for the induction of prothymocyte to thymocyte differentiation is the production, by the thymus gland, of one or more thymic hormones. Several candidates have been isolated and proposed as the putative hormone, including thymopoietin, facteur thymique serique (FTS), thymic humoral factor (THF), and thymosin. This hormone programs lymphoid induction, maturation, and migration from thymic cortex to medulla. The mature *T-lymphocytes* (T-LY) then disseminate with characteristic homing patterns to peripheral lymphoid organs.

Anatomically, the thymus reaches its maximal percentage of total body weight at birth with gradual involution to less than 0.02% of total body weight by age 15. Sensitive assays of serum thymosin levels have shown a gradual, but later than anatomical, decay with age. After migration from the thymus, T-LY characteristically are found in splenic periarteriolar and white pulp areas and in subcortical areas of lymph nodes or lymphoid aggregates. T-LY tend to be long lived and have characteristic recirculatory patterns through lymph and venous channels. They circulate in large volume through the thoracic duct; diversion of this pathway to the outside has been used to modulate T-LY immune responses. The traffic pattern characteristics of T-LY can be altered drastically by various agents and diseases. Under these circumstances, the results of random measurement of peripheral T-LY populations are quite misleading if they are used to monitor the suppressive effects of immunotherapy.

T-LY have many highly diverse immunobiologic functions. They provide a primary defense mechanism against selected viral, fungal, protozoal, and chronic- or facultative-type bacterial infections (eg, tuberculosis) and play an important, but not absolute, role in preventing the emergence or survival of neoplastic cells. In these roles, the T-LY is an amplifier cell that recruits uncommitted LY and macrophages to migrate to an area of inflammatory or immunologic interest. T-LY amplify inflammatory reactions by producing and releasing minihormones, lymphokines, that not only attract but also restrict other cells, especially monocytes and neutrophils, to the site of a reaction (eg, a PPD positive skin test, pulmonary area of tuberculous infection).

The other primary lymphoid effector cell, the *B-lymphocyte* (B-LY), does not yet have an identifiable, restricted site of maturation. The bone marrow seems to be the most likely primary staging area for B-LY. B-LY tend to have shorter biologic half-lives than T-LY and are found in the germinal follicles and subcapsular regions of lymphatic glands or the red pulp of the spleen. The ultimate differentiation of most B-LY, after appropriate antigen stimulation, is to an antibody-producing plasma cell. The production of these highly specific proteins is critical to facilitate phagocytosis of encapsulated organisms, inhibit the dissemination of enteroviruses and probably other viral infections, and mediate certain types of cytotoxic responses. IgA is the predominant antibody defense mechanism of most host-environmental interfaces, especially in the gut and bronchial tree. IgE, normally a minor immunoglobulin, mediates many of the allergic diseases, such as asthma and hay fever. IgD may have an important role in recognition of antigen and the initiation of antibody synthesis. Phylogenetically, IgM is the most primitive and IgG is the major immunoglobulin in human serum.

Recently, two non-T, non-B lymphocyte lines have been identified. One, the killer or *K-lymphocyte*, requires antibody assistance to effect cell destruction. The other, the natural killer or *NK-lymphocyte*, does not require antibody participation. Their significance in host responses, especially to tumor cells, is being explored.

Another major cell involved in the immunologic response is the *tissue macrophage*, which populates all important areas of reticuloendothelial prominence, especially the lung, liver, spleen, and lymph nodes. Although the most important functions of the macrophage and its monocyte precursor are phagocytosis and cytotoxicity against appropriate targets, they also play a pivotal role in both initiating and regulating almost all immune responses. Macrophages appear to be necessary for the proper alteration of certain antigens prior to lymphoid responses and occasionally may provide an alternate route for disposal of foreign material without requiring an immune response from the lymphoid series. They are essential for the appropriate response of T-LY to antigenic

stimuli. The monocyte-macrophage cell is a highly efficient and adaptable phagocyte and possesses many lysosomal hydrolytic enzymes. This cell line is efficiently recruited and concentrated by T-cell amplifying signals or focused by appropriate types of antibody at inflammatory sites. Once recruited, they provide highly effective cytotoxic activity against tumor cells or cells infected by a virus, protozoan, fungus, or bacterium.

Cellular Interactions During Immunologic Responses: Two novel concepts have confounded the simplistic dual lymphocyte theory of immunologic responses in man. There is now clear evidence of the existence of multiple subpopulations of T-LY. One T-LY subpopulation simply provides a basis for memory. These cells are critical for the retention of specific information necessary for future host responses to similar antigens. Amplifier LY constitute another subpopulation; their lymphokines attract nonimmunologically committed cells, usually monocytes, into the area of a T-LY response and thus provide a large population of effective phagocytic and killer cells in the area of appropriate stimulus. This population, in concert with other cells, mediates delayed hypersensitivity responses, allograft rejection, and resistance to fungal and protozoal diseases. Another T-LY subpopulation can be directly cytotoxic to histoincompatible or neoplastic cells.

It is now apparent that the most important role of the T-LY is to regulate immunologic and inflammatory responses (Miller, 1978). Two recently described T-LY subpopulations appear to be of primary importance in establishing an effective host response. One, helper T-LY, promote optimal differentiation of B-LY to plasma cells; thus, helper T-LY ultimately increase the quantity of IgM, IgG, IgA, IgD, or IgE produced. If not regulated, excess antibody production ensues and may lead to immune complex formation or autoimmune diseases.

A counterbalance mechanism is provided by a subpopulation of regulatory or suppressor T-LY. These T-LY can suppress not only other T-LY responses but also an effective B-LY response to an antigen. They may play critical roles in the clinical expression of certain viral-mediated diseases, resistance to neoplastic growth, autoimmune disease, and acquired immunodeficiencies. Clinically, the low titers of many autoantibodies that appear in the aged reflect diminished activity or number of regulatory cells.

Another closely related and equally significant concept is that immune responses are controlled by a gene complex located on chromosome 6 (Bach and Bach, 1978). These genes express their effects through the suppressor cell system. Therefore, heredity can directly affect the quality and quantity of responses to various tumor and microbial antigens. The significance of genetic control of immune responses in man is already evident. A human population immunized with influenza vaccine will develop highly diverse antibody responses. Only the low responders have an unexpectedly high incidence of certain histocompatibility antigens. This suggests that the basis for their deficient antibody production rests with similar immune response gene(s). Heredity also may alter responses to streptococcal antigens.

In summary, an effective immune response represents an orchestration of multiple cells interacting with an inciting stimulus and with each other. The interaction can be physical (cell to cell) or mediated by molecular signals in a programmed sequence that involves recognition, proliferation, and a final effect. The conductor appears to be an individual's genetic makeup. Any drug that alters the immune response may act on one or any combination of the sequence steps, and even though a drug is cytotoxic, if its lethal effects are selectively directed towards suppressor cells, the *net* result may be an enhanced immune response (Broder and Waldmann, 1978).

Laboratory Identification of Effector Cells and Molecules: In recent years, several laboratory assays that identify lymphocyte subpopulations have gained wide acceptance. As a rule, these assays measure lymphocyte populations in the peripheral blood and can provide useful diagnostic and prognostic information in patients with leukemias and lymphomas. They have only limited usefulness when LY traffic patterns are changed or certain drugs, especially corticosteroids, are being used. In these situations, peripheral lymphocyte values may have no relationship to actual events and may be seriously misleading. Lymphocyte populations are measured and expressed as percentage ratios (B-LY/T-LY); they should always be converted to absolute values by calculation from the leukocyte total and differential counts.

B-LY have multiple surface markers and receptor sites. Changes in B-LY receptors are not universally linked to disease states. If B-LY need quantification in individuals being treated with drugs that affect immune responses, at least two surface receptors should be measured. The most prevalent and useful surface-marker assays available on a limited basis in clinical laboratories are determination of B-LY membrane immunoglobulin and the receptor sites for activated components of complement.

The ultimate measurement of B-LY function is their ability to differentiate into plasma cells and produce antibody. Widely accepted, reproducible, and routinely available assays for quantitative determination of immunoglobulins, immunoelectrophoretic analysis of monoclonal or polyclonal immunoglobulins, or assays for specific antibodies (eg, ASO titers, viral titers) can be used as indices of B-LY function.

The identification of T-LY is somewhat simpler. T-LY bind sheep erythrocytes to their surface and can be measured as sheep erythrocyte T-LY rosettes. The assay, done on small amounts of blood containing heparin or ethylenediaminotetraacetate (EDTA), is widely used and results are reproducible. T-LY predominate in normal peripheral blood, comprising approximately 60% to 80% of all lymphocytes; values are also available for bone marrow, lymph nodes, and biologic fluids such as cerebrospinal, pleural, and peritoneal fluid.

T-LY function can be measured in several ways. Ability of the patient's T-LY to recall past immunologic encounters can be evaluated by routine skin testing with candidin, PPD, trichophytin, and streptodornase-streptokinase. More than 90% of the normal population will have a typical delayed hypersensitivity reaction to one or more antigens within 72 hours. Before absolute anergy can be documented, the ultimate test of T-LY function is to challenge the patient with a "new" antigen; those most commonly used are dinitrochlorbenzene (DNCB) or dinitrofluorbenzene (DNFB). After topical application, both low-molecular-weight compounds diffuse rapidly into the dermis and combine with protein, becoming an effective T-LY antigen. A normal response is evidenced by development of a contact hypersensitivity reaction; lack of a response indicates anergy.

DISORDERS AFFECTING IMMUNE AND INFLAMMATORY RESPONSES

Autoantibody-Mediated Diseases: Diseases that are theoretically amenable to immunomodulatory therapy can be categorized by their immunopathogenesis. Autoimmune diseases are characterized by destructive reactions during which antibodies attach to cell surface antigens and activate complement or macrophages or effector T-lymphocytes to attack target organ tissue directly. Cell destruction is limited to the target tissue affected. Unlike immune complex diseases, signs and symptoms of systemic inflammation are rare.

The most common target tissue affected by autoantibodies is the thyroid. Graves' disease, primary myxedema, or Hashimoto's thyroiditis are the sequelae, depending upon the type of effector mechanism present. Autoantibodies can cause hemolytic anemia, thrombocytopenia, pemphigus, or glomerulonephritis as isolated diseases. Large doses of corticosteroids are used to treat these immune disorders. Methotrexate and azathioprine [Imuran] have also been administered in severe pemphigus and pemphigoid skin diseases.

Myasthenia gravis is characterized by an autoantibody-mediated antagonism or destruction of the acetylcholine receptor. Corticosteroids, plasmapheresis, and immunosuppressants are used only in refractory cases; anticholinesterase agents and, possibly, thymectomy are the major components in a management program (see Chapter 18, Drugs Used in Myasthenia Gravis).

Immune Complex Diseases: This group of diseases, the prototype of which is systemic lupus erythematosus, is characterized by a clinical picture of diffuse vasculitis. The hallmark of these diseases is the presence of appropriately sized antigen-antibody complexes that escape reticuloendothelial phagocytosis and circulate, ultimately lodging in small vessels where they incite an inflammatory vasculitic response via the complement pathway. Although arthralgias, arthritis, rash, pleuropericarditis, and diverse forms of glomerulitis predominate, expression of these diseases can be extremely protean, based entirely on the final anatomical localization of the complexes. The more common diseases include systemic lupus erythematosus, mixed connective tissue disease, some forms of polyarteritis nodosa, chronic active hepatitis and viral hepatitis prodromes, mixed cryoglobulinemia, rheumatoid vasculitis, and many forms of glomerulonephritis.

Therapeutic interference in these immune complex diseases can range from attempts to inhibit antigen-driven lymphoid division or antibody production (cytotoxic drugs); removal of antigen-antibody complexes, antibody, or antigen (plasmapheresis); or inhibition of their final effector pathway, the complement system (corticosteroids).

Granulomatous Diseases: These chronic inflammatory diseases can best be characterized as a state of frustrated mononuclear responses. They often present as fever of undetermined etiology and are often associated with drug reactions, parasitic infections, chronically replicating viruses, or large, poorly degradable antigens. In many instances (eg, allergic granulomatoses, granulomatous hepatitis), a specific etiology is never found. The systemic signs and symptoms are secondary to a persistent T-lymphocytic and monocytic inflammatory response. Nonspecific attempts to reduce the inflammation with corticosteroids are often necessary. Recently, a new approach to treatment has been to attempt to enhance the immune response through the use of immunomodulating agents (eg, levamisole), thereby facilitating elimination of the offending agent and terminating the cycle of chronic inflammatory stimulus. This has the advantage of obviating the need to reduce the inflammatory response that often has resulted in increasing the risk of infection. Occasionally, specific cytotoxic agents are indicated in granulomatous diseases; Wegener's granulomatosis is the prototype.

Inflammatory And Vasculitic Diseases of Unknown Etiology: Polymyositis and dermatomyositis, some forms of polyarteritis nodosa, scleroderma, vasculitides associated with perivascular mononuclear infiltration and necrosis, and Behcet's syndrome are examples of multisystem inflammatory diseases without a known cause. Continuing advances in immunopathology will ultimately relegate most of these diseases to either the immune complex group or a group of T-lymphocytic, nongranulomatous, inflammatory diseases. Until this occurs, nonspecific broad forms of immunosuppression will continue to be used.

Immune Deficiency Diseases: Strictly classified, most of these diseases are secondary to a genetic aberration and can be classified according to the predominant lymphocyte defect. Chromosome X-linked agammaglobulinemia (B-LY), thymic hypoplasia (T-LY), severe combined immunodeficiency (B- and T-LY), or lymphocytic-myeloid deficiencies are examples of specific lymphoid defects. Hematopoietic hypoplasia is complete immunologic bankruptcy but can be treated with bone marrow transplantation from an appropriate donor. One identifiable cause of severe combined immunodeficiency is adenosine deaminase deficiency. Therapeutic attempts to provide this enzyme from exogenous sources (erythrocytes) are now in progress. Restoration of thymic function in patients with hereditary absence of the gland has been attempted by either fetal thymic transplantation or thymosin therapy, and patients with X-linked B-LY deficiencies or common variable immunodeficiency can be effectively treated periodically with pooled immunoglobulin therapy.

Therapeutic reversal of the most common immunodeficiency state, protein-calorie malnutrition, has only recently proved feasible with the advent of enteral and intravenous hyperalimentation. Restoration of protein-calorie intake by hyperalimentation, education, or diet will restore to normal the severely depressed T-LY functions and neutrophil, monocyte, and B-LY responses that occur during malnutrition (Faulk, 1974). The combination of immunologic defects and protein-calorie deprivation can be highly lethal during the postoperative period, in patients with systemic inflammatory diseases, and in those with malignancies who are undergoing chemotherapy or radiation. Since routine skin testing is a good indicator of T-LY function, preintervention determination of the presence and degree of anergy is a good predictor of potential postintervention morbidity and mortality and dictates a need for increased surveillance and improved nutrition.

Suppression Of Allograft Rejection: The most common rejection response to a histoincompatible renal, marrow, or heart graft is the development of cytotoxic T-LY. Monocytes and B-LY also play a role, the latter being especially prominent during accelerated or "white graft" rejection episodes. There is a consensus that corticosteroids are indispensable to attenuate rejection episodes and azathioprine may be helpful. The role of antilymphocyte globulin (ALG), an agent that would seem to be particularly helpful in allotransplantation because of its ability to markedly suppress T-LY mediated immune responses, is not clear. There is a dearth of controlled studies on this agent, and marked differences in potency between batches and source have added to the confusion (Barnes, 1977).

Erythroblastosis Fetalis: Hemolytic anemia in the fetus or neonate is caused by the transplacental transmission of maternal antibody that reacts with Rh$_o$(D)-positive antigen in the fetus. Rh$_o$(D) immune globulin [Gamulin Rh, HypRho-D, RhoGAM] is given to the mother following delivery to inhibit the development of maternal antibody and protect the fetus in any subsequent pregnancy. This prophylactic use of Rh$_o$(D) immune globulin was one of the first successful examples of immunomodulator therapy in man.

DRUG THERAPY

Corticosteroid therapy is the mainstay in the treatment of most immune diseases except immune deficiency diseases and hemolytic anemia in the newborn. Combination therapy with a corticosteroid and the immunosuppressant, azathioprine [Imuran], is used prophylactically and for maintenance therapy to suppress allograft rejection.

The cytotoxic drugs, cyclophosphamide [Cytoxan], chlorambucil [Leukeran], and methotrexate, are effective antineoplastic agents, especially when used in a large dose-pulsed method of administration. The larger doses enhance neoplastic cell cytotoxicity, and pulsed therapy permits interval recovery of the immune response to cancer. Conversely, these drugs are effective when employed conventionally in low doses to maintain immunosuppression with minimal toxicity. In view of their considerable potential toxicity, antineoplastic drugs are usually reserved for autoantibody-mediated, immune complex or granulomatous diseases and vasculitides that do not respond adequately to corticosteroid therapy. They, and some of the investigational agents, may be the only effective drug therapy for certain patients with granulomatous disease, polymyositis, and dermatomyositis.

Pooled immune globulin is the only approved drug for replacement therapy in immunodeficiency diseases. Rh$_o$(D) immune globulin has a long history of successful use in mothers to prevent or decrease the severity of Rh hemolytic disease of the newborn (erythroblastosis fetalis).

The specific uses of the miscellaneous investigational agents administered in immune disorders are discussed in the evaluations. Although their role is not well established, it is a reflection of the diversity of the clinical investigational activities in the treatment of immune disorders.

External diversion of thoracic lymph flow and plasmapheresis are not considered drugs and are not evaluated. The latter method ostensibly removes antigen-antibody complexes, antibody, and possibly even antigen and has been used in systemic lupus erythematosus and myasthenia gravis with varied success (Jones, 1977). Combining pheresis techniques with cytotoxic therapy that kills ultrasensitive lymphoid cells that begin to proliferate in response to decreasing antibody levels has also been tried.

Adverse Reactions and Precautions: Reactions peculiar to each drug are discussed in the evaluations, but certain generalities apply to all immunomodulator therapy. Marrow suppression by cytotoxic agents limits the availability of phagocytic and scavenger neutrophils and, to a lesser degree, monocytes. Regardless of the normal state of the immunologic responses, the lack of these final effector cells makes the danger of overwhelming infection paramount. The more subtle forms of drug-inhibited immunoinflammatory responses emerge clinically as infection with unusual or bizarre pathogens, for example, *Pneumocystis*, *Listeria*, cytomegalovirus, or *Toxoplasma*. More common, and just as dangerous, is gram-negative bacteremia or the inability to cope appropriately with *Streptococcus pneumoniae*.

Although the risk of infection in a compromised host is well appreciated, the risk of an increased incidence of neoplasia in patients undergoing immunomodulatory therapy is less clear but of great importance. There is no debate that the incidence (eg, central nervous system lymphomas) is higher in patients with renal and heart transplants. This may represent a complex situation involving multiple immunosuppressive agents and the stimulatory presence of a foreign graft. Impressive, but entirely anecdotal, data exist concerning the emergence of tumors in patients treated with low-dose, immunosuppressive cytotoxic therapy. Reports of highly malignant lymphomas predominate, but solid tumors in young patients also have been described. The confounding variable is that the diseases being treated have abnormal immune responses and, on that basis alone, are associated with a high risk of neoplasia.

The alkylating agents produce varying degrees of oligospermia and sometimes permanent azoospermia. To assure future childbearing potential, males should be informed of the opportunity for cryogenic storage of spermatozoa prior to the initiation of therapy.

The use of any immunomodulator entails both great theoretical and actual risk to the patient. The risk/benefit ratio should be determined and informed consent should be obtained.

ANTI-INFLAMMATORY CORTICOSTEROIDS

CORTICOSTEROIDS

Corticosteroids have broad effects on both immune and inflammatory responses. Man is relatively steroid-resistant and corticosteroid effects are not based on the cytotoxicity of these agents. Steroids do not prevent the recognition of the antigen by lymphoid cells and have little effect on the subsequent proliferation of the cells. Instead, they weaken or inhibit the soluble lymphocyte (lymphokine) signals needed to initiate and amplify an immune response, and the ability of a monocyte-macrophage cell to migrate into inflammatory sites is significantly affected. The net result, suppression of delayed hypersensitivity reactions, is secondary to the inability of the T-LY, monocytes, and neutrophils to respond efficiently. The ability of corti-

costeroids to suppress immune complex-initiated, granulocyte-amplified vasculitis and granulomatous inflammations is also secondary to their limitation of neutrophil and monocyte access to the reaction.

Corticosteroids markedly alter lymphocyte traffic and induce a peripheral blood lymphopenia. Lymphocytes tend to sequester within lymph nodes and bone marrow, but total body lymphocyte mass is probably not decreased. T-LY assay of peripheral blood samples to monitor this type of therapy or disease response is not useful. Anti-inflammatory dosages of steroids will suppress a delayed hypersensitivity reaction and the response to dinitrochlorbenzene.

Specific adverse reactions become manifest as the host becomes compromised. In most respects, they do not differ from reactions to other immunosuppressive agents, although the incidence of *Listeria* and disseminated fungal infections appears to be greater and patients have a propensity to develop relatively painless colonic perforations with subsequent gram-negative sepsis. Sudden decreases in serum albumin levels during acute inflammation and the presence of the nephrotic syndrome or liver disease will increase the amount of active steroid available and require a reduction of dose. No increased risk of neoplasia in patients receiving corticosteroids for long periods has been reported.

ROUTES, USUAL DOSAGE, AND PREPARATIONS. *Oral, Parenteral*: Prednisone 1 to 2 mg/kg of body weight (or the equivalent) provides tissue and serum concentrations with lymphoid, neutrophil, and monocyte effects. Doses higher than 2 mg/kg probably do not increase the therapeutic effect but do increase drug-related morbidity. In acute necrotizing inflammatory states, morning administration or divided daily doses are preferred to an alternate-day regimen when starting therapy. Once the disease or inflammatory condition is relatively stable, persistent attempts should be made to give the steroid on alternate days, since this reduces most adverse effects (Fauci et al, 1976). Many schedules have been tried. The most popular one is calculating the alternate-day dose as double the daily dosage. The dose also can be reduced gradually on alternate days. When severe drug reactions or the erythema multiforme syndromes that involve mucous membranes are being treated, intravenous administration is preferred because severe gastrointestinal mucosal loss may impair absorption.

For preparations, see Chapter 41.

CYTOTOXIC AGENTS

AZATHIOPRINE
[Imuran]

AZATHIOPRINE SODIUM
[Imuran]

Azathioprine, a purine analogue, is metabolized to its active immunosuppressive component, 6-mercaptopurine. This drug has been extensively administered in allotransplantation, systemic lupus erythematosus, rheumatoid arthritis, polymyositis, Crohn's disease, and many other systemic inflammatory states. The mechanism of immunosuppressive action of azathioprine is unknown. Experimentally, delayed hypersensitivity and cellular cytotoxicity tests are suppressed to a greater degree than are antibody responses. Azathioprine is widely used because its clinical efficacy is at least equal to that of the alkylating agents and it is relatively nontoxic. Clinically, azathioprine decreases the number of mononuclear and granulocytic cells available for migration to an area of inflammation. It also inhibits the proliferation of promyelocytes within bone marrow, thus decreasing the number of blood monocytes that ultimately become macrophages in the periphery (van Furth et al, 1975). Usual daily doses do not have pronounced effects on immunologic responses, per se. The length of time before a clinical response is noted with azathioprine is at least two to four weeks.

Hematologic toxicity is usually limited to mild leukopenia and thrombocytopenia. A limited number of cases of acute idiosyncratic aplastic anemia have occurred shortly after initiation of therapy or have suddenly interrupted a previously stable course.

Enzyme changes characteristic of hepatocellular necrosis and cholestasis may occur relatively early (one to two weeks) but also extremely late (years) during treatment and usually require discontinuing therapy. If administration must be continued, close observation is required, since deaths caused by hepatic decompensation have occurred.

A very important adverse effect is drug fever. If the febrile state is not recognized as being drug-related, extensive, hazardous, and expensive testing soon follows in order to exclude the diagnosis of an infection in the compromised host.

Nausea is common, especially within the first two weeks of therapy, and may necessitate drug withdrawal. Pancreatitis, hypersensitivity-type interstitial pneumonitis, and red cell aplasia have been reported occasionally. Unusually deep suntanning also has been noted frequently by patients on long-term therapy.

Because allopurinol inhibits xanthine oxidase, the enzyme required for 6-mercaptopurine metabolism, the dose of azathioprine should be reduced to one-third or one-fourth of the usual maintenance dose in patients taking the two drugs concomitantly.

Patients with allotransplants on long-term corticosteroid and azathioprine therapy have had normal infants and have had normal semen counts during treatment. To date, there has been no compelling evidence to suggest that fetal abnormalities occur during azathioprine therapy in man, although a significant teratogenic potential has been noted in animals. Azathioprine should be avoided during pregnancy if possible.

ROUTES, USUAL DOSAGE, AND PREPARATIONS. *Oral, Intravenous*: 2 to 3 mg/kg of body weight daily.

AZATHIOPRINE:
Imuran (Burroughs Wellcome). Tablets 50 mg.
AZATHIOPRINE SODIUM:
Imuran [*sodium*] (Burroughs Wellcome). Powder (lyophilized) equivalent to 100 mg of azathioprine.

CHLORAMBUCIL
[Leukeran]

This alkylating agent has been used extensively, in low doses, for immunosuppression in Europe but has not gained wide acceptance in the United States. Behcet's syndrome, systemic lupus erythematosus, and Wegener's granulomatosis have been reported to respond favorably to this drug. The induction time for an immunologic effect is apparently longer than that of cyclophosphamide, but serious hematologic depression appears to occur less frequently and urinary excretion is not involved. Oligospermia has been reported and azoospermia has been observed at cumulative doses of 400 mg.

See also Chapter 68, Antineoplastic Agents.

ROUTE, USUAL DOSAGE, AND PREPARATIONS. *Oral*: 0.05 to 0.1 mg/kg of body weight daily.

Leukeran (Burroughs Wellcome). Tablets 2 mg.

CYCLOPHOSPHAMIDE
[Cytoxan]

Cyclophosphamide is a cyclic mustard with alkylating properties. It is the only agent available that can inhibit an established secondary immune response, which usually is present in patients considered to be candidates for immunomodulatory therapy. Recent immunopharmacologic studies with cyclophosphamide provide a striking example of how this immunosuppressive drug can produce its effect by immunostimulation. Cyclophosphamide may have selective toxicity for regulator cells and, if given at the appropriate time, will increase delayed hypersensitivity reactions.

Since the drug must undergo hepatic microsomal activation prior to any effect on immune responses, it can be given orally. It also is administered intravenously and, if inadvertently given subcutaneously during intravenous injection, cyclophosphamide does not cause severe tissue necrosis. The effects are not immediate; with daily oral administration, 7 to 14 days usually are required before any clinically detectable immunomodulatory effect occurs.

The leukocyte count does not directly relate to immunomodulatory effects, and measuring T-LY and B-LY usually does not predict response because of the effects of the underlying disease and concomitant steroid therapy on lymphocyte kinetics. This observation also applies to most other immunomodulators.

Although never proved by clinical trial, there is a widespread belief that the addition of cyclophosphamide to a high-dose corticosteroid regimen allows gradual reduction of dosage to a less toxic level.

The decision to use cyclophosphamide must be based upon a favorable balance between improvement of the patient's condition versus the risk of drug therapy. This situation exists in patients with Wegener's granulomatosis, selected forms of vasculitis, and renal disease only. Its role in the treatment of systemic lupus erythematosus remains unsettled. Cyclophosphamide produces the usual adverse effects associated with most cytotoxic agents such as reversible alopecia, nausea, and vomiting. More serious reactions are life-threatening bone marrow suppression and acute hemorrhagic cystitis, bladder telangiectasia, and signs of abnormal urinary cytology. Adverse reactions affecting the bladder can be minimized by increasing fluid intake and emptying the bladder prior to sleep. Long-term use is associated with bladder fibrosis and carcinoma. Impaired urinary excretion has been reported with large doses only. The drug should be discontinued if hematuria occurs. Massive urinary bleeding may require supravesicular diversion.

When cyclophosphamide therapy is considered in the young, the probability of drug-induced infertility must be considered (*Br Med J*, 2:785-786, 1978; Sherins et al, 1978). Ovulation is inhibited and permanently impaired in 30% to 50% of women after continuous low-dose therapy; aspermia is also common after three to six months of therapy (Schein and Winokur, 1975). The teratogenic potential of cyclophosphamide appears to be low, but contraception should be encouraged during treatment.

For indications and reactions, see Chapter 68, Antineoplastic Agents.

Cytoxan (Mead Johnson). Powder 100, 200, and 500 mg; tablets, 25 and 50 mg.

METHOTREXATE SODIUM

Methotrexate is a folic acid analogue with marked affinity for dihydrofolic reductase, an enzyme required for thymidine and DNA synthesis. Its major effect is to inhibit cell proliferation. The primary immunotherapeutic use of methotrexate has been in patients with polymyositis or dermatomyositis (Metzger et al, 1974). Methotrexate has been added to drug regimens of patients with inflammatory muscle disease when there has been no clinical response after three to six months of therapy with prednisone 1 mg/kg.

The side effects of methotrexate are minor and include transient stomatitis and, rarely, bone marrow depression. Hypersensitivity pneumonitis has occurred. Severe hepatotoxic reactions observed in patients with psoriasis are related to daily dosage, underlying hepatic disease, and alcohol intake. Such reactions have not occurred in patients with polymyositis on the weekly low-dosage schedule. Routine hepatic enzyme tests do not predict hepatotoxicity. Aminopterin, another antifolic agent, has a strong association with fetal abnormalities and has been used as an abortifacient. Methotrexate has been reported to act as an abortifacient, but patients taking the drug after the first trimester have delivered normal children.

See also Chapter 68, Antineoplastic Agents.

ROUTE, USUAL DOSAGE, AND PREPARATIONS. *Intravenous*: 25 to 50 mg is given weekly until a clinical or enzyme response occurs; the amount is then decreased to 25 to 50 mg monthly. The dose of prednisone can be reduced gradually during once-monthly administration of methotrexate.

Methotrexate Sodium (Lederle). Solution equivalent to 2.5 and 25 mg of base/ml in 2 ml containers.

AGENTS FOR REPLACEMENT THERAPY

IMMUNE GLOBULIN

When the roles of B-LY and T-LY became evident, clinical classification of immunodeficiency states became a reality. Prior to this, therapy with immune globulins (ISG) was used haphazardly and over-enthusiastically in patients with "increased incidence of infection." Repeated patient visits, pain on injection, and unnecessary expense were the result.

It is evident that only certain types of bacterial infection, usually those caused by encapsulated organisms, such as pneumococci, meningococci, or staphylococci, are associated with true B-LY deficiencies. Repeated viral respiratory infections do not suggest the presence of a true B-LY immunodeficiency state. The concurrent development of laboratory tests for precise immunoglobulin quantitation and function has provided a means for documenting antibody deficiency.

An appropriate use of immune globulin is in the treatment of immunodeficiency states characterized by impaired or absent antibody synthesis. This does not include the transient hypogammaglobulinemia of infancy and selective IgA deficiency. IgA deficiency, common in the United States and frequently characterized by recurrent sinopulmonary infection, is not ameliorated by immune globulin therapy. Recurrent systemic infections with encapsulated organisms are not a significant problem and, since IgA-deficient patients can produce IgG, IgM, and, occasionally, IgA antibodies, there is the additional risk of hypersensitivity reactions. Furthermore, parenteral administration of immune globulin containing IgA does not result in transmucosal passage of antibody into bronchial lumina.

Pain at the site of injection is common after intramuscular administration. Systemic reactions, which presumably are secondary to immune globulin aggregates activating vasoactive and complement systems after gaining access to the intravascular space, include anxiety, nausea, vomiting, hypotension, and syncope. Treatment of these reactions is the same as that for any Type I hypersensitivity reaction.

With the increasing use of cell and plasma separators, there may be an increase in the use of plasma infusion therapy. This method is less painful and leads to a more rapid and greater elevation of antibody levels. Disadvantages inherent with the technique include the possibility of transmission of hepatitis virus, IgA reactions, and infusion of viable lymphoid cells or lymphocytotoxic antibody that may cause systemic reactions (Buckley, 1977).

See also Chapter 64, Blood, Blood Components, and Blood Substitutes, and Chapter 67, Vaccines and Antiserums.

ROUTE, USUAL DOSAGE AND PREPARATIONS. *Intramuscular*: 100 mg/kg of body weight (0.6 ml/kg) monthly. The volume required necessitates the use of multiple sites of injection (maximum, 5 ml/injection site), which is associated with pain and possible psychological morbidity, especially in children. In adults, the required volume may exceed the recommendations for a given injection site and more frequent administration of smaller volumes may be required (eg, 10 ml/ injection/week). The optimal dosage is not known. Many patients with antibody deficiency states have responded to approximately one-half the currently recommended dose.

Drug available generically: Concentrated solution containing 16.5 ± 1.5% gamma globulin in 2 and 10 ml containers.

THYMOSIN

Thymosin is a relatively crude low-molecular-weight hormone obtained by purifying bovine thymus extracts. The reported active thymosin fraction V actually contains up to 80 separate electrophoretic components. Blood levels of thymosin appear to be highest in children and young adults; the level begins to fall during the third and fourth decade and is lowest in the elderly. When thymosin is incubated with T-LY that lack surface receptors, their sheep erythrocyte rosetting capability is restored. Significant toxicity has not been reported to date in animal studies.

Early clinical trials with thymosin have produced mixed and mostly negative results. It seems to be of benefit only when there is some pre-existing T-LY function. The indications for thymosin other than in thymosin deficiency disorders remain to be determined. Controlled trials in patients with cancer and selected T-LY mediated immune diseases, such as systemic lupus erythematosus or rheumatoid arthritis, are in progress.

(Investigational drug)

AGENT FOR ERYTHROBLASTOSIS FETALIS

RHo IMMUNE GLOBULIN
[Gamulin Rh, HypRho-D, RhoGAM]

Rho(D) immune globulin is a sterile, concentrated solution of immune globulin prepared from the blood plasma of donors having high Rh antibody titers who are nonreactive for hepatitis B surface antigen. It is used to prevent formation of active antibodies in Rho(D)-negative, D^u-negative mothers after delivery of an Rho(D)-positive or D^u-positive infant, abortion of an Rh-positive fetus, or when Rh-positive blood is erroneously transfused into an Rho-negative woman. The bleeding associated with ectopic pregnancy and the remote possibility that the needle may penetrate the placenta or fetus when amniocentesis is performed also dictate that women with ectopic pregnancy or those undergoing amniocentesis be injected with Rho(D) immune globulin. To be effective, this product must be given within 72 hours after delivery, abortion, or other potentially sensitizing event. When more refined testing reveals that an Rh-negative mother is D^u-positive (Rho(D) factor variant), Rho immune globulin is not needed, since these individuals are not at risk of developing Rh antibodies. The mechanism by which anti-Rh prevents alloimmunization is not completely understood. Direct suppression by specific antibody combining with Rho erythrocyte antigens and enhanced erythrocyte removal from the circulation are probable.

Although the decrease in Rh sensitization resulting from the injection of Rho(D) immune globulin is greater than 90%, use of the globulin is not infallible. Thus, some women develop anti-Rh antibodies several months after delivery despite treatment. Others, who may have been "primed" by a first pregnancy (probably before delivery and treatment), may become sensitized during a subsequent Rho-positive pregnancy through the occurrence of small intrapartum fetal-maternal hemorrhages. Apparently, even with the widespread use of Rho(D) immune globulin, there will continue to be a few sensitized women. To identify these individuals, careful and thorough prenatal testing must still be continued.

Adverse reactions occur infrequently, are mild, and are generally confined to the site of injection. Slight elevations of temperature have been reported following injection. Sensitization due to repeated injection of immune globulins is unusual, and these agents do not appear to transmit serum hepatitis. When a significant number of fetal hemoglobin-positive erythrocytes are detected in maternal postpartum blood or Rho blood has been given to a Rh-negative individual, larger than recommended amounts of Rho(D) immune globulin (approximately one full dose of drug [300 mcg antibody/15 ml of transfused red cells]) must be given.

Rho(D) immune globulin is contraindicated in Rh-positive patients and in Rh-negative patients who have developed Rh antibodies because of a previous delivery, abortion, transfusion of Rh-positive blood, or other sensitizing event. This preparation is to be given only to the postpartum mother. *It must not be given to the infant.* It should be stored at 2 to 8 C and should not be frozen.

ROUTE, USUAL DOSAGE, AND PREPARATIONS. *Intramuscular*: The entire contents of one vial (containing 300 mcg of antibody globulin) is administered.

Drug available generically: Unit-dose vials. *Gamulin Rh* (Parke, Davis), *HypRho-D* (Cutter), *RhoGAM* (Ortho). Package contains a single dose of the drug and a 1:1,000 dilution for crossmatching.

MISCELLANEOUS INVESTIGATIONAL AGENTS OR USES

BCG ADJUVANT

CP ADJUVANT

Bacillus Calmette-Guerin vaccine (BCG), a suspension of viable, attenuated bovine tubercle bacilli, and Corynebacterium Parvum (CP), a killed bacterial suspension, have adjuvant or immunostimulating properties. Monocyte, and to a much lesser extent, T-LY functions are enhanced by these agents. Some animal studies have demonstrated increased resistance to selected tumors after use of CP or BCG in controlled situations. Most clinical trials have been with BCG vaccination of patients with melanomas, leukemia, and various carcinomas; in general, the clinical results have been disappointing. There is no debate, however, concerning the efficacy of intralesional injection of either adjuvant. Both CP and BCG will recruit and activate monocytes at the injection site and lead to tumor rejection by a cytotoxic nonspecific mechanism. This technique may have distinct advantages for use in selected skin lesions with or without regional lymph gland involvement.

The recent realization that CP and BCG therapy may increase lymphocyte suppressor activity and circulating immune complexes and possibly enhance tumor growth has forced a critical re-examination of the basis for their use however (Broder and Waldmann, 1978). BCG is available for vaccination against tuberculosis (see Chapter 67). CP and BCG should be used in the treatment of cancer only by an oncologist or immunologist conducting a clinical trial from which meaningful data can be obtained.

BCG has the additional drawback of being a viable suspension, and adverse effects ranging from influenza-like illnesses to extreme pyrexia and hepatitis have been reported when intralesional BCG vaccination was used in compromised patients (Sparks et al, 1973). Deaths have occurred. The severity of the adverse effects appears to be related to both dose and technique of administration. The multiple-puncture tine technique has had very low morbidity in contrast to intratumor injection. The latter method usually requires hospitalization and prophylactic medication to control adverse reactions. Persistent reactions have responded to isoniazid.

ANTI-HUMAN LYMPHOCYTE GLOBULIN
[Pressimmune]

Antilymphocyte globulin is an antibody produced in horses by human lymphocytes. The antibody is particularly directed toward T-LY and has little effect on antibody production by B-LY. It is very expensive because of the processing necessary to remove undesirable antibodies; however, serum sickness and bone marrow hypoplasia still occur occasionally. Although the agent can be shown to alter the immune response, neither an essential nor adjunctive role for this agent has been conclusively established in organ transplantation or other immune disorders.

DINITROCHLORBENZENE (DNCB)

There is increasing use of dinitrochlorbenzene to assess T-LY function. Ability to sensitize patients with dinitrochlorbenzene may indicate a favorable prognosis in those with malignancy and probable successful reversal of a state of malnutrition. Studies suggest that a negative response to skin testing with this antigen (anergy) is a strong predictor of postintervention, postoperative, or intrachemotherapeutic infection. Therapeutic attempts to reduce the anergic state by improved nutrition are indicated, if possible, prior to intervention.

The following procedure is recommended: 2,000 mcg of dinitrochlorbenzene in 0.1 ml of acetone is dropped within a 1 cm-diameter stainless steel or inert plastic ring on the volar surface of the forearm within two hours after preparation. After air drying, the site of application is covered with a bandage for four to six hours.

Several possible skin reactions can occur: An *immediate* erythematous flare usually indicates a pharmacologic response that has no relevance to the state of lymphocyte function. Within three to five days, a vesicular, erythematous, mildly indurated and pruritic area develops at the original site of application, indicating a *primary* T-LY reaction. If no spontaneous in situ reaction occurs within 10 to 14 days, the subject is challenged with 50 mcg, 100 mcg, and 200 mcg of dinitrochlorbenzene and acetone at separate sites on the volar surface of the opposite forearm; the subsequent *secondary* skin reaction is evaluated within the next 4 to 48 hours.

If the skin response is exaggerated and becomes uncomfortable, topical steroid creams may be applied. Test sites may become hyperpigmented and remain so for two to four months thereafter.

Since dinitrochlorbenzene incites a vigorous T-LY and monocyte reaction at the site of application, topical administration of this chemical in a previously sensitized patient can be used to recruit cytotoxic cells to an area of local tumor, fungus, or viral infection. Currently, this mode of therapy is clearly investigational.

FRENTIZOLE

Frentizole, 1-(6-methoxy-2-benzothiazolyl)-3-phenyl urea, appears to have broad B-LY and T-LY suppressive activity. In preliminary studies, it appears to produce only minimal host-compromising side effects.

INDOMETHACIN
[Indocin]

T-lymphocyte suppressor effects may be mediated in part by prostaglandins. In vitro tests and in vivo trials in normal individuals and patients with hypogammaglobulinemia using indomethacin, a synthetase inhibitor, have shown that antibody recall responses are increased during therapy. Currently, the efficacy of indomethacin is being investigated in common variable immunodeficiency states, severe combined immunodeficiency states, and selected forms of nephritis.

See Chapter 7, Antiarthritic Drugs, and Chapter 8, Drugs Used in Gout, for a discussion of the pharmacology, therapeutic indications, and preparations for indomethacin.

LEVAMISOLE

Levamisole (tetramisole) has been used for a number of years as an oral ascaricide in many parts of the world. Its properties as an immunomodulator have led to its investigation in a number of other diseases states (Symoens and Rosenthal, 1977). In vitro, both monocyte and T-LY functions are stimulated by levamisole, apparently secondary to alteration of intracellular cyclic AMP/GMP ratios. T-LY suppressor functions appear to be consistently enhanced. The drug has been reported to restore delayed hypersensitivity skin tests to normal in patients with cancer (Tripodi et al, 1973) and rheumatoid arthritis (Basch et al, 1977). Some degree of T-LY function is probably necessary for its successful use.

Trials with levamisole in a number of diseases, including those assumed to be secondary to deficient suppressor function, especially systemic lupus erythematosus and rheumatoid arthritis (International Symposium on Levamisole in Rheumatoid Arthritis, *J Rheumatol*, 1978), are now in progress. See also Chapter 7, Antiarthritic Drugs. Results have not been consistent in patients with recurrent aphthous stomatitis, recurrent herpes simplex, and various forms of cancer.

A single anthelmintic dose of levamisole (2.5 mg/kg) may be associated with mild side effects (nervousness, insomnia, gastrointestinal upset, alterations in taste and smell). Repeated administration, which is often required in investigational situations when the drug is used as an immunomodulator, may cause severe adverse reactions in certain patients (skin rash, febrile illness, mouth ulceration, neutropenia, thrombocytopenia, agranulocytosis). Proteinuria and a type of immune complex nephropathy also have been reported. (See also El-Ghobarey et al, 1978 and Symoens et al, 1978.) Generally, severe adverse reactions are more common when steroid therapy is given concomitantly or when doses larger than 150 mg daily are used for two or three days per week. Because of these adverse reactions, some investigators use an initial daily dose of 50 mg, increasing the amount by 50 mg every two weeks to a maximum of 150 mg.

LITHIUM CARBONATE

The elevated peripheral leukocyte counts, which are presumed to be secondary to increased marrow production, that occur during lithium treatment has increased interest in the supportive use of this drug during cytotoxic therapy. Lithium also prevents increases in lymphocyte intracellular cyclic AMP and is capable of enhancing lymphocyte proliferation and decreasing T-LY suppressor activity. Its future role in immunomodulation is being explored.

NIRIDAZOLE
[Ambilhar]

Niridazole is an anthelmintic agent with selective T-LY inhibiting properties and very little B-LY and antibody inhibitory effects. Long-term suppression of graft rejection and delayed hypersensitivity responses have been reported in man when the drug was used in doses much lower than those used for parasitic disease (Webster et al, 1975). When used as an antischistosomal agent in man, it apparently produces few toxic effects (see Chapter 83, Anthelmintics).

TRANSFER FACTOR

Transfer factor (TF) is a very enigmatic, low-molecular-weight, nonsensitizing polyribonucleotide-polypeptide extracted from human leukocytes. It was originally thought to be capable of transferring highly specific immunologic information to a recipient after intramuscular administration. Recent evidence suggests that both nonspecific and specific immunologic stimulation are transferred. Transfer factor has several theoretical advantages, the most obvious being an absence of viable cells and histocompatibility antigens. Any donor with the desired positive delayed hypersensitivity skin test can be used as a source of transfer factor. Transfer of immune information by transfer factor is usually quite rapid; the recipient may develop a positive delayed hypersensitivity skin test within 48 to 72 hours. In most immunodeficiency disorders, repeated administration has been necessary.

The clinical applications of transfer factor have been promising in only a few diseases: disseminated coccidioidomycosis and other disseminated fungal infections and in some patients with chronic mucocutaneous candidosis. The increasing ease of cell separation may increase interest in preparing this substance but, at this time, use of transfer factor is still clearly investigational. Its application and use should not be indiscriminate since there are theoretical disadvantages to nonspecific immunostimulation in certain immune deficiency states.

Selected References

International symposium on levamisole in rheumatoid arthritis. *J Rheumatol* 5(suppl 4):1-153, 1978.

Treatment of childhood cancer: Effects on gonads. *Br Med J* 2:785-786, 1978.

Bach FH, Bach ML: Major histocompatibility complex: Genetic control of antigens eliciting cell-mediated immune reactions, in Samter M, et al (eds): *Immunological Diseases*, ed 3. Boston, Little, Brown and Company, 1978, vol 1, 325-340.

Barnes AD: Clinical use of antilymphocyte globulin, in Thompson RA (ed): *Recent Advances in Clinical Immunology*. New York, Churchill Livingstone, 1977, 203-217.

Basch CM, et al: Cellular immune reactivity in patients with rheumatoid arthritis and effects of levamisole. *J Rheumatol* 4:377-388, 1977.

Broder S, Waldmann TA: Suppressor-cell network in cancer, parts 1 and 2. 299:1281-1284, 1335-1341, 1978.

Buckley RH: Replacement therapy in immunodeficiency, in Thompson RA (ed): *Recent Advances in Clinical Immunology*. New York, Churchill Livingstone, 1977, 219-244.

El-Ghobarey AF, et al: Clinical and laboratory studies of levamisole in patients with rheumatoid arthritis. *Q J Med* 47:385-400, 1978.

Fauci AS, et al: Glucocorticosteroid therapy: Mechanisms of action and clinical considerations. *Ann Intern Med* 84:304-315, 1976.

Faulk WP: Nutrition and immunity. *Nature* 250:283-284, 1974.

Jones JV: Plasmapheresis: Great economy in use of horses. *N Engl J Med* 297:1173-1175, 1977.

Metzger AL, et al: Polymyositis and dermatomyositis: Combined methotrexate and corticosteroid therapy. *Ann Intern Med* 81:182-189, 1974.

Miller JFAP: Cellular basis of immune responses, in Samter M, et al (eds): *Immunological Diseases*, ed 3. Boston, Little Brown and Company, 1978, vol 1, 35-48.

Schein PS, Winokur SH: Immunosuppressive and cytotoxic chemotherapy: Long-term complications. *Ann Intern Med* 82:84-95, 1975.

Sherins RJ, et al: Gynecomastia and gonadal dysfunction in adolescent boys treated with chemotherapy. *N Engl J Med* 299:12-16, 1978.

Sparks FC, et al: Complications of BCG immunotherapy in patients with cancer. *N Engl J Med* 289:827-830, 1973.

Symoens J, Rosenthal M: Levamisole in modulation of immune response: Current experimental and clinical state. *J Reticuloendothel Soc* 21:175-221, 1977.

Symoens J, et al: Adverse reactions to levamisole. *Cancer Treat Rep* 62: 1721-1730, 1978.

Tripodi D, et al: Drug-induced restoration of cutaneous delayed hypersensitivity in anergic patients with cancer. *N Engl J Med* 289:354-357, 1973.

van Furth R, et al: Effect of azathioprine (Imuran) on cell cycle of promonocytes and production of monocytes in bone marrow. *J Exp Med* 141:531-546, 1975.

Webster LT Jr, et al: Suppression of delayed hypersensitivity in schistosome-infected patients by niridazole. *N Engl J Med* 292:1144-1147, 1975.

Vaccines and Antiserums | 67

Vaccines are biological agents used to induce active immunity against infectious diseases. Bacterial vaccines are prepared from whole bacteria (eg, pertussis vaccine) or from purified capsular polysaccharides of certain bacteria (eg, pneumococcal vaccine) and toxoids from formaldehyde-treated bacterial toxins (eg, diphtheria toxoid). Bacterial vaccines and toxoids may be single agents (eg, typhoid vaccine, tetanus toxoid) or combined (eg, diphtheria and tetanus toxoids and pertussis vaccine). With the exception of BCG for tuberculosis, they are composed of nonliving agents. Viral vaccines are composed of live, attenuated viruses (eg, measles) or inactivated nonliving viruses (eg, influenza). They may be used as single agents or in various combinations; inactivated virus vaccines are not combined with live virus vaccines.

Antiserums are used to produce passive immunity prophylactically, such as following exposure to an infectious agent (eg, hepatitis B, rabies, tetanus). Diphtheria and tetanus antiserums (antitoxins) can be used either prophylactically or therapeutically. Botulism antitoxin is only used therapeutically (see Chapter 87). The source of these preparations may be man or animal; they consist of antibody concentrated in the gamma globulin fraction of serum.

Agents discussed in this chapter include those used for routine basic immunizations, those used for special immunization procedures (ie, related to direct exposure or enhanced susceptibility to infection, recommended for foreign travel), and those used therapeutically in special situations.

The Center for Disease Control (CDC), U.S. Public Health Service, Atlanta, Ga. 30333, provides a number of services related to infectious disease control. Although the Center serves principally as a resource for state and local health departments, it also offers direct and indirect services to hospitals and practicing physicians in the United States. Its range of services includes reference laboratory diagnosis and epidemiologic consultation (both generally arranged through state health departments) and supply of special prophylactic or therapeutic drugs and biologicals. It maintains 24-hour telephone coverage, and inquiries are routed to appropriate specialty areas during working hours. Sufficient staff is available during off-duty hours to respond promptly to emergency needs. The Center's telephone numbers are: weekdays (8:00 am to 5:00 pm, EST) (404) 329-3676; off-duty hours, (404) 329-3644.

Immunization requirements for foreign travel vary from time to time in various countries. Local and state health departments can advise travelers on the best sequence of inoculations, including those that may be required for re-entry into the United States. The Center publishes a useful guide, *Vaccination Certificate Requirements for International Travel.*

Although routine immunization programs have controlled or virtually eliminated some infectious diseases in the United States, outbreaks of diseases for which effective vaccines exist continue

to occur, especially in deprived socio-economic and remote geographic areas. Tables 1 and 2 present schedules for basic immunization and recall doses for infants and those who did not receive immunization during infancy.

Parents and older patients should be informed of the proposed immunizations and of the necessity of maintaining a suitable record of vaccinations. For medical and legal reasons, it is desirable for the physician to record the vaccine used, manufacturer, lot number, volume injected, site used, and any reported reactions. If the time sequence of a recommended schedule is interrupted, it is not necessary to start the series over again.

The dose and concentration of biologi-

TABLE 1.
RECOMMENDED SCHEDULE FOR ACTIVE IMMUNIZATION
OF NORMAL INFANTS AND CHILDREN

2 mo	DTP[1]	TOPV[2a]
4 mo	DTP	TOPV
6 mo	DTP	2b
1 yr		Tuberculin Test[3]
15 mo	Measles,[4] Rubella[4]	Mumps[4]
1½ yr	DTP	TOPV
4-6 yr	DTP	TOPV
14-16 yr	Td[5]—repeat every 10 years	

[1] DTP—diphtheria and tetanus toxoids and pertussis vaccine.

[2a] TOPV—trivalent oral poliovirus vaccine. This recommendation is suitable for breast-fed as well as bottle-fed infants.

[2b] A third dose of TOPV is optional but may be given in areas of high endemicity of poliomyelitis.

[3] Frequency of repeated tuberculin tests depends on risk of exposure of the child and on the prevalence of tuberculosis in the population group. For the pediatrician's office or outpatient clinic, an annual or biennial tuberculin test, unless local circumstances clearly indicate otherwise, is appropriate. The initial test should be done at the time of, or preceding, the measles immunization.

[4] May be given at 15 months as measles-rubella or measles-mumps-rubella combined vaccines (see evaluations on Mumps Virus Vaccine Live and Rubella Virus Vaccine Live for further discussion of age of administration).

[5] Td—tetanus and diphtheria toxoids adsorbed for adult use for those more than 7 years of age, in contrast to diphtheria and tetanus (DT) toxoids which contain a larger amount of diphtheria antigen. *Tetanus toxoid at time of injury:* For clean, minor wounds, no booster dose is needed by a fully immunized child unless more than 10 years have elapsed since the last dose. For contaminated wounds, a booster dose should be given if more than 5 years have elapsed since the last dose.

Concentration and Storage of Vaccines
Because the concentration of antigen varies in different products, the manufacturer's package insert should be consulted regarding the volume of individual doses of immunizing agents.

Because biologics are of varying stability, the manufacturer's recommendations for optimal storage conditions (eg, temperature, light) should be carefully followed. Failure to observe these precautions may significantly reduce the potency and effectiveness of the vaccines.

Adapted from Report of the Committee on Infectious Diseases, American Academy of Pediatrics, 1977.

cals may vary with the manufacturer, and it is important to be familiar with the package inserts of all products used.

Intramuscular injections should be deep into the chosen site, either deltoid, mid-lateral thigh, or upper outer quadrant of the buttock, with care exercised to avoid the sciatic nerve.

Adverse Reactions and Precautions

Any of the commonly used immunizing agents can produce undesirable, some-times life-threatening, reactions. Adverse reactions may result either from the in-jected agents or from a foreign protein incorporated with the agent during its manufacture (eg, egg protein in rabies vac-cine prepared in embryonated duck eggs); they often can be avoided with appropriate precautions or minimized with immediate therapy. A syringe containing epinephrine should be readily available.

If a severe febrile reaction, somnolence, or convulsion occurs, subsequent inocula-tions should be given cautiously. When

DTP (diphtheria, tetanus, pertussis) com-bined antigen is believed to be involved, further pertussis antigen should be avoided. Resumption of injections depends upon the anticipated risk of exposure and the patient's clinical condition.

Vaccination with most live virus vaccines is contraindicated in patients with im-paired cellular immunity (eg, those receiv-ing corticosteroids, antineoplastic agents, immunosuppressive agents, radiation therapy); those with leukemia, lymphoma, generalized malignancy, or dysgamma-globulinemia; and during pregnancy. However, the newly developed live at-tenuated varicella-zoster vaccine may be an exception; if preliminary findings are confirmed, this vaccine will be recom-mended for use in children with leukemia. Routine immunizations generally should be deferred if the patient has an active in-fection. When required by circumstances, poliomyelitis and yellow fever live virus vaccines may be used during pregnancy.

When an antiserum must be used, one prepared from human sources is preferred. The two major reactions that follow injec-

TABLE 2.
PRIMARY IMMUNIZATION FOR CHILDREN NOT IMMUNIZED IN INFANCY*

Under 7 Years of Age

First visit	DTP, TOPV, Tuberculin Test
Interval after first visit	
1 mo	Measles,† Mumps, Rubella
2 mo	DTP, TOPV
4 mo	DTP, TOPV‡
10 to 16 mo or preschool	DTP, TOPV
Age 14-16 yr	Td—repeat every 10 yr

7 Years of Age and Over

First visit	Td, TOPV, Tuberculin Test
Interval after first visit	
1 mo	Measles, Mumps, Rubella
2 mo	Td, TOPV
8 to 14 mo	Td, TOPV
Age 14-16 yr	Td—repeat every 10 yr

*Physicians may choose to alter the sequence of these schedules if specific infections are prevalent at the time. For example, measles vaccine might be given on the first visit if an epidemic is underway in the community.

†Measles vaccine is not routinely given before 15 months of age (see Table 1).

‡Optional

Adapted from Report of the Committee on Infectious Diseases, American Academy of Pediatrics, 1977.

tion of hyperimmune serum of animal origin are anaphylaxis and serum sickness. A scratch, intradermal, or conjunctival test to determine sensitivity should precede injection, regardless of whether or not the patient previously received an injection of animal serum. *A syringe containing 1 ml of epinephrine 1:1,000 should be readily available.* A 1:1,000 dilution of the serum is injected intradermally, employing just enough to raise a visible bleb. The test is positive if a wheal appears within 30 minutes. The same fluid may be used for a scratch test, which may be safer. For the conjunctival test, one drop of a 1:10 dilution of serum in isotonic sodium chloride solution is instilled in one eye and one drop of sodium chloride solution in the other eye to serve as a control. If lacrimation and conjunctivitis occur within 30 minutes, the test is positive.

If the sensitivity test is positive and the need for serum is imperative, desensitization can be performed by injecting small, graded doses of the serum. For example, if no reaction occurs, the following doses are injected at 15-minute intervals: (1) 0.05 ml of 1:20 dilution, subcutaneously; (2) 0.1 ml of 1:10 dilution, subcutaneously; (3) 0.3 ml of 1:10 dilution, subcutaneously; (4) 0.1 ml of undiluted serum, subcutaneously; (5) 0.2 ml of undiluted serum, intramuscularly; (6) 0.5 ml of undiluted serum, intramuscularly; and (7) remaining dose, intramuscularly.

If anaphylactic reactions occur, epinephrine 1:1,000 (adults, 0.5 ml; children, 0.01 ml/kg of body weight [maximum, 0.5 ml]) is immediately injected subcutaneously or intramuscularly. If there is no improvement, epinephrine 1:1,000 diluted 1:10 in physiologic saline is injected slowly intravenously. The dose may be repeated in 1 to 15 minutes if necessary. Antihistamines may be given intramuscularly to treat severe urticaria or edema of the larynx. Vasopressors, positive-pressure oxygen, and corticosteroids may be useful.

Serum sickness, manifested by urticaria, lymphadenopathy, arthralgia, and fever, usually appears a few days or weeks after injection of serum. The symptoms usually can be alleviated by use of salicylates, antihistamines, and corticosteroids.

ROUTINE IMMUNIZING AGENTS

The use of single antigens is recommended only when there is a definite contraindication to the other components in a combined antigen preparation.

Diphtheria, Tetanus, and Pertussis

DIPHTHERIA TOXOID ADSORBED

Diphtheria is primarily a disease of childhood but may occur in all age groups. Although it is now uncommon in the United States, localized outbreaks are reported occasionally. In recent years (1971-1975), respiratory diphtheria occurred more often in children than adults, but cutaneous diphtheria was recognized much more commonly in adults. Diphtheria antitoxin is given with appropriate antibiotics to treat clinical diphtheria, but the antitoxin is probably of no value for cutaneous lesions.

Diphtheria toxoid is a preparation of detoxified growth products of *Corynebacterium diphtheriae*. It is not generally available alone because it usually is given in combination with tetanus toxoid and pertussis vaccine (DTP) for primary immunization of infants and young children. Diphtheria toxoid also is combined with tetanus toxoid without pertussis vaccine in pediatric preparations (DT) and, in reduced amounts, in adult preparations (Td).

Tenderness at the site of injection and, rarely, fever, malaise, myalgia, or sterile abscess may occur.

ROUTE AND USUAL DOSAGE.
Intramuscular: For primary immunization of children between 6 weeks and 7 years, the manufacturers' recommended dose of DTP should be given at four- to eight-week intervals for three doses. Ideally, immunization should begin at 2 to 3 months of age. A fourth dose should be given one year later at about 18 months of age and a booster dose given prior to entry in school (4 to 6 years of age).

For primary immunization of older children (7 years or more), two doses of Td should be given at four- to six-week intervals, and a booster dose should be given six months to one year after the second dose.

DIPHTHERIA ANTITOXIN

This sterile solution of concentrated antitoxin is obtained from the blood of horses hyperimmunized against diphtheria toxin. It is used to treat diphtheria or for prophylaxis in exposed, nonimmunized, susceptible individuals who are not under close surveillance. Antitoxin should be administered on the basis of a clinical diagnosis of diphtheria without waiting for bacteriologic confirmation. The dose depends upon the site and extent of the diphtheritic membrane, degree of toxicity, and duration of illness. Appropriate antimicrobial therapy (eg, penicillin, tetracyclines, erythromycin) helps eliminate bacteria from the infected sites but is of no value against the toxin.

Serum sickness (urticaria, fever, pruritus, malaise, arthralgia) may occur in 7 to 12 days. Before injecting diphtheria antitoxin, it is essential to obtain a history of previous injection of serum as well as of pre-existing asthma or allergy. A skin or conjunctival test for sensitivity should be performed in all patients. If a positive reaction occurs, the antitoxin should be administered according to the procedure on desensitization outlined in the section on Adverse Reactions and Precautions in the Introduction. Preparation for immediate administration of epinephrine 1:1,000 is essential before testing for sensitivity or administering diphtheria antitoxin. Active immunization with diphtheria toxoid, using a different site, should be initiated at the same time that diphtheria antitoxin is given.

ROUTES AND USUAL DOSAGE.
The entire dose required should be given at one time if possible.

Intramuscular: *Adults and children*, for prophylaxis, 1,000 to 10,000 units.

Intravenous: *Adults and children*, dosage is empiric, for treatment, 20,000 to 80,000 units or more, depending upon duration of illness, degree of toxicity, and site and size of membrane.

PERTUSSIS VACCINE

Immunization against pertussis early in life is strongly recommended because this disease is highly communicable and most deaths occur in infants less than 1 year of age. The widespread use of pertussis vaccine during the past 25 years has been associated with a marked reduction in morbidity and mortality from this disease. Pertussis vaccine is usually given in combination with diphtheria and tetanus toxoids (DTP).

Convulsions in infants following use of DTP are believed to be caused by the pertussis component; no further pertussis antigen should be used in this instance. Other contraindications include severe alteration of consciousness, focal neurologic signs, screaming episodes, collapse, and thrombocytopenic purpura. Severe reactions have occurred rarely following administration of pertussis vaccine to individuals of any age. However, the incidence is lower than that of similar effects produced by the disease itself. About 80% of cases of pertussis occur in the first five years of life, and fatalities are rare in older patients. Because of this pattern of morbidity and mortality and an apparent increase in the incidence of adverse reactions with age, use of the vaccine after the seventh birthday generally is not advisable. Other common adverse reactions include induration, local tenderness, fever, and malaise. Formation of sterile abscesses is rare.

See also the evaluation on Diphtheria and Tetanus Toxoids and Pertussis Vaccine (DTP).

ROUTE AND USUAL DOSAGE.
Intramuscular: *Children 2 months to 6 years*, 4 protective units (0.5 ml) at four- to eight-week intervals for three doses (total of 12 protective units); a reinforcing fourth injection should be given about one year after completion of the initial course and a recall injection upon entry into school. Recall injections upon intimate exposure may be given to children up to 7 years of age.

TETANUS TOXOID ADSORBED

An immunizing course of tetanus toxoid is highly effective, produces few adverse reactions, and provides long lasting protection against tetanus. Tetanus toxoid is a sterile preparation of detoxified growth products of *Clostridium tetani*. It is available in fluid or adsorbed form; *the latter is preferred*. This agent usually is given in combination with diphtheria toxoid and pertussis vaccine (DTP) for primary immunization of infants and young children. For primary immunization of adults, Td (tetanus and diphtheria toxoids adsorbed for adult use) or tetanus toxoid alone may be used. For children in whom the pertussis component is contraindicated, DT is recommended.

Tetanus toxoid is used prophylactically for wound management in patients not completely immunized. Considerations in treatment are the condition of the wounds and whether to use tetanus toxoid for active immunization or tetanus immune globulin for passive immunization. A guide to wound management is given in Table 3.

Adverse reactions occur infrequently and include erythema, induration, and tenderness at the site of injection; fever and malaise occur more rarely. The incidence of adverse reactions may be higher in persons over 25 years of age. High tetanus antibody levels following too frequent booster doses of tetanus toxoid have been associated with hypersensitivity reactions. (See also the evaluations on the combinations of tetanus toxoid with diphtheria toxoid and pertussis vaccine.)

TABLE 3.
RECOMMENDED USE OF TETANUS TOXOID AND TETANUS IMMUNE GLOBULIN (HUMAN)—TIG—IN WOUND MANAGEMENT

TYPE OF WOUND	IMMUNIZATION STATUS
Unimmunized, Uncertain, or Incomplete (one or two doses of toxoid)	
Low-risk wound	One dose of Td* or DT† followed by completion of immunization; booster every 10 years thereafter.
Tetanus-prone wounds and wounds neglected for > 24 hr	One dose of Td* or DT† plus 250-500 U TIG followed by completion of immunization. Note: Use separate syringe and sites for TIG and toxoid.
Full Primary Immunization with Booster Dose Within 10 Years of Wound	
Low-risk wounds	No toxoid necessary.
Tetanus-prone wounds	If more than 5 years since last dose, one dose of Td.* If less than 5 years, no toxoid necessary.
Wound neglected > 24 hr	One dose of Td plus 250-500 U TIG.
Full Primary Immunization with No Booster Doses or Last Booster Dose > 10 Years	
Low-risk wounds	One dose of Td.
Tetanus-prone wounds	One dose of Td.
Wounds neglected > 24 hr	One dose of Td plus 250-500 U TIG.

Wound definition—It is impossible to categorize all clinical situations by any terminology. In this scheme "tetanus-prone" refers to wounds which yield anaerobic conditions or were incurred in circumstances yielding the probability of exposure to tetanus spores. Examples include severe necrotizing machinery injuries, puncture wounds, wounds heavily contaminated with animal excreta, and so forth. All others are to be considered low-risk from the standpoint of tetanus. Neglected wounds are at greater risk.

*Td—(adult) should be used in individuals more than 6 years old.

†DT—(pediatric) should be used individuals less than 6 years old.

From Report of the Committee on Infectious Diseases, American Academy of Pediatrics, 1977.

ROUTE AND USUAL DOSAGE.
Intramuscular: The adsorbed form is preferred to the fluid preparation. For *adults and children* not previously immunized, 0.5 ml for three injections; the second injection is given four to six weeks after the first and the third injection six months to one year after the second. A booster dose is given every ten years.

DIPHTHERIA AND TETANUS TOXOIDS AND PERTUSSIS VACCINE ADSORBED (DTP)

This combination of diphtheria and tetanus toxoids with pertussis vaccine is the recommended preparation for routine primary immunization and recall (booster) injections in children under 7 years of age. It is available both in fluid form and in precipitated or adsorbed form; *the latter is preferred* because its slower absorption increases immunogenicity.

The combined triple antigens are not recommended after the seventh birthday because of the increased possibility of severe local and, sometimes, generalized reactions; pertussis antigen is the ingredient most often suspected. Tetanus and diphtheria toxoids, adult type (Td), may be used for primary immunization of older patients (7 years or more); diphtheria and tetanus toxoids, pediatric type (DT), may be used in younger children. (See the evaluations.)

The most common untoward effects include transient fever with tenderness, erythema, and induration at the site of injection. Reactions involving the central nervous system may occur after any injection in a course and may be manifested by convulsions, uncontrollable screaming, infantile massive spasm, hypsarrhythmia, pseudotumor cerebri, or acute disseminated encephalomyelitis. Any central nervous system reaction is generally regarded as a contraindication to further use of pertussis antigen (see that evaluation and the Introduction).

ROUTE AND USUAL DOSAGE.
Intramuscular: *Infants 2 months of age*, initially, 0.5 ml, followed by two more doses at four- to eight-week intervals. A reinforcing fourth dose is given 7 to 12 months after the third, and a booster dose is given when the child is 5 to 6 years old. This preparation should not be used after the seventh birthday. (See the manufacturer's recommendations for volume dose of preparation used.)

DIPHTHERIA AND TETANUS TOXOIDS ADSORBED (Pediatric) (DT)

Diphtheria and tetanus toxoids pediatric (DT) may be used for primary immunization and recall injections in children up to 7 years of age when pertussis vaccine must be given separately or omitted.

As with other routine immunization procedures, use of combined diphtheria and tetanus toxoids should be deferred in the presence of active infection or febrile acute respiratory tract disease. (See the Introduction.)

ROUTE AND USUAL DOSAGE.
Intramuscular: *Infants and children up to 7 years*, two 0.5-ml doses of adsorbed DT at intervals of at least four weeks. A reinforcing injection to complete primary vaccination is given one year later and repeated at the time the child enters school.

TETANUS AND DIPHTHERIA TOXOIDS ADSORBED FOR ADULT USE (Td)

Tetanus and diphtheria toxoids adsorbed for adult use (Td) is used for primary immunization or recall (booster) injections in adults and children over 7 years of age. It contains the same amount of tetanus toxoid as in DTP but only 10% to 25% of the diphtheria toxoid. For use in wound management, see Table 3.

Reactions to Td are usually mild in patients under 20 years. They include erythema, induration, and tenderness at the site of injection; fever and malaise also may occur. See also the Introduction and evaluations on the individual toxoids.

ROUTE AND USUAL DOSAGE.
Intramuscular: *Adults and children 7 years and older*, two injections of 0.5 ml with an interval of at least four weeks

between injections. A reinforcing dose to complete basic immunization is given 6 to 12 months later and every ten years thereafter.

TETANUS IMMUNE GLOBULIN

Tetanus immune globulin is a sterile solution of globulins obtained from the plasma of adults hyperimmunized with tetanus toxoid. It is thought to be effective prophylactically in patients with wounds contaminated with *Clostridium tetani*. This agent is preferred to tetanus antitoxin for passive immunization and is used if the patient has received less than two immunizing doses of tetanus toxoid, if the wound is unattended for more than 24 hours, or if the history of immunization is uncertain.

Because tetanus immune globulin is of human origin, it is relatively free from risk of hypersensitivity reactions. As with other gamma globulin preparations, pain and erythema may occur at the site of injection. Tetanus immune globulin should be used intramuscularly only. Active immunization with tetanus toxoid should be initiated concomitantly and a different site and different syringe should be used for the injection.

ROUTE AND USUAL DOSAGE.
Intramuscular: For prophylaxis, *adults and children*, 250 units as a single dose. For treatment, the optimal therapeutic dose has not been established; 3,000 to 5,000 units usually are cited in the literature, but doses as large as 10,000 units and as small as 500 units have been used.

TETANUS ANTITOXIN EQUINE

Tetanus antitoxin is a sterile solution of concentrated antibody proteins obtained from the blood of horses hyperimmunized with tetanus toxin or toxoid. It is used prophylactically in nonimmunized patients with tetanus-prone wounds and as a part of therapy in patients with active tetanus. Because of the risk of hypersensitivity reactions, tetanus immune globulin is pre-

ferred; tetanus antitoxin should be used only when the former is not available.

Appropriate conjunctival and skin tests for sensitivity to equine serum should always precede use of tetanus antitoxin (see the section on Adverse Reactions and Precautions in the Introduction). Epinephrine 1:1,000 should be available for prompt treatment of any severe reactions that may occur. When given for prophylaxis, tetanus antitoxin should be administered intramuscularly to lessen the severity of reactions, which range from pain at the site of injection to serum sickness (arthralgia, urticaria, fever, malaise) and anaphylactic shock. For therapy, the intravenous route is preferred. Active immunization with tetanus toxoid should be initiated at the same time that tetanus antitoxin is given; a different site and a different syringe should be used.

ROUTES AND USUAL DOSAGE.
Intramuscular: *Adults and children*, for prophylaxis, 3,000 to 5,000 units within 24 hours after injury. If 48 hours have elapsed between the time of injury and treatment, 10,000 to 20,000 units should be given.
Intravenous: *Adults and children*, for treatment, 40,000 to 100,000 units or more.

Measles, Mumps, and Rubella

MEASLES VIRUS VACCINE LIVE

Widespread use of measles virus vaccines had reduced the overall incidence of measles by 95%, but more recently immunization efforts have lapsed in some areas with a consequent resurgence of cases. At present, it is generally believed that inoculation with live measles virus vaccine confers prolonged protection.

Live measles virus vaccine is a bacteriologically sterile preparation containing modified measles (rubeola) virus, attenuated strains derived from the original Edmonston B strain, grown in chick embryo cell cultures. It is capable of producing active immunity in a high percentage of recipients after a single dose and produces a noncommunicable, mild, or inapparent measles infection. Combinations of measles virus vaccine with live mumps and rubella virus vaccines are available.

Rarely, convulsions associated with fever have occurred after use of live measles virus vaccine. Other reactions observed rarely are thrombocytopenia, purpura, and central nervous system effects. No allergic reactions have been reported after administration of vaccine prepared from chick embryo tissue to persons with known allergy to egg protein; however, the risk should be considered in patients with known sensitivity to eggs.

Measles virus vaccine is contraindicated in the presence of any severe febrile illness and during pregnancy. It also is contraindicated in patients with leukemia, lymphoma, or generalized malignancy and those being treated with agents that may interfere with immune mechanisms (eg, corticosteroids, irradiation, antineoplastic agents). Vaccination should be postponed for three months after administration of immune globulin, whole blood, or plasma, since the measles virus antibody content in these materials may be sufficient to neutralize the vaccine virus.

ROUTE AND USUAL DOSAGE.
Subcutaneous: *Children 15 months or older*, a single dose of 0.5 ml of reconstituted vaccine is given, preferably into the outer aspect of the upper arm. It is essential that only the diluent supplied with the vaccine be used for reconstitution. If measles vaccine was given prior to 1 year of age, vaccination should be repeated at or after 15 months of age because maternal immunity may interfere with the development of active immunity.

MUMPS VIRUS VACCINE LIVE

Live mumps virus vaccine is a suspension of the Jeryl Lynn strain of mumps virus grown in chick embryo tissue culture. It provides active immunity in about 97% of children and about 93% of adults following a single subcutaneous injection. Circulating antibodies provide continuing protection against mumps for at least ten years after immunization. Children 1 year

or older and adults may be vaccinated. The vaccine is of particular value in susceptible individuals approaching puberty and in adolescents and adults. Combinations of mumps vaccine with live measles and rubella virus vaccines are available.

Fever or tenderness at the site of injection has been reported. Parotitis has occurred occasionally. The vaccine is contraindicated during pregnancy, in patients with hypogammaglobulinemia or dysgammaglobulinemia, in those receiving immunosuppressive therapy (eg, corticosteroids, irradiation, antineoplastic agents), in those with acute active infection, or in those with blood dyscrasias, leukemia, lymphomas, or malignant neoplasms affecting the bone marrow or lymphoid system.

ROUTE AND USUAL DOSAGE.
Subcutaneous: *Adults and children 15 months or older*, the total volume (0.5 ml) of reconstituted vaccine is administered. The reconstituted vaccine retains potency for eight hours at 2 to 8 C in the dark and should be discarded if not used within that period. Only the diluent supplied should be used for reconstitution.

RUBELLA VIRUS VACCINE LIVE

Live rubella virus vaccine is a suspension of attenuated rubella virus derived from the Wistar Institute RA 27/3 strain, which is grown in human diploid cell (WI-38) culture.

Vaccination against rubella is recommended for children between 15 months of age and puberty and in nonpregnant adolescent girls and women *if they agree to prevent pregnancy for three months*. Circulating rubella antibody levels are detectable in 96% to 98% of patients within four to six weeks following vaccination and persist for as long as nine years, suggesting active immunity of long duration. Reinfection following exposure to wild rubella virus, as evidenced by increased antibody levels without viremia or disease, occurs in some vaccinees. Although the monovalent rubella vaccine should not be given routinely within three months after receiving plasma or blood transfusion or immune globulin therapy, it may be administered in the postpartum period prior to the patient's discharge from the hospital (see the manufacturer's literature). Combinations of rubella virus vaccine with live measles and mumps virus vaccines also are available.

Adverse reactions include fever; rash, induration, erythema, and tenderness at the site of injection; and regional adenopathy. Transient arthritis-like symptoms, arthralgia, and polyneuritis may occur within two months after immunization. Encephalitis also has been reported very rarely. The incidence of untoward reactions seems to increase with age and is probably higher in females.

Vaccination should be avoided in patients with leukemia, lymphomas, or generalized malignancy and in those being treated with immunosuppressive therapy (corticosteroids, antineoplastic drugs, or irradiation). Vaccination should be postponed in the presence of a febrile illness. Rubella virus vaccine is contraindicated in pregnant women. Susceptible women of childbearing age may be considered for vaccination only if they agree to prevent pregnancy during the following three months. If vaccination is contemplated, a serologic test for susceptibility may be performed.

ROUTE AND USUAL DOSAGE.
Subcutaneous: *Adults and children 15 months or older*, the total volume of reconstituted vaccine (0.5 ml) is injected in the outer aspect of the upper arm. It should not be injected intravenously or intramuscularly. The vaccine should be refrigerated and protected from light. It must remain refrigerated after reconstitution and should be discarded if not used within eight hours. Only the diluent supplied should be used to reconstitute the vaccine.

MEASLES, MUMPS, AND RUBELLA VIRUS VACCINE LIVE

Live measles, mumps, and rubella virus vaccine is a suspension of the same attenuated viruses present in the monovalent vaccines. It is indicated for simultaneous routine immunization of children 15 months of age or older and may be used up to the age of puberty in patients who have not previously been vaccinated against or experienced any of the natural infections. Clinical studies have shown that the vaccine produces antibody levels comparable to those obtained with use of each monovalent vaccine given at properly spaced intervals.

Adverse reactions generally are the same as those associated with the individual monovalent vaccines (see the evaluations).

ROUTE AND USUAL DOSAGE.
Subcutaneous: *Children 15 months to puberty*, the total volume of reconstituted vaccine (0.5 ml) is injected in the outer aspect of the upper arm.

MEASLES AND RUBELLA VIRUS VACCINE LIVE

Live measles and rubella virus vaccine is a suspension of the same attenuated viruses present in equivalent monovalent vaccines. Available evidence indicates that it produces antibodies against measles and rubella in 95% of susceptible children.

Adverse reactions and precautions are the same as those associated with the monovalent vaccines (see the evaluations).

ROUTE AND USUAL DOSAGE.
Subcutaneous: *Adults and children 15 months of age to puberty*, 0.5 ml in the outer aspect of the upper arm.

RUBELLA AND MUMPS VIRUS VACCINE LIVE

Live rubella and mumps virus vaccine is a suspension of the same attenuated viruses present in equivalent monovalent vaccines. The vaccine is used for simultaneous routine immunization of children 15 months of age to puberty who have been vaccinated against measles or experienced the natural disease but who have no history of immunizing exposure to rubella and mumps viruses. The vaccine produces antibody levels comparable to those stimulated by the monovalent vaccines given separately; the degree of protection against natural disease is also comparable.

Contraindications, precautions, and adverse reactions are the same as those associated with the individual monovalent vaccines (see the evaluations).

ROUTE AND USUAL DOSAGE.
Subcutaneous: *Children 15 months of age to puberty*, the total volume of reconstituted vaccine (0.5 ml) is injected in the outer aspect of the upper arm. The reconstituted vaccine should be stored at 2 to 8 C and discarded if not used within eight hours.

Poliomyelitis

POLIOVIRUS VACCINE INACTIVATED

This vaccine consists of the three serotypes of poliovirus propagated in monkey kidney cell culture and rendered noninfectious by formalin treatment. Protection from paralytic poliomyelitis derives from the development of serum antibodies following a series of injections. Formaldehyde-inactivated vaccine induces humoral immunity without the hazard of inducing paralysis. This vaccine may be used to immunize immunodeficient patients and their household contacts. The protective immune response to inactivated poliovirus vaccine in the immunodeficient patient cannot be assured. However, the vaccine is safe and therefore should be administered in an attempt to provide some protection. Physicians may elect to give a primary series of vaccinations or, when constrained by time, at least two doses one month apart to susceptible adults who (1) by reason of travel are at risk of exposure to poliomyelitis, or (2) are likely to come into contact with vaccine virus following routine immunization of their children. Primary immunization for persons of all ages consists of four doses; the volume and route of injection are specified by the manufacturer.

This vaccine is no longer manufactured in the United States but is available through a U.S. distributor (Elkins-Sinn, Inc, 2 Easterbrook Lane, Cherry Hill, N.J. 08802, (800) 257-8349).

POLIOVIRUS VACCINE LIVE ORAL TRIVALENT

This vaccine is now the agent of choice because it is easier to administer than the inactivated vaccine and produces immunity resembling that induced by natural poliovirus infection (ie, it stimulates intestinal immunity as well as circulating antibodies).

This vaccine contains attenuated poliovirus Types I, II, and III grown in monkey kidney tissue culture or human diploid cell culture. Poliovirus vaccine is easily administered *but it must not be injected*; immunity is achieved rapidly and is long lasting. In susceptible individuals, the type-specific serum neutralizing antibody titer begins to increase about one week after ingestion and reaches a peak about three weeks later. A primary series of three adequately spaced doses of trivalent oral poliovirus vaccine produces an immune response to the three virus types in over 90% of recipients.

Live oral poliovirus vaccine is recommended routinely for all infants and children who do not have, or live with persons who have, immune deficiency diseases or altered immune states. Routine immunization for adults living in the continental United States is considered unnecessary because most adults are immune, exposure to wild virus is unlikely, and there may be a slightly greater risk of vaccine-associated paralysis among adults than among children receiving this vaccine. However, any nonimmunized adult who might come into contact with a known case by traveling to epidemic or endemic areas should receive trivalent oral poliovirus vaccine or the inactivated poliovirus vaccine according to the schedule outlined for children and adolescents. If there is not sufficient time for a complete series, one dose of oral poliovirus vaccine is preferred.

Rarely, paralysis has occurred in individuals receiving oral poliovirus vaccine or those who had close contact with vaccine recipients within two months after administration. Tonsillectomy, adenoidectomy, and pregnancy are not contraindications to its use when immunization is required, as during an epidemic. The vaccine should not be administered if the patient has diarrhea. Immunization is contraindicated when the immune state of the recipient may be altered, such as in those with dysgammaglobulinemia, lymphoma, leukemia, and generalized malignancies, as well as in those receiving therapeutic regimens that may impair cellular immunity (eg, corticosteroids, antineoplastic agents, immunosuppressive agents, irradiation).

ROUTE AND USUAL DOSAGE.

Oral: Each dose of trivalent poliovirus vaccine contains approximately 800,000 tissue culture infective doses (TCID$_{50}$) of Type I virus, 100,000 of Type II, and 500,000 of Type III. For primary immunization, three doses are administered. *Infants*, the first dose is given at 2 months of age and the second at 4 months; a third dose at 6 months is optional. Another dose should be given at approximately 18 months of age. *Children and adolescents*, the first two doses should be given at six- to eight-week intervals and the third 8 to 12 months after the second dose. All children who have completed the series should be given a single booster dose at 4 to 6 years of age.

MISCELLANEOUS VACCINES

BCG VACCINE

This vaccine, used for active immunization against tuberculosis, is derived from an attenuated strain of the bovine tubercle bacillus *(Mycobacterium bovis)* and is commonly referred to as BCG (Bacillus Calmette-Guerin) vaccine. All of the BCG vaccines available in the world have been derived from the original strain; however, they vary in immunogenicity, efficacy, and reactogenicity. Available data from the use of these vaccines are mostly from other countries and do not necessarily pertain to the vaccines currently available in the United States. The efficacy of the current vaccines has not been demonstrated directly and can only be inferred. Since most cases of tuberculosis in the United States

do not reflect high rates of primary infection, the use of BCG vaccine is not recommended for routine immunization against tuberculosis.

The vaccine should be reserved for persons who have a negative reaction to a tuberculin skin test and who have repeated exposure to persistently untreated or ineffectively treated, sputum-positive pulmonary tuberculosis or are members of well-defined groups with excessive rates of new infections and ineffective control or treatment measures. The tuberculin skin test should be repeated two to three months following administration of the vaccine.

Adverse reactions are usually mild and uncommon but may occur as long as a year or more after vaccination. The vaccine should not be given to persons with impaired immune responses, skin infections or burns, or during pregnancy. It should not be given during therapy with isoniazid because the drug inhibits multiplication of BCG.

The manufacturer's literature should be consulted for route of administration and dosage; no other schedule should be employed.

CHOLERA VACCINE

This vaccine is a sterile suspension of killed cholera organisms *(Vibrio cholerae)* containing eight billion killed organisms per milliliter; higher concentrations produce severe local and systemic reactions. The vaccine presently available provides limited protection for three to six months but does not prevent transmission of the disease. The U.S. Public Health Service does not require cholera vaccination for entry into the United States from cholera-infected areas, and the World Health Organization no longer recommends routine vaccination for travel to or from cholera-infected areas. Nevertheless, many countries still require evidence of cholera vaccination for entry.

Malaise, fever, and induration and erythema at the site of injection may occur. The vaccine is contraindicated in individuals who have had a serious reaction to previous injections.

ROUTES AND USUAL DOSAGE.
Intramuscular, Subcutaneous: Primary immunization consists of two doses one week to one month or more apart; booster doses should be given at six-month intervals but are effective regardless of the length of the interval after the primary series. The amounts given in each dose are: for *adults and children over 10 years*, 0.5 ml; for *children 5 to 10 years*, 0.3 ml; and for *children 6 months through 4 years*, 0.2 ml.

Intradermal: For persons 5 years of age and older, two doses of 0.2 ml given one week to one month apart for primary immunization; booster doses of 0.2 ml are given at six-month intervals if necessary.

INFLUENZA VIRUS VACCINE

Influenza virus vaccine is a monovalent or polyvalent product prepared from type A or B influenza virus grown in embryonated chicken eggs. It is available as an inactivated "whole virus" or "split virus" product. The split-virus vaccine is recommended for persons less than 13 years of age because it is associated with fewer side effects than the whole virus vaccine in this age group. Influenza vaccines should contain strains that are prevalent in the community. For example, the 1978-1979 formulation consisted of three strains: A/USSR/77 (H1N1), A/Texas/77 (H3N2), and B/Hong Kong/72.

Annual vaccination is recommended for children and adults in the following high-risk categories: (1) congenital or acquired heart disease, (2) chronic renal disease, (3) chronic bronchopulmonary disease, (4) diabetes mellitus and other metabolic diseases, (5) chronic, severe anemia (eg, sickle cell disease), (6) immunocompromised persons; and (7) those over 65 years of age.

Fever, malaise, myalgia, and other systemic symptoms occur less commonly in adults than in children. Reactions may appear within 6 to 12 hours and disappear within one to two days. Currently available purified vaccines are fairly well tolerated. Allergic reactions are rare because current influenza vaccines contain very small quantities of egg protein; nevertheless, persons who are hypersensitive to eggs should not be given the vaccine. During the large-scale influenza immunization program in 1976, the Guillain-Barre syndrome developed in excess frequency among persons who received the Swine influenza vaccine; the overall incidence for the 10 weeks following vaccination was five to six times higher than in unvaccinated persons.

ROUTE AND USUAL DOSAGE.
See the manufacturer's literature. Recommendations for vaccine composition and administration are widely publicized each year.

PLAGUE VACCINE

Plague vaccine is prepared from *Yersinia pestis* grown on artificial media, killed with formaldehyde, and preserved with 0.5% phenol. Its use generally is restricted to persons traveling to Vietnam, Cambodia, or Laos; those whose work brings them into frequent contact with wild rodents in plague enzootic areas, eg, Southwestern United States; and laboratory personnel working with *Yersinia pestis* or infected rodents. Immunization apparently reduces the incidence and severity of plague.

Adverse reactions include myalgia, fever, pain at the site of injection, and lymphadenopathy.

ROUTE AND USUAL DOSAGE.
Intramuscular: Adults and children over 10 years, for primary vaccination, two 0.5-ml doses four or more weeks apart, followed by a third dose of 0.2 ml 4 to 12 weeks after the second injection. Previously vaccinated individuals need only two 0.2-ml doses, 28 days apart. *Children under 10 years* receive the same series but at a reduced dosage as follows: *infants under 1 year*, 0.1 ml; *1 to 4 years*, 0.2 ml; *5 to 10 years*, 0.3 ml. Booster doses of 0.1 to 0.2 ml may be given at three-month intervals as long as the risk of plague infection exists.

RABIES VACCINE

Rabies vaccine is a sterile suspension of killed, fixed rabies virus obtained from duck embryo tissue infected with fixed rabies virus. The virus is inactivated with beta-propiolactone. Rabies vaccine prepared in human diploid cell tissue culture is available through the Center for Disease Control on a limited, experimental basis. Persons may be eligible to receive the vaccine if (1) they have a serious allergy to duck embryo vaccine; (2) they do not develop adequate antibody titer to duck embryo vaccine; or (3) they have been bitten by an animal proved to be rabid. Requests for the vaccine should be made to the Center for Disease Control, (404) 633-3311, extension 3727.

Pre-exposure immunoprophylaxis with rabies vaccine (duck embryo) is recommended for persons with an unusually high risk of exposure (eg, veterinarians, animal handlers, persons engaged in experimental canine or feline surgery, laboratory personnel working with rabies virus, spelunkers).

Both laboratory data and clinical experience indicate that postexposure prophylaxis against rabies is usually effective when properly applied, although failures do occur. This procedure is based on the assumption that every animal capable of carrying rabies should be considered rabid until proved otherwise; thus, each case must be evaluated individually. Dogs and cats should be isolated and observed by a veterinarian for ten days after the bite. If no clinical signs of rabies develop during this period, it can be considered that no exposure to rabies occurred. However, if the animal is killed or dies, the head should be sent to the local health authorities for confirmatory diagnosis. According to the U.S. Public Health Service Advisory Committee on Rabies, carnivorous animals (especially skunks, foxes, coyotes, raccoons, dogs, and cats) and bats are more likely to be infective than other animals; bites of rabbits, squirrels, chipmunks, rats, and mice rarely, if ever, call for rabies prophylaxis, because rabies is rare in rodents and no human rabies has resulted from the bite of a rodent. Properly immunized domestic animals are not likely to develop rabies. In doubtful or unusual cases, the local health authority should be consulted. Even in areas where rabies is enzootic, if adequate data indicate that infection is not present in the particular species, the local authority may recommend that no specific rabies immunoprophylaxis be given.

As part of the postexposure prophylactic treatment, all bite wounds, as well as scratches and skin abrasions exposed to licks of animals, should be immediately and thoroughly flushed with copious amounts of soap and water. If debridement is necessary, the wound area may be infiltrated with a local anesthetic. If possible, bite wounds should not be sutured immediately. Antibiotics may be given and appropriate tetanus prophylaxis initiated if indicated. The management of patients exposed to possibly rabid animals should follow the guides given in Table 4.

Mild to severe local erythematous reactions occur in approximately one-third of patients receiving either vaccine. Some patients develop inflammation and induration at the site of injection, regional lymphadenopathy, and, occasionally, urticaria or serum sickness. Severe abdominal distress with nausea and vomiting occasionally occurs within a few minutes after receiving the vaccine. A systemic reaction characterized by malaise, febrile episodes, and chills has been observed rarely.

Rabies vaccine should be used with caution in patients with known sensitivity to avian protein. Antihistamines may help prevent or ameliorate reactions in these patients. Although cross sensitization between duck protein and chicken protein has occurred only rarely, caution should be observed in administering duck embryo vaccine to persons known to be highly sensitive to chicken eggs. Epinephrine should be available immediately in case of an anaphylactic reaction. Vaccine administration should be stopped if neurologic reactions develop.

ROUTE AND USUAL DOSAGE.
Subcutaneous: Adults and children, for

pre-exposure immunoprophylaxis (duck embryo vaccine), two 1-ml doses administered in the outer aspect of the upper arm at approximately one-month intervals, followed by a booster dose after six or seven months. A detectable antibody response does not develop in all individuals; therefore, a blood sample should be collected one month after the booster dose is given and submitted to the local health authority for serum antibody determination. If necessary, booster doses may be repeated until an antibody response is detectable. Persons in high-risk occupations should be given a booster dose at least every two years. Those with a demonstrated antibody response to pre-exposure rabies vaccine need only a single booster dose after a nonbite exposure; if bitten by a rabid animal, these people should receive a course of five daily doses of vaccine, followed by a booster dose 20 days after the last injection. For *postexposure* immunoprophylaxis (duck embryo vaccine), when given with-

out rabies immune globulin or antiserum, 14 daily injections should be administered, using the dose recommended by the manufacturer. When given with rabies immune globulin or antiserum, 21 doses are administered; these may be given as 21 daily doses or 14 doses during the first seven days and then seven daily doses. Two supplemental booster doses of vaccine should be given 10 and 20 days after completion of the 21-day course. Serum should be drawn for rabies antibody determination at the time of the second booster injection.

ANTIRABIES SERUM EQUINE (ARS)

This hyperimmune equine serum is useful in the prevention of rabies, although rabies immune globulin is preferable. It should be used in combination with rabies vaccine for postexposure treatment in persons who have not been previously immunized and shown to have an adequate

TABLE 4.
POSTEXPOSURE ANTIRABIES GUIDE

The following recommendations are only a guide. They should be used in conjunction with knowledge of the animal species involved, circumstances of the bite or other exposure, vaccination status of the animal, and presence of rabies in the region.

ANIMAL AND ITS CONDITION		TREATMENT	
		Kind of Exposure	
Species	Condition at Time of Attack	Bite	Non-Bite
WILD Skunk Fox Raccoon Bat	Regard as Rabid	RIG + DEV	RIG + DEV[1]
DOMESTIC Dog	Healthy	None[2]	None[2]
	Escaped (unknown)	RIG + DEV	DEV[3]
Cat	Rabid	RIG + DEV	RIG + DEV[1]

DEV = Duck Embryo Vaccine

RIG = Rabies Immune Globulin

[1]Discontinue vaccine if fluorescent antibody (FA) tests of animal killed at time of attack are negative.

[2]Begin RIG + DEV at first sign of rabies in biting dog or cat during holding period (10 days).

[3]14 doses of DEV when no RIG used.

rabies antibody titer. As with all equine serums, tests for sensitivity and precautionary desensitization procedures should be carried out prior to use (see the Introduction and the evaluation on Rabies Vaccine).

ROUTE AND USUAL DOSAGE.
Intramuscular: *Adults and children*, 40 IU/kg of body weight; up to one-half of the total dose should be infiltrated around the wound. A full course of 21 doses of rabies vaccine also should be initiated immediately.

RABIES IMMUNE GLOBULIN (RIG)

This sterile solution of antirabies gamma globulin concentrated by fractionation of plasma from donors hyperimmunized with rabies vaccine *is much preferred to the equine antirabies serum* for postexposure prophylaxis.

ROUTE AND USUAL DOSAGE.
Intramuscular: 20 IU/kg of body weight; half of the material should be infiltrated around the wound if possible. Rabies immune globulin is used as soon as possible after a possible exposure to rabies in conjunction with 14 or 21 doses of rabies vaccine (see the evaluation and Table 4).

SMALLPOX VACCINE

Routine smallpox vaccination has been discontinued in the United States and many other countries. Because of the extraordinary success of the World Health Organization's eradication program, the vaccine should only be administered to travelers to countries that still require proof of vaccination.

TYPHOID VACCINE

Typhoid vaccine is a sterile suspension of killed typhoid bacilli (*Salmonella typhi*) of a strain selected for high antigenicity. It protects 70% to 90% of recipients, depending upon the intensity of subsequent exposure. Routine immunization is not indicated under existing conditions in the United States, but it is recommended for persons exposed to a carrier in the household or subject to unusual exposure because of occupation or travel. Flood conditions are not considered an indication for immunization.

Adverse reactions to typhoid vaccine include local erythema, tenderness at the site of injection, malaise, myalgia, headache, and fever. The vaccine is contraindicated in the presence of acute illness or in patients with chronic debilitating disease.

ROUTE AND USUAL DOSAGE.
Subcutaneous: *Adults and children over 10 years*, two 0.5-ml doses four or more weeks apart or three doses at weekly intervals; *children 6 months to 10 years*, two 0.25-ml doses four or more weeks apart or three doses at weekly intervals. If there is continued or repeated exposure, a booster dose of 0.5 ml should be given at least every three years to adults and children over 10 years and 0.25 ml to children under 10 years.

TYPHUS VACCINE

Typhus vaccine is a sterile suspension of killed epidemic typhus rickettsiae (*Rickettsia prowazekii*) grown in chick embryo culture. It affords protection against louse-borne (epidemic) typhus only; it does not protect against murine or scrub typhus. Vaccination is suggested only for persons traveling to or working in countries where typhus is still endemic and who will be in close contact with the indigenous population or for special-risk groups, ie, medical personnel who care for patients in areas where louse-borne typhus occurs, laboratory personnel who work with the organism.

Vaccination is contraindicated in patients highly allergic to eggs. Sensitivity testing is required prior to use of the vaccine (see the Introduction). Allergic or systemic reactions are minimal, but the possibility of an anaphylactic reaction should be borne in mind. The vaccine is contraindicated in the presence of active illness or in patients with debilitating diseases (eg, tuberculosis).

ROUTE AND USUAL DOSAGE.
Subcutaneous: *Adults and children over 10 years*, two doses at intervals of four weeks using amounts recommended by the manufacturer. A single subcutaneous injection should be administered as a booster dose at intervals of 6 to 12 months for as long as opportunity for exposure exists.

YELLOW FEVER VACCINE

Yellow fever vaccine used in the United States is a suspension of live, attenuated virus prepared from 17D strain which is grown in chick embryo. It is highly effective and provides immunity lasting ten years or more. Vaccination is recommended for persons 6 months of age or older traveling to or living in countries in which yellow fever is endemic and for laboratory personnel who might be exposed to virulent yellow fever virus.

Yellow fever vaccine must meet standards established by the World Health Organization and must be administered at WHO-approved yellow fever vaccination centers located in most cities in the United States; specific information may be obtained from city or county public health officers.

Adverse reactions are generally mild and consist of headache, myalgia, or low-grade fever. The vaccine is contraindicated in individuals highly sensitive to eggs; patients with febrile illnesses or dysgammaglobulinemia; or those receiving corticosteroid, antineoplastic, or immunosuppressive drugs.

ROUTE AND USUAL DOSAGE.
Subcutaneous: *Adults and children over 6 months*, 0.5 ml of reconstituted vaccine. International Regulations do not require revaccination more frequently than every ten years.

MENINGOCOCCAL POLYSACCHARIDE VACCINES

Three meningococcal polysaccharide vaccines have been licensed for use: monovalent serogroup A, monovalent serogroup C, and bivalent serogroups A-C. These vaccines contain the specific purified bacterial capsular polysaccharides for each group.

Each antigen produces a good antibody response in most adults and children over 2 years of age. Monovalent A vaccine has been effective in preventing group A meningococcal disease in outbreaks in Brazil and Finland. Monovalent serogroup C vaccine has been used effectively for the routine immunization of American military recruits since October, 1971; it also was effective in preventing cases in children 2 years and over during an epidemic in Brazil, but it does not appear to be effective in children under 2 years. Bivalent A-C vaccine currently is used for military recruits.

Routine immunization with meningococcal polysaccharide vaccines is not recommended, but it should be considered for the following special groups: (1) travelers to countries where meningococcal disease is epidemic, (2) persons living in institutions in which there is an outbreak, (3) as an adjunct to antibiotic chemoprophylaxis for household contacts of an individual with meningococcal group A or C disease, and (4) military recruits.

Adverse reactions include localized erythema and possibly low-grade fever that usually subsides within one to two days.

ROUTE AND USUAL DOSAGE.
Subcutaneous: One inoculation of the volume specified by the manufacturer. The lyophilized vaccine is reconstituted in 0.5 ml of the sterile diluent provided.

PNEUMOCOCCAL POLYSACCHARIDE VACCINES

Pneumococcal polysaccharide vaccines contain purified polysaccharide antigens of the following 14 types of pneumococcus most frequently associated with disease in adults and children: 1, 2, 3, 4, 6, 8, 9, 12, 14, 19, 23, 25, 51(7F), and 56(18C). These 14 types cause about 80% of pneumococcal disease in the United States. Each 0.5-ml dose of vaccine contains 50 mcg of the purified capsular material from each type dissolved in isotonic saline solution containing 0.25% phenol as preservative.

Each antigen produces a good antibody response in most adults, and protection against infection is achieved in about two weeks. Detectable antibody levels persist for five to eight years. Children less than 2 years of age have an unsatisfactory antibody response, but older children respond similarly to adults.

Immunization with pneumococcal polysaccharide vaccines should be considered for the following special groups: (1) persons over 2 years with chronic conditions that may be complicated by pneumococcal disease, such as sickle cell anemia and other causes of functional or anatomical splenic dysfunction (eg, splenectomy); (2) persons over 2 years with certain chronic diseases associated with increased risk of pneumococcal disease, such as chronic cardiac, pulmonary, hepatic, and renal disease; and metabolic diseases such as diabetes mellitus; and (3) persons living in nursing homes and other closed institutions where there is an increased risk of systemic pneumococcal disease, either in endemic or epidemic form.

Serious adverse effects are rare. The most common untoward effect has been local erythema and soreness at the injection site, usually subsiding within one to two days. Contraindications include febrile respiratory illness or active infection, children under 2 years, and pregnancy.

ROUTES AND USUAL DOSAGE.
Subcutaneous, Intramuscular: A single 0.5-ml dose. Intravenous inoculation should be avoided.

INVESTIGATIONAL VACCINES

HAEMOPHILUS INFLUENZAE TYPE B VACCINE

This vaccine is a highly purified form of type b capsular polysaccharide which has induced an excellent antibody response in adults and children over 2 years of age. The vaccine has been less immunogenic in infants under the age of 2. Protection against meningitis has been related to the immunogenicity of the vaccine. However, since type b *H. influenzae* meningitis occurs most often in young infants, the immunogenicity of the vaccine must be improved for this age group before licensure.

VARICELLA-ZOSTER VACCINE LIVE ATTENUATED

A live attenuated vaccine has been prepared from varicella-zoster virus cultivated in human embryonic fibroblasts and passaged in guinea pig embryo cells and WI-38 cells. Preliminary studies in Japan in about 500 children revealed that the antibody response exceeded 90% and that this vaccine was well tolerated. Side effects were limited to mild, transient fever and rash that occurred in 1% to 2% of vaccinees. Administration of the vaccine to 45 children in remission from acute leukemia revealed mild fever and/or papules in 7 (15%).

Clinical studies are currently in progress in the United States to evaluate further the safety and efficacy of this vaccine.

HEPATITIS B VACCINE INACTIVATED

An inactivated hepatitis B vaccine has been prepared from purified hepatitis B surface antigen (HBsAg) from HBsAg-positive donor blood. The purified HBsAg is the noninfectious component of hepatitis B virus which contains an outer coat (HBsAg) and an inner core containing the infectious core component. The purified HBsAg, which is essentially free of the infectious inner core, is inactivated by formalin and tested in chimpanzees for lack of infectivity.

Inactivated hepatitis B vaccine has been shown to be safe and effective when tested in chimpanzees. Preliminary studies in adult volunteers revealed that the vaccine is well tolerated and immunogenic. In initial studies with an alum-adsorbed inactivated hepatitis B vaccine, the antibody response was 85% after two doses given one month apart.

Clinical studies to determine the safety and efficacy of the inactivated hepatitis B vaccine are currently in progress.

ANTISERUMS (IMMUNE GLOBULINS) FOR SPECIFIC INFECTIONS

Antiserums for therapeutic or prophylactic use consist of the immunoglobulin fraction of serum in which the specific antibodies are concentrated. They may be of human or animal origin; when available, preparations from human source are preferred.

Unlike the active immunity conferred either by natural infection or vaccines, antibodies contained in antiserums remain in the circulation for a limited half-life, especially those derived from nonhuman sources, and provide passive immunity only. When the serum is prepared by injecting the animal or human source with a purified toxin or toxoid, it is referred to as an antitoxin.

IMMUNE GLOBULIN

Immune globulin, commonly called gamma globulin, is prepared from a fraction of pooled plasma from normal donors. It consists primarily of the IgG fraction which contains concentrated antibodies and is used primarily to modify or prevent measles and to prevent type A hepatitis.

Reactions following use of immune globulin have occurred infrequently. *The preparation must not be given intravenously.*

ROUTE AND USUAL DOSAGE.
Intramuscular: Adults and children, for persons exposed to type A (infectious) hepatitis, 0.02 to 0.04 ml/kg of body weight. For prevention of measles in nonimmune individuals, 0.25 ml/kg given within the first six days after exposure. For modification of measles, 0.05 ml/kg (maximum, 15 ml) given within the first six days after exposure.

HEPATITIS B IMMUNE GLOBULIN (HBIG)

This sterile solution of immunoglobulin is prepared from pooled plasma obtained from donors with high titers of antibody to hepatitis B surface antigen (anti-HBs).

Hepatitis B immune globulin is indicated for postexposure prophylaxis following either parenteral exposure (eg, accidental "needle-stick," direct mucous membrane contact [accidental splash]) or oral ingestion (pipetting accident) of HBsAg-positive materials such as blood, plasma, or serum. Its use may also be considered for infants born to mothers who had hepatitis B infection during the last trimester of pregnancy, although its efficacy in this situation has not been established.

Adverse reactions include local pain and tenderness at the injection site, urticaria, and angioedema. Allergic reactions are very rare.

ROUTE AND USUAL DOSAGE.
Intramuscular: 0.06 ml/kg of body weight; the usual adult dose is 3 to 5 ml administered as soon as possible (not later than seven days) after exposure and repeated 25 to 30 days after the first dose. Intravenous administration should be avoided.

PERTUSSIS IMMUNE GLOBULIN

This solution of gamma globulin is prepared from venous blood of humans hyperimmunized with pertussis vaccine. Pertussis immune globulin has been used in an effort to attenuate pertussis, but controlled studies have not shown that it has an appreciable clinical therapeutic effect. It does not prevent clinical pertussis in susceptible infants intimately exposed to pertussis.

ROUTE AND USUAL DOSAGE.
See the manufacturer's literature.

VARICELLA-ZOSTER IMMUNE GLOBULIN (HUMAN)

Limited quantities of this preparation (VZIG) are available for immunodeficient children exposed to chicken pox who have leukemia, lymphoma, or generalized malignancy or who are not immunocompetent, either congenitally or through the use of immunosuppressive therapy. Neonates whose mothers develop varicella four days prior to or 48 hours after delivery also are eligible for VZIG administration.

For availability, consult the Division of Clinical Microbiology, Sidney Farber Cancer Institute, 44 Binney Street, Boston, MA ([617] 732-3121) or the Center for Disease Control ([404] 329-3745).

Selected References

American Academy of Pediatrics: *Report of the Committee on Infectious Diseases*, ed 18. Evanston, Ill, American Academy of Pediatrics, 1977.

Krugman S, Katz SL: Childhood immunization procedures. *JAMA* 237:2228-2230, 1977.

Nightingale EO: Recommendations for national policy on poliomyelitis vaccination. *N Engl J Med* 297:249-253, 1977.

Rimland D, et al: Immunization for the internist. *Ann Intern Med* 85:622-629, 1976.

Rothstein RJ, Baker FJ II: Tetanus: Prevention and treatment. *JAMA* 240:675-676, 1978.

Stiehm ER: Standard and special human immune serum globulins as therapeutic agents. *Pediatrics* 63:301-319, 1979.

Antineoplastic Agents | 68

The treatment of cancer continues to be one of the greatest challenges in medicine. Although great efforts have been made in cancer research and major developments have occurred in molecular and cellular biology, many fundamental questions remain unanswered and the etiology and pathogenesis of the basic neoplastic process are still unknown.

A major improvement in the strategy of cancer treatment during the last 30 years has been the development of effective antineoplastic agents. Until recently, chemotherapy was used primarily in hematologic malignancies and only secondarily in the treatment of solid tumors unresponsive to surgery and radiation therapy. With a better understanding of the pharmacology and mechanisms of action of several empirically discovered antitumor drugs, a more rational application of these agents, often in combination with other agents or treatment modalities, and the synthesis of new and more effective drugs have evolved.

The underlying principle of curative cancer therapy is the removal or eradication of the last neoplastic cell, since it appears that a single clonogenic malignant cell is capable of multiplying and eventually killing the host by the volume of its progeny. Surgical extirpation or irradiation of malignant tissue only removes localized and regional disease. At present, only one-third of patients are cured with surgery or radiation therapy alone; in the remaining patients, the tumor is already microscopically disseminated at the time of diagnosis and local therapy will fail.

On the basis of cell kinetics, it is assumed that, at the time of discovery, a palpable tumor 1 cm in diameter contains approximately one billion (10^9) cells and that the original tumor cell may have undergone 30 doublings to reach a mass of 1 g. Thirty cell doublings are equivalent to two-thirds of the lifespan of the tumor and, assuming exponential growth, ten more will increase the mass to over 1 kg or 10^{12} cells, a tumor burden that is considered incompatible with life. It is highly probable that viable tumor cells already have been shed into the lymphatic system or blood stream with resulting metastatic disease long before the primary lesion is evident. At present, only systemic therapy with antineoplastic drugs or immunotherapy can control tumor cell growth anywhere in the body.

It has been demonstrated that chemotherapy alone can be curative in choriocarcinoma, acute lymphocytic leukemia, some cases of Hodgkin's disease, Burkitt's lymphoma, diffuse histiocytic lymphoma, certain testicular tumors, and perhaps osteogenic sarcoma. Objective tumor regression and enhanced survival have been achieved in acute myelocytic leukemia, non-Hodgkin's lymphoma, multiple myeloma, chronic leukemias, and adenocarcinomas of the breast and ovary. Surgery and radiation therapy in conjunction with chemotherapy have been effective in Wilms' tumor, embryonal rhabdomyosarcoma, and Ewing's sarcoma. Adjuvant chemotherapy is being used in breast cancer and other tumors to achieve total cell kill of residual microscopic disease that remains after surgical removal of most of the tumor. (See Table 1.) Immunotherapy also is being investigated and is expected to play a major role in the treatment of cancer.

The rationale for cancer chemotherapy is based on certain concepts regarding cell cycle kinetics, total cell kill, pharmacokinetics, and host factors. All living cells have an inherent capacity to multiply and, in normal growing tissue, the rate of cell birth equals the rate of cell loss. This steady state is disturbed in tumor tissue, and uncontrolled cell proliferation continues until the death of the host. In the early phases of growth, tumor cell populations grow in an exponential fashion. However, with the increasing volume of the tumor, successive doublings occur at increasingly longer intervals, and the tumor growth curve reaches a plateau (Gompertzian growth). The prolongation of the doubling time with increase of tumor volume is probably due to crowding of cells, a smaller growth fraction (ratio of proliferating cells in mitotic cycle to total number of cells), and increased cell loss caused by impaired vascular and nutritional supply. It appears that sensitivity to treatment depends upon the growth rate of the tissue. Since smaller tumors have a greater growth rate, it has been postulated that "small is sensitive." Based on a mathematical model, the point of maximum sensitivity has been calculated to be the point of maximum growth rate (37% of the final plateau volume).

The volume of the tumor consists of three types or compartments of cells. In most slowly growing solid tumors, a great number of cells are permanently nondividing and will eventually die. A substantial number of cells are temporarily nondividing and are partially or completely insensitive to antineoplastic drugs. A small fraction of cells, probably 5% to 10%, are actively dividing and proliferating and are

TABLE 1.
CLINICAL RESPONSE TO CHEMOTHERAPEUTIC AGENTS

Disease	Effective Drugs (Used as Single Agents or in Combination)
NEOPLASMS USUALLY RESPONDING TO CHEMOTHERAPY WITH IMPROVEMENT IN SURVIVAL:	
Acute Lymphocytic Leukemia of Childhood	Vincristine, prednisone, methotrexate, mercaptopurine, doxorubicin, cyclophosphamide, asparaginase, cytarabine, thioguanine
Hodgkin's Disease	Mechlorethamine, vincristine, prednisone, procarbazine, doxorubicin, bleomycin, vinblastine, dacarbazine, carmustine, lomustine, chlorambucil, thiotepa
Non-Hodgkin's Lymphoma	Cyclophosphamide, vincristine, prednisone, doxorubicin, bleomycin, methotrexate, cytarabine, chlorambucil, carmustine, lomustine

Disease	Effective Drugs (Used as Single Agents or in Combination)
Testicular Carcinoma	Vinblastine, bleomycin, cisplatin, doxorubicin, dactinomycin, cyclophosphamide, chlorambucil, mithramycin
Embryonal Rhabdomyosarcoma	Doxorubicin, cyclophosphamide, vincristine, dactinomycin, methotrexate
Ewing's Sarcoma	Vincristine, cyclophosphamide, dactinomycin, doxorubicin, carmustine
Wilms' Tumor	Dactinomycin, vincristine, cyclophosphamide, doxorubicin
Burkitt's Lymphoma	Cyclophosphamide, vincristine, methotrexate, carmustine
Choriocarcinoma	Methotrexate, dactinomycin, vinblastine, mercaptopurine
Neuroblastoma	Cyclophosphamide, vincristine, doxorubicin, prednisone, dacarbazine, vinblastine

NEOPLASMS OFTEN RESPONDING TO CHEMOTHERAPY WITH POSSIBLE IMPROVEMENT IN SURVIVAL:

Carcinoma of Ovary	Melphalan, chlorambucil, cyclophosphamide, fluorouracil, thiotepa, doxorubicin, cisplatin, progestins
Carcinoma of Breast	Estrogens, androgens, progestins, tamoxifen, cyclophosphamide, methotrexate, fluorouracil, vincristine, prednisone, doxorubicin, melphalan, chlorambucil, vinblastine, thiotepa, mitomycin
Acute Myelogenous Leukemia	Cytarabine, thioguanine, doxorubicin, mercaptopurine, methotrexate, cyclophosphamide, vincristine
Multiple Myeloma	Melphalan, cyclophosphamide, prednisone, carmustine, doxorubicin, chlorambucil
Carcinoma of the Endometrium	Progestins, doxorubicin, fluorouracil, cyclophosphamide, tamoxifen
Carcinoma of the Prostate	Estrogens, cyclophosphamide, doxorubicin, fluorouracil, progestins, tamoxifen, cisplatin
Adrenal Cortical Carcinoma	Mitotane
Oat Cell Carcinoma of the Lung	Cyclophosphamide, methotrexate, procarbazine, doxorubicin, vincristine, lomustine, carmustine
Sarcoma (Soft Tissue and Osteosarcoma)	Dactinomycin, cyclophosphamide, doxorubicin, dacarbazine, methotrexate, vincristine

NEOPLASMS RESPONDING TO CHEMOTHERAPY WITH QUESTIONABLE IMPROVEMENT IN SURVIVAL:

Chronic Lymphocytic Leukemia	Chlorambucil, cyclophosphamide, prednisone
Chronic Myelocytic Leukemia	Busulfan, hydroxyurea, mercaptopurine, thioguanine, melphalan
Squamous Cell Carcinoma of Head and Neck	Methotrexate, cisplatin, bleomycin, vinblastine, cyclophosphamide, fluorouracil, doxorubicin
Carcinoma of the Colon	Fluorouracil, lomustine, vincristine, mitomycin
Carcinoma of the Stomach	Fluorouracil, doxorubicin, mitomycin, nitrosoureas
Carcinoma of the Pancreas	Fluorouracil, doxorubicin, mitomycin
Brain Neoplasms, Primary and Metastatic	Carmustine, lomustine, procarbazine, dexamethasone (for cerebral edema)
Malignant Melanoma	Dacarbazine, lomustine, cyclophosphamide, melphalan
Renal Cell Carcinoma	Progestins, hydroxyurea, vinblastine, lomustine
Bladder Carcinoma	Thiotepa (topical), doxorubicin, cisplatin, mitomycin, fluorouracil, cyclophosphamide
Thyroid Carcinoma	Doxorubicin
Hepatocellular Carcinoma	Fluorouracil, doxorubicin, carmustine, lomustine
Carcinoma of the Cervix	Mitomycin, methotrexate, cyclophosphamide, bleomycin, fluorouracil, vincristine

very sensitive to drugs optimally employed.

Actively dividing cells pass through certain phases from one mitosis to the next. The first part of the interphase after completion of cell division is called the G_1 phase. When the proliferative cycle continues, a burst of RNA synthesis occurs at the end of the presynthetic G_1 period and the S phase begins, during which DNA replication takes place. After completion of the S phase (usually six to eight hours), the cells enter the G_2 period, in which the cell has a diploid number of chromosomes and twice the DNA content. During this phase, DNA synthesis ceases but RNA and protein synthesis continue. The cells remain in G_2 for a relatively short period (two to three hours) and then enter mitosis, during which the rates of protein and RNA synthesis diminish abruptly, while genetic material is segregated into daughter cells. The period of mitosis and cell division generally lasts less than one hour.

After completion of mitosis, the cells enter one of the aforementioned three compartments. They may re-enter the G_1 phase and continue to proliferate actively, enter a resting state (G_0) and be reversibly out of cycle, or lose their ability to proliferate and be irreversibly out of cycle. Some cycling cells have a limited capacity to divide after several generations, whereas others have the potential to produce an unlimited line of descendants; the latter are the so-called clonogenic or stem cells. Cells in the G_0 phase also may have clonogenic potential and will be recruited into the proliferating cell compartment upon receiving an appropriate stimulus.

It appears that actively dividing normal and tumor cells are extremely sensitive to the cytotoxic effect of chemotherapeutic agents, including the constantly renewing population in the bone marrow, the gastrointestinal tract, and the epidermis. The ideal antineoplastic drug would destroy only cancer cells without harming normal cells. However, no definite selectivity for tumor cells has been demonstrated, and drug susceptibility of some tumors can be explained by the premise that tumor cells proliferate more rapidly than normal ones

or that tumors have more cells in the drug-sensitive phases of the cell cycle.

Most antineoplastic drugs vary in their effect during the cell cycle, and their actions may be separated into phase-dependent lethal effects and nonlethal delay of progression through the cell cycle. Lethal effects can result from depriving the proliferating cell of essential metabolites, preventing repair of damaged cells, or promoting abnormal mitosis that produces cells incapable of survival.

Cytarabine [Cytosar], thioguanine, and hydroxyurea [Hydrea] are probably S-phase specific. Methotrexate, fluorouracil, and mercaptopurine [Purinethol] exert their major effects during the S phase but, because they inhibit RNA and protein synthesis and delay entry into the S phase, their effects are self-limiting. The plant alkaloids, vinblastine [Velban] and vincristine [Oncovin], are considered to be cell cycle-specific because they interfere with mitosis.

Cells that are not in cycle (G_0 or prolonged G_1 phase) are almost completely insensitive to S-phase specific drugs but may be affected by cycle-phase nonspecific agents. Alkylating agents, such as cyclophosphamide [Cytoxan] and carmustine [BiCNU], are called cycle-phase nonspecific because they react with DNA during any phase of the cell cycle, leading to cell death or to a delayed effect at mitosis. Dactinomycin [Cosmegen] and the anthracyclines, daunorubicin and doxorubicin [Adriamycin], bind to DNA and interfere with transcription and are also cycle-phase nonspecific.

Normal tissue with large growth fractions (eg, bone marrow) may have fewer resting cells in G_0 than a slowly growing tumor with a small growth fraction. In this situation, chemotherapy with S-phase specific drugs is probably ineffective, because life-threatening marrow suppression would occur before the development of significant antineoplastic effects. In contrast, tumors that have responded best to presently available cytotoxic agents probably have a larger growth fraction of clonogenic cells than the marrow stem cells of the host. In these patients, careful scheduling of selected antitumor agents can progressively destroy neoplastic cells while sparing sufficient numbers of marrow stem cells in G_0.

Another aspect of antineoplastic drug action is the hypothesis of fractional cell kill. Animal experiments reveal that a given dose of a given drug kills a constant percentage of cells, regardless of the number of cells present at the time of therapy (first-order kinetics). At the time of diagnosis of malignant neoplastic disease, the body burden of tumor cells may be as many as 10^{12} cancer cells. A drug capable of killing 99.9% of cancer cells would reduce their number by only three logs (from 10^{12} to 10^9 cells). Only by giving repeated doses in intermittent courses, using multiple drugs sequentially, or administering combination chemotherapy can regrowth of the tumor mass be prevented and larger percentages of the surviving tumor cells be killed. This effect occurs only in a metabolically homogeneous population of tumor cells and assumes that the exposure to the drug(s) is equal in concentration and duration in all tumor cells. However, large tumors probably have a variable blood supply and pharmacologic sanctuaries (eg, central nervous system, cerebrospinal fluid) are known to exist. Small tumors or microscopic foci of tumor cells are more likely to be metabolically homogeneous and have a larger growth fraction (ie, a high percentage of cells actively synthesizing DNA) than large tumors. Therefore, after the primary tumor has been removed by surgery or ablated by radiation, the likelihood of accomplishing a cure with drugs is probably greater because the tumor cell burden is small. This assumption provides the rationale for the use of adjuvant chemotherapy in breast cancer and osteogenic sarcoma. It is not clear to what extent the immune mechanism of the host participates in the eradication of the last tumor cells, but it is assumed that the tumor cell population must be reduced to an order of magnitude of approximately 10^5 cells, the level at which the host's defensive mechanisms are presumably able to assume control.

The effectiveness of an antineoplastic agent is related directly to its pharmacologic disposition in the patient. Tumoricidal concentrations must reach the tumor cell and remain there for a sufficient time to kill the tumor cells. These pharmacologic considerations apply also to critical normal tissue (bone marrow and gastrointestinal epithelium), and optimum therapy should kill the maximum number of tumor cells with minimum lethal effect on cells of normal tissue.

The problem of drug resistance was recognized soon after chemotherapy was introduced. After repeated exposure to antineoplastic agents, a population of inherently resistant tumor cells may continue to proliferate or biochemical resistance may develop. Some of the mechanisms identified are decreased cellular uptake; increased target enzyme (dihydrofolate reductase) or altered affinity for target enzyme (methotrexate); decreased activation of drug (mercaptopurine and fluorouracil); increased deactivation of drug (cytarabine); increased DNA repair (alkylating agents); and increased utilization of salvage pathways (antimetabolites).

To overcome drug resistance, combinations of drugs with different mechanisms of action that are individually effective in the specific tumor when used alone have been employed empirically. More recently, protocols for combination chemotherapy have been designed on the basis of cell cycle phase specificity of the drugs used. The scheduling of antineoplastic agents is complex and may attempt to promote synchronization of cycling cells or recruit temporarily nondividing cancer cells in G_0 phase. Careful scheduling might allow normal tissue cells to regenerate and the host's immunologic mechanisms to recover, thus preventing prohibitive toxicity. (See the discussion on Combination Therapy.)

Adverse Reactions

Hematologic and gastrointestinal toxicity may be dose limiting. Nausea and vomiting often are central nervous system effects.

Alopecia and sterility may occur but cannot be considered dose limiting in the treatment of a potentially lethal disease. The dose-limiting toxic effects of some drugs (eg, neurotoxicity of vincristine [Oncovin], cardiotoxicity of doxorubicin [Adriamycin], pulmonary and cutaneous toxicity of bleomycin [Blenoxane], renal toxicity of methotrexate) are probably not related to the cell cycle. The acute and delayed toxic effects of the antineoplastic agents are summarized in Table 2.

Drug Interactions

The toxicity and efficacy of antineoplastic agents also can be influenced by drugs administered concomitantly for other disorders. The xanthine oxidase inhibitor, allopurinol [Zyloprim], also inhibits the enzymatic oxidation of mercaptopurine; consequently, the dose of the latter must be reduced when both drugs are used together. Phenobarbital induces hepatic microsomal enzymes that activate cyclophosphamide, whereas chloramphenicol inhibits them. Drug interactions may cause either underdosage or overdosage with detrimental results and must be considered carefully whenever antineoplastic agents are used.

ALKYLATING AGENTS

Alkylating agents are highly reactive compounds that covalently attach electrophilic (positively charged) "alkyl" groups to nucleophilic (negatively charged) cellular substances, such as phosphate, amino, sulfhydryl, hydroxyl, car-

TABLE 2.
TOXICITY OF COMMERCIALLY AVAILABLE ANTINEOPLASTIC AGENTS

Drug	Acute Toxicity	Delayed Toxicity
ALKYLATING AGENTS		
Nitrogen Mustards		
Chlorambucil [Leukeran]	Mild nausea and vomiting	Bone marrow depression; acute leukemia
Cyclophosphamide [Cytoxan]	Nausea and vomiting	Bone marrow depression; alopecia; hemorrhagic cystitis
Mechlorethamine Hydrochloride [Mustargen]	Nausea; vomiting; local irritant effect	Bone marrow depression; alopecia; diarrhea; oral ulcers; jaundice; effect on gonads
Melphalan [Alkeran]	Mild nausea and vomiting	Bone marrow depression; acute leukemia
Ethyleneamine Derivative		
Thiotepa	Mild nausea and vomiting	Bone marrow depression
Alkyl Sulfonates		
Busulfan [Myleran]	Mild nausea and vomiting	Bone marrow depression; hyperpigmentation; pulmonary fibrosis; acute leukemia
Nitrosoureas		
Carmustine [BiCNU]	Nausea; vomiting; local phlebitis	Delayed bone marrow depression, cumulative; pulmonary fibrosis
Lomustine [CeeNU]	Nausea and vomiting	Delayed bone marrow depression, cumulative; alopecia
Triazenes		
Dacarbazine [DTIC-Dome]	Nausea; vomiting; local irritant effect	Bone marrow depression; flu-like syndrome; alopecia; renal impairment; transient elevation of liver enzymes

Drug	Acute Toxicity	Delayed Toxicity
ANTIMETABOLITES		
Folic Acid Analogues		
Methotrexate	Nausea and vomiting	Bone marrow depression; stomatitis; ulcerations; diarrhea; hepatic and renal toxicity; pulmonary infiltrates; osteoporosis; alopecia
Pyrimidine Analogues		
Cytarabine [Cytosar]	Nausea and vomiting	Bone marrow depression; megaloblastosis; diarrhea; oral ulcerations; hepatic damage
Floxuridine [FUDR]	Nausea and vomiting	Same as Fluorouracil
Fluorouracil [Adrucil]	Nausea and vomiting	Bone marrow depression; stomatitis; diarrhea; alopecia; pigmentation; cerebellar ataxia
Purine Analogues		
Mercaptopurine [Purinethol]	Nausea and vomiting	Bone marrow depression; hepatic damage; oral ulcers; potentiated by allopurinol
Thioguanine	Occasional nausea and vomiting	Bone marrow depression; possible hepatic damage
NATURAL PRODUCTS		
Vinca Alkaloids		
Vinblastine Sulfate [Velban]	Nausea; vomiting; local irritant effect	Bone marrow depression; alopecia; stomatitis; loss of deep tendon reflexes; jaw pain; paralytic ileus
Vincristine Sulfate [Oncovin]	Local irritant effect	Peripheral neuropathy; neuritic pain; alopecia; constipation; paralytic ileus; mild bone marrow depression
Antibiotics		
Bleomycin Sulfate [Blenoxane]	Nausea; vomiting; anaphylaxis; hypotension	Pneumonitis and pulmonary fibrosis; cutaneous reactions; alopecia; stomatitis
Dactinomycin [Cosmegen]	Nausea; vomiting; local irritant effect	Bone marrow depression; stomatitis; proctitis; diarrhea; alopecia; erythema in irradiated area
Doxorubicin Hydrochloride [Adriamycin]	Nausea; vomiting; local irritant effect	Bone marrow depression; alopecia; cardiotoxicity (may be irreversible); stomatitis; diarrhea; erythema in irradiated area
Mithramycin [Mithracin]	Nausea; vomiting; local irritant effect	Bone marrow depression; hemorrhagic diathesis; stomatitis; diarrhea; hepatic damage; hypocalcemia
Mitomycin [Mutamycin]	Nausea; vomiting; local irritant effect	Bone marrow depression (cumulative); stomatitis; alopecia; renal toxicity
HORMONES		
Adrenal Corticosteroids		
Prednisone and Similar Preparations	None	Hyperadrenocorticism; fluid retention; increased susceptibility to infections; mental aberrations
Estrogens		
Chlorotrianisene	Occasional nausea	Same as Diethylstilbestrol

Drug	Acute Toxicity	Delayed Toxicity
Conjugated Estrogens	Occasional nausea	Same as Diethylstilbestrol
Diethylstilbestrol	Occasional nausea	Hyperadrenocorticism; fluid retention; increased susceptibility to infections; mental aberrations
Diethylstilbestrol Diphosphate	Occasional nausea	Same as Diethylstilbestrol
Ethinyl Estradiol	Occasional nausea	Same as Diethylstilbestrol
Androgens		
Calusterone [Methosarb]	None	Fluid retention; masculinization; hypercalcemia
Dromostanolone Propionate [Drolban]	None	Same as Calusterone
Fluoxymesterone	None	Same as Calusterone and cholestatic jaundice
Testolactone [Teslac]	None	Fluid retention; hypercalcemia
Testosterone Propionate	None	Same as Calusterone
Testosterone Enanthate	None	Same as Calusterone
Progestins		
Hydroxyprogesterone Caproate [Delalutin]	None	Fluid retention; hypercalcemia; cholestatic jaundice
Medroxyprogesterone Acetate [Depo-Provera]	None	Fluid retention
Megestrol Acetate [Megace]	None	Fluid retention
Antiestrogen		
Tamoxifen Citrate [Nolvadex]	Occasional nausea	Hot flushes; vaginal bleeding; pruritus vulvae
ENZYMES		
Asparaginase [Elspar]	Nausea; fever; anaphylaxis	Hypersensitivity; abdominal pain; coagulation defects; renal and hepatic damage; pancreatitis; hyperglycemia; central nervous system depression
MISCELLANEOUS AGENTS		
Substituted Urea		
Hydroxyurea [Hydrea]	Mild nausea and vomiting	Bone marrow depression; hyperkeratosis and hyperpigmentation; stomatitis
Methyl Hydrazine Derivative		
Procarbazine Hydrochloride [Matulane]	Nausea and vomiting	Bone marrow depression; stomatitis; dermatitis; peripheral neuropathy; central nervous system depression
Adrenocortical Suppressant		
Mitotane [Lysodren]	Nausea and vomiting	Central nervous system depression; dermatitis; diarrhea; visual disturbances; adrenal insufficiency
Heavy Metal Complex		
Cisplatin [Platinol]	Nausea and vomiting	Bone marrow depression; renal damage; ototoxicity

boxyl, and imidazole groups. The alkylation of purines and pyrimidines of DNA seems to be most destructive to the cell. The 7-nitrogen of the purine base, guanine, is strongly nucleophilic and its alkylation may lead to chain scission, depurination, and miscoding. Polyfunctional alkylating agents can cause cross linking of two nucleic acid chains or the linking of a nucleic acid to a protein that would prevent separation of the strands of DNA. Monofunctional alkylating agents may cause nonlethal mutagenic and carcinogenic cell damage that can be reproduced as an inherited mutation. They all have immunosuppressive properties.

Although cells in late G_1 or S phase are most susceptible, nonproliferating cells in G_0 also may be destroyed by alkylating agents. Accordingly, alkylating agents are considered to be cell cycle-nonspecific and can be used clinically in tumors with small growth fractions.

The major types of clinically useful alkylating agents are the nitrogen mustards (chlorambucil [Leukeran], cyclophosphamide [Cytoxan], mechlorethamine [Mustargen], melphalan [Alkeran]), ethyleneimines (thiotepa), alkyl sulfonates (busulfan [Myleran]), nitrosoureas (carmustine [BiCNU], lomustine [CeeNU]), and triazenes (dacarbazine [DTIC-Dome]).

BUSULFAN
[Myleran]

$$CH_3SO_2O(CH_2)_4OSO_2CH_3$$

Busulfan is a cell cycle-nonspecific bifunctional alkylating agent. Its cytotoxic action is selective in that it primarily affects granulocytes and, to some extent, platelets. This is the drug of choice in chronic myelocytic leukemia but is of no value in acute leukemia or in the blastic crisis of chronic myelocytic leukemia. Busulfan may be useful in polycythemia vera and myelofibrosis with myeloid metaplasia.

Toxic effects primarily affect the hematologic system and leukopenia may be dose limiting. The reduction in white blood cell count begins after about ten days

of therapy and continues for about two weeks after discontinuation of the drug. Thrombocytopenia and anemia also are observed occasionally; therefore, blood cell counts should be performed frequently. Hyperpigmentation may develop during prolonged therapy and may be part of an Addisonian-like wasting syndrome manifested by asthenia, hypotension, nausea, vomiting, and weight loss. Usually there is no objective evidence of adrenal hypofunction. Long-term delayed effects, such as cataract formation, ovarian fibrosis, amenorrhea, testicular atrophy, aspermia, and gynecomastia, may occur. A rare and potentially fatal complication is the "busulfan lung" syndrome manifested by persistent cough and progressive dyspnea due to intra-alveolar exudation of fibrin with subsequent organization. Serum uric acid levels should be monitored frequently; hyperuricemia, which may result in nephropathy and acute renal failure, can be treated by hydration, alkalization of the urine, and administration of allopurinol.

ROUTE, USUAL DOSAGE, AND PREPARATIONS. *Oral*: For chronic intermittent therapy, 4 to 8 mg daily until the white blood count decreases to 10,000/microliter; treatment is discontinued until the white blood count increases to 50,000/microliter and then is resumed as before.

For chronic continuous therapy, 4 to 6 mg daily until the white blood count decreases to 10,000 to 20,000/microliter; the dose then is reduced as necessary to maintain the white blood count at this level (usually about 2 mg daily).

Myleran (Burroughs Wellcome). Tablets 2 mg.

CARMUSTINE (BCNU)
[BiCNU]

$$\underset{ClCH_2CH_2N-C-NHCH_2CH_2Cl}{\overset{NO\ O}{\overset{|\ \ ||}{}}}$$

Carmustine is a nitrosourea. It alkylates DNA and RNA and, since it contains two chlorethyl groups, is capable of cross linking DNA. Carmustine also inhibits several enzymes by carbamoylation of amino acids in protein. Outstanding features of carmustine are its high lipid solubility and relative lack of ionization at physiologic pH, which enable it to cross the blood-brain barrier quite effectively.

Carmustine is used alone or in combination with other chemotherapeutic agents as palliative therapy in the treatment of central nervous system tumors (primary and metastatic), in multiple myeloma (in combination with prednisone), and in Hodgkin's disease and non-Hodgkin's lymphomas. In lymphomas, it is used as secondary therapy in combination with other drugs in patients who relapse or fail to respond to primary therapy. Carmustine also is effective in melanoma, gastric and colorectal adenocarcinoma, and hepatoma.

This agent causes delayed bone marrow suppression; therefore, complete blood counts should be performed frequently for at least six weeks after a dose. Platelet nadirs occur four to five weeks and leukocyte nadirs five to six weeks after therapy is begun. Thrombocytopenia is usually more severe than leukopenia, and both may be dose limiting. Carmustine should not be given more often than every six weeks. Since the effect on the bone marrow is cumulative, dosage adjustments must be made on the basis of nadir blood counts obtained after the prior dose.

Nausea and vomiting are noted frequently and are dose related. They occur within two hours and usually last four to six hours. With large doses, reversible hepatotoxicity, manifested by increased transaminase, alkaline phosphatase, and bilirubin levels, has been reported in a small percentage of patients. There also have been isolated reports of optic neuritis following use of carmustine. Pulmonary toxicity has been reported. The nitrosoureas may have mutagenic, teratogenic, and carcinogenic potential. Accidental skin contact with the reconstituted drug has caused transient hyperpigmentation.

A burning sensation at the site of injection is common and can be alleviated by slowing the rate of infusion.

ROUTE, USUAL DOSAGE, AND PREPARATIONS. *Intravenous:* Carmustine is dissolved in 3 ml of the sterile diluent supplied and then 27 ml of sterile water for injection is added aseptically. Each milliliter of the resulting solution contains 3.3 mg of carmustine. The reconstituted solution may be further diluted with sodium chloride for injection or 5% dextrose for injection and should be infused intravenously over a one- to two-hour period. Infusion over shorter periods of time may produce intense pain and burning at the site of injection.

As a single agent in previously untreated patients, 200 mg/M^2 of body surface is administered every six weeks. This may be given as a single dose or divided into daily injections of 100 mg/M^2 on two successive days. When carmustine is used with other myelosuppressive agents or in patients with impaired bone marrow function, the dose should be adjusted accordingly. Subsequent dosage should be determined by the hematologic response to the preceding dose. The course of carmustine should not be repeated until circulating blood elements have returned to acceptable levels (platelet count above 100,000/microliter; leukocyte count above 4,000/microliter), usually within six weeks.

BiCNU (Bristol). Powder (lyophilized) 100 mg with 3 ml of sterile diluent (absolute alcohol).

CHLORAMBUCIL
[Leukeran]

Chlorambucil is an aromatic derivative of mechlorethamine and is the slowest-acting, least toxic nitrogen mustard in clinical use. It is cell cycle-nonspecific and has a marked lympholytic effect.

Chlorambucil is the drug of choice in chronic lymphocytic leukemia and is also effective in Hodgkin's disease and non-Hodgkin's lymphomas, multiple myeloma, and particularly in primary macroglobulinemia (Waldenstrom's). This agent also is useful in carcinoma of the ovary, breast, and testes, usually in combination with other agents. It has been used in non-neoplastic diseases, with good responses reported in the treatment of vasculitis as a complication of rheumatoid arthritis and in autoimmune hemolytic anemias associated with cold agglutinins.

Hematologic toxicity is most prominent. Myelosuppression is usually moderate, gradual, and rapidly reversible. Leukopenia develops after the third week of treatment and continues for up to ten days after the last dose. Chlorambucil is usually withheld for about four weeks after a course of radiation therapy or other chemotherapy that depresses bone marrow function. When the white blood cell count decreases suddenly or is reduced to 50% of the pretreatment level, the dose must be reduced or the drug discontinued until leukocyte and platelet counts stabilize or return to a satisfactory level. Gastrointestinal, dermatologic, and hepatic toxicity are seldom encountered with usual doses.

Serum uric acid levels should be monitored frequently to detect hyperuricemia that could lead to renal failure.

ROUTE, USUAL DOSAGE, AND PREPARATIONS. *Oral*: For Hodgkin's disease, initially, 0.2 mg/kg of body weight daily. For nodular lymphomas or chronic lymphocytic leukemia, initially, 0.1 mg/kg daily. The dose is given daily for three to six weeks. When maintenance therapy is necessary, the daily dose should not exceed 0.1 mg/kg and as little as 0.03 mg/kg may be the largest amount tolerated. The drug should be taken one hour before breakfast or two hours after the evening meal.

Leukeran (Burroughs Wellcome). Tablets 2 mg.

CYCLOPHOSPHAMIDE
[Cytoxan]

$$CICH_2CH_2 \diagdown \underset{N-P}{\overset{O}{\uparrow}} \diagup O \diagdown$$
$$CICH_2CH_2 \diagup \qquad \underset{H}{N} \diagup \quad \cdot H_2O$$

This is the most widely used alkylating agent and can be administered orally or intravenously. Cyclophosphamide does not have a vesicant action. It was originally designed as an inactive transport form of nitrogen mustard that would be activated by neoplastic tissue containing high concentrations of phosphatase and phosphamidase that would cause the cyclic phosphamide to cleave at the phosphorus-nitrogen linkage. However, no evidence for this selective activity has been demonstrated and the drug is apparently activated in the liver through its drug-metabolizing microsomal oxidase system. Cyclophosphamide is metabolized to phosphoramide mustard, which is highly cytotoxic. Since it is activated in the liver, its metabolism can be affected by other drugs, depending upon the mixed-function oxidase system. Corticosteroids and sex hormones appear to inhibit these enzymes and would decrease the action and toxicity of cyclophosphamide, whereas barbiturates stimulate this system and would have the opposite effect.

The major indications for cyclophosphamide are in the treatment of lympho- and myeloproliferative disorders. It is a primary drug for induction and maintenance therapy in non-Hodgkin's lymphoma. Burkitt's lymphoma is highly responsive and cyclophosphamide is very beneficial in acute lymphocytic leukemia in children. It also is useful in multiple myeloma and chronic lymphocytic leukemia. Solid tumors that often respond to this drug are carcinoma of the ovary, breast, and lung; neuroblastoma; and sarcomas.

Cyclophosphamide has a marked immunosuppressive action and has been used in non-neoplastic diseases, such as rheumatoid arthritis, nephrotic syndrome in children, and Wegener's granulomatosis.

A variety of toxic effects have been observed. Bone marrow depression and gastrointestinal disturbances are common. Thrombocytopenia is probably less severe than with other alkylating agents. More than 50% of patients receiving intensive or prolonged therapy experience alopecia, which is usually reversible. One dose-limiting toxic effect resulting from the high concentration of active metabolites in the urinary tract is sterile hemorrhagic cystitis. This can be ameliorated by ample fluid intake and frequent voiding. Bladder fibrosis and carcinoma of the bladder have been reported after long-term use of cyclophosphamide.

Other toxic effects are impaired liver function, hyperpigmentation, oral ulceration, amenorrhea, azoospermia, irreversible pulmonary fibrosis, and a syndrome of inappropriate secretion of antidiuretic hormone (SIADH). After use of large doses of cyclophosphamide, myocarditis and congestive heart failure have been observed and the cardiotoxic effect of doxorubicin was potentiated.

ROUTES, USUAL DOSAGE, AND PREPARATIONS.
Intravenous: For patients with no hematologic deficiency, initially, 40 to 50 mg/kg of body weight given in divided doses over a period of two to five days. Marked leukopenia frequently occurs with this dose, but recovery usually begins after seven to ten days. The dose is reduced in patients with impaired bone marrow function. For maintenance therapy, 10 to 15 mg/kg every seven to ten days or 3 to 5 mg/kg twice weekly.

> *Cytoxan* (Mead Johnson). Crystalline powder 100, 200, and 500 mg.

Oral: For maintenance therapy, 1 to 5 mg/kg of body weight daily.

> *Cytoxan* (Mead Johnson). Tablets 25 and 50 mg.

DACARBAZINE
[DTIC-Dome]

The mechanism of action of dacarbazine is uncertain. It was originally considered an antimetabolite, acting as a purine analogue. It has demonstrated alkylating activity and is cell cycle-nonspecific. Dacarbazine is effective in malignant melanoma, Hodgkin's disease, neuroblastoma, and soft tissue sarcomas.

Myelosuppression is usually dose limiting. This effect is delayed, with leukopenia generally reported after 10 days of therapy

and thrombocytopenia after 10 to 15 days, but they may appear two to four weeks after the last dose. Nausea and vomiting usually occur within one to three hours after administration and last for up to 12 hours. Most patients develop tolerance after one to two days of treatment. An "influenza-like" syndrome consisting of fever, myalgia, and malaise has been described. Other untoward effects are pain at the infusion site, facial flushing and paresthesia, alopecia, and elevation of hepatic enzyme levels.

ROUTE, USUAL DOSAGE, AND PREPARATIONS.
Intravenous: 2 to 4.5 mg/kg of body weight daily for 10 days every 28 days or 250 mg/M^2/day for five days every three weeks.

> *DTIC-Dome* (Dome). Powder 100 and 200 mg.

LOMUSTINE (CCNU)
[CeeNU]

This nitrosourea may inhibit several key enzymatic processes leading to DNA synthesis. There is evidence to suggest that lomustine does not function solely as an alkylating agent, since cross resistance with conventional alkylating agents has not been observed and apparently it acts in a different phase of the cell cycle. Because of the high lipid solubility and relative lack of ionization at physiologic pH, lomustine readily crosses the blood-brain barrier.

Lomustine has shown good activity against central nervous system tumors (overall response rate, 41%), Hodgkin's disease (response rate, 46%), and lung cancer (response rate, 16%). Fair activity has been reported in breast cancer, renal cell tumors, and melanoma. The properties of lomustine that permit oral administration, infrequent schedules of administration because of its delayed myelosuppression, lack of toxicity on other major organs, and ability to cross the blood-brain barrier in central nervous system diseases have been major factors stimulating interest in combining it with other drugs in the treatment of certain tumors.

The most serious toxic effect is bone marrow suppression, which is delayed, dose related, dose limiting, and cumulative. Thrombocytopenia develops about four weeks and leukopenia about six weeks after a dose of lomustine; both persist for one to two weeks. Gastrointestinal disturbances (nausea and vomiting) occur two to six hours after administration and last less than 24 hours. Other reactions include stomatitis, alopecia, anemia, and hepatotoxicity manifested by transient, reversible elevation of liver function tests. Neurologic reactions, such as disorientation, lethargy, ataxia, and dysarthria, have been noted in some patients. However, their relationship to medication is unclear.

ROUTE, USUAL DOSAGE, AND PREPARATIONS. *Oral: Adults and children,* 130 mg/M² of body surface is given as a single dose every six weeks. In patients with impaired bone marrow function, the dose should be reduced to 100 mg/M² every six weeks. When used with other myelosuppressive drugs, the dose must be reduced. Blood counts should be monitored weekly and the dose should not be repeated before six weeks; circulating blood elements should return to acceptable levels (platelet count above 100,000/microliter; leukocyte count above 4,000/microliter).

   CeeNU (Bristol). Capsules 10, 40, and 100 mg (stable for at least two years when stored at room temperature in tightly closed containers).

MECHLORETHAMINE HYDROCHLORIDE
[Mustargen]

$$\underset{ClCH_2CH_2}{\overset{ClCH_2CH_2}{\diagdown}} \underset{+NHCH_3}{N} \quad Cl^-$$

The major indications for this alkylating agent are in the treatment of disseminated Hodgkin's disease and other lymphomas. Mechlorethamine also may be useful in chronic myelocytic leukemia, polycythemia vera, bronchogenic carcinoma, and other solid tumors. Malignant pleural effu-

sions can be effectively palliated by intracavitary instillation.

The most common reactions following administration of the drug are nausea and vomiting, which are direct central nervous system effects. These reactions usually can be controlled by premedication with a short-acting barbiturate and an antiemetic. Anorexia, weakness, and diarrhea also may occur.

The most serious toxic effect is bone marrow depression. Lymphopenia is usually apparent within 24 hours. The nadir of the fall in granulocytes and thrombocytes usually occurs within 7 to 21 days after administration of the drug. Hematologic recovery is usually adequate after four weeks, and rebound hyperplasia may be present from the fifth to seventh week. Myelosuppression may be more marked in patients who have previously received chemotherapy or radiation and the dose of mechlorethamine must be adjusted accordingly. Other toxic effects are maculopapular skin eruptions, alopecia, hearing loss and tinnitus, vertigo, jaundice, menstrual irregularities, impaired spermatogenesis, and total germinal aplasia. Rarely, hemolytic anemia associated with such diseases as lymphomas and chronic lymphocytic leukemia may be precipitated by treatment with alkylating agents, including mechlorethamine.

Thrombosis and thrombophlebitis may result from direct contact of the drug with the intima of the injected vein. Extravasation into subcutaneous tissue can cause severe, brawny induration and slough may result. If accidental extravasation has occurred, the involved area should be infiltrated with sterile isotonic sodium thiosulfate solution (1/6 molar), and an ice compress should be applied intermittently for 6 to 12 hours. Various chromosomal abnormalities have been reported in association with nitrogen mustard therapy. It should be borne in mind that use of mechlorethamine may predispose the patient to bacterial, viral, or fungal infection. This is more likely to occur when concomitant steroid therapy is employed. Erythema multiforme was observed in one patient. Herpes zoster, a common complicating infection in patients with lymphomas, may first appear after therapy is instituted and on occasion may be precipitated by treatment.

ROUTES, USUAL DOSAGE, AND PREPARATIONS. This highly reactive agent has a marked vesicant action. Therefore, it is usually injected into the tubing of a freely flowing intravenous infusion. Since the compound undergoes chemical transformation rapidly and decomposes on standing, it must be prepared immediately before administration and the use of surgical gloves is advised to protect the hands of the physician preparing the solution. A few minutes after administration, mechlorethamine is no longer present in active form and less than 0.01% of the drug is recovered in the urine.

Intravenous: For disseminated Hodgkin's disease and other lymphomas, 6 mg/M^2 of body surface on days one and eight given as a component of the MOPP regimen; the course is repeated every 28 days. For bronchogenic carcinoma and other solid tumors, 0.4 mg/kg of body weight (10 mg/M^2) as a single dose or in divided doses on successive days.

Intracavitary: For malignant pleural effusions, 0.2 to 0.4 mg/kg of body weight. See published articles for more specific data.

> *Mustargen* (Merck Sharp & Dohme). Powder (crystalline) 10 mg with sodium chloride q.s. 100 mg.

MELPHALAN
[Alkeran]

This phenylalanine derivative of nitrogen mustard is a cell cycle-nonspecific agent. Melphalan is given orally and is very effective in the treatment of multiple myeloma; cross resistance with cyclophosphamide apparently does not occur. It also has been used extensively as an adjuvant in the treatment of stage II breast carcinoma. Ovarian carcinoma and testicular semi-noma have responded to this agent. Melphalan also has been used for arterial infusion of extremities affected by malignant melanoma.

Melphalan produces dose-related depression of bone marrow function that results in leukopenia, thrombocytopenia, and anemia. Nausea and vomiting have occurred after large doses. Since its safety during early pregnancy has not been established, melphalan should not be used during this period.

ROUTE, USUAL DOSAGE, AND PREPARATIONS. *Oral*: 0.25 mg/kg of body weight for four consecutive days every six weeks, or 0.1 to 0.15 mg/kg daily for two to three weeks, then 2 to 4 mg daily following a rest period of up to four weeks. The dosage is adjusted to produce mild leukopenia (less than 3,500/microliter) and thrombocytopenia (less than 100,000/microliter).

> *Alkeran* (Burroughs Wellome). Tablets 2 mg.

THIOTEPA

This drug is a cell cycle-nonspecific trifunctional alkylating agent. It is used only parenterally and is effective in the palliative management of carcinoma of the breast and ovary. It has limited usefulness in lymphomas. Intracavitary instillation may control pleural or peritoneal effusions. Intravesical instillation is sometimes useful in small papillary carcinomas of the urinary bladder.

Thiotepa may produce nausea, anorexia, and headache. It has a dose-related toxic effect on the hematopoietic system. Initial effects on the bone marrow may not become evident for 5 to 30 days (median, 15 days). As with other alkylating agents, the white blood cell and platelet counts are reliable guides. All of these elements should be monitored weekly during maintenance therapy and for at least four weeks after therapy is terminated.

Patients with impaired renal function may not tolerate this drug. Thiotepa is contraindicated during the first trimester of pregnancy. Concomitant radiation therapy should be carried out cautiously, for the depressant effect on bone marrow is additive.

ROUTES, USUAL DOSAGE, AND PREPARATIONS. Dosage must always be carefully individualized. To avoid too frequent administration, one has to bear in mind that the clinical response to thiotepa is slow and that the drug has a cumulative bone marrow depressant effect.

Intravenous: 0.2 mg/kg of body weight is given daily for five days every four weeks, blood count permitting.

Topical: For bladder instillation, 60 mg in 30 to 60 ml of distilled water is instilled into the bladder by catheter and retained for two hours. The patient may be positioned every 15 minutes for maximum area contact.

Thiotepa (Lederle). Powder 15 mg.

ANTIMETABOLITES

These compounds are so chemically similar to normally occurring metabolites that they enter the same metabolic system, but they differ enough to interfere with normal metabolic pathways. Antimetabolites interfere with normal biosynthesis by competing for important enzymatic reactions in the synthesis of purines, pyrimidines, and their precursors. They also may be incorporated into nucleic acids in place of the corresponding normal nucleotides. This leads to an imbalance in the growth of cells or to errors in coding, transcription, or translation after incorporation into DNA and RNA. Antimetabolites with recognized clinical value are folic acid, pyrimidine, and purine analogues. They act primarily during the DNA synthetic phase of the cell cycle (S phase), some exclusively (eg, cytarabine) and others (eg, methotrexate) by preventing further entry of the cells into the DNA synthetic phase.

CYTARABINE (Cytosine Arabinoside)
[Cytosar-U]

This pyrimidine analogue is a synthetic nucleoside that differs from the normal nucleosides, cytidine and deoxycytidine, in that the sugar moiety is arabinose rather than ribose or deoxyribose. It interferes with DNA synthesis by inhibiting DNA polymerase, and its effects are exerted during the DNA synthetic phase of the cell cycle (S phase). It is rapidly deaminated in the blood to an inactive metabolite, uracil arabinoside, and disappears from the blood in approximately 20 minutes. After intrathecal injection, it may persist for several hours because of low levels of deaminase in the cerebrospinal fluid. Cytarabine has a marked immunosuppressive effect and can suppress either humoral or cellular responses or both, depending upon the dosage schedules used. The schedule of administration influences the antitumor effect and toxicity of this drug. Although cytarabine has not proved effective against solid tumors, it is very useful in acute myelogenous leukemia, especially in combination with thioguanine and daunoubicin or doxorubicin.

The major toxic effect of cytarabine is bone marrow depression manifested by megaloblastosis of the red cell precursors, reticulocytopenia, leukopenia, and thrombocytopenia, generally in that order. The leukopenia is caused primarily by granulocyte depression, and normal lymphoid elements are only minimally affected. The white blood cell count may continue to fall after the drug is stopped and reach the nadir after drug-free intervals of five to seven days. Recovery occurs after two to three weeks but may take longer if administration is prolonged. Gastrointestinal disturbances, stomatitis, thrombophlebitis, hepatic dysfunction, and fever also have been reported.

ROUTES, USUAL DOSAGE, AND PREPARATIONS. Only physicians experienced in cancer chemotherapy should use cytarabine. For induction therapy, patients should be hospitalized in a facility with laboratory and supportive resources available to monitor drug tolerance and protect and maintain the patient compromised by drug toxicity. *Intravenous*: Although larger total doses are tolerated when given by rapid intravenous injection rather than by slow infusion, the optimal dosage schedule is still to be determined. The most frequently used dosage schedules are: For rapid injection continuous treatment, initially, 2 mg/kg of body weight daily for ten days. Blood counts should be performed daily and, if neither an antileukemic effect nor toxicity is apparent after ten days, the dose is increased to 4 mg/kg/day. This dose is maintained until toxicity or a therapeutic response is evident.

For intravenous infusion continuous treatment, 0.5 to 1 mg/kg daily, initially. This may be given in an infusion of any desired duration (1, 4, 12, or 24 hours). Results with one-hour infusions have been satisfactory and are most convenient for many patients. This dosage is continued for ten days, with the peripheral blood count monitored daily. If there is no toxic or therapeutic response, the dose is increased to 2 mg/kg/day until toxicity or remission occurs. *Subcutaneous*: To maintain remissions, 1 mg/kg of body weight is injected once or twice weekly.

Cytosar-U (Upjohn). Powder (freeze-dried) 100 and 500 mg with diluent.

FLUOROURACIL (5 FU)
  [Adrucil]

This fluorinated pyrimidine was developed as a potential antineoplastic agent

because of the observation that tumor cells utilized the normal pyrimidine base, uracil, for biosynthesis of DNA more effectively than did nontumor cells. Fluorouracil is converted in vivo to the deoxynucleotide that inhibits thymidylate synthetase, an enzyme that promotes methylation of deoxyuridilic acid to thymidylic acid. By blocking thymidylate synthetase, DNA synthesis is prevented. In addition, fluorouracil is incorporated as the nucleotide into RNA, probably depressing RNA synthesis directly by blocking incorporation of uracil and orotic acid into RNA. Localization of the action of fluorouracil at the precise step in the cell cycle has not been possible, and the drug acts as a self-limiting inhibitor of S phase.

Fluorouracil is extensively used in the treatment of colorectal carcinoma. It also is effective in gastric and pancreatic adenocarcinoma (sometimes in conjunction with radiation therapy). Other responsive tumors are carcinoma of the breast, bladder, ovary, and uterine cervix and hepatoma. Objective evidence of a palliative effect has been noted in 40% of patients with carcinoma of the breast, in 10% to 15% of those with carcinoma of the rectum, and in 20% of those with carcinoma of the colon. The variations in the reported incidence of remissions are primarily due to differences in dosage, selection and condition of patients, and criteria used to evaluate objective signs of response. The average duration of remissions induced by repeated courses of therapy at monthly intervals is five to six months, but responses lasting as long as four years have been reported.

The major toxic effects of fluorouracil affect the gastrointestinal and hematologic systems. Anorexia, nausea, and vomiting are common. Stomatitis and diarrhea serve as indications that therapy should be interrupted. Leukopenia is the major dose-limiting effect, with the nadir of the white blood cell count commonly occurring between day 7 and 14 after the first dose. Thrombocytopenia is much less prominent and may be observed between days 7 and 17. Other adverse effects are alopecia, dermatitis, and hyperpigmentation. Reversible cerebellar ataxia occurs in 1% of patients. This is probably dose related but may occur at any time during therapy, usually after several months. Cerebellar signs may persist for several weeks after discontinuing the drug.

Drug catabolism may be impaired in patients with extensive liver metastases, resulting in increased anabolism of fluorouracil to toxic compounds.

The use of slow intravenous infusions lasting two to eight hours markedly decreases the toxicity of fluorouracil. However, results of clinical studies have indicated that rapid injections may be more effective. It has been reported that the weekly administration of fluorouracil without an initial loading dose has produced clinical responses with significantly less toxicity. There also is some evidence that fluorouracil administered orally once weekly produces antineoplastic effects and is well tolerated, but absorption is erratic after this route.

ROUTE, USUAL DOSAGE, AND PREPARATIONS. *Intravenous*: The original regimen consisted of a loading dose of 12 mg/kg of body weight daily for four successive days, followed (if no toxicity is observed) by 6 mg/kg every other day until the 12th day, with a single daily dose not exceeding 800 mg. However, all untoward effects are markedly increased and can be very dangerous when this regimen is used. Therefore, many oncologists administer weekly doses of 15 mg/kg (maximum single dose, 1 g). Treatment is continued as long as there is evidence of clinical improvement. The dosage and frequency of each successive course should be regulated on the basis of the patient's tolerance to the drug.

Recent studies comparing the loading regimen, the weekly regimen, and the oral route have demonstrated that a loading dose of 12 mg/kg/day for five days, followed by weekly maintenance doses of 10 to 15 mg/kg as a single dose (maximum,

1 g/week) produces the highest rate of objective remissions.

Adrucil (Adria), *Fluorouracil* (Roche). Solution 50 mg/ml in 10 ml containers.

TOPICAL FLUOROURACIL
[Efudex]

Topical preparations containing 1% or 2% fluorouracil are used for the treatment of multiple actinic (solar) keratoses on the head and neck and the 5% concentration is used on keratoses in other areas. The 5% concentration also is useful in the treatment of superficial basal cell carcinomas when conventional methods are impractical, such as in patients with multiple lesions or difficult treatment sites. The diagnosis should be established before treatment is begun, since this new method has not been proved effective in other types of basal cell carcinomas. If the lesions are isolated and easily accessible, conventional techniques are preferred because of their higher success rate (almost 100% versus approximately 93% with fluorouracil). For a description of the mechanism of action, see the preceding evaluation on Fluorouracil.

Efudex is contraindicated in patients with known hypersensitivity to any of its components. If an occlusive dressing is used, the incidence of inflammatory reactions in adjacent normal skin may be increased. A porous gauze dressing may be applied for cosmetic reasons without increasing the frequency of reactions. Prolonged exposure to ultraviolet rays should be avoided while this preparation is being used, because this may intensify the severity of reactions. The safety of the use of topical fluorouracil during pregnancy has not been established.

If this preparation is applied with the fingers, the hands should be washed immediately thereafter. It should be applied with care near the eyes, nose, and mouth. Unresponsive solar keratoses should be biopsied to confirm the diagnosis. Patients should be informed that the treated areas may be unsightly during therapy and, in some cases, for several weeks following cessation of treatment. Follow-up biopsies should be performed as indicated in the management of superficial basal cell carcinoma.

The most frequently encountered local reactions are pain, pruritus, hyperpigmentation, and burning at the site of application. Other local reactions include dermatitis, scarring, soreness, tenderness, suppuration, scaling, and swelling. A topical corticosteroid cream may be employed to hasten the involution of severe inflammation following cessation of topical fluorouracil therapy. Insomnia, stomatitis, irritability, medicinal taste, photosensitivity, lacrimation, and telangiectasia also have been reported, although a causal relationship is remote. Laboratory abnormalities reported are leukocytosis, thrombocytopenia, toxic granulation, and eosinophilia.

ROUTE, USUAL DOSAGE, AND PREPARATIONS.
Topical: The response to application occurs in the following sequence: erythema, usually followed by vesiculation, erosion, ulceration, necrosis, and epithelialization. For superficial basal cell carcinoma, the 5% concentration is applied twice daily in an amount sufficient to cover the lesions. Treatment should be continued for at least three to six weeks and may be required for as long as 10 or 12 weeks before the lesions are obliterated. As in any neoplastic condition, the patient should be followed for a reasonable period of time to determine if a cure has been obtained.

For actinic keratoses, the medication is applied twice daily. The stage of ulceration and necrosis is usually attained within two to four weeks, and complete healing is usually evident within one to two months after cessation of therapy.

> *Efudex* (Roche). Solution 2% and 5% with propylene glycol, tris(hydroxymethyl)aminomethane, hydroxypropyl cellulose, methylparaben, propylparaben, and edetate disodium in 10 ml containers; cream 5% in a vanishing cream base consisting of white petrolatum, stearyl alcohol, propylene glycol, polysorbate 60, methylparaben, and propylparaben in 25 g containers.

FLOXURIDINE
[FUDR]

Floxuridine is the deoxyriboside derivative of fluorouracil. Intra-arterial administration of this drug has a palliative effect in certain malignancies that do not respond to surgery or other forms of treatment. These include carcinoma of the rectum, colon, and gastrointestinal tract and liver metastases from these sites.

The usefulness of floxuridine is based upon its distinctive metabolism, which depends upon the rate of administration. Following rapid intravenous injection, floxuridine is rapidly broken down to fluorouracil and then to urea, and its efficacy and adverse effects are the same as those of fluorouracil. However, when floxuridine is given by slow, continuous intra-arterial infusion, it is anabolically converted to the active agent, floxuridine monophosphate, which blocks DNA synthesis. With this method of administration, the dose can be reduced (30 mg/kg to 1 mg/kg) and the drug is three times more effective than with rapid intravenous injection; therefore, intra-arterial infusion is used exclusively.

Local reactions (eg, aphthous stomatitis, erythema) are more prominent than systemic reactions after intra-arterial injection. Systemic reactions are similar to those seen with fluorouracil. The most common of these are nausea, vomiting, diarrhea, and enteritis. Anemia and leukopenia also occur. Other adverse effects include gastrointestinal disorders (anorexia, cramps, duodenal ulcer, gastritis, glossitis, pharyngitis) and dermatologic reactions (alopecia, dermatitis, pruritus, rash, ulceration). Elevated alkaline phosphatase, serum transaminase, serum bilirubin, and lactic dehydrogenase values have been noted.

Because of its toxicity and low therapeutic index, floxuridine should be given under the supervision of a physician who is experienced not only in cancer chemotherapy, but in the technique of intra-arterial infusion. Ambulatory patients must be hospitalized during the first course of treatment and should be informed about toxic manifestations. White blood cell and platelet counts should be performed regularly.

As with fluorouracil, floxuridine should be discontinued immediately when any of the following signs and symptoms appear: stomatitis, esophagopharyngitis, gastrointestinal ulcerations and bleeding, diarrhea (five or more loose stools daily), intractable vomiting, leukocyte count less than 3,500/microliter or a rapidly decreasing count, thrombocytopenia with a platelet count under 100,000/microliter, or hemorrhage from any site. Floxuridine is contraindicated in patients with poor nutritional status or bone marrow depression, and it should be avoided in pregnant women, particularly during the first trimester, because of its potential teratogenicity.

ROUTE, USUAL DOSAGE, AND PREPARATIONS. *Intra-arterial*: The specialized nature of this technique requires the combined skill of a surgeon and oncologist. *Adults*, with the patient under general anesthesia, the artery supplying the tumor is surgically exposed and the catheter is inserted into the lumen and sutured to the vessel wall. A suitable infusion pump is then used to administer 0.1 to 0.6 mg/kg of body weight continuously over a 24-hour period. For hepatic artery infusion, the dosage is 0.4 to 0.6 mg/kg because the drug is metabolized immediately by the liver. Infusion is continued until a local toxic reaction (eg, cutaneous erythema, mucositis) occurs over the region of infusion. The infusion is stopped until the reaction subsides; additional courses then are given for as long as the response continues. Adequate courses of therapy have varied from one month to several years.

FUDR (Roche). Powder 500 mg.

MERCAPTOPURINE
[Purinethol]

Mercaptopurine is the thio-analogue of hypoxanthine, which is part of the synthetic pathway of adenine and guanine. It interferes with purine synthesis and is cell cycle-specific for the S phase. The drug also is an immunosuppressant.

Mercaptopurine produces complete remission in 30% of children with acute lymphoblastic or stem cell leukemia. When administered after a prednisone-induced remission, the incidence of prolonged complete bone marrow remissions approaches 80%. Mercaptopurine is less effective in acute myeloblastic leukemia in adults; complete remissions occur in less than 20% of patients and the duration is shorter than in the lymphoblastic type. In the early phase of chronic myelocytic leukemia, the drug produces remissions in 80% of adults, but busulfan is the drug of choice for initial therapy. In the acute blastic phase, remissions are rarely attained. The drug is generally used with other drugs to treat acute leukemia.

Toxic effects include leukopenia, thrombocytopenia, hemorrhage, nausea, vomiting, anorexia, aphthous stomatitis, and cholestatic jaundice. Myelosuppression can be delayed and leukocyte counts should be performed weekly; mercaptopurine should be discontinued if an abnormal reduction occurs. The leukocyte count is used to establish a maintenance dose. Smaller doses are recommended in patients with impaired renal or hepatic function to avoid accumulation. Since mercaptopurine is metabolized by xanthine oxidase, the dose should be reduced to 33% to 50% of the usual amount if allopurinol, a xanthine oxidase inhibitor, is used concomitantly. Mercaptopurine should be avoided during the first trimester of pregnancy.

ROUTE, USUAL DOSAGE, AND PREPARATIONS.
Oral: *Adults and children over 5 years*, 2.5 mg/kg of body weight daily in single or divided doses. If clinical improvement does not occur and leukocyte depression is not observed within four weeks, the dose may be increased to a maximum of 5 mg/kg daily. The total daily dosage may be given at one time. It is calculated to the closest multiple of 25 mg. Once a remission is achieved, administration may be continued for a prolonged period. Therapy should be discontinued if serious toxic effects occur; it may be reinstituted at one-half the previous dosage after toxic manifestations disappear. Appropriate dosage modifications are required when mercaptopurine is used with other cytotoxic drugs.

> *Purinethol* (Burroughs Wellcome). Tablets 50 mg.

METHOTREXATE

METHOTREXATE SODIUM

This folic acid analogue competitively binds to dihydrofolate reductase, the enzyme that reduces folic acid to tetrahydrofolic acid (THF). THF is critically important to the metabolic transfer of one-carbon units in a variety of biochemical reactions. These include biosynthesis of thymidylic acid (the nucleoside specific to DNA) and inosinic acid, the precursor of adenine and guanine nucleotides in de novo purine biosynthesis. Methotrexate is cell cycle-specific for the S phase. The block of dihydrofolate reduction can be bypassed clinically by the use of leucovorin calcium (citrovorum factor). This "rescue" agent may allow the preferential recovery of normal tissue and thus permit the use of larger doses of methotrexate.

Methotrexate has been very effective in women with choriocarcinoma and related trophoblastic tumors; cures have been reported in approximately 75% of cases. It induces complete remissions in acute lymphoblastic leukemia of childhood but is of more value for maintenance therapy. Methotrexate is effective in Burkitt's lymphoma; mycosis fungoides; carcinomas of the head and neck region, breast, testis, and uterine cervix; and embryonal rhabdomyosarcoma. Large doses of methotrexate with leucovorin rescue have been used in bronchogenic carcinoma and osteogenic sarcoma. Methotrexate is a component of combination chemotherapeutic regimens used to treat breast, lung, testicular, and ovarian carcinoma. It also has been used in severe psoriasis (see Chapter 61, Dermatologic Preparations).

Toxicity usually involves the gastrointestinal tract, bone marrow, and oral mucosa. Stomatitis is common and is an indication for interruption of therapy. Diarrhea also is an indication to discontinue methotrexate. Hemorrhagic enteritis and intestinal perforation can occur if therapy is continued after the appearance of diarrhea. Hepatic dysfunction has been observed after long-term use; it is usually reversible and subclinical but may lead to fibrosis and cirrhosis.

Myelosuppression is very common and is dose limiting. Since methotrexate is excreted principally by the kidneys, its use in the presence of impaired renal function may result in renal tubular necrosis. Even moderate degrees of prerenal azotemia enhance toxicity. Therefore, renal function should be monitored prior to and during methotrexate therapy. Adequate hydration and alkalization of the urine (using sodium bicarbonate or acetazolamide) will enhance excretion of methotrexate. Alopecia and dermatitis have been reported, and osteoporosis is observed occasionally in children on long-term maintenance therapy. An acute reversible allergic pneumonitis may develop, especially with intermittent therapy. It is characterized by fever, cough, shortness of breath, peripheral eosinophilia, and patchy pulmonary infiltrates. Central nervous system toxicity has been observed when methotrexate is given intrathecally. This drug has been reported to act as an abortifacient and should not be used during the first trimester of pregnancy.

Vinca alkaloids increase the cellular uptake of methotrexate while penicillin, kanamycin, corticosteroids, bleomycin, and asparaginase decrease cellular uptake.

ROUTES, USUAL DOSAGE, AND PREPARATIONS. *Oral, Intravenous*: 2.5 to 5 mg orally daily, or 0.4 mg/kg of body weight intravenously (maximum, 25 mg daily) for four to five days, or 0.4 mg/kg intravenously twice weekly. When used with cyclophosphamide and fluorouracil, the dose of methotrexate is 40 mg/M^2 (30 mg/M^2 if over 60 years) intravenously on days one and eight every 28 days.

Oral, Intramuscular: For choriocarcinoma and similar trophoblastic disease, 15 to 30 mg daily for five days, with the course repeated three to five times.

Oral: For lymphomas (Burkitt's tumor, stages I and II), 10 to 25 mg daily for four to eight days.

Intrathecal: 0.2 to 0.5 mg/kg of body weight (maximum, 12 mg) every two to five days until the cell count of cerebrospinal fluid returns to normal.

  Methotrexate (Lederle). Tablets 2.5 mg.
  Methotrexate Sodium (Lederle). Powder 20 mg; solution 2.5 and 25 mg/ml in 2 ml containers (strengths expressed in terms of the base).

THIOGUANINE

Thioguanine is an analogue of guanine and is metabolized along pathways similar to those used by mercaptopurine. Its growth-inhibiting action seems to be in its substitution for guanine in nucleic acid synthesis, producing functionally altered polynucleotides. It is cell cycle-specific for the S phase.

Thioguanine also is an analogue of mercaptopurine and is effective in the treatment of the same types of leukemia. It is preferred to mercaptopurine because it causes fewer gastrointestinal reactions; in addition, it may be used with allopurinol without an adjustment of dose. The rate and duration of responses induced by thioguanine and mercaptopurine in acute leukemias are similar. As with other antineoplastic agents of the same class, cross resistance occurs between the two drugs. The combination of thioguanine and cytarabine is active against acute myelogenous leukemia in adults and in the blast crisis of chronic myelogenous leukemia.

Thioguanine depresses bone marrow function and causes leukopenia, thrombocytopenia, and hemorrhage. Hemoglobin levels and white blood cell and platelet counts should be determined at weekly intervals. Thioguanine should be discontinued if leukocyte or platelet counts decrease suddenly. Therapy may be reinstituted at the same or reduced dosage when the cell counts return to normal levels. Occasionally, nausea, vomiting, anorexia, and aphthous stomatitis may develop if large doses are used.

Thioguanine should not be given during the first trimester of pregnancy because of its potential teratogenic effects.

ROUTE, USUAL DOSAGE, AND PREPARATIONS. *Oral*: *Adults*, 2 mg/kg of body weight daily. The total daily dose is calculated to the closest multiple of 20 mg. If there is no response to this dose after four weeks, the amount may be increased cautiously to 3 mg/kg daily. If no clinical or laboratory evidence of improvement with the larger dose is observed, another class of drugs should be substituted for thioguanine.

For dosage in acute myeloblastic leukemia, see the section on Combination Therapy.

  Thioguanine (Burroughs Wellcome). Tablets 40 mg.

MISCELLANEOUS AGENTS

ASPARAGINASE
[Elspar]

Asparaginase is an enzyme derived from cultures of either *Escherichia coli* or *Erwinia carotovora*. The trademarked product is derived from *E. coli*. It inhibits asparagine synthetase and catalyzes the hydrolysis of the amino acid, asparagine, to aspartic acid and ammonia, thus depleting the amount of asparagine in tumor cells. Certain leukemic cells apparently cannot convert aspartic acid to asparagine via the asparagine synthetase reaction and depend upon an exogenous source of asparagine. Normal cells, however, are able to synthesize asparagine. Asparaginase was considered to be a unique antitumor agent that exploited this biochemical difference between normal and neoplastic cells. The asparagine-depleting action interferes with protein and also DNA and RNA synthesis in tumor cells. Asparaginase probably is cell cycle-specific for the postmitotic G_1 phase. It is effective in patients with acute lymphocytic leukemia and is most often combined with other chemotherapeutic agents to induce remissions of the disease in children. This agent should not be used as the sole induction agent unless combination therapy is deemed inappropriate, and it is not recommended for maintenance therapy. It is less effective in solid tumors.

The usefulness of asparaginase is limited by a variety of toxic effects. Despite its immunosuppressive properties, hypersensitivity reactions ranging from urticaria to anaphylactic shock occur in approximately 10% of patients during the initial course and more frequently when the drug is readministered. Allergic reactions are not completely predictable on the basis of an intradermal skin test.

Neurotoxic reactions are observed primarily in adults; approximately 25% of patients exhibit a decreased level of consciousness ranging from confusion to coma. Seizures or focal neurologic signs are rare. Since the drug does not cross the blood-brain barrier, the central nervous system toxicity is probably related to elevated levels of ammonia and aspartic or glutamic acid or to inhibited protein synthesis.

Decreased protein synthesis may result in hypoalbuminemia leading to edema. In addition to hypofibrinogenemia, other clotting factors, notably V, VII, VIII, and IX, may be decreased. Reduction of circulating platelets also has occurred. This, together with increased levels of fibrin degradation products in the serum, may indicate the development of disseminated intravascular coagulation (consumption coagulopathy). Myelosuppression is rare and usually not severe.

Hepatotoxicity, with abnormal results of liver function tests, occurs in approximately 50% to 75% of patients. Hyperglycemia is probably secondary to decreased insulin production. Pancreatitis, sometimes fulminant, has been observed in about 5% of patients. Azotemia, usually prerenal, occurs frequently. Acute renal shutdown and fatal renal insufficiency have been reported during treatment. Fatal hyperthermia also has been observed.

ROUTES, USUAL DOSAGE, AND PREPARATIONS. When administered intravenously, this enzyme should be injected into the tubing of an already running infusion of sodium chloride injection or 5% dextrose in water over a period of at least 30 minutes. Because of the occurrence of allergic reactions, an intradermal skin test should be performed prior to initial administration and when the drug is readministered after a week or more has elapsed between courses. However, negative results of the skin test do not preclude the possibility of the development of an allergic reaction.

Intravenous: Doses range from 200 IU/kg/day for 28 days when given as the sole induction agent in *adults and children* to 1,000 IU/kg/day for 10 days when used following therapy with prednisone and vincristine in *children*.

Intramuscular (children only): 6,000 IU/M² given intermittently on days 4, 7, 10, 13, 16, 19, 22, 25, and 28 in a combination regimen with prednisone and vincristine. The administration of asparaginase intravenously concurrently with or immediately before a course of vincristine and prednisone may be associated with increased toxicity.

Elspar (Merck Sharp & Dohme). Lyophilized plug or powder containing 10,000 IU with 80 mg of mannitol in 10 ml containers. For reconstitution, 5 ml of sterile water for injection or sodium chloride injection are added. The solution may be used within an eight-hour period following reconstitution if it remains clear.

CISPLATIN (CPDD)
[Platinol]

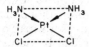

Cisplatin is a heavy metal complex containing a central atom of platinum surrounded by two chloride atoms and two ammonia molecules in the cis position. It has biochemical properties similar to those of bifunctional alkylating agents in that it produces interstrand and intrastrand cross-links in DNA and is apparently cell-cycle nonspecific.

Cisplatin is indicated in the treatment of metastatic testicular tumors and ovarian carcinoma. Patients with bladder carcinoma and carcinoma of the prostate also have responded to this agent. An effective combination for the treatment of patients with metastatic testicular carcinoma includes cisplatin, bleomycin, and vinblastine. In metastatic ovarian carcinoma, the combination of cisplatin and doxorubicin has produced good results.

The most frequent and serious toxicity produced by cisplatin is renal insufficiency, probably caused by renal tubular damage. This is manifested by elevations in BUN, creatinine, and serum uric acid levels and/or a decrease in creatinine clearance. It is first noted during the second week of therapy after the initial dose. Nephrotoxicity is dose related and cumulative, and renal function must return to normal before another dose of cisplatin can be given. Intravenous infusion, hydration, and administration of diuretics have been used to reduce nephrotoxicity.

Other major dose-related manifestations of toxicity are myelosuppression, nausea, and vomiting. Myelosuppression occurs in 25% to 30% of patients treated with cisplatin and is most pronounced with larger doses (more than 50 mg/M^2 of body surface). The nadirs in circulating platelet and leukocyte counts occur between days 18 and 23 (range, 7.5 to 45), with most patients recovering by day 39 (range, 13 to 62). Decreased hemoglobin levels of more than 2 g Hb/dl parallel the occurrence of leukopenia and thrombocytopenia.

Nausea and vomiting occur in almost all patients treated with cisplatin and are occasionally so severe that the drug must be discontinued. These reactions usually begin within one to four hours after treatment and last up to 24 hours. Nausea and anorexia may persist for up to one week after treatment.

Ototoxicity, manifested by tinnitus and/or hearing loss in the high frequency range (4,000 to 8,000 Hz), has been observed in up to 31% of patients treated with a single dose of 50 mg/M^2 of cisplatin. Hearing loss may be unilateral or bilateral and tends to become more severe with repeated doses. Occasionally decreased ability to hear normal conversational tones may occur.

Neurotoxicity, usually characterized by peripheral neuropathies, has occurred and may be irreversible. Loss of taste and seizures also have been reported. Decreases in serum calcium, magnesium, potassium, and sodium concentrations have been observed in patients receiving cisplatin. In some cases, these effects may be related to the intravenous infusion of large volumes of fluid. In other cases, decreased levels of electrolytes may persist for several weeks, apparently due to inappropriate electrolyte excretion resulting from renal tubular damage.

In patients previously treated with cisplatin, anaphylactoid reactions (facial edema, wheezing, tachycardia, and hypotension) have been observed within a few minutes after readministration.

ROUTE, USUAL DOSAGE, AND PREPARATIONS. *Intravenous*: When given as a single agent, 100 mg/M^2 once every four weeks. Pretreatment hydration with 1 to 2 L of 5% dextrose in 0.5% normal saline infused for 8 to 12 hours is recommended. Cisplatin is then diluted in 2 L of 5% dextrose in 0.5% or 0.33% normal saline containing 37.5 g of mannitol and infused over a six- to eight-hour period. Adequate hydration and urinary output must be maintained during the following 24 hours. The course should not be repeated until the serum creatinine level is below 1.5 mg/dl and/or the BUN level is below 25 mg/dl and circulating blood elements are at an acceptable level (platelet count above 100,000/microliter, leukocyte count above 4,000/ microliter). Subsequent doses also should be withheld until an audiometric analysis indicates that auditory acuity is within normal limits.

Platinol (Bristol). Powder (lyophilized) 10 mg/vial.

HYDROXYUREA
[Hydrea]

$$NH_2$$
$$|$$
$$C=O$$
$$|$$
$$NHOH$$

Hydroxyurea directly inhibits DNA synthesis by inhibiting ribonucleoside diphosphate reductase, an enzyme that catalyzes the conversion of ribonucleotides to deoxyribonucleotides, a crucial step in the biosynthesis of DNA. Hydroxyurea is an S phase-specific agent and does not block RNA or protein synthesis. It is effective in chronic granulocytic leukemia refractory to busulfan and mercaptopurine. This agent has produced temporary remissions in melanoma and renal cell carcinoma and also is a component of some maintenance regimens used in acute myelogenous leukemia. Hydroxyurea has been given with radiation therapy in squamous cell carcinoma of the head and neck region and uterine cervix.

Hematologic reactions (leukopenia, thrombocytopenia, anemia, megaloblastosis) are most prominent. This toxicity is dose limiting, but recovery is usually rapid when hydroxyurea is discontinued. Anorexia, nausea, and vomiting are uncommon and stomatitis is seen only rarely. Dermatologic reactions (maculopapular rash, pruritus, and alopecia) are mild and reversible. Less common are central nervous system disturbances (headache, dizziness, disorientation, hallucinations, convulsions). Impairment of renal function with hyperuricemia, uric acid calculi, and elevated BUN levels has been reported.

Blood, bone marrow, renal, and hepatic function should be evaluated prior to and at weekly intervals during therapy. The drug should be discontinued if the white blood cell count falls below 2,500/microliter or the platelet count below 100,000/microliter. Administration may be resumed when the counts return to satisfactory levels. Anemia can be corrected by blood transfusions without discontinuing hydroxyurea. Because the drug is excreted primarily by the kidneys, it must be used with caution in patients with impaired renal function. Hydroxyurea is contraindicated in patients with bone marrow depression or thrombocytopenia resulting from recent exposure to radiation or chemotherapy. Since this drug has caused teratogenic effects in experimental animals, it should not be used in women of childbearing age.

ROUTE, USUAL DOSAGE, AND PREPARATIONS.
Oral: For solid tumors, 80 mg/kg of body weight as a single dose every three days or 20 to 30 mg/kg daily. The dose should be decreased in patients with impaired marrow or renal function.

For carcinoma of the head and neck region, hydroxyurea is administered with irradiation according to the following schedule: 80 mg/kg as a single dose every third day at least seven days before initiating radiation therapy. This dose is continued during radiation therapy as well as indefinitely afterwards, provided the patient is adequately observed and experiences no unusual or severe reactions. Irradiation should be given at the maximal dose considered appropriate for the particular therapeutic situation; adjustment of irradiation dosage is usually not necessary when hydroxyurea is used concomitantly.

Hydrea (Squibb). Capsules 500 mg.

MITOTANE
[Lysodren]

Mitotane is the ortho para isomer of the insecticide, chlorophenothane (DDT). In toxicology studies in dogs, related insecticides damaged the adrenal cortex. The drug produces selective atrophy of the zona fasciculata and reticularis. It interferes with the synthesis of cortisol and alters its extra-adrenal metabolism.

Mitotane is indicated in the palliative treatment of both functional and nonfunctional inoperable carcinoma of the adrenal cortex. A significant reduction in tumor mass is seen in 34% to 54% of patients, with a mean duration of tumor regression of about ten months. Administration of the drug rapidly decreases the level of corticosteroids and their metabolites in blood and urine. This response is useful both in adjusting the dose and in monitoring the response to hyperadrenocorticism due to an adrenal tumor or adrenal hyperplasia.

Anorexia, nausea and vomiting, or diarrhea occurs in 80% of patients. About 40% of patients experience lethargy, somnolence, dizziness, or vertigo, and 15% to 20% develop dermatitis. Less frequent adverse effects are blurred vision, diplopia, lens opacities, retinopathy, albuminuria, hemorrhagic cystitis, flushing, hyperpyrexia, orthostatic hypotension, and hypertension. Hypersensitivity to mitotane has been reported and is a contraindication to use.

ROUTE, USUAL DOSAGE, AND PREPARATIONS.
Oral: 6 to 15 mg/kg of body weight daily in three or four divided doses. Small doses should be given initially with a gradual increase to the maximum tolerated amount. This may vary from 2 to 16 g but is usually 8 to 10 g daily. If adverse reactions occur, the dose is reduced until the maximal tolerated amount is determined. Therapy should be supervised by a physician familiar with the use of mitotane, and patients should be hospitalized until a maintenance dose is established. Treatment should be continued as long as clinical benefit is apparent. If no improvement is observed after three months of therapy using the maximal tolerated dose, the drug should be discontinued.

Lysodren (Bristol) Tablets 500 mg.

PROCARBAZINE HYDROCHLORIDE
[Matulane]

$$CH_3\overset{+}{N}H_2NHCH_2 - \underset{}{\bigcirc} - \underset{\underset{CH_3}{|}}{\overset{\overset{O}{||}\ \overset{CH_3}{|}}{CNHCH}} \quad Cl^-$$

The mechanism of action of this methylhydrazine derivative is uncertain. It inhibits the synthesis of protein, RNA, and DNA by alkylation. Oxidation of nucleic acids and inhibition of transmethylation have also been postulated. Procarbazine is cell cycle-specific for the S phase.

Procarbazine is effective in primary and metastatic brain tumors, bronchogenic carcinoma, and non-Hodgkin's lymphoma. The standard treatment in advanced Hodgkin's disease is the combination of procarbazine, mechlorethamine, vincristine, and prednisone (the MOPP regimen).

Bone marrow depression and gastrointestinal disturbances are the primary toxic manifestations. Leukopenia and thrombocytopenia are usually dose limiting and may be delayed for several weeks after the start of treatment. Like other hydrazine derivatives, procarbazine also may cause hemolysis. Nausea and vomiting occur frequently and may be dose limiting but tolerance may develop with continued administration of the drug. Stomatitis, dysphagia, and diarrhea are less common. Neurologic reactions (eg, peripheral neuropathy with paresthesia, nystagmus, ataxia, lethargy, drowsiness, depression) have been noted. Other untoward effects include myalgia, arthralgia, dermatitis, pruritus, hyperpigmentation, and alopecia.

The effects of central nervous system depressants may be enhanced and a disulfiram-like reaction may occur when alcohol is ingested concomitantly. Since procarbazine inhibits monoamine oxidase, sympathomimetics, tricyclic antidepressants, phenothiazines, and beverages or food with a high tyramine content (eg, bananas, ripe cheese) should be avoided.

ROUTE, USUAL DOSAGE, AND PREPARATIONS.
Oral: Initially, 100 mg/M² of body surface is given daily; the dose is increased over a one-week period to 150 to 200 mg/M². This

amount is maintained for three weeks and then reduced to 100 mg/M² daily until toxicity develops. The dose is decreased in patients with hepatic, renal, or bone marrow dysfunction. As a component of the MOPP regimen, 100 mg/M² is given daily for 14 days every four weeks.

Matulane (Roche). Capsules 50 mg.

Antibiotics

BLEOMYCIN SULFATE
[Blenoxane]

The bleomycins are a group of complex glycopeptides extracted from a strain of *Streptomyces verticillus*. Bleomycin binds to DNA, leading to single-strand breaks and double-stranded scissions. Cells are most sensitive to bleomycin during the G₂ and M phases of the cell cycle. Most studies suggest that noncycling cells are more sensitive than cycling cells. Testicular tumors, malignant lymphomas, uterine cervix carcinoma, and squamous cell carcinomas of the head and neck region (eg, buccal mucosa, tongue, tonsil, pharynx) are most responsive.

Because of its lack of significant myelosuppressive activity, bleomycin has been used extensively with other drugs. The combination of bleomycin, vinblastine, and cisplatin is very effective in testicular tumors. In Hodgkin's disease, bleomycin has been added to the MOPP regimen, and the combination of doxorubicin, bleomycin, vinblastine, and dacarbazine (ABVD) is probably equally effective. Responses also have been observed in non-Hodgkin's lymphoma. The combination of bleomycin, mitomycin, and vincristine is active in the treatment of carcinoma of the cervix. Bleomycin also has been administered intravesically to treat recurrent superficial bladder tumors.

The usual dose-limiting toxic effect of bleomycin is pulmonary fibrosis, which occurs in approximately 10% of patients. The incidence and severity of pulmonary toxicity are related to the age of the patient and the total dose given. Patients older than 70 years or those receiving a total dose of more than 400 units are clearly at greater risk than younger patients treated with lower doses. Radiation therapy to the thorax probably increases the risk of pulmonary toxicity. The development of pulmonary toxicity is usually delayed, and may occur four to ten weeks after initiation of therapy. The radiographic appearance is typical of interstitial pneumonitis that may progress to pulmonary fibrosis. Rales, rhonchi, and, occasionally, pleural friction rubs usually precede radiographic changes. The lesions are found most frequently in the lower lobes and subpleural areas and consist of a fibrinous exudate, atypical proliferation of alveolar cells, hyaline membranes, interstitial and intra-alveolar fibrosis, and squamous metaplasia of the distal air spaces. Pulmonary function tests are not necessarily predictive. The most sensitive method for early detection of pulmonary toxicity may be serial determination of carbon monoxide diffusion capacity.

Other reactions include fever, which is noted in 20% to 50% of patients treated, and mucocutaneous changes (eg, alopecia, cutaneous hyperpigmentation, erythema, hyperkeratosis, mucositis). Neither clinically significant myelosuppression nor immunosuppression has been reported.

The safety of bleomycin during pregnancy or lactation is unknown.

ROUTES, USUAL DOSAGE, AND PREPARATIONS. *Intramuscular, Intravenous, Subcutaneous*: For squamous cell carcinomas, lymphomas, and testicular carcinoma, 0.25 to 0.5 units/kg of body weight (10 to 20 units/M²) once or twice weekly. Because of the possible occurrence of anaphylactic reactions, patients with lymphomas should be started with 2 units or less for the first two doses. If no acute reaction is observed, the regular dosage schedule may be used. For Hodgkin's disease, after a 50% response, a maintenance dose of 5 units is given once weekly.

For intramuscular or subcutaneous use, the contents of the ampul are dissolved in 1 to 5 ml of sterile water for injection, sodium chloride injection, or 5% dextrose injection. For intravenous use, the contents of the ampul are dissolved in 5 ml or more of sodium chloride injection or 5% dextrose injection and administered slowly over a period of ten minutes.

Blenoxane (Bristol). Powder 15 units.

DACTINOMYCIN (Actinomycin D)
[Cosmegen]

Dactinomycin is an antibiotic derived from *Streptomyces parvullus*. It forms a stable complex with DNA, causing inhibition of DNA-dependent RNA synthesis. It is cell cycle-specific for the G_1 and S phases.

Dactinomycin is effective in gestational trophoblastic tumors and, in combination with surgery and radiation therapy, in Wilms' tumor. It also is active in testicular tumors, embryonal rhabdomyosarcoma, Ewing's sarcoma, osteosarcoma, and other sarcomas.

Toxicity is manifested primarily by hematologic and gastrointestinal reactions; the former usually do not become apparent until two to four days after treatment is stopped and may not be maximal before one to two weeks have passed. Bone marrow depression occurs one to seven days after completion of therapy. Thrombocytopenia is often seen first and leukopenia may be dose limiting. Anorexia, nausea, and vomiting usually occur within a few hours after administration and may be ameliorated by use of phenothiazine antiemetics prior to therapy. Stomatitis, cheilitis, glossitis, and proctitis are also commonly dose limiting.

Dermatologic reactions include alopecia and acneiform eruption. Cutaneous erythema, desquamation, and hyperpigmentation also are seen, especially in previously irradiated areas.

Dactinomycin is a local irritant if extravasation occurs. Anaphylactic reactions have been reported. The drug should be avoided in the presence of infections and should be given cautiously to those with liver disease or impaired bone marrow function.

ROUTES, USUAL DOSAGE, AND PREPARATIONS. *Intravenous*: *Adults*, the usual dose is 500 mcg (0.5 mg) daily for a maximum of five days. *Children*, 15 mcg (0.015 mg)/kg of body weight daily for five days, or a total dose of 2,500 mcg (2.5 mg)/M² of body surface given over a one-week period. In both adults and children, a second course may be administered after at least three weeks have elapsed, provided all signs of toxicity have disappeared. Dactinomycin is administered through a running intravenous infusion or, if the drug is given directly into the vein without the use of an infusion, the "two-needle technique" should be used.

Isolation Perfusion Technique: The dosage schedules and technique vary from one investigator to another; the published literature should be consulted for details. In general, the following doses are suggested: 50 mcg (0.05 mg)/kg of body weight for lower extremity or pelvis; 35 mcg (0.035 mg)/kg for upper extremity. After bone marrow function has recovered (three to four weeks), the course is repeated.

Cosmegen (Merck Sharp & Dohme). Powder (lyophilized) 0.5 mg with mannitol 20 mg.

DOXORUBICIN HYDROCHLORIDE
[Adriamycin]

Doxorubicin is an anthracycline glycoside antibiotic isolated from *Streptomyces peucetius*. It inhibits DNA-dependent synthesis of RNA due to intercalation between base pairs of DNA and is cell cycle-specific for the S and/or G_2 phase.

Doxorubicin is one of the most effective antineoplastic agents and has been useful in acute lymphocytic and acute myelogenous leukemia; Hodgkin's disease and non-Hodgkin's lymphoma; sarcomas (Ewing's, osteogenic, rhabdomyosarcoma, and soft tissue); neuroblastoma; Wilms' tumor; carcinoma of the breast, lung, bladder, prostate, ovary, testes, and thyroid; squamous cell carcinoma of the head and neck; and hepatoma. The combination of cisplatin and doxorubicin appears to be very effective in genitourinary tumors (including bladder, prostate, testicular, and ovarian carcinoma).

The toxic effects are hematologic, cardiac, and dermatologic. Leukopenia is the major dose-limiting reaction, with the nadir occurring 10 to 15 days after initial administration. Blood counts usually return to normal levels approximately 21 days after administration. Thrombocytopenia and anemia follow a similar pattern but are of relatively smaller magnitude.

Both acute and cumulative dose-dependent cardiotoxicity may occur. The acute effects after a single intravenous dose can take place within a few minutes and may persist for as long as two weeks. They consist of electrocardiographic changes such as sinus tachycardia, voltage reduction, flattening of the T-wave, depression of the S-T segment, and arrhythmias. Consideration regarding suspension of doxorubicin therapy should include the overall status of the patient as well as these findings. Doxorubicin must be discontinued when congestive heart failure secondary to diffuse cardiomyopathy develops; this may occur during or up to several weeks after completion of treatment. The total cumulative dose should not exceed 550 mg/M2 of body surface, since the risk of congestive cardiac failure increases markedly with larger amounts. This drug should not be given to patients with significantly impaired cardiac function. If it is used with cyclophosphamide, the total dose should not exceed 400 mg/M2, since cyclophosphamide-induced hemorrhagic cystitis may be exacerbated. Cardiotoxicity may be potentiated in patients who had received radiation therapy to the mediastinum.

Doxorubicin also may cause a recurrence of radiation-induced skin reactions and exacerbates tissue changes due to irradiation in mucous membranes and the liver.

Nausea and vomiting are usually mild to moderate; diarrhea and stomatitis also may develop. Alopecia is seen in about 80% of patients and usually there is complete regrowth of hair two to five months after cessation of therapy. Fever, chills, and urticaria have been observed and anaphylaxis may occur.

The urine may turn red after administration of doxorubicin but the discoloration is transient and is of no clinical significance. Erythematous streaking along the vein proximal to the site of injection may be observed. Extravasation causes severe tissue necrosis; thus, great care in administration is needed.

Doxorubicin and related compounds have been shown to have mutagenic and carcinogenic properties when tested in experimental models.

ROUTE, USUAL DOSAGE, AND PREPARATIONS.

Intravenous: 60 to 75 mg/M² of body surface given as a single dose every three weeks, or 30 mg/M² daily for three days, repeated every four weeks. The drug is administered slowly by direct intravenous administration into the side arm of a freely running intravenous infusion. The dose is reduced in patients with impaired hepatic function. If daunorubicin has been given previously, the total cumulative dose of the two drugs should not exceed 500 mg/M².

Adriamycin (Adria). Powder (lyophilized) 10 and 50 mg with 50 and 250 mg of lactose, respectively.

MITHRAMYCIN
[Mithracin]

Mithramycin is an antibiotic produced by *Streptomyces plicatus*. Like dactinomycin, it inhibits DNA-dependent synthesis of RNA but apparently does not affect the synthesis of DNA itself. It is cell cycle-specific for the S phase. Mithramycin has an effect on calcium metabolism and probably suppresses osteoclasts and also may block parathyroid hormone production.

The primary indication for mithramycin is embryonal cell carcinoma of the testes. Since other cell types are much less responsive, use of mithramycin in other types of tumors is not recommended at the present time. Mithramycin also has been effective in the treatment of severe hypercalcemia that does not respond to conventional therapy (see Chapter 54, Agents Affecting Calcium Metabolism).

The most important toxic effect associated with mithramycin is a bleeding syndrome that usually begins with an episode of epistaxis. Severe thrombocytopenia, coagulation defects resulting in hemorrhagic diathesis, and even death have been reported after use of mithramycin. The drug should be administered only to hospitalized patients and those who can be observed carefully with frequent monitoring of platelet count and prothrombin time during and after therapy. Leukopenia occurs less frequently.

Most patients experience anorexia, nausea, and vomiting, which may begin one to two hours after initiation of therapy and persist for 12 to 24 hours. The prior use of antiemetics may be helpful. If facial flushing occurs, administration of mithramycin should be discontinued. Other adverse effects are fever, facial edema, increased pigmentation, acneiform rashes, stomatitis, drowsiness, lethargy, malaise, headache, and depression. Abnormal results of liver and renal function tests have been observed and a reduction of the serum calcium level is common. Before each dose, the lactic dehydrogenase and blood urea nitrogen levels, prothrombin time, and platelet count must be monitored. Mithramycin is contraindicated in those with impaired liver and kidney function, coagulation disorders, or thrombocytopenia.

ROUTE, USUAL DOSAGE, AND PREPARATIONS. *Intravenous*: 0.025 to 0.05 mg/kg of body weight is given every two days for up to eight doses. This schedule is less toxic than daily administration. The dose is diluted in 1,000 ml of 5% dextrose in water or normal saline and infused slowly over a period of four to six hours. Extravasation can cause local irritation and cellulitis. For the dosage used in hypercalcemia, see Chapter 54.

  Mithracin (Dome). Powder (freeze-dried) 2,500 mcg with mannitol 100 mg and sufficient disodium phosphate to adjust to pH 7.

MITOMYCIN
[Mutamycin]

Mitomycin is an antibiotic isolated from *Streptomyces caespitosus*. After activation by intracellular reductases, the drug functions as an alkylating agent, cross linking with DNA. At high concentrations, RNA and protein synthesis also are inhibited.

Mitomycin is cell cycle-nonspecific but appears to be most active in the G_1 and S phases.

This drug is effective against tumors resistant to other alkylating agents. The major indications are colorectal, gastric, and pancreatic adenocarcinoma; most commonly, mitomycin is given with other drugs. Activity also has been reported in carcinoma of the breast, head and neck region, lung, and cervix and in hepatoma and malignant melanoma.

The most significant toxic effect is myelosuppression. Characteristically, this is delayed and unpredictable. After a single dose of 20 mg/M² of body surface, the average time to nadir is three and one-half weeks for leukopenia and four weeks for thrombocytopenia. Leukopenia persists for one to two weeks and thrombocytopenia for two to three weeks. The blood count recovers in most patients within eight weeks; however, in about 25% of patients, the blood count does not return to within normal limits. There also is a cumulative effect and greater and more prolonged myelosuppression is noted in subsequent courses.

Adverse reactions include nausea, vomiting, anorexia, and stomatitis. Alopecia and skin rashes are seen frequently.

Renal toxicity, in the form of glomerular sclerosis, has been observed after several months of therapy in about 2% of patients. It does not appear to be dose related and is manifested clinically by increased levels of BUN and serum creatinine. Abnormalities in liver function tests also have been reported. Severe pulmonary toxicity may occur. Other rare manifestations of toxicity include fever, dyspnea and hemoptysis, drowsiness, and diarrhea.

Extravasation causes severe cellulitis and ulceration.

ROUTE, USUAL DOSAGE, AND PREPARATIONS. *Intravenous*: 10 to 20 mg/M² of body surface every six to eight weeks, administered through a running intravenous infusion. Alternatively, 2 mg/M² daily for five days, followed by a drug-free interval of two days, and then 2 mg/M² for an additional five days (total dose, 20 mg/M² given over a 12-day period). Subsequent doses should not be administered until the leukocyte count has returned to 3,000 and the platelet count to 75,000. Doses greater than 20 mg/M² are more toxic and not more effective. The dose must be reduced appropriately when this drug is used with other myelosuppressive agents.

Mutamycin (Bristol). Powder 5 and 20 mg.

Plant Alkaloids

VINBLASTINE SULFATE
[Velban]

Vinblastine is the sulfate salt of a dimeric alkaloid derived from the periwinkle plant, *Vinca rosea*. It appears to bind or crystallize critical microtubular proteins of the mitotic spindle, leading to metaphase arrest. Interference with metabolic pathways of amino acids from glutamic acid to the citric acid cycle and to urea has been suggested. It is cell cycle-specific for the M phase.

Vinblastine produces beneficial responses in Hodgkin's disease and non-Hodgkin's lymphomas, mycosis fungoides, histiocytosis X (Letterer-Siwe disease), and neuroblastoma. It also is effective in choriocarcinoma and carcinoma of the breast. For testicular carcinoma, vinblastine is usually administered with bleomycin and cisplatin.

Leukopenia is the most common toxic effect caused by vinblastine, with the nadir occurring within four to ten days; recovery is observed within 7 to 14 days. With larger doses, the white blood cell count may not return to normal levels until three weeks have elapsed. Thrombocytopenia and anemia are uncommon. Neurotoxic effects have been reported in 5% to 20% of patients and include paresthesias, loss of deep tendon reflexes, peripheral neuritis, mental depression, headache, and convulsions. Gastrointestinal disturbances occur frequently. Nausea and vomiting are common but usually are readily controlled by antiemetic agents. Other manifestations are stomatitis and constipation or diarrhea.

Alopecia may develop and is reversible. Regrowth of hair may occur while maintenance therapy continues. Extravasation can cause phlebitis and severe cellulitis. Local injection of hyaluronidase and the application of moderate heat to the area of leakage help to disperse the drug and are thought to minimize discomfort and the possibility of cellulitis. Caution is necessary when vinblastine is used during pregnancy, and animal studies suggest that teratogenic effects may occur.

ROUTE, USUAL DOSAGE, AND PREPARATIONS. Vinblastine should be given no more frequently than once every seven days. Dosage is determined by body weight and the results of weekly white blood cell counts. Dosage should be decreased in the presence of liver disease.
Intravenous: Initially, 0.1 mg/kg of body weight is given as a single dose. Successive weekly doses are increased by increments of 0.05 mg/kg until the white blood cell count falls to 3,000/microliter, a decrease in tumor size occurs, or a maximal dose of 0.5 mg/kg is reached. Thereafter, a maintenance dose one increment smaller than the final dose is given at 7- to 14-day intervals. The requirements of individual patients vary; in most cases, the desired response is achieved when a dose of 0.15 to 0.2 mg/kg has been given. Once a remission is induced, some clinicians administer 10 mg once or twice monthly. In combination with bleomycin, vinblastine is often given

in a dose of 0.4 mg/kg on two successive days every three weeks, depending upon the blood count and other signs of toxicity.
Velban (Lilly). Powder (lyophilized) 10 mg.

VINCRISTINE SULFATE
[Oncovin]

Vincristine is the sulfate salt of a dimeric alkaloid derived from the periwinkle plant, *Vinca rosea*. It is cell cycle specific and blocks mitosis with metaphase arrest due to crystallization of microtubular and spindle protein. The vinca alkaloids do not appear to be cross resistant.

Vincristine is particularly effective in inducing remissions in children with acute lymphoblastic leukemia. When used with prednisone, it induces complete remissions in 80% to 90% of patients and is probably even more effective in combination with daunorubicin. It also is very effective in malignant lymphomas, and the combination of mechlorethamine, vincristine, procarbazine, and prednisone (MOPP regimen) is considered the treatment of choice in advanced Hodgkin's disease. Breast carcinoma, Ewing's sarcoma, neuroblastoma, rhabdomyosarcoma, Wilms' tumor, and soft tissue sarcomas also have responded to vincristine.

In contrast to vinblastine, vincristine does not produce bone marrow depression, which makes it particularly useful in combination with myelosuppressive agents. Neurologic toxic effects are dose limiting; manifestations include paresthesia (occasionally severe), loss of deep tendon reflexes, ataxia, foot drop, slapping gait, and muscle wasting. Mild sensory neuropathy is common. The loss of the Achilles tendon reflex is the first sign of peripheral neuropathy. The primary muscle groups involved include the dorsiflexors of hands and wrists and the extensors of the feet. Cranial nerve deficits with ptosis, diplopia, abducens nerve palsy, and vocal cord paralysis have been reported.

Constipation and abdominal pain occur frequently and usually respond well to such measures as enemas and laxatives but, if severe, may be dose limiting. Alopecia is observed in over 20% of patients. Vincristine is a local irritant, and extravasation causes severe cellulitis and phlebitis. Liver impairment increases the drug's toxicity.

ROUTE, USUAL DOSAGE, AND PREPARATIONS. *Intravenous*: 1 to 2 mg/M2 of body surface every week. Individual doses in adults should not exceed 2 mg. The therapeutic effect does not appear to be dose related, and significantly greater toxic reactions without increased benefit occur with larger doses. The drug is administered through a running intravenous infusion or injected with care to prevent extravasation. The dose should be reduced in those with liver disease.

> *Oncovin* (Lilly). Powder 1 and 5 mg with diluent and 10 and 50 mg of lactose, respectively.

Hormones

Although their precise mechanism of action is not known, hormones have been used empirically for decades to treat endocrine-related tumors (carcinoma of the breast, prostate, endometrium, ovary, kidney, and thyroid) and nonendocrine malignant neoplasms responsive to hormone therapy (eg, leukemia, lymphomas).

It was established recently that steroid hormones must bind to receptor proteins in tumor cells in order to exert their antitumor effects; the absence or loss of specific hormone receptor proteins can be correlated with a lack of antineoplastic effects. The steroid hormones apparently form a mobile complex with the receptor protein that binds directly to DNA in the nucleus and alters the transcription of structural or regulatory genes, thus affecting RNA and protein synthesis. Highly specific receptor proteins have been identified for estradiol, cortisol, dexamethasone, stanolone, and progesterone.

The most frequently used hormones are estrogens, androgens, progestins, and the adrenal corticosteroids. More recently, compounds with antiestrogenic and antiandrogenic activity have been developed. Estrogen linked to nitrogen mustard and similar agents is being investigated for antitumor effects.

Adrenal corticosteroids also are useful as adjunctive therapy in the treatment of hypercalcemia and cerebral edema, and androgens occasionally are used for their anabolic effect.

ADRENAL CORTICOSTEROIDS

Adrenal corticosteroids affect specific cell types through unknown modes of action. In vitro studies indicate that they inhibit RNA and protein synthesis. They also interfere with lymphoid proliferation, have a lympholytic effect, cause regression of lymphatic tissue, inhibit growth of certain mesenchymal tissues, and have antiinflammatory and immunosuppressive activities.

Major indications are acute and chronic lymphocytic leukemia, Hodgkin's disease and non-Hodgkin's lymphomas, breast carcinoma, prostatic carcinoma, and multiple myeloma. Adrenal corticosteroids usually are given with other chemotherapeutic agents. They may be indicated for specific complications, such as hypercalcemia and intracranial metastases, and are used in conjunction with radiation therapy to reduce edema in critical areas (eg, superior mediastinum, brain, spinal cord). They are particularly useful in the symptomatic palliation of severe myelosuppression due to bone marrow involvement or previous radiation or chemotherapy. They may minimize bleeding caused by thrombocytopenia and reduce autoimmune hemolysis. The corticosteroids may produce temporary symptomatic improvement in critically ill patients by suppressing fever, sweating, and pain and by restoring appetite, lost weight, strength, and a sense of well-being.

Long-term therapy can lead to characteristic Cushingoid features with accumulation of fat on the trunk and face. Metabolic effects include sodium retention, which may result in edema, heart failure, and hypertension; potassium loss, which may produce muscle weakness; and decreased glucose tolerance, which may result in glycosuria and overt diabetes mellitus. Loss of skin collagen can result in "paper thin" skin and cutaneous striae. Proximal myopathy, osteoporosis, and vertebral compression fractures can develop. Peptic ulcerations may occur. Pituitary-adrenal suppression and retardation or interruption of growth have been observed in children. Euphoria is common and some patients may develop psychoses. Caution should be exercised in patients receiving long-term steroid therapy, since they are more susceptible to severe infections, and sudden withdrawal of medication or development of stress may result in acute adrenocortical insufficiency. In order to minimize the complications of corticosteroid therapy, an attempt should be made to reduce the dosage required to control the manifestations of the disease.

For a further discussion on adrenal corticosteroids, see Chapter 41.

ROUTES AND USUAL DOSAGE.
PREDNISONE:
Oral: 10 to 100 mg daily. For dosage used in combination therapy, see the discussion on the treatment of leukemia, lymphoma, and breast carcinoma.
DEXAMETHASONE, DEXAMETHASONE SODIUM PHOSPHATE:
Oral, Intramuscular, Intravenous: To reduce cerebral edema, 4 to 16 mg daily in divided doses.

For preparations, see Chapter 41.

ESTROGENS

Estrogens are effective in the treatment of metastatic breast carcinoma in postmenopausal patients and in carcinoma of the prostate. In breast carcinoma, ablation of endogenous estrogen production by oophorectomy and adrenalectomy or the administration of estrogen induces tumor regression in approximately 30% of patients. Additive estrogen therapy is more effective as the number of years since menopause increases. A remission rate of 13% has been reported during the first five years after menopause as compared with 20% to 35% after the fifth year. In patients with tumors containing estrogen receptors, the response rate is approximately 65%. Evidence of tumor regression may not be apparent for several weeks, and it is necessary to continue therapy for 8 to 12 weeks before effectiveness can be evaluated. If the response is favorable, estrogen therapy should be continued until there is evidence of progression of the neoplasm. Occasionally, the tumor may again regress when estrogen is withdrawn. Remission may last a few months to several years, with an average duration of 15 months. The duration of survival is longer in responsive patients than in nonresponsive patients.

Disseminated prostatic carcinoma can be controlled by orchiectomy or estrogen therapy. Successful treatment is manifested almost immediately by reduced bone pain and decreased acid phosphatase levels.

When estrogens are used to treat breast carcinoma, adverse effects include edema, nausea, anorexia, changes in libido, breast tenderness, abdominal cramps, dizziness, irritability, and urinary frequency. Fluid retention may be a serious problem, especially in patients with cardiovascular disease. Pigmentation of nipples and areola occurs in almost all patients. Occasionally, patients experience an exacerbation of bone pain and the neoplastic process. Hypercalcemia is a potentially fatal complication. Estrogens should be discontinued and appropriate treatment for hypercalcemia must be instituted. Since the liver inactivates estrogens, toxic effects tend to be more severe in the presence of hepatic damage. Rarely, cholestatic jaundice may occur. Urinary incontinence when coughing or straining is a frequent complaint of older women. Postmenopausal patients should be warned that uterine bleeding often occurs with prolonged high-dose estrogen therapy or upon withdrawal of estrogen. Vaginal carcinoma has been reported rarely in the offspring of women who used diethylstilbestrol during pregnancy.

When estrogens are used for prostatic carcinoma, gynecomastia and impotence are expected adverse effects. Fluid retention may be hazardous and should be treated appropriately. The risk of cardiovascular complications increases with larger doses. Diethylstilbestrol diphosphate can cause pruritus and burning pain in the anogenital region or in metastatic sites during or after administration of the drug. These may be ameliorated by slowing the rate of intravenous infusion and administering antihistamines or sedatives simultaneously.

ROUTES AND USUAL DOSAGE.
CHLOROTRIANISENE:
Oral: For prostatic carcinoma, 12 to 25 mg daily.
CONJUGATED ESTROGENS:
Oral: For breast carcinoma, 10 mg three times daily; for prostatic carcinoma, 3.75 to 7.5 mg daily.
DIETHYLSTILBESTROL:
Oral: For breast carcinoma, 5 mg three times daily (range, 5 to 15 mg daily); for prostatic carcinoma, 1 to 3 mg daily.
DIETHYLSTILBESTROL DIPHOSPHATE:
Intravenous: For prostatic carcinoma, 500 mg dissolved in 300 ml of saline or 5% dextrose on the first day; 1 g in 300 ml of saline or dextrose is then given daily for five days or more, depending upon the response of the patient. The infusion should be administered slowly (20 to 30 drops/min) during the first 10 to 15 minutes and then the rate of flow adjusted so that the entire amount is given within one hour. Following the first intensive course of therapy, 250 to 500 mg may be administered in a similar manner once or twice

weekly, or oral maintenance therapy may be instituted.
Oral: For prostatic carcinoma, 50 mg three times daily, increased to 200 mg or more if necessary.
ESTERIFIED ESTROGENS:
Oral: For breast carcinoma, 10 mg three times daily; for prostatic carcinoma, 1.25 mg or more three times daily.
ETHINYL ESTRADIOL:
Oral: For breast carcinoma, 0.5 to 1 mg three times daily; for prostatic carcinoma, 0.15 to 0.3 mg daily.
POLYESTRADIOL PHOSPHATE:
Intramuscular (deep): For prostatic carcinoma, initially, 40 mg every two to four weeks or less frequently. If the response is not satisfactory, up to 80 mg may be given.

For preparations, see Chapter 43, Estrogens and Progestins.

ANDROGENS

Large doses of androgens produce objective signs of regression of disseminated carcinoma of the breast in about 20% of patients, with the median period of regression being eight months. Androgens are progressively more effective as the period after menopause increases. The tumor remission rate is only 8% in the first year after menopause, about 15% from the second through the fifth postmenopausal year, and 25% thereafter. Skin and lymph node metastases are most responsive, followed by osseous lesions; metastases to viscera are least responsive. Calusterone has been claimed to be somewhat more effective but an insufficient number of comparative studies have been performed. Testolactone is relatively inert hormonally, produces a lesser degree of virilization, and has a similar tumor remission rate as the other androgens. The prototype parenteral androgen preparations, testosterone propionate and enanthate, although as effective as other androgens, are now rarely used because of their marked virilizing effect. Fluoxymesterone and dromostanolone are less virilizing than testosterone.

Adverse effects caused by androgens include fluid retention, masculinization with clitoral enlargement, hirsutism, deepening of the voice, increased libido, acne, alopecia, and erythrocythemia.

Androgens are contraindicated in patients with cardiorenal disease or hypercalcemia and in pregnant women or nursing mothers. If hypercalcemia develops, the androgen should be discontinued immediately and appropriate corrective measures instituted (eg, forced hydration, administration of diuretics, adrenal corticosteroids, oral or intravenous phosphate therapy, mithramycin). Cholestatic jaundice has been noted with oral therapy. Hepatocellular neoplasms have rarely been associated with long-term therapy. Rarely, exacerbation of the malignant process may occur.

ROUTES, USUAL DOSAGE, AND PREPARATIONS.
CALUSTERONE:
Oral: 50 mg four times daily; doses of 150 to 300 mg have been used successfully.
    Methosarb (Upjohn). Tablets 50 mg.
DROMOSTANOLONE PROPIONATE:
Intramuscular: 100 mg three times weekly for 8 to 12 weeks or as long as there is objective evidence of remission.
    Drolban (Lilly). Solution 50 mg/ml in 10 ml containers.
FLUOXYMESTERONE:
Oral: 20 to 30 mg daily.
    See Chapter 42, Androgens and Anabolic Steroids, for preparations.
METHYLTESTOSTERONE:
Oral: 200 mg.
Buccal: 100 mg daily.
    See Chapter 42 for preparations.
TESTOLACTONE:
Intramuscular: 100 mg three times weekly.
    Teslac (Squibb). Suspension (sterile, aqueous) 100 mg/ml in 5 ml containers.
Oral: 250 mg four times daily.
    Teslac (Squibb). Tablets 50 and 250 mg.
TESTOSTERONE ENANTHATE, TESTOSTERONE PROPIONATE:
Intramuscular: 100 mg three times weekly.
    See Chapter 42 for preparations.

PROGESTINS

Progestins have been used successfully to treat carcinoma of the endometrium,

breast, prostate, and kidney. A recent report suggests that high-dose progestin therapy may be of benefit in ovarian carcinoma.

Adverse reactions are usually minimal; anorexia, fluid retention, and pain at the site of injection may occur.

ROUTES, USUAL DOSAGE, AND PREPARATIONS.
HYDROXYPROGESTERONE CAPROATE:
Intramuscular: 1 g twice weekly.
    Delalutin (Squibb). Solution 125 mg/ml (in sesame oil) in 2 and 10 ml containers and 250 mg/ml (in castor oil) in 1 and 5 ml containers.
MEDROXYPROGESTERONE ACETATE:
Intramuscular: Initially, 400 mg to 1 g weekly; for maintenance, 400 mg monthly.
    Depo-Provera (Upjohn). Suspension (aqueous) 100 mg/ml in 5 ml containers and 400 mg/ml in 1, 2.5, and 10 ml containers.
MEGESTROL ACETATE:
Oral: For breast cancer, 160 mg/day in four divided doses. For endometrial carcinoma, 40 to 320 mg daily in divided doses.
    Megace (Mead Johnson). Tablets 20 and 40 mg.

Antiestrogen

TAMOXIFEN CITRATE
[Nolvadex]

Tamoxifen, a nonsteroidal antiestrogenic agent, is the citrate salt of the trans-isomer of a triphenylethylene derivative. It is reported to have oncogenic activity in animals and is teratogenic in rats and rabbits with evidence of skeletal abnormalities. The antiestrogenic effects may be related to the drug's ability to compete with estradiol for estrogen receptor protein.

Tamoxifen is useful in the palliative treatment of advanced breast cancer in postmenopausal women; objective remissions also have been achieved in premenopausal patients. Recently, a number of studies have been initiated using tamoxifen as an adjuvant after surgery for carcinoma of the breast. Response rates in women with advanced breast cancer ranged from 16% to 52% (average, 32%) with a mean duration of response ranging from more than 6.7 to more than 17.5 months. The longest remission lasted more than four years. Previous cytotoxic therapy did not reduce the rate and previous hormonal therapy with or without previous cytotoxic treatment did not preclude a response. Patients who benefited from previous hormonal therapy had a significantly greater chance of responding to administration of tamoxifen (67%) than nonresponders (15%). It has been reported that more than 70% of patients receiving antiestrogen treatment who responded and then relapsed were able to benefit from further hormonal therapy. The response rate to tamoxifen seems to increase with age and number of years past menopause. The rate was 32% in patients 41 to 50 years and was 48% in those over 70 years. Soft tissue lesions respond better than either bone or visceral disease. In the presence of cytoplasmic estrogen receptor protein, the rate was 50%, but only 7% to 12% of patients with estrogen receptor-negative tumors responded.

Increased bone and tumor pain and exacerbation of local disease have been observed, sometimes in association with good tumor response.

No life-threatening adverse reactions have been reported, and less than 3% of patients could not tolerate tamoxifen. Those who temporarily withdrew from therapy or required dosage reduction because of side effects were able to tolerate reduced dosage or resumption of therapy. Adverse effects occur less frequently and are significantly milder than with androgens or estrogens.

The most common reactions with tamoxifen therapy were nausea or vomiting and hot flashes. The platelet count decreased temporarily but never resulted in hemorrhage; leukopenia was transient, even with continued therapy. Less frequently reported adverse reactions were vaginal bleeding or discharge, menstrual irregularities, and skin rash. Other untoward effects observed infrequently were hypercalcemia, peripheral edema, loss of appetite, pruritus vulvae, depression, dizziness, lightheadedness, and headache. Abnormal results of liver function tests have been reported rarely.

Four cases of retinal and corneal damage were reported following overdosages of 120 to 160 mg twice a day for periods in excess of 17 months. This would be equivalent to 20 to 30 years of therapy at recommended dosage levels.

ROUTE, USUAL DOSAGE, AND PREPARATIONS. *Oral*: 10 to 20 mg twice daily.

> *Nolvadex* (Stuart). Tablets 15.2 mg (equivalent to 10 mg of the base). (Protect from heat and light.)

Radioactive Isotopes

GOLD AU 198
[Aureotope]

Radioactive gold is used principally to treat pleural effusions and ascites secondary to cancer. Its effectiveness in pleural effusions apparently is comparable to that of mechlorethamine. Because radiation sickness may occur in some patients, the dose should be adjusted to ensure minimal radiation exposure to the patient and laboratory personnel.

Gold Au 198 is contraindicated in patients with ulcerative tumors, unhealed surgical wounds, exposed cavities, or evidence of loculation. It should not be administered during pregnancy and lactation or to persons less than 18 years of age and should not be given more often than once every four weeks unless there is accumulation of fluid. Gold Au 198 is restricted for use by physicians licensed by the Nuclear Regulatory Commission.

ROUTES, USUAL DOSAGE, AND PREPARATIONS. *Intrapleural, Intraperitoneal*: For pleural effusions, 25 to 100 millicuries. For ascites, 35 to 100 millicuries.

> *Aureotope* (Squibb). 25 to 250 millicuries.

SODIUM PHOSPHATE P 32
[Phosphotope]

Sodium phosphate P 32 is used principally to treat the proliferative phase of polycythemia vera; it reduces the erythrocyte count, packed red blood cell volume, and hypervolemia. It is as effective as the alkylating agents for the palliative treatment of chronic myelocytic leukemia. When used with local irradiation, radioactive phosphorus may control enlargement of the spleen in the early stages. It also may be helpful in some patients with chronic lymphocytic leukemia, but this type of leukemia usually responds more readily to other chemotherapeutic agents.

Although usual doses rarely cause radiation sickness, dosage should be adjusted individually to ensure minimal radiation exposure to the patient and laboratory personnel. Excessive amounts can cause leukopenia, thrombocytopenia, and anemia. Periodic blood cell counts are required. Sodium phosphate P 32 and the alkylating agents cannot be used in sequence to treat chronic myelocytic leukemia, for once resistance has developed to one agent there is no further response to the other. This agent is contraindicated in polycythemia vera when the leukocyte count is less than 5,000/microliter or the platelet count less than 150,000/microliter and in chronic myelocytic leukemia when the leukocyte count is less than 20,000/microliter and the red blood cell count less than 2,500,000/microliter.

Treatment with sodium phosphate P 32 is restricted for use by physicians licensed by the Nuclear Regulatory Commission.

ROUTES, USUAL DOSAGE, AND PREPARATIONS. *Oral*: For polycythemia vera, initially, 6 millicuries.

> *Phosphotope* (Squibb). Solutions available in several potencies up to 30 millicuries.
> *Sodium Phosphate P 32* (Abbott). Solutions in same concentrations as injection.

Intravenous: For polycythemia vera, 3 to 5 millicuries (75% of oral dose), depending upon the initial erythrocyte, leukocyte, and platelet counts and the patient's weight. Phlebotomy may be used adjunctively. For chronic myelocytic leukemia, the initial dose is calculated on the basis of the leukocyte count (less than 40,000/microliter, 3 millicuries; 40,000 to 100,000/microliter, 4 millicuries; more than 100,000/microliter, 5 millicuries); subsequent doses are based upon the response of the patient.

> *Phosphotope* (Squibb). Available in several potencies up to 30 millicuries.
> *Sodium Phosphate P 32* (Abbott). 1.5 millicuries/ml in 20, 25, and 30 millicurie containers.

COMBINATION CHEMOTHERAPY

It was soon recognized that tumors responding to a single chemotherapeutic agent often recurred or that drug-induced toxicity was intolerable. Recurrences were thought to be caused by regrowth of tumor cells between the therapeutic intervals required to allow recovery of normal tissues but which permitted emergence of drug-resistant cell lines. Resistance is the result of the presence of cells inherently and originally nonresponsive to the drug used or the result of a stepwise induction of biochemical resistance.

Various mechanisms of biochemical resistance have been proposed. A decreased cellular uptake apparently is responsible for resistance to methotrexate, dactinomycin, the anthracyclines, and mechlorethamine. The alkylating agents and anthracyclines may be less effective because of increased DNA repair. Resistance to antimetabolites may be the result of the utilization of alternate pathways by tumor cells or decreased enzymatic activation of drug. An increase of target enzyme, such as dihydrofolate reductase, alters the effectiveness of methotrexate; an increase in asparagine synthetase interferes with the action of asparaginase; and increased levels of deaminase could increase deactivation of cytarabine.

Based on such observations, it was proposed that use of two or more drugs in combination might increase the antitumor effect and minimize the development of resistant tumor cells. By combining drugs that are effective as single agents but that have different biochemical actions at different phases of the cell cycle, a synergistic or additive antitumor effect may be possible. Although the toxic reactions produced by the individual agents used in combination chemotherapy should not overlap, the possible additive toxicity with combination therapy must be weighed against the anticipated benefits.

Useful combinations include drugs that bind to DNA with or without cross linkage and thus alter DNA replication or RNA transcription and subsequent protein synthesis (eg, alkylating agents [including nitrosoureas], antitumor antibiotics, cisplatin [Platinol], dacarbazine [DTIC-Dome], procarbazine [Matulane]), drugs that inhibit enzymes used in purine, pyrimidine, DNA, or RNA synthesis (eg, antimetabolites), and mitotic inhibitors (eg, plant alkaloids).

The effectiveness of combination chemotherapy has been demonstrated in acute leukemia; Hodgkin's disease; non-Hodgkin's lymphoma; carcinoma of the breast, testis, and ovary; childhood neuroblastoma; Wilms' tumor; and osteogenic sarcoma. As a result, many protocols of combination chemotherapy are presently being investigated in gastrointestinal, pulmonary, and prostatic carcinoma and soft tissue sarcomas.

Leukemias: Combination chemotherapy has produced excellent remissions in acute lymphocytic leukemia in children. Treatment is both intensive and complicated and requires sophisticated support facilities (replacement of blood components, control of infections). Management consists of induction therapy, consolidation therapy, central nervous system prophylaxis, maintenance therapy, and intensification therapy (or periodic reinduction).

Induction therapy with vincristine (1.5 mg/M² intravenously weekly for four to six weeks) and prednisone (40 mg/M² orally daily in divided doses for four to six weeks) leads to complete clinical remission in 80% to 90% of children with acute lymphocytic leukemia. Neither of these drugs is myelosuppressive to normal hematopoietic stem cells and toxicity is attributed to vincristine, which causes peripheral neuropathy, alopecia, and gastrointestinal disturbances (constipation and intestinal colic). If patients do not respond to initial therapy, daunorubicin or asparaginase [Elspar] may be added to the regimen. Since complete remission is not identical with complete eradication of the leukemic cell population, intensive therapy with craniospinal irradiation or cranial irradiation along with intrathecal doses of methotrexate is added to prevent meningeal or central nervous system leukemic involvement. Maintenance therapy with methotrexate (20 mg/M² intravenously weekly) plus mercaptopurine (50 mg/M² orally daily) prolongs the period of remission. Cyclophosphamide also has been utilized in this situation, but cystitis may occur. The optimal duration of maintenance therapy required to achieve tumor control is not known. With appropriate treatment and adequate supportive care, the projected five-year survival rate for children with acute lymphocytic leukemia is approaching 50%.

Leukemia in adults is predominantly acute myelogenous leukemia, and responses to therapy occur much less frequently and are of shorter duration than in children with acute lymphocytic leukemia. The most effective drugs are cytarabine [Cytosar], daunorubicin, and thioguanine.

Induction with intravenous administration of cytarabine and oral use of thioguanine (both drugs given in doses of 100 mg/M² every 12 hours on days one through ten) repeated every 30 days, blood count permitting, achieves a response rate of approximately 50%. The combination of cytarabine (100 mg/M² infused intravenously daily for seven days) plus daunorubicin (45 mg/M² intravenously daily for three days) is effective in more than 80% of patients under the age of 60 years. Doxorubicin [Adriamycin] may be substituted for daunorubicin in patients resistant to the latter.

Optimal maintenance therapy is still being investigated; one schedule employs repeated cycles of sequential administration of vincristine, followed after a rest period by methotrexate plus carmustine [BiCNU], followed by thioguanine plus cyclophosphamide, followed by hydroxyurea [Hydrea] plus daunorubicin. More intensive intermittent courses of various drugs and the use of immunotherapy are currently being investigated.

In active chronic lymphocytic leukemia, chlorambucil or cyclophosphamide, with or without steroids, is employed most frequently. In chronic myelogenous leukemia, busulfan [Myleran] is the most commonly used single drug, although hydroxyurea and mercaptopurine are also effective for palliation. Combination chemotherapy as used in acute myelogenous leukemia is given in blast crisis.

Lymphomas: The most impressive progress has been achieved in Hodgkin's disease. Chemotherapy is the treatment of choice for systemic disease. A number of agents are active in Hodgkin's disease and the combination of mechlorethamine [Mustargen], vincristine [Oncovin], procarbazine [Matulane], and prednisone (MOPP regimen) induces complete remission in more than 80% of treated patients, with a subsequent long duration of remission and disease-free survival. The dose employed every four weeks for six courses is: mechlorethamine 6 mg/M² intravenously on days one and eight; vincristine 1.4 mg/M² intravenously on days one and eight; procarbazine 100 mg/M² orally on days one to fourteen; and prednisone 40 mg/M² orally on days one to fourteen (of cycles one and four only). The value of maintenance therapy in prolonging the duration of remission has been confirmed, but the optimal interval and duration of therapy is still to be determined.

Although the MOPP regimen is still the treatment of choice, another combination of four drugs, ABVD (doxorubicin [Adriamycin], bleomycin [Blenoxane], vinblastine [Velban], and dacarbazine [DTIC-Dome]), has produced similar remission rates. There is no cross resistance between the combinations of MOPP and ABVD, and either regimen may be used if the other fails. The dosage schedule for ABVD is: doxorubicin 25 mg/M² intravenously on days one and fourteen; bleomycin 10 units/M² intravenously on days one and fourteen; vinblastine 6 mg/M² intravenously on days one and fourteen; and

dacarbazine 150 mg/M² intravenously on days one to five. This cycle is repeated every four weeks for six courses. In addition to the blood count, electrocardiogram, chest x-rays, and lung function studies should be performed.

Single drugs effective in Hodgkin's disease are lomustine [CeeNU], chlorambucil, thiotepa, streptozocin, and epipodophyllotoxin VM 26.

The responses to chemotherapy in non-Hodgkin's lymphomas (undifferentiated, histiocytic, mixed histiocytic-lymphocytic, and lymphocytic) are less impressive. With single agents, the overall complete remission rate is usually below 20%, whereas the response rate in favorable histologic types after use of a combination of cyclophosphamide, vincristine, and prednisone (CVP) is 40%. The doses employed are: cyclophosphamide 400 mg/M² orally on days one to five; vincristine 1.4 mg/M² intravenously on day one; and prednisone 100 mg/M² orally on days one to five. This cycle is repeated every three weeks for six courses.

In unfavorable histologic types, the most effective combinations are cyclophosphamide, doxorubicin [Adriamycin], vincristine [Oncovin], and prednisone (CHOP) and bleomycin, doxorubicin [Adriamycin], cyclophosphamide, vincristine [Oncovin], and prednisone (BACOP). The dose of CHOP is: cyclophosphamide 750 mg/M² intravenously on day one; doxorubicin 50 mg/M² intravenously on day one; vincristine 1.4 mg/M² intravenously on day one; and prednisone 25 mg four times daily orally on days one to five. The dose of BACOP is: bleomycin 5 units/M² intravenously on days fifteen and twenty-two; doxorubicin 25 mg/M² intravenously on days one and eight; cyclophosphamide 650 mg/M² intravenously on days one and eight; vincristine 1.4 mg/M² intravenously on days one and eight; and prednisone 60 mg/M² orally on days fifteen to twenty-eight. With both regimens, the cycle is repeated every four weeks for six courses.

Other drugs effective in non-Hodgkin's lymphomas are carmustine, procarbazine, vinblastine, chlorambucil, methotrexate, and mechlorethamine.

Breast Carcinoma: Many regimens of nonhormonal combination chemotherapy have been developed in recent years for use in breast carcinoma. A number of drugs with differing mechanisms of action have significant activity as single agents. One of the first combinations used was methotrexate plus thiotepa. The Cooper regimen (CMFVP), which consists of cyclophosphamide, methotrexate, fluorouracil, vincristine, and prednisone, was initially reported to be effective in 90% of treated patients. However, the overall cumulative response rate is approximately 50%. A similar response rate can be achieved using cyclophosphamide, methotrexate, and fluorouracil (CMF). The recommended dosage schedule of CMF is: cyclophosphamide 100 mg/M² orally on days one to fourteen; methotrexate 40 mg/M² intravenously on days one and eight; and fluorouracil 500 mg/M² intravenously on days one and eight. The cycle is repeated every four weeks.

Other effective combinations are doxorubicin 40 mg/M² intravenously on day one plus cyclophosphamide 200 mg/M² orally on days three to six, repeated every 21 days, or cyclophosphamide 100 mg/M² orally on days one to fourteen, doxorubicin 25 mg/M² intravenously on days one and eight, and fluorouracil 500 mg/M² intravenously on days one and eight, repeated every 28 days. These combinations are effective in approximately 70% of patients, but the cardiotoxicity of doxorubicin must be taken into account.

A new concept in the treatment of breast cancer is the use of adjuvant chemotherapy after curative surgery. Unfortunately, the disease is disseminated with micrometastases in many patients at the time of diagnosis and surgery is often not curative. Within ten years, 76% of patients with axillary node involvement and 86% of those with four or more regional nodes containing a tumor will have recurrent disease. The five-year survival rate after the onset of chemotherapy for recurrent metastases is less than 5%. In an effort to reduce the risk of recurrent disease and improve survival, systemic chemotherapy has been initiated after removal of the primary tumor. At that time, the number of tumor cells in micrometastatic foci is as small as possible and, since smaller tumor cell populations have a larger growth fraction (proliferative pool), they may be more responsive to the action of antineoplastic agents. Preliminary data from ongoing studies seem to support this concept. Patients with stage II disease (positive axillary nodes) who received combination therapy with the CMF regimen for 12 months had a significantly lower failure rate after surgery than untreated patients and probably an improved survival rate can be expected. This difference is well documented in premenopausal women but is less evident in postmenopausal patients. The results reported after adjuvant chemotherapy with a single agent (melphalan) also favor the treated group. Many controlled clinical trials are in progress using the CMF regimen plus the antiestrogen, tamoxifen [Nolvadex], and immunotherapy with BCG.

Miscellaneous Carcinomas: Several other types of tumors respond to combination chemotherapy and combined modality treatment (surgery, radiation, chemotherapy, and immunotherapy) with prolonged survival times.

The concept of combining antitumor drugs had one of its first applications almost 20 years ago in the treatment of testicular tumors. The three-drug combination of chlorambucil, methotrexate, and dactinomycin produced an overall response rate of 50%. The combination of bleomycin and vinblastine also was found to be very effective, and the addition of cisplatin to the regimen produced a 100% response rate in 20 evaluable patients when the following schedule was used: cisplatin 20 mg/M² intravenously daily for five days every three weeks, vinblastine 0.2 mg/kg intravenously daily for two days every three weeks, and bleomycin 30 units intravenously weekly for 12 consecutive weeks.

The combination of hexamethyl-melamine, cyclophosphamide, fluorouracil, and methotrexate appears to be more effective in ovarian carcinoma than melphalan [Alkeran] alone. The combination of cyclophosphamide, vincristine, doxorubicin, and dacarbazine (Cy-VA-DIC) has been beneficial in metastatic sarcoma in the following schedule: cyclophosphamide 400 to 500 mg/M² intravenously on day two; vincristine 1.5 mg/M² intravenously on days one, eight, and fifteen; doxorubicin 50 mg/M² intravenously on day two; and dacarbazine 250 mg/M² intravenously on days one to five. This cycle is repeated every three weeks.

In colorectal carcinoma, the combinations of fluorouracil, semustine, and vincristine or fluorouracil, doxorubicin, and mitomycin are being investigated.

Nonoat cell carcinoma of the lung reportedly responds to various combinations of cyclophosphamide, methotrexate, doxorubicin, and either lomustine or procarbazine.

The concept of combined modality therapy has been applied successfully to pediatric tumors. The addition of chemotherapy with dactinomycin and vincristine to surgery and radiation therapy has greatly increased the cure rate of Wilms' tumor from 30% to over 80%. Encouraging results were reported in children with osteogenic sarcoma who were given large doses of methotrexate with leucovorin rescue. Combined modality treatment also has been beneficial in rhabdomyosarcoma and Ewing's sarcoma.

The combination of radiation therapy and chemotherapy frequently is used in gastric, colon, and pancreatic carcinoma and appears to be beneficial in many cases. Hydroxyurea [Hydrea] has increased the effectiveness of radiation therapy in cervical carcinoma, exerting a possible radiosensitizing effect.

Several protocols using immunotherapy are being actively investigated, and it is hoped that this modality will have a specific role in the general treatment strategy employed against malignant diseases.

Although great progress has been made in the field of chemotherapy, many questions remain unanswered, eg, the duration, intensity, and schedules of therapy. Further improvement in survival of cancer patients can be expected with a better understanding of the natural history of the various tumors, improved histologic classifications, and newer techniques to define the extent of disease accurately.

INVESTIGATIONAL DRUGS

AZACITIDINE

This antimetabolite, an analogue of cytidine, is rapidly phosphorylated and incorporated into both RNA and DNA. By disrupting the process of translation of nucleic acid sequences into protein, protein synthesis is inhibited. Moreover, it affects de novo pyrimidine synthesis by inhibiting orotidylic acid decarboxylase. It is cell cycle-specific for the S phase. The major indication for azacitidine is in the treatment of acute granulocytic leukemia.

Toxicity is mainly hematologic, manifested by leukopenia, thrombocytopenia, and anemia. Nausea and vomiting are dose related and antiemetics appear to be most helpful if used 24 to 48 hours before starting therapy. Other toxic effects are neuromuscular disturbances, fever, hypotension, and skin rash.

ROUTE AND USUAL DOSAGE.
Intravenous: A continuous infusion is given in a dose of 50 to 200 mg/M² for five days every 14 to 25 days.

DAUNORUBICIN HYDROCHLORIDE

Daunorubicin is an antitumor antibiotic, an anthracycline glycoside isolated from *Streptomyces peucetius*. It forms a stable complex with DNA, thereby inhibiting DNA-dependent RNA synthesis. It is cell cycle-specific for the S phase. The major indications for daunorubicin are in acute granulocytic and lymphocytic leukemia and neuroblastoma.

Toxicity is mainly manifested by hematologic reactions. Myelosuppression is dose limiting and severe aplasia may develop. Leukopenia is more significant than thrombocytopenia. Nausea and vomiting are usually mild. Stomatitis typically begins as a burning sensation with erythema of the oral mucosa leading to ulceration in two or three days. Alopecia develops in about 80% of patients; it often has a sudden onset ofter three to four weeks of therapy but is usually reversible. Febrile reactions also may occur.

Cardiotoxicity with transient, reversible changes in the electrocardiogram may occur, and the risk of congestive heart failure increases when the total cumulative dose exceeds 550 mg/M². Cardiotoxicity may occur one to six months after treatment is discontinued. The total dose of daunorubicin should be limited to 450 mg/M² with concomitant use of cyclophosphamide or when radiation therapy to the mediastinum has been administered previously.

Severe local tissue necrosis may develop if extravasation occurs. Daunorubicin causes transient red discoloration of the urine, which is of no clinical significance.

ROUTE AND USUAL DOSAGE.

Intravenous: 30 to 60 mg/M² daily for three days, repeated at three- to six-week intervals. The drug is administered through a running intravenous infusion. It is contraindicated in patients with significant heart disease.

FTORAFUR

This pyrimidine antimetabolite is structurally similar to floxuridine [FUDR] and acts as a weak inhibitor of DNA thymine and RNA pyrimidine synthesis. The clinical and experimental antitumor activity of ftorafur is similar to that of fluorouracil, with greatest activity seen in gastrointestinal and breast carcinoma, and there is a suggestion that ftorafur has greater activity than fluorouracil in rectal carcinoma.

The minimal toxicity of ftorafur in comparison to fluorouracil appears to be its greatest advantage and is explained by the slow release of small amounts of fluorouracil during metabolism of the chemically unstable ftorafur molecules.

Of 16 evaluable patients with metastatic adenocarcinoma, particularly of the gastrointestinal tract, who received intravenous doses of 1 to 3 g/M²/day for five days every two to four weeks, objective regressions were observed in four patients, and the disease remained stable in four patients. Dose-limiting gastrointestinal and neurologic toxicity occurred with doses of more than 2 g/M²/day for five days but myelosuppression was not observed. This lack of significant myelosuppression at an active dose level makes the drug attractive for combination use. In 66 courses, nausea and vomiting were observed in 56 (85%), chills and fever in 10 (15%), ataxia in 4 (6%), dizziness in 2 (3%), mucositis in 2 (3%), and phlebitis in 1 (2%).

HEXAMETHYLMELAMINE

Hexamethylmelamine is a synthetic agent with a structure that closely resembles that of triethylenemelamine, an alkylating agent. Results of studies in man suggest that the metabolism of this compound differs from that of triethylenemelamine. It has been suggested that hexamethylmelamine may have the properties of an antimetabolite as well as an alkylating agent. In preliminary trials, this agent has been reported to have produced an objective regression rate of 20% in bronchogenic carcinoma and carcinoma of the cervix. Activity also has been shown in carcinoma of the ovary.

Nausea and vomiting with moderate, reversible leukopenia and occasional thrombocytopenia have occurred. With repeated courses, peripheral neuropathy has been reported; two cases were irreversible. Other adverse reactions include numbness, paresthesia, depression, confusion, drowsiness, and hallucinations. It is still uncertain whether this drug shows cross resistance with alkylating agents.

ISOPHOSPHAMIDE

When activated enzymatically in the liver, this derivative of cyclophosphamide exerts a cytotoxic alkylating effect that has been shown to be more pronounced than that of cyclophosphamide in the treatment of some tumors in animals. In foreign studies, preliminary responses have been reported in carcinoma of the ovary, pancreas, colon, and breast. Evidence from studies in the United States suggests that isophosphamide is useful for the following cell types of lung cancer: epidermoid (squamous), adenocarcinoma, and large cell. Antineoplastic activity against other human cancers, such as small cell lung cancer, leukemia, and non-Hodgkin's lymphoma, may also exist. The drug has been used in both single and fractionated dose regimens. A high level of fluid intake should be maintained.

In large doses (50 to 80 mg/kg of body weight), isophosphamide has caused azotemia, hematuria, and urinary frequency. Severe hemorrhagic cystitis also has been reported.

MITOLACTOL (Dibromodulcitol)

This orally administered alkylating agent has been evaluated in patients with carcinoma of the breast. Clinical activity has been reported in chronic myelocytic leukemia, Hodgkin's disease, squamous cell carcinoma of the upper respiratory tract, and adenocarcinoma of the breast. The combination of doxorubicin and mitolactol has produced responses in patients who have not responded to combination chemotherapy with cyclophosphamide, methotrexate, and fluorouracil.

Mitolactol is myelosuppressive and produces leukopenia and thrombocytopenia which are generally reversible. No gastrointestinal reactions or abnormalities of liver or renal function have been reported in patients receiving this drug in therapeutic trials.

PORFIROMYCIN

This antibiotic isolated from culture filtrates of *Streptomyces* is the N-methyl analogue of mitomycin. The two compounds have the same degree of activity and effectiveness against tumors in animals, but porfiromycin is about one-fourth as toxic. The biological effect of the drug appears to depend upon its ability to methylate DNA, RNA, and ribosomes. This agent has not received extensive trials in the management of malignant diseases, but objective responses have been reported in patients with cervical, ovarian, and hepatocellular carcinoma and gastrointestinal neoplasms.

Toxicity is primarily hematologic and is manifested by leukopenia and thrombocytopenia. The drug seems to have a cumulative effect in that toxicity is more pronounced with succeeding courses. The toxicity of porfiromycin with doses of 500 mcg/kg of body weight twice weekly has been reported to be comparable to that encountered with mitomycin in doses of 125 mcg/kg twice weekly. This tends to agree with animal data which show that the maximum tolerated dose of porfiromycin in dogs was four or five times that of mitomycin. Extreme care must be taken to avoid extravasation, for extensive local tissue necrosis will occur.

RAZOXANE

This *bis*-diketopiperazine compound inhibits the DNA metabolism in the G_2-M phase of the cell cycle. It was selected for clinical trials on the basis of antitumor activity in L 1210 and Lewis lung tumor. Its action is dependent upon the schedule of administration in the L 1210 system. Razoxane is more active when given intermittently than when given daily.

Tumor regressions were induced in 4 of 5 patients with squamous cell carcinoma of the lung and in 2 of 11 patients with adenocarcinoma of the colon. No objective remissions were noted in oat cell carcinoma of the lung. In large bowel cancer, a phase II evaluation at the Mayo Clinic has shown evidence that razoxane was active in 3 of 13 previously untreated patients and further study in this area is indicated.

Hematologic adverse effects are dose limiting.

SEMUSTINE (Methyl CCNU)

Semustine is unique among the nitrosoureas in its high degree of effectiveness in Lewis lung carcinoma, an extremely resistant animal tumor with growth characteristics and cellular kinetics similar to those of some human malignant tumors. Like the other nitrosoureas, this agent has the dual mode of action of alkylation and protein modification. Its overall action is cell cycle-nonspecific. Therapeutic responses have been observed in patients with brain tumors, colorectal and gastric adenocarcinomas, Hodgkin's disease, non-Hodgkin's lymphoma, and malignant melanoma. Combination therapy with fluorouracil has proved to be of some value in the management of gastrointestinal malignancies, particularly those of the stomach, colon, and pancreas.

The acute adverse effects of semustine are gastrointestinal disturbances. Nausea and vomiting occur four to six hours after drug administration and last six to eight hours. The dose-limiting toxicity is bone marrow suppression with delayed leukopenia (nadir of white blood cell count occurring six weeks after administration) and thrombocytopenia (nadir occurs after about four weeks). This myelosuppression is cumulative. Anemia is less apparent. Alopecia is observed occasionally.

ROUTE AND USUAL DOSAGE.
Oral: 200 mg/M² as a single dose every six weeks.

STREPTOZOCIN

Streptozocin (1-methyl nitrosourea glucosamine) is an antibiotic derived from *Streptomyces acromogenes*. It has been shown to be a specific beta cell toxin and therefore useful in the treatment of malignant islet cell adenomas. The principal therapeutic use of streptozocin has been in metastatic, insulin-secreting islet cell tumors of the pancreas; this agent has produced significant tumor regression and a return to a normal glycemic state in patients with this disease. More recently, responses in patients with carcinoid tumors, squamous cell carcinomas, and lymphomas, including Hodgkin's disease, have been reported. Streptozocin may be a desirable addition to combination therapy with agents that are predominantly myelosuppressive for use in the treatment of advanced lymphomas and sarcomas.

Most serious reactions encountered with this drug are those affecting the kidneys. Renal effects vary from proteinuria and azotemia to Fanconi syndrome. Azotemia occurs frequently and proteinuria is the first manifestation of renal toxicity. Unfortunately, there is a poor correlation between pretreatment renal function, total dose of streptozocin, and appearance of renal toxicity. Patients with pre-existing impaired renal function should not receive streptozocin. Urinary output should be maintained during and following treatment to ensure maximum dilution of the drug while passing through renal tubules.

Hematologic toxicity is encountered only rarely. Miscellaneous untoward effects include fever and eosinophilia. Hepatotoxicity has been reported in animal toxicity studies but has not been a serious problem clinically. Hepatotoxicity has been manifested by transient elevation in serum transaminase in some clinical trials.

Podophyllotoxins

Podophyllotoxins are natural products isolated from the roots of *Podophyllum peltatum* (commonly known as May Apple or Mandrake). The resin, podophyllin, has been used to treat condyloma acuminatum. The mechanism of action is inhibition of mitosis. A series of semisynthetic compounds have recently been shown to have antineoplastic activity in experimental animals and are undergoing clinical investigation.

EPIPODOPHYLLOTOXIN VM 26

This semisynthetic derivative of podophyllotoxin is a spindle poison, inhibits DNA synthesis, and lyses cells in mitosis.

Responses have been observed in non-Hodgkin's lymphoma, Hodgkin's disease, bladder cancer, brain tumors, and neuroblastoma. In European studies, this agent has been reported to have significant activity in Hodgkin's disease (27% to 56%), histiocytic lymphoma (23% to 52%), and lymphocytic lymphoma (32% to 36%).

Hematologic reactions have been most frequently dose limiting. After weekly doses of 100 mg/M² intravenously, both the white blood cell and platelet count nadirs occurred between 7 and 14 days and recovered within one week. Gastrointestinal disturbances consisting of nausea and vomiting or diarrhea are usually mild. Hypotension can occur following intravenous push injection. Alopecia and, rarely, anaphylaxis have been reported.

EPIPODOPHYLLOTOXIN VP 16

This is also a semisynthetic derivative of podophyllotoxin and its mechanism of action as a mitotic inhibitor is similar to that of VM 26. It is effective in acute granulocytic leukemia and histiocytic lymphoma.

Toxicity is manifested primarily by myelosuppression. Anorexia, nausea, vomiting, and alopecia have been reported with doses of 50 mg/M² intravenously daily for five days and 100 mg/M² orally daily for five days. VP 16 and VM 26 apparently are not cross resistant.

Selected References

Cancer chemotherapy. *Med Lett Drugs Ther* 20:81-88, 1978.

Pharmacologic basis of cancer chemotherapy. *Semin Oncol* 4:131-262, (June) 1977.

Calabresi P, Parks RE Jr: Chemotherapy of neoplastic diseases, in Goodman LS, Gilman A (eds): *The Pharmacological Basis of Therapeutics*, ed 5. New York, Macmillan Publishing Co, Inc, 1975, 1248-1307.

Carter SK, et al: *Chemotherapy of Cancer*. New York, John Wiley & Sons, 1977.

Chabner BA, et al: Clinical pharmacology of antineoplastic agents, parts 1 and 2. *N Engl J Med* 292:1107-1113, 1159-1168, 1975.

Clarysse A, et al: *Cancer Chemotherapy*. Berlin, Springer-Verlag, 1976.

Cline MJ, Haskell CM: *Cancer Chemotherapy*, ed 2. Philadelphia, WB Saunders Co, 1975.

Holland JF, Frei E (eds): *Cancer Medicine*, ed 2. Philadelphia, Lea & Febiger, 1973.

Livingston RB, Carter SK: *Single Agents in Cancer Chemotherapy*. New York, Plenum Press, 1970.

Sather MR, et al: *Cancer Chemotherapeutic Agents*. Boston, GK Hall & Co, 1978.

ANTIBACTERIAL SPECTRUM AND INDICATIONS

ADVERSE REACTIONS AND PRECAUTIONS

 Allergic Reactions

 Tests for Hypersensitivity

 Miscellaneous Reactions

INDIVIDUAL EVALUATIONS

 Penicillin G and Closely Related Compounds

 Semisynthetic Penicillins That Are Not Penicillinase Resistant

 Penicillinase-Resistant Penicillins (Antistaphylococcal Penicillins)

A unique combination of high efficacy and relatively low toxicity, even in immature infants (Eichenwald and McCracken, 1978), makes the penicillins one of the most commonly prescribed and generally useful group of antibiotics. Both natural and semisynthetic penicillins are available. The natural compounds are extracted from cultures of *Penicillium chrysogenum*, whereas the semisynthetic agents are prepared by chemical modification of a natural penicillin or by synthesis from the basic penicillin nucleus, 6-aminopenicillanic acid.

The penicillins interfere with the cross linkage of mucopeptides that are structural components of the bacterial cell wall and may cause the release of autolysins. Thus, their action appears to involve both inhibition of synthesis and increased cell wall breakdown. Nevertheless, these drugs primarily affect growing cells and have minimal or no activity against intracellular microorganisms, dormant bacteria (so-called persisting forms), or those organisms that lack cell walls.

ANTIBACTERIAL SPECTRUM AND INDICATIONS

In patients who are not allergic to these drugs, penicillin G (benzyl penicillin) remains the drug of choice to treat infections caused by susceptible cocci, including nonpenicillinase-producing *Staphylococcus aureus*; group A, group B, and non-enterococcal group D streptococci; gonococci (1% to 2% are resistant because of beta lactamase production); pneumococci (rare strains are resistant); and meningococci. Penicillin G also is preferred for infections caused by *Treponema pallidum*, *Clostridium*, *Bacillus anthracis*, most strains of *Corynebacterium diphtheriae* (some experts prefer erythromycin), several species of *Actinomyces*, fusobacteria, most species of *Bacteroides* except *B. fragilis*, *Actinomyces israelii*, *Streptobacillus moniliformis*, and *Pasteurella multocida*. Most species of *Leptospira* are moderately susceptible to penicillin G, but the drug is ineffective against amebae, plasmodia, rickettsiae, fungi, and viruses.

Penicillin V potassium [Compocillin VK, Ledercillin VK, Pen-Vee K, Uticillin VK, V-Cillin K, Veetids] is more acid stable than penicillin G and equivalent oral doses produce higher blood levels, but it has no proved therapeutic advantage over larger oral doses of buffered penicillin G.

The penicillinase-resistant penicillins (oxacillin sodium [Bactocill, Prostaphlin], cloxacillin sodium [Cloxapen, Tegopen], dicloxacillin sodium [Dycill, Dynapen], methicillin sodium [Celbenin, Staphcillin], and nafcillin sodium [Nafcil, Unipen]) are the drugs of choice when treating infections caused by penicillin G-resistant organisms (eg, hospital-acquired staphylococcal infections). Therapy usually should be instituted immediately while bacterial susceptibility studies are in progress, since delay in administration may contribute to increased mortality in serious infections. If bacterial susceptibility tests demonstrate sensitivity to penicillin G, use of the penicillinase-resistant penicillins may be discontinued because of their greater expense, their greater potential for serious toxicity, and to reduce the risk of increasing bacterial resistance to the anti-staphylococcal penicillins. Originally, it was anticipated that widespread use of penicillinase-resistant penicillins would result in rapid emergence of resistant strains of S. aureus in the United States, since this had occurred in areas of Western Europe several years ago. Fortunately, this has not become a serious problem in this country yet, although resistant strains have been increasing in frequency during the past few years and now represent 5% to 15% of isolates in many hospitals. Vancomycin [Vancocin] usually is effective against these organisms.

Ideally, bacterial susceptibility to any penicillin should be determined by appropriate in vitro tests before the agent is administered; practically, this is not always convenient. Sensitivity studies generally are not necessary if initial culture indicates that the causative organism is a streptococcus or meningococcus, but they should be conducted if the organism is a staphylococ-cus or enterococcus. In pneumococcal infections, an oxacillin (not penicillin) disc should be used to determine resistance to penicillin G. Tests should be conducted when treating patients who acquire gonorrhea in the Orient or those who recently returned from the Orient. Also, the United States Public Health Service recommends that gonococci unresponsive to penicillin G be tested.

Another group of semisynthetic penicillins (ampicillin [Amcill, Omnipen, Penbritin, Polycillin, Principen], hetacillin [Versapen], amoxicillin [Amoxil, Larotid, Polymox, Trimox], carbenicillin disodium [Geopen] or indanyl sodium [Geocillin], and ticarcillin disodium [Ticar]), often designated as broad spectrum penicillins, are ineffective against penicillinase-producing organisms. However, their gram-positive antibacterial spectrum is similar to that of penicillin G, and they are more active than penicillin G against several gram-negative organisms, especially *Haemophilus influenzae* (however, about 10% of these bacteria produce beta lactamase), *Escherichia coli*, and *Proteus mirabilis*.

Aqueous penicillin G administered intravenously is still the drug of choice in bacterial meningitis caused by susceptible strains of *Neisseria meningitidis* or *Streptococcus pneumoniae*. Since meningitis occurring in adults under the age of 60 is rarely caused by *H. influenzae*, large doses of penicillin G often are preferred in these patients even before the results of culture and sensitivity tests are available. In patients over 60 years, the incidence of meningitis caused by penicillin-resistant, gram-negative organisms is increasing. Large doses of ampicillin also are effective against susceptible organisms causing meningitis; it is considered a drug of first choice in children with meningitis caused by *H. influenzae*. In infants up to 2 or 3 months of age, an aminoglycoside is given in addition to penicillin G or ampicillin because of the frequency of coliform meningitis in this age group. Because ampicillin-resistant strains of *H. influenzae* have been reported throughout most of the United States, it is currently recommended that chloramphenicol be given intravenously (100 mg/kg/day) with ampicillin for initial treatment of children with meningitis before the results of culture and sensitivity tests are known. If ampicillin-sensitive organisms alone are cultured from the cerebrospinal fluid, chloramphenicol can be discontinued. Some specialists recommend that patients with meningitis who are allergic to penicillin still be given the drug cautiously (see the section on Adverse Reactions and Precautions) if they have never had an immediate reaction to the antibiotic. If penicillin is contraindicated for other reasons, chloramphenicol should be given initially.

Dosage and Administration: Oral administration is indicated in mild infections, in infections requiring prolonged treatment, or for prophylaxis. This route should not be used for the initial treatment of syphilis, subacute bacterial endocarditis, or actinomycosis. Oral preparations may be given for prophylaxis of rheumatic fever, but the intramuscular injection of benzathine penicillin G is preferred when patient compliance is in doubt.

Oral preparations tend to be absorbed erratically and many are susceptible to destruction by gastric acid. Therefore, to ensure adequate blood and tissue levels, large doses of penicillin G and ampicillin should be given frequently (one hour before or two hours after meals) or a preparation that is less susceptible to acid destruction (penicillin V, cloxacillin, oxacillin, dicloxacillin, and nafcillin) may be used. When given with meals, penicillin V potassium (which is better absorbed than the acid) produces blood levels almost as high as those obtained when the drug is taken on an empty stomach.

Transient high blood concentrations can be produced by injecting an aqueous solution of penicillin G intravenously or intramuscularly every three to six hours; however, with the latter route, the drug is irritating and administration can be very painful. When large doses (eg, 10 million units or more daily) are required, penicillin G must be given intravenously. High tissue levels can be obtained by continuous or intermittent intravenous infusion. Intrathecal injection should never be used

because of the irritant effect of even small doses on the central nervous system.

When more sustained effects are needed, less soluble preparations are given intramuscularly. Procaine penicillin G in water may be given every 8 to 12 hours or even once daily, depending upon the dosage needed. An aqueous preparation of benzathine penicillin G provides detectable drug levels for as long as four weeks after a single intramuscular injection. However, because the blood levels produced are low, these forms of penicillin are effective against only very susceptible bacteria.

Penicillin preparations for topical use are no longer marketed in the United States, since hypersensitization is a frequent complication of their use.

Plasma protein binding of the penicillins varies, and its clinical significance is largely unknown and still controversial. Only the free drug has antibacterial activity. About 20% of ampicillin and amoxicillin, 35% to 60% of penicillin G, 40% of methicillin, 45% of ticarcillin, 50% of carbenicillin, 50% to 70% of penicillin V, and 90% or more of oxacillin, cloxacillin, and dicloxacillin are bound. The protein-penicillin complex dissociates readily and as free drug is withdrawn from plasma additional penicillin is unbound from protein stores. When initiating therapy with any penicillin that is protein bound in excess of 70%, a loading dose double the usual dose may be given to provide therapeutic blood levels more rapidly.

The claims for clinical superiority of one penicillin over another based on in vitro sensitivity are questionable, because such testing does not take into account factors such as stability in gastric acid, rates of absorption and excretion, degree of protein binding, diffusion into abscesses or body cavities, and minimal effective blood and tissue concentrations.

Most penicillins are rapidly excreted in the urine as unchanged drug or metabolites. The rate of elimination in very young infants is slow because of their reduced renal function. Some penicillins, especially ampicillin and nafcillin, are present in the bile in concentrations that are well above the minimal inhibitory levels for most sensitive organisms and are reabsorbed from the intestine. Diffusion into cerebrospinal, synovial, and other body fluids is poor unless very large doses are given or inflammation (eg, meningitis, pleuritis, arthritis) is present. The penicillins cross the placenta, but at a slow rate.

Treatment of Syphilis and Gonorrhea

The management of venereal diseases is an important public health problem because these diseases are widespread and many organisms, such as *Neisseria gonorrhoeae*, are becoming increasingly resistant to drug therapy. The United States Public Health Service has made the following recommendations for the treatment of syphilis and gonorrhea. Although these recommendations represent carefully formulated regimens based on current knowledge, they do not preclude the use of new agents as they become available.

SYPHILIS:

I. Primary, secondary, and latent syphilis of less than one year's duration. Intramuscular: Adults, benzathine penicillin G 2.4 million units (1.2 million units in each buttock) in a single dose; or aqueous procaine penicillin G 600,000 units daily for eight days to a total of 4.8 million units; or procaine penicillin G in oil with aluminum monostearate 2% 2.4 million units initially, usually administered as above, followed by two subsequent injections of 1.2 million units at three-day intervals to a total of 4.8 million units. (The latter preparation is not available in the United States.) Benzathine penicillin G is the drug of choice because it provides effective treatment in a single visit.

Patients allergic to penicillin can be given tetracycline hydrochloride 500 mg orally four times a day one hour before or two hours after meals for 15 days, or erythromycin 500 mg as the base, stearate, or ethylsuccinate orally four times a day for 15 days.

II. Syphilis of more than one year's duration (latent, cardiovascular, late benign, or neurosyphilis). Intramuscular: Adults, ben-

zathine penicillin G 2.4 million units injected weekly as for primary syphilis for three successive weeks to a total of 7.2 million units; or aqueous procaine penicillin G 600,000 units daily for 15 days to a total of 9 million units. Cerebrospinal fluid examination is mandatory in patients with suspected asymptomatic neurosyphilis and is desirable in other patients with syphilis of more than one year's duration to exclude asymptomatic neurosyphilis.

Patients allergic to penicillin can be given the same tetracycline or erythromycin preparations as for primary syphilis, but therapy should be continued for 30 days instead of 15 days. There are no published studies that adequately document the efficacy of drugs other than penicillin for syphilis of more than one year's duration. Cerebrospinal fluid examinations are highly recommended before therapy with these regimens is begun.

III. Syphilis in pregnancy. All pregnant women should have a nontreponemal serologic test for syphilis, such as the VDRL or RPR test, at the time of the first prenatal visit. The treponemal tests (eg, the FTA-ABS test) should not be used for routine screening. In women suspected of being at high risk for syphilis, a second nontreponemal test should be performed during the third trimester. Seroreactive patients should be evaluated expeditiously, including a history, physical examination, quantitative nontreponemal test, and a confirmatory treponemal test.

If the treponemal test is nonreactive and there is no clinical evidence of syphilis, treatment may be withheld. Both the quantitative nontreponemal test and the confirmatory test should be repeated within four weeks. If there is clinical or serologic evidence of syphilis or if the diagnosis of syphilis cannot be excluded with reasonable certainty and the patient is not allergic to penicillin, she can be treated as outlined for nonpregnant patients.

Pregnant patients allergic to penicillin may be given erythromycin as the base, stearate, or ethylsuccinate in dosage schedules appropriate for the stage of syphilis as recommended for nonpregnant patients. Although the schedules for erythromycin appear safe for mother and fetus, their efficacy is not well established. Therefore, documentation of penicillin allergy is particularly important before erythromycin is used during pregnancy. Erythromycin estolate and tetracycline are not recommended for syphilitic infections in pregnant women because of potential adverse effects on mother and fetus.

IV. Congenital syphilis. All children with congenital syphilis should have a cerebrospinal fluid examination before treatment. Those with normal cerebrospinal fluid should be given an intramuscular dose of benzathine penicillin G 50,000 units/kg of body weight in a single dose; children with abnormal cerebrospinal fluid should be · given aqueous crystalline penicillin G intramuscularly or intravenously 50,000 units/kg daily in two divided doses for a minimum of ten days; or aqueous procaine penicillin G 50,000 units/kg once daily intramuscularly for a minimum of ten days. Other antibiotics are not recommended.

GONORRHEA:

Physicians are cautioned to use no less than the recommended doses. When administering tetracycline orally, it must be remembered that food and some dairy products interfere with absorption. Oral forms of tetracycline should be given one hour before or two hours after meals.

I. Uncomplicated gonococcal infections in men and women.

Drug Regimens of Choice: (a) Aqueous procaine penicillin G 4.8 million units injected intramuscularly at two sites given with 1 g of probenecid orally; or (b) tetracycline hydrochloride 0.5 g orally four times daily for five days (total dosage, 10 g) [other tetracyclines are no more effective than tetracycline hydrochloride; all are ineffective as single-dose therapy]; or (c) ampicillin 3.5 g or amoxicillin 3 g, either with 1 g of probenecid orally. Evidence shows that the latter regimens are slightly less effective than the first two regimens. Patients who are allergic to the penicillins or probenecid should be treated with oral tetracycline as above. Patients who cannot tolerate tetracycline may be treated with spectinomycin hydrochloride 2 g in one intramuscular injection.

Special considerations are: (a) Single-dose treatment is preferred in patients who are unlikely to complete the multiple-dose tetracycline regimen. (b) The aqueous procaine penicillin G regimen is preferred in men with anorectal infection. (c) Pharyngeal infection is difficult to treat. High failure rates have been reported with ampicillin and spectinomycin. (d) Tetracycline treatment results in fewer cases of postgonococcal urethritis in men. It may eliminate coexisting chlamydial infections in men and women. (e) Patients with incubating syphilis (seronegative, without clinical signs of syphilis) are likely to be cured by all of the above regimens except spectinomycin. All patients should have a serologic test for syphilis at the time of diagnosis. (f) Patients with gonorrhea who also have syphilis or are established contacts of syphilitic patients should be given additional treatment appropriate to the stage of syphilis.

Treatment of Sexual Partners: Men and women exposed to gonorrhea should be examined, cultured, and treated at once with one of the regimens above.

Follow-up: Follow-up cultures should be obtained from the infected site(s) three to seven days after completion of treatment. Cultures should be obtained from the anal canal of all women who have been treated for gonorrhea.

Treatment Failures: The patient who does not respond to therapy with penicillin, ampicillin, amoxicillin, or tetracycline should be treated with spectinomycin 2 g intramuscularly. Most recurrent infections after treatment with the recommended schedules are caused by *reinfection* and indicate a need for improved contact tracing and patient education. Since infection by penicillinase (β-lactamase)-producing *Neisseria gonorrhoeae* is a cause of treatment failure, post-treatment isolates should be tested for penicillinase production.

Not Recommended: Although long-acting forms of penicillin (eg, benzathine penicillin G) are effective in syphilis therapy, they have *no* place in the treatment of gonorrhea. Oral penicillin preparations (eg, penicillin V) are not recommended for the treatment of gonococcal infection.

II. Penicillinase-producing *Neisseria gonorrhoeae* (PPNG). Patients with uncomplicated PPNG infections and their sexual contacts should receive spectinomycin 2 g intramuscularly in a single injection. Because gonococci are very rarely resistant to spectinomycin and reinfection is the most common cause of treatment failure, patients with positive cultures after spectinomycin therapy should be retreated with the same dose. A PPNG isolate that is resistant to spectinomycin may be treated with cefoxitin 2 g in a single intramuscular injection with probenecid 1 g orally.

III. Treatment in pregnancy. All pregnant women should have endocervical culture for gonococci as an integral part of prenatal care at the time of the first visit. A second culture late in the third trimester should be obtained from women at high risk of gonococcal infection. Drug regimens of choice are aqueous procaine penicillin G, ampicillin, or amoxicillin, each with probenecid as described above. Women who are allergic to penicillin or probenecid should be treated with spectinomycin. See the sections on acute salpingitis and disseminated gonococcal infections for the treatment of these conditions during pregnancy. Tetracycline should not be used in pregnant women because of potential toxic effects on the mother and fetus.

IV. Acute salpingitis (pelvic inflammatory disease). There are no reliable clinical criteria to distinguish gonococcal from nongonococcal salpingitis. Endocervical cultures for *N. gonorrhoeae* are essential. Therapy should be initiated immediately. In the following situations, hospitalization should be strongly considered: uncertain diagnosis, in which surgical emergencies such as appendicitis and ectopic pregnancy must be excluded; suspicion of pelvic abscess; severe illness; pregnancy; inability of patient to follow or tolerate an outpatient regimen; or failure of patient to respond to outpatient therapy.

For *outpatients*, tetracycline 0.5 g orally four times a day for ten days (should not be used in pregnant patients); or aqueous procaine penicillin G 4.8 million units intramuscularly, ampicillin 3.5 g, or amoxicillin 3 g, each with probenecid 1 g. Each regimen is followed by ampicillin 0.5 g or amoxicillin 0.5 g orally four times a day for ten days.

For *hospitalized patients*, aqueous crystalline penicillin G 20 million units intravenously daily until improvement occurs, followed by ampicillin 0.5 g orally four times a day to complete ten days of therapy; or tetracycline 0.25 g intravenously four times a day until improvement occurs, followed by 0.5 g orally four times a day to complete ten days of therapy. This regimen should not be used for pregnant women. The dosage may have to be adjusted if renal function is depressed. Since optimal therapy for hospitalized patients has not been established, other antibiotics in addition to penicillin are frequently used.

Special considerations are: (a) Failure of the patient to improve on the recommended regimens does not indicate the need for stepwise additional antibiotics but requires clinical reassessment. (b) The intrauterine device is a risk factor for the development of pelvic inflammatory disease. The effect of removing an intrauterine device on the response of acute salpingitis to antimicrobial therapy and on the risk of recurrent salpingitis is unknown. (c) Adequate treatment of women with acute salpingitis must include examination and appropriate treatment of their sexual partners because of the high incidence of nonsymptomatic urethral infection. Failure to treat sexual partners is a major cause of recurrent gonococcal salpingitis. (d) Follow-up of patients with acute salpingitis is essential during and after treatment. All patients should be recultured for *N. gonorrhoeae* after treatment.

V. Acute epididymitis. Acute epididymitis can be caused by *N. gonorrhoeae*, *Chlamydia*, or other organisms. If gonococci are demonstrated by Gram stain or culture of urethral secretions, aqueous procaine penicillin G 4.8 million units, ampicillin 3.5 g, or amoxicillin 3 g, each with probenecid 1 g, is given. Each regimen is followed by ampicillin 0.5 g or amoxicillin 0.5 g orally four times a day for ten days, or tetracycline 0.5 g orally four times a day for ten days. If gonococci are not demonstrated, the tetracycline regimen should be used.

VI. Disseminated gonococcal infection. One of the following equally effective treatment schedules may be administered in the arthritis-dermatitis syndrome: (a) ampicillin 3.5 g or amoxicillin 3 g orally, each with probenecid 1 g, followed by ampicillin 0.5 g or amoxicillin 0.5 g four times a day orally for seven days; or (b) tetracycline 0.5 g orally four times a day for seven days (tetracycline should not be used for complicated gonococcal infection in pregnant women); or (c) spectinomycin 2 g intramuscularly twice a day for three days (treatment of choice for disseminated infections caused by PPNG); or (d) erythromycin 0.5 g orally four times a day for seven days; or (e) aqueous crystalline penicillin G 10 million units intravenously daily until improvement occurs, followed by ampicillin 0.5 g four times a day to complete seven days of antibiotic treatment.

Special considerations are: (a) Hospitalization is indicated in patients who may be unreliable, have uncertain diagnosis, or have purulent joint effusions or other complications. (b) Open drainage of joints other than the hip is not indicated. Intra-articular injection of antibiotics is unnecessary.

Meningitis and Endocarditis: Meningitis and endocarditis caused by gonococci require high-dose intravenous penicillin therapy. In penicillin-allergic patients with endocarditis, desensitization and administration of penicillin are indicated. Chloramphenicol may be used in penicillin-allergic patients with meningitis.

VII. Gonococcal infections in pediatric patients. With gonococcal infections in children beyond the newborn period, the possibility of sexual abuse must be considered. Genital, anal, and pharyngeal cultures should be obtained from all patients before antibiotic treatment. Appropriate cultures should be obtained from individuals who have had contact with the child.

VIII. Prevention of gonococcal ophthalmia. When required by state legislation or indicated by local epidemiologic considerations, effective and acceptable regimens for prophylaxis of neonatal gonococcal ophthalmia include ophthalmic ointment or drops containing tetracycline or erythromycin *or* a 1% silver nitrate solution.

Special considerations are: (a) Bacitracin is not recommended. (b) The value of irrigation after application of silver nitrate is unknown.

IX. Management of infants born to mothers with gonococcal infection. The infant born to a mother with symptomatic gonorrhea is at high risk of infection and requires treatment with a single intravenous or intramuscular injection of aqueous crystalline penicillin G 50,000 units to full-term infants or 20,000 units to low-birth-weight infants. Topical prophylaxis for neonatal ophthalmia is not adequate. Clinical illness requires additional treatment.

X. Neonatal disease.

Gonococcal Ophthalmia: Patients should be hospitalized and isolated for 24 hours after initiation of treatment. Untreated gonococcal ophthalmia is highly contagious. Aqueous crystalline penicillin G 50,000 units/kg/day in two doses intravenously should be administered for seven days. Saline irrigation of the eyes should be performed as needed. Topical antibiotic preparations alone are not sufficient or required when appropriate systemic antibiotic therapy is given.

Complicated Infection: Patients with arthritis and septicemia should be hospitalized and treated with aqueous crystalline penicillin G 75,000 to 100,000 units/kg/day intravenously in two or three divided doses for seven days. Meningitis should be treated with aqueous crystalline penicillin G 100,000 units/kg/day divided into three or four intravenous doses and continued for at least ten days.

XI. Childhood disease. Children who weigh 100 lbs (45 kg) or more should receive adult regimens. Children who weigh less than 100 lbs should be treated as follows:

Uncomplicated Disease: Uncomplicated vulvovaginitis, urethritis, proctitis, or pharyngitis can be treated at one visit with amoxicillin 50 mg/kg of body weight orally with probenecid 25 mg/kg (maximum, 1 g), or aqueous procaine penicillin G 100,000 units/kg intramuscularly plus probenecid 25 mg/kg (maximum, 1 g).

Special considerations are: (a) Topical and/or systemic estrogen therapy is of no benefit in vulvovaginitis. (b) Long-acting penicillins, such as benzathine penicillin G, are not effective. (c) All patients should have follow-up cultures, and the source of infection should be identified, examined, and treated.

Gonococcal Ophthalmia: Ophthalmia in children is treated as in neonates, but the dose of penicillin is increased to 100,000 units/kg/day intravenously.

Complicated Infections: Patients with peritonitis or arthritis require hospitalization and treatment with aqueous crystalline penicillin G 100,000 units/kg/day intravenously for seven days. Aqueous crystalline penicillin G 250,000 units/kg/day intravenously in six divided doses for at least ten days is recommended for meningitis.

Allergy to Penicillins: Children who are allergic to penicillins should be treated with spectinomycin 40 mg/kg intramuscularly. Children older than 8 years may be treated with tetracycline 40 mg/kg/day orally in four divided doses for five days. For treatment of complicated disease, the alternative regimens recommended for adults may be used in appropriate pediatric dosages.

Adverse Reactions and Precautions

Hypersensitivity Reactions: The incidence of hypersensitivity to the penicillins has been estimated to be between 1% and 5%. Among the antimicrobials, this group of drugs causes the largest number of allergic reactions. This appears to reflect the wide usage of the penicillins rather than any specific potential for sensitization. Topical application or exposure to dust or aerosol containing a penicillin formerly was the most common source of hypersensitization. Today, parenteral and oral preparations probably are chiefly responsible, although it is possible that an individual who has never been given a penicillin may develop a reaction through previous exposure to normal environmental sources of penicillium molds or penicillins (eg, in milk). Once a hypersensitivity reaction occurs to any penicillin, it should be assumed that the patient will react to all other drugs in the class. Nevertheless, the occurrence of an untoward reaction does not necessarily imply repetition of the effect on subsequent exposures. Allergic reactivity can be lost or the reaction may not have been hypersensitive in nature (see below).

Penicillins may cause hypersensitivity reactions by any one of four immune mechanisms:

Type I reactions are mediated by IgE antibodies. These reaginic antibodies fix to the surface of the tissue mast cells, resulting in release of vasoactive compounds (eg, histamine). Manifestations include urticaria, angioedema, and anaphylaxis, as well as rhinitis, asthma, and laryngeal edema. Reactions may be accompanied by fever; approximately 40% of penicillin reactions are manifested by fever alone. This reaction usually resolves within 48 hours after the drug is stopped but may persist for up to five days.

Type I responses often are immediate (occurring within one hour after administration of the drug), but accelerated urticaria and other reactions that develop 1 to 72 hours after the drug is given also may be seen. However, severe anaphylaxis, hypotension, and death are rare. Type I reactions are the most commonly reported adverse effects of penicillin and, like all undesirable responses to these drugs, may occur following either oral or parenteral administration; they are more prevalent after parenteral injection.

The belief has been held for years that allergic reactions to penicillin, especially anaphylaxis, are observed more commonly in atopic patients, but this point is controversial. Some authorities still believe this to be true, whereas others believe there is no greater frequency of allergic reactions to penicillin in atopic individuals than in the rest of the population. Certainly, an individual should not be denied penicillin on the basis of other allergic manifestations when there is no history or clearcut evidence of hypersensitivity to penicillin. Nevertheless, it would seem prudent to test such individuals more rigorously for penicillin allergy than those with no evidence of allergic phenomena.

Type II reactions are caused by cytotoxic antibodies of the IgG or IgM class. Penicillin acts as a hapten on the cell surface and reacts with antipenicillin antibodies, resulting in the destruction of the cell. Complement may enter into the reaction but is not required. Hemolytic anemia is an example of an adverse reaction mediated by this mechanism.

Type III reactions involve the formation of immune complexes of IgG or IgM antibodies and penicillin (or a metabolite) which, in turn, act as antigens. These complexes are deposited in tissue spaces or on cells of skin, kidneys, or other organs. There is complement fixation. Polymorphonuclear leukocytes are attracted by the resultant immune reactant, and an inflammatory response occurs. Interstitial nephritis, vasculitis, serum sickness, and some late urticarial reactions probably are caused by this mechanism.

Type IV reactions are classified as delayed (occurring 72 hours or more following administration of the drug) and are mediated by T lymphocytes. Fixed drug eruptions and other rashes, including contact dermatitis, are manifestations of type IV reactions. Rarely, Stevens-Johnson syndrome, serum sickness, hemolytic anemia, or thrombocytopenia may occur.

Hypersensitive-type rashes can be seen following the administration of any penicillin but, at least in the case of ampicillin, the vast majority are not allergic in nature. These mildly pruritic maculopapular eruptions usually occur within 1 to 28 days, are not associated with positive skin tests, and resolve whether or not ampicillin administration is continued. They do not preclude the future use of a penicillin.

The recurrence of allergic reactions upon subsequent administration of a penicillin to an individual who exhibited an initial reaction is not always constant. There is no doubt that penicillins should be used with extreme care, if at all, in most patients suspected or known to be hypersensitive to this group of antibiotics. Yet, this approach should be tempered with the knowledge that urticaria (particularly accelerated or late forms) may improve with continued therapy. This effect appears to be caused by an increase of benzylpenicilloyl-specific IgG that behaves as a blocking antibody.

Since hypersensitivity reactions to the penicillins may occur at any time, members of this class of antibiotics should not be administered unless appropriate drugs and resuscitative equipment are immediately available. In acute anaphylactic reactions, epinephrine (subcutaneously or intramuscularly for mild reactions and intravenously for more serious reactions) can be lifesaving. Parenteral administration of antihistamines may be valuable. In addition, prompt administration of oxygen, placement of an endotracheal tube, or tracheostomy (if laryngeal edema occurs) may be indicated. After the immediate reaction has been controlled, a corticosteroid may be given parenterally to prevent relapse and also may be useful in more prolonged reactions (eg, serum sickness). Corticosteroids are not useful in immediate reactions. Accelerated and late urticarial reactions may be treated with antihistamines. Maculopapular rashes are self-limiting, but antihistamines relieve pruritus.

Toxic Reactions: The penicillins per se are essentially nontoxic in man. Most reactions are caused by the irritant effects of excessive concentration or reactions to a related molecule (eg, procaine toxicity from injection of procaine penicillin G). Pain and sterile inflammation may occur at the site of intramuscular injection, and phlebitis or thrombophlebitis is sometimes seen when these drugs are given intravenously. Nausea, vomiting, and mild to severe diarrhea may result from irritation of the gastrointestinal tract. However, the most serious consequences of the irritant properties of the penicillins involve the nervous system. Accidental injection into a peripheral nerve causes pain and dysfunction of that part of the body innervated by the nerve. This effect usually is slowly reversible. High concentrations of penicillin in the central nervous system may cause arachnoiditis, convulsions, or, possibly, fatal encephalopathy.

Miscellaneous Reactions: Serious superinfections with resistant organisms, especially gram-negative bacteria (eg, *Pseudomonas, Proteus*) and *Candida*, may occur following long-term therapy with any of the penicillins, particularly with extended spectrum derivatives such as ampicillin.

Nephropathy, a sensitivity reaction manifested as interstitial nephritis, has been reported. Kidney damage usually is accompanied by proteinuria, hematuria, and acute renal failure. Fever and eosinophilia also are observed frequently and pyuria occasionally. Nephropathy occurs most frequently with methicillin but may be caused by any of the penicillins, except that there have been no well-documented cases of nephrotoxicity caused by nafcillin. This may be related to the fact that nafcillin is principally (approximately 80% to 85%) excreted by the liver rather than the kidneys. Patients usually recover when the drug is discontinued, but fatalities have occurred.

Massive intravenous doses of penicillin G potassium (1.7 mEq of potassium/million units) may cause hyperkalemia and, rarely, convulsions in patients with impaired renal function. Convulsions also may follow rapid intravenous injection of a large single dose (5 million units or greater in an adult), especially in epileptics, infants, or other susceptible individuals. Because of their central nervous system irritant properties, the intrathecal administration of the penicillins is not justified.

Although bone marrow depression has been observed after use of methicillin, oxacillin, and other penicillinase-resistant penicillins, no fatalities have been reported to date. Ampicillin has caused agranulocytosis with peripheral cytosis and bone marrow histiocytosis.

Several semisynthetic penicillins induce platelet dysfunction which may lead to bleeding. This effect is seen with methicillin, carbenicillin, ticarcillin, and even with penicillin itself, but has not been reported with dicloxacillin. Coombs' positive anemia occurs rarely following penicillin therapy.

Tests for Hypersensitivity: Earliest attempts to test for penicillin hypersensitivity involved injecting a small amount of penicillin G intradermally. This procedure is unreliable and dangerous, since even a small amount of penicillin can cause serious reactions or death in sensitive individuals.

Two preparations have been developed that more accurately predict reactions to the penicillins, particularly when they are used concomitantly. One of these, benzylpenicilloyl-poly-L-lysine (BPO-PL) [Pre-Pen], is a major antigenic determinant of benzylpenicillin; a concentration of 6×10^{-5} M is used. The second is a benzylpenicillin minor determinant mixture containing penicillin breakdown products, such as penilloates and penicilloates (BP-MDM), prepared by the method of Levine et al (1969) and used in a concentration of 2×10^{-2} M. The minor determinants must be freshly prepared, since they are unstable and no satisfactory technique has been developed to market them. Both major and minor determinants possess a greater margin of safety than penicillin G itself. Nevertheless, it is advisable to perform prick tests prior to intradermal injection because the risk of anaphylaxis is greater when a larger amount is injected.

When BPO-PL and BP-MDM are used as a combined testing procedure, greater than 95% of penicillin IgE-mediated hypersensitivity probably can be predicted. In one study of 86 adults and 167 children (Warrington et al, 1978), it was found that of 169 patients with negative skin tests, only two children showed mild reactions when challenged with penicillin, an incidence of 1.2%. The same study showed that when BPO-PL was used alone, up to 31% of allergic patients would have false-negative tests for hypersensitivity. Also, reactivity to BP-MDM is more frequently associated with severe anaphylactic reactions than reactivity to BPO-PL (Levine and Redmond, 1969). Skin tests are of no value in predicting late urticarial reactions or non-IgE hypersensitivity, such as interstitial nephritis.

When minor determinants of ampicillin, cloxacillin, and methicillin were used to screen for allergy, they were not significantly more sensitive than those derived from benzylpenicillin. Only 4 of 181 patients tested with cloxacillin or methicillin demonstrated greater reactivity to those reagents than to BPO-PL or BP-MDM, and no patient had a greater reactivity to the ampicillin derivative than to the benzylpenicillin derivative (Warrington et al, 1978). All patients with skin reactivity to the minor determinants of ampicillin, cloxacillin, and methicillin also reacted to BP-MDM.

When conducting a skin test for penicillin sensitivity, it is important that a careful history be taken relative to previous reactions. Several investigators (Finke et al, 1965; Bierman and VanArsdel, 1969; Van Dellen and Gleich, 1970) have shown that skin tests for penicillin allergy may be negative shortly after a reaction to penicillin.

PENICILLIN G AND CLOSELY RELATED COMPOUNDS

PENICILLIN G

Penicillin G preparations are drugs of first choice in nonallergic patients with infections caused by susceptible organisms (see the Introduction for antibacterial spectrum).

Since oral preparations are absorbed erratically and penicillin G is destroyed by gastric acid, this route should be used only for mild or stabilized infections or long-term prophylaxis. Parenteral use of the short-acting salts produces transient high blood levels. When massive doses are indicated, the intravenous route is preferred. If sustained, low-level blood concentrations are desirable, procaine penicillin G in water or benzathine penicillin G in water may be injected intramuscularly. Intravenous injection of procaine penicillin G must be avoided.

Allergic reactions are the most common adverse effects caused by penicillin G (see the Introduction), and this drug is contraindicated in patients known to be hypersensitive to penicillins. Whenever possible, another antibacterial agent such as erythromycin should be given to patients with a history of allergic conditions. If allergic reactions occur, penicillin G should be discontinued immediately and, if necessary, appropriate ameliorative treatment given (see the Introduction). In most instances, discontinuation of penicillin G is sufficient. Another antibacterial agent should be substituted if further treatment is necessary. Intrathecal administration of 10,000 units or more, high-dose therapy in neonates or in patients with renal disease, or rapid intravenous administration of more than 20 million units daily may produce convulsions, although intravenous doses larger than this are sometimes used to treat staphylococcal bacterial endocarditis caused by sensitive organisms.

ROUTES, USUAL DOSAGE, AND PREPARATIONS. PENICILLIN G SODIUM, POTASSIUM:

Oral: *Adults and children over 12 years,* 600,000 to 1.6 million units (375 mg to 1 g) daily in divided doses three or four times daily (in adults, amounts of 3.2 million units [2 g] daily in divided doses are not uncommon for severe infections); *children under 12 years,* 40,000 (25 mg) to 80,000 units (50 mg)/kg of body weight daily in divided doses every six to eight hours.

Intramuscular, Intravenous: *Adults,* 300,000 to 1.2 million units daily; very large doses (10 to as much as 100 million units daily) have been infused intravenously for certain serious infections. This represents heroic therapy, however. *Children,* 50,000 to 250,000 units/kg of body weight daily in divided doses every four hours; doses up to 10 million units daily have been infused intravenously. *In-*

fants over 7 days, 75,000 units/kg daily in divided doses every eight hours; for meningitis, 150,000 to 250,000 units/kg daily in divided doses every six to eight hours; *under 7 days*, 50,000 units/kg daily in divided doses every 12 hours; for meningitis, 100,000 to 150,000 units/kg daily in divided doses every 8 to 12 hours.

PROCAINE PENICILLIN G:

Intramuscular: Adults and children, 600,000 to 1 million units daily in one or two doses depending upon the condition being treated. Ten days to two weeks of therapy is usually sufficient. *Infants*, 50,000 units/kg of body weight once daily. For treatment of venereal infections, see the Introduction.

BENZATHINE PENICILLIN G IN WATER:

Intramuscular: Adults, 1.2 million units in a single dose; *older children*, a single injection of 900,000 units; *infants and children under 60 lb (27.3 kg)*, a single dose of 50,000 units/kg of body weight. For treatment of venereal infections, see the Introduction. For prophylaxis of rheumatic fever, 1.2 million units once each month or 600,000 units every two weeks on a continuing basis.

Oral: For prophylaxis of rheumatic fever, *adults and older children*, 200,000 units (125 mg) twice daily on a continuing basis. Before dental procedures or minor upper respiratory tract surgery (to prevent bacterial endocarditis in patients with congenital and/or rheumatic heart lesions), 1.2 million units (750 mg) one hour before the procedure and 600,000 units (375 mg) every six hours for the next two and one-half days.

Drug available generically: Powder; suspension for injection; suspension (oral) 125 and 250 mg/5 ml; tablets (buffered, plain) 125, 250, and 500 mg.

Available Trademarks.

BENZATHINE PENICILLIN G:
Bicillin, Bicillin LA (Wyeth).

PENICILLIN G POTASSIUM:
Pentids (Squibb), *Pfizerpen, Pfizerpen G* (Pfipharmecs).

PROCAINE PENICILLIN G:
Crysticillin A.S. (Squibb), *Duracillin A.S.* (Lilly), *Wycillin* (Wyeth).

COMBINATIONS OF PENICILLIN G.

Combinations of procaine penicillin G and benzathine penicillin G are marketed for the convenience of physicians who believe that they may be helpful in situations in which both immediate and long-term effects are desired and the patient cannot conveniently return for care. The incidence of local reactions to the combination is lower than might be expected from the increased dosage of either agent alone. In general, however, it is preferable to administer penicillins as single-entity preparations for specific indications.

Bicillin C-R Injection (Wyeth). Solution containing benzathine penicillin G and procaine penicillin G 150,000 units/ml each in 10 ml containers or 300,000 units/ml each in 1, 2, and 4 ml containers.

Bicillin C-R 900/300 (Wyeth). Solution containing benzathine penicillin G 900,000 units and procaine penicillin G 300,000 units/2 ml (450,000 units and 150,000 units/ml respectively) in 2 ml containers.

PENICILLIN V
[V-Cillin]

POTASSIUM PENICILLIN V
[Compocillin-VK, Ledercillin VK, Pen-Vee K, Uticillin VK, V-Cillin K, Veetids]

These phenoxymethyl congeners of penicillin G are available only for oral administration. They have the same antibacterial spectrum as penicillin G (see the Introduction) but are more resistant to destruction by gastric acid. When taken in a fasting state, blood levels of penicillin V are somewhat higher than those produced by an equal quantity of oral penicillin G; when taken with food, the blood levels of penicillin V are considerably higher. However, penicillin V has no proven advantage over larger oral doses of buffered penicillin G taken on an empty stomach, and even large oral doses of penicillin V do not produce blood levels higher than those easily achieved by parenteral administration of penicillin G.

Allergic reactions are the most common adverse effects (see the Introduction).

ROUTE, USUAL DOSAGE, AND PREPARATIONS.
Oral: *Adults*, 125 to 500 mg four to six
times daily. *Children*, 25 to 50 mg/kg of
body weight daily in divided doses every
six to eight hours. For prophylactic treatment of rheumatic fever, *adults*, 125 to 250
mg daily.

PENICILLIN V:
Drug available generically: Suspension 125
and 250 mg/5 ml; tablets 125, 250, and 500 mg.
V-Cillin (Lilly). Powder for drops 125 mg/0.6
ml.

POTASSIUM PENICILLIN V:
Drug available generically: Powder for oral
solution (plain, buffered) 125 and 250 mg/ml;
solution 125 and 250 mg/5 ml; tablets 125, 250,
and 500 mg.
Ledercillin VK (Lederle), *Veetids* (Squibb).
Powder for oral solution 125 and 250 mg/5 ml;
tablets 250 and 500 mg.
Compocillin-VK (Ross), *Pen-Vee K* (Wyeth),
V-Cillin K (Lilly). Powder for oral solution 125
and 250 mg/5 ml; tablets 125, 250, and 500 mg.
Uticillin VK (Upjohn). Granules for oral solution 125 and 250 mg/5 ml; tablets 250 and 500
mg.

Additional Trademarks.
Betapen-VK (Bristol), *Penapar VK* (Parke,
Davis), *Pfizerpen VK* (Pfipharmecs), *Robicillin
VK* (Robins).

SEMISYNTHETIC PENICILLINS THAT
ARE NOT PENICILLINASE RESISTANT

AMPICILLIN
[Amcill, Omnipen, Penbritin, Polycillin,
Principen]

AMPICILLIN SODIUM
[Amcil-S, Omnipen-N, Penbritin-S,
Polycillin-N, Principen/N]

Ampicillin, a semisynthetic penicillin for
oral and parenteral use, has the same general spectrum of activity as penicillin G
against gram-positive organisms (see the
Introduction) and is more effective against
gram-negative bacteria. In vitro, it is active
against *Haemophilus influenzae, Bordetella pertussis, Neisseria gonorrhoeae,
N. meningitidis, Salmonella typhi*, non-
penicillinase-producing strains of *Proteus
mirabilis*, many strains of *Escherichia coli*,
and several strains of *Shigella*. Present
clinical experience indicates that ampicillin may be effective against some strains of
Klebsiella (most strains of *K. pneumoniae*
are resistant). *Despite this broader spectrum, ampicillin should not be substituted
routinely for penicillin G when treating
infections caused by penicillin G-
susceptible bacteria*. Both urinary tract infections and bacterial endocarditis caused
by *Streptococcus faecalis* respond to this
drug, but there are no definitive data to
support the routine use of ampicillin,
either alone or combined with streptomycin, in preference to the concomitant administration of penicillin G and an aminoglycoside in the treatment of subacute
bacterial endocarditis. Infections caused by
Listeria monocytogenes also may respond
to ampicillin.

Ampicillin is inactivated by penicillinase
and therefore is ineffective against penicillin G-resistant staphylococci. Enteric
bacilli, especially *E. coli* and *Proteus*, have
become resistant to ampicillin by selective
elimination of strains that do not produce
penicillinase (some strains of *E. coli* also
may be resistant to ampicillin through a
different mechanism). Many infections
caused by *H. influenzae* still respond to
ampicillin, but resistance is becoming a
serious problem. *Pseudomonas* organisms
are resistant but streptococci and
pneumococci are not.

Because ampicillin has an antibacterial
spectrum similar to that of the tetracyclines, it is often used instead of these
agents, particularly in young children and
pregnant women for whom tetracyclines
are inappropriate. It also may be used in
place of more potentially toxic agents such
as chloramphenicol.

The primary clinical indications for ampicillin are urinary, respiratory, and gastrointestinal tract infections and bacterial
otitis and meningitis in children. Urinary
tract infections caused by susceptible bacteria, especially *E. coli, P. mirabilis*,

nonhemolytic streptococci, and penicillin G-resistant enterococci, appear to respond rapidly to ampicillin. Ampicillin is used in the treatment of gonorrhea, but penicillin G is still the drug of choice (see the Introduction); the latter is also preferred in infections caused by *Streptococcus pneumoniae*, but respiratory tract infections in which *H. influenzae* and *S. pneumoniae* occur together may be highly responsive to ampicillin.

Ampicillin is useful occasionally in biliary tract and intestinal infections caused by sensitive strains of *E. coli*, penicillin G-resistant enterococci, salmonellae, and shigellae, because relatively high concentrations appear in the bile. However, an increasing number of ampicillin-resistant *Salmonella* and *Shigella* species are emerging (50% or more of *Shigella* strains throughout the United States are now resistant to ampicillin). The results of treatment of enteritis caused by salmonellae (eg, *S. typhi, S. typhimurium*) have been somewhat disappointing. Even chloramphenicol has not produced consistently satisfactory results, but it continues to be the drug of choice except in typhoid carriers with resistant infections who require prolonged treatment (see Chapter 71, Chloramphenicol and Derivatives). In these individuals, ampicillin and amoxicillin have been used with some success. Ampicillin is a drug of choice for treating typhoid fever resistant to chloramphenicol. It can be administered orally or parenterally, but there is a higher failure rate after oral administration.

Parenteral administration of large doses of ampicillin is effective, reliable, and relatively nontoxic in children with bacterial meningitis caused by susceptible strains of *N. meningitidis, S. pneumoniae* (pneumococci), or *H. influenzae*, although large doses of penicillin G may be preferred for sensitive organisms. Because resistant strains of *H. influenzae* are increasing in frequency, ampicillin should not be used routinely as the drug of choice for meningitis unless the strain is known to be susceptible. Bacterial meningitis in adults has responded to treatment with ampicillin (see the Introduction).

Ampicillin is water soluble, acid stable, and readily absorbed from the gastrointestinal tract when given orally (absorption is decreased if taken with food). Approximate peak serum levels after a single 500-mg dose are: intravenous, 45 mcg/ml within five minutes; intramuscular, 8 mcg/ml within one hour; and oral, 2.5 to 5 mcg/ml within two hours. Low levels of ampicillin persist for six hours after intravenous administration and for eight hours after intramuscular or oral administration. About 20% is bound to plasma protein. The minimal inhibitory concentrations against susceptible bacteria in vitro range from 0.02 to 5 mcg/ml. Ampicillin is excreted rapidly in the urine; urinary levels of 0.25 to 2.5 mg/ml are attained.

Ampicillin is usually well tolerated. Adverse reactions are generally mild and consist most often of skin rashes or diarrhea. The incidence of diarrhea has been reported to be as great as 11% in adults and 20% in children, although these figures may be high. Diarrhea usually is not severe enough to require discontinuing the drug. Rarely, antibiotic-associated colitis caused by *Clostridium difficile* may occur during ampicillin therapy. This almost always resolves quickly if the penicillin is stopped and vancomycin is administered (see Chapter 72, Macrolide and Lincosamide Antibiotics, and Chapter 76, Miscellaneous Antibacterial Agents). Rashes develop more often with ampicillin than with penicillin G, especially in patients with infectious mononucleosis. Approximately 1% to 5% of the rashes are allergic in nature and require discontinuing the antibiotic. This incidence presumably is about the same as for other penicillins. Other rashes, which may have a slower onset than allergic rash, are not regarded as a true penicillin allergy and disappear at the same rate whether ampicillin is continued or not. These rashes are not contraindications to the use of penicillin G, nor should they be considered an indication that the patient is allergic to penicillin. Other hypersensitivity reactions include pruritus, urticaria, eosinophilia, fever, and angioedema. Ampicillin is contraindicated in patients with a history of sensitivity to other penicillins.

Local phlebitis has occurred after intravenous infusion, and local pain is common after intramuscular injection. When given orally, ampicillin also may cause cramping, nausea, vomiting, and diarrhea.

A moderate elevation of the serum glutamic oxaloacetic transaminase (SGOT) level has been observed in a few infants after intramuscular administration. It has not been determined that this reaction is caused by liver disease.

There have been a few reports of nephropathy associated with ampicillin therapy. In two cases, this appeared to be an allergic reaction; in other cases, the renal function of patients with renal disease or prerenal azotemia had deteriorated during therapy. There also have been reports of anemia, eosinophilia, thrombocytopenia, leukopenia, and agranulocytosis, which are believed to be hypersensitivity phenomena.

Superinfections, especially in the gastrointestinal tract, have been noted, particularly when large doses were given or therapy was prolonged. *Enterobacter, Pseudomonas, Candida,* and, rarely, *Cl. difficile* are some of the organisms involved. If superinfection occurs, the dosage may have to be reduced or another antibacterial agent substituted.

Definitive information on the toxicity of ampicillin during pregnancy is not available; however, the penicillins in general appear to be nonteratogenic in man.

ROUTES, USUAL DOSAGE, AND PREPARATIONS.
AMPICILLIN (TRIHYDRATE OR ANHYDROUS):
Oral: Adults and children weighing more than 20 kg, 250 to 500 mg four times daily at six-hour intervals; *less than 20 kg,* 50 to 100 mg/kg of body weight daily in divided doses every six hours. The larger dose is administered for severe infections. The stomach need not be empty when this drug is given orally, but peak plasma levels may be higher in fasting patients.

Drug available generically: Capsules 250 and 500 mg; powder for suspension 125, 250, and 500 mg/5 ml; suspension 125 and 250 mg/5 ml; tablets 125 mg.

AMPICILLIN (ANHYDROUS):
Omnipen (Wyeth). Capsules 250 and 500 mg; powder for suspension 125, 250, and 500 mg/5 ml.

AMPICILLIN (TRIHYDRATE):
Principen (Squibb). Capsules 250 and 500 mg; powder for suspension 125 and 250 mg/5 ml.
Amcill (Parke, Davis). Capsules 250 and 500 mg; drops for suspension (pediatric) 100 mg/ml; powder for suspension 125 and 250 mg/5 ml; tablets (chewable) 125 mg.
Penbritin (Ayerst), *Polycillin* (Bristol). Capsules 250 and 500 mg; drops for suspension (pediatric) 100 mg/ml; powder for suspension 125 and 250 mg/5 ml.
Additional Trademarks.
A-Cillin (Hauck), *Alpen* (Lederle), *Pensyn* (Upjohn), *SK-Ampicillin* (Smith Kline & French), *Supen* (Reid-Provident), *Totacillin* (Beecham).
AVAILABLE MIXTURES.
Generic: Powder for suspension containing ampicillin 3.5 g and probenecid 1 g.
Amcill-GC (Parke, Davis), *Polycillin-PRB* (Bristol). Powder for suspension containing ampicillin 3.5 g (as the trihydrate) and probenecid 1 g.
Principen w/Probenecid (Squibb). Nine capsules per package, each containing ampicillin trihydrate equivalent to ampicillin 389 mg and probenecid 111 mg.

AMPICILLIN SODIUM:
Intramuscular: Adults and children over 20 kg, 250 to 500 mg four times daily at six-hour intervals; *less than 20 kg,* 100 to 200 mg/kg of body weight daily in divided doses every six hours. *Infants less than 7 days,* 50 mg/kg daily in divided doses every 12 hours; *over 7 days,* 75 mg/kg daily in divided doses every eight hours.
Intravenous: Adults and children over 20 kg, 250 to 500 mg four times daily at six-hour intervals. For severe infections, doses up to 2 g every six hours may be used. For bacterial meningitis, 8 to 14 g daily (150 to 250 mg/kg of body weight daily) in divided doses every three to four hours. *Children under 20 kg,* 100 to 200 mg/kg daily in divided doses every six hours. For bacterial meningitis, 150 to 250 mg/kg daily (doses as high as 400 mg/kg have been used) in divided doses every four to six hours. *Infants under 7 days,* 50 mg/kg daily in divided doses every 12 hours; for meningitis, 100 mg/kg daily in divided doses every 12 hours. *Infants over 7 days,* 75 mg/kg daily in divided doses every eight hours; for meningitis, 150 to 200 mg/kg daily in divided doses every six to eight hours.
For dosage used in gonorrhea, see the Introduction.

(Strengths expressed in terms of the base)

Amcill-S (Parke, Davis). Powder 125, 250, and 500 mg and 1 g.

Omnipen-N (Wyeth), *Polycillin-N* (Bristol), *Principen/N* (Squibb). Powder 125, 250, and 500 mg and 1 and 2 g.

Penbritin-S (Ayerst). Powder 125, 250, and 500 mg and 1, 2, and 4 g.

Additional Trademarks.

Alpen-N (Lederle), *Totacillin-N* (Beecham).

HETACILLIN
[Versapen]

HETACILLIN POTASSIUM
[Versapen-K]

Hetacillin, a semisynthetic penicillin for oral use, has no demonstrated antibacterial activity itself, but is converted in the body to ampicillin and acetone. Therefore, hetacillin must be considered another form of ampicillin with the same antibacterial spectrum, indications, lack of effect on penicillinase-producing bacteria, precautions, and adverse reactions (see the Introduction and the evaluation on Ampicillin). It has not been shown to be superior to ampicillin in any respect.

Oral preparations are fairly stable in acid and, although food retards absorption, hetacillin is consistently absorbed from the gastrointestinal tract. The half-life for conversion of hetacillin to ampicillin at pH 7.1 is approximately 20 minutes.

ROUTE, USUAL DOSAGE, AND PREPARATIONS. The dosage recommendations of the manufacturer are low. Since the active moiety of hetacillin is ampicillin, the dosages used should be in the same range as those for ampicillin (see that evaluation) or larger, since 1 g of hetacillin yields less than 1 g of ampicillin.

(Strengths expressed in terms of ampicillin)

HETACILLIN:
Versapen (Bristol). Powder for suspension (pediatric) 112.5 mg/ml; powder for suspension 112.5 and 225 mg/5 ml.
HETACILLIN POTASSIUM:
Versapen-K (Bristol). Capsules 225 and 450 mg.

AMOXICILLIN TRIHYDRATE
[Amoxil, Larotid, Polymox, Trimox]

Amoxicillin is a semisynthetic penicillin used orally. Its in vitro antibacterial spectrum is essentially identical to that of ampicillin (see the Introduction and the evaluation on Ampicillin). Both amoxicillin and ampicillin are absorbed at the same rate, but identical doses of the two drugs result in higher peak serum levels of amoxicillin. There is evidence (Eichenwald and McCracken, 1978) that absorption of amoxicillin may be greater and less variable in children than that of ampicillin. Like ampicillin, amoxicillin is not effective against penicillinase-producing organisms. It usually is indicated for treating infections of the skin, soft tissues, or lower respiratory and urinary tracts caused by susceptible strains of nonpenicillinase-producing staphylococci, streptococci (including *S. faecalis*), *Streptococcus pneumoniae*, *Haemophilus influenzae*, *Escherichia coli*, and *Proteus mirabilis*. Since *Neisseria gonorrhoeae* is sensitive to amoxicillin, the drug also can be used to treat acute, uncomplicated anogenital and urethral gonorrheal infections in men and women. Like ampicillin, amoxicillin may be useful in treating typhoid fever resistant to chloramphenicol; there is some evidence to suggest that large doses (100 mg/kg/day) of amoxicillin may eliminate the postinfective carrier state, whereas approximately 10% of patients may become carriers following treatment with chloramphenicol. Amoxicillin does not penetrate into cerebrospinal or synovial fluid unless severe inflammation is present, and it should not be used to treat meningitis or joint infections.

This penicillin is readily absorbed following oral administration. It is resistant to destruction by gastric acid and absorption does not appear to be substantially affected by the presence of food in the stomach. Approximately 20% is bound to plasma protein. Serum levels after a single 500-mg dose are: 3 mcg/ml after one-half hour, 7 to 7.5 mcg/ml after one to two hours, and traces (0.2 mcg/ml) after eight hours. These levels vary somewhat, depending upon the dosage form used. After eight hours, about 60% of the dose is excreted almost entirely unchanged in the urine.

Amoxicillin appears to be well tolerated. The most common adverse reactions are mild nausea, vomiting, and diarrhea, which may have a lower incidence and severity at therapeutic dosage than that reported for ampicillin. Like other penicillins, amoxicillin may cause hypersensitivity reactions that occasionally can be severe. Rashes of varying intensity, fever, a serum sickness-like response, anemia, eosinophilia, thrombocytopenia, thrombocytopenic purpura, leukopenia, and agranulocytosis, all believed to be hypersensitivity phenomena, have been reported. These reactions usually subside when the drug is discontinued.

Life-threatening anaphylactic reactions occur much less frequently with use of orally administered penicillins than parenterally administered agents. Anaphylaxis that might endanger life has not been reported following use of amoxicillin.

This drug may cause a moderate increase in the level of serum glutamic oxaloacetic transaminase (SGOT), but the clinical significance of this finding has not been determined.

Overgrowth of nonsusceptible organisms may occur with prolonged use of amoxicillin; the organisms most commonly involved are *Enterobacter*, *Pseudomonas*, or *Candida*. If superinfections occur, amoxicillin should be discontinued and

appropriate corrective therapy instituted.

The effect of amoxicillin on the fetus has not been determined, but the penicillins in general appear to be nonteratogenic in man.

ROUTE, USUAL DOSAGE, AND PREPARATIONS. *Oral: Adults and children weighing more than 20 kg, 250 to 500 mg; less than 20 kg, 20 to 40 mg/kg of body weight. These amounts are administered daily in divided doses at eight-hour intervals.*
For the dosage used in gonorrhea, see the Introduction.

> Drug available generically: Capsules 250 and 500 mg; oral suspension and powder for suspension 125 and 250 mg/ml.
> *Amoxil* (Beecham), *Larotid* (Roche), *Polymox* (Bristol), *Trimox* (Squibb). Capsules 250 and 500 mg; drops for suspension (pediatric) 50 mg/ml; powder for suspension 125 and 250 mg/5 ml.
> **Additional Trademarks.**
> *Robamox* (Robins), *Sumox* (Reid-Provident), *Utimox* (Parke, Davis), *Wymox* (Wyeth).

CARBENICILLIN DISODIUM
[Geopen]

CARBENICILLIN INDANYL SODIUM
[Geocillin]

Carbenicillin disodium is a semisynthetic penicillin for parenteral use; it is not absorbed by the oral route. The indanyl sodium form is acid stable and is readily absorbed following oral administration; once absorbed, it is rapidly hydrolyzed to carbenicillin. It is indicated only for the treatment of urinary tract infections and is one of the few drugs with documented efficacy in chronic bacterial prostatitis. The antibacterial spectrum of carbenicillin is similar to that of ampicillin except that carbenicillin is active against *Pseudomonas aeruginosa*, some ampicillin-resistant strains of *Haemophilus influenzae*, and infections caused by susceptible *Proteus* (particularly indole-positive strains) and anaerobic bacteria; unlike other penicillins, both carbenicillin and ticarcillin are active against most strains of *Bacteroides fragilis*. Some pathogenic strains of microorganisms that have become more important clinically in recent years (eg, *Actinobacter* species, *Citrobacter*, *Serratia*) also are susceptible. Most species of *Klebsiella* are resistant, and some strains of *Pseudomonas* that were originally sensitive have developed resistance rapidly, although the majority of strains remain sensitive. Carbenicillin is inactivated by penicillinase-producing staphylococci.

The main clinical indications for carbenicillin are systemic infections caused by susceptible anaerobic bacteria, *Pseudomonas*, indole-positive *Proteus* (eg, *P. vulgaris*), *P. mirabilis*, and certain strains of *Escherichia coli*. It is commonly given with gentamicin, tobramycin, or amikacin for deep tissue or systemic infections (including pneumonia) caused by *Pseudomonas*, because these combinations have synergistic effects against many strains of *Pseudomonas* both in vitro and in vivo. However, since the aminoglycosides are inactivated by carbenicillin when the drugs are mixed together in solution, they should be given concomitantly but separately. Carbenicillin is effective in urinary tract infections caused by *Pseudomonas*, *E. coli*, *Enterobacter*, *Proteus* species, and enterococci (*S. faecalis*). Because carbenicillin may be more expensive than many of the other penicillins (particularly penicillin G), its use should be restricted to those situations in which it has a distinct advantage over less expensive antibacterial agents.

Peak blood levels usually are reached in one hour following intramuscular injection and 15 to 30 minutes after intravenous use. Peak serum levels of up to 500 mcg/ml can be achieved following the rapid (15 to 30 minutes) intravenous administration of 5 g. Serum levels of 10 to 25 mcg/ml usually are effective against most susceptible organisms; however, 100 mcg/ml or more is needed for infections caused by *Pseudo-*monas and *B. fragilis*. Carbenicillin is 50% bound to plasma proteins and is excreted unchanged by the kidney. Urinary levels of 1 to 5 mg/ml are achieved after intramuscular injection of 1 to 2 g.

Carbenicillin is relatively well tolerated, but hypersensitivity reactions (eg, pruritus, rash, urticaria, fever) occur. Serious and, rarely, fatal anaphylactic reactions may develop.

Large doses of carbenicillin may cause hematologic abnormalities similar to those observed with several other penicillins, including anemia, thrombocytopenia, leukopenia, neutropenia, and eosinophilia. Hypokalemia has been observed in patients receiving large doses of the drug. Several uremic patients given large amounts of carbenicillin disodium (24 g daily) developed hemorrhagic conditions associated with abnormal clotting and prothrombin times; the bleeding stopped when therapy was discontinued.

As with other penicillins, convulsions can occur if serum levels are excessive. Local pain at the site of injection and phlebitis following intravenous administration may occur. Nausea has been reported. Elevated serum transaminase (SGOT, SGPT) levels also have been seen.

Carbenicillin usually is contraindicated in patients with a history of allergic reactions to other penicillins, and it should be given cautiously to those with other known or suspected allergies. If superinfection with a resistant organism occurs, another antibacterial agent should be substituted.

Definitive information on the toxicity of carbenicillin during pregnancy is not available; however, the penicillins in general appear to be nonteratogenic in man.

Large doses of the disodium salt may contribute significantly to the sodium load in patients with impaired sodium excretion mechanisms (eg, renal, cardiac, or liver disease). Each gram of carbenicillin contains 5.5 to 6.5 mEq of sodium.

ROUTES, USUAL DOSAGE, AND PREPARATIONS. *Intramuscular*: For uncomplicated urinary tract infections, *adults*, 1 to 2 g every six hours; *children*, 50 to 200 mg/kg of body weight daily in divided doses every four to six hours.

Intravenous: The drug can be administered in divided doses or by continuous or intermittent infusion. For uncomplicated urinary tract infections, *adults and children*, the same dosage and time sequence as for the intramuscular route.

For serious urinary tract infections, *adults*, 200 mg/kg of body weight given by continuous or intermittent infusion.

For septicemia and severe systemic, respiratory, or soft tissue infections, *adults*, 300 to 500 mg/kg daily (20 g to a maximum of 40 g); *children*, 400 to 600 mg/kg daily. *Infants less than 7 days*, 200 mg/kg daily in divided doses every 12 hours; *over 7 days*, 300 to 400 mg/kg daily in divided doses every six to eight hours.

For infections other than urinary tract infections complicated by renal insufficiency (creatinine clearance less than 5 ml/min), *adults*, 2 g every 8 to 12 hours; during peritoneal dialysis, 2 g every six hours; during hemodialysis, 2 g every four hours. Clinical data are insufficient to recommend a dose for *children with impaired renal function*.

CARBENICILLIN DISODIUM:

Geopen (Roerig). Powder 1, 2, and 5 g containers (for intravenous and intramuscular use) and 10 and 30 g containers (for intravenous use only).

Oral: *Adults*, one to two tablets four times daily. Clinical data are insufficient to recommend a dose for *children*. (See also the manufacturer's literature.)

CARBENICILLIN INDANYL SODIUM:

Geocillin (Roerig). Tablets equivalent to 382 mg of carbenicillin.

TICARCILLIN DISODIUM
[Ticar]

Ticarcillin is a semisynthetic penicillin closely related to carbenicillin. Since it is not absorbed orally, it must be given either intravenously or intramuscularly. Its antibacterial spectrum, indications, and pattern of adverse reactions are the same as those of carbenicillin (see that evaluation) except that ticarcillin is more active in vitro against *Escherichia coli, Klebsiella, Enterobacter, Proteus*, and *Pseudomonas aeruginosa* (Eickhoff and Ehret, 1976). Some strains of *Pseudomonas* develop resistance fairly rapidly. Ticarcillin also is active in vitro against *Bacteroides fragilis* (Roy et al, 1977; Henderson et al, 1977), and recent clinical studies (Webb et al, 1978 and others) indicate that it is useful in anaerobic infections caused by this organism. It is inactivated by penicillinase-producing organisms.

Ticarcillin is 45% protein bound. Its half-life is approximately 70 minutes in normal individuals, and peak blood levels in excess of 60 mcg/ml can be achieved one-half to one hour following intramuscular doses of 2 g. Intravenous doses of 5 g produce blood levels greater than 300 mcg/ml in 15 minutes. As with other penicillins, ticarcillin is excreted by the kidney; urinary concentrations of 2 to 4 mg/ml are obtained in individuals with normal renal function following intramuscular injection of 1 to 2 g. Both serum half-life and urinary concentration are increased in patients with decreased renal function, and dosage adjustments may be required in the presence of severe renal impairment (see below).

Reproductive studies performed in mice and rats have shown no impairment of fertility or teratogenic effects. Studies in pregnant women currently are inadequate to evaluate the dangers to the human fetus, although the penicillins in general do not appear to have significant teratogenic effects in man. Nevertheless, ticarcillin should be given during pregnancy only if the potential benefit clearly justifies the potential risk to the fetus.

ROUTES, USUAL DOSAGE, AND PREPARATIONS. *Intramuscular*: For uncomplicated urinary tract infections, *adults*, 1 g every six hours; *children under 40 kg*, 50 to 100 mg/kg of body weight daily in divided doses every six to eight hours.

Intravenous (by infusion over a period of 10 to 20 minutes): For systemic infections, including those of the skin, soft tissue, and respiratory tract, or bacterial septicemia, *adults,* 200 to 300 mg/kg of body weight daily in divided doses every three, four, or six hours; *children under 40 kg (88 lb),* 200 to 300 mg/kg/day in divided doses every four or six hours (the daily dose should not exceed that used for adults); *infants over 7 days,* 200 to 300 mg/kg daily in divided doses every six to eight hours; *under 7 days,* 100 to 200 mg/kg daily in divided doses every 12 hours.

For uncomplicated urinary tract infections, *adults,* 1 g every six hours; *children over 40 kg,* 50 to 100 mg/kg/day in divided doses every six or eight hours. For urinary tract infections with complications, *adults and children,* 150 to 200 mg/kg/day in divided doses every four or eight hours.

Patients with renal insufficiency should be given ticarcillin according to the following schedule (see also the manufacturer's literature):

An initial loading dose of 3 g followed by:

Creatinine Clearance (ml/min)	Dosage
>60	3 g every four hours
30—60	2 g every four hours
10—30	2 g every eight hours
<10	2 g every 12 hours (or 1 g intramuscularly every 6 hours)
<10 (with hepatic dysfunction)	2 g every 24 hours (or 1 g intramuscularly every 12 hours)

Patients on peritoneal dialysis should be given 3 g every 12 hours. Patients on hemodialysis should be given 3 g after each dialysis.

Ticar (Beecham). Powder 1, 3, and 6 g (equivalent to base).

PENICILLINASE-RESISTANT PENICILLINS (Antistaphylococcal Penicillins)

METHICILLIN SODIUM
[Celbenin, Staphcillin]

Methicillin sodium is a water-soluble, penicillinase-resistant, semisynthetic salt of penicillin for parenteral use. It is effective against infections caused by nonpenicillinase-producing staphylococci, pneumococci, and beta-hemolytic streptococci; however, penicillin G is still the preferred agent for use against these organisms. Methicillin should be reserved for infections in which penicillin G-resistant staphylococci are suspected or identified. It is used most frequently for infections of the skin, soft tissues, and respiratory tract (eg, bacterial endocarditis, suppurative osteomyelitis, pseudomembranous enterocolitis) caused by penicillin G-resistant staphylococci. Levels adequate for the management of staphylococcal meningitis can be achieved when large doses (12 g or more daily) are used.

Staphylococci may develop resistance to methicillin by a nonpenicillinase mechanism. This drug also is a powerful inducer of penicillinase in inducible bacteria. In recent years, methicillin-resistant strains of *Staphylococcus aureus* have been increasing in frequency in the United States and now comprise 5% to 15% of isolates in many hospitals. Some strains of *S. aureus* in the hospital environment have *natural* resistance to methicillin. These strains also are usually resistant to other penicillinase-resistant penicillins and most cephalosporins or are susceptible only at relatively high concentrations, but they generally are susceptible to vancomycin.

Peak plasma levels produced by usual intramuscular doses occur in 30 minutes to one hour, and therapeutic concentrations last three to four hours. Approximately 40% of methicillin is bound to plasma proteins and 35% to 50% or more is rapidly excreted unaltered in the urine. The dose should be reduced in the presence of renal disease. Like penicillin G, methicillin is found in the bile and enters other body fluids slowly.

Methicillin is generally well tolerated; untoward effects are usually mild and most commonly consist of the allergic reactions typical of all penicillins (see the Introduction). A serious effect that has been reported rarely is reversible bone marrow depression manifested by anemia, neutropenia, or granulocytopenia.

Fatal superinfections with nonsusceptible organisms, especially gram-negative bacteria, have occurred. Other reactions include diarrhea, edema, vomiting, fever, chills, albuminuria, hematuria, azotemia, eosinophilia, leukocytosis, and hemolytic anemia.

Phlebitis has occurred after repeated intravenous injections. Following intramuscular injection, methicillin produces about the same degree or slightly more pain as injections of other penicillins. However, a smaller volume of methicillin is required to provide an equivalent dose than with oxacillin or nafcillin, which may be an advantage. If large doses of penicillin are needed, it may be impractical to use oxacillin or nafcillin because of the large volume that would have to be injected. Sterile abscesses have developed at the site of intramuscular injection of all penicillins, including methicillin.

Interstitial nephritis has been associated with use of methicillin. Nephrotoxicity is reported more frequently with use of this drug than other penicillins given parenterally. This may be a reflection of the greater use of methicillin than oxacillin or nafcillin. Cystitis, which can result in hematuria, is most likely to occur in patients with low urine output given large doses of methicillin (or related drugs) and is probably a direct irritant effect of the large concentration of the antibiotic in the urine on the bladder mucosa. Like other penicillins, methicillin is eliminated

slowly in very young infants because of their reduced renal function. Therefore, high blood concentrations following even a single dose persist for a longer period in infants than in older children or adults. Recent studies have indicated that most of an administered dose is eliminated within 12 hours in normal older children and adults.

A history of sensitization to other penicillins is usually a contraindication to the use of methicillin. In addition, this drug should be given cautiously to patients with other known allergies. Because bone marrow depression may occur, blood cell studies may be indicated periodically, especially during prolonged therapy.

The effect of this drug on the fetus is not known, but the penicillins in general do not appear to produce teratogenic effects in man.

ROUTES, USUAL DOSAGE, AND PREPARATIONS. Although methicillin is stable in dry form, it is very sensitive to heat when dissolved. Therefore, solutions for intramuscular administration must be used within 24 hours if stored at room temperature or within four days if refrigerated. Solutions for intravenous use must be used within eight hours. Moreover, since the drug is extremely unstable in acidic solutions and is destroyed in solutions containing certain basic antibiotics, solutions for parenteral use ideally should have an approximately neutral pH and no other drugs should be added. To help prevent destruction while in solution, methicillin can be administered from an auxiliary "piggy-back" infusion container rather than being dissolved in the intravenous fluid package. Dextrose solutions with a pH below 5.5 (many commercial solutions may have a pH as low as 3.5) particularly should not be used with methicillin. Staphcillin preparations contain a citrate buffer that will modify the pH of some unbuffered dextrose solutions sufficiently enough to allow safe storage of the mixed solution for up to eight hours. However, if the pH of a solution or buffering capacity of a methicillin preparation is not known, sodium chloride injection should be used as the diluent; this preparation also should be used promptly.

Intramuscular: *Adults*, 1 g in 1.5 ml of water for injection or sodium chloride injection every four to six hours (maximum, 1 g every three hours); *children*, 100 to 200 mg/kg of body weight daily in divided doses every six hours. *Infants over 7 days*, 75 to 100 mg/kg daily in divided doses every six to eight hours; *less than 7 days*, 50 to 75 mg/kg daily in divided doses every 8 to 12 hours. Since methicillin must be injected frequently, its use for long-term therapy may be inadvisable.

Intravenous (slow): *Adults*, 1 to 2 g in 50 ml of sodium choride injection every four to six hours infused at a rate of 10 ml/min. For serious infections (eg, severe bacterial endocarditis), 12 g or more daily. *Children*, 100 to 200 mg/kg of body weight daily in divided doses every six hours; *infants*, same as intramuscular dosage.

> **Celbenin** (Beecham). Powder (buffered) 1, 2, 4, and 6 g (900 mg methicillin base/g).
> **Staphcillin** (Bristol). Powder (buffered) 1, 4, and 6 g (900 mg methicillin base/g).

OXACILLIN SODIUM
[Bactocill, Prostaphlin]

Oxacillin sodium is a semisynthetic, penicillinase-resistant penicillin with actions and efficacy similar to those of methicillin and nafcillin (see the evaluations). Its antibacterial spectrum is similar to that of penicillin G (see the Introduction and the evaluation on Penicillin G); in addition, large doses are effective in the treatment of staphylococcal infections that are resistant to penicillin G.

Oxacillin is useful in staphylococcal infections of the skin and soft tissues, in respiratory and genitourinary tract infections caused by susceptible organisms, in suppurative osteomyelitis and pseudomembranous enterocolitis caused by penicillin G-resistant staphylococci, and in mixed infections caused by penicillin G-resistant staphylococci and pneumococci or beta-hemolytic streptococci.

This penicillin is more resistant to destruction by gastric acid than penicillin G or methicillin but is somewhat less resistant than penicillin V. Oxacillin also is less susceptible to rapid deterioration in acidic intravenous fluids than methicillin.

The presence of food in the stomach interferes with the absorption of orally administered oxacillin; when the stomach is empty, approximately 60% of a dose is absorbed, and doses of 500 mg to 1 g produce average peak plasma concentrations of 4 to 8 mcg/ml in one hour. Intramuscular doses of 500 mg to 1 g produce blood concentrations of 7 to 13 mcg/ml, but only a negligible amount remains after four to six hours.

Oxacillin also appears in bile, pleural and amniotic fluids, and human breast milk. Effective antibacterial levels are not achieved in the central nervous system unless the meninges are inflamed. Oxacillin has been effective in staphylococcal meningitis. It is excreted rapidly by the kidney, although not as rapidly as penicillin G.

Oxacillin is generally well tolerated. Untoward effects are similar to those produced by other penicillins (see the Introduction) and include rash, urticaria, and pruritus ani and vulvae. Nausea, vomiting, diarrhea, hairy tongue, fever, and eosinophilia have occurred occasionally. A few serious anaphylactic reactions have been reported, but there have been no deaths. Increased levels of serum glutamic oxaloacetic transaminase (SGOT) have been noted in a few patients, as has interstitial nephritis. Some infants receiving large doses have developed transient hematuria, albuminuria, and azotemia. Hepatic and renal function tests should be performed at regular intervals during prolonged therapy.

A history of allergic reactions to other penicillins is usually a contraindication to use of oxacillin, although cross reactions do not always occur. In addition, this drug should be administered cautiously to patients with other known or suspected allergies.

The effect of this drug on the fetus has not been determined, but the penicillins in general appear to be nonteratogenic in man.

ROUTES, USUAL DOSAGE, AND PREPARATIONS. *Oral*: Oxacillin should be taken at least one hour before or two hours after meals, and administration should be continued for at least five days. *Adults and children weighing more than 40 kg*, 500 mg to 1 g every four to six hours; *less than 40 kg*, 50 to 100 mg/kg of body weight daily in divided doses every six hours.

> (Strengths expressed in terms of the base)
> *Bactocill* (Beecham). Capsules 250 and 500 mg.
> *Prostaphlin* (Bristol). Capsules 250 and 500 mg; solution 250 mg/5 ml.

Intramuscular: Adults and children weighing more than 40 kg, 250 mg to 1 g every four to six hours (up to 8 g daily may be given for severe infections); *less than 40 kg*, 50 to 100 mg/kg of body weight daily (or more in severe infections) in equally divided doses every four to six hours. *Infants over 7 days*, 75 to 100 mg/kg daily in divided doses every six to eight hours; *under 7 days*, 50 to 75 mg/kg daily in divided doses every 8 to 12 hours.

Intravenous: When administered by intravenous infusion, the dose should be well diluted (20 mg/ml) and given over a period of approximately 10 to 15 minutes. Doses are comparable to those administered intramuscularly; for severe infections *in adults and older children*, 1 g or more may be given every three to four hours.

> (Strengths expressed in terms of the base)
> *Bactocill* (Beecham). Powder 500 mg and 1, 2, and 4 g.
> *Prostaphlin* (Bristol). Powder 250 and 500 mg and 1, 2, and 4 g.

CLOXACILLIN SODIUM
[Cloxapen, Tegopen]

This semisynthetic penicillin salt is used orally and is similar to oxacillin sodium in its in vitro activity against both penicillin G-resistant and penicillin G-sensitive staphylococci, streptococci, and pneumococci. It is used to treat staphylococcal infections of the skin, soft tissues, and respiratory tract; infections of the genitourinary tract or joint spaces; and suppurative osteomyelitis caused by penicillin G-resistant staphylococci. However, penicillin G is preferred for infections caused by sensitive organisms since equivalent doses are more effective than cloxacillin. Mixed infections caused by penicillin G-resistant staphylococci and pneumococci or beta-hemolytic streptococci respond to cloxacillin.

Absorption of cloxacillin from the gastrointestinal tract is rapid but variable; doses may be absorbed inadequately, eg, food in the stomach or small intestine reduces absorption and decreases the ultimate plasma level obtainable from a given dose. Although cloxacillin is more resistant to destruction by gastric acid than many other penicillins, it is degraded to some extent in the stomach.

At equivalent oral doses, somewhat higher plasma levels have been reported with cloxacillin than with either oxacillin or nafcillin. Peak serum levels occur approximately one hour after administration of the capsule form and somewhat sooner after use of the oral solution. Effective plasma levels can be maintained for four to six hours after a single dose.

Cloxacillin is distributed throughout the body, but the highest concentrations appear in the kidney and liver. Plasma protein binding is high (90% to 94%). Between 30% and 45% of a single dose is excreted in the urine, and significant amounts are excreted in the bile.

This penicillin is generally well tolerated. Adverse reactions are essentially the same as those observed with other penicillins (see the Introduction). It may produce allergic reactions (rash, urticaria), epigastric fullness or abdominal discomfort, diarrhea, nausea, and vomiting. A few cases of eosinophilia, mild leukopenia, and elevated serum glutamic oxaloacetic transaminase (SGOT) levels have been reported. Cloxacillin has little effect on the liver, kidney, or cell-forming elements of bone marrow.

Superinfections with gram-negative organisms have occurred occasionally. If they are severe, therapy must be discontinued.

Cloxacillin generally is contraindicated in patients with a history of sensitivity to any penicillin, and it should be used cautiously in patients with other known allergies.

The effect of this drug on the fetus has not been determined, but the penicillins in general appear to be nonteratogenic in man.

ROUTE, USUAL DOSAGE, AND PREPARATIONS. *Oral*: *Adults and children weighing 20 kg or more*, 500 mg to 1 g every four to six hours given one hour before or two hours after meals (250 mg every six hours is recommended by the manufacturer for mild to moderate respiratory tract infections or localized skin and soft tissue infections). *Children less than 20 kg*, 50 to 100 mg/kg of body weight daily in four equal doses every six hours. The larger dose is reserved for severe infections; if this does not control the infection, it is advisable to substitute a penicillinase-resistant penicillin that can be given parenterally (eg, methicillin).

(Strengths expressed in terms of the base)
Cloxapen (Beecham). Capsules 250 and 500 mg.
Tegopen (Bristol). Capsules 250 and 500 mg; powder for solution 125 mg/5 ml.

DICLOXACILLIN SODIUM
[Dycill, Dynapen]

This semisynthetic, penicillinase-resistant penicillin is claimed to produce higher blood levels more rapidly than the other penicillins, but there is little definitive evidence that this offers a practical clinical advantage. Dicloxacillin is closely related to cloxacillin in its chemistry, indications, adverse reactions, serum binding, onset and duration of action, and bacterial spectrum (see the Introduction and the evaluation on Cloxacillin Sodium). It is not clinically superior to oxacillin, cloxacillin, or any of the other semisynthetic penicillins.

Experience with this drug in newborn infants is limited; therefore, dicloxacillin should not be used in neonates until additional information becomes available. The effect of this drug on the fetus has not been determined, but the penicillins in general appear to be nonteratogenic in man.

ROUTE, USUAL DOSAGE, AND PREPARATIONS. *Oral*: The following doses are given one hour before or two hours after meals. *Adults and children weighing 40 kg or more*, 250 mg to 1 g every four to six hours; *less than 40 kg*, 25 to 100 mg/kg of body weight daily in four equal doses every six hours. The larger dose is for severe infections. For minor infections caused by susceptible organisms, *adults and children weighing 40 kg or more*, 125 to 250 mg every four to six hours; *less than 40 kg*, 25 to 50 mg/kg daily in four equal doses.

(Strengths expressed in terms of the base)
Dycill (Beecham). Capsules 250 and 500 mg.
Dynapen (Bristol). Capsules 125 and 250 mg; powder for suspension 62.5 mg/5 ml.

NAFCILLIN SODIUM
[Nafcil, Unipen]

This semisynthetic penicillin is effective against beta-hemolytic streptococci and pneumococci, and is the most potent of the penicillinase-resistant penicillins against staphylococci (including penicillin G-resistant strains). It probably is the penicillin of choice for treating life-threatening staphylococcal infections. It also has been used in mixed infections caused by penicillin G-resistant staphylococci with streptococci or pneumococci and as initial therapy for serious staphylococcal infections in which penicillin G resistance is suspected but not yet verified by in vitro tests.

Nafcillin is effective in infections of the respiratory tract, soft tissues, and skin caused by susceptible organisms and in suppurative osteomyelitis. It also has been of some benefit in urinary tract infections.

Nafcillin is used both orally and parenterally. It is stable in gastric acid, but is absorbed more slowly after oral administration than some of the other penicillins; therefore, the oral route should be used only for mild infections. The minimal concentration necessary for in vitro activity against staphylococci ranges from 0.2 to 2 mcg/ml. After oral administration of 500 mg to 1 g, a maximal blood concentration of 1.5 to 5 mcg/ml is attained in one hour. After intramuscular administration of 500 mg, the average maximal blood level is 5 to 8 mcg/ml in one to two hours, and some of the drug persists for four to six hours.

A high concentration of nafcillin is attained in the bile, which represents the major route of excretion for this drug. A portion is reabsorbed from the gastrointestinal tract, and a small amount is found in synovial fluid after parenteral administration. Only about 10% is excreted in the urine; therefore, urinary levels are never very great. There is some evidence that nafcillin penetrates into the cerebrospinal fluid better than methicillin.

Nafcillin is generally well tolerated. Allergic reactions, principally rash, occur most commonly (see the Introduction). Nausea and diarrhea are noted occasionally. Nafcillin may cause pain and tissue irritation when given intramuscularly, and the total volume injected is greater than for methicillin. An increase in the level of serum glutamic oxaloacetic transaminase (SGOT) occasionally is observed after intramuscular injection; however, since this reaction subsides rapidly after therapy is discontinued, it may be caused by local tissue injury. The incidence of nephrotoxicity is low when compared to methicillin, a possible advantage over the latter drug. Thrombophlebitis has been reported in a few patients after intravenous administration of nafcillin; this effect is presumably due to vessel injury.

Since cross sensitivity with other penicillins exists, nafcillin is usually contraindicated in those with a history of sensitivity to any penicillin, and it must be administered cautiously to patients with other known or suspected allergies.

ROUTES, USUAL DOSAGE, AND PREPARATIONS. *Oral: Adults,* 250 mg to 1 g every four to six hours, preferably two hours before meals; *children,* 50 to 100 mg/kg of body weight daily in four divided doses every six hours.

> *Unipen* (Wyeth). Capsules 250 mg; powder for solution 250 mg/5 ml; tablets 500 mg (strengths expressed in terms of the base).

Intramuscular: Adults, 500 mg every four to six hours; *children,* 150 mg/kg of body weight daily in two divided doses every six hours.

Intravenous: Adults, 500 mg to 1 g in 15 to 30 ml of water for injection or sodium chloride injection infused over a 10-minute period every four hours or dissolved in 150 ml of sodium choride injection and given by slow intravenous drip. Up to 8 g daily can be given for serious infections. *Children,* 150 mg/kg of body weight daily in four divided doses every six hours.

> (Strengths expressed in terms of the base)
> *Nafcil* (Bristol). Powder (buffered) 500 mg and 1, 2, and 4 g.
> *Unipen* (Wyeth). Powder (buffered) 500 mg and 1 and 2 g.

Selected References

Altman LC, Tompkins LS: Toxic and allergic manifestations of antimicrobials. *Postgrad Med* 64:157-167, (Sept)v1978.

Appel GB, Neu HC: Antimicrobial agents in patients with renal disease. *Med Times* 105:109-129, (Sept) 1977.

Bierman CW, VanArsdel PP Jr: Penicillin allergy in children: Role of immunological tests in its diagnosis. *J Allergy Clin Immunol* 43:267-272, 1969.

Cama LD, Chistensen BG: Structure-activity relationships of "non-classical" beta-lactam antibiotics, in Clarke FH (ed): *Annual Reports in Medicinal Chemistry.* New York, Academic Press, 1978, vol 13, 149-158.

Downham TF II, et al: Systemic toxic reactions to procaine penicillin G. *Sex Transmit Dis* 5:4-9, 1978.

Eichenwald HF, McCracken GH Jr: Antimicrobial therapy in infants and children. Part I. Review of antimicrobial agents. *J Pediatr* 93:337-356, 1978.

Eickhoff TC, Ehret JM: Comparative activity in vitro of ticarcillin BL-P1654, and carbenicillin. *Antimicrob Agents Chemother* 10:241-244, 1976.

Finke SR, et al: Results of comparative skin tests with penicilloyl-polylysine and penicillin in patients with penicillin allergy. *Am J Med* 38:71-82, 1965.

Greenburg RN: Syphilis: Review and overview. *Clin Med* 85:14-22, (July) 1978.

Grieco MH, Rosenzweig D: Mechanisms and management of penicillin allergy. *Med Times* 105:1d-9d, (Sept) 1977.

Hagan DG: Comprehensive review of gonorrhea. *Clin Med* 85:27-37, (July) 1978.

Henderson DK, et al: Comparative susceptibility of anaerobic bacteria to ticarcillin, cefoxitin, metronidazole, and related antimicrobial agents. *Antimicrob Agents Chemother* 11:679-682, 1977.

Jabbar A, et al: Use of oral carbenicillin in urinary tract infection. *Curr Ther Res* 23:22-26, 1978.

Lambert HP: Use of antibiotics: Meningitis. *Br Med J* 2:259-261, 1978.

Levine BB, Redmond AP: Minor haptenic determinant-specific reagins of penicillin hypersensitivity in man. *Int Arch Allergy Appl Immunol* 35:445-455, 1969.

McCracken GH Jr, Eichenwald HF: Antimicrobial therapy in infants and children. Part II. Therapy of infectious conditions. *J Pediatr* 93:357-377, 1978.

Nelson JD: *Pocketbook of Pediatric Antimicrobial Therapy*, ed 2. Dallas, Clarke and Courts, Inc, 1977-1978.

Nolan CM, White PC Jr: Treatment of typhoid carriers with amoxicillin: Correlates of successful therapy. *JAMA* 239:2352-2354, 1978.

Petersdorf RG: Antimicrobial prophylaxis of bacterial endocarditis: Prudent caution or bacterial overkill? *Am J Med* 65:220-223, 1978.

Pratt WB: *Chemotherapy of Infection*. New York, Oxford University Press, 1977, 22-84.

Roy I, et al: In vitro activity of ticarcillin against anaerobic bacteria compared with that of carbenicillin and penicillin. *Antimicrob Agents Chemother* 11:258-261, 1977.

Van Dellen RG, Gleich GJ: Penicillin skin tests as predictive and diagnostic aids in penicillin allergy. *Med Clin North Am* 54:997-1007, 1970.

Warrington RJ, et al: Diagnosis of penicillin allergy by skin testing: The Manitoba experience. *Can Med Assoc J* 118:787-791, 1978.

Webb D, et al: Ticarcillin disodium in aerobic infections. *Arch Intern Med* 138:1618-1620, 1978.

The beta-lactam antibiotics include the penicillins, cephalosporins, and cephamycins. Each of these families of compounds contains a beta-lactam ring. The penicillins and cephalosporins differ primarily in that the penicillins are derivatives of 6-aminopenicillanic acid (6-APA), whereas the cephalosporins are characterized by substituent groups added to 7-aminocephalosporanic acid (7-ACA). The 7-ACA nucleus was derived initially from cephalosporin C, a fermentation product of *Cephalosporium acremonium*. The cephamycins also are related chemically to cephalosporin C (cefoxitin is actually derived from cephamycin C, which is elaborated by *Streptomyces lactamdurans*) but possess a 7-alpha-methoxy group that imparts considerable resistance to all beta lactamases. In addition to being closely related chemically, the three groups of drugs have similar pharmacologic properties and mechanisms of action: They interfere with a terminal step in bacterial wall synthesis and, perhaps, increase cell wall breakdown (there is evidence that

penicillin may have this latter action), thereby exerting a bactericidal effect on susceptible organisms.

Antibacterial Spectrum: The cephalosporins have similar spectra that encompass both gram-positive and gram-negative bacteria, but there is considerable variation among these agents; the newer cephalosporins have greater activity against gram-negative enteric bacilli. Cephalosporins are active in vitro against most staphylococci, including both penicillin-sensitive and penicillinase-producing *Staphylococcus aureus*; most streptococci, including group A beta-hemolytic streptococci and *Streptococcus pneumoniae*; *Clostridium* species; *Escherichia coli*; nonhospital-acquired *Klebsiella*; *Proteus mirabilis*; *Neisseria gonorrhoeae*; and some species of *Salmonella* and *Shigella*. Most of these drugs are active against *Treponema pallidum*. The susceptibility of *Haemophilus influenzae* and *Bacteroides* species is quite variable; generally, cephalosporins are less active against *H. influenzae* than ampicillin or penicillin G.

They are ineffective against *Pseudomonas*, many species of indole-positive *Proteus* (eg, *P. morganii*, *P. rettgeri*, *P. vulgaris*), *Serratia marcescens*, *Bordetella*, *Bacteroides fragilis*, and many strains of hospital-acquired *Klebsiella*. Most species of enterococci (eg, *Streptococcus faecalis*) and *Enterobacter* are highly resistant.

The cephamycins, represented by cefoxitin [Mefoxin], have the same spectrum as the cephalosporins but, because of increased resistance to cephalosporinases, they also are active against *P. morganii*, *P. vulgaris*, *P. rettgeri*, *Serratia* species, *Bacteroides* species (including *B. fragilis*), and many strains of *E. coli* and *Klebsiella* that have become resistant to the cephalosporins.

Indications: Although the cephalosporins have a broad antibacterial spectrum (somewhat greater than many of the penicillins) and can be administered with relative safety (except for a few circumstances discussed below), they should not be regarded as antibiotics of first choice for treatment of presumed infections. They have been shown to reduce the incidence of surgical wound infections after a wide variety of surgical procedures, but their very active promotion and wide therapeutic usage is out of proportion to their importance in anti-infective therapy. Cephalosporins are very effective in reducing surgical wound infections *if used properly*. Such usage may constitute the greatest value of this group of drugs. The prophylactic use of antibiotics in surgery does not necessarily create a problem per se. The problem arises when antibiotics are misused (eg, not given preoperatively, continued for too long a period postoperatively, used for trivial infections).

Penicillin G is still preferred to treat infections caused by pneumococci, group A or viridans streptococci, and non-penicillinase-producing staphylococci, because it is usually effective and is less expensive than the cephalosporins. Ampicillin is the drug of choice for enterococcal urinary tract infections and infections caused by sensitive strains of *H. influenzae*, *E. coli*, *Salmonella*, or *Shigella*; however, cephalosporins generally are resistant to beta lactamases that inactivate ampicillin, which occasionally makes them superior to that drug. The cephalosporins may be used as primary drugs when treating nonhospital-acquired *Klebsiella* infections (especially those caused by *K. pneumoniae*). Their spectrum is not broad enough to allow their use empirically as the sole antibiotic in suspected gram-negative sepsis, but they may be administered with an aminoglycoside to treat serious conditions presumed to be caused by gram-negative organisms (eg, severe intra-abdominal infections) before the results of bacteriologic studies are obtained. Because of chemical incompatibility, these two classes of drugs should never be mixed in the same container and should be given at different sites. Also, concomitant use of an aminoglycoside (eg, gentamicin) and a cephalosporin appears to increase the risk of nephrotoxicity; therefore, combined therapy should be avoided or undertaken with great caution in patients who are likely to have reduced renal function (eg, the elderly). Once the infecting organism has been identified, the least expensive and least toxic anti-infective agent likely to be effective should be given.

There is laboratory and clinical evidence that cross allergenicity exists between the cephalosporins and penicillins. Cross sensitivity has been demonstrated by both serum and skin tests; however, most patients assumed to be allergic to penicillin usually can tolerate a cephalosporin. The exact incidence of cross reactivity is not known. It has been estimated that 5% to 30% of patients who are hypersensitive to penicillin will experience an allergic reaction to a cephalosporin, with the true incidence probably falling between 5% and 10% (Pratt, 1977); the risk is greatly influenced by the severity of the prior reaction to penicillin. In children, the incidence of clinical cross reactivity is less than 5%. Therefore, although cross allergenicity with the penicillins is possible, the cephalosporins still are effective substitutes for the latter drugs in patients with an equivocal history of penicillin allergy or a history of mild reactions, such as transient morbilliform rash, in whom less expensive and relatively nontoxic alternative antibiotics (eg, erythromycin) are not appropriate or are contraindicated. Cephalosporins should *not* be used in individuals with immediate hypersensitivity reactions to the penicillins (eg, urticaria, angioedema, bronchospasm, anaphylaxis). Since there is risk involved whenever a cephalosporin is given to a patient who is sensitive to penicillin, the physician must be fully prepared to treat any hypersensitivity reactions that occur.

As alternative antibacterial drugs, the cephalosporins may be used to treat susceptible infections of the respiratory and urinary tracts, skin, soft tissues, bone, and joints. Selected cases of septicemia, peritonitis, septic abortion, and bacterial endocarditis caused by sensitive organisms also have responded to these drugs, although bacterial endocarditis usually does not respond as favorably to the cephalosporins as to penicillin, even with concurrent use of streptomycin. Despite the in vitro susceptibility of *N. gonorrhoeae* to several cephalosporins and some therapeutic action of these drugs against *T. pallidum*, the clinical usefulness of the cephalosporins in gonorrhea and syphilis has been limited. Cefoxitin may be considered an alternative drug for the treatment of gonorrhea in pregnant women who are allergic to penicillin. It also may be especially suitable for treating intra-abdominal or pelvic infections caused by *B. fragilis*.

Pharmacology: The cephalosporins are administered by various routes. Those resistant to acid hydrolysis (cephalexin [Keflex], cephaloglycin [Kafocin], cefadroxil [Duricef], and cefaclor [Ceclor]) can be given orally. Absorption from the gut is variable, but therapeutic blood levels usually can be attained with all agents except cephaloglycin, which has limited absorption and cannot be used to treat systemic infections. Cephalosporins that are more susceptible to gastric acid destruction or are not absorbed well (cephalothin [Keflin], cephaloridine [Loridine], cephapirin [Cefadyl], cephacetrile [Celospor], cefazolin [Ancef, Kefzol], and cefamandole [Mandol]) must be adminis-

tered parenterally. Cefoxitin is given only parenterally and is considered with this group of cephalosporins. Cephradine [Anspor, Velosef] has physical characteristics (eg, resistance to gastric acid secretion) that permit it to be administered either orally or parenterally.

Once absorbed, the cephalosporins are bound to protein to varying degrees. Although the unbound drug is the active portion, protein binding is not a major factor affecting therapeutic action, since the degree of protein binding generally is low (a range of 20% to 90%, with most less than 70%, except for cefazolin, which is greater than 90%).

The cephalosporins penetrate most tissues well with two notable exceptions. It is questionable whether therapeutic concentrations can be attained easily in the eye (large doses of cephalothin and cephaloridine produce therapeutic levels) and, unlike the penicillins, the cephalosporins are unpredictable in the manner in which they cross the blood-brain barrier; penetration into cerebrospinal fluid is poor even when the meninges are inflamed. The cephalosporins, therefore, never should be considered an adequate substitute for the penicillins in the treatment of meningitis. Chloramphenicol is probably the drug of choice in patients with life-threatening allergy to penicillin who develop meningitis, especially that caused by *H. influenzae, S. pneumoniae,* or *N. meningitidis*.

Most cephalosporins are excreted unchanged by both glomerular filtration and proximal tubular secretion. Therefore, like the penicillins, the concurrent administration of probenecid delays the excretion of the cephalosporins and prolongs serum half-life. Similarly, renal impairment may delay excretion of these antibiotics. Dosage adjustments may be necessary in individuals with impaired renal function but need not be as precise as those required for the aminoglycosides, since the threat of serious toxicity is not as great.

Some cephalosporins (eg, cephalothin, which is appreciably metabolized to a desacetyl form) are metabolized in the body. However, these compounds and their metabolites are primarily excreted in the urine. Consequently, high biliary levels are not easily achieved for most drugs in this class (exceptions are cefazolin and cefamandole), and they are minimally excreted by the gastrointestinal tract.

Resistance: Beta lactamases capable of hydrolyzing penicillins (penicillinases) or cephalosporins (cephalosporinases) into microbiologically inactive products are elaborated by many bacteria resistant to these antibiotics. Although the susceptibility of individual penicillins to the penicillinases varies widely, these enzymes are more specific for the penicillins than for the cephalosporins. Conversely, the beta lactamases that hydrolyze cephalosporins are generally specific for cephalosporins. As with the penicillins, the affinity of an enzyme for a particular cephalosporin varies considerably. The beta lactamases elaborated by gram-positive bacteria (eg, staphylococcal strains) are usually penicillinases, whereas those produced by gram-negative organisms (eg, *Enterobacter* species, *K. pneumoniae*) are most frequently cephalosporinases. Some microorganisms (eg, *P. aeruginosa*) include strains that produce penicillin-specific beta lactamases, while other strains form enzymes that attack the cephalosporins.

Bacterial cross resistance between cephalosporins and other antibacterial agents has not been clearly demonstrated, except that strains of *S. aureus* and *S. albus* that are naturally resistant to methicillin are generally resistant to the cephalosporins also; their use to treat infections caused by methicillin-resistant staphylococci has failed in most cases.

General Comparative Evaluations: There are currently 11 cephalosporins and one cephamycin marketed in the United States. Other cephalosporins are entering final stages of clinical investigation. In Europe, 17 or 18 compounds are available. Yet the cephalosporins are recognized as therapeutic drugs of first choice only in the treatment of nonhospital-acquired *Klebsiella* infections and, as alternatives to the penicillins, the cephalosporins can be valuable despite the substantial danger of cross sensitization in patients

allergic to the penicillins. There appears to be little doubt, therefore, that this group of anti-infective drugs is overpromoted and overused. It would seem wise for physicians to familiarize themselves with one orally administered and one parenterally administered cephalosporin and use these two agents when appropriate and with proper precautions to the exclusion of all other drugs in this class. The following information may be useful in formulating guidelines:

Cephalothin, cephapirin, cephacetrile, cefazolin, and cefamandole are all similar and there appears to be little basis for choosing one over the other. Cefamandole may be more effective against certain cephalosporinase-producing gram-negative organisms and is active against some ampicillin-resistant strains of *H. influenzae*. Cefazolin and cefamandole may be less painful when injected intramuscularly than the other parenterally administered drugs, especially cephalothin.

Cephaloridine is nephrotoxic when given in large doses and has been largely replaced by safer agents.

The orally administered compounds, cephalexin, cefadroxil, cefaclor, and cephradine, are similar in their actions, toxicity, and rate of absorption. However, cefaclor is the only orally administered cephalosporin that is effective both in vitro and clinically against beta-lactamase negative and positive *H. influenzae*. Because cephaloglycin is poorly absorbed and cannot be used to treat systemic infections, it has been rendered obsolete.

Cephradine has the possible advantage of being able to be administered both orally and parenterally.

Adverse Reactions and Precautions: Rash, urticaria, fever, and eosinophilia have been associated with use of the cephalosporins. The incidence of these mild allergic reactions is highest in patients who are hypersensitive to the penicillins. Severe hypersensitivity reactions, including anaphylaxis, have been reported infrequently. Rarely, fatal anaphylaxis has resulted from parenteral injection of a cephalosporin.

Leukopenia, thrombocytopenia, and neutropenia have been observed following administration of the cephalosporins, and both direct and indirect positive Coombs' tests have been noted. Hemolytic anemia has occurred after the use of cephalothin, but it is not common or severe.

Gastrointestinal symptoms include anorexia, nausea, vomiting, and diarrhea. Diarrhea may be the most common and often the most severe untoward effect noted, and it can be severe enough to warrant discontinuing therapy. It occurs least often with administration of cephalexin.

The intramuscular injection of cephalothin frequently causes pain, which is not commonly observed following injection of the other cephalosporins. Intravenous administration of these drugs may cause thrombophlebitis. Phlebitis usually can be prevented by alternating veins or slowly injecting a solution diluted with sodium chloride or dextrose injection. Intrathecal injection is not recommended because data in animals and limited clinical observations indicate that administration by this route may be toxic to the nervous system; a variety of effects, including nystagmus, hallucinations, and convulsions, have been observed.

The most serious adverse effect produced by cephaloridine is renal tubular necrosis. This reaction has been shown to be dose-dependent and may occur most commonly in dehydrated individuals with low cardiac output and in those receiving diuretics concomitantly. Reversible renal injury also has been reported following administration of cephalothin, but the incidence is much lower than with cephaloridine. Possible modification of kidney function, usually manifested as a transient increase in blood urea nitrogen levels, has been attributed to cefamandole, cephapirin, cefazolin, and cephacetrile, but definitive evidence of significant nephrotoxicity is lacking. There may be synergistic nephrotoxicity when a cephalosporin and an aminoglycoside are administered concomitantly. This reaction is more likely to occur in the elderly and others with decreased renal function. Some signs of hepatic dysfunction (transient increases in blood SGOT, SGPT, and alkaline phosphatase levels) also have been noted following administration of the cephalosporins.

Some patients receiving cephalosporin therapy may show a false-positive reaction for glucose in the urine when tested with Benedict's or Fehling's solution or Clinitest tablets. The drugs apparently do not interfere with results obtained with enzyme-based tests such as Tes-Tape or Clinistix.

Overgrowth of resistant organisms, notably *Pseudomonas*, often occurs at multiple sites after long-term use of the cephalosporins. Candidosis also may occur, usually in the mouth, when orally administered cephalosporins are given for prolonged periods. Therefore, patients receiving the cephalosporins should be watched very closely for signs of superinfection, particularly if therapy is prolonged or if the patient is severely ill and being exposed to invasive devices such as urethral catheters and endotracheal tubes.

The risk to the fetus when the cephalosporins are administered to pregnant women has not been fully assessed but, as with the penicillins, there is no evidence of teratogenicity in man. Although evaluations of the safety of cephalosporins in infants (particularly premature infants and those under 1 month of age) are limited, the incidence and severity of reactions appear to be similar to those noted with the penicillins (see the evaluations). There is presently no primary indication for the use of any cephalosporin in newborn infants.

PARENTERALLY ADMINISTERED CEPHALOSPORINS

CEPHALOTHIN SODIUM
[Keflin]

Cephalothin was the first cephalosporin derivative marketed and has the same antibacterial spectrum as the other cephalosporins (see the Introduction). It should be restricted to the treatment of serious infections caused by susceptible organisms (eg, *Klebsiella pneumoniae*) or to use in patients who are hypersensitive to the penicillins. It may be given with an aminoglycoside for severe intra-abdominal infections before the results of culture studies are known, but there is increased danger of nephrotoxicity in the elderly and others with impaired renal function. Cephalothin is highly resistant to penicillinase and, therefore, is useful against penicillinase-producing bacteria. It has been effective in bacteremias and infections of the respiratory tract, skin, soft tissues, bones, joints, and cardiovascular system. Cephalothin also is suitable for treating urinary tract infections, since a high concentration of active drug is excreted in the urine. This drug may be of value in treating peritonitis and septic abortion, although other drugs (eg, clindamycin) are preferred. Cephalothin is not very active against *B. fragilis* or non-group A streptococci in the gut. Its activity against clostridia, anaerobic staphylococci, and fusobacteria is reasonably good. For the use of cephalothin in the eye, see Chapter 24, Ocular Anti-infective and Anti-inflammatory Agents.

This drug is administered either intravenously or intramuscularly, but the severe pain occurring after intramuscular injection markedly restricts use of this route. Occasionally local induration or, rarely, sterile abscess or necrosis and slough may follow intramuscular administration. In the rare instances when use of the intramuscular route is deemed essential, injections must be made deep into the muscle. Local thrombophlebitis may occur after intravenous administration. Intrathecal use is not recommended.

Approximately 65% of cephalothin is bound to protein in the blood. Between 60% and 90% of a single dose is excreted by the renal tubules, largely unchanged; excretion is delayed by probenecid. Peak urinary concentrations may reach several hundred micrograms per milliliter following usual doses, and the serum half-life is approximately 30 minutes. In adults with normal renal function, 60% of the dose is excreted in six hours; therefore, the drug must be administered every four to six hours to maintain effective plasma concentrations. Although cephalothin has been reported to cause renal tubular necrosis, the danger of nephrotoxicity usually is minimal. It is well tolerated and can be used in patients with kidney disease if adjustments in dosage are made. Many physicians believe that the nephrotoxic potential is greater in patients with pre-existing renal disease.

Adverse effects are similar to those produced by the penicillins and other cephalosporins and include rash, urticaria, fever, and eosinophilia. A direct positive Coombs' test is sometimes observed, particularly in azotemic patients, but true hemolytic anemia has occurred rarely. Other reactions seen only rarely include anaphylactic shock, neutropenia, and leukopenia. Elevated SGOT levels have been noted. Blood urea nitrogen (BUN) levels may increase but frequently return to normal during therapy. Overgrowth of resistant organisms has been observed; various organisms, including *Pseudomonas*, can replace pre-existing pathogens in the urinary tract.

Hematologic studies and hepatic and renal function tests should be performed periodically during prolonged therapy. Dosage should be reduced in patients with impaired renal function to avoid excessive accumulation of the drug (see below).

Because cerebrospinal fluid levels are unpredictable, even in the presence of infection, cephalothin should never be used to treat meningitis. Although this antibiotic crosses the placenta, results of limited trials indicate that it may be safe for use during pregnancy and in both premature and full-term infants; however, there are few, if any, indications for its use in these patients.

ROUTES, USUAL DOSAGE, AND PREPARATIONS. *Intravenous*: *Adults*, 4 to 12 g daily, dissolved in sodium chloride or dextrose injection, is administered slowly (over a period of up to 60 minutes) in divided doses. *Infants and children*, 80 to 160 mg/kg of body weight daily in divided doses.

Intramuscular (deep): *Adults*, 500 mg to 1 g four to six times daily (up to 2 g every four hours to a total of 12 g daily may be given for serious infections); *infants and children*, 80 to 160 mg/kg of body weight daily in divided doses.

The following guidelines may be used for patients with impaired renal function receiving cephalothin by either parenteral route (after a loading dose of 1 to 2 g): Mild impairment (creatinine clearance, 50 to 80 ml/min), up to 2 g every six hours; moderate impairment (creatinine clearance, 25 to 50 ml/min), up to 1.5 g every six hours; severe impairment (creatinine clearance, 10 to 25 ml/min), up to 1 g every six hours; very severe impairment (creatinine clearance, 2 to 10 ml/min), up to 0.5 g every six hours; essentially no function (creatinine clearance less than 2 ml/min), up to 0.5 g every eight hours when dialysis is not being performed.

Keflin (Lilly). Powder (equivalent to base) 1, 2, and 4 g.

CEPHALORIDINE
[Loridine]

The in vitro spectrum and clinical applications of cephaloridine are similar to those of the other cephalosporins (see the Introduction and the evaluation on Cephalothin). It can be administered either intramuscularly or intravenously. Because of the potential nephrotoxicity of cephaloridine, the desirability of determining the causative organism and its sensitivity to this agent before initiating therapy cannot be overemphasized.

Although cephaloridine has been used to treat infections caused by gram-positive staphylococci, it is less resistant to staphylococcal penicillinase than cephalothin, and, therefore, is less effective against penicillinase-producing organisms and should not be used to treat infections caused by penicillinase-positive strains of *S. aureus*. This agent also is readily degraded by cephalosporinases produced by some gram-negative bacteria (eg, *Enterobacter, Pseudomonas*). Cephaloridine should be reserved for use in infections caused by susceptible gram-negative bacilli when penicillin cannot be tolerated. However, even under these circumstances, other parenterally administered cephalosporins and cefoxitin are preferred. The drug should be used with caution in patients hypersensitive to penicillin. Except for cefoxitin or, possibly, cefamandole, cephaloridine appears to be more active than the other cephalosporins against anaerobic bacteria and penetrates into the cerebrospinal fluid more consistently. However, accumulation in cerebrospinal fluid is poor unless the meninges are inflamed; therefore, this drug should never be used to treat meningitis. For the use of cephaloridine in the eye, see Chapter 24, Ocular Anti-infective and Anti-inflammatory Agents.

Injection of cephaloridine is less painful than that of cephalothin; when similar doses of the two drugs are administered, cephaloridine produces higher blood levels because its half-life in patients with normal renal function (approximately 1.5 hours) is about three times that of cephalothin. The rate of excretion is retarded to a limited extent by probenecid. Approximately 20% of cephaloridine is bound to protein in the blood.

Doses of cephaloridine larger than 4 g daily may cause acute renal tubular necrosis, resulting in fatal uremia; therefore, assessment of renal function before and during treatment is essential. Cephaloridine should not be used with other potentially nephrotoxic drugs such as the aminoglycoside antibiotics (eg, kanamycin, gentamicin). This precaution is particularly important in elderly patients or others with reduced renal function. Also, it should not be given with intravenous boluses of loop diuretics, such as furosemide, because these agents enhance the nephrotoxicity of cephaloridine. Renal toxicity also may be enhanced in dehydrated patients with low cardiac output.

Other adverse reactions are similar to those produced by cephalothin. Direct and indirect positive Coombs' tests and elevated levels of SGOT and alkaline phosphatase have been reported. Leukopenia has been associated with cephaloridine therapy, but evidence is insufficient to establish a clearcut causal relationship. Thus, it is advisable to monitor hepatic and hematopoietic function, especially when therapy is continued for more than ten days.

Hypersensitivity reactions (urticaria, pruritus, maculopapular or erythematous rash, and fever) may develop during therapy. Anaphylaxis has been reported. Some patients who are sensitive to penicillin also may be sensitive to cephaloridine. Nausea and vomiting occur rarely.

Colonization by resistant organisms, notably *Pseudomonas*, may be noted at multiple sites, particularly following long-term administration. Patients receiving any cephalosporin, particularly those with serious illness, should be carefully observed for signs of superinfection.

Pain at the site of intramuscular injection and thrombophlebitis at the site of intravenous injection have been noted infrequently. Intrathecal administration is not recommended.

Information is inadequate to assess the risk to the fetus when this drug is given to pregnant women. For the same reason, it is not recommended for use in premature infants or those under 1 month of age.

ROUTES, USUAL DOSAGE, AND PREPARATIONS. *Intramuscular*: *Adults*, 500 mg to a maximum of 1 g three or four times daily at equally spaced intervals. *Children over 1 month*, 30 to 50 mg/kg of body weight daily in three divided doses at equally spaced intervals; up to 100 mg/kg daily has been given in severe infections, but these doses should be used with caution.

Intravenous: *Adults and children*, 500 mg to 1.5 g (for serious infections, 2 to 4 g/day are recommended by the manufacturer for *adults*; 1 g/day is usually considered a maximum dose for *children*) dissolved in 5 or 10 ml of diluent (water for injection, sodium chloride injection, or 5% dextrose injection) and administered slowly as a continuous infusion or by intermittent injections over a period of three to four minutes. The cephaloridine solution should not be mixed with solutions containing other antibiotics.

Because large amounts may produce renal tubular necrosis, dosage must be reduced in patients with impaired renal function. The following guidelines should be used: slight impairment (creatinine clearance, 60 to 80 ml/min), up to 1 g every eight hours; mild impairment (creatinine clearance, 40 to 60 ml/min), up to 1 g every 12 hours; moderate impairment (creatinine clearance, 20 to 40 ml/min), up to 600 mg every 12 hours; marked impairment (creatinine clearance, 5 to 20 ml/min), up to 600 mg every 24 hours; essentially no function (creatinine clearance, less than 5 ml/min), up to 600 mg every 48 hours when dialysis is not being performed. (See the manufacturer's literature for further information.)

Loridine (Lilly). Powder 500 mg and 1 g.

CEPHAPIRIN SODIUM
[Cefadyl]

Cephapirin is one of the newer semisynthetic cephalosporins. Its in vitro spectrum is essentially identical to that of cephalothin (see the Introduction). Like the other cephalosporins, cephapirin should be reserved for use in infections caused by susceptible organisms when there is a definite reason to use the drug (eg, when the patient is hypersensitive to penicillin) (see the Introduction).

Cephapirin is effective in urinary tract infections and infections of the respiratory tract, skin, soft tissues, and bone. Septicemia, bacteremia, and cardiovascular, intra-abdominal, and joint infections have responded. Because cephapirin does not penetrate cerebrospinal fluid unless the meninges are inflamed, and then not as readily as some other antibiotics, this agent should not be used in meningitis. However, it is probably as effective as cephalothin in *Staphylococcus aureus* infections or septic arthritis caused by susceptible organisms.

Serum levels following intramuscular or intravenous injection are comparable to those attained with cephalothin. Approximately 50% of the drug is bound to serum proteins, and it has a serum half-life of about 35 minutes. Since cephapirin is excreted primarily by the kidney, antibacterial concentrations can be achieved in the urine.

Cephapirin causes pain on intramuscular injection, but neither the severity nor the incidence is as great as that following administration of cephalothin, although it appears to be greater than that observed after injection of cephaloridine or cefazolin. Like the other parenterally administered cephalosporins, this drug occasionally may cause phlebitis. Because of possible neurotoxicity, it should not be given intrathecally.

The adverse effects reported for cephapirin are the same as those produced by the other cephalosporins. Common reactions include mild hypersensitivity, manifested most frequently as fever or rash; eosinophilia; leukopenia; neutropenia; and transient increases in SGOT, SGPT, alkaline phosphatase, bilirubin, and BUN levels. These reactions usually disappear when the drug is discontinued. Occasionally, severe hypersensitivity reactions, manifested as urticaria, a serum sickness-like illness, or anaphylaxis have been observed. Unlike cephaloridine, this antibiotic has not been reported to cause significant nephrotoxicity.

A false-positive response for glycosuria may be observed with certain tests (see the Introduction). Overgrowth of nonsusceptible organisms can occur after prolonged use.

The safety of cephapirin in pregnant women has not been established. Preliminary studies indicate that the drug may be safe for use in infants under 3 months of age, but the benefit-to-risk ratio should always be carefully considered before administering cephapirin to infants of this age or to pregnant women since there is no primary indication for its use in these groups.

ROUTES, USUAL DOSAGE, AND PREPARATIONS. *Intramuscular, Intravenous: Adults,* 500 mg to 1 g every four to six hours; in severe infections, up to 12 g daily in divided doses. *Children,* 40 to 80 mg/kg of body weight in four equally divided doses. In patients with renal impairment, the following guidelines may be useful in determining dosage: Moderate impairment (creatinine clearance, 25 to 50 ml/min; serum creatinine, greater than 5 mg/dl), 7.5 to 15 mg/kg of body weight every 12 hours; severe impairment (creatinine clearance, less than 5 ml/min), 7.5 to 15 mg/kg just before dialysis and at 12-hour intervals thereafter.

Cefadyl (Bristol). Powder (equivalent to base) 1, 2, 4, and 20 g.

CEPHACETRILE SODIUM
[Celospor]

Cephacetrile can be administered either intramuscularly or intravenously. Its antibacterial spectrum resembles that of cephalothin and cephaloridine (see the Introduction); the minimum inhibitory concentration in vitro against *Staphylococcus aureus* is slightly higher than that for either of these agents and, against *Escherichia coli,* intermediate between that of the other two drugs. This cephalosporin can be used to treat respiratory tract infections caused by group A beta-hemolytic streptococci, *S.*

pneumoniae, nonhospital-acquired *Klebsiella pneumoniae*, *E. coli*, and *S. aureus*. It also may be effective against respiratory infections caused by *Haemophilus influenzae*, but most authorities believe it is indicated only rarely for this purpose, since more specific drugs are available. Infections of the skin and soft tissues caused by group A beta-hemolytic streptococci and *S. aureus* have responded, as have infections of the urinary tract caused by *E. coli*, *K. pneumoniae*, *Proteus mirabilis*, and a few strains of *Streptococcus faecalis* (it is ineffective against most strains).

Approximately 30% of cephacetrile is bound to protein, and the plasma half-life is 30 to 55 minutes after intravenous administration and 60 to 85 minutes after intramuscular administration. Approximately 95% to 97% of this drug is excreted by the kidneys as free drug or as the desacetyl derivative.

Cephacetrile generally is well tolerated. Administration occasionally has caused hypersensitivity reactions (pruritus, maculopapular or urticarial rash, eosinophilia, and drug fever). Headache, vertigo, blurred vision, leukopenia, neutropenia, and monocytosis also have been reported. Elevated SGOT, SGPT, and alkaline phosphatase levels and transitory increases in BUN and serum creatinine levels may occur. A direct positive Coombs' test is sometimes observed.

Intramuscular injection of cephacetrile can be painful, and phlebitis and thrombosis may occur after intravenous administration. If large intravenous doses (greater than 6 g daily) are necessary for more than three days, thrombophlebitis may be avoided by alternating the sites of infusion.

A false-positive response for glycosuria may be observed in patients receiving cephacetrile with some testing procedures (see the Introduction).

The safety of cephacetrile during pregnancy has not been established, although no teratogenic effects have been reported clinically.

Prolonged use of this cephalosporin may result in overgrowth of nonsusceptible organisms. Like other cephalosporins, cephacetrile should be used cautiously in patients known to be sensitive to the penicillins.

ROUTES, USUAL DOSAGE, AND PREPARATIONS. *Intramuscular, Intravenous*: *Adults*, 500 mg to 1 g every four to six hours; in severe infections, 1.5 to 2 g every four hours (maximum, 12 g daily). Dosage for *children under 12 years* has not been established. In patients with renal impairment, cephacetrile should be administered at 12-hour intervals in doses that achieve a steady-state serum concentration of approximately 15 mcg/ml. The following guideline may be useful: Mild impairment (creatinine clearance, 50 ml/min or greater), a loading dose of 1 g, followed by a maintenance dose of 1 g; moderate impairment (creatinine clearance, 25 to 50 ml/min), a loading dose of 1 g, followed by a maintenance dose of 850 to 925 mg; severe impairment (creatinine clearance, 5 to 25 ml/min), a loading dose of 750 mg, followed by a maintenance dose of 350 to 650 mg; essentially no function (creatinine clearance less than 5 ml/min), a loading dose of 500 mg, followed by a maintenance dose of 125 to 350 mg.

Celospor (Ciba-Geigy). Not available in the United States.

CEFAZOLIN SODIUM
[Ancef, Kefzol]

Like other cephalosporins, cefazolin sodium is active in vitro against many gram-positive and gram-negative organisms (see the Introduction). It was the first cephalosporin to be marketed that had both reasonable ease of administration and a good margin of safety when given intramuscularly or intravenously. Cefazolin rarely causes the severe pain that has made intramuscular administration of cephalothin impractical, and it lacks the nephrotoxic potential of cephaloridine. It should not be used intrathecally. Cefazolin produces higher and more sustained serum levels than cephalothin. Approximately 85% is bound to serum proteins and the serum half-life is 1.8 hours. Up to 95% of a single dose is excreted unchanged in the urine, usually within 24 hours; the remainder appears in the bile.

Cefazolin should be reserved primarily for treatment of infections caused by sensitive organisms (especially gram-negative pathogens) in patients hypersensitive to penicillin. Cefazolin can be used to treat infections of the respiratory tract, soft tissue, skin, and bone. Because most of it is excreted in the urine, this agent may be useful in urinary tract infections, particularly when ampicillin-resistant organisms are suspected or demonstrated, since some of these strains will respond to cefazolin. Depending upon the mechanism of ampicillin resistance, both ampicillin and cefazolin may be essentially useless in some infections caused by species of *Serratia, Providencia, Pseudomonas*, or indole-positive *Proteus*. Cefazolin will not penetrate cerebrospinal fluid unless inflammation is present and even then adequate antimicrobial concentrations may not be obtained. Therefore, it should never be used to treat meningitis. Bacterial endocarditis and bacteremia may respond to cefazolin, but therapeutic failures in endocarditis caused by *S. aureus* have occurred and have been attributed to the susceptibility of this drug to beta lactamases. Following repeated doses, concentrations in the bile may be greater than those found in the serum, which may indicate that cefazolin is of benefit in biliary tract infections. Although *Neisseria gonorrhoeae* is susceptible to cefazolin in vitro, this agent is not useful clinically in patients with gonorrhea.

A greater serum concentration is achieved after parenteral administration of this antibiotic than after use of the other cephalosporins. The concentration is approximately two times that obtained with comparable doses of cephaloridine and four times that obtained with cephalothin. However, cefazolin is probably the most labile of the cephalosporins to cephalosporinases or penicillinases and may not be as useful as other agents in infections caused by penicillin-resistant strains of *Staphylococcus*.

The usual adverse reactions ascribed to the cephalosporins have been reported for cefazolin. Hypersensitivity reactions (eg, fever, rash) and hematologic reactions (eg, leukopenia, thrombocytopenia) have been observed. Direct and indirect positive Coombs' tests and transient elevations of SGOT, SGPT, and alkaline phosphatase levels have been noted; these reactions disappear and test results return to normal when the antibiotic is discontinued.

Pain on intramuscular injection and phlebitis following intravenous injection occur less frequently and are not as severe as with cephalothin. A false-positive response for glycosuria has been reported using the reducing tests but not after use of enzyme tests.

Overgrowth of nonsusceptible organisms may occur with prolonged use of cefazolin. The safety of this agent in pregnant women and in infants less than 1 month of age has not been established.

ROUTES, USUAL DOSAGE, AND PREPARATIONS. *Intramuscular, Intravenous: Adults*, for mild infections caused by susceptible gram-positive organisms, 250 to 500 mg every eight hours; in severe infections, 500 mg to 1 g may be given every six to eight hours. In life-threatening infections (eg, endocarditis, septicemia), 6 to 8 g daily may be given intravenously. Doses of 500 mg to 1 g every 12 hours may be given for pneumococcal pneumonia or acute uncomplicated urinary tract infections if the maximum doses are not exceeded. *Children and infants over 1 month*, 25 to 50 mg/kg of body weight daily in three or four divided doses (total daily dose should not exceed 100 mg/kg even for severe infections).

The following guidelines may be used for patients with impaired renal function: After an initial loading dose appropriate for the infection has been given: In patients with creatinine clearance of 40 to 70 ml/min or greater, the usual dose for normal individuals is given at 12-hour intervals; creatinine clearance of 20 to 40 ml/min, 125 to 250 mg is given every 12 hours for mild to moderate infections and 250 to 600 mg is given for moderate to severe infections; creatinine clearance of 5 to 20 ml/min, 75 to 150 mg every 24 hours is given for mild to moderate infections and 150 to 400 mg is given every 24 hours for moderate to severe infections; severe impairment (creatinine clearance, less than 5 ml/min), 37.5 to 75 mg may be given every 24 hours for mild to moderate infections and 75 to 200 mg every 24 hours for moderate to severe infections.

In *children with impaired renal function*, a usual therapeutic dose can be given as a loading dose, followed by a maintenance dose every 12 hours according to the following schedule: creatinine clearance 40 to 70 ml/min, 60% of the usual daily dose; 20 to 40 ml/min, 25% of usual daily dose; 5 to 20 ml/min, 10% of normal daily dose.

Ancef (Smith Kline & French). Powder (lyophilized, sterile) 250 and 500 mg and 1, 5, and 10 g (strengths expressed in terms of base). *Kefzol* (Lilly). Powder (sterile) 250 and 500 mg and 1 and 10 g (strengths expressed in terms of base).

CEFAMANDOLE NAFATE
[Mandol]

This newer cephalosporin antibiotic has an antibacterial spectrum similar to that of the other cephalosporins (see the Introduction); however, because it is purported to be more resistant than most other cephalosporins to the cephalosporinases produced by gram-negative bacilli, it often has greater activity against *Escherichia coli*, indole-positive *Proteus* strains, members of the *Enterobacteriaceae* family, and *Haemophilus influenzae*. It also is active against many ampicillin-resistant strains of *H. influenzae*. Cefamandole appears to be slightly less effective in vitro than cephaloridine and cefazolin against alpha-hemolytic streptococci, pneumo-

cocci, and almost all strains of beta-hemolytic streptococci, but this difference is probably insignificant clinically. Like the other cephalosporins, it has no effect on *Pseudomonas* or the enterococci, and its activity against *B. fragilis* is poor.

This agent can be administered intravenously or intramuscularly, but the pain produced on intramuscular injection may somewhat restrict the use of the latter route. The pain is less severe than that caused by injection of cephalothin. Cefamandole may cause phlebitis when given intravenously, but this effect is not common and is not necessarily an indication for discontinuing therapy. Cefamandole should not be injected intrathecally.

Cefamandole is bound to protein to a greater extent than most cephalosporins (70% to 90%). Between 65% and 80% of a single dose is excreted primarily by the kidneys over an eight-hour period, largely as unmetabolized drug. Administration of probenecid prolongs the excretion time and maintains high blood levels for longer periods. Peak serum concentrations can be achieved within one-half to two hours following intramuscular injection and within ten minutes after intravenous injection. The serum half-life is approximately 40 minutes. Since the half-life is prolonged in patients with decreased renal function, dosage adjustments are necessary in these individuals.

The adverse reactions reported for cefamandole are similar to those observed following use of the penicillins and other cephalosporins. Hypersensitivity reactions consisting of maculopapular rash, urticaria, eosinophilia, and drug fever have been noted. These reactions are most common in patients with a history of allergy (particularly to penicillin). Cefamandole is contraindicated in those allergic to other cephalosporins and should be used with caution in any individual who has demonstrated some form of allergy, particularly drug allergy. Neutropenia and thrombocytopenia occur rarely, and direct positive Coombs' tests have been reported. Transient elevations of SGOT, SGPT, and alkaline phosphatase levels sometimes occur. Although BUN levels have been

Creatinine clearance ml/min/1.73 M²	>80	50-80	25-50	10-25	2-10	<2
Renal function	normal	mild impairment	moderate impairment	marked impairment	severe impairment	zero
Life-threatening infections (maximum dose)	2 g every 4 hours	1.5 g every 4 hours or 2 g every 6 hours	1.5 g every 6 hours or 2 g every 8 hours	1 g every 6 hours or 1.25 g every 8 hours	0.67 g every 8 hours or 1 g every 12 hours	0.5 g every 8 hours or 0.75 g every 12 hours
Less severe infections	1-2 g every 6 hours	0.75-1.5 g every 6 hours	0.75-1.5 g every 8 hours	0.5 to 1 g every 8 hours	0.5-0.75 g every 12 hours	0.25-0.5 g every 12 hours

elevated and creatinine clearance has decreased following cefamandole administration, the evidence does not substantiate the fact that this drug is primarily nephrotoxic. Safe use of this antibiotic in infants under 3 months of age or in pregnant women has not been established.

ROUTES, USUAL DOSAGE, AND PREPARATIONS. *Intramuscular, Intravenous: Adults,* 500 mg to 1 g every four to eight hours; in life-threatening infections, up to 2 g may be given every four hours. *Infants and children,* 50 to 100 mg/kg of body weight daily in equally divided doses every four to eight hours; doses up to 150 mg/kg daily (not to exceed the maximal adult dose) may be given for serious infections.

In patients with impaired renal function, dosage must be reduced. Doses given in the table above may be used as a guideline if creatinine clearance can be determined. When serum creatinine values are the only available data, the following formulas may be helpful:

$$\text{dose for adult males} = \frac{\text{Weight (kg)} \times (146 - \text{age})}{72 \times \text{serum creatinine}}$$

dose for adult females = 0.9 × male dose

Mandol (Lilly). Powder (sterile) 500 mg and 1 and 2 g (strengths expressed in terms of base).

CEFOXITIN SODIUM
[Mefoxin]

Cefoxitin, a beta-lactam antibiotic closely related to the cephalosporins, is classified as a cephamycin. It is derived from cephamycin C, which is produced by *Streptomyces lactamdurans*, and contains a methoxy group in the 7-alpha position; this imparts a high degree of stability in the presence of beta lactamases (both penicillinases and cephalosporinases). This drug is available only for parenteral use since it is not absorbed to any appreciable extent from the gastrointestinal tract. Intramuscular injection is less painful than with cephalothin but more painful than with cefamandole. Dilution with 0.5% lidocaine solution may reduce discomfort to an acceptable level for some patients. Cefoxitin is more prone to cause phlebitis when given intravenously than cefamandole.

Following intramuscular administration, cefoxitin is readily absorbed, with peak serum concentrations occurring as soon as 20 minutes following injection. Once absorbed, the drug is 50% to 60% bound to serum proteins. The biological half-life of cefoxitin is 45 minutes to one hour. Over a six-hour period after injection, approximately 85% of a given dose is excreted in the urine, mostly as unchanged drug (only 1.5% to 4.5% is degraded in the body).

The antibacterial spectrum of cefoxitin is similar to that of cefamandole and somewhat broader than that of the older cephalosporins (see the Introduction), but this drug has only moderate activity against *H. influenzae* and should not be used to treat infections caused by this organism. In vitro, it is equivalent or slightly less active against the gram-positive cocci than the cephalosporins and, like all cephalosporins, is inactive against enterococci (eg, *Streptococcus faecalis*); however, it is more active than most cephalosporins against *Escherichia coli*, *Klebsiella* species, and *Proteus mirabilis*. Some strains of gram-negative bacilli that are highly resistant to cephalothin are sensitive to cefoxitin. Other *Proteus* strains, as well as some strains of *Providencia* and *Serratia* resistant to the cephalosporins, may be sensitive to cefoxitin. Up to 80% of *Bacteroides fragilis* and a high percentage of other enteric anaerobes, many of which generally are resistant to the cephalosporins, also are susceptible to cefoxitin. Organisms that are resistant include *Pseudomonas*, most *Enterobacter* species, and methicillin-resistant staphylococci.

Cefoxitin has been effective in infections caused by susceptible organisms involving the lower respiratory or urinary tracts; bone and joints; skin and soft tissues; intra-abdominal infections such as peritonitis or intra-abdominal abscess; gynecological infections, including endometritis and pelvic cellulitis; and septicemia. It appears to be most useful in treating infections caused by susceptible aerobic gram-negative rods resistant to the cephalosporins; in polymicrobial infections caused by two or more resistant gram-negative aerobic rods or several aerobic gram-positive bacteria; or in mixed infections involving aerobic gram-negative and gram-positive bacteria or several species of anaerobic pathogens with or without aerobic bacteria. However, penicillin G is still preferred for the parenteral treatment of group A streptococcal or pneumococcal infections because it is more effective and less expensive. Similarly, a penicillinase-resistant penicillin or, possibly, a cephalosporin is preferred in staphylococcal infections. Although the antibacterial spectrum of cefoxitin is wider than that of most cephalosporins, aerobic gram-negative enteric pathogens are more likely to be susceptible to gentamicin, tobramycin, or amikacin than to cefoxitin,

and anaerobes are more likely to be sensitive to clindamycin or chloramphenicol. Therefore, the primary indication of cefoxitin appears to be the treatment of infection caused by susceptible organisms in individuals allergic to penicillin or in those who are unable to tolerate the older and often more potent but potentially more toxic antibiotics.

Cefoxitin is usually well tolerated. Adverse reactions resemble those observed with the cephalosporins. Skin rash, drug fever, and eosinophilia have been recorded and probably represent allergic manifestations. Cross allergenicity with penicillin in individuals allergic to penicillin has been noted, and the risk factor is similar to that for the cephalosporins. Other reactions include a direct positive Coombs' test; a transient increase in SGOT, SGPT, and BUN levels; and neutropenia. A false-positive response for glycosuria may be observed when testing with reagents sensitive to reducing substances. Cefoxitin has not been shown to be teratogenic in mice or rats, but there are no well-controlled studies in pregnant women. Therefore, before cefoxitin is given to pregnant women, the anticipated benefits must be weighed against the possible risk to the fetus.

ROUTES, USUAL DOSAGE, AND PREPARATIONS. Large doses should be given only by the intravenous route because of the large volumes or high concentrations required.

Intramuscular, Intravenous: *Adults*, for mild uncomplicated infections, 1 g every six to eight hours (total daily dose, 3 to 4 g); for moderate or severe infections, 1 g every four hours or 2 g every six to eight hours (total daily dose, 6 to 8 g); for life-threatening infections, 2 g every four hours or 3 g every six hours (total daily dose, 12 g). *Infants and children*, 50 to 150 mg/kg of body weight daily divided into four to six doses.
Dosage must be adjusted in patients with renal impairment. In adults, after a loading dose of 1 to 2 g, the following maintenance doses may be given: For those with mild impairment (creatinine clearance, 50 to 30 ml/min), 1 to 2 g every 8 to 12 hours; for

moderate impairment (creatinine clearance, 29 to 10 ml/min), 1 to 2 g every 12 to 24 hours; for severe impairment (creatinine clearance, 9 to 5 ml/min), 0.5 to 1 g every 12 to 24 hours; for those with essentially no function (creatinine clearance less than 5), 0.5 to 1 g every 24 to 48 hours.

In patients undergoing hemodialysis, a loading dose of 1 to 2 g can be given after each hemodialysis session, followed by a maintenance dose as indicated above.

Mefoxin (Merck Sharp & Dohme). Powder (equivalent to base) 1 and 2 g.

ORALLY ADMINISTERED CEPHALOSPORINS

CEPHALEXIN MONOHYDRATE
[Keflex]

Cephalexin, which is administered only orally, has an in vitro antibacterial spectrum similar to that of the other cephalosporins (see the Introduction). As with other cephalosporins, staphylococci that are resistant to methicillin are almost always resistant to cephalexin.

Cephalexin can be used to treat a variety of systemic infections as well as those of the urinary tract, but it usually is not a drug of choice for systemic infections. This cephalosporin is useful primarily against susceptible bacteria in the respiratory and urinary tracts, skin, and soft tissues. In the treatment of otitis media in children, it is important to use large doses (100 mg/kg daily); lower doses have been associated with failure rates of up to 25% to 50%. Because some organisms usually sensitive to the cephalosporins can be resistant, sensitivity tests should be performed prior to initiating therapy with cephalexin. For its use in the eye, see Chapter 24, Ocular Anti-infective and Anti-inflammatory Agents.

Cephalexin is acid stable and the presence of food in the stomach does not interfere with its absorption, although peak serum and urine levels may be somewhat delayed.

Renal function should be determined periodically in patients receiving cephalexin for prolonged periods. The drug should be administered with care and in reduced doses in patients with severe renal impairment.

Long-term use can result in overgrowth of nonsusceptible organisms, usually *Pseudomonas*. Genital and vaginal candidosis also is seen. The safety of this drug in pregnant women has not been established. A direct positive Coombs' test and a false-positive response for glycosuria have been observed.

Adverse reactions resemble those observed with cephaloglycin. Although diarrhea is observed less frequently with cephalexin than the other cephalosporins, it is still the most frequent untoward effect noted and occasionally is severe enough to necessitate discontinuation of therapy. Pyrosis, nausea, vomiting, and abdominal pain also have been observed. Allergic manifestations, which are uncommon, include rash, genital and anal pruritus, urticaria, angioedema, and anaphylactic reactions. Slight elevations of SGOT and SGPT levels have been reported. Eosinophilia and neutropenia, as well as cross sensitivity to the penicillins, have been observed.

ROUTE, USUAL DOSAGE, AND PREPARATIONS. *Oral: Adults*, 250 mg every six hours (maximum, 4 g daily in divided doses). If more than 4 g is needed, a parenteral cephalosporin preparation should be substituted. *Children*, 25 to 50 mg/kg of body weight in four divided doses; for severe infections, this dose may be doubled.

The dose should be reduced in those with impaired renal function.

Keflex (Lilly). Capsules 250 and 500 mg; drops (pediatric) 100 mg/ml (after reconstitution); suspension 125 and 250 mg/5 ml (after reconstitution).

CEPHALOGLYCIN
[Kafocin]

Cephaloglycin is administered only orally. Its in vitro spectrum is similar to that of the other cephalosporins (see the Introduction) and includes many pathogens that infect the urinary tract (eg, *Escherichia coli*, certain species of *Klebsiella*, *Staphylococcus aureus*). Cephaloglycin is ineffective against *Pseudomonas* and most species of enterococci, *Enterobacter*, and indole-positive *Proteus*. Because of its limited absorption, serum levels adequate to treat systemic infections cannot be attained clinically. The usefulness of this drug is very limited, and it has been superseded by other cephalosporins. Although it is excreted almost entirely by the kidney as desacetylcephaloglycin, an active metabolite, it is not even a drug of choice for treating urinary tract infections. The availability of cephalexin and cephradine, which also are excreted by the kidney and produce higher bactericidal concentrations in the urine than cephaloglycin, has rendered cephaloglycin obsolete.

The presence of food in the stomach does not significantly alter the total amount of cephaloglycin absorbed but will delay the onset of peak serum and urine levels.

Diarrhea is the most common adverse effect and, occasionally, has been severe enough to require discontinuation of therapy. Nausea and vomiting also may occur. These symptoms usually subside rapidly after discontinuing the drug. Other reactions include rash, urticaria, fever, headache, and vertigo. Eosinophilia occurs infrequently.

Cephaloglycin usually can be administered safely to patients sensitive to penicillin, although there is laboratory evidence of cross allergenicity. The safety of this drug in pregnant women, premature infants, and those under 1 year of age has not been established. Prolonged use may result in overgrowth of nonsusceptible organisms, especially *Pseudomonas*. A false-positive response for glycosuria may be observed in patients receiving this drug. Cephaloglycin should be administered with caution in patients with severe renal impairment.

ROUTE, USUAL DOSAGE, AND PREPARATIONS.
Oral: *Adults*, 250 to 500 mg four times daily, depending upon the severity of the infection. If larger doses are necessary, a parenteral cephalosporin should be considered. *Children over 1 year*, 25 to 50 mg/kg of body weight daily in four divided doses.
   Kafocin (Lilly). Capsules 250 mg.

CEFADROXIL MONOHYDRATE
[Duricef]

This newer cephalosporin is administered only orally. Its in vitro spectrum is similar to that of the other cephalosporins (see the Introduction) but, because its lability to beta lactamases is very low, it may be more active than some of the other cephalosporins against organisms that elaborate penicillinases or cephalosporinases. Definitive clinical data are not yet available to substantiate this supposition.

Cefadroxil is readily absorbed from the gastrointestinal tract; peak serum concentrations are achieved within 1.5 to 2 hours following oral administration. The half-life is approximately 1.5 hours with normal therapeutic doses, and minimal inhibitory concentrations for some common gram-negative urinary tract pathogens (*E. coli*, *P. mirabilis*, *Klebsiella* species) may be maintained in the urine for 20 to 22 hours. Peak serum concentrations are comparable or slightly higher than those attained with cephalexin and cephradine, persist for approximately twice as long as with these agents, and appear to be unaffected by the presence of food in the gut. The drug can be used as an alternative agent for treating urinary tract infections.

Adverse effects do not appear to be a serious problem with cefadroxil. The most common side effects reported involve the gastrointestinal tract, with nausea and vomiting being mentioned most often. Gastritis, bloating, cramps, and diarrhea also have been noted. Candidal vaginitis and other vaginal infections have occurred in patients receiving this drug, but not as often as with cephalexin. Less common reactions include rash, swollen eyes, chills, nervousness, and dizziness. Cefadroxil is contraindicated in individuals hypersensitive to any of the cephalosporins. Safe use of this drug during pregnancy and in infants and children has not been established.

ROUTE, USUAL DOSAGE, AND PREPARATIONS. *Oral: Adults,* for urinary tract infections, 1 g every 12 hours; for infections of the skin and related structures, 500 mg every 12 hours or 1 g every 24 hours.

In patients with renal impairment, a loading dose of 1 g is followed by the usual dosage at the following intervals: Creatinine clearance, 50 to 25 ml/min, every 12 hours; 25 to 10 ml/min, every 24 hours; 10 to 0 ml/min, every 36 hours. Patients with a creatinine clearance value over 50 ml/min may be considered to have normal renal function for purposes of administering cefadroxil.

Duricef (Mead Johnson). Capsules 500 mg.

CEFACLOR
[Ceclor]

This newer, orally effective cephalosporin has an in vitro spectrum similar to that of the other cephalosporins (see the Introduction). It is more active than many of the cephalosporins against *Haemophilus influenzae*, including ampicillin-resistant strains. Rare strains of staphylococci have a natural resistance to cefaclor, and all staphylococci resistant to methicillin-type

penicillins exhibit cross resistance to this antibiotic.

Cefaclor may be used as an alternative to penicillin and other antibiotics when these preferred agents cannot be tolerated or are contraindicated. It is effective in infections of the respiratory tract including pneumonia, bronchitis, pharyngitis, and tonsillitis. Otitis media, infections of skin and soft tissues, and urinary tract infections caused by susceptible organisms also usually respond. Although cefaclor generally eradicates streptococci from the nasopharynx, data are not sufficient to establish the usefulness of this drug as a substitute for penicillin in the prophylaxis of rheumatic fever.

Cefaclor is well absorbed following oral administration. The presence of food in the gastrointestinal tract delays absorption somewhat and reduces peak serum levels but does not alter the total amount of drug absorbed. When taken on an empty stomach, peak serum levels are attained in 30 to 60 minutes, and approximately 60% to 85% of a given dose is excreted unchanged in the urine within eight hours. The serum half-life in normal individuals is 36 to 54 minutes. In patients with reduced renal function, the half-life is prolonged since cefaclor is not appreciably metabolized. The half-life is 2.3 to 2.8 hours in patients who are anuric or even anephric.

Diarrhea is the most frequent adverse effect noted with cefaclor but only rarely is it severe enough to warrant discontinuation of therapy. Nausea and vomiting also may occur. Allergic reactions include urticaria and morbilliform eruptions, which usually subside when the drug is stopped. Eosinophilia has been reported. Slight elevations of SGOT and SGPT levels sometimes occur.

Cefaclor is contraindicated in patients allergic to other cephalosporins and should be used with caution in those sensitive to penicillin. Safe use of this product during pregnancy has not been established.

ROUTE, USUAL DOSAGE, AND PREPARATIONS. *Oral: Adults,* 250 mg every eight hours; for severe infections, this amount may be increased to a maximum of 4 g daily. *Chil-*

dren, 20 to 40 mg/kg of body weight daily in equally divided doses every eight hours (the larger dosage is recommended for otitis media). For severe infections, 40 mg/kg/day or more (maximum, 1 g daily). Cefaclor may be administered to patients with marked renal impairment without modification of the usual dosage. Hemodialysis shortens the serum half-life by 50%.

> *Ceclor* (Lilly). Capsules 250 and 500 mg; powder (for suspension) 125 and 250 mg/5 ml.

ORALLY OR PARENTERALLY ADMINISTERED CEPHALOSPORIN

CEPHRADINE
[Anspor, Velosef]

Cephradine is the only cephalosporin currently available in the United States that can be administered both orally and parenterally. It is acid stable and rapidly absorbed when administered orally in a fasting state; the presence of food delays the rate of absorption somewhat but does not affect the total amount of drug absorbed, except in young infants. Usual oral doses (250 to 500 mg) produce peak serum levels of approximately 9 and 17 mcg/ml, respectively, usually within one hour. A single intravenous [Velosef] dose of 1 g produces a serum level of 86 mcg/ml in 5 minutes that declines to 50 mcg/ml in 15 minutes, 26 mcg/ml in 30 minutes, and 12 mcg/ml in 60 minutes. After four hours, 1 mcg/ml can be detected. This drug is excreted unchanged in the urine.

The antibacterial spectrum of cephradine is essentially the same as that of the other cephalosporins (see the Introduction). It is active in vitro against many gram-positive organisms, including penicillinase-producing strains, and many gram-negative organisms. It is inactive against *Pseudomonas* or *Acinetobacter* species and most strains of *Enterobacter*, *Proteus morganii*, and *P. vulgaris*. Organisms resistant to methicillin also are resistant to cephradine.

This cephalosporin can be given orally to treat infections of the respiratory and urinary tracts, skin, and soft tissues caused by susceptible organisms. Intravenous administration can be used for severe infections of these organ systems and for septicemia.

As with the other cephalosporins, gastrointestinal disturbances and hypersensitivity phenomena are the most common adverse reactions. Abdominal pain, heartburn, glossitis, nausea, vomiting, and diarrhea that may be severe enough to require discontinuation of therapy have been reported. Pruritus, rash or urticaria, edema, erythema, joint pain, and drug fever, as well as mild, transient eosinophilia, leukopenia, and neutropenia have been observed. Other adverse effects include headache, dizziness, tightness in the chest, dyspnea, paresthesia, and candidal vaginitis. Isolated cases of hepatomegaly have occurred. Transitory increases in SGOT, SGPT, total bilirubin, alkaline phosphatase, and BUN levels have occurred, but there have been no reports of frank hepatic or renal damage.

Prolonged administration of cephradine may promote the overgrowth of nonsusceptible organisms. False-positive tests for glycosuria may be observed in patients receiving cephradine (see the Introduction). A false-positive direct Coombs' test also has been reported. Cephradine is contraindicated in patients hypersensitive to the cephalosporins and should be used with caution in individuals with markedly impaired renal function.

The safety of cephradine during pregnancy has not been established, but neither the cephalosporins nor the penicillins appear to be teratogenic in man. However, before cephradine is given, the benefits of drug therapy should be weighed against the possible risk to the fetus. This agent should not be used in neonates.

Pain and occasional sterile abscesses have been experienced by some patients following intramuscular injection. Thrombophlebitis has occurred during intravenous infustion, most frequently when high concentrations were infused for long periods into the same vein. This reaction usually can be avoided by alternating the sites of infusion.

ROUTES, USUAL DOSAGE, AND PREPARATIONS. *Intramuscular (deep), Intravenous*: *Adults*, 2 to 4 g daily in equally divided doses every six hours. In severe infections, the dose may be increased to a maximum of 8 g. For pneumococcal pneumonia and acute uncomplicated urinary tract infections, 500 mg four times daily may be sufficient. *Infants and children*, 50 to 100 mg/kg of body weight daily in equally divided doses every six hours.

> *Velosef* (Squibb). Powder 250 and 500 mg and 1 g (intramuscular), and 25 and 500 mg and 1, 2, and 4 g (intravenous).

Oral: *Adults*, 250 mg every six hours or 500 mg every 12 hours for respiratory tract infections (other than lobar pneumonia) and most other infections; for lobar pneumonia or urinary tract infections, 500 mg every 6 hours or 1 g every 12 hours. Severe infections may require larger doses. *Infants over 9 months and children*, 25 to 50 mg/kg of body weight daily in four divided doses. The maximum daily dose should not exceed 4 g.

Based on an initial loading dose in adults of 750 mg, followed by 500 mg (regardless of the route used), the doses may be given to patients with renal insufficiency according to the following guide: Creatinine clearance greater than 20 ml/min, every 6 to 12 hours; 15 to 19 ml/min, every 12 to 24 hours; 10 to 14 ml/min, every 24 to 40 hours; 5 to 9 ml/min, every 40 to 50 hours; less than 5 ml/min, every 50 to 70 hours. Longer time intervals may be necessary in children.

> *Anspor* (Smith Kline & French), *Velosef* (Squibb). Capsules 250 and 500 mg; suspension 125 and 250 mg/5 ml.

Selected References

Cefamandole and cefoxitin. *Med Lett Drugs Ther* 21:13-16, 1979.

Prophylactic use of antibiotics. *South Med J* 70(suppl):1-71, (Oct) 1977.

Acar JF, et al: Methicillin-resistant staphylococcemia: Bacteriologic failure of treatment with cephalosporins. *Antimicrob Agents Chemother* 10:280-285, 1970.

Barza M: Nephrotoxicity of cephalosporins: Overview. *J Infect Dis* 137(suppl):60-73, (May) 1978.

Barza M, Miao PV: Antimicrobial spectrum, pharmacology, and therapeutic use of antibiotics. III. Cephalosporins. *J Maine Med Assoc* 68:156-165, (May) 1977.

Bill NJ, Washington JA II: Comparison of in vitro activity of cephalexin, cephradine, and cefaclor. *Antimicrob Agents Chemother* 11:470-474, 1977.

Brogden RN, et al: Cefoxitin: Review of its antibacterial activity, pharmacological properties and therapeutic use. *Drugs* 17:1-37, 1979.

EORTC International Antimicrobial Therapy Project Group: Three antibiotic regimens in treatment of infection in febrile granulocytopenic patients with cancer. *J Infect Dis* 137:14-29, 1978.

Foglesong MA, et al: Stability and blood level determinations of cefaclor, a new oral cephalosporin antibiotic. *Antimicrob Agents Chemother* 13:49-52, 1978.

Jones RN, et al: In vitro antimicrobial activity comparison of cefaclor (compound 99638), cephradine, and cephalothin. *J Antibiot* 30:1-3, 1977.

Kammer RB, et al: Rapid detection of ampicillin-resistant *Haemophilus influenzae* and their susceptibility to sixteen antibiotics. *Antimicrob Agents Chemother* 8:91-94, 1975.

Katz E, Schlamowitz S: Savings achieved through cephalosporin surveillance. *Am J Hosp Pharm* 35:1521-1523, 1978.

McCloskey RV: Answers to your questions on Mefoxin--new antibiotic. *Mod Med* 47:82-87, (Feb 15-28) 1979.

Moellering RC Jr: Cefamandole: Status report based on symposium on cefamandole. *J Infect Dis* 137(suppl):190-194, (May) 1978.

Moellering RC Jr, Swartz MN: Newer cephalosporins, *N Engl J Med* 294:24-28, 1976.

Neu HC: Cefoxitin: Overview of clinical studies in United States. *Rev Infect Dis* 1:233-239, 1979.

Neu HC: New beta-lactam antibiotic: Is it a major advance? *Drugs* 17:153-156, 1979.

Petz LD: Immunologic cross-reactivity between penicillins and cephalosporins: Review. *J Infect Dis* 137(suppl):74-79, (May) 1978.

Pratt WB: *Chemotherapy of Infection*. New York, Oxford University Press, 1977, 52-56.

Root RK, Hierholzer WJ Jr: Cephalosporins, in Melmon KL, Morrelli HF (eds): *Clinical Pharmacology: Basic Priniciples in Therapeutics*, ed 2. New York, Macmillan Publishing Co, Inc, 1978, 752-754.

Ross S, et al: Cephalosporin antibiotics in pediatric practice. *South Med J* 70:855-861, 1977.

Santoro J, Levison ME: In vitro activity of cefaclor, a new orally administered cephalosporin antibiotic. *Antimicrob Agents Chemother* 12:442-443, 1977.

Schönfeld H (ed): *Antibiotics and Chemotherapy: Pharmacokinetics.* New York, S Karger, 1978, vol 25.

Sutter VL, Finegold SM: Susceptibility of anaerobic bacteria to carbenicillin, cefoxitin, and related drugs. *J Infect Dis* 131:417-422, 1975.

Weinstein L: Cephalosporins, in Goodman LS, Gilman A (eds): *The Pharmacological Basis of Therapeutics,* ed 5. New York, Macmillan Publishing Co, 1975, 1158-1164.

Chloramphenicol and Derivatives | 71

Chloramphenicol [Chloromycetin, Mychel], originally derived from the soil actinomycete *Streptomyces venezuelae*, is now produced synthetically. It is effective clinically against many strains of gram-positive and gram-negative bacteria, rickettsiae, chlamydiae (the psittacosislymphogranuloma group), and mycoplasma. Its wide antibacterial spectrum and generally good tolerance by patients make this a valuable agent for treating life-threatening, overwhelming infections caused by susceptible organisms. However, because chloramphenicol can cause fatal aplastic anemia, it should not be used to treat infections that respond to other potentially less toxic agents. It also should not be used in unidentified infections, with the possible exception of certain extremely serious conditions (eg, infection in an immunosuppressed host when aminoglycosides cannot be used) or in trivial infections. This drug should never be used for prophylaxis.

Chloramphenicol usually is bacteriostatic, but it may be bactericidal to some organisms under special conditions. It acts by binding the 50S subunit of the bacterial 70S ribosome (Vazquez, 1964), thereby inhibiting protein synthesis. This binding is readily reversible; thus, if in vitro growth of a culture has been stopped by the addition of chloramphenicol, growth will begin again if the culture is replenished with new growth medium. The binding of chloramphenicol to ribosomes is inhibited by the macrolide antibiotics (eg, erythromycin), lincomycin, and clindamycin (Vazquez, 1966). Evidence indicates that binding sites for these drugs are in close proximity to each other or are partially shared in some fashion. They do not all bind to the same receptor as has been postulated by some authorities because the binding of the macrolides, lincomycin, and clindamycin is not inhibited by chloramphenicol (Oleinick et al, 1968).

Spectrum of Activity: Chloramphenicol is still the most effective antibiotic for treating acute typhoid fever and other serious *Salmonella* infections caused by sensitive organisms. (Resistant strains of *S. typhi* have been identified [Gonzales-Cortez et al, 1973]; infections with these strains usually can be treated with ampicillin, the combination of sulfamethoxazole and trimethoprim [Bactrim, Septra], or possibly amoxicillin.) Typhoid relapses respond to retreatment with chloramphenicol, but this compound is not effective in typhoid carriers who should be treated with sulfamethoxazole and trimethoprim, ampicillin (if the strain is sensitive), or, if cholecystitis or cholelithiasis is present, by cholecystectomy. Also, there is recent evidence that large doses of amoxicillin (100 mg/kg/day) may eliminate the postinfective carrier state, whereas approximately 10% of patients may become carriers following treatment with chloramphenicol. In gastroenteritis caused by *Salmonella* other than *S. typhi*, administration of an antimicrobial agent may not shorten the duration of illness and may even prolong the convalescent carrier state.

Chloramphenicol sometimes is used to treat life-threatening infections caused by *Bacteroides*, since some strains are sensitive only to this drug. It is the drug of choice for treating *Bacteroides* infections of the central nervous system.

Since ampicillin generally is as effective as chloramphenicol against most strains of type b *Haemophilus influenzae*, it is preferred for treating these infections. Use of chloramphenicol should be reserved for ampicillin-resistant organisms. If severe infections (eg, meningitis, epiglottitis, cellulitis) occur in areas where ampicillin-resistant strains of *H. influenzae* are widespread and treatment must be started before results of susceptibility tests become available, penicillin G or ampicillin and chloramphenicol may be used initially. Once the results of culture and sensitivity tests are available, treatment should be continued with the single most appropriate agent. Even when susceptibility tests show that chloramphenicol is the most effective drug, however, some physicians still prefer to use ampicillin if the organism is not resistant. Chloramphenicol also may be administered to treat meningitis caused by *Neisseria meningitidis* or *Staphylococcus pneumoniae*, particularly in patients hypersensitive to penicillin.

Occasional strains of *Proteus*, *Escherichia coli*, and *Serratia* are susceptible only to chloramphenicol. This antibiotic is as effective as the tetracyclines for treating Rocky Mountain spotted fever and other rickettsial infections and can be used when the tetracyclines are contraindicated because of renal or hepatic disease in infants and young children. Chloramphenicol may be given for melioidosis (*Pseudomonas pseudomallei* infection) if sulfonamides or tetracyclines cannot be used.

Strains of certain organisms have become resistant to chloramphenicol. One mechanism is the acquisition of R-factors (Benveniste and Davies, 1973), particularly by enteric bacteria, governing the production of an acetyltransferase, which inactivates chloramphenicol by acetylation of a hydroxyl group. Resistance to chloramphenicol can be passed, for example, from a resistant *Salmonella* to a sensitive *Escherichia coli* and even transferred back from an induced-resistant *E. coli* to a sensitive *Salmonella*.

Pharmacology: Chloramphenicol is readily absorbed from the gastrointestinal tract with peak blood levels achieved in approximately two hours. It diffuses into cerebrospinal fluid (a level approximately one-half that in plasma can be obtained) and into aqueous and vitreous humors, synovial fluid, pleural fluid, ascitic fluid, and bile, a desirable characteristic not easily achieved with other antibiotics. Chloramphenicol also readily crosses the placenta, and it appears in appreciable quantities in the milk of nursing mothers. Because this antibacterial drug readily penetrates ocular tissue, it is effective when administered systemically in ocular infections caused by susceptible organisms, including some strains of *Pseudomonas* other than *P. aeruginosa*. It is also used topically in the eye but not as commonly today as in the past (see Chapter 24, Ocular Anti-infective and Anti-inflammatory Agents).

In patients with normal hepatic function, 90% of chloramphenicol is conjugated to the glucuronide in the liver, 2% is deacetylated and dehalogenated, and 8% is excreted unchanged. The dose of chloramphenicol, therefore, should be reduced or the interval between doses lengthened in patients with impaired hepatic function. Unfortunately, good therapeutic guidelines have not as yet been established for modifying dosage.

If the capacity of the liver to conjugate substances with glucuronic acid is not impaired, the dosage of chloramphenicol does not require reduction in patients with impaired renal function for, although the nontoxic, bacteriologically inactive glucuronide of chloramphenicol accumulates in these individuals, the biologically active form of the drug does not. In patients with renal impairment complicated by hepatic insufficiency, the usual dosage must be reduced to prevent toxicity.

Adverse Reactions and Precautions

Chloramphenicol causes two types of hematopoietic abnormalities. The first, a true toxic reaction manifested by bone marrow depression, is dose related, progressive, and reversible upon discontinuation of therapy. It is associated with anemia, reticulocytopenia, elevated serum iron and iron-binding capacity, and decreased uptake of iron by the erythrocyte. There is vacuolization of erythroid precursors as well as increased cellularity of bone marrow. The ratio of myeloid/erythroid elements is increased and leukopenia may be present. This reaction occurs to some extent in everyone given chloramphenicol and is most likely to be serious in patients receiving large doses and/or prolonged therapy or in those with hepatic or renal insufficiency. It is not a prodrome to aplastic anemia. The mechanism of this toxic effect is not completely understood, but there is evidence that the reaction occurs as a result of inhibition of mitochondrial protein synthesis.

A second, more serious type of bone marrow depression, which may occur after a single dose as well as following prolonged therapy, is aplastic anemia. This condition is not dose related and may occur weeks or even months after administration of the drug. In its most severe form, it is characterized by pancytopenia with an aplastic marrow. Aplastic anemia does not appear to be the result of drug hypersensitivity; rather, it is believed to be an idiosyncratic response that may be caused by a genetically determined biochemical lesion (Yunis, 1969). Because it occurs rarely, the incidence is difficult to establish precisely. Values ranging from 1 in 24,000 to 1 in 50,000 have been extrapolated from the available data (Wallerstein et al, 1969). The prognosis is very poor, since the anemia usually is irreversible.

Because the incidence of aplastic anemia appears to be lower after parenteral than after oral administration, some clinicians believe that the drug can be injected without incurring this blood dyscrasia. There are, however, four reported cases of aplastic anemia associated with injection of chloramphenicol (Domart et al, 1961; Restrepo and Zambrano, 1968; Wallerstein et al, 1969; Grilliat et al, 1966), and two cases which occurred when the drug was administered topically in the form of eye drops (Rosenthal and Blackman, 1965; Carpenter, 1975). It has been argued that complicating conditions in most of these cases cloud the validity of the findings. For example, one young woman receiving low doses of chloramphenicol intramuscularly was also being given other drugs, including phenylbutazone, that are known to cause blood dyscrasias. Because definitive data are lacking and because of the dire consequences of aplastic anemia, it must be assumed that this drug is capable of causing aplastic anemia when administered by *any* route until proven otherwise.

Other blood dyscrasias noted, especially following use of large doses, include thrombocytopenia with no change in red or white blood cells, transient leukopenia, neutropenia, and agranulocytosis that can be precipitous and severe. Aplastic anemia without pancytopenia as well as leukemia following what appeared to be aplastic anemia also have been reported. Chloramphenicol increases the rate of bone marrow suppression in uremic patients when compared to that in normal individuals, a condition that aggravates existing anemia. It also inhibits the normal function of developing white blood cells in these patients.

Before administering a drug known to cause blood dyscrasias, it is advisable to perform appropriate pretreatment blood counts to obtain baseline values for later comparison. Thereafter, periodic blood studies may reveal early peripheral changes caused by the dose-related, direct marrow-depressant effects of chloramphenicol. Such studies, however, cannot predict the future occurrence of aplastic anemia or of precipitous agranulocytosis. Some authorities recommend that leukocyte and differential counts be performed every 48 hours during chloramphenicol therapy and that prolonged or repeated use of the drug be avoided. In view of the prodigious number of routine hemograms that are performed and the rarity of diagnosing a potentially fatal blood disorder by such means, the chance of benefiting any given patient by routine examination is remote. Whether to conduct periodic blood counts on a routine basis is an individual decision that must be made by each physician. Careful observation for sudden sore throat or development of additional infection may be more important than routine studies. If such signs appear, immediate laboratory evaluation is then indicated.

Allergic reactions (eg, rash, angioedema, urticaria) have been observed following administration of chloramphenicol. Rarely, anaphylactic and Herxheimer-like reactions have been reported during treatment of typhoid. Sensitization to chloramphenicol may occur after topical use. Hypersensitivity reactions are uncommon.

Adverse gastrointestinal symptoms include nausea, vomiting, glossitis, stomatitis, diarrhea, and enterocolitis. Mild fever, headache, depression, delirium, or confusion is not uncommon. Optic neuropathy or peripheral neuritis occurs infrequently.

The plasma concentration of chloramphenicol is higher in premature infants and neonates under 2 weeks of age than in older infants because of inadequate metabolic inactivation in the immature liver and depressed rates of glomerular filtration and tubular secretion. High blood levels in premature and full-term infants frequently cause a toxic reaction referred to as the grey syndrome; in rare instances, this condition has occurred in infants up to 25 months of age who have high blood levels of chloramphenicol (Craft et al, 1974). The exact biochemical basis for this reaction is unknown, but it is characterized by abdominal distention, progressive pallid cyanosis, vomiting, irregular respiration, hypothermia, and acute circulatory failure. Since it can be fatal, administration of chloramphenicol to infants during the first two weeks of life is not recommended except under unusual circumstances. In these infants, the recommended dosage should not be exceeded and, if possible, plasma levels should be monitored.

Chloramphenicol can inhibit the primary immune response in mice and certain other animals, possibly by suppressing the growth rate of antigen-stimulated lymphocytes that are rapidly dividing. There is no evidence, however, that this immunosuppressive effect is clinically important. Therapeutic doses of chloramphenicol may interfere with the anamnestic response to tetanus toxoid in man. Thus, concomitant administration of this antibiotic and active immunizing agents should probably be avoided. Therapeutic doses also inhibit the biotransformation of tolbutamide [Orinase], phenytoin [Dilantin], dicumarol, and other drugs metabolized by hepatic microsomal enzymes. This action may enhance the toxicity of these drugs when they are administered with chloramphenicol.

Bacterial and fungal superinfections can occur during administration of chloramphenicol, especially if therapy is prolonged. The possibility of developing a superinfection in addition to the increased danger of toxicity are two reasons why long-term therapy with chloramphenicol is discouraged.

CHLORAMPHENICOL
[Chloromycetin, Mychel]

CHLORAMPHENICOL PALMITATE
[Chloromycetin Palmitate]

CHLORAMPHENICOL SODIUM SUCCINATE
[Chloromycetin Sodium Succinate, Mychel-S]

$$O_2N-\langle\ \rangle-\underset{\underset{OH}{|}}{\overset{\overset{H}{|}}{C}}-\underset{\underset{H}{|}}{\overset{\overset{NHCCHCl_2}{|}}{C}}-CH_2OH$$

Since high blood levels of chloramphenicol are achieved rapidly following oral administration, this route is preferred except in cases of overwhelming sepsis. Parenteral preparations should be used only when oral administration is contraindicated or impractical, and oral forms should be substituted as soon as feasible. The sodium succinate ester may produce a bitter taste for a few minutes after injection. It has been demonstrated that chloramphenicol sodium succinate is ineffective when given intramuscularly, and use of this route may cause moderate local pain; therefore, this drug should be injected only intravenously. As with other antibiotics that are effective systemically, topical use of chloramphenicol generally should be avoided, except by local instillation into the eye or ear.

For indications, adverse reactions, and precautions, see the Introduction.

ROUTES, USUAL DOSAGE, AND PREPARATIONS. If doses larger than those recommended are required to treat severe infections, they should be reduced as soon as clinical improvement occurs.

CHLORAMPHENICOL:

Oral: Adults, children, and full-term infants over 2 weeks, 50 mg/kg of body weight daily in divided doses every six or eight hours. In typhoid and paratyphoid fevers, some authorities recommend that this dosage schedule be continued for at least two weeks and, in severe illness, the dose may be doubled initially until clinical improvement occurs. In patients in whom the half-life of the drug may be increased (eg, those with impaired hepatic function), the interval between doses may be lengthened and/or the dose reduced. *Premature infants,* 25 mg/kg daily in divided doses, usually at 12-hour intervals. *Full-term infants under 2 weeks,* 25 mg/kg daily in divided doses every four to six hours. For all infants, it is advisable, if possible, to monitor chloramphenicol blood levels frequently; the concentration of the drug should be maintained between 5 and 20 mcg/ml.

> Drug available generically: Capsules 250 mg.
> *Chloromycetin* (Parke, Davis). Capsules 50, 100, and 250 mg.
> *Mychel* (Rachelle). Capsules 250 mg.

Intravenous: Adults may be given the same dosage on a weight basis as that used orally. This drug should not be used parenterally in *children* except to initiate therapy for meningitis or severe sepsis, when 100 mg/kg of body weight daily can

be given. (The sodium succinate ester is most commonly used in children.)

> *Chloromycetin* (Parke, Davis). Solution 250 mg/ml in 2 ml containers.

Topical: This route generally should be avoided except in the eye or ear (for dose and preparations, see Chapters 24 and 27).

CHLORAMPHENICOL PALMITATE:

Oral: The palmitate is hydrolyzed to chloramphenicol base before absorption from the gastrointestinal tract, but it yields lower blood levels dose-for-dose than the base. The dosage recommended by the manufacturer is the same as that for the parent compound.

> *Chloromycetin Palmitate* (Parke, Davis). Suspension equivalent to chloramphenicol 150 mg/5 ml.

CHLORAMPHENICOL SODIUM SUCCINATE:

Intravenous: A solution is prepared for intravenous use by dissolving the drug in a suitable aqueous diluent (eg, water for injection, 5% dextrose injection) to make a solution containing the equivalent of 100 mg/ml of chloramphenicol base. The dosage for *adults and children* is the same as that for the base, although blood levels may be attained somewhat less rapidly than when the base is used orally because the succinate salt must be hydrolyzed to free chloramphenicol.

> *Chloromycetin Sodium Succinate* (Parke, Davis), *Mychel-S* (Rachelle). Powder 1 g (equivalent to 100 mg of chloramphenicol/ml when reconstituted).

Selected References

Beneviste R, Davies J: Mechanisms of antibiotic resistance in bacteria. *Annu Rev Biochem* 42:471-506, 1973.

Carpenter G: Chloramphenicol eye drops and marrow aplasia. *Lancet* 2:326-327, 1975.

Craft AW, et al: The "grey toddler." Chloramphenicol toxicity. *Arch Dis Child* 49:235-237, 1974.

Domart A, et al: Aplasie médullaire mortelle après administration de chloramphénicol par voie intra-musculaire chez duex adultes. *Sem Hop Paris* 37:2256-2258, 1961.

Gonzalez-Cortez A, et al: Water-borne transmission of chloramphenicol-resistant *Salmonella typhi* in Mexico. *Lancet* 2:605-607, 1973.

Grilliat JP, et al: Cytopénie mortelle après thérapeutique par hemisuccinate de chloramphenicol. *Ann Med Nancy* 5:754-762, 1966.

Martelo OJ, et al: Chloramphenicol and bone marrow mitochondria. *J Lab Clin Med* 74:927-940, 1969.

Oleinick NL, et al: Nonidentity of site of action of erythromycin A and chloramphenicol on *Bacillus subtilis* ribosomes. *Biochim Biophys Acta* 155:290-292, 1968.

Restrepo A, Zambrano F: Anemia aplastica tardia secundaria a cloranfenicol. Descripcion de diez casos. *Antioquia Medica* 18:593-606, 1968.

Rosenthal RL, Blackman A: Bone-marrow hypoplasia following use of chloramphenicol eye-drops. *JAMA* 191:148-149, 1965.

Vazquez D: Binding of chloramphenicol by ribosomes from *Bacillus megaterium*. *Biochem Biophys Res Commun* 15:464-468, 1964.

Vazquez D: Binding of chloramphenicol to ribosomes: Effect of a number of antibiotics. *Biochim Biophys Acta* 114:277-288, 1966.

Wallerstein RO, et al: Statewide study of chloramphenicol therapy and fatal aplastic anemia. *JAMA* 208:2045-2050, 1969.

Yunis AA: Drug-induced bone marrow injury. *Adv Intern Med* 15:357-376, 1969.

Macrolide and Lincosamide Antibiotics | 72

The macrolide group of antibiotics is composed of erythromycin and troleandomycin. These drugs contain a large lactone ring to which sugars are attached. Erythromycin and its derivatives are antibacterial agents of major clinical importance, while troleandomycin is an obsolete drug of little use in the treatment of infectious disease. The lincosamide antibiotics, lincomycin and clindamycin, are considered with the macrolides because their antibacterial spectrum, mechanism of action, and clinical applications are similar (Pratt, 1977).

MACROLIDES

Spectrum and Indications: Erythromycin is produced by a strain of *Streptomyces erythreus* and is considered to be one of the safest antibiotics in use today. Its antimicrobial spectrum is similar to that of penicillin G (Nicholas, 1977, part I); the drug is active in vitro against most gram-positive bacteria, including many strains of *Listeria. Staphylococcus aureus, Streptococcus pyogenes, S. pneumoniae,* the viridans streptococci, and many strains of *S. faecalis* also are sensitive. Clinically,

occasional strains of these organisms, particularly *S. aureus,* may be resistant in a nosocomial setting, for example, when patients have been treated recently with erythromycin or are undergoing immunosuppressive therapy. Gram-positive bacilli that are most often sensitive include *Clostridium tetani, Cl. perfringens (welchii), Corynebacterium diphtheriae,* and *Actinomyces israelii. Nocardia asteroides* has variable sensitivity to erythromycin alone, but a combination of erythromycin and ampicillin appears to act synergistically against the majority of strains.

Most species of *Neisseria* and some species of *Bordetella, Brucella, Yersinia,* and *Haemophilus* are sensitive. Only a few strains of *Bacteroides fragilis* are affected by usual therapeutic blood levels of erythromycin. The majority of other gram-negative organisms are resistant. The sensitivity of all gram-negative organisms is increased in an alkaline medium; erythromycin is a weak base which is ionized to a lesser degree at high pH values, making relatively more drug available in a form that can more readily enter the cell. Thus, alkalization of the urine may be of clinical importance in the rare case when erythromycin is used to treat a urinary tract infection.

Erythromycin is active against *Mycoplasma pneumoniae* (PPLO, Eaton agent), certain *Actinomyces* and *Treponema* species, and many species of *Rickettsia* and *Chlamydia*. Based on laboratory and clinical data, this drug appears to be active against *Legionella pneumophila*, the bacterium causing Legionnaires' disease, and currently is the drug of choice in the therapy of pneumonia caused by this bacillus. The usual dose of erythromycin (2 g orally) may be inadequate to effect a cure (Sanford, 1979). It has been suggested that intravenous injection of 2 to 4 g daily is more likely to be effective. Regardless of the route used, organisms may persist despite therapy, and radiographic resolution is slow, often requiring many weeks.

Erythromycin inhibits bacterial protein synthesis by binding to the 50S microsomal subunits (Mao and Putterman, 1969). Experiments investigating the competitive effects of antibiotics indicate that these binding sites overlay the binding sites for chloramphenicol and the lincosamides but are not identical to them. Nevertheless, because competitive inhibition may occur when two or more of these agents (ie, erythromycin, lincomycin, clindamycin, chloramphenicol) are administered simultaneously, combined therapy with these drugs should be avoided. Erythromycin, like chloramphenicol, inhibits protein synthesis on ribosomes from mammalian mitochondria but does not bind to mammalian 80S ribosomes, which accounts in part for its selective toxicity (Mao et al, 1970).

Erythromycin is most often employed to treat mild infections of the skin, soft tissues, and body cavities caused by grampositive organisms (Nicholas, 1977, part II). It is used primarily as an alternative to penicillin for mild to moderately severe infections caused by susceptible organisms in which high blood levels of penicillin are not required or in patients who cannot tolerate penicillin. This use of the drug may be more conservative than is warranted; 25 years of clinical experience with erythromycin has demonstrated a lack of widespread bacterial resistance and a relative freedom from significant toxicity.

Erythromycin may be used to treat pa-tients with nonfulminating staphylococcal infections caused by either penicillin-sensitive or penicillin-resistant strains; however, this is not a drug of first choice for severe infections since it may not be bactericidal, depending upon the nature of the organism and the tissue concentration of drug that can be obtained. Erythromycin is not generally administered for infections caused by *S. aureus* but may be employed in the treatment of pharyngitis, scarlet fever, cellulitis, and erysipelas caused by group A *Streptococcus pyogenes*. It also may be given as an alternative to penicillin in the prophylaxis of endocarditis or recurrent attacks of rheumatic fever in individuals with demonstrable sequelae of rheumatic fever who are allergic to penicillin; prophylaxis is particularly indicated in patients with cardiac abnormalities during tooth extraction, oral surgery, or other dental procedures. Pneumonia, otitis media, and meningitis may respond to full therapeutic doses of erythromycin, but penicillin continues to be the drug of choice. The combined action of erythromycin and sulfonamides usually is more effective than erythromycin alone in children with otitis media caused by *H. influenzae*. This enhanced effect is useful when the patient is allergic to ampicillin or when erythromycin alone is not effective, but such therapy may not be a preferred alternative to the combination of sulfamethoxazole and trimethoprim [Bactrim, Septra] (see Chapter 77, Sulfonamides and Related Compounds). When erythromycin is combined with a sulfonamide, however, the dose of each component should be determined individually for best results, because such factors as age, body weight, and severity of the disease must be considered. Although it is not a preferred alternative, erythromycin may be used instead of penicillin for treating gas gangrene, but debridement remains the most essential therapeutic procedure; erythromycin also rapidly eradicates *Cl. tetani* from wounds.

Patients with acute diphtheria, sometimes including those who have previously failed to respond to penicillin, have been treated successfully with erythromycin and diphtheria antitoxin. Erythromycin is preferred therapy for the carrier state of this disease.

Erythromycin is an acceptable alternative to penicillin for treating all stages of syphilis and is as effective as penicillin in early stages of the infection. It may be the drug of choice in syphilitic patients allergic to penicillin and in uncomplicated gonorrhea in pregnant women because of its safety; however, the patient must be followed carefully to assure eradication of the organisms. (See also Chapter 69, Penicillins.)

Primary atypical pneumonia caused by *M. pneumoniae* and chlamydial infections may respond to erythromycin equally well or better than to the tetracyclines (*Scott Med J*, 1977) and the drug is safer in children under 8 years of age in whom the latter agents cause mottling and staining of teeth. Erythromycin may be useful in treating erythrasma, intestinal amebiasis, and prostatitis caused by *Staphylococcus epidermidis*. It is effective in blepharitis (see also Chapter 24, Ocular Anti-infective and Anti-inflammatory Agents) and, like the tetracyclines, is used in some forms of acne.

Many gram-positive organisms, especially certain strains of *Staphylococcus*, are capable of developing resistance to erythromycin, but widespread resistance to this drug has not materialized, although the greater use of clindamycin for treating both outpatient and nosocomial infections appears to be increasing somewhat the overall frequency of erythromycin resistance. One reason for the lack of erythromycin-resistant organisms has only recently become apparent (Lacey, 1977): Many bacteria that acquire resistance to an antibiotic are at a disadvantage in the normal environment when compared to nonresistant organisms, and the resistant bacteria often are quickly replaced by sensitive bacteria when administration of the antibiotic is discontinued. It does not necessarily follow, therefore, that development of a resistant bacterial colony caused by extensive use of an antibacterial agent in the hospital renders that agent obsolete. Withdrawal of the drug for a few weeks or months may

allow replacement of a resistant flora with one composed largely of sensitive organisms. This might be an argument for a policy that involves the rotational use of effective antibiotics to retard or even prevent the development of certain resistant nosocomial strains of bacteria.

An unusual type of erythromycin-induced resistance occurs in *Staphylococcus aureus* infections (Weisblum et al, 1971): When organisms are exposed to low concentrations of this drug (about 10^{-8} M), they become resistant to all macrolides and lincosamides. This effect appears to be mediated through the acquisition of a plasmid that contains a gene for an RNA methylase. When there is too little erythromycin to inhibit protein synthesis, this enzyme is induced, which modifies bacterial RNA; subsequently, usual bacteriostatic concentrations of macrolides or lincosamides are no longer effective. In contrast, if the organism is exposed to high concentrations of erythromycin (greater than 10^{-7} M), staphylococcal growth is inhibited and induced resistance is blocked because protein synthesis is inhibited. In a similar manner, beta-lactamase producing staphylococci resistant to penicillin and indirectly (but not constitutively) resistant to erythromycin can be eradicated by a combination of erythromycin and penicillin, the former inhibiting the synthesis of the beta lactamase that is mediating resistance to the latter (Allen and Epp, 1978).

When given orally, erythromycin and its derivatives are inactivated to varying degrees by gastric acid (Nicholas, 1977, part I). This effect can be minimized by giving these preparations before meals, by using enteric- or film-coated preparations (eg, E-Mycin, Ilotycin), or by using an ester form of the drug (eg, erythromycin estolate, erythromycin ethylsuccinate). The gluceptate and lactobionate esters may be given intravenously when large doses are required.

The in vitro antibacterial spectrum of troleandomycin [TAO] is similar to that of erythromycin, but this agent is less active and has no clinical advantage over erythromycin. Troleandomycin should be used only when it has been established that the organism is not sensitive to more effective agents.

Adverse Reactions and Precautions: Except for erythromycin estolate [Ilosone], erythromycin and its derivatives seldom cause serious adverse reactions. When given orally, they infrequently produce mild gastrointestinal disturbances (nausea, vomiting, pyrosis, diarrhea), usually only after large doses (2 g or more daily). Tablets with acid-resistant coating may be given with meals to reduce the possibility of these untoward effects, but serum levels will be reduced. Mild allergic reactions such as urticaria and other rashes have occurred, but serious reactions (eg, severe abdominal pain, drug fever, eosinophilia) are rare.

Sensorineural hearing loss, although extremely rare, has been associated with use of large doses of erythromycin (Nicholas, 1977, part I). It occurs within a few hours to several days and is manifested as marked bilateral hearing loss that gradually reverses on discontinuation of the drug.

The parenteral dosage forms of the erythromycins may be physically and/or chemically incompatible with solutions containing vitamin B complex, ascorbic acid, cephalothin, tetracycline, colistin, chloramphenicol, heparin, metaraminol, and phenytoin. Such mixing should be avoided.

Erythromycin estolate is the erythromycin ester that has been associated with hepatotoxicity (ie, cholestatic jaundice) most often, although other esters and erythromycin base itself also have caused hepatic dysfunction. Hepatotoxicity occurs most frequently and rapidly (two to three days) in patients who have previously received erythromycin estolate. The jaundice appears to be a hypersensitivity reaction and is reversible when the antibiotic is discontinued. There may be accompanying upper right quadrant pain, fever, and changes in hepatic function tests suggesting choledocholithiasis. Other forms of erythromycin are preferred in patients with a history of liver disease, in those with pre-existing liver disease, or in those suspected of having impaired liver function.

Troleandomycin may cause hepatic changes (eg, jaundice, hyperbilirubinemia, abnormal liver function tests) if administered for two weeks or longer. These changes are usually reversible if the drug is discontinued promptly. The most common adverse effects are hypersensitivity reactions, nausea, vomiting, diarrhea, anal burning, and headache. Anaphylactic reactions also have occurred. Because of its potential toxicity, troleandomycin is contraindicated in chronic conditions such as acne or pyoderma, in patients with hepatic disease or dysfunction, and in those sensitive to the drug.

INDIVIDUAL EVALUATIONS

ERYTHROMYCIN
[E-Mycin, Ilotycin, Robimycin, RP-Mycin]

ERYTHROMYCIN ESTOLATE
[Ilosone]

ERYTHROMYCIN ETHYLSUCCINATE
[E.E.S., Pediamycin]

ERYTHROMYCIN GLUCEPTATE
[Ilotycin Gluceptate]

ERYTHROMYCIN LACTOBIONATE
[Erythrocin Lactobionate-IV]

ERYTHROMYCIN STEARATE
[Bristamycin, Erythrocin Stearate, Erypar, Ethril, Pfizer-E]

All of the erythromycins have the same spectrum of antibacterial activity and uses; adverse reactions also are similar, except that erythromycin estolate has a greater propensity to cause hepatotoxicity. See the foregoing section on Macrolides for a detailed discussion.

ROUTES, USUAL DOSAGE, AND PREPARATIONS.
All doses and preparation strengths are
expressed in terms of the base. For streptococcal infections, therapy should be continued for at least ten days.

Oral: (Base) *Adults*, initially, 500 mg, followed by 250 mg every six hours.
(Estolate) *Adults and children over 25 kg
of body weight*, 250 mg every six hours.
(Ethylsuccinate) *Adults*, 400 mg four times
daily.
(Stearate) *Adults*, 250 mg every six hours or
500 mg every 12 hours given on an empty
stomach or immediately before meals.
(All forms) For severe infections in *adults*,
4 g may be given daily in divided doses.
Children, 30 to 50 mg/kg of body weight
daily in four divided doses; for severe
infections, the dose may be doubled.

ERYTHROMYCIN:
Drug available generically: Tablets 250 and
500 mg; tablets (enteric-coated) 250 mg.
E-Mycin (Upjohn), *Ilotycin* (Dista), *Robimycin*
(Robins), *RP-Mycin* (Reid-Provident). Tablets
(enteric-coated) 250 mg.

ERYTHROMYCIN ESTOLATE:
Ilosone (Dista). Capsules 125 and 250 mg;
drops 100 mg/ml; granules for suspension 125
mg/5 ml after reconstitution; suspension 125
and 250 mg/5 ml; tablets (chewable) 125 and
250 mg; tablets 500 mg.

ERYTHROMYCIN ETHYLSUCCINATE:
Drug available generically: Granules for suspension 200 mg/5 ml after reconstitution.
E.E.S. (Abbott), *Pediamycin* (Ross). Granules
for drops 100 mg/2.5 ml after reconstitution;
granules for suspension 200 mg/5 ml after reconstitution; suspension 200 and 400 mg/5 ml;
tablets (chewable) 200 mg.
E.E.S. 400 (Abbott). Tablets 400 mg.

ERYTHROMYCIN STEARATE:
Drug available generically: Tablets 250 and
500 mg.
Bristamycin (Bristol). Tablets 250 mg.
Erythrocin Stearate (Abbott). Tablets 125, 250,
and 500 mg.
Erypar (Parke, Davis), *Ethril* (Squibb),
Pfizer-E (Pfipharmecs).Tablets 250 and 500 mg.

Intravenous: For severe infections in
adults and children, 15 to 20 mg/kg of body
weight daily. Larger doses may be given in
very severe infections (maximum dose of
the lactobionate salt is 4 g daily). Continuous infusion is preferable, but administration in divided doses no less frequently
than every six hours is also effective. If the
drug is given by intermittent injection,
one-fourth of the total dose can be given in
20 to 60 minutes by infusion of a solution
containing 250 to 500 mg in 100 to 250 ml
of 0.9% sodium chloride or 5% dextrose
injection. The infusion should be sufficiently slow to avoid pain along the vein.
An oral dosage form of erythromycin
should be substituted as soon as possible.

ERYTHROMYCIN GLUCEPTATE:
Ilotycin Gluceptate (Dista). Powder 250 and
500 mg and 1 g.
ERYTHROMYCIN LACTOBIONATE:
Erythrocin Lactobionate-IV (Abbott). Powder
(lyophilized) 500 mg and 1 g.

Topical: Use of this route is discouraged
because of the danger of sensitization,
which precludes subsequent administration of erythromycin. When selected for
use, the preparation is applied to the affected area three or four times daily. For
use in the eye, see Chapter 24, Ocular
Anti-infective and Anti-inflammatory
Agents.

ERYTHROMYCIN:
Ilotycin (Dista). Ointment 1% in ½ and 1 oz and
1 lb containers.

TROLEANDOMYCIN
[TAO]

Troleandomycin should rarely be used
because more effective and potentially less
toxic agents are available. For information
on uses, adverse reactions, and precautions, see the foregoing section on Macrolides.

ROUTE, USUAL DOSAGE, AND PREPARATIONS.
Oral: *Adults*, 250 to 500 mg four times
daily; *children*, 6.6 to 11 mg/kg of body
weight every six hours. For streptococcal
infections, therapy should be continued for
at least ten days.

TAO (Roerig). Capsules equivalent to 250 mg of oleandomycin; suspension equivalent to 125 mg of oleandomycin/5 ml.

LINCOSAMIDES

Spectrum and Indications: Lincomycin hydrochloride monohydrate [Lincocin], an antibacterial agent produced by *Streptomyces lincolnensis* var. *lincolnensis*, and its semisynthetic derivatives, clindamycin hydrochloride, clindamycin palmitate hydrochloride, and clindamycin phosphate [Cleocin], have a spectrum of activity similar to that of erythromycin (Pratt, 1977), except clindamycin generally is considered to be a drug of choice for serious infections caused by anaerobic organisms, especially *Bacteroides fragilis*, often considered the most resistant of the anaerobic pathogens (Finegold et al, 1975). Although lincomycin is the parent lincosamide, it is no longer the agent of first choice in treating infections susceptible to this group of drugs. Clindamycin differs chemically from lincomycin by the substitution of a chlorine atom for a hydroxyl group on the parent compound. With this slight molecular modification, clindamycin is better absorbed, more potent, and probably less toxic than lincomycin (McGehee et al, 1968). Also, it is purported to cause less diarrhea than lincomycin following oral administration, but this has not been proved.

Like erythromycin, the lincosamides are active against the common gram-positive pathogens, including staphylococci (although some resistant strains have been reported), streptococci (including *S. pneumoniae* but excluding *S. faecalis*), and pneumococci. Anaerobic organisms susceptible to clindamycin in vitro include *Bacteroides* species, *Fusobacterium* species, *Propionibacterium*, *Eubacterium*, *Peptococcus* species, *Peptostreptococcus* species, microaerophilic streptococci, clostridia (most *Cl. perfringens* [*welchii*] and *Cl. tetani* are susceptible, but *Cl. sporogens* and *Cl. tertium* frequently are resistant), several *Actinomyces* species, and some *Nocardia* species. With few exceptions (eg, some strains of *Mycoplasma pneumoniae*), gram-negative organisms are not sensitive to the lincosamides.

Clindamycin often is the most effective antibiotic in the treatment of some anaerobic infections and is especially useful in those caused by certain species of *Bacteroides* (eg, *B. fragilis*) not sensitive to the penicillins. Primary lung abscesses may respond, although penicillin G (10 to 12 megaunits/day) or carbenicillin (8 to 12 weeks of therapy) is preferred if the organism is penicillin sensitive. Intra-abdominal sepsis and endocarditis also may be treated successfully with this drug. Certain obstetric, gynecologic, soft tissue, bone, and joint infections may be resolved with clindamycin, but culturing is frequently necessary to determine if a penicillin (eg, carbenicillin, ticarcillin) or chloramphenicol might be preferred. Clindamycin also may be indicated in infections caused by susceptible gram-positive organisms resistant to the penicillins and erythromycins or in patients who cannot tolerate these drugs. Both lincomycin and clindamycin may be effective in acute and chronic osteomyelitis caused by susceptible gram-positive organisms. Lincomycin and clindamycin are not suitable for treating brain abscesses caused by anaerobic bacteria because of poor penetration of the blood-brain barrier.

Staphylococci, especially *S. aureus*, may develop resistance slowly to lincomycin and clindamycin. *Streptococcus pneumoniae* also is rarely resistant to both drugs. The frequency with which resistance develops has not been determined, but natural resistance occurs in less than 1% of patients. When cross resistance occurs between lincomycin and clindamycin, it develops for *all* resistant strains. Since erythromycin-resistant strains of *S. aureus* also may be resistant to lincomycin or clindamycin, neither drug should be used to treat infections caused by erythromycin-resistant staphylococci unless in vitro tests show that the organism is sensitive. Cross resistance between lincomycin or clindamycin and most other antibacterial agents has not been encountered clinically, although it has been demonstrated in vitro.

Food may interfere with the absorption

of orally administered lincomycin, but the absorption of clindamycin does not appear to be appreciably retarded by the presence of food in the stomach.

Adverse Reactions and Precautions: Lincomycin and clindamycin are usually well tolerated, but they may cause fatal colitis (Tedesco, 1977). Some authorities contend that the incidence of serious colitis is great enough to restrict use of these compounds to the treatment of a few specific, serious infections in hospitalized patients.

Nausea, vomiting, flatulence, bloating, cramping, tenesmus, anorexia, and weight loss may occur following administration of the lincosamides. More frequent evacuation of softer than normal stools is common, and occasionally persistent severe diarrhea has been observed. The stool may contain blood, mucus, and pus and be associated with a potentially fatal pseudomembranous colitis. The incidence of diarrhea associated with clindamycin therapy has been reported to be as low as 2% and as high as 21%, and pseudomembranous colitis has been estimated to occur in from less than 1% to more than 10% of patients (Tedesco, 1977; Swartzberg et al, 1977; Gurwith et al, 1977; Lusk et al, 1977; Neu et al, 1977). Diarrhea occurs most often within a few days to two weeks after therapy is begun, but its onset may be delayed for two or three weeks after completion of therapy. Diarrhea that develops during administration usually will cease 7 to 14 days after the medication is discontinued. If the lincosamide is continued in spite of diarrhea or if the diarrhea begins after the medication is stopped, the disorder may become protracted (two to four weeks' duration) and debilitating. Therefore, the drug should be discontinued as soon as is practical. The patient should be warned about possible complications.

Diarrhea (and pseudomembranous or candidal colitis or staphylococcal enterocolitis) is associated with either oral or parenteral administration of lincomycin or clindamycin, but the incidence is several times greater when these drugs are given orally. Individuals over 20 years of age are approximately twice as likely to develop diarrhea as those under 20, and the incidence in women is slightly greater than in men. The risk appears to be unrelated to the duration of therapy, total drug dosage, or underlying disease. However, there is a correlation between the severity of illness and the tendency to develop diarrhea (Lusk et al, 1977).

The pseudomembranous colitis that occurs with lincosamides also has been observed following treatment with tetracyclines, chloramphenicol, ampicillin, and other antibiotics (Fekety, 1978). It appears to be noted more commonly with lincosamide therapy, but the general term, antibiotic-associated colitis (AAC), is now used to define this entity. The syndrome has been studied in detail using Syrian hamsters as an animal model (Rifkin et al, 1977; Rifkin et al, 1978 A; Lusk et al, 1978). The syndrome in the hamster is caused by an enterotoxin produced by *Clostridium difficile*. Passive immunization of hamsters with *Cl. sordellii* antitoxin protects them from AAC after administration of clindamycin. A heat-labile toxin has been demonstrated in the feces of patients with AAC induced by clindamycin and ampicillin (Larson and Price, 1977; Larson et al, 1977; Rifkin et al, 1978 B; Bartlett et al, 1978), and enterotoxigenic strains of *Cl. difficile* usually can be found in the feces of patients with this syndrome (Fekety, 1978; Tedesco et al, 1978). Isolation of the organism from stools usually takes several days, but initiation of treatment of seriously ill patients is justified once the pseudomembranous lesions have been demonstrated by sigmoidoscopy. Toxigenic *Cl. difficile* isolates have been found to be very sensitive to vancomycin (minimal inhibitory concentration usually less than 1 mcg/ml) and also may respond to metronidazole or cholestyramine resin.

If severe diarrhea occurs while a lincosamide is being given, the drug should be discontinued and therapy initiated to restore and maintain normal fluid and electrolyte balance. Vancomycin (500 mg every six hours for adults with normal renal function) may be given and at the present time is considered the antibiotic of choice. Serum albumin also may be administered.

Although steroids have been used systemically, there is little evidence that they are beneficial. Cholestyramine resin [Questran] has been shown to be of some use in treating diarrhea caused by antibacterial agents; the mechanism of action is not clear, but it appears that this anion-binding resin may bind and neutralize the toxin. Occasionally, additional aggressive supportive treatment also may be necessary, particularly in elderly patients. (See Chapter 58, Antidiarrheal Agents.) The antidiarrheal mixture, diphenoxylate hydrochloride with atropine sulfate [Colonil, Lomotil], has been given to treat lincosamide-induced diarrhea. The effectiveness of this mixture has been questioned, however, since the clinical course of experimentally induced shigellosis has been prolonged with its use. Furthermore, in a double-blind study of healthy volunteers, the incidence of diarrhea was higher when the mixture was administered with parenteral lincomycin than when the lincomycin was given with a placebo. In addition, some cases of toxic megacolon have been anecdotally linked to the use of diphenoxylate and atropine in AAC. Therefore, unless favorable definitive data become available, the mixture should not be used in lincosamide-induced diarrhea.

When given intramuscularly, clindamycin may cause pain, induration, and sterile abscesses; pain is less severe with lincomycin. These reactions usually can be minimized or avoided by injection deep into the muscle. Hypotension has occurred after intramuscular injection of both drugs. Intravenous administration may cause thrombophlebitis, particularly with prolonged infusion through an indwelling venous catheter. Rapid intravenous injection of lincomycin has resulted in cardiac arrest.

Leukopenia (chiefly neutropenia) has been reported rarely following administration of the lincosamides. In addition, agranulocytosis, thrombocytopenic purpura, and eosinophilia have been associated with their use. These effects are reversible following withdrawal of the drugs. Hypersensitivity reactions are rare with either drug. They are generally mild and most often consist of pruritus, rash, and urticaria. However, angioedema, exfoliative dermatitis, anaphylactic reactions, and serum sickness have been noted. Some patients may experience dizziness, headache, generalized myalgia, proctitis, and vaginitis with either drug. Superinfections caused by nonsusceptible organisms also have occurred, especially when the duration of therapy exceeded ten days.

The safety of these drugs during pregnancy has not been established, although several hundred pregnant women have been given lincomycin or clindamycin during all stages of pregnancy with no harmful effects reported.

Because significant amounts of lincomycin and clindamycin are excreted unchanged in the urine, serum levels in patients with severe renal impairment may be double or triple those observed in patients with normal kidney function receiving the same dose. Serum levels should be determined at frequent intervals in patients with impaired renal function and the dosage adjusted to produce levels comparable to those observed in patients with normal renal function (an average of 1 to 2 mcg/ml after oral administration, 4 to 10 mcg/ml after intramuscular administration, and 8 to 20 mcg/ml after intravenous administration). Transitory changes in many liver function tests have occurred after administration of these drugs, and both have caused jaundice.

INDIVIDUAL EVALUATIONS

LINCOMYCIN HYDROCHLORIDE MONOHYDRATE
[Lincocin]

The spectrum of activity of lincomycin is similar to that of erythromycin. It is primarily reserved for use in infections caused by susceptible organisms that are resistant to the penicillins and erythromycin or in patients who cannot tolerate other antibacterial agents.

For specific uses, adverse reactions, and precautions, see the foregoing section on Lincosamides.

ROUTES, USUAL DOSAGE, AND PREPARATIONS. *Oral: Adults,* 500 mg three or, for more severe infections, four times daily; *children and infants over 1 month,* 30 to 60 mg/kg of body weight daily in three or four divided doses. For streptococcal infections, therapy should be continued for at least ten days.

> *Lincocin* (Upjohn). Capsules 250 (pediatric) and 500 mg; syrup 250 mg/5 ml (strengths expressed in terms of the base).

Intramuscular: For serious infections, *adults,* 600 mg every 24 hours; *children and infants over 1 month,* 10 mg/kg of body weight every 24 hours. The dose may be administered every 12 hours or more often in severe infections.

Intravenous: For serious infections, *adults,* 600 mg to 1 g every 8 to 12 hours; dosage may be increased to a maximum of 8 g daily for more severe infections. *Children and infants over 1 month,* 10 to 20 mg/kg of body weight daily in two or three divided doses. The solution is added to 0.9% sodium chloride injection or 5% dextrose injection and infused slowly.

> *Lincocin* (Upjohn). Solution (sterile) 300 mg/ml in 2 and 10 ml containers (strength expressed in terms of the base).

CLINDAMYCIN HYDROCHLORIDE
[Cleocin Hydrochloride]

CLINDAMYCIN PALMITATE HYDROCHLORIDE
[Cleocin Pediatric]

CLINDAMYCIN PHOSPHATE
[Cleocin Phosphate]

Clindamycin is a semisynthetic derivative of lincomycin with the same indications for use as the parent compound. It may be better absorbed, more potent, and less toxic than lincomycin. For specific uses, adverse reactions, and precautions, see the foregoing section on Lincosamides.

ROUTES, USUAL DOSAGE, AND PREPARATIONS. For streptococcal infections, treatment should be continued for at least ten days. *Oral:* (Hydrochloride) *Adults,* for serious infections, 150 to 300 mg every six hours; for more severe infections, 300 to 450 mg every six hours. *Children and infants over 1 month,* for moderate to severe infections, 8 to 16 mg/kg of body weight daily in three or four divided doses; for more severe infections, 16 to 20 mg/kg daily in three or four divided doses.

(Palmitate Hydrochloride) *Adults and older children,* for serious infections, 8 to 12 mg/kg of body weight daily in three or four divided doses; for severe infections, 13 to 16 mg/kg daily in three or four divided doses; for life-threatening infections, 17 to 25 mg/kg daily in three or four divided doses. *Children weighing 10 kg or less,* 37.5 mg three times daily is the minimum dose.

> CLINDAMYCIN HYDROCHLORIDE:
> *Cleocin Hydrochloride* (Upjohn). Capsules 75 and 150 mg (strengths expressed in terms of the base).
> CLINDAMYCIN PALMITATE HYDROCHLORIDE:
> *Cleocin Pediatric* (Upjohn). Granules for suspension 75 mg/5 ml (strength expressed in terms of the base).

Intramuscular: Adults, for moderate to severe infections, 600 mg to 2.7 g daily in two, three, or four equally divided doses. Injection of more than 600 mg at a single site is not recommended. *Children over 1 month,* for moderate to severe infections, 15 to 25 mg/kg of body weight daily in three or four equally divided doses; for severe infections, 25 to 40 mg/kg daily (minimum, 300 mg daily). Oral therapy should be substituted as soon as possible.

Intravenous: Adults, for serious infections, 600 mg to 1.2 g daily in two, three, or four equally divided doses; for more severe infections, 1.2 to 2.7 g daily in two, three, or four equally divided doses; for life-threatening infections, as much as 4.8 g daily has been given. The initial dose may be administered as a single rapid infusion, followed by continuous infusion. *Children over 1 month*, for serious infections, 15 to 25 mg/kg of body weight daily in three or four equally divided doses; for more severe infections, 25 to 40 mg/kg daily (minimum, 300 mg). Oral therapy should be substituted as soon as possible.

CLINDAMYCIN PHOSPHATE:
Cleocin Phosphate (Upjohn). Solution (sterile) 150 mg/ml in 2 and 4 ml containers (strength expressed in terms of the base).

Selected References

Erythromycin symposium. *Scott Med J* 22(suppl 1):349-407, 1977.

Allen NE, Epp JK: Mechanism of penicillin-erythromycin synergy on antibiotic-resistant *Staphylococcus aureus*. *Antimicrob Agents Chemother* 13:849-853, 1978.

Bartlett JG, et al: Antibiotic-associated pseudomembranous colitis due to toxin-producing clostridia. *N Engl J Med* 298:531-534, 1978.

Fekety R: Antibiotic-associated pseudomembranous colitis. *Clin Microbiol Newslett* (preview issue, Oct 1978)

Finegold SM, et al: Management of anaerobic infections. *Ann Intern Med* 83:375-389, 1975.

Gurwith MJ, et al: Diarrhea associated with clindamycin and ampicillin therapy: Preliminary results of cooperative study. *J Infect Dis* 135 (suppl):104-110, 1977.

Lacey RW: New look at erythromycin. *Postgrad Med J* 53:195-200, 1977.

Larson HE, Price AB: Pseudomembranous colitis: Presence of clostridial toxin. *Lancet* 2:1312-1314, 1977.

Larson HE, et al: Undescribed toxin in pseudomembranous colitis. *Br Med J* 1:1246-1248, 1977.

Lusk RH, et al: Clindamycin-induced enterocolitis in hamsters. *J Infect Dis* 137:464-475, 1978.

Lusk RH, et al: Gastrointestinal side effects of clindamycin and ampicillin therapy. *J Infect Dis* 135(suppl):111-119, 1977.

Mao JCH, Putterman M: Intermolecular complex of erythromycin and ribosome. *J Mol Biol* 44:347-361, 1969.

Mao JCH, et al: Biochemical basis for selective toxicity of erythromycin. *Biochem Pharmacol* 19:391-399, 1970.

McGehee RF Jr, et al: Comparative studies of antibacterial activity in vitro and absorption and excretion of lincomycin and clindamycin. *Am J Med Sci* 256:279-292, 1968.

Neu HC, et al: Incidence of diarrhea and colitis associated with clindamycin therapy. *J Infect Dis* 135(suppl):120-125, 1977.

Nicholas P: Erythromycin: Clinical review. I. Clinical pharmacology. II. Therapeutic uses. *NY State J Med* 77:2088-2094, 2243-2246, 1977.

Pratt WB: *Chemotherapy of Infection*. New York, Oxford University Press, 1977, 142-149.

Rifkin GD, et al: Gastrointestinal and systemic toxicity of fecal extracts from hamsters with clindamycin-induced colitis. *Gastroenterology* 74:52-57, 1978 A.

Rifkin GD, et al: Neutralization by *Clostridium sordellii* antitoxin of toxins implicated in clindamycin-induced cecitis in hamster. *Gastroenterology* 75:422-424, 1978 B.

Rifkin GD, et al: Antibiotic-induced colitis: Implication of toxin neutralized by *Clostridium sordellii* antitoxin. *Lancet* 2:1103-1106, 1977.

Sanford JP: Legionnaires' disease—first thousand days. *N Engl J Med* 300:654-656, 1979.

Swartzberg JE, et al: Clinical study of gastrointestinal complications associated with clindamycin therapy. *J Infect Dis* 135(suppl):99-103, 1977.

Tedesco FJ: Clindamycin and colitis: A review. *J Infect Dis* 135 (suppl):95-98, 1977.

Tedesco FJ, et al: Oral vancomycin for antibiotic-associated pseudomembranous colitis. *Lancet* 2:226-228, 1978.

Weisblum B, et al: Erythromycin-inducible resistance in *Staphylococcus aureus*: Requirements for induction. *J Bacteriol* 106:835-847, 1971.

Tetracyclines | 73

The discovery and development of penicillin and streptomycin created an awareness of the potential therapeutic value of other antibacterial substances that might be extracted from cultures of microorganisms. As a result, several extensive screening programs were undertaken. One of these, conducted by Benjamin M. Duggar, culminated in the discovery in 1948 of the first of the tetracyclines, chlortetracycline [Aureomycin]. Subsequently, thousands of related compounds were examined, a few of which have been developed for clinical use to treat infectious diseases.

The tetracyclines are broad spectrum antibacterial agents extracted from species of *Streptomyces* or produced by chemical manipulation of the naturally occurring materials. All members of this class are closely related chemically and, therefore, bacteria have almost identical patterns of susceptibility and resistance to each drug.

Mechanism of Action: The tetracyclines block the attachment of aminoacyl transfer RNA to the messenger RNA ribosome complex, thereby interfering with protein synthesis (Pratt, 1977). Binding of the antibiotic occurs chiefly at the 30S ribosomal subunit and is largely reversible. The tetracyclines, therefore, are bacteriostatic agents at blood levels commonly achieved with administration of normal therapeutic doses. They may be bactericidal experimentally when high concentrations are used in vitro. Because tetracyclines do not inhibit bacterial cell wall synthesis, they are effective against cell wall-deficient organisms (specifically *Mycoplasma pneumoniae*) and bacterial variants (protoplasts and L-forms) that may develop and persist during treatment with cell wall-inhibiting antibiotics (eg, penicillins, cephalosporins, cephamycins).

Antibacterial Spectrum and Indications: Tetracyclines are effective in vitro against a great variety of bacteria, including both gram-positive and gram-negative organisms (Ory, 1974; Siegel, 1978, part II). They are among the antibiotics of first choice in infections caused by *Francisella tularensis, Pseudomonas pseudomallei, Vibrio cholerae, V. fetus, Haemophilus ducreyi, Calymmatobacterium granulomatis*, and *Mycoplasma pneumoniae*; all rickettsial infections; relapsing fever due to *Borrelia novyi* or *B. recurrentis*; and all infections caused by *Chlamydia* (ie, psittacosis, lymphogranuloma venereum, trachoma, inclusion conjunctivitis, keratoconjunctivitis). Tetracyclines are also drugs of choice in severe brucellosis (sometimes given with streptomycin 1 g daily) and in granuloma inguinale and nonspecific urethritis. They are usually combined with streptomycin, which some authorities consider the antibiotic of choice, to treat plague caused by *Yersinia pestis*.

The tetracyclines may be used as alternative antibiotics when the infecting organism is susceptible and the agent of first choice is ineffective or not tolerated. Organisms that are usually susceptible include *Streptococcus pneumoniae* and group A and B streptococci (some strains of these organisms are resistant to all tetracyclines); *S. pyogenes*; most anaerobic streptococci; *Listeria monocytgenes*; *Bacillus anthracis*; *Erysipelothrix insidiosa*; *Fusobacterium fusiforme*; some strains of *Escherichia coli* (resistant strains may emerge rapidly); *Haemophilus influenzae*; *Neisseria gonorrhoeae* (tetracyclines may be drugs of first choice under certain circumstances); *Treponema pallidum*; *Pseudomonas mallei*; some strains of *Mima-Herellae*; *Clostridium tetani*; *Bordetella pertussis*; *Bacteroides* (many strains of *B. fragilis* are resistant); *Actinomyces israelii*; *Nocardia asteroides*; and some indole-producing strains of *Proteus* (most *Proteus* and *Pseudomonas* are resistant).

Tetracyclines may be useful adjunctively in acute intestinal amebiasis, as ancillary agents in *Plasmodium falciparum* infections resistant to the antimalarial agents, and as alternative drugs in bacillary dysentery caused by susceptible strains of *Shigella*.

Although the role of infection in the pathogenesis of chronic bronchitis and emphysema and the place of antibiotics in their treatment have yet to be clarified, it has been customary to prescribe antibiotics for chronic bronchitis, bronchiectasis, and chronic obstructive lung disease. The tetracyclines often are given to adults and children over 8 years of age to treat exacerbations of bronchitis. In severe bronchitis with chronic purulent infection, tetracyclines can be administered continuously or intermittently for years as a prophylactic measure or they may be alternated with ampicillin. Bronchiectasis also may respond to the judicious use of tetracyclines or other broad spectrum antibiotics. In severe infections, therapy should be based upon the results of sputum cultures and susceptibility studies. The tetracyclines may be given as supportive therapy for certain chronic lung problems (eg, cystic fibrosis). Such usage represents one of the very few instances in which they may be given, even chronically, to children under 8 years of age. Their use in children also may be warranted in life-threatening infection when the preferred anti-infective agents are not effective or are toxic. However, tetracyclines should be used only as a last resort in young children and infants. Sinusitis occurring as a mixed bacterial infection is often helped by the use of the tetracyclines.

The efficacy of tetracycline in acne is well documented (Ad Hoc Committee on Use of Drugs in Dermatology, 1975). To provide lasting benefit, the drug must be given for weeks, months, or even years. Maintenance doses as small as 250 mg daily may control lesions after treatment with usual therapeutic doses has brought about maximum improvement. At these low dosage levels, adverse effects are rare. Because treatment is suppressive rather than curative, use of tetracycline should be restricted to the treatment of chronic, severe, inflammatory lesions refractory to other methods of treatment.

A topical form of tetracycline [Topicycline] for the treatment of acne is supplied as a powder with a liquid carrier that must be mixed before use. The liquid portion is a solution of *n*-decyl methyl sulfoxide and sucrose esters in 40% alcohol. The manufacturer claims that the sulfoxide, which is related chemically to dimethyl sulfoxide (DMSO), enhances cutaneous penetration of the tetracycline. This topical preparation does not appear to be as effective as systemic tetracyclines for treating acne (see Chapter 61, Dermatologic Preparations).

A tetracycline-susceptible pleomorphic organism may be involved in the malabsorption of Whipple's disease, and treatment with tetracycline often brings about remission. Although therapy must be continued indefinitely, intermittent administration may be adequate after remission has been maintained for 9 to 12 months. Tetracycline also may be indicated in other diseases of malabsorption characterized by bacterial overgrowth in the small bowel. Since organisms tend to become refractory during prolonged treatment, several different broad spectrum antimicrobial agents should be given alternately.

Doxycycline [Vibramycin] has been claimed to prevent travelers' diarrhea caused by enteropathogenic bacteria, primarily enterotoxigenic *E. coli* (Sack et al, 1978), with single daily doses as low as 100 mg. Protection appears to persist for at least one week after the drug is stopped.

It should be emphasized that many infections responsive to tetracyclines are serious and some are prone to relapse. In prescribing tetracyclines, it is important to individualize treatment; the agent selected should be given in a dose that is truly therapeutic, with therapy continued as long as it is safe and desirable.

Clinical Pharmacology: The tetracyclines are incompletely and variably absorbed from the stomach and upper portion of the intestinal tract; doxycycline and minocycline [Minocin] are more completely absorbed than the other agents. Tetracyclines form insoluble complexes in the gut with calcium, magnesium, iron, aluminum, and other bivalent and trivalent cations. Therefore, the presence of food, milk and milk products, vitamin and mineral preparations, or cathartics and antacids containing metal salts may result in decreased and erratic absorption. The absorption of doxycycline and minocycline appears to be affected only slightly by the presence of food. Sodium bicarbonate, which contains no polyvalent cations and which cannot chelate with tetracyclines, also interferes with the gastrointestinal absorption of these drugs, possibly through an effect on gastric pH.

A parenteral route is used in patients who are unable to take tetracyclines orally. Intravenous administration is used initially in serious infections, malabsorption syndromes, and critically ill or comatose patients. Rapid intravenous administration (less than one to five minutes) should be avoided and oral medication should be substituted as soon as possible. Prolonged intravenous infusion may cause thrombophlebitis and the high blood levels obtained may be hepatotoxic (with the possible exception of doxycycline), particularly in individuals with renal impairment. The tetracyclines probably should not be given to patients with severe renal impairment. Intramuscular injection also can be employed but is extremely painful, even when the preparation contains 2% lidocaine and is injected into a large muscle mass. Furthermore, the serum concentrations attained tend to be low, even with maximum doses; this route should be used only as a last resort. Tetracyclines should never be injected intrathecally.

Topical application of the tetracyclines in an ointment or cream base is of little value except in some ocular infections (see Chapter 24, Ocular Anti-infective and Anti-inflammatory Agents) and occasionally produces hypersensitivity. Topical use of these agents, therefore, is not recommended except for use in the eye and possibly for acne.

When administered in doses sufficient to provide adequate serum levels, the tetracyclines diffuse readily into most fluids and tissues, including cerebrospinal fluid (even when meninges are not inflamed) and ischemic tissue. They cross the placenta and are present in the milk of lactating women.

The rates of absorption, peak blood concentrations, and durations of action vary among the tetracyclines. Peak serum levels are generally attained two to four hours after oral administration. Approximate mean serum half-lives and peak blood levels appear in the Table. Because tetracycline is considered to be the basic moiety, the half-lives of derivatives are often evaluated in terms of tetracycline equivalents. The longer half-life of the newer tetracyclines allows administration of smaller doses at longer intervals. The convenience of once or twice daily use facilitates consistent treatment and smaller doses are less likely to cause gastrointestinal disturbances.

Tetracyclines have an affinity for rapidly growing or metabolizing tissue and tend to localize in the liver, tumors, new bone, and teeth, particularly before birth and during the first three years of life. They fluoresce bright yellow when exposed to ultraviolet radiation of 3,600 Angstrom units. Fluorescence may be detected within 24 hours in all tissues except the brain after a single dose of 3 to 4 g. Since tetracycline remains visible in bone and neoplastic tissue for several weeks, it has been used experimentally to study the formation of cortical bone and urinary calculi and clinically to detect new growths.

Most tetracyclines are excreted primarily by the kidneys and can be recovered unchanged from the urine. Variable amounts are eliminated in the feces. All tetracyclines are concentrated in the liver and excreted in bile, with considerable reabsorptive cycling from the gastrointestinal tract. Because of enterohepatic circulation, tetracyclines may be detected in the blood for several days after treatment is discontinued.

Resistance: The development of bacterial resistance can severely limit the usefulness of an antibiotic. Several species of bacteria, especially *E. coli*, beta-hemolytic streptococci, *S. pneumoniae*, *N. gonorrhoeae*, and strains of *Bacteroides* and *Shigella*, have become increasingly resistant to the tetracyclines (Siegel, 1978, part I). Some strains of *S. aureus* are resistant to all tetracyclines. Since there is evidence that resistance develops in direct proportion to usage, the prevalence of resistant organisms is likely to increase in the future unless usage of tetracyclines is curtailed.

Resistance may occur through several mechanisms. Strains of mutant *E. coli* with tetracycline-resistant ribosomes have been isolated in the laboratory, and there is evidence that some bacteria may be induced to produce enzymes that degrade the antibiotic. The major mechanism of resistance, however, is believed to be decreased permeability of the bacterial cell surface to the drug. This may explain why strains of staphylococci and possibly other organisms resistant to most tetracyclines are sensitive in vitro to minocycline and doxycycline (the most lipid soluble of the tetracyclines); therefore, these derivatives may penetrate the tetracycline-resistant bacterial cell wall to reach the ribosome that remains drug sensitive. This observation is of doubtful clinical value, however, since the antimicrobial spectra of the tetracyclines are so similar that bacterial cross resistance occurs almost invariably.

Resistance can be passed from one organism to another by transfer of small plasmids of extrachromosomal DNA called R-factors that contain genetic information for the development of resistance. An R-factor often induces resistance to several antibiotics simultaneously. *E. coli* have been shown to acquire resistance by conjugation, that is, the direct passage of genetic material between bacteria. Staphylococci may transfer resistance when a bacteriophage (a virus capable of infecting bacteria) carries the plasmid into the cell.

Adverse Reactions and Precautions

All tetracyclines have relatively low toxicity at usual dosage levels (Kurylowicz,

SOME PHARMACOKINETIC VALUES FOR THE TETRACYCLINES

Drug	Percentage of Oral Dose Absorbed	Commonly Reported Serum Half-Life (Hours)
Chlortetracycline	30	5.5-6
Demeclocycline	66	12
Doxycycline	90-100	15-17
Methacycline	low	14-15
Minocycline	90-100	15-20
Oxytetracycline	58	9.5
Tetracycline	77	8-10

1976; Pratt, 1977; Siegel, 1978, part I). Gastrointestinal disturbances (anorexia, heartburn, nausea, vomiting, flatulence, and, most often, diarrhea) occur in about 10% of patients receiving 2 g or more of tetracycline or the equivalent daily; this increases somewhat after prolonged administration. These reactions usually are not disabling but, when severe, treatment must be discontinued or at least interrupted and resumed later with lower doses. When diarrhea persists or is severe, it is important to determine whether it is nonspecific or is caused by overgrowth of *Staphylococcus aureus*. The latter condition can be life-threatening and is most likely to occur in elderly or debilitated patients and in those who are receiving several antibiotics, immunosuppressive agents, or corticosteroids.

Other undesirable reactions of the various tetracyclines include dryness of the mouth; hoarseness; stomatitis, including vesiculopapular oral lesions; glossitis, including black hairy tongue; pharyngitis; dysphagia; enterocolitis; proctitis; and inflammatory lesions caused by candidal overgrowth of the vulvovaginal and perianal regions. Most of these reactions result from suppression of normal enteric flora with overgrowth of other organisms. Prolonged therapy may result in replacement of normal oral and intestinal flora by resistant strains of *S. aureus*, *Pseudomonas*, *Klebsiella*, *Enterobacter*, *Proteus*, *Candida*, and *Clostridium difficile*. Severe staphylococcal enterocolitis has occurred during oral and, rarely, during intravenous or intramuscular administration.

Hypersensitivity reactions, which occur infrequently, include urticaria, angioedema, exfoliative dermatitis, idiopathic nonthrombocytopenic purpura, exacerbation of systemic lupus erythematosus, and anaphylactic shock, which has occasionally caused death. Cross sensitization among the tetracyclines is common.

Photosensitivity reactions also have been noted occasionally, most commonly after use of demeclocycline [Declomycin]; photosensitivity has been reported very rarely after use of minocycline [Minocin]. The reaction is usually manifested as exaggerated sunburn upon exposure to ultraviolet light; marked erythema and, rarely, bullae may occur in exposed areas of the body. Photosensitivity is reversible over a period of days or weeks. A few cases of papular eruption have been reported. Onycholysis occurs in about 25% of those affected.

Except for doxycycline [Vibramycin] and possibly minocycline, the tetracyclines are thought to have an antianabolic effect, which may produce negative nitrogen balance and increase blood urea nitrogen levels. This is of no clinical importance when usual doses are given to patients with normal renal function. When renal function is impaired, tetracyclines may increase azotemia. Tetracyclines may be administered to patients with renal disease if the total daily dose is reduced in proportion to renal insufficiency and the interval between doses is increased.

A smaller amount of doxycycline and minocycline is excreted by the kidney than of other tetracyclines, possibly because these two analogues are very lipid soluble, a characteristic that is thought to interfere with renal clearance. Studies indicate that these tetracyclines may not accumulate significantly in the serum of patients with renal insufficiency and may not increase the severity of azotemia. Therefore, doxycycline and minocycline have been advocated to treat these patients, particularly for extrarenal infections.

Insult to the proximal renal tubules can be caused by degradation products of the tetracyclines that accumulate in outdated preparations. Albuminuria, glycosuria, aminoaciduria, hypophosphatemia, hypokalemia, and renal tubular acidosis are manifestations of this condition. The damage usually is reversible after withdrawal of the responsible agent, although a few fatalities have occurred. In all of the cases reported, outdated capsules containing citric acid, an excipient which supposedly increased the absorption of tetracycline, were ingested. (This type of product was discontinued several years ago.) The use of outdated tetracycline also has caused a systemic lupus erythematosus-like syndrome. It is, therefore, important that both physician and patient be aware of the necessity of adhering strictly to the expiration date of all medicinals and of avoiding excessive heat and humidity when storing drugs for any length of time.

Fatalities attributable to renal complications have been reported when tetracyclines were used with methoxyflurane [Penthrane]. No other anesthetic is known to be contraindicated during treatment with these antibiotics.

The tetracyclines may cause liver damage that is sometimes associated with pancreatitis, particularly when large doses (2 g or more daily) are administered intravenously. The damage is detectable by liver function studies. Diffuse, fine vacuolar fatty metamorphosis of the liver has been demonstrated histologically. Significant hepatotoxicity is most likely to occur when the tetracyclines are administered with other hepatotoxic drugs or when pre-existing hepatic or renal insufficiency exists. A number of deaths have been reported, most of them occurring when doses greater than 1 g daily were given intravenously to pregnant or postpartum women with pyelonephritis or other renal disease. Because kidney infections are common and diffuse fatty metamorphosis of the liver may occur as a complication of pregnancy, tetracyclines should be prescribed only when absolutely necessary and with great caution in pregnant women.

Tetracyclines also should be avoided during pregnancy because they are attracted to embryonic and growing osseous tissue where they form a tetracycline-calcium orthophosphate complex. Although no teratogenic effects have been reported in humans, temporary depression of bone growth occurs in the fetus and young children. The danger is greatest from midpregnancy to 3 years of age, but it may continue to age 7 and possibly longer. The incidence of adverse effects is influenced more by the total quantity of tetracycline ingested by mother or child than by the duration of treatment.

Changes occur in both deciduous and permanent teeth during the time of tooth development and include dysgenesis, staining, and increased tendency to caries. Discoloration may be progressive and varies from yellowish brown to dark gray. Thus, tetracyclines should not be used in children under 8 years (see statement of Committee on Drugs, American Academy of Pediatrics, *Pediatrics*, 1975) unless there are compelling reasons to do so. Discoloration of the nails and onycholysis also may occur upon exposure to ultraviolet light.

The tetracyclines can cause a rare condition known as pseudotumor cerebri. Tense bulging of the fontanelles caused by increased intracranial pressure occurs in infants and meningeal irritation with papilledema is observed in adults. There are no abnormalities of the spinal fluid and the diagnosis, chiefly one of exclusion, may require careful neurologic appraisal. When the antibiotic is discontinued, spinal fluid pressure returns to normal over a period of days or weeks.

Vertigo may be observed after use of most tetracyclines, especially minocycline. This effect usually is not serious but may persist for one or two days.

Tetracyclines delay blood coagulation and may potentiate the effect of coumarin-type anticoagulants. In addition to chelating calcium, they may cause physicochemical changes in plasma lipoproteins. Interference with bacterial synthesis of vitamin K in the intestine, particularly in elderly people with marginal hepatic function, also may be a factor. Patients receiving tetracyclines intravenously have decreased prothrombin activity and impaired thromboplastin regeneration.

Blood dyscrasias, including neutropenia and hemolytic anemia, have occurred rarely following administration of the tetracyclines. Oxytetracycline [Terramycin] has been suspected of causing thrombocytopenia, either by depressing platelet formation or through an immunologic reaction. Tetracyclines are irritating when given intravenously and, with the possible exception of doxycycline, can cause thrombophlebitis.

Metabolic effects, which are rarely of clinical importance, include increased excretion of riboflavin, folic acid, and

N-methylnicotinamide. Large oral doses (2 to 4 g daily) of tetracyclines are reported to interfere with the absorption of iron.

Because there is evidence that tetracyclines interfere with the bactericidal action of the penicillins after concomitant parenteral administration, such use should be avoided. There is no definitive evidence that similar interference of sufficient magnitude to be important clinically occurs in ambulatory patients given the drug orally.

INDIVIDUAL EVALUATIONS

DEMECLOCYCLINE
[Declomycin]

DEMECLOCYCLINE HYDROCHLORIDE
[Declomycin Hydrochloride]

The indications, actions, and adverse effects of demeclocycline are comparable to those of the other tetracyclines (see the Introduction). Its half-life (12 hours) is somewhat longer than several of the other agents in this group (see the Table); therefore, longer intervals between doses produce equivalent therapeutic blood levels, resulting in less gastrointestinal irritation. The only commonly used tetracyclines with a longer half-life are doxycycline and minocycline.

Demeclocycline is the tetracycline most frequently associated with photosensitivity reactions at therapeutic dosage levels and, possibly, with the largest number of anaphylactoid reactions, although allergic reactions to all tetracyclines are rare. Demeclocycline has been implicated in a few cases of nephrogenic diabetes insipidus, all of which were reversible within four weeks after medication was discontinued; degradation products resulting from improper or prolonged storage may have caused the disorder.

ROUTE, USUAL DOSAGE, AND PREPARATIONS. *Oral: Adults,* 600 mg daily in two or four divided doses.*Infants and young children* (under special circumstances, see the Introduction) and *children over 8 years,* 6 to 12 mg/kg of body weight daily in two or four divided doses; in severe infections, the dose may be doubled for the first few days. Therapy should be continued for at least 24 to 48 hours after signs and symptoms have subsided. For streptococcal infections, therapy should be continued for at least ten days.

DEMECLOCYCLINE:
Declomycin (Lederle). Syrup 75 mg/5 ml (strength expressed in terms of the hydrochloride salt).
DEMECLOCYCLINE HYDROCHLORIDE:
Declomycin Hydrochloride (Lederle). Capsules 150 mg; tablets 75, 150, and 300 mg.

DOXYCYCLINE CALCIUM
[Vibramycin Calcium]

DOXYCYCLINE HYCLATE
[Vibramycin Hyclate]

DOXYCYCLINE MONOHYDRATE
[Vibramycin Monohydrate]

Doxycycline, a synthetic analogue of oxytetracycline, has the same indications, actions, and adverse effects as other tetracyclines (see the Introduction). Its antimicrobial spectrum also is similar to that of other tetracyclines, although there is evidence that some strains of *Bacteroides fragilis* resistant to other tetracyclines are susceptible to doxycycline in vitro.

Doxycycline is almost completely absorbed from the gastrointestinal tract, with average peak serum levels of 2.6 mcg/ml achieved within two hours after ingestion of a single 200-mg dose. Therefore, parenteral administration is seldom necessary for rapid production of therapeutic blood levels. Intravenous administration is indicated primarily when oral administration is not feasible; infusion of 200 mg over a period of two hours will produce an average serum concentration of 3.6 mcg/ml.

Doxycycline is long-acting, having a serum half-life of 15 to 17 hours after the initial dose and about 22 hours after the fourth day of treatment. A small oral dose given once or twice daily produces therapeutic serum levels with little danger of dose-related side effects. Although most studies have shown no significant difference in the serum half-life of doxycycline in normal subjects compared to those with impaired renal function, there are some reports of increased serum urea nitrogen levels and prolonged half-life in patients with renal failure (eg, Morgan and Ribush, 1972). Nevertheless, many authorities believe that doxycycline can be administered to patients with renal insufficiency without exacerbating azotemia. Hemodialysis and peritoneal dialysis do not appreciably alter the serum half-life, whereas other drugs (eg, phenytoin, carbamazepine) may significantly decrease it.

The affinity of doxycycline for metallic ions may not be as great as that of other tetracyclines, since this drug can be given with food or milk without significant inactivation or impairment of absorption.

The toxic potential of doxycycline appears to be low, being largely limited to photosensitivity and allergic reactions. Gastrointestinal disturbances include nausea, vomiting, and diarrhea, which can be severe. Like other tetracyclines, doxycycline should not be administered to pregnant women and young children unless there is some compelling reason to do so.

ROUTES, USUAL DOSAGE, AND PREPARATIONS. *Oral*: *Adults and children over 8 years weighing 45 kg or more*, 100 mg at 12-hour intervals for two doses, followed by 100 mg once daily. *Children weighing less than 45 kg over 8 years of age or under special circumstances if younger* (see the Introduction), 5 mg/kg of body weight daily at 12-hour intervals. In severe infections in both adults and children, the initial daily dose may be given every 12 hours for as long as necessary. Therapy should be continued for at least 24 to 48 hours after signs and symptoms have subsided. For streptococcal infections, therapy should be continued for at least ten days.

DOXYCYCLINE CALCIUM:
Vibramycin Calcium (Pfizer). Syrup equivalent to 50 mg of base/5 ml.
DOXYCYCLINE HYCLATE:
Drug available generically: Capsules 50 and 100 mg.
Vibramycin Hyclate (Pfizer). Capsules equivalent to 50 and 100 mg of base.
DOXYCYCLINE MONOHYDRATE:
Vibramycin Monohydrate (Pfizer). Powder for suspension equivalent to 25 mg of base/5 ml after reconstitution.

Intravenous: *Adults and children over 8 years weighing 45 kg or more*, initially, 200 mg daily given in one or two infusions, followed by 100 to 200 mg daily (depending upon the severity of infection) in one or two infusions. *Children under 45 kg or 8 years* (only under special circumstances, see the Introduction), 5 mg/kg of body weight daily in one or two infusions.

DOXYCYCLINE HYCLATE:
Vibramycin Hyclate (Pfizer). Powder equivalent to 100 or 200 mg of base with ascorbic acid 480 or 960 mg, respectively.

METHACYCLINE HYDROCHLORIDE
[Rondomycin]

Methacycline is an analogue of oxytetracycline, and its indications, antibacterial spectrum, and degree of effectiveness are similar to those of the other tetracyclines (see the Introduction). Although it is not well absorbed from the gastrointestinal tract, the half-life is approximately 15 hours because of its slow renal excretion and poor distribution in body tissues. This must be considered when calculating dosage. Methacycline is extensively bound to plasma proteins (about 80%).

Methacycline produces the same adverse reactions as other tetracyclines, except that it is somewhat less likely to cause photosensitivity.

ROUTE, USUAL DOSAGE, AND PREPARATIONS. *Oral: Adults,* 600 mg daily in two or four doses; *children over 8 years,* 10 mg/kg of body weight daily in divided doses every 6 to 12 hours. Therapy should be continued for at least 24 to 48 hours after signs and symptoms have subsided. For streptococcal infections, therapy should be continued for at least ten days.

> *Rondomycin* (Wallace). Capsules 150 and 300 mg (equivalent to 140 mg and 280 mg of base, respectively); syrup 75 mg (equivalent to 70 mg of base)/5 ml.

MINOCYCLINE HYDROCHLORIDE
[Minocin]

Minocycline, a semisynthetic derivative of tetracycline, has some superiority over the earlier analogues. Its absorption from the gastrointestinal tract is rapid, nearly complete, and is usually not significantly affected by the presence of food or milk products. Serum levels are higher and persist longer than those of the other tetracyclines, except perhaps doxycycline.

Usual initial oral or intravenous doses of 200 mg produce a serum concentration of approximately 2.25 mcg/ml after one hour and 1.25 mcg/ml after 12 hours. In patients with normal renal function given a single dose of 200 mg, the serum half-life is approximately 15 to 20 hours, regardless of route. Intravenous use, therefore, is seldom necessary unless oral administration is not possible or desirable.

Nearly equal amounts are excreted in the urine after either oral or intravenous administration. Because minocycline appears to be more completely metabolized than other tetracyclines, the percentage of drug excreted unchanged is only one-half to one-third that of most other tetracyclines. Although the unchanged drug does not accumulate to the same extent as most other tetracyclines in patients with impaired renal function, even usual oral doses may lead to excessive systemic accumulation and possible hepatotoxicity in these patients. Under such conditions, lower than usual doses are indicated and, if therapy is prolonged, serum levels should be determined. Minocycline is widely distributed in the body.

The antimicrobial spectrum of minocycline is the same as that of other analogues (see the Introduction), although it has greater in vitro activity against many bacterial species. Thus, it is moderately active against some strains of staphylococci resistant to tetracycline, but this effect has not been demonstrated clinically. It has been effective in infections caused by *Mycobacterium marinum.* Clinical trials comparing the sensitivity of minocycline and tetracycline showed that therapeutic results were as good or probably better with the newer analogue and the incidence of side effects was lower. The decreased frequency of administration for minocycline was considered to be a definite advantage.

Adverse reactions are similar to those produced by other tetracyclines. Gastrointestinal disturbances (nausea, vomiting) are observed most commonly. Hypersensitivity reactions in the form of rash, fever, or both occur. Pigmentation of the skin and mucous membranes has been reported. Minocycline apparently has a greater propensity to cause transient, reversible vestibular reactions (dizziness, vertigo, ataxia) than other tetracyclines. Because the incidence of these reactions has not been precisely determined, the United States Public Health Service recommends that minocycline not be used for the prophylaxis of meningococcal disease, although there is evidence that it may be effective for this use. Patients should be informed of the possibility of vestibular side effects and advised to take all precautions if dizziness or vertigo occurs.

Photosensitivity has been reported very rarely. As with all tetracyclines, minocycline may affect the teeth and skeletal development in children and should not be used unless essential during pregnancy and early childhood. Minocycline should be prescribed cautiously, usually in reduced doses, in patients with renal or hepatic insufficiency.

ROUTES, USUAL DOSAGE, AND PREPARATIONS. *Oral*: *Adults and children over 12 years*, 200 mg initially, followed by 100 mg every 12 hours. *Children 8 to 12 years*, 4 mg/kg of body weight daily in divided doses every 12 hours. Therapy should be continued for at least 24 to 48 hours after signs and symptoms have subsided. For streptococcal infections, therapy should be continued for at least ten days.

> *Minocin* (Lederle). Capsules equivalent to 50 and 100 mg of base; syrup equivalent to 50 mg of base/5 ml.

Intravenous: *Adults*, 200 mg, followed by 100 mg every 12 hours (maximum, 400 mg daily). The drug should be diluted before administration (see the manufacturer's literature). *Children over 8 years*, 4 mg/kg of body weight initially, followed by 2 mg/kg every 12 hours.

> *Minocin* (Lederle). Powder equivalent to 100 mg of base.

OXYTETRACYCLINE
[Terramycin]

OXYTETRACYCLINE CALCIUM
[Terramycin Calcium]

OXYTETRACYCLINE HYDROCHLORIDE
[Terramycin Hydrochloride]

This agent has a spectrum of activity similar to that of the other tetracyclines and it may produce similar adverse reactions (see the Introduction).

Gastrointestinal disturbances, particularly diarrhea, are believed to occur more frequently with therapeutic doses of oxytetracycline than with other tetracyclines. Also, it has been claimed that oxytetracycline is the least likely to cause discoloration of the teeth when administered to pregnant women and children during odontogenesis; when staining does occur, it is said that the color is creamy white in contrast to the yellowish brown or dark discoloration produced by other tetracyclines. None of these claims have been substantiated positively.

ROUTES, USUAL DOSAGE, AND PREPARATIONS. *Oral*: *Adults*, 1 to 2 g daily in four equally divided doses, depending upon the severity of the infection; a total of 2 to 4 g may be given to severely ill patients. *Children over 8 years* (except under special circumstances, see the Introduction), 25 to 50 mg/kg of body weight daily in four equally divided doses.

> OXYTETRACYCLINE:
> Drug available generically: Capsules 250 mg.
> *Terramycin* [*base*] (Pfizer). Tablets 250 mg.
> OXYTETRACYCLINE CALCIUM:
> *Terramycin* [*calcium*] (Pfizer). Syrup equivalent to 125 mg of base/5 ml.
> OXYTETRACYCLINE HYDROCHLORIDE:
> Drug available generically: Capsules 250 mg.
> *Terramycin* [*hydrochloride*] (Pfizer). Capsules equivalent to 125 and 250 mg of base.

Intramuscular: Intramuscular therapy should be reserved for situations in which oral or intravenous therapy is not feasible. Injection by this route can be extremely painful. *Adults*, 250 mg once every 24 hours or 300 mg in divided doses at 8- to 12-hour intervals, depending upon the severity of illness; *children over 8 years* (except under special circumstances, see the Introduction), 15 to 25 mg/kg of body weight daily up to a maximum of 250 mg in a single daily injection. The dosage may be given at 8- to 12-hour intervals.

> OXYTETRACYCLINE:
> *Terramycin* [*base*] (Pfizer). Solution 50 mg/ml in 2 and 10 ml containers and 125 mg/ml in 2 ml containers with lidocaine 2%.

Intravenous: *Adults*, 500 mg to 1 g daily in two doses (250 mg dissolved in 10 ml of sterile water for injection and then diluted to a final volume of 100 ml with 5% dextrose or sodium chloride injection). *Children over 8 years* (except under special circumstances, see the Introduction), 10 to 20 mg/kg of body weight daily in two divided doses; the drug is diluted as described for adults.

> OXYTETRACYCLINE HYDROCHLORIDE:
> *Terramycin* [*hydrochloride*] (Pfizer). Powder 250 and 500 mg with ascorbic acid.

TETRACYCLINE
[Achromycin V, Panmycin, Robitet, SK-Tetracycline, Sumycin, Tetracyn]

TETRACYCLINE HYDROCHLORIDE
[Achromycin, Achromycin V, Panmycin, Robitet, Sumycin, Tetracyn]

TETRACYCLINE PHOSPHATE COMPLEX
[Tetrex]

Tetracycline is the most widely used member of its class and is available as the base, hydrochloride salt, and phosphate complex. Tetracycline hydrochloride is one of the analogues of choice for parenteral administration. Studies have shown that it penetrates tissues better than oxytetracycline and causes less frequent and less severe gastrointestinal disturbances. The phosphate complex was developed in an attempt to increase gastrointestinal absorption, but there is no definitive evidence that it is any more effective than other oral forms when administered in comparable doses.

All forms of tetracycline have essentially the same spectrum of antibacterial activity, and their effectiveness is similar to that of the other tetracyclines. The incidence of serious toxicity is relatively low (see the Introduction). Tetracycline appears to be one of the analogues least likely to cause photosensitivity. When given in a dose of 250 mg every six hours, therapeutic serum levels (2 to 4 mcg/ml) may not be attained until the second or third day of treatment (or sometimes longer); steady state serum concentrations usually are reached after multiple doses within five half-lives. Therefore, it is often desirable to initiate treatment with a large loading dose or to prescribe a larger than usual maintenance dose for the first two days of therapy. The serum half-life of tetracycline is 8 to 10 hours.

ROUTES, USUAL DOSAGE, AND PREPARATIONS. *Oral: Adults,* 250 to 500 mg every six hours; the larger dose should be reserved for severe infections. *Children over 8 years,* 25 to 50 mg/kg of body weight daily in four divided doses. Therapy should be continued for at least 24 to 48 hours after signs and symptoms have subsided. Streptococcal infections should be treated for at least ten days.

TETRACYCLINE (strengths expressed in terms of the hydrochloride salt):
Drug available generically: Syrup 125 mg/5 ml.
Achromycin V (Lederle), *Panmycin* (Upjohn), *Robitet* (Robins), *SK-Tetracycline* (Smith Kline & French), *Tetracyn* (Pfipharmecs). Syrup 125 mg/5 ml.
Sumycin (Squibb). Syrup (buffered with potassium metaphosphate) 125 mg/5 ml.
TETRACYCLINE HYDROCHLORIDE:
Drug available generically: Capsules 250 and 500 mg.
Achromycin V (Lederle), *Tetracyn* (Pfipharmecs). Capsules 250 and 500 mg.
Panmycin (Upjohn). Capsules 250 mg; tablets 250 and 500 mg.
Robitet (Robins), *Sumycin* (Squibb). Capsules, tablets 250 and 500 mg.

Additional Trademarks.
Bristacycline (Bristol), *Cyclopar* (Parke, Davis).
TETRACYCLINE PHOSPHATE COMPLEX (strengths expressed in terms of the hydrochloride salt):
Tetrex (Bristol). Capsules 250 and 500 mg.

Intramuscular: Intramuscular administration should be reserved for situations in which oral or intravenous therapy is not feasible. Injection can be extremely painful. *Adults and children over 8 years weighing more than 40 kg,* 250 mg once every 24 hours or 300 mg in divided doses at 8- to 12-hour intervals. *Children weighing less than 40 kg over 8 years or under special circumstances if younger* (see the Introduction), 15 to 25 mg/kg of body weight daily up to a maximum of 250 mg in a single daily injection or in divided doses at 8- to 12-hour intervals.

Intravenous: Adults, 250 to 500 mg twice daily at 12-hour intervals (maximum, 500 mg every six hours); *children over 8 years* (except under special circumstances, see the Introduction), 20 to 30 mg/kg of body weight daily in divided doses every 8 to 12 hours. Contents of the vial should be diluted before administration (see the manufacturers' literature) and injected at a rate not exceeding 2 mg/min (normally a two-hour infusion). Parenteral therapy is indicated only when oral therapy is inadequate or not tolerated. Oral therapy should be instituted as soon as possible.

TETRACYCLINE HYDROCHLORIDE:
Achromycin [*hydrochloride*] (Lederle), *Tetracyn* [*hydrochloride*] (Pfizer). Powder (intramuscular) 100 and 250 mg with procaine hydrochloride, magnesium chloride, and ascorbic acid; powder (intravenous) 250 and 500 mg with ascorbic acid.

Topical: See Chapter 24, Ocular Anti-infective and Anti-inflammatory Agents, and Chapter 61, Dermatologic Preparations.

MIXTURES

There is little justification for the use of fixed combinations of tetracyclines and other agents. The convenience of such products may be greatly outweighed by the dangers of inappropriate or excessive dosage (especially in small or elderly patients or in those with impaired hepatic or renal function), hypersensitivity to one agent in the combination, or administration of superfluous drugs. The following preparations are evaluated briefly for the sake of completeness, and no recommendation is made for any of them.

AZOTREX

UROBIOTIC

These products contain a tetracycline, a sulfonamide, and a urinary analgesic and are promoted for the treatment of urinary tract infections, although tetracyclines are not primary drugs of choice for this indication. Since no synergistic action has been demonstrated between the tetracyclines and sulfonamides, the use of either agent alone is preferred. Phenazopyridine is contraindicated in patients with renal insufficiency and hepatitis.

Because proof of efficacy is lacking, no dosage recommendation is made.

Azotrex (Bristol). Each capsule contains tetracycline phosphate complex equivalent to tet-

racycline hydrochloride 125 mg, sulfamethizole 250 mg, and phenazopyridine hydrochloride 50 mg.

Urobiotic (Roerig). Each capsule contains oxytetracycline hydrochloride equivalent to oxytetracycline 250 mg, sulfamethizole 250 mg, and phenazopyridine hydrochloride 50 mg.

ACHROSTATIN V

DECLOSTATIN

MYSTECLIN-F

TERRASTATIN

TETRASTATIN

These mixtures contain tetracycline and an antifungal agent (amphotericin B or nystatin). They are designed to prevent the overgrowth of intestinal fungi, but the rationale for use of these fixed-ratio combinations is weak. Intestinal candidosis does not occur frequently, and there is no clinical evidence that the routine prophylactic administration of an antifungal agent reduces its incidence. Furthermore, in most therapeutic regimens using these mixtures, the fixed combinations provide the minimal or less than the minimal dosage of the antifungal agent. If use of an antifungal drug is indicated to treat intestinal candidosis in a patient receiving an antibacterial agent, it is preferable to give the antibacterial and antifungal compounds separately.

Because proof of efficacy is lacking, no dosage recommendation is made.

Achrostatin V (Lederle). Each capsule contains tetracycline hydrochloride 250 mg and nystatin 250,000 units.

Declostatin (Lederle). Each capsule contains demeclocycline hydrochloride 150 mg and nystatin 250,000 units; each tablet contains demeclocycline hydrochloride 300 mg and nystatin 500,000 units.

Mysteclin-F (Squibb). Each capsule contains tetracycline equivalent to tetracycline hydrochloride 125 or 250 mg and amphotericin B 25 or 50 mg; each 5 ml of syrup contains tetracycline equivalent to tetracycline hydrochloride 125 mg and amphotericin B 25 mg. Preparations buffered with potassium metaphosphate.

Terrastatin (Pfizer). Each capsule contains oxytetracycline 250 mg and nystatin 250,000 units.

Tetrastatin (Pfipharmecs). Each capsule contains tetracycline hydrochloride 250 mg and nystatin 250,000 units.

Selected References

Topicycline: Topical tetracycline for acne. *Med Lett Drugs Ther* 20:35-36, 1978.

Ad Hoc Committee on Use of Antibiotics in Dermatology, American Academy of Dermatology: Systemic antibiotics for treatment of acne vulgaris: Efficacy and safety. *Arch Dermatol* 111:1630-1636, 1975.

Committee on Drugs, American Academy of Pediatrics: Requiem for tetracyclines. *Pediatrics* 55:142-143, 1975.

Kurylowicz W (ed): *Antibiotics: A Critical Review.* Warsaw, Polish Medical Publishers, 1976, 125-127.

Morgan T, Ribush N: Effect of oxytetracycline and doxycycline on protein metabolism. *Med J Aust* 1:55-58, 1972.

Ory EM: Tetracyclines, in Kagan BM (ed): *Antimicrobial Therapy*, ed 2. Philadelphia, WB Saunders Company, 1974, 95-104.

Pratt WB: *Chemotherapy of Infection.* New York, Oxford University Press, 1977, 152-156.

Sack DA, et al: Prophylactic doxycycline for travelers' diarrhea: Results of prospective double-blind study of Peace Corps volunteers in Kenya. *N Engl J Med* 298:758-763, 1978.

Siegel D: Tetracyclines: New look at old antibiotic: I. Clinical pharmacology. II. Clinical uses. *NY State J Med* 78:950-956, 1115-1120, 1978.

Aminoglycosides | 74

The aminoglycoside antibiotics are so named because they are composed of amino sugars connected by glycosidic linkages. Most aminoglycosides are prepared by natural fermentation from various species of *Streptomyces*. The exceptions are gentamicin [Garamycin], which is fermented from *Micromonospora purpurea*, and amikacin [Amikin], the first semisynthetic aminoglycoside, which is produced by the chemical modification of kanamycin (Bint, 1978). Other drugs in this group include streptomycin, kanamycin [Kantrex], neomycin [Mycifradin, Myciguent, Neobiotic], paromomycin [Humatin], tobramycin [Nebcin], and spectinomycin [Trobicin]. The last compound is not discussed in this chapter because its chemical configuration and mechanism of action differ from the other compounds in this class (see Chapter 76, Miscellaneous Antibacterial Agents). The aminoglycosides have a similar antibacterial spectrum and toxicity profile.

The aminoglycosides are bactericidal. They appear to act on the 30S ribosomal subunit to stop synthesis of bacterial cell protein and distort the fidelity of messenger ribonucleic acid (mRNA) translation of the genetic code (Pratt, 1977). Misreading the code originally was thought to account for the lethality of the aminoglycosides, but subsequent investigation does not appear to substantiate this concept. Their exact bactericidal mechanism of action is unknown.

Bacterial Spectrum and Indications

The aminoglycosides are active against gram-negative rods, principally sensitive strains of *Enterobacteriaceae* (including *Proteus*), *Pseudomonas*, and *Serratia*. Gentamicin, tobramycin, and amikacin are particularly active against *P. aeruginosa* and amikacin is often effective against gentamicin- and tobramycin-resistant strains. *Neisseria gonorrhoeae* and *N. meningitidis* also are susceptible to some aminoglycosides, but these drugs are not used to treat infections caused by these gram-negative cocci, with the exception of spectinomycin, a drug that has a specific indication for treating gonorrhea under certain circumstances. Several genera of organisms (eg, *Salmonella*, *Shigella*) are reported to be susceptible to the aminoglycosides both in vitro and in vivo but, because less toxic antibacterial agents with equal or greater clinical effectiveness are available, the aminoglycosides are seldom, if ever, used to treat diseases caused by these organisms.

Some gram-positive organisms (most notably staphylococci) are inhibited by the aminoglycoside antibiotics; however, there is very limited clinical experience with the use of these antibiotics as sole agents in the treatment of serious staphylococcal infections. Other antibiotics with less potential toxicity (penicillins, cephalosporins, and clindamycin) are available to treat these infections and the aminoglycoside antibiotics are used only in unusual clinical circumstances. The gram-positive rods of *Bacillus* and *Corynebacterium* are sensitive to gentamicin, tobramycin, and amikacin, but the aminoglycosides are not indicated for infections caused by these organisms.

Aminoglycoside antibiotics generally are inactive against streptococci (including the pneumococcus), clostridia, *Bacteroides*, *Rickettsia*, fungi, and viruses.

The aminoglycosides are indicated for the treatment of serious systemic infections caused by susceptible organisms. Gentamicin, kanamycin, tobramycin, and amikacin are used parenterally to treat bacteremias and pulmonary, soft tissue, osseous, or complicated urinary tract infections caused by sensitive gram-negative rods. Streptomycin is seldom administered alone except, possibly, in tularemia or bubonic plague. Because of a synergistic effect when given with certain other drugs, streptomycin often is used in combination regimens in the management of several diseases (eg, tuberculosis, endocarditis). Kanamycin also may be given with other drugs to treat tuberculosis.

Kanamycin, neomycin, and paromomycin may be given preoperatively to suppress some enteric aerobic flora. Because aminoglycosides reduce the bacterial production of ammonia, they have been used orally as adjuncts in the management of hepatic coma. They also have been administered orally in an effort to control diarrhea caused by enteropathogenic *Escherichia coli*, but definitive proof of efficacy is lacking. Paromomycin is directly amebicidal and is used alone or with other drugs in intestinal amebiasis (see Chapter 83, Antiprotozoal Agents).

Neomycin and gentamicin have been applied topically to treat serious wound and burn infections caused by gram-negative organisms. Their effectiveness in serious wound infections appears to be minimal and the potential for the rapid development of drug-resistant organisms is considerable; this appears to obviate their usefulness in this setting. The use of neomycin as a peritoneal or pleural irrigant following surgery is of questionable value and may even be dangerous since sufficient drug may be absorbed to cause serious ototoxicity and nephrotoxicity (Davia et al, 1970; Masur et al, 1976; Weinstein et al, 1977) or neuromuscular blockade, particularly when used with muscle relaxants. In addition, neomycin is a common ingredient of over-the-counter preparations used for minor lacerations, abrasions, or burns, but its usefulness in such a setting has not been established.

Pharmacology

Poor absorption following oral administration is a general characteristic of the aminoglycosides. Nevertheless, oral administration of quantities sufficient to reduce bacterial flora in the bowel or to treat hepatic coma may result in detectable serum levels. Aminoglycosides are very poorly absorbed through intact skin, but considerable absorption may occur following their topical use on large denuded or burned areas. They also are absorbed in variable amounts during irrigation of closed body cavities or infected wounds. After intramuscular injection, almost 100% of an injected dose is absorbed.

The aminoglycosides are poorly bound to serum protein but are widely distributed throughout the body except for the central nervous system and the eye where penetration into the cerebrospinal fluid and the humors of the eye may be inadequate for antibacterial purposes, even in the presence of inflammation. Concentrations approximating 25% to 50% of serum levels are achieved in pleural and pericardial fluid. The aminoglycosides also cross the placenta (Weinstein et al, 1976), and effects upon the developing fetus or newborn infant must be considered if the mother is given an aminoglycoside during pregnancy.

The aminoglycosides are concentrated in the kidney where they are excreted unchanged by glomerular filtration; there is negligible tubular reabsorption. It has been recommended that the urine be alkalized for best results when treating urinary tract infections, but this procedure has not been proved to be clinically important except when using streptomycin. The other drugs in this class produce urinary concentrations higher than those found in the serum without alkalization. Therefore, use of this technique to augment the activity of the aminoglycosides appears to be neither practical nor necessary.

Resistance

Clinically, the most important type of bacterial resistance to the aminoglycosides develops when extrachromosomal genes (plasmids) are transmitted by bacterial conjugation. These plasmids govern the production of enzymes that inactivate the aminoglycosides by acetylation of amino groups or phosphorylation or adenylation of hydroxyl groups (Benveniste and Davies, 1973). There are, however, different patterns of drug resistance. Some enzymes will inactivate certain aminoglycosides but not others, and an enzyme that can chemically modify several aminoglycosides may inhibit the antibacterial action of some but not all of the drugs so modified. Thus, acetylation of kanamycin A and gentamicin will inactivate kanamycin but leave the modified gentamicin with substantial antibacterial activity. The clinical implications are obvious: If an organism becomes resistant to one aminoglycoside, it is possible that another drug from this class may be an effective substitute. For example, *Pseudomonas* resistant to amikacin is often resistant to all of the aminoglycosides, whereas strains resistant to gentamicin or tobramycin may be sensitive to amikacin. Nevertheless, when cross resistance among aminoglycosides does occur, it usually is complete.

Bacterial resistance to streptomycin is common and develops rapidly. Resistance to the other aminoglycosides occurs at a much slower rate. Cross resistance between streptomycin and other aminoglycosides occurs frequently but is highly variable and unpredictable. Aminoglycoside-resistant bacteria are more likely to emerge when these antibiotics are widely used. Thus, it is advisable to consider the indications for their use carefully prior to selecting one of these agents.

Adverse Reactions and Precautions

All aminoglycosides are potentially toxic to both branches of the eighth cranial nerve. There is evidence (Matz et al, 1965; Shapiro, 1968; Root and Hierholzer, 1978; and others) that sensory receptor portions of the inner ear (eg, hair cells of the cochlea) are affected and not the nerve itself, but the end result can be the same as if the nerve were destroyed. Ototoxicity may be manifested as tinnitus or any degree of hearing loss from temporary inability to detect certain (usually high frequency) tones to total, permanent deafness. In fact, tinnitus or a feeling of "fullness" in the ear may be early signs of potential hearing loss. Patients receiving aminoglycosides should be instructed to report such sensations as soon as they occur. If practicable, an audiometric test should be performed regularly in patients receiving an aminoglycoside since, by the time hearing loss can be detected by inability of the patient to react to normal conversational tones, considerable permanent damage can have occurred. This is obviously more important in patients taking large doses and/or long-term therapy than for those receiving usual therapeutic doses for short periods. Symptoms of vestibular toxicity include dizziness and vertigo; if toxicity is severe, ataxia and a Meniere-like syndrome may be seen.

The ototoxic potential of the aminoglycosides depends upon the characteristics of the drug, magnitude of the dose, duration of therapy, renal function of the patient, and, perhaps, other parameters such as age and individual susceptibility. Some aminoglycosides (eg, kanamycin) impair auditory acuity most frequently, while others (eg, streptomycin, gentamicin) primarily affect vestibular function. All of these agents affect both functions if the concentration attained in the inner ear is high enough and maintained for a long enough period of time. Evidence exists that ethacrynic acid [Edecrin] and furosemide

[Lasix] potentiate the ototoxicity of the aminoglycosides (Cooperman and Rubin, 1973). This effect is particularly prominent in patients with uremia (Mathog and Klein, 1969). If loss of hearing or diminished balance acuity is not extensive, normal function may return upon discontinuance of the drug.

Nephrotoxicity may occur (Brewer, 1977) during or following use of an aminoglycoside antibiotic and is most often manifested as transient proteinuria or increased serum creatinine level. Severe azotemia may be observed. In general, nephrotoxic reactions are not serious and are usually completely reversible upon cessation of therapy; they should not be deterrents to the use of these drugs. Nevertheless, aminoglycosides should not be used without a clear indication and routine serum creatinine determinations are warranted during therapy. In addition to furosemide and ethacrynic acid, some cephalosporins (eg, cephaloridine, cephalothin) and, possibly, cyclopropane or methoxyflurane may potentiate the nephrotoxicity of the aminoglycosides (Avery, 1976), particularly when large doses are administered. Accordingly, concomitant use of these drugs should be avoided unless unusual clinical circumstances warrant the risk.

The aminoglycoside antibiotics rarely may cause neuromuscular blockade that can lead to paralysis and potentially fatal respiratory arrest. Apnea may occur after rapid (bolus) intravenous injection, administration to patients with myasthenia gravis, or concomitant use of general anesthetics or neuromuscular blocking agents such as tubocurarine or succinylcholine. The risk is greatest after intravenous administration, but a curare-like paralysis also may occur following intramuscular injection or absorption from local sites in patients already compromised by other drugs or diseases that affect neuromuscular transmission. The blockade usually can be counteracted by the prompt administration of a drug with anticholinesterase effects (eg, neostigmine); if there is no (or minimal) response, calcium gluconate may be given.

Allergic or local hypersensitivity reactions have been observed occasionally following use of aminoglycosides. Usually these reactions are serious only in patients previously sensitized to an aminoglycoside or with a history of allergy. Changes in reticulocyte count, transaminase (SGOT·or SGPT) levels, and granulocytopenia have been reported.

Superinfection with fungi or other organisms occur during therapy.

Dosage must be adjusted in patients with impaired renal function, in azotemic patients on dialysis (aminoglycosides are dialyzable molecules), and in neonates. Accurate measurement of drug blood level samples obtained at proper intervals after parenteral administration is particularly useful for adjusting the maintenance dosage. Although this modification is desirable, it must be remembered that the serum level measurement is influenced by many factors. For example, peak serum levels are obtained at different times following intravenous or intramuscular administration. Furthermore, the duration of an intravenous dose must be known in order to interpret the peak value. Although some investigators have reported that serum levels of certain aminoglycosides are reasonably predictable, unexpected variations can occur, and it is advisable to monitor peak and valley serum levels. The physician also should be familiar with the antibiotic assay methods used in a particular hospital and the factors that may affect its accuracy.

If aminoglycoside serum levels cannot be measured periodically, dosage guidelines based upon sound pharmacokinetic principles can be used to assist in determining the dosage of these antibiotics. Gentamicin, tobramycin, kanamycin, and amikacin are similar pharmacokinetically and a single dosage guideline may be applied to each (Sarubbi and Hull, 1978). The guideline suggested (see the evaluation on Amikacin Sulfate) is actually a modification of the principle of replacing a percentage of the loading dose at the half-life. It allows for administration of the maintenance dose at convenient intervals (8, 12, and 24 hours), which circumvents the disadvantage of awkward dosing intervals and the potential for long subtherapeutic periods sometimes associated with certain other dosage schedules. Thus, the physician can select an appropriate loading dose and plan maintenance doses based on an estimated body weight-corrected creatinine clearance value. This method (as is true for other dosage guidelines) does not obviate the need to monitor antibiotic serum levels, but it does allow the physician to plot a rational treatment course if results of blood level measurements are pending or are unavailable. Other acceptable dosage schedules (some using nomographs) also are available.

Aminoglycosides cross the placenta, and streptomycin has been associated with functional eighth nerve damage in infants born to mothers given the drug during pregnancy (Conway and Birt, 1965). Although there is no conclusive evidence that the aminoglycosides are teratogenic or cause ototoxicity or nephrotoxicity in the fetus, it must be assumed that such effects are possible. These agents should be given to pregnant women only in the presence of life-threatening infections that do not respond to other antibiotics.

INDIVIDUAL EVALUATIONS

GENTAMICIN SULFATE
[Garamycin]

Gentamicin	R	R´
C$_1$	CH$_3$	CH$_3$
C$_2$	CH$_3$	H
C$_{1A}$	H	H

Gentamicin sulfate is a mixture of three closely related antibacterial agents obtained from cultures of *Micromonospora purpurea*. Preparations are available for both parenteral and topical use; the drug is not given orally to treat systemic infections since it is poorly absorbed from the gastrointestinal tract. It has been used orally as part of a prophylactic regimen in patients undergoing chemotherapy for cancer while the leukocyte count is less than or equal to 1,000. The in vitro antibacterial spectrum of gentamicin is similar to that of the other aminoglycosides. It is active against *Enterobacter aerogenes*, *Escherichia coli*, *Klebsiella pneumoniae*, *Proteus mirabilis*, indole-positive *Proteus* species, *Pseudomonas aeruginosa*, some species of *Neisseria* and nonpigmented *Serratia*, and *Shigella*. It has limited activity against some gram-positive bacteria (eg, staphylococci) and is rarely used as a single agent in the treatment of penicillin-resistant S. *aureus* infections since other antibiotics (eg, semisynthetic penicillins such as methicillin, nafcillin; clindamycin; cephalosporins; vancomycin) are usually preferred.

Microorganisms resistant to gentamicin include the pneumococcus, certain other streptococci, anaerobic bacteria (eg, clostridia, *Bacteroides*), *Rickettsia*, mycobacteria, fungi, and viruses.

Gentamicin is somewhat more potent on a weight basis than kanamycin or amikacin and it is more effective against *Pseudomonas aeruginosa* than kanamycin. Furthermore, it appears to be less ototoxic than kanamycin.

The systemic use of gentamicin should be restricted to the treatment of serious infections caused by susceptible gram-negative bacteria. If gram-negative bacterial septicemia is suspected, gentamicin may be given empirically while awaiting identification of the bacteria and determination of bacterial sensitivity. Demonstration of susceptibility is important, however, since not all strains of susceptible genera are sensitive to gentamicin.

Although mild infections caused by *P. aeruginosa* may be treated satisfactorily with carbenicillin alone (see Chapter 69,

Penicillins), severe infections are often treated with carbenicillin and gentamicin or tobramycin. These combinations often act in a synergistic fashion and may eliminate bacteria more rapidly and reduce the likelihood of the emergence of carbenicillin-resistant organisms. Combined use of carbenicillin and gentamicin has been useful in serious pulmonary, blood stream, and heart valve infections.

Serious problems associated with drug-resistant organisms have occurred after use of topical preparations. It is thus generally advisable not to use this drug topically, except in special circumstances for burns infected with *P. aeruginosa* or in certain eye infections (see Chapter 61, Dermatologic Preparations, and Chapter 24, Ocular Anti-infective and Anti-inflammatory Agents).

Bacterial resistance to gentamicin usually develops infrequently, although it may be more common in hospitals where the drug is used extensively. In fact, epidemics of gentamicin-resistant *Klebsiella*, *Serratia*, and *Proteus rettgeri* have been reported in hospitals. Resistance is most likely to occur following widespread topical use, and organisms frequently show cross resistance to other aminoglycosides (eg, kanamycin, tobramycin), but usually not to amikacin.

Gentamicin can cause renal damage as well as functional damage to both the cochlear and vestibular portions of the eighth cranial nerve, particularly in patients with impaired renal function, in those also receiving other potentially nephrotoxic or ototoxic drugs, or in patients taking certain potent diuretics (eg, furosemide, ethacrynic acid).

Auditory impairment is maximal in the high-tone range, although patients usually retain normal conversational hearing. Vestibular damage occurs more often than auditory damage, and complete loss of vestibular function has been reported. Ototoxicity is most likely to occur in patients with impaired renal function, especially those receiving gentamicin for longer periods or in larger doses than usually recommended. To minimize this possibility, the dosage schedule must be modified in proportion to the degree of renal impairment. Dosage adjustments are preferably made on the basis of gentamicin serum concentrations or use of an appropriate dosing guideline that incorporates the weight-corrected creatinine clearance of the patient. Peak therapeutic serum levels usually range from 4 to 10 mcg/ml 60 minutes after intramuscular injection or 30 minutes after intravenous infusion. Gentamicin serum concentrations exceeding 12 mcg/ml are generally considered to be hazardous. Trough concentrations (amount of drug present just prior to the next dose) should be less than 2 mcg/ml. The average half-life of gentamicin after intramuscular injection is slightly more than two hours in most individuals with normal renal function. Most of the antibiotic is excreted unchanged in the urine.

Infrequently reported adverse reactions include anemia, purpura, fever, hypotension, nausea, vomiting, arthralgia, and convulsions. Laboratory abnormalities include increased transaminase (SGOT, SGPT) and unbound serum bilirubin levels.

This drug is incompatible with heparin in solution with which it reacts to form a precipitate. Gentamicin acts synergistically with several penicillins, particularly carbenicillin, but is slowly inactivated when the two drugs are mixed and allowed to stand. Because gentamicin is incompatible with certain other drugs as well, it usually should not be premixed with any drug (there are some exceptions, see Trissel, 1977), but should be administered separately using the recommended route of administration and usual dosage schedule. For other interactions, see the Introduction.

ROUTES, USUAL DOSAGE, AND PREPARATIONS. *Intramuscular, Intravenous: Patients with normal renal function: Adults,* 3 to 5 mg/kg of body weight daily in three equally divided doses every eight hours. The larger dose is used only for life-threatening infections. *Children,* 6 to 7.5 mg/kg daily in three equally divided doses every eight hours. *Infants 1 week or older,* 7.5 mg/kg daily in three equally divided doses every eight hours. *Premature or full-term neonates less than 1 week*, 5 mg/kg daily in two divided doses every 12 hours.

Patients with impaired renal function: Whenever possible, the gentamicin serum concentration should be obtained to help determine dosage. If serum levels are unavailable or unreliable, adults may be given gentamicin according to an appropriate dosing schedule that takes into consideration the ideal body weight-corrected creatinine clearance and extension of dosing interval to avoid unnecessarily elevated trough levels of the drug. For one suggested chart, see the dosage statement in the evaluation on Amikacin Sulfate.

Patients undergoing hemodialysis: *Adults*, in most cases, 1 to 1.7 mg/kg of body weight (depending upon the severity of infection) given at the end of each six-hour dialysis period. *Children*, 2 mg/kg at the end of each six-hour dialysis period. It is of considerable importance to measure gentamicin serum levels in patients undergoing dialysis.

When administered intravenously, gentamicin can be given in 5% dextrose or isotonic sodium chloride injection. The dose should be administered over a period of approximately 30 minutes. The total duration of therapy by either the intramuscular or intravenous route generally should not exceed ten days.

> *Garamycin* (Schering). Solution 10 (pediatric) and 40 mg/ml in 2 ml containers and 40 mg/ml in 1.5 and 2 ml disposable syringes (strengths expressed in terms of the base).

Topical: The availability of numerous alternative topical agents obviates the need for topical application of gentamicin except in rare situations (eg, certain infections of the eye). When use is appropriate, a small quantity of ointment or cream is carefully applied to the lesion three or four times daily. The treated area may be covered with a loose gauze dressing if indicated. For ophthalmic use, see Chapter 24, Ocular Anti-infective and Anti-inflammatory Agents.

> *Garamycin* (Schering). Cream and ointment equivalent to 0.1% of base in 15 g containers.

TOBRAMYCIN SULFATE
[Nebcin]

This water-soluble aminoglycoside derived from *Steptomyces tenebrarius* is closely related to gentamicin in its bacterial spectrum, degree of effectiveness, and toxicity. Tobramycin is primarily employed in the treatment of moderate to severe infections caused by susceptible aerobic gram-negative bacilli, including strains of *Pseudomonas aeruginosa*, *Klebsiella*, *Enterobacter*, indole-positive and indole-negative *Proteus*, *Citrobacter* species, and *Providencia*. Tobramycin generally appears to be more active than gentamicin against *P. aeruginosa* (Laxer et al, 1975) and it may be the aminoglycoside of choice for such infections. However, it is usually less active than gentamicin against *Serratia*. Tobramycin is not considered a drug of choice against staphylococci and such organisms as streptococci (including the pneumococcus). Resistant organisms include anaerobic bacteria (eg, clostridia, *Bacteroides*), rickettsiae, fungi, and viruses.

Tobramycin, alone or in combination with other antibiotics, such as the penicillins or cephalosporins, is used to treat infections of the blood stream, soft tissue (including burns), bone, lung, and urinary tract. As with all aminoglycosides, bacterial resistance can develop and cross resistance between tobramycin and other related agents has been noted.

Although animal studies indicate that gentamicin is more ototoxic than tobramycin, the two drugs appear to have a similar potential to cause eighth cranial nerve damage clinically (Bendush et al, 1977). Both auditory and vestibular function can be affected; the vestibular portion is more susceptible, particularly if renal function is impaired or large doses are given for long periods. Symptoms include dizziness, vertigo, tinnitus, and hearing loss, usually in the high frequency range.

Tobramycin also is potentially nephrotoxic. Renal injury usually is reflected as rising serum creatinine levels and may actually progress to nonoliguric renal failure. Nephrotoxicity is particularly likely to develop in patients with pre-existing renal impairment. These effects are potentiated by other nephrotoxic drugs and some diuretics (eg, ethacrynic acid, furosemide). For other interactions, see the Introduction.

Adverse reactions reported infrequently are anemia, granulocytopenia, thrombocytopenia, fever, rash, pruritus, urticaria, nausea, vomiting, headache, and lethargy. Increased levels of serum transaminase (SGOT, SGPT) and bilirubin also have been observed. Overgrowth of nonsusceptible organisms can occur when tobramycin is given for long periods.

ROUTES, USUAL DOSAGE, AND PREPARATIONS. *Intramuscular, Intravenous: Adults, children, and older infants with normal renal function*, 3 to 5 mg/kg of body weight daily according to the severity of the infection. To prevent toxicity due to excessive blood levels, dosage should not exceed 5 mg/kg/ day unless serum levels are monitored. The total daily dose is usually given in equally divided amounts every eight hours. *Neonates up to 1 week of age with normal renal function*, up to 4 mg/kg daily in two divided doses every 12 hours. The duration of therapy should not exceed seven to ten days.

For *adults and children with impaired renal function*, dosage modification is indicated. Tobramycin serum levels should be monitored if possible or the aminoglycoside dosing chart proposed by Sarubbi and Hull (see the dosage statement in the evaluation on Amikacin Sulfate) can be used as a guide for adults.

> *Nebcin* (Lilly). Solution 10 (pediatric) and 40 mg/ml in 2 ml containers and 40 mg/ml in 1.5 and 2 ml disposable syringes (strengths expressed in terms of the base).

KANAMYCIN SULFATE
[Kantrex]

The in vitro antibacterial spectrum of kanamycin is similar to that of other aminoglycosides. This antibiotic once demonstrated considerable activity against most aerobic gram-negative bacilli, but a steady increase in the number of kanamycin-resistant organisms in recent years has resulted in a substantial reduction in the efficacy of this drug. However, many strains of *Escherichia coli, Enterobacter, Klebsiella*, and *Proteus* and mycobacteria have remained susceptible. Organisms that become resistant to kanamycin may demonstrate cross resistance to other aminoglycoside antibiotics. Certain microorganisms, among which are the streptococci (including the pneumococcus), *Pseudomonas aeruginosa*, anaerobic bacteria, rickettsiae, fungi, and viruses, should be considered resistant. Kanamycin is less active on a weight basis than gentamicin or tobramycin and appears to have a greater potential for causing ototoxicity than either of these drugs.

Kanamycin is used parenterally to treat infections caused by susceptible organisms and orally to diminish the aerobic bacterial content of the gastrointestinal tract preoperatively and to treat enteritis caused by susceptible organisms. It reduces bacterial production of ammonia and may be useful in cirrhotic patients with gastrointestinal bleeding in whom hepatic coma is a threat. Although intestinal absorption is poor, caution must be exercised when this drug is given orally to patients with renal insufficiency, since some absorption occurs and toxic levels may result.

As with all aminoglycosides, parenteral use of kanamycin may be associated with ototoxicity, particularly if other potentially ototoxic agents are given concurrently. This complication, which may affect both cochlear and vestibular function, has been particularly noted in elderly patients and in those with impaired renal function. Ototoxicity has been related to overall dosage and duration of therapy, as well as to blood levels. Excessive amounts of drug given for either short or long periods, as well as usual therapeutic amounts administered for prolonged periods, probably increase the incidence of ototoxicity. Kanamycin should be discontinued if tinnitus, dizziness, or vertigo occurs, and it may be contraindicated in patients with pre-existing drug-induced damage of the eighth cranial nerve. For other interactions, see the Introduction.

Hypersensitivity reactions (eg, fever, pruritus, rash, eosinophilia), renal damage, headache, and paresthesias have been reported. Stomatitis, diarrhea, and proctitis may result from oral administration. Pain and, occasionally, sterile abscesses may occur when kanamycin is injected.

ROUTES, USUAL DOSAGE, AND PREPARATIONS. Daily parenteral doses of 15 mg/kg of body weight probably should not be exceeded; the maximum daily dose for adults is 1.5 g. Dosage for adults with impaired renal function is determined on the basis of serum levels or according to an appropriate dosage schedule. One such schedule proposed by Sarubbi and Hull appears in the dosage

statement in the evaluation on Amikacin Sulfate.

Intramuscular: *Adults and children* may be given a total daily dose of 15 mg/kg of body weight daily in two equally divided doses every 12 hours (occasionally, an 8-hour interval is used). *Infants* may be given kanamycin according to the following table*: (The total daily dose in mg is given in two or three divided doses at 8- or 12-hour intervals.)

| WEIGHT | | DAILY DOSAGE |
Lb	Kg	(mg)
2.2	1.00	15.0
2.8	1.25	18.8
3.3	1.50	22.5
3.9	1.75	26.2
4.4	2.00	30.0
5.0	2.25	33.8
5.5	2.50	37.5
6.0	2.75	41.2
6.6	3.00	45.0
7.7	3.50	52.5
8.8	4.00	60.0
9.9	4.50	67.5
11.0	5.00	75.0

*Data from manufacturer's literature.

Intravenous: When it is necessary to administer kanamycin intravenously, the drug should be diluted to 2.5 mg/ml in normal sodium chloride injection or 5% dextrose injection and infused at a rate of 2 to 3 ml/min.

Kantrex (Bristol). Solution 37.5 (pediatric) and 250 mg/ml in 2 ml containers and 333 mg/ml in 3 ml containers (strengths expressed in terms of the base).

Oral (not for systemic effects): *Adults*, up to 8 g daily in divided doses (eg, for reducing the bacterial flora in the bowel, 1 g every hour for four hours, followed by 1 g every six hours for up to 48 hours). *Infants and children*, 50 mg/kg of body weight daily in four to six divided doses for five to seven days.

Kantrex (Bristol). Capsules 500 mg (strengths expressed in terms of the base).

AMIKACIN SULFATE
[Amikin]

Amikacin, the first semisynthetic aminoglycoside, is a water-soluble acylated derivative of kanamycin A. This chemical manipulation prevents inactivating bacterial enzymes from gaining access to susceptible hydroxyl and amino groups on the molecule, thereby making amikacin resistant to most of the enzymes that inactivate kanamycin, gentamicin, and tobramycin. Amikacin is susceptible to only one of the nine well-characterized aminoglycoside-inactivating enzymes, an acetyltransferase.

Amikacin is active in vitro against a wide variety of gram-negative organisms, including some species that are resistant to gentamicin and tobramycin. Susceptible organisms include *Escherichia coli*, *Pseudomonas aeruginosa*, indole-positive and indole-negative *Proteus*, *Klebsiella pneumoniae*, *Enterobacter* species, *Serratia* species, *Acinetobacter*, *Citrobacter freundii*, and *Providencia stuartii*. Gram-positive penicillinase-producing and nonpenicillinase-producing staphylococci also are susceptible, but amikacin should not be used to treat infections caused by these organisms since less toxic antibiotics

are available that have equal or greater effectiveness. *Streptococcus pneumoniae*, *S. pyogenes*, and *S. faecalis* are uniformly insensitive, as are certain strains of the aforementioned gram-negative organisms. Of the gram-negative organisms, however, *P. aeruginosa* is the only species of major clinical importance that includes a notable number of amikacin-resistant strains.

Amikacin is generally less active in vitro on a weight basis than gentamicin or tobramycin. However, therapeutic serum levels are easily achieved after intramuscular or intravenous injection. This agent can be used to treat serious aerobic gram-negative bacillary infections caused by susceptible gentamicin- or tobramycin-resistant organisms. Amikacin is not absorbed following oral ingestion but must be administered parenterally.

Amikacin has been effective in acute and chronic genitourinary tract infections, including pyelonephritis; respiratory, bone, joint, and intra-abdominal infections; skin and soft tissue infections, including third-degree burns; omphalitis in infants; and septicemia. It may be the parenterally administered drug of choice for burns infected with gentamicin- or tobramycin-resistant strains of *Pseudomonas aeruginosa* or *Providencia stuartii*.

The pharmacologic and pharmacokinetic properties of kanamycin and amikacin are virtually identical. The average serum half-life of both drugs is approximately two hours. In adults, peak serum levels of 18 to 25 mcg/ml are achieved approximately one hour after intramuscular injection of 7.5 mg/kg of body weight; newborn infants given this same dose have peak blood levels of 17 to 20 mcg/ml after one-half to one hour. A peak serum concentration of approximately 25 mcg/ml is achieved one-half hour following a 30-minute infusion of 7.5 mg/kg of body weight in adults.

In vitro, more than 90% of sensitive bacterial strains are inhibited by concentrations of 2 to 4 mcg/ml. Although peak blood levels are several times greater than these values when amikacin is given intramuscularly or intravenously, trough levels at 8 or 12 hours may fall below 2 mcg/ml. For this reason, administration every eight hours may be necessary for serious infections. Some clinicians have administered amikacin as a continuous intravenous infusion, but the advantage of this method over intermittent administration is yet to be proved.

Amikacin is excreted unchanged in the urine and is filtered almost entirely by the glomerulus; there is limited tubular reabsorption. In adults with normal renal function, 94% to 98% of a parenteral dose is excreted within 24 hours.

As with kanamycin, only a negligible amount is protein bound and amikacin does not appreciably displace serum-bound bilirubin. This drug does not penetrate readily into the cerebrospinal fluid in therapeutic amounts, even when the meninges are inflamed, and must be given intrathecally for gram-negative bacillary meningitis.

As with the other aminoglycosides, ototoxicity and nephrotoxicity have been reported clinically, most commonly in association with large doses, prolonged therapy, impaired renal function, previous therapy with another aminoglycoside antibiotic, or administration with certain potent diuretics (eg, furosemide, ethacrynic acid). The incidence and severity of reactions are roughly equivalent for gentamicin and amikacin.

Both unilateral and bilateral high frequency hearing loss, tinnitus, and even complete hearing loss have been observed clinically. Vestibular disturbances, manifested as dizziness, vertigo, and nystagmus, have been associated with amikacin therapy; partial or complete recovery frequently occurs when amikacin is discontinued. The incidence of both vestibular and auditory disorders is notably higher in patients who previously received aminoglycosides. During prolonged therapy with amikacin, patients should be questioned regularly about hearing or vestibular irregularities (eg, tinnitus, "fullness" in the ear) and periodic audiometric tests should be performed if practicable.

Nephrotoxic reactions range from mild renal injury to frank renal failure. Elevation of the blood urea nitrogen or serum creatinine level during therapy with amikacin may reflect drug-induced nephrotoxicity. These parameters usually return to baseline values after discontinuation of therapy. Periodic measurements of amikacin serum concentrations, serum creatinine levels, and creatinine clearance are useful to monitor for nephrotoxicity.

Other toxic effects, some of which may be hypersensitivity-type reactions, include nausea and vomiting, headache, drug fever, skin rash, tremors, paresthesias, arthralgia, eosinophilia, anemia, and hypotension. With the possible exception of nausea and vomiting, these reactions are rare. Prolonged use may result in overgrowth of nonsusceptible organisms.

Cross allergenicity between amikacin and other aminoglycosides has been demonstrated. Because of the danger of incompatibilities or drug inactivation, amikacin usually should not be mixed with other drug solutions for combined administration (there are some exceptions depending upon the nature of the drug involved, see Trissel, 1977).

ROUTES, USUAL DOSAGE, AND PREPARATIONS. *Intramuscular: Adults, children, and older infants with normal renal function,* 15 mg/kg of body weight daily in two or three equally divided doses at 12- or 8-hour intervals. The total daily dose for adults should not exceed 1.5 g except in unusual clinical conditions such as some burn-wound infections. Uncomplicated urinary tract infections in adults frequently respond to doses of 250 mg given twice daily. *Neonates with normal renal function* should be given a loading dose of 10 mg/kg, followed by 7.5 mg/kg every 12 hours. Infections usually respond in 24 to 48 hours, but if a response is not observed in three to five days, bacterial sensitivity should be redetermined and therapy reevaluated. For both adults and children, except in unusual circumstances, the duration of administration should not exceed ten days.

Patients with impaired renal function should receive the usual loading dose of amikacin (7.5 mg/kg), but maintenance doses must be modified. It is particularly important to measure serum amikacin levels in these patients; peak levels should be approximately 25 mcg/ml and trough levels 5 to 8 mcg/ml. Amikacin serum concentrations have been shown to be reasonably predictable (Sarubbi and Hull, 1978) and, if serum level measurements are not readily available, dosage can be modified according to the weight-corrected creatinine clearance of the patient. This value for males is arrived at by the following equation:

$$\text{corrected clearance} = \frac{140 - \text{age}}{\text{serum creatinine}}$$

For females, 85% of the calculated value is used. Maintenance dosage is then calculated as a percentage of the loading dose according to the corrected clearance determination (see the following dosage chart). The interval between doses can be extended to 12 or 24 hours to avoid unnecessarily elevated trough serum levels.

It also should be noted that the initial loading dose is calculated using the lean (or ideal) body weight of the patient. The aminoglycoside antibiotics are not particularly well distributed in adipose tissue. Patients of even moderate obesity should have an ideal (nonobese) body weight calculated as follows:

Male Ideal Weight = 50 kg + 2.3 kg
for every inch over 5 feet
Female Ideal Weight = 45.5 kg + 2.3 kg
for every inch over 5 feet

Many dosing guidelines have been designed and presented in tabular or nomograph form. The guideline proposed by Sarubbi and Hull incorporates essential factors, including loading dose, ideal weight, corrected creatinine clearance [C(c)cr] and maintenance dosing, and it is applicable to amikacin, kanamycin, gentamicin, and tobramycin. For the sake of simplicity and consistency, it is referred to throughout this chapter. The procedure is as follows.

1. Select Loading Dose in mg/kg [IDEAL WEIGHT] to provide peak serum levels in range listed below for desired aminoglycoside.

Aminoglycoside	Usual Loading Doses	Expected Peak Serum Levels
Tobramycin Gentamicin	1.5 to 2.0 mg/kg	4 to 10 mcg/ml
Amikacin Kanamycin	5.0 to 7.5 mg/kg	15 to 30 mcg/ml

2. Select Maintenance Dose (as percentage of chosen loading dose) to continue peak serum levels indicated above according to desired dosing interval and the patient's corrected creatinine clearance.

Percentage of Loading Dose Required For Dosage Interval Selected

C(c)cr(ml/min)	half life† (hrs)	8 hrs	12 hrs	24 hrs
90	3.1	84%	—	—
80	3.4	80	91%	—
70	3.9	76	88	—
60	4.5	71	84	—
50	5.3	65	79	—
40	6.5	57	72	92%
30	8.4	48	63	86
25	9.9	43	57	81
20	11.9	37	50	75
17	13.6	33	46	70
15	15.1	31	42	67
12	17.9	27	37	61
10‡	20.4	24	34	56
7	25.9	19	28	47
5	31.5	16	23	41
2	46.8	11	16	30
0	69.3	8	11	21

†*Alternatively, one half of the chosen loading dose may be given at an interval approximately equal to the estimated half life.*

‡*Dosing for patients with C (c) cr ≤10 ml/min should be assisted by measured serum levels.*

From Sarubbi FA Jr, Hull JH: Amikacin serum concentrations: Prediction of levels and dosage guidelines. *Ann Intern Med* 89:612-618, 1978.

Intravenous: The dosage regimens are identical to those for intramuscular use. The solution should be injected over a 30- to 60-minute period in adults and a one- to two-hour period in infants.

Amikin (Bristol). Solution 50 and 250 mg/ml.

NEOMYCIN SULFATE
[Mycifradin Sulfate, Myciguent, Neobiotic]

Neomycin has an antibacterial spectrum essentially identical to that of kanamycin, but it appears to be the most toxic aminoglycoside antibiotic. In vitro testing shows it to be effective against *Escherichia coli*, *Enterobacter aerogenes*, and many strains of *Klebsiella* and *Proteus*. Many strains of *Staphylococcus aureus* also show in vitro sensitivity to neomycin. Microorganisms resistant to neomycin include various streptococci (including the pneumococcus), *Pseudomonas*, some *Enterobacter* species, anaerobic bacteria (including *Bacteroides*), *Rickettsia*, fungi, and viruses.

Neomycin is most commonly applied topically to treat superficial skin infections, although much of this use is unjustified since definitive evidence of effectiveness is lacking. Topical application usually is not associated with toxicity, but sensitization to neomycin occurs frequently, sometimes causing contact dermatitis similar to the condition being treated. For use in the eye, see Chapter 24, Ocular Anti-infective and Anti-inflammatory Agents.

Neomycin can be used orally in patients threatened with hepatic coma, since the drug reduces the number of ammonia-producing bacteria in the gastrointestinal tract. It also is given prophylactically in combination with oral erythromycin to prepare the bowel prior to intestinal surgery. Neomycin has been administered in an attempt to control diarrhea caused by enteropathogenic *E. coli*, but the evidence for its effectiveness is far from conclusive. Although only small amounts are absorbed following oral administration, this antibiotic may accumulate, particularly in patients with renal impairment, and result in toxicity (Ward and Rounthwaite, 1978). Diarrhea and malabsorption are the most common adverse reactions following oral administration, and superinfections may occur after prolonged oral use.

Although parenteral preparations of neomycin are still marketed, their use should be universally condemned since safer, equally effective antibiotics are available. When given parenterally, neomycin is highly ototoxic and nephrotoxic; these effects are dose related. The nephrotoxicity may be reversible, but ototoxicity involving the cochlear portion of the eighth cranial nerve is usually irreversible and may progress insidiously after the drug is discontinued. Intraperitoneal or intravenous use has caused apnea.

Neomycin should not be administered with other drugs that are potentially ototoxic or nephrotoxic, since effects may be additive. For other interactions, see the Introduction.

ROUTES, USUAL DOSAGE, AND PREPARATIONS. *Topical*: An appropriate preparation is applied one or two times daily.

Drug available generically: Ointment 5 mg/g in ½ and 1 oz containers.
Myciguent (Upjohn). Cream 5 mg (equivalent to 3.5 mg of the base)/g in ½ oz containers; ointment 5 mg (equivalent to 3.5 mg of the base)/g in ½, 1, and 4 oz containers.

Oral: For hepatic coma, *adults*, 4 to 8 g daily in four divided doses for five or six days. For diarrhea caused by enteropathogenic *E. coli*, *adults*, 50 mg/kg of body weight daily in four divided doses; *newborn and premature infants*, 10 to 50 mg/kg daily in four divided doses; *older infants and children*, 50 to 100 mg/kg daily in four divided doses.

Drug available generically: Tablets 500 mg.
Mycifradin Sulfate (Upjohn). Solution 125 mg/5 ml; tablets 500 mg.
Neobiotic (Pfipharmecs). Tablets 500 mg.

Intramuscular: The parenteral administration of neomycin is not recommended and no useful dosage regimen is recognized.

> Drug available generically: Powder (sterile) 500 mg.
> *Mycifradin Sulfate* (Upjohn). Powder (sterile) 500 mg (equivalent to 350 mg of the base).

STREPTOMYCIN SULFATE

Streptomycin, like other aminoglycosides, is bactericidal against a variety of aerobic gram-negative bacilli and certain mycobacteria. The antibiotic has been used to treat infections caused by *Escherichia coli, Brucella, Francisella, Yersinia*, and *M. tuberculosis*. Resistant microorganisms include *Pseudomonas aeruginosa*, various streptococci, anaerobic bacteria, rickettsiae, fungi, and viruses. Streptomycin is not commonly used today since more effective aminoglycoside antibiotics (ie, gentamicin, tobramycin, kanamycin, amikacin) are available and other antituberculosis agents (eg, isoniazid, ethambutol, rifampin) are preferred. Indications include tuberculosis (see Chapter 79, Antimycobacterial Agents), tularemia, bubonic and pneumonic plague, glanders, and severe cases of brucellosis. Physicians usually prefer not to use streptomycin to treat plague because it is so rapidly bactericidal that it virtually always precipitates a Herxheimer-like reaction, which can be fatal. Streptomycin also is used with large doses of penicillin in the treatment of certain types of streptococcal (particularly enterococcal) endocarditis.

Streptomycin is rarely used today to treat urinary tract infections. However, if used for this indication, the urine should be alkalized to pH 8 or higher, since this drug is more active in an alkaline medium. Alkalization can be accomplished by giving 500 mg each of sodium citrate and sodium bicarbonate every three hours.

Many organisms develop resistance to streptomycin rapidly; in fact, some become streptomycin-dependent. Cross resistance between streptomycin and neomycin has been reported, and similar resistance between streptomycin and gentamicin, kanamycin, tobramycin, or amikacin is possible.

The intramuscular route is used most commonly; injection should be deep into the muscle since pain and sterile abscesses have occurred with more superficial injection. Administration of streptomycin by the intrapleural or intrathecal route is rarely if ever employed any longer. However, if used intrathecally, a preservative-free preparation is needed. The topical appplication of streptomycin is contraindicated because of the high risk of sensitization and rapidly developing bacterial resistance.

Streptomycin causes hypersensitivity reactions ranging from rash to exfoliative dermatitis and anaphylactic shock; hematopoietic damage, including neutropenia, agranulocytosis, aplastic anemia, and, rarely, thrombocytopenic purpura; renal damage; and neurologic changes, including peripheral neuritis, damage to the cochlear and vestibular portions of the eighth cranial nerve (a fairly common occurrence), and, less commonly, damage to the optic nerve. Dizziness is the usual warning sign of labyrinthine dysfunction and tinnitus the sign of auditory damage. Administration to pregnant women has been reported to damage eighth cranial nerve function in the fetus. Streptomycin should not be given with other ototoxic drugs because effects may be additive. For other interactions, see the Introduction.

Intrathecal administration has produced radiculitis, transverse myelitis, arachnoiditis, nerve root pain, and even paraplegia. The more serious adverse reactions usually occur after large doses and prolonged administration.

ROUTES, USUAL DOSAGE, AND PREPARATIONS. All doses are expressed in terms of the base.

Intramuscular: Adults, 15 to 25 mg/kg of body weight daily in two divided doses for seven to ten days and 1 g daily thereafter; *premature and newborn infants,* 20 to 30 mg/kg daily in two divided doses; *children,* 20 to 40 mg/kg daily in two divided doses.

Intrathecal: Adults, 75 to 100 mg dissolved in 10 ml of isotonic sodium chloride injection and given over a ten-minute period after withdrawal of 10 ml of cerebrospinal fluid. *Children,* 1 mg/kg of body weight daily. Dosage for patients with renal impairment must be based upon creatinine clearance and decreased in direct proportion to the degree of renal dysfunction.

> Drug available generically: Powder (for solution) 1 and 5 g; solution 400 mg/ml in 2.5 and 12.5 ml containers, and 500 mg/ml in 2 and 10 ml containers. (Strengths expressed in terms of the base.)

PAROMOMYCIN SULFATE
[Humatin]

The antimicrobial spectrum of paromomycin is essentially identical to that of neomycin. The drug is poorly absorbed following oral administration; almost 100% of an ingested dose can be recovered from the stool. Therefore, paromomycin has been administered orally to treat diarrheal disease caused by enteropathogenic *Escherichia coli*, but conclusive evidence of effectiveness is still lacking. Paromomycin is effective in reducing the population of susceptible enteric bacteria and can be used in the management of hepatic coma or preoperatively for bowel preparation, but it is not a primary drug of choice in these situations.

Paromomycin is directly amebicidal and, since its action is confined to the intestinal lumen, it can be given alone and with other drugs to treat asymptomatic as well as acute and chronic intestinal amebiasis (see Chapter 82, Antiprotozoal Agents). It is not useful for the treatment of extraintestinal amebiasis.

Paromomycin may cause nausea, abdominal cramps, and diarrhea, particularly in patients receiving over 3 g daily. Overgrowth of nonsusceptible organisms may occur if the drug is administered for prolonged periods.

ROUTE, USUAL DOSAGE, AND PREPARATIONS. *Oral: Adults and children,* for diarrhea, 25 mg/kg of body weight daily in three divided doses.

Adults, for hepatic coma, 3 to 4 g daily in divided doses at regular intervals for five to six days.

Paromomycin may be better tolerated if taken with meals.

> *Humatin* (Parke, Davis). Capsules 250 mg; syrup 125 mg/5 ml.

Selected References

Advances in aminoglycoside therapy: Amikacin. *J Infect Dis* 134(suppl):242-460, (Nov) 1976.

Avery GS (ed): *Drug Treatment: Principles and Practice of Clinical Pharmacology and Therapeutics*. Acton, Mass, Publishing Sciences Group, Inc, 1976, 932.

Bendush CL, et al: Evaluation of nephrotoxic and ototoxic effects of tobramycin in worldwide study. *Med J Aust* 2(suppl): 22-26, 1977.

Benveniste R, Davies J: Mechanisms of antibiotic resistance in bacteria. *Annu Rev Biochem* 42:471-506, 1973.

Bint AJ: Guide to new antibiotics. *Br J Hosp Med* 19:335-342, 1978.

Brewer NS: Antimicrobial agents. II. Aminoglycosides. *Mayo Clin Proc* 52:675-679, 1977.

Chung CW, Carson TR: Cross-sensitivity of common aminoglycoside antibiotics. *Arch Dermatol* 112:1101-1107, 1976.

Conway N, Birt BD: Streptomycin in pregnancy: Effect on foetal ear. *Br Med J* 2:260-263, 1965.

Cooperman LB, Rubin IL: Toxicity of ethacrynic acid and furosemide. *Am Heart J* 85:831-834, 1973.

Davia JE, et al: Uremia, deafness, and paralysis due to irrigating antibiotic solutions. *Arch Intern Med* 125: 136-139, 1970.

Jackson GG: Present status of aminoglycoside antibiotics and their safe, effective use. *Clin Ther* 1:200-215, 1977.

Laxer RM, et al: Antimicrobial activity of tobramycin against gram-negative bacteria and the combination of ampicillin/tobramycin against *E. coli. Chemotherapy* 21:90-98, 1975.

Masur H, et al: Neomycin toxicity revisited. *Arch Surg* 111:822-825, 1976.

Mathog RH, Klein WJ Jr: Ototoxicity of ethacrynic acid and aminoglycoside antibiotics in uremia. *N Engl J Med* 280:1223-1224, 1969.

Matz GJ, et al: Ototoxicity of kanamycin: Comparative histopathological study. *Laryngoscope* 75:1690-1698, 1965.

Pratt WB: *Chemotherapy of Infection*. New York, Oxford University Press, 1977, 89-94.

Root RK, Hierholzer WJ Jr: Infectious disease, in Melmon KL, Morrelli HF (eds): *Clinical Pharmacology: Basic Principles in Therapeutics*, ed 2. New York, Macmillan Publishing Co, Inc, 1978, 756.

Sarubbi FA Jr, Hull JH: Amikacin serum concentrations: Prediction of levels and dosage guidelines. *Ann Intern Med* 89:612-618, 1978.

Shapiro SL: Antibiotic deafness. *EENT Monthly* 47:679-683, 1968.

Siber GR, et al: Pharmacokinetics of gentamicin in children and adults. *J Infect Dis* 132:637-651, 1975.

Trissel LA: *Handbook on Injectable Drugs*. Washington, DC, American Society of Hospital Pharmacists, Inc, 1977.

Ward KM, Rounthwaite FJ: Neomycin ototoxicity. *Ann Otol Rhinol Laryngol* 87:211-215, 1978.

Weinstein AJ, et al: Systemic absorption of neomycin irrigating solution. *JAMA* 238:152-153, 1977.

Weinstein AJ, et al: Placental transfer of clindamycin and gentamicin in term pregnancy. *Am J Obstet Gynecol* 124:688-691, 1976.

Young LS: Aminoglycosides. *J Surg Pract* 7:22-28, (March-April), 1978.

The polymyxins are a group of related polypeptides elaborated by strains of *Bacillus polymyxa*. Only polymyxins B and E have a sufficient therapeutic margin of safety to be useful clinically. Polymyxin E is commonly known as colistin; colistimethate sodium, its sulfomethyl derivative, is the parenteral form of the drug. The polymyxins have pronounced in vitro activity against *Pseudomonas aeruginosa* and a number of other gram-negative organisms, the most prominent of which are *Escherichia, Haemophilus, Klebsiella, Enterobacter, Salmonella, Shigella, Bordetella*, and *Vibrio*. They are bactericidal in vitro at concentrations attainable in plasma or urine with therapeutic doses. Most species of *Proteus, Neisseria*, and *Providencia* are resistant, and many strains of *Serratia marcescens* are usually resistant. *Brucella* is only moderately affected. Polymyxins are ineffective against gram-positive bacteria.

Clinically, neither polymyxin B nor the colistins are drugs of first choice for treating gram-negative bacterial infections. With the development of more effective, less toxic antibiotics, therapeutic indications for the polymyxins have become limited. They are administered primarily to treat infections caused by *P. aeruginosa* strains that are resistant to carbenicillin [Geopen], ticarcillin [Ticar], gentamicin [Garamycin], tobramycin [Nebcin], and amikacin [Amikin], and infections caused by susceptible strains of *Escherichia, Enterobacter*, and *Klebsiella*. Severe urinary tract infections and bacteremia caused by susceptible organisms arising from the urinary tract may be suitable indications for the use of the polymyxins.

Polymyxin B has been injected intrathecally to treat bacillary meningitis caused by gram-negative organisms. Since the drug does not enter cerebrospinal fluid to any appreciable extent even when the meninges are inflamed, adequate concentrations cannot be attained by parenteral routes alone. Severe toxicity has occurred with intrathecal administration, however, and this route should be considered for use only in carefully selected patients. Colistimethate sodium should not be administered intrathecally.

Colistin sulfate is given orally to treat diarrhea caused by enteropathic *E. coli* in children with acute or refractory enteritis. This is the only acceptable oral use of the polymyxins, since these agents are absorbed to a very limited extent from the gastrointestinal tract.

The polymyxins exert their antibiotic activity by interacting with phospholipid components in the cytoplasmic membrane of susceptible bacteria. The structure of the cell surface is distorted, a change that can be observed with the electron microscope. Although the precise biochemical mechanism of action remains obscure, it is known that the polymyxins cause leakage of small molecules (eg, phosphate, nucleosides) from susceptible bacteria proportional to their lethal effect. The polymyxins behave as cationic surface-active compounds at physiologic pH. Their antibacterial activity is inhibited, therefore, in the presence of anionic compounds such as soap.

Bacterial resistance to the polymyxins develops slowly. The overall efficacy of these drugs has remained fairly constant. Cross resistance between polymyxin B and colistin usually is complete.

Polymyxin B and the colistins are excreted principally by the kidneys. After a single intramuscular dose of colistimethate sodium, peak levels of excretion occur in the urine within two hours, and 40% to 80% of the dose is recovered within eight hours. Renal excretion of polymyxin B is slower; very little appears in the urine within the first 12 hours after a single dose. When polymyxin B is given to patients who are in renal failure, dangerously high blood levels may occur and the drug may persist for long periods.

Adverse Reactions and Precautions

The incidence and severity of adverse reactions produced by polymyxin B and the colistins are essentially the same except that the risk of nephrotoxicity is greater with polymyxin B. This reaction and neuromuscular blockade are the most serious adverse effects produced by the polymyxins. Irritation and severe pain are associated with intramuscular injection of polymyxin B, but colistimethate sodium is practically nonirritating to tissue.

Transient neurologic disturbances such as dizziness, ataxia, slurred speech, blurred vision, circumoral paresthesias, and numbness of the extremities have been observed following administration of the polymyxins and occur most often in patients with impaired renal function. These reactions disappear as the drugs are excreted. Muscular weakness, paresis, and complete paralysis have been reported also and may delay recovery from anesthesia or may even progress to respiratory arrest and death. The neuromuscular blockade produced by the polymyxins is resistant to the action of

neostigmine and is not easily reversed, although the intravenous injection of calcium gluconate may be beneficial. Neurotoxicity may constitute a serious potential danger, especially when polymyxin B or colistimethate sodium is administered to individuals with neuromuscular disease (eg, myasthenia gravis); to patients receiving a neuromuscular blocking drug (eg, tubocurarine), other potentially neurotoxic drugs (eg, kanamycin [Kantrex]), or an anesthetic with a prominent muscle relaxing action (eg, ether); or to those given magnesium, quinidine, or quinine parenterally.

Nephrotoxicity is usually manifested as oliguria with increased levels of blood urea nitrogen (BUN) or serum creatinine. The colistins and polymyxin B, therefore, must be used cautiously and in reduced doses in patients with impaired renal function because they are primarily excreted by the kidneys.

Significant absorption of polymyxin B may occur when solutions are used to wash the peritoneum or other membrane surfaces. If toxic blood levels are attained, the adverse reactions may be similar to those observed with parenteral administration, especially if renal function is impaired.

Careful animal studies (Craig and Kunin, 1973) have shown that tissue binding of the polymyxins is the major determinant of the distribution and persistence of these antibiotics in the body. These investigators found that the polymyxin antibiotics accumulated in tissues even when serum levels were undetectable, a characteristic that may explain the cumulative toxicity of these drugs. Therefore, since the pharmacokinetic behavior of the polymyxins is complex, it is not possible to make definite dosage recommendations for patients with renal failure. When polymyxins must be used in these patients, serial determination of drug plasma levels is the only truly reliable method of determining whether a therapeutic, relatively nontoxic blood level is being maintained. For practical dosage guidelines in patients with impaired renal function, see the evaluations and the manufacturers' literature.

INDIVIDUAL EVALUATIONS

COLISTIMETHATE SODIUM
[Coly-Mycin M]

L-DAB=α,γ-diaminobutyric acid

This compound is the sodium salt of the sulfomethyl derivative of colistin. Its in vitro antibacterial spectrum includes many gram-negative bacilli (see the Introduction); it is not active against gram-positive bacteria. Colistimethate may be useful for treating infections caused by *Pseudomonas aeruginosa*, especially in the urinary tract. With the development of carbenicillin, ticarcillin, gentamicin, and other aminoglycoside antibiotics, however, it is no longer the drug of choice for serious *Pseudomonas* infections but remains an alternative drug for treating susceptible infections when a more effective or potentially less toxic antibiotic cannot be used. Cures have been reported when colistimethate was administered with carbenicillin for *Pseudomonas* sepsis in children with acute leukopenia. Treatment of intestinal infections also has been attempted with colistimethate, but the infections frequently do not respond to intramuscular injection. Hence, orally administered colistin sulfate is preferred over colistimethate for treating bacterial enteritis.

Bacterial resistance to colistimethate sodium and cross resistance to polymyxin B develop slowly in vitro and perhaps in vivo as well. The in vitro antibacterial potency of colistimethate is one-third to one-fifth that of polymyxin B on a weight basis. Its half-life in blood is approximately two to three hours. Colistimethate sodium is not irritating to tissues when injected intramuscularly and is preferred to polymyxin B when this route is used. Therapeutic concentrations do not appear in cerebrospinal fluid following intramuscular injection.

Colistimethate sodium may adversely affect the kidneys and nervous system. Elevated blood urea nitrogen levels, usually reversible, have been reported in adults and a few infants. Symptoms of uremia and acute renal failure as a result of overdosage in patients with impaired renal function also have been observed. In patients with acute renal failure or chronic nephropathies, the dosage of colistimethate must be adjusted according to the degree of renal impairment. Because they may have inadequate renal reserves, the dosage for infants and elderly patients should be carefully regulated. Blood urea nitrogen or serum creatinine levels should be determined periodically, and close attention should be given to urinary output, since oliguria may be a sign of impending renal damage.

Fever, dysphonia, gastrointestinal disturbances, dermatoses, pain at the site of injection, and a few possible cases of neutropenia and granulocytopenia have been reported.

Secondary infections caused by nonsusceptible bacteria may occur during therapy. Cross sensitivity between colistimethate sodium and polymyxin B has been observed.

See the Introduction for further information on adverse reactions and precautions.

ROUTES, USUAL DOSAGE, AND PREPARATIONS. *Intramuscular, Intravenous*: The intravenous dose must be administered slowly over a period of three to five minutes or given by intravenous drip. *Adults and children with normal renal function*, 2.5 to 5 mg/kg of body weight daily in two to four divided doses (maximum, 300 mg daily). *Adults with impaired renal function*, following an initial dose of 2.5 to 5 mg/kg, the dosage should be modified according to the following schedule (see the manufacturer's literature for further information):

	RENAL IMPAIRMENT		
	Mild	Moderate	Marked
Serum Creatinine (mg/dl)	1.3-1.5	1.6-2.5	2.6-4.0
Daily Dose (mg/kg)	2.5-3.8	2.5	1.5
Dosage interval (hours)	12	12-24	36

Coly-Mycin M Parenteral (Parke, Davis). Powder (lyophilized) equivalent to 20 or 150 mg colistin base.

COLISTIN SULFATE
[Coly-Mycin S]

L-DAB=α,γ-diaminobutyric acid
polymyxin B₁; R=(+)-6-methyloctanoyl
polymyxin B₂; R=6-methylheptanoyl

Colistin sulfate is the water-soluble salt of colistin. Its in vitro antibacterial potency is approximately the same as that of polymyxin B. This drug is only slightly absorbed from the gastrointestinal tract and is used orally in infants and children to treat diarrhea associated with acute or refractory bacterial enteritis caused by enteropathic *Escherichia coli* and other susceptible gram-negative bacilli (see the Introduction for the bacterial spectrum). The use of colistin sulfate should be restricted to those species shown to be refractory to other antimicrobial agents. When systemic acid-base imbalance is associated with severe enteritis, appropriate concomitant parenteral therapy should be employed.

Large doses of colistin, like polymyxin B, may be both nephrotoxic and neurotoxic. Because it is poorly absorbed from the gastrointestinal tract, usual oral doses rarely produce adverse effects. Frequent measurements of renal function should be made when this drug is used in infants and children with chronic renal failure.

ROUTE, USUAL DOSAGE, AND PREPARATIONS. *Oral*: *Infants and children*, 5 to 15 mg/kg of body weight daily in three divided doses.

Coly-Mycin S (Parke, Davis). Powder equivalent to 300 mg of colistin base, providing the equivalent of 25 mg of colistin base/5 ml when suspended in 37 ml of distilled water.

POLYMYXIN B SULFATE
[Aerosporin]

L-DAB=α,γ-diaminobutyric acid
colistin A (polymyxin E₁); R=(+)-6-methyloctanoyl
polymyxin E₂; R=6-methylheptanoyl

Polymyxin B sulfate is active against many gram-negative bacilli (see the Introduction) and is used primarily to treat infections caused by *Pseudomonas* species, especially in the urinary tract. This agent also can be used to treat meningitis but must be given intrathecally, which may be hazardous. Polymyxin B should be reserved for treatment of susceptible infections that do not respond to other antibiotics. It can be administered by all parenteral routes and by topical application to the eye and skin. Administration of polymyxin B by inhalation has been abandoned because of its marginal effectiveness and because it led to the selection of resistant *Pseudomonas*.

The half-life of polymyxin B in the blood is approximately six hours. Following absorption, very little of the drug is excreted during the first 12 hours. Thereafter, concentrations of 20 to 100 mcg/ml are excreted in the urine. Elimination continues for one to three days after administration is stopped.

Caution is mandatory when polymyxin B is used in patients with impaired renal function, since the drug is nephrotoxic and neurotoxic. Parenteral doses that produce blood levels of 1 to 2 mcg/ml can cause flushing of the face and dizziness that may progress to ataxia, drowsiness, and paresthesias. Neuromuscular blockade also has been reported following therapeutic doses (see the Introduction for a more detailed discussion of adverse reactions).

ROUTES, USUAL DOSAGE, AND PREPARATIONS. *Intravenous*: *Adults and children with normal renal function*, 15,000 to 25,000 units/kg of body weight daily. Total daily dose should not exceed 25,000 units/kg, although *infants* usually tolerate up to 40,000 units/kg daily if needed. Dextrose injection 5% may be used as a vehicle and one-half of the daily dose should be given by intravenous drip every 12 hours. To avoid widespread neuromuscular blockade, this drug should not be injected rapidly as a single bolus injection.

Intramuscular: This route is not recommended routinely because of marked pain at the site of injection. The drug may be injected in a 1% procaine hydrochloride solution to help reduce the pain. Otherwise, either water for injection or sodium chloride solution for injection may be used as a vehicle.
Adults and children with normal renal function, 25,000 to 30,000 units/kg of body weight daily in divided doses at four- or six-hour intervals. *Infants* may tolerate up to 40,000 units/kg daily, and *premature or newborn infants* with *P. aeruginosa* infections may be given 45,000 units/kg daily.

Intrathecal: *Adults and children over 2 years with normal renal function*, 50,000 units once daily for three to four days, followed by 50,000 units once every other day; *children under 2 years with normal renal function*, 20,000 units once daily for three to four days, or 25,000 units once every other day. These amounts are given for at least two weeks after cultures of the cerebrospinal fluid are negative and sugar content has returned to normal.

The dose should be reduced in patients with impaired renal function in direct proportion to the degree of renal impairment as determined by an acceptable measuring guide such as the creatinine clearance test or blood creatinine levels.

> Drug available generically: Powder 500,000 units equivalent to 63.7 mg of polymyxin B standard.
>
> *Aerosporin* (Burroughs Wellcome). Powder 500,000 units equivalent to 63.7 mg of polymyxin B standard.

Topical: See Chapter 24, Ocular Antiinfective and Anti-inflammatory Agents, and Chapter 61, Dermatologic Preparations.

MIXTURES

A number of mixtures for topical application contain polymyxin B in combination with other antibiotics, most frequently neomycin and/or bacitracin. Liquid and ointment formulations are available for application to the skin, eye, ear, or for use as a bladder rinse. The proposed rationale for these mixtures is that they have a wide antibacterial spectrum that includes both gram-positive and gram-negative organisms. A few mixtures also contain an adrenal corticosteroid. There is no evidence, however, that the addition of a corticosteroid enhances the efficacy of these combinations.

Fixed-ratio mixtures for topical use containing polymyxin B have reasonable therapeutic value but have disadvantages as well. It is possible for sufficient amounts of any drug in the mixture to be absorbed from abraded or burn-damaged skin or mucous membranes to cause systemic toxicity if applied to extensive areas. The antibiotics in these mixtures are also capable of causing hypersensitization following topical application.

Cortisporin (Burroughs Wellcome). Each gram of ointment contains polymyxin B sulfate 5,000 units, zinc bacitracin 400 units, neomycin sulfate 5 mg equivalent to neomycin 3.5 mg, and cortisol 10 mg; each gram of cream contains polymyxin B sulfate 10,000 units, neomycin sulfate 5 mg equivalent to neomycin base 3.5 mg, gramicidin 0.25 mg, and cortisol acetate 5 mg.

Neo-Polycin (Dow). Each gram of ointment contains polymyxin B sulfate 5,000 units, zinc bacitracin 400 units, and neomycin sulfate equivalent to neomycin 3.5 mg.

Neosporin (Burroughs Wellcome). Each gram of ointment or powder contains polymyxin B sulfate 5,000 units, zinc bacitracin 400 units, and neomycin sulfate 5 mg equivalent to neomycin 3.5 mg; each 90 g of aerosol contains polymyxin B sulfate 100,000 units, zinc bacitracin 8,000 units, and neomycin sulfate 100 mg equivalent to neomycin base 70 mg.

Neosporin G (Burroughs Wellcome). Each gram of cream contains polymyxin B sulfate 10,000 units, neomycin sulfate 5 mg equivalent to neomycin 3.5 mg, and gramicidin 0.25 mg.

Neosporin G.U. Irrigant (Burroughs Wellcome). Each milliliter of solution contains polymyxin B sulfate 200,000 units and neomycin sulfate equivalent to neomycin 40 mg.

Polysporin Ointment (Burroughs Wellcome). Each gram of ointment contains polymyxin B sulfate 10,000 units and zinc bacitracin 500 units.

Selected References

Craig WA, Kunin CM: Dynamics of binding and release of polymyxin antibiotics by tissues. *J Pharmacol Exp Ther* 184:757-765, 1973.

Kagan BM (ed): *Antimicrobial Therapy*, ed 2. Philadelphia, WB Saunders Co, 1974.

Kurylowicz W (ed): *Antibiotics, A Critical Review*. Warsaw, Polish Medical Publishers, 1976.

Pratt WB: *Chemotherapy of Infection*. New York, Oxford University Press, 1977.

Miscellaneous Antibacterial Agents | 76

BACITRACIN
[Baciguent]

BACITRACIN COMBINATIONS

Bacitracin, a mixture of polypeptide antibiotics produced by a strain of *Bacillus subtilis*, is bactericidal against gram-positive organisms, especially common skin pathogens such as staphylococci and streptococci, and *Neisseria*; it is inactive against most gram negative organisms. Bacterial resistance occurs rarely, although some strains of *Staphylococcus* are naturally resistant. Bacitracin interferes with bacterial cell wall synthesis by preventing the formation of the peptidoglycan chains that are cross linked to form the rigid bacterial cell wall (Siewert and Strominger, 1967).

Parenteral use of bacitracin has been abandoned almost entirely because nephrotoxicity, primarily manifested as tubular degeneration, may occur and because safer, more effective agents with similar antibacterial spectra are available. A parenteral preparation is still marketed, however, and may be used as a drug of last resort in infants with pneumonia and empyema caused by susceptible staphylococci. Since the drug is not absorbed from the gastrointestinal tract, the major use of bacitracin is limited to the topical treatment of superficial gram-positive infections. The base is available as a single-entity product and as a component of mixtures, while the zinc salt is used only in mixtures.

The rationale for use of combination preparations containing bacitracin and other antibacterial agents (eg, neomycin, polymyxin B) is that, by a judicious choice of at least two antibiotics with complementary antibacterial spectra, activity against most pathogens can be assured. Such use appears justified because of the difficulty of identifying the dominant organisms and because of the relative safety of these topical agents. A corticosteroid may be included in these preparations to reduce local inflammation and pruritus. Steroid-containing preparations suppress the healing process, however, and may increase susceptibility to other infections.

These topical mixtures are effective in a variety of dermatitides infected with susceptible bacteria (eg, ulcers, sycosis, external otitis), but they are of doubtful value in pyodermas, such as impetigo, which require systemic therapy. Ophthalmic preparations are useful in treating superficial bacterial infections of the eye (see Chapter 24, Ocular Anti-infective and Anti-inflammatory Agents).

Hypersensitivity reactions, usually manifested as allergic dermatitis, may be serious but occur only rarely when bacitracin is applied topically. Superinfections, especially with fungi, have been observed after use of mixtures containing bacitracin, and this possibility should be considered if an initial improvement is followed by relapse. Even use of combination preparations containing an antifungal agent frequently does not prevent superinfection.

ROUTE, USUAL DOSAGE, AND PREPARATIONS.
BACITRACIN:

Topical: *Adults and children*, ointment is applied to lesions once or twice daily.

> Drug available generically: Ointment, solution for parenteral injection.
> *Baciguent* (Upjohn). Ointment 500 units/g in ½, 1, and 4 oz containers (nonprescription).

BACITRACIN COMBINATIONS:

Topical: The following preparations are among the better known and more frequently prescribed topical antibacterial mixtures containing bacitracin. They are applied to the affected area two to five times daily.

> *Bacimycin* (Merrell-National). Each gram of ointment contains bacitracin 500 units and neomycin sulfate 5 mg in ½ oz containers (nonprescription).
> *Mycitracin* (Upjohn). Each gram of ointment contains bacitracin 500 units, neomycin sulfate 5 mg equivalent to neomycin 3.5 mg, and polymyxin B sulfate 5,000 units in 1/32, ½, and 1 oz containers (nonprescription).
> *Neo-Polycin* (Dow). Each gram of ointment contains bacitracin zinc 400 units, neomycin sulfate equivalent to neomycin 3.5 mg, and polymyxin B sulfate 5,000 units in 1/32, ½, and 1 oz containers (nonprescription).
> *Neosporin* (Burroughs Wellcome). Each gram of ointment contains bacitracin zinc 400 units, polymyxin B sulfate 5,000 units, and neomycin sulfate 5 mg equivalent to neomycin 3.5 mg in 1/32, ½, and 1 oz containers (nonprescription); each 90 g container of powder (aerosol) contains bacitracin zinc 8,000 units, polymyxin B sulfate 100,000 units, and neomycin sulfate 100 mg equivalent to neomycin 70 mg; each gram of powder contains bacitracin zinc 400 units, polymyxin B sulfate 5,000 units, and neomycin sulfate 5 mg equivalent to neomycin 3.5 mg in 10 g containers.
> *Polysporin* (Burroughs Wellcome). Each gram of ointment contains bacitracin zinc 500 units and polymyxin B sulfate 10,000 units in 1/32, ½, and 1 oz containers (nonprescription).

VANCOMYCIN HYDROCHLORIDE
[Vancocin Hydrochloride]

Vancomycin, a glycopeptide of unknown chemical structure, exerts its antimicrobial action by inhibiting bacterial cell wall synthesis. The exact mechanism of action remains unknown. It is bactericidal for gram-positive cocci and is the most potent available antibiotic against staphylococci.

Because of its toxicity, vancomycin generally should be reserved for use when less toxic antibiotics are ineffective or not tolerated. It remains a drug of major importance in the treatment of bacterial endocarditis, either alone or with an aminoglycoside (eg, gentamicin). If the penicillins and cephalosporins cannot be given to treat serious infections caused by staphylococci, streptococci, or enterococci because of patient hypersensitivity to these drugs, vancomycin may be an acceptable alternative. Methicillin-resistant staphylococci also are frequently susceptible to vancomycin. Since the drug is poorly absorbed, it may be administered orally to treat staphylococcal enteritis or enterocolitis. It is a drug of choice in treating antibiotic-induced colitis (see Chapter 58, Antidiarrheal Agents, and Chapter 72, Macrolide and Lincosamide Antibiotics). The drug may be administered through a nasogastric tube that has been passed beyond the pylorus if vomiting develops. For use of vancomycin in the eye, see Chapter 24, Ocular Anti-infective and Anti-inflammatory Agents.

Intravenous use of vancomycin may produce thrombophlebitis. The frequency of this reaction can be reduced by administration through a catheter inserted under sterile conditions (eg, in the operating room) into the subclavian vein; this procedure dilutes the drug in a large volume of blood as it enters the circulation.

Patients receiving vancomycin often experience circumoral paresthesia. Skin rash, renal damage, eosinophilia, and high fever also are common reactions to intravenously administered vancomycin, and marked hypotension and anaphylactic shock have been reported. Vancomycin can cause severe ototoxicity and nephrotoxicity. Large doses, prolonged therapy, or use in patients with impaired renal function has caused permanent deafness and fatal uremia. If possible, audiograms should be obtained before or early during the course of therapy and repeated at the slightest subjective sign of hearing impairment. The daily use of a simple bedside test such as the response of the patient to a whisper or the ticking of a wristwatch usually can detect the beginning of hearing loss. Renal function should be assessed at least twice weekly, preferably by measuring creatinine clearance, if treatment is continued for more than one week.

ROUTES, USUAL DOSAGE, AND PREPARATIONS. Solutions are stable for 96 hours (intravenous) or one week (oral) if refrigerated. *Intravenous: Adults with normal renal function*, 2 g daily in two to four divided doses; 3 to 4 g daily may be used in seriously ill patients. *Children and infants older than four weeks with normal renal function*, 40 mg/kg of body weight daily in two to four divided doses. The total dose should be diluted with 100 to 200 ml of sodium chloride injection or 5% dextrose injection and given slowly to lessen the risk of thrombophlebitis.

The dosage interval should be increased in adults with renal impairment according to the following schedule:

	Creatinine Clearance ml/min		
	80-50	50-10	<10
Dosage Intervals	24-72 hours	3-10 days	1 g every 7 days

Vancocin Hydrochloride (Lilly). Powder 500 mg.

Oral: Adults, an aqueous solution containing 500 mg to 1 g may be given every six hours (maximal daily dose, 4 g). *Children*, the dosage is reduced.

Vancocin Hydrochloride (Lilly). Powder 10 g.

SPECTINOMYCIN DIHYDROCHLORIDE PENTAHYDRATE
[Trobicin]

Spectinomycin is an aminocyclitol produced by a strain of *Streptomyces spectabilis*. It interacts with the bacterial 30S ribosomal subunit (Anderson et al, 1967) to inhibit protein synthesis by an unknown mechanism. This effect is reversible if the drug is discontinued.

Spectinomycin is active against most strains of *Neisseria gonorrhoeae* in vitro. Clinically, it may be used to treat acute gonorrheal urethritis and proctitis in men and acute cervicitis and proctitis in women when the strain of the organism is susceptible and the primary effective drugs cannot be used. It is not a drug of first choice in uncomplicated gonorrhea caused by penicillin-susceptible organisms when patients are not allergic to penicillin. The resistance of the gonococcus to penicillin is still relative and many strains become susceptible by increasing the dose of penicillin G. Tetracycline usually is the drug of second choice when a patient is allergic to penicillin, is over 8 years of age, and is not pregnant. Spectinomycin may be used in place of tetracycline if the patient cannot tolerate tetracycline or the gonococcus is resistant to it. Spectinomycin becomes a drug of first choice in pregnant women with gonorrhea who are allergic to penicillin or probenecid and in infected children 8 years of age or younger. It also is preferred in disseminated gonococcal infection in penicillin-sensitive individuals (see also Chapter 69, Penicillins). This agent is not effective in syphilis.

Adverse effects occur infrequently and include pain at the site of injection, nausea, chills, fever, insomnia, urticaria, and oliguria. Abnormal results of laboratory tests may be seen following multiple doses of the drug and include decreased hemoglobin, hematocrit, and creatinine clearance and elevated alkaline phosphatase, blood urea nitrogen (BUN), and serum glutamic pyruvic transaminase (SGPT) levels.

Effects on the fetus when the drug is used during pregnancy and the safety of its use in infants and children have not been established.

ROUTE, USUAL DOSAGE, AND PREPARATIONS. *Intramuscular: Adults*, 2 to 4 g; the dose usually should be divided between two gluteal sites. The larger amounts are indicated for retreatment after other antibiotic therapy has failed or for patients living in areas where resistance to penicillin is known to be prevalent.

Trobicin (Upjohn). Powder (for solution) 2 and 4 g with 3.2 and 6.2 ml of diluent, respectively.

GRAMICIDINS AND TYROCIDINES

There are a number of antibiotic substances known to affect bacterial membrane permeability. Most of them are too toxic to be used clinically. One group, the polymyxins, are administered both orally and parenterally to combat bacterial infections caused by gram-negative organisms and, although still useful, these drugs largely have been superceded by the broad spectrum penicillins and the aminoglycosides (see Chapter 75, Polymyxins). Two other classes of compounds that act by altering membrane permeability are the gramicidins and the tyrocidines. These agents are too toxic for systemic use but are applied topically in the form of a mixture called tyrothricin. This mixture was first isolated from *Bacillus brevis* and contains approximately 20% gramicidin A and 80%

tyrocidines; it is bactericidal. Its bactericidal effect appears to occur as a result of changes in cellular cation content, primarily the loss of potassium ion.

Gramicidin A and the tyrocidines are active against many gram-positive organisms. Tyrocidines are less active in this respect but also inhibit some gramnegative bacilli.

Tyrothricin is used to treat infected surface ulcers, wounds, and pyodermas and infections of the eye, nose, and throat. It may be applied as an ointment containing 0.5 mg/g or a solution containing 0.5 mg/ml.

When properly applied, tyrothricin is relatively free from adverse reactions. Strong concentrations may be irritating. When used at normal therapeutic levels, tissue toxicity is remarkably low and sensitization does not occur. The gramicidins and tyrocidines are potent hemolytic agents and must not be used in any way that would allow them access to the blood stream.

Selected References

Handbook of Antimicrobial Therapy. New Rochelle, NY, The Medical Letter, Inc, 1976.

Anderson P, et al: Effect of spectinomycin on polypeptide synthesis in extracts of *Escherichia coli. J Mol Biol* 29:203-215, 1967.

Kurylowicz W (ed): *Antibiotics: A Critical Review.* Warsaw, Polish Medical Publishers, 1976.

Pratt WB: *Chemotherapy of Infection*. New York, Oxford University Press, 1977.

Siewert G, Strominger JL: Bacitracin: An inhibitor of dephosphorylation of lipid pyrophosphate, an intermediate in biosynthesis of peptidoglycan of bacterial cell walls. *Proc Natl Acad Sci USA* 57:767-773, 1967.

Sulfonamides and Related Compounds | 77

The modern chemotherapeutic era of infectious disease began in 1935 when Domagk demonstrated that a dye, prontosil, was able to combat streptococcal infection in mice. It was discovered subsequently that prontosil is metabolized to para-aminobenzene sulfonamide. Using this knowledge, thousands of sulfonamide compounds have been synthesized, many of which are used successfully in the treatment of infection.

Bacterial synthesis of purine and, ultimately, DNA is dependent upon the presence of folic acid derivatives. Bacterial cells are impermeable to folic acid and most of them synthesize it from aminobenzoic acid (PABA). The anti-infective sulfonamides usually have a free amino group on the benzene ring and produce a bacteriostatic effect by competitively blocking the bacterial synthesis of folic acid from aminobenzoic acid. It is this mechanism of action that makes sulfonamides useful in the treatment of infectious disease. Because bacterial replication and growth are not suppressed immediately, the bacteriostatic action becomes apparent only after the existing stores of bacterial folic acid are depleted. There is evidence that a second mechanism also is involved whereby the enzyme systems of some bacteria incorporate a small amount of sulfonamide into a sulfonamide-containing analogue of folic acid that may be a self-inhibitor of the enzyme system. Since humans absorb preformed folic acid from their diet, the inhibition of folic acid synthesis has a minimal effect on human cells.

Inhibition of bacterial cell growth by sulfonamides can be reversed in vitro if certain products (eg, thymidine, purines, methionine, serine) are added to the growth medium. This may be important clinically since pus is a rich source of the protein residues that can inhibit the effectiveness of these drugs in purulent infections. Also, when determining in vitro bacterial sensitivity to the sulfonamides, it is essential that the culture medium be free of aminobenzoic acid, for trace amounts of this compound may interfere with results.

The sulfonamides may be bactericidal rather than bacteriostatic in vitro when bacteria are grown on a medium containing amino acids and purines but lacking thymine. This effect can be reversed by adding thymine. Since a similar effect has been demonstrated in blood and urine, it may be that sulfonamides are bactericidal in tissue and other body fluids that contain little or no thymine.

In addition to the anti-infective compounds, other sulfonamide derivatives used therapeutically include those with diuretic, antidiabetic, and antithyroid effects (see Chapters 15, Anticonvulsants; 22, Agents Used to Treat Glaucoma; 39, Diuretics; 47, Agents Used to Regulate Blood Glucose; and 48, Agents Used to Treat Thyroid Disease).

The anti-infective sulfonamides are usually given orally. When parenteral administration is indicated, sulfisoxazole diolamine [Gantrisin Diolamine] may be given subcutaneously, intramuscularly, or intravenously or a sodium salt (eg, sulfadiazine sodium) may be administered intravenously. When the intravenous route is used, the drug must be well diluted and injected slowly to avoid extravasation. Irritation caused by the alkaline sodium salts precludes intramuscular or subcutaneous administration.

Estimates of effective blood concentrations vary between 6 and 15 mg/dl. Because the sulfonamides are concentrated in the urine, however, blood levels effective for urinary tract infections may be lower than those needed for systemic infections. Some bacterial strains may require higher blood levels than others. Drugs that are metabolized are inactivated primarily in the liver by acetylation or conjugation with glucuronic acid. Either process may increase or decrease the solubility of the drug

in the urine, the major route of excretion. Acetylated metabolites and many of the conjugates are inactive therapeutically.

The sulfonamides can be classified as short-, intermediate-, or long-acting, according to their duration in the body. The extent of binding of sulfonamides to serum protein (albumin) influences the rate of renal excretion; therefore, the shorter-acting compounds are usually less bound than the longer-acting ones. A fourth category, ultralong-acting, has been applied to two drugs (sulfadoxine, sulfametopyrazine) that are available in the United Kingdom but not in the United States. It is claimed that these products (half-life, 150 and 65 hours, respectively) maintain adequate blood levels with weekly administration. Poorly absorbed sulfonamides, those used topically, and the sulfapyridines are not classified according to duration of action.

Short-Acting Sulfonamides: Sulfisoxazole [Gantrisin], sulfamethizole [Thiosulfil], sulfacytine [Renoquid], and sulfachlorpyridazine [Sonilyn] are rapidly absorbed following oral administration and have half-lives of four to seven hours. Although sulfadiazine (half-life, 17 hours) is not short-acting, it traditionally has been used in the same manner and, therefore, is included in this category. Other short-acting compounds (eg, sulfamerazine, sulfamethazine) are relatively insoluble or weakly anti-infective and are rarely used except in combination with other drugs. Sulfamerazine and sulfamethazine are combined with sulfadiazine to form a short-acting combination known as trisulfapyrimidines (see the section on Mixtures).

Because the short-acting agents produce high urinary levels, they are usually the sulfonamides of choice for urinary tract infections. The newer compounds in this group are relatively safe, well tolerated, and have a low risk of crystalluria. They also can be used for systemic therapy, in which they have an advantage over long-acting sulfonamides in that exposure can be terminated rapidly if serious adverse reactions develop. Dosage intervals of four to eight hours usually maintain adequate antimicrobial activity in the blood.

Intermediate- and Long-Acting Sulfonamides: The intermediate-acting sulfonamides are absorbed and excreted somewhat more slowly following oral administration than the short-acting compounds. The half-life usually is 10 to 12 hours. Therapeutic blood levels can be maintained with administration once or twice daily. Sulfamethoxazole [Gantanol] is a representative of this class. It is useful in urinary tract infections or other infections requiring prolonged courses of therapy and also may be administered to prevent recurrence of nonobstructive infections. Sulfamethoxazole is used alone or in combination with trimethoprim (see the section on Mixtures).

The long-acting sulfonamides are absorbed fairly rapidly but are excreted so slowly that it takes several days for elimination of a single dose. Their half-lives range between 17 and 40 hours. Sulfameter [Sulla] is a representative of this class; a small oral dose given once daily may maintain an adequate antibacterial blood level. Although this dosage schedule may be convenient for the patient, the low urinary concentration of active drug may render it less effective than the short-acting compounds for urinary tract infections. Because the excretion rate is prolonged, excessive blood concentrations may accumulate if sulfameter is given frequently, in large doses, or to patients with impaired renal function.

Topical Sulfonamides: Topical preparations containing sulfonamides (eg, sulfacetamide sodium) are used on the skin and mucous membranes and in the eye; however, with the exception of mafenide [Sulfamylon], these compounds are ineffective when applied to wounds, probably because pus and cellular debris readily inhibit their action. Their primary clinical uses are to treat certain mild ocular infections (see Chapter 24, Ocular Anti-infective and Anti-inflammatory Agents) and to prevent sepsis in patients with severe burns. Silver sulfadiazine [Silvadene] and mafenide often are used for burns, but mafenide may cause pain on application, particularly when applied to second- or third-degree burns.

Intravaginal insertion of sulfonamides constitutes their main use on mucous membrane surfaces. Appropriate preparations of sulfisoxazole (eg, sulfisoxazole diolamine) and triple sulfonamide combinations are used alone and with other drugs to treat nonspecific vaginitis and cervicitis. One triple sulfonamide preparation [Sultrin] has some effectiveness in *Corynebacterium vaginale* (*Haemophilus vaginalis*) vaginitis.

Poorly Absorbed Sulfonamides: Relatively insoluble sulfonamides have been used to reduce normal bacterial flora within the gut before colonic surgery and as adjunctive therapy for ulcerative colitis. The only compound currently available for this purpose is phthalylsulfathiazole [Sulfathalidine].

Sulfapyridines: The two drugs in this category are sulfapyridine and sulfasalazine [Azulfidine, S.A.S.-500]. Sulfapyridine is quite toxic and must be used with caution but is still the preferred drug for treating dermatitis herpetiformis. Sulfasalazine is given orally to treat ulcerative colitis and is particularly useful in preventing relapses. Some authorities believe that it can be used to treat diverticulitis, but most of the evidence appears to be anecdotal. The action of sulfasalazine in these conditions may be completely independent of its anti-infective properties (see also Chapter 58, Antidiarrheal Agents).

Indications

The sulfonamides were once a mainstay in the treatment of infectious diseases, but their importance has diminished as bacterial resistance has increased and more effective antimicrobial agents have been developed. Nevertheless, because of the established effectiveness, low cost, and relative lack of toxicity of the newer compounds, sulfonamides are among the drugs of choice for treating acute, uncomplicated urinary tract infections caused by susceptible bacterial strains, particularly *Escherichia coli* and *Proteus mirabilis*. For greatest effectiveness, it is desirable to use a sulfonamide that is excreted in high antibacterial concentration (largely in the active rather than in the acetylated form), is reasonably soluble in acidic urine, and maintains adequate antibacterial levels in the blood and tissues during the period in which high concentrations are excreted. The short-acting drugs that most nearly meet these criteria are sulfisoxazole, sulfamethizole, sulfacytine, and sulfachlorpyridazine. Sulfacetamide or sulfamethoxazole alone or sulfamethoxazole combined with trimethoprim [Bactrim, Septra] also are used. The combination often is more effective than a single sulfonamide (see the section on Mixtures). Prompt reduction of bacteriuria (eg, sterile urine culture within four days after initiation of therapy) is a clinical indication of effectiveness; therapy should then be continued for seven to ten days (usually no longer than 14 days) for upper tract infections. Lower tract infections may respond sooner.

The sulfonamides (particularly sulfadiazine) are drugs of choice for treating nocardiosis and can be used to treat chancroid, trachoma, and inclusion conjunctivitis. These compounds have been used to treat lymphogranuloma venereum but are not drugs of first choice.

Respiratory infections (including bronchitis), otitis media, tonsillitis, and pharyngitis caused by susceptible streptococci, pneumococci, *Haemophilus influenzae*, and *Neisseria* may respond to the sulfonamides, but other antimicrobials are clearly superior and are preferred. Although penicillin is the drug of choice for the long-term prophylaxis of streptococcal infections (eg, rheumatic fever), sulfonamides can be used in patients who cannot tolerate penicillin. However, they are not effective in streptococcal pharyngitis.

Other indications for the sulfonamides include preoperative suppression of normal intestinal flora; treatment of dermatitis herpetiformis and ulcerative colitis; adjunctive therapy in malaria caused by chloroquine-resistant strains of *Plasmodium falciparum*; and in toxoplasmosis (in conjunction with pyrimethamine) or *Pneumocystis carinii* infections (in conjunction with trimethoprim).

Because there are few controlled clinical studies and because studies in normal subjects may not correlate well with clinical efficacy or safety, it is difficult to recommend specific drugs. The antibacterial spectrums of the various sulfonamides are comparable and it is not known to what degree, if any, bacterial sensitivities to each drug differ. Although disc sensitivity tests have some value in determining which sulfonamide may be most useful in a given situation, clinical response does not always correlate well with results of such tests. In general, use of the older sulfonamides (eg, sulfanilamide, sulfathiazole) has been largely discontinued since the newer compounds are better tolerated, safer, and more effective.

Resistance: Many bacteria become highly resistant to the sulfonamides during therapy. Once resistance develops, cross resistance to other sulfonamides is usual. Resistance may be minimized by initiating treatment promptly with adequate doses and continuing treatment for a sufficient period to eradicate the infection.

Although some strains of *Klebsiella, Enterobacter*, or *Proteus* are readily inhibited by the sulfonamides, particularly in vitro, other strains are totally resistant. Resistance has been reported in strains of *H. influenzae, Streptococcus pneumoniae, Pseudomonas* species, *S. faecalis*, and other enterococci, as well as staphylococci, spirochetes, clostridia, gonococci, and shigellae. The sulfonamides are seldom used to treat meningococcal meningitis because of the increase in resistant strains. They should be used in meningococcal carriers or to prevent meningococcal meningitis only when the infecting strains have been proved to be sensitive in vitro.

Adverse Reactions and Precautions

The short-acting sulfonamides generally are as effective as the long-acting agents, and their more rapid elimination is an advantage if toxic reactions occur.

Hypersensitivity reactions affecting the skin and mucous membranes include urticaria and maculopapular rashes that are often accompanied by pruritus and fever. Contact dermatitis is common. Photosensitivity and more serious dermatologic reactions (eg, exfoliative dermatitis, toxic epidermal necrolysis, erythema nodosum) are observed occasionally. The sulfonamides may provoke Stevens-Johnson syndrome, especially in children. This syndrome involves both the skin and mucous membranes and is fatal·in approximately 25% of susceptible patients. Therefore, if a rash develops after use of a sulfonamide, therapy should be stopped and the illness re-evaluated. Most sulfonamides produce sensitization which may preclude the later use of any sulfonamide derivative, including those not used for their anti-infective properties.

Anorexia, nausea, vomiting, and diarrhea are common side effects of sulfonamide therapy. Reactions involving the central nervous system include headache, lethargy, dizziness, and mental depression. Peripheral neuritis, psychoses, ataxia, vertigo, tinnitus, and convulsions have been reported rarely.

Sulfonamides may cause toxic nephrosis with oliguria and anuria, crystalluria, and gross or microscopic hematuria with or without crystalluria. Since these agents are primarily excreted by the kidneys, there must be a reasonable urinary output (1,000 to 1,500 ml/day for individuals with normal kidney function) before therapy is begun, and appropriate hydration should be continued throughout the treatment period. The solubility of the sulfonamides is highest in alkaline urine; therefore, efforts to achieve and maintain an alkaline urine may be beneficial. If renal function is normal, even patients with one kidney may be given the more soluble sulfonamides (eg, sulfisoxazole) with relatively little danger of crystalluria. However, sulfonamides must be used cautiously in those with impaired renal function. Dosage requirements in these patients have not been well defined and periodic determination of sulfonamide levels in blood and urine is essential to assure that therapeutic levels of the drug are being maintained without toxic accumulation. Similarly, frequent,

even daily, urinalyses are advisable in all patients receiving sulfonamides intravenously. Severe sulfonamide-induced hypersensitivity reactions may cause renal damage. Sulfonamides are contraindicated in any situation in which adequate urine volume cannot be maintained to prevent toxic effects on the kidney.

Hepatitis with focal or diffuse necrosis and cholestatic jaundice may occur. The conjugation of sulfonamides is reduced in patients with impaired liver function, and toxic reactions may follow usual therapeutic doses.

The sulfonamides are capable of causing blood dyscrasias (leukopenia, granulocytopenia, thrombocytopenia, hypoprothrombinemia, agranulocytosis, and hemolytic or aplastic anemia). Hemolytic anemia has been observed in patients with and without a deficiency of erythrocytic glucose-6-phosphate dehydrogenase (G6PD), particularly when therapy is first initiated. This hazard should be borne in mind if there is a family history of G6PD deficiency, which occurs most commonly in blacks and people of Mediterranean ethnic groups. Blood studies performed at regular intervals may be of value during prolonged therapy with any sulfonamide, since they detect the milder leukopenias. Clinical signs such as sore throat, fever, pallor, purpura, or jaundice also may be early indications of serious blood disorders.

Nonspecific reactions include malaise and a serum sickness-like syndrome. The sulfonamides have been implicated in precipitating polyarteritis nodosa, systemic lupus erythematosus, and goiter.

Sulfonamides cross the placenta and are excreted in milk. Since they compete with bilirubin for albumin binding, high levels of free bilirubin (and kernicterus) can occur in infants born to mothers who take sulfonamides near term and in nursing neonates whose mothers are taking sulfonamides. Therefore, the use of long-acting sulfonamides in pregnant women near term is particularly inadvisable, since these drugs may persist in the infant after birth. In addition, sulfonamides should not be given to infants less than 2 months of age.

Interactions: Because sulfamethizole [Thiosulfil] and sulfathiazole may form insoluble precipitates with formaldehyde in the urine, their concomitant administration with methenamine compounds (eg, methenamine mandelate [Mandelamine]) should be avoided. Hypoglycemia has been reported after antibacterial sulfonamides were given to a few patients receiving tolbutamide [Orinase]; therefore, these agents should be given cautiously to patients receiving any oral hypoglycemic agent. Sulfonamides also should be used cautiously in those receiving coumarin anticoagulants or methotrexate, since they have been reported to enhance the action of these agents.

SHORT-ACTING SULFONAMIDES

SULFACHLORPYRIDAZINE
[Sonilyn]

The actions of this compound are similar to those of sulfisoxazole. Sulfachlorpyridazine is used primarily to treat urinary tract infections caused by susceptible organisms. Frequent administration is necessary to maintain constant blood levels and adequate urinary concentrations. Although sulfachlorpyridazine is more soluble than most sulfonamides and the potential for crystalluria is low, such an occurrence is still possible because of the high concentrations that can be attained in the urine.

For the antibacterial spectrum, adverse reactions, and precautions, see the Introduction.

ROUTE, USUAL DOSAGE, AND PREPARATIONS. *Oral*: Dosage depends upon the severity of the infection. *Adults*, 2 to 4 g initially, then 2 to 4 g daily in three to six divided doses. *Children and infants over 2 months*, 75 mg/kg of body weight initially, then 150 mg/kg daily (maximum, 6 g) in four to six divided doses.

Sonilyn (Mallinckrodt). Tablets 500 mg.

SULFACYTINE
[Renoquid]

Sulfacytine is rapidly absorbed following oral administration. It has a biological half-life of approximately four hours and is 86% bound to serum proteins. More than 90% of a given dose is excreted by the kidneys, almost entirely in the free, active form. This drug is highly soluble in urine within the normal acidic pH range.

Sulfacytine is used to treat acute urinary tract infections caused by susceptible strains of *Escherichia coli*, the *Klebsiella-Enterobacter* group, *Staphylococcus aureus*, *Proteus mirabilis*, and, less frequently, *P. vulgaris*. Compared to sulfisoxazole, which has a similar half-life, sulfacytine is two to three times more active against mutually susceptible organisms.

Sulfacytine is generally well tolerated but may cause any of the toxic manifestations produced by the sulfonamides, including kernicterus and Stevens-Johnson syndrome (see the Introduction). Common adverse reactions are headache, gastrointestinal disturbances, and allergic rash. Although the risk of crystalluria apparently is minimal, fluid intake should be increased when sulfacytine is prescribed and the drug should be used with caution in patients with impaired renal function.

Teratogenic studies in rats and rabbits have revealed no evidence of impaired fertility or fetal damage following use of sulfacytine. Nevertheless, because no well-controlled clinical studies exist, this sulfonamide should not be used during pregnancy unless the expected benefits outweigh the possible adverse effects. Because the drug crosses the placenta and is excreted in milk, it may cause kernicterus. Therefore, it should not be given to nursing mothers or infants less than 2 months of age. Sulfacytine is contraindicated in individuals allergic to the sulfonamides.

ROUTE, USUAL DOSAGE, AND PREPARATIONS.
Oral: Adults, 500 mg initially, followed by
250 mg four times daily for up to ten days.
Patients under 14 years probably should
not be given this drug, since experience
with this sulfonamide in children is lacking.
    Renoquid (Parke, Davis). Tablets 250 mg.

SULFADIAZINE

SULFADIAZINE SODIUM

Sulfadiazine is the sulfonamide of choice
for treating nocardiosis. It may be used in
the short- or long-term treatment of urinary
tract infections but is no longer preferred
for this purpose, since large doses and
alkalization of the urine are needed for
effective therapy. This drug may be administered for prophylaxis (eg, to prevent
recurrences of rheumatic fever) when other
anti-infective agents cannot be used and is
a preferred sulfonamide for general use in
susceptible systemic infections.

The low solubility of sulfadiazine necessitates the maintenance of an adequate
urinary volume (at least 1,500 ml daily);
concomitant alkalization of the urine reduces the tendency to cause crystalluria
but accelerates the urinary excretion of the
drug.

The sodium salt is highly alkaline and
irritating. When parenteral administration
is necessary, the drug may be given intravenously after it is well diluted with
isotonic sodium chloride injection. Intrathecal, subcutaneous, or intramuscular
administration is contraindicated.

For the antibacterial spectrum, adverse
reactions, and precautions, see the Introduction.

ROUTES, USUAL DOSAGE, AND PREPARATIONS.
The blood level should be maintained at 10
to 15 mg/dl.
Oral: Adults, 2 to 4 g initially, then 1 g
every four to six hours. *Children and infants over 2 months,* 75 mg/kg of body
weight initially, then 150 mg/kg daily in
four to six divided doses. The total daily
dose should not exceed 6 g. For
prophylaxis of rheumatic fever, 500 mg
once daily for patients under 30 kg and 1 g
daily for those over 30 kg.
    SULFADIAZINE:
        Drug available generically: Tablets 325, 450,
        and 500 mg.
Intravenous: Adults, initially, 100 mg/kg of
body weight up to a total of 5 g, then 30 to
50 mg/kg every six to eight hours. *Children
over 2 months,* 50 mg/kg initially, then 100
mg/kg daily in four divided doses. Oral
therapy should be substituted as soon as
possible.
    SULFADIAZINE SODIUM:
        Drug available generically: Powder; solution
        250 mg/ml in 10 ml containers.

SULFAMETHIZOLE
[Thiosulfil]

The actions and uses of this highly soluble, rapidly excreted sulfonamide are
similar to those of sulfisoxazole and sulfadiazine. It is one of the preferred sulfonamides for the treatment of urinary tract
infections caused by susceptible organisms. Approximately 90% of sulfamethizole is excreted by the kidneys in
the active form, which is readily soluble
even in acidic urine. Thus, the risk of
crystalluria is minimal and alkalization of
the urine usually is unnecessary; nevertheless, adequate fluid intake should be maintained.

For the antibacterial spectrum, adverse
reactions, and precautions, see the Introduction.

ROUTE, USUAL DOSAGE, AND PREPARATIONS.
Oral: Adults and children over 34 kg, 500
mg to 1 g three or four times daily. *Infants
over 2 months weighing up to 9 kg,* 50 to 60
mg/kg of body weight daily in four divided
doses. *Children 9 to 23 kg,* a maximum of
600 mg daily in four divided doses; *23 to 34
kg,* a maximum of 1.2 g daily in four
divided doses.

Drug available generically: Tablets 500 mg. *Thiosulfil* (Ayerst). Suspension 250 mg/5 ml; tablets 250 and 500 mg (Forte).

SULFISOXAZOLE
[Gantrisin]

SULFISOXAZOLE ACETYL
[Gantrisin Acetyl]

SULFISOXAZOLE DIOLAMINE
[Gantrisin Diolamine]

In general, the actions and uses of sulfisoxazole are similar to those of sulfadiazine. Sulfisoxazole is one of the most effective sulfonamides for treating urinary tract infections and is of some value in systemic infections. Small doses are effective for the prophylaxis of recurrent otitis media. A vaginal cream containing sulfisoxazole may be beneficial in vaginitis caused by sensitive bacterial strains.

Sulfisoxazole acetyl is a tasteless soluble derivative for oral use. It is converted to the base in the intestine. Sulfisoxazole diolamine also is soluble and, since this form has minimal tissue irritant effects, it may be injected or applied topically to the eye.

Sulfisoxazole is rapidly absorbed and excreted. Both the base and acetylated forms are relatively highly soluble even in acidic urine when compared to most other sulfonamides. Thus, the risk of crystalluria is low and alkalization of the urine usually is unnecessary; nevertheless, adequate fluid intake should be maintained.

Topical application of sulfonamides can cause sensitization and these agents are inactivated by blood and pus when used by this route. For the antibacterial spectrum, adverse reactions, and precautions, see the Introduction.

ROUTES, USUAL DOSAGE, AND PREPARATIONS. All concentrations are expressed in terms of the base.
Oral: *Adults*, 2 to 4 g initially, then 1 to 2 g every four to six hours. *Children over 2 months*, 75 mg/kg of body weight initially, then 150 mg/kg daily in divided doses every four hours (maximum, 6 g daily). A concentrated, timed-release preparation (Lipo Gantrisin) is given in approximately the same milligram doses every 12 hours.
SULFISOXAZOLE:
Drug available generically: Tablets 450 and 500 mg.
Gantrisin (Roche). Tablets 500 mg.
SULFISOXAZOLE ACETYL:
Gantrisin [*acetyl*] (Roche). Liquid (timed-release) 1 g/5 ml (Lipo Gantrisin); suspension (pediatric) 500 mg/5 ml; syrup 500 mg/5 ml.
Topical (vaginal): 2.5 to 5 ml (one-half to one applicatorful) of cream applied intravaginally twice daily.
SULFISOXAZOLE:
Gantrisin (Roche). Cream (vaginal) 10% in 3 oz containers.
SULFISOXAZOLE DIOLAMINE:
See Chapter 24, Ocular Anti-infective and Anti-inflammatory Agents.
Intravenous, Subcutaneous: *Adults*, same as oral dosage. *Children over 2 months*, 50 mg/kg of body weight initially, then 100 mg/kg daily in three (intravenous) or four (subcutaneous) divided doses.
SULFISOXAZOLE DIOLAMINE:
Gantrisin [*diolamine*] (Roche). Solution 400 mg/ml in 5 and 10 ml containers.

INTERMEDIATE- AND LONG-ACTING SULFONAMIDES

SULFAMETHOXAZOLE
[Gantanol]

This compound is classified as an intermediate-acting sulfonamide and resembles sulfisoxazole in its therapeutic effectiveness, but absorption and excretion of the unconjugated drug are slower. During therapy, it is important to maintain an adequate urinary output (at least 1,500 ml daily in adults) by ensuring adequate fluid intake, but alkalization of the urine usually is unnecessary.

Sulfamethoxazole is useful for treating infections of the lower urinary tract caused by susceptible organisms. It also is used with trimethoprim for urinary tract and systemic infections (see the section on Mixtures).

For the antibacterial spectrum, adverse reactions, and precautions, see the Introduction.

ROUTE, USUAL DOSAGE, AND PREPARATIONS. *Oral*: *Adults*, 2 g initially, then 1 g two or three times daily. *Children over 2 months*, initially, 50 to 60 mg/kg of body weight (maximum, 75 mg/kg/24 hours), then one-half of this amount every 12 hours.

> Drug available generically: Tablets 500 mg and 1 g.
> *Gantanol* (Roche). Suspension 500 mg/5 ml; tablets 500 mg and 1 g (Gantanol DS).

SULFAMETER
[Sulla]

Sulfameter is classified as a long-acting sulfonamide. It may be effective in urinary tract infections caused by susceptible strains of bacteria, especially *Escherichia coli*. Although about 60% to 70% of this drug is excreted in the urine in the unchanged, active form, its slow elimination produces a lower urinary concentration than that attainable with the short-acting compounds. In addition, its slow excretion increases the hazard to the patient if a serious adverse reaction occurs. Therefore, the use of sulfameter instead of a short-acting sulfonamide is only rarely justified and should be limited to those situations in which a once daily dosage schedule is necessary. Sulfameter should not be used to treat acute infections.

For the antibacterial spectrum, adverse reactions, and precautions, see the Introduction.

ROUTE, USUAL DOSAGE, AND PREPARATIONS. *Oral*: *Adults and children over 12 years*, 1.5 g initially, then 500 mg once daily. Sulfameter should be used with consider-able care in *children under 12 years*.

> *Sulla* (Robins). Tablets 500 mg.

TOPICAL SULFONAMIDES AND RELATED COMPOUNDS

MAFENIDE ACETATE
[Sulfamylon]

Mafenide is not a true sulfonamide chemically but has essentially the same antibacterial spectrum as silver sulfadiazine. It is used topically to prevent sepsis and reduce morbidity and mortality in patients with burns and is particularly effective against susceptible strains of *Pseudomonas aeruginosa*. Unlike most sulfonamides, the action of mafenide is not inhibited by pus and body fluids. It is highly soluble and diffuses into burn tissue where it is metabolized to compounds devoid of antimicrobial action.

Unlike silver sulfadiazine, mafenide causes pain at the site of application, which can be severe. Allergic skin reactions and acid-base disturbances (hyperchloremic acidosis with tachypnea and hyperventilation) also may develop.

ROUTE, USUAL DOSAGE, AND PREPARATIONS. *Topical*: Following cleansing and debriding of the wound, the cream is applied with a sterile gloved hand to the burned area two or three times daily to a thickness of 1 mm. It should be applied more frequently to burned areas from which the cream might be removed by movement of the patient. Therapy is continued until satisfactory healing has occurred or until the burn site is ready for grafting. Dressings can be applied over the cream, although this is unnecessary. Concomitant daily hydrotherapy and mechanical debridement are advisable, especially in patients with third-degree burns.

> *Sulfamylon* (Winthrop). Cream (water-miscible) equivalent to 85 mg of base/g in 2, 4, and 14.5 oz containers.

SILVER SULFADIAZINE
[Silvadene]

This sulfonamide is used to prevent and treat infections in patients with second- and third-degree burns. In vitro sensitivity tests indicate that it is at least as active and, in most cases, more active against common gram-positive and gram-negative bacteria than sulfadiazine base. The drug is effective against *Pseudomonas* species, the most common pathogen in fatal burn sepsis. It also inhibits the growth of *Enterobacter*, *Klebsiella*, *Escherichia coli*, *Proteus*, *Staphylococcus*, and *Streptococcus* (including enterococci). Some strains of *Candida albicans* and, possibly, herpes virus also are sensitive. The antibacterial action of this compound does not appear to be entirely attributable to its sulfonamide content. Silver also is thought to have bacteriostatic properties.

Silver sulfadiazine reduces morbidity and mortality in patients with extensive second- and third-degree burns. By inhibiting the growth of pathogenic bacteria, the drug may help prevent partial-thickness burns from progressing to full-thickness wounds. In favorable cases, epithelialization of second-degree burns is apparent after about ten days. The cream base also appears to soften eschar; however, by decreasing local bacterial action, silver sulfadiazine decreases autolysis of eschar and, therefore, should be combined with daily hydrotherapy and debridement to enhance rapid removal of eschar in patients with third-degree burns.

Application of silver sulfadiazine is usually painless, and it does not cause electrolyte disturbances even after prolonged contact with the burned area. Approximately 2.5% of patients experience rash, pruritus, or a burning sensation when the cream is applied.

Significant quantities of sulfadiazine can be absorbed following prolonged treatment of extensive burns; serum levels infrequently approach those observed following systemic therapy with sulfadiazine. Accordingly, all adverse reactions attributable to systemic sulfonamides are possible (see the Introduction). However, it is not necessary to monitor serum levels during prolonged treatment except, possibly, in patients with impaired renal or hepatic function.

Safe use of silver sulfadiazine during pregnancy has not been established. On theoretical grounds, the drug probably should be withheld from sensitive or pregnant patients but, in view of the hazards of sepsis with severe burns, the use of silver sulfadiazine in such patients must be determined individually.

ROUTE, USUAL DOSAGE, AND PREPARATIONS. *Topical*: Following cleansing and debriding of the wound, the cream is applied with a sterile gloved hand to the burned surface once or twice daily to a thickness of 1 mm. Care should be taken to get the cream into all interstices and crevices of the irregular burn surface since application of the cream is not painful. The drug should be applied more frequently to burned areas from which the cream might be removed by movement of the patient. Therapy is continued until satisfactory healing has occurred or until the burned site is ready for grafting. Dressings can be applied over the burn and, although this is unnecessary, a layer of fine mesh gauze covered with a mildly firm roller bandage will help ensure contact of the drug with the wound. This covering will be more comfortable than no dressing to most patients. The low solubility of the drug facilitates the maintenance of antimicrobial action for many hours. For this reason, once daily application of cream and dressing usually suffices. Concomitant daily hydrotherapy and mechanical debridement also are advisable, especially in patients with third-degree burns.

Silvadene (Marion). Cream (water-miscible) 10 mg/g in 50 and 400 g containers.

MISCELLANEOUS SULFONAMIDES

PHTHALYLSULFATHIAZOLE
[Sulfathalidine]

Since this sulfonamide is poorly absorbed, its actions are essentially confined to the gut where it produces soft stools. Phthalylsulfathiazole is used as an adjunct in the treatment of ulcerative colitis, as well as to reduce bacterial flora in the pre- and postoperative management of patients undergoing bowel surgery.

See Chapter 58, Antidiarrheal Agents, for a discussion of adverse reactions, usual dosage, and preparations.

SULFAPYRIDINE

This compound is relatively insoluble and is slowly absorbed following oral administration. Unlike many of the newer sulfonamides, there is a high risk of crystalluria when sulfapyridine is given. It is quite toxic and would be considered obsolete except that it is probably still the preferred drug for treating dermatitis herpetiformis. Its mechanism of action in this condition is unknown.

For adverse reactions and precautions, see the Introduction.

ROUTE, USUAL DOSAGE, AND PREPARATIONS.
Oral: Adults, 500 mg four times daily until definite improvement is noted. The daily dose is then decreased by 500 mg at three-day intervals until symptom-free maintenance is achieved. The dosage may be increased if there is a recurrence.
    Drug available generically: Tablets 500 mg.

SULFASALAZINE
[Azulfidine, S.A.S.-500]

Sulfasalazine (salicylazosulfapyridine) often is effective as an adjunct in the management of ulcerative colitis, particularly to prevent relapses, and possibly in diverticulitis. Sulfasalazine is converted to sulfapyridine in the intestine, but its effect in ulcerative colitis is apparently not due to its antibacterial action, since this drug does not alter the intestinal flora.

See Chapter 58, Antidiarrheal Agents, for a discussion of adverse reactions, usual dosage, and preparations.

MIXTURES

Mixtures Containing Only Sulfonamides

The rationale for combining several sulfonamides in a single preparation for systemic use is that the solubilities of the sulfonamides are independent of each other but their therapeutic effects are additive. Use of combination therapy thereby decreases the risk of crystalluria. Similar reasoning is used for combinations of sulfonamides used topically. However, although mixtures of sulfonamides still enjoy some degree of popularity, they are used less frequently today than formerly because the availability of newer single-entity agents that are more soluble in urine (eg, sulfisoxazole) has made the logic for their existence obsolete.

SULFATHIAZOLE, SULFACETAMIDE, AND SULFABENZAMIDE
[Sultrin]

This combination of sulfathiazole, sulfacetamide, and sulfabenzamide (each at a different concentration and, apparently, each most active at a pH different from that found in the vagina) is promoted for the prophylaxis or treatment of cervical and vaginal infections caused by sensitive organisms. Most organisms responsible for vaginitis are not sensitive to the sulfonamides, although this mixture has some effectiveness in *Corynebacterium vaginale* (*Haemophilus vaginalis*) vaginitis. Therefore, the combination is of limited usefulness. Sensitization may occur from topical application of sulfonamides.

ROUTE, USUAL DOSAGE, AND PREPARATIONS. *Topical (vaginal)*: One applicatorful of cream inserted twice daily for four to six days; the dosage may then be reduced by one-quarter to one-half. Alternatively, one vaginal tablet may be inserted at bedtime and on arising for ten days; this course may be repeated if necessary.

> *Sultrin* (Ortho). Cream containing sulfathiazole 3.42%, sulfacetamide 2.86%, and sulfabenzamide 3.7% with urea 0.64% in 78 g containers; each vaginal tablet contains sulfathiazole 172.5 mg, sulfacetamide 143.75 mg, and sulfabenzamide 184 mg.

TRISULFAPYRIMIDINES
[Sulfose, Terfonyl]

This combination of equal parts of sulfadiazine, sulfamerazine, and sulfamethazine appears to produce somewhat higher total blood levels of sulfonamide than equal doses of sulfadiazine alone, but the effectiveness remains the same.

The incidence of crystalluria (but not of other untoward effects) is reduced with trisulfapyrimidines. For indications, adverse reactions, and precautions, see the Introduction.

ROUTE, USUAL DOSAGE, AND PREPARATIONS. *Oral*: *Adults*, 3 to 4 g initially, then 1 g every six hours. *Children and infants over 2 months*, 75 mg/kg of body weight initially, then 150 mg/kg daily in four to six divided doses.

> Drug available generically: Tablets 500 mg.
> *Sulfose* (Wyeth), *Terfonyl* (Squibb). Suspension 500 mg/5 ml; tablets 500 mg.

Mixtures Containing a Sulfonamide and Another Drug

Fixed-ratio combinations of sulfonamides and antibiotics have been popular in practice but, in general, the rationale for their use is questionable. There is no substantial evidence that there are any significant mixed infections requiring administration of the fixed-ratios available. Use of such combinations exposes patients to the potential adverse reactions of two potent drugs and frequently increases the cost of medication when compared to individual doses of each drug alone. Most older products have been removed from the market, the main notable exception being mixtures of a sulfonamide combined with phenazopyridine alone or phenazopyridine and a tetracycline. A fixed-ratio combination containing sulfamethoxazole and trimethoprim [Bactrim, Septra] appears to be one of the few rational fixed-ratio mixtures. A demonstrable synergism exists between the two agents in this mixture at the ratio in which they are present.

In contrast to fixed-ratio combinations, use of more than one single-entity antibacterial agent may be indicated in severe infections when treatment must be initiated empirically pending determination of the specific etiologic organism; however, when the causative organism has been identified, the drug that best meets the needs of the patient should be given.

Other mixtures containing sulfonamides are listed in Chapter 24, Ocular Anti-infective and Anti-inflammatory Agents.

SULFAMETHOXAZOLE AND TRIMETHOPRIM
[Bactrim, Septra]

Trimethoprim

A fixed-ratio combination containing sulfamethoxazole and trimethoprim is effective in vitro against a wide variety of gram-positive and gram-negative organisms, including staphylococci, streptococci, *Escherichia coli, Haemophilus influenzae*, and *Proteus, Salmonella*, and *Shigella* species. Some *Klebsiella-Enterobacter* species are sensitive to the combination, despite the fact that many are completely resistant to sulfamethoxazole alone. The mixture also has some antiprotozoal effects (eg, in *Pneumocystis* and *Plasmodium* infections) and is active against *Nocardia*.

This combination is a primary medication for treating both acute and chronic urinary tract infections and may be particularly useful when the infection is associated with prostatitis. Also, it is effective prophylactically in individuals prone to recurrent urinary tract infections, an action attributed to the properties of the combination or, perhaps, to trimethoprim alone. Work by Kunin et al (1978) indicates that trimethoprim may be as effective as the combination for treating recurrent urinary tract infections. These authors suggest that trimethoprim has an additional advantage in that it can be used with relative safety in patients with impaired renal function or in those who cannot tolerate sulfonamides. However, the value of long-term suppressive therapy of urinary tract infections with antibiotics remains unproven.

The combination of sulfamethoxazole and trimethoprim also may be a therapy of choice for treating shigellosis, particularly in individuals living in areas where antibiotic-resistant shigellae are common. This mixture may be as effective as chloramphenicol in treating typhoid and paratyphoid fevers and is the preparation of choice for typhoid fever that is resistant to both chloramphenicol and ampicillin. Trimethoprim and sulfamethoxazole is useful for children with acute otitis media caused by susceptible strains of *H. influenzae* and *Streptococcus pneumoniae*. This mixture has been used successfully to treat *Pneumocystis carinii* infections in children 9 months to 16 years of age whose host defenses have been suppressed by cancer

therapy; adults also may respond (Lau and Young, 1976), and the combination may be used for the prophylaxis of this disease in immunosuppressed patients (Hughes et al, 1977).

Experimentally, the combination has been effective in subacute bacterial endocarditis. Susceptible infections of the nose, throat, ear, skin, soft tissues, and bone, as well as septicemias, brucellosis, enteric fever, and uncomplicated gonorrhea also may respond to this mixture.

Resistance to trimethoprim develops in vitro when strains of certain bacteria are cultured serially in increasing concentrations of the drug. Clinically, emergence of strains resistant to the combination has been uncommon, and cross resistance between the combination and other anti-infective agents has not been reported.

This mixture is usually well tolerated; however, because it contains a sulfonamide, any adverse effect reported with use of this group of drugs may occur following administration of the combination (see the Introduction). Because blood dyscrasias have been reported, periodic blood tests are probably indicated in patients receiving long-term therapy, but the sudden appearance of sore throat, fever, pallor, purpura, or jaundice may be more reliable indications of the imminent appearance of a blood disorder than routine blood studies. Crystalluria can occur; therefore, patients taking this medication should maintain an adequate fluid intake. Glossitis and renal and liver damage have been reported infrequently.

Since trimethoprim is a folate antagonist that can inhibit the normal development of purines, it might be expected to cause teratogenic effects. Fetal malformations have occurred in several animal species but have not as yet been reported clinically. Nevertheless, because of the lack of published data on use of the drug in pregnant women and because folate levels are probably marginal during pregnancy, the combination of trimethoprim and sulfamethoxazole is generally contraindicated in pregnant women or should be used only with full knowledge of the potential danger. Similarly, use of the mixture should be restricted in all patients considered to have marginal levels of folates.

ROUTE, USUAL DOSAGE, AND PREPARATIONS. *Oral:* The following dosages are given to patients with normal renal function: *Adults,* for urinary tract infections, two tablets or four teaspoonsful (20 ml) of suspension every 12 hours for 10 to 14 days. For shigellosis, the same dose is administered for five days. *Children,* for urinary tract infections or acute otitis media, 8 mg/kg of body weight of trimethoprim and 40 mg/kg of sulfamethoxazole daily in two divided doses every 12 hours for 10 days. The same dose can be given for five days to treat shigellosis. The following table may be used as a *guideline in children 2 months of age or older:*

WEIGHT		DOSE (every 12 hours)	
lb	kg	teaspoonsful	tablets
22	10	1 (5 ml)	½
44	20	2 (10 ml)	1
66	30	3 (15 ml)	1½
88	40	4 (20 ml)	2
			(or 1 DS tablet)

For severe infections, the daily amount may be increased by one-half and given in three divided doses.

The dosage for patients with *Pneumocystis carinii* pneumonitis is 20 mg/kg of trimethoprim and 100 mg/kg of sulfamethoxazole daily in equally divided doses every six hours for 14 days. The following table *can be used as a guideline in children:*

WEIGHT		DOSE (every 6 hours)	
lb	kg	teaspoonsful	tablets
18	8	1 (5 ml)	½
35	16	2 (10 ml)	1
53	24	3 (15 ml)	1½
70	32	4 (20 ml)	2
			(or 1 DS tablet)

For patients with impaired renal function, it is recommended that the usual dose be given if creatinine clearance is above 30 ml/min; that the dose be reduced to one-half the usual amount if creatinine clearance is between 15 and 30 ml/min; and that the drug not be used if creatinine clearance is below 15 ml/min. All patients should maintain an adequate urine volume to prevent crystalluria.

Bactrim (Roche), *Septra* (Burroughs Wellcome). Each 5 ml of suspension contains sulfamethoxazole 200 mg and trimethoprim 40 mg; each tablet contains sulfamethoxazole 400 mg and trimethoprim 80 mg; each double-strength tablet contains sulfamethoxazole 800 mg and trimethoprim 160 mg (Bactrim-DS, Septra-DS).

SULFONAMIDES AND PHENAZOPYRIDINE

Phenazopyridine, a urinary tract analgesic, is combined with sulfonamides, most commonly sulfamethoxazole, in fixed-ratio preparations promoted for the treatment of urinary tract infections. Since phenazopyridine may relieve such symptoms as pain, burning, urgency, and frequency, its concomitant use with a sulfonamide is regarded as possibly beneficial. However, this analgesic preferably is given separately rather than in a fixed-combination product so that it can be eliminated from the regimen as soon as symptoms are controlled. Some preparations also contain a tetracycline.

ROUTE, USUAL DOSAGE, AND PREPARATIONS. *Oral:* Dosage is the same as that for the sulfonamide without phenazopyridine (see the evaluation on the appropriate sulfonamide).

Azo Gantanol (Roche). Each tablet contains sulfamethoxazole 500 mg and phenazopyridine hydrochloride 100 mg.

Azo Gantrisin (Roche). Each tablet contains sulfisoxazole 500 mg and phenazopyridine hydrochloride 50 mg.

Azotrex Capsules (Bristol). Each capsule contains sulfamethizole 250 mg, tetracycline phosphate complex equivalent to tetracycline hydrochloride activity 125 mg, and phenazopyridine hydrochloride 50 mg.

Thiosulfil A, Thiosulfil A Forte (Ayerst). Each tablet contains sulfamethizole 250 or 500 mg (Forte) and phenazopyridine hydrochloride 50 mg.

Urobiotic-250 (Roerig). Each capsule contains sulfamethizole 250 mg, oxytetracycline hydrochloride 250 mg equivalent to oxytetracycline, and phenazopyridine hydrochloride 50 mg.

Selected References

Trimethoprim-sulphamethoxazole. *Drugs* 1:7-53, 1971.

Baxter CR: Topical use of 1.0% silver sulfadiazine, in Polk HC Jr, Stone HH (eds): *Contemporary Burn Management*. Boston, Little, Brown and Company, 1971, 217-225.

Finland M, Kass EH (eds): Trimethoprim-sulfamethoxazole. *J Infect Dis* 128(suppl):425-816, (Nov) 1972.

Fox CL Jr: Silver sulfadiazine: New topical therapy of *Pseudomonas* infection in burns. *Arch Surg* 96:184-188, 1968.

Garrod LP: Trimethoprim: Its possible place in antibacterial therapy. *Drugs* 1:3-6, 1971.

Hughes WT, et al: Successful chemoprophylaxis for *Pneumocystis carinii* pneumonitis. *N Engl J Med* 297:1419-1426, 1977.

Kunin CM, et al: Trimethoprim therapy for urinary tract infection. *JAMA* 239:2588-2590, 1978.

Lau WK, Young LS: Trimethoprim-sulfamethoxazole treatment of *Pneumocystis carinii* pneumonia in adults. *N Engl J Med* 295:716-718, 1976.

Lloyd JR: Thermal trauma: Therapeutic achievements and investigative horizons. *Surg Clin North Am* 57:121-138, 1977.

Urinary Tract Antiseptics | 78

Any anti-infective agent excreted primarily in the urine is potentially useful in the treatment of uncomplicated urinary infections caused by susceptible organisms. Because of important variations in the rates of absorption and excretion, extent of protein binding, attainable urinary drug levels, and mechanism of action, some compounds are more effective than others. Primary drugs include ampicillin, the tetracyclines, the soluble sulfonamides, and a combination product containing sulfamethoxazole and trimethoprim [Bactrim, Septra]. Also useful, but usually under somewhat restricted conditions, are the aminoglycosides, cephalosporins, and carbenicillin [Geocillin, Geopen]. Most of these drugs have other, more general applications and are discussed in detail in other chapters.

A few drugs (nitrofurantoin, nalidixic acid, oxolinic acid, methenamine) are used only for treating urinary infections. These agents usually demonstrate good activity against the pathogens that commonly infect the urinary tract and, since they are concentrated in the urine, have been classified broadly as urinary tract antiseptics. A fifth compound, phenazopyridine hydrochloride [Pyridium], has been used in the past as a urinary antiseptic, but it has little or no action against the organisms responsible for urinary tract infections. It is of value, however, as a urinary tract analgesic to relieve the pain, burning, urgency, and frequency of urination associated with cystitis, prostatitis, and urethritis, whether caused by infection or related to other disorders.

Urinary antiseptics frequently are not drugs of first choice for treating urinary infections and often cannot be used as the sole therapeutic agent. Nevertheless, because they are fairly nontoxic, they may be important drugs in the management of urinary infections, particularly those that persist despite vigorous therapy or recur with frustrating regularity. Therefore, unless bacterial resistance develops, they may be useful for long-term therapy.

Drug therapy cannot be completely successful if the underlying cause of the urinary tract infection remains. Therefore, the physician must have a working knowledge of the pathophysiology of urinary infection, since etiology and drug usage must be considered together when planning a therapeutic regimen to avoid persistent or recurrent infection.

Factors that alter host resistance are more important in the development of infection than the route by which the organism gains access to the urine. Bacteria introduced into the urinary tract will not flourish unless there is also a breakdown in host resistance. Thus, successful therapy must be a two-step process: The factor decreasing host resistance is identified and removed and the organism is eradicated with appropriate antibacterial medication. For more complete discussions on the pathogenesis of urinary tract infections, see specialty texts or available literature (eg,

Adatto et al, 1979; Burke et al, 1979; Lapides, 1976; Lohr et al, 1977; Roland, 1979).

Most urinary tract infections follow ischemic episodes involving the bladder and are caused by overdistention of the bladder and high intravesical pressure. In young girls, uninhibited or infantile bladder and, to a lesser extent, infrequent voiding are the main factors impairing host resistance, whereas, in women, uninhibited neurogenic bladder and infrequent voiding are responsible (Lapides, 1976; Addato et al, 1979). Frequent voiding in conjunction with appropriate medication may prevent recurrent episodes of urinary infections. Sexual intercourse, the use of bubble baths, the degree of cleanliness of the female perineum, and changes in the vaginal flora are of minimal or no importance in the development of such infections.

In male infants and young boys, stenosis of the urethral meatus and posterior urethral valves commonly precipitates urinary infection, while obstructive uropathy in the prostatic urethra is the leading cause in adult males. Recurrent urinary infections in elderly men often are misdiagnosed as chronic prostatitis, a situation which has led to the belief that chronic bacterial prostatitis is commonly responsible for recurrent urinary infections. True chronic prostatitis occurs infrequently, is rarely symptomatic, and is usually secondary to urethrocystitis. It is often easily cured if the cause of host resistance can be eliminated. In many men with recurrent urinary infections, early obstructive uropathy is the cause of infection.

Less frequently, a variety of genitourinary diseases can lead to urinary tract infections, including bladder exstrophy, epispadias, ureterocele, and ectopic ureter; carcinoma of the urethra, bladder, and pelvis; prostatic, vesical, ureteral, and kidney calculus disease; enterovesical fistulas; supravesical urinary diversion; intersex problems; urethral diverticula; condyloma acuminata of the urethra; cystitis produced by interstitial, radiation, and cancer chemotherapy; and polycystic kidney disease (Lapides, 1976).

INDIVIDUAL EVALUATIONS

NITROFURANTOIN
[Cyantin, Furadantin, Macrodantin]

Nitrofurantoin is used orally as a urinary antiseptic. It has a wide in vitro spectrum of antibacterial activity against both gram-positive and gram-negative organisms, including some that commonly cause urinary tract infections (eg, *Streptococcus faecalis*, *Escherichia coli*) and others that are responsible for urinary tract infections only rarely or not at all (eg, *Salmonella*, *Shigella*, *Staphylococcus pyogenes*). Most strains of *Klebsiella*, *Enterobacter*, *Serratia*, indole-positive *Proteus* species, and *Streptococcus pyogenes* also are susceptible. *Pseudomonas aeruginosa* and most strains of *Proteus* are resistant. Although many bacterial enzyme systems are inhibited by nitrofurantoin, its exact mechanism of action is unknown (Paul and Paul, 1964).

Nitrofurantoin is effective in the treatment of bacteriuria associated with infection of the lower genitourinary tract. It is used to treat uncomplicated urinary tract infections in men, women, and especially in children (Burke et al, 1979). Administration for periods longer than 14 days is rarely necessary for acute uncomplicated infections. Nitrofurantoin also is one of the more effective agents available for short-term prophylaxis or long-term suppressive therapy of chronic urinary infections after bacteria have been eliminated or markedly reduced by therapy with other, more effective agents (Lohr et al, 1977). Insufficient evidence is available to ascertain its usefulness in other types of genitourinary tract infections (eg, prostatitis).

Nitrofurantoin is available in a microcrystalline [eg, Furadantin] and a macrocrystalline [Macrodantin] form. Following oral administration, it is readily absorbed from the gastrointestinal tract.

Clinical studies on absorption and excretion indicate that, in normal fasting individuals, less nitrofurantoin is absorbed and at a slower rate from the macrocrystalline than the microcrystalline form (Bates et al, 1974). The presence of food in the intestine delays the absorption of both forms appreciably, increases peak levels of the macrocrystalline but not the microcrystalline compound, enhances bioavailability of both forms, and prolongs the duration of therapeutic urinary concentrations. Nitrofurantoin is the first drug for which it has been shown that food in the gastrointestinal tract increases bioavailability (Bates et al, 1974). This finding is important because most physicians recommend that the drug be taken with meals to diminish the incidence and severity of nausea and vomiting.

There is some evidence that decreased gastric acidity interferes with the absorption of nitrofurantoin and, therefore, excessive use of antacids should be avoided. Prolonged therapy does not appear to alter normal intestinal microflora significantly (Stamey, 1972).

Once absorbed, 60% of nitrofurantoin is reversibly bound to serum proteins and the drug is rapidly excreted by the kidneys. Thus, antibacterial concentrations of unbound drug in the serum are ineffective, but levels of 100 to 125 mcg/ml, which are bactericidal to sensitive organisms, are easily attained in the urine of patients with normal renal function. Alkalizing the urine increases the urinary concentration of the drug but decreases antibacterial efficacy. Efforts to increase the pH of the urine, therefore, have no therapeutic advantage (Pratt, 1977). If creatinine clearance is less than 40 ml/min, antibacterial concentrations of nitrofurantoin attained in the urine are inadequate and elevated blood levels of the drug with an increased danger of toxicity result. The hazard increases with the degree of renal insufficiency. Therefore, nitrofurantoin is contraindicated when renal function is markedly diminished.

The overall incidence of adverse effects is relatively high (as much as 10% or more). The most common reactions are nausea, vomiting, diarrhea (the severity of these effects is dose related), and fever. The incidence of adverse effects has been reported to be significantly lower with the macrocrystalline than with the microcrystalline form (Kalowski et al, 1974).

Occasionally, pulmonary complications can develop within a few days after therapy is initiated. This iatrogenic syndrome represents a hypersensitivity reaction and is manifested as an acute pneumonitis with cough, dyspnea, wheezing, and fluid infiltration, often associated with eosinophilia (Hailey et al, 1969). Usually, discontinuing the drug relieves symptoms but, in severe cases, corticosteroid therapy may be indicated. Chronic interstitial pneumonitis resulting in pulmonary fibrosis also has occurred in patients receiving long-term (more than six months) nitrofurantoin therapy. This disorder may not respond to discontinuation of the drug or steroid therapy, and permanent pulmonary damage may result.

Other types of hypersensitivity reactions occur less frequently but may be severe. Rash and urticaria are most common, but chills and fever are sometimes seen. Rarely, hepatotoxicity manifested as hepatitis and cholestatic jaundice may develop. Angioedema and anaphylaxis also have been reported (Pratt, 1977).

Neurotoxicity is sometimes observed. Most of the effects are mild and consist of malaise, myalgia, headache, dizziness, drowsiness, or vertigo. Polyneuropathy, including severe peripheral neuritis, may occur, particularly if nitrofurantoin is given to patients with renal insufficiency, anemia, diabetes, electrolyte imbalance, vitamin B-complex deficiency, or in larger than recommended doses.

The systemic administration of nitrofurantoin occasionally may cause bone marrow depression. Hemolytic anemia has been reported in patients with congenital erythrocytic glucose-6-phosphate dehydrogenase (G6PD) deficiency (Pratt, 1977), and megaloblastic anemia has bee observed rarely (Bass, 1963).

Large doses of nitrofurantoin depress spermatogenesis by acting directly on seminiferous tubules. Usual therapeutic doses appear to have no such effect (Pratt, 1977).

Although fetal toxicity has not been reported, the possibility should be considered. Nitrofurantoin should be used in pregnant women only when benefits outweigh the potential hazard (see Chapter 2). Adequate information on the use of this drug in newborn infants is lacking. The drug should not be given to infants under 1 month of age because it may cause hemolytic anemia.

Nitrofurantoin has an advantage over many other antimicrobial agents in that bacterial resistance develops slowly and to a limited degree in vivo, and bacterial cross resistance and cross sensitization occur infrequently. Organisms isolated from the urine of women with recurring infections who were treated with nitrofurantoin remain sensitive, even after many courses of therapy (Kunin, 1974).

ROUTE, USUAL DOSAGE, AND PREPARATIONS.
Oral: *Adults*, 50 to 100 mg four times daily. *Children*, 5 to 7 mg/kg of body weight every 24 hours given in four divided doses. These doses should be reduced by one-half if administration is continued for more than ten days; after 20 days, the amounts should be reduced to one-quarter.
For prophylaxis of frequently recurring urinary tract infections in women, 50 to 100 mg at bedtime.
> Drug available generically: Capsules, tablets 50 and 100 mg.
> *Cyantin* (Lederle). Tablets 50 and 100 mg.
> *Furadantin* (Norwich-Eaton). Suspension 25 mg/5 ml; tablets 50 and 100 mg.
> *Macrodantin* (Norwich-Eaton). Capsules 25, 50, and 100 mg.

NALIDIXIC ACID
[NegGram]

Nalidixic acid rapidly inhibits DNA synthesis in susceptible bacteria (Goss et al, 1965), but bacterial RNA and protein synthesis continues for some time after exposure to the drug. Mammalian DNA synthesis is unaffected by nalidixic acid.

This depression of bacterial DNA synthesis apparently is reversible since normal growth resumes when bacteria are no longer exposed to the drug.

Nalidixic acid is administered orally, primarily to treat recurrent urinary infections. It is effective against the majority of gram-negative organisms that infect the urinary tract, especially *Escherichia coli* and most species of *Proteus*; treatment of infections caused by *Proteus* organisms resistant to other antibacterial agents is a major indication for use of this drug. Nalidixic acid also is active against other coliform bacteria such as *Klebsiella* and *Enterobacter aerogenes*. Most *Pseudomonas* species and *Streptococcus faecalis* are resistant (Stamey, 1971). This drug is relatively ineffective against gram-positive bacteria.

Nalidixic acid has a narrow antibacterial spectrum, and bacterial sensitivity tests are important in determining when this agent should be used. Since urinary infections caused by *Pseudomonas* and *S. faecalis* are uncommon, this drug may be administered when *Proteus* infection is suspected pending the results of bacterial culture. Nalidixic acid also may be used in acute uncomplicated cystitis without prior sensitivity testing, because this condition is almost always caused by sensitive organisms. Antibacterial concentrations of nalidixic acid are not obtained in prostatic fluid. As with any antibacterial agent used to treat urinary infections, follow-up cultures are desirable to determine if the infection has been cured.

Nalidixic acid is not suitable for treating systemic infections, since effective antibacterial blood and tissue levels cannot be attained at safe dosage levels and the drug is highly bound (93% or greater) by plasma proteins. Even hydroxynalidixic acid, the chief active metabolite of nalidixic acid which accounts for one-third of the biologically active drug in the plasma, is 68% bound to plasma proteins.

Some organisms develop resistance to nalidixic acid so rapidly (often within 48 hours) that the drug is useless as a therapeutic agent against them. If the infecting pathogen is sensitive initially and does not develop resistance, therapy should be continued for two weeks; if the urine does not become sterile 48 to 72 hours following initiation of treatment, another drug must be substituted. Cross resistance to oxolinic acid has been reported.

The incidence of untoward effects associated with nalidixic acid is low. The most common reactions are nausea, vomiting, rash, and urticaria. Diarrhea, abdominal pain, fever, eosinophilia, and photosensitivity occur occasionally. Superinfection with fungal organisms has not been noted. Patients taking this drug should be warned against excessive exposure to sunlight. Hemolytic anemia has been reported (Beutler, 1969); patients with a deficiency of glucose-6-phosphate dehydrogenase (G6PD) seem most susceptible. Leukopenia and thrombocytopenia also have occurred.

Nalidixic acid occasionally causes neurologic reactions (headache, malaise, paresthesias, drowsiness, dizziness, myalgia, muscular weakness, visual abnormalities, excitement, confusion, hallucinations). Convulsions have occurred in children and adults after overdosage; therefore, care must be exercised when children are treated on an outpatient basis or when any patient with a history of convulsive disorders or central nervous system damage receives this drug. Because nalidixic acid may accumulate in patients with renal or hepatic insufficiency, it should be used very cautiously in these patients, especially if neurologic damage is present. Patients with a creatinine clearance of 2 to 8 ml/min have received full therapeutic doses, however, without signs of overt toxicity (Stamey et al, 1969).

Nalidixic acid may increase intracranial pressure, causing papilledema and bulging fontanelles in infants (Rao, 1974). False-positive reactions to chemical tests for urinary glucose also occur. Caution is indicated if this drug is used during pregnancy, although it has been administered during the second and third trimesters without adversely affecting mother or fetus. Nalidixic acid should not be given to infants under 1 month of age.

ROUTE, USUAL DOSAGE, AND PREPARATIONS. *Oral*: *Adults,* 4 g daily in four divided doses for two weeks; one week of therapy may be sufficient to treat uncomplicated lower urinary tract infections. The dosage is then reduced to 2 g daily if long-term treatment is indicated. *Children under 12 years,* 55 mg/kg of body weight daily in four divided doses; for prolonged therapy, the daily dose may be reduced to 33 mg/kg.

NegGram (Winthrop). Suspension 250 mg/5 ml; tablets 250 and 500 mg and 1 g.

OXOLINIC ACID
[Utibid]

Oxolinic acid is closely related chemically to nalidixic acid. It has a similar antibacterial spectrum and probably an identical mechanism of antibacterial action, although this has not been proved. Because oxolinic acid, like nalidixic acid, has a narrow spectrum, bacterial culture and sensitivity tests generally should be performed prior to its use. Nevertheless, since its spectrum includes most of the gram-negative pathogens that commonly cause urinary infections, this agent may be used initially in selected cases (eg, when indole-positive *Proteus* is suspected as the infecting organism) before the results of sensitivity tests become available.

When bacterial resistance develops to oxolinic acid, it is usually rapid (Mohring and Madsen, 1971). If follow-up cultures indicate that the urine is not sterile within 48 to 72 hours, it is likely that the organism will have developed resistance. Cross resistance to nalidixic acid has been reported.

Following oral administration, oxolinic acid is rapidly absorbed, but peak blood and tissue levels are inadequate for effective systemic use. Urinary concentrations of approximately 40 to 75 mcg/ml are attained in 8 and 12 hours, respectively. The in vitro and in vivo potency of oxolinic acid is greater on a weight basis than that of nalidixic acid and, because oxolinic acid has a longer duration of action, adequate urinary levels can be maintained with administration twice daily (Mohring and Madsen, 1971). This appears to be its chief advantage over nalidixic acid, since the latter agent must be taken four times daily to be effective.

Oxolinic acid is usually well tolerated. The most common adverse effects are insomnia, restlessness, dizziness, nervousness, headache, and nausea. The incidence of central nervous system effects is greater with oxolinic acid than with nalidixic acid. Occasional reactions include anorexia, abdominal pain or cramps, vomiting, diarrhea or constipation, weakness, and pruritus. Increased values for liver function tests and reduced leukocyte counts have been reported. Rarely, the drug may cause swelling of the extremities, urticaria, soreness of the mouth and gums, a metallic taste, palpitation, decreased hematocrit levels, and eosinophilia. Visual disturbances may occur, including photophobia, blurred vision, changes in color perception, interference with accommodation, and diplopia. Vision usually returns to normal when the drug is discontinued (Pratt, 1977). Because oxolinic acid may stimulate the central nervous system, especially in the elderly, it should be used with caution in patients receiving other drugs that may have a similar effect; it is contraindicated in those with a history of convulsive disorders.

The safety of oxolinic acid during pregnancy has not been established. Its use is contraindicated in infants and, since it is excreted in milk, it should not be administered to nursing mothers.

ROUTE, USUAL DOSAGE, AND PREPARATIONS.
Oral: *Adults*, 750 mg twice daily; if bacterial resistance does not develop, therapy should be 'continued for two weeks. Dosage for *children* has not been established.
Utibid (Parke, Davis). Tablets 750 mg.

METHENAMINE

METHENAMINE HIPPURATE
[Hiprex, Urex]

METHENAMINE MANDELATE
[Mandelamine]

METHENAMINE SULFOSALICYLATE
[Hexalet]

Methenamine is an orally administered urinary antiseptic available as the free compound, as one of several salts, or as a component of a drug combination. It is readily absorbed from the gastrointestinal tract and rapidly excreted, almost entirely in the urine. This drug has no antibacterial action itself, but acts by liberating formaldehyde in an acid medium. Formaldehyde apparently acts by denaturing protein. Methenamine may be either bacteriostatic or bactericidal, depending upon the amount of formaldehyde produced by its hydrolysis; this, in turn, is largely dependent upon the urinary pH. Thus, an acid urine is essential for antibacterial action; effectiveness is maximal at pH 5.5 or below. To assure an acidic pH, patients should be instructed to severely restrict or avoid ingestion of most fruits (especially citrus fruits and juices), milk and milk products, or antacids containing sodium carbonate or bicarbonate. A protein-rich diet with liberal amounts of cranberries (usually as vitamin C-enriched cranberry juice), plums, and prunes should be consumed. If this diet does not produce a sufficiently acid pH, it may be supplemented with large amounts of ascorbic acid. Alternatively, ammonium chloride may be given three or four times daily or methionine may be used. Caution must be exercised when using these acidifying chemicals, however, since large doses of ammonium chloride may induce metabolic acidosis in patients with impaired renal function and large doses of methionine may provoke symptoms of cerebral dysfunction when administered to children.

Like the parent compound, methenamine mandelate, hippurate, and sulfosalicylate are effective only in acid urine, a condition the salts themselves help establish. Additionally, the mandelate and hippurate salts combine the antibacterial activity of methenamine and the weak antibacterial effects of mandelic or hippuric acid. Nevertheless, urinary pH may not be lowered sufficiently by these salts alone and, in many patients, additional measures must be taken to decrease urinary pH.

Methenamine is active against a variety of gram-positive and gram-negative organisms, most notably *Escherichia coli*, that commonly cause urinary infections. Because it is active only in acid media, effectiveness is markedly diminished in infections caused by urea-splitting organisms that increase urinary pH, such as *Proteus* and some *Pseudomonas* species. Methenamine is most commonly used for prophylactic or suppressive therapy between episodes of recurrent infection more properly treated with other drugs and against infections refractory to more effective antibacterial agents because of such problems as anatomical abnormalities or indwelling catheters. This drug is never indicated for upper urinary tract infections because it is eliminated too rapidly to allow therapeutic amounts of formaldehyde to be generated (Pratt, 1977). Furthermore, since it is difficult clinically to distinguish between upper and lower tract infections, methenamine should not be used as the sole therapeutic agent in the treatment of acute urinary tract infections.

Methenamine is a relatively safe drug. Release of formaldehyde by acid hydrolysis in the gastrointestinal tract may account for the mild gastric irritation that sometimes occurs; enteric-coated preparations do not completely prevent this reaction (Goodman and Gilman, 1975). Large doses may cause acute inflammation of the urinary tract. If this occurs, the drug should be discontinued and an alkalizing salt (eg, sodium bicarbonate) given. Hypersensitivity reactions (usually manifested as rash)

have occurred rarely.

Methenamine salts can be given for prolonged periods without the development of resistant organisms. These salts generally are well tolerated but have caused nausea, gastric distress, rash, and dysuria in some patients. They are contraindicated in dehydrated patients and in those with severe renal disease or hepatic insufficiency. Methenamine mandelate should not be given to those with markedly decreased urinary output (Pratt, 1977).

If these agents are to be used effectively, patients should be taught to measure urinary pH and to adjust urine acidity.

Because sulfamethizole and sulfathiazole may form insoluble precipitates with formaldehyde in the urine, methenamine compounds should not be used with these sulfonamides.

ROUTE, USUAL DOSAGE, AND PREPARATIONS. METHENAMINE, METHENAMINE MANDELATE: *Oral: Adults,* 1 g four times daily after each meal and at bedtime; *children under 6 years,* 50 mg/kg of body weight daily divided into three doses; *children 6 to 12 years,* 500 mg four times daily.

METHENAMINE:
Drug available generically: Tablets 300 and 450 mg.
METHENAMINE MANDELATE:
Drug available generically: Suspension 250 and 500 mg/5 ml; tablets (plain, enteric-coated) 250 and 500 mg and 1 g.
Mandelamine (Parke, Davis). Granules 500 mg and 1 g; suspension 250 and 560 (Forte) mg/5 ml; tablets (enteric-coated) 250 and 500 mg and 1 g.

METHENAMINE HIPPURATE:
Oral: Adults and children over 12 years, 1 g twice daily; *children 6 to 12 years,* 500 mg to 1 g twice daily.
Hiprex (Merrell-National), *Urex* (Riker). Tablets 1 g.

METHENAMINE SULFOSALICYLATE:
Oral: Adults, 1 g four times daily, preferably after meals and at bedtime; *children 6 to 12 years,* 500 mg four times daily.
Hexalet (Webcon). Tablets 500 mg and 1 g.

AVAILABLE MIXTURES.
The following combinations are listed only to acknowledge their availability. The ratios of drugs in these mixtures prevent proper dosage adjustment of individual ingredients. In addition, some are too com-

plex to provide rational therapy, and some also contain ingredients of dubious merit. Those that contain phenazopyridine are not suitable for long-term administration.

> *Azo-Mandelamine* (Parke, Davis). Each tablet (enteric-coated) contains methenamine mandelate 500 mg and phenazopyridine hydrochloride 50 mg.
>
> *Trac Tabs* (Hyrex). Each tablet contains methenamine 40.8 mg, atropine sulfate 0.03 mg, hyoscyamine 0.03 mg, methylene blue 5.4 mg, phenyl salicylate 18.1 mg, gelsemium 6.1 mg, and benzoic acid 4.5 mg; Trac Tabs 2X contains the same formulation in double strength.
>
> *Urised* (Webcon). Each tablet contains methenamine 40.8 mg, atropine sulfate 0.03 mg, benzoic acid 4.5 mg, hyoscyamine 0.03 mg, methylene blue 5.4 mg, and phenyl salicylate 18.1 mg.

METHENAMINE AND SODIUM BIPHOSPHATE

This product has the same indications and essentially the same efficacy as other methenamine preparations (see the preceding evaluation). Sodium biphosphate is added to provide an acid urine, but additional acidification may be needed.

ROUTE, USUAL DOSAGE, AND PREPARATIONS.
Oral: One tablet four times daily.

> Mixture available generically: Each tablet contains 325 each of methenamine and sodium biphosphate.

PHENAZOPYRIDINE HYDROCHLORIDE
[Pyridium]

Phenazopyridine, an azo dye once believed to be a urinary antiseptic (an effect no longer attributed to the drug), is now used to relieve the pain, burning, urgency, and frequency of urination associated with cystitis, prostatitis, and urethritis. It is absorbed from the gastrointestinal tract and excreted in the urine where it exerts a topical analgesic effect on the urinary tract mucosa. Because it provides only symptomatic relief, prompt appropriate treat-ment of the cause of the pain must be instituted. Phenazopyridine should be discontinued when symptoms are controlled (usually within four to six days). Many fixed-dose combinations containing antibacterial agents and phenazopyridine are available, but separate drug administration is preferred since phenazopyridine therapy should not be prolonged.

Following oral administration, approximately 90% of the dose is eliminated in the urine within 24 hours, about 40% as unchanged drug and 50% as aniline and its metabolites, mainly p-aminophenol and N-acetyl-p-aminophenol (acetaminophen).

The principal adverse reactions are gastrointestinal disturbances and headache, which occur occasionally. A few cases of hemolytic anemia, hyperpigmentation, acute renal failure, and hepatitis have been reported. Overdosage or prolonged use in patients with diminished renal function may produce methemoglobinemia. The use of phenazopyridine is contraindicated in patients with renal insufficiency or severe hepatitis. The drug colors the urine red or orange and clothing is likely to be stained. The stain is difficult to remove from fabric.

ROUTE, USUAL DOSAGE, AND PREPARATIONS.
Oral: *Adults*, 200 mg three times daily after meals; *children 6 to 12 years*, 100 mg three times daily after meals.

> Drug available generically: Tablets 100 and 200 mg.
>
> *Pyridium* (Parke, Davis). Tablets 100 and 200 mg.

Selected References

Adatto K, et al: Behavioral factors and urinary tract infection. *JAMA* 241:2525-2526, 1979.

Bass BH: Megaloblastic anaemia due to nitrofurantoin. *Lancet* 1:530-531, 1963.

Bates TR, et al: Effect of food on nitrofurantoin absorption. *Clin Pharmacol Ther* 16:63-68, 1974.

Beutler E: Drug-induced hemolytic anemia. *Pharmacol Rev* 21:73-103, 1969.

Burke EC, et al: Urinary tract infections in children. *Mayo Clin Proc* 54:131-132, 1979.

Goodman LS, Gilman A (eds): *The Pharmacological Basis of Therapeutics*, ed 5. New York, Macmillan Publishing Co, Inc, 1975, 1006-1007.

Goss WA, et al: Mechanism of action of nalidixic acid on *Escherichia coli*: II. Inhibition of deoxyribonucleic acid synthesis. *J Bacteriol* 89:1068-1074, 1965.

Hailey FJ, et al: Pleuropneumonic reactions to nitrofurantoin. *N Engl J Med* 281:1087-1090, 1969.

Kalowski S, et al : Crystalline and macrocrystalline nitrofurantoin in treatment of urinary tract infection. *N Engl J Med* 290:385-387, 1974.

Kunin CM: *Detection, Prevention, and Management of Urinary Tract Infections: A Manual for the Physician, Nurse and Allied Health Worker*, ed 2. Philadelphia, Lea & Febiger, 1974, 1-230.

Lapides J (ed): *Fundamentals of Urology*. Philadelphia, WB Saunders Co, 1976.

Lohr JA, et al: Prevention of recurrent urinary tract infections in girls. *Pediatrics* 59:562-565, 1977.

Mohring K, Madsen PO: Treatment of urinary tract infections with oxolinic acid in patients with normal and impaired renal function. *Del Med J* 43:376-380, 1971.

Paul HE, Paul MF: Nitrofurans: Chemotherapeutic properties, in Schnitzer RJ, Hawking F (eds): *Experimental Chemotherapy*. New York, Academic Press, 1964, vol 2, 307-370.

Pratt WB: *Chemotherapy of Infection*. New York, Oxford University Press, 1977.

Ronald AR: Treating urinary tract infections in women. *Drug Ther* 9:51-63, (May) 1979.

Rao KG: Pseudotumor cerebri associated with nalidixic acid. *Urology* 4:204-207, 1974.

Stamey TA: *Urinary Infections*. Baltimore, Williams & Wilkins Company, 1972.

Stamey TA: Observations on clinical use of nalidixic acid. *Postgrad Med J* 47(suppl):21-26, (Sept) 1971.

Stamey TA, et al: Clinical use of nalidixic acid: A review and some observations. *Invest Urol* 6:582-592, 1969.

Antimycobacterial Agents | 79

Tuberculosis and leprosy (Hansen's disease) are caused by mycobacteria. Traditionally throughout history, attempts have been made to isolate infected individuals who were shunned by the nonaffected populace. As a better understanding of the causes, methods of infection transmission, and possible regimens of therapy developed, it became apparent that isolation is not required routinely as a benefit either to those who were diseased or to society. As a result, the tuberculosis sanatorium and the leprosy colony have been replaced by the treatment of affected individuals as outpatients as long as they are ambulatory, cooperative, and able to manage their own meals and medication. Only occasional patients require hospitalization, usually when there are complications, coexisting unrelated illnesses, or when surgery is indicated.

TUBERCULOSIS CHEMOTHERAPY

Tuberculosis is caused by *Mycobacterium tuberculosis*, a bacillus that can remain dormant in the human host for years. Normal immunologic defense mechanisms are thought to render the tubercle bacillus quiescent (Davidson, 1977), and most infected individuals never develop disease. When active tuberculosis develops, it can become progressive, is potentially fatal, and may be transmitted to susceptible individuals. Modern chemotherapy, the only known effective form of treatment, has the dual goal of preventing the development and transmission of the disease. Because effective bactericidal agents are available, tuberculosis is now classified among those diseases that are potentially curable.

The successful treatment of tuberculosis depends upon prompt diagnosis. About one-third of all cases are discovered in patients with febrile pulmonary disease, another third in patients with unrelated complaints, and a final third in those undergoing routine medical examinations (Buckingham, 1978). Detailed records of therapy, including changes in regimen, all bacteriologic reports, and results of drug susceptibility tests, must be kept. Every new case of tuberculosis should be reported to the proper health authorities.

In tuberculosis chemotherapy, certain basic principles must be followed. Except for prophylaxis and some cases of primary tuberculosis in which a single drug may be used because the bacterial population is small, both pulmonary and extrapulmonary disease are always treated with multiple drugs. Any large population of wild strain *M. tuberculosis* (encountered in widespread disease) will have naturally occurring mutants resistant to each of the antituberculosis drugs. Although use of a single drug destroys susceptible organisms, the resistant mutants then become dominant. The administration of additional drugs inhibits the growth of organisms spontaneously resistant to the first drug. The possibility of selecting within a population of tubercle bacilli a mutant simultaneously resistant to two or more drugs is highly remote. In the United States, the incidence of primary drug resistance, particularly to streptomycin and isoniazid, is much greater among children from households where a family member has received treatment for tuberculosis and the therapy has failed, in some large inner cities, and in the foreign-born, especially those who came to this country during the last two decades from areas with a high

incidence of tuberculosis. This is a factor to be considered when treating primary tuberculosis, particularly in children who have been associated with individuals with tuberculous meningitis and in children of immigrants who had lived in high-incidence areas.

The choice of agents depends primarily upon whether the strain of organism is known or can be presumed to be susceptible to the major antituberculosis drugs. Most strains are highly susceptible. However, if there is any possibility of previous treatment with an antituberculosis drug or if infection with drug-resistant strains is suspected, the possibility of bacterial resistance must be considered. If drug therapy was given previously, it is prudent to use agents for retreatment that have never before been used in the patient until results of sensitivity studies are available.

In addition to use of multiple drugs, adequate doses must be administered for sufficient periods of time to effect a cure. Consistency of drug administration and reliable patient compliance are keystones of successful therapy. With optimal treatment, the rate of cure approaches 100%.

Regimens of Chemotherapy: Although effective antituberculosis agents have been available for 30 years, there is no general agreement on optimal regimens of therapy or duration of treatment in tuberculosis. Expanded knowledge of pharmacodynamics and the introduction of additional major drugs have led to new approaches to treatment, especially with respect to duration of therapy. The various points of view on this subject are presented below. Authorities agree that the best chance of bringing about rapid and complete recovery is when the diagnosis is first made, when the organisms are multiplying rapidly, and before chronic, often irreversible, changes occur.

Isoniazid [INH, Nydrazid] and rifampin [Rifadin, Rimactane] are the most potent antituberculosis drugs available, and a regimen that includes both drugs may be superior to other commonly used combinations. The bactericidal effect of the combination in infected mice has been demonstrated experimentally. The most effective initial regimen usually consists of isoniazid, rifampin, and ethambutol [Myambutol] given simultaneously in doses sufficient to provide peak serum concentrations and maximum suppression of infection. All three drugs are considered to be primary antituberculosis agents. There is little evidence that ethambutol enhances the efficacy of isoniazid and rifampin, but it is included to preclude monotherapy in case the strain proves to be resistant to isoniazid, the patient is unable to tolerate one of these more potent agents, or it becomes desirable to discontinue rifampin. This combination is particularly beneficial in older patients with normal liver function or abnormal kidney function. Rifampin can be discontinued after sputum cultures become negative, but isoniazid and ethambutol should be continued for 24 months. In primary tuberculosis caused by drug-resistant bacilli, rifampin should be prescribed initially and combined with ethambutol or even two additional effective agents if the severity of clinical or roentgenographic abnormalities indicates the need for intensive chemotherapy.

Largely because of expense, rifampin is not universally advocated in initial treatment. However, when the possibility of producing a lasting cure is taken into account, rifampin may not be expensive if the total period of chemotherapy is reduced, and particularly if the need for frequent, long-term follow-up is eliminated. Although the cost of rifampin is higher than that of other oral agents, it is less than that of injectable drugs when the expense of administration is included. In addition, since rifampin, isoniazid, and ethambutol are administered orally, initial hospitalization and frequent visits to the physician can be avoided in most cases, assuming that the patient remains cooperative and his physician is knowledgeable in tuberculosis chemotherapy. Rifampin is not necessarily indicated in every case of active tuberculosis. If a patient is asymptomatic, has minimal pulmonary tuberculosis, limited tuberculous lymphadenitis, pleural effusion, or even extensive tuberculosis, a regimen that does not include rifampin may provide definitive results if the drugs chosen are administered correctly for a minimum of two years.

Therapeutic response appears to be almost as good with combinations of streptomycin, ethambutol, and isoniazid (particularly in younger patients or those with abnormal liver function but normal kidney function); streptomycin, aminosalicylic acid, and isoniazid; or even ethambutol and isoniazid. Streptomycin may be discontinued when sputum cultures become negative, but ethambutol and isoniazid should be continued for 24 months.

Excellent results have been obtained when rifampin and isoniazid were given for 18 to 24 months to patients with cavitary or extensive pulmonary tuberculosis. This regimen, given for nine months and supplemented initially by ethambutol, appears to be as useful as regimens used for longer periods for treating minimal or noncavitary disease.

A single drug should never be added to an initial regimen that proves to be ineffective. In this situation (which occurs rarely if optimal treatment is prescribed initially), two effective agents not previously administered should be added. It may be best to substitute an entirely new regimen on the basis of dependable bacterial susceptibility studies. Such specialized studies are readily available through many state health departments or large independent laboratories (particularly east of the Mississippi River). A telephone call to a state health department laboratory will quickly determine whether a given state will perform the service. In areas where testing is not available, susceptibility studies will be performed by the Center for Disease Control.

Regimens that are generally no longer selected for initial treatment include streptomycin and isoniazid; streptomycin and aminosalicylic acid (PAS); and, in adults, aminosalicylic acid and isoniazid (this combination is still widely used in infants and children). The first is unsatisfactory because streptomycin must be given daily for weeks or months to prevent bacterial resistance. This is a costly, painful process and is potentially toxic for the eighth cranial nerve. The second and third regimens are inferior mainly because of the possible gastrointestinal distress caused by aminosalicylic acid and the fact that it is poorly tolerated by adults.

Other drugs used to treat tuberculosis include capreomycin [Capastat], cycloserine [Seromycin], ethionamide [Trecator-SC], kanamycin [Kantrex], and pyrazinamide. These secondary drugs are less useful from the standpoint of therapeutic efficacy, potential toxicity, or patient acceptance and are reserved for use in retreatment or when the primary drugs are not tolerated.

Adrenal Corticosteroids: Steroids have a mixed effect on tuberculosis. Although they inhibit delayed-type hypersensitivity and thus may activate a latent infection, they also ameliorate the symptoms of the disease (Kasik, 1979). In fulminating pulmonary tuberculosis, treatment with steroids can be a lifesaving adjunct to intensive chemotherapy. Even unconscious patients may be saved by the immediate application of all measures indicated, including administration of large intravenous doses of methylprednisolone [Solu-Medrol] or equivalent agent until the patient is no longer comatose. Therapy should begin with a daily dose of 80 to 120 mg; 30 to 40 mg is injected initially and the remainder may be added to intravenous fluids. If the patient is conscious, 40 mg daily is a reasonable dose.

Corticosteroids may be indicated in patients with tuberculous meningitis. In conscious patients, parenteral administration may be limited to the first few days of treatment or omitted altogether; prednisone 30 to 40 mg daily may be given orally.

Corticosteroids may be used in combination with adequate chemotherapy to treat tuberculosis when widespread disease is accompanied by fever, anorexia, marked weakness, and debility. Steroids may be required for days or weeks until control of the disease is established but, to avoid complications, the duration of treatment usually should be limited to four to six weeks. Prednisolone (15 to 40 mg daily) frequently brings about rapid improvement. To avoid a rebound phenomenon, the total daily dose should be decreased very gradually (usually by 2.5 mg of prednisolone every three days) as soon as the patient shows definite signs of improvement, usually within a week after beginning treatment. Administration of a larger dose is resumed if the patient develops symptoms or signs such as fever or anemia.

For preparations, see Chapter 41, Adrenal Corticosteroids.

Length of Treatment: The actual time necessary to produce a cure in any given patient is highly variable and depends upon many factors, such as the type of disease, age of the patient, and duration of the disease before therapy was begun. Accordingly, standard lengths of time have been recommended (usually 18 to 24 months) that are broad enough to cover the needs of all patients. Because patient compliance with these long regimens is variable, experimental and clinical studies are being conducted in an effort to establish effective short-term regimens that will produce better compliance, reduce the workload of the physician, and save a substantial amount of money for the patient.

Experimental short-term programs were undertaken first by the English (see Fox and Mitchison, 1975 and 1976, and Fox, 1977) and later by other workers (eg, Pilheu, 1977). Studies in this country are being conducted under the direction of the U.S. Public Health Service (PHS), the Center for Disease Control (CDC), and the Arkansas State Department of Health. In the Arkansas program, direct supervision is utilized to ensure that potentially unreliable patients (eg, institutionalized patients, some alcoholics) comply with prescribed therapy; otherwise, supervision is the same as for other outpatient populations. This procedure is claimed to be highly successful. It appears that the program is less expensive than conventional therapy because the money saved through short-term therapy easily makes up for the added expense of direct supervision when necessary. The PHS program uses standard daily doses of rifampin and isoniazid for six months, followed by isoniazid and ethambutol in some patients and placebos in others for various lengths of times from a few weeks to a few months. This program has been less successful, with delinquency rates as high as 43% at some participating centers. However, the PHS directors believe they are still achieving much better results with the usual 18- to 24-month treatment programs. The cooperative study sponsored by the CDC is based on earlier studies by Dr. Wallace Fox and the World Health Organization (WHO), which show that the same cure rates may be achieved by giving isoniazid and rifampin for six months rather than for two years.

It seems likely that the results of studies such as those described above will revise the recommended length of therapy. However, until further definitive evidence is available, it is still best to give intensive, combined chemotherapy for a minimum of two years in nearly all cases of active pulmonary or extrapulmonary tuberculosis. Treatment with rifampin, ethambutol, and isoniazid for 6 to 12 months, followed by ethambutol and isoniazid for a total period of two years, has provided definitive treatment in almost every case in which the organisms were originally susceptible and in which the patient took medication consistently.

Intermittent Chemotherapy: Combined chemotherapy can be administered intermittently with little or no loss of therapeutic effect provided the mean daily dose of each agent is not significantly decreased. In most clinical studies, medication was given two or three times a week. Results have been best when intermittent therapy was preceded by daily treatment with the same agents in the usual doses for one to three months.

Intermittent outpatient chemotherapy is most practical in areas with a high incidence of tuberculosis and limited facilities for treatment, as in developing countries. In the United States, the intermittent administration of drugs may be effective in recalcitrant patients, alcoholics, and others

who cannot be depended upon to adhere to a daily regimen. The drugs *must* be given under the close supervision of a visiting nurse who ascertains ingestion. The intermittent administration of rifampin is not currently recommended because of several reports of apparent immunologic reactions attributed to such usage.

Retreatment: For various reasons, treatment is not always optimal and retreatment is frequently necessary. It is then even more important to prescribe the best available chemotherapy. A single new drug should not be added to the combination of agents administered previously unless there is proof that the strains are still susceptible to these agents. Since it is usually necessary to resume treatment before new sensitivity studies are available, the regimen should be dictated by the patient's previous treatment, therapeutic response, results of earlier susceptibility studies, and need for intensive chemotherapy.

When effective combined chemotherapy is discontinued prematurely (eg, after one month), the same regimen often can be resumed with satisfactory results. If the patient has received a number of courses of chemotherapy (eg, three months' duration or longer), often interspersed with isoniazid alone, it is wise to prescribe both rifampin and ethambutol with one or two other agents most likely to be effective as determined by the patient's record. For critically ill patients with a poorly documented chemotherapeutic history, rifampin, ethambutol, capreomycin, and one or two of the older agents least likely to have been prescribed previously (eg, ethionamide, pyrazinamide, possibly cycloserine) should be given. In desperate situations, patients may tolerate a number of potentially toxic drugs amazingly well.

Preventive Treatment: On the basis of studies carried out by the Public Health Service, it was formerly recommended that any person with a positive Mantoux test be given a course of chemoprophylaxis with isoniazid alone for a year. As a result, isoniazid was given indiscriminately to thousands of individuals. After the risk of isoniazid-induced hepatitis became apparent, the indications for preventive treatment were curtailed. At present, prophylactic chemotherapy is recommended for all household contacts and other close associates of patients with active pulmonary tuberculosis, particularly those with grossly positive sputum tests; persons with a positive Mantoux and an abnormal chest x-ray, including those with a past history of tuberculosis and inadequate chemotherapy; individuals whose Mantoux is known to have converted from negative to positive during the previous two years; infected individuals at special risk of developing active tuberculosis because of treatment with adrenal corticosteroids or immunosuppressive agents; and patients with diseases that lower resistance to the tubercle bacillus (particularly leukemia, Hodgkin's disease, diabetes, and silicosis). In addition, preventive treatment is considered mandatory for all positive tuberculin reactors under 6 years of age and is still recommended for individuals under 35 years, with the exception of pregnant women. Among older reactors, the risk of developing active tuberculosis must be weighed against the risk of isoniazid-induced hepatitis.

Therapy with isoniazid alone is indicated only when the mycobacterial population is believed to be small, a factor often difficult to assess. In cases of old tuberculosis, preventive therapy should not be started until active tuberculosis has been ruled out by bacteriologic and roentgenographic studies. If there is any evidence of active disease, the patient should receive combined chemotherapy of sufficient duration to prevent the emergence of drug-resistant strains of tubercle bacilli.

Adverse Reactions

Although most antituberculosis agents are well tolerated, all have some potential toxicity. The most serious error made by physicians is failure to recognize true toxicity promptly. A more common error is failure to distinguish between true toxicity and the plethora of patient's symptoms and unrelated abnormalities. The physician who makes a false diagnosis of drug toxicity may delete one drug after another from the patient's regimen, sometimes making inappropriate substitutions. Loss of drug susceptibility and therapeutic failure may be the end result.

Hypersensitivity reactions occur most often between the third and eighth week of treatment. If a patient tolerates a drug or group of drugs well for at least four months, he usually can complete a full course of chemotherapy. The most common early symptoms of hypersensitivity are fever, which increases over a period of several days, tachycardia, anorexia, and malaise. At this time, laboratory studies are usually within normal limits, but eosinophilia and other abnormalities are observed on rare occasions. If the offending drug is discontinued promptly, the patient soon recovers. If not, the reaction becomes progressively worse and is often accompanied by cutaneous reactions, including exfoliative dermatitis; hepatitis; renal abnormalities; and, occasionally, acute blood dyscrasias. Severe reactions can be fatal.

Patients who develop hypersensitivity to one antituberculosis drug may be at greater than usual risk of reacting to other drugs. When such reactions occur, all chemotherapy should be discontinued unless the tuberculosis is life-threatening (in which case drugs least likely to produce these reactions are given, possibly with corticosteroids if indicated). When the reaction has subsided, treatment should be resumed with one drug at a time, beginning with a test dose, then adding other drugs as rapidly as they can be tolerated until the patient is again receiving adequate chemotherapy. Desensitization to streptomycin and some other drugs usually is successful. However, with the number of effective agents available, it is not advisable to risk resuming treatment with a drug that has caused a serious reaction (eg, hepatitis).

Many of the adverse reactions reported in the literature have been noted infrequently, sometimes only once and without verification. Also, in combined chemotherapy, toxicity ascribed to one drug may actually have been caused by another or by an incompatible combination of drugs. In the evaluations that follow, emphasis is placed on those toxic effects and adverse reactions that are well documented and occur with some frequency. Significant infrequent reactions also are noted, and adverse reactions that have been reported but not verified are so designated.

Precautions

Many toxic effects of the antituberculosis agents, particularly those related to dosage, can be avoided by taking into account the patient's age, weight, and general health. Renal status is especially important, since impaired function may lead to proportionately high serum concentrations with increased danger of toxicity unless the doses are reduced.

Relatively small doses of drugs may produce therapeutic serum concentrations in elderly or unusually small adults. Some antimycobacterial agents are prescribed routinely on the basis of body weight and consideration should be given to this factor in prescribing all drugs, especially those administered to children.

Although most agents are metabolized in the liver, evidence of hepatic dysfunction is seldom a deterrent in selecting a regimen. Alcoholic patients, who constitute a considerable reservoir of tuberculosis infection in the United States, tolerate the usual regimens well, even when cirrhosis is present. Nevertheless, when there is a history of alcoholism, infectious hepatitis, jaundice, or other hepatic disease, it is advisable to obtain a complete profile of liver function before beginning treatment. In fact, in any new case in which the patient has not been under regular medical supervision, it is wise to obtain preliminary studies of the renal, hepatic, and hematopoietic systems for baseline purposes.

Since most or all treatment is now given on an outpatient basis, the patient should receive thorough instructions regarding the potential toxicity of the drugs administered to him. Patients also must be monitored at regular intervals throughout treatment; weekly interviews should be scheduled for the first month or two. Laboratory studies, including serum enzymes, should be obtained promptly if indicated.

PRIMARY DRUGS

ETHAMBUTOL HYDROCHLORIDE
[Myambutol]

$$CH_3CH_2 \text{---} \overset{\overset{\displaystyle CH_2OH}{|}}{\underset{\underset{\displaystyle H}{|}}{C}} \text{---} \overset{+}{N}H_2CH_2CH_2\overset{+}{N}H_2 \text{---} \overset{\overset{\displaystyle H}{|}}{\underset{\underset{\displaystyle CH_2OH}{|}}{C}} \text{---} CH_2CH_3 \quad 2Cl^-$$

This synthetic compound is a highly effective orally administered adjunct to the more potent antimycobacterial agents, isoniazid and rifampin. Because of its relative lack of toxicity and good patient acceptance, ethambutol has supplanted aminosalicylic acid for initial treatment. In retreatment and cases of primary resistance, ethambutol is of great value when combined with other effective antimycobacterial agents. *Mycobacterium tuberculosis*, *M. bovis*, and most strains of *M. kansasii* are highly susceptible to ethambutol, and some nonphotochromogens (mycobacterial group III organisms) are appreciably susceptible to this drug in vitro.

Like other antimycobacterial agents, ethambutol interferes with the protein metabolism of mycobacteria, apparently by inhibiting the synthesis of ribonucleic acid. The drug is absorbed rapidly from the gastrointestinal tract and is excreted mainly by the kidneys; only 10% is converted to therapeutically inactive metabolites. Ethambutol does not pass through intact meninges but can be detected in presumably therapeutic concentrations in the cerebrospinal fluid of patients with tuberculous meningitis.

Because no practicable method of determining serum concentrations exists, ethambutol must .be prescribed on the basis of body weight, and the drug should not be used in patients with impaired renal function. The dose must be calculated carefully and adjusted if there are appreciable changes in the patient's weight. However, in the interest of simplicity for the patient, dosages should be rounded off to the nearest whole tablet.

The only significant adverse effect produced by ethambutol is ocular toxicity, which is dose related and generally reversible over a period of weeks or months. In rare cases, recovery may be delayed for up to one year or more and the effect may be irreversible. Signs and symptoms are bilateral and are consistent with retrobulbar neuritis; they include decreased visual acuity, loss of color discrimination, constriction of visual fields, and central and peripheral scotomata. With currently recommended doses, ocular toxicity is rare in patients with normal renal function. Regular ophthalmologic examinations are not necessary during treatment, but the patient should be instructed to report any visual changes promptly and be questioned about his vision during each regularly scheduled visit. Symptoms often precede objective evidence of toxicity. If a patient complains of blurring or fading of vision, a complete ophthalmologic examination should be performed at once. Treatment with ethambutol should be stopped immediately if symptoms persist or there is a significant decrease in visual acuity. When ocular toxicity is detected early and therapy stopped, color discrimination is not lost and visual acuity soon returns to pretreatment levels.

In the past, a complete ophthalmologic examination was recommended to establish a baseline before beginning treatment with ethambutol. This still is mandatory if the patient has cataracts or other ocular abnormalities which make changes in vision difficult to detect or evaluate. Pretreatment examinations are not routinely indicated, however, in patients with normal vision or simple errors of refraction corrected by glasses.

In the earliest clinical studies, patients receiving very large doses of ethambutol occasionally had symptoms of peripheral neuritis. This condition rarely, if ever, occurs with the doses used presently.

The incidence of hypersensitivity to ethambutol is very low (about 0.1%) and reactions tend to be mild.

Patients treated with ethambutol have included many pregnant women, most of whom were already on chemotherapy before conception and therefore received ethambutol during the first trimester. No teratogenic effects definitely attributable to ethambutol have been reported. Likewise, no toxic effects have been observed in children receiving therapeutic doses of the drug but, because of the difficulty of determining visual acuity in small children and because aminosalicylic acid is usually well tolerated in this group, few children have been treated with ethambutol. However, in serious cases of tuberculosis, particularly disseminated tuberculosis caused by highly drug-resistant strains of tubercle bacilli, young children have received ethambutol for up to five years without evidence of toxicity.

ROUTE, USUAL DOSAGE, AND PREPARATIONS. *Oral*: 15 to 25 mg/kg of body weight; the total amount must be given in one dose each day to produce therapeutic serum concentrations. In one suggested regimen, 15 mg/kg is given throughout treatment. In another, 25 mg/kg is administered for two months, followed by 15 mg/kg thereafter for the duration of therapy. In a third regimen, 20 mg/kg is given throughout treatment; this program is both safe and effective in patients with normal renal function.

Myambutol (Lederle). Tablets 100 and 400 mg.

ISONIAZID
[INH, Nydrazid]

This synthetic compound probably remains the best single antimycobacterial agent with respect to therapeutic efficacy, toxicity, cost, ease of administration, and patient acceptance. It is used most often in combination with other effective agents, which has resulted in pronounced improvement in all aspects of this disease. Even the introduction of rifampin has not diminished the importance of isoniazid. Neither drug alone is bactericidal in the strictest sense, but the combination is definitely bactericidal.

Isoniazid may be administered as a single drug to treat uncomplicated primary tuberculosis and for prophylaxis. For maximum therapeutic effect and convenience, isoniazid should be administered orally. It can be given parenterally (using oral dosage levels) if oral administration is not practical. In critical cases, both routes may be used until clinical improvement occurs.

Approximately 16% of all individuals given isoniazid are rapid inactivators of the drug. This is rarely of clinical significance, even with usual therapeutic doses, because the drug has a wide therapeutic range.

The metabolism of isoniazid is characterized by increased excretion of pyridoxine, which may cause peripheral neuritis, particularly when large doses are prescribed. The incidence is about 10% when 8 to 10 mg/kg of body weight is given. Peripheral neuritis occasionally produces bizarre symptoms and therefore may not be recognized promptly. It is treated with pyridoxine (up to 300 mg daily) given orally; in severe cases, parenteral administration may be more effective. Since peripheral neuritis is not always completely reversible, some clinicians consider it advisable to administer pyridoxine (25 to 50 mg daily) concurrently to patients receiving usual doses of isoniazid, especially those with diabetes mellitus, alcoholism, or malnutrition. Those receiving larger doses or those with pre-existing symptoms of peripheral neuritis should receive 100 to 300 mg of pyridoxine daily.

Convulsions have occurred in patients treated with isoniazid (less than 1%). However, this drug has been administered without difficulty to many individuals receiving treatment for convulsive disorders. Since the action of phenytoin may be potentiated by isoniazid, the dose of the anticonvulsant should be reduced or blood levels of phenytoin monitored when the two drugs are given simultaneously, particularly in slow isoniazid inactivators. Reversible psychotic episodes may be precipitated in a small percentage of patients treated with very large doses of isoniazid.

An arthralgic or arthritic reaction has been noted infrequently. Optic neuropathy has been reported rarely in the literature, but a causal relationship has not been established. This is true also of many diverse abnormalities listed in the package inserts of isoniazid preparations, which enumerate everything from severe hematologic disturbances to gynecomastia (which occurs with some frequency among alcoholics, whether or not they have tuberculosis and are receiving isoniazid). It is probable that the severe abnormalities reported, including vasculitis accompanied by antinuclear antibodies, are manifestations of a hypersensitivity reaction simulating disseminated lupus erythematosus.

Isoniazid can cause hepatic necrosis; although the mechanism is not yet known, it is probably not a hypersensitivity reaction. The incidence of hepatitis increases with age; it is negligible in individuals less than 35 years of age, increases to about 1% between the ages of 35 to 49, and may be almost 2.5% after the age of 50. The daily consumption of alcohol increases the risk of isoniazid-related hepatitis.

Patients should be monitored periodically to detect signs or symptoms of hepatitis or other significant adverse reactions, but routine laboratory studies are not recommended. It is well known that serum transaminase levels are elevated during the first few months of treatment in at least 10% of patients, and sometimes there is more specific evidence of liver dysfunction. However, all values tend to return to normal and are not an indication for discontinuing treatment without clinical evidence of hepatitis.

ROUTES, USUAL DOSAGE, AND PREPARATIONS. *Oral, Intramuscular: Adults,* 4 to 5 mg/kg of body weight daily or 300 mg daily is given orally in a single dose with other antimycobacterial agents. For disseminated tuberculosis (particularly tuberculous meningitis) and pulmonary disease caused by atypical mycobacteria, 10 to 20 mg/kg daily. In critical cases, 100 to 200 mg daily may be given parenterally to supplement oral administration. When chemotherapy is given twice a week, isoniazid is often prescribed in a dose of 15 mg/kg combined with 50 mg/kg of ethambutol and 25 to 30 mg/kg of streptomycin. *Infants and children,* for active tuberculosis, 10 to 20 mg/kg daily in one or more doses; for preventive therapy, approximately 10 mg/kg daily in one dose.

> Drug available generically: Powder; tablets 50, 100, and 300 mg.
>
> *INH* (Ciba). Dual pack preparation containing 30 isoniazid tablets 300 mg and 60 rifampin capsules 300 mg (Rimactane/INH).
>
> *Nydrazid* (Squibb). Syrup 50 mg/5 ml; tablets 100 mg; solution (parenteral) 100 mg/ml in 10 ml containers.

RIFAMPIN
[Rifadin, Rimactane]

This semisynthetic antibiotic represents the greatest contribution to the chemotherapy of tuberculosis since the introduction of isoniazid. In vitro and in vivo, rifampin has a marked inhibitory effect against *Mycobacterium tuberculosis, M. bovis,* and nearly all strains of *M. kansasii.* Some strains of scotochromogens (mycobacterial group II) and a few strains of nonphotochromogens (mycobacterial group III) are also inhibited by low concentrations of the drug. Rifampin is most active during cell multiplication, but it also appears to have some effect on resting cells. Electron microscopy has revealed changes in the cytoplasm and disappearance of ribosomes in tubercle bacilli exposed to rifampin, which indicates inhibition of DNA-dependent RNA polymerase.

Rifampin diffuses freely into body tissues and fluids, including cerebrospinal fluid. At currently recommended doses, peak serum levels occur in two to four hours and levels above the minimal inhibitory concentration persist for at least six hours. The drug is metabolized by the liver and excreted mainly in the bile, although therapeutic concentrations appear in the urine. Rifampin and its metabolites impart a reddish-orange color to urine, feces, saliva, sweat, and tears; there also is at least one report (Lyons, 1979) of discoloration of soft contact lenses in patients taking rifampin. Patients should be informed of these problems to prevent anxiety.

Rifampin is active against many bacteria and some viruses. Because of the rapid emergence of resistant strains, its use is not generally recommended in nontuberculous infections; however, it can be administered to meningococcal carriers and is being used to treat leprosy (see the section on Chemotherapy of Leprosy). In addition, rifampin is being used investigationally for chemoprophylaxis in carriers of *Haemophilus influenzae.* When treating tuberculosis, bacterial resistance to rifampin can be prevented by combination therapy with streptomycin, isoniazid, ethambutol, or other effective antimycobacterial agents administered in therapeutic doses. Therefore, it is useful in both initial and retreatment regimens (see the Introduction).

Most patients tolerate and accept rifampin well. Abdominal distress, aching in muscles and joints, or cramping in the legs occurs occasionally, especially duing the first few weeks of treatment. During this period, clinically apparent, asymptomatic jaundice also may be noted but tends to subside without interruption of therapy. The jaundice, substantiated by laboratory evidence of liver dysfunction, may be alleviated by reducing the dose of rifampin but, if accompanied by symptoms of hepatitis, therapy should be discontinued. Since both rifampin and bile are excreted by hepatic cells, jaundice may be caused by the displacement of bilirubin which then enters the blood, chiefly in conjugated form. This is most likely to occur when the patient has impaired liver function or when rifampin is combined with other drugs, particularly isoniazid and other agents that are potentially hepatotoxic. The incidence of liver dysfunction caused by rifampin, as determined by elevation of serum transaminase levels and other abnormalities, varies from 4% to 35%. When rifampin is administered to patients with impaired liver function, they should be kept under close medical supervision, including the monitoring of serum enzyme levels in alcoholics and those with pre-existing liver disease for at least the first two or three months of treatment. In a USPHS cooperative study, marked elevation of SGPT (more that 100 units/ml) occurred in 4.2% of patients treated with rifampin in combination with isoniazid or isoniazid and ethambutol, but jaundice was not observed in any patient.

Pruritus with or without rash has been noted in less than 3% of patients.

A serious reaction, assumed to be immunologic in nature, has occurred during intermittent treatment with large doses of rifampin or when treatment was resumed after a lapse of days or weeks. The mechanism is unknown but rifampin-dependent antibodies have been demonstrated in the serum of some patients who experienced the reaction. It is characterized by a severe flu-like syndrome with dyspnea, sometimes accompanied by wheezing; purpura associated with thrombocytopenia; leukopenia; and, occasionally, a state similar to true anaphylaxis. Rarely, hemolysis, hemoglobinuria, hematuria, and renal insufficiency also occurred. Treatment with rifampin had to be discontinued in only 3% of cases, and most patients were able to tolerate the drug when the dose was reduced during intermittent therapy or when daily treatment was substituted for intermittent therapy. In fact, regimens of intermittent treatment with rifampin and other agents have been used for years without significant toxicity.

A number of other questions about rifampin await further experience and investigation. The drug does not appear to have teratogenic effects in man, even when inadvertently administered during the first trimester of pregnancy. No adverse effects have been reported when rifampin was given to children, although routine administration to young children is not presently recommended. Rifampin has been shown to have immunosuppressive properties; these have no clinical significance in tuberculosis but could interfere with certain immunization procedures or with the treatment of patients receiving immunosuppressive drugs. It has been found that patients receiving coumarin-type anticoagulants require larger doses to maintain the desired prothrombin time when rifampin is given concomitantly. Aminosalicylic acid may interfere with the absorption of rifampin, and it has been reported that rifampin may interfere with the effectiveness of oral contraceptives.

ROUTE, USUAL DOSAGE, AND PREPARATIONS. *Oral: Adults,* 600 mg or 10 to 20 mg/kg of body weight daily; *children,* 10 to 20 mg/kg (maximum, 600 mg daily). The drug should be given in a single dose one hour before a meal (usually breakfast) or two hours afterward.

   Rifadin (Dow), *Rimactane* (Ciba). Capsules 300 mg.

SECONDARY DRUGS

AMINOSALICYLIC ACID
[Parasal]

AMINOSALICYLATE CALCIUM
[Parasal Calcium]

AMINOSALICYLATE SODIUM
[Parasal Sodium]

Until ethambutol became available, aminosalicylic acid (para-aminosalicylic acid, PAS) was widely used in combination chemotherapy to deter emergence of streptomycin- and isoniazid-resistant strains of tubercle bacilli. Used alone, the antimycobacterial effect of aminosalicylic acid is scarcely discernible. Furthermore, patient acceptance and tolerance of the drug are poor. Therapy must be discontinued in approximately 20% of patients (15% because of intolerable adverse effects, particularly nausea, vomiting, and diarrhea, and 4% because of hypersensitivity reactions that occasionally may be very serious or even fatal). Furthermore, investigators have estimated that 20% to 50% of patients who appear to tolerate aminosalicylic acid do not take this bulky medication consistently.

Aminosalicylic acid is now seldom included in initial regimens and is used almost exclusively as a second or third drug in antituberculosis regimens given to children under 2 years of age. (These patients are unable to participate correctly in eye testing procedures required when ethambutol is administered.) Also, the inclusion of aminosalicylic acid in retreatment regimens may prevent the emergence of bacterial resistance to more potent agents.

This drug is usually administered as a salt of the active compound; the sodium salt is used most often, although a calcium salt is available. When the former is used, the usual total daily dose of 12 g includes large amounts of sodium ion which may be contraindicated in some patients.

ROUTE, USUAL DOSAGE, AND PREPARATIONS. *Oral*: *Adults*, 150 to 200 mg/kg of body weight daily (maximum, 12 g) in two or three doses always given after meals. There is evidence that a single dose of 6 g may be equally effective when combined with isoniazid or other potent agents administered once daily. *Children*, 200 to 300 mg/kg daily in three or four divided doses given after meals.

AMINOSALICYLIC ACID:
Drug available generically: Powder (bulk); tablets (plain) 500 mg.
Parasal (Panray). Powder (bulk); tablets (plain, buffered) 500 mg.

AMINOSALICYLATE CALCIUM:
Parasal Calcium (Panray). Capsules, tablets 500 mg; powder (bulk).

AMINOSALICYLATE SODIUM:
Drug available generically: Powder (bulk); tablets (plain) 500 mg and 1 g.
Parasal Sodium (Panray). Crystals; powder (bulk); tablets 500 and 690 mg and 1 g.

CAPREOMYCIN SULFATE
[Capastat Sulfate]

Capreomycin is a polypeptide antibiotic isolated from a species of *Streptomyces*. It is chemically and pharmacologically related to viomycin and has similar potential toxicity; bacterial susceptibility studies show that cross resistance between the two drugs is common.

Capreomycin has a marked suppressive effect against *Mycobacterium tuberculosis* and *M. bovis* in vitro and in vivo. Most strains of *M. kansasii* also are susceptible, but other atypical mycobacteria are often resistant. This agent usually is reserved for use in the retreatment of tuberculosis when parenteral chemotherapy is indicated; it is given by deep intramuscular injection.

When compared with kanamycin (an antibiotic derived from another species of *Streptomyces*), capreomycin is less toxic and has a somewhat greater antimycobacterial effect. Capreomycin approaches streptomycin in therapeutic efficacy and, since there is no cross resistance between the two, it is useful in patients with streptomycin-resistant strains of tubercle bacilli. Nevertheless, because of its potential nephrotoxicity, capreomycin cannot be routinely substituted for streptomycin.

Extensive experimental and clinical investigations have demonstrated that renal damage is the most consistent and significant toxic effect caused by capreomycin; this is manifested by elevated urea nitrogen levels, decreased creatinine clearance, albuminuria, and cylindruria. Fatal toxic nephritis was reported in one patient given both capreomycin and aminosalicylic acid for one month. However, capreomycin must be discontinued because of nephrotoxicity in fewer than 10% of all patients, and renal abnormalities nearly always disappear with cessation of treatment. Hypokalemia also is a significant side effect of this drug and blood potassium levels should be monitored. When capreomycin is used with other effective agents that are administered orally every day, its prolonged daily use is rarely necessary. After two to four weeks, it can be given two or three times a week with much less risk of permanent renal damage and without an appreciable reduction in total chemotherapeutic effect.

Capreomycin is potentially toxic to the eighth cranial nerve. However, even when administered every day for two to four months, vestibular toxicity occurred infrequently and auditory toxicity rarely.

Eosinophilia occurs frequently during treatment and occasionally has been marked. Definite hypersensitivity reactions, manifested by fever and rash, apparently are uncommon and are not severe.

Because of its potential toxicity for the kidneys and eighth cranial nerve, capreomycin is rarely prescribed for patients with renal disease and should not be administered with other potentially nephrotoxic or ototoxic antimicrobial agents (eg, colistin, gentamicin). It is advisable to obtain pertinent baseline laboratory data before beginning treatment with capreomycin, and all patients should have a monthly clinical workup and a weekly complete blood count, urinalysis, and SMA-12 screening. There is no evidence that previous damage to the eighth nerve precludes treatment with capreomycin, but impaired renal function must be considered, particularly with respect to dosage and frequency of administration.

ROUTE, USUAL DOSAGE, AND PREPARATIONS. *Intramuscular (deep): Adults,* 20 mg/kg of body weight (approximately 1 g) daily for two to four weeks, followed by 1 g two or three times weekly for 6 to 12 months or longer, if necessary. Most patients tolerate doses of 1 g daily for two to four months and occasionally for as long as six months. Information is inadequate to establish a dosage for *children.* The drug should be dissolved in 2 ml of sodium chloride injection or sterile water for injection; two to three minutes should be allowed for complete dissolution.

   Capastat Sulfate (Lilly). Powder equivalent to 1 g capreomycin activity in 5 ml containers.

CYCLOSERINE
[Seromycin]

Cycloserine, an antibiotic derived from a species of *Streptomyces,* is administered orally and has proved to be an effective antimycobacterial agent when tolerated. It is used in problem retreatment programs and for urinary tract tuberculosis. Amounts that provide serum concentrations higher than the minimal inhibitory concentrations in vitro must be used for retreatment purposes; this is probably necessary for all antimycobacterial agents, but it is particularly important for agents used in retreatment regimens. Because the drug is highly concentrated in the urine, large doses need not be used in urinary tract tuberculosis.

The limiting factor in the use of cycloserine is its potential central nervous system toxicity, including both neurologic and psychic disturbances. Neurologic reactions vary from muscular twitching to convulsive seizures and may be prevented by administering large doses of pyridoxine concomitantly (at least 100 mg three times daily). Psychic disturbances range from nervousness to frank psychotic episodes. Such toxicity is occasionally related to excessive serum concentrations but more often cannot be predicted or prevented. Patients with a history of mental illness often tolerate cycloserine unusually well, whereas apparently stable individuals may develop a psychotic reaction soon after initiation of treatment, sometimes before therapeutic serum levels are achieved.

Psychotic episodes occur in nearly 10% of patients treated with cycloserine and require prompt cessation of treatment. These reactions are nearly always reversible within two weeks; large doses of chlorpromazine may hasten recovery. Until the patient's condition returns to normal, he should be watched closely and security measures taken if necessary. Suicide has occurred occasionally during a drug-induced psychotic reaction.

Hypersensitivity reactions to cycloserine are rare. Isoniazid should not be given with cycloserine because of possible additive central nervous system toxicity. Ingestion of alcohol is inadvisable while the patient is receiving cycloserine, although many alcoholics have experienced no difficulty (presumably during periods of abstinence).

ROUTE, USUAL DOSAGE, AND PREPARATIONS. *Oral:* Initially, 15 mg/kg of body weight, increased by increments of 250 mg every few days (if well tolerated) until therapeutic serum levels are produced. Best results occur with trough serum concentrations of

25 to 30 mcg/ml. These levels usually can be attained by giving 1 to 2 g daily in three divided doses after meals. It may be possible to administer cycloserine once a day in a smaller total dose when it is used with other agents prescribed once a day without loss of therapeutic effect. Blood used to determine serum drug concentrations should be drawn before the patient's first dose of the day.

Seromycin (Lilly). Capsules 250 mg.

ETHIONAMIDE
[Trecator-SC]

This drug is the thioamide of isonicotinic acid and is related to isoniazid, but there is no cross resistance between the two agents. Ethionamide is about one-tenth as active as isoniazid and, like the latter drug, is widely distributed in the body, including the cerebrospinal fluid. It is effective against human and bovine strains of *Mycobacterium tuberculosis* and against *M. kansasii*.

The usefulness of ethionamide in tuberculosis is limited because many patients cannot tolerate therapeutic doses. In approximately one-third of cases, ethionamide must be discontinued or the dose reduced. Most patients tolerate one-half to two-thirds of the usual total daily dose, but the therapeutic efficacy of these amounts is uncertain, particularly since ethionamide is used in retreatment regimens, often in combination with drugs having marginal antimycobacterial activity.

Ethionamide almost invariably causes gastrointestinal disturbances, most frequently, anorexia, nausea, and vomiting, which are thought to be caused by its central nervous system effects rather than direct gastric irritation.

Ethionamide is potentially toxic to the liver. Abnormal results of liver function studies are noted during treatment in 9% of patients, and jaundice occurs in 1% to 3%. However, recovery is usually rapid when ethionamide is discontinued.

Hypersensitivity reactions are infrequent. Like isoniazid, ethionamide may cause peripheral neuritis, particularly in susceptible patients. Mental depression has occasionally been attributed to treatment with this agent.

ROUTE, USUAL DOSAGE, AND PREPARATIONS.
Oral: 0.5 to 1 g daily in one to three doses after meals. Variations in dosage and timing of administration may be tried. Some patients tolerate the drug best when given as a single dose at bedtime, whereas others prefer a single dose after the evening meal. When the total amount can be given in one dose, serum concentrations are higher and a therapeutic effect more likely than when small doses are administered two or three times a day.

Trecator-SC (Ives). Tablets 250 mg.

KANAMYCIN SULFATE
[Kantrex]

This antibiotic is administered only parenterally when treating tuberculosis and has been shown to have variable cross resistance with capreomycin. Its potential to cause eighth cranial nerve damage is greater than that of capreomycin. Although kanamycin is sometimes incorporated into multiple-drug regimens, it has no prominent place in the treatment of human tuberculosis.

Kanamycin can cause severe and permanent hearing loss (see Chapter 74, Aminoglycosides); the deafness sometimes is associated with loss of labyrinthine function. Therefore, close clinical supervision is required, including monthly audiometric tests at least during the first three months of use. Kanamycin also is moderately nephrotoxic. Urinalysis, complete blood count, and SMA-12 screening should be performed weekly.

ROUTE, USUAL DOSAGE, AND PREPARATIONS. *Intramuscular (deep): Adults and children,* 15 mg/kg of body weight (maximum, 1 g), usually in a single dose three to five times weekly.

> *Kantrex* (Bristol). Solution 37.5 mg/ml (pediatric) and 250 mg/ml in 2 ml containers, and 333 mg/ml in 3 ml containers (strengths expressed in terms of the base).

PYRAZINAMIDE

Pyrazinamide, an analogue of nicotinamide, is not water soluble and is active against mycobacteria in vitro only in an acid medium, making routine susceptibility studies impossible. It has been used in the United States primarily for retreatment and only when the disease is a greater threat than the potential drug toxicity, but there are indications that it may have much wider value (Fox and Mitchison, 1975), particularly in short-term therapy. When administered with other agents in therapeutic doses, it may contribute to the total antimycobacterial effect.

Sophisticated studies of altered enzyme activity and other aspects of host metabolism have not explained the mode of action of pyrazinamide. This drug is most effective against intracellular tubercle bacilli, which may explain its efficacy in murine tuberculosis, primarily an intracellular disease.

Pyrazinamide can cause hepatotoxicity, which apparently is dose related. A dose of 3 g daily has been found to be effective adjunctively when given with isoniazid in the initial treatment of tuberculosis, but the incidence of hepatotoxicity is approximately 14% and deaths have occurred rarely from acute yellow atrophy of the liver. Doses of 1.5 g daily allow the development of isoniazid resistance in approximately 14% of patients; liver damage, although rarely serious, is noted in about 10% of these patients. Pretreatment laboratory studies should include a complete profile of liver function. It is usually recommended that serum transaminases be determined every two to four weeks throughout treatment.

Pyrazinamide almost routinely causes hyperuricemia, which is usually asymptomatic; serum uric acid levels of 12 to 14 mg/dl are not uncommon. If symptoms of gout develop and continued treatment with pyrazinamide is necessary, the patient may be given a uricosuric agent (eg, probenecid 0.5 g twice daily). A complete blood count, urinalysis, and SMA-12 screening should be performed monthly.

ROUTE, USUAL DOSAGE, AND PREPARATIONS. *Oral: Adults,* 20 to 35 mg/kg of body weight daily in one or more doses (maximum, 3 g daily); *children,* information is inadequate to establish dosage.

> Drug available generically: Tablets 500 mg (available to hospitals only).

STREPTOMYCIN SULFATE

Streptomycin was the first chemotherapeutic agent of undeniable efficacy in the treatment of tuberculosis. It must be administered intramuscularly, which limits its usefulness in long-term chemotherapy, especially today, when highly effective oral regimens are available and the vast majority of patients are treated as outpatients. Streptomycin is the most valuable and least toxic of the parenterally administered antibiotics derived from *Streptomyces*. The only other highly effective agent available for parenteral use is isoniazid. The combination of streptomycin and isoniazid administered intramuscularly has an immediate, marked suppressive effect upon susceptible organisms and often has been lifesaving in critical situations.

Streptomycin is of greatest value in the early weeks or months of therapy. Possibly because it is administered parenterally and high serum concentrations are produced rapidly, this drug appears to enhance the effect of agents administered orally, even such effective agents as ethambutol and isoniazid.

The fact that streptomycin is administered parenterally is a definite asset in the treatment of comatose patients, those unable to take oral medication, or patients with poor gastrointestinal absorption. In some cases, it may be advisable to give streptomycin on an outpatient basis twice a week in combination with two oral agents prescribed daily. Streptomycin also is a major agent in intermittent therapy (see the Introduction), and it is one of the few agents that is effective in vitro against nonphotochromogens (myobacterial group III organisms) in vitro.

Most individuals tolerate streptomycin well. Occasionally, transient headache or malaise occurs soon after injection. Clinically unimportant facial paresthesia, particularly around the mouth, is noted in approximately 15% of patients and may be accompanied by a tingling sensation in the hands.

When administered correctly, streptomycin is rarely toxic. Hypersensitivity reactions occur occasionally during the early weeks of treatment but are less frequent than with aminosalicylic acid and usually less serious than with aminosalicylic acid or isoniazid. Although streptomycin is related to a family of potentially nephrotoxic drugs, it has been given daily for up to six months with little or no evidence of renal toxicity.

Streptomycin has a selective neurotoxic effect upon the eighth cranial nerve when large doses are administered for long periods (see Chapter 74, Aminoglycosides), although some patients may develop eighth nerve damage on a total dosage of 10 to 12 g. Usually, however, when this agent is prescribed correctly, damage to the eighth nerve almost never occurs. If usual adult doses are administered daily to young children for two months or more, permanent loss of labyrinthine function is almost a certainty.

A few reports of anaphylactic and hematopoietic reactions, including agranulocytosis and aplastic anemia, have appeared in the literature.

ROUTE, USUAL DOSAGE, AND PREPARATIONS. (All doses and strengths expressed in terms of the base)
Intramuscular: *Adults*, 20 mg/kg of body weight (maximum, rarely more than 1 g) once a day for two to three weeks. Thereafter, the frequency of administration can usually be decreased to 1 g every other day or three times weekly and then to 1 g twice a week; patients with normal renal function can tolerate this regimen well for months. The dose should be reduced in elderly patients, children, small adults, and individuals with impaired renal function.

Drug available generically: Powder 1 and 5 g; solution 400 mg/ml in 2.5 and 12.5 ml containers and 500 mg/ml in 2 and 10 ml containers.

MIXTURES

There is no justification for the use of commercial combinations of antimycobacterial agents. In the interest of maximum therapeutic efficacy and minimal potential toxicity, such factors as age, body weight, and renal function must be considered in prescribing each agent of a chemotherapeutic regimen. Even pyridoxine should be prescribed separately in an appropriate dose.

ATYPICAL MYCOBACTERIAL INFECTIONS

Drug susceptibility of atypical mycobacteria ranges from those that are completely susceptibile to those that are markedly resistant. Some strains of *M. kansasii* may be as susceptible to chemotherapy as *M. tuberculosis*, whereas others are resistant.

Since any degree of bacterial resistance can facilitate emergence of highly drug-resistant strains, the initial treatment of photochromogenic (mycobacterial Group I) infections should be vigorous. The most effective regimen usually consists of the daily administration of rifampin, isoniazid, and ethambutol. When the results of susceptibility studies are obtained, it may be necessary to alter the regimen. When photochromogenic infections are treated initially with the best possible regimen, definitive results are almost the rule. In cases of reactivation (nearly always a result of poor initial therapy), the regimen of retreatment should be based on the results of tests of susceptibility to all available agents. In difficult cases it may be necessary to administer five or six agents simultaneously, including those having less potency and greater potential toxicity than the major antituberculosis agents. It may be necessary to employ surgical resection in conjunction with chemotherapy in selected patients with atypical mycobacterial infections.

The only other group of atypical mycobacteria causing disease with any frequency are the nonphotochromogens (mycobacterial group III organisms), including *M. avium-intracellulare* complex. Unfortunately, most strains frequently are resistant to all antituberculosis agents. Nevertheless, with individualized multiple drug regimens chosen on the basis of susceptibility tests, 35% to 75% of cases still may be treated successfully. When the disease is sufficiently limited, resectional surgery carried out soon after conversion of sputum provides the best chance of cure.

The only member of Group II of clinical significance is *M. scrofulaceum*, so named because it may cause cervical lymphadenitis in children. Chemotherapy is of little help in this condition; surgical excision is the recommended treatment.

Members of Group IV, including *M. fortuitum*, are highly resistant to all available antituberculosis drugs. Fortunately, the organisms are ubiquitous saprophytes which rarely cause disease. Treatment with large doses of broad spectrum antibiotics to which the organisms are susceptible in vitro has apparently been helpful in isolated cases.

LEPROSY

It is estimated that 12 to 20 million people worldwide have leprosy (Hansen's disease). The majority of these individuals are in India, China, and Africa, although approximately 3,000 known cases exist in the United States. Therefore, while the possibility is still remote, the likelihood of a physician encountering a patient with leprosy is greater today than ever before because of the ease of intercontinental travel, the fact that servicemen have been stationed in countries where leprosy is endemic, and the steady influx of immigrants from endemic areas.

It is beyond the scope of this book to discuss the treatment of leprosy in detail, but certain general observations may be useful since the myths, superstitions, and legends surrounding leprosy still persist. Generally, leprosy is best managed by specialists who, in the United States, are almost always associated with U.S. Public Health Service hospitals or outpatient clinics. Indeed, it is usually necessary to use the resources of these facilities to establish a diagnosis. Biopsies taken from a suspected lesion will be examined, at no cost, at the U.S. Public Health Service Hospital at Carville, Louisiana. The biopsy should be taken entirely from within the lesion and preserved in neutral formalin. Once leprosy has been positively diagnosed, the attending physician must report the case to local health officials whether he decides to treat the patient himself or refers the case to a specialist. The Center for Disease Control in Atlanta, Georgia, or the U.S. Public Health Service Hospital at Carville also should be notified.

Leprosy is an infectious disease caused by the bacillus, *Mycobacterium leprae*. Active infection was once thought to be extremely contagious, but there is now evidence that the vast majority of people are partially or completely resistant to the bacillus and, even though there might be contact with the organism, active disease occurs only rarely. Although the mode of transmission has not yet been clearly defined, it is now generally believed that bacilli from skin lesions or nasal discharges of infected persons enter the body through the skin or respiratory tract but that only susceptible individuals will develop the disease. Except, perhaps, while awaiting confirmation of positive diagnosis, hospitalization is unnecessary and no special isolation is required.

The four forms of leprosy are: indeterminate, tuberculoid, lepromatous, and dimorphous (borderline). Indeterminate leprosy is the earliest recognizable form, and symptoms may be no more severe than localized hypopigmentation and some sensory loss. Although it is always treated if diagnosed, this condition may resolve spontaneously without therapy. When treatment is not given or healing does not occur, the condition may progress to tuberculoid leprosy in those with the greatest relative degree of resistance to the infection or to lepromatous leprosy in those with the least resistance. Dimorphous leprosy has some of the features of both the tuberculoid and lepromatous types.

Chemotherapy is the mainstay in the treatment of leprosy. Dapsone [Avlosulfon], a sulfone, is the drug of choice and the agent most commonly used for all forms of leprosy. The other available sulfone, sulfoxone [Diasone], is seldom used because its absorption is erratic, it is more expensive, and its therapeutic action occurs as a result of hydrolysis to dapsone. An investigational repository sulfone, acedapsone (DADDS), is being studied and may have some use in the general prophylaxis and treatment of tuberculoid leprosy.

Some strains of *M. leprae* have become resistant to the sulfones and occasional cases of primary sulfone resistance are now being found. Clofazimine (Lamprene, B663), which is available only for investigational use in the United States, and rifampin [Rifadin, Rimactane] have been used successfully to treat these patients. Ethionamide also may be useful in combined drug regimens.

With increasing frequency, experts are recommending that all lepromatous and more active cases of dimorphous leprosy be treated with combination drug regimens similar to the approach used in tuberculosis. The fifth report of the Expert Committee on Leprosy of the World Health Organization (1977) recommends 100 mg of dapsone daily combined with either 100 mg of clofazimine daily for six months or 600 mg of rifampin daily for at least two weeks, followed in both cases by the usual dapsone monotherapy. It is hoped that such an approach would diminish the chances of the eventual development of sulfone-resistant strains of *M. leprae* and/or shorten the treatment period for lepromatous patients from life to some finite number of years. Unfortunately, none of the studies to date have clearly established which combination of drugs is best, what dosage is optimal, or how long therapy should be given. Long-term trials of various combinations by the World Health Organization should ultimately provide answers to these questions.

Leprosy reactions represent a very complex problem in the management of patients with leprosy in up to 50% of cases. In general, two types of reactions are seen: reversal reactions in the dimorphous and tuberculoid forms and erythema nodosum leprosum (ENL) in the lepromatous and, occasionally, dimorphous forms. Both conditions are characterized by fever, which may be accompanied by neuritis, malaise, arthralgia, elevated white blood cell count, and edema. During reversal reactions, pre-existing lesions become erythematous and edematous; they occasionally ulcerate and new lesions may appear. In erythema nodosum leprosum, characteristic erythematous nodules may appear anywhere on the skin.

Mild leprosy reactions can be treated with aspirin; however, no treatment may be required in some patients. Antimonials (stibophen [Fuadin] and antimony potassium tartrate) have been used but, because of their toxic effects and the fact that better drugs are available, it is highly questionable whether the antimonials have a place in the treatment of these reactions.

Severe leprosy reactions of either type always respond to corticosteroids; prednisone 60 mg daily is usually sufficient for initial control and the dose usually can be reduced gradually to an alternate-day schedule if prolonged therapy is required. Corticosteroids should be used whenever neuritis that is causing a progressive neural deficit is observed.

Thalidomide, available only for extremely restricted investigational use in the United States, is the treatment of choice for erythema nodosum leprosum. It is of no value in reversal reactions. After an initial dose of up to 400 mg daily (adults), the amount can be decreased over a period of two weeks to 100 mg daily. The course can be repeated if reactions recur. Thalidomide is contraindicated in women of childbearing age who might conceive during therapy, except under unusual circumstances. Clofazimine (300 mg daily) also slowly controls most leprosy reactions of either type. Information on both drugs can be obtained from the U.S. Public Health Service Hospital at Carville, Louisiana.

In general, antileprosy therapy should be continued despite the appearance of a leprosy reaction. Stopping or reducing the dose of dapsone or any other medication will not immediately ameliorate the reactive episode. Such approaches in the past may have been responsible, at least in part, for the appearance of sulfone-resistant strains of *M. leprae*.

It must be remembered that, at best, the treatment of leprosy or leprosy reactions is difficult and complex and should only be undertaken by specialists or in consultation with them. Assistance is available at all times from the experts at Carville.

Adverse Reactions and Precautions

The adverse reactions produced by the sulfones are usually mild and occur infrequently with the doses used to treat leprosy. Nausea, vomiting, headache, dizziness, and tachycardia are uncommon, and methemoglobinemia, leukopenia, agranulocytosis, and allergic dermatitis (sometimes exfoliative with concurrent liver damage, fever, and lymphadenitis) have been observed only rarely with therapeutic doses. Hemolysis and significant hemolytic anemia also occur infrequently except in patients with erythrocyte glucose-6-phosphate dehydrogenase (G6PD) deficiency. Peripheral neuritis has been reported rarely after large doses.

Clofazimine, a red-colored compound that is deposited in the tissues, may discolor the skin and conjunctivae. The skin first develops a reddish hue that may progress to a mahogany brown, while the leprosy lesions themselves become even more pigmented and appear mauve, slate-gray, or black. The degree of pigmentation varies from patient to patient; generally the larger the dose and the more advanced the disease, the more pronounced the pigmentation will be. The conjunctivae become varying shades of red-brown. In addition, a red tint may appear in the urine, sputum, and sweat. All of these effects clear slowly after therapy is discontinued. Diminished sweating and tear production may be noted and photosensitivity reactions have been reported. Nausea, vomiting, and diarrhea may occur but are uncommon if the dose is less than 100 mg daily. Larger doses sometimes produce abdominal pain and, because of extensive deposition of the drug in the wall of the small bowel which may become edematous, symptoms suggesting bowel obstruction occasionally develop.

The adverse effects following use of rifampin [Rifadin, Rimactane] in the treatment of leprosy are the same as those observed when the drug is used to treat tuberculosis (see the section on Tuberculosis Chemotherapy).

INDIVIDUAL EVALUATIONS

DAPSONE
[Avlosulfon]

$$H_2N - \bigcirc - SO_2 - \bigcirc - NH_2$$

Dapsone is the sulfone of choice for the treatment of all forms of leprosy. Continuous treatment with this drug assures a negative bacterial state in almost all patients with lepromatous leprosy; however, five years or more will be required to achieve this condition. Most authorities recommend that administration be continued in lepromatous cases for life. Patients with indeterminate or tuberculoid leprosy, which are milder forms of the disease, probably should receive dapsone for two years and those with the dimorphous form, for ten years after an "inactive" status has been obtained. An "inactive" state is achieved when skin scrapings and/or biopsy are negative for bacteria and there has been no clinical evidence of activity for at least one year.

The adverse reactions produced by dapsone are similar to those of the sulfones as a group (see the introduction to this section).

ROUTE, USUAL DOSAGE, AND PREPARATIONS.
Oral: *Adults*, for dimorphous and lepromatous leprosy, 100 mg daily; for tuberculoid and indeterminate cases, 50 mg daily. It is advisable to screen the patient for a G6PD deficiency prior to initiation of therapy. If deficiency is found, the drug should be given more cautiously, starting with small doses of 25 mg twice weekly. If the patient cannot tolerate the drug and severe hemolysis occurs, clofazimine should be used as an alternative agent. *Children*, 1.4 mg/kg of body weight daily.
Avlosulfon (Ayerst). Tablets 25 and 100 mg.

SULFOXONE SODIUM
[Diasone Sodium]

$$Na^+ {}^-O_2SCH_2NH-\bigcirc-SO_2-\bigcirc-NHCH_2SO_2^- Na^+$$

This sulfone can be used to treat all forms of leprosy and dermatitis herpetiformis. It is hydrolyzed in the gut to dapsone; a 165-mg enteric-coated tablet of sulfoxone sodium makes available approximately 25 mg of dapsone. However, it is seldom used because its absorption is erratic (165 mg of sulfoxone may be equivalent to more or less than 25 mg of dapsone in a given

patient). Sulfoxone also is more costly than dapsone.

The adverse reactions produced by sulfoxone are similar to those of the sulfones as a group (see the introduction to this section).

ROUTE, USUAL DOSAGE, AND PREPARATIONS.
Oral: *Adults*, for leprosy, 330 mg daily. For dermatitis herpetiformis, *adults*, 330 mg daily for one week; the dose then may be increased to 660 mg daily if necessary. For maintenance, the dose is 330 mg daily.
Diasone Sodium (Abbott). Tablets (enteric-coated) 165 mg.

CLOFAZIMINE (B663)
[Lamprene]

Clofazimine is apparently as effective as dapsone for the treatment of leprosy and is the treatment of choice for those infected with sulfone-resistant *M. leprae*. It also will slowly control most associated reactions. Its use is investigational in the United States, however, and it may be obtained only through the U.S. Public Health Service Hospital at Carville.

Although no strains of *M. leprae* resistant to clofazimine have yet appeared, many investigators believe that this drug, like dapsone, should be used in a combination regimen for the treatment of all lepromatous and very active dimorphous cases. In addition to its use with dapsone in sulfone-sensitive infections, trials utilizing clofazimine plus either rifampin or ethionamide for varying periods are under investigation for the management of infections due to sulfone-resistant bacilli.

ROUTE, USUAL DOSAGE, AND PREPARATIONS.
Oral: *Adults*, for all forms of leprosy, 100 mg daily. Control of reactions may require 100 mg three times daily, but the dose must

be reduced at once if symptoms of gastrointestinal toxicity develop.

Lamprene (Geigy). Capsules 100 mg (Investigational drug).

RIFAMPIN

[Rifadin, Rimactane]

Although not an FDA-approved indication for rifampin in the United States, this drug is effective in the treatment of leprosy. It appears to be bactericidal for *M. leprae* while other drugs currently in use are considered to be bacteriostatic. Reports indicate that rifampin in oral doses of 300 to 600 mg daily (adult) renders bacilli noninfective for the mouse footpad and, therefore, presumably noninfectious for contacts more rapidly than dapsone or clofazimine (several days versus two to three months). However, the clinical response, as measured by clearance of skin lesions and reduction in the number of bacilli, does not appear to improve. Some patients have taken rifampin (as monotherapy) for as long as eight years without problems. On the other hand, resistant strains of *M. leprae* may appear within three to four years in others and, for this reason, it is now recommended that rifampin be used only in combination drug regimens. Trials are now underway utilizing rifampin plus dapsone for infections with sulfone-sensitive *M. leprae* and rifampin plus either clofazimine or eithionamide for infections with sulfone-resistant *M. leprae*.

ROUTE, USUAL DOSAGE, AND PREPARATIONS. *Oral: Adults*, for all forms of leprosy, 600 mg daily. Regimens utilizing 300 mg daily or intermittent therapy with 1.2 to 1.5 g are being investigated.

Rifadin (Dow), *Rimactane* (Ciba). Capsules 300 mg.

Selected References

Drugs for treatment of tuberculosis. *Med Lett Drugs Ther* 19:97-99, 1977.

Acocella G: Clinical pharmacokinetics of rifampin. *Clin Pharmacokinet* 3:108-127, 1978.

Avery GS (ed): *Drug Treatment: Principles and Practice of Clinical Pharmacology and Therapeutics*. Acton, Mass, Publishing Sciences Group, Inc, 1976.

Buckingham WB: Right drugs on right schedule can cure or prevent TB. *Mod Med* 46:110-118, (October 15-30) 1978.

Davidson PT: Changing concepts in tuberculosis chemotherapy. *Comp Ther* 3:38-44, (Dec) 1977.

Elliott J: Will short-term TB therapy regimens work? *JAMA* 240:2526, 1978.

Fox W: Modern management and therapy of pulmonary tuberculosis. *Proc R Soc Med* 70:4-15, 1977.

Fox W, Mitchison DA: Short-course chemotherapy for tuberculosis. *Lancet* 2:1349-1350, 1976.

Fox W, Mitchison DA: Short-course chemotherapy for pulmonary tuberculosis. *Am Rev Res Dis* 111:325-353, 1975.

Johnston RF, Audet PR: Antituberculosis chemotherapy. *Am Fam Physician* 17:136-139, (June) 1978.

Kasik JE: Tuberculosis and other mycobacterial disease, in Conn HF (ed): *Current Therapy 1979*. Philadelphia, WB Saunders Co, 1979, 155-160.

Lyons RW: Orange contact lenses from rifampin. *N Engl J Med* 300:372-373, 1979.

Pilheu JA: Short-duration treatment of pulmonary tuberculosis. *Chest* 71:583-586, 1977.

Van Scoy RE: Antituberculosis agents: Isoniazid, rifampin, streptomycin, ethambutol. *Mayo Clin Proc* 52:694-700, 1977.

Antifungal Agents | 80

For therapeutic purposes, fungal infections may be divided into three categories: dermatophytic, systemic, and candidal. Dermatophytic infections occur most commonly and involve the skin, hair, and nails. Approximately 20 species of *Epidermophyton*, *Trichophyton*, and *Microsporum* cause these infections, which are treated orally with griseofulvin [Fulvicin P/G, Fulvicin-U/F, Grifulvin V, Grisactin, Gris-PEG] or topically by the application of agents such as tolnaftate [Aftate, Tinactin], haloprogin [Halotex], clotrimazole [Lotrimin, Mycelex], or miconazole [MicaTin].

Systemic fungal infections may be subdivided into two classes. The first group is caused by organisms that are opportunistic and occur most commonly but not exclusively in debilitated or immunosuppressed patients or in those in whom bacterial flora is modified by prolonged or massive antibiotic therapy. Examples of such mycoses are cryptococcosis, aspergillosis, and zygomycosis. Other systemic fungal infections vary widely in incidence and most often include histoplasmosis, blastomycosis, coccidioidomycosis, paracoccidioidomycosis, and sporotrichosis. There also are many other less common systemic mycoses, examples of which are chromomycoses, mycetoma, penicilliosis, and geotrichosis. Systemic mycotic infections frequently constitute a serious medical problem. They may be chronic in nature, difficult to diagnose, and a major therapeutic challenge to both physician and patient. Drugs used in their treatment include amphotericin B [Fungizone], flucytosine [Ancobon], hydroxystilbamidine, and potassium iodide.

The remaining mycotic category includes only candidosis. *Candida albicans* most commonly causes human disease, but *C. tropicalis*, *C. paropsilosis*, and, more rarely, other species have been implicated as well. Candidosis usually affects moist skin or mucous membranes, including the gastrointestinal tract, and may cause systemic disease but only rarely involves the intact skin or nails of normal individuals. Patients with intertrigo or chronic paronychia, diabetes mellitus, or those recently given immunosuppressive drugs, antibacterial agents, or oral contraceptives are most susceptible to candidal infection. Drugs effective in mucocutaneous candidosis are amphotericin B, candicidin [Candeptin, Vanobid], nystatin [Candex, Mycostatin, Nilstat, O-V Statin], clotrimazole, and miconazole [Monistat]. Systemic candidosis generally responds to intravenous amphotericin B alone or with flucytosine. Use of the combination is justified only if in vitro testing documents susceptibility of the organism to both drugs. Flucytosine should not be used alone since candidal species often are resistant to it or, if susceptible, may become resistant.

Other Infections: The organisms causing actinomycosis (*Actinomyces israelii*) and nocardiosis (*Nocardia* species), although once considered fungi, are bacteria that do not respond to antifungal agents. The drug of choice for actinomycosis is penicillin G (2 to 20 million units daily for at least six weeks). In patients allergic to penicillin, tetracyclines are the primary alternative drugs. Other less established agents include lincomycin [Lincocin], clindamycin [Cleocin], and erythromycin. For nocardiosis, treatment with absorbable systemic sulfonamides (eg, triple sulfonamides, sulfadiazine 4 to 8 g daily in four divided doses, adjusted to maintain a plasma level of 10 to 15 mg/dl) for 6 to 12 months is often curative. With some strains (as guided by in vitro susceptibility testing), concomitant use of another antibacterial agent (eg, tetracycline, gentamicin) may be helpful. Drainage of abscesses and debridement are essential. Also, surgical removal of some of the lesions is sometimes the only satisfactory treatment.

Adverse Reactions and Precautions

Some topical preparations used to treat dermatophytoses are irritating or potentially sensitizing and should be discontinued if evidence of these effects develops. This is particularly true of preparations that also contain salicylic acid. Amphotericin B and nystatin administered orally for their local action in the gut are not absorbed and produce few adverse effects. Agents that are absorbed from the gastrointestinal tract, whether metabolized or excreted unchanged, cause adverse reactions ranging in severity from those that are mild and inconsequential to effects that are dangerous or potentially fatal. See the evaluations for a detailed description of the possible adverse effects.

An etiologic diagnosis should be made before initiating treatment with any antifungal drug. Most of these agents are not active against bacteria, and it is not always possible to differentiate between bacterial, fungal, or mixed infections solely on the basis of symptoms. Usually it is necessary to identify the kind of fungus involved, because most antifungal agents are not effective against both the dermatophytes and *Candida*, with the possible exception of the imidazole compounds (eg, clotrimazole, miconazole).

INDIVIDUAL EVALUATIONS

ACRISORCIN
[Akrinol]

Acrisorcin is used in the treatment of chromophytosis, a chronic fungal infection of the skin caused by *Pityrosporon orbiculare*. The drug is not effective in any other infection. Acrisorcin is applied to visible lesions and relapses are common because clinically undetected foci remain untreated. Therefore, the drug seldom produces permanent cure and has been replaced by newer, more effective agents.

A few local reactions (eg, blisters, erythematous vesicular eruptions, urticaria) have been reported. Acrisorcin should not be used near the eyes, and treatment should be discontinued if signs of irritation or sensitization develop.

ROUTE, USUAL DOSAGE, AND PREPARATIONS. *Topical*: The manufacturer recommends that a small quantity of cream be applied to lesions morning and night. Before the evening application, lesions should be scrubbed with a stiff brush and soap and the area rinsed thoroughly to avoid inactivation of the drug by residual soap. Treatment should be continued for at least six weeks.

Akrinol (Schering). Cream 0.2% in 50 g containers.

AMPHOTERICIN B
[Fungizone]

Amphotericin B is a polyene antibiotic produced by *Streptomyces nodosus*. Low concentrations inhibit the growth of fungi, protozoa, and algae. High concentrations (near the upper limits of tolerance in man) exert a fungicidal effect on some strains. The polyenes bind to cellular membranes, thereby altering their selective permeability. Unlike penicillin, which attacks only growing organisms, amphotericin B is active against both growing and resting cells. The ability of an organism to bind amphotericin B appears to depend upon the presence of ergosterol in the cellular membrane. Since bacterial membranes do not contain sterols, bacteria do not bind the drug and are insensitive to it.

Amphotericin B must be injected intravenously for systemic fungal infections and intrathecally at lumbar, cisternal, or cerebral ventricular sites for meningitis. Topical application is effective in candidosis of the skin, nails, or mucous membranes (including perleche and paronychia). Although it is not absorbed from the gastrointestinal tract, amphotericin B is sometimes given orally to decrease intestinal candidal colonization. It also may be administered intra-articularly or into the bladder and renal pelvis.

Amphotericin B may be lifesaving in almost all systemic fungal infections and is the only effective drug available for histoplasmosis, mucormycosis, and aspergillosis, although *Aspergillus* species frequently are naturally resistant and respond poorly. Iodides are indicated for cutaneous sporotrichosis, but amphotericin B may be used in patients who cannot tolerate or do not respond to iodides and is preferred in the systemic or extracutaneous form of the disease. Amphotericin B is the drug of choice for systemic blastomycosis; hydroxystilbamidine is a less effective alternative that may be used in patients with nonprogressive cutaneous disease if amphotericin B cannot be tolerated. Amphotericin B also is the drug of choice for cryptococcosis and candidosis. It has some effect in mucocutaneous leishmaniasis caused by the protozoan, *Leishmania braziliensis*, and in certain other protozoal diseases (see Chapter 82, Antiprotozoal Agents).

Investigationally, amphotericin B has been effective in mycotic keratitis by topical application, in some cases of fungal endophthalmitis by intravenous or even intraorbital injection (although recovery of vision has generally been poor), and in pulmonary aspergillosis by intrabronchial administration. The activity of amphotericin B in geotrichosis is usually poor since *Geotrichum* species are generally resistant to the drug. It is ineffective in penicilliosis.

Preparations combining amphotericin B with broad spectrum antibiotics have been promoted to prevent candidal overgrowth in the intestine during antibacterial therapy. The rationale for use of this combination is weak. Intestinal candidosis occurs primarily in patients with hematologic malignancy and is observed only infrequently in other patient populations. Furthermore, there is no evidence that oral amphotericin B counteracts the infection, that routine prophylactic administration of an antifungal agent reduces its frequency, or that amphotericin B is an effective or even desirable adjunct to antibacterial therapy. If the simultaneous use of an antifungal agent and an antibacterial agent is indicated, the compounds should be given separately. (See the section on Mixtures of Antifungal Drugs with Other Agents, and Chapter 73, Tetracyclines.)

Fungal resistance to amphotericin B has not been a serious problem, although clinical evidence of acquired resistance by *Coccidioides immitis* and some *Candida* species has been reported. Coccidioidomycosis may be difficult or impossible to cure and blastomycosis may relapse. Some species of *Zygomycetes* are highly resistant.

ADVERSE REACTIONS AND PRECAUTIONS.

When given parenterally, amphotericin B causes unpleasant and potentially dangerous reactions in most patients. These effects may be minimized by appropriate management, including ancillary therapy with heparin and antipyretics. Use of corticosteroids or anti-inflammatory agents also may be indicated.

Adverse reactions following intravenous administration include chills, sweats, fever, myalgia, malaise, anorexia, nausea, vomiting, headache, and azotemia. Reactions occurring rarely are thrombocytopenia, leukopenia, hypotension, cardiac arrest (after rapid injection), polyneuropathy, convulsions, and anaphylactic reactions. Anemia often occurs during prolonged therapy (0.5 to 0.6 mg/kg for four weeks or more).

Evidence of renal damage (increased blood urea nitrogen, serum creatinine, and nonprotein nitrogen levels; decreased glomerular filtration, renal plasma flow, and creatinine clearance; appearance of granular and hyaline casts) develops in almost all patients. Permanent renal damage has been reported when large doses were used for prolonged periods, especially when the total dosage exceeded 3 g. Renal tubular necrosis and nephrocalcinosis have been observed. Hypokalemia is common and potassium levels should be determined at least twice weekly. If hypokalemia occurs, potassium salts should be administered orally. It has been claimed that nephrotoxicity and febrile reactions may be lessened if the initial dose of amphotericin B is small and the amount gradually increased to the desired level.

Determinations of blood urea nitrogen or serum creatinine levels should be made on alternate days while the dosage is being increased and weekly thereafter during therapy. If levels exceed 50 mg/dl or 3.5 mg/dl, respectively, the dosage should be reduced until the levels are below these limits. Weekly determinations of creatinine clearance may provide a more sensitive evaluation of renal function than serum creatinine levels.

Intrathecal injection may cause nausea and vomiting; urinary retention; pain in the back, legs, or abdomen; headache, radiculitis; paresis (usually transient); paresthesias; tinnitus and diminished hearing; vertigo; and, rarely, impaired vision that may progress to blindness. However, intrathecal administration of amphotericin B to treat meningitis caused by *Coccidioides immitis* is more effective than the intravenous route. The drug is excreted primarily in the bile. Since urinary excretion is of minor importance, renal insufficiency does not appreciably influence serum levels. Blood levels are demonstrable for one to two weeks after termination of therapy.

Amphotericin B is essentially devoid of toxicity during oral or topical use. The infrequent reactions have been mild and transitory and consist mainly of nausea, vomiting, and diarrhea following oral administration and pruritus, mild local irritation, and allergic dermatitis after topical application.

Systemic therapy should be employed only in patients who are under close observation and have a confirmed diagnosis of a progressive, potentially fatal mycosis caused by a susceptible fungus. There is no justification for use of this drug in vague and undiagnosed conditions merely on the basis of a positive skin or serologic test.

Therapy must be continued for a sufficient period, usually two to four months. Antineoplastic agents or large doses of corticosteroids should not be given with amphotericin B unless they are needed to treat an underlying disease or, in the case of steroids, to control reactions to amphotericin B.

Systemic fungal infections that occur during pregnancy have been treated successfully with amphotericin B without obvious adverse effects on the fetus, but the number of cases reported has been small.

ROUTES, USUAL DOSAGE, AND PREPARATIONS.

Detailed instructions for the storage, preparation, and administration of amphotericin

B should be closely followed, because this drug is unstable under unfavorable conditions (eg, exposure to heat, low pH). Since the intravenous preparation is a colloidal suspension, membrane filters in intravenous infusion lines may remove clinically significant amounts of the drug. If an in-line membrane filter is used, the mean pore diameter should be no less than 1 micron.

Since amphotericin B is heat labile, the powder should be stored in the refrigerator. Solutions for parenteral injection should be used promptly. These solutions are prepared by adding 10 ml of water for injection to 50 mg of amphotericin B and shaking the vial until the solution is clear. The contents are then added to dextrose injection.

Intravenous (infusion): Dosage must be adjusted individually according to the severity of the disease and tolerance of the patient. Concentrations should not exceed 0.2 mg/ml in 5% dextrose injection and should have a pH of 4.2 or above. Antibacterial agents, potassium chloride, and sodium chloride must not be added to the solution because they cause the drug to precipitate. The infusion usually is given slowly over a period of two to six hours, and the initial dose should not exceed 0.25 mg/kg of body weight (an initial total dose of 1 mg daily is often preferred). The total amount may be increased by 5 to 10 mg daily to a maximum of 1.5 mg/kg given every other day. The total dose of 30 mg/kg (1.5 to 2.5 g) usually can be administered over a period of six to ten weeks, but several months of therapy may be necessary to achieve a cure; shorter periods may produce an inadequate response and lead to relapse. Therapy should be resumed gradually according to the above schedule whenever administration is interrupted for longer than seven days.

Intrathecal: A total of 50 mg is diluted with at least 150 ml of 5% dextrose injection (for intracisternal or intraventricular injection) or 10% dextrose without preservative (for hyperbaric translumbar injection) to a final concentration of about 0.25 mg/ml. Therapy is initiated with 0.1 ml (0.025 mg) and the dose is gradually increased until the patient can tolerate 0.5 mg, the usual maximum dose, without excessive discomfort. The minimal tolerated dose is given at 48- to 72-hour intervals.

Fungizone (Squibb). Powder 50 mg.

Topical: For dermatomycoses caused by *Candida* species, preparations are applied by rubbing well into the affected area two to four times daily; the duration of treatment varies from one to two weeks for intertrigo (diaper rash) to many weeks for more tenacious conditions such as interdigital (erosio) lesions. Persistent or recurrent infection may be due to continued fecal contamination and oral administration of an anticandidal agent such as nystatin may be required. For use in the eye, see Chapter 24, Ocular Anti-infective and Anti-inflammatory Agents.

Fungizone (Squibb). Cream 3% in 20 g containers; lotion 3% in 30 ml containers; ointment 3% in 20 g containers.

CANDICIDIN
[Candeptin, Vanobid]

This polyene antibiotic is derived from a soil actinomycete similar to *Streptomyces griseus*. It is fungistatic or fungicidal depending upon the concentration achieved at the site of therapy. It is used topically only for the treatment of vaginal candidosis. So that the male partner will not become a source of reinfection, coitus should be avoided or a condom should be used during therapy and for a few weeks following an apparent cure. Consideration should be given to treating the male sexual partner with appropriate therapy simultaneously.

During pregnancy, manual insertion of the tablet is preferable to use of the tablet inserter. Also, care should be exercised when ointment is applied with the applicator. Untoward effects have been mild and infrequent. Slight irritation of the vulvar and perivulvar area occurs most commonly. Sensitization has been reported only rarely.

1358

ROUTE, USUAL DOSAGE, AND PREPARATIONS.
Intravaginal: One applicatorful of ointment or one capsule or tablet is inserted high in the vagina morning and night for 14 days. The course is repeated if symptoms persist or reappear.

> *Candeptin* (Schmid). Capsules; ointment 0.06% in 75 g containers; tablets. Activity in each capsule, applicatorful of ointment (5 g), or tablet is equivalent to 3 mg of candicidin.
> *Vanobid* (Merrell-National). Ointment 0.06% in 75 g containers; tablets. Activity in each applicatorful of ointment (5 g) or tablet is equivalent to 3 mg of candicidin.

CARBOL-FUCHSIN SOLUTION

This dye has been used topically to treat dermatophytic infections but causes staining and has been made obsolete by more effective agents. It should no longer be used.

> Drug available under the name Castellani's Paint: The original formulation contained basic fuchsin 0.3%, phenol 4.5%, resorcinol 10%, acetone 5%, and ethyl alcohol 10%. In most instances, the currently available preparations of Castellani's Paint no longer contain phenol. This solution is available in 1 and 4 oz, pt, and gal containers.

CLIOQUINOL (Iodochlorhydroxyquin)
[Vioform]

This preparation may be useful in localized dermatophytoses, especially if bacteria also are present, since the drug has both antibacterial and antifungal activity. Clioquinol should not be used near the eyes. It infrequently causes irritation of sensitized skin.

ROUTE, USUAL DOSAGE, AND PREPARATIONS.
Topical: A 3% concentration is applied several times daily.

> Drug available generically: Cream and ointment 3% in 1 oz and 1 lb containers; powder in ½, 1, and 4 oz containers.
> *Vioform* (Ciba). Cream and ointment 3% in 1 oz containers (nonprescription).

CLOTRIMAZOLE
[Lotrimin, Gyne-Lotrimin, Mycelex, Mycelex-G]

Clotrimazole is closely related chemically to miconazole and has a broad in vitro antifungal spectrum that includes *Petriellidium boydii*, *Sporothrix schenckii*, *Histoplasma capsulatum*, *Blastomyces dermatitidis*, *Cryptococcus neoformans*, *C. immitis*, and species of *Aspergillus* and *Candida*. It is applied topically to the skin and vaginal mucosa and is a drug of choice in infections caused by the pathogenic dermatophytes (*Epidermophyton*, *Microsporum*, and *Trichophyton* species), *Candida albicans*, and *Malassezia furfur*. Clinical improvement, including relief from pruritus, usually occurs within one week. If no significant improvement is seen following one month of therapy, the diagnosis should be redetermined.

In Europe, clotrimazole is used systemically as well as topically. In the United States, only topical and vaginal preparations are marketed commercially, but a topical oral form (troche) is available for investigational use in oropharyngeal candidosis. The troche acts locally in the oropharynx by impregnating the mucosa. Most clinical studies indicate that systemic clotrimazole has little efficacy and considerable toxicity.

Adverse effects after topical use include erythema; stinging, blistering, and peeling of the skin; edema; pruritus; and urticaria. If general irritation becomes intolerable, treatment should be discontinued and appropriate corrective measures instituted. Gastrointestinal effects (abdominal cramping, midepigastric pain, nausea, vomiting, diarrhea) are common if the drug is swallowed following oral administration. Mental disturbances that may include hallucinations and disorientation have been observed in up to 25% of patients if the drug is administered orally for systemic use. Preparations of clotrimazole are not intended for ophthalmic use and should be used with caution around the eyes.

ROUTES, USUAL DOSAGE, AND PREPARATIONS. *Topical*: A sufficient amount of cream or solution to cover the affected and surrounding area is applied twice daily (morning and evening).

> *Lotrimin* (Schering), *Mycelex* (Dome). Cream 1% in 15 and 30 g containers; solution 1% in 10 and 30 ml containers.

Intravaginal: One tablet is inserted into the vagina nightly for 7 days or one applicatorful of cream is inserted into the vagina nightly for 7 to 14 days.

> *Gyne-Lotrimin* (Schering). Tablets (vaginal) 100 mg with applicator.
> *Mycelex-G* (Dome). Cream (vaginal) 1% with applicator; tablets (vaginal) 100 mg with applicator.

FLUCYTOSINE
[Ancobon]

This synthetic antifungal agent is administered orally only for the treatment of serious systemic infections caused by susceptible *Candida* species or *Cryptococcus neoformans*, particularly endocarditis caused by *Candida* or meningitis attributable to *C. neoformans*. Some *Cladosporium* and *Torulopsis* species also may be susceptible.

Resistance may develop during therapy, and 40% to 50% of the pretreatment clinical isolates of *Candida* species are resistant to flucytosine. Therefore, susceptibility tests must be performed initially and at frequent intervals during treatment of candidal and cryptococcal infections. Care must be taken to assure that erroneous results are not obtained. The commonly used media (including those used for testing amphotericin B sensitivity) interfere with the in vitro activity of flucytosine. Reproducible, reliable results can be obtained using synthetic media free of cytosine and uridine.

Flucytosine is well absorbed from the gastrointestinal tract and peak serum levels are achieved in four to six hours. It is widely distributed in body water. Levels achieved in the liver, kidney, spleen, heart, and lung are equal to those in the serum. Levels in the cerebrospinal fluid and central nervous system are about 80% of those obtained in the serum.

Flucytosine is less toxic than amphotericin B, but it may cause nausea, vomiting, diarrhea, rash, anemia, headache, drowsiness, confusion, vertigo, and hallucinations. The most common blood dyscrasia associated with the drug is a reversible neutropenia; eosinophilia, leukopenia, and thrombocytopenia also have been observed. Elevation of hepatic enzymes (SGOT, SGPT), blood urea nitrogen, and creatinine levels may occur. Bowel perforation has been reported rarely.

This antifungal agent must be used with caution in patients with impaired renal function, since approximately 90% of the drug is excreted by the kidneys. However, since flucytosine appears to cause no renal toxicity, it can be used safely in these patients if the dosage is modified. This can be an advantage over amphotericin B, for which renal impairment may be a relative contraindication.

Flucytosine also must be administered with care to those with bone marrow depression (eg, patients with certain hematologic diseases, those being treated with radiation or drugs that depress bone marrow function), and it is contraindicated in patients known to be hypersensitive to the drug itself.

The safety of flucytosine during pregnancy has not been established. Therefore, the potential benefits must be weighed against the possible hazards if flucytosine is considered for use in women of childbearing age.

Route, Usual Dosage, and Preparations. *Oral*: *Adults and children with normal renal function*, 150 to 200 mg/kg of body weight daily in divided doses at six-hour intervals. Lower doses have been recommended, but they often are inadequate and continued use may lead to the colonization of drug-resistant fungi. The pharmacokinetics of flucytosine in normal individuals and those with renal insufficiency form the basis for proposed guidelines to modify dosage in patients with renal impairment. One such schedule follows:

DOSAGE SCHEDULE FOR 5-FLUOROCYTOSINE (FLUCYTOSINE) IN RELATION TO CREATININE CLEARANCE*

Creatinine Clearance (ml/min)	Individual Dose (mg/kg)	Dose Interval (hours)	Daily Dose (mg/kg
>40	25-50	6	100-200
40-20	25-50	12	50-100
20-10	25-50	24	25-50
<10	50	>24†	—

*From Schonebeck J, et al: Studies on oral antimycotic agent 5-fluorocytosine in individuals with normal and impaired kidney function. Chemotherapy 18:321-326, 1973.

†Interval according to serum concentrations of the drug which must be measured regularly

Ancobon (Roche). Capsules 250 and 500 mg.

GENTIAN VIOLET

This dye has been used topically to treat intertriginous candidosis but causes staining and, because more effective agents are available, it is now obsolete.

Drug available generically: Solution 1% and 2%; powder.

AVAILABLE TRADEMARKS.

Genapax (Key), *GVS* (Savage), *Hyva Gentian Violet* (Holland-Rantos).

GRISEOFULVIN

[Fulvicin P/G, Fulvicin-U/F, Grifulvin V, Grisactin, Gris-PEG]

Griseofulvin is an antibiotic derived from a species of *Penicillium*. It can be fungistatic or fungicidal. For this drug to exert a fungicidal effect, the organism must be actively growing, since one of the major cellular effects of griseofulvin is to inhibit fungal mitosis. It is the only drug effective orally against species of *Epidermophyton*, *Microsporum*, and *Trichophyton* that cause dermatophytic infections. Griseofulvin is ineffective against bacteria and other fungi, including *Candida* species. If mixed infections occur, concomitant use of a drug active against the second organism is necessary. Griseofulvin is most effective in dermatophytic infections of the scalp and glabrous skin, although several weeks of therapy may be required to effect a cure. It is less active in chronic infections of the feet and palms. Adjunctive therapy with keratolytic agents may be indicated in areas of hyperkeratosis. Dermatophytic infections of the fingernails usually respond within six months, although nine months of therapy may be necessary. Treatment for toenail infections usually must be continued for nine months or until a normal nail is present, which can take 15 months or longer. Reinfection of toenails occurs frequently. It is important to establish that a dermatophytic fungus is the cause of the onychomycosis since infections of the fingernails and especially toenails may have other causes. Some forms of onychomycosis are almost completely resistant to therapy. Treatment of these infections with griseofulvin must be continued for several months beyond the schedules given above before a beneficial effect is observed, if indeed therapy is successful at all. In stubborn infections, concomitant treatment with topical antifungal agents may be helpful.

The absorption rate of griseofulvin is enhanced after a high-fat meal, but the total amount of drug absorbed is not affected. Therapy should be continued until infected keratinous structures have been completely eradicated, as determined by clinical and laboratory examination.

During long-term administration, griseofulvin is deposited in the skin, hair, and nails and is actively secreted from eccrine sweat glands. Originally, it was postulated that griseofulvin was incorporated into cells and then carried into the stratum corneum to explain the delay of two to three weeks in healing of cutaneous fungal infections. However, more careful observations in recent years indicate that the drug appears to move in and out of the stratum corneum more rapidly than was believed formerly and that lesions began to heal within a few days after initiating treatment. The stratum corneum can be cleared of drug within two days after therapy is discontinued, which is much faster than would be expected if the drug were tightly bound to the cells from where it would have to migrate to the tissue surface. Plasma levels remain measurable for four days after therapy has been stopped. Although keratin containing the drug is quite resistant to certain fungal infections, the effectiveness of this compound as a prophylactic agent has not been established.

Serious reactions associated with the use of griseofulvin occur infrequently. Leukopenia is sometimes seen and granulocytopenia may occur when the drug is administered in large doses and/or given for a long period of time. Therefore, it may be advisable to perform blood counts occasionally during therapy with this drug. The most common minor reaction is headache, which may develop in up to 15% of patients; this usually disappears within a few days, even with continued therapy. Other reactions include dysgeusia, dryness of the mouth, gastrointestinal disturbances (nausea, vomiting, diarrhea), arthralgia, peripheral neuritis, vertigo, and fever. Griseofulvin occasionally causes syncope,

blurred vision, photosensitivity, insomnia, and rash. Rarely, it may cause serum sickness, angioedema, confusion, lapses of memory, and impaired judgment that may affect the performance of routine tasks. This compound also may produce estrogen-like effects in children. Patients sensitive to penicillin rarely may be sensitive to griseofulvin.

Griseofulvin may cause hepatotoxicity and is contraindicated in patients with acute intermittent porphyria or a history of that condition, hepatocellular failure, and in those who are hypersensitive to the drug itself. It should not be used for trivial infections that usually respond to a topical agent alone. Griseofulvin decreases the activity of warfarin-type anticoagulants, requiring dosage adjustments. Conversely, barbiturates depress griseofulvin activity and an increase in dosage of the latter may be required.

The safe use of griseofulvin during pregnancy has not been established. Therefore, potential benefits must be weighed against the possible hazards if griseofulvin is considered for use in women of childbearing age.

ROUTE, USUAL DOSAGE, AND PREPARATIONS. Griseofulvin was originally marketed in a macrocrystalline form which required the use of large doses to achieve and maintain effective blood levels. A microcrystalline form was subsequently developed that replaced the macrocrystalline preparations because the same blood levels could be achieved with smaller doses. More recently, an ultramicrocrystalline product has been marketed; this form is claimed to produce the same blood levels as the microcrystalline form at a further reduction in dosage, but there is no convincing evidence that further reducing the particle size confers any significant advantage in efficacy or safety and, therefore, there appears to be no practical therapeutic difference between these two forms.

MICROCRYSTALLINE FORM:

Oral: *Adults*, 500 mg daily in single or divided doses after meals; 1 g or more daily in divided doses has been recommended for stubborn infections. *Children*, approximately 10 mg/kg of body weight daily in single or divided doses after meals.

Divided dosage regimens usually are indicated only if the patient cannot tolerate a single daily dose. Because griseofulvin is absorbed over a relatively long period of time, once-a-day administration will maintain adequate blood levels.

> Drug available generically: Capsules 250 mg.
> *Fulvicin-U/F* (Schering). Tablets 250 and 500 mg.
> *Grifulvin V* (McNeil). Suspension 125 mg/5 ml; tablets 125, 250, and 500 mg.
> *Grisactin* (Ayerst). Capsules 125 and 250 mg; tablets 500 mg.

ULTRAMICROCRYSTALLINE FORM:
Oral: *Adults*, 250 mg daily in single or divided doses after meals; 500 mg or more can be given for stubborn infections. *Children*, approximately 5 mg/kg of body weight daily in single or divided doses after meals.

> *Fulvicin P/G* (Schering). Tablets 125 and 250 mg.
> *Gris-PEG* (Dorsey). Tablets 125 mg.

HALOPROGIN
[Halotex]

Haloprogin is a synthetic topical antifungal agent used in the treatment of superficial fungal infections of the skin caused by several *Trichophyton* species, *Microsporum* species, and *Epidermophyton floccosum*. It also has been used to treat infections caused by *Pityrosporon orbiculare*, and there is some evidence of activity against cutaneous candidal infections. The cure rate may be slightly higher and relapses may occur less frequently with haloprogin than with tolnaftate.

Adverse reactions include local irritation, burning sensation, and vesicle formation. Haloprogin may increase pruritus and maceration and exacerbate pre-existing lesions. If sensitization is noted, the drug should be discontinued and not used again. Contact with the eyes must be avoided.

ROUTE, USUAL DOSAGE, AND PREPARATIONS.
Topical: The preparation is applied liberally to the affected area twice daily for two or three weeks. Interdigital lesions may require up to four weeks of therapy. If there is no improvement after four weeks, haloprogin should be discontinued and the diagnosis redetermined.

> *Halotex* (Westwood). Cream 1% in 15 and 30 g containers; solution 1% in 10 and 30 ml containers.

HYDROXYSTILBAMIDINE ISETHIONATE

Hydroxystilbamidine is administered intravenously to treat blastomycosis. It appears to be most effective in patients with dermal or noncavitary pulmonary disease who have adequate host defenses. Patients with significantly impaired host response, such as those receiving immunosuppressive therapy, require amphotericin B. Amphotericin B is more effective than hydroxystilbamidine in disseminated blastomycosis, and relapses probably occur less frequently after its use. Hydroxystilbamidine is a minor alternative drug in the treatment of leishmaniasis.

Blastomycosis has been reported to recur several months to several years following arrest of symptoms by either hydroxystilbamidine or amphotericin B. Remissions, therefore, should not be interpreted as cures until patients have been symptom-free for prolonged periods.

Serious adverse reactions, including hypotension and tachycardia, have been observed during or immediately following intravenous administration of hydroxystilbamidine. They may be minimized by slow infusion of a dilute solution. Common untoward effects are anorexia, nausea, vomiting, malaise, and headache. Reactions noted occasionally are dizziness, flushing, hyperhidrosis, dyspnea, formication, salivation, syncope, paresthesias, fecal and urinary incontinence, and edema of the face and eyelids. These reactions usually disappear within 30 minutes. The parent compound, stilbamidine, produces neuropathies (eg, trigeminal neuropathy) fairly often, but only rare and questionable occurrences have been reported with hydroxystilbamidine. Impaired hepatic function is sometimes noted, and the presence of hepatic disease is a relative contraindication to the use of this drug.

ROUTE, USUAL DOSAGE, AND PREPARATIONS. *Intravenous (infusion)*: A total course of 8 g is given in daily doses of 225 mg in 200 ml of 5% dextrose injection or sodium chloride injection. Freshly prepared solutions must be protected from light and heat during administration and infused immediately over a period of two to three hours. If necessary, the dose may be given intramuscularly in 10 ml of sodium chloride or 5% dextrose injection, but the drug causes pain when given by this route.
Drug available generically: Powder 225 mg.

MICONAZOLE NITRATE
[MicaTin, Monistat]

Miconazole is a synthetic imidazole derivative with broad spectrum in vitro antifungal activity. Sensitive genera in vitro include *Ctenomyces, Trichophyton, Microsporum, Epidermophyton, Blastomyces, Streptomyces, Madurella, Alternaria, Cladosporium, Phialophora, Basidiobolus, Entomophthora, Nocardia, Sporothrix, Allescheria, Aureobasidium, Cephalosporium,* and *Candida*. It also is active in vitro against gram-positive (but not gram-negative) bacteria, and high concentrations are trichomonicidal. When applied topically on the skin, miconazole is effective in dermatophytic infections caused by *Epidermophyton, Microsporum,* and

Trichophyton species, but its efficacy in fungal infections of the nails is unknown; studies adequate to assess its value in onychomycosis have not been conducted. Along with clotrimazole, miconazole may ultimately prove to be a primary drug of choice in cutaneous dermatophytic infections. It also is effective in candidal infections of the skin and mucosal surfaces and may be significantly more effective than nystatin in vulvovaginal candidosis. Recent clinical experience also has confirmed that miconazole is effective against chromophytosis. Because of its broad spectrum, it is particularly useful in mixed skin infections.

Intravenous administration of miconazole may produce good results in systemic infections caused by *Candida albicans, Cryptococcus,* and *Aspergillus*. The rate of initial failures and relapses is unacceptably high in coccidioidomycosis.

The exact biochemical mechanism of action of miconazole is not known, but there is evidence that it affects the permeability of fungi by acting directly on the cell wall or plasma membrane. The drug is fungistatic or fungicidal, depending upon the concentration attained at a given site. Thus, topical application may produce a fungicidal effect, whereas systemic (intravenous) administration usually is fungistatic. Fungicidal concentrations are not attained in urine or cerebrospinal fluid following intravenous injection.

Adverse reactions to topical application consist of irritation, burning sensation, or maceration. If these reactions appear to be caused by hypersensitivity or undue discomfort occurs, the drug should be discontinued. Miconazole should be used cautiously around the eyes. Intravenous injection may cause thrombophlebitis, pruritus, rash, nausea, vomiting, diarrhea, anemia, thrombocytopenia, hyperlipidemia (hypercholesterolemia, hypertriglyceridemia), hyponatremia, and bronchospasm (presumably a hypersensitivity reaction).

ROUTES, USUAL DOSAGE, AND PREPARATIONS. *Intravenous*: 25 to 30 mg/kg of body weight in two or three equally divided doses at 8- or 12-hour intervals. Generally, therapy should be continued until laboratory and clinical tests indicate that active fungal infection is no longer present.

> *Monistat-I.V.* (Ortho). Solution (sterile) 10 mg/ml in 20 mg containers.

Topical: For dermatophytoses and candidal infections, a sufficient amount of cream to cover the affected area is applied twice daily (morning and evening). Chromophytosis may be treated once daily. Miconazole should be applied sparingly to intertriginous areas. In most dermatophytic and candidal infections, two weeks of therapy are usually sufficient. Patients with infections of the feet should be treated for four weeks to prevent recurrence. If no improvement is seen after one month of therapy, the diagnosis should be redetermined.

> *MicaTin* (Johnson & Johnson). Cream 2% in 15, 28, and 85 g containers; lotion 2% in 12 and 30 ml containers.

Intravaginal: One applicatorful of cream is inserted high in the vagina nightly for seven days. In resistant cases, the course of therapy may be repeated after the diagnosis has been reconfirmed.

> *Monistat 7* (Ortho). Cream 2% in 47 g containers.

NYSTATIN

[Candex, Mycostatin, Nilstat, O-V Statin]

Nystatin is a polyene antibiotic derived from *Streptomyces noursei*. It is fungistatic or fungicidal, depending upon the concentration, route of administration, and infecting organism. This drug is active in vitro against a variety of fungi, including all *Candida* species that cause infections in man. Clinically, its use is usually limited to the treatment of candidal infections of the skin, mucous membranes, gastrointestinal tract, and vagina. Nystatin is too toxic for parenteral use and is not absorbed from the gastrointestinal tract.

Oral preparations combining nystatin with broad spectrum antibiotics have been promoted to prevent candidal overgrowth in the intestine during antibacterial therapy. Use of these mixtures is unwarranted since intestinal candidosis does not occur often, and there is no clinical evidence that routine prophylactic administration of an antifungal agent reduces its incidence. (See the section on Mixtures of Antifungal Drugs with Other Agents, and Chapter 73, Tetracyclines.)

The infrequent reactions to nystatin have been mild and transitory. The drug may cause nausea, vomiting, and diarrhea after oral administration. Irritation occurs rarely after topical application, but hypersensitivity has not been observed. Resistance to nystatin has not been reported clinically.

ROUTES, USUAL DOSAGE, AND PREPARATIONS.
Oral: *Adults* (tablets), 500,000 to 1,000,000 units three times daily. *Adults and children* (suspension), 400,000 to 600,000 units four times daily (one-half of dose in each side of mouth), held in the mouth for a time before swallowing; *infants*, 200,000 units four times daily; *premature and low-birth-weight infants*, 100,000 units four times daily. Treatment should be continued for at least 48 hours after disappearance of symptoms.

> Drug available generically: Tablets 500,000 units.
> *Mycostatin* (Squibb), *Nilstat* (Lederle). Drops (suspension) 100,000 units/ml; tablets 500,000 units.
> *O-V Statin* (Squibb). Oral/vaginal therapy pack containing 21 tablets (oral) 500,000 units and 14 tablets (vaginal) 100,000 units.

Vaginal: 100,000 to 200,000 units daily for two weeks or longer.

> Drug available generically: Tablets (vaginal) 100,000 units.
> *Mycostatin* (Squibb), *Nilstat* (Lederle). Tablets (vaginal) 100,000 units.

Topical: Ointment or cream is applied to lesions twice daily or as directed. Powder is preferred for moist lesions and is applied two or three times daily. For use in the eye, see Chapter 24, Ocular Anti-infective and Anti-inflammatory Agents.

> Drug available generically: Cream 100,000 units/g in 15 g containers.
> *Candex* (Dome). Cream 100,000 units/g in 15 g containers; lotion 100,000 units/ml in 30 ml containers.
> *Mycostatin* (Squibb). Cream and ointment 100,000 units/g in 15 and 30 g containers; powder 100,000 units/g in 15 g containers.
> *Nilstat* (Lederle). Cream 100,000 units/g in 15 g containers; ointment 100,000 units/g in 15 and 240 g containers.

POTASSIUM IODIDE

Potassium iodide is the therapy of choice for cutaneous lymphatic sporotrichosis in patients who can tolerate the drug and do not have a history of iodism. It is not effective against systemic or extracutaneous sporotrichosis, which should be treated with amphotericin B; the latter drug also has been used successfully in a few cases of the lymphocutaneous disease that did not respond to iodine. Chromomycosis may respond to potassium iodide.

If symptoms of iodism (brassy taste in the mouth, rhinitis, coryza, salivation, lacrimation, sneezing, burning of mouth and throat, ocular irritation, sialadenitis, and dermal lesions) occur, administration may have to be discontinued for a few days or the dosage decreased. Heartburn, nausea, and diarrhea also occur occasionally. Hypothyroidism may develop in patients with goiter (see Chapter 48, Agents Used to Treat Thyroid Disease).

ROUTE, USUAL DOSAGE, AND PREPARATIONS. *Oral*: 1 ml of a saturated solution (1 g/ml) is given three times daily; the amount is increased by 1 ml daily, depending upon tolerance, to a maximal daily dose of 12 to 15 ml. Cure requires at least six to eight weeks of treatment. Therapy should be continued for a minimum of four weeks after the disappearance or stabilization of the lesions.

Drug available generically: Solution 1 g/ml.

SELENIUM SULFIDE
[Exsel, Selsun]

Selenium sulfide may have some use in the treatment of chromophytosis, a chronic fungal infection of the skin caused by *Pityrosporon orbiculare*, although superior agents are available. It also is used to treat seborrheic dermatitis of the scalp (see Chapter 61, Dermatologic Preparations).

Contact with the eyes and genital area should be avoided because of the irritant properties of the drug. The detergent component of the lotion may cause sensitization.

ROUTE, USUAL DOSAGE, AND PREPARATIONS. *Topical*: Affected areas are covered with the lotion and lathered; the preparation is thoroughly rinsed off after 10 to 15 minutes. The lotion is applied once daily for four days. Therapy may be repeated in one week if needed.

Drug available generically: Lotion 2.5%.
Exsel (Herbert), *Selsun* (Abbott). Lotion 2.5% in 120 ml containers.

TOLNAFTATE
[Aftate, Tinactin]

Tolnaftate is effective topically against *Epidermophyton*, *Microsporum*, and *Trichophyton* species, which cause dermatophytic infections, and *Pityrosporon orbiculare*, which causes chromophytosis. It is not effective in candidal or bacterial infections; therefore, microscopic or cultural identification of the infecting organism is necessary before tolnaftate is used. Fungal infections of the scalp, nails, soles, and palms usually do not respond well to tolnaftate, since they are frequently chronic and often refractory to topical medication. However, tolnaftate may be given adjunctively with griseofulvin for local benefit. Relapses are common in *T. rubrum* infections but a second course of tolnaftate may be beneficial.

There have been some subjective claims that tolnaftate is irritating, but no confirmed adverse reactions have been reported.

ROUTE, USUAL DOSAGE, AND PREPARATIONS. *Topical*: One or two drops of solution or a small amount of cream or powder is rubbed into lesions twice daily for two to three weeks; treatment for four to six weeks may be required in some cases. The powder or powder aerosol may be used following the original treatment period to help maintain remission in patients susceptible to tinea.

Aftate (Plough). Gel 1% in ½ oz containers; powder 1% in 2 ¼ oz containers; powder (aerosol) 1% in 5 oz containers; liquid 1%

(aerosol) in 5 oz containers (all forms nonprescription).
Tinactin (Schering). Cream 1% in 15 g containers; powder 1% in 45 g containers; powder (aerosol) 1% in 120 g containers; solution 1% in 10 ml containers (all forms nonprescription).

TRIACETIN
[Enzactin]

$$
\begin{array}{c}
\overset{\displaystyle O}{\underset{\displaystyle \|}{}} \\
H_2COCCH_3 \\
\overset{\displaystyle O}{\underset{\displaystyle \|}{}} \\
HCOCCH_3 \\
\overset{\displaystyle O}{\underset{\displaystyle \|}{}} \\
H_2COCCH_3
\end{array}
$$

Triacetin is used topically to treat superficial fungal infections. Controlled clinical trials have not proved that this agent has a therapeutic effect greater than that provided by the alteration of pH and the keratolytic action of acetic acid, which is released slowly from triacetin by esterases present in fungi, skin, and serum.

ROUTE, USUAL DOSAGE, AND PREPARATIONS.
No useful dosage regimen can be recommended, since this compound may be no more effective than the acetic acid it releases.

Enzactin (Ayerst). Aerosol 15% in 3 oz containers; cream 250 mg/g in 1 oz containers; powder 33.3% in 1½ oz containers (all forms nonprescription).

UNDECYLENIC ACID

$$
CH_2 = CH(CH_2)_8COH
$$

Clinical results suggest that this compound is a useful proprietary agent for the treatment of dermatophytic infections. It is well tolerated and may be worth a trial in localized mild infections.

ROUTE, USUAL DOSAGE, AND PREPARATIONS.
Topical: The concentration should not exceed 10% for application to skin or 1% to mucous membranes. Dosage recommendations vary with different manufacturers. A common practice is to apply powder or aerosol in the morning and an ointment or

aerosol at night (see the evaluation on Compound Undecylenic Acid).

AVAILABLE TRADEMARK.
Desenex Solution, Soap (Pharmacraft) (nonprescription).
SIMILAR PREPARATIONS.
Caldesene Medicated Powder (nonprescription), *Cruex Medicated Cream, Powder* (Pharmacraft) (nonprescription).

MIXTURES OF ANTIFUNGAL DRUGS

BENZOIC AND SALICYLIC ACIDS OINTMENT

This mixture contains benzoic acid 6% and salicylic acid 3%. It has no significant antifungal action but is an effective keratolytic agent. Prior treatment with this preparation makes infections in deeper layers accessible to more potent antifungal agents. Its use should be discontinued if irritation occurs. See also Chapter 61, Dermatologic Preparations.

ROUTE, USUAL DOSAGE, AND PREPARATIONS.
Topical: The ointment is applied once or twice daily to the involved area.

Mixture available under the name Whitfield's Ointment in 1 oz and 1 lb containers (nonprescription).

COMPOUND UNDECYLENIC ACID

This mixture of undecylenic acid and zinc undecylenate is used topically to treat dermatophytoses and, like the individual ingredients, may be effective in minor lesions. Its use should be discontinued if sensitization or irritation develops.

ROUTE, USUAL DOSAGE, AND PREPARATIONS.
Topical: Ointment or powder is applied once or twice daily to the involved area.

Mixture available generically: Ointment containing undecylenic acid 5% and zinc undecylenate 20%.
AVAILABLE TRADEMARK.
Desenex Powder, Foot Powder (spray), Ointment (Pharmacraft) (nonprescription).

SPOROSTACIN

Sporostacin, a combination of chlordantoin and benzalkonium chloride, is promoted for topical use in the treatment of candidal infections of the vulvovaginal area. In vitro, chlordantoin inhibits *Candida albicans*, and a combination of chlordantoin and benzalkonium chloride acts synergistically. Cure rates have ranged from less than 50% to 70% after a 14-day course of treatment to 90% or more after three courses. Adequate controlled studies to confirm these findings have not been published. Use of this mixture may be justified in patients who do not tolerate or respond to more effective agents such as amphotericin B, nystatin, or miconazole.

Irritation and sensitization occur (usually in less than 1% of patients). The drug should be discontinued promptly if erythema (an uncommon side effect) or dermatitis is noted.

ROUTE, USUAL DOSAGE, AND PREPARATIONS. *Topical*: For candidal infections of the vulvovaginal area, the cream is applied to the affected area once or twice daily as required. For mycotic vaginitis, one applicatorful of cream is applied twice daily for 14 days; the course of therapy may be repeated if necessary.

> *Sporostacin* (Ortho). Cream containing chlordantoin 1% and benzalkonium chloride 0.05% in 95 g containers.
> ADDITIONAL MIXTURES.
> *Nystaform* (Dome). Each gram of ointment contains nystatin 100,000 units and clioquinol 1% in ½ oz containers.
> *Propion Gel* (Wyeth). Gel containing calcium propionate 10% and sodium propionate 10% in 95 g containers.
> *Verdefam* (Texas Pharmacal). Cream containing sodium propionate 1%, sodium caprylate 1%, propionic acid 3%, and copper undecylenate 0.5% in 1 oz containers; solution containing sodium propionate 2%, sodium caprylate 2%, propionic acid 3%, undecylenic acid 5%, salicylic acid 5%, and copper undecylenate 0.5% in 2 oz containers.

MIXTURES OF ANTIFUNGAL DRUGS WITH OTHER AGENTS

Several topical antifungal agents are incorporated into mixtures with antibiotics, corticosteroids, local anti-infectives, coal tar derivatives, local anesthetics, or other antifungal agents. Some dermatophytoses represent mixed infections of dermatophytes, *Candida* species, and/or bacteria and may not respond unless treated with an agent specific for each organism. Corticosteroids have been included to combat inflammation. In such instances, use of a single topical preparation combining appropriate amounts of the indicated drugs may be rational and more convenient than use of the agents separately. However, such preparations should be used selectively and not routinely. If irritation or sensitization occurs, the responsible ingredient must be found by a process of trial and error after application of the mixture is stopped. The rationale for inclusion of local anesthetics and coal tar derivatives in antifungal preparations is highly questionable. These agents lack anti-infective action and, like other topically applied drugs, may cause sensitization. Also, pruritus due to infection is rapidly controlled as inflammation, edema, and swelling subside.

Oral mixtures of a broad spectrum antibacterial agent (tetracycline or oxytetracycline) and an antifungal drug (amphotericin B or nystatin) have been promoted to prevent the overgrowth of intestinal fungi during antibacterial therapy. The rationale for use of such combinations is difficult to justify. Intestinal candidosis is an uncommon complication of broad spectrum antibiotic therapy, and there is no clinical evidence that routine administration of an antifungal agent reduces the incidence. The use of an antifungal agent is indicated if symptomatic intestinal candidosis occurs in a patient receiving an antibacterial drug or if asymptomatic colonization of *Candida* occurs in a patient for whom fungal disease represents a special risk (eg, patients with diabetes mellitus, those receiving antineoplastic agents or corticosteroids, debilitated patients, infants or elderly patients). However, in these situations, it is preferable to give the antibacterial and antifungal agents separately, since the amounts of antifungal agents in fixed combinations may be suboptimal. (For a listing of available mixtures containing a tetracycline and an antifungal agent, see Chapter 73, Tetracyclines.)

Caldecort (Pennwalt). Each gram of ointment contains calcium undecylenate 30 mg and cortisol acetate 10 mg in 7 and 28 g containers.

Racet (Lemmon). Cream containing clioquinol 3% and cortisol 0.5% in 15, 30, and 454 g containers.

Racet LCD (Lemmon). Cream containing clioquinol 3%, cortisol 0.5%, and coal tar solution 5% in 30 and 454 g containers.

Vioform-Hydrocortisone (Ciba). Cream, ointment, or lotion containing clioquinol 3% and cortisol 1% in 5 and 20 g (cream), 20 g (ointment), or 15 ml (lotion) containers; cream or ointment (mild) containing clioquinol 3% and cortisol 0.5% in ½ and 1 oz (cream) or 1 oz (ointment) containers.

Selected References

Barrett WE, Hanigan JJ: Bioavailability of griseofulvin PEG ultramicrosize (Gris-PEG) tablets in man under steady-state conditions. *Curr Ther Res* 18:491-500, 1975.

Bennett JE: Systemic mycoses and antifungal therapy, in Cluff LE, Johnson JE (eds): *Clinical Concepts of Infectious Disease*, ed 2. Baltimore, Williams & Wilkins Company, 1978, 412-419.

Cartwright RY: Antifungal agents, in Clarke FH (ed): *Annual Reports in Medicinal Chemistry*. New York, Academic Press, 1978, vol 13, 113-119.

Goldstein E, Hoeprich PD: Candidosis, in Hoeprich PD (ed): *Infectious Diseases*, ed 2. Hagerstown, Md, Harper and Row, Publishers, 1977, 372-382.

Hoeprich PD: Chemotherapy of systemic fungal diseases. *Annu Rev Pharmacol Toxicol* 18:205-231, 1978.

Holt RJ: New antifungal drugs. *Drugs* 9:401-405, 1975.

Ipp MM, et al: Clotrimazole: Intermittent therapy in chronic mucocutaneous candidiasis. *Am J Dis Child* 131:305-307, 1977.

Sawyer PR, et al: Clotrimazole: Review of its antifungal activity and therapeutic efficacy. *Drugs* 9:424-447, 1975.

Sawyer PR, et al: Miconazole: Review of its antifungal activity and therapeutic efficacy. *Drugs* 9:406-423, 1975.

Stretcher GS, Smith JG Jr: Diagnosis and treatment of cutaneous fungus diseases. *DM* 2-40, (Sept) 1975.

Wallace SM, et al: Topically applied antifungal agents: Percutaneous penetration and prophylactic activity against *Trichophyton mentagrophytes* infection. *Arch Dermatol* 113:1539-1542, 1977.

During the past 20 years, hundreds of chemicals have been reported to possess antiviral activity in various laboratory models. Yet, the development of clinically useful antiviral drugs has lagged far behind that of antibacterial agents. This difference may be explained in part by the realization that what was often thought to be an antiviral effect was instead an action on host cells, often toxic in nature, that made the host less susceptible to viral attack. It was of little practical importance that this "pseudo" antiviral action frequently occurred at drug concentrations well below those causing an easily detectable, overt effect on the host since even extensive clinical trial of many of these agents did not yield useful antiviral drugs.

Another deterrent to the development of antiviral drugs is the concept that the growth and multiplication of viruses is so intimately interwoven with the metabolism of the host cell that specificity of antiviral action is impossible. Although it is true that host and virus use similar substrate and enzyme systems, some viruses contain enzymes distinct from those of the host cell and others carry information in their genetic code for synthesizing virus-specific enzymes. One approach to specificity of action, therefore, might be the selective inhibition of enzyme systems unique to virus-infected cells that are absent in the normal host cell (eg, virus-induced nucleic acid polymerases). An example of a compound undergoing laboratory and clinical investigation that may be highly specific in inhibiting the enzymes of herpes viruses is acyclovir (9-[2-hydroxyethoxymethyl]-guanine). Even when specificity of action is not possible because a drug may inhibit nucleic acid synthesis in both the virus and host cell, antiviral action may occur at concentrations below those that markedly affect the host. Vidarabine [Vira-A] exerts its effect in this manner.

CLASSIFICATION AND BIOLOGY OF VIRUSES

Viruses are rudimentary organisms capable of parasitizing the cells of man, animals, plants, and bacteria. Their genetic material consists of either ribonucleic acid (RNA) or desoxyribonucleic acid (DNA), but never both. Viruses may be further subdivided by other characteristics such as gross morphology, serology, whether the virus shell has an envelope, and whether viral multiplication occurs in the nucleus or cytoplasm of the infected cell (Pratt, 1977; Bauer, 1977). Most viruses survive outside the host cell for only a short period of time and depend upon the metabolic process of the host for replication.

At the onset of infection, viruses usually are adsorbed onto the surface of a host cell by an electrostatic interaction. In a few instances (eg, influenza virus, polio virus), the cell membrane contains receptor sites specific for the virus. In man, infection begins with entry of the viral cell (virion) into the host cell. Although diverse and often elaborate mechanisms exist by which viruses gain access to the interior of the cell, entry into human or animal tissue is accomplished either by fusion of the outer viral coat with the cellular plasma membrane or ingestion by a phagocytic vacuole (pinocytosis). When fusion takes place, the entire nucleocapsid may pass into the cell before uncoating occurs. If the virion is engulfed by pinocytosis, its outer membrane is stripped away by cellular enzymes. In either case, the genetic material is exposed.

Following uncoating, the genome is replicated in sufficient quantity to form a new generation of virions, and viral protein is synthesized on host cell ribosomes. The processes involved are complex and often utilize not only cellular enzyme systems but also viral enzymes produced for specialized functions.

Once the viral components have been manufactured, they are assembled and released as mature virions to begin the cycle again. Release may occur quickly by lysis and death of the host cell or over a period of time by a process known as budding, in which the cellular membrane remains intact and the cell may be preserved.

It is apparent from the above discussion that virus multiplication is heavily dependent on host cell mechanisms. An effective antiviral agent must, therefore, (1) act intracellularly, and (2) inhibit virus mechanisms to a greater extent than similar mechanisms in normal cells.

NONDRUG TREATMENT OF VIRAL INFECTIONS

When treating viral diseases, it is important to remember that chemotherapeutic approaches are still limited and other measures may be more effective. Controlling insect populations responsible for spreading certain diseases (eg, yellow fever) may be of value in some parts of the world. Prophylactic immunization enlisting the normal defense mechanisms of the body is the most effective known means of controlling many viral diseases (eg, measles, smallpox, mumps, polio). The passive assistance mechanisms afforded by the use of immune globulin, equine antisera, or antiserum from vaccinated humans are useful adjuncts to immunization.

Interferon is another host-resistant mechanism that may have significant value in the treatment of viral diseases. Interferon is a general term applied to a group of carbohydrate-containing proteins produced by nearly all diploid mammalian cells infected with viruses. Human interferon has a molecular weight of about 21,000. Once released, these proteins inhibit viral multiplication in other cells. The exact mechanism is unknown, but it is well established that interferon does not interact directly with viruses or affect their adsorption onto or penetration into the host cell. Nevertheless, it blocks virion replication at a stage prior to assembly.

There are two approaches to the use of interferon as an antiviral agent: the administration of purified interferon or the use of agents that induce interferon production endogenously. Until recently, the latter appeared to hold the greatest promise, since only limited quantities of human interferon had been extracted for pilot studies and species specificity is of great importance in the effectiveness of this compound. Obtaining material from human leukocytes is a time-consuming and somewhat expensive procedure. Current studies involving the culturing of human-foreskin fibroblasts on microscopic dextran beads (Leff, 1978) may lead to a practical and less expensive method of harvesting human interferon in quantities sufficient for practical use. At this time, interferon is not of practical importance as an antiviral drug. Its potential usefulness is great, however, because it has a wide spectrum of effect against viral infections (eg, zoster) and cancerous tumors with suspected viral etiology (eg, osteosarcoma).

Agents that induce interferon production include certain microorganisms (eg, viruses themselves, *Chlamydia, Rickettsia, Mycoplasma, Escherichia coli, Haemophilus influenzae, Trypanosoma cruzi*), microbial extracts, certain dyes (eg methylene blue, acridine orange), some synthetic polymers (eg, polyvinylsulfate), and a series of substituted polycyclic aromatic compounds. The most potent of the synthetic inducers is a compound with the designation rI:rC, a double-stranded homopolymer of inosine and cytosine. Unfortunately, one of the greatest deterrents to developing a practical interferon inducer is that the most promising agents often have considerable toxicity.

DRUG THERAPY FOR VIRAL INFECTIONS

Mechanisms of Action

Many antiviral drugs have a mechanism of action similar to that of the compounds used in the chemotherapy of cancer. Both groups of drugs compete with the cell for the building blocks of nucleic acids (thymine, cytosine, guanine, adenine). As a result, the synthesis of DNA and RNA may be inhibited. Most clinically useful antiviral drugs that act in this manner inhibit DNA production or cause the formation of abnormal DNA and, therefore, have variable effectiveness against DNA viruses. Vidarabine [Vira-A], idoxuridine [Dendrid, Herplex, Stoxil], and trifluridine [Viroptic] are examples of such drugs. In contrast, methisazone is thought to cause the formation of abnormal messenger RNA by altering the function of RNA polymerases.

Viral multiplication also can be slowed by preventing virion penetration into the cell and subsequent uncoating. Amantadine has this effect on influenza viruses. This action can be explained by the fact that amantadine is a primary amine; ammonium ions have a similar, though weaker, action. However, uncoating may not be the only action of amantadine; there is some evidence that it may inhibit RNA synthesis as well.

Classification

Pyrimidine and Purine Derivatives and Related Drugs: Idoxuridine [Dendrid, Herplex, Stoxil] was one of the first compounds to be recognized as having clinically useful antiviral activity. Although originally introduced into medicine as an antitumor compound, this drug has been administered since the mid 1960's to treat herpes virus infections. Idoxuridine is used in this country primarily to treat herpes simplex keratitis (see Chapter 24, Ocular Anti-infective and Anti-inflammatory Agents) but is available in England and some other countries as a topical preparation containing idoxuridine and dimethylsulfoxide (DMSO) to treat cutaneous herpes simplex and herpes zoster virus lesions. It also has been given parenterally in an effort to treat herpes encephalitis and cytomegalic inclusion disease, but parenteral forms of the drug are not available commercially and there is no proof that it is effective in these infections.

Other related compounds being investigated for antiherpetic activity include acyclovir [Zovirax], ribavirin, and trifluridine [Viroptic]. Acyclovir is a new nucleoside analogue under experimental and clinical investigation (Schaeffer et al, 1978). In vitro, it inhibits multiplication of varicella-zoster virus, cytomegalovirus, and B virus but has no effect on vaccinia virus, adenovirus type 5, and a range of RNA viruses including those that cause yellow fever, measles, and some forms of influenza. In vitro activity is said to be 160 times greater than vidarabine and 10 times greater than idoxuridine.

Good results have been obtained when acyclovir was used in vivo against type 1 herpes virus injected intracerebrally in mice, worked into the cornea of the rabbit eye with a microtrephine, or inoculated into the skin of guinea pigs. Acyclovir also has been effective in uncomplicated dendritic corneal epithelial ulcers in man (Jones et al, 1979).

In mice, approximately 95% of a single dose of acyclovir is excreted as unmetabolized drug and it has an oral LD_{50} of over 10 g/kg. Thus, because of an apparently high antiviral activity when compared to other antiherpetic compounds, good activity in animal models, demonstrated activity in man, relatively low toxicity, and lack of metabolic breakdown, acyclovir appears to be potentially useful against the various manifestations of herpes virus infections.

Ribavirin appears to have a fairly broad spectrum of action: It inhibits herpetic keratitis in rabbits and herpes, vaccinia, or vesicular stomatitis virus infections in mice. The splenomegaly and hepatomegaly induced by Friend leukemia virus, as well as infections caused by influenza A and B viruses and parainfluenza 1 virus in various animal species also are alleviated. Recent studies indicate that ribavirin also is efficacious in man; however, it probably is not effective clinically against influenza A and has only marginal effects against influenza B. Ribavirin is commercially available under the trade name Virazol in several Latin American countries but is not marketed in the United States.

Trifluridine has been used to treat ocular herpetic infections; it appears to be more effective than idoxuridine and is active against strains of herpes virus resistant to the latter drug. Trifluridine is still being used experimentally and is not commercially available.

Several compounds related to vidarabine, including metabolic breakdown products and synthetic analogues, are being investigated both experimentally and clinically for antiviral activity. An example of one such drug is a 5'-monophosphate compound referred to as ara-AMP. A consideration of these compounds and the research involving them is beyond the scope of this chapter. The interested reader is referred to the proceedings of the First, Second, and Third Conferences on Antiviral Substances published by the New York Academy of Sciences, 1965, 1970, and 1977.

Amantadine and Derivatives: Amantadine [Symmetrel] is an antiviral drug with a narrow spectrum of action. It is used prophylactically against influenza A and also can reduce the severity and duration of fever and intensity of other symptoms of influenza caused by A strains. Amantadine is most widely used, however, in treating parkinsonism (see Chapter 16, Drugs Used in Extrapyramidal Movement Disorders).

Early reports on rimantadine, an amantadine analogue marketed in the USSR, indicated that this compound was more active than amantadine against influenza viruses both in vitro and in vivo, but subsequent investigations have refuted this claim. Cyclooctylamine, another related compound investigated for use in influenza, is clearly less active than either amantadine or rimantadine. Although active research is being conducted on these and other related agents, none have demonstrated a greater activity against influenza viral infections than amantadine.

Thiosemicarbazones: Several isatin 3-thiosemicarbazones have undergone extensive laboratory and clinical testing as antiviral agents. One of these, methisazone

[Marboran], is effective in preventing smallpox. It is not marketed in the United States. This drug has been used to treat smallpox, eczema vaccinatum, vaccinia gangrenosa, and generalized vaccinia. With the virtual eradication of smallpox, however, methisazone is of little clinical importance today.

Agents with Immunopotentiating Action: Still another approach to the therapy of viral infections is the use of chemicals that may enhance the normal immune response. Two potentially useful compounds being investigated for such activity are levamisole (see also Chapter 66, Immunomodulators) and inosiplex [Isoprinosine].

Levamisole was developed initially as an anthelmintic but was found to have immunopotentiating activity in mice infected with *Brucella* or immunized with sheep erythrocytes. It reverses certain depressed cellular immune responses in cancer-bearing animals and man and induces remission or delays the occurrence of cancer to a limited degree. Clinically, levamisole has an ameliorating action against infections caused by intracellular bacteria (eg, *Brucella, Listeria, Pseudomonas*) and may modify the course of herpes virus infection in animals and possibly in man. Yet, this drug has no direct antiviral action and does not induce interferon production.

Inosiplex has been tried clinically in the treatment of herpes and rhinovirus infections and infections caused by influenza virus. Prophylactic use of the drug has been disappointing. Neither levamisole nor inosiplex is marketed in the United States.

Antimetabolite: For 20 years, it has been known that the glucose derivative, 2-deoxy-D-glucose, will inhibit the multiplication of certain viruses (Kilbourne, 1959), but clinical use of this compound has not been extensively investigated. It appears to be a relatively nontoxic agent that is easily administered and readily penetrates into most tissues. Recently, it has been used successfully in the treatment of human genital herpes infections (Blough and Giuntoli, 1979).

Resistance

Viruses can become resistant to antiviral medication (Herrmann and Herrmann, 1977). For example, herpes virus grown on tissue culture and exposed to increasing concentrations of idoxuridine eventually develops resistant strains, and the resistance persists through subsequent passages. Clinically, some cases of herpetic keratitis may become refractory to idoxuridine because of the development of resistant viral strains, but the resistant organism often responds to vidarabine.

Resistance is not yet an important medical problem since most major viral infections are not treated with antiviral agents or the courses of chemotherapy are short. As the development and use of antiviral drugs become more prevalent, the number and incidence of resistant strains undoubtedly will increase.

Adverse Reactions

The toxic manifestations of antiviral drugs vary widely and are highly dependent upon the manner in which the compound interacts with the metabolism of the host cell. Most antiviral agents used in medicine today and those compounds undergoing serious clinical trial generally have minimal toxicity against host cells and usually are well tolerated. The more common adverse reactions are mild and include stomatitis, anorexia, nausea (although sometimes nausea is severe enough to warrant discontinuation of the drug), vomiting, and weight loss. More severe effects (eg, alopecia, tissue necrosis, blood dyscrasias, bone marrow depression, kidney and liver impairment, convulsions) are seen only occasionally. Chromosomal breakage is observed rarely, as are neurologic disorders manifested as insomnia, dizziness, and depression. For reactions attributable to a specific drug, see the evaluations.

INDIVIDUAL EVALUATIONS

AMANTADINE HYDROCHLORIDE
[Symmetrel]

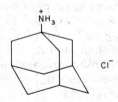

Amantadine, a water-soluble primary amine, inhibits the replication of certain orthomyxoviruses by impeding penetration of the viruses into the host cells and subsequent uncoating. Most important among the organisms affected are influenza A viruses. This drug is inactive against influenza B viruses. Prophylactically, amantadine protects 50% to 70% of recipients exposed to influenza A viruses and is indicated for patients over 1 year of age during influenza A outbreaks, especially individuals for whom influenza would entail a grave risk, such as the elderly. It may be most effective in individuals who already have antibodies against influenza A virus strains; therefore, previous vaccination does not interfere with and may augment its effect. Amantadine also may have therapeutic value if given promptly after the first symptoms of infection appear.

Amantadine also has been used to treat parkinsonism. Its mechanism of action in this disorder apparently involves the release of dopamine and other catecholamines from neuronal storage sites or the delay in reuptake of these neurotransmitters into synaptic vesicles (see Chapter 16, Drugs Used in Extrapyramidal Movement Disorders).

Amantadine is well tolerated. Adverse effects usually occur only at the higher dosage levels (400 mg daily or more) used to treat parkinsonism. These doses are approximately double those used in influenza. The most common reactions are irritability, nervousness, inability to concentrate, tremor, slurred speech, ataxia, mental depression, insomnia, blurred vision, lethargy, and dizziness. Occasional untoward effects include anorexia, nausea, vomiting, and orthostatic hypotension. Rarely, leukopenia and neutropenia are observed but other hematologic disorders have not been reported.

Livedo reticularis is commonly associated with the use of amantadine in parkinsonism, particularly in women given the drug for one month or longer. This reaction has not been observed in patients receiving the drug for prophylaxis of influenza. Symptoms may subside during continued administration or persist throughout the period of therapy but disappear gradually over a period of 2 to 12 weeks in all patients after drug therapy is discontinued. Laboratory studies have not revealed an association between livedo reticularis and any underlying systemic disorder.

Edema of the ankles (usually associated with livedo reticularis) has been noted in some patients. The manufacturer reports that congestive heart failure has developed in a few patients receiving amantadine.

The peripheral and central adverse effects of anticholinergic drugs are increased by the concomitant use of amantadine, and acute psychotic reactions, which may be identical to those caused by atropine poisoning, may occur when large doses of anticholinergic agents are used. Psychotic reactions also have developed occasionally in patients receiving amantadine and levodopa. If signs of central toxicity develop, the dose of the anticholinergic drug or levodopa should be reduced while the patient is receiving amantadine.

Caution must be exercised when this drug is administered to patients with impaired renal function, liver disease, epilepsy, and psychosis or severe psychoneurosis not controlled by chemotherapeutic agents. Patients who become dizzy after taking amantadine should avoid activities requiring mental alertness (eg, driving). Those with cerebral arteriosclerosis should be given amantadine only under close medical supervision.

Since amantadine has not been investigated extensively in pregnant women, young children, and infants, careful monitoring is required in women of childbearing age and children less than 1 year old (if it is used at all in this latter group). Amantadine is excreted in milk and should not be given to nursing mothers.

ROUTE, USUAL DOSAGE, AND PREPARATIONS. *Oral*: For prophylaxis, *adults*, 100 mg twice daily; *children 1 to 9 years*, 4 to 9 mg/kg of body weight daily in two or three equal doses (maximum, 150 mg daily); *9 to 12 years*, 100 mg twice daily. Administration should be started in anticipation of contact or as soon as possible after exposure to influenza A viruses. In a planned program of prophylaxis, amantadine should be given daily for at least 10 days following known exposure, up to 30 days for possible repeated and unknown exposures, and up to 90 days for possible uncontrolled, repeated, and unknown exposures.

For treatment of established influenza A, the same doses used for prophylaxis should be administered as soon as possible after the onset of illness; therapy should be continued for ten days.

    Symmetrel (Endo). Capsules 100 mg; syrup 50 mg/5 ml.

IDOXURIDINE
[Dendrid, Herplex, Stoxil]

Idoxuridine, a halogenated synthetic nucleoside containing the natural sugar, deoxyribose, is a derivative of deoxyuridine and an analogue of thymidine. It is incorporated as a constituent of both cellular and viral DNA and irreversibly inhibits the incorporation of up to 90% of the thymidine normally found in viral DNA.

Idoxuridine is used in the United States only topically to treat herpes simplex infections of the cornea, conjunctiva, and eyelids. It improves the course of acute dendritic keratitis and also has been used to treat ocular vaccinia infections (see Chapter 24, Ocular Anti-infective and Anti-inflammatory Agents). Topical preparations for application on the skin and mucous membranes (combined with dimethylsulfoxide [DMSO] as a carrier) are used in England and other countries and their efficacy in treating varicella zoster and herpes simplex infections of the skin and mucous membranes appears to be good. In one study (Kaufman, 1977), idoxuridine was reported to be effective in the treatment of recurrent genital herpes when applied topically in a solution of DMSO, but subsequent controlled trials have cast doubt on this finding. Favorable subjective effects, sometimes including dramatic relief from pain as well as accelerated healing, have been reported.

Idoxuridine may cause slight local irritation, photophobia, mild edema of the eyelids and cornea, and small punctate defects in the corneal epithelium when used topically in the eye. This agent may interfere with corneal epithelial regeneration and inhibit stromal healing. If blood levels high enough to produce systemic toxicity are attained, idoxuridine can cause stomatitis, anorexia, nausea, vomiting, and, occasionally, mild signs of iodism. Alopecia, leukopenia, and thrombocytopenia also have been reported after systemic administration. Idoxuridine is hepatotoxic and can cause cholestatic jaundice.

For ophthalmic dosage and preparations, see Chapter 24.

VIDARABINE
[Vira-A]

Vidarabine (adenine arabinoside) is a purine nucleoside that inhibits a variety of DNA viruses in vitro at concentrations below those toxic to the host cell. Its primary mechanism of action has not been clearly established but it appears to inhibit DNA polymerase. The in vitro antiviral spectrum includes the herpesviruses (herpes simplex types 1 and 2, pseudorabies, *Herpesvirus saimiri*, varicella-zoster), some pox viruses (myxoma and, possibly, vaccinia), and the Rouse sarcoma leukovirus. It is not effective against RNA viruses, bacteria, or fungi.

Vidarabine is used topically to treat ocular herpes simplex (see Chapter 24, Ocular Anti-infective and Anti-inflammatory Agents). It also has been shown (Whitley et al, 1976) to have some efficacy against herpes zoster in immunosuppressed patients and has been used topically to treat herpetic infections of the skin and mucous membranes, although some workers (eg, Adams et al, 1976; Goodman et al, 1975) have observed no effect on either primary or recurrent genital infection with *Herpesvirus*. In general, usage other than in the eyes has met with variable success and is still being evaluated.

Vidarabine has been given parenterally for herpes encephalitis. In one study, mortality was reduced from 70% to 28%, and debilitating neurologic sequelae were prevented (Whitley et al, 1977) when intravenous infusion was started early in the course of disease. Vidarabine apparently does not alter morbidity or the occurrence of serious neurologic damage if the patient is already comatose, which emphasizes the need for early diagnosis and treatment. After severe neurologic impairment has occurred, use of vidarabine may prevent death but cannot reverse the damage, although many such patients show significant recovery over a long period of convalescence. Herpes simplex virus encephalitis should be suspected whenever there is a history of febrile encephalopathy, disordered mental state, altered level of consciousness, and focal cerebral signs. Examination of the cerebrospinal fluid and a brain scan using electroencephalography or computerized axial tomography may support the suspected diagnosis, but brain biopsy and viral isolation in cell cultures or the use of specific fluorescent antibody techniques are required to confirm the disease.

Following intravenous administration, vidarabine is rapidly metabolized by deamination to the less active ara-hypoxanthine (Ara-Hx); 41% to 53% of the daily dose is recovered in the urine as Ara-Hx within 24 hours and only 1% to 3% is excreted unchanged. Because of its poor solubility and absorption, the drug cannot be given subcutaneously or intramuscularly and probably is not suitable for oral administration.

Adverse effects observed when vidarabine is used in the eye are similar to those for idoxuridine but the incidence is lower; reported effects include lacrimation; burning sensation, irritation, and a sensation of foreign body in the eye; conjunctival and corneal edema; and photophobia. Vidarabine and idoxuridine have similar efficacy and toxicity when used topically in previously untreated patients. There appears to be little cross resistance between the two drugs and patients allergic or resistant to idoxuridine may respond to vidarabine.

When therapeutic doses are given by intravenous infusion, the most commonly reported adverse reactions are anorexia and nausea. Larger doses cause more severe nausea, vomiting, and diarrhea, but these reactions seldom require cessation of therapy. Central nervous system disturbances have been noted occasionally at therapeutic levels and include dizziness, tremor, confusion, ataxia, psychosis, and hallucinations. The first indication of hepatotoxicity may be elevated SGOT or total bilirubin levels. Hematologic changes, which are manifested as decreased hemoglobin or hematocrit levels, thrombocytopenia, reticulocytopenia, and leukopenia, are uncommon; nevertheless, appropriate hematologic monitoring may be indicated (complete blood count and platelet count twice weekly during therapy). Other reactions include weight loss, malaise, pruritus, rash, hematemesis, and pain at the site of injection.

Vidarabine should be administered with special care to patients at risk from fluid overload (eg, those with impaired renal function) or cerebral edema (eg, those with central nervous system infections). Patients with impaired renal or hepatic function must be observed closely, since toxic effects may occur at lower dosage levels; adjustments in dosage may be necessary.

The safe use of vidarabine during pregnancy has not been established. The drug has been shown to have some tumorigenic activity in mice and rats, teratogenic effects in rats and rabbits, and, possibly, mutagenic effects in mice. Therefore, until more clinical data are available, it is advisable to restrict the systemic use of vidarabine in pregnant patients to life-threatening illnesses in which the possible benefits outweigh the potential risks.

ROUTES, USUAL DOSAGE, AND PREPARATIONS. *Intravenous*: *Adults and children*, 15 mg/kg of body weight daily for ten days. The drug must be diluted and given by slow continuous infusion over a period of 12 to 24 hours. Rapid or bolus injection must be avoided.

> *Vira-A* (Parke, Davis). Suspension (sterile) 200 mg (equivalent to 187.4 mg of base)/ml in 5 ml containers.

Topical: See Chapter 24, Ocular Anti-infective and Anti-inflammatory Agents.

Selected References

Amantadine for high-risk influenza. *Med Lett Drugs Ther* 20:25-26, 1978.

Adams HG, et al: Genital herpetic infection in men and women: Clinical course and effect of topical application of adenine arabinoside. *J Infect Dis* 133(suppl):151-159, (June) 1976.

Bauer DJ: *The Specific Treatment of Virus Diseases*. Baltimore, University Park Press, 1977.

Blough HA, Giuntoli RL: Successful treatment of human genital herpes infections with 2-deoxy-D-glucose. *JAMA* 241:2798-2801, 1979.

Goodman EL, et al: Prospective double-blind evaluation of topical adenine arabinoside in male herpes progenitalis. *Antimicrob Agents and Chemother* 8:693-697, 1975.

Herrmann EC Jr (ed): Proceedings of the Third Conference on Antiviral Substances. *Ann NY Acad Sci* 284:1-720, 1977.

Herrmann EC Jr, Herrmann JA: Working hypothesis: Virus resistance as indicator of specific antiviral activity. *Ann NY Acad Sci* 284:632-637, 1977.

Herrman EC Jr, Stinebring WR (eds): Proceedings of Second Conference on Antiviral Substances. *Ann NY Acad Sci* 173:1-844, 1970.

Hoffmann CE: Antiviral agents, in Clarke FH (ed): *Annual Reports in Medicinal Chemistry*. New York, Academic Press, 1978, vol 13, 139-148.

Jones BR, et al: Efficacy of acycloguanosine (Wellcome 248U) against herpes-simplex corneal ulcers. *Lancet* 1:243-244, 1979.

Kaufman HE: Antiviral agents. *Int J Dermatol* 16:464-475, 1977.

Kilbourne ED: Inhibition of influenza virus multiplication with a glucose antimetabolite (2-deoxy-D-glucose). *Nature* 183:271-272, 1959.

Leff DN: Interferon: Breaking the production bottleneck. *Med World News* 19:82-92, (Oct 16) 1978.

Melmon KL, Morrelli HF (eds): *Clinical Pharmacology: Basic Principles in Therapeutics*, ed 2. New York, Macmillan Publishing Co, Inc, 1978, 709-801.

Merigan TC (ed): Antivirals with clinical potential. *J Infect Dis* 133(suppl):1-285, (June) 1976.

Merigan TC, et al: Human leukocyte interferon for treatment of herpes zoster in patients with cancer. *N Engl J Med* 298:981-987, 1978.

Pratt WB: *Chemotherapy of Infection*. New York, Oxford University Press, 1977, 409-441.

Schaeffer HJ, et al: 9-(2-hydroxyethoxymethyl) guanine activity against viruses of herpes group. *Nature* 272:583-585, 1978.

Whipple HE (ed): Proceedings of First Conference on Antiviral Substances. *Ann NY Acad Sci* 130:1-482, 1965.

Whitley RJ, Alford CA: Current status of antiviral chemotherapy. *South Med J* 71:1134-1140, 1978.

Whitley RJ, et al (eds) and NIAID Collaborative Antiviral Study Group: Adenine arabinoside therapy of biopsy-proved herpes simplex encephalitis. *N Engl J Med* 297:289-294, 1977.

Whitley RJ, et al (eds) and NIAID Collaborative Antiviral Study Group: Adenine arabinoside therapy of herpes zoster in immunosuppressed. *N Engl J Med* 294:1193-1199, 1976.

Antiprotozoal Agents | 82

Protozoal infections contend with worm infections as the most common disease known to mankind. In past centuries, afflic- tions such as amebic dysentery have been widespread, particularly during times of famine and war. Despite generally better worldwide sanitation today, the incidence of parasitic disease remains high, especially in the developing or crowded nations of Africa, Asia, and South America.

Before global travel became commonplace, many protozoal diseases were considered by physicians in the United States to be medical curiosities unlikely to be encountered in a lifetime of medical practice. The advent of jet flight and the involvement of American military forces in many parts of the world have increased the probability that a physician will be asked to diagnose and treat an uncommon parasitic disease. Some protozoal infections formerly confined to tropical areas now occur so commonly in northern latitudes that they are no longer considered to be purely tropical diseases.

All four classes of protozoa include pathogenic organisms: The *Sarcodina*, represented by *Entamoeba histolytica*, cause amebic disease. The *Mastigophora* (flagellates) produce trichomoniasis, giardiasis, leishmaniases, and trypanosomiases. The *Ciliophora* (ciliates) include at least one organism, *Balantidium coli*, that infects man. The *Sporozoa* cause malaria, toxoplasmosis, pneumocystosis, isosporosis, and sarcosporidiosis, the latter being one of the least studied and understood protozoal infections.

Therapy for protozoal infections presents a number of difficulties not usually encountered in treating other infections or parasitic diseases. Currently, there are no known effective immunization procedures in man. The physician, therefore, must rely on chemotherapeutic techniques that often are less than ideal, are frequently toxic to the host, and are almost always too expensive to be used on a single-patient basis in poor countries with a low standard of living. Programs of mass chemotherapy involving large numbers of people have been undertaken with only limited success. More effective measures include control of the insect vector (when one exists), elimination of the reservoir of infection, and improvement of sanitation and living conditions. Unfortunately, the number of people at risk in some parts of the world is large and is spread over large geographical

areas that may be quite inaccessible. These people often are not educated well enough or motivated sufficiently to comply with instructions given by a physician or health worker whom they may consider to be an outsider threatening well-established life patterns. Moreover, they are frequently infected with several organisms which makes diagnosis, therapy, and follow-up complex. Even when individual cures are effected, the patient returns to an environment where reinfection is almost a certainty.

MALARIA

Worldwide, malaria is the most common cause of morbidity and mortality from infection. Virtually all cases of malaria in the United States result from exposure in malarious regions. Most indigenous cases are acquired congenitally or are induced by accidental intravenous blood inoculation among drug addicts or by transfusion of infected blood. Diminution in spraying programs, emergence of insecticide-resistant strains of mosquitoes, and development of drug-resistant strains of *Plasmodium falciparum* have resulted in resurgence of this disease. Several strains of *P. falciparum*, which causes the lethal form of malaria, have become resistant not only to chloroquine [Aralen] but to other antimalarial drugs; this resistance has been documented in many malarious areas. Cases of chloroquine-resistant malaria developing in the United States have to date all been acquired elsewhere in the world.

Falciparum infection in a nonimmune individual can be treated successfully if appropriate antimalarial therapy is initiated before overwhelming parasitemia develops. Complications include hemolytic anemia, toxic encephalopathy with confusion or coma ("cerebral malaria"), renal failure, or noncardiac pulmonary edema. Prompt ancillary treatment in addition to specific antimalarial therapy may determine survival. Transfusion of packed red cells, exchange transfusions, use of plasma volume expanders, administration of adrenal corticosteroids or low-molecular-weight dextran, promotion of diuresis with mannitol, or dialysis may be necessary.

Parasite Life Cycle and Clinical Course: The four species of *Plasmodium* that cause malaria in man are *P. falciparum*, *P. vivax*, *P. ovale*, and *P. malariae*. The human phase of the life cycle begins when an infected female anopheline mosquito bites the host and injects sporozoites from her salivary glands. The sporozoites enter the circulation and rapidly reach the liver where they invade cells, develop into primary tissue schizonts (the primary exoerythrocytic forms), and mature into tissue merozoites. This asymptomatic (prepatent) period lasts 8 to 21 days, varying with the species of plasmodia. At the end of the prepatent period, the merozoites of all four species enter the blood stream, invade red cells, and begin the erythrocytic cycle of asexual reproductive development. In individuals infected with *P. vivax* or *P. ovale*, parasites persist in hepatic cells and produce secondary exoerythrocytic forms; this does not occur with *P. falciparum*. Most authorities believe that *P. malariae* does not have persisting exoerythrocytic forms and, thus, delayed attacks are due to persistent erythrocytic forms. The erythrocytic cycle ends when the infected red cells rupture, releasing parasites (that reinvade other red cells), fragmented erythrocytes, pigments, and other products. The clinical attack of malaria (ie, chills, fever, profound sweating) occurs at this time. After several cycles, some erythrocytic parasites develop into gametocytes, the sexual forms of the organism. If the infected person is then bitten by a female anopheline mosquito and gametocytes enter the mosquito, the cycle from human host to vector is completed and the disease is perpetuated with the sexual stage of parasite reproduction occurring in the mosquito.

Diagnosis: Diagnosis of malaria is made on the basis of clinical history and the presence of parasites on peripheral blood films. The classical cycles of malarial paroxysms take place when the maturation phase of erythrocytic parasites becomes synchronized, although this may not be observed until after several attacks have occurred. In falciparum malaria, cyclic fever may not occur at all. Hence, although the fever is useful for diagnosis, this characteristic is not invariably observed during the early stages of the malarial infection.

If a patient has been in a malarious area recently (even if only at an airport) and complains of having symptoms of "the flu," a diagnosis of malaria is suggested and examination of thick and thin peripheral blood films is indicated. In addition, individuals who intend to travel to malarious areas should receive appropriate prophylactic drugs during and after the trip.

Therapy: Antimalarial agents are classified principally on the basis of their action against the plasmodial organism at different stages in its life cycle. Drugs used to cure the clinical attack of malaria (ie, drugs that attack the asexual forms of the parasite) are known as schizonticidal agents. These include quinine, chloroquine [Aralen], amodiaquine [Camoquin], hydroxychloroquine [Plaquenil], pyrimethamine [Daraprim], tetracycline, and the combination of a long-acting sulfonamide with a folic acid antagonist such as pyrimethamine. These agents achieve clinical cure by eliminating asexual parasitemia.

Radical cure refers to complete elimination of all asexual blood forms and all residual exoerythrocytic forms from the body. Patients who have achieved radical cure may safely give blood for transfusion. It is difficult at times to be sure a patient has achieved a radical cure. In falciparum and perhaps malariae malaria, no secondary exoerythrocytic forms are produced, and elimination of blood forms achieves both clinical and radical cure. Radical cure of the other forms of malaria requires additional therapy to eliminate residual exoerythrocytic forms; the drug of choice is primaquine. Untreated or inadequately treated patients who survive initial attacks become partially immune. Such individuals may have recrudescences or relapses and can transmit malaria by blood transfusion. The natural duration of infection with *P. vivax*, *P. ovale*, and *P. falciparum* is limited to one to four years, and after the expiration of such intervals, patients then will be essentially cured. Untreated infections with *P. malariae* are known to last for many years, although cure is just as readily achieved as with the other species.

The specific antimalarial drugs chosen for treatment of a clinical attack of malaria depend upon the area visited (ie, malarious areas with or without known chloroquine-resistant falciparum malaria), the probability of exposure to infection, whether the patient is pregnant, and whether drug allergy or intolerance exists. (The Center for Disease Control of the U.S. Public Health Service, Atlanta, Ga 30333, publishes a Malaria Surveillance Report annually; this includes a detailed list of areas where there is a risk of infection with malaria. [Day phone (404) 329-3670; other times (404) 329-3644]

Clinical cure of an acute attack of malaria caused by *P. vivax*, *P. ovale*, *P. malariae*, or chloroquine-sensitive strains of *P. falciparum* is readily accomplished with a three-day course of chloroquine phosphate or amodiaquine hydrochloride. If the oral phosphate salt is not tolerated or the attack is severe, chloroquine hydrochloride may be administered intramuscularly or, rarely, intravenously until an oral preparation can be used. Alternatively, quinine dihydrochloride can be given by slow intravenous infusion. No additional treatment is usually required in patients infected with chloroquine-sensitive *P. falciparum*, but to prevent relapses and to achieve radical cure in *P. vivax* and *P. ovale* infections, a two-week course of primaquine also is given (see that evaluation).

Treatment of chloroquine-resistant falciparum malaria should be initiated with quinine orally, if possible, or by slow intravenous infusion in severe cases. A sulfonamide (eg, sulfadoxine, sulfadiazine) and pyrimethamine should be given either simultaneously or within three days. Alternatively, tetracycline may be substituted for the sulfonamide-pyrimethamine combination. These regimens are also effective in the treatment of chloroquine-sensitive strains.

Occasionally, mixed infections occur, but the only ones of therapeutic significance are those of *P. falciparum* with one of the other three species. Treatment of the clinical attack with chloroquine or a similar agent eliminates parasitemia caused by all sensitive species, but relapses caused by species other than *P. falciparum* and *P. malariae* will occur unless a course of primaquine is given. Hence, if a mixed infection is suspected, after treatment of the clinical attack, the patient should be available for long-term observation or given a course of primaquine.

Prevention of malaria while traveling in malarious areas is termed prophylaxis. Causal prophylaxis implies elimination of the exoerythrocytic forms of the parasite before they can invade the red cells. Primaquine has true causal prophylactic activity against all four species of malaria but, because of its potential toxicity, controversy exists concerning this use of the drug.

Suppressive agents inhibit the erythrocytic stage of parasite development and thus prevent clinical attacks. Use of suppressive agents for prophylaxis is known as clinical or field prophylaxis. The drugs of choice for this type of prophylaxis for persons entering endemic areas are the 4-aminoquinolines, chloroquine phosphate, amodiaquine hydrochloride, or hydroxychloroquine. They are administered weekly two weeks before, during, and six to eight weeks after visiting a malarious area.

Travelers who use this form of prophylaxis during their stay in malarious areas may take primaquine on return to prevent subsequent development of malaria. Because of its potential for hemolysis, some experts advise using primaquine in this manner only for patients who have had heavy exposures for extended periods of time. This agent is administered daily for two weeks immediately after the individual has left the malarious area. There is evidence that amodiaquine may be somewhat more effective than chloroquine against some strains of chloroquine-resistant falciparum malaria and the same dosage schedule is used. In areas of known chloroquine resistance, neither drug may provide complete protection. A combination tablet of pyrimethamine 25 mg and sulfadoxine 500 mg [Falcidar, Fansidar, Methipox], which is available almost everywhere but in the United States, is preferred in these areas. Travelers should be informed that any regimen of prophylaxis may not be absolutely complete and instructed to consult a physician if any symptoms appear, even though suppressive drugs were taken.

Pyrimethamine also exerts prophylactic effects, especially against falciparum malaria and, to a lesser degree, against vivax malaria. Resistant strains are known to be present in all areas where pyrimethamine has been widely used.

The dosages employed in the prophylaxis and treatment of malaria are summarized in Table 1. The drugs evaluated include only those that are readily available and have been studied in the treatment of malaria. Notable omissions include the following:

Quinacrine (mepacrine) [Atabrine], although historically important, is obsolete and has been superseded by the 4-aminoquinolines. This agent is not effective against chloroquine-resistant malaria and was used in the past only as a reserve agent when no other drugs were available.

Dapsone, 4-4 diaminodiphenyl sulfone, was useful for the treatment and prophylaxis of chloroquine-resistant falciparum malaria; however, it induced hemolytic anemia and methemoglobi-

TABLE 1.
AGENTS USED IN PROPHYLAXIS AND TREATMENT OF MALARIA
DOSAGE (BASE)[1]

| DRUG | Prophylaxis[2] | | Treatment | |
	Adults	Children	Adults	Children
Chloroquine Phosphate	300 mg weekly	<1 yr, 37.5 mg 1-3 yrs, 75 mg 4-6 yrs, 100 mg 7-10 yrs, 150 mg 11-16 yrs, 225 mg	600 mg initially, then 300 mg at 6, 24, and 48 hrs	10 mg/kg initially, then 5 mg/kg at 6, 24, and 48 hrs
Chloroquine Hydrochloride	—	—	3 mg/kg initially, given intramuscularly or intravenously,[2] then 3 mg/kg every 6 hrs (maximum, 900 mg/24 hrs)	2-3 mg/kg initially, given intramuscularly or intravenously,[2] repeated if necessary in 6 hrs (maximum, 5 mg/kg/24 hrs). Avoid intravenous use in children under 7.
Hydroxychloroquine Sulfate	310 mg weekly	<1 yr, 37.5 mg 1-3 yrs, 75 mg 4-6 yrs, 100 mg 7-10 yrs, 150 mg 11-16 yrs, 225 mg	620 mg initially, then 310 mg at 6, 24, and 48 hrs	10 mg/kg initially, then 5 mg/kg at 6, 24, and 48 hrs
Amodiaquine Hydrochloride	400 mg weekly	<1 yr, 50 mg 2-4 yrs, 50-100 mg 5-8 yrs, 150-200 mg 9-12 yrs, 300 mg	600 mg initially, then 400 mg at 6, 24, and 48 hrs	10 mg/kg initially, then 5 mg/kg at 6, 24, and 48 hrs
Primaquine Phosphate	15 mg daily for 14 days after leaving endemic area *or* 45 mg weekly for 8 weeks	0.3 mg/kg daily for 14 days after leaving endemic area *or* 0.9 mg/kg weekly for 8 weeks	15 mg daily for 14 days	0.3 mg/kg daily for 14 days

TABLE 1. (continued)

DOSAGE (BASE)[1]

DRUG	Prophylaxis[2]		Treatment	
	Adults	Children	Adults	Children
Pyrimethamine	25 mg weekly	2 yrs and under, 6.25-12.5 mg 3-10 yrs, 12.5-25 mg over 10 yrs, adult dose weekly	—	—
Quinine Sulfate	—	—	650 mg every 8 hrs for 10-14 days	25 mg/kg every 8 hrs for 10-14 days
Quinine Dihydrochloride[4]	—	—	600 mg intravenously[3] and repeated in 6-8 hrs (maximum, 1.8 g daily)	25 mg/kg intravenously,[3] one-half in 1 hr infusion, the other half 6-8 hrs later (see the evaluation)
Chloroquine and Primaquine Phosphates	300 mg of chloroquine and 45 mg of primaquine weekly	5-7 kg, 2.5 ml 8-11 kg, 5 ml 12-15 kg, 7.5 ml 16-20 kg, 10 ml 21-24 kg, 12.5 ml 25-45 kg, ½ tablet weekly (see also evaluation)	—	—
Pyrimethamine-Sulfadoxine (not available in U.S.A.)	50 mg pyrimethamine and 1 g sulfadoxine every other week for 6 weeks	in terms of sulfadoxine: 6-11 mos, 125 mg 1-3 yrs, 250 mg 4-8 yrs, 500 mg 9-14 yrs, 750 mg	—	—

[1]*All doses oral unless specified otherwise. Slight variations in dosage may exist between table and text.*
[2]*See text regarding initiation of prophylaxis prior to entering malarious area, continuation during stay, and for six to eight weeks following return from such an area.*
[3]*Drug should be given by slow intravenous infusion over a period of at least one hour; blood pressure and ECG should be monitored frequently.*
[4]*Dose reduced in patients with impaired renal function.*

nemia, and several cases of agranulocytosis were reported to be associated with its antimalarial use. Less toxic drugs are available for treatment of chloroquine-resistant falciparum malaria. Thus dapsone no longer needs to be used.

The combination of trimethoprim, a folic acid antagonist, and sulfalene, a long-acting sulfonamide not yet released for general use in the United States, has been tried but has not been uniformly effective in the treatment of chloroquine-resistant fal-

ciparum malaria. Trimethoprim is marketed in this country only in combination with sulfamethoxazole in a fixed-dosage ratio intended only for antibacterial use.

The combination of pyrimethamine and sulfadoxine [Falcidar, Fancidar, Methipox], taken biweekly and continued for six to eight weeks after leaving the malarious area, is considered the treatment of choice for suppression of chloroquine-resistant malaria. Some authorities prescribe weekly doses of chloroquine in addition in case pyrimethamine-resistant strains of *P. vivax* are present also. Unfortunately, this treatment cannot be initiated in the United States, so chloroquine may be started one to two weeks before reaching the endemic area and taken until the combination is substituted.

A new quinoline-methanol, mefloquine, has been used successfully to treat infections with chloroquine-resistant and chloroquine-sensitive falciparum and vivax malaria. Mefloquine also appears to be an effective, long-acting suppressive agent for use in prophylaxis. It has not been released for general use.

Adverse Reactions and Precautions

Certain antimalarial drugs induce hemolytic anemia in individuals with glucose-6-phosphate dehydrogenase (G6PD) deficiency. This X-linked condition occurs principally in people from regions that historically were endemic for malaria, including those of Mediterranean, African, and Southeast Asian ancestry. The Caucasian and Oriental variants of G6PD deficiency usually precipitate more severe reactions than the African variant. Antimalarial drugs that cause hemolytic anemia in these patients are primaquine and sulfonamides. Chloroquine does not cause hemolysis in G6PD-deficient individuals. Quinine and quinidine have been implicated when given to individuals with the Caucasian variant. Therefore, although the evidence is scanty, those with the Caucasian or Oriental variants of G6PD deficiency who receive quinine or quinidine should be observed closely for evidence of possible hemolysis.

Chloroquine or another 4-aminoquinoline is best suited for use during pregnancy, since teratogenic effects have not been noted with their administration. Pyrimethamine should be avoided because anomalies in the offspring of animals given this drug have been encountered. Use of primaquine probably should be postponed until after delivery.

The 4-aminoquinolines and pyrimethamine (alone or with a long-acting sulfonamide) are well tolerated by children. Dosage should be adjusted according to weight. Because chloroquine tablets are extremely bitter, a syrup or elixir form of chloroquine or amodiaquine has been used in some areas. Chloroquine tablets can be pulverized and mixed with chocolate syrup to make an acceptable preparation for children. Death due to poisoning has occurred in children after accidental ingestion of antimalarial agents.

INDIVIDUAL EVALUATIONS

AMODIAQUINE HYDROCHLORIDE
[Camoquin Hydrochloride]

This 4-aminoquinoline derivative is effective for the prophylaxis and treatment of acute attacks of malaria caused by *Plasmodium vivax*, *P. ovale*, *P. malariae*, and susceptible strains of *P. falciparum*.

Adverse reactions include nausea, vomiting, diarrhea, fatigue, lassitude, and vertigo; reversible pigmentation of the palate, nail beds, and skin may occur when weekly antimalarial doses are given for prolonged periods (five weeks to six years). Most gastrointestinal reactions can be minimized by administering the drug with meals.

ROUTE, USUAL DOSAGE, AND PREPARATIONS. All doses are expressed in terms of the base.
Oral: For treatment of malaria, *adults*, 600 mg initially, followed by 400 mg at 6, 24, and 48 hours. *Children*, 10 mg/kg of body weight initially, and 5 mg/kg at 6, 24, and

48 hours. For prophylaxis of malaria, *adults*, 400 mg; *children less than 1 year*, 50 mg; *2 to 4 years*, 50 to 100 mg; *5 to 8 years*, 150 to 200 mg; *9 to 12 years*, 300 mg. Adjustments within age groups should be based on weight. This dose is given once weekly on the same day of the week beginning two weeks before the individual enters the malarious area and is continued for eight weeks after his return. Primaquine may be added to the regimen immediately after the individual has left an endemic area, particularly if exposure has been heavy and prolonged (see that evaluation).

> *Camoquin Hydrochloride* (Parke, Davis). Tablets equivalent to 200 mg of base.

CHLOROQUINE PHOSPHATE
[Aralen Phosphate]

CHLOROQUINE HYDROCHLORIDE
[Aralen Hydrochloride]

Chloroquine, a 4-aminoquinoline, is the drug of choice for treatment of acute attacks (clinical cure) of malaria caused by *Plasmodium vivax, P. ovale, P. malariae*, and susceptible strains of *P. falciparum*. It also is a component of the combination, Aralen Phosphate with Primaquine Phosphate, which may be used for prophylaxis of all susceptible species of malaria. The combination is no more effective against resistant falciparum strains and has no advantage over the individual drugs used in sequence.

Chloroquine can be administered orally, intramuscularly, or, rarely, intravenously. The hydrochloride salt is given parenterally instead of the oral phosphate salt when severe nausea or vomiting occurs, when absorption of the drug is in question, or when the infection is particularly severe. Special caution is necessary in using the parenteral form in children. Oral adminis-

tration should be substituted as soon as practicable.

Most adverse effects resulting from antimalarial doses of chloroquine are relatively mild, since the amounts used for clinical prophylaxis are small and the larger doses employed to treat acute attacks are given only for short periods. Adverse effects are dose related and include gastrointestinal discomfort with nausea and diarrhea, pruritus, rash, headache, central nervous system stimulation, and reversible interference with visual accommodation. Most gastrointestinal reactions can be minimized by administering the drug with meals. Rapid intravenous injection causes dizziness, nausea, disturbance of vision, and a transient fall in blood pressure. Acute overdosage can cause acute circulatory failure, convulsions, respiratory and cardiac arrest, and death.

ROUTES, USUAL DOSAGE, AND PREPARATIONS. All doses are expressed in terms of the base.
For Treatment of Malaria:
CHLOROQUINE PHOSPHATE:
Oral: *Adults*, 600 mg, followed by 300 mg in six hours and 300 mg daily for the next two days. *Children*, 10 mg/kg of body weight initially, followed by 5 mg/kg in six hours and 5 mg/kg daily for the next two days.

> Drug available generically: Tablets 250 mg (equivalent to 150 mg of base).
> *Aralen Phosphate* (Winthrop). Tablets 500 mg (equivalent to 300 mg of base).

CHLOROQUINE HYDROCHLORIDE:
Intramuscular: *Adults*, 3 mg/kg of body weight initially, repeated, if necessary, at intervals of six hours (maximum, 900 mg in 24 hours). The usual dose for adults is 200 mg every six hours for three days. An oral preparation should be substituted as soon as possible. *Children*, 2 to 3 mg/kg of body weight initially, repeated if necessary in six hours. The total dose should not exceed 5 mg/kg/24 hrs. This route should be used in infants and children only when absolutely necessary.
Intravenous: *Adults*, 3 mg/kg of body weight diluted in 500 ml of sodium chloride injection is administered over a period of one hour. This route should be

avoided in *children under 7 years*.

Aralen Hydrochloride (Winthrop). Solution 50 mg/ml (equivalent to 40 mg/ml of base) in 5 ml containers.

For Prophylaxis of Malaria:

CHLOROQUINE PHOSPHATE:

Oral: Adults, 300 mg; *children*, 5 mg/kg of body weight. The dose is given once weekly on the same day of the week beginning two weeks before the individual enters the malarious area and is continued for eight weeks after his return. Primaquine may be added to the regimen immediately after the individual has left an endemic area, particularly if exposure has been heavy and prolonged (see that evaluation).

Drug available generically: Tablets 250 mg (equivalent to 150 mg of base).

Aralen Phosphate (Winthrop). Tablets 500 mg (equivalent to 300 mg of base).

HYDROXYCHLOROQUINE SULFATE

[Plaquenil Sulfate]

Hydroxychloroquine, a 4-aminoquinoline, is used orally for both prophylaxis and clinical cure of malarial attacks caused by *Plasmodium vivax, P. malariae, P. ovale,* and susceptible strains of *P. falciparum.* It has not been shown to have any therapeutic advantage over chloroquine. Adverse reactions to hydroxychloroquine are the same as those for chloroquine (see the evaluation).

ROUTE, USUAL DOSAGE, AND PREPARATIONS. All doses are expressed in terms of the base.

Oral: For treatment of malaria, *adults*, 620 mg initially, followed by 310 mg in six hours and 310 mg daily for the next two days. *Children*, 10 mg/kg of body weight initially, followed by 5 mg/kg in six hours and 5 mg/kg daily for the next two days. For prophylaxis of malaria, *adults*, 310 mg and *children*, 5 mg/kg of body weight; the dose is given once weekly on the same day of

the week beginning two weeks before the individual enters the malarious area and is continued for eight weeks after his return. Primaquine may be added to the regimen immediately after the individual has left an endemic area, particularly if exposure has been heavy and prolonged (see that evaluation).

Plaquenil Sulfate (Winthrop). Tablets 200 mg (equivalent to 155 mg of base).

PRIMAQUINE PHOSPHATE

Primaquine is the most effective and least toxic of the available 8-aminoquinolines. It is used for prophylaxis or to prevent relapses and to provide radical cure of malaria caused by *Plasmodium vivax* or *P. ovale.* Patients recovering from falciparum malaria may also receive primaquine for its gametocytocidal effect.

The most serious adverse effect is intravascular hemolysis manifested as acute hemolytic anemia in patients with glucose-6-phosphate dehydrogenase (G6PD) deficiency. Primaquine may also induce hemolysis in individuals with other defects of the erythrocytic pentose phosphate pathway of glucose metabolism and in patients with certain hemoglobinopathies. In healthy individuals with G6PD deficiency, the severity of the hemolysis varies directly with the dose and degree of erythrocytic deficiency. There are many molecular variations and degrees of G6PD deficiency found among all races. In individuals with the African variant, the hemolytic anemia induced by the standard course of primaquine therapy is relatively mild, self-limited, and often asymptomatic. In those with the Mediterranean variant, clinically evident hemolysis with the usual dosage schedule is likely. Thus, in patients whose ethnic origin indicates the possibility of G6PD deficiency, screening for this deficiency prior to administering primaquine is advisable.

The hemolytic effect is lessened by use of the following alternative regimens which are as effective as the standard regimen against relapsing forms of malaria. For those with the African variant of G6PD deficiency, 45 mg of primaquine base is given once a week for eight weeks; for those with the Caucasian or Oriental variants, 30 mg of primaquine base is given once weekly for 15 weeks. Monitoring of the hemogram, including reticulocyte counts, is recommended, especially during the first and second weeks. The urine should be examined for hemolysis as well.

Primaquine also may cause abdominal discomfort, nausea, headache, interference with visual accommodation, and pruritus. Methemoglobinemia is common but rarely necessitates interruption of therapy. Leukopenia and agranulocytosis occur rarely.

ROUTE, USUAL DOSAGE, AND PREPARATIONS.
All doses are expressed in terms of the base.
Oral: To prevent relapses, *adults*, 15 mg; *children*, 0.3 mg/kg of body weight. This dose is given daily for 14 days concomitantly or consecutively with chloroquine, hydroxychloroquine, or amodiaquine, which are given on the first three days of an acute attack (see the evaluations). For prophylaxis of malaria, *adults*, 15 mg; *children*, 0.3 mg/kg of body weight. These doses are given daily for 14 days beginning immediately after the individual has left the malarious area, particularly if the exposure has been heavy and prolonged. A daily dose of 30 mg given for 14 days may be necessary in adults exposed to some of the more virulent Southwest Pacific strains (eg, Chesson) of *P. vivax.*
No pediatric formulation of primaquine is available and it may be more convenient to use the combination ablet containing chloroquine and primaquine in children. These tablets are not readily available. (See the evaluation on Chloroquine and Primaquine Phosphates.)

　　Primaquine Phosphate (Winthrop). Tablets 26.3 mg (equivalent to 15 mg of base).

PYRIMETHAMINE
[Daraprim]

Pyrimethamine is a potent dihydrofolate reductase inhibitor that is used for the prophylaxis of malaria caused by susceptible species of *Plasmodium.* Unfortunately, when used on a large scale, parasites readily develop resistance to this drug. It also is used in combination with sulfonamides to treat chloroquine-resistant strains of *P. falciparum.* Sulfonamides and folic acid antagonists should always be given together, for their combined activity is many times greater than that of either drug alone. Furthermore, the number of strains resistant to either agent is thought to be greatly decreased with use of the combination. This combination acts by sequential blockade of two consecutive steps in the formation of folinic acid from aminobenzoic acid (PABA) by the parasite. The sulfonamide prevents the parasite from utilizing PABA to synthesize folic acid and the folic acid antagonist inhibits the enzyme, dihydrofolate reductase, thus preventing formation of tetrahydrofolic acid (folinic acid). For treatment of acute malaria, quinine is usually also administered initially to control symptoms (see that evaluation).

The hazards from small, suppressive antimalarial doses of pyrimethamine are minimal. However, large daily doses or prolonged administration may produce toxicity. Symptoms are mainly a manifestation of interference with folic acid metabolism. The effects, therefore, are most evident in rapidly dividing cells. Pyrimethamine is teratogenic in animals, and its use is contraindicated during pregnancy.

If hematologic abnormalities appear, administration should be stopped and leucovorin (folinic acid) 3 to 9 mg should be administered intramuscularly until the blood cell count returns to safe levels. Alternatively, concomitant administration of 3 to 9 mg of leucovorin usually prevents the anemia, thrombocytopenia, and leukopenia without interfering with the antimalarial action of pyrimethamine.

ROUTE, USUAL DOSAGE, AND PREPARATIONS. *Oral*: For prophylaxis of malaria, *adults and children over 10 years*, 25 mg once weekly; *children 2 years and under*, 6.25 to 12.5 mg weekly; *3 to 10 years*, 12.5 to 25 mg weekly. The dose is given once weekly on the same day of the week. Since adequate blood levels are obtained within a few hours after ingestion, administration need not be started until the day before entering an endemic area and should be continued for six to eight weeks after return.

Primaquine may be added to the regimen immediately after the individual has left the endemic area, particularly if the exposure has been heavy and prolonged (see that evaluation).

For use with quinine and a sulfonamide in the treatment of chloroquine-resistant strains of *P. falciparum*, see the evaluation on Quinine.

    Daraprim (Burroughs Wellcome). Tablets 25 mg.

QUININE SULFATE

QUININE DIHYDROCHLORIDE

Quinine is used with tetracycline or with pyrimethamine and a sulfonamide (eg, sulfadoxine, sulfadiazine) to treat chloroquine-resistant strains of *Plasmodium falciparum*. Unless they are unavailable, the safer and more rapid-acting 4-aminoquinolines should be used instead of quinine in malaria caused by other species or drug-sensitive *P. falciparum*.

Quinine can be administered orally (quinine sulfate) or intravenously (quinine dihydrochloride). The dihydrochloride salt is used in patients with severe attacks of *P. falciparum* when absorption of quinine sulfate cannot be assured.

The usual therapeutic antimalarial doses of quinine sulfate frequently cause symptoms of mild to moderate cinchonism (tinnitus, headache, altered auditory acuity, blurred vision, nausea, diarrhea), but these symptoms seldom are severe enough to necessitate cessation of treatment. Severe symptoms develop only rarely, but occur most often when plasma levels exceed 10 mg/dl. Asthma may be precipitated in susceptible individuals. Urticaria is the most frequent allergic reaction and pruritus may develop with or without rash. Signs of hematologic toxicity include acute hemolysis, hypoprothrombinemia, thrombocytopenic purpura, and agranulocytosis. The precise role played by quinine in precipitating blackwater fever is unknown.

Intravenous administration of the dihydrochloride salt may produce hypotension and acute circulatory failure. It should be injected slowly in very dilute solutions, and oral administration of the sulfate salt should be substituted as soon as possible. Any adverse reactions associated with quinine sulfate must be considered when using the dihydrochloride salt. Quinidine hydrochloride has been substituted for quinine in emergencies when intravenous administration for falciparum malaria is required and the intravenous form of quinine is not available. However, because cardiotoxicity may be induced by quinidine, careful monitoring of the heart should accompany use of this drug. Since parenteral forms of quinine and chloroquine may be obtained from the Center for Disease Control in emergencies, quinidine is rarely needed.

Quinine has been used in the treatment of nocturnal leg cramps and myotonia congenita, in the diagnosis of myasthenia gravis, as an antipyretic-analgesic, to induce labor, and as a local anesthetic or sclerosing agent. More effective drugs are currently available for these uses, except for nocturnal leg cramps. Any reputation this agent may have as an efficient abortifacient is undeserved. Quinine should be given with caution to patients who have atrial fibrillation and to those who manifest idiosyncrasy to it in the form of cutaneous angioedema or visual or auditory symptoms. This drug is contraindicated in the presence of optic neuritis and tinnitus.

ROUTES, USUAL DOSAGE, AND PREPARATIONS. All doses are expressed in terms of the base.

QUININE SULFATE:
Oral: For treatment of malaria, *adults*, 650 mg every eight hours for 10 to 14 days. *Children*, 25 mg/kg of body weight every eight hours for 10 to 14 days. For treatment of chloroquine-resistant *P. falciparum* malaria, pyrimethamine 50 mg daily for the first three days and sulfadiazine 2 g daily for the first six days should be added to the regimen. Alternatively, administration of quinine may be limited to three to five days and tetracycline 1 g daily may be given concurrently for ten days.

Drug available generically: Capsules 120, 200, 300, and 325 mg; tablets 300 mg.

QUININE DIHYDROCHLORIDE:
Intravenous: For treatment of severe malaria, *adults*, 600 mg in 300 ml of sodium chloride injection infused over at least a one-hour period. This dose is repeated in six to eight hours, (maximum total daily dose, 1.8 g). Following clinical response, quinine sulfate should be given orally as soon as practicable. *Infants and children*, 25 mg/kg of body weight administered by slow (over a one-hour period) intravenous infusion; one-half of this dose is given initially and the other half is given six to eight hours later if the oral dose cannot be tolerated. If the infection is caused by chloroquine-resistant *P. falciparum*, pyrimethamine and sulfadiazine or tetracycline should be added as described above.

Drug available generically: Powder 500 mg. If unavailable locally, the drug may be obtained from the Parasitic Disease Drug Service, Center for Disease Control, Atlanta, Ga. (See the Introduction to this section for telephone numbers.)

MIXTURES

CHLOROQUINE AND PRIMAQUINE PHOSPHATES
[Aralen Phosphate with Primaquine Phosphate]

This combination of chloroquine and primaquine is suitable and safe for the prophylaxis of malaria, provided its use is continued for at least eight weeks after the individual has left a malarious area. It has been especially effective in the long-term prophylaxis of vivax malaria in military personnel. It has never achieved widespread acceptance for civilian use.

This combination is also more easily tolerated by individuals susceptible to the adverse effects of primaquine. The same adverse effects and precautions apply to the combination as for either drug used alone. See the evaluations for details.

ROUTE, USUAL DOSAGE, AND PREPARATIONS.
Oral: For prophylaxis of malaria, *adults and children over 45 kg*, one tablet weekly on the same day of each week, starting two weeks before entering the malarious area and continuing for eight weeks after leaving. For younger children, a suspension of the tablets is made in chocolate syrup or fruit juice so that each 5 ml contains 40 mg of chloroquine base and 6 mg of primaquine base. The following amounts are then given once weekly on the same day of each week: *Children 5 to 7 kg*, 2.5 ml; *8 to 11 kg*, 5 ml; *12 to 15 kg*, 7.5 ml; *16 to 20 kg*, 10 ml; *21 to 24 kg*, 12.5 ml; and *25 to 45 kg*, one-half tablet. These doses should not be exceeded.

Aralen Phosphate with Primaquine Phosphate (Winthrop). Tablets containing chloroquine phosphate 500 mg (equivalent to 300 mg base) and primaquine phosphate 79 mg (equivalent to 45 mg base).

TRICHOMONIASIS

Infections of the vagina caused by *Trichomonas vaginalis* are common and occur most frequently during the reproductive years when estrogen levels are high. Infections often recur, which indicates that trichomonads may persist in extravaginal foci, particularly in the urethra. *T. vaginalis* has been found in the urine when it has been absent in the vaginal mucus and may be present in the male urethra, the periurethral glands and ducts of both sexes, and in the rectum.

Diagnosis should be made by microscopic examination of a hanging drop preparation containing fresh exudate from the vagina, semen, or prostatic fluid obtained by massage or urinary sediment. Trichomonal flagella usually are identified easily in fresh preparations, but special stains are required to identify them in fixed smears. When symptoms are suggestive of trichomoniasis (eg, wet inflamed vagina; "strawberry" cervix; thin, yellow, frothy malodorous discharge) but parasites cannot be identified, cultures should be used to confirm the diagnosis. Cultures are usually required to establish a positive diagnosis in men. When signs and symptoms disappear and results of microscopic examination of appropriate samples are negative, it may be assumed that the initial infection has been controlled, although cultures are mandatory for the evaluation of "cures" in patients of either sex.

Until the development of metronidazole [Flagyl], antitrichomonal therapy depended solely on the use of locally acting agents. Metronidazole is the first systemically acting trichomonacide and has become the drug of choice. Other potentially useful systemic trichomonacides are undergoing clinical trial. At least two of these agents (tinidazole, nimorazole) are available in other countries.

Locally acting anti-infective preparations (eg, povidone-iodine [Betadine], aminacrine) may be useful in vaginal infections caused by susceptible organisms, including *T. vaginalis*, when extravaginal sources of reinfection are not present. However, objective evidence of their value is sparse and the patient will not be cured if extravaginal sites of reinfection persist. High concentrations of clotrimazole [Gyne-Lotrimin, Lotrimin, Mycelex, Mycelex-G] also may be trichomonacidal when applied topically (Sawyer et al, 1975). See Chapter 80, Antifungal Agents, for more information on this drug.

Adjuvants are combined with topical trichomonacides to assist penetration into mucus, pus, and detritus. Some are wetting agents, such as sodium lauryl sulfate, docusate sodium (dioctyl sodium sulfosuccinate), or a nonoxynol, whereas others (eg, white vinegar, boric acid, lactic acid) help restore the slightly acidic vaginal pH.

It has been claimed that the vaginal instillation of lactobacilli is beneficial in the treatment of vaginitis, regardless of etiology, by reducing the vaginal pH. However, lactobacilli do not restore vaginal flora to normal or eradicate specific pathogens and, therefore, have limited value.

Adverse Reactions and Precautions

Hypersensitivity reactions are the principal adverse effects associated with use of the locally active trichomonacides. They may cause burning, pruritus, or staining at the site of treatment, but these effects rarely necessitate discontinuation of therapy. Topical preparations that contain iodine rarely cause iodism and have been reported to modify the results of the protein-bound iodine (PBI) test.

The adverse reactions produced by metronidazole are discussed in the following evaluation.

INDIVIDUAL EVALUATIONS

METRONIDAZOLE
[Flagyl]

$$O_2N - \text{(imidazole ring)} \quad CH_2CH_2QH, \ N, \ CH_3, \ N$$

Metronidazole, a systemic trichomonacide, is highly effective in the treatment of *Trichomonas vaginalis* infections in men and women. The drug is biologically active in semen and urine and, therefore, is active against trichomonads in extravaginal as well as vaginal foci. It is inactive against *Candida albicans* and other yeast or bacteria that cause vaginitis.

Despite its broad application in treating trichomonal infections, many authorities recommend that metronidazole be reserved for use in infections confirmed by either examination of a hanging drop preparation or by culture and when locally acting agents are not effective. The rationale for this cautious approach is that metronidazole is carcinogenic in mice and, possibly, rats under certain experimental conditions and is mutagenic to some bacteria in concentrations found in the body fluids of individuals receiving therapeutic doses of the drug. Conversely, because the drug has not been shown to be carcinogenic in hamsters and other animal species so far studied or in man, other authorities believe that the risk of using the drug is justified and that topical therapy is only necessary in those who do not tolerate oral therapy or who have persistent infections that may respond to topical preparations. In the final analysis, the approach to therapy may be dictated to a large extent by the type of patient being treated. The sexually active woman and her male partner who is likely to be a source of reinfection would seem to be likely candidates for systemic therapy since both must be treated simultaneously. A single oral dose of 2 g is preferred, if it can be tolerated, since it achieves a cure rate comparable to other systemic regimens; can be given under supervision, thereby assuring compliance; and is more likely to be accepted by the male partner who is often asymptomatic and may not comply with a multiple-dose regimen or prolonged topical therapy.

Because latent candidal infections may be activated either during or following treatment of a trichomonal infection with metronidazole, it usually is advisable to treat both infections at the same time if laboratory tests confirm the presence of both organisms. (For information on agents used to treat candidal infections, see Chapter 80, Antifungal Agents.) Although metronidazole is active against anaerobic bac-

teria in various areas of the body, it does not affect the normal vaginal bacterial flora, including the Doderlein bacillus.

The incidence of adverse effects with metronidazole is low and no serious reactions have been reported clinically. The most frequent reaction is nausea. For other adverse effects and use of metronidazole during pregnancy (usually the drug is contraindicated), see the evaluation on Metronidazole in the section on Amebiasis.

ROUTE, USUAL DOSAGE, AND PREPARATIONS. *Oral*: *Adults*, 250 mg three times daily for seven to ten days. If a second course of treatment is needed, there should be a four- to six-week interval between courses. Alternatively, a single dose of 2 g, or 1 g morning and evening may be preferred if tolerated.

Flagyl (Searle). Tablets 250 mg.

POVIDONE-IODINE
[Betadine]

$$\left[\begin{array}{c} -CHCH_2- \\ | \\ N \\ \end{array} \diagup\hspace{-6pt}O \right]_n \cdot xI$$

Clinical evidence indicates that this water-soluble complex of polyvinylpyrrolidone and iodine may be beneficial in vaginal infections not complicated by the presence of extravaginal foci of infection. Although povidone-iodine does not produce the degree of local irritation associated with the use of tincture of iodine, reactions may occur in patients allergic to iodine. Serum protein-bound iodine levels increase temporarily in some patients using the drug.

ROUTE, USUAL DOSAGE, AND PREPARATIONS. *Topical (vaginal)*: After swabbing the cervix and vulvovaginal area with a povidone-iodine solution in the office, one applicatorful of the gel is inserted nightly, followed by use of the douche preparation the next morning. Daily applications of gel and douche should be continued for at least two weeks and possibly throughout the menstrual cycle, including the days of menses. Infections may resolve in 10 to 15 days, or therapy may be required for two or three menstrual cycles.

Drug available generically: Douche in 8 oz containers; solution in 4, 8, and 16 oz and 1 gal containers.

Betadine (Purdue Frederick). Douche 10% in ½ and 8 oz and 1 gal containers; gel 10% in 18 g and 3 oz containers; solution 10% in ½, 1, 8, 16, and 32 oz and 1 gal containers. (In all preparations, the percentage indicates the amount of povidone-iodine.)

MIXTURES

A number of combination products are available for local application in the treatment of trichomoniasis. Their suitability varies with the ingredients and the goal of treatment in a specific patient. Objective evidence of their efficacy is sparse. Some preparations are recommended not only for trichomoniasis but also for other vaginal infections characterized as bacterial, candidal, mixed, or "nonspecific." None of these mixtures is as effective as metronidazole for trichomoniasis.

Preparations containing antibiotics may be effective against susceptible bacteria, although sulfonamides are undesirable for topical use because of their sensitizing properties. The quinoline derivatives present in some mixtures may have a degree of usefulness, but aminacrine is of doubtful value. Organic mercurial compounds have very limited anti-infective activity clinically. Estrogens are of value only if atrophic vaginitis complicates the infection. Adrenal corticosteroids are occasionally included for their anti-inflammatory action. Some preparations contain alleged debriding agents (eg, allantoin) as a therapeutic gesture, but these drugs have little value. Detergents and surfactants may exert some cleansing effect and improve the action of other ingredients, but this has not been proved. The vehicles for some vaginal preparations have soothing or cleansing properties that may be useful in the presence of inflammation or pathologic exudation.

Following is a listing of mixtures available for trichomonal and other vaginal in-fections. They are listed only for the sake of completeness rather than for any claimed therapeutic advantage. Those containing a sulfonamide may produce sensitization and preclude future systemic use of sulfonamides.

AVC (Merrell-National). Cream containing aminacrine hydrochloride 0.2%, allantoin 2%, and sulfanilamide 15%; each suppository contains aminacrine hydrochloride 14 mg, allantoin 140 mg, and sulfanilamide 1.05 g.

AVC/Dienestrol (Merrell-National). Cream containing aminacrine hydrochloride 0.2%, allantoin 2%, dienestrol 0.01%, and sulfanilamide 15%; each suppository contains aminacrine hydrochloride 14 mg, allantoin 140 mg, dienestrol 0.7 mg, and sulfanilamide 1.05 g.

Vagisec (Schmid). Liquid containing nonoxynol 9, edetate sodium, and docusate sodium (dioctyl sodium sulfosuccinate).

Vagisec Plus (Schmid). Each suppository contains aminacrine hydrochloride 6 mg, nonoxynol 9 5.25 mg, edetate sodium 0.66 mg, and docusate sodium (dioctyl sodium sulfosuccinate) 0.07 mg.

Vagitrol (Syntex). Cream containing aminacrine hydrochloride 0.2%, allantoin 2%, and sulfanilamide 15%; each suppository contains aminacrine hydrochloride 14 mg, allantoin 140 mg, and sulfanilamide 1.05 g.

GIARDIASIS

The terms giardiasis and lambliasis have both been applied to infection of the gastrointestinal tract caused by *Giardia lamblia.* Man is the principal host and main source of infection. The concept has been held that there is no intermediate host for this parasite, but recent evidence indicates that the disease may be transmitted by beavers (a source of contamination high in mountainous watershed areas) and, possibly, dogs. The motile trophozoite of *G. lamblia* inhabits the small intestine where it attaches to the intestinal mucosa. It is passed as the trophozoite only in individuals with frank diarrhea; it is passed as a cyst, the usual infective stage, in formed stools. The majority of individuals harboring *G. lamblia* are asymptomatic and excrete cyst forms, as do those with obvious active disease.

G. lamblia is the most common flagellate to inhabit the gastrointestinal tract of man worldwide. It is becoming one of the most common protozoans infecting those returning to the United States following foreign travel, especially young children, and has occurred in endemic form in the United States.

Positive diagnosis of giardiasis requires identification of trophozoites or cysts in fresh stool specimens. Symptoms of the disease are nonspecific and commonly include diarrhea (with or without bouts of constipation), abdominal distention, flatulence, nocturnal borborygmi, vomiting, colicky pain related to food ingestion, profound malaise, anemia, and cholecystitis. Weight loss is common due to malabsorption of food. Because vitamin A is poorly absorbed and steatorrhea may be present, the infection may resemble celiac syndrome or kwashiorkor. The pain associated with giardiasis also may mimic that of appendicitis or cholelithiasis.

One of the more serious problems of giardiasis is concomitant (secondary) infection with other parasites or bacteria. It is frequently associated with amebiasis, helminthiasis, or, sometimes, more exotic parasitic diseases or bacterial infections such as those caused by the enterotoxic *Escherichia coli*.

For years, quinacrine [Atabrine] has been considered the drug of choice for treating giardiasis in individuals who could tolerate it. Metronidazole [Flagyl] and the other nitroimidazole compounds are now replacing quinacrine because they appear to have superior therapeutic activity and usually are less toxic. Furazolidone [Furoxone] also is a primary antigiardial agent.

Metronidazole usually is given in a dose of 250 mg three times daily for one week when treating giardiasis. Better cure rates are achieved with a single daily dose of 2 g for three days, but toxicity is common with this schedule. Metronidazole is discussed more completely in the sections on Amebiasis and Trichomoniasis.

Quinacrine still may be preferred for initial therapy in adults or when therapy with metronidazole has failed in children, but children do not tolerate quinacrine well. Severe nausea and vomiting or other toxic effects occasionally preclude its use in both adults and children. Prolonged administration stains the skin yellow, a condition occasionally confused with hepatitis. The usual dose for giardiasis is 100 mg three times daily for one week. For more detailed information on this drug, see Chapter 83, Anthelmintics.

INDIVIDUAL EVALUATION

FURAZOLIDONE
[Furoxone]

This nitrofuran is one of the more potent, effective agents employed in the treatment of giardiasis. Cure rates in excess of 90% with few relapses have been reported, but the drug has not been widely used for treating giardiasis in the United States. In addition to its antigiardial activity, it is moderately effective against a variety of gram-positive and gram-negative enteric organisms, including *Salmonella*, *Shigella*, *Escherichia coli*, staphylococci, and enterococci. It has been used to treat bacterial enteritis and dysentery and shigellosis and may be effective in the treatment of cholera.

Furazolidone usually is well tolerated, even by children; however, nausea and vomiting occur frequently and vesicular or morbilliform pruritic rash has been reported. It may cause agranulocytosis and, in people with G6PD deficiency, acute hemolysis. The drug is incompletely absorbed; traces appear in the urine and metabolic degradation products may tint the urine brown. Other toxic effects characteristic of the nitrofurans also may occur (see Chapter 78, Urinary Tract Antiseptics, for additional information).

Furazolidone produces a disulfiram-type reaction in some patients after ingestion of alcohol. A metabolite of furazolidone markedly inhibits the activity of monoamine oxidase, and a hypertensive reaction may occur if the drug is given with adrenergic agents, tricyclic compounds, or foods containing significant amounts of tyramine (eg, cheese, liver, pickled herring, wines [especially chianti], yeast extracts, broad beans, chocolate).

ROUTE, USUAL DOSAGE, AND PREPARATIONS. *Oral: Adults,* 100 mg four times daily. *Children,* 6 mg/kg of body weight daily divided into four doses. The drug should not be given to *infants under 1 month.*

 Furoxone (Norwich-Eaton). Liquid 50 mg/15 ml; tablets 100 mg.

BALANTIDIASIS

Balantidiasis is caused by the ciliate protozoan, *Balantidium coli,* an organism that infects the large intestine. It also can attack pigs, which are considered possible reservoirs of infection. Although people handling these animals may acquire the infection from them, it also is possible for the disease to be transmitted by man. The incidence of balantidiasis in man is low in comparison to most other protozoal infections. Many individuals are asymptomatic, although some have diarrhea and abdominal pain. In severe infections, a dysenteric syndrome similar to that observed in amebiasis develops. Balantidiasis is treated with metronidazole or other nitroimidazoles; for dosage, see the section on Amebiasis.

LEISHMANIASES AND TRYPANOSOMIASES

Although leishmaniases and trypanosomiases affect large numbers of people, these diseases remain largely tropical and subtropical in distribution because they are transmitted by blood-sucking insect vectors primarily indigenous to the tropics. Consequently, neither infection is observed very often in temperate areas such as the United States.

Leishmaniases: These infections result from invasion of the reticuloendothelial system by *Leishmania,* which is transmitted to the human host by sandflies of the genus *Phlebotomus* or *Lutzomyia* from a reservoir of organisms present in rodents or other small animals. In man, the three types of infection range from mild conditions that may be self-limiting to severe or even fatal disease. Visceral leishmaniasis, widely known as kala-azar, is caused by *L. donovani.* It usually has a gradual onset and is characterized by fever, weight loss, hepatosplenomegaly and hepatic dysfunction, anemia, hemorrhage, and lymphadenopathy. If untreated, it often is fatal. Mucocutaneous leishmaniasis results from invasion by *L. brasiliensis.* It occurs in South America in several different forms. Marked disfiguration is a prominent feature of the disease due to progressive and extensive ulceration of the mucous membranes of the mouth, palate, pharynx, and nose. Cutaneous leishmaniasis, sometimes called oriental sore, is caused by *L. tropica* (Old World cutaneous leishmaniasis) and *L. brasiliensis, L. mexicana,* or *L. peruviana* (New World cutaneous leishmaniasis). A nodule, which may crust or ulcerate and is very slow to bleed, develops at the point of the insect bite. *Leishmania* organisms usually can be identified in tissue samples taken from the borders of the skin ulcerations.

Few drugs are uniformly effective in leishmaniases. The pentavalent antimonial compounds (eg, sodium stibogluconate [Pentostam], meglumine antimoniate) are used most commonly. The diamidines (eg, pentamidine) and certain antimicrobial agents (eg, amphotericin B [Fungizone]) may be suitable alternatives if the antimonial agents are not effective or cannot be tolerated. Metronidazole [Flagyl] also may be beneficial. Berberine chloride, emetine, and quinacrine [Atabrine] have been used locally. All have various shortcomings that involve relative effectiveness, toxicity, or both. Several of these drugs are available to physicians in the United States only from the Center for Disease Control of the U.S. Public Health Service, Atlanta, Ga 30333.

Trypanosomiases: There are two types of trypanosomiases, African and South American. African trypanosomiasis (sleeping sickness) is caused by the bite of an infected *Glossina* (tsetse fly). Two forms of African trypanosomiasis have been identified: the first is caused by *Trypanosoma gambiense*, the second by *T. rhodesiense*. Both have similar clinical features, but the onset of symptoms and progression of disease is more rapid with *T. rhodesiense* infection. In the earlier stages of disease, the organism localizes in the lymphatic system and causes intermittent attacks of fever, lymphadenopathy, hepatosplenomegaly, dyspnea, and tachycardia. When the organisms reach the central nervous system, the chronic, so-called sleeping sickness state begins, characterized by headache, disturbances in coordination, mental dullness, and apathy. As the disease progresses, the patient sleeps constantly, becomes emaciated, and, if untreated, will die.

The hemolymphatic stage of African trypanosomiasis can be treated with pentamidine or suramin. When the parasite is entrenched within the central nervous system, melarsoprol is the drug of choice.

South American trypanosomiasis (Chagas' disease) is transmitted to man by the bite of reduviid bugs infected with *T. cruzi*. Despite the name "South American trypanosomiasis," these parasites have been found in reservoir hosts as far north as Texas (two cases have been reported). *T. cruzi* is regarded as distinct from the organisms causing African trypanosomiasis and has some characteristics similar to *Leishmania*. Symptoms of Chagas' disease vary from region to region. Early signs are local swelling (chagoma) at the site of the bite associated with severe inflammation. Other symptoms that are allergic in nature include rash, fever, and edema of the eyelids and face. The chronic form of the disease may be asymptomatic or may produce organomegaly, particularly megaesophagus and megacolon. *T. cruzi* has extraordinary affinity for cardiac parenchymal cells and also attacks nerve cells in the mesenteric plexus; chronic cardiopathies are usually the cause of death when Chagas' disease is of long-standing duration. Some forms of the disease may include both organomegaly and cardiac involvement. Central nervous system involvement, such as meningoencephalitis, is a severe complication of Chagas' disease and is often fatal, especially in small children.

Chagas' disease has remained resistant to most forms of therapy. Primaquine may be effective against extracellular trypanosomes in the blood but is ineffective against intracellular forms. Recently, nifurtimox [Lampit, Bayer 2502] has been shown to have some activity against both intracellular and extracellular parasites. Toxicity limits the usefulness of these compounds. Like the drugs used to treat leishmaniases, many of the agents used in trypanosomiases are available only from the Center for Disease Control of the U.S. Public Health Service, Atlanta, Ga 30333.

INDIVIDUAL EVALUATIONS

MEGLUMINE ANTIMONIATE

Meglumine antimoniate is a drug of choice in treating cutaneous and mucocutaneous leishmanial infections. It has some effect on visceral leishmaniasis (kala-azar); although East African and Mediterranean forms of the disease are relatively resistant to the antimonials, Indian, Chinese, and Brazilian forms are more susceptible. This compound also is useful in the management of post kala-azar dermal leishmaniasis.

This antimonial is relatively safe and usually is well tolerated but, like sodium stibogluconate, is capable of causing antimony poisoning (see the following evaluation).

Meglumine antimoniate is not available in the United States.

SODIUM STIBOGLUCONATE
[Pentostam]

This pentavalent antimonial compound is a drug of choice in treating visceral leishmaniasis and also exerts an effect against the cutaneous and mucocutaneous forms. The antimonial compounds inhibit various enzymes in *Leishmania* and may act on parasite ribosomes, but their exact mode of action has not been fully established.

Although sodium stibogluconate is usually well tolerated, adverse reactions can be severe. The most common and serious effect is cardiotoxicity manifested as cardiac irregularities, including severe bradycardia. Vasodilation and shock have been observed. Liver and kidney function also may be impaired. Milder reactions include nausea, vomiting, rash, headache, syncope, dyspnea, facial edema, and abdominal pain. Pain in joints and muscles may occur toward the end of a therapeutic course. Nevertheless, pentavalent antimonials are less toxic than trivalent ones. Pentavalent antimonials are generally contraindicated in the presence of cardiac, hepatic, or renal disease, pneumonia, tuberculosis, pregnancy, or in infants under 18 months of age.

Dosage information and preparations of sodium antimonyl gluconate (sodium stibogluconate) are available from the Center for Disease Control (see the introduction to this section).

MELARSOPROL
[MEL-B]

Melarsoprol, a trivalent arsenical compound, is the drug of choice for treating meningoencephalitis associated with the late stages of African trypanosomiasis. It has some effectiveness in the earlier stages as well but, because of its potential to cause encephalopathy, is not used until later in the course of the disease. The drug is given intravenously but is irritating to tissues and care must be taken to avoid extravasation.

Melarsoprol is very toxic and many of the adverse effects are those of arsenic poisoning. Serious, potentially fatal reactive encephalopathy develops in approximately 12% of patients. Other reactions include abdominal pain, vomiting, hypotension, albuminuria, peripheral neuropathy, arthralgia, angioedema, and rashes. A Herxheimer-like reaction may occur following the first dose of melarsoprol. Pa-

tients receiving this drug should be hospitalized and closely monitored.

Information on dosage and precautions for therapeutic use are available from the Center for Disease Control (see the introduction to this section).

NIFURTIMOX
[Lampit, Bayer 2502]

This nitrofuran derivative is effective in the acute stage of Chagas' disease because it rapidly reduces parasitemia. It inhibits both the extracellular mastigote and intracellular amastigote stages of *Trypanosoma cruzi*, but its mechanism of action is unknown. It is more effective against Argentinean and Chilean strains of the parasite than against Brazilean strains. Following absorption after oral administration, nifurtimox is extensively metabolized; the metabolites are excreted primarily by the kidney.

Adverse reactions are generally mild and are more common in adults than in children. They usually consist of anorexia, nausea, vomiting, abdominal pain, excitation, vertigo, headache, myalgia, insomnia, and skin rashes. Peripheral neuritis and psychoses also may be seen.

Information on dosage and preparations is available from the Center for Disease Control (see the introduction to this section).

PENTAMIDINE

Like the related diamidine compounds, propamidine and stilbamidine, pentamidine has trypanosomicidal and leishmanicidal activity but is quite toxic. Its mechanism of action has not been defined. Since this drug is poorly absorbed from the gastrointestinal tract, it must be administered intramuscularly.

Pentamidine may cause pain at the site of injection, followed by abscess formation and tissue necrosis. Other reactions include vomiting, hypotension, tachycardia, and hypoglycemia. A large percentage of patients experience impairment of renal and hepatic function that is usually reversible when the drug is discontinued. Blood dyscrasias also have been reported.

ROUTE, USUAL DOSAGE, AND PREPARATIONS. *Intramuscular*: *Adults*, 4 mg/kg of body weight daily for 12 to 14 days. For prophylaxis of African trypanosomiasis, 4 mg/kg is given as a single dose every three to six months.

Pentamidine is available from the Center for Disease Control (see the Introduction).

SURAMIN

[Bayer 205]

Suramin, a trypanosomicidal drug developed from a nonmetallic dye group of which trypan blue is a member, is useful in treating both types of African trypanosomiasis. It is the drug of choice for Rhodesian trypanosomiasis when the central nervous system is not involved and also is used for the destruction of adult worms in onchocerciasis. This drug appears to be selectively absorbed into trypanosomes, perhaps by pinocytosis, where it binds with enzymes, often in a reversible fashion. The exact mechanism of action has not been explained. Suramin is not taken into host cells with equal ease or it would be too toxic to be used as a drug. It is tightly bound to proteins and persists in the circulation for long periods, is released slowly from plasma proteins, and is excreted slowly by the kidney; this allows the drug to be effective for chemoprophylaxis of African trypanosomiasis when given every two weeks.

Suramin should be administered only in a hospital under close medical supervision. Adverse effects involving the central nervous system are common following injection and include paresthesias, hyperesthesia of the palms and soles, peripheral neuropathy, and photophobia. Pruritus and urticaria may develop quickly, even with therapeutic doses, and other types of rashes, including exfoliative dermatitis, may develop later. Suramin is nephrotoxic, causing proteinuria or even hematuria and cylindruria if the damage is pronounced. Rarely, blood dyscrasias and hemolytic anemia have been reported. Occasionally, a shock-like reaction characterized by nausea, vomiting, hypotension, and unconsciousness occurs immediately after injection. Because of this possibility, a 100- to 200-mg test dose should be administered before the first full therapeutic injection is given. In the absence of a severe reaction, therapy can be initiated.

ROUTE, USUAL DOSAGE, AND PREPARATIONS. *Intravenous*: *Adults*, following a test dose of 100 to 200 mg, 1 g is given on days 1, 3, 7, 14, and 21. The dose for *children* is 20 mg/kg of body weight given on the same days as for adults. Since suramin is a poorly soluble powder, a fresh solution must be prepared before each injection.

Suramin is available from the Center for Disease Control (see the introduction to this section).

AMEBIASIS

Amebiasis usually refers to an infection caused by *Entamoeba histolytica*, which causes intermittent disease among millions of people worldwide, including an estimated 2% to 20% of the population of the United States. The disease is transmitted when mature cysts are ingested. Each cyst develops into eight trophozoites, usually in the ileocecal region of the intestine; a colony is established in the cecum and later extends throughout the colon. Trophozoites can penetrate the mucosa, causing ulceration of the intestinal wall which may simulate ulcerative colitis. Diarrhea and abdominal pain are common features, although some individuals do not develop any of these symptoms. Such patients remain asymptomatic but continue to spread the disease by passing mature cysts in formed stools. *E. histolytica* occasionally invades the liver, where it may cause abscesses. The liver is the major site of extraintestinal infection; amebic abscesses rarely occur in other organs.

Classification of Amebicides: Some drugs act upon amebae only within the lumen of the bowel, whereas others affect the parasite within the intestinal wall or in other organs of the body. A few act at more than one site.

The amides (eg, diloxanide [Furamide]) and iodoquinol (diiodohydroxyquin) [Yodoxin] are active in the intestinal lumen. They are referred to as oral luminal or contact amebicides. Of these two agents, diloxanide is most useful.

Emetine and its analogue, dehydro-emetine (which is as effective as emetine and probably less toxic), and chloroquine [Aralen] are tissue amebicides. The emetines are given parenterally and affect amebae in the intestinal wall and liver. Chloroquine is given orally and acts principally in the liver; it is appreciably less effective than the emetines but also is less toxic. Chloroquine probably is inadequate as sole therapy for amebic abscess but can be combined with the emetines.

Metronidazole [Flagyl] is effective against amebae at all sites where they are commonly found, but its actions are more pronounced in the tissue because most of the compound is absorbed during passage through the small intestine. Only the small portion that remains unabsorbed is available to act as a luminal amebicide. For this reason, metronidazole often is classified as an orally effective tissue amebicide. Nevertheless, following its introduction into medicine, metronidazole quickly became a useful agent for treating both intestinal and hepatic amebiasis because of its relatively low toxic potential and high degree of effectiveness, a condition that still persists despite the fact that resistant organisms are becoming more prevalent.

Studies are available that indicate metronidazole is carcinogenic in mice and, possibly, rats, but not in hamsters, and it is mutagenic to certain bacteria. Since metronidazole has not been implicated in causing cancer in man, the potential risks associated with its use are justified in patients with serious or persistent

amebiasis, although it should not be used during the first trimester and should be avoided, if possible, during the entire pregnancy.

Some antibiotics, such as paromomycin [Humatin] and erythromycin, have a direct amebicidal action. Others, such as tetracycline and oxytetracycline [Terramycin], act indirectly in the intestinal lumen and wall by modifying the flora necessary for survival of the amebae. None of these antibiotics are effective as sole therapy in amebiasis but may be used as adjunctive drugs.

Therapy: Chronic, nondysenteric, asymptomatic amebiasis (cyst carrier state) is treated with a luminal amebicide. The drug of choice is probably diloxanide. Iodoquinol is a suitable alternative and should be used when diloxanide cannot be tolerated or is not readily available. Because the asymptomatic cyst passer is not treated in areas where amebiasis is endemic and because metronidazole is less effective as a luminal amebicide than as a tissue amebicide, this agent is not a drug of first choice to treat asymptomatic amebiasis but is useful as an alternative.

In intestinal amebiasis, *E. histolytica* organisms are present in the intestinal lumen, on the mucosal surface of the bowel, and in the walls of the intestine; therefore, the drug or combination of drugs must be active against the organism in tissue as well as in the intestinal lumen. Metronidazole is the drug of choice and often is effective alone. In mild to moderate disease, alternative therapy may include a tetracycline or paromomycin in conjunction with iodoquinol. For severe disease, a tetracycline plus iodoquinol or, more commonly, emetine or dehydroemetine combined with iodoquinol are alternatives to metronidazole.

Amebic abscesses can be treated with metronidazole. Alternative therapy consists of emetine or dehydroemetine plus chloroquine. A luminal amebicide also may be indicated if amebae are present in the colon in order to eliminate the primary source of infection.

Liver abscesses usually must be drained, preferably by closed aspiration when there is a palpable mass, persistent localized tenderness, or markedly raised hemidiaphragm. Liver scanning techniques using rose bengal, sodium iodide I 131, or gold Au 198; sonarography; or computerized axial tomography are useful in locating the abscesses. Amebic liver abscesses sometimes rupture into the lungs, pleura, pericardium, or peritoneum. These complications are treated by drainage and administration of the same regimen used for hepatic amebiasis.

Complications of intestinal amebiasis include ameboma (a tumor-like mass of granulomatous tissue) and stricture, peritonitis, or intussusception. When they occur, these conditions are treated with metronidazole or the concomitant administration of emetine or dehydroemetine, a luminal amebicide, and a tetracycline. Intussusception must be reduced surgically during therapy. Peritonitis is usually fatal in spite of treatment. Ulcerative postdysenteric colitis may respond to maintenance of an adequate fluid and electrolyte balance, correction of anemia by blood transfusion, and a high-calorie diet. Sulfasalazine [Azulfidine, S.A.S.-500] or phthalylsulfathiazole [Sulfathalidine] has been administered, but their effectiveness is unpredictable.

Dosage recommendations for treating the various forms of amebiasis appear in

TABLE 2.
RECOMMENDED THERAPY FOR AMEBIASIS*

Type of Infection	Drug of Choice	Alternate Drugs
Asymptomatic	Diloxanide Furoate[1]	Iodoquinol[2] or Metronidazole[3]
Mild to Moderate Intestinal Disease	Metronidazole[3]	A Tetracycline[4] *plus* Iodoquinol[2] or Paromomycin[5] *plus* Iodoquinol[2]
Severe Intestinal Disease	Metronidazole[3]	A Tetracycline[4] *plus* Iodoquinol[2] or Emetine[6] *plus* Iodoquinol[2] or Dehydroemetine[7] *plus* Iodoquinol[2]
Hepatic Abscess	Metronidazole[3]	Dehydroemetine[7] *plus* Chloroquine Phosphate[8] or Emetine[6] *plus* Chloroquine Phosphate[8]

*From the Parasitic Disease Division, Center for Disease Control. Except for emetine and dehydroemetine, all drugs are given orally.

[1] *Adult Dose:* 500 mg tid X 10d. *Pediatric Dose:* 20 mg/kg/day in 3 doses X 10d.

[2] *Adult Dose:* 650 mg tid X 20d. *Pediatric Dose:* 30-40 mg/kg/day in 3 doses X 20d (maximum, 2 g/day).

[3] *Adult Dose:* 750 mg tid X 5-10d. *Pediatric Dose:* 35-50 mg/kg/day in 3 doses X 10d.

[4] *Adult Dose:* 500 mg qid X 10d. *Pediatric Dose:* 10 mg/kg qid X 10d (maximum, 2 g/day).

[5] *Adult Dose:* 25-35 mg/kg/day in 3 doses X 5-10d. *Pediatric Dose:* Same as adult.

[6] *Adult Dose:* 1 mg/kg/day (maximum, 60 mg/day) for up to 5d. *Pediatric Dose:* 0.5 mg/kg bid (maximum, 60 mg/day) for up to 5d.

[7] *Adult Dose:* 1-1.5 mg/kg/day (maximum, 90 mg/day) for up to 5d. *Pediatric Dose:* 1-1.5 mg/kg/day (maximum, 90 mg/day) in 2 doses for up to 5d.

[8] *Adult Dose:* 1 g (500 mg base) daily X 2 then 500 mg (250 mg base) daily X 2-3 weeks. *Pediatric Dose:* 10 mg (base)/kg/day X 21d (maximum, 600 mg/day).

the evaluations and are summarized in Table 2.

Adverse Reactions and Precautions

The adverse reactions produced by the amebicides and the precautions necessary in their use vary. All drugs may cause gastrointestinal disturbances (eg, anorexia, nausea and vomiting, epigastric burning and pain, increased gastrointestinal motility, diarrhea, constipation).

The halogenated hydroxyquinolines (eg, iodoquinol [Yodoxin]) are neurotoxic. The degree of toxicity is related to the compound used, the dose administered, and the duration of therapy. Clioquinol (iodochlorhydroxyquin), a drug no longer available in this country, is the hydroxyquinoline most likely to be associated with serious toxicity. Large doses, even when given for short periods, may cause subacute myelo-optic neuropathy (SMON) and acute cerebral illness, including agitation and retrograde amnesia. Therapeutic doses seldom cause serious toxicity when given for brief periods but permanent optic atrophy and blindness have occurred, particularly when administration has been prolonged. Between 1956 and 1970, an epidemic of SMON involving more than 10,000 cases was recorded in Japan, presumably caused by clioquinol. Children appear to be most susceptible.

For a more detailed discussion of adverse reactions, precautions, and contraindications, see the evaluations.

INDIVIDUAL EVALUATIONS

METRONIDAZOLE
[Flagyl]

This nitroimidazole compound is amebicidal at both intestinal and extraintestinal sites and currently is preferred for all amebic infections except asymptomatic intestinal amebiasis; its effectiveness in asymptomatic cyst carriers remains to be fully evaluated. This drug appears to be effective as a luminal amebicide and is a suitable alternative to iodoquinol or diloxanide. Metronidazole can be used alone or with other drugs. See also the introduction to this section.

The incidence of adverse effects is low and no serious reactions have been reported clinically. The most frequent reaction is nausea; diarrhea occurs less commonly. Other untoward effects include unpleasant taste, furry tongue, glossitis, stomatitis, anorexia, epigastric distress, vomiting, abdominal cramping, constipation, dizziness, ataxia, headache, urticaria, vaginal and urethral burning or discomfort, and, rarely, an unexplained darkening in the color of the urine.

When taken with alcoholic beverages, metronidazole may produce a disulfiram [Antabuse]-type reaction (abdominal distress, nausea, vomiting, headache, and modification of the taste of the alcoholic beverage) caused by accumulation of acetaldehyde due to the ability of metronidazole to interfere with the oxidation of alcohol to carbon dioxide.

Temporary decreases in total leukocyte (particularly polymorphonuclear) counts have been reported following metronidazole therapy; therefore, total and differential white cell counts should be performed once a week if the drug is given for longer than seven days, especially in very young, very old, or debilitated patients or if a second course of therapy is necessary because of relapse or reinfection. Metronidazole should be used with caution in individuals with or prone to blood dyscrasias, since the parent nitroimidazole nucleus has a potential for depressing bone marrow activity. Similarly, it should be used cautiously in individuals with pronounced central nervous system disorders.

Metronidazole has been found to be carcinogenic in mice and, probably, rats but not in hamsters and other animal species thus far tested. It has not been shown to be carcinogenic in man. Since amebiasis can be life-threatening and metronidazole is generally well tolerated, use of the drug is justified, particularly when alternative combination therapy may expose the patient to a greater risk of toxicity.

Metronidazole has been effective in the treatment of amebiasis and trichomoniasis during pregnancy. No complications have been observed and no adverse reactions affecting the fetus have been reported. There is evidence, however, that the drug readily crosses the placenta and it may be the only known drug not used for cancer chemotherapy that has mutagenic activity against certain bacteria at concentrations readily obtainable in body fluids following therapeutic doses. Therefore, it is recommended that metronidazole not be used during the first trimester and be avoided throughout pregnancy if possible until additional data on hazards to the fetus become available. Metronidazole is excreted in breast milk, but no adverse effects have been observed in nursing infants.

ROUTE, USUAL DOSAGE, AND PREPARATIONS. *Oral: Adults*, 750 mg three times daily for five to ten days; *children*, 35 to 50 mg/kg of body weight daily in three divided doses for ten days.

Flagyl (Searle). Tablets 250 mg.

DEHYDROEMETINE DIHYDROCHLORIDE

EMETINE HYDROCHLORIDE

These salts of an ipecac alkaloid are directly amebicidal in the intestinal lumen against trophozoites of *Entamoeba histolytica* but are not active against cysts. They also are used, often in conjunction with other drugs, to treat hepatic abscesses.

The emetines most often are administered by subcutaneous or deep intramuscular injection. Although they are irritating to the gastrointestinal tract, an English preparation of emetine bismuth iodide (EBI) for oral administration is available abroad. No oral preparation is available in the United States. These drugs are not given intravenously since administration by this route may produce severe toxic reactions. The emetines are concentrated in the liver, kidney, spleen, and lung, which may contribute to their efficacy in hepatic amebiasis. It is assumed that the kidney is the major route of excretion in man, but documentation for this is not adequate.

Data on mechanism of action suggest that emetines inhibit polypeptide chain elongation, thereby blocking protein synthesis in eukaryotic but not in prokaryotic cells. Therefore, protein synthesis is inhibited in parasitic and mammalian cells but not in bacteria.

Adverse reactions are observed in 50% to 75% of individuals treated with the emetines. Both drugs have a similar incidence of toxicity, although dehydroemetine may be slightly less cardiotoxic than emetine. The drugs accumulate in the body, and untoward effects occur with increasing frequency as repeated courses are administered. Cardiovascular reactions are the most serious and include precordial pain, dyspnea, tachycardia, hypotension, gallop rhythm, cardiac dilatation, congestive failure, and death. Electrocardiographic changes are those of conduction delay and can be of long duration (average, six weeks); those reported include widening of the QRS complex, prolongation of the P-R and Q-T intervals, changes in the S-T segment, and flattening or inversion of the T wave. If these changes are observed, the drug should be discontinued immediately. Injury to the myocardium, as well as other organs, may occur.

Nausea, vomiting, and diarrhea are sometimes seen even when the drugs are administered parenterally. Because the drugs themselves occasionally cause diarrhea, it may be difficult to assess the response to therapy in patients being treated for amebic dysentery. Headache, debilitating skeletal muscle weakness, stiffness, pain and muscle weakness at the site of injection, as well as eczematous, urticarial, or purpuric lesions also have been observed.

Patients receiving the emetines should be hospitalized and remain in bed during treatment. An electrocardiogram should be performed before therapy is initiated and repeated daily; the heart rate and blood pressure also should be monitored. The emetines should not be used during pregnancy, in patients with heart or kidney disease, or in children unless other therapy is ineffective. These drugs must be used with caution in debilitated or aged patients. If a ten-day course of therapy is not successful, six weeks to two months should elapse before a second course is started to prevent cumulative toxicity.

ROUTES, USUAL DOSAGE, AND PREPARATIONS. EMETINE HYDROCHLORIDE:
Intramuscular (deep), Subcutaneous: *Adults*, 1 mg/kg of body weight daily (maximum, 60 mg daily) in one dose (alternatively, two divided doses may be given if the patient cannot tolerate one dose) for not more than five days; three days usually are sufficient to produce an improvement and allow the use of other drugs (eg, metronidazole). One-half of this amount should be given to underweight, aged, or debilitated patients. *Children*, 1 mg/kg daily (maximum, 10 mg daily for children under 8 years, and 20 mg daily for those over 8 years) in two doses for not more than five days. Multiple injection sites should be used to avoid abscesses.
Drug available generically: Solution 65 mg/ml in 1 ml containers.
DEHYDROEMETINE DIHYDROCHLORIDE:
Intramuscular (deep), Subcutaneous: *Adults*, 1 to 1.5 mg/kg of body weight (maximum, 90 mg) daily in one dose for up to five days; *children*, 1 to 1.5 mg/kg daily in two divided doses for up to five days.
Drug available from the Parasitic Disease Drug Service, Center for Disease Control, Atlanta, Ga 30333.

TETRACYCLINES

These broad spectrum antibiotics are partially active against amebae in the intestinal lumen and wall. They are indirectly amebicidal in that they modify the intestinal flora necessary for amebic viability. Tetracycline and oxytetracycline are the most effective members of this group. They may be used with other drugs to treat invasive intestinal amebiasis but are ineffective in the treatment of asymptomatic cyst carriers (see also the Introduction).

For adverse reactions, precautions, and other uses, see Chapter 73, Tetracyclines.

ROUTE, USUAL DOSAGE, AND PREPARATIONS. OXYTETRACYCLINE, TETRACYCLINE:
Oral: *Adults*, 250 to 500 mg every six hours for up to two weeks; *children*, 10 mg/kg of body weight (maximum, 600 mg) four times daily for ten days.
See Chapter 73 for preparations.

CHLOROQUINE PHOSPHATE
[Aralen Phosphate]

This 4-aminoquinoline compound is amebicidal and is useful in treating hepatic amebic infections, usually in conjunction with emetine or dehydroemetine. Chloroquine is less effective than the emetines but is preferred when it is effective alone because it is less toxic.

Adverse reactions and precautions associated with use of chloroquine in amebiasis are similar to those associated with its use in malaria, except that daily use for a longer period of time may increase the frequency of gastrointestinal disturbances (see the section on Malaria).

ROUTE, USUAL DOSAGE, AND PREPARATIONS.
All doses are expressed in terms of the salt.
Oral: *Adults*, 1 g daily for two days, followed by 500 mg daily for two to three weeks; *children*, 10 mg/kg of body weight (maximum, 600 mg) daily for three weeks.
Drug available generically: Tablets 250 mg (equivalent to 150 mg of base).
Aralen Phosphate (Winthrop). Tablets 500 mg (equivalent to 300 mg of the base).

DILOXANIDE FUROATE
[Furamide]

Diloxanide is an amebicide with limited antibacterial, antifungal, and anthelmintic activity. It is highly effective in the therapy of asymptomatic or mildly symptomatic cyst passers. It is less effective in patients with symptomatic intestinal amebiasis who are passing trophozoites or in those with acute amebic dysentery, and it is of no value in extraintestinal amebiasis. The mechanism of action of this drug is unknown.

Diloxanide is relatively safe. Excessive flatulence is the most common side effect. Infrequently reported adverse reactions include esophagitis, nausea, vomiting, persistent or recurrent diarrhea, abdominal cramps, vague tingling sensations, pruritus, urticaria, and albuminuria. Hematologic and blood chemistry abnormalities have not been noted. Discontinuation of therapy because of adverse reactions is rarely necessary.

Since the safety of diloxanide in pregnancy has not been determined, it should not be given to pregnant women. Also, it should not be administered to children under 2 years.

ROUTE, USUAL DOSAGE, AND PREPARATIONS. *Oral: Adults,* 500 mg three times daily for ten days. *Children 2 years or older,* 20 mg/kg of body weight daily in three divided doses for ten days. The course of treatment may be repeated if the initial course is unsuccessful.

> *Furamide* (The Boots Co. Ltd., Nottingham, England). Tablets 500 mg.
> In the United States, this preparation is available from the Center for Disease Control of the U.S. Public Health Service, Atlanta, Ga 30333.

PAROMOMYCIN SULFATE
[Humatin]

This aminoglycoside is active against amebae in the intestinal lumen. It is directly amebicidal and can be used with other drugs (eg, iodoquinol) to treat mild to moderate intestinal amebiasis (see the Introduction).

Frequently reported adverse reactions include nausea, increased gastrointestinal motility, abdominal pain, and diarrhea. Rash, headache, vertigo, and vomiting have occurred occasionally. Patients should be observed for signs of superinfection. Paromomycin is poorly absorbed from the intact gastrointestinal tract, and most of a single dose is eliminated in the feces. Nevertheless, to avoid absorption (which may cause ototoxicity and nephrotoxicity), the drug should be used with caution in patients with intestinal inflammation or ulcerative lesions.

ROUTE, USUAL DOSAGE, AND PREPARATIONS. *Oral: Adults and children,* 25 to 35 mg/kg of body weight daily in three divided doses with meals for five to ten days. The course may be repeated after a two-week interval.

> *Humatin* (Parke, Davis). Capsules 250 mg; syrup (pediatric) 125 mg/5 ml (strengths expressed in terms of the base).

IODOQUINOL (Diiodohydroxyquin)
[Yodoxin]

This organic iodine compound acts against amebae in the intestinal lumen. It can be used alone in the treatment of asymptomatic intestinal amebiasis or combined with other drugs in other common forms of amebiasis (see the introduction to this section). Iodoquinol also has been used in the prophylaxis of "travelers' diarrhea," but there is no evidence that it is effective and the possible adverse effects greatly outweigh any questionable benefit. It should not be used to treat nonspecific diarrhea, particularly in children, because of its potential toxicity.

Occasional adverse reactions include nausea, abdominal cramps, pruritus ani, rash, acne, and slight enlargement of the thyroid gland. Iodoquinol has caused subacute myelo-optic neuropathy (SMON) but not as often as clioquinol (iodochlorhydroxyquin), a drug no longer available in the United States. SMON is characterized by muscle pain and weakness, usually below the T-12 vertebra; painful dysesthesias, especially of the limbs, often associated with significant alteration of gait; and, in some instances, optic atrophy.

SMON can occur when moderate to large doses are given for three weeks or more. While these symptoms regress following discontinuation of the drug, they are not always completely reversible. Iodoquinol interferes with the results of some thyroid function tests (eg, protein-bound iodine) for several months and is contraindicated in patients hypersensitive to iodine or in those with liver disease.

ROUTE, USUAL DOSAGE, AND PREPARATIONS. *Oral: Adults,* 650 mg three times daily after meals for up to three weeks; *children,* 30 to 40 mg/kg of body weight daily in two or three doses (maximum, 2 g daily) for up to three weeks. If required, the course may be repeated after a two- or three-week interval.

> Drug available generically: Tablets 650 mg.
> *Yodoxin* (Glenwood). Tablets 210 mg; powder 25 g.

CARBARSONE

This organic arsenic compound is active against amebae in the lumen of the intestine. It has been used alone in chronic amebiasis without hepatic involvement and as an adjunct in other common forms of the disease. Although carbarsone is still available for medicinal use, it is obsolete as an amebicide because less toxic and more effective drugs are available.

> Drug available generically: Capsules 250 mg.

TOXOPLASMOSIS

Toxoplasmosis is caused by the obligate intracellular parasite, *Toxoplasma gondii*. This protozoan is worldwide in distribution and shows a remarkable lack of specificity for host, infecting a wide variety of creatures ranging from poikilotherms to man. Felines are known to be definitive hosts harboring the enteric sexual cycle (oocysts are shed in the feces) and extraintestinal asexual forms. Other animals, including man, are intermediate hosts in which only the asexual forms (ie, the tachyzoites or proliferative forms, the bradyzoites or encysted forms). Many of these animals and man may harbor and pass the parasite without clear evidence of disease. The infection can be contracted by ingestion of cysts, usually from inadequately cooked or raw meat or accidental ingestion of oocysts from cat feces.

When proliferative disease develops, it may vary from an almost inapparent condition to a severe systemic disease that may progress to encephalitis and death. The severity of the disease and the danger it poses appears to depend in large part upon whether the infection is congenital (a rare occurrence in the United States) or acquired. Congenital toxoplasmosis usually is more hazardous; the eyes, brain, and other organs may be severely damaged. Congenital toxoplasmosis displays a characteristic syndrome of hydrocephalus, occasionally microcephaly with cerebral calcification, hepatosplenomegaly with jaundice, and bilateral retinochoroiditis. The disease may not be apparent at birth and appear later in life. When present in its complete form, the congenital disease usually is fatal.

In adults, acquired infection often is subclinical. The most common symptomatic manifestations are retinochoroiditis (although eye involvement in the United States is uncommon), lymphadenopathy, fever, and, occasionally, a rash on the palms and soles. The most serious consequence of the disease is meningoencephalitis. Since tissues other than the eye and nervous system may be involved, toxoplasmosis may mimic other diseases, including atypical pneumonia, and may cause myocarditis that can result in heart failure. A mononucleosis-like syndrome (prolonged low-grade fever, malaise, and enlargement of multiple lymph nodes) may occur in adults as a form of mild infection.

The treatment of choice for toxoplasmosis is the combination of sulfadiazine and pyrimethamine [Daraprim], which seems to have synergistic effects. These compounds alter the folic acid cycle of *Toxoplasma*; pyrimethamine modifies the utilization of folic acid, whereas sulfadiazine interferes with the biosynthesis of this compound. For adults, pyrimethamine usually is given in an initial dose of 100 mg, followed by a maintenance dose of 25 mg daily. Sulfadiazine may be given in an initial dose of 2 to 4 g, followed by 1 g every four to six hours. If the eyes are involved, therapy is continued for about five weeks.

Pyrimethamine may deplete folic acid stores to the extent that reversible bone marrow depression occurs. Folinic acid (leucovorin), which does not reduce the effectiveness of pyrimethamine but does reduce the incidence of bone marrow depression, may be given orally three times each week to patients receiving pyrimethamine. For information on the sulfonamides, see Chapter 77. Pyrimethamine is discussed in the section on Malaria in this chapter.

PNEUMOCYSTOSIS

Pneumocystosis is caused by the sporozoan parasite *Pneumocystis carinii*. It is an opportunistic organism that usually does not cause infection unless immune responses are impaired and was not recognized as a disease entity until 1942. Children are more susceptible than adults, and individuals receiving immunosuppressive drugs are most susceptible. The infection may be diagnosed by identification of the organism or serological testing. The organism is most readily apparent in lung biopsy material or tracheal brushing.

The symptoms of early pneumocystosis are usually generalized and vague and include frequent dry cough, dyspnea and/or tachypnea, chest discomfort, and marked pallor. The most common and consistent finding is cyanosis, particularly of the perioral region. Infants will have various feeding difficulties, fail to thrive, and occasionally will have a foamy saliva in the mouth.

In overt disease, a condition designated as interstitial plasma cell pneumonia occurs in which there is infiltration of the lungs and the lung tissue takes on a honeycombed appearance. If untreated, interstitial plasma cell pneumonia may be fatal in more than 50% of patients. Death is often sudden with few, if any, premonitory signs.

Some of the diamidine drugs (eg, pentamidine) are known to have appreciable value in treating pneumocystosis (see the section on Leishmaniases and Trypanosomiases for a discussion of pentamidine and related compounds). Early stages of the disease usually respond more readily to these drugs than does interstitial plasma cell pneumonia. Many antibiotics have been tried in this latter condition without much success. However, the combination of sulfamethoxazole and trimethoprim [Bactrim, Septra] has been used with good results. Some authorities are beginning to consider this preparation as the possible therapy of choice (see Chapter 77, Sulfonamides and Related Compounds, for a discussion of this mixture).

ISOSPOROSIS

Infections by most coccidial parasites are of far greater concern in fowl and animals, in whom they may cause diseases that are serious and potentially fatal, than in man, in whom the disease is relatively benign. A type of human coccidiosis (isosporosis) is caused by *Isospora belli* or *I. hominis* (intracellular parasites that are harbored in the gut after transmission by contact with contaminated fowl, animals, or their excreta) and is self-limiting, resolving in two to four weeks without treatment. It is

characterized by a subacute febrile syndrome, headache, anorexia, and a variety of gastrointestinal symptoms including diarrhea, abdominal tenderness, and abdominal distention.

Bismuth salicylate has been used with some success in the symptomatic treatment of isosporosis. All other compounds commonly used to treat protozoal disease characterized by gastrointestinal disturbances have little, if any, beneficial effect and do not appear to shorten the duration of this disease.

Selected References

Chemoprophylaxis of malaria. *Morbid Mortal Week Rep* 27(suppl):81-90, (March 10) 1978.

Drugs for parasitic infections. *Med Lett Drugs Ther* 20:17-24, 1978.

Beck JW, Davies JE: *Medical Parasitology*, ed 2. St Louis, CV Mosby Co, 1976.

Botero D: Chemotherapy of human intestinal parasitic diseases. *Annu Rev Pharmacol Toxicol* 18:1-15, 1978.

Fisher MH, Wang CC: Antiparasitic agents, in Clarke FH (ed): *Annual Reports in Medicinal Chemistry*. New York, Academic Press, 1978, vol 13, 130-138.

Gazder AJ, Banerjee M: Single-dose treatment of giardiasis in children: Comparison of tinidazole and metronidazole. *Curr Med Res Opin* 5:164-168, 1977.

Hunter GW III, et al: *Tropical Medicine*, ed 5. Philadelphia, WB Saunders Co, 1976.

Krogstad DJ, et al: Amebiasis. *N Engl J Med* 298:262-265, 1978.

Krupp IM: A pet disease: Visceral larva migrans. *Drug Ther* 8:143-151, (May) 1978.

Marsden PD (ed): Intestinal parasites. *Clin Gastroenterol* 7:1-243, 1978.

Pratt WB: *Chemotherapy of Infection*. New York, Oxford University Press, 1977, 347-372.

Rozman RS: Chemotherapy of malaria. *Annu Rev Pharmacol Toxicol* 13: 127-152, 1973.

Schantz PM, Glickman LT: Toxocaral visceral larva migrans. *N Engl J Med* 298:436-439, 1978.

Schultz MC: Antiprotozoan agents, in Kagen BM (ed): *Antimicrobial Therapy*, ed 2. Philadelphia, WB Saunders Co, 1974, 162-169.

Singh G, Kumar S: Short course of single daily dosage treatment with tinidazole and metronidazole in intestinal amoebiasis: Comparative study. *Curr Med Res Opin* 5:157-160, 1977.

Steck EA: Current approaches in the chemotherapy of leishmaniases. Paper read before the first meeting of the WHO Scientific Working Group on Leishmaniases held in Geneva, Dec 13-20, 1977.

Steck EA: *The Chemotherapy of Protozoan Diseases.* Washington, DC, Division of Medicinal Chemistry, Walter Reed Army Institute of Research, vols 1-4, 1974.

Steck EA: Leishmaniases. *Prog Drug Res* 18:289-351, 1974.

Swami B, et al: Tinidazole and metronidazole in treatment of intestinal amoebiasis. *Curr Med Res Opin* 5:152-156, 1977.

Zaman V (ed): Symposium on common diseases. I. Amoebiasis, giardiasis, and trichomoniasis. *Drugs* 15(suppl 1):1-60, 1978.

Parasitic worm infections are a major cause of disease in many areas of the world. Helminthiasis is often associated with squalid living conditions, but poor sanitation is not an absolute prerequisite to infection. Some parasites are so ubiquitous and easily transmitted that infection may be viewed as a social disease. As an example, ascariasis is the most common of all clinically significant human helminthiases. Although it is most prevalent in the tropics, infection occurs worldwide and affects all levels of society. Approximately one-third of the world population (more than a billion people) host this parasite.

Many people harboring worms are asymptomatic or nearly so and frequently are in no physical danger from the parasite. Complete eradication of intestinal helminths is an absolute goal, therefore, only when the worms have a high pathogenic potential or multiply within the human host. Therapy to relieve symptoms and decrease the worm burden may be sufficient in those less seriously affected, and no therapy may be needed in asymptomatic patients with self-limiting infection. Nevertheless, patients living in countries with a relatively high standard of living who can avail themselves of individualized therapy should be treated for all helminthic infections diagnosed unless the side effects of treatment are potentially more dangerous or unpleasant than the infection. Ideally, such individualized treatment should be carried out throughout the world, but often it is not practical to effect radical cures of helminthic diseases in developing countries where members of a community cannot be effectively treated individually or, frequently, even en masse, because of the prohibitive costs of medication, limited medical facilities, and great potential for reinfection. It is apparent, therefore, that successful control of helminthiasis involves more than simple application of chemotherapeutic measures. Equally important adjunctive techniques include removal of patients from the environment in which they were infected or, where possible, cleansing the environment of the offending parasite. Similarly, knowledge of when to treat and what symptoms or problems precede complications is of considerable value to the physician.

The term anthelmintic properly refers not only to those agents that act locally to expel worms from the gastrointestinal tract but also to those that work systemically to eliminate helminths that have migrated into the body tissues. Most common intestinal parasites can be eliminated with reasonable certainty and safety by using an appropriate anthelmintic.

The relative specificity of anthelmintic drugs usually necessitates accurate diagnosis, although this may be less essential with use of the newer, broader spectrum agents (eg, mebendazole [Vermox], pyrantel [Antiminth], thiabendazole [Mintezol]). Parasites occasionally can be identified by gross examination of the stool, but more often it is necessary to submit an appropriate specimen (stool, blood, urine, sputum, aspirate, or biopsy) to a parasitology laboratory for definitive diagnosis.

When treating complex infections such as schistosomiasis, it may be difficult to evaluate the effectiveness of therapy. Criteria for satisfactory progress when treating most helminthic infections include relief of signs and symptoms, absence of

CLASSIFICATION OF THE MAJOR HELMINTHS
AND DRUGS USED TO TREAT HELMINTHIASIS

Phylum Nemathelminthes — Class or Subclass NEMATODA (Roundworms)

Genus and Species	Common Name	Drug(s) of Choice	Alternate Drugs
Ascaris lumbricoides	Roundworm	Pyrantel pamoate Mebendazole	Piperazine Thiabendazole Pyrvinium pamoate Bephenium hydroxynaphthoate
Enterobius (Oxyuris) vermicularis	Pinworm	Mebendazole Pyrantel pamoate	Piperazine Pyrvinium pamoate Thiabendazole
Trichuris trichiura	Whipworm	Mebendazole	Thiabendazole
Strongyloides stercoralis	Threadworm	Thiabendazole	Mebendazole
Necator americanus	New World or American Hookworm (distribution worldwide)	Pyrantel pamoate Mebendazole	Bephenium hydroxynaphthoate Thiabendazole Tetrachloroethylene
Ancylostoma duodenale	Old World, European, or Common Hookworm (distribution worldwide)	Pyrantel pamoate Bephenium hydroxynaphthoate	Mebendazole Thiabendazole Tetrachloroethylene
A. braziliense	Cutaneous Larva Migrans	Thiabendazole (topical)	Thiabendazole (oral) Diethylcarbamazine citrate Ethyl chloride spray Carbon dioxide snow
Wuchereria bancrofti	Filarial Worms	Diethylcarbamazine citrate	None
W. (Brugia) malayi	Filarial Worms	Diethylcarbamazine citrate	None
Loa loa	Filarial Worms	Diethylcarbamazine citrate	None
Onchocerca volvulus	Filarial Worms	Diethylcarbamazine citrate	None
Dracunculus medinensis	Guineaworm	Niridazole	Metronidazole
Trichinella spiralis	Pork Roundworm	Aspirin[1]	Thiabendazole (plus corticosteroids)[2]
Toxocara canis, T. cati	Visceral Larva Migrans	Thiabendazole (plus corticosteroids [eg, 20 to 40 mg prednisone daily] if symptoms are severe or there is ocular involvement)	Diethylcarbamazine citrate

	Genus and Species	Common Name	Drug(s) of Choice	Alternate Drugs
Phylum Platyhelminthes (Flatworms) — **Class or Subclass** TREMATODA (Flukes)	*Schistosoma haematobium*	Blood Flukes	Niridazole Stibocaptate Metrifonate	Antimony potassium tartrate
	S. mansoni		Niridazole Stibocaptate Oxamniquine	Antimony potassium tartrate Hycanthone
	S. japonicum		Antimony potassium tartrate Niridazole	Stibocaptate
	Clonorchis sinensis	Liver Flukes	Chloroquine phosphate	Dehydroemetine
	Fasciola hepatica		Bithionol	Emetine Dehydroemetine
	Paragonimus westermani	Lung Flukes	Bithionol	Chloroquine phosphate (6 weeks or more of therapy)
	P. kellicotti		Bithionol	Chloroquine phosphate (6 weeks or more of therapy)
	Fasciolopsis buski	Intestinal Fluke	Hexylresorcinol[3] Tetrachloroethylene[3]	Bephenium hydroxynaphthoate
CESTODA (Tapeworms)	*Taenia saginata*	Beef Tapeworm	Niclosamide	Paromomycin Mebendazole Quinacrine hydrochloride
	T. solium	Pork Tapeworm	Niclosamide	Paromomycin Mebendazole Quinacrine hydrochloride
	Diphyllobothrium latum	Fish Tapeworm	Niclosamide	Paromomycin Quinacrine hydrochloride
	Hymenolepis nana	Dwarf Tapeworm	Niclosamide	Paromomycin Quinacrine hydrochloride
	Echinococcus granulosus	Hydatid Disease	Mebendazole	None
	E. multilocularis[4]	Alveolar Hydatid Disease	Mebendazole	None

[1]*No specific treatment exists, but aspirin may be the only agent required in most patients.*

[2]*May be lifesaving in severe infections.*

[3]*These agents are so effective that no alternative drug need be considered.*

[4]*Wilson JF, et al: Clinical trial of mebendazole in treatment of alveolar hydatid disease. Am Rev Resp Dis 118:747-757, 1978.*

the parasite in blood or stool, or, if parasites persist, reduction in the fecal parasitic egg count.

When the initial course of therapy using the drug of choice has not effected a cure and alternative therapy is more hazardous, a second attempt at treatment with the first-choice drug should be undertaken before another anthelmintic is prescribed. In mixed infections, the effect of therapy on each species present must be considered. A drug effective against one type of helminth may irritate another and cause it to migrate from the intestines into body tissues where it may pose a grave danger to the host.

The helminths that commonly infect man belong to two different phyla: (1) the Nemathelminthes, which is composed of the class Nematoda, the roundworms, and (2) the Platyhelminthes or flatworms, which encompass the class Trematoda (flukes) and subclass Cestoda (tapeworms). For classification and suggested drug therapy, see the Table. Except where indicated, those compounds not marketed in this country are available from the Parasitic Division, Center for Disease Control, Atlanta, Georgia, 30333, telephone (404) 329-3670.

Parasitic Characteristics Important to Therapy

Ascariasis (Roundworm Infection): This is the most common helminthic disease worldwide; it is most prevalent in tropical countries. Infection occurs following ingestion of embryonated eggs. Larvae hatch in the small intestine and migrate by way of the venous and lymphatic systems to the lungs, where they travel to the air sacs, up the pulmonary tree to the epiglottis, and are swallowed. Upon reaching the small intestinal lumen for the second time, the larvae develop into adult worms.

Symptoms and signs may include vague complaints of abdominal distress (epigastric pain, nausea, vomiting, and anorexia), cough, fever, and pulmonary infiltration. Ascariasis should always be treated since it has the potential for causing serious com-

plications, even in patients who are asymptomatic, as a result of the migration of adult worms into the pancreatic and bile ducts, gallbladder, or liver; complete obstruction of the appendix or intestinal lumen also may occur. Byproducts or breakdown products of worms, both living and dead, may cause severe reactions in individuals who are sensitized to these products.

Enterobiasis (Pinworm Infection): This is the most common parasitic disease in the United States. Principal symptoms are pruritus ani and vulvae that may become severe enough to result in persistent scratching during the day and restlessness or insomnia at night; however, most individuals are asymptomatic. Serious conditions that may be associated with enterobiasis include vaginitis and, rarely, salpingitis, appendicitis, or peritoneal granulomata. Because of the relative ubiquity of *Enterobius vermicularis*, it is important that good personal hygienic techniques, including careful hand washing following defecation or urination (especially for the female), be instituted along with drug therapy to prevent reinfection.

Trichuriasis (Whipworm Infection): This infection seldom produces discernible symptoms, although some individuals (especially children) with a heavy worm burden may develop diarrhea or dysentery. When the worm load is extremely heavy, rectal prolapse may occur exposing a mucosa covered with small white worms. Also, anemia may be observed in malnourished children. Chronic appendicitis, finger clubbing, and severe cachexia have been reported as a result of the infection. Patients with heavy infections must be treated.

Strongyloidiasis (Threadworm Infection): This infection carries a serious potential pathologic risk and should always be treated, even in asymptomatic individuals. If left untreated, a cyclic autoinfection may develop in which larvae penetrate the colon or the perianal mucosa, migrate through the systemic circulation, and reenter the intestine. Such an infection may be maintained for many years and result in a massive worm burden. Diarrhea, malabsorption syndromes, duodenitis (clinically resembling peptic ulcer), eosinophilia, and pneumonia may occur. Severe autoinfection can be fatal, especially in patients receiving corticosteroids or other immunosuppressive drugs. Some asymptomatic infections become overwhelming following the use of such agents. Despite the possible seriousness of strongyloidiasis, the usual case of infection is asymptomatic or has symptoms referable only to duodenitis.

Uncinariasis (Hookworm Infection): Hookworm larvae penetrate the skin or are swallowed (frequently with *Ancylostoma duodenale*) and penetrate the intestinal mucosa. They then pass to the lymphatics and venules and migrate to the lungs, up the bronchi and trachea, and are swallowed. When they reach the small intestine, they attach themselves to the luminal walls by means of a buccal capsule. Ulcerations may be created at the site of attachment as the worms ingest blood from the mucosal vessels. Chronic blood loss is a characteristic of uncinariasis and individuals who have a marginal iron intake or inadequate iron stores (eg, malnourished children, some menstruating women) are especially prone to anemia. Others with satisfactory iron intake may develop anemia if the worm burden is sufficiently great to cause blood loss that cannot be compensated by the normal erythropoietic mechanisms. Those with light worm burdens are asymptomatic and may not require treatment in the absence of anemia.

The main symptoms and signs of severe uncinariasis are the same as those of progressive iron deficiency anemia, a condition that must be corrected at the same time that anthelmintic therapy is begun. Additional symptoms include abdominal fullness, epigastric pain, and cough due to pneumonitis that occurs when large numbers of worms are migrating through the lungs. Local erythema and pruritus ("ground itch") may occur at the site of skin penetration.

Determining which of the two hookworm species is present may be difficult but is desirable, if possible, because of the wide difference in cure rate of the two species. This can be done only by careful examination of the adult worm or by culturing the eggs and examining the infective third-stage larva, since the eggs of the two major species are almost identical. In the United States, there has been a marked reduction in the incidence of hookworm infection (except for some areas in the southern United States) and what remains is almost universally *Necator*. Some cases are imported and the species usually is unknown at the time of treatment.

Cutaneous Larva Migrans (Creeping Eruption): This infection of the skin is caused by a species of hookworm common in cats and dogs. It occurs on the southeastern and gulf coasts of the United States and many tropical and subtropical areas of the world. Filiform larvae penetrate and migrate about in the skin, where they remain for up to several months. An allergic reaction to the worm causes intense pruritus which leads to scratching, possible excoriation of the skin, and secondary infection.

Filariasis: This disease is transferred to man by insect bite. Allergic reactions may occur during therapy due to disintegration of microfilariae, particularly in cases of onchocerciasis and loiasis. These reactions may be serious or even life-threatening when treating onchocerciasis and may cause meningoencephalitis and nephrotic syndrome in patients with loiasis. It has been recommended by some that subcutaneous nodules containing adult worms should be excised before drug therapy is begun in order to minimize allergic manifestations.

Dracunculiasis (Guineaworm Infection): The adult worms emerge, usually from the foot or leg, approximately one year after infection. A few weeks before they appear, patients often develop urticaria. If the condition is recognized before the worms burst through the skin and cause an inflammatory reaction, they can be extracted easily with a forceps. Intense, painful, inflammatory reactions, often with secondary bacterial infections and tetanus, may occur if the disease is untreated or treated improperly.

Trichinosis (Pork Roundworm Infection): This infection may cause gastrointestinal upset followed by temperature elevation, myalgias, periorbital edema, and eosinophilia. The great majority of affected individuals recover following the use of aspirin and supportive therapy but cysts remain in the muscles. A small percentage will develop life-threatening complications such as congestive heart failure, meningitis, neuritis, or a Guillain-Barre type of syndrome.

Visceral Larva Migrans: This condition denotes the prolonged migration of larvae of animal nematodes in human tissue other than the skin. It is commonly caused by dog or cat ascarids, but can be the result of other nematodes. The infection is manifested as persistent hypereosinophilia, hepatomegaly, and, frequently, as pneumonitis, particularly in children. It also rarely causes meningoencephalitis and ocular involvement. It usually is self-limiting over an 18-month period, is diagnosed on suspicion aroused by the eosinophilia, and is confirmed by serologic examination. Generally no specific therapy is required unless the infection is severe or involves the eye.

Schistosomiasis (Blood Fluke Infection): Freshwater snails are the intermediate hosts for these flukes, which penetrate the skin to produce infection. Management and treatment of this disease may be difficult and are still controversial. In the early stages, schistosomiasis may respond well to chemotherapy (see the Table). However, in later stages, intestinal and hepatic fibrosis develop, pathology that cannot be reversed by drug treatment. Under these circumstances, absolute parasitologic cure is not always attainable or even essential; reduction of the fecal egg count often is a more realistic goal. A new drug, prazaquantel, is undergoing clinical investigation for antischistosomal activity. It appears to be potentially valuable, and many experts believe it may become the drug of choice in treating schistosomiasis.

Fascioliasis (Liver Fluke Infection): This is the only fluke infection acquired in the continental United States. It usually results from ingesting watercress and other aquatic plants collected from areas contaminated by animal excreta; a snail is required as an intermediate host. Currently there is no completely safe and effective therapy for fascioliasis. In the past, emetine was used but has been largely abandoned because of toxicity. Oral bithionol and intramuscular dehydroemetine presently are the favored drugs.

Clonorchiasis (Oriental Liver Fluke Infection): This infection is sometimes seen in patients who have been to the Far East and now is commonly seen in the United States in Southeast Asian refugees. The parasite may live for 40 years in man. No satisfactory treatment is available and, because of its probable limited pathogenicity, aggressive chemotherapy with potentially toxic drugs is unwarranted except in heavy infections or in patients with biliary tract symptomatology or disease.

Paragonimiasis (Lung Fluke Infection): *Paragonimus westermani*, which occurs in the Far East, is the primary etiologic agent of disease in man. *P. kellicotti* appears to be limited to the Americas, but it, along with a number of other species that are distributed worldwide, rarely infects man. The primary manifestations of disease are pulmonary, often with hemoptysis, but gastrointestinal and central nervous system involvement also have been reported. Bithionol is an effective drug for treatment except when the parasite is localized in the brain or spinal cord. If the patient cannot tolerate bithionol, chloroquine may be tried, although it is less effective.

Fasciolopsiasis (Intestinal Fluke Infection): The giant intestinal fluke occurs primarily in Southeast Asia (see Table).

Cestodiases (Tapeworm Infections): Cestodiases, which include beef, pork, fish, and dwarf tapeworm infections and infections caused by *Echinococcus granulosus* (hydatid disease), should be treated when diagnosed, with the possible exception of some cases of hydatid infection. Individuals may harbor single or multiple tapeworms for years and remain asymptomatic. Often, infection with the larger species first becomes apparent when a segment (proglottid) is passed in the stool. Of the large tapeworms, only *Taenia solium* (pork tapeworm) infections require special consideration during therapy because the eggs of this tapeworm can develop into the larval (cysticercus) stage in man. Although cysticercosis usually is acquired by the ingestion of *T. solium* eggs, it is possible that during therapy eggs released from the adult tapeworm into the upper levels of the small intestine could be regurgitated into the acid environment of the stomach necessary for hatching the larvae. The hatched larvae then pass back into the small intestine from which they invade tissue and cause cysticercosis. For this reason, drugs that are prone to cause vomiting may be undesirable for the treatment of pork tapeworm infection. Dwarf tapeworm is the most common tapeworm affecting man in this country. Infections involving large numbers of worms (colonies of up to 1,000) have been reported. Since the worms are embedded in intestinal mucosa, infection often is refractory to treatment and intensive therapy is necessary to achieve a cure. Heavy infections of dwarf tapeworm may cause diarrhea. Hydatid disease is preferably treated with surgery, but recent work has shown that mebendazole may be effective, particularly to shrink cysts preoperatively.

INDIVIDUAL EVALUATIONS

ANTIMONY POTASSIUM TARTRATE

Antimony potassium tartrate is the most potent and most toxic trivalent antimony compound. It is one of the drugs of choice for treating infections caused by *Schistosoma japonicum*. Some experts use it for all cases of *S. japonicum* infection, while others use it only when there is schistosomal liver disease and niridazole is contraindicated. Cure rates vary widely and

depend upon the dose that can be tolerated by the patient and the stage of the disease. Less toxic agents are used to treat *S. mansoni* and *S. haematobium* infections. The trivalent antimonials exert their effect by blocking the pathway for anaerobic metabolism of glucose in the parasite by inhibiting the rate-limiting enzyme, phosphofructokinase. Anemia or poor nutritional status should be corrected prior to treatment with antimony potassium tartrate.

Lack of patient compliance is the main cause of therapeutic failure with this compound. Patients will discontinue taking the drug because of adverse effects or discomfort associated with multiple intravenous injections. Adverse reactions include paroxysms of coughing and vomiting during injection of the drug. Nausea and vomiting may persist even after injection. If injection is too rapid, circulatory collapse may occur. Reversible electrocardiographic changes are common during therapy but usually do not necessitate discontinuation of the drug. Other adverse effects reported are pruritus, rashes, colic, headache, facial edema, diarrhea, dizziness, dyspnea, hypotension, syncope, shock, bradycardia, myalgia, severe arthralgia, weakness, renal damage, and, occasionally, jaundice (secondary to hepatitis or hemolytic anemia) and anaphylactoid reactions.

Antiemetics should not be used in conjunction with antimony potassium tartrate because they mask nausea and vomiting, which may be signs of progressive hepatic necrosis caused by toxic doses of the drug. Treatment should be discontinued if vomiting is severe or persistent or if a blood dyscrasia (eg, thrombocytopenia), albuminuria, purpura, fever, or severe dermatitis develops. This drug is contraindicated in the presence of febrile infections, cardiac or renal disease, and hepatic damage not caused by schistosomiasis.

ROUTE, USUAL DOSAGE, AND PREPARATIONS. *Intravenous*: The drug should be given two hours after a light meal, and the patient should remain recumbent for one hour following treatment. Extreme care must be exercised to prevent extravasation of the drug in order to prevent painful cellulitis and necrosis. Antimony potassium tartrate should be given extremely slowly in a 0.5% (5 mg/ml) solution freshly prepared in water for injection or 5% dextrose injection; it is administered on alternate days according to the following schedule: For *S. japonicum* infections, *adults*, 8 ml initially, increased by 4 ml with each subsequent dose until the 11th day, when 28 ml is given; administration of this dose then is continued on alternate days until a total of 500 ml (2.5 g) has been given.

Drug available generically: Powder.

tion is lacking on the safety of bephenium during pregnancy; therefore, the possible risk to the fetus should be weighed against the expected therapeutic benefits if this agent is considered for use in pregnant women.

ROUTE, USUAL DOSAGE, AND PREPARATIONS. *Oral*: *Adults and chilren over 22.5 kg, 5 g twice daily; children under 22.5 kg, 2.5 g twice daily*. This dose is given for one day in *A. duodenale* infections and for three days in *N. americanus* infections.

Alcopar (Burroughs Wellcome). Not available in the United States.

BEPHENIUM HYDROXYNAPHTHOATE
[Alcopar]

DIETHYLCARBAMAZINE CITRATE
[Hetrazan]

Bephenium is one of the drugs of choice for treating hookworm infections. It is active against both species of hookworm but is more effective against *Ancylostoma duodenale* infections, with cure rates of 80% to 98% reported following one-day treatment. Administration on three successive days may be necessary to remove *Necator americanus*. Bephenium also is useful in mixed hookworm and roundworm infections, since usual doses have some effect against *Ascaris lumbricoides*. It has been tried in *Trichuris trichiura* infections with little success.

Bephenium is only slightly absorbed from the gastrointestinal tract, and less than 0.5% of the drug is excreted in the urine following oral administration. It is usually administered in flavored vehicles to mask its bitter taste.

Serious adverse effects have not been reported, but bephenium may cause nausea and vomiting. Dehydration, electrolyte imbalance, and diarrhea should be corrected before the drug is used. Informa-

This synthetic piperazine derivative is the drug of choice in the treatment of filariasis caused by *Wuchereria bancrofti*, *W. (Brugia) malayi, Loa loa, Dipetalonema streptocerca, Mansonella ozzardi*, and *Onchocerca volvulus*. It destroys the microfilariae of all these species. Diethylcarbamazine also either kills or sterilizes adult females of *Wuchereria* species, including *Brugia malayi* and some of the adults of *Loa loa* and *D. perstans*, but has little effect on the microfilariae of *D. perstans*. The adults of *Onchocerca* are not killed and either must be removed surgically or killed by treatment with suramin sodium; otherwise, microfilariae generally reappear a few months after treatment with diethylcarbamazine. There is some evidence that diethylcarbamazine is effective against cutaneous larva migrans caused by the larvae of *Ancylostoma braziliense*.

Diethylcarbamazine is rapidly absorbed from the gastrointestinal tract. Peak blood levels are reached in approximately four hours. Renal excretion of a single dose, both as unchanged compound and metabolites, is complete in 48 hours. The exact mechanism of action is unknown. Although diethylcarbamazine is a derivative of piperazine, unsubstituted piperazine has no filaricidal action.

Adverse reactions directly attributable to diethylcarbamazine are usually mild and consist of headache, dizziness, weakness, nausea, and vomiting. Allergic reactions, caused by substances released when microfilariae are destroyed, are usually mild in patients with wuchereriasis but may be serious in those with onchocerciasis and loiasis. They include pedal edema that may be severe, intense pruritus, dermatitis, fever, colic, and lymphadenitis. In addition, tachycardia is sometimes seen. Allergic encephalopathy (reaction to dead microfilariae) has occurred rarely in patients treated for loiasis. These reactions usually subside within three to seven days, and even larger doses than those that initiated the adverse effects may be administered without further problems. The concomitant administration of antihistamines or corticosteroids is advisable to minimize allergic effects, particularly when there is ocular involvement with onchocerciasis. If reactions are severe, the dosage should be reduced or treatment interrupted.

ROUTE, USUAL DOSAGE, AND PREPARATIONS. *Oral: Adults and children*, for infections caused by *Loa loa, W. bancrofti, B. malayi*, and *D. perstans*, 2 mg/kg of body weight three times daily after meals for 10 to 30 days. Patients with onchocerciasis should receive appropriate additional treatment to kill adult parasites. Because severe Herxheimer-like reactions are more likely when treating *O. volvulus* infections, an alternative *adult* dosage schedule for either systemic or ocular onchocerciasis is: Initially, 25 mg daily for three days, increased by increments of 1 mg/kg daily in divided doses up to a maximum of 3 mg/kg three times daily, which is maintained for 21 days. *Infants and small children* should be given 0.5 mg/kg three times daily (maximum, 25 mg daily) for three days; 1 mg/kg three times daily (maximum, 50 mg

daily) for three days; 1.5 mg/kg three times daily (maximum, 100 mg daily) for three days; and 2 mg/kg three times daily (maximum, 150 mg daily) for two to three weeks.

Some experts believe that *Loa loa* infections should be treated in the same manner as *O. volvulus* infections because of the potential for severe reactions.

Hetrazan (Lederle). Tablets 50 mg.

HYCANTHONE
[Etrenol]

Hycanthone, a metabolite of lucanthone, is useful for treating infections of *Schistosoma mansoni* and *S. haematobium*; cure rates of 65% to 90% have been reported. It is less effective in young children than in older children and adults. Some *S. mansoni* parasites have developed resistance to this compound.

Side effects include pain at the site of injection, nausea, vomiting, anorexia, and dizziness. The drug has been shown to be mutagenic, teratogenic, and carcinogenic under certain experimental conditions in animals. Postnecrotic cirrhosis or death may occur if hycanthone is given to patients with hepatic necrosis and has even been observed after use of this drug in patients without pre-existing liver disease. This anthelmintic is contraindicated in all cases of schistosomal infections in which the patient has a tender, enlarged liver or a history of jaundice and in those with concomitant bacterial or viral infections. Because of the potential severe toxicity of hycanthone, it is a controversial drug but is approved by the World Health Organization and its use is widespread.

ROUTE, USUAL DOSAGE, AND PREPARATIONS. *Intramuscular*: 7.5 mg/kg of body weight as a single dose; this dose may be repeated in three months.

Etrenol (Winthrop). Powder 2 mg in 2 ml containers. Not available in the United States.

MEBENDAZOLE
[Vermox]

Mebendazole has the broadest spectrum of any anthelmintic drug. It is the primary drug of choice in enterobiasis and trichuriasis. Single doses have produced cure rates of 90% and 100% in the former and, after multiple doses, cure rates as high as 94% (particularly in children) have been reported in the latter. However, retreatment may be necessary in massive whipworm infections (more than 40,000 eggs/g of feces). Mebendazole may decrease the whipworm fecal egg count by 70% to 99% even in refractory infections.

Mebendazole is one of the drugs of choice for treating both types of hookworm infections. Cure rates of approximately 95% have been reported after multiple doses, and the fecal egg count is reduced markedly for both species of hookworm that commonly infect man. Mebendazole also is a first choice alternative drug for treating ascariasis (it is very effective in a three-day course); however, since a single dose of pyrantel pamoate is just as effective, the latter agent is the primary drug of choice. In a small number of cases, children with heavy *Ascaris* infections treated with mebendazole have had worms migrate to the mouth. This drug is effective to a lesser degree in stronglyoidiasis and has been used successfully in *Taenia* and *Echinococcus granulosus* infections; large doses usually are required. Because of its wide spectrum, mebendazole may be particularly useful in mixed infections.

Occasional adverse effects include transient abdominal pain and diarrhea. Mebendazole has not caused systemic toxicity, probably because it is poorly absorbed (5% to 10%). It has produced teratogenic effects in rats, but not in dogs, sheep, or horses; nevertheless, since there may be a possible danger to the fetus, this anthelmintic is contraindicated during pregnancy.

ROUTE, USUAL DOSAGE, AND PREPARATIONS. *Oral*: *Adults and children*, 100 mg morning and evening for three consecutive days for most infections; enterobiasis can usually be treated with a single 100-mg dose. If a cure is not achieved with initial therapy, a second course given three weeks later may be beneficial. For *Taenia* infections, doses up to 300 mg three times daily for three days have produced 100% cure rates; 200 mg twice daily for four days also has provided a high cure rate. Mebendazole has not been extensively investigated in *children under 2 years*; therefore, the relative benefit-to-risk ratio must be considered when it is used in these patients.

Vermox (Ortho). Tablets (chewable) 100 mg.

METRIFONATE
[Bilarcil]

Metrifonate is an organophosphorus cholinesterase inhibitor which is very effective in the treatment of *Schistosoma haematobium* infections and *S. mansoni* infections of the urinary tract (cure rate in these conditions is 90% to 95%). It has the added advantage, particularly in developing countries, of being inexpensive, averaging approximately 10% of the cost of other antischistosomal medications.

Most side effects are minimal and transient and include mild abdominal pain, diarrhea, vomiting, weakness, headache, dizziness, and vertigo. Plasma cholinesterase levels are depressed to approximately 5% of pretreatment values within six hours following drug administration and return to normal within four to six weeks. Therefore, metrifonate should be avoided in individuals who already have low levels of cholinesterase such as those with genetic variants, severe liver disease, or who are living in areas where there is extensive use of organophosphorus insecticides. Furthermore, cholinesterase-inhibiting muscle relaxants should be avoided during surgery in any patient taking metrifonate, unless plans have been made for assisted ventilation.

Animal studies have demonstrated mutagenicity and organ damage with prolonged use of this drug in large doses.

ROUTE, USUAL DOSAGE, AND PREPARATIONS. *Intramuscular*: 7.5 to 10 mg/kg of body weight every two to three weeks for three doses.

> *Bilarcil* (Bayer AG). Not available in the United States.

NICLOSAMIDE
[Yomesan]

Niclosamide is the preferred agent for treating tapeworm infections. It is highly effective with reported cure rates greater than 90% for *Taenia saginata*, 86% for *T. solium*, 97% for *Diphyllobothrium latum*, and 90% for *Hymenolepis nana*. This anthelmintic has the convenience of oral administration without intubation, and its use does not require hospitalization. Concomitant use of a laxative is not necessary except for *T. solium* infections. Niclosamide may destroy *T. solium* segments during therapy, thereby releasing viable eggs; therefore, when a laxative is given, it should be administered within one to two hours following use of the athelmintic to avoid the possibility of cysticercosis.

Niclosamide is not absorbed and no serious adverse reactions have been reported. Up to 10% of patients may experience malaise, mild abdominal pain, and nausea on the day the drug is administered. Since tapeworm infections generally are not life-threatening, it is recommended that treatment of pregnant women be postponed until after delivery.

ROUTE, USUAL DOSAGE, AND PREPARATIONS. This drug should be taken on an empty stomach and tablets should be chewed thoroughly.
Qral: *Adults and children over 8 years*, two doses of 1 g each one hour apart; *2 to 8 years*, two doses of 500 mg each one hour apart; *under 2 years*, two doses of 250 mg

each one hour apart. For *H. nana* infections, the drug should be administered for five successive days. The patient should omit breakfast but may eat two hours after the last dose. The tablets should be chewed and then swallowed with water.

> *Yomesan* (Bayer). Tablets 500 mg. Not marketed in the United States but may be obtained by licensed physicians from the Parasitic Disease Drug Service, Center for Disease Control (see the Introduction for the address and telephone number).

NIRIDAZOLE
[Ambilhar]

Niridazole and several other antimonials (eg, metrifonate) all are effective in the treatment of *Schistosoma haematobium* infections but, because niridazole is very effective it is a drug of choice. Although only moderately effective against *S. japonicum*, the comparative lower toxicity of niridazole also makes it a preferred drug for this infection when there is no central nervous system involvement or liver disease. It has become an alternative drug for the treatment of *S. mansoni* infections since the introduction of oxamniquine, because niridazole is only moderately active against this organism whereas oxamniquine is highly effective. It has been postulated that niridazole has some anti-inflammatory properties, and this action makes this anthelmintic effective in the treatment and extraction of *Dracunculus medinensis*.

Niridazole is absorbed by the gastrointestinal tract over a period of 10 to 15 hours, with peak plasma levels at six hours. It is extensively metabolized by the liver and the metabolites are excreted in the urine and feces, resulting in a dark brown urine and feces. The mechanism of action is not completely understood.

Children are usually less prone to experience untoward effects when taking niridazole than adults. Adverse reactions that are reversible upon discontinuation of the drug include gastrointestinal disturbances such as anorexia, abdominal cramping, vomiting, and diarrhea. Headache, dizziness, rashes, and, occasionally, electrocardiographic changes and neuropsychiatric disturbances, including insomnia, anxiety, confusion, hallucinations, and seizures, also have been seen. Transient reduction in spermatogenesis has been reported in animals, but additional studies are needed to determine the effects of niridazole on human spermatozoa. Hemolytic anemia may occur in patients with G6PD deficiency.

The usual recommended dosage of niridazole should not be given to patients with a history of liver disease, neuropsychiatric or convulsive disorders, decompensated heart disease, or renal insufficiency; it also should not be given concurrently with isoniazid. Since experiments using body fluids of humans and mice have demonstrated that niridazole is mutagenically active in small doses against certain bacteria, the drug should not be given to pregnant women. Additional studies are needed to ascertain the risks more completely.

ROUTE, USUAL DOSAGE, AND PREPARATIONS.
Oral: *Adults and children*, 25 mg/kg of body weight daily (maximum, 1.5 g) in two divided doses; this dosage is given for five to seven days in schistosomiasis and for seven to ten days in dracunculiasis.

Ambilhar (Ciba). Tablets 500 mg. Not marketed in the United States but may be obtained by licensed physicians from the Parasitic Disease Drug Service, Center for Disease Control (see the Introduction for the address and telephone number).

OXAMNIQUINE
[Mansil]

Oxamniquine, a tetrahydroquinoline derivative, has schistosomicidal activity against both immature and mature worms. It is becoming the drug of choice in the treatment of *Schistosoma mansoni* infections. It is much less effective, if at all, against *S. haematobium* or *S. japonicum* infections. Its advantages over other antischistosomal medications are that it can be given orally as well as intramuscularly (the oral route is actually preferred) and the course of medication is relatively short. In South America, especially Brazil, 100% cure rates have been reported following single doses. In Africa, the drug must be administered for several days to get a 90% to 100% cure rate. Even patients with decompensated hepatosplenic disease have been cured with brief dosage schedules.

The most common side effects are dizziness and somnolence, but fever, eosinophilia, transient pulmonary infiltration, liver function test abnormalities, EEG changes, hallucinations, and seizures have been seen. It should not be given to patients with decompensated congestive heart failure or renal failure. Use of this compound should be avoided in pregnant women, although there is as yet no evidence of teratogenicity or carcinogenicity; however, these problems have been reported with related compounds.

ROUTES, USUAL DOSAGE, AND PREPARATIONS.
Oral: *Adults* (*western hemisphere*), 15 mg/kg of body weight as a single dose; (*Africa*) 15 mg/kg twice daily for two days. *Children* (*western hemisphere*), 20 mg/kg in two equally divided doses two to eight hours apart; (*Africa*) 15 mg/kg twice daily for two or three days.
Intramuscular: (*South America only*) 7.5 mg/kg of body weight as a single dose.

Mansil (Pfizer). Not available in the United States.

PIPERAZINE CITRATE
[Antepar, Multifuge, Vermizine]

PIPERAZINE TARTRATE

All piperazine salts form piperazine hexahydrate in solution and are equally effective. Piperazine is an alternative drug for the treatment of ascariasis. A single dose cures approximately 70% of infected individuals, and two doses given on successive days increase the cure rate to between 90% and 100%. *Ascaris* worms are passed, paralyzed and alive, usually one to three days after treatment. A laxative is not needed to expel the worms from the gut. Pinworm infections also respond to piperazine. The majority of worms are passed alive and active during the first four days of therapy. A seven-day course of treatment usually is needed for optimal effects. Piperazine is readily absorbed from the gastrointestinal tract and most of an oral dose is excreted in the urine within 24 hours.

In therapeutic doses, adverse reactions are uncommon but may include nausea, vomiting, diarrhea, and allergic reactions. With larger doses, as in inadvertent overdosage or when the drug accumulates in the presence of renal insufficiency, muscular incoordination or weakness, vertigo, speech difficulty, confusion, and myoclonic contractions have been reported. These effects are transient and usually disappear when the drug is discontinued. Piperazine may induce or exacerbate epileptic seizures in predisposed patients. For the above reasons, it is contraindicated in those with renal or hepatic insufficiency and in epileptic patients. There have been no reports of harmful effects to the fetus after use of piperazine in pregnant women.

ROUTE, USUAL DOSAGE, AND PREPARATIONS. (Doses and strengths expressed in terms of the hexahydrate salt.)
Oral: For ascariasis, *adults*, 3.5 g once daily for two consecutive days; *children*, 75 mg/kg of body weight (maximum, 3.5 g) once daily for two consecutive days. For pinworms, *adults and children*, 65 mg/kg (maximum, 2.5 g) once daily for seven consecutive days. (See the manufacturers' literature for dosage tables.) The course should be repeated after a one-week interval. Fasting before treatment is not necessary.

PIPERAZINE CITRATE:
Drug available generically: Syrup 500 mg/5 ml; tablets 250 and 500 mg.
Antepar (Burroughs Wellcome), *Multifuge* (Bluline), *Vermizine* (North American). Syrup 500 mg/5 ml; tablets 500 mg.
PIPERAZINE TARTRATE:
Drug available generically: Tablets 250 and 500 mg.

PYRANTEL PAMOATE
[Antiminth]

Pyrantel is the drug of choice for treating ascariasis. The cure rate is almost 100% after a single dose. Similarly, it is a drug of choice (a position it shares with mebendazole) in enterobiasis, with a cure rate of 90% to 100% following a single dose. The hookworms, *Necator americanus* and *Ancylostoma duodenale*, are also susceptible to pyrantel. Cure rates of 48% to 93% and 92% to 93%, respectively, have been reported. Three consecutive daily doses are generally more effective than a single dose. Despite the possible disadvantage of multiple doses, some authorities who consider pyrantel the agent of choice for treating hookworm infections do so on the basis of its broad spectrum. This drug is ineffective in the treatment of whipworm. Pyrantel acts by paralyzing the worms, which are then expelled from the body, usually without the need of a laxative.

Pyrantel is poorly and incompletely absorbed from the gastrointestinal tract, with 50% of an oral dose excreted unchanged in the feces and 7% excreted unchanged in the urine. Nevertheless, systemic adverse reactions include anorexia, nausea, headache, dizziness, drowsiness, and rash, as well as elevated SGOT levels. Other untoward effects that probably result from local activity in the gut are abdominal pain, vomiting, and diarrhea. Safe usage in pregnancy has not been determined. Pyrantel should be used with caution in patients with pre-existing liver dysfunction. There has been little experience with the drug in children under 2 years of age.

ROUTE, USUAL DOSAGE, AND PREPARATIONS. (Dosage expressed in terms of the base.) *Oral*: *Adults and children*, for roundworms and pinworms, a single dose of 11 mg/kg of body weight (maximum, 1 g); for hookworms, this dose is given for three consecutive days. Fasting before treatment is not necessary. Dosage may be repeated in one month if indicated.

Antiminth (Roerig). Suspension 250 mg/5 ml.

PYRVINIUM PAMOATE
[Povan]

Pyrvinium pamoate is the salt of a cyanine dye. It is regarded as an alternative drug in enterobiasis (pinworm infection). A single oral dose produces cure rates of up to 96%. However, since reinfection is common, a second course of therapy should be given two weeks after the first; a cure cannot be assured until perianal swabs of cellophane tape are free of eggs for five to six weeks. Daily doses of pyrvinium for five to seven consecutive days may be effective in strongyloidiasis.

Pyrvinium is minimally absorbed from the gastrointestinal tract. Adverse reactions consist of nausea, abdominal cramps, vomiting, and, rarely, photosensitivity. Patients should be told that the drug stains stools bright red and will stain clothing if vomited. The tablets should be swallowed immediately and not chewed.

ROUTE, USUAL DOSAGE, AND PREPARATIONS. (Dosage expressed in terms of the base.) *Oral*: *Adults and children*, a single dose of 5 mg/kg of body weight is given for pinworm infections and is repeated in two or three weeks.

Povan (Parke, Davis). Suspension 50 mg/5 ml; tablets 50 mg.

QUINACRINE HYDROCHLORIDE
[Atabrine Hydrochloride]

Quinacrine is an effective alternative drug in the treatment of infections caused by *Taenia saginata* (beef tapeworm), *T. solium* (pork tapeworm), and *Diphyllobothrium latum* (fish tapeworm). It is less active against the dwarf tapeworm, *Hymenolepis nana*. Quinacrine also is effective against animal tapeworms that occasionally cause human infections (eg, *Dipylidium caninum*, *H. diminuta*).

Quinacrine acts on the attachment organs of the worm, causing dislodgement and excretion of the intact worm without expulsion of the eggs. Treatment is followed by the use of a saline laxative to facilitate expulsion of the worms, which are stained yellow by the drug. Large tapeworms frequently are eliminated by a single treatment but, if the scolex is not found, the stools should be examined periodically and shown to be free of worm eggs and segments for three to six months to be certain of cure. *H. nana* infections are usually multiple and require more prolonged treatment than large tapeworm infections.

Because orally administered quinacrine causes vomiting in approximately 25% of patients, a nasogastric tube may be used to deliver the drug directly into the duodenum. This technique also has the advantage of depositing a greater concentration of the drug in closer proximity to the head of the larger tapeworms. Although it is an awkward and uncomfortable route of administration, with proper preparation and purgation of the patient, use of the nasogastric tube may effect cures in greater than 90% of infections treated. Nasogastric intubation should not be used for *H. nana* infections.

Nausea and vomiting are the most common adverse effects after anthelmintic dosages of quinacrine. Vomiting reduces the effectiveness of the drug and, in *T. solium* infections, has the potential danger of producing cysticercosis. Yellowish discoloration of the skin occurs frequently. Other effects include transient dizziness and, less commonly, manifestations of toxic psychosis (eg, hallucinations) and exacerbation of psoriasis. Aplastic anemia and acute hepatic necrosis are rare toxic reactions.

Quinacrine should be used cautiously in patients over 60 years of age and in those with a history of psychosis. Treatment of pregnant women should be postponed until after delivery because tapeworm infections generally are not life-threatening and quinacrine crosses the placenta, thereby posing a potential hazard to the fetus.

ROUTES, USUAL DOSAGE, AND PREPARATIONS. Proper preparation of the patient is important. The diet should be restricted to liquid or semisolid fat-free food on the day before treatment, and no food should be taken after the evening meal. An enema may be given to reduce the amount of stool that must be searched for the scolex on the following day; patients with *H. nana* infection may be given a saline laxative. The drug is administered the following morning. It frequently has a laxative effect, but when it does not, a saline laxative is given one and one-half to two hours after the last dose. To reduce the possibility of nausea and vomiting, sodium bicarbonate (500 to 600 mg) may be given prior to each dose of quinacrine or an antiemetic (eg, prochlorperazine) may be used, particularly when treating *T. solium*.

Oral, Duodenal Tube: Adults, 800 mg; this amount may be given in two divided doses 30 minutes apart or in four or eight divided doses at 10-minute intervals to help prevent vomiting. *Children weighing 18 to 34 kg*, 400 mg in divided doses; *34 to 45.5 kg*, 600 mg in divided doses. Some sources recommend different dosages and more prolonged treatment for *H. nana* infections.

Atabrine Hydrochloride (Winthrop). Tablets 100 mg.

STIBOCAPTATE
[Astiban]

Stibocaptate (antimony sodium dimercaptosuccinate) is an alternative drug for treating infections caused by *Schistosoma haematobium*, *S. mansoni*, and *S. japonicum*. This agent is the least toxic of the trivalent antimony compounds currently in use and fewer injections are necessary than with the other compounds.

Stibocaptate may cause pain at the site of injection. Adverse effects are similar to those produced by the other trivalent antimony compounds. Gastrointestinal effects include anorexia, diarrhea, constipation, nausea, vomiting, and abdominal pain. Patients also may experience asthenia, lassitude, vertigo, headache, fever, arthralgia, myalgia, rash, impaired liver function, and electrocardiographic changes (eg, flattening or inversion of the T wave). Coughing or chest pain occurs rarely. Contraindications to the use of stibocaptate include other antimonial therapy within the previous two months, respiratory infections, tuberculosis, fever, jaundice, severe anemia, and cardiac, hepatic, or renal insufficiency. If intestinal helminths are present, they should be treated two weeks before initiating therapy with this agent. Information is lacking on the safety of stibocaptate during pregnancy and in children less than 10 years of age.

ROUTE, USUAL DOSAGE, AND PREPARATIONS.
Intramuscular: A 10% solution is prepared in water for injection and should be used within 24 hours if unrefrigerated; refrigerated solutions may be used if they are colorless and clear. The total dose is divided into five equal amounts to be given once or twice a week or, in hospitalized patients, as often as every day, depending upon the tolerance of the patient. *Adults*, 40 mg/kg of body weight (total dose) in five divided doses; *children 6 years and older*, 50 mg/kg in five divided doses.

> *Astiban* (Hoffman-LaRoche, Switzerland). Powder 500 mg in 5 ml containers and 10 g in 100 ml containers. Not marketed in the United States but may be obtained by licensed physicians from the Parasitic Disease Drug Service, Center for Disease Control (see the Introduction for address and telephone number).

SURAMIN SODIUM

Suramin, a complex derivative of urea, is used primarily in the treatment and prophylaxis of African trypanosomiasis. It also is used in combination with diethylcarbamazine in the treatment of onchocerciasis when there is ocular involvement or when repeated courses of diethylcarbamazine have not been effective for symptomatic skin disease. Diethylcarbamazine kills the microfilariae of *Onchocerca volvulus* quickly but generally is ineffective against the adults. Multiple doses of suramin cause death and degeneration of the adult female *O. volvulus* within one or two months after treatment, but males remain alive for a longer period. Microfilariae gradually die over a period of several months.

The need for multiple doses and its potentially dangerous adverse reactions limit the usefulness of suramin; close medical supervision during treatment is essential. Suramin may cause nausea, vomiting, colic, urticaria, severe local irritation if ex-travasated, and, in very sensitive persons, shock, syncope, acute circulatory failure, and seizures. Allergic effects due to proteins released by degenerating microfilariae (eg, pruritus, rash, fever, edema, burning and hyperesthesia of the soles of the feet, photophobia, iritis, lacrimation) occur later and generally are less intense than with diethylcarbamazine. The drug may cause albuminuria, casts, and hematuria and, rarely, agranulocytosis or hemolytic anemia, nephritis, and renal failure. It is contraindicated in patients with severe renal or ocular disease.

ROUTE, USUAL DOSAGE, AND PREPARATIONS.
Intravenous: A 10% solution in water for injection is used. For onchocerciasis, *adults*, 200 to 500 mg initially to test tolerance, then 1 g weekly for five weeks; *children*, 100 mg initially to test tolerance, then 10 to 15 mg/kg of body weight weekly for five weeks. The drug may be administered intramuscularly if the intravenous route is impractical. The total dose for adults should not exceed 5.5 g, since larger doses may cause renal toxicity.

> Drug available generically from the Parasitic Disease Drug Service, Center for Disease Control (see the Introduction for address and telephone number).

TETRACHLOROETHYLENE

$$Cl_2C = CCl_2$$

A single oral dose of this drug cures approximately 80% of hookworm infections caused by *Necator americanus* and about 25% of those caused by *Ancylostoma duodenale*. The treatment may be repeated one or more times at intervals of four days or a fecal examination may be made after two weeks and a second dose given if hookworm eggs are present. Tetrachloroethylene also cures most cases of fasciolopsiasis. If *Ascaris lumbricoides* also is present, it is generally recommended that the roundworms be eliminated before tetrachloroethylene is used to avoid the possibility that the drug might stimulate migration of the ascarids.

Nausea, vomiting, dizziness, and inebriation occur occasionally. Syncope has been reported rarely. Tetrachloroethylene has been used in severely anemic patients without causing serious untoward effects.

ROUTE, USUAL DOSAGE, AND PREPARATIONS. *Oral: Adults*, 5 ml; *children* 0.12 ml/kg of body weight (maximum, 5 ml). Only a low-bulk, low-fat meal should be eaten the evening before treatment, and alcohol must be avoided before and for 24 hours after use of tetrachloroethylene. Breakfast is omitted and the drug is given early in the morning; the patient should remain recumbent for the next four hours if possible. No laxative should be given, since this increases the toxic effects and decreases the effectiveness of the drug.

> Drug available only in veterinary preparations (eg, *Nema Worm Capsules* [Parke, Davis]), but these are effective for human use: Capsules 0.2, 0.5, 1, 2.5, and 5 ml.

THIABENDAZOLE
[Mintezol]

Thiabendazole is the drug of choice in the treatment of *Strongyloides stercoralis* infection; cure rates of almost 100% have been achieved. It also is the drug of choice for treating cutaneous larva migrans caused by larvae of *Ancylostoma braziliense*. Although thiabendazole is effective against pinworm infection, untoward effects may occur relatively more frequently than with some of the other effective agents. Hookworms and roundworms are susceptible to this drug, but light infections are more successfully treated than heavy ones and other available preparations are more useful. The number of developing trichina larvae of *Trichinella spiralis* was reduced when thiabendazole was used in experimentally infected pigs, and brief activity also has been demonstrated against the adult *T. spiralis* in the intestine of man. Excellent results were obtained in one instance in which thiabendazole was used in eight of nine people who had consumed infected pork. The individual who rejected

therapy developed severe trichinosis, while the others did not. Results in the treatment of whipworm have been variable, with a cure rate of 33% to 50% reported. Thiabendazole has been tried in the treatment of guineaworm infection, but it is not a drug of choice or a primary alternative drug.

Thiabendazole given orally or applied topically is the drug of choice for cutaneous larva migrans. Freezing the skin with ethyl chloride or carbon dioxide snow also may be useful; this latter technique requires formation of a vesicle so the skin will slough off taking the filiform larva with it. The larvae themselves are unaffected by repeated freezing and thawing.

Common untoward effects are dizziness, anorexia, nausea, and vomiting. Diarrhea, fever, epigastric distress, flushing, chills, angioedema, pruritus, lethargy, rash, malodorous urine and sweat, and headache occur less frequently. Tinnitus, hypotension, syncope, numbness, transient leukopenia, enuresis, hyperglycemia, changes in liver function, and xanthopsia, as well as a few cases of erythema multiforme and Stevens-Johnson syndrome, also have been reported. Adverse reactions are transient and appear to be dose related. Thiabendazole should be used cautiously in patients with impaired liver or kidney function. Although studies in animals have revealed no teratogenic effects, the expected therapeutic benefits should be weighed against the potential harm to the fetus if this drug is used during pregnancy.

ROUTE, USUAL DOSAGE, AND PREPARATIONS. *Oral: Adults and children*, 25 mg/kg of body weight (maximum, 3 g) twice daily after meals. For strongyloidiasis, cutaneous larva migrans, and hookworm, whipworm, and roundworm infection, treatment is given for one or two days; for trichinosis, for two to four days; and for pinworm infection, for one day with the dose repeated in 7 and 14 days. For guineaworm infection, 50 to 100 mg/kg daily for one to three days or 500 mg daily for seven days has been given. For cutaneous larva migrans, thiabendazole also is applied topically four times daily for five days.

When the drug is used to treat trichinosis or ocular visceral larva migrans, concomitant administration of corticosteroids may be needed to minimize the severe inflammatory reaction to the dying larvae.

Mintezol (Merck Sharp & Dohme). Suspension 500 mg/5 ml; tablets (chewable) 500 mg.

Selected References

Drugs for parasitic infections. *Med Lett Drugs Ther* 20:17-24, 1978.

Avery GS (ed): *Drug Treatment: Principles and Practice of Clinical Pharmacology and Therapeutics.* Acton, Mass, Publishing Sciences Group, Inc, 1976, 540-544.

Beck JW, Davies JE: *Medical Parasitology*, ed 2. St Louis, CV Mosby Co, 1976.

Botero D: Chemotherapy of human intestinal parasitic diseases. *Annu Rev Pharmacol Toxicol* 18:1-15, 1978.

Goodman LS, Gilman A: *The Pharmacological Basis of Therapeutics*, ed 5. New York, Macmillan Publishing Co, Inc, 1975, 1036-1044.

Holmstedt B, et al: Metrifonate: Summary of toxicological and pharmacological information available. *Arch Toxicol* 41:3-29, 1978.

Hunter GW III, et al: *Tropical Medicine*, ed 5. Philadelphia, WB Saunders Co, 1976.

James MFM, Jewsbury JM: Schistosomiasis, metriphonate, cholinesterase, and suxamethonium. *Br Med J* 1:442, 1978.

Marsden PD (ed): Intestinal parasites. *Clin Gastroenterol* 7:1-243, 1978.

Melman KL, Morrelli HF (eds): *Clinical Pharmacology: Basic Principles in Therapeutics*, ed 2. New York, Macmillan Publishing Co, Inc, 1978, 444-445.

Omer AHS: Oxamniquine for treating *Schistosoma mansoni* infection in Sudan. *Br Med J* 2:163-165, 1978.

Omer AHS, Teesdale CH: Metrifonate trial in treatment of various presentations of *Schistosoma haematobium* and *S. mansoni* infections in Sudan. *Ann Trop Med Parasitol* 72:145-150, 1978.

Pratt WB: *Chemotherapy of Infection.* New York, Oxford University Press, 1977, 373-407.

Scabicides and Pediculicides | 84

Arthropod infestations cause skin disorders in man and animals. Insect- or mite-produced skin lesions and the secondary infection sometimes associated with them may be nonspecific and mimic nonparasitic dermatoses. Parasitic arthropods causing skin reactions in man are the itch mite, louse, bed bug, human and animal flea, mange mite, red poultry mite, sheep tick, and harvest mite. Nonparasitic arthropods include forage mites, which live in various stored products such as flour, and house dust mites. The reactions caused by these nonparasitic organisms are allergic in nature.

Disease Characteristics

The most common infestations produced by the parasitic arthropods are scabies and pediculosis. Scabies occurs when the itch mite, *Sarcoptes scabiei* var. *hominis*, invades the skin; generally less severe infestations with fewer lesions may be caused by species usually found on fowl, dogs, cats, horses, and other animal species, including more exotic types such as snakes and tigers. Pediculosis in man is caused by three kinds of lice: *Phthirus pubis* (crab louse), which mainly infests the pubic region; *Pediculus humanus* (body louse), which infests the underwear and attacks the trunk and limbs; and *P. capitis* (head louse), which affects the scalp. *P. humanus* and *P. capitis* are sometimes considered to be subspecies, but recent evidence

(Busvine, 1978) suggests that they may qualify as full species.

Scabetic infestations are pandemic. Major epidemics are alleged to occur in a 25- to 30-year cyclic pattern. The cycles may be the result of a form of "herd immunity" that develops in the group currently infested and persists until a "nonimmune" population emerges, but such immunity is not absolute. In support of this concept, there is evidence that reinfestation occurs with greater difficulty than contracting the initial infestation (Mellanby, 1977). If "herd immunity" were the only cause of the cyclic phenomenon, however, a longer cycle would be expected, since the epidemics themselves last for approximately 15 years and it takes about 45 years to build up a nonsensitized population (Christophersen, 1978). The cause of the cyclic scabetic fluctuations, therefore, remains as obscure as for other diseases with a periodic occurrence. Based on extrapolations from information obtained during previous cycles in this century, the present epidemic may abate in the 1980's.

The incidence of head and crab lice infestations is increasing in North American and Western Europe; this may be true for head lice worldwide, but there is no evidence that body lice infestations are increasing. The primary contributing factors responsible for the increase are not apparent. The prevalence of crab lice may be a reflection of increased sexual promiscuity, a factor that has little or no bearing on the occurrence of head and body lice.

Although pediculosis has traditionally been thought to be associated with filth and squalor, regular bathing and shampooing do not ensure that an individual will remain free of louse infestations; nevertheless, poor personal hygiene by those with pediculosis may increase the possibility of secondary bacterial infection. Louse infestations have increased without regard to race or socioeconomic barriers with the exception of blacks, who are rarely infested; the reason for the decreased incidence has not been explained. The longer hair styles and greater prevalence of beards fashionable recently have been blamed for contributing to the increased incidence of pediculosis. This may be a spurious association, since lice live at the hair roots to have ready access to the scalp. It appears that long hair or complex hairdos are of contributory importance, therefore, only when they impede early detection of an infestation. Failure to recognize an infestation quickly delays treatment and increases the opportunity for transmission to other family members or associates.

Pruritus is associated with both parasitic infestations and is sometimes accompanied by papular dermatitis, although neither symptom is invariably present. In scabetic infestations, the mites burrow into the horny layer of the cracks and folds in skin where irritation and pruritus result, probably caused by sensitization to acarine products. Scratching leads to excoriation, which may be followed by secondary infection. During severe infestations, induration and crusting may occur. In louse infestations, symptoms are produced by an allergic reaction to injection of saliva and deposition of excrement by the parasite into the skin.

Louse infestations per se generally are not dangerous or injurious to health. Head and pubic lice usually, represent only a source of physical irritation and social embarrassment, although head lice can harbor typhus and relapsing fever. However, *P. capitis* has never acted as a primary vector in the spread of any disease. Body lice can transmit diseases, primarily typhus, relapsing fever, and, rarely, trench fever. Louse-borne diseases are now much more re-stricted and only occur in a few parts of the world, since these diseases can spread only in areas that have a high proportion of infested individuals. Louse-borne disease has been devastating among armies and civilian populations alike during times of war and other disasters such as flooding and famine.

Classic scabetic infestations usually are diagnosed easily in adults, but diagnosis can be difficult in infants and children and sometimes in adults as well (Shelley and Wood, 1976; Orkin and Maibach, 1978). Classic scabies has been encountered less frequently in the United States during the current epidemic than previously, but may be seen more commonly in developing countries. A detailed discussion of both classic and atypical forms of the disease is found in *Scabies and Pediculosis*, Orkin et al (see the list of Selected References at the end of this chapter). The pathognomonic lesion of scabies is the burrow produced by the gravid female. Secondary lesions include vesicles, pustules, excoriations, and crusts. In adults, burrows are observed most frequently on the sides and webs of fingers, the ulnar border of the hand, the volar aspects of the wrists, the points of the elbows, the axillary folds, the margins of the feet, the areolae of the nipples in women, and the genitalia in men. In infants and children, scabetic eruptions are common on the head, neck, and buttocks, and the symptoms of secondary infection are more likely to obscure the characteristic lesion than in adults.

Since scabetic lesions, particularly those modified by secondary bacterial infections, can mimic almost any skin disease, differential diagnosis must exclude such common conditions as atopic dermatitis, impetigo, ecthyma, animal scabies, seborrheic dermatitis, neurodermatitis, dermatitis herpetiformis, psoriasis, papular urticaria, pediculosis, and chicken pox. Identification of the mite from direct skin scrapings or, occasionally, cutaneous biopsy ensures definitive diagnosis, a goal not always attainable, especially if the physician is inexperienced in searching for the parasite. Mineral oil is preferred to potassium hydroxide solution or water as a medium in which to examine skin scrapings (Muller et al, 1973; Hazelrigg, 1978), since mites adhere to the oil and remain alive and motile; dry scraping kills and fragments the mites. Mineral oil does not digest or dissolve ova or fecal pellets, items that are diagnostic even when mites are not present.

Pediculosis pubis and capitis may be diagnosed by identifying the adult louse or, more commonly, eggs (nits) attached to the hair shaft initially at the hair-skin junction. Pediculosis pubis mainly involves the pubic region but can spread to the trunk, legs, and axillae. Rarely, it may invade the margins of the eyebrows and eyelashes (mainly in children), scalp, and mustache. Children can acquire the disease through contact with infected adults, perhaps through the common use of towels. Pediculosis capitis usually is found only on the scalp and is common in children; the occipital and postauricular regions are the areas most commonly involved. In rare instances, the beard and other exceptionally hairy areas may harbor head lice. Pediculosis corporis can be confirmed by the presence of lice or nits in the seams of clothing, commonly where clothing comes in contact with the axillae, or at the beltline and collar. Except in heavily infested individuals, parasites may be almost absent from the body.

As a first step in the treatment of scabies or pediculosis, the source of infestation must be determined and avoided. All affected members of a family should be treated at the same time. Because scabetic and crab lice infestations, particularly, are spread by intimate physical contact, they can be considered venereal diseases. Therapy of an infected individual may include simultaneous treatment of the sexual partner to avoid a "ping-pong" passing of the disease from one partner to the other. Adults harboring either parasite should be examined for the presence of other sexually transmitted diseases. In pediculosis corporis, all close contacts should be examined and treated if infected.

Finally, decontamination procedures should be instituted in addition to therapy.

These consist of the following (see also Juranek, 1976):

Pediculosis: Since heat is lethal to lice and their eggs, many personal articles can be disinsected by machine washing in hot water and/or drying using the hot cycle of the dryer. Eggs are killed after five minutes at 51.5 C or 30 minutes at 49.5 C, and adult lice succumb to slightly lower temperatures. Combs and brushes can be disinsected by soaking them for one hour in saponated cresol solution 2% or equivalent (eg, Lysol, Pine-Sol) or heating them in water to about 60 C for five to ten minutes. Personal articles of clothing or bedding that cannot be washed may be dry cleaned or placed in a plastic bag and sealed for ten days (head lice and crab lice). This method is effective because head lice die in about 48 hours without a blood meal and nits kept at room temperature for ten days do not hatch. Similarly, when crab lice are separated from the human host, they die in less than 24 hours. Body lice may survive for 4 to 10 days away from the host, and eggs may hatch for up to 30 days after removal from the human host. Shaving or cutting the hair is not necessary. Cleaning of houses, wards, or other rooms inhabited by infested patients should be limited to thorough vacuuming. Fumigation is not recommended.

Scabies: Clothing and bedding should be machine washed and dried using the hot cycles of both washer and dryer. Special environmental clean-up is not indicated.

Comparative Drug Therapy

The object of treatment of scabies and pediculosis is elimination of the offending organism and prevention or treatment of secondary infection. Appropriate antibacterial preparations may be applied topically if indicated; occasionally, systemic antibiotics may be required to counteract severe secondary infection.

One cardinal concept when treating scabies or pediculosis is that medication cures only if correctly utilized. Claims by a patient that he has undergone successful therapy at an earlier date should not lead a physician into misdiagnosing one of these parasitic infestations. Often, on the advice of a friend, pharmacist, or even physician, an individual may undertake self-medication without curing the infestations, even though symptoms may be ameliorated and temporary relief obtained.

Crotamiton [Eurax] and lindane (gamma benzene hexachloride) [Kwell] are the drugs of choice for treating scabies. Benzyl benzoate is effective but rarely used in the United States. No definitive data have been published to prove that either crotamiton or lindane is ovicidal. Therefore, two applications may be required with crotamiton, although only one course of treatment with lindane usually is indicated because of the potential danger of percutaneous absorption leading to systemic toxicity. Sulfur (in ointment form) is still useful even though its origin as a scabicide goes back into antiquity. It is messy, has a bad odor, and stains clothing, but may be a preferred agent for infants, small children, or pregnant women because of its great margin of safety. Thiabendazole, given orally (Hernández-Pérez and Bechelli, 1969) or applied topically as a 10% solution (Hernández-Pérez, 1976) has been used, but not in the United States. An emulsion concentrate (NBIN) containing 6% chlorophenothane, 68% benzyl benzoate, 12% benzocaine, and 14% polysorbate 80 is recommended by the World Health Organization as a relatively inexpensive scabicide that can be compounded from materials readily obtainable even in developing countries. The preparation requires a 1:15 dilution with water before application.

Lindane and chlorophenothane (DDT) are effective against head, body, and pubic lice, but the latter agent is not available in the United States. Head and body lice resistant to these drugs have been identified. Benzyl benzoate and chlorophenothane are preferred drugs to eliminate lice resistant to lindane and vice versa. Benzyl benzoate has been prescribed for pubic lice. Malathion can be used to treat louse infestations resistant to both lindane and chlorophenothane and is an alternative drug for pediculosis capitis

(in a 0.5% concentration) and pubis (in a 0.5% or 1% concentration). Malathion is not readily available in pharmacies in the United States. Strains of malathion-resistant body lice have been discovered but have not yet appeared in the United States. Resistance of *Phthirus pubis* to these insecticides has not been reported. Petrolatum applied thickly twice daily for eight days with mechanical removal of nits safely eliminates crab lice from the eyelashes. An ophthalamic ointment containing physostigmine 0.25% may be used, but undesirable effects on vision, pupillary size, and accommodation have been noted; therefore, it should be reserved for alternative therapy. Mixtures containing pyrethrin 0.165% or 0.3% and piperonyl butoxide are available without prescription [A-200 Pyrinate, RID] and may be useful in treating pediculosis.

Ointments containing mercury or Peruvian balsam and sulfur were once widely used to treat scabies and pediculosis as well as other skin diseases. Because Peruvian balsam can be sensitizing and mercury can be absorbed through intact or damaged skin causing renal toxicity, these preparations have no place in the modern therapy of parasitic infestations.

Adverse Reactions and Precautions

Scabicides and pediculicides may irritate the skin, eyes, and mucous membranes and cause allergic reactions. If signs of intolerance develop, the medication should be discontinued and inflammation allowed to subside before alternative therapy is substituted.

Large-scale use of chlorophenothane (DDT) and lindane (gamma benzene hexachloride) as delousing agents under wartime and disaster conditions did not produce significant toxicity. If appreciable amounts are absorbed, however, systemic toxicity may occur (see the evaluation on Lindane).

Because patients tend to apply topical preparations more freely and for longer periods than prescribed, the physician should give careful instructions on the use

of scabicides and pediculicides and prescribe only the amount needed for a given
course of therapy with no refills. If a preparation is used too often or for too long a
period, it may cause dermatitis that is mistaken for persistence of the parasitic infestation which, in turn, is aggravated by
further application of the drug. The patient
should be instructed not to use topical
preparations other than those prescribed.

INDIVIDUAL EVALUATIONS

CROTAMITON
[Eurax]

$$CH_3CH=CHCNCH_2CH_3$$

Crotamiton is an effective scabicide with
antipruritic properties. It is claimed to be
useful as an antipruritic alone.

This agent rarely may cause allergic contact dermatitis and, occasionally, irritant
contact dermatitis; it is irritating to denuded skin. If these reactions are severe,
the drug should be discontinued and appropriate countermeasures taken.

ROUTE, USUAL DOSAGE, AND PREPARATIONS.
Topical: The preparation should be mas-
saged into the skin of the whole body,
working from the chin down. Particular
attention should be given to the body folds,
hands, feet, and intertriginous areas. Contact with the eyes, mouth, and urethral
meatus should be avoided. Two applications at 24-hour intervals will eradicate
most scabetic infestations. A cleansing bath
should be taken 48 hours following the last
application. In resistant cases, treatment
may be repeated one week later or an
alternative drug used.

Eurax (Geigy). Cream 10% in 60 g containers.

LINDANE (Gamma Benzene Hexachloride)
[Kwell]

Lindane is effective in all forms of
pediculosis and scabies. It is irritating to
the eyes, skin, and mucosa. Allergic contact
dermatitis has not been documented, but
irritant contact dermatitis is common if the
drug is applied liberally, too frequently, or
for extended periods. If irritation becomes
evident, the drug should be washed off and
not used again. Lindane is absorbed
through intact skin and is toxic if absorbed
in excessive amounts. This agent is excreted slowly in the urine (half-life, approximately 26 hours).

If accidental ingestion occurs, prompt
gastric lavage will eliminate much of the
preparation. If a laxative is used, oils
should be avoided since they enhance
absorption. Systemic toxicity is usually
manifested as central nervous system
stimulation progressing to convulsions;
barbiturates may be used to counteract
this effect. There is also clinical evidence
that intravenous diazepam [Valium] is
effective in controlling these convulsions.
Intravenous administration of calcium
gluconate also may be beneficial, but epinephrine should be avoided.

ROUTE, USUAL DOSAGE, AND PREPARATIONS.
Topical: For scabies, *adults and older
children*, following a soap and warm water
bath using a soft brush, no more than 20 to
30 g of lotion or cream is applied to all parts
of the body except the face. The eyes,
eyelashes, and mucous membranes should
be avoided. The medication is washed off
thoroughly after 12 hours. Other scabicides should be used in *infants* when
possible.

For pediculosis capitis, the scalp is first
moistened with water; up to 1 oz of the
shampoo is applied, worked into a lather,
and the scalp thoroughly shampooed for
five minutes. It is then rinsed and dried.

Remaining nits may be removed with a fine-toothed comb or forceps. Treatment may be repeated in one week if viable eggs persist or new eggs are seen, *but not more than twice.*

For pediculosis pubis, therapy is preceded by a bath and drying with a towel. A thin layer of lotion is applied to the affected and adjacent areas, particularly the pubic mons and perianal region. In hairy individuals, the thighs, trunk, and axillary regions should be covered. The lotion is washed off thoroughly after 12 hours. Remaining nits may be removed with a fine-toothed comb or forceps. One application is usually sufficient, but a second application may be repeated in one week if viable eggs persist or new eggs appear at the skin-hair junction. This agent should be applied *no more than twice.* It is not necessary to shave the areas. The shampoo may be applied to the pubic, perineal, and axillary areas as above, but is not as effective as the lotion.

Drug available generically (powder 6%) and as gamma benzene hexachloride (cream 1% in 2 and 16 oz containers).

Kwell (Reed & Carnrick). Cream, lotion, and shampoo 1% in 2 and 16 oz containers.

SULFUR

This compound may be applied topically as a 6% (range, 5% to 10%) ointment of precipitated sulfur in petrolatum to treat scabies. Some physicians prefer to add 3% Peruvian balsam, although this latter agent is of no additional benefit and may be sensitizing. Some authorities consider sulfur to be a preferred scabicide for infants, small children, and pregnant women.

Sulfur ointment has staining properties and an unpleasant odor; rarely, it causes irritation and dermatitis if used frequently. It should not be used with mercury compounds since the two chemicals react to release hydrogen sulfide, which has a foul odor, may be irritating, and stains the skin black.

ROUTE, USUAL DOSAGE, AND PREPARATIONS. *Topical*: Following a cleansing scrub using a soft brush, hot water, and soap, the skin is dried and sulfur ointment is applied nightly for three nights. Bathing may be undertaken each night prior to the application of the drug or once, 24 hours after the last application.

No pharmaceutical dosage form is available; compounding is necessary for prescription. The usual formulation is a 6% ointment of precipitated sulfur in petrolatum.

BENZYL BENZOATE

This agent has been used to treat pediculosis capitis and pubis. It is still widely used outside the United States to treat scabies but has been supplanted by crotamiton and lindane in this country.

Benzyl benzoate is relatively nontoxic but may irritate the skin and eyes. Increased pruritus and burning sensation, particularly of the genitalia and scalp, may occur. Contact with the eyes and urethral meatus should be avoided; subjective irritation (burning and stinging) is not uncommon. There is no evidence that this drug is absorbed through the skin in amounts sufficient to cause systemic toxicity. Benzyl benzoate is converted to hippuric acid following ingestion, but systemic toxic symptoms have not been described in man. In laboratory animals, this agent has been reported to cause progressive incoordination, central nervous system excitation, convulsions, and death.

ROUTE, USUAL DOSAGE, AND PREPARATIONS. *Topical*: Ideally, after thorough cleansing of the affected areas with soap and water for 10 minutes, a preparation containing approximately 25% of the drug is applied; after this application has dried, the medication may be reapplied and the residue washed off 24 hours later. Benzyl benzoate may be applied nightly or every other night for a total of three applications.

Drug available generically: Emulsion 50% in 16 and 64 oz containers; lotion 27% in 16 and 64 oz containers and 50% in 4 and 16 oz containers.

Selected References

Busvine JR: Evidence from double infestations for specific status of human head lice and body lice (Anoplura). *System Entomol* 3:1-8, 1978.

Busvine JR: Pediculosis: Biology of parasites, in Orkin M, et al (eds): *Scabies and Pediculosis.* Philadelphia, JB Lippincott Company, 1977, 143-152.

Christophersen J: Epidemiology of scabies in Denmark, 1900 to 1975. *Arch Dermatol* 114:747-750, 1978.

Fernandez N, et al: Pathologic findings in human scabies. *Arch Dermatol* 113:320-324, 1977.

Hazelrigg DE: Scraping for scabies. *Am Fam Physician* 17:129, (Jan) 1978.

Hernández-Pérez E: Topically applied thiabendazole in treatment of scabies. *Arch Dermatol* 112:1400-1401, 1976.

Hernández-Pérez E, Bechelli CA: Tiabendazol oral en escabiosis. *Dermatol Iberoltinoam* 4:427-432, 1969.

Juranek DD: Nuisance diseases: Pediculosis and scabies. *Assoc Pract Infect Control Newslett* 4:1-5, 1976.

Mellanby K: Immunology of scabies, in Orkin M, et al (eds): *Scabies and Pediculosis.* Philadelphia, JB Lippincott Company, 1977, 84-87.

Muller G, et al: Scraping for human scabies: A better method for positive preparations. *Arch Dermatol* 107:70, 1973.

Nienhuis M, Rowles B: Preventing, controlling and treating pediculosis and scabies. *US Pharmacist*, Oct 1976, 35-42.

Orkin M, Maibach HI: Current concepts in parasitology: This scabies pandemic. *N Engl J Med* 298:496-498, 1978.

Orkin M, et al (eds): *Scabies and Pediculosis.* Philadelphia, JB Lippincott Company, 1977.

Orkin M, et al: Treatment of today's scabies and pediculosis. *JAMA* 236:1136-1139, 1976.

Shelley WB, Wood MG: Larval papule as a sign of scabies. *JAMA* 236:1144-1145, 1976.

General Antidotes | 85

Principles of Poison Therapy

There are four basic guidelines employed in the treatment of the poisoned patient; their sequence of initiation depends upon the circumstances. The following sequence is for an idealized situation when adequate time is available.

Individual Assessment: Consulting an appropriate toxicology reference source is essential, because early identification of the ingredients (most toxic and all other) can save time and lessen the chance of complications. It is important to remember that hazard is not synonymous with potency of a poison, for ingestion of 120 g of turpentine is as threatening as 120 mg of strychnine, and solvents are often more life-threatening than the active ingredient. A list of suggested general references is presented at the end of this chapter. In addition, the microfiche toxicology file, POISINDEX[R] (Rumack et al, 1979), is especially valuable and is available in many hospital emergency rooms. Readily available poison control center telephone numbers complete the suggested minimum list of information resources.

Estimates of the dose, the time elapsed since exposure, and the condition of the patient will determine whether induced vomiting, gastric lavage, supportive care, or specific antidotal therapy is required and the sequence of use indicated. Factors that may affect the patient's response to the poison (ie, the patient's age, possible presence of hereditary and other associated diseases, current drug therapy if any, an allergic drug history) also should be considered prior to institution of therapy (see Chapter 4). Acquisition of a blood sample to determine a baseline for monitoring drug or chemical intoxication can be helpful in assessing the progress of the therapeutic program.

Supportive Care: Hypoventilation is avoided by ensuring an adequate airway with use of suction, oxygenation, and mechanical ventilation if required. Anticonvulsants may be necessary if seizures interfere with ventilation. The maintenance of circulation and prevention of arrhythmias may require cardiac massage, volume replacement, and drug therapy. It is especially important when treating poisoning to avoid unnecessary drug use. Hypotension severe enough to require correction may best be treated with intravenous fluids rather than drugs. This is particularly true when poisoning causes central nervous system depression and a relative hypovolemia in dehydrated patients.

Termination of Exposure: Elimination of the poison from the gut, skin, or eyes before extensive absorption or damage can occur is effective treatment for most cases of acute poisoning. No further therapeutic intervention usually is required.

Use of Specific Drug Antidotes: It is estimated that specific antidotes are required in no more than 2% of the total number of poisonings; however, this represents a substantial number of patients in whom a better than average outcome can be expected when the poisoning is severe.

Agents Used to Terminate Exposure to Poisons

General antidotes are used for supportive care and to terminate exposure to many toxins. The number of agents employed for supportive care is obviously broad, and they have been discussed throughout this text. The number of general antidotes given to terminate exposure is much more limited: The emetics, charcoal adsorbent, and urinary acidifying and alkalizing agents are presented in this chapter; saline cathartics and diuretics are discussed in Chapters 59 and 39, respectively; and drugs that antagonize the toxic action of one agent and possibly a few closely related derivatives appear in the following chapter, Specific Antidotes.

Initially, contaminated clothing should be removed and all routes of exposure should be determined. When the eyes are involved, adequate volumes of water applied immediately can prevent blindness. When the skin is affected, water and, if the poison and/or solvent is lipid soluble, tincture of green soap can be useful to limit absorption. The hair should be shampooed if contaminated (eg, pesticide spray). Adequate ventilation must be assured when the lungs are a major route of elimination of the poison. Emetics, lavage, and an adsorbent limit gastrointestinal absorption of the poison.

Important procedures employed later in the course of treatment may include osmotic catharsis with sodium or magnesium sulfate, diuresis, acidification or alkaliza-tion of the urine, and dialysis. Dialysis should be considered only when hypotension, acid-base disturbance, convulsions, apnea, or hyperthermia persist.

Emetics act directly and/or reflexly on the chemoreceptor trigger zone of the medulla, the latter through stimulation of receptors in the gastrointestinal tract. Their effectiveness is increased by concomitant ingestion of 200 to 300 ml of water, because the fluid-distended stomach is more susceptible to induced vomiting. The amount of water should be limited to 300 ml or 15 ml/kg in children to avoid pyloric emptying. Carbonated drinks or milk should not be used for this purpose.

Ipecac syrup is the most useful emetic because, although slightly slower in action than parenteral apomorphine, it is available for home use and is preferred in infants and children because it produces less central nervous system depression. Considerable variation exists in the amount of stomach contents removed by either drug. Therefore, activated charcoal, if indicated, and a saline cathartic should be administered after use of either ipecac syrup or apomorphine.

Antimony potassium tartrate (tartar emetic) and mustard powder also have been used, but the former is too toxic and the latter usually is ineffective. Cupric or zinc sulfate often is effective, but the potential hemolytic and renal toxicity are too great to recommend use of either agent. Mechanical production of gagging or use of soap or hypertonic sodium chloride solution is relatively ineffective. Sodium chloride may be absorbed in toxic amounts, and deaths have occurred following its use as an emetic or as a hypertonic irrigant for gastric lavage. Tap water usually is used as the lavage irrigant but isotonic or half-isotonic sodium chloride solution is preferred in young children, because even a 5% increase in body fluid volume of electrolyte-free water may be sufficient to cause water intoxication manifested by convulsions.

There is universal agreement that emptying the stomach completely after ingestion of most poisons is desirable (for exceptions, see the discussion on Contraindications). If vomiting does not occur spontaneously, ipecac-induced emesis or lavage is the treatment chosen. Insertion of the lavage tube may cause vomiting, especially in children, but this technique is usually less efficient than induced vomiting, especially when large tablets or capsules are present. Induced emesis also may partially empty the upper small intestine.

If vomiting cannot be induced by emetics, gastric lavage using a large bore tube should be started, preferably within three hours after ingestion, unless it is contraindicated (see the following section). Lavage may be effective even five to six hours after ingestion, depending upon the rate of disintegration and dissolution of the formulation ingested and whether gastrointestinal transit time is lengthened by the poison. To minimize the chances of aspiration, the patient should be placed on his left side with the face near the edge of the table and the legs elevated. In comatose patients, a cuffed endotracheal tube should be used whenever possible. Stomach contents should be aspirated by suction before instilling the lavage solution. Repeated lavage using small amounts of fluid (about 100 to 250 ml in adults; 25 to 50 ml in small children) should be performed until returns are clear. Thereafter, an adsorbent should be instilled through the lavage tube and allowed to remain in the stomach.

Contraindications: Emetics are contraindicated in patients who are unconscious, in shock, semicomatose, or in whom coma may be expected imminently. They should not be used if strongly caustic substances, such as strong alkalis (lye) or acids, have been ingested since additional injury, such as perforation of the esophagus with resultant mediastinitis, may occur. The caustic substance should be diluted with a demulcent instead. If an antiemetic has been ingested recently, gastric lavage generally is preferred to apomorphine, for the latter's action on the chemoreceptor trigger zone of the medulla would be suppressed in such instances; ipecac syrup usually is effective because of its additional reflex action, especially if less than one hour has elapsed since ingestion of the antiemetic. Lavage is contraindicated in strychnine

poisoning unless the airway is protected with an endotracheal tube.

Emetics may be contraindicated after ingestion of certain high viscosity petroleum distillates, eg, (1) mineral seal or signal oils present in furniture and oil polishes, because they have the highest risk of severe aspiration pneumonitis; (2) oils (fuel, diesel, motor, cutting, mineral, suntan, baby oils), because even though they are relatively nontoxic, they may cause lipid pneumonia if aspiration occurs. Emesis generally is recommended for lower viscosity hydrocarbons, because of their inherent central nervous system toxicity and potential for other toxic effects. The same contraindications and recommendation apply to lavage if the patient is comatose; however, lavage should be conducted only after a cuffed endotracheal intubation. When any petroleum distillate is a solvent for a very toxic substance (eg, certain insecticides), the benefits of employing emetics or gastric lavage usually outweigh the risks of aspiration or toxic reactions from the petroleum distillate.

Lavage with boluses of 300 to 500 ml of fluid initially, especially on a full stomach, may force material through the pylorus where it cannot be recovered. Aspiration of vomitus into the bronchial tree is a potential hazard of both gastric lavage and emetic-induced vomiting; however, in conscious patients, the hazard is less with use of emetics.

EMETICS

APOMORPHINE HYDROCHLORIDE

Apomorphine acts directly on the chemoreceptor trigger zone and usually induces vomiting in adults in two to ten minutes. The expelled contents may contain reflux from the upper intestinal tract. Since this emetic is more effective when the stomach is full, 200 to 300 ml of water should be given just before subcutaneous injection. When an adsorbable poison has been ingested, activated charcoal should be given orally either immediately after apomorphine or, if delay in administration of the emetic is anticipated, before the injection to reduce absorption of any poison remaining in the stomach. Apomorphine is as effective as ipecac syrup, but the latter is considerably safer and is recommended as an emetic of first choice, especially in children.

Apomorphine produces some degree of central nervous system depression, but euphoria, restlessness, and tremors may be observed instead. Acute circulatory failure may occur in aged or debilitated patients. Overdosage produces violent vomiting, retching, respiratory depression, acute circulatory failure, and death. Although it is seldom necessary to reverse the depressant actions of apomorphine, it is not unusual to require administration of a narcotic antagonist to terminate protracted vomiting; naloxone (0.01 mg/kg of body weight) is administered for either purpose.

This drug is contraindicated in patients sensitive to morphine derivatives. For other contraindications, see the Introduction. Apomorphine is not stable and should not be used if the solution is green or brown.

ROUTE, USUAL DOSAGE, AND PREPARATIONS. *Subcutaneous*: *Adults*, 0.1 mg/kg of body weight (maximum, 6 mg), and *children*, 0.066 mg/kg; 200 to 300 ml of water should be consumed just before the injection.

Drug available generically: Tablets (hypodermic) 6 mg.

IPECAC SYRUP

This emetic is preferred in young patients because it produces less central nervous system depression than apomorphine. Ipecac alkaloids act both reflexly on the gastric mucosa and centrally on the chemoreceptor trigger zone to induce vomiting. An adequate dose causes vomiting within 30 minutes in about 90% of patients; the average time is usually less than 20 minutes. The emetic action is increased if 200 to 300 ml of water is taken immediately after administration of the syrup. (Neither milk nor carbonated beverages should be substituted for water.) In young and frightened children, giving water prior to the ipecac syrup may be more successful.

Ipecac syrup is available without prescription in a maximum amount of 30 ml. Physicians often recommend that an ounce of the syrup be obtained and stored when children become 1 year old; thus, it is readily available in the home and may be given immediately when a physician prescribes it by telephone.

Activated charcoal should not be given with ipecac syrup, because it adsorbs the ipecac and nullifies the emetic effect; it may, however, be given after vomiting has occurred to reduce absorption of any poison remaining in the stomach. For contraindications, see the Introduction.

ROUTE, USUAL DOSAGE, AND PREPARATIONS. *Oral*: *Adults*, 20 ml, followed by 200 to 300 ml of water; *children over 1 to 12 years*, 15 ml (one tablespoonful), preceded or followed by 240 ml (one full glass) of water; *infants 9 to 12 months*, 10 ml (2 teaspoonsfuls), preceded or followed by 120 to 240 ml (one-half to one full glass) of water. The dose may be repeated once after 20 minutes if vomiting has not occurred. If vomiting does not occur within 30 minutes, gastric lavage should be performed. Absorption of ipecac may cause atrial fibrillation or other serious myocardial conduction disturbances.

Drug available generically: Syrup in 15 and 30 ml (nonprescription) and 120 ml containers.

ADSORBENT

ACTIVATED CHARCOAL

This effective adsorbent is a useful adjunct in the treatment of acute poisoning. Although the adsorptive efficacy of charcoal has not been determined for many drugs in vivo, it is known to reduce the gastrointestinal absorption of drugs that are common causes of poisoning, such as analgesics (salicylates, acetaminophen, propoxyphene), sedative-hypnotics, and tricyclic antidepressants. This agent does not affect the absorption of mineral acids, alkalis, cyanide, methyl or ethyl alcohol, and drugs that are insoluble in aqueous acidic solution; the adsorption of ferrous sulfate is low.

Activated charcoal should be given within 30 minutes after ingestion of the poison, if possible, although it has been shown to be effective even when administration is delayed several hours, particularly if bowel sounds are absent. It is less effective in the treatment of poisoning caused by rapidly absorbed agents. Repeated doses may be effective for drugs that are absorbed slowly or are recycled through the enterohepatic system. There appears to be little desorption of the poison during its passage through the gastrointestinal tract.

Charcoal adsorbs ipecac; thus, syrup of ipecac should be given before activated charcoal is used. Activated charcoal is then given after emesis.

Charcoals from different sources have different adsorption capacities. The most effective are those of small particle size (large total surface area) and low mineral content. Universal antidote, which is a mixture of nonactivated charcoal, magnesium oxide, and tannic acid, is ineffective and may be toxic because of the tannic acid present.

ROUTE, USUAL DOSAGE, AND PREPARATIONS. *Oral*: *Adults and children*, activated charcoal should be administered as a slurry in water. A flavoring agent may be added to improve taste, but ice cream, which has been used to improve palatability, decreases efficacy and should not be used. Although the optimal ratio of charcoal to poison appears to be 5:1 to 10:1, this amount may be impracticable. A dose of 30 g is considered the minimum, and 100 g in 250 ml in water is preferred by many physicians. There is no toxicity and, therefore, no maximum dose limit. Repeated doses can be administered when necessary.

Drug available generically: Powder.
AVAILABLE TRADEMARKS.
Norit A (Pfanstiehl).

URINARY ACIDIFIER

AMMONIUM CHLORIDE

Ammonium chloride is an acidifying salt which temporarily reduces urinary pH. Tolerance develops within two to three days. Ammonium chloride is used in conjunction with the urinary antiseptic, methenamine (see Chapter 78, Urinary Tract Antiseptics). It also can be used to acidify urine in order to impede renal tubular reabsorption of organic bases and thus enhance their urinary excretion when such bases are the cause of poisoning. However, only a few organic bases (eg, quinine, quinidine, chloroquine) that have a pKa close to neutral and are appreciably eliminated via the kidney can be expected to have their excretion hastened to a significant extent by urinary acidifiction. Other measures to terminate exposure are generally much more effective. Ammonium chloride should not be used as a diuretic for forced diuresis to hasten excretion of poisons; furosemide, the thiazides, or osmotic agents (eg, mannitol) are more effective and reliable.

Adequate doses of ammonium chloride frequently cause gastric irritation, nausea, and even vomiting. Absorption also may be erratic, depending upon the poison ingested. This agent is relatively contraindicated in patients with impaired hepatic or renal function because of the risk of ammonium toxicity.

Ascorbic acid (but not sodium ascorbate) can be used as an alternative agent if ammonium chloride is not tolerated or is contraindicated. Doses of 0.5 to 2 g every four hours are recommended; however, the desirable alteration in urinary pH is not always obtained (Naccarto et al, 1979), even at the higher dose levels.

ROUTE, USUAL DOSAGE, AND PREPARATIONS. *Oral*: *Adults*, 1 to 2 g four or six times daily. Urinary pH should be monitored and the dosage adjusted accordingly. The development of tolerance following three consecutive days of therapy will usually necessitate interruption of administration for three to four days.

Drug available generically: Tablets (plain, enteric-coated) 300 and 500 mg (nonprescription).

URINARY ALKALIZER

SODIUM BICARBONATE

Sodium bicarbonate is used principally to treat metabolic acidosis (see Chapter 51, Replenishers and Regulators of Water and Electrolytes). It is eliminated principally in the urine and effectively alkalizes it. Since alkaline urine interferes with the renal tubular reabsorption of organic acids (eg, aspirin, phenobarbital), excretion of such substances is enhanced. Excessive alkalization of the urine may alkalize the plasma to a degree that interferes with the passage of organic acids out of the brain; this, in turn, prolongs the degree and duration of central nervous system toxicity and also aggravates potassium depletion caused by aspirin poisoning. The administration of sodium bicarbonate and dosages selected should be based on the degree of metabolic acidosis, sodium overload, and potassium depletion rather than just measurement of urinary pH (Done, 1977).

Sodium bicarbonate is completely absorbed orally and usually is excreted within three to four hours. Carbon dioxide formation in the stomach may be bothersome; therefore, a preparation containing sodium citrate and citric acid (Shohl's solution) may be substituted.

The maximum sodium tolerance is 250 mEq/M²/24 hours in healthy persons (1 g of sodium bicarbonate contains 11.9 mEq of sodium). Sodium bicarbonate must be used with caution in edematous patients with sodium-retaining disorders. Average doses in those with renal insufficiency or prolonged administration of average doses in patients with normal renal function may cause systemic alkalosis with irritability, neuromuscular excitability, and tetany.

ROUTES, USUAL DOSAGE, AND PREPARATIONS. *Oral*: *Adults*, 300 mg to 1.8 g one to four times daily, usually before meals and at bedtime. In view of the considerable variations among individuals and their diet, the urinary pH of each patient should be monitored and the dosage adjusted accordingly.

Drug available generically: Tablets 300 and 600 mg (nonprescription).
SIMILAR PREPARATION.
Bicitra (Shohl's solution) (Willen). Each 5 ml of liquid contains sodium citrate 500 mg and citric acid 300 mg in 120 and 480 ml containers.

Intravenous: *Adults and children*, 2 to 5 mEq/kg of body weight is administered over a four- to eight-hour period; the specific amount depends upon the degree of metabolic acidosis.

Drug available generically: Solution 4.2% (0.5 mEq/ml) in 10 ml containers, 7.5% (0.89 mEq/ml) and 8.4% (1 mEq/ml) in 50 ml containers.

General References

Physicians Desk Reference, ed 34. Oradell, NJ, Medical Economics Company, 1980.
Arena JM: Poisoning: Treatment and prevention, parts I, II, and III. *JAMA* 232:1272-1275; 233:358-363; 233:900-903, 1975.
Arena JM: *Poisoning: Toxicology, Symptoms, Treatments*, ed 3. Springfield, Ill, Charles C Thomas Publisher, 1974.
Casarett LJ, Doull J: *Toxicology: The Basic Science of Poisons*. New York, Macmillan Publishing Company, Inc, 1975.
Garrettson LK (ed): *Handbook of Common Poisonings in Children*, publication no. (FDA) 76-7004. US Department of Health, Education and Welfare, Food and Drug Administration, 1976.
Gleason MN, et al: *Clinical Toxicology of Commercial Products*, ed 4. Baltimore, Williams & Wilkins Company, 1976.
Rumack BH, Temple AR (eds): *Management of the Poisoned Patient*. Princeton, NJ, Science Press, 1977.
Rumack BH, et al (eds): POISINDEX^R: A Microfiche emergency poison management system. Micromedex, Inc, Englewood, Colo, 1979.

Selected References

Done AK: Aspirin revisited. *Emergency Med* 9:151-160, (Sept) 1977.
Naccarto DV, et al: Appraisal of ascorbic acid for acidifying urine of methenamine-treated geriatric patients. *J Am Geriat Soc* 27:34-37, 1979.

Specific Antidotes | 86

Specific drug antidotes are divided into two categories for discussion in this text: (1) those whose primary clinical use is the treatment of poisoning (the narcotic antagonists, metal antagonists, and a miscellaneous group composed of acetylcysteine [Mucomyst], cyanide antagonists, physostigmine [Antilirium], pralidoxime [Protopam], and protamine), and (2) those used in the treatment of poisoning but having other clinical indications in addition. The latter include vitamin K to counteract the effects of coumarin; potassium salts for digitalis; chlorpromazine for amphetamine and cocaine; oxygen for carbon monoxide; antihistamines for phenothiazine-induced dystonias; leucovorin for methotrexate; thymidine for fluorouracil; purines for mercaptopurine; atropine for bethanechol or other muscarinic stimulants, as well as for organophosphates; and neostigmine or edrophonium for tubocurarine. Not included are pyridoxine and folic acid, which are used to treat specific vitamin deficiencies induced by prolonged therapy with isoniazid and phenytoin, respectively. Evaluations on drugs in this second category may be found in chapters that discuss their main therapeutic indications.

NARCOTIC ANTAGONISTS

Through common usage, the agents discussed in this section have been designated narcotic antagonists. However, because they have been shown to interact with opiate receptors in the brain, thus antagonizing the actions of not only the so-called narcotics but also other substances with an affinity for opiate receptors, the term opioid antagonists may be more appropriate. Therefore, these two terms are used interchangeably in this text.

Antagonists have a stronger affinity for opiate receptors in the brain than agonists and can displace the latter from these sites. If the antagonist is given before the agonist, the latter's effects are blocked since receptor sites are already occupied. Although they bind to the receptor, pure antagonists do not initiate physiologic action as agonists do. However, some agents have mixed antagonist-agonist properties; their affinity for the receptor is intermediate between pure agonists and pure antagonists, but one of these properties predominates and is the basis for the principal clinical use of the drugs. Naloxone has only antagonist properties.

The available narcotic antagonists, nalorphine [Nalline], levallorphan [Lorfan], and naloxone [Narcan], are the N-allyl analogues of morphine, levorphanol [Levo-Dromoran], and oxymorphone [Numorphan], respectively. They are used primarily to counteract the severe respiratory depression, coma, and convulsions produced by excessive doses of opiates or opioids, including heroin. They also may be used to diagnose opioid dependence, and some antagonists are being investigated for the treatment of this type of dependence.

The actions of nalorphine and levallorphan are similar; both possess some agonist properties in addition to antagonist effects, although the latter predominate. When administered in the absence of a narcotic, the agonist properties observed include analgesia, respiratory depression, miosis, and subjective effects described as euphoria similar to that induced by morphine; drowsiness or intoxication similar to that produced by sedatives; and dysphoria and hallucinations. These responses preclude the use of nalorphine and levallorphan as analgesics. Their agonist action, which produces respiratory depression and subjective effects, also has limited their use as antagonists. Unlike these older antagonists, naloxone does not possess agonist properties. Since respiratory depression does not occur with therapeutic doses, it is the drug of choice to counteract this effect in patients with known or suspected narcotic overdosage.

Several opioid antagonists are being investigated for use in the treatment of morphine-type dependence. Since an antagonist administered to former narcotic-dependent subjects blocks the euphorigenic and dependence-producing effects of a narcotic, its use aids in preventing a relapse to addiction. Cyclazocine, which is related chemically to pentazocine, has produced favorable results, but its agonist effects are a disadvantage. Naloxone also has been effective but, because of its short duration of action when administered parenterally and its lack of activity when given orally, its use for this purpose is not practical. Longer-acting derivatives (eg, naltrexone) are under investigation.

INDIVIDUAL EVALUATIONS

NALOXONE
[Narcan]

Naloxone is the drug of choice to treat respiratory depression known or suspected to be caused by an overdose of an opiate or opioid. It promptly increases the respiratory rate and volume. Since naloxone does not produce respiratory depression nor affect that produced by barbiturates, an absence of response suggests that the depression is not the result of narcotic overdose. If the clinical history strongly suggests opiate-induced respiratory depression, some physicians administer an additional 2 to 4 mg of naloxone to ensure the absence of a narcotic overdose. Naloxone effectively reverses the agonist effects of pentazocine and other mixed agonist-antagonist agents (eg, cyclazocine, nalorphine) and, like other narcotic antagonists, precipitates withdrawal symptoms in individuals dependent on morphine-like drugs; therefore, it must be administered cautiously (0.1 to 0.2 mg intravenously, repeated at two- to three-minute intervals) until respiratory depression is reversed in these patients.

The onset of action is rapid; an effect usually is noted within two minutes after intravenous injection and only slightly later after intramuscular or subcutaneous injection, but the former is preferred. Like other narcotic antagonists, its duration of action may be shorter than that of some narcotics. Thus, repeated doses may be necessary to treat respiratory depression effectively, but even large doses do not increase the degree of existing depression.

In addition to antagonizing respiratory depression, coma, and convulsions, naloxone counteracts other actions of the narcotics, such as analgesia, cardiovascular and gastrointestinal effects, pupillary response, release of antidiuretic hormone, and hyperglycemia. Naloxone may precipitate a withdrawal syndrome in dependent patients. Although the syndrome is relatively self-limited (15 to 60 minutes) because of the short serum half-life, naloxone should be administered cautiously to dependent patients.

Naloxone may be administered postoperatively to reverse severe respiratory depression resulting from the use of opioids. However, since it also may decrease the analgesic and sedative effects of these drugs, dosage must be selected carefully to provide the desired effect. Naloxone has been given with various morphine-like analgesics in an attempt to prevent respiratory depression while retaining the analgesic effect, but there is little evidence to support the use of such combined therapy.

Naloxone is effective in the treatment of neonatal respiratory depression resulting from administration of large doses of morphine-like drugs to the mother during labor and delivery. The antagonist should not be administered to the mother before delivery, but it is preferable to inject the drug intravenously if respiratory depression is present in the infant after birth. It should be kept in mind that, if the mother is dependent on morphine-like drugs, the infant is also dependent and may exhibit withdrawal symptoms after birth. Because administration of an antagonist will precipitate a withdrawal reaction in these infants, careful monitoring should be provided after the desired effect is achieved.

Naloxone also may be given to diagnose narcotic addiction, but it must be administered cautiously and in small doses to avoid precipitating a severe withdrawal syndrome in narcotic-dependent individuals. The pupillography test using nalorphine has been useful when employed by trained personnel, but chemical methods to detect the presence of narcotics in the urine is more sensitive and may be preferable.

Naloxone has been reported to reverse the toxic effects of dextromethorphan.

This drug has been notably free from adverse reactions. Tolerance and psychic or physical dependence do not develop. Naloxone is not subject to the narcotic controls of the Controlled Substances Act.

ROUTES, USUAL DOSAGE, AND PREPARATIONS. *Intravenous*: For respiratory depression caused by opioid overdosage, *adults*, 0.4 mg; if an immediate response is not observed, the dose may be repeated at two- to three-minute intervals. If physical dependence is suspected but the patient is not in imminent danger, 0.1 to 0.2 mg may be given at two- to three-minute intervals until the desired therapeutic effect is obtained. *Children*, 0.01 mg/kg of body weight initially, repeated at two- to three-minute intervals as necessary. To reverse narcotic-induced respiratory depression in *newborn infants*, 0.01 mg/kg initially, repeated once in three to five minutes if there is no response. The dose may need to be repeated in 30 to 90 minutes, depending upon the degree of depression in the infant. The drug also has been given by continuous infusion (3.66 mcg/kg/hr has been effective) to counteract the respiratory depression induced by morphine when used in anesthesia (Johnstone et al, 1974). For postoperative respiratory depression caused by narcotic overdosage, *adults*, 0.1 to 0.2 mg intravenously at two- to three-minute intervals until the desired effect is achieved. This dose may be repeated at one- to two-hour intervals as necessary. If necessary, the drug also may be given intramuscularly or subcutaneously.

Narcan (Endo). Solution 0.4 mg/ml in 1 ml containers and 0.02 mg/ml in 2 ml containers (Narcan Neonatal) with methylparaben and propylparaben as preservatives.

METAL ANTAGONISTS

Heavy metal poisoning continues to be a serious toxicologic problem. Metal ions enter the body following parenteral administration for medical use, through ingestion or inhalation, and, occasionally, through abraded or intact skin. The absorption and distribution of organometallic compounds and inorganic metallic compounds usually are quite different.

Heavy metal ions react with two or more ligands of an organic compound through at least one coordinate covalent bond. The resulting product is either a stable compound (heterocycle) and is termed a chelate (claw) or is a less stable, nonheterocyclic compound and is referred to as a complex. Medically useful heavy metal antagonists are nonionic, water soluble, and chemically stable and are eliminated by the kidney. The electrophilic ligands of metal antagonists compete with electrophilic physiologic ligands for the free metal ion in vivo. The stability constant of a metal antagonist is an overall representation of the affinity and dissociation constants. If the metal antagonist has a higher stability constant than the existing physiologic complex or chelate in vivo, the metal antagonist will gradually displace the bound metal. Because none of the metal antagonists have complete specificity for only one metal cation, long-term use may lead to trace element deficiencies. The intensity and type of deficiency depends upon the nature of the metal antagonist.

Other than terminating exposure, the only successful approach to the treatment of acute heavy metal poisoning is inactivation of the metal ion by metal antagonists. The agents administered primarily for this purpose are edetate calcium disodium [Calcium Disodium Versenate], deferoxamine [Desferal], dimercaprol [BAL], and penicillamine [Cuprimine, Depen]. Edetate disodium [Endrate, Sodium Versenate] has high affinity for calcium and is used in severe hypercalcemia and digitalis-induced arrhythmias. It should *not* be used to treat heavy metal poisoning.

Therapy with a metal antagonist is most effective when it is begun immediately after exposure to the heavy metal. If the time elapsed between ingestion of the toxic material and initiation of therapy is sufficiently long to allow incorporation of the metal into certain metal-avid binding sites in tissue and bone, prolonged therapy will be needed.

Because of the increasing use of radioactive isotopes in biomedical and industrial research, the incidence of accidental poisoning with radioactive heavy metals is increasing. Poisoning caused by one of the more conventional radioactive isotopes, such as iron, can be treated with deferoxamine to hasten excretion. However, treatment is more difficult if the toxic agent is one of the more exotic metals such as uranium, radium, strontium, plutonium, or yttrium. Neither radium nor strontium can be removed from the body because their stability constants with various metal antagonists are about the same as those of calcium. However, their rate of excretion can be increased by infusion of calcium salts in conjunction with oral administra-

tion of ammonium chloride. The excretion of plutonium, thorium, and some other radioactive isotopes can be increased considerably by chelation with edetate calcium disodium. Trisodium calcium pentetate (DPTA), currently available only as an investigational drug in this country, hastens the excretion of lanthanum, yttrium, americium, scandium, and plutonium but does not increase the excretion of strontium, polonium, or uranium.

The occasional severe adverse reactions produced by penicillamine and dimercaprol and the pain associated with the intramuscular administration of edetate calcium disodium and dimercaprol have stimulated searches for safer orally effective agents to treat lead poisoning. An investigational drug, 2,3-dimercaptosuccinic acid, which is similar to dimercaprol chemically but is water soluble, may represent such an agent (Friedheim et al, 1978). It is effective clinically in mobilizing and enhancing the excretion of lead; experimentally, it is active against mercury and arsenic as well. Currently, 3 to 5 mg/kg of body weight orally at six-hour intervals is the suggested dosage for lead poisoning.

Some metal antagonists have been tried in conditions other than heavy metal poisoning or in diseases associated with heavy metal retention (eg, penicillamine in Wilson's disease and primary biliary cirrhosis; deferoxamine in hemochromatosis). Penicillamine is also being evaluated in the therapy of cystinuria, rheumatoid arthritis, and chronic active hepatitis. Metal antagonists have been tried unsuccessfully in the treatment of porphyria, scleroderma, angina pectoris, nephrocalcinosis, calcified mitral stenosis, otosclerosis, atherosclerosis, and sarcoidosis.

Adverse Reactions and Precautions

Because of wide variation in toxic manifestations, it is impossible to generalize concerning the adverse reactions and precautions of metal antagonists. Serious toxic effects can occur with use of these compounds; however, adverse reactions are rarely life-threatening, are usually reversible, and generally are less severe than the effects of heavy metal poisoning (see the evaluations).

INDIVIDUAL EVALUATIONS

EDETATE CALCIUM DISODIUM
[Calcium Disodium Versenate]

This drug is used primarily to treat lead poisoning (plumbism). The chelates formed are water soluble, are not easily dissociated, and are readily excreted by the kidneys. Edetate calcium disodium does not produce negative calcium balance. It is capable of binding and increasing the excretion of zinc and copper, but the intensity of this action is thought to be clinically insignificant if therapy is not continued beyond seven days. This agent is of questionable or unproved value in poisoning caused by cadmium, chromium, manganese, gold, and nickel and is ineffective in poisoning caused by mercury or arsenic.

The optimal pH range for the combination of edetate calcium disodium with lead includes all physiologic pH values. When treating lead poisoning in adults, the drug is given intravenously for three to seven days to allow continued chelation and excretion of the heavy metal as it is released from tissues into extracellular fluid. Peak excretion of chelated lead occurs within 24 to 48 hours.

Guidelines recently revised by the Center for Disease Control for the diagnosis and treatment of lead poisoning have been reviewed (Pincus and Saccar, 1979). The upper limit of normal lead blood levels is 29 mcg/dl of whole blood. When lead levels are between 30 and 69 mcg/dl and derangement of heme synthesis is sus-

pected (erythrocyte protoporphyrin whole blood concentration is greater than 50 mcg/dl in children), a 24-hour diagnostic mobilization test is commonly performed. Two variants of this test are used. With the first, a 24-hour urine sample is collected after administration of edetate calcium disodium. If the 24-hour urinary excretion of lead is greater than 1 mcg/mg of edetate calcium disodium administered, the presence of excessive amounts of lead in the body is indicated. With the second variant, the collection of a 24-hour urine control sample is followed by collection of another 24-hour urine sample after administration of edetate calcium disodium. If the lead concentration of the second sample is three times greater than that of the first and contains more than 50 mcg of lead, the test is considered positive.

If the mobilization test is positive, a five-day course of chelation therapy is administered, and the test is then repeated to determine if another course of therapy is necessary. When the urinary lead excretion can be monitored daily, the course of therapy can be terminated when less than 0.5 mcg of lead per mg of edetate calcium disodium is excreted in 24 hours. Results of these tests are valid only when renal function is normal, and their acceptability is limited by the necessity of collecting uncontaminated urine samples.

The Center for Disease Control recommends that the mobilization test be omitted and appropriate chelation be given immediately to symptomatic patients or those having lead levels greater than 70 mcg/dl of whole blood.

Too rapid mobilization of lead with deposition in lead-avid soft tissues at a rate faster than its urinary clearance may exacerbate toxicity. Thus, the preferred treatment for severe lead poisoning, especially lead encephalopathy, is combined therapy with edetate calcium disodium and dimercaprol; this increases the excretion of lead and is less toxic than when either agent is given alone. Penicillamine may be administered orally for follow-up therapy when necessary (see the evaluation).

Edetate calcium disodium is not metabolized and is excreted within 24 hours exclusively by glomerular filtration. Therefore, adequate urine flow should be established before initiating therapy. Use of this drug is contraindicated in anuric or severely oliguric patients.

Edetate calcium disodium is poorly absorbed from the gastrointestinal tract. Furthermore, if lead is present in the intestine, its absorption may be increased because the lead chelate formed is more soluble than the lead itself. After absorption, the chelate dissociates and releases free lead ions, which can produce toxic reactions. Thus, oral administration for prophylaxis may enhance lead absorption in workers exposed to this metal. The most effective way to prevent chronic exposure is to maintain proper industrial hygiene.

Common adverse reactions are gastroenteritis following oral administration and pain at the site of intramuscular injection. Other reactions include transient bone marrow depression, hypotension, cheilosis, chills, fever, and histamine-like reactions (sneezing, nasal congestion, and lacrimation). Very large doses occasionally cause acute renal tubular necrosis and rarely are fatal. Therefore, edetate calcium disodium should be used with caution, if at all, in patients with pre-existing renal disease. Some patients may develop hypercalcemia, since lead displaces calcium from the chelate. Edetate calcium disodium interferes with the duration of action of zinc insulin preparations by forming a chelate with zinc; therefore, these preparations are incompatible in intravenous admixtures.

It is suggested that urinalysis and blood urea nitrogen, serum creatinine, calcium, and phosphorus levels be measured before treatment is begun and on the third and fifth days of therapy.

ROUTES, USUAL DOSAGE, AND PREPARATIONS. *Intravenous*: Since edetate calcium disodium is eliminated by the kidneys and renal function is related to body surface area, some investigators calculate dosage on the basis of body surface area. *Adults*, 1.5 g/M^2/day in two divided doses for three to five days. For mildly symptomatic adults or adults with whole blood levels of 50 to 70 mcg/dl, the total daily dose may be reduced to 1 g/M^2. Each dose is diluted in 250 or 500 ml of sodium chloride injection or 5% dextrose injection and administered over a period of eight hours. Therapy is then interrupted for at least two days (preferably two weeks) and a second course given if necessary. The maximum 24-hour dose should not exceed 50 mg/kg (1.75 g/M^2), even in cases of severe poisoning. For *children*, intramuscular injection is preferred to avoid extravasation at the intravenous injection site or the possibility of lead encephalopathy. If the intravenous route is chosen, treatment courses and doses are the same as those expressed for adults with the following exceptions: The maximum 24-hour dose may be increased to 75 mg/kg of body weight in very severe poisoning, but the total amount of fluid administered per dose must be reduced as required. Generally, although two courses of therapy are adequate in adults, children may require additional courses when mobilization of lead from labile skeletal stores approaches the critical blood level of 70 mcg/dl; therapy should be continued intermittently until the lead blood concentration remains below 50 mcg/dl.

Intramuscular (deep): *Adults*, the dose and treatment course schedule are the same as for intravenous use. The drug is administered as a 20% solution. Generally, procaine is added to a final concentration of 0.5% to 1.5% to minimize pain following injection. In *children* with encephalopathy, combined therapy with dimercaprol is preferred. Dimercaprol is given intramuscularly initially. Four hours later and every four hours thereafter for five to seven days, dimercaprol plus edetate calcium disodium 12.5 mg/kg of body weight is administered; separate sites are used if the latter is also given intramuscularly. The doses of dimercaprol given concomitantly are: for very severe poisoning, 750 mg/M^2/day in divided doses every four hours; for less severe acute poisoning, 500 mg/M^2/day in divided doses every four hours; for mild poisoning, 333 mg/M^2/day in divided doses every four to six hours. Alternatively, 25 mg/kg of edetate calcium disodium is given as the sole agent every 12 hours for three to five days. After five to seven days, the same procedure is followed as for intravenous administration.

For diagnosis, *adults*, 500 mg/M^2 to a maximum of 1 g diluted in 500 ml of 5% dextrose injection and infused over a period of at least one hour. The urine is collected for 24 hours before and after the start of infusion for measurement of total lead output. For diagnosis, *children*, 500 mg/M^2/day to a maximal dose of 1 g in two divided doses at 12-hour intervals, preferably by intramuscular injection. The urine is collected for 24 hours from the start of injection for measurement of total lead output. A 24-hour control urine sample taken prior to drug administration may aid in interpretating test results.

> **Calcium Disodium Versenate** (Riker). Solution 200 mg/ml in 5 ml containers.

Oral: Use of this route is not advisable because it enhances lead absorption.

> **Calcium Disodium Versenate** (Riker). Tablets 500 mg.

DEFEROXAMINE MESYLATE
[Desferal]

$$H_3\overset{+}{N}(CH_2)_5NC(CH_2)_2CNH(CH_2)_5NC(CH_2)_2CNH(CH_2)_5NCCH_3 \quad CH_3SO_3^-$$

Deferoxamine, a compound obtained from *Streptomyces pilosus*, is a potent and highly specific iron chelating agent. It readily complexes with ferric ion to form ferrioxamine, a stable, water-soluble chelate; it also has limited affinity for ferrous ion. In addition to combining with free ionic iron, deferoxamine can remove iron from ferritin and hemosiderin (except in bone marrow). It is much less effective against transferrin and does not remove iron from the cytochromes, myoglobin, or hemoglobin. Deferoxamine binds 8.5 mg iron/100 mg.

This drug is useful in the treatment of acute iron intoxication (Stein, 1976); other measures, such as induced vomiting, airway maintenance, gastric lavage with sodium phosphate or sodium bicarbonate to form nonabsorbable iron salts, and control of metabolic acidosis and shock, are also important. Urinary excretion of the ferrioxamine complex accounts for two-thirds of the iron eliminated; the remainder is excreted in the bile. The ferrioxamine complex has a characteristic reddish color; thus, the appearance of reddish-brown urine after injection of deferoxamine is presumptive evidence of elevated serum iron levels and an indication for further therapy.

The shorter the interval between iron ingestion and deferoxamine administration, the greater the probability of successful recovery without complications or sequelae. The first phase (30 to 120 minutes) of acute iron intoxication includes signs and symptoms caused principally by gastrointestinal irritation and necrosis. An asymptomatic phase may ensue that can mislead the physician as to the severity of the intoxication. Continued aggressive evaluation of the patient must be maintained, and deferoxamine may have to be administered to avoid or lessen the later phases of acidosis, hepatic failure, and pyloric stenosis. The serum iron level is not always an accurate indication of the severity of iron intoxication; potentially fatal necrosis of the gastrointestinal tract can occur even when the serum iron concentration is low.

Deferoxamine is useful in the management of secondary hemochromatosis to promote iron excretion (Pippard et al, 1978; Propper et al, 1977). It usually is administered by slow intravenous or subcutaneous infusion to promote iron excretion in patients with chronic anemia and iron overload secondary to multiple blood transfusions (Cohen and Schwartz, 1978 A and B; Graziano et al, 1978; Weiner et al, 1978). Actual negative net accumulation of iron may be demonstrated in some patients. It is also helpful if patients receive supplemental intravenous deferoxamine therapy during blood transfusion as well. No tolerance to deferoxamine was demonstrated over a period of two years. Total dose and duration of therapy must be determined for each patient on the basis of an initial dose response curve. The goal is to use the minimum amount of deferoxamine that will just prevent net iron accumulation.

Deferoxamine is less effective in primary hemochromatosis (Young et al, 1979); phlebotomy eliminates more iron. However, use of deferoxamine is beneficial when venesection is contraindicated (eg, when the patient is hypoproteinemic or too anemic to tolerate blood loss).

Deferoxamine generally is well tolerated. Rapid intravenous injection can cause hypotension, tachycardia, erythema, and urticaria. Some patients experience a local histamine-like reaction or induration following subcutaneous administration; this reaction is rare when the drug is given intramuscularly. Severe, transient pain at the site of injection may occur. Patients receiving long-term therapy have had mild allergic-type dermatologic reactions, blurred vision, diarrhea, abdominal discomfort, leg cramps, tachycardia, and fever. Anaphylactic reactions are rare.

Cataracts have been observed rarely in patients who received the drug for prolonged periods to treat chronic iron storage diseases. There are no absolute contraindications to the use of deferoxamine when treating acute iron intoxication or hemochromatosis. Since the drug and the ferrioxamine complex are excreted primarily by the kidneys, deferoxamine is contraindicated in patients with severe renal disease or anuria. Exchange transfusion or hemodialysis may have to be considered in patients with acute renal failure, life-threatening symptoms (especially shock) refractory to treatment, or when the amount of iron is so large that maximum recommended doses of deferoxamine cannot be expected to complex with more than a fraction of the free iron available.

ROUTES, USUAL DOSAGE, AND PREPARATIONS.
FOR POISONING:
The intramuscular route of administration is generally preferred for acute poisoning unless the situation necessitates intravenous therapy.

Intramuscular: For *adults and children* not in shock, 20 mg/kg of body weight every four to six hours, depending upon the condition of the patient. Deferoxamine should be prepared by adding 2 ml of sterile water for injection to each vial. The total dose should not exceed 6 g/24 hours. *Intravenous*: For *adults and children* with signs of shock, a serum iron level greater than 350 mcg/dl, or free iron in the plasma, 10 mg/kg/hr is infused for eight hours, followed by 5 mg/kg/hr if needed. Faster rates of administration or boluses may cause severe hypotension. The rate of infusion should never exceed 15 mg/kg/hr, and the total dose should not exceed 6 g/24 hours.

FOR HEMOCHROMATOSES:
Continuous subcutaneous or intravenous infusion is recommended for iron overload associated with hemochromatoses, because more iron is eliminated per unit dose of deferoxamine than with intramuscular bolus administration. The concomitant oral administration of ascorbic acid (0.5 to 1 g twice daily) seems to improve the chelating action of deferoxamine in hemochromatosis, particularly if there is a vitamin C deficiency. Cardiac decompensation may occur, however, with combined deferoxamine and ascorbic acid therapy; ascorbic acid should be discontinued if such symptoms and signs develop.

Intravenous: *Adults*, 1 g of deferoxamine is dissolved in 10 ml of water (isotonic). The average total daily dose is 2 g administered by slow infusion (not to exceed 15 mg/kg/hr) over a 12-hour period. As much as 4 g/24 hours has been administered but there may be little, if any, more iron excreted than 2 g/12 hours, depending upon the individual patient. Deferoxamine can be administered with, but separate from, each unit of blood transfused.

Subcutaneous: 1 g of deferoxamine is dissolved in 10 ml of water (isotonic). The average total daily dose is 2 g administered by slow infusion over a 12-hour period, usually in an anterior abdominal wall site, during the night. As much as 4 g/24 hours has been administered, but there may be little, if any, more iron excreted than 2 g/12 hours, depending upon the individual patient.

    Desferal (Ciba). Powder for solution (lyophilized, sterile) 500 mg.

DIMERCAPROL
[BAL in Oil]

$$\underset{\underset{\text{SH}}{|}\ \underset{\text{SH}}{|}}{CH_2CH_2CH_2OH}$$

By forming chelates or complexes, dimercaprol antagonizes the toxic effects of arsenic, mercury, and gold. It is not useful in treating arsine (AsH_3) poisoning. Therapy is most effective if it is begun within one or two hours after ingestion. Retrospective clinical studies reveal that dimercaprol effectively neutralizes mercury within four hours, but efficacy is reduced after six hours. Dimercaprol should be used only in acute mercury poisoning; in chronic intoxication, excretion of mercury is increased but the clinical condition may not improve. Although this drug also removes lead, edetate calcium disodium or penicillamine is preferred. However, in severe lead poisoning in children, the combination of dimercaprol and edetate calcium disodium is preferred, since some studies suggest that this regimen hastens excretion of lead and reduces the incidence of brain damage. Dimercaprol may increase the rate of copper excretion in Wilson's disease (hepatolenticular degeneration), but penicillamine is the drug of choice.

Dimercaprol is not beneficial in antimony or bismuth poisoning and should not be used in iron, cadmium, or selenium poisoning because the dimercaprol-metal complexes formed are more nephrotoxic than the metal alone.

In usual doses, adverse reactions are generally mild and transitory. They include local pain at the site of injection, paresthesias, lacrimation, blepharal spasm, apprehension, diaphoresis, asthenia, salivation, and vomiting. Many of these effects, as well as symptoms of serum sickness, are relieved by administration of an antihistamine. Dimercaprol has a strong odor and imparts an unpleasant odor to the patient's breath. Fever, which persists throughout therapy, may occur in children.

Large doses cause moderate hypertension followed by hypotension, coma, or convulsions. Dimercaprol also may induce metabolic acidosis associated with elevated serum lactate levels. With continued use of large doses, capillary damage resulting in loss of protein and fluid from the circulation occurs.

Like all metal antagonists, dimercaprol is potentially nephrotoxic. If acute renal failure develops during therapy, dimercaprol should be discontinued or used only with extreme caution, since toxic concentrations may appear in the serum. Since the chelate rapidly dissociates in an acid medium, releasing the bound metal, the urine should be kept alkaline. If dimercaprol is used as a component of lavage fluid to bind metal, the complex or chelate formed must be removed to avoid later dissociation in the intestinal tract.

ROUTE, USUAL DOSAGE, AND PREPARATIONS. *Intramuscular*: *Adults and children*, for mild arsenic or gold poisoning, 2.5 mg/kg of body weight four times daily for two days, two times on the third day, then once daily thereafter for ten days; for severe arsenic or gold poisoning, 3 mg/kg every four hours for two days, four times on the third day, then twice daily thereafter for 4 to 13 days. For mercury poisoning, 5 mg/kg initially, followed by 2.5 mg/kg one or two times daily for ten days. The suggested dosage based on body surface area is: for very severe poisoning, 750 mg/M²/day in divided doses every four hours; for less severe poisoning, 500 mg/M²/day in divided doses every four hours; for mild poisoning, 333 mg/M²/day in divided doses every four to six hours. Dosage is adjusted as described above.

For dosage used in lead poisoning, see the evaluation on Edetate Calcium Disodium.

BAL in Oil (Hynson, Westcott & Dunning). Solution 100 mg/ml in peanut oil in 3 ml containers.

PENICILLAMINE
[Cuprimine, Depen]

$$CH_3-\underset{\underset{CH_3}{|}}{\overset{\overset{SH}{|}}{C}}---\underset{\underset{H}{|}}{\overset{\overset{NH_2}{|}}{C}}---\overset{\overset{O}{||}}{C}OH$$

This synthetic sulfhydryl compound is an inactive degradation product of penicillin. It combines with copper, iron, mercury, lead, and arsenic to form soluble complexes that are readily excreted by the kidneys. Penicillamine itself is oxidized to a disulfide derivative and is also excreted by the kidneys.

This agent is effective orally and is superior to other metal antagonists for chelating copper. Its primary therapeutic use is to remove excess copper in patients with Wilson's disease. Such use, which must be continued indefinitely, promotes long-term survival in these patients; prophylactic administration is now recommended for individuals homozygous for Wilson's disease before clinical symptoms develop.

Penicillamine also is effective in primary biliary cirrhosis (Jain et al, 1977), another disease affecting copper metabolism. Copper accumulates in the liver in both primary biliary cirrhosis and Wilson's disease but does not accumulate in the brain in the former disease. Although hepatic copper levels correlate with the severity of the disease (Fleming et al, 1978), recent data suggest that the beneficial action of penicillamine also may be related in part to an immunologic action, which reduces immune complexes and immunoglobulins present in those with primary biliary cirrhosis (Epstein et al, 1979). It is too early to determine whether the reduction of elevated hepatic copper levels and improved liver function will justify the substantial risk associated with prolonged administration of penicillamine.

Penicillamine chelates lead less effectively than edetate calcium disodium or dimercaprol but has the advantage of being effective orally. This antagonist is not the drug of choice for severe lead intoxication, although it may be given after initial therapy with edetate calcium disodium. Penicillamine is useful in the treatment of asymptomatic patients with moderately elevated blood levels of lead. Unless excessive oral lead exposure is terminated, absorption of lead may be enhanced with penicillamine.

Although dimercaprol is the standard therapy for arsenic poisoning, penicillamine also is reported to be effective (Peterson and Rumack, 1977).

This chelating agent may be useful in treating cystinuria; it combines with cystine to form a soluble, readily excreted disulfide complex.

ADVERSE REACTIONS AND PRECAUTIONS.

The severity of adverse reactions associated with short-term administration is generally acceptable. Most untoward effects occur shortly after therapy is begun. Impairment of taste is usually transient. Erythematous maculopapular rashes with pruritus are common and considered to be hypersensitivity reactions; they often can be alleviated by concomitant administration of cyproheptadine or hydroxyzine. Purpuric or vesicular ecchymoses or rashes accompanied by fever, leukopenia, thrombocytopenia, eosinophilia, arthralgia, and lymphadenopathy may indicate the onset of a penicillamine-induced autoimmune syndrome or bone marrow suppression. Discontinuation of therapy or reduction in dosage, as well as administration of adrenal corticosteroids, may be necessary. If oral mucosal ulcers resembling aphthae and gastrointestinal upset occur, they usually respond to a reduction in dosage. Isolated cases of cholestatic jaundice and pancreatitis, which presumably were induced by penicillamine, have been reported.

Long-term administration is associated with adverse reactions of such severity that the drug must be discontinued in about 20% of patients. The two most common symptoms of serious toxicity are bone marrow suppression and development of immune disorders. Thrombocytopenia may be an early sign of impending bone marrow aplasia, which may be manifested by agranulocytosis, selective red cell aplasia, or erythryomyeloid aplasia. Autoimmune or immune complex disorders associated with and presumably caused by penicillamine include pemphigus, dermatomyositis, polymyositis, lupus erythematosus, diffuse alveolitis, obliterative bronchiolitis, and myasthenia gravis. Nephrotic syndrome may occur after several months of treatment, and a progressive and fatal complication resembling Goodpasture's syndrome has been reported.

Reversible proteinuria develops during therapy with doses of 1.2 g or more daily. If this occurs, the dosage should not be increased further and quantitative urinary protein determinations should be performed periodically. Therapy should be terminated if proteinuria exceeds 2 g/24 hours or hematuria occurs.

Optic neuropathy has been observed in patients given racemic penicillamine, but has not been reported with use of the D isomer; the neuropathy disappeared after administration of pyridoxine. Penicillamine increases the requirement for pyridoxine, and patients taking this chelating agent should receive 25 mg of pyridoxine daily. Use of supplemental multivitamin preparations is unnecessary but, if given, should be copper-free.

Careful examination of the skin, as well as urinalysis, differential and white blood cell counts, direct platelet counts, and hemoglobin determinations should be performed every three days during the first two weeks of therapy, at least every ten days for three or four months, and monthly thereafter for the duration of treatment. If the white blood count falls below 3,000/microliter or the platelet count below 100,000/microliter, the drug should be discontinued until these values become normal; when therapy is resumed, the dose should be small and the amount increased cautiously.

Since penicillamine has been associated with intrauterine growth retardation, it is recommended that the drug be withheld from pregnant patients with rheumatoid arthritis or cystinuria. However, pregnant patients with Wilson's disease or primary biliary cirrhosis may require this agent.

Cross sensitivity between penicillin and penicillamine does not always occur; therefore, penicillamine can be given cautiously to patients who are hypersensitive to penicillin.

ROUTE, USUAL DOSAGE, AND PREPARATIONS. *Oral*: For Wilson's disease and primary biliary cirrhosis (investigational), *older children and adults*, initially, 125 or 250 mg daily, increased gradually over a four- to eight-week period as indicated by side effects and urinary copper excretion. The usual maintenance dose is 250 mg four times daily; however, it is recommended that the total daily dose be limited to 500 to 750 mg to minimize untoward effects if efficacy is not compromised. *Infants over 6 months and young children*, a single daily dose of 250 mg dissolved in fruit juice. Penicillamine should be given on an empty stomach between meals and at bedtime; the last dose should be given at least three hours after the evening meal. Patients also should be maintained on a low-copper diet. Although these guidelines are helpful, dosage must be individualized and can be determined only by measuring the urinary excretion of copper. If the patient is on a low-copper diet and is using an oral cation exchange resin, negative copper balance will result if the urinary excretion of copper is 1 mg or more every 24 hours. For lead poisoning, *adults and children*, 600 mg/M² daily in two divided doses given two hours before meals until the concentration of lead remains below 50 mcg/dl of whole blood (usually four weeks to several months). A low-calcium diet augments the lead sequestering action.

For cystinuria, *adults and older children*, 2 g (range, 1 to 4 g) daily in four divided doses; *young children and infants*, 30 mg/kg of body weight daily in three or four equally divided doses. If equal doses are not possible or if adverse reactions necessitate a reduction in dosage, the largest amount should be given at bedtime. High fluid intake also is required (about 500 ml of water at bedtime and another 500 ml during the night when the urine is more concentrated and more acidic than during the day). Effective therapy is indicated by the urinary excretion of 100 to 200 mg of cystine every 24 hours in patients without a history of renal calculi and less than 100 mg/24 hours in patients with a history of calculi or flank pain.

Cuprimine (Merck Sharp & Dohme). Capsules 125 and 250 mg.
Depen (Wallace). Tablets 250 mg.

MISCELLANEOUS SPECIFIC ANTIDOTES

ACETYLCYSTEINE
[Mucomyst]

$$HSCH_2CHCOH$$
$$\underset{\underset{O}{\overset{\|}{NHCCH_3}}}{}$$

This mucolytic drug is used as an antidote for severe acetaminophen poisoning (Ameer and Greenblatt, 1977; Rumack, 1978) characterized by ingestion of at least 10 to 15 g of acetaminophen and a plasma concentration above a semilogarithmic line connecting 200 mcg/ml at four hours and 50 mcg/ml at 12 hours following ingestion (Rumack and Matthew, 1975). Approximately two-thirds of patients fulfilling these criteria develop symptoms of hepatotoxicity and should benefit from specific antidotal therapy. The incidence of hepatotoxicity is 100% with plasma acetaminophen concentrations above 300 mcg/ml.

Acetaminophen-induced hepatic damage is thought to be produced by an uncharacterized reactive intermediate of a minor metabolite that is normally inactivated by conjugation with glutathione. Overdosage occurs when the glutathione protective mechanism is 70% or more depleted. A number of sulfhydryl compounds have been tried as antidotes: Glutathione does not penetrate cells well, dimercaprol is ineffective, penicillamine is not especially useful and may cause additive or synergistic toxicity, and cysteamine is effective but produces serious adverse effects (Prescott et al, 1977). Oral methionine (Crome et al, 1977) or parenteral acetylcysteine are effective; on the basis of the limited data available, methionine appears to be somewhat less active. Because of the first-pass effect, the oral use of acetylcysteine is hypothetically more effective than parenteral therapy, but nausea and vomiting may be prominent with this route of administration.

Acetylcysteine is hydrolyzed rapidly to cysteine after cellular penetration. Adverse reactions are minor; transient elevation of blood pressure may occur but no arrhythmias have been documented.

ROUTE, USUAL DOSAGE, AND PREPARATIONS. **Oral**: The 10% or 20% solution is diluted to a 5% isotonic solution. A loading dose of 140 mg/kg of body weight is administered; 70 mg/kg is then given every four hours for 17 additional doses. Occasionally the patient may vomit. If this occurs within one hour after a dose, administration is repeated by nasogastric tube if necessary.

> *Mucomyst* (Mead Johnson). Solution (sterile) 10% and 20% in 4, 10, and 30 ml containers.

CYANIDE ANTIDOTE KIT

Cyanide ion combines principally with ferricytochrome oxidase to produce tissue hypoxia. A cyanide antidote kit containing two antagonists is available to treat cyanide poisoning. One antagonist is present in two forms, amyl nitrite pearls for inhalation and sodium nitrite solution for intravenous use. The second antagonist is sodium thiosulfate also for intravenous use. Nitrite ion converts hemoglobin to methemoglobin; the ferric ion formed competes with ferricytochrome oxidase for the available cyanide ion. Cyanide ion is biotransformed to the relatively nontoxic thiocyanate ion by hepatic rhodanase and thiol-containing compounds normally present in the body; sodium thiosulfate enhances the biotransformation by making more sulfur available. Oxygen is an important adjunct in the treatment of cyanide poisoning. It helps to reverse the binding of cyanide and ferricytochrome oxidase, enhances the conversion of cyanide to thiocyanate, and increases the delivery of oxygen to tissues.

Adverse reactions to cyanide antagonists are seldom clinically significant in otherwise healthy individuals at recommended doses. However, reactions may be clinically relevant in some situations (eg, prolonged sodium nitroprusside infusion in a hypertensive patient). Large amounts of methemoglobin decrease the amount of oxygen available for tissues, and nitrites also can produce cardiovascular instability, usually manifested as hypotension, which is especially likely to occur during anesthesia.

The use of the traditional cyanide antagonists is being re-evaluated in light of recent investigations in Europe using cobalt edetate and in the United States using hydroxocobalamin (Graham et al, 1977; Cottrell et al, 1978). Intravenous injection of cobalt edetate 600 mg forms a relatively nontoxic complex with cyanide; a supplemental dose of 300 mg is administered if recovery is delayed. Although some physicians in Britain consider cobalt edetate the treatment of choice (the drug is unavailable in the United States), it often induces vomiting and anaphylactic reactions have been reported occasionally.

The vitamin, hydroxocobalamin [alpha-Redisol] (see Chapter 52), combines with cyanide ion to form cyanocobalamin (vitamin B_{12}). No adverse reactions have been reported at this early stage of investigation. Hydroxocobalamin is given intravenously; however, no commercial parenteral preparation is available which contains the amount of drug required to combat cyanide toxicity without administering undesirable or excessive quantities of fluid. The role of hydroxocobalamin in cyanide poisoning is promising but investigational.

ROUTES, USUAL DOSAGE, AND PREPARATIONS. *Inhalation, Intravenous*: *Adults*, oxygen therapy should be initiated and amyl nitrite inhaled from the crushed pearls for 30 seconds of every minute until an intravenous route is established. Amyl nitrite then is discontinued and all of the sodium nitrite (300 mg) in the 10-ml ampul is administered intravenously. The 12.5 g of sodium thiosulfate contained in the 50-ml ampul is then administered intravenously. If symptoms persist, a second dose of sodium nitrite (one-half the amount of the first dose) should be given 30 minutes later. *Children*, see the manufacturer's literature.

Cyanide Antidote Package (Lilly). Each kit contains 12 amyl nitrite pearls 0.3 ml, two 10-ml containers of sodium nitrite 300 mg, two 50-ml containers of sodium thiosulfate 12.5 g, disposable syringes, stomach tube, and instructions.

PHYSOSTIGMINE SALICYLATE
[Antilirium]

This tertiary amine alkaloid is classified as an anticholinesterase. It has been replaced in the treatment of myasthenia gravis by quaternary amines with similar anticholinesterase activity that do not significantly penetrate the central nervous system. However, this property of physostigmine is useful in the treatment of central anticholinergic toxicity (Rumack, 1973), which is characterized by anxiety, disorientation, delirium, hyperactivity, hallucinations, illusions, impaired consciousness, impaired memory, and seizures. Physostigmine also is capable of antagonizing, although less effectively, the peripheral signs and symptoms (tachycardia; mydriasis; facial flushing; reduced sweating; hyperpyrexia; depressed bronchial, pharyngeal, nasal, and gastrointestinal secretions; decreased gastrointestinal and urinary tract motility). Abnormalities in cardiac conduction and rhythm are most resistant to reversal.

This spectrum of anticholinergic toxicity is most characteristic of poisoning with atropine and scopolamine.

Other classes of drugs have secondary anticholinergic activity. These include antihistamines, tricyclic antidepressants, certain antiemetics, some antiparkinsonism drugs (centrally acting anticholinergic drugs), phenothiazines, and, to a lesser extent, butyrophenones. Physostigmine should not be used routinely for overdosage of these classes of drugs but may be useful adjunctively if severe anticholinergic toxicity is suspected. It may aggravate some cardiac disturbances caused by the nonanticholinergic cardiotoxicity of these agents (eg, bradyarrhythmias).

Physostigmine also has reversed the central nervous system depression associated with the benzodiazepines, lorazepam and diazepam, which have little if any anti-cholinergic activity (Larson et al, 1977). Results of experimental data demonstrate that the central cholinergic system may play a role in regulating central dopamin-ergic activity (Davis et al, 1977), which may account for the nonspecific action of physostigmine. Alternatively, physostigmine may have an effect on the awake-sleep state, for it has been shown to arouse individuals from nonREM to REM sleep or from REM sleep to a fully awake state as if stimulation of the cholinergic system were involved in a continuum of arousal (Sitaram et al, 1976).

Physostigmine is almost completely hydrolyzed by the enzyme that it inhibits. It is relatively short acting (half-life, one to two hours). Renal impairment does not alter dosage.

The decision to initiate physostigmine therapy requires clinical judgment. In some instances (ie, presence of convulsions, hypertension, arrhythmias, severe hallucinations), treatment of anticholinergic toxicity may demand aggressive therapy. A response to physostigmine in a comatose patient can confirm a suspected diagnosis. The drug may improve ventilation in marginal situations when endotracheal intubation and mechanical ventilation are not readily available or could be avoided or improve the care of agitated, disoriented patients. However, if the diagnosis and overdose are well documented, if supportive care has improved and stabilized vital signs, and if urine output is adequate, there may be little value in using physostigmine for arousal.

Hypersensitivity to physostigmine occurs infrequently. The drug can produce slight to moderate bradycardia; severe bradyarrhythmias are more likely to develop if physostigmine is given to overcome the effects of orphenadrine and tricyclic antidepressants. Severe hypotensive episodes are rare, although convulsions have been observed. There is always a danger of excessive salivation, vomiting, urination, and defecation. The most dangerous sequelae of these actions may be aspiration, and adequate suction should always be available. In such instances,

administration of atropine may be necessary. Such adverse reactions are less likely to occur when anticholinergic poisoning is established. In this instance, a return to a more normal level of function occurs.

A dystonic extrapyramidal reaction should not be mistaken for central anticholinergic toxicity. The akinesia, akathisia, and dyskinesia of the former can be confused with the signs and symptoms of hyperactivity caused by the latter; however, there is little or no impaired consciousness associated with dystonic extrapyramidal reactions. Physostigmine worsens the rigidity, tremor, and akinesia of parkinsonism and extrapyramidal dystonic reactions.

Because of its short duration of action, physostigmine often becomes ineffective gradually over a 30- to 60-minute period; therefore, continued observation of the patient is important.

Any cholinergic sign or symptom that is undesirable in a given clinical situation may be considered a relative contraindication (eg, precipitation of an asthmatic attack).

ROUTES, USUAL DOSAGE, AND PREPARATIONS. *Intravenous*: *Adults*, 1 to 2 mg given slowly. The dose may be repeated as life-threatening signs and symptoms recur. The compound should not be administered more rapidly than 1 mg/min but should not be used as a continuous drip. Frequent periodic surveillance is essential to determine the appropriate dosage schedule in any given individual. The response to a single dose seldom lasts longer than 30 to 60 minutes. *Children*, for diagnosis, 0.5 mg given slowly. If toxic effects persist and no cholinergic effects are produced, the drug should be readministered at five-minute intervals until a maximum dose of 2 mg has been given. For therapy, the lowest total effective dose should be repeated if life-threatening signs and symptoms recur.

Intramuscular: *Adults*, 1 to 2 mg every one to two hours as needed. *Children*, 0.03 mg/kg of body weight (0.9 mg/M²) every one to two hours as needed.

Drug available generically: Solution 1 mg/ml in 2 ml containers.

Antilirium (O'Neal, Jones & Feldman). Solution 1 mg/ml in 2 ml containers.

PRALIDOXIME CHLORIDE
[Protopam Chloride]

Pralidoxime is a cholinesterase reactivator used primarily as an adjunct to atropine in the treatment of poisoning caused by pesticides that are organophosphate cholinesterase inhibitors. Atropine must be given first until its effects become apparent and only then should pralidoxime be administered.

In organophosphate poisoning, pralidoxime competes with the phosphorylated inhibited enzyme to form an oxime-phosphonate complex which liberates active cholinesterase. This occurs primarily at the neuromuscular junction in skeletal muscle but also at autonomic effector sites; relatively little reactivation occurs in the central nervous system. This relative specificity in its site of action determines the role of pralidoxime in anticholinesterase poisoning: It is used to reverse muscular paralysis, particularly that of the respiratory muscles. Atropine must be administered to treat symptoms of poisoning originating at sites where pralidoxime is relatively ineffective, especially the respiratory center. Therefore, atropine is given with pralidoxime to control convulsions, improve central respiratory function, and reduce increased bronchopulmonary secretions, hypersalivation, lacrimation, hyperhidrosis, nausea, vomiting, abdominal cramps, bradycardia, miosis, headache, lethargy, and drowsiness. One of the best indices for monitoring therapy is the degree of tracheal secretions.

Pralidoxime is not equally effective against all cholinesterase inhibitors. The most successful use of this agent has been in poisoning caused by the organophosphate pesticide, parathion. Pralidoxime also has been useful in poisoning caused by the related agents mevinphos, isoflurophate, parathion, Azodrin, Diazinon, disulfoton, EPN, methyl demeton, methyl parathion, phosphamidon, TEPP, and sarin. (See the manufacturer's literature for a list of additional substances.) Pralidoxime is not indicated to antagonize the effects of carbamate-type cholinesterase inhibitors (eg, neostigmine, pyridostigmine, ambenonium) that are used in the treatment of myasthenia gravis, since their action is reversible.

Pralidoxime is most effective if administered immediately after poisoning. Generally, little is accomplished if the drug is given more than 36 hours after termination of exposure. When the poison has been ingested, however, exposure may continue for some time due to slow absorption from the lower bowel, and fatal relapses have been reported after initial improvement. Continued administration for several days may be useful in such patients. Close supervision of the patient is indicated for at least 48 to 72 hours. If dermal exposure has occurred, clothing should be removed and the hair and skin washed thoroughly with sodium bicarbonate or alcohol as soon as possible. Diazepam may be given cautiously if convulsions are not controlled by atropine.

Pralidoxime may cause dizziness, diplopia, impaired accommodation, headache, drowsiness, nausea, tachycardia, increased systolic and diastolic blood pressure, hyperventilation, and muscle weakness when given parenterally to those who have not been exposed to anticholinesterase poisons. No significant toxic effects have been reported after prolonged oral administration.

Although therapy should not be delayed pending the results of laboratory tests, red blood cell, plasma cholinesterase, and urinary paranitrophenol measurements (in the case of parathion exposure) may be helpful in confirming the diagnosis and following the course of the illness. Depression of the plasma cholinesterase level does not necessarily reflect nerve cholinesterase activity. The red blood cell cholinesterase concentration provides a more accurate index of intoxication; a reduction below 50% of normal has been seen only with organophosphate ester poisoning. When pralidoxime is administered soon after onset of poisoning, the red blood cell cholinesterase level may be restored more rapidly than the plasma level. However, both plasma and red blood cell levels may remain depressed for a month or longer after intoxication; they may also be depressed in patients with subclinical chronic exposures. Therefore, exposure to anticholinesterase inhibitors should be avoided for several weeks after poisoning.

The dose of pralidoxime should be reduced in patients with impaired renal function because blood levels are increased in these patients.

ROUTES, USUAL DOSAGE, AND PREPARATIONS. *Intravenous*: For severe poisoning (coma, cyanosis, respiratory depression) caused by organophosphate-containing substances, the following treatment program should be instituted: A patent airway is secured and, if necessary, positive pressure artificial respiration is begun, 2 to 4 mg of atropine is then given intravenously to adults and this dose is repeated at intervals until secretions are inhibited or severe signs of atropine toxicity appear. For children, a test dose of atropine 50 mcg/kg of body weight is given initially; doses of 0.5 to 1 mg are then repeated until secretions are inhibited or signs of atropine toxicity occur. Some degree of atropinization should be maintained for at least 48 hours. *Adults*, after atropine, 1 g of pralidoxime, preferably diluted in 100 ml of sodium chloride injection, is infused over a 30-minute period or injected at a rate not exceeding 200 mg/min. If the response is poor, the dose may be repeated in one hour. *Children* may be given 20 to 40 mg/kg using the same procedure. If infusion is not feasible, a 5% solution may be injected over a five-minute period.

For moderately severe poisoning (hyperhidrosis, lacrimation, hypersalivation, diarrhea, and constriction in the chest), the patient is treated as for severe poisoning, except that establishment of a patent airway or institution of artificial respiration is unnecessary; however, the patient should be kept under observation.

Protopam Chloride (Ayerst). Powder 1 g.

Oral: For mild poisoning (headache, blurred vision, mild muscarinic signs), exposure to the poison is terminated and atropine therapy initiated. If necessary, 1 to 2 g of pralidoxime is given; this dose can be repeated in three hours. The patient should remain under the physician's supervision for at least 24 hours.

Protopam Chloride (Ayerst). Tablets 500 mg.

PROTAMINE SULFATE

Protamine sulfate binds and inactivates heparin because of its strong electropositive charge. Paradoxically, it has anticoagulant action of its own and prolongs clotting time. It is a true antithromboplastin, although it is not as active as heparin and is not used clinically as an anticoagulant. Each milligram of protamine sulfate neutralizes 80 to 100 U.S.P. units of heparin activity, depending upon the source of heparin. The reaction is almost instantaneous and the effects of protamine persist for approximately two hours. However, since the effect of heparin may last longer than that of protamine, bleeding may recur, particularly in postoperative patients, and another injection of protamine may be needed.

Protamine is usually well tolerated. Large intravenous doses (up to 200 mg in two hours) have been administered without untoward effects. However, this drug must be used cautiously to prevent thrombotic complications (see Chapter 63, Anticoagulants and Thrombolytics).

Toxic manifestations include acute hypotension, dyspnea, and bradycardia; occasionally, a feeling of warmth and flushing of the face may be observed.

ROUTE, USUAL DOSAGE, AND PREPARATIONS. *Intravenous*: Total dosage is determined by the amount of heparin given over the previous three to four hours (each milligram of protamine sulfate, calculated as dry material, neutralizes not less than 80 U.S.P. units of heparin activity derived from lung tissue and not less than 100 U.S.P. units of heparin activity derived from intestinal mucosa). A 1% solution is injected slowly over a period of one to three minutes. A single dose should not exceed 50 mg.

Drug available generically: Powder 50 mg with 5 ml of diluent; solution 1% in 5 and 25 ml containers.

Selected References

Narcotic Antagonists

Johnstone RE, et al: Reversal of morphine anesthesia with naloxone. *Anesthesiology* 41:361-367, 1974.

Martin WR: Naloxone. *Ann Intern Med* 85:765-768, 1974.

Way EL, Settle AA: Uses of narcotic antagonists. *Ration Drug Ther* 9:1-5, (Feb) 1975.

Metal Antagonists

Cohen A, Schwartz E: Iron chelation therapy with deferoxamine in Cooley anemia. *J Pediatr* 92:643-647, 1978 A.

Cohen A, Schwartz E: Excretion of iron in response to deferoxamine in sickle cell anemia. *J Pediatr* 92:659-662, 1978 B.

Epstein O, et al: Reduction of immune complexes and immunoglobulins induced by D-penicillamine in primary biliary cirrhosis. *N Engl J Med* 300:274-278, 1979.

Fleming CR, et al: Asymptomatic primary biliary cirrhosis: Presentation, histology, and results with D-penicillamine. *Mayo Clin Proc* 53:587-593, 1978.

Friedheim E, et al: Treatment of lead poisoning by 2,3-dimercaptosuccinic acid. *Lancet* 2:1234-1236, 1978.

Graziano JH, et al: Chelation therapy in beta-thalassemia major. I. Intravenous and subcutaneous deferoxamine. *J Pediatr* 92:648-652, 1978.

Jain S, et al: Controlled trial of D-penicillamine therapy in primary biliary cirrhosis. *Lancet* 1:831-834, 1977.

Peterson RG, Rumack BH: D-penicillamine therapy of acute arsenic poisoning. *J Pediatr* 91:661-666, 1977.

Pincus D, Saccar CV: Lead poisoning. *Am Fam Physician* 19:120-124, (June) 1979.

Pippard MJ, et al: Prevention of iron loading in transfusion-dependent thalassaemia. *Lancet* 1:1178-1181, 1978.

Propper RD, et al: Continuous subcutaneous administration of deferoxamine in patients with iron overload. *N Engl J Med* 297:418-423, 1977.

Stein M, et al: Acute iron poisoning in children. *West J Med* 125:289-297, 1976.

Weiner M, et al: Cooley anemia. High transfusion regimen and chelation therapy, results, and perspective. *J Pediatr* 92:653-658, 1978.

Young N, et al: Treatment of primary hemochromatosis with deferoxamine. *JAMA* 241:1152-1154, 1979.

Acetylcysteine

Ameer B, Greenblatt DJ: Acetaminophen. *Ann Intern Med* 87:202-209, 1977.

Crome P, et al: Oral methionine in treatment of severe paracetamol (acetaminophen) overdose. *Lancet* 2:829-830, 1977.

Prescott LF, et al: Treatment of paracetamol (acetaminophen) poisoning with N-acetylcysteine. *Lancet* 2:432-434, 1977.

Rumack BH (ed): Aspirin and acetaminophen: Comparative view for pediatric patient, with particular regard to toxicity, both in therapeutic dose and in overdose. *Pediatrics* 62(suppl): 865-946, (Nov) 1978.

Rumack BH, Matthew HJ: Acetaminophen poisoning and toxicity. *Pediatrics* 55:871-876, 1975.

Cyanide Antagonists

Cottrell JE, et al: Prevention of nitroprusside-induced cyanide toxicity with hydroxocobalamin. *N Engl J Med* 298:809-811, 1978.

Graham DL, et al: Acute cyanide poisoning complicated by lactic acidosis and pulmonary edema. *Arch Intern Med* 137:1051-1055, 1977.

Pralidoxime

Doull J: Treatment of insecticide poisoning, in Wilkinson CF (ed): *Insecticide Biochemistry and Physiology.* New York, Plenum Press, 1976, 649-667.

Hayes WJ Jr: *Toxicology of Pesticides.* Baltimore, Williams & Wilkins Company, 1975.

Physostigmine

Davis KL, et al: Neurotransmitter metabolites in cerebrospinal fluid of man following physostigmine. *Life Sci* 21:933-936, 1977.

Larson GF, et al: Physostigmine reversal of diazepam-induced depression. *Anesth Analg* 56:348-351, 1977.

Rumack BH: Anticholinergic poisoning: Treatment with physostigmine. *Pediatrics* 52:449-451, 1973.

Sitaram N, et al: REM sleep induction by physostigmine infusion during sleep. *Science* 191:1281-1283, 1976.

Antitoxins and Antivenins | 87

ANTITOXIN

 Botulism Antitoxin

ANTIVENINS

 Venom Antibodies for Passive Immunity

  Black Widow Spider Antivenin

  Polyvalent Crotaline Antivenin

  North American Coral Snake
   Antivenin

 Venom Allergens For Immunotherapy

  Bee

  Yellow Jacket

  Yellow Hornet

  White-Faced Hornet

  Wasp

The drugs in this chapter are used in a manner similar to that of the specific antidotes discussed in Chapter 86, but they have a biological rather than a synthetic chemical origin. All contain some form of protein. These biological products are divided into antitoxins and antivenins.

Antitoxins: Antiserums, of which antitoxins are a subgroup, are used primarily for prophylaxis and are discussed in Chapter 67, Vaccines and Antiserums. However, botulism antitoxin is used therapeutically and is included in this chapter.

Antivenins: An antivenin is defined as a proteinaceous material used in the treatment of venom poisoning. Like antitoxins, some antivenins (black widow spider, polyvalent crotaline, and North American coral snake antivenins) contain antibodies and are used only therapeutically. Other antivenins contain venom allergens (specific hymenoptera venom protein allergens of the honeybee, yellow jacket, yellow hornet, white-faced hornet, or

wasp) and are used prophylactically to immunize highly susceptible individuals. Hymenoptera allergens also are used to diagnose hypersensitivity.

Polyvalent crotaline antivenin and North American coral snake antivenin are effective against the venoms of selected poisonous snakes indigenous to the United States. The Oklahoma Poison Information Center ([405] 271-5454) maintains (in cooperation with the Oklahoma City Zoo) an International Antivenin Index (Rappolt et al, 1978) and can be contacted for information on availability of snake antivenins; it also maintains a snakebite consultation service for physicians. The physician also is encouraged to consult the literature (eg, Russell, 1975) and manufacturers of antivenin preparations for recommended methods of management of venomous snakebite and precautions regarding the use of antivenin.

An antibody-type antivenin is not yet available for the management of acute, serious reactions to hymenoptera sting. Individuals suspected or known to be especially sensitive to such stings should possess an Emergency Insect Sting Treatment Kit [ANA-Kit] (Hollister-Stier), which is available on prescription. The kit contains 1 ml of epinephrine 1:1,000 in a syringe designed to administer two measured doses of 0.3 ml each, if required (the syringe is graduated so that smaller doses can be administered to children), a tourniquet, and four chewable tablets of chlorpheniramine maleate (2 mg each).

Sensitivity Testing: Antitoxins and antivenins are prepared from animal sources, and two major reactions can follow injection of hyperimmune serum of animal origin: anaphylaxis and serum sickness. To determine sensitivity, a scratch, intradermal, or conjunctival test must precede injection, regardless of whether or not the patient previously received an injection of animal serum. A syringe containing 1 ml of epinephrine 1:1,000 should be readily available. A 1:1,000 dilution of the serum is injected intradermally, employing just enough to raise a visible bleb. The test is positive if a wheal appears within 30 minutes. The same fluid can be used for a scratch test, which may be safer. For the conjunctival test, one drop of a 1:10 dilution of serum in isotonic sodium chloride solution is instilled in one eye and one drop of sodium chloride solution is instilled in the other eye to serve as a control. The appearance of lacrimation and conjunctivitis within 30 minutes constitutes a positive reaction.

If the sensitivity test is positive and the need for serum is imperative, a desensitization procedure can be performed by injecting small, graded doses of the serum. For example, if no reaction occurs, the following doses are injected at 15-minute intervals: (1) 0.05 ml of 1:20 dilution, subcutaneously; (2) 0.1 ml of 1:10 dilution, subcutaneously; (3) 0.3 ml of 1:10 dilution, subcutaneously; (4) 0.1 ml of undiluted serum, subcutaneously; (5) 0.2 ml of undiluted serum, intramuscularly; (6) 0.5 ml of undiluted serum, intramuscularly; and (7) remaining doses, intramuscularly.

If anaphylactic reactions occur, epinephrine 1:1,000 in a dose of 0.5 ml for adults and 0.01 ml/kg of body weight (maximum, 0.5 ml) for children is immediately injected subcutaneously or intramuscularly. If there is no improvement, epinephrine 1:1,000 diluted 1:10 in physiologic saline is injected slowly intravenously. The dose is repeated in 1 to 15 minutes if necessary. Antihistamines may be given intramuscularly to treat severe urticaria or laryngeal edema. Vasopressors, positive-pressure oxygen, and corticosteroids may be useful.

ANTITOXIN

BOTULISM ANTITOXIN

Botulism antitoxin is a sterile solution of concentrated antitoxins, chiefly globulins, obtained from the blood of horses immunized against toxins of *Clostridium botulinus*: trivalent antitoxin (A, B, E) effective against toxin type A, B, and E and monovalent antitoxin E are available for human use. Its efficacy has not been well documented in humans, but animal studies would imply that if therapy is to be effective, the antitoxin should be given promptly early in the course of the disease. Patients first should be tested for sensitivity to equine serum (see the Introduction). Until the specific type of botulinus toxin has been identified, it is generally prudent to use trivalent ABE antitoxin. Local health officials should be notified of any cases resembling botulism.

Appropriate precautions should be taken to prevent or arrest possible allergic and other untoward reactions (eg, urticaria, fever, pruritus). Serum sickness may occur 5 to 13 days after administration.

See the literature supplied with the antitoxin for dosage and routes of administration.

Botulism Antitoxin, U.S.P. may be obtained from the Center for Disease Control, Atlanta, Georgia 30333. The Center's telephone numbers are: (404) 329-3311; off-duty hours (404) 329-3644.

ANTIVENINS

Venom Antibodies for Passive Immunity

POLYVALENT CROTALINE ANTIVENIN

Polyvalent crotaline antivenin is a suspension of venom-neutralizing antibodies prepared from the serum of horses immunized against the venoms of the pit vipers, *Crotalus adamanteus, C. atrox, C. durissus terrificus,* and *Bothrops atrox.* It is useful against the venom of all 17 species of crotalidae in North and South America. In general, it is effective against North American rattlesnakes, water moccasins, and copperheads but is of no value against true vipers (eg, puff adder, cobra, mamba), other noncrotalid snakes (eg, American coral snake), or any venomous spiders or scorpions. This antivenin should be administered immediately following emergency first-aid procedures. Tests for sensitivity to horse serum should precede administration (see the Introduction). Because of the short latent period (2 to 15 minutes) between the bite and the appearance of clinical symptoms, intravenous administration is probably the most efficient route.

Lyophilized preparations are active for at least five years; they are readily soluble in water for injection and should be reconstituted immediately prior to administration.

ROUTES, USUAL DOSAGE, AND PREPARATIONS. *Intravenous, Subcutaneous, Intramuscular: Adults,* 1 to 15, or even more, containers of reconstituted serum, preferably administered intravenously, depending upon the severity of symptoms and signs, time elapsed since the bite, and size of snake. See the manufacturer's literature for more detailed dosage. For intravenous use, a 1:10 dilution of antivenin in sterile isotonic sodium chloride injection or 5% dextrose injection is administered as a constant drip at a rate of 120 drops/min. *Children* may require twice the adult dosage because they have less resistance and less body fluid with which to dilute the venom.

Antivenin Crotalidae Polyvalent (Equine Origin) (Wyeth). Powder with 10 ml of bacteriostatic water for injection.

NORTH AMERICAN CORAL SNAKE ANTIVENIN
[Antivenin (*Micrurus fulvius*)]

Antivenin (*Micrurus fulvius*) is a concentrated and lyophilized preparation of serum globulins obtained from horses immunized with the venom of eastern coral snakes (*M. fulvius fulvius*). This antivenin will neutralize the venom of the two subspecies of *M. fulvius*: *M.f. fulvius* found in areas from eastern North Carolina through Florida and in the gulf coastal plain to the Mississippi River, and *M.f. tenere* (Texas coral snake) found west of the Mississippi River in Louisiana, Arkansas, and Texas. It will *not* neutralize the venom of *Micruroides euryxanthus* (Arizona or Sonoran coral snake) found only in southeastern Arizona and southwestern New Mexico.

There are relatively few coral snakebites each year, and it is not possible to predict whether envenomation has occurred even when fang punctures are present. The victim of a coral snakebite should be immobilized immediately and completely and carried to the nearest hospital as soon as possible. If complete immobilization is not practical, the bitten extremity should be splinted. If there is any evidence of a break in the skin from the bite, the victim should be hospitalized for observation and treatment.

If symptoms of envenomation occur, the antivenin should be given intravenously as soon as possible. Tests for sensitivity to horse serum should precede administration (see the Introduction). See the manufacturer's literature for dosage.

Antivenin (Micrurus fulvius) (Equine Origin) (Wyeth). Lyophilized preparation with 10 ml of bacteriostatic water for reconstitution.

BLACK WIDOW SPIDER ANTIVENIN
[Antivenin (*Lactrodectus mactans*)]

Black widow spider antivenin is prepared from the serum of horses immunized against the venom of the black widow spider (*Lactrodectus mactans*). Earliest possible use of the antivenin is recommended for greatest effectiveness. If possible, the patient should be hospitalized.

Supportive therapy may include warm baths, intravenous injection of morphine or 10 ml of 10% calcium gluconate solution to control myalgia, and administration of barbiturates to lessen extreme restlessness. Central nervous system depressants must be used with caution, however, because the venom is a neurotoxin that can cause respiratory arrest. Corticosteroids also have been used with varying results. No apparent benefit is gained by local treatment (eg, tourniquets, incision, suction) at the site of the bite.

A test for hypersensitivity to horse serum should be performed prior to use of this preparation. (See the Introduction.)

ROUTES, USUAL DOSAGE, AND PREPARATIONS. *Intramuscular (anterolateral thigh): Adults and children*, entire contents of one container (2.5 ml restored serum). Although one dose usually relieves symptoms in one to three hours, a second dose may be needed.

Intravenous: This is the preferred route in severe cases, in children under 12 years, or for those in shock. The contents of the container is diluted in 10 to 50 ml of saline and administered over a 15-minute period.

> *Antivenin (Lactrodectus mactans) (Equine Origin)* (Merck Sharp & Dohme). Powder (for suspension) containing not less than 6,000 Antivenin Units with 2.5 ml of sterile water for injection.

Venom Allergens for Immunotherapy

HYMENOPTERA VENOM ALLERGENIC EXTRACTS

(Bee Venom, Yellow Jacket Venom, Yellow Hornet Venom, White-faced Hornet Venom, Wasp Venom)
[Albay, Pharmalgen]

Whole-body allergenic extracts of stinging insects (hymenoptera) were formerly used routinely in an attempt to diminish hypersensitivity to the venom of honeybees, wasps, yellow jackets, and hornets. However, recent studies have shown that whole-body preparations were no more effective than a placebo, but that venom allergenic extracts were highly effective for both diagnosis and therapy (Hunt et al, 1976). Venom allergenic extracts presently are recommended for use in a diagnostic skin test to determine the presence of hypersensitivity to hymenoptera venom and to immunize highly susceptible individuals. One controlled study (Hunt et al, 1978) demonstrated a marked decrease in the incidence of systemic reactions in susceptible individuals following immunotherapy with venom preparations. Efficacy approaches 95% and the failure rate may be less than 1% when more rigorous desensitization procedures are employed in individuals who are especially sensitive.

Since insect sting hypersensitivity is primarily an immediate Type I IgE-mediated reaction, the mechanism of action of these allergenic extracts is probably related to their ability to increase venom-specific IgG-blocking antibodies. IgE antibodies also increase initially with hyposensitization therapy but return to normal levels after approximately one year of treatment. Currently, maintenance therapy must be given indefinitely, usually at the rate of one injection per month, in order to retain hyposensitivity.

Individuals who have experienced a potentially life-threatening reaction to an insect sting and who react positively to a skin test are the only candidates for immunotherapy; those who have not received venom therapy have a 60% to 70% chance of reacting severely when stung by the same type of insect. Individuals previously exposed to the now obsolete hyposensitization procedure employing whole-body allergenic extracts should be re-evaluated; if a skin test is positive, hyposensitization can be considered. Those who have experienced a sting that did not produce an allergic reaction but who later are found to have skin-sensitizing antibodies should not receive venom immunotherapy. An Emergency Insect Sting Treatment Kit [ANA-Kit] and instruction in its use should be provided; however, most of these patients will not even have an allergic reaction. Patients with a history of a reaction to previous stings but who do not demonstrate a positive skin test reaction to venom generally are not treated. Since it is not known if sting-sensitive patients who subsequently lose their IgE antivenom antibody can be resensitized by further stings, it is advisable to retest such patients after any subsequent stings. Immunotherapy is not currently recommended for those who exhibit a large local reaction to skin testing but do not have any previous history of systemic response; however, they also should be provided with the insect sting kit and instruction in its use.

Immunotherapy employing more than one extract may be necessary for those who have positive skin tests to more than one venom.

ADVERSE REACTIONS AND PRECAUTIONS.

A potentially severe systemic anaphylactic reaction is always a possibility with use of these agents. For that reason, a tourniquet, epinephrine, and agents to treat shock and bronchospasm always should be available during the use of these materials. In addition, it is recommended that patients remain in the office for 60 minutes after injection and that anyone receiving these allergens should be given an Emergency Insect Sting Treatment Kit [ANA-Kit] for use after leaving the treatment area.

Some form of systemic reaction has been noted in one-sixth of adults during build up of the dose to the maintenance level (100 mcg). These may include any of the following: wheezing, dyspnea, sneezing, hoarseness, tachycardia, gastrointestinal discomfort and nausea, neck or chest pain, cyanosis, sweating, lacrimation, urticaria, angioedema, and pruritus. Systemic reactions commonly occur within a very short time after injection; however, a serum sickness-like reaction manifested by fever, malaise, and joint and muscle pain can appear up to 48 hours following injection. One-half of adults exhibit local swelling and soreness at the site of injection. Both local and systemic reactions occur less frequently in children.

There are no *known* absolute contraindications to the use of hymenoptera venom allergenic extracts either for diagnosis or hyposensitization. Relative contraindica-

tions may include acute infections and immunodeficiency disease. Individuals with negative skin tests to hymenoptera venom should not be treated. The safe use of these materials during pregnancy is unknown.

Appropriate needle and syringe techniques are critical to avoid serum hepatitis, other infections, and intravascular administration. An observation period of one hour is recommended by the manufacturer following the subcutaneous injection of these allergens in immunotherapy.

ROUTES, USUAL DOSAGE, AND PREPARATIONS. *Intradermal (diagnosis), Subcutaneous (immunotherapy):* A scratch test followed by an intradermal test is recommended for diagnostic skin testing. The subcutaneous route of administration is preferred for immunotherapy. It is important to include a negative control with diluent and a positive control with histamine for reactivity in order to interpret correctly the significance of the wheal and flare reaction if it occurs. It is essential to refer to the product information sheet for recommended dilutions and interpretation of the wheal and flare response whether one is using these agents for diagnosis and/or for immunotherapy. Injections are generally given weekly for four months in the initial phase of immunotherapy and then monthly thereafter.

Albay (Hollister-Stier). Each vacuum-sealed vial contains venom protein 500 mcg. When reconstituted with 5 ml of the appropriate diluent, each vial contains 100 mcg/ml of venom protein (honeybee, yellow jacket, yellow hornet, white-faced hornet, or wasp). Diluents for reconstitution are 50% glycerin, normal saline, or Hollister-Stier normal saline with human serum albumin.

Pharmalgen (Pharmacia). Diagnostic kit containing five vacuum-sealed vials of freeze-dried venom/venom protein (one vial each of honeybee, yellow jacket, yellow hornet, white-faced hornet, and wasp venom). When reconstituted with 1.1 ml of diluent supplied in the kit, each vial contains 100 mcg/ml of venom protein. The freeze-dried product is stable at 2 to 8 C for approximately two years. The product instruction sheet should be consulted for the stability of various dilutions, which are considerably less stable than the freeze-dried product. Treatment kit contains six vials of freeze-dried venom/venom protein (one vial each of honeybee, yellow jacket, yellow hornet, white-faced hornet, wasp, or mixed vespid venom; the latter contains equal amounts of venom protein from yellow jacket, yellow hornet, and white-faced hornet). When reconstituted with 1.2 ml of diluent, each vial of a single-venom preparation contains 100 mcg/ml and each vial of the mixed vespid preparation contains 300 mcg/ml.

Selected References

Hunt KJ, et al: Controlled trial of immunotherapy in insect hypersensitivity. *N Engl J Med* 299:157-161, 1978.

Hunt KJ, et al: Diagnosis of allergy to stinging insects by skin testing with hymenoptera venoms. *Ann Intern Med* 85:56-59, 1976.

Rappolt RT, et al: Medical toxicologist's notebook: Snakebite treatment and international antivenin index. *Clin Toxicol* 13:409-438, 1978.

Russell FE: Snake venom poisoning in United States: Experiences with 550 cases. *JAMA* 233:341-344, 1975.

Manufacturers

Abbott Laboratories, Abbott Park, 1400 Sheridan Road, North Chicago, Illinois 60064

Acme United Corp., 100 Hicks Street, Bridgeport, Connecticut 06609

Adria Laboratories, Inc., P.O. Box 16529, Columbus, Ohio 43216

Aeroceuticals Health Care Products, P.O. Box 4, 49 John Street, Southport, Connecticut 06490

Alcon Laboratories, Inc., P.O. Box 1959, 6201 S. Freeway, Fort Worth, Texas 76101

Allergan Pharmaceuticals, 2525 Dupont Drive, Irvine, California 92713

Almay Inc., P.O. Box 748, Apex, North Carolina 27502

Alpha Therapeutic Corp., 820 Mission Street, South Pasadena, California 91030

Alza Corporation, 950 Page Mill Road, Palo Alto, California 94304

American Optical Corp., Soft Contact Lens Division, 14 Mechanic Street, Southbridge, Massachussetts 01550

Arbrook, Inc., P.O. Box 1227, Arlington, Texas 76010

Arch Laboratories, Division of Lewis-Howe Company, 319 S. Fourth Street, St. Louis, Missouri 63102

Armour-Dial, Inc., Armour Research Center, 15101 N. Scottsdale Road, Scottsdale, Arizona 85260

Armour Pharmaceutical Company, Greyhound Tower, Phoenix, Arizona 85077

Arnar-Stone Laboratories, Inc., 1600 Waukegan Road, McGaw Park, Illinois 60085

B. F. Ascher & Company, Inc., 5100 E. 59th Street, Kansas City, Missouri 64130

Astra Pharmaceutical Products, Inc., 7 Neponset Street, Worcester, Massachusetts 01606

Avicon, Inc., 6201 South Freeway, P.O. Box 85, Ft. Worth, Texas 76101

Ayerst Laboratories, Division of American Home Products Corporation, 685 Third Avenue, New York, New York 10017

Barnes-Hind Pharmaceuticals, Inc., 895 Kifer Road, Sunnyvale, California 94086

Baxter Laboratories, One Baxter Parkway, Deerfield, Illinois 60015

Baylor Laboratories, Inc., P.O. Drawer 277, Hurst, Texas 76053

Beach Pharmaceuticals, Division of Beach Products, Inc., 5220 S. Manhattan Avenue, Tampa, Florida 33611

Beecham Laboratories, Division of Beecham, Inc., 501 Fifth Street, Bristol, Tennessee 37620

Beiersdorf, Inc., P.O. Box 529, South Norwalk, Connecticut 06854

Berlex Laboratories Inc., 110 E. Hanover Avenue, Cedar Knolls, New Jersey 07927.

Bird Corp., Mark 7, Palm Springs, California 92262

Blair Laboratories, Inc., 50 Washington Street, Norwalk, Connecticut 06856

Bluline Laboratories, Inc., 302 South Broadway, St. Louis, Missouri 63102

Boehringer Ingelheim Ltd., 90 East Ridge, P.O. Box 368, Ridgefield Connecticut 06877

The Boots Co., Ltd., Thane Road, Nottingham NG-2 3AA, England

Boots Pharmaceuticals, 6540 Line Avenue, Shreveport, Louisiana 71106

John H. Breck, Inc., Berdan Avenue, Wayne, New Jersey 07470

Breon Laboratories, Inc., 90 Park Avenue, New York, New York 10016

Bristol Laboratories, Division of Bristol-Myers Company, P.O. Box 657, Syracuse, New York 13201

Bristol-Myers Products, Division of Bristol-Myers Company, 345 Park Avenue, New York, New York 10022

Buffington Division, Otis Clapp & Sons, Inc., 143 Albany Street, Cambridge, Massachusetts 02139

Burroughs Wellcome Company, 3030 Cornwallis Road, Research Triangle Park, North Carolina 27709

Burton, Parsons & Company, Inc., 120 Westhampton Avenue, Washington, D.C. 20027

C & M Pharmacal, Inc., 1519 E. Eight Mile Road, Hazel Park, Michigan 48030

Carnrick Laboratories, Division of G. W. Carnrick Company, 65 Horse Hill Road, Cedar Knolls, New Jersey 07927

The Central Pharmacal Company, 110-128 E. Third Street, Seymour, Indiana 47274

Century Pharmaceuticals, Inc., 4553 Allisonville Road, Indianapolis, Indiana 46205

Ciba Pharmaceutical Company, Division of Ciba-Geigy Corporation, 556 Morris Avenue, Summit, New Jersey 07901

Comatic Laboratories, Inc., P.O. Box 42300, Houston, Texas 77042

Cooper Laboratories, Inc., Research & Development Division, 110 E. Hanover Avenue, Cedar Knolls, New Jersey 07927

Critikon, Division of McNeil Laboratories, P.O. Box 19154, Irvine, California 92713

Cutter Laboratories, Inc., 4th and Parker Streets, Berkeley, California 94710

Davis & Geck, Division American Cyanamid Company, Middletown Road, Pearl River, New York 10965

Dermik Laboratories, Inc., 500 Virginia Drive, Fort Washington, Pennsylvania 19034

Dista Products Company, Division of Eli Lilly and Company, P.O. Box 1407, Indianapolis, Indiana 46206

Doak Pharmacal Company, Inc., 700 Shames Drive, Westbury, L.I., New York 11590

Dome Laboratories, Division of Miles Laboratories, Inc., 400 Morgan Lane, West Haven, Connecticut 06516

Dooner Laboratories, Inc., Ward Hill, Box 909, Haverhill, Massachusetts 01830

Dorsey Laboratories, Division of Sandoz, Inc., P.O. Box 83288, Lincoln, Nebraska 68501

Dow Chemical U.S.A., 9550 N. Zionsville Road, P.O. Box 68511, Indianapolis, Indiana 46268

The Doyle Pharmaceutical Company, 5320 W. 23rd Street, Minneapolis, Minnesota 55416

Durel Pharmaceutical, Inc., P.O. Box 841, South Norwalk, Connecticut 06856

Paul B. Elder Company, Inc., P.O. Box 31, 705 East Mulberry Street, Bryan, Ohio 43506

Endo Laboratories, Inc., Subsidiary of E.I. du Pont de Nemours & Company, Inc., 1000 Stewart Avenue, Garden City, New York 11530

Fellows Testagar, Inc., Division of Fellows Medical Mfg. Co., Inc., 12741 Capital Avenue, Oak Park, Michigan 48237

Ferndale Laboratories, Inc., 780 W. Eight Mile Road, Ferndale, Michigan 48220

Ferring Pharmaceuticals, Inc., P.O. Box 40, FDR Station, New York, New York 10022

Fisons Corporation, Pharmaceutical Division, Two Preston Court, Bedford, Massachusetts 07130

C. B. Fleet Company, Inc., 4615 Murray Place, P.O. Box 1100, Lynchburg, Virginia 24505

Fleming & Company, 9730 Reavis Park Drive, St. Louis, Missouri 63123

Flint Laboratories, Division of Travenol Laboratories, Inc., One Baxter Parkway, Deerfield, Illinois 60015

E. Fougera & Company, Inc., Cantiague Road, P.O. Box 73, Hicksville, L.I., New York 11802

Geigy Pharmaceuticals, Division of Ciba-Geigy Corporation, Summit, New Jersey 07901

General Mills, Inc., 4620 W. 77th Street, Minneapolis, Minnesota 55435

Gerber Products Company, 445 State Street, Fremont, Michigan 49412

Geriatric Pharmaceutical Corporation, 397 Jericho Turnpike, Floral Park, New York 11001

Glenbrook Laboratories, Division of Sterling Drug Inc., 90 Park Avenue, New York, New York 10016

Glenwood Laboratories, Inc., 83 N. Summit Street, Tenafly, New Jersey 07670

Guardian Chemical Corp., 230 Marcus Blvd., Hauppauge, New York 11787

W. E. Hauck, Inc., P.O. Box 1065, Roswell, Georgia 30075

Herald Pharmacal, Inc., 6503 Warwick Road, Richmond, Virginia 23225

G. S. Herbert Laboratories, Division of Allergan Pharmaceuticals, 2525 Dupont Drive, Irvine, California 92713

Dow B. Hickam, Inc., 5629 Grapevine, P.O. Box 35413, Houston, Texas 77035

Hoechst-Roussel Pharmaceuticals, Inc., Division of American Hoechst Corporation, Route 202-206 North, Somerville, New Jersey 08876

Holland-Rantos Company, Inc., P.O. Box 385, 865 Centennial Avenue, Piscataway, New Jersey 08854

Hollister-Stier Laboratories, 3525 North Regal Street, Box 3145, Terminal Annex, Spokane, Washington 99220

Hyland Laboratories, Division of Travenol Laboratories, Inc., 3300 Hyland Avenue, P.O. Box 2214, Costa Mesa, California 92626

Hynson, Westcott & Dunning, Inc., Charles & Chase Streets, Baltimore, Maryland 21201

Hyrex Pharmaceuticals, P.O. Box 18385, Memphis, Tennessee 38118

ICN Pharmaceuticals, Inc., 2727 Campus Drive, Irvine, California 92664

Ingram Pharmaceutical Company, 202 Green Street, San Francisco, California 94111

Ives Laboratories, Inc., 685 Third Avenue, New York, New York 10017

The Andrew Jergens Company, 2535 Spring Grove Avenue, Cincinnati, Ohio 45214

Johnson & Johnson, 501 George Street, New Brunswick, New Jersey 08903

Jordan-Simner, Inc., 6852 N.W. 12th Avenue, Ft. Lauderdale, Florida 33309

Kay Pharmacal Company, Inc., P.O. Box 50375, 1312 N. Utica, Tulsa, Oklahoma 74150

Key Pharmaceuticals, Inc., 50 N.W. 176th Street, Box 3670, Miami, Florida 33169

Kinney & Company, Inc., 1307 12th Street, P.O. Box 307, Columbus, Indiana 47201

C. F. Kirk Laboratories, Inc., 655 Madison Street, New York, New York 10021

Knoll Pharmaceutical Company, 30 N. Jefferson Road, Whippany, New Jersey 07981

Kremers-Urban Company, 5600 W. County Line Road, P.O. Box 2038, Milwaukee, Wisconsin 53201

Laser, Inc., P.O. Box 207, 2000 North Main Street, Crown Point, Indiana 46307

Lederle Laboratories, A Division of American Cyanamid Company, Pearl River, New York 10965

Leeming Division, Pfizer, Inc., 235 East 42nd Street, New York, New York 10017

Lemmon Pharmacal Company, Temple Avenue, Box 30, Sellersville, Pennsylvania 18960

Lever Brothers Company, Lever Division, 390 Park Avenue, New York, New York 10022

Lewis-Howe Company, 319 S. 4th Street, St. Louis, Missouri 63102

Lilly Research Laboratories, Division of Eli Lilly and Company, Indianapolis, Indiana 46206

Lincoln Laboratories, Inc., Hickory Point Road, Box 1139, Decatur, Illinois 62526

Loma Linda Food Company, 11503 Pierce Street, Riverside, California 92505

Mallard, Inc., 3021 Wabash Avenue, Detroit, Michigan 48216

Mallinckrodt, Inc., Mallinckrodt and Second Streets, St. Louis, Missouri 63147

Marion Laboratories, Inc., Pharmaceutical Division, 10236 Bunker Ridge Road, Kansas City, Missouri 64137

Maurry Biological Co., Inc., 6109 S. Western Avenue, Los Angeles, California 90047

Mayrand Inc., P.O. Box 20246, 1026 E. Lindsay Street, Greensboro North Carolina 27420

McGaw Laboratories, P.O. Box 11887, Santa Ana, California 92711

McNeil Laboratories, Inc., Camp Hill Road, Fort Washington, Pennsylvania 19034

Mead Johnson Laboratories, 2404 W. Pennsylvania Street, Evansville, Indiana 47721

Medicone Company, 225 Varick Street, New York, New York 10014

Menley & James Laboratories, 1500 Spring Garden Street, Philadelphia, Pennsylvania 19101

Merck Sharp & Dohme, Division of Merck & Co., Inc., West Point, Pennsylvania 19486

Merrell-National Laboratories, Division of Richardson-Merrell, Inc., 110 E. Amity Road, Lockland Station, Cincinnati, Ohio 45215

Meyer Laboratories, Inc., 1900 W. Commercial Boulevard, Fort Lauderdale, Florida 33309

Miles Laboratories, Inc., 1127 Myrtle Street, Elkhart, Indiana 46514

Milex Products, Inc., 5915 Northwest Highway, Chicago, Illinois 60631

Muro Pharmacal Laboratories, Inc., 121 Liberty Street, Quincy, Massachusetts 02169

Neutrogena Corporation, 5755 W. 96th Street, Los Angeles, California 90045

Nicholas Laboratories, P.O. Box 500, 2770 S. 171st Street, New Berlin (Milwaukee), Wisconsin 53151

Norcliff Thayer, Inc., 1 Scarsdale Road, Tuckahoe, New York 10707

North American Pharmacal, Inc., 6851 Chase Road, Dearborn, Michigan 48121

Norwich-Eaton Laboratories, Division of Morton-Norwich, P.O. Box 191, Norwich, New York 13815

Obetrol Pharmaceuticals, Division of Rexar Pharmacal Corporation, 396 Rockaway Avenue, Valley Stream, New York 11581

Ohio Medical Products, Division of Air Reduction Company, Inc., 3030 Airco Drive, Madison, Wisconsin 53701

O'Neal, Jones & Feldman, Inc., 2510 Metro Blvd., Maryland Heights, Missouri 60343

Organon Inc., 375 Mt. Pleasant Avenue, West Orange, New Jersey 07502

Ortho Pharmaceutical Corporation, Highway 202, Raritan, New Jersey 08869

Owen-Dara Laboratories, Inc., Division of Alcon Laboratories, Inc., 3737 Belt Line Road, Box 34630, Dallas, Texas 75234

Panray Division, Ormont Drug & Chemical Company, Inc., South Dean Street, Box 150, Englewood, New Jersey 07631

Parke, Davis & Company, 201 Tabor Road, Morris Plains, New Jersey 07950

Pasadena Research Laboratories, Inc., 2107 E. Villa Street, Pasadena, California 91107

Pedinol Pharmacal, Inc., 295 Broadway, Bethpage, New York 11714

Pennwalt Corporation, Pharmaceutical Division, P.O. Box 1710, Rochester, New York 14603

Person & Covey, Inc., 616 Allen Avenue, Glendale, California 91201

Pfanstiehl Laboratories, Inc., 1219 Glen Rock Avenue, Waukegan, Illinois 60085

Pfipharmecs Division, Pfizer Inc., 235 East 42nd Street, New York, New York 10017

Pfizer Laboratories, Division of Pfizer, Inc., 235 E. 42nd Street, New York, New York 10017

Pharmacia Laboratories, Inc., 800 Centennial Avenue, Piscataway, New Jersey 08854

Pharmacraft Consumer Products, Pharmaceutical Division, Pennwalt Corporation, 155 Jefferson Road, Rochester, New York 14623

Philips Roxane Laboratories, Inc., 330 Oak Street, Columbus, Ohio 43216

Plough, Inc., 3022 Jackson Avenue, P.O. Box 377, Memphis, Tennessee 38101

Wm. P. Poythress & Company, Inc., 16 N. 22nd Street, P.O. Box 26946, Richmond, Virginia 23261

Procter & Gamble Company, P.O. Box 39175, Cincinnati, Ohio 45247

Professional Pharmacal Co., Division of Steri-Med Inc., P.O. Box 459, Lindenhurst, New York 11757

The Purdue Frederick Company, 50 Washington Street, Norwalk, Connecticut 06856

Rachelle Laboratories, Inc., Subsidiary of International Rectifier Corporation, 700 Henry Ford Avenue, P.O. Box 2029, Long Beach, California 90801

Reed & Carnrick, 30 Boright Avenue, Kenilworth, New Jersey 07033

Reid-Provident Laboratories, Inc., 25 Fifth Street, N.W., Atlanta, Georgia 30308

Research Industries Corporation, Pharmaceutical Division, 1847 W. 2300 South, Salt Lake City, Utah 84119

Riker Laboratories, Inc., Subsidiary of 3M Company, 19901 Nordhoff Street, Northridge, California 91324

A. H. Robins Company, Inc., 1211 Sherwood Avenue, Richmond, Virginia 23220

Roche Laboratories, Division of Hoffmann-LaRoche, Inc., 340 Kingsland Street, Nutley, New Jersey 07110

Roerig Division of Pfizer Pharmaceuticals, 235 E. 42nd Street, New York, New York 10017

William H. Rorer, Inc., 500 Virginia Drive, Fort Washington, Pennsylvania 19034

Ross Laboratories, Division of Abbott Laboratories, 625 Cleveland Avenue, Columbus, Ohio 43216

Roussel Corporation, 155 E. 44th Street, New York, New York 10017

Rowell Laboratories, Inc., Lake of the Woods, 210 Main Street, W., Baudette, Minnesota 56623

Sandoz Pharmaceuticals, Division of Sandoz, Inc., Route 10, East Hanover, New Jersey 07936

Saron Pharmacal Corporation, 1640 Central Avenue, St. Petersburg, Florida 33712

Savage Laboratories, A Division of Byk-Gulden, Inc., 1000 Main Street, P.O. Box 1000, Missouri City, Texas 77459

Scherer Laboratories, Inc., 14335 Gillis Road, Dallas, Texas 75234

Schering Corporation, Galloping Hill Road, Kenilworth, New Jersey 07033

Schmid Laboratories, Inc., Route 46 West, Little Falls, New Jersey 07424

A. O. Schmidt Company, 2100 Bryant Street, San Francisco, California 94110

Searle Laboratories, Division of G. D. Searle & Company, P.O. Box 5110, Chicago, Illinois 60680

Serono Laboratories, Inc., 607 Boylston Street, Boston, Massachusetts 02116

Sherwood Medical, 1831 Olive Street, St. Louis, Missouri 63103

Smith Kline & French Laboratories, 1500 Spring Garden Street, Philadelphia, Pennsylvania 19101

SMP Division, Cooper Laboratories (P.R.), Inc., P.O. Box 367, San German, Puerto Rico 00753

Spencer-Mead Inc., 270 W. Merrick Road, Valley Stream, New York 11582

E.R. Squibb & Sons, Inc., Georges Road, New Brunswick, New Jersey 08903

Steri-Med, Inc., Division of Ketchum Laboratories, 369 Bayview Avenue, Amityville, New York 11701

Stiefel Laboratories, Inc., Oak Hill, New York 12460

Stuart Pharmaceuticals, Division of ICI Americas, Inc., 3411 Silverside Road, P.O. Box 751, Wilmington, Delaware 19897

Surgikos, A Johnson & Johnson Company, 501 George Street, New Brunswick, New Jersey 08903

Syntex Laboratories, Inc., 3401 Hillview Avenue, Stanford Industrial Park, Palo Alto, California 94304

Texas Pharmacal Company, P.O. Box 1659, San Antonio, Texas 78296

THEX Corporation, 202 Green Street, San Francisco, California 94111

TI-Pharmaceuticals, 201 San Antonio Circle, Suite 114, Mountain View, California 94040

Travenol Laboratories, Inc., One Baxter Parkway, Deerfield, Illinois 60015

Tutag Pharmaceuticals, Inc., 2599 W. Midway Boulevard, Broomfield, Colorado 80020

UAD Laboratories, Inc., 1400 Commerce Street, Minden, Louisiana 71055

The Ulmer Pharmacal Company, Division of Physicians Hospital Supply Company, 1400 Harmon Place, Minneapolis, Minnesota 55403

Union Carbide Corporation, 270 Park Avenue, New York, New York 10017

The Upjohn Company, 7000 Portage Road, Kalamazoo, Michigan 49001

USV Pharmaceutical Corporation, 1 Scarsdale Road, Tuckahoe, New York 10707

Vestal Laboratories, 5075 Manchester Avenue, St. Louis, Missouri 63110

VioBin Corporation, 226 W. Livingston Street, Monticello, Illinois 61856

Wallace Laboratories, Half Acre Road, Cranbury, New Jersey 08512

Warner-Lambert Company, 201 Tabor Road, Morris Plains, New Jersey 07950

Warren-Teed Pharmaceuticals, Inc., Subsidiary of Rohm and Haas Company, 582 W. Goodale Street, Columbus, Ohio 43215

Webcon Pharmaceuticals, Division of Alcon Laboratories, Inc., P.O. Box 1629, 6201 S. Freeway, Fort Worth, Texas 76101

West Chemical Products, Inc., 42-16 West Street, Long Island, New York 11101

Westwood Pharmaceuticals, Inc., 468 Dewitt Street, Buffalo, New York 14213

Wharton Laboratories, Inc., Division of U.S. Ethicals, Inc., 37-02 Forty-Eighth Avenue, Long Island City, New York 11101

Whitehall Laboratories, Division of American Home Products Corporation, 685 Third Avenue, New York, New York 10017

Willen Drug Company, 18 N. High Street, Baltimore, Maryland 21202

Winthrop Laboratories, 90 Park Avenue, New York, New York 10016

Wyeth Laboratories, Division of American Home Products Corporation, P.O. Box 8299, Philadelphia, Pennsylvania 19101